PRINCIPLES OF
SURGERY

FIFTH EDITION

NOTICE

PRINCIPLES OF SURGERY

FIFTH EDITION

EDITOR-IN-CHIEF

SEYMOUR I. SCHWARTZ, M.D.

Professor and Chair
Department of Surgery
University of Rochester School of Medicine and Dentistry

ASSOCIATE EDITORS

G. Tom Shires, M.D.

Professor and Chair
Department of Surgery
Cornell University Medical College

Frank C. Spencer, M.D.

Professor and Director
Department of Surgery
New York University School of Medicine

WITH

Wendy Cowles Husser, M.A.

University of Rochester
School of Medicine and Dentistry

McGraw-Hill Book Company

New York   St. Louis   San Francisco   Colorado Springs   Oklahoma City
Auckland   Bogota   Hamburg   Lisbon   London   Madrid   Mexico   Milan   Montreal
New Delhi   Panama   Paris   San Juan   São Paulo   Singapore   Sydney   Tokyo   Toronto

PRINCIPLES OF SURGERY

1 2 3 4 5 6 7 8 9 0   DOWDOW   8 9 4 3 2 0 9 8

ISBN 0-07-055822-1   1 VOL EDITION
ISBN 0-07-079979-2   2 VOL SET EDITION
ISBN 0-07-055826-4   VOLUME ONE
ISBN 0-07-055829-9   VOLUME TWO

This book was set in Times Roman by York Graphic Services, Inc.
The editors were Ray Moloney and Mariapaz Ramos-Englis.
The production supervisor was Elaine Gardenier.
The index was prepared by Philip James.
The cover was designed by Edward R. Schultheis.
Front cover art courtesy of: Yale Historical Library.
Illustration on back cover is from—An Explanation
of the Fashion and use of three and fifty Instruments
of Chirurgery—gathered out of Ambrosius Pareus.
R. R. Donnelley & Sons Company was printer and binder.

Library of Congress Cataloging-in-Publication Data

Principles of surgery.

    Available as 1 v. and as a 2-v. set.
    Includes bibliographies and index.
    1. Surgery. I. Schwartz, Seymour, I., 1928–
II. Title. [DNLM: 1. Surgery. WO100 P957]
RD31.P88 1989   617   88-9158
ISBN 0-07-079979-2 (set)
ISBN 0-07-055826-4 (v. 1)
ISBN 0-07-055829-9 (v. 2)
ISBN 0-07-055822-1 (single v.)

To students of Surgery, at all levels, in their quest
for knowledge

Contents

Contributors

James T. Adams, M.D.
Professor of Surgery
Department of Surgery
University of Rochester school of
Medicine and Dentistry (35)

R. Peter Altman, M.D.
Rudolph N. Schullinger Professor of Surgery
College of Physicians and Surgeons
Columbia University (39)

Joseph F. Amaral, M.D.
Fellow in Surgery
Brown University (1)

Kathryn D. Anderson, M.D.
Professor of Surgery and Child Health
George Washington University
Attending Surgeon, Children's Hospital
Washington, D.C. (39)

Richard M. Bergland, M.D.
Clinical Professor of Surgery (Neurosurgery)
SUNY Downstate
Beth Israel Hospital (37)

George H. Bornside, Ph.D.
Professor Emeritus of Surgical Research
and Microbiology
Departments of Surgery and Microbiology
Louisiana State University
Medical Center (5)

Richard I. Burton, M.D.
Professor and Chair
Department of Orthopaedics
University of Rochester
School of Medicine and Dentistry (45)

Peter C. Canizaro, M.D.
Professor and Chairman
Department of Surgery
Texas Tech University Health Sciences
Center (2, 4)

C. James Carrico, M.D.
Professor and Chairman of Surgery
University of Washington School of
Medicine (4)

Douglas Chyatte, M.D.
Assistant Professor
Section of Neurological Surgery
Yale University School of Medicine (42)

Isidore Cohn, Jr, M.D.
Professor and Chairman
Department of Surgery
Louisiana State University
School of Medicine (5)

William F. Collins, M.D.
Harvey and Kate Cushing
Professor and Chairman
Department of Surgery
Yale University School of Medicine (42)

Robert E. Condon, M.D.
Ausman Foundation Professor
and Chairman, Department of Surgery
The Medical College of Wisconsin (34)

Alfred T. Culliford, M.D.
Associate Professor
Department of Surgery
New York University Medical Center (19)

Numbers in parentheses refer to contributors' chapters.

P. William Curreri
Professor and Chairman
Department of Surgery
University of South Alabama
College of Medicine (7)

Louis R. M. Del Guercio, M.D.
Professor and Chairman
Department of Surgery
New York Medical College, Valhalla (13)

Eric J. DeMaria, M.D.
Resident in Surgery
Brown University (37)

Charles C. Duncan, M.D.
Associate Professor of Surgery
Section of Neurosurgery
Chief, Pediatric Neurosurgery
Yale University School of Medicine (42)

Robert B. Duthie, M.D. M.B.
Nuffield Professor of Orthopaedic Surgery
Nuffield Orthopaedic Center
Oxford, England (43)

James S. Economou, M.D.
Assistant Professor of Surgery
Division of Surgical Oncology
UCLA School of Medicine and
Jonsson Comprehensive Cancer Clinic (9)

Martin R. Eichelberger, M.D.
Associate Professor of Surgery
and Child Health
George Washington University
Attending Surgeon, Children's Hospital
Washington D.C. (39)

Irwin N. Frank, M.D.
Professor of Surgery
Department of Urology
University of Rochester
School of Medicine and Dentistry (40)

Richard E. Fry, M.D.
Assistant Professor of Surgery
The University of Texas Southwestern Medical
School at Dallas (23)

William J. Fry, M.D.
Professor and Chairman
Department of Surgery
The University of Texas Southwestern Medical
School at Dallas (23)

Donald S. Gann, M.D.
J. Murray Beardsley Professor and
Chairman, Department of Surgery
Brown University (1, 37)

Stanley M. Goldberg, M.D.
Clinical Professor of Surgery
Director, Division of Colon and Rectal Surgery
Department of Surgery
University of Minnesota Medical School (28)

Lazar J. Greenfield, M.D.
Professor and Chairman
Department of Surgery
University of Michigan, Ann Arbor (22)

Philip C. Guzzetta, M.D.
Associate Professor of Surgery
and Child Health
George Washington University,
Attending Surgeon, Children's Hospital
Washington D.C. (39)

Charles M. Haskell, M.D.
Professor of Medicine and Surgery
UCLA School of Medicine
Director, Wadsworth Cancer Center
Chief, Hematology and Oncology Section
of the Medical and Research Services
W. Los Angeles V.A. Medical Center (9)

Richard H. Hatch, M.D.
Assistant Clinical Professor
Department of Obstetrics and Gynecology
University of Utah (41)

Arthur L. Herbst, M.D.
Chairman and Joseph Bolivar DeLee
Distinguished Service Professor
Department of Obstetrics and Gynecology
University of Chicago (41)

Franklin T. Hoaglund, M.D.
Professor of Surgery, Department of
Orthopaedic Surgery
University of California at San Francisco
(43, 44)

Anthony M. Imparato, M.D.
Professor of Surgery
Director, Division of Vascular Surgery
New York University Medical Center (21)

Ronald C. Jones, M.D.
Clinical Professor of Surgery
University of Texas Health Science Center
and Chief of Surgery
Baylor University Medical Center, Dallas (6)

M. J. Jurkiewicz, M.D.
Professor of Surgery
Section of Plastic Surgery
Emory University School of Medicine (46)

Edwin L. Kaplan, M.D.
Professor of Surgery
Pritzker School of Medicine
University of Chicago (38)

Thomas C. King, M.D.
Ferrer Professor of Surgery
Columbia Presbyterian Hospital (17)

Stephen F. Lowry, M.D.
Associate Professor of Surgery
Director, Hyperalimentation Unit
Department of Surgery
Cornell University Medical College (2)

Arnold Luterman, M.D.
Ripps-Meisler Professor of Surgery
Director
University of South Alabama Burn
Center (7)

Robert N. McClelland, M.D.
Professor of Surgery
The University of Texas
Southwestern Medical School at Dallas (6)

James M. McGreevy
Associate Professor of Surgery
University of Utah Medical School (26)

Laura Ment, M.D.
Associate Professor
Department of Pediatrics and Neurology
Yale University School of Medicine (42)

Richard J. Migliori, M.D.
Medical Fellow in Surgery
Department of Surgery
University of Minnesota Medical
Center (10)

Roland D. Miller, M.D.
Professor and Chairman of Anesthesia
and Professor of Pharmacology
Department of Anesthesia
University of California, San Francisco (11)

Thomas A. Miller, M.D.
Professor of Surgery
Department of Surgery
University of Texas Health Science Center
at Houston (26)

Frank G. Moody, M.D.
Denton A. Cooley Professor and Chairman
Department of Surgery
University of Texas Health Science Center
at Houston (26)

Donald L. Morton, M.D.
Professor and Chief, Surgical Oncology
Director, John Wayne Cancer Clinic
UCLA School of Medicine
and Jonsson Comprehensive Cancer
Center (9)

John H. Morton, M.D.
Professor of Surgery
Department of Surgery
University of Rochester School of Medicine
and Dentistry (36)

John S. Najarian, M.D.
Jay Phillips Professor and Chairman
Department of Surgery
University of Minnesota Hospital (10)

Kurt D. Newman, M.D.
Assistant Professor of Surgery and
Child Health
George Washington University
Attending Surgeon, Children's Hospital
Washington D.C. (39)

Santhat Nivatvongs, M.D.
Associate Professor of Surgery
Senior Associate Consultant
General and Colon and Rectal Surgery
Mayo Medical School (28)

Peter C. Pairolero, M.D.
Associate Professor of Surgery
Mayo Medical School (25)

Robert G. Parker, M.D.
Professor and Chairman
Department of Radiation Oncology
UCLA School of Medicine
and Jonsson Comprehensive Cancer
Center (9)

W. Spencer Payne, M.D.
James C. Masson Professor of Surgery
Mayo Medical School (25)

Erle E. Peacock, Jr., M.D.
Chapel Hill
North Carolina (8)

Malcolm O. Perry, M.D.
Professor of Surgery
Vanderbilt University School of Medicine (6)

Joseph M. Piepmeier, M.D.
Associate Professor
Section of Neurological Surgery
Yale University School of Medicine (42)

Judson G. Randolph, M.D.
Professor of Surgery and Child Health
George Washington University
Surgeon-in-Chief, Children's Hospital,
Washington D.C.   (39)

Keith Reemtsma, M.D.
Valentine Mott and Johnson and Johnson
Professor and Chairman
Department of Surgery
Columbia Presbyterian Hospital   (10)

Thomas S. Riles, M.D.
Associate Professor of Surgery
Department of Surgery
New York University Medical Center   (21)

Franklin Robinson, M.D.
Clinical Professor
Section of Neurological Surgery
Yale University School of Medicine   (42)

David A. Rothenberger, M.D.
Associate Professor
Division of Colon and Rectal Surgery
Department of Surgery
University of Minnesota Medical School   (28)

Benjamin F. Rush, Jr., M.D.
Professor and Chairman
Department of Surgery
University of Medicine and Dentistry
of New Jersey at Newark   (15, 16)

Kimberlee J. Sass, M.D.
Associate Research Scientist
Section of Neurological Surgery
Clinical Neuropsychologist
Yale University School of Medicine   (42)

John A. Savino, M.D.
Professor of Surgery
Department of Surgery
New York Medical College   (13)

Seymour I. Schwartz, M.D.
Professor and Chair
Department of Surgery
University of Rochester School of Medicine
and Dentistry   (3, 12, 24, 29, 30, 31, 33, 44)

G. Tom Shires, M.D.
Lewis Atterbury Stimson Professor and Chairman
Department of Surgery
Cornell University Medical College   (2, 4, 6)

G. Tom Shires III, M.D.
Assistant Professor
Department of Surgery
Cornell University Medical College   (2, 4, 6)

William Silen, M.D.
Johnson & Johnson Professor of Surgery
Harvard Medical School   (32)

Richard L. Simmons, M.D.
Professor of Surgery and Microbiology
Department of Surgery
University of Minnesota Medical Center   (10)

Craig R. Smith, M.D.
Assistant Professor of Surgery
Department of Surgery
Columbia Presbyterian Hospital   (10, 17)

William H. Snyder III, M.D.
Professor of Surgery
The University of Texas Southwestern Medical
School at Dallas   (6)

Dennis D. Spencer, M.D.
Nixdorff-German Professor of Neurosurgery
Professor and Chief
Section of Neurological Surgery
Yale University School of Medicine   (42)

Frank C. Spencer, M.D.
Professor and Chairman
Department of Surgery
New York University School of Medicine
(18, 19, 20)

Michael L. Steer, M.D.
Professor of Surgery
Harvard Medical School   (32)

Thomas R. Stevenson, M.D.
Assistant Professor of Surgery
Section of Plastic Surgery
University of Michigan Hospitals   (46)

Erwin R. Thal, M.D.
Professor of Surgery
The University of Texas Southwestern
Medical School at Dallas   (6)

James C. Thompson, M.D.
James Woods Harris Professor and Chairman
of Surgery
Department of Surgery
The University of Texas Medical Branch   (27)

Courtney M. Townsend, Jr., M.D.
Robertson-Poth Professor
Department of Surgery
The University of Texas Medical Branch,
Galveston (27)

Victor F. Trastek, M.D.
Instructor
Mayo Medical School (25)

Alonzo P. Walker, M.D.
Assistant Professor of Surgery
Medical College of Wisconsin (34)

R. Christie Wray, Jr., M.D.
Professor and Chair
Division of Plastic Surgery
University of Rochester School of Medicine
and Dentistry (14)

Preface

The publication of the 5th edition of this textbook constitutes a meaningful milestone. As with many anniversaries, the anniversary of the remaining editors' 25-year association with *Principles of Surgery* prompts reminiscence and reflections. Many events have occurred since six younger surgeons, David Hume, Richard C. Lillehei, G. Tom Shires, Frank C. Spencer, Edward H. Storer, and I, agreed to embark on a new venture—the creation of a new textbook of surgery that would be readily different from those already available. Drs. Hume, Lillehei, and Storer all died tragically during their intellectual prime. The three remaining editors have been privileged to witness extraordinary changes and refinements in the science of surgery. As a consequence, we have felt obliged to impart a presentation of these changes with the publication of subsequent editions. We are particularly gratified by the favorable reception of our extended efforts. The major reward that we have realized from these five editions is the sense that we have contributed to the education of a generation of students of surgery.

Seymour I. Schwartz, M.D.

Preface to the First Edition

The raison d'être for a new textbook in a discipline which has been served by standard works for many years was the Editorial Board's initial conviction that a distinct need for a modern approach in the dissemination of surgical knowledge existed. As incoming chapters were reviewed, both the need and satisfaction became increasingly apparent and, at the completion, we felt a sense of excitement at having the opportunity to contribute to the education of modern and future students concerned with the care of surgical patients.

The recent explosion of factual knowledge has emphasized the need for a presentation which would provide the student an opportunity to assimilate pertinent facts in a logical fashion. This would then permit correlation, synthesis of concepts, and eventual extrapolation to specific situations. The physiologic bases for diseases are therefore emphasized and the manifestations and diagnostic studies are considered as a reflection of pathophysiology. Therapy then becomes logical in this schema and the necessity to regurgitate facts is minimized. In appreciation of the impact which Harrison's PRINCIPLES OF INTERNAL MEDICINE has had, the clinical manifestations of the disease processes are considered in detail for each area. Since the operative procedure represents the one element in the therapeutic armentarium unique to the surgeon, the indications, important technical considerations, and complications receive appropriate emphasis. While we apprecite that a textbook cannot hope to incorporate an atlas of surgical procedures, we have provided the student a single book which will satisfy the sequential demands in the care and considerations of surgical patients.

The ultimate goal of the Editorial Board has been to collate a book which is deserving of the adjective "modern." We have therefore selected as authors dynamic and active contributors to their particular fields. The au courant concept is hopefully apparent throughout the entire work and is exemplified by appropriate emphasis on diseases of modern surgical interest, such as trauma, transplantation, and the recently appreciated importance of rehabilitation. Cardiovascular surgery is presented in keeping with the exponential strides recently achieved.

There are two major subdivisions to the text. In the first twelve chapters, subjects that transcend several organ systems are presented. The second portion of the book represents a consideration of specific organ systems and surgical specialties.

Throughout the text, the authors have addressed themselves to a sophisticated audience, regarding the medical student as a graduate student, incorporating material generally sought after by the surgeon in training and presenting information appropriate for the continuing education of the practicing surgeon. The need for a text such as we have envisioned is great and the goal admittedly high. It is our hope that this effort fulfills the expressed demands.

Seymour I. Schwartz, M.D.

Contents of Volume One

Endocrine and Metabolic Responses to Injury

Donald S. Gann and Joseph F. Amaral

Introduction

INTRODUCTION

Injury occurs in so many forms and is of such varying intensities that it is not surprising that the response to injury may also be quite variable. There are metabolic changes that are common to virtually all injuries and that when taken together constitute one aspect of the body's response to trauma. These metabolic changes may be broadly divided into: (1) those concerned with whole body energy and substrate metabolism; (2) those concerned with fluid and electrolyte metabolism; and (3) those concerned with local wound metabolism. The changes in whole body energy and substrate metabolism and those in fluid and electrolyte metabolism are for the most part the result of the systemic neuroendocrine environment. By contrast, local wound metabolism is to a large extent independent of the systemic neuroendocrine environment.

Although it has been customary to view the neuroendocrine environment consequent to injury as a response to injury per se, it is now clear that the pattern of hormonal response seen is the result of a set of physiological reflexes initiated by specific aspects of the injury. Each of these aspects of injury may be viewed as a stimulus initiating the reflex. The stimuli are alterations in "homeostasis" that are perceived by specialized receptors that are located peripherally and centrally. These receptors transduce the stimulus into a discrete set of neural inputs (afferent signals) that are transmitted to the central nervous system via specific neural pathways. In the central nervous system, these inputs are integrated with other signals, resulting in the production of a discrete set of neural outputs (efferent signals). In turn, the efferent signals result in the stimulation or inhibition of the release of numerous neuroendocrine effectors that produce physiologic changes aimed at correcting the alterations in homeostasis. The response to these stimuli may be modulated by a number of factors including concurrent medical illness, the quality and quantity of fluid replacement, concurrent medications, presence of ethanol or other commonly abused drugs, and the age of the individual.

In the absence of major injury, sepsis, or starvation, the alterations in homeostasis are small and the response is directed at fine tuning and integrating the physiologic functioning of the organism. In the presence of major injury, sepsis, or starvation, the stimuli are multiple and intensified and the reflexes are directed at an integrated attempt by the organism to restore cardiovascular stability, to preserve oxygen delivery, to mobilize energy substrates, to increase the supply of critical substrates, primarily glucose, directed at healing the wound, and to minimize pain.

In order to clarify the mechanisms underlying the response to injury, we will break the injury into its potential components (stimuli), the interactions and modulations of these components in the central nervous system, and the metabolic results of the neuroendocrine effectors. We will separate the metabolic responses of the whole body, of the kidney, and of the wound.

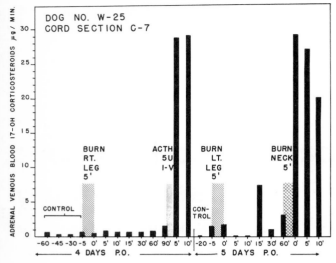

Fig. 1-1. Adrenocortical response to a burn following section of the cord at the level of C_7. A 5-min burn of the right leg, which was below the level of section, produced no increase in adrenocorticosteroid secretion over the control values. Five units of ACTH given intravenously produced an immediate and marked rise in adrenocortical output. With the dog under pentobarbital anesthesia, a burn of the left hindlimb produced no significant increase in adrenocorticosteroid output, but in marked contrast, a burn of the neck, which was above the level of cord section, produced an immediate and marked increase in adrenocortical secretion. (From: *Hume DM, Egdahl RH: Ann Surg 150:697, 1959, with permission.*)

SYSTEMIC NEUROENDOCRINE REFLEXES

Stimuli

In order for a reflex to be initiated, the stimulus must be perceived by specialized receptors that transduce the stimulus into electrical activity and transmit it to the brain. As shown in Fig. 1-1, dogs subjected to a 5-min burn of an area below the level of cord transection do not demonstrate any increase in corticosteroid secretion, whereas the same animals subjected to a 5-min burn above the level of cord transection demonstrate a response similar to that seen following the intravenous injection of five units of ACTH (maximum adrenal stimulation). Similarly, paraplegics do not respond to injuries below the level of the cord transection. As shown in Fig. 1-2, a paraplegic patient, from spinal cord transection at T_4, undergoing gastrectomy fails to release ACTH in response to the operation but is capable of producing corticosteroids in response to intravenously administered ACTH. In both examples, the denervation prevents afferent impulses from reaching the brain. This is exemplified by the experiments of Hume and Egdahl in which one hindlimb of a dog was left attached to the body only by the femoral nerve, artery, and vein (Fig. 1-3). Trauma to the innervated but otherwise detached hindlimb continued to evoke an increased secretion of ACTH and cortisol. When the nerve was severed, however, leaving only the artery and vein intact, the response to trauma was

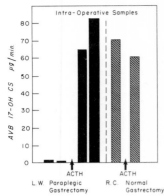

Fig. 1-2. Comparison of the adrenal venous blood content of 17-hydroxycorticosteroid (17-OHCS) in response to a gastric operation in a patient with spinal cord transection at T_4 and in a normal patient. The paraplegic patient fails to demonstrate an increase in 17-OHCS. This presumably results from the absence of ACTH production in response to surgery, since the ability of paraplegic patient's adrenal glands to respond to ACTH is demonstrated by the marked increase in 17-OHCS content of adrenal venous blood in response to intravenously administered ACTH. In contrast, the normal patient shows maximal secretion of 17-OHCS in response to the operation and no further increase is seen with intravenous ACTH. (From: *Hume DM et al: Surgery 52:174, 1962, with permission.*)

eliminated. Similarly, patients undergoing hip replacement under spinal anesthesia do not demonstrate an increase in vasopressin secretion during the procedure when compared with patients undergoing the same procedure under general anesthesia (Fig. 1-4). As the effect of spinal anesthesia wears off, the response for vasopressin is the same in both groups. Laparotomies or burns, in the absence of diminished circulatory volume, do not result in adrenocortical stimulation if the traumatized area is denervated. Similarly, local anesthetics, by blocking the

Fig. 1-3. The effect of limb denervation on ACTH secretion following trauma. The hind leg has been isolated so that it is attached to the body by only one artery, one vein, and one nerve. The burn of the isolated leg produces a marked and immediate response in adrenal venous corticosteroid secretion. During the height of this response the nerve was cut and the secretion dropped promptly to control values. A second burn of the leg now produced no adrenocortical response. ACTH injected subcutaneously into the isolated leg produced a prompt and marked increase in adrenocortical secretion. (From: *Hume DM et al: Surgery 52:697, 1962, with permission.*)

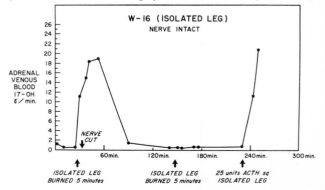

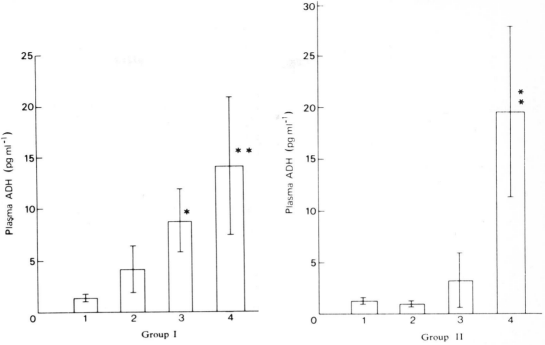

Fig. 1-4. Plasma vasopressin concentrations in 14 patients undergoing total hip replacement under general anesthesia (7 patients—Group I) or epidural anesthesia (7 patients—Group II). Patients who underwent surgery under general anesthesia developed a progressive increase in plasma vasopressin, whereas those under epidural anesthesia demonstrated an increase only 4-h after surgery and presumably as the anesthetic wore off. (From: *Bonnet F et al: Br J Anaesth 54:29, 1982, with permission.*)

transmission of afferent impulses from the area of injury, inhibit the neuroendocrine response to operative trauma elicited by stimuli present at the operative site.

The perception of the stimulus need not be conscious, as evidenced by the ability of individuals to respond to stimuli present in injury despite the presence of general anesthesia. The response may not be the same that would have occurred had anesthesia not been present. This difference arises, at least in part, through the ability of general anesthetics themselves to initiate, inhibit, or augment neuroendocrine reflexes. No operative trauma ought to be thought of without a consideration of the particular anesthetic agent employed and the depth and duration of anesthesia.

The primary stimuli to the neuroendocrine reflexes include (1) changes in effective circulating volume; (2) changes in the concentrations of oxygen, carbon dioxide, or hydrogen ions of tissues or blood; (3) pain; (4) emotional stimuli such as anxiety and pain; (5) alterations in the availability of substrates, particularly glucose; (6) changes in core or ambient temperature; and (7) sepsis (Fig. 1-5).

EFFECTIVE CIRCULATING VOLUME. Virtually all injuries are characterized by the loss of effective circulating volume that may result from the direct loss of blood, as in hemorrhage, from the loss or sequestration of plasma vol-

ume, as in dehydration and third space losses, and from the inability of the body fluids to circulate, as in cardiac failure or pulmonary embolism. The loss of the effective circulating volume is sensed by high-pressure baroreceptors in the aorta, carotid arteries, and renal arteries, which are sensitive to the arterial pressure and its rate of change, and by low-pressure stretch receptors in the atria, which are sensitive to the atrial volume and its rate of change. The total circulating volume and the effective circulating volume are not the same in that the total circulating volume is effective only to the extent that it is sensed by these receptors. Therefore, pump failure or sequestration of fluid behind an obstruction (e.g., tension pneumothorax, cardiac tamponade, and cirrhosis) leads to an effective circulating volume that is less than the total circulating volume. Even though the total circulating volume may be increased, as in congestive heart failure, the effective circulating volume as sensed by high- and low-pressure receptors is decreased. This results in the initiation and maintenance of the baroreceptor reflex such that salt and water continue to be conserved and total peripheral resistance is increased.

The afferent signals from high-pressure baroreceptors and from low-pressure stretch receptors exert a tonic inhibition over the release of many hormones and the activities of the central and autonomic nervous systems (Fig. 1-6). A decrease in effective circulating volume produces a decrease in baroreceptor and stretch receptor activities that leads to a release of the tonic inhibition of the neuroendocrine system. This leads to the increased secretion of ACTH, vasopressin, renin, growth hormone, beta-endorphin, and catecholamines. In turn, these neuroendocrine effectors bring about further neuroendocrine

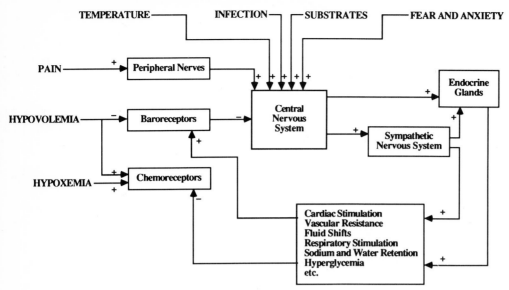

changes, including stimulation of cortisol secretion by the adrenal gland in response to ACTH, stimulation of the conversion of angiotensinogen to angiotensin in the vascular space by renin; stimulation of aldosterone secretion by the adrenal gland in response to ACTH and angiotensin II; stimulation of glucagon secretion by the pancreas in response to epinephrine, and inhibition of insulin secretion by the pancreas in response to epinephrine. Decreases in the effective circulating volume that are sensed by high-pressure stretch receptors in the juxtaglomerular complexes of the kidney also lead to the secretion of renin and, therefore, to the formation of angiotensin and to the secretion of aldosterone. The decrease in baroreceptor

Fig. 1-5. Overview of the neuroendocrine reflexes induced by shock and injury. There are at least seven stimuli consequent to injury that elicit neuroendocrine reflexes. These include hypovolemia; pain; changes in pO_2, pCO_2, pH; infection; emotional arousal; changes in substrate availability; and changes in temperature. The most common of these are hypovolemia and pain.

Fig. 1-6. Efferent limb of baroreceptor and chemoreceptor activation. Inactivation of baroreceptors or activation of chemoreceptors results in the stimulation of the hypothalamus and of the vascular component of the sympathetic nervous system. However, in contrast to the inactivation of baroreceptors, activation of chemoreceptors produces a decrease in cardiac sympathetic nervous system activity and an increase in parasympathetic activity.

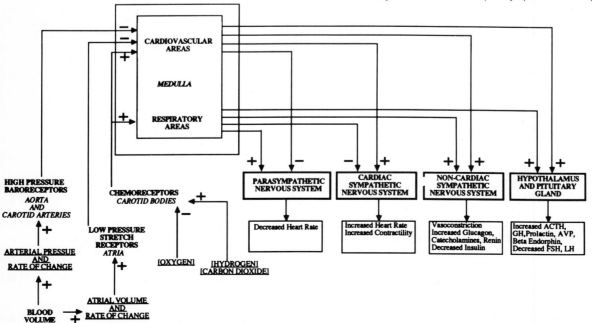

and in stretch receptor discharge also stimulates the vascular component of the sympathetic nervous system, leading to peripheral vasoconstriction and to an increase in cardiac sympathetic and a decrease in cardiac parasympathetic nervous activities, which in turn lead to an increase in heart rate and cardiac contractility.

The neuroendocrine and autonomic responses initiated by a decrease in effective circulating volume are proportional to the magnitude of the decrease. The neuroendocrine response to a 20 percent hemorrhage is greater than that observed following a 10 percent hemorrhage. Many of the neuroendocrine and cardiovascular responses have maximal responses that are achieved usually when the effective circulating volume has been decreased by 30 to 40 percent. Further decreases in the effective circulating volume cannot be compensated for, and hypotension ensues.

CHEMORECEPTOR REFLEX. Changes in the concentration of oxygen, hydrogen ions, and carbon dioxide in the blood initiate cardiovascular, pulmonary, and neuroendocrine responses through the activation of peripheral chemoreceptors. Under normal circumstances, these receptors, which are located in the carotid and the aortic bodies, are not activated. Decreases in the concentration of oxygen or, to a lesser extent, increases in the concentrations of hydrogen ions and carbon dioxide are sensed by these receptors, leading to the activation of neuroendocrine reflexes. As a result of the extremely high blood flow through the chemoreceptors, the pO_2 of arterial blood, chemoreceptor tissue, and venous blood is nearly the same. A decrease in arterial blood flow or in arterial oxygen tension increases the extraction of oxygen by the chemoreceptor tissue, decreases the venous pO_2, and through an unknown mechanism, activates the chemoreceptor.

Similar to the inactivation of baroreceptors and stretch receptors, the activation of chemoreceptors results in the stimulation of the hypothalamus and of the vascular component of the sympathetic nervous system (Fig. 1-6). In contrast to the inactivation of baroreceptors and stretch receptors, the activation of chemoreceptors produces a decrease in cardiac sympathetic nervous system activity and an increase in parasympathetic nervous system activity, thereby leading to a decrease in heart rate and cardiac contractility. Chemoreceptor activation stimulates the respiratory center, leading to an increase in respiratory rate. Hypovolemia is usually accompanied by hyperventilation because the decrease in the effective circulating volume activates the chemoreceptor through a reduction in blood flow.

PAIN AND EMOTION. Pain and emotional arousal are characteristic of any injury and lead to the activation of the neuroendocrine system. Pain, acting through projections of peripheral nociceptive fibers to the central nervous system, results in the stimulation of the thalamus and of the hypothalamus. Emotional arousal is produced by the perception or threat of injury and through the limbic areas of the brain invokes an emotional response resulting in anger, fear, or anxiety. In turn, these emotional changes stimulate the neuroendocrine reflexes through projections from the limbic system to hypothalamic and lower brain stem nuclei. As a result, both pain and emotion arousal produce an increase in the secretion of vasopressin, ACTH, endogenous opiates, catecholamines, cortisol, and aldosterone and changes in the activity of the autonomic nervous system.

Emotional factors have an effect on epinephrine release (sweating, tremor, tachycardia, dry mouth, pallor, etc.), the so-called fight or flight response described by Cannon. This factor may contribute to some of the differences between the effects of injury in the conscious state versus those of the same type of injury in the anesthetized patient. As noted by Wiggers when discussing the role of emotional factors in the investigation of hemorrhagic shock, "The writer cannot be convinced that a subject with an indwelling catheter in his arm vein and auricle and forewarned that an experiment is to be conducted which will probably lead to uncomfortable experiences, is entirely free from psychic reactions which may influence the course of events."

SUBSTRATE ALTERATIONS. Changes in the plasma glucose concentration are the primary substrate alterations that activate neuroendocrine reflexes. The plasma glucose concentration is sensed by receptors in the hypothalamus (ventromedial nucleus) and in the pancreas. A decrease in the plasma glucose concentration stimulates the release of catecholamines, growth hormone, cortisol, ACTH, beta-endorphin, and vasopressin through central pathways (hypothalamus and autonomic nervous system) and stimulates the release of glucagon both by central (autonomic nervous system) and by peripheral pathways (direct pancreatic activation). In addition, the secretion of insulin is inhibited by central pathways (autonomic nervous system) and by the pancreas itself.

Although changes in the concentrations of individual amino acids produce alterations in the secretion of various hormones, their potency varies from amino acid to amino acid and the mechanisms by which they produce these alterations are not entirely understood. For example, arginine is a potent stimulus to the secretion of insulin and of glucagon, but leucine, which also stimulates the secretion of insulin, does not stimulate the secretion of glucagon. The stimulation of hormonal secretion by amino acids is, at least in part, directed through cell surface receptors, since nonmetabolizable analogs of leucine and arginine are effective. The intracellular metabolism of amino acids may also be important. Amino acids also exert an important role in the neuroendocrine response because they are the parent compound for a number of hormonal agents and neurotransmitters (e.g., thyroxine, catecholamines, histamine, serotonin, and all peptide hormones).

TEMPERATURE. Changes in the core temperature of the body are sensed in the preoptic area of the hypothalamus and lead to alterations in the secretion of many hormones including ACTH, vasopressin, cortisol, epinephrine, growth hormone, catecholamines, aldosterone, and thyroxine. The core temperature may change as a result of alterations in ambient temperature, as a result of the loss of the normal thermal insulating barrier (burns), as a result of inadequate hepatic blood flow (hypovolemia) or substrate supply (starvation), or as a result of inadequate peripheral vasoconstriction or vasodilation (sepsis).

Changes in the ambient temperature stimulate neuroendocrine reflexes, either directly or through changes in the core temperature. Similarly, infection may stimulate the neuroendocrine system directly through the action of endotoxin, or indirectly through secondary changes in blood volume, oxygen concentration, substrate concentrations, and pain or through monokines released from inflammatory cells such as tumor necrosis factor and interleukin-1.

Integration of Stimuli and Modulation of Output

As indicated above, the principal signals to initiate the neuroendocrine response to injury are those of hypovolemia and of pain. The hormonal response is diffuse and includes the release of ACTH, cortisol, growth hormone, epinephrine, norepinephrine, glucagon, renin, angiotensin, and aldosterone (Table 1-1). In each case, the prompt initiation of hormonal release depends upon a reflex activated by afferent nerves. Although the reflex initiation of increased sympathetic activity may take place at the level of the medulla or spinal cord alone, it appears that even these reflexes require hypothalamic coordination similar to that observed in the control of the release of the anterior pituitary hormones. The precise pathways from afferent nerve endings to the hypothalamus have been studied in detail primarily for ACTH and to a lesser degree for vasopressin and catecholamines. Data for the control of other hormones, where they are available, seem analogous, and it is highly likely that the afferent pathways are shared to a considerable extent. This provides a basis for a coordinated response of the neuroendocrine system to injury.

The central pathways have been best delineated for the neural control of ACTH and vasopressin in response to hypovolemia and to a lesser extent in response to pain. The principal afferent receptors for blood volume lie in the right atrium and in the carotid arteries and for nociception in the substantia gelatinosa of the dorsal horn

Table 1-1. NEUROENDOCRINE RESPONSE

Increased release		Decreased release or unchanged
Epinephrine	Beta-endorphin	Insulin
Norepinephrine	Growth hormone	Estrogen
Dopamine	Prolactin	Testosterone
Glucagon	Somatostatin	Thyroxine
Renin	Eicosanoids	T_3
Angiotensin	Histamine	TSH
Vasopressin	Kinins	FSH
ACTH	Serotonin	LH
Cortisol	Interleukin-1	IGF
Aldosterone	TNF	

and nucleus caudalis of cranial nerve V. The afferent nerves from volume receptors converge on the nucleus tractus solitarius (NTS) and related structures in the dorsolateral medulla (Fig. 1-7). From this point, they project without synapsing to the nuclei of the locus ceruleus, parabrachial nucleus, and periaqueductal gray area in the dorsal pons, to the locus subceruleus and dorsal raphe nucleus of the dorsal pons and to the A1 region of the caudal, ventrolateral medulla. The pathway to A1 appears to constitute the principal projection from NTS. Nociceptive fibers also project to A1 neurons by nonsynaptic projections from the nucleus caudalis of cranial nerve V and the substantia gelatinosa of the dorsal horn. The A1 region of the medulla appears to be the first possible site for the interaction of pain and volume signals. Nucleus caudalis also projects to the region of the dorsal pons mentioned above, and interaction of nociception and volume stimuli has been observed in this region.

Fibers from A1 project, again without synapsing, to the nuclei of the locus ceruleus, parabrachial nucleus, and periaqueductal gray area in the dorsal pons and via the median forebrain bundle to the ventral hypothalamus and to the paraventricular nucleus. The dorsal pons area is critical to the generation of the classic neuroendocrine response to injury, since a lesion in the periaqueductal gray area of the dorsal pons will eliminate the response. This response appears to arise from fibers that project from the nuclei of the dorsal pons to the hypothalamus in three principal pathways, two stimulatory and one inhibitory. A dorsal stimulatory pathway courses through the dorsal longitudinal fasciculus to end in the dorsal hypothalamus, including the paraventricular nucleus. A ventral stimulatory pathway courses through the ventral tegmental area of the midbrain to enter the medial forebrain bundle and terminate in the anteroventral hypothalamic nuclei, including the suprachiasmatic and ventromedial nuclei and in the dorsal hypothalamus, including the paraventricular nucleus. An intermediate inhibitory pathway passes up the central tegmental tract and mammillary peduncles to terminate in the posterior hypothalamic area. Output from the paraventricular nucleus includes the release of corticotropin releasing factor (CRF), the agent that controls pituitary release of ACTH from the median eminence and arginine vasopressin (AVP). By contrast, output from the posterior hypothalamic area produces inhibition of CRF and AVP release either through the release of a specific factor or through inhibitory projections to the paraventricular nucleus and other hypothalamic areas.

Although the previous discussion has focused on the importance of the paraventricular nucleus in neuroendocrine reflexes, other nuclei in the hypothalamus play a central role in these reflexes by controlling the release of releasing factors, which in turn govern the secretion of various anterior pituitary hormones or autonomic nervous system activity. There is no clear overlap of function among the various hypothalamic nuclei. For example, the posterior hypothalamic area is involved in the control of ACTH and of the descending sympathetic activity. The paraventricular nucleus is involved in the con-

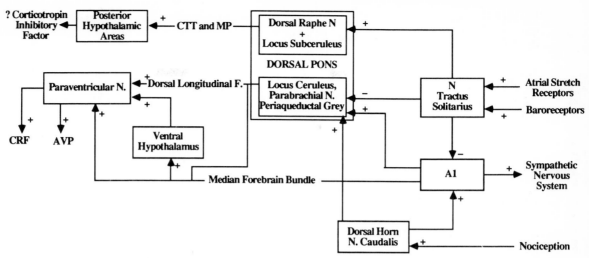

Fig. 1-7. The proposed neural organization for the control of ACTH and vasopressin in response to hemodynamic change and nociception. Three principal areas of the hypothalamus receive signals from the principal pontine areas, projecting through the areas defined in the midbrain to inhibit or facilitate release of vasopressin and of corticotropin releasing factor (CRF) by the median eminence and thus of ACTH. Thus, the principal pathways from atrial and carotid receptors to the median eminence for control of release of CRF and vasopressin are multiple. Symbols: N, nucleus; F, fasiculus; +, stimulates; −, inhibits.

trol of vasopressin, of oxytocin, and of ACTH. The ventromedial nucleus is involved in the control of growth hormone and ACTH. The supraoptic nucleus has been shown to be active in the control of vasopressin and of oxytocin. The suprachiasmatic nucleus appears to control the circadian rhythms of ACTH and of gonadotropins. In turn, hypothalamic control of the anterior pituitary is accomplished by the secretion of neurohormones into the capillary loops in the median eminence. Although this view focuses on the role of the hypothalamus in neuroendocrine control, it is clear that this region of the brain is important in the coordination of other autonomic functions as well as in the control of other hormones that appear to be less affected by injury.

As a result of the similar pathways through which sensory inputs enter into the central nervous system, integration of afferent signals can occur in the CNS with a resultant modulation of efferent signals from the CNS. Consequently, the neuroendocrine response to a given stimulus is not an all or none phenomenon nor is it always the same. The response depends to a large extent upon the intensity and the duration of the stimulus, the presence of simultaneous and sequential stimuli that are qualitatively the same or different, the status of the receptor at the time of stimulation, and the time of day during which the stimulus occurs.

The dependence of the response to a stimulus upon the intensity and duration of the stimulus, as well as the importance of central nervous system integration, is well described for cardiopulmonary reflexes and adrenomedullary secretion of catecholamines. Despite the potent

activation of the sympathetic nervous system by small nonhypotensive hemorrhages, adrenomedullary secretion of catecholamines occurs only when hypotension develops. Since nonhypotensive hemorrhages have little if any effect upon arterial baroreceptors, this finding suggests that inactivation of cardiac stretch receptors alone is not sufficient for the activation of catecholamine release. Similarly, activation of chemoreceptors alone or inactivation of baroreceptors in isolation produces potent sympathetic nervous system activity but little adrenal catecholamine secretion. Adrenal catecholamine secretion does occur during hypotensive hemorrhages in which both receptors are activated, suggesting that high-pressure baroreceptors and low-pressure volume receptors both must be inactivated for adrenomedullary stimulation to occur. Afferent fibers from baroreceptors travel via the sinus branch of the glossopharyngeal nerve and via the vagus nerve to the nucleus tractus solitarius (NTS). Similarly, the afferent fibers from the cardiac stretch receptors travel via the vagus nerve to the NTS, from which secondary projections are sent to higher brain centers. Therefore, the interaction of arterial baroreceptor and cardiac stretch receptor inputs may occur as early as the NTS.

In addition to the intensity and the duration, the rate at which a stimulus is presented is also an important parameter in the modulation of efferent signals that are elicited by the stimulus. For example, Bereiter et al. have demonstrated that the serum epinephrine concentration in the cat following hemorrhage is a function of the rate and the magnitude of the hemorrhage (Fig. 1-8). Whereas small hemorrhages, equivalent to 10 to 20 percent of the blood volume, elicited the same increase in serum epinephrine concentrations independent of the rate of hemorrhage, large hemorrhages, equivalent to 30 percent of the blood volume, elicited a greater response when they were performed rapidly (10 percent/min) than when they were performed slowly (2 percent/min). Similar findings have also been reported for aldosterone, renin, and vasopressin (Fig. 1-9). Thus the neuroendocrine response of a trauma-

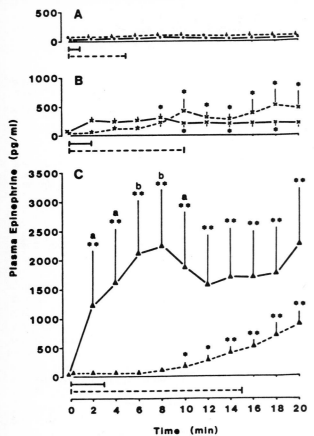

Fig. 1-8. Plasma epinephrine concentrations in response to graded blood loss in the cat at rapid and slow rates of hemorrhage. *A.* 10 percent hemorrhage, rapid rate = ●———● (*n* = 6), slow rate = ●—–—–● (*n* = 7). *B.* 20 percent hemorrhage, rapid rate = ×———× (*n* = 11), slow rate = ×–—–—× (*n* = 7). *C.* 30 percent hemorrhage, rapid rate = Δ———Δ (*n* = 8), slow rate = Δ–—–—Δ (*n* = 8). The horizontal bars under each figure represent the period of blood removal for each hemorrhage magnitude. *$p < 0.05$, **$p < 0.01$ vs. control group. a. $p < 0.05$; b. $p < 0.01$ vs. slow rate of hemorrhage. (From: *Bereiter DA et al: Am J Physiol 1986, with permission.*)

tized individual with a ruptured spleen who loses 30 percent blood volume in 1 h may be considerably different from the response seen in a patient with multiple long bone fractures who loses 30 percent blood volume over 1 day.

The responsiveness of receptors themselves to the transduction of the stimulus into neural activity is itself variable. For example, central osmoreceptors located in the hypothalamus, near the third ventricle, change their set point in response to other neural inputs. Alterations both of plasma osmolality and of effective circulating volume are potent stimuli to the secretion of vasopressin. Inputs from receptors monitoring these parameters interact in the central nervous system such that a change in the set point of the osmoreceptor occurs when the secretion of vasopressin is altered by neural inputs from baroreceptors. As a result, changes in the effective circulating vol-

ume do not eliminate the influence of the osmoregulatory system. Instead, the change in the set point of the osmoreceptor makes it more or less sensitive to a given osmotic stimulus. Clinically, this situation is observed in the hypervolemic, hyponatremic patient who despite an increased effective circulating volume produces vasopressin in response to the low plasma osmolality.

Similarly, the set point and the gain of baroreceptors may be altered by the convergence of other sensory inputs, such as viscerosomatic and somatosensory afferents, with baroreceptor inputs in the cardiovascular areas of the medulla. The responsiveness of baroreceptors themselves may be increased by the response they initiate, since baroreceptor responsiveness is increased by catecholamines, vasopressin, and angiotensin. Furthermore, the sensitivity of some receptors, such as those of the adrenal cortex, changes as a function of the time of day. For example, despite a similar response of ACTH to hemorrhage when it occurs in the morning or at night, the secretory response of cortisol to ACTH is significantly greater at night (Fig. 1-10). The latter finding may have particular significance for the traumatized patient, since severe trauma is much more likely to occur at night than during the day, but its importance in recovery from injury remains unknown. A particular stimulus of the same magnitude, rate, and duration may have less effect under certain circumstances than under others.

The stimuli accompanying injury, sepsis, and starvation rarely occur singly. Upon injury, the individual is likely to perceive multiple stimuli simultaneously. The neuroendocrine response to injury is the summation of all the stimuli the individual perceives and processes, and it is often different from the response to any single stimulus given alone (Fig. 1-11). For example, Egdahl and coworkers found hypothermic dogs responded with smaller increases in the secretions of ACTH, corticosteroids, and catecholamines than did normothermic dogs; Redding and Mueller found an increase in the survival of dogs that were hemorrhaged at lower ambient temperatures than dogs at normal or increased temperatures; Bereiter et al. demonstrated that the secretion of ACTH was greater to hemorrhage and noxious stimulation than to hemorrhage or noxious stimulation alone (Fig. 1-12); Wood et al. have demonstrated that dogs with an elevated rectal temperature (and presumably infection) respond with a greater decrease in blood pressure and a greater increase in the secretion of ACTH, corticosteroids, and vasopressin than do dogs who are normothermic; and Overman and Wang reported that although a 40 percent hemorrhage alone produced a 50 percent mortality, a 30 percent hemorrhage produced a similar mortality only when combined with sciatic nerve stimulation.

In addition to multiple stimuli occurring simultaneously, it is not uncommon for multiple stimuli to occur sequentially as well. A patient involved in a motor vehicle accident may first experience pain from fractured ribs, then hypovolemia from a ruptured spleen, and then hypoxia from a slowly developing tension pneumothorax. According to classic endocrine feedback mechanisms, one might expect that the elevation of serum cortisol, for

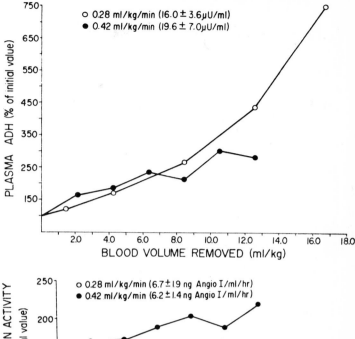

Fig. 1-9. The effect of rate of hemorrhage on vasopressin secretion and renin activity. There was no difference in plasma vasopressin when hemorrhages of 12 percent or less were performed either slowly (0.28 mL/kg/min) rapidly (0.42 mL/kg/min) in dogs. However, hemorrhages of greater than 12 percent were associated with a greater plasma vasopressin concentration if they were performed slowly. In contrast, renin activity was greater for fast hemorrhages. (From: *Claybaugh JR, Share L: Am J Physiol 224:519, 1973, with permission.*)

example, resulting from one set of stimuli would inhibit the release of ACTH by the second set. Under most circumstances this is not true and the response is unchanged or may actually be greater than the initial response (potentiation). The mechanism of this physiologic facilitation is not known, but it appears to take 60 to 90 min to offset the feedback inhibition of cortisol, and it lasts for at least 24 h. Gann, Lilly, and colleagues have demonstrated physiologic facilitation and potentiation for cortisol and catecholamines in response to sequential hemorrhages of the same magnitude and to sequential operations (Fig. 1-13). Similarly, Raff et al. have demonstrated potentiation of the adrenocortical response to hypoxia when an operation has been performed 2 h prior to the hypoxic stimulus but not 24 h prior (Fig. 1-14). The neuroendocrine response to trauma, shock, and sepsis may modify the response to subsequent operation, and the response to a second injury, such as posttraumatic operation, may

be considerably different from what it would have been had it occurred first.

The response to the stimuli consequent to injury may be modified by a variety of factors present in the individual prior to injury such as (1) ethanol and other recreational drugs, (2) concurrent medications, (3) drug withdrawal, (4) preexistent illness, and (5) the age of the individual.

Of these modifiers ethanol deserves special emphasis, since ethanol intoxication is a common finding in the multiply injured patient. According to *The Injury Fact Book* by Baker, O'Neill, and Karpf, over 75 percent of fatally injured motorcycle and auto accident victims between the ages of fifteen to sixty are intoxicated (blood ethanol > 100 mg percent) when the accident occurs at night and over 50 percent when it occurs during the day. Furthermore, over 50 percent of nighttime and 25 percent of daytime pedestrian deaths among people fifteen to sixty-five years old involves an intoxicated individual.

The significance of alcohol intoxication on the overall response to injury has not been well studied but the ability of alcohol to alter metabolic and endocrine events is well recognized. For example, ethanol impairs hepatic gluconeogenesis by decreasing the concentration of NAD+ in the liver and thereby producing a more reduced state. This action of ethanol probably explains the find-

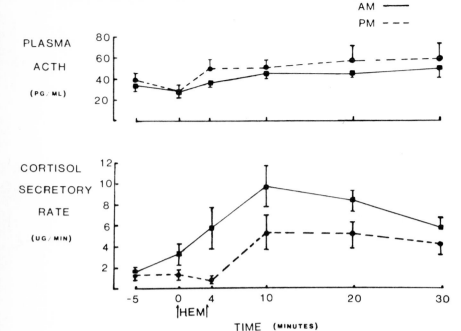

Fig. 1-10. Plasma ACTH concentration and cortisol secretory rates in dogs after a 10 mL/kg hemorrhage for 3 min in the morning (*n* = 9) or at night (*n* = 7). Although there was difference in plasma ACTH when the hemorrhage was performed in the morning or at night, cortisol secretion was greater in the morning. (From: *Engeland WC et al: Endocrinology 110:1856, 1982, with permission.*)

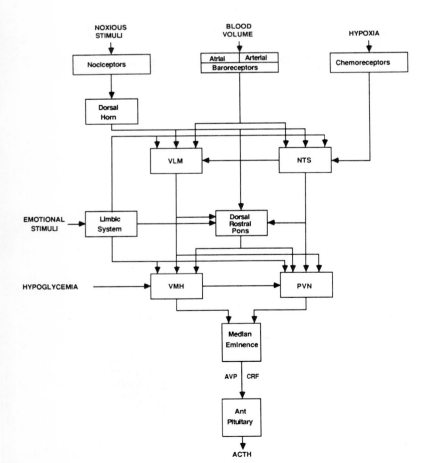

Fig. 1-11. Possible sites for the integration of the various stimuli elicited by injury are schematically represented. For example, noxious stimuli, hypovolemia, and hypoxia may first interact at NTS. Symbols: NTS, nucleus tractus solitarius; PVN, paraventricular nucleus; VLM, ventrolateral medulla; VMN, ventromedial hypothalamus (dorsomedial, arcuate, suprachiasmatic, periventricular, and premammillary nuclei). The dorsal rostral pons contains the loci ceruleus and subceruleus, the parabrachial nucleus, the periaqueductal gray and the dorsal raphe nucleus. Although this figure shows the release of ACTH, it is likely that other anterior pituitary hormones are controlled in a similar manner.

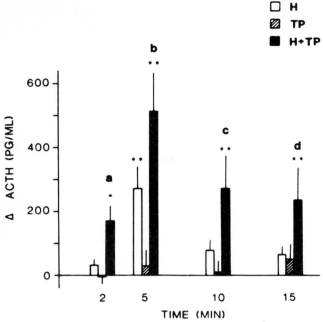

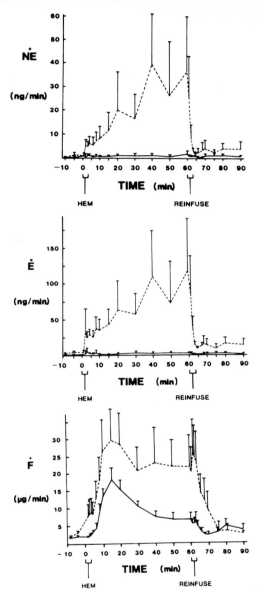

Fig. 1-12. Potentiation of the ACTH response to hemorrhage by nerve stimulation. H = hemorrhage, TP = tooth pulp, * = $p < 0.05$ vs. baseline, ** = $p < 0.01$ vs. baseline. (Letters above each sample time point denote intragroup individual comparisons: a = $p < 0.05$ H + TP vs. TP, b = $p < 0.01$ H + TP vs. TP or H, c = $p < 0.05$ H + TP vs. H, d = $p < 0.05$ H + TP vs. TP or H.) At all time points, the response of ACTH to hemorrhage and tooth pulp stimulation was greater than the response to either hemorrhage or tooth pulp stimulation alone. (From: *Bereiter DS et al: Endocrinology 113:1439, 1983, with permission.*)

Fig. 1-13. Potentiation of the secretory rates of epinephrine (E), norepinephrine (NE), and cortisol (F) to a 7.5 mL/kg hemorrhage in dogs when a hemorrhage of the same magnitude was performed on the previous day. The pattern of response between E and NE is the same, but that for NE is at a lower absolute rate than that for E. Hemorrhages took place at 0 min; reinfusion occurred at 60 min. ———— = mean response on day 1; — — — — = mean response on day 2. (From: *Lilly MP et al: Endocrinology 111:1917, 1982; 112:681, 1983, with permission.*)

ings of Stoner et al. in which the plasma glucose and pyruvate concentrations were lower and the plasma lactate concentrations were higher in intoxicated than in nonintoxicated patients at a given injury severity score. In addition, ethanol is capable of altering the neuroendocrine response as evidenced by an increase in central and urinary catecholamines, an increase in adrenal medullary catecholamine turnover, and by increasing plasma concentrations of cortisol and ACTH. Similarly, narcotics such as heroin and other recreational drugs such as cocaine produce potent metabolic and endocrine alterations and because of their anesthetic properties may serve to alter the response to injury. Withdrawal from these agents in the postinjury period may have profound metabolic and endocrine consequences that serve to prolong or alter the response to the injury. The latter is also true for commonly used drugs such as insulin which may be withheld from an unconscious patient who is not known to be diabetic.

Efferent Output

There are three major branches to the efferent limb of the reflex neuroendocrine response to injury, the autonomic response, the hormonal response, and the local tissue response. The former two responses arise in two distinct areas of the brain: the autonomic regions of the brain stem and the hypothalamic-pituitary axis. Output from the former changes the activities of the sympathetic and parasympathetic nervous systems, whereas outputs from both areas change the rates of hormonal secretion. As such, the endocrine response may be divided into hor-

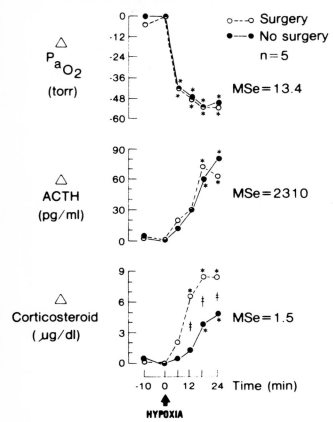

Fig. 1-14. Potentiation of plasma corticosteroids in dogs who are made hypoxic after surgery when compared with dogs made hypoxic without previous surgery. (* = different from 0 min sample; ‡ = difference between surgery and no surgery.) (From: *Raff H et al: Proc Soc Exp Biol Med 172:400, 1983, with permission.*)

mones whose secretion is primarily under hypothalamic-pituitary control (cortisol, thyroxine, growth hormone, and vasopressin) and hormones whose secretion is primarily under autonomic control (insulin, glucagon, and catecholamines). The local tissue response is composed of numerous small peptides (tissue factors, monokines, and autocoids) whose release may be mediated by the local inflammatory response in an injured area or by the injured tissue itself.

The hormones secreted by endocrine organs, the autocoids and monokines produced by tissues and inflammatory cells, and the neurotransmitters released at nerve terminals fall into one of five chemical classes. These are the fatty acid derivatives of cholesterol (cortisol, aldosterone) or arachidonic acid (prostaglandins, leukotrienes), proteins (insulin, glucagon), glycoproteins (thyroid stimulating hormone, follicle stimulating hormone), small polypeptides (vasopressin, enkephalin), and the amines (catecholamines, thyroxine, serotonin). All these agents act as cellular receptors that are either on the surface of cell membranes or in the cytoplasm of the cell. These cellular receptors are neither fixed nor unchangeable. Instead, they are in a dynamic state in which the number of recep-

tors on cells can be increased (up regulation) or decreased (down regulation) according to need. In addition, the affinity of these receptors for their specific hormone can also be changed.

By and large, the chemical nature of these agents determines the mechanism through which they exert their effects. Steroid hormones and possibly thyroxine, which are freely permeable to cell membranes, bind to cytosolic receptors in target cells. Although there are some rapid actions of steroid hormones that may be mediated by their binding to receptors on the plasma membrane, for the most part the interaction of steroid hormones and of thyroid hormones with receptors on the cell surface does not appear to be an important step in the initiation of the actions of these hormones since they appear to diffuse rapidly and freely across the cell membrane. Upon entering the cell, steroid hormones bind to cytosolic receptors that are specific for each hormone in a process that may be modulated by vitamin B_6. Once bound to the receptor, the receptor-hormone complex is activated and translocated to the nucleus. In the nucleus, the receptor-hormone complex binds to the nonhistone protein of nuclear chromatin, thereby modulating the transcription of genes into specific mRNA molecules that ultimately direct the synthesis of enzymatic, structural, and regulatory proteins (Fig. 1-15). This explains the 1- to 2-h delay in onset of most of the primary actions of steroid hormones. In addition, recent evidence suggests that the receptor hormone complex binds tRNA species. This may be a posttranscriptional mechanism through which steroid hormones are capable of modulating gene expression, i.e., by altering the efficiency of the translation of mRNA to proteins.

In contrast to steroid hormones, the action of most peptide and amine hormones, which generally bind to cell surface receptors, is faster and of shorter duration. In general, these hormones act either through alterations in the intracellular concentrations of cyclic adenosine monophosphate (cAMP) or calcium, the so-called second messengers, or through other intermediates (growth hormone via somatomedins). The second messenger system of hormonal action operates primarily through the activation and inactivation of regulatory proteins and enzymes rather than through the synthesis of new proteins (Fig. 1-16); this explains the faster onset of action and shorter duration of the effect of hormones that operate via this system versus those of steroid and other lipid soluble hormones.

The adrenergic receptor system may be considered the prototype for examining the mechanisms of action of second messengers since all the second messenger pathways known are represented in the four adrenergic receptors (alpha$_1$, alpha$_2$, beta$_1$, beta$_2$). Beta$_1$ and beta$_2$ receptors (differentiated on the basis of radioligand binding affinity) both function via the activation of membrane bound adenylate cyclase, which in turn leads to the production of cAMP. The increased intracellular concentration of cAMP activates an inactive protein kinase that then phosphorylates an inactive phosphorylase kinase to an active form. In turn, the active phosphorylase kinase phosphory-

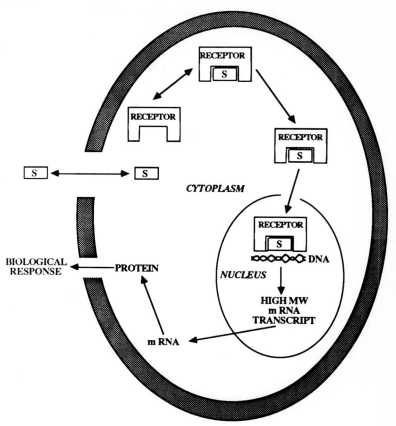

Fig. 1-15. The mechanism of action of steroid hormones. Steroids, which permeate the cell membrane freely, bind to cytosolic receptors and are then translocated to the nucleus, where the receptor hormone complex interacts with DNA to modulate transcription.

Fig. 1-16. Hormonal action mediated by cAMP or calcium. Alpha-1 receptors, through activation of phosphatidylinositol turnover, increase the intracellular concentration of calcium. Beta receptors, through activation of adenylate cyclase, increase the intracellular concentration of cAMP. An increase in either cAMP or calcium is then able to convert inactive protein kinase to active protein kinase.

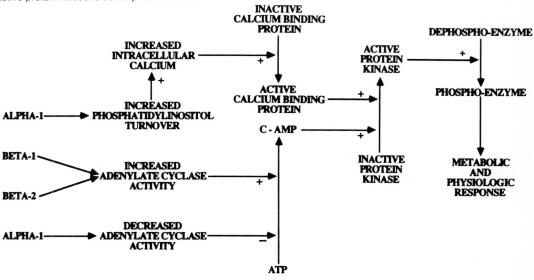

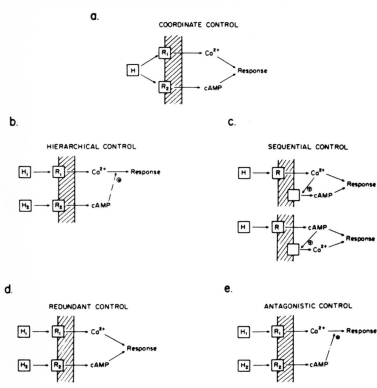

Fig. 1-17. The patterns of synarchic regulation by calcium and cAMP second messengers. See text for description of these patterns. (From: *Rassmusen H: Calcium and c-AMP as Synarchic Messengers. New York, Wiley Intersciences, 1981, Chap 4, with permission.*)

lates dephosphoregulatory enzymes, which may result in the activation of the regulatory enzyme (e.g., glycogen phosphorylase) or in its inactivation (e.g., glycogen synthetase). By contrast, alpha$_2$ receptor activation inhibits membrane bound adenylate cyclase, thereby decreasing the concentration of cAMP and active protein kinase.

Alpha$_2$ receptor activation results in an increase in phosphatidylinosital turnover that then mediates an increase in intracellular calcium concentration from intracellular and extracellular sources. The increase in intracellular calcium activates a calcium binding protein, calmodulin, which in turn activates an inactive protein kinase or phosphorylase kinase. It should also be noted that calcium is utilized as a second messenger for stimulus-response coupling of many other key biological processes including excitation-contraction coupling in muscle, excitation-secretion coupling at nerve endings and in exocrine and endocrine glands, maintenance of oxidative phosphorylation, activation of contractile and motile cell systems (microtubules and microfilaments), platelet activation, regulation of plasma membrane permeability, tight gap junction, and cell-to-cell communication.

The actions of intracellular cAMP and calcium in the coupling of receptor activation with hormonal action (stimulus-response coupling) are not independent. Instead, the actions of calcium and cAMP in stimulus-response coupling are highly interrelated and have been termed synarchic by Rassmusen. There are five basic patterns to the synarchic control of hormone-response coupling that cAMP and calcium (Fig. 1-17). In coordinate control, a hormone activates both a calcium activating receptor and a cAMP activating receptor, either one of which may produce the response alone. In hierarchical control, separate stimuli activate independently the calcium and cAMP pathways that are both necessary for a given response. In sequential control, the activation of one of the two limbs of the system leads to the activation of the other limb. Although the first limb can produce the response, activation of the second limb augments the response. In redundant control, two separate stimuli independently activate the two different limbs of the messenger system, either one of which can produce the response. Finally, in antagonist control one stimulus activates one limb of the messenger system that leads to the response and a second stimulus activates the second limb, which inhibits the ability of the first limb to produce the response. Although each of these control mechanisms can occasionally be found in cells in pure form, most of the presently known hormone-response coupling mechanisms involve mixed patterns.

HORMONAL REPONSE TO INJURY

CRF-ACTH-CORTISOL. Most types of trauma are characterized by an increased secretion of CRF, ACTH, and

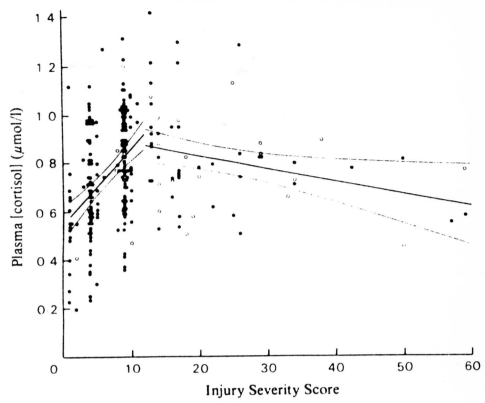

Fig. 1-18. The relationship between plasma cortisol and injury severity score (ISS) in initial samples from multiply injured patients studied within 8-h of injury. The regression lines and their 95 percent confidence limits between ISS 1 to 12 and ISS 13 to 59 are shown for ethanol negative (●) and ethanol positive (○) patients combined. (From: *Stoner HB et al: Clin Sci 56:563, 1979, with permission.*)

Fig. 1-19. There is a strong correlation between the extent of thermal injury, as determined by the percentage of body surface area burned and the plasma cortisol concentration in human beings. (From: *Vaughn GM et al: J Trauma 22:263–273, 1982, with permission.*)

cortisol that correlates with the severity of the injury (Fig. 1-18) and with the body surface area that is burned (Fig. 1-19). The plasma concentration of cortisol, which loses its normal circadian rhythm after injury, remains elevated for up to 4 weeks following thermal injury, for less than 1 week following soft tissue trauma, and for a few days following hemorrhage. In fact, in pure hypovolemia the plasma cortisol concentration returns rapidly to normal once the blood volume has been restored. Super-

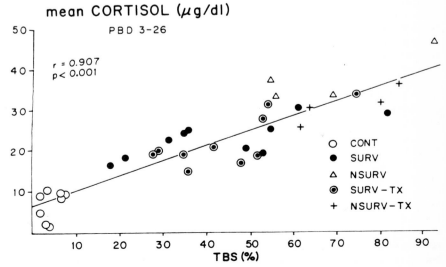

vening infection, however, will prolong the increase in plasma cortisol in all these injuries.

The synthesis and the release of cortisol from cells of the adrenal zona fasciculata is primarily under the control of adrenocorticotropin (ACTH) and is mediated by an increase in the intracellular concentration of cAMP that is produced by the binding of ACTH to surface receptors on the adrenal cells. ACTH is synthesized and stored in chromophobe cells of the anterior pituitary gland as a fragment of a larger molecule, pro-opiomelanocortin, that also contains gamma- and beta-lipotrophin, alpha-melanocyte stimulating hormone and beta-endorphin. The release of ACTH from these cells is stimulated by corticotropin releasing factor (CRF) from the paraventricular nucleus of the hypothalamus and may be potentiated by angiotensin II, vasopressin, and possibly oxytocin. Recent evidence also suggests that interleukin-1 may stimulate the production of ACTH by pituitary cells. By contrast, the release of ACTH is inhibited by cortisol (long feedback) and by ACTH itself (short feedback). In general, ACTH is increased following injury in a pattern that closely parallels that observed for cortisol. Cortisol may remain elevated for prolonged periods following injury despite an early return of ACTH to normal as demonstrated in the studies of burn victims by Vaughan and colleagues.

Corticotropin releasing factor is synthesized primarily in cells of the paraventricular nucleus that are near but distinct from those that secrete vasopressin. The release of CRF into the hypophyseal-portal venous system is induced primarily by neurogenic inputs into the hypothalamic cells. Vasopressin potentiates the release of CRF, as well as its action on the anterior pituitary gland; the release of both CRF and vasopressin may be potentiated by angiotensin II.

Cortisol has widespread effects upon the metabolism and utilization of glucose, amino acids, and fatty acids. In the liver, cortisol inhibits the pentose phosphate shunt, the action of insulin, and several regulatory glycolytic enzymes, including glucokinase, phosphofructokinase, and pyruvate kinase, and it stimulates the uptake of amino acids, the activities of amino acid transaminases, the activity of glycogen synthetase, and the activities and de novo synthesis of several regulatory gluconeogenic enzymes, including pyruvate carboxylase, phosphoenol-pyruvate carboxykinase, fructose-1,6-bisphosphatase and glucose-6-phosphatase. Cortisol also potentiates the actions of glucagon and epinephrine on the liver. In skeletal muscle tissue, cortisol appears to have no direct effect on glucose uptake or glucose metabolism but it does inhibit insulin mediated glucose uptake. In addition, cortisol reduces the uptake and increases the release of amino acids by skeletal muscle. In the absence of cortisol, amino acid release and tissue concentrations of amino acids are decreased. Therefore, cortisol appears to exert an important role in maintaining, at least, euglycemia during stressful conditions by increasing the availability of gluconeogenic substrates to the liver. As a result of these actions, it is no surprise that there is a close correlation between the plasma concentrations of glucose and cortisol following injury.

In adipose tissue, cortisol increases lipolysis directly and indirectly through the potentiation of other lipolytic hormones such as epinephrine and growth hormone. As a result, the concentrations of free fatty acids in the plasma increase. Cortisol also decreases glucose uptake in adipose tissue.

Cortisol, at least in excess concentrations, inhibits immunologic and inflammatory responses, as reflected by impaired lymphocyte, monocyte, and polymorphonuclear cell functioning. In particular, the administration of corticosteroids increases the circulating concentrations of lymphocytes and neutrophils and decreases the circulating concentrations of monocytes and eosinophils. At inflammatory sites, corticosteroids reduce markedly the number of polymorphonuclear cells, monocytes, macrophages, and lymphocytes that accumulate. The reduction of the inflammatory response is, at least in part, the result of these alterations in white cell mobilization and migration. In addition, cortisol decreases glucose uptake and amino acid release by lymphocytes, inhibits phospholipase A (an enzyme necessary for prostaglandin and leukotriene synthesis), and stabilizes lysosomal membranes, actions that may alter the function of inflammatory cells by decreasing their metabolism and their release of prostaglandins and of proteolytic enzymes. Therefore, it is not surprising that patients receiving steroids have impaired wound healing and that they may frequently have a serious infection with little systemic manifestation.

Because of their potent anti-inflammatory properties, corticosteroids are administered for a variety of inflammatory disease states. The exogenous administration of corticosteroids partially inhibits ACTH, as described previously, and leads to decreased adrenal stimulation, atrophy, and finally very little production of corticosteroid. If the adrenal is sufficiently atrophic, even a large dose of ACTH, such as that which might occur following severe injury, will fail to stimulate the adrenal cortex acutely to produce an increased output of corticosteroids. Patients who have been on steroid administration for prolonged periods of time, whose adrenals have become atrophic, and who are not given corticosteroids to support them during an operation or following trauma may die because of the failure of cortisol to be released from an adrenal rendered temporarily inactive by atrophy. If acute adrenal insufficiency does occur, the most prominent features are fever and hypotension. In the past, when bilateral adrenalectomy was attempted prior to the availability of cortisone, it was universally fatal as a result of adrenal insufficiency. Similarly, if a patient with unsuspected adrenal insufficiency is operated upon without being supported with exogenous corticosteroids, death is likely to ensue. Thus, cortisol is necessary for the normal response to trauma.

Death resulting from adrenal insufficiency in an injured patient is generally associated with hypoglycemia, hyponatremia, and hyperkalemia. The latter two findings result from the loss of the sodium retaining and kaliuretic properties of aldosterone and to a lesser extent of cortisol. Hyponatremia in posttraumatic adrenal insufficiency is also exaggerated by increased concentrations of vasopressin (and therefore decreased free water clearance)

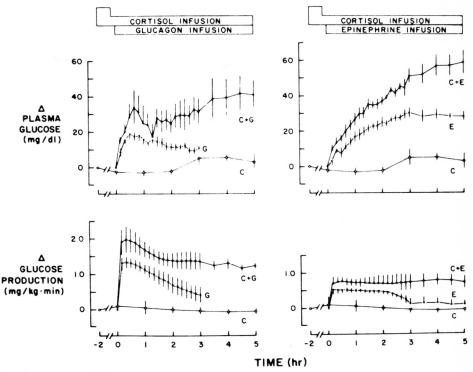

Fig. 1-20. The influence of cortisol (C) on the response of plasma glucose and glucose production to glucagon (G) or epinephrine (E). Cortisol, which by itself did not alter plasma glucose or glucose production, had the effect of increasing and more importantly prolonging the stimulatory effects of glucagon and epinephrine on glucose production. As a result, the effects of the combined hormone infusions on plasma glucose were more than additive. (From: *Eigler NJ et al: Clin Invest 63:114, 1979, with permission.*)

consequent to injury. Hypoglycemia arises because of the important effects cortisol exerts on hepatic glucose production. It is noteworthy that despite the major effects of cortisol on hepatic carbohydrate metabolism, adrenalectomized animals and man do not exhibit marked alterations in carbohydrate metabolism if food is constantly available. However, in the presence of injury or of starvation, adrenalectomized animals and man do exhibit marked alterations in hepatic carbohydrate metabolism that result in rapid and fatal hypoglycemia. The absence of cortisol mediated induction of de novo synthesis of hepatic enzymes is not sufficient to explain the reduction in serum glucose, since enzyme synthesis requires several hours. Perfusion of the livers of adrenalectomized animals in the absence of any gluconeogenic hormones, such as epinephrine or glucagon, reveals no difference in the gluconeogenic conversion of lactate or alanine to glucose when compared with normal animals. Total glucose release is impaired and glycogen stores are virtually absent. In the presence of glucagon or epinephrine, the perfused livers of adrenalectomized animals do exhibit a marked impairment in gluconeogenesis. Thus, stress-induced hypoglycemia in adrenalectomized animals and man appears to be, at least in part, the result of the inability to store glycogen and the absence of the permissive

action of corticosteroids on glucagon and epinephrine mediated gluconeogenesis.

The permissive action of cortisol was first proposed by Ingle to explain the finding that adrenalectomized animals given maintenance doses of corticosteroids showed some of the metabolic changes formerly ascribed to an increased secretion of corticosteroids. He proposed that the primary role of cortisol in trauma was to permit or augment the action of other hormones. Glucagon and epinephrine stimulated hepatic gluconeogenesis are markedly enhanced in the presence of cortisol, lending credence to this hypothesis (Fig. 1-20). Not all the beneficial effects of cortisol following trauma can be ascribed to their permissive action. For example, studies of blood volume restitution following hemorrhage have demonstrated that maintenance concentrations of cortisol are not sufficient for complete blood volume restitution and that increased concentrations of cortisol are necessary (Fig. 1-21).

Paraplegic patients who fail to respond to the operative trauma with an increase in cortisol secretion generally tolerate the operative procedure well. There are at least three possible explanations for this apparent paradox. First and foremost, the secretion of cortisol remains low in the paraplegic patient despite trauma because of the absence of afferent nerve impulses from the area of injury, but the response to uncompensated hemorrhage, supervening infection, or hypothalamic stimulation from hypoglycemia remains intact. Paraplegic patients are able to respond to a reduction in the effective circulating volume should it occur because the baroreceptor reflexes are mediated by cranial nerves. In severe trauma, the hepatic

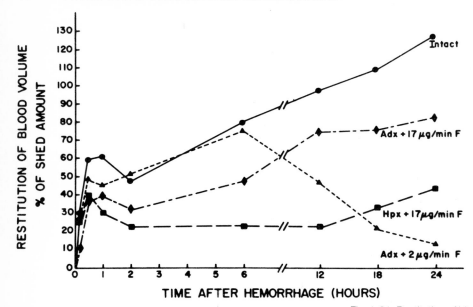

Fig. 1-21. Restitution of blood volume after 10 percent hemorrhage in four groups of splenectomized dogs: intact (●) adrenalectomized infused with cortisol at 2 μg/min (Δ); adrenalectomized infused with cortisol at 2 μg/min prior to hemorrhage, then at 17 μg/min (◆); hypophysectomized infused with cortisol at 17 μg/min (°). The response of each group differed significantly from that of each other group ($P < 0.01$, analysis of variance). (From: *Gann et al: Recent Prog Horm Res 34:357, 1978, with permission.*)

conjugation of corticosteroids to inactive forms may be reduced, so that larger amounts of the unconjugated (active) form are suddenly available even though the rate of secretion remains constant. An operative trauma is far better tolerated in patients whose body cells have not been deprived of the adrenal corticosteroids preoperatively than in those in whom preexisting deficiency is present.

Adrenal exhaustion, which was once thought to occur following prolonged trauma, probably never occurs, and isolated instances of adrenal insufficiency after severe injury are most likely the result of pituitary infarction secondary to hypotension. By contrast, most patients who die following injury, sepsis, burns, infection, and other forms of severe prolonged trauma die with very high blood levels of corticosteroids (Fig. 1-22). The very existence of continued high concentrations of plasma corticosteroids in the severely burned patient is usually a bad prognostic sign, suggesting that the trauma of burns is continuing and severe and that death may ensue.

TSH-THYROXINE. Since most injuries are associated with hypermetabolism in the immediate postoperative or posttraumatic period, it would be reasonable to postulate that the activity of thyroid hormones, agents known to dramatically increase the metabolic rate, would be increased following injury. This is not the case, however, and in most injuries the concentrations of thyroid hormones are normal or decreased (Fig. 1-23). Therefore, even though the presence of thyroid hormones is necessary for the normal functioning of organs in response to a traumatic stress, an increased secretion is not necessary.

The thyroid hormones, thyroxine (T_4) and triiodothyronine (T_3), are synthesized and released from the thyroid gland in response to thyroid stimulating hormone (TSH). Inhibition of thyroid hormone release occurs through the actions of T_4 and T_3 themselves on the hypothalamus and pituitary and thyroid glands. Upon stimulation by TSH,

the thyroid gland releases primarily T_4 which, in turn, is converted in the periphery to T_3. As a result, most of the circulating T_4 is derived from the thyroid gland and most of the circulating T_3 from peripheral conversion. Both T_4 and T_3 are bound to plasma proteins so that free and bound forms exist in the circulation. Following injury, burns, and a major operation the peripheral conversion of T_4 to T_3 is impaired, resulting in reduced circulating concentrations of both free and total T_3. In part this is the result of a cortisol mediated block of the conversion of T_4 to T_3 and of an increased conversion of T_4 to the biologically inactive molecule, reverse T_3. An increase in reverse T_3 is also characteristic of injury (Fig. 1-24). The plasma concentrations of total T_4 also are frequently decreased after injury, but free T_4 concentrations usually remain normal. In fact, depressed concentrations of free T_4 appear to be an ominous clinical finding associated with death in traumatized, burned, and critically ill medical patients (Fig. 1-23).

TSH is synthesized and released by basophilic cells of the anterior pituitary in response to the stimulatory action of the hypothalamic hormone, thyrotropin releasing hormone (TRH). Inhibition of TSH release is the result of the inhibitory influences of T_4 and T_3 on the pituitary gland and hypothalamus. The release of TSH is also stimulated by estrogens and inhibited by corticosteroids, somatostatin, growth hormone, and fasting. Physiologically, T_3 is much more potent than T_4. In addition, available evidence suggests that the inhibition of TSH secretion by the anterior pituitary gland occurs primarily through T_3.

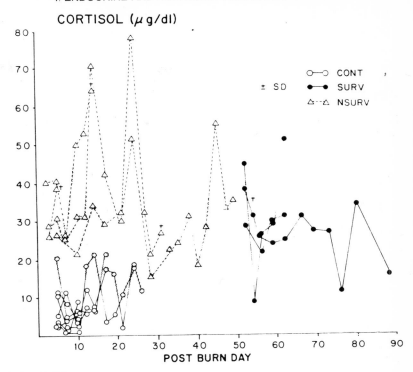

Fig. 1-22. There appears to be a negative correlation between survival after major thermal injury and plasma cortisol concentration with survivors (surv) having plasma cortisol concentrations below those of nonsurvivors (nsurv). Both groups had cortisol concentrations greater than controls. (From: *Vaughan GM et al: J Trauma 22:263–273, 1982, with permission.*)

However, despite this, TSH secretion is not increased after injury or surgery even though the plasma concentrations of free and total T_3 are frequently decreased. This appears to result from the rapid conversion of T_4 to T_3 by pituitary cells, such that T_4 and T_3 are equipotent inhibitors of TSH secretion. It appears that following injury the normal circulating concentrations of free T_4 are sufficient to inhibit the secretion of TSH. Burn patients, however, have recently been noted to have a reduction in the serum concentration of TSH that paradoxically is associated with low serum concentrations of both free T_4 and free T_3. This situation is similar to the euthyroid sick syndrome observed in critically ill nonsurgical patients and may be the result of an impairment in the pituitary's ability to secrete TSH, the hypothalamus's ability to secrete TRH, or an alteration in the peripheral binding of these hormones to their carrier molecules. The exact etiology is not known.

The synthesis of TRH is not limited to the hypothalamus and TRH is not specific for the release of TSH. TRH appears to be the primary agent responsible for the secretion of TSH by the pituitary gland. Recent evidence suggests TRH may be important in the response to shock, as evidenced by the improvement of blood pressure, respiratory rate, heart rate, and survival in animals who have been administered TRH during hemorrhagic shock. These improvements are thought to be mediated by TRH

stimulation of central pathways that modulate sympathoadrenal function, but the precise mechanisms for these phenomena are not known.

The thyroid hormones have numerous effects on cellular metabolism, growth, and differentiation. Among these are their ability to increase oxygen consumption, heat production, and the activities of the sympathetic nervous system. The thyroid hormones may also have profound metabolic effects when present in excess, including an increase in glucose oxidation, gluconeogenesis, glycogenolysis, proteolysis, lipolysis, and ketogenesis. Despite these actions, thyroid hormones do not appear to be important in the moment-to-moment regulation of plasma substrates, such as glucose.

GROWTH HORMONE. As is the case for most pituitary hormones, the secretion of growth hormone is under the control of a number of inputs including neural, hormonal, and nonneuroendocrine signals, such as substrate supply. The hypothalamic mechanisms controlling the synthesis and the release of growth hormone from acidophilic cells of the adenohypophysis involve both stimulation and inhibition. Pituitary release of growth hormone is stimulated by growth hormone releasing factor, a substance produced in the ventromedial, arcuate, and possibly dorsomedial nuclei of the hypothalamus. Inhibition of growth hormone release is primarily mediated by somatostatin, which is derived from the preoptic area and the amygdyla. Despite the presence of both stimulatory and inhibitory properties, the primary influence of the hypothalamus upon the release of growth hormone is stimulatory. This is evidenced by the inhibition of growth hormone secretion when the hypophyseal-portal circulation con-

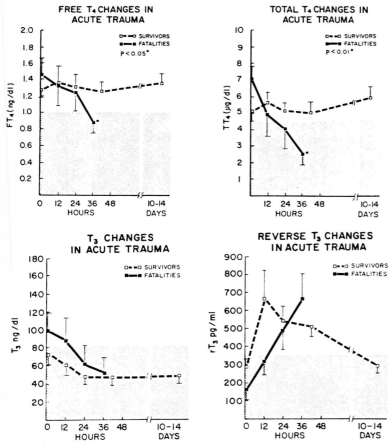

Fig. 1-23. Alterations in total T_4, free T_4, total T_3, and reverse T_3 in 19 acutely traumatized patients. Results are reported as mean ± SEM and statistically significant deviations are noted at matched time samples. Shaded regions denote subnormal levels of free T_4, total T_4, and total T_3 and normal range of reverse T_3. All patients had subnormal values of total T_3 and elevated values of reverse T_3 at some time point. Patients who died had subnormal values of total and free T_4, whereas survivors did not. (From: *Phillips RH et al: J Trauma 24:116, 1984, with permission.*)

necting the hypothalamus and pituitary gland is transected or injured. Other hormonal agents capable of stimulating growth hormone release include thyroxine, vasopressin, ACTH, alpha-MSH, testosterone, estrogen, and alpha-adrenergic stimulation. By contrast, only cortisol, growth hormone itself, and beta-adrenergic stimulation, in addition to somatostatin, suppress growth hormone release. Growth hormone secretion can also be stimulated by nonhormonal stimuli such as decreased effective circulating volume, fasting hypoglycemia, decreasing plasma fatty acid concentrations, increasing amino acid concentrations, exercise, and stress or inhibited by nonhormonal stimuli such as hyperglycemia and rising plasma fatty acid concentrations.

The ability of a decrease in effective circulating volume to stimulate growth hormone production results in the increased secretion of growth hormone following virtually all forms of injury. For example, Carey et al. found war wounds as well as hemorrhage to be potent stimuli for growth hormone release in human beings, and Chartiers et al. demonstrated an increased secretion of growth hormone following surgical stress such as an operation and anesthesia. Plasma concentrations of growth hormone remain elevated for approximately 24 h following these injuries and then return to normal (Fig. 1-25).

Growth hormone has numerous metabolic functions

that lead to an increase in plasma glucose, by an inhibition of glucose transport in liver and skeletal muscle; an increase in plasma fatty acids and ketone bodies, by stimulation of lipolysis in adipose tissue and potentiation of the actions of catecholamines on adipose tissue; an increase in plasma ketone bodies, by stimulation of ketogenesis in the liver, and in the accumulation of nitrogen by the synthesis of proteins in skeletal muscle and in liver. In addition, growth hormone promotes linear growth. Thus the actions of growth hormone on protein metabolism are anabolic whereas on carbohydrate and lipid metabolism they are catabolic.

Although not completely understood, growth hormone appears to produce its effects either through direct action on target cells or through the release of a group of intermediary compounds, the somatomedins, which act as second messengers in a manner somewhat analogous to calcium and cAMP.

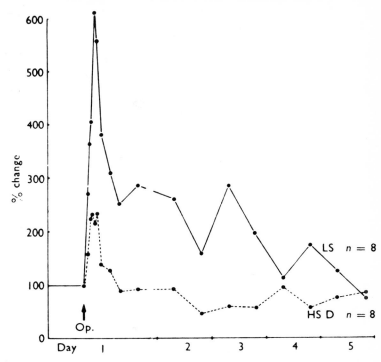

Fig. 1-28. Plasma aldosterone values in patients undergoing routine cholecystectomy. Patients who either had a conventional preoperative salt intake (LS) or a high salt intake (HS) both demonstrated an increase in plasma aldosterone secretion at the time of surgery. However, only patients with a normal salt intake preoperatively demonstrated a persistent elevation in plasma aldosterone, whereas patients on a high salt diet demonstrated an immediate return to normal values in the postoperative period. (From: *Cochrane JPS: Br J Surg 774, 1978, with permission.*)

crease in the release of nonesterified fatty acids from adipose tissue of starved rats in the presence of vasopressin. Vasopressin may act to lower the plasma concentrations of ketone bodies and nonesterified fatty acids following injury, but its role in lipid metabolism in man remains uncertain.

ALDOSTERONE. Plasma aldosterone concentrations, like those of cortisol, demonstrate a circadian rhythm in which the peak concentrations occur at midmorning and the lowest concentrations at late afternoon and night. Following injury, the circadian rhythm is lost and elevated concentrations of both these hormones are observed during the entire 24-h period. Plasma concentrations of aldosterone also increase following anesthesia alone but not to the extent seen following injury and a major operation (Fig. 1-28). The highest concentrations of aldosterone have been noted in the agonal period following injury.

Cells of the adrenal zona glomerulosa synthesize and secrete aldosterone in response to at least three stimuli. Angiotensin II stimulates aldosterone secretion through a calcium dependent, cAMP independent enhancement of the conversion of cholesterol to pregnenolone and of corticosterone to 18-hydroxycorticosterone and aldosterone. ACTH stimulates aldosterone secretion through a cal-cium dependent, cAMP dependent pathway that enhances the early conversion of cholesterol to pregnenolone. Elevation of the serum potassium concentration stimulates the release of aldosterone through a calcium dependent, cAMP independent increase in the conversion of cholesterol to pregnenolone. There is also evidence suggesting the existence of a pituitary produced aldosterone stimulating factor (ASF) in human beings (not similar to ACTH) that is a glycoprotein present in the urine of normal but not of hypophysectomized human beings. This factor produces hypertension and hyperaldosteronism when given to rodents.

Following injury, the two most important mechanisms for aldosterone secretion appear to be through ACTH and angiotensin. ACTH is considerably more potent on a molar basis than angiotensin with regard to aldosterone secretion. For example, nephrectomized dogs produce aldosterone in response to hemorrhage despite the absence of angiotensin. Stress-induced elevations in aldosterone are probably mediated primarily through ACTH. The stimulatory effects of ACTH on aldosterone production are short-lived. As a result of this short-lived potency, ACTH probably has a minor role in the overall control of aldosterone secretion in chronic states during which angiotensin II is probably the most important stimulus. Angiotensin II appears to exert a role in early as well as late aldosterone production following injury, since hypophysectomy does not completely abolish aldosterone secretion following injury, aldosterone concentrations are elevated well after ACTH concentrations have returned to normal, plasma concentrations of aldosterone demonstrate a strong correlation with angiotensin II fol-

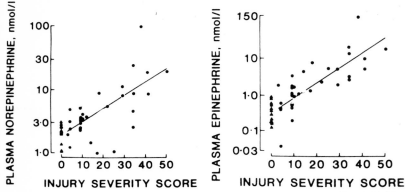

Fig. 1-29. The relationship between plasma concentrations of norepinephrine and of epinephrine with injury severity score in 40 multiply injured patients. There was a positive correlation between injury severity score, plasma norepinephrine, and plasma epinephrine. (From: *Frayn KN, Little RA, Maycock PF: Circ Shock 16:229, 1985, with permission.*)

lowing injury, and nephrectomized dogs produce only 50 percent of the aldosterone they normally produce in response to hemorrhage when the kidneys are intact.

In addition to the three or four stimulatory pathways for the synthesis and the secretion of aldosterone, there is considerable evidence suggesting the presence of an inhibitory pathway that appears to involve a tonic inhibition terone secretion by dopamine. For example, metaclopropramide, a dopamine antagonist, produces an increased secretion of aldosterone, whereas bromocriptine, a dopamine agonist, decreases the secretion of aldosterone stimulated by ACTH or by angiotensin II but does not alter the basal secretory rate of aldosterone. This pathway may be important in mediating changes in the secretion of aldosterone in response to alterations in the plasma sodium concentration or the effective circulating volume.

The primary actions of aldosterone are related to fluid and electrolyte metabolism. In the early distal convoluted tubule, aldosterone increases the reabsorption of sodium and of chloride and in the late distal convoluted tubules and in the early collecting ducts it promotes the reabsorption of sodium and the secretion of potassium. The latter process is not an obligatory, one to one exchange of sodium ions for potassium ions and of sodium ions for hydrogen ions as has been previously thought. Instead, experimental evidence suggests that the secretion of potassium and of hydrogen ions results from an increase in the electronegativity of the luminal tubular fluid as sodium reabsorption is stimulated by aldosterone. In turn, the increase in tubular electronegativity drives potassium and hydrogen ions across the tubular membrane into the tubular fluid in order to restore electrical neutrality.

CATECHOLAMINES. Catecholamines increase immediately after injury and achieve peak concentrations at about 24 to 48 h after injury, from which time they decrease to base line. This increase appears to be related to the severity of injury (Fig. 1-29) and changes in norepinephrine and epinephrine are qualitatively and quantitatively the same. Changes in norepinephrine are generally thought to reflect changes in the activity of the sympathetic nervous system, i.e., spillover into the blood, whereas changes in epinephrine are generally thought to reflect changes in the activity of the adrenal medulla. In this regard, epinephrine, produced almost exclusively by the adrenal medulla, functions primarily as a hormone whereas dopamine and norepinephrine, produced for the most part by nerve terminals, function primarily as neurotransmitters.

Plasma catecholamine concentrations have been extensively studied in numerous forms of injury in human beings. Among the most extensive studies are those of Benedict and Grahame-Smith, who examine plasma catecholamine concentrations in patients with shock due to septicemia, trauma, and hemorrhage (Figs. 1-30 and 1-31). In these studies, plasma norepinephrine (noradrenaline) and epinephrine (adrenal) concentrations were increased above normal irrespective of the type of shock (septic, hemorrhagic, and traumatic) whereas there was no difference in the plasma dopamine concentration between patients with shock and normal controls. In most of the nonsurvivors, irrespective of the type of shock, high plasma norepinephrine and, to a lesser extent, epinephrine concentrations were sustained until just before death, when they rapidly declined. The association between sustained norepinephrine concentrations and death is not well established, however, and was not seen in the studies of Davies et al. in which plasma catecholamine concentrations were measured in accident victims.

Numerous stimuli have been identified that lead to an increase in catecholamine secretion including hypovolemia, hypoglycemia, hypoxemia, pain, and fear, which are all present to some degree following injury. Among these stimuli, plasma catecholamine concentrations following injury are best correlated with the volume of blood lost. It is also important to note that part of the response following injury appears to be psychologically mediated since plasma catecholamine concentrations are greater in patients who sustained minor injuries in a motor vehicle accident than in those who sustained minor injuries by other means.

The exact mechanisms involved in the adrenomedullary control of catecholamine secretion remain poorly

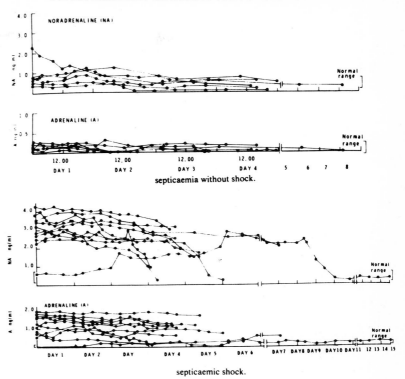

Fig. 1-30. Plasma noradrenaline and adrenalin concentrations in septic patients with or without shock. The concentrations of noradrenaline and adrenalin were greater in patients with shock than in those without. (From: *Benedict CR, Grahame-Smith DG: Q J Med 185:1, 1978, with permission.*)

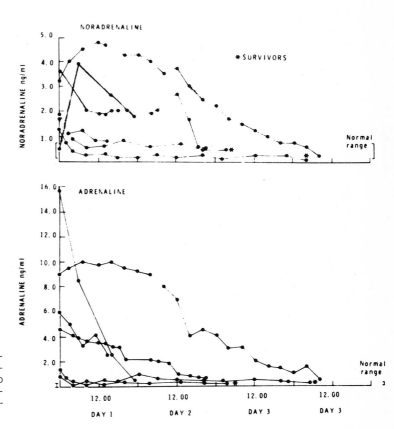

Fig. 1-31. Plasma noradrenaline and adrenalin concentrations in patients with hypovolemic shock. The concentrations of noradrenaline and adrenalin returned to normal values in survivors whereas they remained elevated in nonsurvivors. (From: *Benedict CR, Grahame-Smith DG: Q J Med 185:1, 1978, with permission.*)

understood. In this regard, it is of note that the activation of the sympathetic nervous system does not occur in an all or none fashion and that is not equivalent to adrenomedullary activation. Adrenomedullary activation is not equivalent to complete activation of the sympathetic nervous system. For example, sympathetically mediated adrenomedullary secretion of catecholamines can occur in the absence of increased cardiac or renal sympathetic nervous system activity. Conversely, small nonhypotensive hemorrhages lead to activation of the sympathetic nervous system but do not increase the adrenomedullary secretion of catecholamines. The latter occurs only when some degree of hypotension develops.

The actions of epinephrine and norepinephrine as hormones may be broadly classified as metabolic, hemodynamic, or modulatory. Metabolic actions of epinephrine include stimulation of glycogenolysis (alpha$_1$), gluconeogenesis (alpha$_1$), lipolysis (beta$_1$), and ketogenesis (beta$_1$) in the liver; stimulation of lipolysis (beta$_1$) in adipose tissue; and stimulation of glycogenolysis (alpha$_1$) and inhibition of insulin stimulated glucose uptake (beta$_2$ and alpha$_1$) in skeletal muscle. As a result of these actions, epinephrine appears to exert a major role in stress-induced hyperglycemia by increasing glucose production by the liver and by decreasing glucose uptake in peripheral tissues. There is a strong correlation between plasma glucose concentrations following injury and plasma catecholamine concentrations (Fig. 1-32).

Hormonal modulations produced by catecholamines include a beta receptor mediated increase in the release of renin and parathyroid hormone and an alpha receptor mediated inhibition and beta receptor mediated stimulation of insulin and glucagon secretion. The hormonal modulations produced by catecholamines are to a large extent dependent upon the adrenergic receptor density present on the secretory cells they act upon. For example, alpha and beta islets cells in the pancreas that secrete

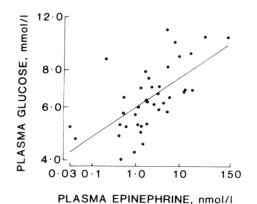

Fig. 1-32. The relationship between plasma concentrations of glucose and of epinephrine in 40 multiply injured patients. There was a positive correlation between plasma glucose and plasma epinephrine ($r = 0.64$, $p < 0.001$). (From: *Frayn KN, Little RA, Maycock PF: Circ Shock 16:229, 1985, with permission.*)

glucagon and insulin, respectively, contain both alpha- and beta-adrenergic receptors but beta islet cells have a greater number of alpha-adrenergic receptors than do alpha islet cells. As a result stimulation of the pancreas by catecholamines and by the sympathetic nervous system results in an increased secretion of glucagon and a decreased secretion of insulin (Fig. 1-33).

Hemodynamic effects of catecholamines include alpha$_1$ mediated venous and arterial vasoconstriction; beta$_2$ mediated arterial vasodilation; and beta$_1$ mediated increases in myocardial rate, contractility, and conductivity. Pharmacologically, the particular hemodynamic effect produced by catecholamines is dose dependent. For example, in low doses epinephrine acts primarily at beta$_1$ and beta$_2$ receptors whereas at high doses it acts primarily at alpha$_1$ receptors. Physiologically, it appears that

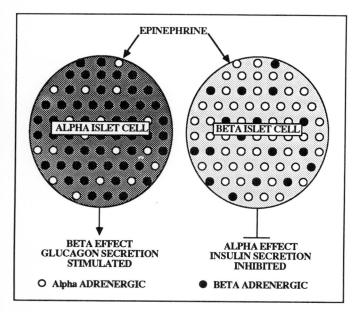

Fig. 1-33. Adrenergic receptor density of alpha and beta pancreatic islets. Beta islet cells have a greater density of alpha-adrenergic receptors and alpha islets have a greater density of beta-adrenergic receptors. As a result, stimulation of pancreatic islets by epinephrine or norepinephrine results in a decreased secretion of insulin and an increased secretion of glucagon.

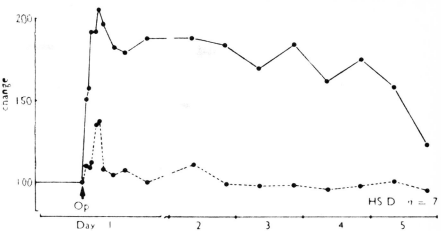

Fig. 1-34. Plasma renin activity in patients undergoing routine cholecystectomy. Patients who either had a conventional preoperative salt intake (LS) or a high salt intake (HS) both demonstrated an increase in plasma renin activity at the time of surgery. However, only patients with a normal salt intake preoperatively demonstrated a persistent elevation in plasma renin activity whereas patients on a high salt diet demonstrated an immediate return to normal values in the postoperative period. (From: *Cochrane JPS: Br J Surg 65:744, 1978, with permission.*)

norepinephrine is most important in the beta$_1$ and alpha$_2$ actions of catecholamines, whereas epinephrine is responsible for the beta$_2$ effects. The hemodynamic effects of dopamine are mediated through dopaminergic receptors as well as adrenergic receptors. In low circulating concentrations (<10 μg/mL), dopamine acts primarily through dopaminergic receptors, but at higher concentrations it acts at beta and eventually at alpha receptors. Because of dopamine's renal vasodilating effects at low concentrations, low-dose dopamine is frequently used following injury to improve urine output.

RENIN-ANGIOTENSIN. Plasma renin activity demonstrates a circadian rhythm in which the peak activity occurs at midmorning and the lowest activity at late afternoon and night. Following injury, the circadian rhythm is lost and an increased renin activity is observed during the entire 24-h period. The highest activity of renin has been noted in the agonal period following injury. It can be suppressed in the immediate postoperative period by salt and water loading (Fig. 1-34).

Renin exists in an inactive form, prorenin, in the myoepithelial cells of the renal afferent arterioles. The proteolytic cleavage of the zymogen and the release of renin are under the control of three intrarenal receptors (the macula densa, the juxtaglomerular neurogenic receptor, and the juxtaglomerular cell) and the influences of several hormones and ions (ACTH, vasopressin, prostaglandins, glucagon, potassium, magnesium, and calcium). The macula densa receptor senses the concentration of chloride in tubular fluid as it passes through the distal nephron such that a decrease in the concentration of chloride in the tubular fluid results in an increase in the release of renin. The neurogenic receptor of the juxtaglomerular apparatus responds to beta-adrenergic stimulation by in-

creasing the release of renin and the juxtaglomerular cell itself, which acts as a stretch receptor, responds to a decrease in stretch (and therefore blood pressure) with an increased secretion of renin.

In the circulation renin converts renin substrate, which is produced by the liver, into angiotensin I. Angiotensin I acts primarily as the precursor for the formation of angiotensin II, a process mediated in the pulmonary circulation by the carboxypeptidase, angiotensin converting enzyme. In addition, it potentiates the release of catecholamines by the adrenal medulla and it redistributes renal blood flow to the cortex by decreasing blood flow to the medullary areas of the kidney.

The actions of angiotensin II may be broadly classified according to its effects upon hemodynamics, fluid and electrolyte balance, hormonal regulation, and metabolism. Angiotensin II is a potent vasoconstrictor with additional hemodynamic activity including an increase in heart rate and contractility and an increase in vascular permeability. Angiotensin II affects fluid and electrolyte homeostasis through its potent stimulation of aldosterone synthesis and secretion, its ability to increase vasopressin secretion, and its participation in the regulation of thirst. Endocrine modulatory effects of angiotensin II, in addition to those noted on the secretion of aldosterone and vasopressin, include potentiation of the release of epinephrine by the adrenal medulla, increase in the release of CRF, and increase in sympathetic neurotransmission. Metabolic actions of angiotensin II include the stimulation of glycogenolysis and gluconeogenesis in the liver.

Plasma concentrations of angiotensin II are elevated immediately after injury. During slow hemorrhages, angiotensin levels are elevated prior to alterations in blood pressure or catecholamines. Angiotensin II production is increased during hemorrhage in baroreceptor deinnervated animals, presumably by the activation of renal receptors. The presence of angiotensin II during shock has been thought to be essential to survival, since nephrectomized animals do not withstand hypovolemia as well as nonnephrectomized animals. Recent studies with renin-angiotensin inhibitors suggest that inhibition of

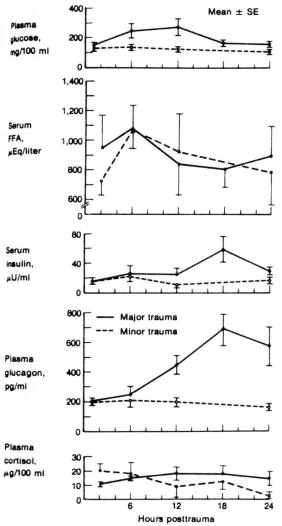

Fig. 1-35. Plasma concentrations of insulin, glucagon, cortisol, glucose, and free fatty acids in seven major and seven minor trauma patients observed over 24-h. The most significant findings were an early elevation of plasma glucose in association with a low-normal insulin concentration and a normal but gradually rising glucagon concentration that reached three times the normal value in 18-h. (From: *Meguid MM et al: Arch Surg 109:776, 1974, with permission.*)

the renin-angiotensin system may improve survival during severe hemorrhage. In part, the benefits obtained from inhibition of the renin-angiotensin system may be related to an improvement in renal blood flow and cardiac output consequent to a reduction in vascular resistance.

INSULIN. Studies examining the plasma concentration of insulin following injury in human beings have noted a biphasic pattern of insulin release (Fig. 1-35). The first period, lasting only a few hours, is characterized by the suppression of insulin secretion, which is mediated by the high concentrations of catecholamines released by stress. This is followed by a period of normal to increased insulin secretion, the so-called phase of insulin resistance. Early

increases in plasma insulin concentrations after injury in human beings have been noted by some investigators. For example, Vitek et al. in a study of road traffic accidents noted a 31.5 percent increase in the insulin concentration above controls by 3 h after injury and a 51.7 percent increase approximately 6 h after injury. As a result of the inconsistent response of the plasma insulin concentration to injury, plasma insulin concentrations correlate poorly with injury severity. In this regard, the insulin-glucose ratio appears to be a better predictor of survival than either the plasma glucose or plasma insulin concentration alone.

The synthesis and secretion of insulin by beta islet cells of the pancreas are controlled by the concentration of circulating substrate (glucose, amino acids, and free fatty acids), the activity of the autonomic nervous system, and the direct and indirect effects of several hormones. Increases in the plasma concentration of glucose, amino acids, free fatty acids, and ketone bodies stimulate the secretion of insulin. Under normal physiologic conditions, the plasma concentration of glucose is the most important stimulus for insulin secretion. During injury and stress, however, the effect of glucose is blunted by neural and humoral mechanisms, so-called insulin resistance. As noted previously, the effect of the autonomic nervous system on a target cell depends to a large extent on the adrenergic receptor density present. Beta islet cells have a greater density of alpha-adrenergic receptors, which inhibit insulin secretion, than of beta-adrenergic receptors, which stimulate insulin secretion. Stimulation of the sympathetic innervation of the pancreas or an increase in the circulating concentration of epinephrine or norepinephrine produce an inhibition of insulin secretion. Hormonal modulators of insulin secretion include somatostatin, glucagon, gastrointestinal hormones, and beta-endorphin, which act through a direct action on the B-islet cells, and cortisol, estrogen, and progesterone, which act indirectly by interfering with the peripheral actions of insulin.

Insulin is the primary anabolic hormone in human beings that promotes the storage of carbohydrate, protein, and lipid through its actions primarily on the liver, skeletal muscle, and adipose tissue, and secondarily on almost all other tissues in the body. Notable exceptions include hemopoietic, central nervous system, and wounded tissues. The major actions of insulin on carbohydrate metabolism are to promote the entry of glucose into cells by stimulating membrane transport of glucose, to promote glycogenesis and glycolysis, and to inhibit gluconeogenesis in the liver. The major action of insulin in protein metabolism is to promote protein synthesis, which is accomplished by increasing the transport of amino acids into the liver and other peripheral tissues and by inhibiting gluconeogenesis and amino acid oxidation. The actions of insulin on lipid metabolism are directed toward the stimulation of lipid synthesis and inhibition of lipid degradation.

GLUCAGON. Although an immediate increase in the plasma glucagon concentration that correlated with the plasma glucose concentration has been noted by Wilmore and colleagues following thermal injury, most studies of

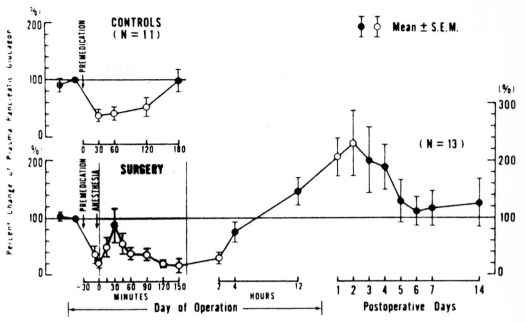

Fig. 1-36. Changes in plasma glucagon during and after elective surgery in 13 patients. Open circles represent significant differences when compared with the fasting value on the day of surgery. (From: *Miyata M, Yamamoto T, Nakao K: Horm Metab Res 8:239, 1976, with permission.*)

glucagon metabolism following nonthermal injury and hypovolemia have noted no increase in the plasma concentration of glucagon until 12 h after injury. During an operation, the plasma concentration of glucagon has been shown to decrease followed by a return to base line 12 h after injury, an increase above base line at 1 day, and a return to base-line values by 3 days (Fig. 1-36). Similarly, Meguid and colleagues, in a study of 14 injured patients, noted no increase in the plasma glucagon concentration immediately after injury, a peak increase at 18 h, and a return to base line by 36 h (Fig. 1-35). Following hemorrhage, portal venous delivery of glucagon also does not increase until well after hyperglycemia has ensued (Fig. 1-37). Despite the apparent difference between thermal and nonthermal injury, glucagon concentrations are generally increased at some point in the immediate postinjury period for all forms of injury.

The synthesis and secretion of glucagon by the alpha islet cells of the pancreas are under the control of the concentrations of circulating substrates (glucose, amino acids, and fatty acids), the activity of the autonomic and the central nervous systems, and the action of circulating and local hormones. Under normal conditions, the primary stimuli are the plasma concentrations of glucose and of amino acids and exercise. Glucose alters glucagon secretion in an inverse manner that appears to result primarily from a direct action of glucose on the alpha cell.

The potency of different amino acids to stimulate glucagon secretion is variable and unrelated to their ability to stimulate insulin secretion, but, in general, the gluconeo-

genic amino acids have a greater stimulatory effect than the nongluconeogenic amino acids. The ability of amino acids to stimulate glucagon secretion is critical for the maintenance of euglycemia when a protein meal is ingested. If this did not occur, the unopposed stimulation of insulin secretion by amino acids after a protein meal would result in hypoglycemia. In the presence of glucagon, however, the liver increases its production of glucose, thereby allowing the action of insulin to be opposed and glucose homeostasis to be maintained. Unger has proposed the insulin/glucagon (I/G) ratio in plasma as a quantitative measure of hepatic glucose balance. When the I/G ratio is greater than 5, glycogenesis, lipogenesis, and protein synthesis are favored. When the I/G ratio is less than 3, glycogenolysis, gluconeogenesis, and lipolysis are favored. The validity of this relationship in vivo is not certain.

The potency of glucose and of amino acids in altering glucagon and insulin secretion depends upon the route of administration, with a greater increase in glucagon and insulin secretion occurring following the ingestion of a protein meal than following the intravenous administration of similar concentrations of amino acids. Similarly, the ingestion of glucose results in a greater increase in insulin and decrease in glucagon than a similar glucose load administered intravenously. This phenomenon may be mediated through the presentation of a greater concentration of substrate to the pancreas when the substrates enter through the gastrointestinal tract, through the potentiation by gastrointestinal hormones of substrate induced pancreatic secretion, or through the effects of neural inputs to the pancreas that are activated by eating.

The autonomic nervous system mechanisms controlling glucagon release are similar to those for insulin; i.e., activation of alpha-adrenergic receptors stimulates gluca-

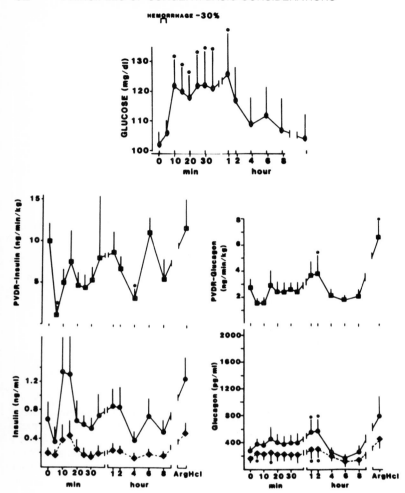

Fig. 1-37. Arterial (circles) and portal venous (diamonds) concentrations of glucagon and insulin, portal venous delivery (squares) of glucagon and insulin and arterial concentrations of glucose (ovals) in response to a 30 percent hemorrhage in dogs. These results suggest that alterations in glucagon occurred too late to participate in the immediate hyperglycemia that followed hemorrhage. (From: *McLeod MK, Carlson DE, Gann DS: Am J Physiol 251:E597, 1986, with permission.*)

gon secretion whereas the activation of beta-adrenergic receptors or the parasympathetic efferents to the pancreas inhibit glucagon release. Unlike the beta islet cell, however, the alpha islet has a much greater density of alpha-adrenergic receptors than of beta-adrenergic receptors. As a result, increased circulating concentrations of epinephrine or norepinephrine, or sympathetic nervous system stimulation of the pancreas, increase rather than decrease the secretion of glucagon.

The physiologic actions of glucagon are limited primarily to the liver and include stimulation of glycogenolysis and gluconeogenesis. The net result is an increase in hepatic glucose production that under basal conditions accounts for approximately 75 percent of the glucose produced by the liver. Although in the absence of cortisol the peak action of glucagon is very brief, in the presence of cortisol the action of glucagon is longer and the initial increase in hepatic glucose production is greater. Nevertheless, the effects of glucagon are not long-lasting and after 30 to 60 min the activity assigned to glucagon decreases, even if the plasma glucagon concentration remains elevated. If the concentration of glucagon increases further, however, the activity of glucagon does

increase because it appears that an increase in the concentration of glucagon rather than the absolute amount of glucagon present is what determines its physiologic activity.

Despite the increase in hepatic glucose production under normal circumstances, glucagon does not appear to exert an important role in the immediate hyperglycemia that follows injury. For example, McLeod et al. noted an immediate increase in plasma glucose following hemorrhage that was not associated with increases in peripheral glucagon concentrations or in the delivery of glucagon to the liver by the portal vein. In addition, Lautt and co-workers have demonstrated the abolition of the hyperglycemic response to hemorrhage in adrenalectomized and hepatic denervated cats and the restitution of this response when either the adrenals or the liver are left intact.

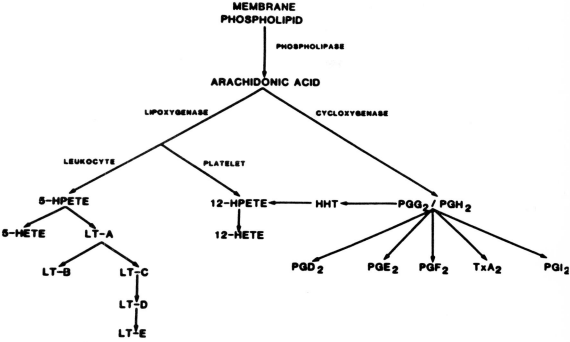

Fig. 1-38. Eicosanoid synthesis. Cortisol inhibits phospholipase A. As a result, the synthesis of all eicosanoids is decreased. In contrast, aspirin and indomethacin inhibit cyclooxygenase. As a result, the synthesis of leukotrienes may be increased. (From: *Gann DS, Amaral JF: The pathophysiology of trauma and shock, in Zuidema GD et al (eds): The Management of Trauma. Philadelphia, Saunders, 1985, with permission.*)

In addition to its effects on carbohydrate metabolism, glucagon stimulates lipolysis in liver and adipose tissue and stimulates ketogenesis in the liver. As a result, glucagon is very important during starvation and injury because of its ability to mobilize fatty acids and to increase ketogenesis.

SOMATOSTATIN. Somatostatin, which is present in pancreatic D cells, hypothalamus, limbic system, brain stem, spinal cord, other neural tissue, salivary glands, parafollicular thyroid cells, kidney, and gastrointestinal tissue, is a potent inhibitor of both insulin and glucagon secretion. Although somatostatin was originally named for its ability to inhibit growth hormone secretion, it is now recognized to also inhibit the secretion of TSH, renin, calcitonin, gastrin, secretin, and cholecystokinin as well as insulin and glucagon.

EICOSANOIDS. Plasma concentrations of eicosanoids, which compose a group of 20 carbon, cyclic fatty acids derived primarily from arachidonic acid, are increased during hemorrhagic, septic, and endotoxic shock and following thermal and nonthermal injury. The presence of these substances in increased concentrations has been implicated in pathologic conditions such as ARDS and renal failure.

The arachidonic acid used in eicosanoid synthesis is derived from cell membrane phospholipids (phosphatidylcholine and phosphatidylinositol) and is converted by a series of enzymatic reactions into four major eicosanoid groups composed of the classic prostaglandins (PGE, PGF), the prostacyclins (PGI), the thromboxanes (TxB), and the leukotrienes (Fig. 1-38). Cortisol inhibits phospholipase A and therefore inhibits the synthesis of all eicosanoids. By contrast, aspirin and indocin inhibit cyclooxygenase and therefore prostaglandin synthesis but they may increase leukotriene synthesis.

The eicosanoids are tissue-specific. For example, vascular endothelium converts arachidonic acid primarily to prostacyclin (PGI_2) whereas platelets convert it primarily to thromboxane (TxA_2). The eicosanoids have a very short half-life and duration of action of 30 s to 5 min once released. Their metabolism into inactive fragments occurs primarily at the site of release and secondarily in the lung. Since they are not stored in cells, the release of these agents requires de novo synthesis. Although there are numerous stimuli for prostaglandin synthesis and release, many of which are not recognized at present, the better-known stimuli include hypoxia, ischemia, tissue injury, pyrogen, endotoxin, collagen, thrombin, neural stimulation, and hormonal stimulation (serotonin, acetylcholine, histamine, norepinephrine, vasopressin, angiotensin II, and bradykinin). These stimuli are relatively nonspecific because they result in the release of several prostaglandins whose structures depend upon the tissue stimulated and not the stimulus itself.

Prostaglandin synthesis has been linked to phosphatidylinositol breakdown in calcium-dependent hormonal regulation ($alpha_1$). The increase in prostaglandins may, in turn, increase the breakdown of phosphatidylinositol, thereby augmenting the hormonal response. The biological actions of prostaglandins are closely linked to alterations in the intracellular concentration of cAMP. In general, a prostaglandin mediated increase in the concentration of cAMP in a target cell results in stimulation of a target cell action, whereas a prostaglandin mediated decrease in cAMP results in inhibition of a target cell action. In this regard, the most potent prostaglandins capable of producing changes in cAMP are prostacyclin and thromboxane. A specific prostaglandin does not always lead to a specific change in the intracellular cAMP concentration of all target tissues, so that the same prostaglandin that inhibits cAMP formation in one tissue may stimulate it in another.

The eicosanoids have widespread effects on systemic and pulmonary vasculature, on neurotransmission, and on the local effects of hormones. For every action produced by a given eicosanoid there is another that produces an antagonistic action. For example, thromboxane A_2 is a potent vasoconstrictor released by platelets that stimulates platelet aggregation, whereas prostacyclin is a potent vasodilator released by vascular endothelium that inhibits platelet aggregation. Because of their antagonistic actions, an increase in the release of TxA_2 or a decrease in the production of PgI_2 would favor platelet aggregation and vasoconstriction. These features are characteristic of the adult respiratory distress syndrome, and in fact, the ratio of TxB_2 (the major metabolite of TxA_2) to 6-keto-$F_{1\alpha}$ (the major metabolite of PgI_2) is greater in the plasma of patients with sepsis and ARDS than in patients with sepsis alone. Some investigators believe that the primary event in ARDS is platelet aggregation and thromboxane release that in turn produce pulmonary vasoconstriction, leukocyte trapping, free oxygen radical release, and endothelial damage.

The E family of prostaglandins, PGE_1 and PGE_2, produce bronchodilation, whereas $PGF_{2\alpha}$ produces bronchoconstriction. PgE_2 and $PgF_{2\alpha}$ increase pulmonary vascular resistance and capillary permeability, whereas they decrease systemic vascular resistance. These agents have also been implicated in the development of systemic sepsis, since the major hemodynamic feature of sepsis is an increase in pulmonary vascular resistance with a concomitant decrease in systemic vascular resistance.

The prostaglandins are major components of the inflammatory response, whose importance has been repeatedly documented by the resolution of inflammatory conditions such as bursitis, arthritis, and tenosynovitis with treatment with antiprostaglandin agents. The inflammatory response is characterized by increased vascular permeability, leukocyte migration, vasodilation, which lead to the classic manifestations of rubor, dolor, tumor, and calor (redness, pain, swelling, and heat). PgE compounds are capable of inducing all these local changes as well as systemic manifestations such as fever and headache. Prostaglandins of the PgD and PgG families also participate in the response, but members of the PgF family probably do not because they are venoconstrictors and much weaker than members of the PgE group. The PgF group is thought to be involved in the termination of the inflammatory response.

The leukotrienes are also important mediators of the inflammatory response, produced by a variety of cell types (pulmonary parenchymal cells, macrophages, mast cells, leukocytes, smooth muscle cells, and connective tissue cells) that may exert an important role in the development of cell and tissue injury during shock and ischemia. Included in this group of compounds is the slow-releasing substance of anaphylaxis. These compounds increase postcapillary leakage with 1000 times the potency of histamine and also produce leukocyte adherence, bronchoconstriction, and vasoconstriction. Although the concentrations of leukotrienes in the plasma increase only moderately during shock, their intense biologic activities suggest they may exert an important role in the pathophysiology of shock.

KALLIKREINS-KININS. There are two kinins in human beings, bradykinin and kallidin, that are produced through the action of the serine protease kallikrein on high (Fitzgerald factor) and low molecular weight kininogens in plasma and in tissues, respectively. As a result, bradykinin is present primarily in the circulation and kallidin in tissues. Kallikrein itself exists in plasma in an inactive form as prekallikrein (Fletcher factor), whose activation depends upon activation of the clotting system through Hageman factor. The plasma kinins are rapidly broken down by two enzymes: kinase I and kinase II. Kinase I is a carboxypeptidase that is identical to the anaphylatoxin inactivator that degrades C_{3a}, C_{4a}, and C_{5a} anaphylatoxins, and kinase II is a dipeptidase that is identical to angiotensin converting enzyme, which converts angiotensin I to angiotensin II. During ARDS, the resultant endothelial damage may inhibit the formation or action of kinase II, thereby producing an accumulation of bradykinin and a reduction of angiotensin II. These changes may be important in the systemic as well as the local manifestations of ARDS.

Increased plasma concentrations of kallikrein and bradykinin and decreased plasma concentrations of prekallikrein have been noted during hemorrhagic shock, endotoxic shock, septic shock, and tissue injury. For example, Aasen and colleagues have demonstrated in septic patients that the plasma concentration of prekallikrein decreases and the activity of kallikrein increases. Furthermore, these changes appeared to correlate with survival and severity of injury, since there was a gradual increase in the concentrations of prekallikrein in survivors but not in nonsurvivors and a greater activity of kallikrein in patients with septic shock than in patients with sepsis but no hypotension.

The kinins are potent vasodilators that increase capillary permeability, produce edema, evoke pain, increase bronchial resistance, and enhance glucose clearance. As such they appear to be important mediators of the inflammatory response. They have been implicated in the regulation of fluid and electrolytes by the kidney by causing renal vasodilation, a reduction in renal blood flow, an increase in the formation of renin, and an increase in sodium and water retention when administered in pharmacologic doses.

SEROTONIN. Serotonin (5-hydroxytryptamine), which is released by enterochromaffin cells of the gut and by platelets, is a neurotransmitter formed from tryptophan that acts primarily on smooth muscle and nerve endings. It is a potent vasoconstrictor and bronchoconstrictor that increases platelet aggregation, myocardial inotropy, and myocardial chronotropy. The action of serotonin on smooth muscle is considerably greater on venous smooth muscle than on precapillary sphincter muscle. As a result it is primarily a venoconstrictor rather than an arterial constrictor. It is released by tissue injury and is an important mediator of the inflammatory response.

HISTAMINE. Histamine has long been implicated in the pathophysiology of tissue injury and shock and elevated concentrations have been demonstrated after hemorrhagic shock, septic shock, endotoxemia, and thermal and nonthermal injury. The highest levels of histamine seem to occur with sepsis and endotoxemia. Following the administration of endotoxin to dogs, there is an immediate explosive release of histamine that correlates with the amount of endotoxin administered and with the decline in arterial blood pressure and circulating platelets consequent to the administration of endotoxin. Histamine levels have been inversely correlated with survival in patients with septic shock and after endotoxin administration in rats. By contrast, there is no association between the concentration of histamine and survival following thermal injury.

Histamine is synthesized from histidine and stored primarily in mast cells in tissue and in basophils in blood. It is also stored in the gastric mucosa, neurons, platelets, and epidermis. Release of histamine from these tissues is associated with a decrease in the intracellular concentration of cAMP and an increase in intracellular calcium. Histamine acts on cell surface receptors that are divisible into H_1 and H_2. Receptors of the H_1 type mediate an increase in the uptake of L-histidine (precursor of histamine) into cells as well as actions such as bronchoconstriction, increased myocardial contractility, and intestinal contraction, whereas receptors of the H_2 type inhibit histamine release and mediate changes in gastric secretion cardiac rate and immunologic function. Both receptor types appear to mediate small vessel vasodilation and increased vascular permeability. Exogenously administered histamine leads to a variety of effects common to septic shock including hypotension, peripheral pooling of blood, increased capillary permeability, decreased venous return, and myocardial failure.

SOMATOMEDINS AND THE INSULINLIKE GROWTH FACTORS. The somatomedins are a family of polypeptides that stimulate proteoglycan synthesis in cartilage and DNA synthesis and cell replication in a variety of cell types and that demonstrate insulinlike activity including increasing glucose uptake and protein synthesis in skeletal muscle, increasing glucose uptake, glucose oxidation, and lipid synthesis in adipose tissue, and increasing protein synthesis and glycogenesis in the liver. Human plasma also contains large amounts of insulinlike activity that does not reside in insulin itself, so-called nonsuppressible insulinlike activity, NSILA. It is divisible into two chemically and biologically related polypeptides, NSILA-I and NSILA-II, which in addition to their in-

sulinlike effects have marked effects on cell growth. They are now referred to as insulinlike growth factor I (IGF-I) and insulinlike growth factor II (IGF-II), and it appears that somatomedin-C, somatomedin-A, and IGF-I are the same molecule.

The plasma concentration of IGF-I is decreased after injury. This may be the result of the starvation that accompanies injury, since the plasma concentration of IGF-I is also depressed during fasting. Nonetheless, the concentration of insulinlike growth factors is increased during the late stages of endotoxicosis. This increase may explain the paradoxical increase in peripheral glucose utilization and depression in hepatic gluconeogenesis that has been noted during late endotoxicosis in association with a reduction in the plasma concentration of insulin.

INTERLEUKIN-1. Interleukin-1, or leukocyte endogenous mediator as it was called in the past, is a proteinlike molecule with a molecular weight of approximately 15,000 that is released primarily by activated monocyte-macrophage cell types. (It is also probably the same molecule as lymphocyte activating factor and endogenous pyrogen.) Activation of these cell types may result from the ingestion of cellular and tissue debrides, from contact with immune complexes, or by an interaction with chemicals such as endotoxin. Thus, nearly all infections, immunological reactions, and inflammatory processes stimulate the synthesis and release of leukocyte endogenous mediator by phagocytic cells. Once released, it circulates to various tissues in the body, having a profound influence upon the metabolism of the reticuloendothelial system, the liver, the brain, and skeletal muscle. For example, the fever that accompanies the acute phase response to injury or infection is thought to be the result of an interleukin-1 mediated alteration in the set point of the hypothalamic thermoregulatory center. As such, it can be considered a hormone. Many of the primary actions of interleukin-1 occur in the tissues from which it originates.

In the liver, interleukin-1 stimulates protein synthesis, resulting in the production of acute phase reactants, the accumulation of iron and zinc, and the release of copper. As a result, the plasma concentrations of iron and of zinc decrease, whereas the concentration of copper increases. The copper is released primarily with ceruloplasmin, a protein that is important in clearing oxygen radicals from injured and infected tissues and in donating copper groups to copper-dependent enzymes. An example of the latter is lysyl oxidase, an enzyme that is critical in wound healing because of its ability to form cross links between collagen molecules. The decrease in serum iron is thought to be important in the inhibition of bacterial growth and in the genesis of anemia in chronic infections. Other acute phase reactants that increase in response to interleukin-1 include fibrinogen, haptoglobin, C-reactive protein, and components of complement and alpha$_2$ macroglobin. The latter is a protease inhibitor that may exert an important role at the site of injury or infection by inhibiting the proteases that are released by leukocytes and by macrophages.

It is apparent that this burst in hepatic protein synthesis requires a great deal of energy and amino acid. This, in

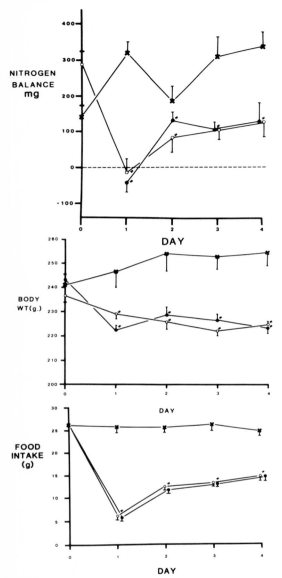

Fig. 1-39. Effect of wounding on food intake, nitrogen balance, and body weight. Food intake by wounded animals (●) was considerably less than that of animals allowed to eat ad libitum (×). When animals were pair-fed (○) to the reduced food intake of the wounded animals, negative nitrogen balance and weight loss were the same in these two groups. In contrast, there was a marked difference in nitrogen balance and body weight between wounded animals and animals allowed to eat ad libitum. (From: *Shearer JD et al: Am J Surg 147:456, 1984, with permission.*)

part, may be provided by an interleukin-1 mediated increase in protein degradation and amino acid release from skeletal muscle tissue that precedes the increase in hepatic protein synthesis. The amino acids released appear to be used by the liver for energy as well as for protein synthesis, since an appreciable amount of the amino acids released is oxidized. The skeletal muscle wasting and negative nitrogen balance that accompanies injury may be

a direct result of interleukin-1. In addition, the increase in hepatic protein synthesis produced by interleukin-1 is not global. Albumin synthesis decreases during the acute phase response, and there is suggestive evidence that overall protein synthesis in the liver is decreased.

TUMOR NECROSIS FACTOR. Tumor necrosis factor (TNF), or cachectin, is a monokine released by macrophages that is capable of inducing hemorrhagic necrosis of tumors. In addition, it may be in large part responsible for the wasting associated with chronic illness and malignancy. Recent evidence suggests that TNF may exert an important role in the response to injury and infection. For example, the lethal effects of endotoxin including fever, hypotension, metabolic acidosis, hemoconcentration, hyperglycemia, and hypokalemia appear to be mediated by TNF. Tumor necrosis factor also mediates a decrease in the transmembrane potential of skeletal muscle that may be important in the sequestration of fluid and electrolytes during injury.

METABOLIC CHANGES INDUCED BY INJURY

The immediate postinjury period is characterized by starvation, immobilization, restoration of homeostasis, and repair. The metabolic events consequent to injury are the result of stimuli present in the injury and starvation and are presumably directed at restoration of homeostasis and at repair. For example, the nitrogen balance and weight loss that follow injury appear to be, in large part, the result of the starvation that accompanies the injury (Fig. 1-39). Recent evidence from our laboratories also suggests that the metabolic response to injury may be altered to some degree by the inflammatory response to the injury. For example, temporal alterations in plasma ketone body and lactate concentrations of wounded animals appear to correlate with the inflammatory infiltrate of wounded tissue. Tumor necrosis factor appears to be responsible for many of the manifestations of endotoxemia. An understanding of the metabolic response consequent to starvation and the metabolic alterations produced by the inflammatory infiltrate is central to an understanding of the metabolic response to injury.

Metabolic Response Consequent to Starvation

SUBSTRATE METABOLISM. The average resting, 70-kg human being using 1800 kcal/day of energy requires 180 g of glucose for the metabolism of the nervous tissue (144 g) and other glycolytic tissue (RBC, WBC, renal medulla) (36 g) (Fig. 1-40), energy for obligate daily activity, amino acids for protein synthesis, and fatty acids for lipid synthesis. In the absence of food, a fasting human being must supply these substrates from existing body stores.

Glucose and energy are obtained from the 75 g of glycogen stored in the liver (Table 1-2). However, this is not sufficient for the energy or the glucose requirements of a fasting human being. Free glucose cannot be provided to the circulation from the 150 g of glycogen present in skel-

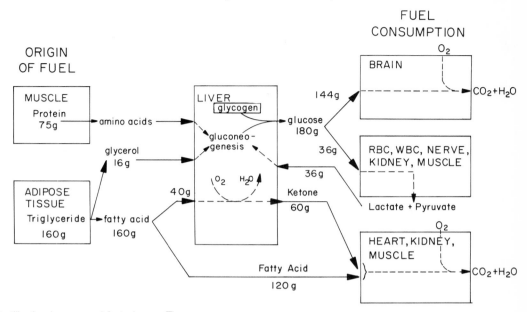

Fig. 1-40. Scheme of fuel utilization in a normal fasted man. The two primary sources are muscle protein and fat. The brain oxidizes glucose completely, the glycolyzers break down glucose by aerobic or anaerobic glycolysis into lactate and pyruvate, which are then remade in the liver in glucose, and the rest of the body burns fatty acids and ketones. (Adapted from: *Cahill GF: N Engl J Med 282:668, 1970, with permission.*)

etal muscle since it lacks glucose-6-phosphatase, the enzyme necessary for the release of free glucose from a cell. Thus, the primary stimulus to the metabolic events that occur during fasting and starvation is a reduction in the serum glucose concentration that occurs as the glucose needs of glucose-dependent tissues can no longer be met by the breakdown of glycogen (Fig. 1-41). The reduction in serum glucose, which occurs within 15 h of fasting, results in a decrease in the secretion of insulin and an increase in the secretion of glucagon, cortisol, growth hormone, and catecholamines, changes that stimulate an increase in hepatic gluconeogenesis and glycogenolysis. The changes in insulin and glucagon secretion appear to be the primary response, since significant increases in the secretion of the counterregulatory hormones, particularly catecholamines, are not usually seen until the reduction in the serum glucose concentration is severe. Furthermore, an increase in the secretion of catecholamines, growth hormone, and cortisol is not necessary, since the basal concentrations of the counterregulatory hormones will be unopposed by the reduction in insulin. The glucose required for glucose-dependent tissues during starvation is provided by glycogenolysis and gluconeogenesis (Fig. 1-42). This requires the provision of gluconeogenic precursors to the liver.

There are three primary gluconeogenic precursors used by the liver and to a lesser extent by the kidney for the synthesis of glucose. These are lactate, glycerol, and amino acids such as alanine and glutamine (Table 1-3). There are two main sources for lactate. The first is from the metabolism of glucose by erythrocytes and white cells that do not oxidize the glucose they require. Although most cells that require glucose such as the brain and nervous tissue metabolize glucose completely to carbon dioxide, erythrocytes and white cells convert glucose to lactate by aerobic glycolysis and release the newly formed lactate into the circulation. In turn, this lactate can be reconverted to glucose in the liver and again made available for use by peripheral tissues, a process described by the Coris (Fig. 1-43). The lactate made available from these sources does not provide any new carbon skeleton for glucose synthesis, since the carbon is derived from preexistent molecules of glucose. If glucose use by

Table 1-2

Fuel	Weight, kg	Calories
Tissues:		
Fat (adipose triglyceride)	15	141,000
Protein (mainly muscle)	6	24,000
Glycogen (muscle)	0.150	600
Glycogen (liver)	0.075	300
Total		165,900
Circulating fuels:		
Glucose (extracellular fluid)	0.020	80
Free fatty acids (plasma)	0.0003	3
Triglycerides (plasma)	0.003	30
Total		113

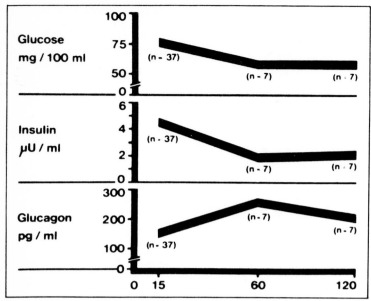

Fig. 1-41. The primary stimulus to the neuroendocrine response to fasting and starvation is hypoglycemia. Arterial concentrations of glucose, insulin, and glucagon after 15-, 60-, and 120-h of fasting are shown. (From: *Ahnefeld FW, Burri C, Dick W, Halmagyi M: Parenteral Nutrition. Heidelberg, Springer-Verlag, 1976, with permission.*)

Fig. 1-42. The five phases of glucose homeostasis. This represents the origin of blood glucose in a 70-kg man who ingests 100 g of glucose and then fasts for 40 days. Phase I is the absorptive phase in which the 100 g of glucose enters the circulation by absorption from the gut. Phase II is the postabsorptive phase in which glucose is stored as glycogen in response to increased secretion of insulin and decreased secretion of glucagon. Phase III represents early starvation in which the fall in blood sugar leads to a decrease in insulin secretion and an increase in glucagon and catecholamine secretion. The latter results in an increase in gluconeogenesis and glycogenolysis. Phase IV is intermediary starvation in which hepatic glycogen stores have been depleted and the sole source of glucose is gluconeogenesis. Phase V represents prolonged starvation in which ketone bodies become the primary fuel, thereby resulting in a decrease in gluconeogenesis. (From: *Ruderman NB: Annu Rev Med 248, 1975, with permission.*)

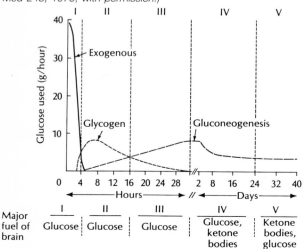

white cells increases, glucose must still be provided from some other carbon source. In part, this demand may be met by the release of lactate from the second major source in the body, skeletal muscle. Although skeletal muscle cannot release free glucose, as noted previously, it can release lactate by the breakdown of its endogenous glycogen stores.

Gluconeogenesis from lactate of skeletal muscle origin is also not sufficient to maintain glucose homeostasis. As a result, approximately 75 g of protein is degraded daily during fasting and starvation to provide the required gluconeogenic amino acids to the liver. These amino acids are noted in Table 1-4. Proteolysis results primarily from a decrease in insulin and an increase in cortisol and is associated with a rapid increase in the urinary nitrogen

Table 1-3. GLUCOSE AVAILABLE IN EARLY STARVATION STATE IN A 70-KG MAN

Origin	Amount of glucose, g/24 h
New glucose (gluconeogenesis):	
Fat (glycerol)	16
Protein	43
Stores or recycled glucose:	
Glycogen	85
Recycled glucose	36
Total	180

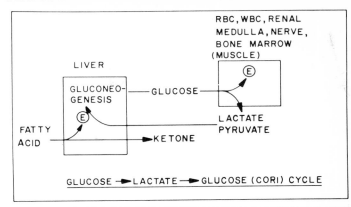

Fig. 1-43. The Cori cycle (top) provides for the transfer of energy from the liver to the periphery. Glucose gives up energy to the periphery by anaerobic or aerobic glycolysis to lactate and pyruvate. The latter are then remade into glucose in the liver, utilizing energy derived from the metabolism of fatty acids. In the glucose to alanine cycle (bottom) described by Felig et al, glucose is metabolized to pyruvate in muscle; pyruvate is then converted to alanine, which is then transported to the liver, where it is remade into glucose.

excretion from the normal 5 to 7 g/day to approximately 8 to 11 g during the first 2 to 4 days of fasting. Although the protein mobilized in starvation is derived primarily from skeletal muscle, the loss of protein from other organs (liver, pancreas, gastrointestinal tract, and kidneys) is proportionately much greater (Fig. 1-44). In the liver this protein loss appears to be somewhat selective since the enzymes necessary for gluconeogenesis and lipolysis are spared; those required for the synthesis of urea and serum proteins are not. In the pancreas, exocrine function is lost by a reduction in the production of gastrointestinal hor-

mones and enzymes, and in the gastrointestinal tract, digestive function is impaired by a reduction in the production of digestive enzymes and the regeneration of epithelial cells. For these reasons, starved patients often become paradoxically food intolerant, as manifested by the development of diarrhea and malabsorption when small amounts of food or enteral feedings are given.

The use of amino acids by the liver for gluconeogenesis creates a problem in handling the ammonia that is formed during the deamination of the amino acid, a necessary

Fig. 1-44. The percentage of protein lost from various tissues during starvation. Although the greatest amount is derived from skeletal muscle, the tissue with the largest loss is the liver. (Modified from: *Addis T, Poo LJ, Lew W: J Biol Chem 115:111, 1936, with permission.*)

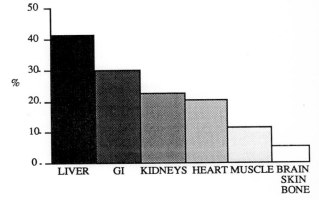

Table 1-4

Gluconeogenesis	Ketogenesis	Gluconeogenesis and ketogenesis
Alanine	Leucine*	Isoleucine*
Arginine*		Lysine*
Aspartic acid		Phenylalanine*
Asparagine		Tyrosine*
Cystine		Tryptophan*
Glutamic acid		
Glycine		
Histidine*		
Hydroxyproline		
Methionine*		
Proline		
Serine		
Threonine*		
Valine*		

*Essential AA.

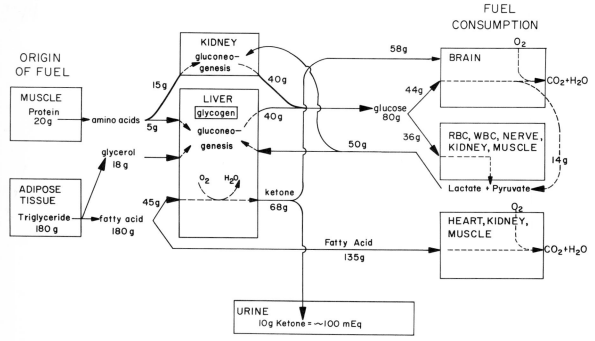

FASTING MAN ADAPTED (5-6 wks.)
(24 hours, basal : ~1500 calories)

Fig. 1-45. Schema of fuel metabolism after 5 to 6 weeks of starvation. Liver glycogen sources are depleted, there is a diminished utilization of muscle protein, the brain is burning ketones, and gluconeogenesis from amino acids is taking place to a large extent in the kidney. (Adapted from: *Cahill GF: N Engl J Med 282:668, 1970, with permission.*)

process before the carbon skeleton can be made available for gluconeogenesis. Although under normal circumstances, urea synthesis is the primary mechanism, the synthesis of urea in the liver requires a considerable amount of energy and the enzymes required for ureagenesis are decreased during prolonged starvation. Consequently, the renal excretion of ammonium ion becomes the primary route of elimination of alpha amino nitrogen during starvation. Additionally, the kidney also assumes an increasing role in gluconeogenesis since glutamine and glutamate serve as the primary amino acids for transport of the amino groups to the kidney for ammonia formation and for gluconeogenesis in the kidney. The kidney may account for up to 45 percent of glucose production during late starvation.

The rapid proteolysis of body protein cannot proceed at a rate of 75 g/day for very long. The total amount of protein in a 70-kg man is approximately 6000 g, and the continued degradation of protein results in continued loss of function such that death will ensue well before all the protein is broken down. Fortunately, proteolysis does slow down by about the fifth day of starvation and eventually reaches a nadir of 20 g of protein per day. This is reflected in a decline in urinary excretion of nitrogen to a minimum of approximately 2 to 4 g of nitrogen per day.

The reduction in protein breakdown is in large part made possible through ketoadaptation of the brain. Although the brain can metabolize ketone bodies, the limited transport of ketone bodies through the blood-brain barrier under normal conditions limits their utilization. In the presence of adequate glucose concentrations, glucose is used preferentially. During starvation, transport systems in the blood-brain barrier increase the rate of ketone body transport, and the metabolism of the brain is adapted to utilize ketone bodies. Consequently, there is a significant reduction in the amount of glucose needed by the brain and therefore in the amount of protein that must be degraded for gluconeogenesis (Fig. 1-45 and Table 1-5).

Table 1-5. GLUCOSE AVAILABLE IN LATE STARVATION STATE IN A 70-KG MAN

Origin	Amount of glucose, g/24 h
New glucose (gluconeogenesis):	
Fat (glycerol)	18
Protein	12
Stored or recycled glucose:	
Glycogen	0
Recycled glucose	50
Total	80

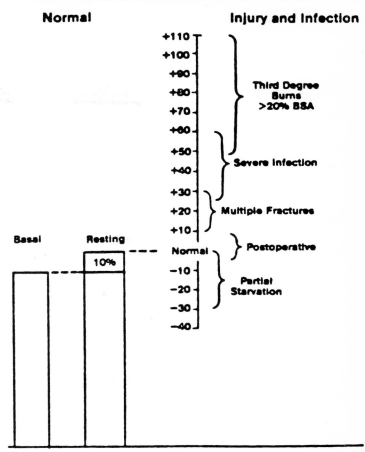

Fig. 1-48. Resting energy expenditure of adult patients during injury, stress, and starvation. The highest resting energy expenditures are seen following thermal injuries and severe infections. (From: *Kinney JM: The application of indirect calorimetry to clinical studies, in Assessment of Energy Metabolism in Health and Disease. Columbus, OH, Ross Laboratories, 1980, p 42, with permission.*)

process itself since it persists for as long as inflammation is present. The most severe injury is a thermal burn, in which sustained increases in resting energy expenditure of greater than 100 percent have been noted.

In large part, the increase in energy expenditure following injury appears to result from the increased activity of the sympathetic nervous system and the increased circulating concentrations of catecholamines. Wilmore and colleagues have demonstrated that the metabolic rate can be decreased in severely burned patients by the administration of alpha- and beta-adrenergic blockers or beta-adrenergic blockers alone. Conversely, the administration of epinephrine or norepinephrine to normal human beings increases the basal metabolic rate.

The increase in resting energy expenditure is also dependent upon the size of the individual and to some extent upon the environmental temperature. The largest increases in energy expenditure are seen in heavily muscled, well-nourished young men who have large body cell masses, and the smallest increases are in elderly, poorly nourished women who have small body cell masses. This is a reflection of the linear relationship between body cell mass and resting energy expenditure.

Although energy can be derived from carbohydrates, proteins, or fat, following injury the available stores of carbohydrate are small, nutritional intake of carbohydrates and proteins is reduced or absent, glucose required for glucose-dependent tissues persists, and degradation of protein for energy will require the loss or reduction of some body function. As a result, the primary source for energy during injury is fat, a finding that is reflected in the low respiratory quotients (0.7 to 0.8) that are noted after injury and sepsis. There is also evidence to suggest that the dependence on lipids after septic injury is greater than that observed following nonseptic injury. These findings argue in favor of the use of intralipids during parenteral nutrition.

ENERGY METABOLISM IN TISSUES. A significant reduction in energy charge and ATP content has been noted

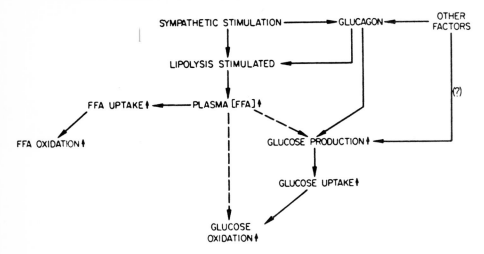

Fig. 1-49. The role of sympathetic stimulation in substrate kinetics during stress. (From: *Lefer AM, Schumer W: Molecular and Cellular Aspects of Shock and Trauma. New York, Alan R. Liss, 1983, with permission.*)

during severe hemorrhagic shock; hypoxia; total ischemia in the liver, kidney, skeletal muscle, and cardiac muscle; sepsis; and following wounding. The reduction in energy charge and high-energy phosphates is proportional to the severity of the injury.

The reduction in high-energy phosphates may be the result of anaerobic metabolism consequent to hypoperfusion or hypoxia or to a dilutional effect from inflammatory cells. For example, hypovolemia and sepsis demonstrate a reduction in tissue high-energy phosphate concentrations that appear to result from anaerobic metabolism in poorly perfused and hypoxemic tissues. The reduction in high-energy phosphates during shock usually occurs in the liver and kidneys prior to the reductions in cardiac and skeletal muscle and is related to the severity of the hemorrhagic, septic, or hypoxic insult. The different response between tissue types, in part, may be the result of the differences in blood flow and in the resting metabolic activity of the specific tissue examined. A reduction in the energy charge ATP and creatine phosphate content of all tissues eventually occurs if there is insufficient compensation to the hemorrhage or septic insult.

Wounded tissue also demonstrates a reduction in its energy charge, ATP, and creatine phosphate content during early healing that traditionally has been attributed to a decrease in the production of high-energy phosphate compounds from anaerobic metabolism in wounded tissue. Recent evidence suggests that the metabolism of wounded tissue is aerobic rather than anaerobic, a finding that implies wounded tissue has the same capacity for the production of high-energy phosphates as nonwounded tissue. A reduction in the energy charge of wounded tissue could be an artifact resulting from varying high-energy phosphate contents in the component cells of wounded tissue. Inflammatory cells that account for up to 50 percent of the DNA (and therefore 50 percent of the cells) present in wounded tissue contain very few high-energy compounds. As a result, the presence of these

cells in wounded tissue can dilute the overall high-energy phosphate content measured in wounded tissue even though the high-energy phosphate content of the resident tissue is normal or actually increased. That is, the muscle present in wounded skeletal muscle may have the same high-energy phosphate content as that seen in normal skeletal muscle. This appears to be the case since the addition of macrophages to normal skeletal muscle results in a high-energy phosphate content similar to that observed in wounded muscle. Similarly, the high-energy phosphate content of septic tissue is usually reduced. Although this reduction also has been attributed to a decrease in high-energy phosphate production secondary to anaerobic metabolism, this reduction also may be dilutional, since septic tissue as well as wounded tissue has a marked inflammatory cell infiltrate.

LIPID METABOLISM DURING INJURY

LIPOLYSIS. The primary source of energy following injury is lipids. It is not surprising that rate of lipolysis is generally increased immediately following injury and during the reparative phase. Immediately after injury, elevated concentrations of cortisol, catecholamines, glucagon, growth hormone, and ACTH, increased sympathetic nervous system activity, and depressed concentrations of insulin favor lipolysis. Among these agents, the best-known stimulus for hormone-sensitive lipase is catecholamines. The sympathetic nervous system is of paramount importance in the lipolytic response to stress, since adrenergic blockade produces a marked reduction in lipolysis (Fig. 1-49). Evidence suggests that norepinephrine released by the sympathetic nervous system is more important in this response than the release of adrenal epinephrine, since the response appears to be primarily mediated through beta₁ receptors.

The net lipolysis observed during the ebb phase results in elevated concentrations of glycerol and free fatty acids in plasma. If the reduction in effective circulating volume is severe, such as might be seen in severe hemorrhage or sepsis, an elevation in plasma free fatty acids may not occur. This may result from intense vasoconstriction in peripheral tissues and therefore minimal blood flow in adipose tissue, such that neuroendocrine agents cannot act on adipose tissue. Because the net production of free fatty acids is dependent upon the balance between lipolysis and reesterification of fatty acids, an increase in the reesterification rate, such as that seen in the presence of high concentrations of lactate, may decrease net free fatty acid release. The latter is supported by the rise in plasma concentrations of glycerol noted after injury, which suggests that lipolysis is occurring, and by increased concentrations of lactate in studies in which there is no change in the concentration of free fatty acids. Other factors that may alter the mobilization of lipids after injury include a decrease in pH, hyperglycemia, and the anesthesia received. For example, lipolysis is directly inhibited by pentobarbital anesthesia, and hemorrhage in the presence of pentobarbital usually results in a fall in the plasma free fatty acid and ketone body concentrations. By contrast, hemorrhage experiments using other types of anesthesia or in awake animals produce a rise in the free fatty acid and ketone body concentrations.

During the reparative or flow phase, net lipolysis persists despite an increase in the concentration of insulin. This is reflected by an increased concentration of plasma free fatty acids and increased clearance of fatty acids. In the presence of oxygen, the fatty acids released can be oxidized by most tissues in the body, including cardiac and skeletal muscle, to produce energy, and normal or elevated rates of fatty acid oxidation have been noted during sepsis, endotoxemia, wounding, and thermal injury. If the rate of clearance of fatty acids is equal to or greater than their rate of appearance, no change or a decrease in the plasma fatty acid concentration may be noted. Even though there is an increase in the rate of appearance and oxidation of free fatty acids during sepsis and endotoxemia, a rise in the plasma free fatty acid concentration is not always noted. An analogous situation is also true for the hypertriglyceridemia that is characteristic of sepsis and endotoxemia. The latter may either be the result of an increase in the release of triglycerides that is in excess of the ability of tissues to clear them or the result of a normal rate of release in the face of a decrease in the ability of tissues to break down the molecules.

Controversy exists whether fatty acids can inhibit glycolysis following injury. Wolfe and colleagues have recently provided evidence in conscious burned dogs that the Randle effect does occur and that it may be a major mechanism for the reduction in glycolysis that occurs in nonseptic injury during the flow phase. An increase in the cytoplasmic concentration of citrate is seen during mild inflammation and injury but not after shock and major injury such as sepsis. Since fatty acid induced inhibition

of glycolysis is mediated through citrate, the absence of an increase in citrate may in part explain the persistence of glycolysis and net proteolysis after injury.

KETOGENESIS. The high concentrations of intracellular fatty acids and the elevated concentration of glucagon during the ebb and flow phases inhibit fatty acid synthesis. In hepatocytes, this also stimulates the transport of acetyl CO-A into the mitochondria for oxidation and ketogenesis. The activity of ketogenesis after shock, injury, and sepsis is variable and correlates inversely with the severity of injury. After major injury, severe shock, and sepsis, ketogenesis is low or absent, whereas after minor injury or mild infection, it is increased but to a lesser extent than that seen during nonstressed starvation. Injuries in which ketogenesis is low also appear to be associated with a small or absent increase in plasma free fatty acid concentrations, suggesting that the absence of ketogenesis in these situations results from the absence of an increase in the intracellular concentrations of free fatty acids.

CARBOHYDRATE METABOLISM DURING INJURY

GLUCOSE METABOLISM. By contrast to fasting and starvation, characterized by hypoglycemia, injury, sepsis, and stress are characterized by hyperglycemia. Hyperglycemia following hemorrhage was first reported by Claude Bernard in 1877 and has subsequently been confirmed in different species such as the dog, cat, pig, rat, and human beings and for different injuries such as sepsis, trauma, and thermal injury. It occurs immediately after injury and persists into the reparative period. The increase in plasma glucose is proportional to the severity of injury as reflected in a positive correlation between injury severity score and glucose concentration trauma victims (Fig. 1-50).

The presence of hyperglycemia provides a ready source of energy to the brain and may be important to early survival. It also appears quite possible that, as suggested by Jarhult and by ourselves, the principal homeostatic significance of increased plasma glucose may be the resulting osmotic transfer of fluids from cells to the interstitium that it induces leading to the restitution of blood volume. Elevated concentrations of glucose may be necessary for adequate delivery of this substrate to wounded tissue.

The alterations in carbohydrate metabolism that occur during injury include an increased hepatic glucose production and an impaired peripheral uptake of glucose that result from an increase in the secretion of catecholamines, cortisol, glucagon, growth hormone, vasopressin, angiotensin II, and somatostatin and a reduction in the secretion of insulin. The primary source of glucose that is released immediately after injury is hepatic glycogen. By contrast, glucose production during the flow phase appears to result primarily from hepatic and renal gluconeogenesis.

Differences also exist in the mechanism through which these alterations occur. Although an immediate increase in the plasma glucagon concentration that correlated with

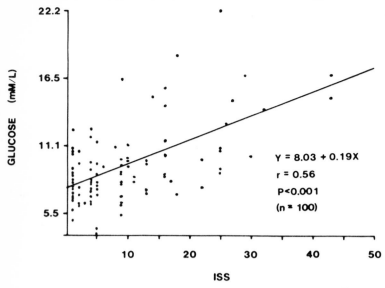

$$Y = 8.03 + 0.19X$$
$$r = 0.56$$
$$P < 0.001$$
$$(n = 100)$$

Fig. 1-50. There is a positive correlation between the serum glucose concentration and the severity of injury in multiply injured patients. (From: *Kenney PR, Allen-Rowlands CF, Gann DS: J Trauma 23:712, 1983, with permission.*)

the plasma glucose concentration following thermal injury was noted by Wilmore and colleagues, most studies of glucagon metabolism following nonthermal injury and hypovolemia have noted no increase in the plasma concentration of glucagon immediately after injury. This suggests that an increase in the peripheral concentration of glucagon or the delivery of glucagon to the liver is not required for the initial hyperglycemia after hemorrhage and injury. This is further supported by the studies of Lautt and coworkers who demonstrated the abolition of the hyperglycemic response to hemorrhage in adrenalectomized and hepatic denervated cats and the restitution of this response when either the adrenals or the liver were left intact. These data imply a redundant system for the control of the hyperglycemic response to hemorrhage and injury in which either of two effectors (hepatic nerves or adrenals) can effectively produce the hyperglycemic response. Thus, the immediate hyperglycemia that occurs following injury appears to be related primarily to the actions of catecholamines and cortisol with little contribution from glucagon, whereas during the flow phase, glucagon becomes more important.

The hyperglycemia that occurs following injury in diabetic patients may be different. Cryer and colleagues have documented the relevance of the counterregulatory hormones in patients with diabetes mellitus. Diabetic patients with insulin-dependent diabetes (IDDM) exhibit greater hyperglycemic responses to counterregulatory hormones, including glucagon, epinephrine, and cortisol, than nondiabetic patients; and acquired deficiencies in the secretion of some of the counterregulatory hormones occur commonly in patients with IDDM. For example, glucagon secretory responses to decrements in plasma glucose concentration occur early in the course of IDDM and deficiencies in epinephrine secretory responses frequently occur late in the disease. Patients with IDDM who have deficiencies in counterregulatory response may develop hypoglycemia following injury and patients with

normal responses may develop marked hyperglycemia as a result of the greater response to counterregulatory hormones when present.

INSULIN RESISTANCE. Another important difference in the mechanism of hyperglycemia following injury is related to the secretion of insulin. Immediately after injury, the plasma insulin concentration is depressed in relation to the degree of hyperglycemia. This results from a reduction in beta islet cell sensitivity to glucose that is mediated by catecholamines, somatostatin, reduced pancreatic blood flow, and the increased activity of the sympathetic nervous system. An intact adrenal gland is also necessary for this response since the blunting of the insulin secretion can be eliminated by adrenalectomy. During the flow phase, beta islet cell sensitivity returns to normal and insulin concentrations rise to more appropriate values but hyperglycemia still persists.

In part this is related to the delayed rate of assimilation of a glucose load, glucosuria, and a resistance to exogenously administered insulin noted in both the ebb and flow phases of injury. This diabetes of injury, first noted by Drucker, should not be interpreted as an actual reduction in glucose uptake and utilization, since glucose uptake and utilization by peripheral tissues in both the ebb and the flow phases is consistently greater than under normal circumstances. Instead the resistance to insulin is manifested in a decreased glucose clearance. The high-plasma glucose concentration and the attendant increase in the plasma to tissue glucose concentration gradient appear to overcome the resistance of peripheral tissues to glucose entry, thereby allowing for normal or increased rates of glucose uptake in peripheral tissues.

During the flow phase, gluconeogenesis persists despite near normal concentrations of insulin, another mani-

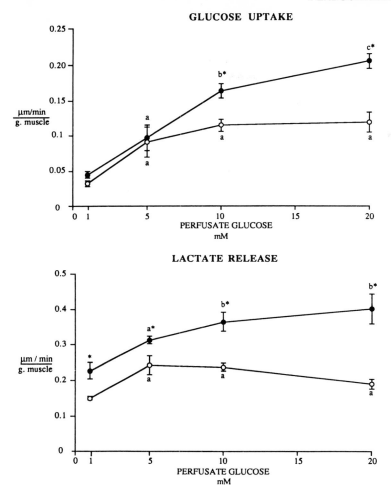

Fig. 1-51. Glucose uptake and lactate production by wounded (●) and nonwounded (○) hindlimbs of rats in response to increasing external glucose supply. Glucose uptake and lactate production by wounded hindlimbs increased as the concentration of external glucose increased. In contrast, glucose uptake and lactate production by nonwounded hindlimbs reached a plateau at an external glucose concentration of 5 mmol. $*p < 0.05$ wounded vs. nonwounded; a. = $p < 0.05$ intragroup difference vs. 1 mmol; b. = $p < 0.05$ intragroup difference vs. 5 mmol; c. = $p < 0.05$ intragroup difference vs. 10 mmol. (From: *Amaral JF et al: in preparation.*)

festation of the insulin resistance that occurs with injury. Therefore, the hyperglycemia that occurs after injury results from a combination of increased hepatic glucose production and release and from a peripheral resistance to the entrance of glucose. Since production supersedes utilization, hyperglycemia persists. If the rate of gluconeogenesis decreases through a reduction either in gluconeogenic precursors or in gluconeogenic enzymatic function, hepatic glucose production will decrease and hypoglycemia will ensue, a finding of terminal injuries and prolonged sepsis.

The insulin resistance that develops following injury is thought to arise from a reduction in the release of insulin from the pancreas and from an inhibition of insulin action on peripheral tissue that is mediated by the sympathetic nervous system, catecholamines, and cortisol. In vitro and in vivo studies have consistently demonstrated the ability of these agents to blunt the release and action of insulin; other unidentified factors are thought to be involved in this response. A reduction in insulin action on adipose tissue by a macrophage mediated monokine suggests a possible role of the inflammatory response in the diabetes of injury. This would not be surprising, since hyperglycemia is one of the earliest and best-recognized features of sepsis.

GLUCOSE METABOLISM IN WOUNDED TISSUE. Glucose must be provided not only to red cells, white cells, renal medulla, and neural tissues following injury, but also to wounded tissue. In fact, glucose uptake and lactate production in wounded tissue are increased by up to 100 percent and are proportional to the circulating concentration of glucose present (Fig. 1-51). The increase in glucose uptake in wounded tissue is associated with an increase in the activity of phosphofructokinase, a major rate limiting enzyme in glycolysis. Despite the increase in glucose uptake and phosphofructokinase activity, wounded and

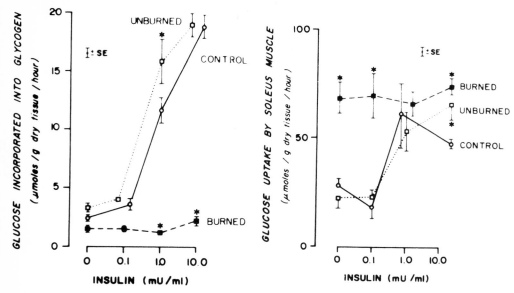

Fig. 1-52. Glucose uptake and glycogen synthesis by the soleus muscles from the burned and unburned limbs of rats 3 days after scald injury. Soleus muscles from the injured limb did not respond to insulin, whereas muscles from the uninjured limb responded to insulin in a dose-dependent fashion with an increase in glucose uptake and glycogen synthesis. (From: *Nelson KM, Turinsky J: J Surg Res 31:292, 1981, with permission.*)

burned tissues demonstrate a lack of insulin sensitivity and do not increase their glucose uptake or glycogenesis in response to insulin (Fig. 1-52).

The accelerated glucose uptake in wounded and burned tissue correlates with the degree of inflammatory cellular infiltrate present. It has been shown that much of the increase above the resting rate of glucose uptake in nonwounded muscle can be explained by glucose uptake in the inflammatory cells. The inflammatory infiltrate may actually mediate an increase in glucose uptake of the wounded noninflammatory tissue itself since the uptake of glucose by muscle in the presence of macrophages is greater than that of muscle not exposed to macrophages.

The increase in glucose uptake and lactate production by wounded, burned, and septic tissue has been attributed to anaerobic glycolysis that results from local tissue hypoxia and a reduction in local tissue perfusion. Although early after injury disruption of blood flow in the injured area may lead to aerobic glycolysis, glucose metabolism in wounded and burned tissue 3 to 5 days after injury appears to be primarily aerobic since oxygen consumption and CO_2 production are normal but lactate production is increased. Aerobic glycolysis is characteristic of the cellular inflammatory infiltrate that accompanies wounds and burns. Metabolic derangements suggestive of aerobic glycolysis have also been observed in septic and endotoxic tissue. An important source of glucose consumption following injury of all types may be the activation of white cells.

LACTATE METABOLISM. There is an increase in the plasma concentration of lactate following most injuries that correlates with the severity of injury (Fig. 1-53). The accumulation of lactate following shock accounts in part for the progressive acidosis of shock and derives from anaerobic metabolism in ischemic tissues. Under these circumstances, the likelihood of survival of patients in profound shock can be estimated from the excess levels of lactate present in the blood. For example, Broder and Weil noted an 82 percent survival in patients in shock with an initial excess lactate concentration of 1 mmol/L, a 60 percent survival with 2 mmol/L, and a 26 percent survival when the excess lactate was 2 to 4 mmol/L. A better prognosticator of survival appears to be the serial change in total plasma lactate. Excess lactate should not be confused with total plasma lactate since the excess lactate is the amount of lactate present in the blood that increases the lactate-pyruvate ratio from normal.

Elevated plasma lactate concentrations may result from local tissue ischemia such as in mesenteric infarction, from diminished hepatic clearance of lactate, and from increased lactate production by inflammatory cells. The latter mechanism may account for the elevation in plasma lactate concentrations seen in burned and wounded tissue well after the effective circulating blood volume has been restored. The differential diagnosis of any injured patient with hyperlactacidemia should include systemic hypoperfusion, regional hypoperfusion, hepatic dysfunction, and severe inflammation.

PROTEIN METABOLISM DURING INJURY

NITROGEN BALANCE. The daily intake of protein for a healthy young adult is usually about 80 to 120 g, or 13 to 20 g of nitrogen. About 2 to 3 g of this nitrogen is excreted per day in the stool and 13 to 20 g in the urine. Following injury, nitrogen excretion in the urine increases greatly and rises to 30 to 50 g of nitrogen per day. This is nearly all in the form of urea nitrogen and results from net proteolysis since nitrogen intake immediately

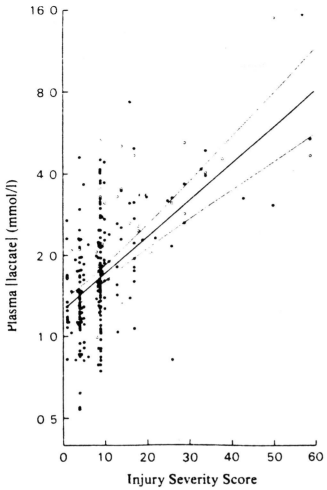

Fig. 1-53. Relationship between plasma lactate and the injury severity score in multiply injured patients. There was a positive correlation between ISS and plasma lactate in both patients who had ingested ethanol (○) and those who had not (●). (From: *Stoner HB, Frayn KN, et al: Clin Sci 56:563, 1979, with permission.*)

tein content and the incorporation of radiolabeled amino acids in visceral tissues and skeletal muscle confirm that it is skeletal muscle that is depleted while visceral tissues (liver, kidney) are spared, a finding contrary to starvation, in which visceral protein is used to a greater extent than muscle.

The net catabolism of protein can result from either increased catabolism, decreased synthesis, or a combination of these factors. Available data on total body protein turnover suggest that after injury, the net changes in catabolism and synthesis depend on the severity of the injury. Elective operations and minor injury appear to result in a decreased rate of synthesis with a normal rate of protein catabolism. Severe trauma, burns, and sepsis appear to be associated with increases in both synthesis and catabolism, but a greater increase in the catabolism occurs resulting in net catabolism. Accelerated proteolysis and a high rate of gluconeogenesis persist after major injury and during sepsis. This appears to result from an inhibition of ketoadaptation after major injury and sepsis since, unlike starvation, ketogenesis is not prominent and does not fuel the brain in significant amounts. As a result, a high requirement for glucose and therefore for gluconeogenesis persists. The mechanisms for inhibition of ketoadaptation are not known. Barocos et al., based on in vitro muscle incubations, have proposed that interleukin-1 may be responsible for the accelerated proteolysis that accompanies fever and sepsis, and Clowes et al. have presented evidence suggesting the involvement of a circulating peptide (proteolysis inducing factor-PIF) containing 33 amino acids in this response that may also represent interleukin-1 or that may be distinct.

The rise in urinary nitrogen and negative nitrogen balance begins shortly after injury, reaches a peak about the first week, and may continue for 3 to 7 weeks. The degree and duration of negative nitrogen balance is related to the severity of injury with elective operative procedures having a brief period of small degree and thermal injuries having long periods of major negative nitrogen balance. The degree of negative nitrogen balance and net protein catabolism also depends on the age, sex, and physical condition of the patient. Young healthy males lose more protein in response to an injury than do women or the elderly, presumably as a result of the smaller body cell mass present in the latter group. In addition, the urinary excretion of nitrogen is less after a second operation if it closely follows the first, presumably the result of a reduction in available protein stores consequent to the first operation. Negative nitrogen balance can be reduced or virtually eliminated by high caloric nitrogen supplementation as with enteral or parenteral nutrition. The loss of protein that occurs after injury is not entirely obligatory to the injury, and it is in large part a manifestation of acute starvation and the increased need for gluconeogenetic precursors during periods of stress.

The evidence that increased nitrogen metabolism following injury is related to the need for carbohydrates has been summarized by Kinney et al. as follows: (1) the caloric contribution of protein to the fuel mixture of normal and injured human beings is less than 20 percent; (2) two-

after injury is minimal or absent. Despite the large amount of protein that is broken down, only 20 percent is used for calories even with major increases in nitrogen excretion. The remainder is used by the liver and the kidneys to produce glucose and is reflected in the accelerated ureagenesis that is noted after injury. This results primarily from an increase in the circulating concentrations of cortisol, glucagon, and catecholamines and the decreased effectiveness of insulin.

The increased excretion of urea following injury is also associated with the urinary loss of sulfur, phosphorus, potassium, magnesium, and creatinine. This suggests the breakdown of intracellular materials. Isotope dilution studies point to a decrease in cell mass rather than in cell number as the source of the protein breakdown. The nitrogen-sulfur and nitrogen-potassium ratios suggest that this loss occurs mainly from muscle. Analysis of the pro-carbon fragments are readily available from adipose tissue as the major energy source; (3) the body has a continuous requirement for carbohydrate intermediates for synthetic purposes, for which the deamination of amino acids is the primary endogenous source; and (4) fatty acids cannot directly yield a net gain of carbohydrate intermediates, glucose, or glycogen.

AMINO ACID METABOLISM. The alterations in plasma amino acids in response to injury are not well defined. Immediately after injury there is little or no change in the total amino acid concentration. Increases have been noted, however, in the concentrations of alanine, cystine, taurine, and the aromatic acids. This may be the result of varying levels of nutrition prior to the insult, of hypoperfusion, of starvation, and of physical activity. Negative nitrogen balance, weight loss, and plasma amino acid concentrations of wounded animals are in the same direction and of the same magnitude as those that occur in nonwounded animals pair-fed to the reduced food intake of the wounded group. Although this suggests that the alterations in proteolysis and in amino acid metabolism are solely the result of starvation, in the same study, the intracellular skeletal muscle concentrations of specific amino acids differed markedly between groups. During the flow phase of injury, alterations in plasma amino acids also appear to be related to the time from injury when they are measured. This is best exemplified by the plasma concentration of alanine, which early in the flow phase is increased but as the injury persists is decreased, presumably as a result of lack of its availability in peripheral tissues and its continued hepatic uptake. This pattern for alanine is noted in most forms of injury.

The type and severity of injury may also have an effect on the alterations seen in amino acid metabolism, although no consensus is established. On the one hand, the direction of changes in the plasma concentrations of specific amino acids are similar in many studies of thermal injury, elective operations, trauma, and sepsis, but the degree of their magnitude is often greater in sepsis. This suggests that changes in amino acid metabolism are not dependent upon the type or the severity of injury. By contrast, other studies have noted marked differences in plasma and muscle amino acid patterns during sepsis and other injuries that suggest the changes seen are related to the severity of the injury or infection and to the offending microorganism.

Despite these opposing points of view, the intracellular muscle concentrations and the muscle to plasma ratios of glutamine are reduced markedly in most studies of sepsis, wounding, and thermal injury. In general, the release of glutamine is greater than can be predicted from its relative abundance in muscle tissue protein, and evidence for its synthesis in muscle has been presented. Glutamine release from wounded and nonwounded muscle is not different and if the release of glutamine is expressed as a ratio to the phenylalanine released, there is a lower release rate in wounded than in nonwounded tissue. Since phenylalanine is neither catabolized nor synthesized in muscle, a lower glutamine-phenylalanine ratio suggests that either the synthesis of glutamine in wounded tissue is

reduced or the local catabolism in wounded muscle is increased. Glutamine is a major energy source for lymphocytes and fibroblasts. As a result, the accelerated utilization of glutamine by the cellular infiltrate in wounded or in septic tissue could explain the decreased concentrations noted at the site of injury and in the plasma. Souba and colleagues have recently shown that the gastrointestinal tract is a major consumer of glutamine following injury. The increased use of glutamine by the gastrointestinal tract may contribute further to the reduction in plasma glutamine concentrations during injury.

The importance of leukocyte and lymphocyte interactions with parenchymal cells in protein metabolism has been demonstrated by Keller, West, and colleagues. In their studies, isolated hepatocytes cultured in the presence of nonparenchymal hepatic (Kupffer) cells, peritoneal macrophages, or conditioned media in which nonparenchymal cells had been previously cultured demonstrated a marked reduction in protein synthesis as evidenced by a reduced rate of incorporation of radiolabeled leucine. This response was even greater when the hepatocyte–nonparenchymal cell mixture was coincubated with endotoxin. These data suggest that there may be a macrophage–Kupffer cell mediated factor that alters protein metabolism in hepatocytes.

WOUND HEALING. It is particularly astounding that most wounds heal despite the presence of negative nitrogen balance, negative energy balance, and reduced tissue and plasma concentrations of zinc, thiamine, riboflavin, vitamin C, and vitamin A. Moore has termed this ability of wound healing to proceed in the presence and absence of abundant substrate supply the biologic priority of wound healing. Levenson has noted that, ''whereas the healing of a wound after injury appears satisfactory, it may be neither normal nor optimal.'' For example, there is a distinct delay in the wound healing of an incisional wound on burned animals when compared with incisional wounds on normal animals, and rodents with a fractured femur do not heal a skin incision as well as rodents with a skin incision alone. The biologic priority of wound healing does not mean that wound healing is normal in the severely injured patient.

The biologic priority of wound healing also does not mean that wound healing cannot be improved in severely injured patients. For example, large open wounds, such as burns, are associated with an inhibition of nitrogen anabolism of the host and may result in protein malnutrition and death if the substrate demands of the wounds are not met exogenously. Although it is not clear if the administration of protein improves wound healing per se, it has been shown to reduce negative nitrogen balance. Some investigators have also noted an improvement in wound healing with protein supplementation, but others have been unable to document any change.

SUMMARY. Generalized catabolism, hyperglycemia, persistent gluconeogenesis, protein wasting, negative nitrogen balance, heat production, and loss of body mass are characteristic of all significant injuries. The degree of these metabolic alterations is directly related to the severity of injury, with the largest and most sustained changes

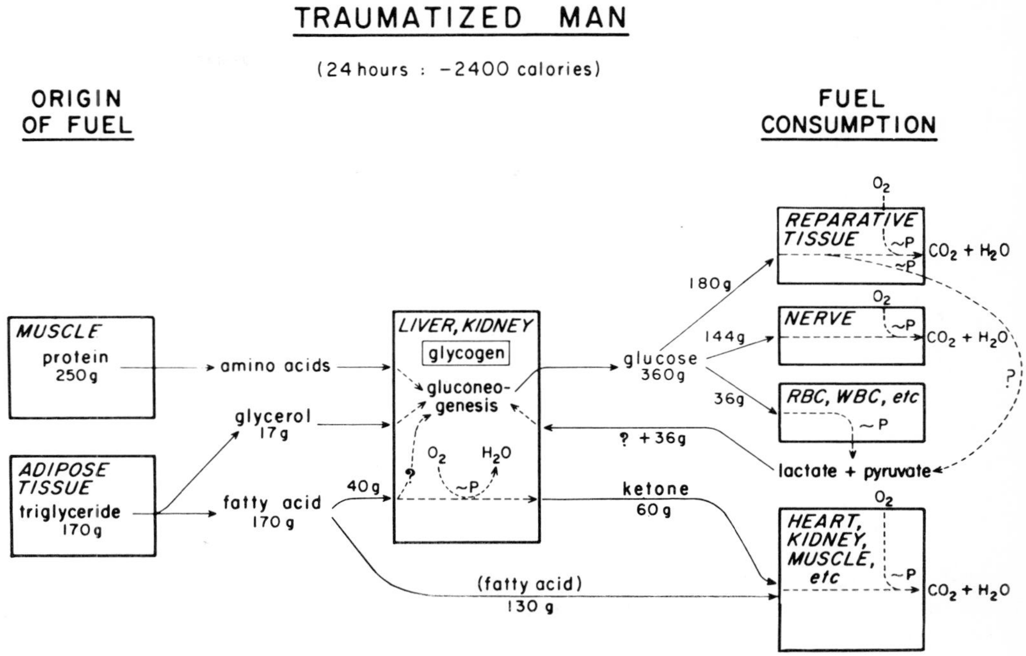

TRAUMATIZED MAN

(24 hours : −2400 calories)

Fig. 1-54. Hypothetical scheme of rates of substrate flow in a traumatized individual excreting 40 g of nitrogen per day. Presumably reparative tissues are glucose utilizers, but the amount of glucose terminally combusted to carbon dioxide and that metabolized to lactate would depend both on the maturity of the tissue and on adequate perfusion and oxygenation. Fat still provides the bulk of the calories. (From: *Cahill GF et al, in Fox CL Jr, Nahas GG (eds): Body Fluid Replacement in the Surgical Patient, New York, Grune and Stratton, 1970, p 286, with permission.*)

being noted after sepsis and burns. Most of the energy required during the posttraumatic period is obtained from the oxidation of lipids; the net catabolism of 300 to 500 g of lean body cell mass per day is required as a source of amino acids for gluconeogenesis (Fig. 1-54). The persistence of the injury, particularly sepsis, through unknown mechanisms produces inhibition of the usual adaptive mechanisms that occur in starvation to reduce the amount of glucose needed per day. As a result, a highly catabolic state persists that in turn leads to protein wasting and malnutrition and ultimately to multiple organ failure and death if the stimuli are not eliminated.

FLUID AND ELECTROLYTE METABOLISM DURING INJURY

Almost all acute injuries are associated with changes in fluid and electrolyte metabolism, acid-base status, and renal function. In part, these alterations arise because patients do not usually have free access to water and electrolytes and frequently do not perceive thirst as a result of sedation, anesthesia, or head injury. A reduction in the effective circulating volume is characteristic of almost all injuries as a result of blood loss as in hemorrhage, loss of vascular tone as in sepsis, pump failure as in cardiac tam-

ponade, excessive unreplaced extrarenal losses as in diarrhea, vomiting, and the drainage of fistulae or from the sequestration of fluids.

The sequestration of fluids or third space is the result of an alteration in capillary permeability consequent to injury, ischemia, or inflammation. Since the fluid present in the third space has the same composition as the extracellular fluid (150 meq of sodium, 112 meq of chloride, 4.6 meq of potassium), one might think of this as an obligatory expansion of the total extracellular space. Although it is true that the total extracellular fluid space is expanded, the functional extracellular volume (that which can contribute to the maintenance of the effective circulating volume) is actually reduced because the fluid present in the third space is itself derived from the functional extracellular volume. Therefore, a liter of fluid trapped in the third space cannot be used, for example, during hemorrhage to replace the effective circulating volume lost. For this reason, the use of diuretics to mobilize fluid in an edematous postoperative patient who is not in congestive heart failure is pointless and potentially harmful, since it will result in a further reduction in the functional or exchangeable extracellular space and effective circulating volume but not in the volume of the third space. "Exchangeable" is not synonymous with "equilibrium" since the constituents of the third space are in dynamic equilibrium with those of the functional extracellular fluid volume. For example, fluid and electrolytes in a pleural effusion are in a constant state of recycling with the plasma and antibiotics administered to a patient will enter the pleural effusion. The volume of the third space cannot be used to replace the volume of the functional extracellular space.

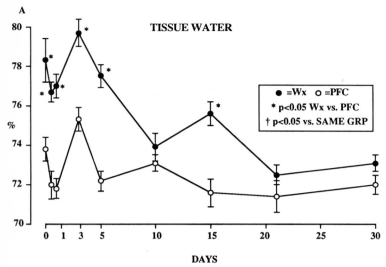

A

TISSUE WATER

● =Wx   o =PFC
* p<0.05 Wx vs. PFC
† p<0.05 vs. SAME GRP

DAYS

Fig. 1-55. The tissue water content of wounded hindlimbs was greater than that of the hindlimbs from pair-fed control animals at 0, $\frac{1}{2}$, 1, 3, 5, and 15 days. The water content of wounded hindlimbs reached its maximum on day 3 (79.7 ± 0.7 percent). It then decreased to control values at day 10, from which time no further differences were noted between the two groups after day 15. (From: *Amaral JF et al: J Trauma, in press.*)

Blalock was the first to demonstrate that traumatic injury to an extremity resulted in the mobilization of fluid and electrolytes to an area of injury, thereby reducing the functional extracellular fluid volume. As shown in Fig. 1-55, even though the formation of the third space after nonthermal traumatic injury occurs immediately and is maximal by 5 to 6 h, the resolution of the third space is slower and may take longer than 10 days. Since the volume of third space is directly proportional to the severity of injury, minor operative procedures, such as an appendectomy, are associated with considerably less fluid sequestration than are major operative procedures such as an extensive retroperitoneal dissection. Similarly, minor traumatic injuries, such as an isolated simple limb fracture, are associated with less fluid sequestration than are those seen following major injuries, such as burns. If there is no intake of fluid into the functional extracellular space by either the oral or the intravenous route, the effective circulating volume will decline to a point at which hypotension ensues.

Hypovolemic shock is also associated with a reduction in the functional extracellular fluid volume in excess of the amount lost from the body by hemorrhage or by dehydration. Shires and colleagues have demonstrated that even though the return of shed blood alone after hemorrhage results in the return of the red cell mass and blood volume to normal, a deficit in the functional extracellular fluid volume persists. This deficit can be eliminated by the return of crystalloid solutions as well as shed blood. For this reason, patients who have sustained a major blood loss should receive blood or packed cells and crystalloid during their resuscitation. The site of this third space formation appears to be the intracellular space as evidenced by a contraction of the intercellular space and an increase in the intracellular volume following hemorrhages of greater than 30 percent of the total blood volume and is thought to be the reason for the irreversible shock encountered in some patients. The mechanism for its formation remains unknown.

Major burns produce an alteration in the capillary permeability of the burned tissue that results in an exudation of plasma and an evaporative loss of water. There is also an increase in fluid flux across capillaries in nonburned tissue that appears to result from hypoproteinemia rather than an alteration in capillary permeability. The formation of edema occurs primarily in the first 24 h with the greatest losses being incurred during the first 8. It is for this reason that thermally injured patients should receive 50 percent of their estimated fluid losses in the first 8 h. Colloid should be given on the second day to minimize edema formation in the nonburned tissue.

Sepsis produces a generalized capillary leak that again produces an increase in the total extracellular fluid volume but a decrease in the functional or exchangeable extracellular fluid volume. As sepsis persists, protein malnutrition produces hypoproteinemia, which in turn may increase the formation of edema. Therefore, the administration of colloid solutions during early sepsis when a capillary leak is present in the absence of hypoproteinemia may be unadvisable, since it may serve to further increase tissue edema. Once hypoproteinemia ensues, colloid administration may theoretically be helpful.

Any traumatic injury produces rapid changes in the functional extracellular fluid volume, effective circulating volume, extracellular osmolality, and electrolyte composition that result in the stimulation of the neuroendocrine system. In turn, the neuroendocrine response induces alterations in renal and circulatory function aimed at improving salt and water balance. Ultimately, the degree of impairment in fluid and electrolyte balance incurred following injury depends in part upon the amount of functional extracellular volume lost, the ability of the neuroendocrine, renal, and circulatory systems to respond, the severity of the injury, the quality and quantity of fluid given, the age of the patient, preexistent illness, concurrent medications, and the anesthetic agents used.

Despite the potentially large number of variables noted, the overall response to the loss of effective circulating volume and electrolytes may be simplified as a coordinated physiologic effort to prevent further unnecessary losses of circulating volume and to replace the volume lost. The former involves the renal conservation of salt and water to minimize excretion and the latter the restoration of blood volume.

Renal Conservation of Salt and Water Following Injury

SODIUM REABSORPTION. The regulation of fluid and electrolytes by the kidney involves the formation of a large glomerular ultrafiltrate from which variable amounts of these substances are reabsorbed or into which they are secreted. The formation of tubular fluid at the glomerulus is dependent upon the forces described in Starling's hypothesis of capillary equilibrium (Fig. 1-56). Thus, the quantity of filtrate formed is dependent upon the renal perfusion pressure at the glomerulus. Under normal circumstances approximately 25 percent of the cardiac output is directed to the kidneys, resulting in the filtration of approximately 180 L of plasma water per day from the 1584 L of blood that pass through the kidneys. Although a reduction in the effective circulating volume and therefore in renal perfusion pressure should result in a reduction in the amount of glomerular ultrafiltrate that is formed, glomerular filtration remains unchanged despite a reduction in the renal perfusion pressure to 80 mmHg (Fig. 1-57). This occurs through the maintenance of renal blood flow, a process referred to as intrinsic autoregulation. The latter is thought to involve tubuloglomerular feedback in which individual nephrons sense their tubular fluid flow and alter the rate of glomerular filtration by changing the glomerular capillary pressure, primarily at the efferent arteriole. Decreases in tubular fluid flow lead to an increase in the efferent arteriolar resistance that, in turn, results in an increase in the fraction of peritubular blood that is filtered at the glomerulus. Thus, the rate of glomerular filtration is maintained.

An increase in the amount of blood filtered at the glomerulus relative to the amount that passes through it produces an increase in the oncotic pressure of the peritubular capillary blood perfusing the proximal tubule (Fig. 1-58). This results from the impermeability of the glomerular basement membranes to protein such that the glomerular filtrate is an ultrafiltrate of plasma. The increase in peritubular oncotic pressure, in turn, produces an increase in the net transfer of water, sodium, chloride, and bicarbonate from the proximal tubular filtrate to the peritubular blood. Sympathetic nervous system activity may directly increase the proximal tubular transport of sodium and suppress the release of cerebral natriuretic hormone and atrial natriuretic factor.

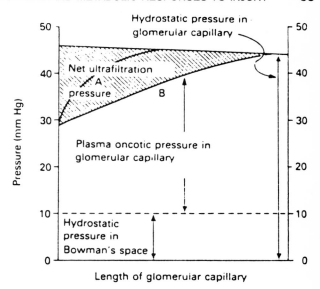

Balance of Mean Values

Hydrostatic pressure in glomerular capillary	45 mm Hg
Hydrostatic pressure in Bowman's space	10
Plasma oncotic pressure in glomerular capillary	27
Oncotic pressure of fluid in Bowman's space	0*
Net ultrafiltration pressure	8 mm Hg

Fig. 1-56. The Starling forces involved in the formation of the glomerular ultrafiltrate. Glomerular filtration pressure declines in the glomerular capillaries primarily as a result of a decrease in plasma oncotic pressure. In contrast, a decrease in the filtration pressure of extrarenal capillaries results primarily from a decrease in hydrostatic pressure. (From: *Valtin H: Renal Function: Mechanisms Preserving Fluid and Solute Balance in Health. Boston, Little, Brown, 1983, with permission.*)

Fig. 1-57. Despite a reduction in renal arterial pressure to 90 mmHg, renal blood flow and glomerular filtration rate are maintained through intrinsic autoregulation. (From: *Powers RS: In Sabiston DC (ed): Davis-Christopher Textbook of Surgery. Philadelphia, Saunders, with permission.*)

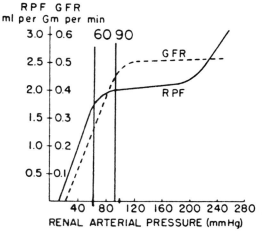

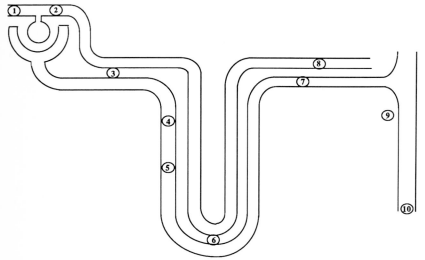

Fig. 1-58. Alterations in nephron function during injury.   1. Decreased renal perfusion pressure.   2. Increased efferent arteriolar resistance leading to a maintenance of GFR (autoregulation). 3. Increased peritubular capillary oncotic pressure from an increase in filtration of blood leads to increased proximal tubular reabsorption.   4. Shift from cortical nephrons to juxtamedullary nephrons. 5. Increased proximal reabsorption leads to decreased delivery of chloride to loop of Henle.   6. Diminished medullary gradient secondary to impaired sodium reabsorption.   7. Increased presentation of sodium to the distal tubules.   8. Increased exchange of sodium for hydrogen and potassium that is enhanced by aldosterone. 9. Increased free water reabsorption mediated by vasopressin that may be impaired by a fall in medullary osmotic gradient. 10. Kaliuesis, acid urine, and possibly loss of free water if action of vasopressin is impaired.

The net result of these alterations is that the delivery of sodium, chloride, and filtered fluid to the loop of Henle is decreased. Since the maintenance of the normal medullary osmotic gradient requires the adequate delivery of sodium and particularly of chloride to the long loops of Henle, a fall in medullary hyperosmolality frequently follows injury. A fall in medullary hyperosmolality may produce a defect in the ability of the kidneys to concentrate urine since the medullary gradient is essential to the renal countercurrent mechanism and the proper functioning of vasopressin. As a result, a larger amount of urine is necessary to eliminate the same amount of solute. This paradoxical increase in free water clearance secondary to a defect in the inner medullary interstitial solute has been termed polyuric prerenal failure and has been implicated in the genesis of nonoliguric renal failure.

Concomitant with the increase in filtration fraction, there is a redistribution of blood flow from glomeruli of the superficial cortical nephrons to those in the juxtamedullary region that further increases sodium reabsorption. The ability of the juxtamedullary nephrons to further increase sodium reabsorption is related to the much longer loops of Henle they possess when compared with those in the superficial cortical area (Fig. 1-59). The ability of the loops of Henle to reabsorb sodium is dependent on the presence of chloride, since the reabsorption of sodium in the loops of Henle passively follows the active reabsorption of chloride. The increase in the filtration fraction consequent to a reduction in the renal perfusion pressure produces an increased movement of sodium and of chloride to the peritubular fluid. As a result, the amount of chloride in the loop of Henle is low following injury and a large amount of sodium is delivered to the distal tubules. The increase in the distal delivery of sodium produces potassium wasting and metabolic alkalosis as sodium is reabsorbed and potassium and hydrogen ions secreted, a process that is augmented by the increased secretion of aldosterone that accompanies hypovolemia and injury. Conversely, if sodium delivery to the distal tubules is in-

adequate as a result of a marked decrease in glomerular filtration, potassium will not be excreted, even in the presence of aldosterone, and hyperkalemia and metabolic acidosis may ensue.

Sodium retention is a hallmark of injury that results in part from the increased secretion of corticosteroids and aldosterone. It is also clear that the larger the sodium load given to the postoperative patient the greater the amount retained. The amount of sodium retained depends more on the amount of sodium given than on the magnitude of injury. Sodium retention after injury cannot be solely explained on the basis of increased aldosterone and cortisol secretion since positive sodium balance persists well after the return of these hormones to normal concentrations (Fig. 1-60). Other factors that are known to contribute to positive sodium balance include an increase in the glomerular filtration fraction with an attendant increase in the proximal reabsorption of sodium and an increased blood flow to juxtamedullary nephrons.

ALKALOSIS. The increased delivery of sodium to the distal tubules is in part responsible for the metabolic alkalosis that commonly accompanies injury. Lyons and Moore have pointed out that the most common acid base disturbance in mild to moderately injured patients who have not deteriorated to severe renal circulatory or pulmonary decompensation is either metabolic or respira-

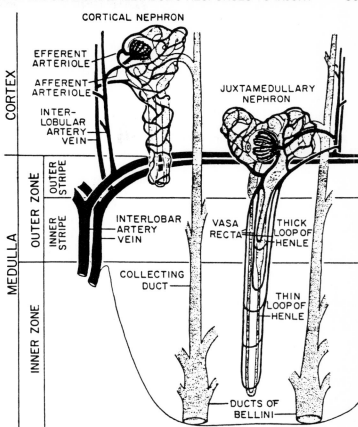

Fig. 1-59. The juxtamedullary nephrons have much longer loops of Henle than those of the cortical area. As a result they have a much longer surface area for reabsorption of sodium chloride and water. (From: *Pitts RF: Physiology of the Kidney and Body Fluids, Chicago, Yearbook Medical, 1974, with permission.*)

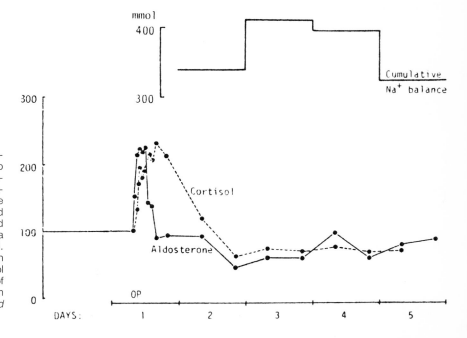

Fig. 1-60. Relationship of plasma aldosterone and plasma cortisol responses to postoperative sodium retention. The results are the median values for eight patients undergoing cholecystectomy at the start of day 1. All patients were in Na+ and K+ balance at the time of operation and the hormone changes are expressed as a percentage of the basal preoperative level. Intravenous intake was 259 mmol Na+ on day 2, and 152 mmol Na+ and 80 mmol K+ on days 3 to 5, with a total of 3 L of water on each day. The periods run from 0800 h. (From: *LeQuesne LP et al: Br Med Bull 1985, with permission.*)

tory alkalosis. In their study, 64 percent of the 105 patients who were operated on developed alkalosis on at least one determination in the postoperative period. It is important to prevent severe alkalosis in the surgical patient because of its potential hazards. These include the production of tissue hypoxia through the effect of alkalosis on the oxygen-hemoglobin dissociation curve, hypokalemia, and alterations in vasomotor tone such as the cerebral vasoconstriction seen with respiratory alkalosis.

ACIDOSIS. The most common acid base disturbance in severely injured patients or those who deteriorated to severe renal circulatory or pulmonary decompensation is either metabolic or respiratory alkalosis. Foremost among the etiologies for acidosis for following injury is shock. The metabolic acidosis that ensues is the result of tissue hypoperfusion and anaerobic metabolism and not the cause of it. Metabolic acidosis may also ensue in patients who have a respiratory alkalosis if hypoventilation suddenly occurs, since the rise in blood lactate that accompanies respiratory alkalosis will be unbuffered. Acidosis has profound effects on the cardiovascular system, producing a decrease in myocardial contractility, a decreased response of the myocardium and peripheral vasculature to catecholamines, and a predisposition to cardiac arrhythmias.

WATER REABSORPTION. Injury and hypotension are also characterized by an increase in water reabsorption. In part, this is related to the increase in sodium reabsorption since the reabsorption of sodium is associated with the passive reabsorption of water. The increase in water reabsorption is also the result of the stimulation of vasopressin secretion during hypotension and injury by osmotic and nonosmotic (baroreceptor) pathways. The increase in plasma vasopressin usually lasts for 3 to 5 days after injury. Under most circumstances it results in water retention and in oliguria unless specific steps are taken to prevent it. Postoperative oliguria was originally believed to be a normal accompaniment of injury that did no particular harm. Although it is certainly well tolerated in most forms of mild to moderate surgical trauma, it is a potentially harmful condition in two ways: the first is that it predisposes to acute tubular necrosis in patients with severe trauma in whom hypovolemia and hypotension are apt to occur, and the second is that it sets the stage for the development of water intoxication (severe hyponatremia) if large volumes of non-solute-containing fluids are given to the patient before, during, or immediately after the operative event. The most common electrolyte abnormality seen following surgery and injury is hyponatremia as a result of the administration of hypotonic fluids under conditions that favor salt and water retention.

The action of vasopressin in effecting water retention requires the presence of an intact countercurrent mechanism in the loop of Henle. If the countercurrent mechanism is disrupted by a fall in medullary osmolality, the action of vasopressin is impaired, resulting in a defect in urinary concentrating ability. Consequently, a normal or increased urine output in a hypotensive or injured patient does not necessarily reflect an adequate blood volume. In order to prevent a fall in the medullary gradient following

injury, adequate tubular fluid flow must be ensured and maximal sodium reabsorption in the proximal nephron must be avoided. This is accomplished by the administration of liberal amounts of salt solutions such as Ringer's lactate or normal saline in the postoperative period. The administration of the solutions may result in marked positive sodium and solute balance and in edema as noted previously. During this period of increased vasopressin secretion the urine volume cannot be increased by the administration of water alone. It is the solute load that determines urine volume, and free water clearance will occur only when the extracellular fluid space has been expanded (Fig. 1-61). By increasing the solute load and the extracellular fluid volume, the urine output can be maintained. Although this may result in a "puffy" patient postoperatively, it will maximize the protection of renal function. The effectiveness of treatment can be monitored by the maintenance of urine output at a rate of 30 mL/h or greater.

The return of vasopressin secretion to normal is signaled by the brisk diuresis of free water and resolution of tissue edema that is usually seen in most surgical patients on the third to fifth postoperative days. This is the so-called fluid mobilization phase of injury. This period may take considerably longer in the presence of pain, hypoxia, or other stimuli to vasopressin secretion. The presence of a diminished urine output and hyponatremia several days after injury is not necessarily related to the inappropriate secretion of vasopressin. The diagnosis of inappropriate secretion of vasopressin cannot be established until all possible stimuli to the secretion of vasopressin have been ruled out.

POSTOPERATIVE PATTERNS. The two patterns most commonly seen in the postoperative period are illustrated in Figs. 1-62 and 1-63. The first is that of a mild to moderate dilutional hyponatremia with hyperkalemia. This is primarily brought about by the secretion of vasopressin plus the overhydration of the patient with non-solute-containing fluids. The potassium level may be somewhat elevated, because potassium is lost from cells as a consequence of corticosteroid and starvation-induced catabolism, is infused in the form of high-potassium-containing old blood, is absorbed from blood left in the peritoneal cavity or wound, and is not well excreted because of impaired renal perfusion.

The hyponatremia and hyperkalemia are made much worse if the trauma is severe and prolonged or if the patient has had a chronic wasting illness prior to operation. Other factors that can make the response worse include starvation, which as previously noted can itself produce hyponatremia through natriuresis, preexisting renal impairment, which predisposes to a further elevation of potassium level and depression of sodium level, cardiac disease with edema, preexisting hyponatremia, a pronounced shift of sodium into the cell with severe trauma, and episodes of hypotension, which further impair renal function. Consequently, cardiac patients may still need sodium replacement postoperatively, even though they may have an elevated total body sodium and total body water.

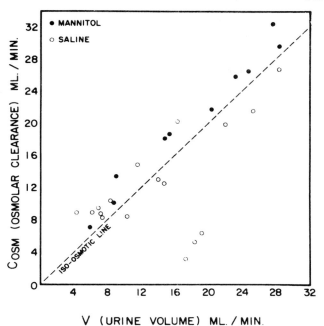

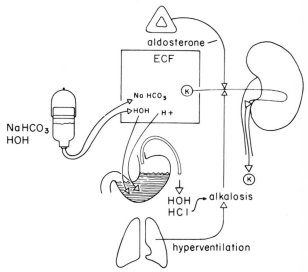

Fig. 1-61. Postoperative patients failed to excrete a water load when given 5 percent dextrose in water. These patients were then given either saline or mannitol. As shown, patients with high urine flow rates given saline were able to excrete free water whereas those with mannitol did not. This suggests that acute expansion of ECF volume in postoperative patients leads to suppression of the high antidiuretic hormone activity normally seen during this period, and thus to excretion of hypotonic urine. (From: *Wright HK, Gann DS: Ann Surg 158:70, 1963, with permission.*)

Fig. 1-62. Pattern of hyponatremia in the postoperative patient. Solute is diluted principally by excessive administration of water without salt. In addition, in severe trauma sodium will move into cells in exchange for potassium. The hyperkalemia may be further aggravated by acidosis, by the action of cortisol, and by the breakdown of blood and may be opposed by the action of aldosterone.

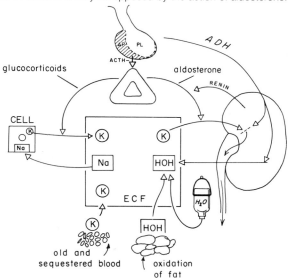

Fig. 1-63. Pattern of hypokalemic alkalosis in the postoperative patient. This is most commonly seen in patients who are alkalotic at the time of operation. The alkalosis produces an additional potassium loss in the urine. Hyperventilation increases the alkalosis and promotes further potassium loss. The administration of sodium bicarbonate, sometimes given in circumstances that are thought likely to be the result of acidosis, may further augment the alkalosis. These events then conspire to produce a severe hypokalemic alkalosis that, if renal function is good, may be made worse by the action of aldosterone in promoting potassium excretion.

These changes can be prevented or minimized by the use of sodium chloride–containing solutions in the preoperative, intraoperative, and postoperative periods and by the replacement of third space losses with normal saline. Potassium administration should be avoided unless the patient has unusual potassium losses or a declining serum potassium concentration.

The second pattern is one of hypokalemic alkalosis, classically seen in the patient with obstructing duodenal ulcer on continuous nasogastric suction or in the infant with hypertrophic pyloric stenosis with protracted vomiting. The alkalosis created by the loss of hydrogen ion from the stomach and the dehydration produced by the loss of water produces marked potassium losses in the urine since sodium reabsorption in the distal tubule must occur primarily in exchange for potassium rather than bicarbonate. The large quantities of chloride lost in the gastric juice limit the ability of the kidney to proximally reabsorb sodium. As a result, a large amount of sodium is delivered to the distal tubules for reabsorption there. Because of the large amount of sodium presented to the distal tubules and the increased secretion of aldosterone, patients with this condition usually have a paradoxically acidic urine from the exchange of hydrogen ion for sodium.

This condition is made worse by starvation, the intravenous administration of non-chloride- and non-potassium-containing solutions, the administration of proximal or loop diuretics, the administration of corticosteroids, the presence of diarrhea or a fistula, hyperventilation al-

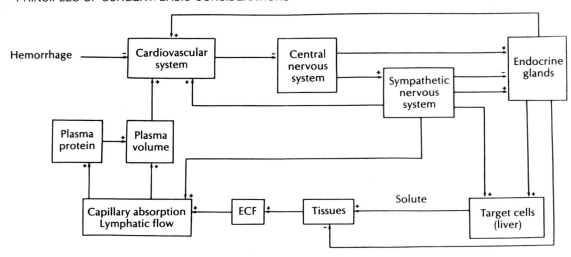

Fig. 1-64. Schematic representation of the restitution of blood volume. [From: *Gann DS, Amaral JF: The pathophysiology of trauma and shock, in Zuidema GD et al (eds). The Management of Trauma. Philadelphia, Saunders, 1985, with permission.*]

kalosis, the preexistence of hypokalemia, or the administration of sodium bicarbonate. These changes can be eliminated by the administration of potassium chloride. Chloride is the most important of these two electrolytes, since without chloride the delivery of sodium to the distal tubules will remain increased and potassium and bicarbonate will be continued to be wasted.

Blood Volume Restitution

Despite the renal conservation of salt and water following injury, an increase in the functional extracellular fluid volume cannot occur even in the complete absence of renal excretion. In order for the functional extracellular fluid volume and effective circulating volume to return to normal following injury, the blood volume must be restored.

The restitution of blood volume can be brought about by exogenous or endogenous fluids. The exogenous restitution of blood volume involves the administration of fluids. These fluids may be given intravenously, in which case the increase in blood volume is direct or they may be given orally, in which case the increase in blood volume is indirectly mediated through intestinal absorption. The endogenous restitution of blood volume involves the movement of fluids present in the interstitial fluid and in cells to the effective circulating volume. This process may be thought of as occurring in two overlapping phases: the first involves the movement of essentially protein-free fluid from the interstitium to the plasma and the second involves the restitution of plasma protein which in turn mediates the movement of additional fluid from the interstitium to the vascular space (Fig. 1-64).

A fall in capillary pressure mediates the net movement of protein-free fluid from the interstitium to the vascular space. The decrease in capillary pressure is initiated by hypotension and augmented by reflex sympathetic vasoconstriction. As capillary hydrostatic pressure decreases, the steady-state flux of fluid described in Starling's hypothesis of capillary equilibrium is changed. This results in the net movement of fluid into the capillary bed and in the restoration of approximately 20 to 50 percent of the blood volume lost. Because this fluid is protein-free, interstitial colloid oncotic pressure and interstitial hydrostatic pressure also decrease, resulting in the establishment of a new steady state in which further net movement of fluid into the vascular space cannot occur.

The further movement of fluid and ultimately the complete restitution of blood volume depends upon the movement of protein from the interstitium to the vascular space. The resultant increase in capillary oncotic pressure and decrease in interstitial oncotic pressure, in turn, mediates a shift of fluid from cells via the interstitial space to the capillary bed. The protein involved in this process is primarily in the form of albumin. This albumin must derive from the interstitium itself, since the restitution of blood volume is complete by 24 h, whereas albumin synthesis takes at least 48 h. The movement of albumin and protein from the interstitium to the capillary space may occur through either the lymphatics or the fenestrae of the capillary membrane. In order for either to be effective, interstitial pressure must increase. The latter can be accomplished through an increase in interstitial volume, since the compliance of the interstitium is fixed. The increase in interstitial volume cannot be derived from the plasma volume since it is already decreased. Water will

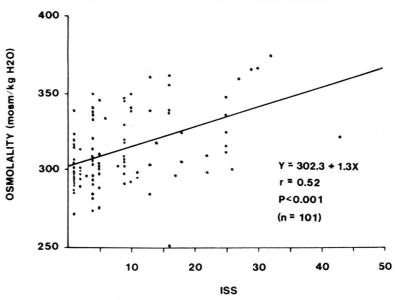

Fig. 1-65. There is a positive correlation between the plasma osmolality and the injury severity score in multiply injured patients. (From: *Kenney PR et al: J Trauma 23:712, 1983, with permission.*)

move out of cells only down an osmotic gradient. Thus, an osmotic gradient between the intracellular and the extracellular space must exist in order for the interstitial volume to increase.

The movement of water from cells to the interstitium appears to be mediated by a hormonally induced increase in extracellular osmolality that was first described by Bergentz and Brief in experimental animals and later confirmed in human beings by Boyd and Mansberger. The increase in serum osmolality occurs promptly after hemorrhage and correlates with the rate and degree of hemorrhage and the severity of the injury (Fig. 1-65). An increase in cortisol is necessary but not sufficient to produce the increase in osmolality. An adrenal factor (probably catecholamines), a pituitary factor (probably vasopressin), and glucagon are required. The solutes, which are derived primarily from the liver, include glucose, phosphate, lactate, and pyruvate. Since these molecules are permeable to the capillary membrane but relatively impermeable to cell membranes, an osmotic gradient is established between interstitium and cells that moves fluid from the cells to the interstitium. In turn, the increase in interstitial volume results in an increase in interstitial pressure, thereby allowing protein to move through the capillary membrane and the lymphatics. The rise in osmolality also appears to contribute to the phase of transcapillary refill, since the increase in interstitial pressure requires the movement of water to the vascular space in order for the equilibrium between the interstitium and capillaries to be maintained.

Nutritional status plays an important role in the hyperosmolality seen after hemorrhage. Fasted animals exhibit a lower degree of hyperglycemia and a slower rise in plasma osmolality than fed animals. As a result, the capacity for blood volume restitution is greater in animals who are fed than in those who are fasted. This difference presumably results from the depletion of hepatic glycogen stores during fasting since the difference can be eliminated by the administration of hyperosmolar glucose to the fasted animals.

One would predict that the higher the serum glucose the more favorable the response. This is in marked contrast to the studies of combat victims by Carey et al. in which a high glucose concentration was associated with a high mortality. It is important to recognize that the changes described result from an increase in the production of solute by the liver and its subsequent delivery to the interstitium bathing skeletal muscle. Given the same increase in solute production, changes in plasma solute concentrations will be smaller if muscle perfusion is adequate than if it is decreased by intense vasoconstriction. A very high increase in the serum glucose may be the result of inadequate tissue perfusion rather than an accelerated rate of glucose production. In this setting, restitution would be significantly impaired and an increase in mortality would be expected. Although the second phase of restitution is present during all hemorrhages, the restitution in very large hemorrhages (>25 percent of the total blood volume) is no greater than that seen in small hemorrhages of 10 percent. This finding correlates with the appearance of a decrease in transmembrane potential, cell swelling, and eventually cell death.

Bibliography

NEUROENDOCRINE REFLEXES
Stimuli, Integration, and Modulation
Achtel RA, Downing SE: Ventricular responses to hypoxemia following chemoreceptor denervation and adrenalectomy. *Am Heart J* 84:377, 1972.

Baertschi AJ, Ward DG, Gann DS: Role of atrial receptors in the control of ACTH. *Am J Physiol* 231:692, 1976.

Bereiter DA, Plotsky PM, Gann DS: Tooth pulp stimulation potentiates the ACTH response to hemorrhage in cats. *Endocrinology* 111:1127, 1982.

Bereiter DA, Zaid AM, Gann DS: Adrenocorticotropin response to graded blood loss in the cat. *Am J Physiol* 247:E398, 1984.

Bereiter DA, Zaid AM, Gann DS: The effect of rate of hemorrhage on sympathoadrenal catecholamine release in the cat. *Am J Physiol* 250:E69, 1985.

Bereiter DA, Gann DS: Caudolateral areas of medulla-mediating release of ACTH in cats. *Am J Physiol* 251:R934, 1986.

Blessing WW: Central neurotransmitter pathways for baroreceptor-initiated secretion of vasopressin. *NIPS* 1:90, 1986.

Brown AM: Receptors under pressure: an update on baroreceptors. *Circ Res* 46:1, 1980.

Claybaugh JR, Share L: Vasopressin, renin, and cardiovascular responses to continuous slow hemorrhage. *Am J Physiol* 224:519, 1973.

Egdahl RH: Pituitary-adrenal response following trauma to the isolated leg. *Surgery* 46:9, 1959.

Egdahl RH: The differential response of the adrenal cortex and medulla to bacterial endotoxin. *J Clin Invest* 38:1120, 1959.

Egdahl RH, Nelson DH, Hume DM: Adrenal cortical function in hypothermia. *Surg Gynecol Obstet* 101:15, 1955.

Engeland WC, Byrnes GJ, Gann DS: The pituitary adrenocortical response to hemorrhage depends on the time of day. *Endocrinology* 110:1856, 1982.

Gann DS, Cryer GL, Pirkle JC Jr: Physiological inhibition and facilitation of adrenocortical response to hemorrhage. *Am J Physiol* 232:R5, 1977.

Gann DS, Dallman MF, Engeland WC: Reflex control and modulation of ACTH and corticosteroids, in McCann SM (ed): *Endocrine Physiology,* III International Review of Physiology. University Park Press, Baltimore, 1981, vol 24, pp 157–199.

Gann DS, Berieter DA, et al: Neural interaction in control of adrenocorticotropin. *Fed Proc* 44:161, 1985.

Goldman WF, Saum WR: A direct excitatory action of catecholamines on rat aotic baroreceptors in vitro. *Circ Res* 55:18, 1984.

Grizzle WE, Dallman MF, et al: Inhibitory and facilitatory hypothalamic areas mediating ACTH release in the cat. *Endocrinology* 95:1450, 1974.

Hensel H: Neural processes in thermoregulation. *Physiol Rev* 53:948, 1973.

Heymans C, Neil E: *Reflexogenic Areas of the Cardiovascular System.* Boston, Little, Brown and Company, 1958.

Holmes AE, Ledsome JR: Effect of norepinephrine and vasopressin on carotid sinus baroreceptor activity in the anesthetized rabbit. *Experentia* 40:825, 1984.

Hume DM, Egdahl RH: The importance of the brain in the neuroendocrine response to injury. *Ann Surg* 150:697, 1959.

Hume DM, Egdahl RH: Effect of hypothermia and of cold exposure on adrenal cortical and medullary secretion. *Ann NY Acad Sci* 80:435, 1959.

Hume DM, Bell CL, Bartter FC: Direct measurement of adrenal secretion during operative trauma and convalescence. *Surgery* 52:174, 1962.

Kircheim HR: Systemic arterial baroreceptor reflexes. *Physiol Rev* 56:100, 1976.

Korner PI: Integrative neural cardiovascular control. *Physiol Rev* 51:312, 1971.

Lambertson CJ: Neural control of respiration, in Mountcastle, VB (ed): *Medical Physiology.* St Louis, Mosby, 1980, 114th ed, p 1749.

Lefcort AM, Ward DG, Gann SD: Electrolytic lesions of the dorsal rostral pons prevents adrenocorticotropin increases after hemorrhage. *Endocrinology* 114:2148, 1984.

Lilly MP, Engeland WC, Gann DS: Adrenomedullary responses to repeated hemorrhage in the anesthetized dog. *Endocrinology* 111:1917, 1982.

Lilly MP, Engeland WC, Gann DS: Responses of cortisol secretion to repeated hemorrhage in the anesthetized dog. *Endocrinology* 112:681, 1983.

Longnecker DE, McCoy S, Drucker WR: Anesthetic influence on response to hemorrhage in rats. *Circ Shock* 6:55, 1979.

O'Berg B, White S: Circulatory effects of interruption and stimulation of cardiac vagal afferents. *Acta Physiol Scand* 80:383, 1970.

Overman RR, Wang SG: The contributory role of the afferent nervous factor in experimental shock: sublethal hemorrhage and sciatic nerve stimulation. *Am J Physiol* 148:289, 1947.

Quest JA, Gebber GL: Modulation of baroreceptor reflexes by somatic afferent nerve stimulation. *Am J Physiol* 222:1251, 1972.

Raff H, Shinsako J, Dallman MF: Surgery potentiates adrenocortical responses to hypoxia in dogs. *Proc Soc Exp Bio Med* 172:400, 1983.

Redding M, Mueller CB: Effect of ambient temperature upon responses to hypovolemic insult in the unanesthetized unrestrained albino rat. *Surgery* 64:110, 1968.

Sato A, Schmidt RF: Somatosympathetic reflexes: Afferent fibers, central pathways, discharge characteristics. *Physiol Rev* 53:916, 1973.

Wigger CJ: *Physiology of Shock.* New York, Commonwealth Fund, 1950.

Wood CE, Shinsako J, et al: Hormonal and hemodynamic responses to 15mL/kg hemorrhage in conscious dogs: Responses correlate to body temperature. *Proc Soc Exp Biol Med* 167:15, 1981.

Zimpfer M, Manders WT, et al: Pentobarbital alters compensatory neural and humoral mechanisms in response to hemorrhage. *Am J Physiol* 243:H713, 1982.

Mechanism of Hormone Action

Ali M, Vedeckis WV: The glucocorticoid receptor protein binds to transfer RNA. *Science* 235:467, 1987.

Cheung WY: Calmodulin. *Sci Am* 7:62, 1982.

Compton MM, Cidlowski JA: Vitamin B6 and glucocorticoid action. *Endocr Rev* 7:140, 1986.

Fain JN: Involvement of phosphatidylinositol breakdown in elevation of cytosol Ca^{++} by hormones and relationship to prostaglandin formation, in Kohn LD (ed): *Hormone Receptors.* New York, Wiley, 1982, vol 6, p 237.

Fain JN, Garcia-Sainz JA: Adrenergic regulation of adipocyte metabolism. *J Lipid Res* 24:945, 1983.

Farese RV: Phosphoinositide metabolism and hormone action. *Endocr Rev* 4:78, 1983.

Greengard P: Phosphorylated proteins as physiological effectors. *Science* 199:146, 1978.

Jensen EV: Interaction of steroid hormones with the nucleus. *Pharmacol Rev* 30:477, 1979.

Means AR, Lagace L, et al: Calmodulin as a mediator of hormone action and cell regulation. *J Cell Biochem* 20:317, 1982.

Motulsky JJ, Insel PA: Adrenergic receptors in man: Direct identification, physiologic regulations and clinical alterations. *N Engl J Med* 307:18, 1982.

Muldoon TG: Regulation of steroid hormone receptor activity. *Endocr Rev* 1:339, 1980.

O'Malley BW, Schrader WT: The receptors of steroid hormones. *Sci Am* 234:32, 1976.

Oppenheimer JH: Thyroid hormone action at the cellular level. *Science* 203:97, 1979.

Rassmusen H: *Calcium and C-amp as Synarchic Messengers.* New York, Wiley Intersciences, 1981.

Spiegel AM, Gierschik P, et al: Clinical implications of guanine nucleotide binding proteins as receptor effector couplers. *N Engl J Med* 312:26, 1985.

Sterling K: Thyroid hormone action at the cell level. *N Engl J Med* 300:117, 173, 1979.

Endocrine Effectors

Aasen AO, Smith-Erichsen N, Amundsen E: Plasma kallikrein-kinnin system in septicemia. *Arch Surg* 118:343, 1983.

Aguilera G, Mendelsohn AO, Catt KJ: Dopaminergic regulation of aldosterone secretion, in Martini L, Ganong WF: *Frontiers in Neuroendocrinology.* New York, Raven, 1984, p 265.

Amir S, Berstein M: Endogeneous opiates interact in stress-induced hyperglycemia in mice. *Physiol Behav* 28:575, 1982.

Aono T et al: Influence of surgical stress under general anesthesia on serum gonadotropin levels. *J Clin Endocrinol Metab* 42:144, 1976.

Aun F, Medeiros-Neto GA, et al: The effect of major trauma on the pathways of thyroid hormone metabolism. *J Trauma* 23:104, 1983.

Averill DB, Scher AM, Feigl ED: Angiotensin causes vasoconstriction during hemorrhage in baroreceptor-denervated dogs. *Am J Physiol* 245:H667, 1983.

Baer PG, McGiff JC: Hormonal systems and renal hemodynamics. *Annu Rev Physiol* 42:589, 1980.

Barakos V, Rodemann HP, et al: Stimulation of muscle protein degradation and prostaglandin E2 release by leukocyte pyrogen (interleukin-1). *N Engl J Med* 308:553, 1983.

Barton RN: Neuroendocrine mobilization of body fuels after injury. *Br Med Bull* 41:218, 1985.

Bauer WE, Vigar SNM, et al: Insulin response during hypovolemic shock. *Surgery* 66:80, 1969.

Baylis PH, Zepre RL, Robertson GL: Arginine vasopressin response to insulin-induced hypoglycemia in man. *J Clin Endocrinol Metab* 53:935, 1981.

Becker RA, Wilmore DW, et al: Free T4, free T3 and reverse T3 in critically ill, terminally injured patients. *J Trauma* 20:713, 1980.

Benedict CR, Grahame-Smith DG: Plasma noradrenaline and adrenaline concentrations and dopamine-B-hydroxylase activity in patients with shock due to septicaemia, trauma and hemorrhage. *Q J Med* 47:1, 1978.

Bernton EW, Long JB, Holaday JW: Opioids and neuropeptides; mechanisms in circulatory shock. *Fed Proc* 44:290, 1985.

Berry HE, Collier JG, Vane JR: The generation of kinins in the blood of dogs during hypotension due to hemorrhage. *Clin Sci* 39:349, 1970.

Besedovsky H, DelRey A, et al: Immunoregulatory feedback between interleukin-1 and glucocorticoid hormones. *Science* 233:652, 1986.

Beutler B, Cerami A: Cachectin and tumour necrosis factor as two sides of the same biological coin. *Nature* 320:584, 1986.

Bie P: Osmoreceptors, vasopressin and control of renal water excretion. *Physiol Rev* 60:961, 1980.

Bonnet F, Harari A, et al: Suppression of antidiuretic hormone hypersecretion during surgery by extradural anaesthesia. *Br J Anesth* 54:30, 1982.

Brizio-Molteni L, Molteni A, et al: Prolactin, corticotropin and gonadotropin concentrations following thermal injury in adults. *J Trauma* 24:1, 1984.

Buckingham J: Hypothalamic-pituitary responses to trauma. *Br Med Bull* 41:203, 1985.

Caldwell MD, Lacy WW, Exton JH: Effects of adrenalectomy on the amino acid and glucose metabolism of perfused rat hindlimbs. *J Biol Chem* 253:6837, 1978.

Carey LC, Cloutier CT, Lowery BD: Growth hormone and adrenal cortisol response to shock and trauma in the human. *Ann Surg* 174, 1971.

Carey LC, Lowery BD, Cloutier CT: Blood sugar and insulin response in human shock. *Ann Surg* 172:342, 1970.

Carey RM, Sen S: Aldosterone-stimulating factor: a new aldosterone secretagogue, in Ganong WF, Martini L: *Frontiers in Neuroendocrinology.* New York, Raven, 1986, p 191.

Caromona RH, Tsao RC, Trunkey DD: The role of prostacyclin and thromboxane in sepsis and septic shock. *Arch Surg* 119:189, 1984.

Carretero OA, Scicli AG: The renal kallikrein-kinin system, in Dunn MJ (ed): *Renal Endocrinology.* Baltimore, Williams and Wilkins, 1983, p 96.

Carstensen H, et al: Testosterone, luteinizing hormone and growth hormone in blood following surgical trauma. *Acta Chir Scand* 138:1, 1972.

Cavalieri RR, Rappooport B: Impaired peripheral conversion of thyroxine to triiodothyronine. *Ann Rev Med* 28:57, 1977.

Chaisson JL, Shikama H, et al: Inhibitory effect of epinephrine on insulin-stimulated glucose uptake by rat skeletal muscle. *J Clin Invest* 68:706, 1981.

Chan TM: The permissive effects of glucocorticoids on hepatic gluconeogenesis. *J Biol Chem* 259:7426, 1984.

Charters AC, O'Dell MWD, Thompson JC: Anterior pituitary function during surgical stress and convalescence. *J Clin Endocrinol Metab* 29:63, 1969.

Clowes GHA, George BC, et al: Muscle proteolysis induced by a circulating peptide in patients with sepsis or trauma. *N Engl J Med* 308:545–552, 1983.

Cochrane JPS, Forsling ML, et al: Arginine vasopressin release following surgical operations. *Br J Surg* 68:209, 1981.

Cooper CE, Nelson DH: ACTH levels in plasma in preoperative and surgically stressed patients. *J Clin Invest* 41:1599, 1962.

Cowley AW, Quitlen EW, Skelton MM: Role of vasopressin in cardiovascular regulation. *Fed Proc* 42:3170, 1983.

Cox BM, Baizman ER: Physiological functions of endorphins, in Malick JB, Bell RMS (eds): *Endorphins: Chemistry, Physiology, Pharmacology and Clinical Relevance.* New York, Marcel Dekker, 1982, p 116.

Cryer, PE: Physiology and pathophysiology of the human sympathoadrenal neuroendocrine system. *N Engl J Med* 303:436, 1980.

Cryer PE: Diseases of the adrenal medulla and sympathetic nervous system, in Felig P, Baxter JD, Broadus AE, Frohman LA (eds): *Endocrinology and Metabolism,* 2d ed. New York, McGraw-Hill, 1987, p 651.

Curtis T, Lefer A: Protective actions of naloxone in hemorrhagic shock. *Am J Physiol* 239:H416, 1980.

Daughaday WH: The adenohypophysis, in Williams RH: *Textbook of Endocrinology*. Philadelphia, Saunders, 1981, p 73.

Davies CL, Newman RJ, et al: The relationship between plasma catecholamines and severity of injury in man. *J Trauma* 24:99, 1984.

Dinarello CA: Interleukin-1 and the pathogenesis of the acute phase response. *N Engl J Med* 311:1413, 1984.

Edelman IS, Ismail-Beigi F: Thyroid thermogenesis and active sodium transport. *Rec Prog Horm Res* 30:235, 1974.

Eigler N, Sacca L, Sherwin RS: Synergistic interactions of physiologic increments of glucagon, epinephrine and cortisol in the dog. *J Clin Invest* 63:114, 1979.

Emerson TW: Participation of endogenous vasoactive agents in the pathogenesis of endotoxic shock. *Adv Exp Med Biol* 23:25, 1974.

Engeland WC, Demsher DP, et al: The adrenal medullary response to graded hemorrhage in awake dogs. *Endocrinology* 109:1539, 1981.

Engeland WC, Bereiter DF, Gann DS: Sympathetic control of adrenal secretion after hemorrhage in awake dogs. *Am J Physiol* 251:R341, 1986.

Engels FL, Fredricks J: Contribution to understanding of mechanism of permissive action of corticoids. *Proc Soc Exp Biol Med* 95:593, 1957.

Fater DC, Sundet WD, et al: Arterial baroreceptors have minimal physiological effects on adrenal medullary secretion. *Am J Physiol* 244:H194, 1983.

Feldman M, Kiser RS, et al: Beta-endorphin and the endocrine pancreas. *N Engl J Med* 308:350, 1983.

Felig P: The endocrine pancreas: Diabetes mellitus, in Felig P, Baxter JD, Broadus AE, Frohman LA (eds): *Endocrinology and Metabolism,* 2d ed. New York, McGraw-Hill, 1987, p 1043.

Felig P, Sherwin RS, et al: Hormonal interactions in the regulation of blood glucose. *Recent Prog Horm Res* 35:501, 1979.

Fletcher JR, Ramwell PW, Herman CW: Prostaglandins and the hemodynamic course of endotoxin shock. *J Surg Res* 20:589, 1976.

Fletcher JR, Short BL, et al: Prostaglandins as mediators of the hemodynamic abnormalities in endotoxemia and sepsis, in McConn R (ed): *Role of Chemical Mediators in the Pathophysiology of Acute Illness and Injury*. New York, Raven, 1982.

Franchimont P: The regulation of follicle stimulating hormone and lutenizing hormone secretion in humans, in Martini L, Ganong WF (eds): *Frontiers in Neuroendocrinology*. New York, Oxford University Press, 1971, p 3331.

Fray JCS, Lush DJ, Valentine AND: Cellular mechanisms of renin secretion. *Fed Proc* 3250, 1983.

Frayn KN, Prete DA, et al: Plasma somatomedin activity after injury in man and its relationship to other hormonal and metabolic changes. *Clin Endocrinol* 20:179, 1984.

Frayn KN, Little RA, et al: The relationship of plasma catecholamines to acute metabolic and hormonal responses to injury in man. *Circ Shock* 16:229, 1985.

Frohman LA: CNS peptides and glucoregulation. *Annu Rev Physiol* 45:95, 1983.

Gann DS, Amaral JF: The pathophysiological response to injury, in Zuidema G, Rutherford R, Ballinger WF: *The Management of Trauma*. Philadelphia, Saunders, 1985, pp 35–100.

Gerich JE, Charles MA, et al: Regulation of pancreatic insulin and glucagon secretion. *Ann Rev Physiol* 38:353, 1976.

Goetel EJ: Leukocyte recognition and metabolism of leukotrienes. *Fed Proc* 42:3128, 1983.

Guillmen R, Vargo T, et al: B-Endorphin and adrenocorticotropin are secreted concomitantly by the pituitary gland. *Science* 197:1367, 1977.

Haberich FJ: Osmoreception in the portal circulation. *Fed Proc* 27:1137, 1968.

Haberland GL: The role of kininogenases, kinin formation and kininogenase inhibition in post traumatic shock and related conditions. *Klin Nochenschr* 56:325, 1978.

Halmagyi DFJ, Gillet DJ, et al: Blood glucose and serum insulin in reversible and irreversible post hemorrhagic shock. *J Trauma* 6:623, 1966.

Halmagyi DFJ, Neering IR, et al: Plasma glucagon in experimental posthemorrhagic shock. *J Trauma* 9:320–326, 1969.

Hammarstrom S: Leukotrienes. *Annu Rev Biochem* 52:355, 1983.

Handlers JS, Orloff J: Antidiuretic hormone. *Annu Rev Physiol* 43:611, 1981.

Hass M, Glick SM: Radioimmunoassayable plasma vasopressin associated with surgery. *Arch Surg* 113:597, 1978.

Hiebert JM, Kieler E, et al: Species differences in insulin secretion responses during hemorrhagic shock. *Surgery* 79:451, 1976.

Holaday JW, Black LE, Long JB: Neuropeptides in shock and trauma, in Gelhoed GW, Chernow B (eds): *Endocrine Aspects of Acute Illness*. Churchill Livingstone, 1985, p 257.

Hollt V: Multiple endogenous opioid peptides. *Trends Neurosci* 6:24, 1983.

Ingenbleck Y: Thyroid function in non-thyroid illness, in DeVisscher M (ed): *The Thyroid Gland*. New York, Raven, 1980.

Ippe E, Dobbs R, Unger RH: Morphine and beta endorphin influence the secretion of the endocrine pancreas. *Nature* 276:190, 1978.

Jackson I: Thyrotropin-releasing hormone. *N Engl J Med* 306:245, 1982.

Kampschmidt RF: Leukocytic endogenous mediator. *J Reticuloendothel Soc* 23:287, 1978.

Kaplan AP: Hageman factor-dependent pathways: mechanisms of initiation and bradykinin formation. *Fed Proc* 42:3123, 1983.

Kendler KS, Weitzman RE, Fisher DA: The effect of pain on plasma arginine vasopressin concentrations in man. *Clin Endocrinol* 8:89, 1978.

Kraus-Friedmann N: Hormonal regulation of hepatic gluconeogenesis. *Physiol Rev* 51:312, 1984.

Landgraf R, Landgraf-Leurs MMC: Prolactin: a diabetogenic hormone. *Diabetologia* 13:99, 1977.

Lang RE, Bruckner UB, et al: Effect of hemorrhagic shock on the concomitant release of endorphin and enkephalin like peptides from the pituitary and adrenal gland in the dog, in Costa E, Trabucchi R (eds): *Regulatory Peptides: From Molecular Biology to Function*. New York, Raven, 1982.

Larsen PR: Thyroid-pituitary interaction. *N Engl J Med* 23:32, 1982.

Lautt WW, Dwan PD, Singh RR: Control of the hyperglycemic response to hemorrhage in cats. *Can J Physiol Pharmacol* 60:1630, 1982.

Lautt WW, Martens ES, Legare: Insulin and glucagon response during hemorrhage induced hyperglycemia. *Can J Physiol Pharmacol* 60:1624, 1982.

Lee JB: The prostaglandins, in Williams RH (ed): *Textbook of Endocrinology*. Philadelphia, Saunders, 1981, p 1047.

Lefer AM: Eicosanoids as mediators of ischemia and shock. *Fed Proc* 44:275, 1985.

Levinsky NG: The renal kallikrein-kinin system. *Circ Res* 44:441, 1978.

McIntosh TK, Faden AI: Thyrotropin-releasing hormone and circulatory shock. *Circ Shock* 18:241, 1986.

McLeod MK, Carlson DE, Gann DS: Hormonal responses associated with early hyperglycemia after graded hemorrhage in dogs. *Am J Physiol* 251:E597, 1986.

Markley K, Horakova Z, et al: The role of histamine in burn, tourniquet and endotoxic shock in mice. *Eur J Pharmacol* 33:255, 1975.

Meguid MM, Brennan MF, et al: Hormone-substrate interrelationships following trauma. *Arch Surg* 109:776, 1974.

Merimer TJ, Zapf MJ, Froesch ER: Insulin-like growth factors in the fed and fasted states. *J Clin Endocrinol Metab* 55:999, 1982.

Miyata M, Yamomoto T, Nakao K: Suppression of glucagon secretion during surgery. *Horm Metab Res* 8:239, 1976.

Molteni A, Warphea RL, et al: Circadian rhythms of serum aldosterone, cortisol and plasma renin activity in burn injuries. *Ann Clin Lab Sci* 9:518, 1979.

Moran WH, Miltenberger FW, et al: Relationship of antidiuretic hormone to surgical stress. *Surgery* 56:99, 1964.

Morgan RJ, Martyn JAJ, et al: Water metabolism and antidiuretic hormone response following thermal injury. *J Trauma* 20:468, 1980.

Mortensen RF, Johnson AA, Eurenius K: Serum corticosteroid binding following thermal injury. *Proc Soc Exp Biol Med* 139:877, 1979.

Moss GS, Cerchio GM, et al: Serum insulin response in hemorrhagic shock in baboons. *Surgery* 68:34, 1970.

Munck A, Guyre PM, Holbrook NJ: Physiological functions of glucocorticoids in stress and their relation to pharmacological actions. *Endocr Rev* 5:25, 1984.

Nagy S, Nagy A, et al: Histamine level changes in the plasma and tissues in hemorrhagic shock. *Circ Shock* 18:227, 1986.

Nakao K, Nakai Y, et al: Substantial rise of plasma beta endorphin levels after insulin-induced hypoglycemia in human subjects. *J Clin Endocrinol Metab* 49:838, 1979.

Nelson DH: Corticosteroid-induced changes in phospholipid membranes as mediators of their action. *Endocr Rev* 1:180, 1980.

Newsome HH, Rose JC: The response of adrenocorticotrophic hormone and growth hormone to surgical stress. *J Clin Endocrinol Metab* 33:481, 1971.

Novelli GP, Marsili M, Pieraccioli E: Anti-shock action of steroids other than cortisone. *Eur Surg Res* 5:169, 1973.

Ono N, Lumpkin MD, et al: Intrahypothalamic action of corticotropin-releasing factor to inhibit growth hormone and LH release in the rat. *Life Sci* 35:118, 1984.

Otsuki M, Dakoda M, Baba S: Influence of glucocorticoids on TRF-induced TSH response in man. *J Clin Endocrinol Metab* 36:945, 1973.

Parrillo JE, Fauci AS: Mechanisms of glucocorticoid action on immune processes. *Annu Rev Pharmacol Toxicol* 19:179, 1979.

Paterson SJ, Robson LE, Kosterlitz HW: Classification of opioid receptors. *Br J Med* 39:31, 1983.

Peach MJ: Renin-angiotensin system: Biochemistry and mechanisms of action. *Physiol Rev* 57:313–370, 1977.

Perdue JF: Chemistry structure and function of insulin-like growth factors and their receptors: A review. *Can J Biochem Cell Biol* 62:1237, 1984.

Pfeffer MA, Pfeffer JM, et al: Systemic hemodynamic effects of leukotrienes C4 and D4 in the rat. *Am J Physiol* 244:H628, 1983.

Pfeiffer A, Herz A: Endocrine action of opioids. *Horm Metab Res* 16:386, 1984.

Phillips LS, Vassilopoulou-Sellin R: Somatomedins. *N Engl J Med* 302:371, 1980.

Phillips RH, Valente WA, et al: Circulating thyroid hormone changes in acute trauma: Prognostic implications for clinical outcome. *J Trauma* 24:116, 1984.

Porte D Jr, Smith PH, Ensinck JW: Neurohumoral regulation of the pancreatic islet A and B cells. *Metabolism* 25:1453, 1976.

Powanda MC, Bersil WR: Hypothesis: Leukocytic endogenous mediator/endogenous pyrogen/lymphocyte activating factor modulates the development of nonspecific and specific immunity and affects nutritional status. *Am J Clin Nutr* 35:762, 1982.

Raptis S, Dollinger HC, et al: Differences in insulin, growth hormone and pancreatic enzyme secretion after intravenous and intraduodenal administration of mixed amino acids in man. *N Engl J Med* 288:1199, 1973.

Rees M, Bowen JC, et al: Plasma beta endorphin immunoreactivity in dogs during anesthesia surgery, escherichia coli sepsis, and naloxone therapy. *Surgery* 93:386, 1983.

Regoli D, Barabe J: Pharmacology of bradykinin and related kinins. *Pharmacol Rev* 32:1, 1980.

Reichlin S: Somatostatin. *N Engl J Med* 309:1495, 1983.

Rizza RA, Mandarino LJ, Gerich JE: Cortisol-induced insulin resistance in man: Impaired suppression of glucose production and stimulation of glucose utilization due to a postreceptor defect of insulin action. *J Clin Endocrinol Metab* 54:131, 1982.

Samuelsson B: Prostaglandins and thromboxanes. *Recent Prog Horm Res* 34:239, 1978.

Sawchenko PE, Friedman MI: Sensory functions of the liver—a review. *Am J Physiol* 236:R5, 1979.

Schachter M: Kallikreins (kinninogenases)—a group of serine proteases with bioregulatory actions. *Pharmacol Rev* 31:1, 1980.

Schrier RW, Berl WT, Anderson RJ: Osmotic and non-osmotic control of vasopressin release. *Am J Physiol* 236:F321, 1979.

Share L: Control of plasma ADH titer in hemorrhage: Role of atrial and arterial receptors. *Am J Physiol* 215:1384, 1968.

Shirani KZ, Vaughan GM, et al: Inappropriate vasopressin secretion in burned patients. *J Trauma* 23:217, 1983.

Shirani KZ, Vaughan GM, et al: Reduced serum T4 and T3 and their altered transport binding after burn injury in rats. *J Trauma* 25:953, 1985.

Silverberg AB, Shah SD, et al: Norepinephrine: Hormone and neurotransmitter in man. *Am J Physiol* 234:E252, 1978.

Skillman JJ, Hedley-White J, Pallotta JA: Hormonal, fuel and respiratory relationships after acute blood loss in man. *Surg Forum* 21:23, 1970.

Skillman JJ, Lauler DP, et al: Hemorrhage in normal man: Effect on renin, cortisol, aldosterone, and urine composition. *Ann Surg* 166:865, 1967.

Sklar AH, Schrier RW: Central nervous system mediators of vasopressin release. *Physiol Rev* 63:1243, 1983.

Slotman GJ, Burchard KW, Gann DS: Thromboxane and prostacyclin in clinical acute respiratory failure. *J Surg Res* 1986.

Swerlick RA, Drucker NA, McCoy S: Insulin effectiveness in hypovolemic dogs. *J Trauma* 21:1013, 1981.

Tracey KJ, Lowry SF, et al: Cachectin/tumor necrosis factor

mediates changes of skeletal muscle plasma membrane potential. *J Exp Med* 164:1368, 1986.

Tracey KJ, Beutler B, et al: Shock and tissue injury induced by recombinant human cachectin. *Science* 234:470, 1986.

Unger RH, Dobbs RE: Insulin, glucagon and somatostatin secretion in the regulation of metabolism. *Annu Rev Physiol* 40:307, 1978.

Vaughan GM, Becker RA, et al: Cortisol and corticotrophin in burned patients. *J Trauma* 22:263, 1982.

Vitek V, Lang DJ, Cowley RA: Admission serum insulin and glucose levels in 247 accident victims. *Clin Chim Acta* 95:93, 1979.

Vitek V, Shatney CH, et al: Thyroid hormone responses in hemorrhagic shock: Study in dogs and preliminary findings in humans. *Surgery* 93:768, 1983.

Wahl R, Grusseudorf M, et al: Changes of thyroid hormone concentrations after severe trauma and in hemorrhagic shock. *Eur Surg Res* 9:suppl 1, 1977.

Williams GH: Aldosterone, in Dunn MJ (ed): *Renal Endocrinology*. Baltimore, Williams and Wilkins, 1983, p 205.

Williamson DH: Regulation of ketone body metabolism and the effects of injury. *Acta Chir Scand* 22-9, 1981.

Wilmore DW, Long JM, et al: Catecholamines: mediators of the hypermetabolic response to thermal injury. *Am Surg* 180:653, 1974.

Wilmore DW, Mason AD, Pruitt BA: Insulin response to glucose in hypermetabolic burn patients. *Ann Surg* 183:314, 1976.

Wilmore WD, Moylan DA, et al: Hyperglucagonemia after burns. *Lancet* 1:73, 1974.

Wise L, Margraf HW, Ballinger WF: Adrenal cortical function in severe burns. *Arch Surg* 105:213, 1972.

Woloski BM, Smith EM, et al: Corticotropin releasing activity of monokines. *Science* 230:1035, 1985.

Wright PD, Henderson K: Cellular glucose utilization during hemorrhagic shock in the pig. *Surgery* 77:322, 1975.

Wright PD, Johnston IDA: The effect of surgical operation on growth hormone levels in surgery. *Surgery* 77:479, 1975.

Yates FE, Marsh DJ, Maran JW: The adrenal cortex, in Mountcastle, VB (ed): *Medical Physiology*. St Louis, Mosby, 1980, 14th ed, pp 1588–1601.

SUBSTRATE METABOLISM FOLLOWING INJURY

Amaral JF, Shearer JD, et al: The temporal characteristics of the metabolic and endocrine response to trauma. *J Trauma*, 1988. (In press.)

Cuthbertson DP: The metabolic response to injury and its nutritional implications: Retrospect and prospect. *J Parenter Enter Nutr* 3:108, 1979.

Engels FL: The significance of the metabolic changes during shock. *Ann NY Acad Sci* 55:383, 1956.

Frayn KN: Substrate turnover after injury. *Br Med Bull* 41:232, 1985.

Moore FD, Brennan MF: Surgical injury: Body composition, protein metabolism and neuroendocrinology, in Ballanger WF, Collins JA, Drucker WR (eds): *Manual of Surgical Nutrition*. Philadelphia, Saunders, 1975, p 169.

Oppenheim W, Williamson D, Smith R: Early biochemical changes and severity of injury in man. *J Trauma* 20:135, 1980.

Siegel JH, Cerra FB, et al: Physiological and metabolic correlations in human sepsis. *Surgery* 86:163, 1979.

Stoner HB, Frayn KN, et al: The relationships between plasma substrates and hormones and the severity of injury in 277 recently injured patients. *Clin Sci* 56:563, 1979.

Stoner HB: Metabolism after trauma and sepsis. *Circ Shock* 19:75, 1986.

Volenec FJ, Clark GM, et al: Metabolic profiles of thermal trauma. *Ann Surg* 190:694, 1979.

Wilmore DW: Hormonal responses and their effect on metabolism. *Surg Clin North Am* 56:999–1018, 1976.

Starvation

Abbott NE, Anderson K: The effect of starvation, infection and injury on the metabolic processes and body composition. *Ann NY Acad Sci* 110:941, 1963.

Addis T, Poo LJ, Lew W: The quantities of protein lost by the various organs and tissues of the body during a fast. *J Biol Chem* 115:111, 1936.

Ahnefeld FW, Burri C, et al: *Parenteral Nutrition*. Springer-Verlag, New York, 1976.

Ashour B, Hansford RG: Effect of fatty acids and ketones on the activity of pyruvate dehydrogenase in skeletal muscle mitochondria. *Biochem J* 214:715, 1983.

Cahill GF: Starvation in man. *N Engl J Med* 235:668, 1970.

Cahill GF: Ketosis *J Parenter Enterol Nutr* 5:281, 1981.

Carter WJ, Shakir KM, et al: Effect of thyroid hormone on the metabolic adaptation to fasting. *Metabolism* 24:1177, 1975.

Chaisson JL, Liljenquist JE, et al: Gluconeogenesis from alanine in normal postabsorptive man: Intrahepatic stimulatory effect of glucagon. *Diabetes* 24:574, 1975.

Chopra IJ, Smith SR: Circulating thyroid hormones and thyrotropin in adult patients with protein caloric malnutrition. *J Clin Endocrinol Metab* 40:221, 1975.

Exton JH: Gluconeogenesis. *Metabolism* 21:945, 1972.

Felig P: The glucose-alanine cycle. *Metabolism* 22:17, 1973.

Hems DA, Whitton PD: Control of hepatic glycogenolysis. *Physiol Rev* 60:1, 1980.

Hers HG: The control of glycogen metabolism in the liver. *Annu Rev Biochem* 45:167, 1976.

Keys A, Brozek J, et al: *The Biology of Human Starvation*. University of Minnesota Press, 1950.

Korchak HM, Masoro EJ: Changes in the level of the fatty acids synthesizing enzymes during starvation. *Biochem Biophys Acta* 58:354, 1962.

Krebs HA: The metabolic fate of amino acids, in Munro HN, Allison JB (eds): *Mammalian Protein Metabolism*. New York, Academic, 1964, vol 1, p 125.

McGarry JD, Foser DW: Hormonal control of ketogenesis: Biochemical considerations. *Arch Intern Med* 137:495, 1977.

Mallette LE, Exton JH, Park CR: Control of gluconeogenesis from amino acids in the perfused rat liver. *J Biol Chem* 244:5713, 1969.

Masoro EJ: Lipids and lipid metabolism. *Annu Rev Physiol* 39:301, 1977.

Morgan HE, Earl DCN, et al: Regulation of protein synthesis in heart muscle. *J Biol Chem* 251:2151, 1971.

Munro HN, Crim MC: The proteins and amino acids, in Goodhart RS, Shils ME (eds): *Modern Nutrition in Health and Disease*. Philadelphia, Lea & Febiger, 1980, p 51.

Newsholme EA, Start C: *Regulation in Metabolism*. New York, Wiley, 1973.

Owen OE, Organ AP, et al: Brain metabolism during fasting. *J Clin Invest* 46:1589, 1967.

Palmblad J, et al: Effects of total energy withdrawal (fasting) on the level of growth hormone, thyrotropin, cortisol, adrenaline, noradrenaline, T4, T3 and rT3 in healthy males. *Acta Med Scand* 201:16, 1977.

Pozefsky T, Tancredi RG, et al: Effect of brief starvation on muscle amino acid metabolism in non-obese man. *J Clin Invest* 57:444, 1976.

Randle PJ, Newsholme EA, Garland PB: Regulation of glucose uptake by muscle: B. Effects of fatty acids, ketone bodies and pyruvate, and of alloxan-diabetes and starvation on the uptake and metabolic fate of glucose in rat heart and diaphragm muscles. *Biochem J* 93:652, 1964.

Sherwin RS, Hendler RG, Felig P: Effect of ketone infusion on amino acid and nitrogen metabolism in man. *J Clin Invest* 55:1382, 1975.

Energy Metabolism following Injury

Atkinson DE: The energy charge of the adenylate pool as a regulator parameter interaction with feedback modifiers. *Biochemistry* 7:4030, 1966.

Chaudry IH, Sayeed MM, Baue AE: Depletion and restoration of tissue ATP in hemorrhagic shock. *Arch Surg* 108:208, 1974.

Chaudry IH, Wichterman KA, Baue AE: Effect of sepsis on tissue adenine nucleotide levels. *Surgery* 85:205, 1979.

Dubois EF: The mechanism of heat loss and temperature regulation, in Dubois EF (ed): *Lane Medical Lectures,* Stanford University Press, 1937.

Duke JH, Jorgensen SB, et al: Contribution of protein to caloric expenditure following injury. *Surgery* 68:168, 1970.

Hems DA, Brosnan JT: Effects of ischemia on content of metabolites in rat liver and kidney in vivo. *Biochem J* 120:105, 1970.

Illner HP, Shires T: Membrane defect and energy status of rabbit skeletal muscle cells in sepsis and septic shock. *Arch Surg* 116:1302, 1981.

Im MJC, Hoopes JE: Energy metabolism in healing skin wounds. *J Surg Res* 10:459, 1970.

Kinney JM: Energy metabolism in Fischer JE (ed): *Surgical Nutrition.* Boston, Little, Brown and Co., 1983, p 97.

Kinney JM, Roe CF: Caloric equivalents of fever. Patterns of postoperative response. *Ann Surg* 156:610, 1962.

Kinney JM, Lister J, Moore FD: Relationship of energy expenditure to total exchangeable potassium. *Ann NY Acad Sci* 110:722, 1963.

Kinney JM, Long CL, et al: Tissue composition of weight loss in surgical patients. I. Elective operations. *Ann Surg* 168:459, 1968.

LePage GA: Biological energy transformations during shock as shown by tissue analysis. *Am J Physiol* 146:267, 1946.

Liaw KY, Askanazi J, et al: Effect of injury and sepsis on high energy phosphates in muscle and red cells. *J Trauma* 20:755, 1980.

Moore FD: Bodily changes during surgical convalescence. *Ann Surg* 137:289, 1953.

Moore FD: Energy and the maintenance of the body cell. *J Parenter Enterol Nutr* 4:22, 1980.

Morris A, Henry W, et al: Macrophage interaction with skeletal muscle: a potential role of macrophages in determining the energy state of healing wounds. *J Trauma* 25:751, 1985.

Nanni G, Siegel JH, et al: Increased lipid fuel dependence in the critically ill septic patient. *J Trauma* 24:14, 1983.

Pass LJ, Schloerb PR, et al: Liver adenosine triphosphate (ATP) in hypoxia and hemorrhagic shock. *J Trauma* 22:730, 1982.

Pruitt BA: Postburn hypermetabolism and nutrition in burn patients, in Ballinger WF, Collins JA, Drucker WR, Dudrick SJ, Zeppa R (eds): *Manual of Surgical Nutrition.* Philadelphia, Saunders, 1975, p 396.

Ryan NT: Metabolic adaptations for energy production during trauma and sepsis. *Surg Clin North Am* 56:1073, 1976.

Wilmore DW, Aulick LH, et al: Influence of the burn wound on local and systemic responses to injury. *Ann Surg* 186:444, 1977.

Wilmore DW, Long JM, et al: Catecholamines: Mediators of the hypermetabolic response to thermal injury. *Am Surg* 180:653, 1974.

Lipid Metabolism following Injury

Allison SP, Hinton P, Chamberlain MJ: Intravenous glucose tolerance, insulin and free fatty acid levels in burn patients. *Lancet* 2:1118, 1968.

Bagby GJ, Corll CB, Martinez RR: Triglyceride and free fatty acid turnover in E. coli endotoxin treated rats. *Circ Shock* 16:76, 1985.

Birkhahn RN, Long CL, et al: A comparison of the effects of skeletal trauma and surgery on the ketosis of starvation in man. *J Trauma* 513, 1981.

Froholm BB: The effect of lactate in canine subcutaneous adipose tissue in situ. *Acta Physiol Scand* 81:110, 1971.

Kaufman RL, Matson CE, Beisel WR: Hypertriglyceridemia produced by endotoxin: Role of impaired triglyceride disposal mechanisms. *J Infect Dis* 133:548, 1976.

Kovach AGB, Russell S, et al: Blood flow, oxygen consumption and free fatty acid release in subcutaneous adipose tissue during hemorrhagic shock in control and phenoxybenzamine-treated dogs. *Circ Res* 26:733, 1970.

Smith R, Fuller DJ, et al: Initial effect of injury on ketone bodies and other blood metabolites. *Lancet* 1:1, 1975.

Wolfe RR, Shaw HF, Durkot MJ: Energy metabolism in trauma and sepsis: the role of fat, in *Molecular and Cellular Aspects of Shock and Trauma.* New York, AR Liss, 1983, p 89.

Carbohydrate Metabolism following Injury

Amaral JF, Shearer J, Caldwell M: Kinetics of glucose uptake in wounded tissue. *Fed Proc* (Abst), 1986.

Amaral JF, Shearer JD, et al: High dose endotoxin decreases glucose uptake in skeletal muscle. *Arch Surg* 1988. (In press.)

Amaral JF, Shearer J, et al: Macrophage insulin like activity increases glucose uptake and hepatic production in skeletal muscle. *Circ Shock* 1988. (In press.)

Amaral JF, Shearer JD, et al: Can lactate be used as a fuel by wounded tissue? *Surgery* 100:252, 1986.

Askanazi J, Elwyn DH, et al: Respiratory distress secondary to a high carbohydrate load. *Surgery* 86:596, 1980.

Black PR, Brooks DC, et al: Mechanisms of insulin resistance following injury. *Ann Surg* 196:420, 1982.

Caldwell MD, Shearer J, et al: Evidence for aerobic glycolysis in λ-carrageenan wounded skeletal muscle. *J Surg Res* 37:63, 1984.

Cannon WB: *The Wisdom of the Body.* New York, W.W. Norton, 1939.

Clark EJ, Rossiter R: Carbohydrate metabolism after burning. *Q J Exp Physiol* 32:279, 1944.

Cryer PE, White NH, Santiago JV: The relevance of glucose counterregulatory systems to patients with insulin-dependent diabetes mellitus. *Endocr Rev* 7:131, 1986.

Drucker WR, Dekieweit JC: Glucose uptake by diaphragms from rats subjected to hemorrhagic shock. *Am J Physiol* 206:317, 1964.

Drucker WR, Gallie BL, et al: In Kovach AGB, Stoner HB,

Spitzer JJ (eds): *Neurohumoral and Metabolic Response to Injury*. New York, Plenum, 1978, p 1870.

Filkins JP: Insulin-like activity (ILA) of a macrophage mediator on adipose tissue glucose oxidation. *J Reticuloendothel Soc* 25:595, 1979.

Forster J, Morris AS, et al: Increased PFK activity in wounded tissue. *Am J Physiol* 1988. (In press.)

Halmagyi DFJ, Irving MH, Varga D: Effect of adrenergic blockade on the metabolic response to hemorrhagic shock. *J Appl Physiol* 25:384, 1968.

Hiebert JM, Celik Z, et al: Insulin response to hemorrhagic shock in the intact and adrenalectomized primate. *Am J Surg* 125:501, 1973.

Hinton P, Allison SP, et al: Insulin and glucose to reduce catabolic response to injury in burned patients. *Lancet* 1:767, 1971.

Hunt TK, Conolly WB, et al: Anaerobic metabolism and wound healing: An hypothesis for the initiation and cessation of collagen synthesis in wounds. *Am J Surg* 135:328, 1978.

Jordan GL, Fischer EP, Lefiak EA: Glucose metabolism and traumatic shock in the human. *Ann Surg* 175:685, 1972.

Kahn CR: Insulin resistance, insulin insensitivity and insulin unresponsiveness: a necessary definition. *Metabolism* 27:1893, 1973.

Long CL, Spencer JL, et al: Carbohydrate metabolism in men: Effect of elective operations and major injury. *J Appl Physiol* 31:110, 1971.

Morris AS, Shearer J, Caldwell MD: The role of the cellular infiltrate on glucose metabolism in wounded tissue. *Surg Forum* 36:95, 1985.

Nelson KM, Turinsky J: Local effect of burn on skeletal muscle insulin responsiveness. *J Surg Res* 31:288, 1981.

Palmer BQ, Brooks DC, et al: Epinephrine acutely mediates skeletal muscle insulin resistance. *Surgery* 94:172, 1983.

Pekala P, Kawakami M, et al: Studies of insulin resistance in adipocytes induced by a macrophage mediator. *J Exp Med* 157:1360, 1983.

Romanosky AJ, Bagby GJ, et al: Increased muscle glucose uptake and lactate release after endotoxin administration. *Am J Physiol* E311, 1980.

Ryan NT, George BC, et al: Chronic tissue insulin resistance following hemorrhagic shock. *Ann Surg* 80:402, 1974.

Shangraw RE, Turinsky J: Local response of muscle to burns: Relationship of glycolysis and amino acid release. *J Parenter Enterol Nutr* 5:193, 1981.

Stoner HB: Studies on the mechanism of shock: The quantitative aspects of glycogen metabolism after limb ischemia in the rat. *Br J Exp Pathol* 39:635, 1958.

Swerlick RA, Drucker NA, McCoy S: Insulin effectiveness in hypovolemic dogs. *J Trauma* 21:1013, 1981.

Turinsky J: Glucose metabolism in the region recovering from burn injury. *Endocrinology* 113:1370, 1983.

Wilmore DW, Mason AD, Pruitt BA: Insulin response to glucose in hypermetabolic burn patients. *Ann Surg* 183:314, 1976.

Protein Metabolism following Injury

Albina JE, Shearer JD, et al: Amino acid metabolism following λ-carrageenan injury to rat skeletal muscle. *Am J Physiol* 250:E24, 1986.

Albina JE, Henry W, et al: Glutamine metabolism in rat skeletal muscle wounded with λ-carregeenan. *Am J Physiol* 250:E24, 1986.

Andrews RP, Morgan HC, Jhrkiewitz MJ: Relationship of dietary protein to the healing of experimental burns. *Surg Forum* 6:72, 1955.

Ardawi MSM, Newsholme EA: Glutamine metabolism in lymphoid tissue, in Haussinger D, Sies H (eds): *Glutamine Metabolism in Mammalian Tissues*. New York, Springer-Verlag, 1984, p 235.

Askanazi S, Elwyn DH, et al: Muscle and plasma amino acids after injury: The role of inactivity. *Ann Surg* 188:797, 1978.

Askanazi I, Carpentier YA, et al: Muscle and plasma amino acids following injury: Influence of intercurrent infection. *Ann Surg* 192:78, 1980.

Aulick LH, Wilmore DH: Increased peripheral amino acid release following burn injury. *Surgery* 85:560, 1979.

Bilmazer C, et al: Quantitative contribution by skeletal muscle to elevated ratio of whole-body protein breakdown in burned children as measured by 3-MEH output. *Metabolism* 27:671, 1978.

Birkhain RH, et al: Effects of major skeletal trauma on whole body protein turnover in man measured by [14C] leucine. *Surgery* 888:294, 1980.

Calloway DH, Grossman MI, et al: Effect of previous level of protein feeding on wound healing and on metabolic response to injury. *Surgery* 37:935, 1955.

Calwell FT Jr: Metabolic responses to thermal trauma. II: Nutritional studies with rats at two environmental temperatures. *Ann Surg* 155:119, 1962.

Chassin JL, McDougall HA, et al: The effect of adrenalectomy on wound healing in normal and in stressed rats. *Proc Soc Exp Biol Med* 86:446, 1954.

Clowes G, Randall H, Cha C: Amino acid and energy metabolism in septic and traumatized patients. *J Parenter Enterol Nutr* 4:195, 1980.

Crane CW, et al: Protein turnover in patients before and after elective orthopedic operations. *Br J Surg* 64:129, 1977.

Crowley CV, Seifter E, et al: Effects of environmental temperature and femoral fracture on wound healing in rats. *J Trauma* 17:436, 1977.

Cuthbertson DP: Observations on the disturbances of metabolism by injury to the limbs. *Q J Med* 1:233, 1932.

Cuthbertson DP, Tilstone WJ: Effects of environmental temperature on the closure of full thickness skin wounds in the rat. *Q J Exp Physiol* 52:249, 1967.

Dale G, et al: The effect of surgical operation on venous plasma free amino acids. *Surgery* 81:295, 1977.

Elwyn DH, Parikh HC, et al: Inter-organ transport of amino acids in hemorrhagic shock. *Am J Phys* 231:377, 1976.

Engels FL, Winton MG, Long CNH: Biochemical studies on shock. I. The metabolism of amino acids and carbohydrates during hemorrhagic shock in the rat. *J Exp Med* 77:397, 1942.

Frawley JP, Artz CP, Howard JM: Muscle metabolism and catabolism in combat casualties. *Arch Surg* 71:612, 1955.

Freund HR, Ryan JA, Fischer JE: Amino acid derangements in patients with sepsis: Treatment with branched chain amino acid rich infusions. *Ann Surg* 188:423, 1978.

Furst P, Bergstrom S, Chao L: Influence of amino acid sulphur on nitrogen and amino acid metabolism in severe trauma. *Acta Chir Scand Suppl* 494:136, 1979.

Howard JE, Bingham RS Jr, Mason RE: Studies on convalescence: In nitrogen and mineral balances during starvation and graduated feeding in healthy young males at bed rest. *Trans Assoc Am Physicians* 59:242, 1946.

Keller GA, West MA, et al: Multiple systems organ failure: Modulation of hepatocyte protein synthesis by endotoxin activated Kuppfer cells. *Ann Surg* 201:87, 1985.

Kien CL, et al: Increased rates of whole body protein synthesis and breakdown in children recovering from burns. *Ann Surg* 187:383, 1978.

Kinney JM, Elwyn DH: Protein metabolism and injury. *Ann Rev Nutr* 3:433, 1983.

Kline DL: The effect of hemorrhage on the plasma amino acid nitrogen of the dog. *Am J Physiol* 146:654, 1946.

LaBrosse EH, Beech JA, et al: Plasma amino acids in normal humans and patients with shock. *Surg Gynecol Obstet* 125:516, 1967.

Levenson SJ, Howard J, Rosen J: Studies of the plasma amino acids and amino conjugates in patients with several battle wounds. *Surg Gynecol Obstet* 101:35, 1955.

Levenson SM, Green RW, et al: Ascorbic acid, riboflavin, thiamine, and nicotinic acid in relation to severe injury, hemorrhage and infection in the human. *Ann Surg* 124:840, 1946.

Levenson SM, Pirani CL, et al: The effect of thermal burns on wound healing. *Surg Gynecol Obstet* 99:74, 1954.

Levenson SM, Seifter E, Van Winkle W: Nutrition, in Hunt TK, Dunphy JE (eds): *Fundamentals of Wound Management.* New York, Appleton Century Croft, 1979, p 286.

Long CL, Schiller WR, et al: Muscle protein catabolism in the septic patient as measured by 3-methylhistidine exertion. *Am J Clin Nutr* 30:1349, 1977.

Lund CL, Levenson SM, et al: Ascorbic acid, thiamine, riboflavin and nicotinic acid in relation to acute burns in man. *Arch Surg* 55:557, 1947.

McCoy S, Case SA, et al: Determinants of blood amino acid concentration after hemorrhage. *Ann Surg* 43:787, 1977.

Miller JDB, Bistran BR, Blackburn GL: Failure of postoperative infection to increase nitrogen excretion in patients maintained on peripheral amino acids. *Am J Clin Nutr* 30:1523, 1977.

Moore RN, Goodrum KJ, Berry LJ: Mediation of an endotoxic effect by macrophages. *J Reticuloendothel Soc* 17:187, 1976.

Odessey R, Khairallah EA, Goldberg AL: Origin and probable significance of alanine production by skeletal muscle. *J Biol Chem* 249:7623, 1974.

O'Donnell TF, Clowes GHA, et al: Proteolysis associated with a deficit of peripheral energy fuel substrates in septic man. *Surgery* 80:192, 1976.

O'Keefe SJD, Sender PM, James WPT: Catabolic loss of body nitrogen in response to surgery. *Lancet* 2:1035, 1974.

Ruderman NB, Berger M: The formation of glutamine and alanine in skeletal muscle. *J Biol Chem* 249:5500, 1974.

Russell JA, Long CH, Engel FL: Biochemical studies of shock: The role of peripheral tissues on the metabolism of protein and carbohydrate during hemorrhagic shock in the rat. *J Exp Med* 79:1, 1944.

Shearer J, Morris A, et al: Effect of starvation on the local and systemic metabolic effects of the λ-carrageenan wound. *Am J Surg* 147:456, 1984.

Shizgal HM, Milne CA, Spainer HA: The effect of nitrogen-sparing intravenously administered fluids on postoperative body composition. *Surgery* 86:60, 1979.

Souba WW, Wilmore DW: Postoperative alteration of arteriovenous exchange of amino acids across the gastrointestinal tract. *Surgery* 94:342, 1983.

Stein TP, Leskin MJ, et al: Changes in protein synthesis after trauma: Importance of nutrition. *Am J Physiol* 233:E348, 1976.

Vinnars E, Bergstrom J, Furst P: Influence of postoperative state in the intracellular free amino acids in human muscle tissue. *Ann Surg* 182:665, 1975.

West MA, Keller GA, et al: Mechanism of hepatic insufficiency in septic multiple system organ failure. *Surg Forum* 35:44, 1984.

Williamson MB, McCarthy TH, Fromm HJ: Relation of protein nutrition to the healing of experimental wounds. *Proc Soc Exp Biol Med* 77:302, 1957.

Williamson OH, et al: Muscle-protein catabolism after injury in man, as measured by urinary excretion of 3-methyl histidine. *Clin Sci Mol Med* 52:527, 1977.

Wilmore DM, Goodwin CW, et al: Effect of injury and infection on visceral metabolism and circulation. *Ann Surg* 192:491, 1980.

Woolfe LIU: Arterial plasma amino acids in patients with serious postoperative infections and in patients with major fractures. *Surgery* 79:283, 1976.

FLUID AND ELECTROLYTE METABOLISM

Andersson B: Regulation of body fluids. *Ann Rev Physiol* 39:185, 1977.

Arturson G: Microvascular permeability to macromolecules in thermal injury. *Acta Physiol Scand* 463:111.

Baxter CR, Shires T: Physiological response to crystalloid resuscitation of severe burns. *Ann NY Acad Sci* 150:874, 1968.

Blalock A: Experimental shock: The cause of low blood pressure caused by muscle injury. *Arch Surg* 20:959, 1930.

Demling RH, Kramer G, Harms B: Role of thermal injury-induced hypoproteinemia on fluid flux and protein permeability in burned and unburned tissue. *Surgery* 136–143, 95.

Elder JM, Miles AA: The action of the lethal toxins of gas gangrene clostridia on capillary permeability. *J Pathol* 74:133–145, 1957.

Harms B, Bodai B, et al: Microvascular fluid and protein flux in pulmonary and systemic circulations after thermal injury. *Microvas Res* 23:77, 1982.

Shires GT, Carrico J, Cannizaro P: Response of the extracellular fluid, in *Shock. Modern Problems in Clinical Surgery.* Philadelphia, Saunders, 1973.

Shires GT III, Peitzman AB, et al: Change in red blood cell transmembrane potential in hemorrhagic shock. *Surg Forum* 32:5, 1981.

Shires T, Williams J, Brown L: Acute changes in extracellular fluids associated with major surgical procedures. *Ann Surg* 154:803, 1961.

Tom WW, Villalba M, et al: Fluorophotometric evaluation of capillary permeability in gram negative-shock. *Arch Surg* 118:636, 1983.

Renal Salt and Water Conservation

Anderson RJ, Gordon JA, et al: Renal concentration defect following nonoliguric acute renal failure in the rat. *Kidney Int* 21:583, 1979.

Anderson RJ, Linas SL, et al: Nonoliguric renal failure. *N Engl J Med* 296:1134, 1977.

Cantin M, Genest J: The heart and atrial natiuretic factor. *Endocr Rev* 6:1, 1985.

Cochrane JPS: The aldosterone response to surgery and the relationship of this response to postoperative sodium retention. *Br J Surg* 65:744, 1978.

Gill JR Jr, Casper AGT: Role of sympathetic nervous system in the renal response to hemorrhage. *J Clin Invest* 48:915.

Gill JR Jr, Casper AGT: Effect of renal alpha-adrenergic stimulation on proximal sodium resorption. *Am J Physiol* 223:1201, 1972.

Hall JE, Guyton AC, Cowley AW Jr: Control of glomerular filtration rate by renin-angiotensin system. *Am J Physiol* 232:F215, 1979.

Itskovitz HD, McGriff JC: Hormonal regulation of renal circulation. *Circ Res* 34/35 (suppl I), 1974.

Johnson MD, Park CS, Malrin RL: Antidiuretic hormone and the distribution of renal cortical blood flow. *Am J Physiol* 232:F111, 1977.

LeQuesne LP, Cochrane JPS, Fieldman NR: Fluid and electrolyte disturbances after trauma: the role of adrenocortical and pituitary hormones. *Br Med Bull* 41:212, 1985.

Miller PD, Krebs RA, et al: Polyuric prerenal failure. *Arch Intern Med* 140:907, 1980.

Navar AG: Renal autoregulation; perspectives from whole kidney and single nephron studies. *Am J Physiol* 234:F357, 1978.

Navar LG, Ploth DW, Bell PD: Distal tubular feedback control of renal hemodynamics and autoregulation. *Ann Rev Physiol* 42:557, 1980.

Schrier RW: Effects of adrenergic nervous system and catecholamines on systemic and renal hemodynamics, sodium and water excretion and renin secretion. *Kidney Int* 6:291, 1974.

Stein JH, Boonjaren S, et al: Mechanism of the redistribution of renal cortical blood flow during hemorrhagic hypotension in the dog. *J Clin Invest* 52:3, 1973.

Valtin H: *Renal Function: Mechanisms Preserving Fluid and Solute Balance in Health.* Little, Brown and Company, 1983, 2d ed.

Blood Volume Restitution

Bergentz SE, Brief DD: The effect of pH and osmolality on the production of canine hemorrhagic shock. *Surgery* 58:412, 1965.

Boyd DR, Mansberger AR: Serum water and osmolal changes in hemorrhagic shock. *Am Surg* 34:744, 1968.

Brooks DK, Williams WG, et al: Osmolar and electrolyte changes in hemorrhagic shock. *Lancet* 1:521, 1963.

Byrnes GJ, Pirkle JC Jr, Gann DS: Cardiovascular stabilization after hemorrhage depends upon restitution of blood volume. *J Trauma* 18:623, 1978.

Casley-Smith JR: The functioning and interrelationships of blood capillaries and lymphatics. *Experientia* 32:1, 1976.

Chien S: Role of the sympathetic nervous system in hemorrhage. *Physiol Rev* 47:214, 1967.

Cope O, Litwin SB: Contribution of the lymphatic system to the replenishment of plasma volume following a hemorrhage. *Ann Surg* 156:655, 1962.

Drucker WR, Chadwick CDJ, Gann DS: Transcapillary refill in hemorrhage and shock. *Arch Surg* 116:1344, 1981.

Friedman SG, Pearce FJ, Drucker WR: The role of blood glucose in the defense of plasma volume during hemorrhage. *J Trauma* 22:86, 1982.

Gann DS: Endocrine control of plasma protein and volume. *Surg Clin North Am* 56:1135, 1976.

Gann DS, Carlson DE, et al: Impaired restitution of blood volume after large hemorrhage. *J Trauma* 21:598, 1981.

Gann DS, Carlson DE, et al: Role of solute in the early restitution of blood volume after hemorrhage. *Surgery* 94:439–446, 1983.

Haddy FJ, Scott JB, Molnar JJ: Mechanisms of volume replacement and vascular constriction following hemorrhage. *Am J Physiol* 208:169, 1965.

Jarhult J: Osmotic fluid transfer from tissue to blood during hemorrhagic hypotension. *Acta Physiol Scand* 1973.

Jarhult J, Lundvall J, et al: Osmolar control of plasma volume during hemorrhagic hypotension. *Acta Physiol Scand* 85:142, 1972.

Kenney PR, Allen-Rowlands CF, Gann DS: Glucose and osmolality as predictors of injury severity. *J Trauma* 23:712, 1983.

Leaf A, Cotran R: *Renal Pathophysiology.* New York, Oxford University Press, 1976.

Menguay R, Master YF: Influence of hyperglycemia on survival after hemorrhagic shock. *Adv Shock Res* 1:43, 1979.

Pirkle JC Jr, Gann DS: Expansion of interstitial fluid is required for full restoration of blood volume. *J Trauma* 16:937, 1977.

Pitts RF: *Physiology of the Body Fluids.* Chicago, Yearbook Medical Publishers, 3d ed, 1974.

Quiros G, Ware J: Modification of cardiovascular responses to hemorrhage by induced hyperosmolality in the rat. *Acta Physiol Scand* 117:391, 1983.

Ware J, Ljanquist O, et al: Osmolar changes in hemorrhage. The effect of an altered nutritional status. *Acta Chir Scand* 148:8, 1982.

Weil M, Afifi AA: Experimental and clinical studies on lactate and pyruvate as indicators of the severity of acute circulatory failure. *Circulation* XLI: 989–1001, 1970.

Wright FS, Briggs JP: Feedback control of glomerular blood flow, pressure and filtration rate. *Physiol Rev* 59:958, 1979.

Wright HK, Gann DS: A defect in urinary concentrating ability during postoperative anti-diuresis. *Surgery Gynecol Obstet* 121:47, 1965.

Wright HK, Gann DS: Correction of defect in free water excretion in postoperative patients by extracellular fluid volume expansion. *Ann Surg* 158:70, 1963.

Chapter 2

Fluid, Electrolyte, and Nutritional Management of the Surgical Patient

G. Tom Shires, Peter C. Canizaro, G. Tom Shires III, and Stephen F. Lowry

ANATOMY OF BODY FLUIDS

One of the most critical aspects of patient care is management of the body composition of fluid and electrolytes. Most diseases, many injuries, and even operative trauma impose a great impact on the physiology of fluid and electrolytes within the body. These changes often exceed those brought about by acute lack of alimentation. Therefore, a thorough understanding of the metabolism of salt, water, and electrolytes and of certain metabolic responses is essential to the care of surgical patients.

The anatomy of body fluids and the physiologic principles that maintain normal fluid and electrolytes will be defined. In addition, a classification of derangements will be outlined to allow an organized therapeutic approach.

A prerequisite to the understanding of fluid and electrolyte management is knowledge of the extent and composition of the various body fluid compartments. Early attempts to define these compartments were relatively accurate, but a more precise definition has been obtained by many investigators through the use of isotope tracer techniques. The wide range of normal values is a function of body size, weight, and sex, but these compartments are relatively constant in the individual patient in the normal steady state. The figures used in this section, therefore, are approximate and presented as a percentage of body weight.

Total Body Water

Water constitutes between 50 and 70 percent of total body weight. Using deuterium oxide or tritiated water for

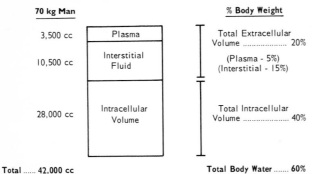

Fig. 2-1. Functional compartments of body fluids.

measurement of total body water, the average normal value for young adult males is 60 percent of body weight and 50 percent for young adult females. A normal variation of ±15 percent applies to both groups. The actual figure for each healthy individual is remarkably constant and is a function of several variables, including lean body mass and age. Since fat contains little water, the lean individual has a greater proportion of water to total body weight than the obese person. The lower percentage of total body water in females correlates well with a relatively large amount of subcutaneous adipose tissue and small muscle mass. Moore et al. have shown that total body water, as a percentage of total body weight, decreases steadily and significantly with age to a low of 52 and 47 percent in males and females, respectively. Con-

versely, the highest proportion of total body water to body weight is found in newborn infants, with a maximum of 75 to 80 percent. During the first several months following birth there is a gradual "physiologic" loss of body water as infants adjust to their environment. At one year of age, the total body water averages approximately 65 percent of the body weight and remains relatively constant throughout the remainder of infancy and childhood.

The water of the body is divided into three functional compartments (Fig. 2-1). The fluid within the body's diverse cell population represents between 30 and 40 percent of the body weight. The extracellular water represents 20 percent of the body weight and is divided between the intravascular fluid, or plasma (5 percent of body weight), and the interstitial, or extravascular, extracellular fluid (15 percent of body weight).

Intracellular Fluid

Measurement of intracellular fluid is determined indirectly by subtraction of the measured extracellular fluid from the measured total body water. The intracellular water is between 30 and 40 percent of the body weight, with the largest proportion in the skeletal muscle mass. Because of the smaller muscle mass in the female, the percentage of intracellular water is lower than in the male.

The chemical composition of the intracellular fluid is shown in Fig. 2-2, with potassium and magnesium the

Fig. 2-2. Chemical composition of body fluid compartments.

PLASMA — 154 meq/L / 154 meq/L

CATIONS		ANIONS	
Na⁺	142	Cl⁻	103
		HCO₃⁻	27
		SO₄⁻⁻	3
		PO₄⁻⁻⁻	
K⁺	4		
Ca⁺⁺	5	Organic Acids	5
Mg⁺⁺	3	Protein	16

INTERSTITIAL FLUID — 153 meq/L / 153 meq/L

CATIONS		ANIONS	
Na⁺	144	Cl⁻	114
		HCO₃⁻	30
K⁺	4	SO₄⁻⁻	3
		PO₄⁻⁻⁻	
Ca⁺⁺	3	Organic Acids	5
Mg⁺⁺	2	Proteins	1

INTRACELLULAR FLUID — 200 meq/L / 200 meq/L

CATIONS		ANIONS	
K⁺	150	HPO₄	150
		SO₄⁻⁻	
		HCO₃⁻	10
Mg⁺⁺	40	Protein	40
Na⁺	10		

principal cations, and phosphates and proteins the principal anions. This is an approximation, since so few data concerning the intracellular fluid are available.

Extracellular Fluid

The total extracellular fluid volume represents approximately 20 percent of the body weight. The extracellular fluid compartment has two major subdivisions. The plasma volume comprises approximately 5 percent of the body weight in the normal adult. The interstitial, or extravascular, extracellular fluid volume comprises approximately 15 percent of the body weight.

The interstitial fluid is further complicated by having a rapidly equilibrating functional component, as well as several more slowly equilibrating nonfunctioning components. The nonfunctioning components include connective tissue water as well as water that has been termed *transcellular,* which includes cerebrospinal and joint fluids. This nonfunctional component normally represents only 10 percent of the interstitial fluid volume (1 to 2 percent of body weight) and is not to be confused with the *relatively* nonfunctional extracellular fluid, often called a "third space," found in burns and soft tissue injuries.

The normal constituents of the extracellular fluid are shown in Fig. 2-2, with sodium the principal cation, and chloride and bicarbonate the principal anions. There are minor differences in ionic composition between the plasma and interstitial fluid that are primarily due to the difference in protein concentration. Because of the higher protein content (organic anions) of the plasma, the total concentration of cations is higher and the concentration of inorganic anions somewhat lower than in the interstitial fluid, as explained by the Gibbs-Donnan equilibrium equation (i.e., the product of the concentrations of any pair of diffusible cations and anions on one side of a semipermeable membrane will equal the product of the same pair of ions on the other side). For practical consideration, however, they may be considered equal. The total concentration of intracellular ions exceeds that of the extracellular compartment and would seem to violate the concept of osmolar equilibrium between the two compartments. This apparent discrepancy is due to the fact that the concentration of ions is expressed in milliequivalents (meq) without regard to osmotic activity. In addition, some of the intracellular cations probably exist in undissociated form.

Osmotic Pressure

The physiologic and chemical activity of electrolytes depend on (1) the *number of particles* present per unit volume [moles or millimoles (mmol) per liter], (2) the *number of electric charges* per unit volume (equivalents or milliequivalents per liter), and (3) the *number of osmotically active particles* or ions per unit volume [osmoles or milliosmoles (mO) per liter]. The use of the terms *grams* or *milligrams per 100 milliliters* expresses the weight of the electrolytes per unit volume but does not allow a physiologic comparison of the solutes in a solution.

A mole of a substance is the molecular weight of that substance in grams, and a millimole is that figure expressed in milligrams. For example, a mole of sodium chloride is 58 grams (Na—23, Cl—35), and a millimole is 58 milligrams. The expression, however, gives no direct information as to the number of osmotically active ions in solution or the electric charges that they carry.

The electrolytes of the body fluids then may be expressed in terms of chemical combining activity, or "equivalents." An equivalent of an ion is its atomic weight expressed in grams divided by the valence, whereas a milliequivalent of an ion is that figure expressed in milligrams. In the case of univalent ions, a milliequivalent is the same as a millimole. In the case of divalent ions, such as calcium or magnesium, one millimole equals two milliequivalents. The importance of this expression is that a milliequivalent of any substance will combine chemically with a milliequivalent of any other substance; in any given solution, the number of milliequivalents of cations present is balanced by precisely the same number of milliequivalents of anions.

When the osmotic pressure of a solution is considered, it is more descriptive to employ the terms osmole and milliosmole. These terms refer to the actual number of osmotically active particles present in solution, but are not dependent on the chemical combining capacities of the substances. Thus, a millimole of sodium chloride, which dissociates nearly completely into sodium and chloride, contributes two milliosmoles, and one millimole of sodium sulfate (Na_2SO_4), which dissociates into three particles, contributes three milliosmoles. One millimole of an un-ionized substance such as glucose is equal to one milliosmole of the substance.

The differences in ionic composition between intracellular and extracellular fluid are maintained by the semipermeable cell membrane. The total number of osmotically active particles is 290 to 310 mO in each compartment. Although the total osmotic pressure of a fluid is the sum of the partial pressures contributed by each of the solutes in that fluid, the *effective* osmotic pressure is dependent on those substances which fail to pass through the pores of the semipermeable membrane. The dissolved proteins in the plasma, therefore, are primarily responsible for effective osmotic pressure between the plasma and the interstitial fluid compartments. This is frequently referred to as the *colloid oncotic pressure*. The effective osmotic pressure between the extracellular and intracellular fluid compartments would be contributed to by any substance that does not traverse the cell membranes freely. Thus, while sodium as the principal cation of the extracellular fluid contributes a major portion of the osmotic pressure, other substances that fail to penetrate the cell membrane freely, such as glucose, also increase the effective osmotic pressure.

Since the cell membranes are completely permeable to water, the effective osmotic pressures in the two compartments are considered to be equal. Any condition that alters the effective osmotic pressure in either compartment will result in redistribution of water between the compartments. Thus, an increase in effective osmotic pressure in the extracellular fluid, which would occur most frequently as a result of increased sodium concentration, would cause a net transfer of water from the intracellular to the extracellular fluid compartment. This transfer of water would continue until the effective osmotic pressures in the two compartments were equal. Conversely, a decrease in the sodium concentration in the extracellular fluid will cause a transfer of water from the extracellular to the intracellular fluid compartment. Depletion of the extracellular fluid volume without a change in the concentration of ions will not result in transfer of free water from the intracellular space.

Thus, the intracellular fluid shares in losses that involve a change in concentration or composition of the extracellular fluid but shares only slowly in changes involving loss of isotonic volume alone. For practical consideration, most losses and gains of body fluid are directly from the extracellular compartment.

NORMAL EXCHANGE OF FLUID AND ELECTROLYTES

Knowledge of the basic principles governing both the internal and external exchanges of water and salt is mandatory for care of the patient undergoing major operative surgery. The stable internal fluid environment, which is maintained by the kidneys, brain, lungs, skin, and gastrointestinal tract, may be compromised by severe surgical stress or direct damage to any of these organs.

Water Exchange

The normal individual consumes an average of 2000 to 2500 mL water/day; approximately 1500 mL water is taken by mouth, and the rest is extracted from solid food, either from the contents of the food or as the product of oxidation (Table 2-1). The daily water losses include 250

mL in stools, 800 to 1500 mL as urine, and approximately 600 mL as insensible loss. A patient deprived of all external access to water must still excrete a minimum of 500 to 800 mL urine/day in order to excrete the products of catabolism, in addition to the mandatory insensible loss through the skin and lungs.

Insensible loss of water occurs through the skin (75 percent) and the lungs (25 percent) and is increased by hypermetabolism, hyperventilation, and fever. The insensible water loss through the skin is not from evaporation of water from sweat glands but from water vapor formed within the body and lost through the skin. With excessive heat production (or excessive environmental heat), the capacity for insensible loss through the skin is exceeded, and sweating occurs. These losses may, but seldom do, exceed 250 mL/day per degree of fever. An unhumidified tracheostomy with hyperventilation increases the loss through the lungs and results in a total insensible loss up to 1.5 L/day.

A frequently overlooked source of gain is the water of solution, which is the water that holds carbohydrates and proteins in solution in the cell. Normally, gain of water from this source is zero, but after 4 to 5 days without food intake, the postoperative patient may begin to gain significant quantities of water (up to 500 mL daily) from excessive cellular catabolism.

Salt Gain and Losses

In the normal individual, the salt intake per day varies between 50 and 90 meq (3 and 5 g) as sodium chloride (Table 2-2). Balance is maintained primarily by the normal kidneys that excrete the excess salt. Under conditions of reduced intake or extrarenal losses, the normal kidney can reduce sodium excretion to less than 1 meq/day within 24 h after restriction. In the patient with salt-wasting kidneys, however, the loss may exceed 200 meq/L of urine. Sweat represents a hypotonic loss of fluids with an average sodium concentration of 15 meq/L in the acclimatized patient. In the unacclimatized individual, the sodium concentration in sweat may be 60 meq/L or more. Insensible fluid lost from the skin and lungs, by

Table 2-1. WATER EXCHANGE (60- to 80-KG MAN)

Routes	Average daily volume, mL	Minimal, mL	Maximal, mL
H₂O gain:			
Sensible:			
Oral fluids	800–1500	0	1500/h
Solid foods	500–700	0	1500
Insensible:			
Water of oxidation	250	125	800
Water of solution	0	0	500
H₂O loss:			
Sensible:			
Urine	800–1500	300	1400/h (diabetes insipidus)
Intestinal	0–250	0	2500/h
Sweat	0	0	4000/h
Insensible:			
Lungs and skin	600	600	1500

Table 2-2. SODIUM (SALT) EXCHANGE (60- to 80-KG MAN)

Sodium exchange	Average	Minimal	Maximal
Sodium gain:			
Diet	50–90 meq/day	0	75–100 meq/h (oral)
Sodium loss:			
Skin			
(sweat)	10–60 meq/day*	0	300 meq/h
Urine	10–80 meq/day	<1 meq/day†	110–200 meq/L‡
Intestines	0–20 meq/day	0	300 meq/h

* Depending on the degree of acclimatization of the individual.
† With normal renal function.
‡ With renal salt wasting.

Table 2-3. COMPOSITION OF GASTROINTESTINAL SECRETIONS

Type of secretion	Volume (mL/24h)	Na (meq/L)	K (meq/L)	Cl (meq/L)	HCO₃ (meq/L)
Salivary	1500	10	26	10	30
	(500–2000)	(2–10)	(20–30)	(8–18)	
Stomach	1500	60	10	130	
	(100–4000)	(9–116)	(0–32)	(8–154)	
Duodenum		140	5	80	
	(100–2000)				
Ileum	3000	140	5	104	30
	(100–9000)	(80–150)	(2–8)	(43–137)	
Colon		60	30	40	
Pancreas		140	5	75	115
	(100–800)	(113–185)	(3–7)	(54–95)	
Bile		145	5	100	35
	(50–800)	(131–164)	(3–12)	(89–180)	

definition, is pure water. For practical considerations, then, normal losses may be relatively free of salt in the healthy individual with normal renal function.

The volume and composition of various types of gastrointestinal secretions are shown in Table 2-3. Gastrointestinal losses are usually isotonic or slightly hypotonic, although there is considerable variation in the composition. These should be replaced by an essentially isotonic salt solution. It is also important to reiterate that distributional or sequestration losses of extracellular fluid at any point in the operative or postoperative course also represent isotonic losses of salt and water.

CLASSIFICATION OF BODY FLUID CHANGES

The disorders in fluid balance may be classified in three general categories: disturbances of (1) volume, (2) concentration, and (3) composition. Of primary importance is the concept that although these disturbances are interrelated, each is a separate entity.

If an isotonic salt solution is added to or lost from the body fluids, only the *volume* of the extracellular fluid is changed. The acute loss of an isotonic extracellular solution, such as intestinal juice, is followed by a significant decrease in the extracellular fluid volume and little, if any, change in the intracellular fluid volume. Fluid will not be transferred from the intracellular space to refill the depleted extracellular space as long as the osmolarity remains the same in the two compartments.

If water alone is added to or lost from the extracellular fluid, the *concentration* of osmotically active particles will change. Sodium ions account for 90 percent of the osmotically active particles in the extracellular fluid and generally reflect the tonicity of body fluid compartments. If the extracellular fluid is depleted of sodium, water will pass into the intracellular space until osmolarity is again equal in the two compartments.

The concentration of most other ions within the extracellular fluid compartment can be altered without significant change in the total number of osmotically active particles, thus producing only a *compositional* change. For instance, a rise of the serum potassium concentration from 4 to 8 meq/L would have a significant effect on the myocardium, but it would not significantly change the effective osmotic pressure of the extracellular fluid compartment. Normally functioning kidneys minimize these changes considerably, particularly if the addition or loss of solute or water is gradual.

An internal loss of extracellular fluid into a nonfunctional space, such as the sequestration of isotonic fluid in a burn, peritonitis, ascites, or muscle trauma, is termed a *distributional* change. This transfer or functional loss of extracellular fluid internally may be extracellular (e.g., peritonitis) or intracellular (e.g., hemorrhagic shock) or both (e.g., major burns). In any event, all distributional shifts or losses result in a contraction of the *functional* extracellular fluid space.

Volume Changes

Volume deficit or excess generally must be diagnosed by clinical examination of the patient. There are no readily available laboratory tests of benefit in the acute phase except measurement of the plasma volume. Changes secondary to long-standing derangements in volume, however, may be discernible by laboratory tests. For example, the blood urea nitrogen (BUN) level slowly rises with a long-standing extracellular fluid deficit of sufficient magnitude to reduce glomerular filtration. The concentration of serum sodium is *not* related to the volume status of extracellular fluid; a severe volume deficit may exist with a normal, low, or high serum level.

VOLUME DEFICIT. Extracellular fluid volume deficit is by far the most common fluid disorder in the surgical patient. The loss of fluid is not water alone, but water and electrolytes in approximately the same proportion as they exist in normal extracellular fluid. The most common disorders leading to an extracellular fluid volume deficit include losses of gastrointestinal fluids due to vomiting, nasogastric suction, diarrhea, and fistular drainage. Other common causes include sequestration of fluid in soft tissue injuries and infections, intraabdominal and retroperi-

Table 2-4. EXTRACELLULAR FLUID VOLUME

Type of sign	Deficit		Excess	
	Moderate	*Severe*	*Moderate*	*Severe*
Central nervous system	Sleepiness Apathy Slow responses Anorexia Cessation of usual activity	Decreased tension re- flexes Anesthesia distal ex- tremities Stupor Coma	None	None
Gastrointestinal	Progressive decrease in food consumption	Nausea, vomiting Refusal to eat Silent ileus and dis- tention	At operation: Edema of stomach, colon, lesser and greater omenta, and small bowel mesentery	
Cardiovascular	Orthostatic hypotension Tachycardia Collapsed veins Collapsing pulse	Cutaneous lividity Hypotension Distant heart sounds Cold extremities Absent peripheral pulses	Elevated venous pressure Distention of peripheral veins Increased cardiac output Loud heart sounds Functional murmurs Bounding pulse High pulse pressure Increased pulmonary 2d sound Gallop	Pulmonary edema
Tissue	Soft, small tongue with longitudinal wrinkling Decreased skin turgor	Atonic muscles Sunken eyes	Subcutaneous pitting edema Basilar rales	Anasarca Moist rales Vomiting Diarrhea
Metabolic	Mild decrease temperature, 97–99°R	Marked decrease tem- perature, 95–98°R	None	None

toneal inflammatory processes, peritonitis, intestinal obstruction, and burns. The signs and symptoms of this state are easily recognized and are listed in Table 2-4. The central nervous system and cardiovascular signs occur early with acute rapid losses, whereas tissue signs may be absent until the deficit has existed for at least 24 h. The central nervous system signs are similar to barbiturate intoxication and may be missed by the casual observer if the volume deficit is mild. The cardiovascular signs are secondary to a decrease in plasma volume and may be associated with varying degrees of hypotension in the patient with a severe extracellular fluid volume deficit. Skin turgor may be difficult to assess in the elderly patient or in the patient with recent weight loss and is not diagnostic in the absence of other confirmatory signs. The body temperature tends to vary with the environmental temperature. In a cool room, the patient may be slightly hypothermic and the febrile response to illness may be suppressed. This occurs frequently and can be very misleading during clinical evaluation of the septic patient. After partial correction of the volume deficit, the temperature will generally rise to the appropriate level.

VOLUME EXCESS. Extracellular fluid volume excess may be generally iatrogenic or secondary to renal insufficiency, cirrhosis, or congestive heart failure. Both the plasma and interstitial fluid volumes are increased. In the healthy young adult, the signs are generally those of cir-

culatory overload, manifested primarily in the pulmonary circulation, and of excessive fluid in other tissue (Table 2-4). In the elderly patient, congestive heart failure with pulmonary edema may develop rather quickly with a moderate volume excess.

Concentration Changes

Sodium is primarily responsible for the osmolarity of the extracellular fluid space: determination of the serum concentration of sodium generally indicates the tonicity of body fluids. Hyponatremia and hypernatremia can be diagnosed on clinical grounds (Table 2-5), but signs and symptoms are not generally present until the changes are severe. Clinical signs of hyponatremia or hypernatremia tend to occur early and with greater severity if the rate of change in extracellular sodium concentration is very rapid. Changes in concentration should be noted early by laboratory tests and corrected promptly.

HYPONATREMIA. Acute symptomatic hyponatremia (sodium less than 130 meq/L) clinically is characterized by central nervous system signs of increased intracranial pressure and tissue signs of excessive intracellular water. The hypertension is probably induced by the rise in intracranial pressure, since the blood pressure generally returns to normal with the administration of hypertonic solutions of sodium salts. Of importance with severe

Table 2-5. ACUTE CHANGES IN OSMOLAR CONCENTRATION

Type of signs	Hyponatremia (water intoxication)		Hypernatremia (water deficit)	
	Moderate:	Severe:	Moderate:	Severe:
Central nervous system	Muscle twitching Hyperactive tendon reflexes Increased intra-cranial pressure (compensated phase)	Convulsions Loss of reflexes Increased intra-cranial pressure (decompensated) phase)	Restlessness Weakness	Delirium Maniacal be-havior
Cardiovascular	Changes in blood pressure and pulse secondary to increased intracranial pressure		Tachycardia Hypotension (if severe)	
Tissue	Salivation, lacrimation, watery diarrhea "Fingerprinting" of skin (sign of intracellular volume excess)		Decreased saliva and tears Dry and sticky mucous membranes Red, swollen tongue Skin flushed	
Renal	Oliguria progressing to anuria		Oliguria	
Metabolic	None		Fever	

hyponatremia is the relatively rapid development of oliguric renal failure, which may not be reversible if therapy is delayed.

Many chronic hyponatremic states are asymptomatic until the serum sodium level falls below 120 meq/L. One important exception is the patient with increased cerebrospinal fluid pressure, following closed head injury, in whom mild hyponatremia may be fatal, because of the progressive increase in intracellular water as the extracellular fluid osmolarity falls.

HYPERNATREMIA. Central nervous system and tissue signs characterize acute symptomatic hypernatremia. This is the only state in which dry, sticky mucous membranes are characteristic. This sign does not occur with pure extracellular fluid volume deficit alone, and may be misleading in the patient who breathes through his mouth. Body temperature is generally elevated and may approach a lethal level, as in the patient with heatstroke.

While volume changes occur frequently without a change in serum sodium, the reverse is not true. The disease states that cause a significant acute alteration in the serum sodium frequently produce a concomitant change in the extracellular fluid volume.

Mixed Volume and Concentration Abnormalities

Mixed volume and concentration abnormalities may develop as a consequence of the disease state or occasionally may result from inappropriate parenteral fluid therapy. Moyer noted that the clinical picture associated with a combination of fluid abnormalities will tend to be an algebraic composite of the signs and symptoms of each state. Like signs produced by both abnormalities will be additive, and opposing signs will tend to nullify one an-

other. For example, the tendency for the body temperature to fall with an extracellular volume deficit may be counteracted by the tendency for it to rise with severe hypernatremia.

One of the more common mixed abnormalities is an extracellular fluid deficit and hyponatremia. This state is readily produced in the patient who continues to drink water while losing large volumes of gastrointestinal fluids. It may also occur in the postoperative period when gastrointestinal losses are replaced with inadequate volumes of only 5% dextrose in water or a hypotonic sodium solution. An extracellular volume deficit accompanied by hypernatremia may be produced by the loss of a large amount of hypotonic salt solution, such as sweat, in the absence of fluid intake.

The prolonged administration of excessive quantities of sodium salts with restricted water intake may result in an extracellular volume excess and hypernatremia. This may also occur when pure water losses (such as insensible loss of water from the skin and lungs) are replaced with sodium-containing solutions only. Similarly, the excessive administration of water or hypotonic salt solutions to the patient with oliguric renal failure may rapidly produce an extracellular volume excess and hyponatremia.

Normally functioning kidneys may minimize these changes to some extent and compensate for many of the imprecise replacements associated with parenteral fluid administration. In contrast, the patient in anuric or oliguric renal failure is particularly prone to develop these mixed volume and osmolar concentration abnormalities. Fluid and electrolyte management in these patients, therefore, must be precise. Unfortunately, the fact that a patient with normal kidneys who develops a significant volume deficit may be in a state of "functional" renal failure is often not appreciated. As the volume deficit progresses, the glomerular filtration rate falls precipitously, and the kidneys' unique functions for maintaining fluid homeostasis are lost. These changes may occur with only a mild volume deficit in the elderly patient with borderline renal function. In these elderly patients, the blood urea nitrogen level may rise higher than 100 mg/dL in response to the fluid deficit with a concomitant rise in the serum creatinine level. Fortunately, these changes are usually reversible with early and adequate correction of the extracellular fluid volume deficit.

Composition Changes

Compositional abnormalities of importance include changes in acid-base balance and concentration changes of potassium, calcium, and magnesium.

ACID-BASE BALANCE

The pH (the negative logarithm of the hydrogen ion concentration) of the body fluids is normally maintained within narrow limits in spite of the large load of acid produced endogenously as a by-product of body metabolism. The acids are neutralized efficiently by several buffer systems and subsequently excreted by the lungs and kidneys.

The important buffers include proteins and phosphates, which play a primary role in maintaining intracellular pH, and the bicarbonate–carbonic acid system, which operates principally in the extracellular fluid space. The proteins and hemoglobin have only minor influence in the extracellular fluid space, but the latter is of prime significance as an intracellular buffer in the red cell.

A buffer system consists of a weak acid or base and the salt of that acid or base. The buffering effect is the result of the formation of an amount of weak acid or base equivalent to the amount of strong acid or base added to the system. The resultant change in pH is considerably less than if the substance were added to water alone. Thus, inorganic acids (e.g., hydrochloric, sulfuric, phosphoric) and organic acids (e.g., lactic, pyruvic, keto acids) combine with base bicarbonate producing the sodium salt of the acid and carbonic acid:

$$HCl + NaHCO_3 \longrightarrow NaCl + H_2CO_3$$

The carbonic acid formed is then excreted via the lungs as CO_2. The inorganic acid anions are excreted by the kidneys with hydrogen or as ammonium salts. The organic acid anions generally are metabolized as the underlying disorder is corrected, although some renal excretion may occur with high levels.

The functions of the buffer systems are expressed in the Henderson-Hasselbalch equation, which defines the pH in terms of the ratio of the salt and acid. The pH of the extracellular fluid is defined primarily by the ratio of the amount of base bicarbonate (majority as sodium bicarbonate) to the amount of carbonic acid (related to the CO_2 content of alveolar air) present in the blood:

$$pH = pK + \log\frac{BHCO_3}{H_2CO_3} = \frac{27 \text{ meq/L}}{1.33 \text{ meq/L}} = \frac{20}{1} = 7.4$$

pK represents the dissociation constant of carbonic acid in the presence of base bicarbonate and by measurement is 6.1. At a body pH of 7.4, the ratio must be 20:1, as depicted. From a chemical standpoint, this is an inefficient buffer system, but the unusual property of CO_2 to behave as an acid or change to a neutral gas subsequently excreted by the lungs makes it quite efficient biologically.

As long as the 20:1 ratio is maintained, regardless of the absolute values, the pH will remain at 7.4. When an acid is added to the system, the concentration of bicarbonate (the numerator in the Henderson-Hasselbalch equation) will decrease. Ventilation will immediately increase to eliminate larger quantities of CO_2 with a subsequent decrease in the carbonic acid (the denominator in the Henderson-Hasselbalch equation) until the 20:1 ratio is reestablished. Slower, more complete compensation is effected by the kidneys with increased excretion of acid salts and retention of bicarbonate. The reverse will occur if an alkali is added to the system. Respiratory acidosis and alkalosis are produced by disturbances of ventilation, with an increase or decrease in the denominator and a resultant change of the 20:1 ratio. Compensation is primarily renal, with a retention of bicarbonate and increased excretion of acid salts in respiratory acidosis and the reverse process in respiratory alkalosis.

The four types of acid-base disturbances are listed in Table 2-6. Use of the CO_2 combining power (approximates the plasma bicarbonate) or CO_2 content (includes bicarbonate, carbonic acid, and dissolved CO_2) and knowledge of the patient's disease may allow an accurate diagnosis in the uncomplicated case. Use of the serum CO_2 content or CO_2 combining power alone is generally inadequate as an index of acid-base balance. This test principally reflects the level of plasma bicarbonate, since dissolved CO_2 and carbonic acid contribute no more than a few millimoles under most circumstances. In the acute phase, therefore, respiratory acidosis or alkalosis may exist without any change in the serum CO_2 content; determinations of the pH and P_{CO_2} from a freshly drawn arterial blood sample are necessary for diagnosis.

Unfortunately, more complex acid-base disturbances are frequently encountered. Combinations of respiratory and metabolic changes occur and may represent compensation for the initial acid-base disturbance or may indicate two or more coexisting primary disorders (Table 2-7).

As previously noted, a knowledge of the pH, bicarbonate concentration, and P_{CO_2} will allow an accurate diagnosis of most acid-base disturbances. However, the clinical interpretation of these measurements is associated with some inherent problems. Although the arterial P_{CO_2} is considered an accurate index of primary respiratory disturbances, changes in the level may represent compensation for a primary metabolic alteration. Thus, a depressed P_{CO_2} (below 40 mmHg) is characteristic of respiratory alkalosis but also represents the normal compensatory response to a metabolic acidosis. Similarly, the level of plasma bicarbonate cannot be regarded exclusively as an index of metabolic disturbances. An elevated plasma bicarbonate level may indicate a primary metabolic alkalosis or a compensatory response to chronic respiratory

Table 2-6. ACIDOSIS-ALKALOSIS

Type of acid-base disorder	Defect	Common causes	$\dfrac{BHCO_3}{H_2CO_3} = \dfrac{20}{1}$	Compensation
Respiratory acidosis	Retention of CO_2 (Decreased alveolar ventilation)	Depression of respiratory center—morphine, CNS injury Pulmonary disease—emphysema, pneumonia	↑ Denominator Ratio less than 20:1	Renal Retention of bicarbonate, excretion of acid salts, increased ammonia formation Chloride shift into red cells
Respiratory alkalosis	Excessive loss of CO_2 (increased alveolar ventilation)	Hyperventilation: Emotional, severe pain, assisted ventilation, encephalitis	↓ Denominator Ratio greater than 20:1	Renal Excretion of bicarbonate, retention of acid salts, decreased ammonia formation
Metabolic acidosis	Retention of fixed acids or Loss of base bicarbonate	Diabetes, azotemia, lactic acid accumulation, starvation Diarrhea, small bowel fistulae	↓ Numerator Ratio less than 20:1	Pulmonary (rapid) Increase rate and depth of breathing Renal (slow) As in respiratory acidosis
Metabolic alkalosis	Loss of fixed acids Gain of base bicarbonate Potassium depletion	Vomiting or gastric suction with pyloric obstruction Excessive intake of bicarbonate Diuretics	↑ Numerator Ratio greater than 20:1	Pulmonary (rapid) Decrease rate and depth of breathing Renal (slow) As in respiratory alkalosis

acidosis. Astrup and colleagues proposed the use of the standard bicarbonate and base excess values. Base excess (or deficit) directly expresses, in meq/L, the amount of fixed base (or acid) added to each liter of blood. This defines the *metabolic* component of acid-base disorders.

One useful approach to defining pure, combined, or compensated disturbances relates measured changes in P_{CO_2} and pH to calculated changes that would be expected from pure etiologies. Within reasonable physiologic ranges, a 10-torr change in P_{CO_2} yields a 0.08 change in pH from the normal values of P_{CO_2} (40 torr) and pH (7.4).

RESPIRATORY ACIDOSIS. This condition is associated with retention of CO_2 secondary to decreased alveolar

Table 2-7. RESPIRATORY AND METABOLIC COMPONENTS OF ACID-BASE DISORDERS

Type of acid-base disorder	Acute (uncompensated)			Chronic (partially compensated)		
	pH	P_{CO_2} (respiratory component)	Plasma HCO_3^-* (metabolic component)	pH	P_{CO_2} (respiratory component)	Plasma HCO_3^-* (metabolic component)
Respiratory acidosis	⇊	⇈	N	↓	⇈	↑
Respiratory alkalosis	⇈	⇊	N	↑	⇊	↓
Metabolic acidosis	⇊	N	⇊	↓	↓	↓
Metabolic alkalosis	⇈	N	⇈	↑	↑?	↑

* Measured as standard bicarbonate, whole blood buffer base, CO_2 content, or CO_2 combining power. The *base excess value* is positive when the standard bicarbonate is above normal and negative when the standard bicarbonate is below normal.

ventilation. The more common causes are listed in Table 2-6. Initially, the arterial P_{CO_2} is elevated (usually above 50 mmHg), and the serum bicarbonate concentration (measured as CO_2 content) is normal. In the chronic form, the P_{CO_2} remains elevated, and the bicarbonate concentration rises as renal compensation occurs.

This problem may be particularly serious in the patient with chronic pulmonary disease in whom preexisting respiratory acidosis may be accentuated in the postoperative period. A number of conditions resulting in inadequate ventilation (e.g., airway obstruction, atelectasis, pneumonia, pleural effusion, pain from an upper abdominal incision, or abdominal distention limiting diaphragmatic excursion) may exist singly or in combination to produce respiratory acidosis. Although restlessness, hypertension, and tachycardia in the immediate postoperative period may be due to pain, similar signs indicate inadequate ventilation with hypercapnia. The use of narcotics in this situation will compound the problem by depressing respiration.

Management involves prompt correction of the pulmonary defect, when feasible, and measures to ensure adequate ventilation. Endotracheal intubation and mechanical ventilation are occasionally necessary to achieve this objective. Strict attention to tracheobronchial hygiene during the postoperative period is an important preventive measure in all patients, particularly those with chronic pulmonary disease. Encouraging deep breathing and coughing, using humidified air to prevent inspissation of secretions, and avoiding oversedation are all indicated.

RESPIRATORY ALKALOSIS. Respiratory alkalosis is a more common problem in the surgical patient than previously recognized. Hyperventilation due to apprehension, pain, hypoxia, central nervous system injury, and assisted ventilation are all common causes. Any of these conditions may cause a rapid decrease in the arterial P_{CO_2} and increase in serum pH. The serum bicarbonate concentration is normal in the acute phase, but falls with compensation if the condition persists.

The majority of patients who require ventilatory support in the postoperative period will develop varying degrees of respiratory alkalosis. This may be inadvertent, due to improper use of the mechanical respirator, or it may occur during attempts to raise the P_{O_2} in a hypoxic patient. Proper management of the patient on a mechanical ventilator requires frequent measurements of blood gases and appropriate corrections of the ventilatory pattern when indicated. The arterial P_{CO_2} should not be allowed to fall below 30 mmHg, as serious complications may occur, particularly in the presence of a complicating hypokalemia or metabolic alkalosis. Generally, the P_{CO_2} can be maintained at an acceptable level by proper adjustments of the ventilatory rate and volume.

The dangers of a severe respiratory alkalosis are those related to potassium depletion and include the development of ventricular arrhythmias and fibrillation, particularly in patients who are digitalized or have preexisting hypokalemia. Other complications include a shift of the oxyhemoglobin dissociation curve to the left, which limits the ability of hemoglobin to unload oxygen at the tissue level except at low tissue oxygen tensions, and the development of tetany and convulsions if the level of ionized calcium is significantly depressed. The development of hypokalemia may be quite sudden and is related to entry of potassium ions into the cells in exchange for hydrogen and an excessive urinary potassium loss in exchange for sodium. Severe and persistent respiratory alkalosis is often difficult to correct and may be associated with a poor prognosis because of the underlying cause of hyperventilation. Treatment is primarily directed toward preventing the condition by the proper use of mechanical ventilation and correcting preexisting potassium deficits.

METABOLIC ACIDOSIS. Metabolic acidosis results from the retention or gain of fixed acids (diabetic ketoacidosis, lactic acidosis, azotemia) or the loss of base bicarbonate (diarrhea, small bowel fistula, renal insufficiency with inability to resorb bicarbonate). The excess of hydrogen ion results in lower pH and serum bicarbonate concentration. The initial compensation is pulmonary, with an increase of the rate and depth of breathing and depression of the arterial P_{CO_2}.

Renal damage may interfere with the important role of the kidneys in the regulation of acid-base balance. The kidneys serve a vital function in this regard through the excretion of nitrogenous waste products and acid metabolites and the resorption of bicarbonates. If renal damage occurs and these functions are lost, metabolic acidosis develops rapidly and may be difficult to control.

With normal kidneys, metabolic acidosis may develop when the capacity of the kidneys for handling a large chloride is exceeded. This is particularly common in patients who have excessive losses of alkaline gastrointestinal fluids (biliary, pancreatic, small bowel secretions) and are maintained on parenteral fluids for an extended period of time. Continued replacement of these losses with fluids having an inappropriate chloride-bicarbonate ratio, such as isotonic sodium chloride solution, will not correct the pH change; the use of a balanced salt solution, such as lactated Ringer's, is indicated.

One of the most common causes of severe metabolic acidosis in surgical patients is acute circulatory failure with accumulation of lactic acid. This is a reflection of tissue hypoxia due to inadequate perfusion, although it is only one of the manifestations of cellular dysfunction. Acute hemorrhagic shock may result in a rapid and profound drop in the pH, and attempts to raise the blood pressure with vasopressors will simply compound the problem by further compromising tissue perfusion. Similarly, attempts to correct the acidosis by the infusion of large quantities of sodium bicarbonate without restoration of flow are futile. Following restoration of adequate tissue perfusion by proper volume replacement, the lactic acid is quickly metabolized and the pH returned to normal. The use of lactated Ringer's solution to replace the extracellular fluid deficit incurred with hemorrhagic shock concomitant with administration of whole blood does not accentuate the lactic acidosis. Instead, there is a rapid decrease in the serum lactate and return of pH toward normal, which is not the case when whole blood alone is used.

The indiscriminate use of sodium bicarbonate during the resuscitation of patients in hypovolemic shock is discouraged for several reasons. A mild metabolic alkalosis is a common finding following resuscitation, in part due to the alkalinizing effects of blood transfusions and the administration of lactated Ringer's solution. After infusion (and partial restoration of hepatic blood flow), the citrate contained in the transfused blood and the lactate in lactated Ringer's solution are metabolized and bicarbonate is formed. The organic acidosis (lactic acid) that developed during the shock episode is rapidly cleared once adequate tissue perfusion is restored. Lactic acid production ceases, the hydrogen ion load is buffered and excreted via the lungs as CO_2, and the organic anion, lactate, is metabolized to bicarbonate by the liver. If excessive quantities of sodium bicarbonate are administered simultaneously, severe metabolic alkalosis can result. An alkaline pH may be highly undesirable in this situation, particularly in patients with hypoxia or low fixed cardiac outputs, because it shifts the oxyhemoglobin dissociation curve to the left. Other factors that tend to shift the oxygen dissociation curve to the left in this situation include the depressed level of erythrocyte 2,3-diphosphoglycerate in the transfused blood and the development of hypothermia. If the curve shifts far enough to the left, significant interference with oxygen unloading at the tissue level may occur.

The treatment of metabolic acidosis, therefore, should be directed toward correction of the underlying disorder when possible. Bicarbonate therapy properly may be reserved for the treatment of severe metabolic acidosis, particularly following cardiac arrest, when partial correction of the pH may be essential to restore myocardial function. Recent studies indicate that the acidosis accompanying cardiac arrest is well compensated for a significant period of time if the patient is well ventilated and not previously acidotic. In addition, the administration of bicarbonate in the usual recommended doses may induce an acute and severe hypernatremia and hyperosmolarity. Thus bicarbonate should be used judiciously during cardiac arrest, the initial dose of bicarbonate not exceeding 50 mL of 7.5% solution (45 meq $NaHCO_3$ containing 90 mO) and the decision for additional doses being based on measurements of pH and P_{CO_2} when possible.

Similarly, pH correction of more protracted states of metabolic acidosis may be indicated but should be accomplished slowly. Frequent measurements of serum electrolytes and blood pH are the best guides to therapy, since a satisfactory formula to estimate the amount of alkali needed has not been devised.

METABOLIC ALKALOSIS. Metabolic alkalosis results from the loss of fixed acids or the gain of bicarbonate and is aggravated by any preexisting potassium depletion. Both the pH and plasma bicarbonate concentration are elevated. Compensation for metabolic alkalosis is primarily by renal mechanisms, since respiratory compensation is generally small and cannot be detected in most patients. Rarely, hypercapnia may represent a compensatory response to metabolic alkalosis in patients without chronic pulmonary disease. When this is suspected, rapid reduction in P_{CO_2} by mechanical ventilation should be avoided. Rather, the P_{CO_2} will fall as the metabolic alkalosis is corrected.

The majority of patients with metabolic alkalosis have some degree of hypokalemia, due in part to influx of potassium ions into the cells, as hydrogen ions efflux into the serum. The dangers of metabolic alkalosis are the same as discussed with respiratory alkalosis.

A problem commonly encountered in the surgical patient is hypochloremic, hypokalemic metabolic alkalosis resulting from persistent vomiting or gastric suction in the patient with pyloric obstruction. Unlike vomiting with an open pylorus involving a combined loss of gastric, pancreatic, biliary, and intestinal secretions, this entity results in loss of fluid with high chloride and hydrogen ion concentrations in relation to sodium. Initially, the urinary excretion of bicarbonate increases to compensate for the alkalosis. This increase in urinary bicarbonate excretion results from net hydrogen ion resorption by the renal tubular cells, with accompanying potassium ion excretion. As the volume deficit progresses, aldosterone-mediated sodium resorption is accompanied by potassium excretion. The resulting hypokalemia leads to excretion of hydrogen ion in place of potassium ion by this mechanism, producing paradoxic aciduria. The net result is a self-perpetuating alkalosis with hypokalemia. Proper management includes replacement of the extracellular fluid volume deficit with isotonic sodium chloride solution in addition to replacement of potassium. Volume repletion should be started and a good urine output obtained before potassium is administered.

Rarely, severe hypokalemic metabolic alkalosis in a patient with pyloric outlet obstruction may be refractory to standard therapy. This occurs most often in patients who also have severe hypochloremia and several liters of nasogastric drainage daily. In the past, the infusion of ammonium chloride or arginine hydrochloride was the usual method for increasing the level of nonvolatile acids. However, infusion of the first may produce ammonia toxicity, and the latter solution is no longer available commercially. Recently, the use of $0.1N$ to $0.2N$ hydrochloric acid has been shown to be safe and effective therapy for correction of severe, resistant metabolic alkalosis. The infusion should be administered over a 6- to 24-h period, with measurements of pH, P_{CO_2}, and serum electrolytes every 4 h. Generally, 1 or 2 L of solution over a period of 24 h is sufficient, although one should not hesitate to infuse additional hydrochloric acid when the need is based on appropriate clinical and laboratory evidence. Temporary control of the alkalosis with this method is usually successful, but the underlying cause should be controlled as soon as possible.

POTASSIUM ABNORMALITIES

The normal dietary intake of potassium is approximately 50 to 100 meq daily, and in the absence of hypokalemia, the majority of this is excreted in the urine. Ninety-eight percent of the potassium in the body is located within the intracellular compartment at a concentration of approximately 150 meq/L, and it is the major cation of intracellular water. Although the total extracellular potassium in a 70-kg male would approximate only 63 meq (4.5 meq/L × 14 L), this small amount is critical to cardiac and neuromuscular function. In addition, the turnover rate in the extracellular fluid compartment may be extremely rapid.

The intracellular and extracellular distribution of potassium is influenced by many factors. Significant quantities of intracellular potassium are released into the extracellular space in response to severe injury or surgical stress, acidosis, and the catabolic state. A significant rise in serum potassium may occur in these states in the presence of oliguric or anuric renal failure, but dangerous hyperkalemia (greater than 6 meq/L) is rarely encountered if renal function is normal. After severe trauma, however, normal or excessive urinary volumes may not reflect the ability of the kidney to clear solutes or to excrete potassium. (See the section High-Output Renal Failure.)

HYPERKALEMIA. The signs of a significant hyperkalemia are limited to the cardiovascular and gastrointestinal systems. The gastrointestinal symptoms include nausea, vomiting, intermittent intestinal colic, and diarrhea. The cardiovascular signs are apparent on the electrocardiogram initially, with high peaked T waves, widened QRS complex, and depressed ST segments. Disappearance of T waves, heart block, and diastolic cardiac arrest may develop with increasing levels of potassium.

Treatment of hyperkalemia consists of immediate measures to reduce the serum potassium level, withholding of exogenous potassium, and correction of the underlying cause if possible. Temporary suppression of the myocardial effects of a sudden rapid rise of potassium level can be accomplished by the intravenous administration of 1 g of 10 percent calcium gluconate under ECG monitoring. Serum potassium levels may be transiently decreased by administration of bicarbonate and glucose with insulin (45 meq $NaHCO_3$ in 1000 mL/$D_{10}W$ with 20 units regular insulin), both of which promote cellular uptake of potassium. However, the definitive treatment of hyperkalemia requires either the enteral administration of cation exchange resins (kayexalate) or dialysis.

HYPOKALEMIA. The more common problem in the surgical patient is hypokalemia, which may occur as a result of (1) excessive renal excretion, (2) movement of potassium into cells, (3) prolonged administration of potassium-free parenteral fluids with continued obligatory renal loss of potassium (20 meq/day or more), (4) total parenteral hyperalimentation with inadequate potassium replacement, and (5) loss in gastrointestinal secretions.

Potassium plays an important role in the regulation of acid-base balance. Increased renal excretion occurs with both respiratory and metabolic alkalosis. Potassium is in competition with hydrogen ion for renal tubular excretion in exchange for sodium ion. Thus, in alkalosis, the increased potassium ion excretion in exchange for sodium ion permits hydrogen ion conservation. Hypokalemia itself may produce a metabolic alkalosis, since an increase in excretion of hydrogen ions occurs when the concentra-

tion of potassium in the tubular cell is low. In addition, movement of hydrogen ions into the cells as a consequence of potassium loss is partly responsible for the alkalosis. In metabolic acidosis the reverse process occurs, and the excess hydrogen ion exchanges for sodium with retention of greater amounts of potassium.

Renal tubular excretion of potassium ion is increased when large quantities of sodium are available for excretion. The more sodium ion available for resorption, the more potassium is exchanged for it in the lumen. Potassium requirements for prolonged or massive isotonic fluid volume replacement are increased, probably on this basis.

The renal excretion of potassium may be small when compared with the amount of potassium that may be lost in gastrointestinal secretions. The amount per liter in various types of gastrointestinal fluids is shown in Table 2-3. Although the average potassium concentration of some of these fluids is relatively low, significant hypokalemia will result if potassium-free fluids are used for replacement.

Hypokalemia also may be a serious problem in the patient maintained on intravenous nutrition. Large quantities of supplemental potassium generally are necessary to restore depleted intracellular stores and to meet the requirements for tissue synthesis during the anabolic phase.

In summary, most of the factors that tend to influence potassium metabolism result in excess excretion, and a tendency toward hypokalemia occurs frequently in the surgical patient except when shock or acidosis interferes with the normal renal handling of potassium.

The signs of potassium deficit are related to failure of normal contractility of skeletal, smooth, and cardiac muscle and include weakness that may progress to flaccid paralysis, diminished to absent tendon reflexes, and paralytic ileus. Sensitivity to digitalis with cardiac arrhythmias and electrocardiographic signs of low voltage, flattening of T waves, and depression of ST segments are characteristic. Signs of potassium deficit may be masked by those of a severe extracellular fluid volume deficit. Repletion of the volume deficit may further aggravate the situation by lowering the serum potassium level secondary to dilution.

The treatment of hypokalemia involves, first, prevention of this state. In the replacement of gastrointestinal fluids, it is safe to replace the upper limits of loss, since an excess is readily handled by the patient with normal renal function. No more than 40 meq should be added to a liter of intravenous fluid, and the rate of administration should not exceed 40 meq/h unless the electrocardiogram is being monitored. In the absence of specific indications, potassium should not be given to the oliguric patient or during the first 24 h following severe surgical stress or trauma.

CALCIUM ABNORMALITIES

The majority of the 1000 to 1200 g of body calcium in the average-sized adult is found in the bone in the form of phosphate and carbonate. Normal daily intake of calcium is between 1 and 3 g. Most of this is excreted via the gastrointestinal tract, and 200 mg or less is excreted in the urine daily. The normal serum level is between 8.5 and 10.5 mg/dL, and approximately half of this is not ionized and is bound to plasma protein. An additional nonionized fraction (5 percent) is bound to other substances in the plasma and interstitial fluid, whereas the remaining 45 percent is the ionized portion that is responsible for neuromuscular stability. Determination of the plasma protein level, therefore, is essential for proper analysis of the serum calcium level. The ratio of ionized to nonionized calcium is also related to the pH; acidosis causes an increase in the ionized fraction, whereas alkalosis causes a decrease.

Disturbances of calcium metabolism generally are not a problem in the uncomplicated postoperative patient, with the exception of skeletal loss during prolonged immobilization. Routine administration of calcium to the surgical patient, therefore, is not needed in the absence of specific indications.

HYPOCALCEMIA. The symptoms of hypocalcemia may be seen at serum levels less than 8 mg/dL, and include numbness and tingling of the circumoral region and the tips of the fingers and toes. The signs are of neuromuscular origin and include hyperactive tendon reflexes, positive Chvostek's sign, muscle and abdominal cramps, tetany with carpopedal spasm, convulsions (with severe deficit), and prolongation of the Q-T interval on the electrocardiogram.

The common causes include acute pancreatitis, massive soft tissue infections (necrotizing fasciitis), acute and chronic renal failure, pancreatic and small intestinal fistulas, and hypoparathyroidism. Transient hypocalcemia is a frequent occurrence in the hyperparathyroid patient following removal of a parathyroid adenoma, owing to atrophy of the remaining glands and avid bone uptake. Asymptomatic hypocalcemia may occur with hypoproteinemia (normal ionized fraction), whereas symptoms may appear with a normal serum calcium level in a patient with severe alkalosis. The latter is due to a decrease in the physiologically active or ionized fraction of total serum calcium. Calcium levels also may fall with a severe depletion of magnesium.

Treatment is directed toward correction of the underlying cause with concomitant repletion of the deficit. Acute symptoms may be relieved by the intravenous administration of calcium gluconate or calcium chloride. Calcium lactate may be given orally, with or without supplemental vitamin D, in the patient requiring prolonged replacement. The routine administration of calcium during massive transfusions of blood remains controversial and reflects a paucity of studies where calcium *ion* levels are measured. In the majority of studies, calcium ion concentrations have been estimated from measured *total* serum calcium levels. Presently, available data indicate that the majority of patients receiving blood transfusions do not require calcium supplementation. The binding of ionized calcium by citrate is generally compensated for by the mobilization of calcium from body stores. For patients receiving blood as rapidly as 500 mL every 5 to 10 min, however, calcium administration is recommended. An

appropriate dose, from the data of Moore, is 0.2 g of calcium chloride (2 mL of 10% calcium chloride solution), administered intravenously in a separate line, for every 500 mL of blood transfused. To avoid dangerous levels of hypercalcemia, this dose of calcium is recommended only while blood is being transfused at the rate noted above. Additionally, the total dose of calcium generally should not exceed 3 g unless there is objective evidence of hypocalcemia. Larger doses are rarely indicated since there is some mobilization of calcium and citrate breakdown with release of calcium ion even with shock and inadequate peripheral perfusion. During massive transfusions, some attempt should be made to monitor the calcium level. A rough approximation of calcium ion concentration can be obtained by monitoring the Q-T interval on the ECG, although techniques for the rapid measurement of calcium ion concentration are now available.

HYPERCALCEMIA. The symptoms of hypercalcemia are rather vague and of gastrointestinal, renal, musculoskeletal, and central nervous system origin. The early manifestations of hypercalcemia include easy fatigue, lassitude, weakness of varying degree, anorexia, nausea, vomiting, and weight loss. With higher serum calcium levels, lassitude gives way to somnambulism, stupor, and finally coma. Other symptoms include severe headaches, pains in the back and extremities, thirst, polydipsia, and polyuria. The critical level for serum calcium is between 16 and 20 mg/100 mL, and unless treatment is instituted promptly, the symptoms may rapidly progress to death. The two major causes of hypercalcemia are hyperparathyroidism and cancer with bony metastasis. The latter is most frequently seen in the patient with metastatic breast cancer who is receiving estrogen therapy.

The treatment of acute hypercalcemia crisis is an emergency. Measures to lower the serum calcium level are instituted immediately while preparations are being made for more definitive treatment. Rapid correction of the associated extracellular fluid volume deficit will immediately lower the serum calcium level by dilution and by increased renal clearance that may be augmented by furosemide administration. Other measures that may be of temporary benefit include the use of calcitonin, mithramycin, steroids, or hemodialysis. The definitive treatment of acute hypercalcemic crisis in patients with hyperparathyroidism is immediate surgery.

Treatment of hypercalcemia in the patient with metastatic cancer is primarily that of prevention. The serum calcium level is checked frequently; if it is elevated, the patient is placed on a low-calcium diet, and measures to ensure adequate hydration are instituted.

MAGNESIUM ABNORMALITIES

The total body content of magnesium in the average adult is approximately 2000 meq, about half of which is incorporated in bone and only slowly exchangeable. The distribution of magnesium is similar to that of potassium, the major portion being intracellular. Serum magnesium concentration normally ranges between 1.5 and 2.5 meq/L. The normal dietary intake of magnesium is approximately 20 meq (240 mg) daily. The larger part is excreted in the feces, and the remainder in the urine. The kidneys show a remarkable ability to conserve magnesium; on a magnesium-free diet, renal excretion of this ion may be less than 1 meq/day.

MAGNESIUM DEFICIENCY. Magnesium deficiency is known to occur with starvation, malabsorption syndromes, protracted losses of gastrointestinal fluid, and prolonged intravenous fluid therapy with magnesium-free solutions, and during total parenteral nutrition when inadequate quantities of magnesium have been added to the solutions. Other causes include acute pancreatitis, treatment of diabetic ketoacidosis, primary aldosteronism, chronic alcoholism, amphotericin B therapy, and a protracted course following thermal injury.

The magnesium ion is essential for proper function of most enzyme systems, and depletion is characterized by neuromuscular and central nervous system hyperactivity. The signs and symptoms are quite similar to those of calcium deficiency, including hyperactive tendon reflexes, muscle tremors, and tetany with a positive Chvostek sign. Progression to delirium and convulsions may occur with a severe deficit. A concomitant calcium deficiency occasionally is noted, and will be refractory to treatment in the absence of magnesium repletion.

The diagnosis of magnesium deficiency depends on an awareness of the syndrome and clinical recognition of the symptoms. Laboratory confirmation is available but not reliable, as the syndrome may exist in the presence of a normal serum magnesium level. The possibility of magnesium deficiency should always be considered in the surgical patient who exhibits disturbed neuromuscular or cerebral activity in the postoperative period. This is particularly important in patients who have had protracted dysfunction of the gastrointestinal tract with long-term maintenance on parenteral fluids and in patients on parenteral hyperalimentation. Routine magnesium is always indicated in the management of these patients.

Treatment of magnesium deficiency is by the parenteral administration of magnesium sulfate or magnesium chloride solution. If renal function is normal, as much as 2 meq of magnesium/kg of body weight can be administered daily by the intravenous or intramuscular route in the face of severe depletion. The intravenous route is preferable for the initial treatment of a severe symptomatic deficit. The solution is prepared by the addition of 80 meq of magnesium sulfate (20 mL of 50% solution containing 4 meq/mL magnesium) to a liter of intravenous fluid and is administered over a 4-h period. If the patient is not symptomatic, the infusion should be given over a longer period of time. The possibility of acute magnesium toxicity should be kept in mind when giving this ion intravenously. When large doses are given, the heart rate, blood pressure, respiration, and ECG should be monitored closely for signs of magnesium toxicity, which could lead to cardiac arrest. It is advisable to have calcium chloride or calcium gluconate available to counteract any adverse effects of a rapidly rising serum magnesium level.

Partial or complete relief of symptoms may follow this infusion as a result of increased concentration of magnesium ion in the extracellular fluid compartment, although continued replacement over a 1- to 3-week period is necessary to replenish the intracellular compartment. For this purpose and for the asymptomatic patient who may have significant magnesium depletion, 10 to 20 meq of 50% magnesium sulfate solution may be given daily by the intramuscular route, in intravenous fluids, or orally as magnesium oxide (800 mg). When intramuscular magnesium sulfate is used, it should be given in divided doses or at multiple sites, since the intramuscular injection of this salt is painful. Following complete repletion of intracellular magnesium and in the absence of abnormal loss, balance may be maintained by the administration of as little as 4 meq of magnesium ion daily. The amount of magnesium supplementation required for patients on parenteral hyperalimentation varies but approximates 12 to 24 meq daily for the average patient.

Magnesium ion should not be given to the oliguric patient or in the presence of severe volume deficit unless actual magnesium depletion is demonstrated. If given to a patient with renal insufficiency, considerably smaller dosages are used, and the patient is carefully observed for signs or symptoms of toxicity.

MAGNESIUM EXCESS. Symptomatic hypermagnesemia, although rare, is most commonly seen with severe renal insufficiency. Retention and accumulation of magnesium may occur in any patient with impaired glomerular or renal tubular function, and the presence of acidosis may rapidly compound the situation. Serum magnesium levels tend to parallel changes in potassium concentration in these cases. In patients on ordinary dietary intakes of magnesium, increased serum concentrations of the ion do not occur until the glomerular filtration rate falls below 30 mL/min. Magnesium-containing antacids and laxatives (milk of magnesia, epsom salts, Gelusil, Maalox) are commonly administered in quantities sufficient to produce toxic serum levels of magnesium where impaired renal function is present. Other conditions that may be associated with symptomatic hypermagnesemia include early thermal injury, massive trauma or surgical stress, severe extracellular volume deficit, and severe acidosis.

The early signs and symptoms include lethargy and weakness with progressive loss of deep tendon reflexes. Interference with cardiac conduction occurs with increasing levels of magnesium and changes in the electrocardiogram (increased P-R interval, widened QRS complex, and elevated T waves) resemble those seen with hyperkalemia. Somnolence leading to coma and muscular paralysis occur in the later stages, and death is usually caused by respiratory or cardiac arrest.

Treatment consists of immediate measures to lower the serum magnesium level by correcting coexisting acidosis, replenishing preexisting extracellular volume deficit, and withholding exogenous magnesium. Acute symptoms may be temporarily controlled by the slow intravenous administration of 5 to 10 meq of calcium chloride or calcium gluconate. If elevated levels or symptoms persist, peritoneal dialysis or hemodialysis is indicated.

A readily available isotonic salt solution for replacing gastrointestinal losses and repairing preexisting volume deficits, in the absence of gross abnormalities of concentration and composition, is lactated Ringer's solution. This solution is "physiologic" and contains 130 meq/L sodium balanced by 109 meq/L chloride and 28 meq/L lactate. This fluid has minimal effects on normal body fluid composition and pH even when infused in large quantities. In a study of 52 patients in hemorrhagic shock, Canizaro et al. demonstrated a significant decrease in serum lactate levels and a return toward normal in serum pH during resuscitation with Ringer's lactate solution. The chief disadvantage of lactated Ringer's solution is the slight hyposmolarity with respect to sodium. Each liter of lactated Ringer's solution furnishes approximately 100 to 150 mL free water. This rarely presents a clinical problem if it is considered in calculating water replacement.

Normal saline is an isotonic solution of 0.9 percent sodium chloride and contains 154 meq/L sodium and 154 meq/L chloride. The high concentration of chloride above the normal serum concentration of 103 meq/L imposes on the kidneys an appreciable load of excess chloride that cannot be rapidly excreted. As such, infusion of a large volume of isotonic sodium chloride solution may induce or aggravate a preexisting acidosis by reducing the amount of bicarbonate anion in the body relative to the carbonic acid content. This solution is ideal, however, for the initial correction of an extracellular fluid volume deficit in the presence of hyponatremia, hypochloremia, and metabolic alkalosis.

A frequent choice for maintenance fluid in the postoperative period, 0.45% sodium chloride in 5% dextrose, provides free water for insensible losses and some sodium for renal adjustment of serum concentration. Potassium (10 to 30 meq/L) may be easily added and is increasingly provided as a prepackaged infusion with this solution for easy administration in the uncomplicated patient requiring a short period of parenteral fluids.

Solutions of 3% sodium chloride, 5% sodium chloride, or molar sodium lactate may be used to correct symptomatic hyponatremic states. The choice of anion (lactate or chloride) is determined by the accompanying acid-base derangement. The need for hydrochloric acid solutions in the treatment of an uncompensated metabolic alkalosis is extremely rare. Indications for its use include very shallow or slow breathing with cyanosis, severe tetany, or pH

greater than 7.55. Following the correction of concentration or compositional abnormalities using specific electrolyte solutions, a balanced salt solution is used to replenish the remaining volume deficit.

FLUID AND ELECTROLYTE THERAPY

Parenteral Solutions

There are many electrolyte solutions of varied compositions that are available for parenteral administration (Table 2-8). Several of the more commonly used solutions are discussed below. Choice of a particular fluid depends on the volume status of the patient and the type of concentration or compositional abnormality present.

Preoperative Fluid Therapy

Preoperative evaluation and correction of existing fluid disorders is an integral part of surgical care. An orderly approach to these problems requires an understanding of the common fluid disturbances associated with surgical illness and adherence to a few simple guidelines.

The analysis of a particular fluid disorder may be facilitated by categorizing the abnormalities into volume, concentration, and compositional changes. Although some disease states produce characteristic changes in fluid balance, much confusion may be avoided by regarding each disturbance as a separate entity. There are no shortcuts; close observation of the patient and frequent reevaluation of the clinical situation is the most rewarding approach. For example, volume changes cannot be accurately predicted from a knowledge of the level of serum sodium, since an extracellular fluid volume deficit or excess may exist with a normal, low, or high sodium concentration. Similarly, any of the four primary acid-base disturbances may be associated with any combination of volume and concentration abnormalities.

CORRECTION OF VOLUME CHANGES

Changes in the volume of extracellular fluid are the most frequent and important abnormalities encountered in the surgical patient. Depletion of the extracellular fluid

Table 2-8. COMPOSITION OF PARENTERAL FLUIDS
(Electrolyte Content, meq/L)

Solutions	Cations				Anions		Osmolality, mO
	Na	K	Ca	Mg	Cl	HCO₃	
Extracellular fluid	142	4	5	3	103	27	280–310
Lactated Ringer's	130	4	3	—	109	28*	273
0.9% sodium chloride	154	—	—	—	154	—	308
D₅ 45% sodium chloride	77	—	—	—	77	—	407
D₅W	—	—	—	—	—	—	253
M/6 sodium lactate	167	—	—	—	—	167*	334
3% sodium chloride	513	—	—	—	513	—	1026

* Present in solution as lactate that is converted to bicarbonate.

compartment without changes in concentration or composition is a common problem. The diagnosis of volume changes is made almost entirely on clinical grounds. The signs that will be present in an individual patient depend not only on the relative or absolute quantity of extracellular fluid that has been lost but also on the rapidity with which it is lost and the presence or absence of signs of associated disease.

Volume deficits in the surgical patient may result from external loss of fluids or from an internal redistribution of extracellular fluid into a nonfunctional compartment. Generally, it involves a combination of the two, but the internal redistribution is frequently overlooked.

The phenomenon of internal redistribution or translocation of extracellular fluid is peculiar to many surgical diseases; in the individual patient, the loss may be quite large. Although the concept of a "third space" is not new, it is generally considered only in relation to patients with massive ascites, burns, or crush injuries. Of more importance, however, is the "third space" loss into the peritoneum, the bowel wall, and other tissues with inflammatory lesions of the intraabdominal organs. The magnitude of these losses may not be fully appreciated without realization of the fact that the peritoneum alone has approximately 1 m^2 of surface area. A slight increase in thickness from sequestration of fluid, which would not be appreciated on casual observation, may result in a functional loss of several liters of fluid. Swelling of the bowel wall and mesentery and secretion of fluid into the lumen of the bowel will cause even larger losses. Similar deficits may occur with massive infection of the subcutaneous tissues (necrotizing fasciitis) or with severe crush injury.

These "parasitic" losses remain a part of the extracellular fluid space and may be measured as a slowly equilibrating volume. The term *nonfunctional* is used because the fluid is no longer able to participate in the normal functions of the extracellular compartment and may just as well have been lost externally. Any transfer of intracellular fluid to the extracellular compartment for replenishment of the loss is insignificant in the acute phase. The patient with ascites may have an enormous total extracellular fluid volume although the functional component is severely depleted. The same is true of extensive inflammatory or obstructive lesions of the gastrointestinal tract, although the loss is not as obvious. These losses will evoke the signs and symptoms of an extracellular fluid volume deficit with or without the concomitant external loss of fluids.

Exact quantification of these deficits is impossible and, at the present time, probably unnecessary. The defect can be estimated on the basis of the severity of the clinical signs. A mild deficit represents a loss of approximately 4 percent of body weight, a moderate loss is 6 to 8 percent of body weight, and a severe deficit is approximately 10 percent of body weight. It is important to reemphasize the fact that cardiovascular signs predominate when there is acute rapid loss of fluid from the extracellular fluid compartment with few or no tissue signs. In addition to the

estimated deficit, fluids lost during the period of treatment must be replaced.

Immediately following diagnosis of a volume deficit, prompt fluid replacement with a balanced salt solution should be started. Continuing thereapy is tailored to the response of the patient, based on frequent clinical examination. Reliance on a formula or single clinical sign to determine adequacy of resuscitation is fraught with danger. Rather, reversal of the signs of the volume deficit, combined with stabilization of the blood pressure and pulse, and an hourly urine volume of 30 to 50 mL are used as general guidelines. An adequate hourly urine output, although usually a reliable index of volume replacement, may be totally misleading. The excessive administration of glucose (over 50 g in a 2- to 3-h period) may result in osmotic diuresis, while an osmotic agent such as mannitol tends to produce urine at the expense of the vascular volume. Patients with chronic renal disease or incipient acute renal damage from shock and injury also may have inappropriately high urinary volumes. In addition, the rapid administration of salt solutions may transiently expand the intravascular volume, increase the glomerular filtration rate, and result in an immediate outpouring of urine, although the total extracellular fluid space remains quite depleted.

The choice of the proper fluid for replacement depends on the existence of concomitant concentration or compositional abnormalities. With pure extracellular fluid volume loss or when only minimal concentration or compositional abnormalities are present, the use of a balanced salt solution, such as lactated Ringer's, is desirable.

RATE OF FLUID ADMINISTRATION. This varies considerably, depending on the severity and type of fluid disturbance, the presence of continuing losses, and the cardiac status. In general, the most severe volume deficits may be safely replaced initially with isotonic solutions at rates up to 2000 mL/h, reducing the rate as the fluid status improves. Constant observation by a physician is mandatory when the administration exceeds 1000 mL/h. At these rates, a significant portion may be lost as urinary output owing to a transient overexpansion of the plasma volume.

In elderly patients, associated cardiovascular disorders do not preclude correction of existing volume deficits, but they do require slower, more careful correction with constant monitoring of the cardiopulmonary system. If urinary output is not promptly restored, this may require measurements of central filling pressures and cardiac output to prevent ongoing renal injury from overcautious volume restoration.

CORRECTION OF CONCENTRATION CHANGES

If severe *symptomatic* hyponatremia or hypernatremia complicates the volume loss, prompt correction of the concentration abnormality to the extent that symptoms are relieved is necessary. Volume replenishment should be accomplished with slower correction of the remaining concentration abnormality. For immediate correction of severe hyponatremia, 5% sodium chloride solution or molar sodium lactate solution is used, depending on the patient's acid-base status. In any case, the sodium deficit can be estimated by multiplying the decrease in serum sodium concentration below normal (in milliequivalents per liter) by the liters of total body water. Initially, up to one-half of the calculated amount of sodium may be administered slowly, followed by clinical and chemical reevaluation of the patient before any additional infusion of sodium salts.

Note that this estimate is based on total body water, since the effective osmotic pressure in the extracellular compartment cannot be increased without increasing this function proportionally in the intracellular compartment. Although absolute reliance on any formula is undesirable, proper use of this estimate will allow a safe quantitative approximation of the sodium deficit. Generally, only a portion of the total deficit is replaced initially to relieve acute symptoms. Further correction is facilitated when renal function is restored by correction of the volume deficit. If the total calculated deficit were given rapidly, severe hypervolemia might occur particularly in patients with limited cardiac reserve. In practice, the infusion of small, successive increments of hypertonic saline solution with frequent evaluation of the clinical response and serum sodium concentration is recommended.

In the treatment of moderate hyponatremia with an associated volume deficit, volume replacement can be started immediately with concomitant correction of the serum sodium deficit. Isotonic sodium chloride solution (normal saline) is used initially in the presence of metabolic alkalosis, whereas M/6 sodium lactate (167 meq/L each of sodium and lactate) is used to correct an associated acidosis. Only a few liters of these solutions may be necessary to correct the serum sodium concentration; the remainder of the volume deficit may be replaced with lactated Ringer's solution.

Treatment of hyponatremia associated with volume excess is by restriction of water. In the presence of severe symptomatic hyponatremia, a small amount of hypertonic salt solution may be infused cautiously to alleviate symptoms. As this will cause additional volume expansion, it is contraindicated in patients with limited cardiac reserve; peritoneal dialysis or hemodialysis is preferred in this situation.

For the correction of severe, symptomatic hypernatremia with an associated volume deficit, 5% dextrose in water may be infused slowly until symptoms are relieved. If the extracellular osmolarity is reduced too rapidly, however, convulsions and coma may result. For this reason, correction of hypernatremia concomitant with repletion of the volume deficit by half-strength sodium chloride or half-strength lactated Ringer's solution is safer in most cases. In the absence of a significant volume deficit, water should be administered cautiously since dangerous hypervolemia may result; constant observation and frequent determinations of the serum sodium concentration are indicated. The problem is somewhat simplified once a sufficient quantity of fluid has been given to permit renal excretion of the solute load.

COMPOSITION AND MISCELLANEOUS CONSIDERATIONS

Correction of existing potassium deficits should be started *after* an adequate urine output is obtained, particularly in the patient with metabolic alkalosis since this may be secondary to or aggravated by potassium depletion. Calcium and magnesium rarely are needed during preoperative resuscitation but should be given as indicated, particularly to patients with massive subcutaneous infections, acute pancreatitis, or chronic starvation.

Fluid abnormalities also must be suspected in the patient for whom an elective procedure is planned. Chronic illnesses frequently are associated with extracellular fluid volume deficits, and concentration and compositional changes are not uncommon. Correction of anemia and recognition of the fact that a concentrated blood volume may exist in the chronically debilitated patient is of obvious importance. The hematocrit increases approximately 3% following the infusion of one unit of packed cells into the adult of average size. The increase may be significantly greater in the patient with a contracted intravascular volume, indicating the need for concurrent volume replacement. Of additional importance is the prevention of volume depletion during the preoperative period. Prolonged periods of fluid restriction in preparation for various diagnostic procedures, the use of cathartics and enemas for preparation of the bowel, and osmotic diuresis from contrast agents may cause a significant acute loss of extracellular fluid. Prompt recognition and treatment of these losses before surgery is necessary to prevent complications during the operative period.

Of additional importance is the prevention of volume depletion during the preoperative period. Prolonged periods of fluid restriction in preparation for various diagnostic procedures, and the use of cathartics and enemas for preparation of the bowel may cause a significant acute loss of extracellular fluid. Prompt recognition and treatment of these losses is necessary to prevent complications during the operative period.

Intraoperative Fluid Management

If preoperative replacement of extracellular fluid volume has been incomplete, hypotension may develop promptly with the induction of anesthesia. This can be quite insidious, as the ability of the awake patient to compensate for mild volume deficit is revealed only when the compensatory mechanisms are abolished with anesthesia. This problem is prevented by maintaining base-line requirements and replacing abnormal losses of fluids and electrolytes by intravenous infusions in the preoperative period.

Blood lost during the operative procedure should be replaced steadily. It is usually unnecessary to replace blood loss of less than 500 mL, but after the loss has exceeded this, replacement should begin. The warnings against the use of a single transfusion during operation have been somewhat confusing. There may be a very definite need for a single-unit transfusion in the patient who loses between 500 and 1000 mL of blood during operation.

In addition to blood losses during operation, there appear to be extracellular fluid losses during major operative procedures. Some of these, including edema from extensive dissection, collections within the lumen and wall of the small bowel, and accumulations of fluid in the peritoneal cavity, are clinically discernible and well recognized. They generally are felt to represent distributional shifts, in that the functional volume of extracellular fluid is reduced but not externally lost from the body. These functional losses are often referred to as "parasitic losses, third space edema, or sequestration" of extracellular fluid. Another source of extracellular fluid loss during major operative trauma is the wound itself. This is a relatively smaller loss and very difficult to quantify except in extensive and major operative procedures.

At the beginning of this century, surgeons became aware that many changes occurred in urinary output, blood volume, and fluid and electrolyte composition during and after surgery. Assessment of these changes, however, awaited the development of analytic techniques and their application to patient studies. In the following 25 years, saline solutions in varying combinations were given to patients undergoing operation, often in excessive amounts. Work in the late 1930s and early 1940s by Moyer and by many others indicated that during and after operative procedures, saline and water solutions should be withheld entirely, because most of the fluid administered was retained.

The possibility existed that the operative and postoperative retention of salt and water administered in relatively small amounts might simply be physiologic retention to replace a deficit of salt and water incurred by the operative procedure. Subsequent studies have revealed that functional extracellular fluid decreases with major abdominal operations, largely as sequestered loss into the operative site. This extracellular fluid volume deficit can be replaced during the operative procedure. These data have led to the conclusion that the need for an extracellular "mimic" in the form of balanced salt solution now can be clinically estimated. Intraoperative correction of the volume deficit with salt solution markedly reduces postoperative oliguria, but is not intended to substitute for blood replacement. Rather, it is felt to be a physiologic supplement, or adjunct, to replace sequestered losses.

Thus, the pendulum has swung from indiscriminate use of salt solutions in the first quarter of this century to almost total withholding of fluid and electrolytes from surgical patients in the second quarter of the century; indications at present are that proper management lies somewhere between these two extremes. Some guidelines are necessary for the intraoperative administration of saline solutions as a "mimic" for the sequestered extracellular fluid. Since this varies from an almost imperceptible minimum to a high of approximately 3 L during

an uncomplicated procedure, quantification is extremely difficult with the presently available means of measuring functional extracellular fluid. Consequently, no accurate formula for intraoperative fluid administration can yet be derived. Some arbitrary but clinically useful guidelines are the following: (1) Blood should be replaced as lost, irrespective of any additional fluid and electrolyte therapy. (2) The replacement of extracellular fluid should begin during the operative procedure. (3) Balanced salt solution needed during operation is approximately 0.5 to 1 L/h, but only to a maximum of 2 to 3 L during a 4-h major abdominal procedure, unless there are other measurable losses.

Using a similar fluid regimen, Thompson and associates reported experiences in a series of 670 patients undergoing major aortoiliac reconstructive procedures. In this group of patients, the average amount of Ringer's lactate solution administered was 3555 mL, giving an average intraoperative replacement of salt solution of 677 mL/h of operative procedure. In the last 6 years of this study there were only two deaths in 298 operations, an operative mortality of 0.67 percent. Among the entire 670 patients, only two patients died of renal failure, an incidence of 0.3 percent. No patient died of pulmonary insufficiency. This extremely low incidence of renal failure, even in the presence of extensive operative trauma, is similar to the authors' data for major abdominal operative procedures.

Data by Virgilio and others have indicated that in the previously healthy surgical patient, the addition of albumin to intraoperative blood and extracellular fluid replacement is not only unnecessary but potentially harmful. Operative measurements of cardiac function and extravascular lung water indicate optimal function with replacement of blood and an extracellular "mimic" without the addition of extra albumin.

In summary, the addition of crystalloid fluid resuscitation, in appropriate volume, to blood replacement in the last quarter century has markedly improved the ability to maintain intraoperative homeostasis and avoid organ injury associated with inadequate volume replacement.

Postoperative Fluid Management

IMMEDIATE POSTOPERATIVE PERIOD

Orders for postoperative fluids are not written until the patient is in the recovery room and the fluid status has been assessed. Evaluation at this point should include a review of preoperative fluid status, the amount of fluid loss and gain during operation, and clinical examination of the patient with assessment of the vital signs and urinary output. Initial fluid orders are written to correct any *existing* deficit, followed by maintenance fluids for the remainder of the day. For the patient with complications who has received or lost large amounts of fluid, it is frequently difficult to estimate the fluid requirements for the ensuing 24 h. In this situation, intravenous fluids are ordered 1 L at a time and the patient is checked frequently until the situation is clarified. Proper replacement of fluids during this relatively short period will facilitate subsequent fluid management.

Immediately after operation, extracellular fluid volume depletion may occur as a result of continued losses of fluid at the site of injury or operative trauma—for example, into the wall or lumen of the small intestine. Several liters of extracellular fluid may be slowly deposited in such areas within a few hours or more during the first day or so from the time of the injury. Unrecognized deficits of extracellular fluid volume during the early postoperative period are manifest primarily as circulatory instability. The signs of volume deficiency in other organ systems may be delayed for several hours with this type of fluid loss. Postoperative hypotension and tachycardia require prompt investigation, followed by appropriate therapy. The generally accepted adequate blood pressure of 90/60 and a pulse of less than 120 in postoperative patients may not be sufficient to prevent renal ischemia unless, in addition to lack of signs of shock, urine flow is adequate. Evaluation of the level of consciousness, pupillary size, airway patency, breathing patterns, pulse rate and volume, skin warmth, color, body temperature, and a 30- to 50-mL hourly urine output, combined with critical review of the operative procedure and the operative fluid management, usually is recommended. Since operative trauma frequently involves loss or transfer of significant quantities of whole blood, plasma, or extracellular fluid that can be only grossly estimated, circulatory instability is most commonly caused by underestimated initial losses or insidious, concealed continued losses. Operative blood loss is usually estimated by the operating surgeon to be 15 to 40 percent less than the isotopically measured blood loss from that patient. For a patient with circulatory instability, further volume replacement of an additional 1000 mL isotonic salt solution, while determining whether continuing losses or other causes are present, often resolves the problem.

It is unnecessary and probably unwise to administer potassium during the first 24 h postoperatively, unless a definite potassium deficit exists. This is particularly important for the patient subjected to prolonged operative trauma involving one or more episodes of hypotension and for the posttraumatic patient with hemorrhagic hypotension. Oliguric renal failure or the more insidious high-output renal failure may develop, and the administration of even a small quantity of potassium may be quite detrimental.

LATER POSTOPERATIVE PERIOD

The problem of volume management during the postoperative convalescent phase is one of accurate measurement and replacement of all losses. In the otherwise healthy individual, this involves the replacement of measured sensible losses, which are generally of gastrointestinal origin, and the estimation and replacement of insensible losses.

The insensible loss is usually relatively constant and will average 600 mL/day. This may be increased by hypermetabolism, hyperventilation, and fever to a maxi-

mum of approximately 1500 mL/day. The estimated insensible loss is replaced with 5% dextrose in water. This loss may be partially offset by an insensible gain of water from excessive tissue catabolism in the complicated postoperative patient, particularly if associated with oliguric renal failure.

Approximately 1 L of fluid should be given to replace that volume of urine required to excrete the catabolic end products of metabolism (800 to 1000 mL/day). In the individual with normal renal function, this may be given as 5% dextrose in water, since the kidneys are able to conserve sodium with excretion of less than 1 meq daily. It is probably unnecessary to stress the kidneys to this degree, however, and a small amount of salt solution may be given in addition to water to cover urinary loss. In the elderly patient with salt-losing kidneys or in patients with head injuries, an insidious hyponatremia may develop if urinary losses are replaced with water. Urinary sodium in these circumstances may exceed 100 meq/L and result in a daily loss of significant amounts of sodium. Measurement of urinary sodium will facilitate accurate replacement.

Urine volume is not replaced on a milliliter-for-milliliter basis. A urinary output of 2000 to 3000 mL on a given day may simply represent diuresis of fluids given during surgery or may represent excessive fluid administration. If these large losses are completely replaced, the urine output will progressively increase, and this may logically progress to a unique situation resembling diabetes insipidus with urinary outputs in excess of 10 L/day.

Sensible losses, by definition, can be measured or, as in the case of sweating, the amount can be estimated. Gastrointestinal losses are usually isotonic or slightly hypotonic, and they are replaced with an essentially isotonic salt solution. When the estimated loss is slightly above or below isotonicity, appropriate corrections can be made in the daily water administration, while isotonic salt solutions are used to replace these losses volume for volume. Sweating is not usually a problem except with the febrile patient in whom losses may, but seldom do, exceed 250 mL/day per degree of fever. Excessive sweating may, in addition, represent a considerable loss of sodium in the unacclimatized individual.

Determination of serum electrolyte levels is generally unnecessary in the patient with an uncomplicated postoperative course maintained on parenteral fluids for 2 to 3 days. A more prolonged period of parenteral replacement or one complicated by excessive fluid losses requires frequent determinations of the serum sodium, potassium, and chloride levels, and carbon dioxide combining power. Adjustments then can be made with intravenous fluids of appropriate composition.

Daily maintenance fluid should be administered at a steady rate as the losses are incurred. If given over a shorter period of time, renal excretion of the excess salt and water may occur while the normal losses continue over the full 24-h period. For the same reason, fluids of different composition are alternated, and additives to intravenous fluids (e.g., potassium chloride and antibiotics) are evenly distributed in the total volume of fluid given.

In summary, daily fluid orders should begin with an assessment of the patient's volume status and a check for possible concentration or compositional disorders as reflected by proper laboratory determinations. All measured and insensible losses are replaced with fluids of appropriate composition, allowing for any preexisting deficit or excess. The amount of potassium replacement is 40 meq daily for renal excretion of potassium in addition to approximately 20 meq/L for replacement of gastrointestinal losses. Inadequate replacement may prolong the usual postoperative ileus and contribute to the insidious development of a resistant metabolic alkalosis. Calcium and magnesium are replaced when needed, as previously discussed.

SPECIAL CONSIDERATIONS IN THE POSTOPERATIVE PATIENT

VOLUME EXCESSES. The administration of isotonic salt solutions in excess of volume losses (external or internal) may result in overexpansion of the extracellular fluid space. The otherwise normal person in a postoperative state tolerates an acute overexpansion extremely well. Excesses administered over a period of several days, however, will soon exceed the kidney's ability to excrete sodium. Therefore, it is important to determine as accurately as possible from intake and output records and serum sodium concentrations the actual needs of the patient managed over several postoperative days. Attention to the signs and symptoms of overload usually prevents this fluid abnormality. It arises most frequently with attempts to meet excessive volume losses that are not measurable, such as those occurring from incompletely controlled fistula drainage.

The earliest sign is a weight gain during the catabolic period, when the patient should be losing ¼ to ½ lb day. Heavy eyelids, hoarseness, or dyspnea on exertion may rapidly appear. Circulatory and pulmonary signs of overload appear late and represent a rather massive overload. Peripheral edema may be a sign, but it does not necessarily indicate volume excess. In the absence of additional evidence for volume overload, other causes for peripheral edema should be considered. Overexpansion of the *total* extracellular fluid may coexist with *depletion* of the functional extracellular fluid compartment, along with decreased effective circulating plasma volume.

HYPONATREMIA. Significant postoperative alterations in serum sodium concentration are infrequent if the fluid resuscitation during operation has included adequate volumes of isotonic salt solutions. The kidneys retain the ability to excrete moderate excesses of salt water administered in the early postoperative period if functional extracellular fluid has been adequately replaced during the operative or immediate postoperative period. Previous studies of sodium balance have revealed that patients do excrete sodium after the functional deficit incurred by the shift of extracellular fluid has been replaced. Wright and Gann have demonstrated normal capacity to excrete water postoperatively when isotonic salt solutions are administered prior to a challenge with a water load. Thus, the commonly described hyponatremia associated with surgical procedures and traumatic injury is prevented by the replacement of extracellular fluid deficits. The daily maintenance of normal osmolarity is simplified by the replacement of observable losses of known sodium content.

Hyponatremia may easily occur when water is given to replace losses of sodium-containing fluids or when water administration consistently exceeds water losses. The latter may occur with oliguria or in association with decreased water loss through the skin and lungs, intracellular shifts of sodium, or the cellular release of excessive amounts of endogenous water. Severe or refractory hyponatremia, however, is difficult to produce if renal function remains normal.

In the presence of hyperglycemia, determination of the glucose concentration is necessary to evaluate the significance of a depressed serum sodium level. Since glucose does not enter cells by passive diffusion, it exerts an osmotic force in the extracellular compartment. This contribution to osmotic pressure is normally small, but with an elevated glucose concentration, the increased osmotic pressure causes the transfer of cellular water into the extracellular compartment, resulting in a dilutional hyponatremia. Hyponatremia may therefore be observed when the total effective osmotic pressure in the extracellular compartment is normal or even above normal. Each 100 mg/dL rise in the blood glucose above normal results in a decrease in the serum sodium concentration of approximately 1.6 to 3 meq/L.

Endogenous Water Release. The patient maintained on intravenous fluids without adequate caloric intake will, between the fifth and tenth days, gain significant quantities of water (maximum, 500 mL/day) from excessive cellular catabolism, thus decreasing the quantity of exogenous water required per day.

Intracellular Shifts. Systemic bacterial sepsis is often accompanied by a precipitous drop in serum sodium concentration. This sudden change is poorly understood but usually accompanies loss of extracellular fluid as either interstitial or intracellular sequestrations. This can be treated by withholding free water, restoring extracellular fluid volume, and initiating treatment of the sepsis.

HYPERNATREMIA. Hypernatremia (serum sodium concentration above 150 meq/L), although uncommon, is a dangerous abnormality. In contradistinction to decreased serum sodium concentration, hypernatremia is easily produced when renal function is normal. The extracellular fluid hyperosmolarity results in a shift of intracellular water from within the cell to the extracellular fluid compartment; in this situation, a high serum sodium level may indicate a significant deficit of total body water. In surgical patients hypernatremia arises most often from excessive or unexpected water losses, although it may result from use of salt-containing solutions to replace water losses. Classification of water losses may be helpful in preventing and treating this abnormality.

Excessive Extrarenal Water Losses. With increased metabolism from any cause, but particularly associated with fever, the water loss through evaporation of sweat may reach several liters daily. Patients with tracheostomy in dry environments can (with high minute volumes) lose as much as 1 to 1.5 L of water/day by this route. Increased water evaporation from a granulating surface is of significant magnitude in the thermally injured patient, and losses may be as great as 3 to 5 L/day.

Increased Renal Water Losses. Extremely large volumes of solute-poor urine may result from hypoxic damage to the distal tubules and collecting ducts or loss of antidiuretic hormone stimulation from damage to the central nervous system. In both instances, facultative water resorption is impaired. The former occurs in high-output renal failure; in our experience, this is the most common type of renal failure following severe injury or operative trauma. The latter occurs with extensive head injuries accompanied by temporary diabetes insipidus.

Solute Loading. High protein intake may produce an increased osmotic load of urea, which necessitates the excretion of large volumes of water. Hypernatremia, azotemia, and extracellular fluid volume deficits follow. In general, these can be prevented by an intake of 7 mL of water/g of dietary protein.

Excessive glucose administration results in the need for a large volume of water for excretion. Osmotic diuretics such as mannitol and urea also result in the obligatory excretion of a large volume of water as well as increasing urinary sodium losses. In addition, isotonic salt solutions, if used to replace pure water losses, rapidly produce hypernatremia.

HIGH-OUTPUT RENAL FAILURE. Acute renal insufficiency following trauma or surgical stress is a highly lethal complication. The diagnosis is based on persistent oliguria and chemical evidence of uremia after stabilization of the circulation. The clinical course is characterized by oliguria lasting from several days to several weeks, followed by a progressive rise in daily urine volume until both the excretory and concentrating functions of the kidney are gradually restored.

Uremia, occurring without a period of oliguria and accompanied by a daily urine volume greater than 1000 to 1500 mL/day, is a more frequent but less well recognized entity. Clinical experience and laboratory experiments suggest that high-output renal failure represents the renal response to a less severe or modified episode of renal injury than that required to produce classic oliguric renal failure. It is a milder form of renal insufficiency and its presence, by serial measurement of blood urea nitrogen and serum electrolytes, permits intelligent chemical and fluid volume management with a much greater latitude because of the daily urine volume excretion. Normal extracellular fluid volume and normal serum sodium concentration, therefore, are quite easily maintained when accurate daily outputs of each are obtained and replaced accordingly. The sodium-containing fluids may be administered as lactate to control the mild metabolic acidosis that occurs. Severe acidosis may develop if isotonic losses from the gastrointestinal tract or renal excretion of sodium are replaced with sodium chloride.

The chief danger of high-output renal failure is the failure to recognize its existence because of normal output.

The inappropriate administration of intravenous potassium in this setting may result in hyperkalemia. Good urinary output and gastrointestinal involvement requiring suction usually indicate the need for daily potassium replacement. With this type of renal failure, however, potassium intoxication may be produced. As little as 20 meq of potassium chloride given intravenously may rapidly produce myocardial potassium intoxication requiring exchange resin or hemodialysis treatment.

The typical course of high-output renal failure begins without a period of oliguria. The daily urine volumes are normal or greater than normal, often reaching levels of 3 to 5 L/day while blood urea nitrogen is increasing. An attempt to decrease urine output by water restriction rapidly results in hypernatremia without a change in urine volume. On the average, urea nitrogen continues to increase for 8 to 12 days before a downward trend occurs. The blood urine urea ratio is about 1:10 until a decrease occurs in the blood urea concentration.

Functionally, the lesion is characterized by a glomerular filtration rate of less than 20 percent of normal and complete resistance to vasopressin for 1 to 3 weeks after the blood urea nitrogen has declined. During the next 6 to 8 weeks, the glomerular filtration rate gradually rises, and the response to vasopressin becomes normal.

NUTRITION IN THE SURGICAL PATIENT
Stephen F. Lowry

The majority of patients undergoing elective surgical operations withstand the brief period of catabolism and starvation without noticeable difficulty. Maintaining an adequate nutritional regimen may be of critical importance in managing seriously ill surgical patients with preexisting weight loss and depleted energy reserves. Between these two extremes are patients for whom nutritional support is not essential for life but may serve to shorten the postoperative recovery phase and minimize the number of complications. Not infrequently a patient may become ill or even die from complications secondary to starvation rather than the underlying disorder. Therefore, it is essential that the surgeon have a sound grasp of the fundamental metabolic changes associated with surgery, trauma, and sepsis and an awareness of the methods available to reverse or ameliorate these events. A detailed discussion of the neuroendocrine and metabolic response to injury has been presented in Chap. 1.

Body Fuel Reserves

The body must mobilize appropriate nutrients from fuel reserves in order to withstand the necessary periods of partial or complete starvation and to meet the additional requirements imposed by surgery, trauma, or sepsis. The extent and availability of these reserves may be of critical importance for successful recovery from an illness. Available information concerning body fuel composition and

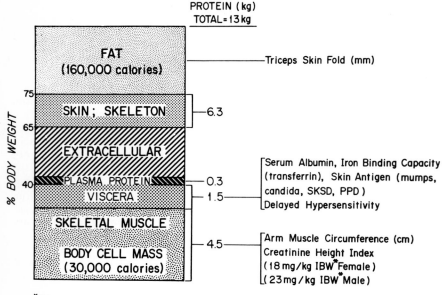

*Ideal Body Weight

Fig. 2-3. Body fuel composition, exclusive of glycogen (900 kcal), in a normal individual. Nutritional assessment techniques corresponding to components of body composition. (From: *Blackburn GL, Bothe A Jr: Cancer Bulletin 30:90, 1978, with permission.*)

the rate of fuel consumption in human beings has recently been reviewed by Cahill and is summarized below.

Carbohydrates, proteins, and fats are the three sources of fuel in human beings. Their relative contributions by both weight and caloric potential are illustrated in Fig. 2-3. Carbohydrate stores, primarily in the form of liver and muscle glycogen, are relatively small and could supply basal caloric requirements for less than 1 day. However, this relatively small quantity is absolutely essential in the emergency situation for the production of high-energy phosphates during anaerobic metabolism. Although glucose yields approximately 4 kcal/g, its storage as glycogen requires the addition of 1 or 2 g of intracellular water and electrolytes. Therefore, it yields only 1 or 2 kcal/g of wet weight.

Protein represents a considerably larger source of fuel, but, as emphasized by Cahill, every molecule of protein in the body has a specific purpose, such as an enzyme, a structural component, or a contractile protein in muscle. Thus, any protein loss represents loss of an essential function. Additionally, the amount of total body protein is relatively fixed in the normal healthy individual, and any additional protein is metabolized, the excess calories being stored as fat. Protein, like glycogen, represents an inefficient energy source relative to its wet weight, since it exists in an aqueous environment.

In contrast to glycogen and protein, fat is stored in a relatively anhydrous state. By weight, then, it is a relatively rich source of energy, supplying approximately 9 kcal/g. Most of the fat in the body serves as a readily available energy source; the few areas where fat serves a specific function (e.g., mechanical fat pads) are the last to be mobilized during starvation.

In summary, protein and fat are the only major sources of fuel. Total protein mass is relatively fixed in amount, and caloric excess or deficiency is met by an increase or decrease in the body's fat mass. Fat depots serve as sources of energy, protein stores represent *potential* sources of energy but only through the loss of some important function, and the small stores of carbohydrates are generally protected except for emergency use during anaerobic glycolysis.

Starvation

During the first several days of complete starvation, caloric needs are supplied by body fat and proteins: the small glycogen reserve is largely spared. Previous studies have shown an obligatory loss of approximately 10 to 15 g of nitrogen daily in the urine during this period, indicating the utilization of approximately 60 to 90 g of protein (each gram of nitrogen represents approximately 6.25 g of muscle protein). The majority of this protein, which is largely derived from skeletal muscle, is converted to glucose in the liver by the process of gluconeogenesis; most of this endogenously produced glucose is used by the brain. The remainder is used by certain tissues such as red blood cells and leukocytes which convert the glucose to lactate and pyruvate. These are returned to the liver and resynthesized into glucose (the Cori cycle). This obligatory nitrogen loss, then, reflects the use of amino acids derived from muscle protein for gluconeogenesis to supply glucose to the brain. No patient, however, should be allowed to starve completely. The administration of at least 100 g of glucose will obviate most of this gluconeogenesis and reduce the nitrogen loss by at least one-half—the well-known "protein-sparing effect" described by Gamble.

Available evidence from Cahill indicates that this protein-sparing effect is regulated by insulin, which is released when exogenous glucose is infused for use by the brain. The slightly elevated insulin level reduces amino acid release from the muscle, amino acid extraction by the liver, and gluconeogenesis. In the diabetic with an absolute or relative lack of insulin, the infusion of glucose does not inhibit gluconeogenesis, and muscle breakdown to amino acids continues unabated. The liver derives its energy by oxidizing fatty acids to ketones, and the remainder of the body utilizes both fatty acids and ketones to meet caloric requirements. Generally a small quantity of the ketones is excreted into the urine.

If complete starvation continues for more than a few days, the obligatory nitrogen loss progressively decreases, as the brain begins to use fat as its fuel source. Unlike other body tissues, however, the brain cannot utilize free fatty acids, since they do not cross the blood-brain barrier. Instead, use of keto acids that are produced by the liver and readily cross the blood-brain barrier gradually displaces the use of glucose by the brain. After prolonged starvation, the net effect of this adaptation to ketone utilization is a protein-sparing effect with reduction of urinary nitrogen excretion to approximately 4 g/day. This 4 g of nitrogen represents approximately 25 g of protein, or about 100 g of lean wet muscle. Thus, the normal individual with an average supply of fat and muscle may survive total starvation for several months. Insulin again may be the signal for the reduction in muscle catabolism and gluconeogenesis (coincident with the increased use of keto acids by the brain), according to Cahill. However, changes in the blood level of alanine, which is quantitatively one of the more important amino acids, may also play a role. A fall in the blood level of this amino acid appears to decrease gluconeogenesis and glucose production by the liver.

Surgery, Trauma, Sepsis

In contrast to the whole-body and tissue-specific energy and protein conservation response exhibited during unstressed starvation, the injured patient manifests variable, but obligatory, increases in energy expenditure and nitrogen excretion (Fig. 2-4, Table 2-9). While the extent and duration of this response to injury are modified by a variety of factors, including the adequacy of resuscitation, infection, and medication, the inability to downregulate body energy expenditure and nitrogen losses may rapidly deplete both labile and functional energy stores. The postinjury metabolic environnment precludes the efficient oxidation of fat and ketone production, thereby promoting the continued erosion of protein pools. This enhanced net protein catabolic process, if unchecked by effective disease-specific therapy and allowed to progress for an extended period without nutritional intervention, eventuates in critical organ failure.

The sequence of metabolic and endocrine events occasioned by surgery, trauma, or sepsis may be divided into several phases. As pointed out by Moore (1960), the magnitude of the changes and the duration of each phase vary

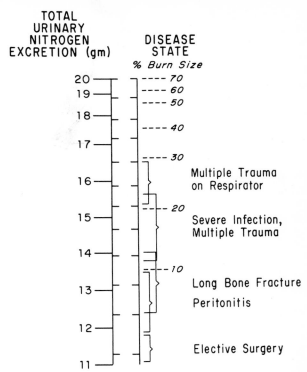

Fig. 2-4. The *minimum* anticipated daily urinary nitrogen excretion of adult patients in relation to the injury stimulus. These losses may be modulated by a number of variables including the age and nutritional status of the patient. (Adapted from: *Grant JP: Handbook of Total Parenteral Nutrition, Philadelphia, Saunders, 1980,* with permission.)

considerably and are directly related to the severity of the injury.

CATABOLIC PHASE. This phase has also been termed the *adrenergic-corticoid phase* since it corresponds to the period during which changes induced by adrenergic and adrenal corticoid hormones are most striking. Immediately following surgery or trauma, there is a sudden in-

Table 2-9. CORRELATION OF INCREASED ENERGY EXPENDITURE AND URINARY NITROGEN EXCRETION AFTER INJURY AND ILLNESS

	% Increase above basal energy expenditure	*Daily urinary N excretion per kg*
Normal	—	0.09
Elective, major surgery	24	0.21
Skeletal trauma	32	0.32
Blunt trauma	37	0.32
Head trauma/steroids	61	0.34
Sepsis	79	0.37
40% thermal injury	132	0.37

SOURCE: Adapted from Long CL et al: *J Parenter Enteral Nutr* 3:452, 1979.

crease in metabolic demands and urinary excretion of nitrogen beyond the levels associated with simple starvation. Patients generally cannot eat, cannot lower their metabolic rate, and cannot effectively alter the source of endogenous fuels to spare protein utilization. This is in distinct contrast to events in the normal individual subjected to prolonged starvation, where most body tissues use fat as their main source of fuel, thereby sparing protein. Trauma apparently results in an obligatory and excessive mobilization of protein in an attempt to provide skeletons for gluconeogenesis, acute phase, and wound repair proteins. The administration of moderate amounts of glucose to these individuals produces little or no change in the rate of protein catabolism, although recent evidence using isotopic determinations of protein kinetics suggests that provision of sufficient nonprotein calories in combination with amino acids does reduce the rate of body protein breakdown.

Glucose turnover is increased, while Cori cycle activity is stimulated and three-carbon intermediates are converted back to glucose in the liver by pyruvate carboxylase and phosphoenolpyruvate carboxylase. Increased synthesis of these two enzymes occurs in the presence of elevated levels of glucagon, glucocorticoids, and catecholamines and low concentrations of insulin—the hormonal environment present during the catabolic phase of injury. Lipolysis also is stimulated by this hormonal milieu, and an obligatory oxidation of fatty acids is evident.

Efforts directed at interruption of afferent neurogenic stimuli by extradural anesthesia have met with partial success in attenuating some of these abnormalities of energy substrate turnover. The impact of such therapy upon nitrogen loss has been far less dramatic, suggesting that circulating or tissue paracrine factors other than classical neuroendocrine hormones are of major importance in early postinjury metabolic responses. Recent evidence would suggest that a class of macrophage and lymphocyte-produced peptides (cytokines), some of which, such as cachectin/tumor necrosis factor and interleukin-1, are already known to enhance hepatic acute-phase protein mRNA and tissue glucose transporter protein production, are likely participants in the derangements of catabolic phase responses. The extent of the negative nitrogen balance in these patients varies considerably and is largely related to the magnitude of the injury.

EARLY ANABOLIC PHASE. Depending on the severity of injury, the body turns from a catabolic to an anabolic phase. This may occur within 3 to 8 days after uncomplicated elective surgery or after weeks in patients with extensive cross-sectional tissue injury, sepsis, or ungrafted thermal injury. This turning point, also known as the *corticoid-withdrawal phase,* is characterized by a sharp decline in nitrogen excretion and restoration of appropriate potassium-nitrogen balance. Generally, this transition period lasts no more than a day or two and coincides with diuresis of retained free water. Renewed interest in oral nutrition and the patient's immediate environment promotes greater muscular activity.

The early anabolic phase may last from a few weeks to a few months depending upon the capacity to ingest adequate nutrition and the extent to which erosion of protein stores has occurred. Nitrogen balance is positive, indicating synthesis of proteins, and there is a rapid and progressive gain in weight and muscular strength. Positive nitrogen balance reaches a maximum of approximately 4 g/day, which represents the synthesis of approximately 25 g of protein and the gain of over 100 g of lean body mass day. The total amount of nitrogen gain will ultimately equal the amount lost during the catabolic phase, although the rate of gain will be much slower than the rate of initial loss.

LATE ANABOLIC PHASE. The final period of convalescence or the late anabolic phase may last from several weeks to several months after a severe injury. This phase is associated with the gradual restoration of adipose stores as the previously positive nitrogen balance declines toward normal. Weight gain is much slower during this phase because of the higher caloric content of fat and can be realized only if intake is in excess of caloric expenditure. In most individuals, the phase ends with a gradual return to the previously normal body weight. The patient who is partially immobilized during this period of time, however, may exhibit a marked gain in weight due to decreased energy expenditure.

Assessment and Requirements

Nutritional homeostasis presupposes that proper timing and administration of nutrients will impact favorably upon the outcome of therapy. Muller has reported a randomized, prospective trial documenting a significant reduction of postoperative morbidity and mortality following intravenous nutritional support. Similar reductions in the complication rate following nutritional support have been observed by other groups in a variety of surgical and traumatic illnesses. Reports that up to 50 percent of selected surgical populations may manifest evidence of protein-calorie malnutrition underscores the importance of identifying patients at increased risk from nutritional morbidity.

Nutritional assessment is undertaken to determine the severity of nutrient deficiencies or excess and to aid in predicting nutritional requirements (Fig. 2-3). Important information is obtained by determining the presence of weight loss and of chronic illnesses or dietary habits that influence the quantity and quality of food intake. Social habits predisposing to malnutrition and the use of medications that may influence food intake or utilization should also be investigated. Physical examination seeks to assess loss of muscle and adipose tissues, organ dysfunction, and subtle change in skin, hair, or neuromuscular function reflecting a frank or impending nutritional deficiency. Anthropometric data (weight change, skin fold thickness, and arm circumference muscle area) and biochemical determinations (creatinine excretion, albumin, and transferrin) may be used to substantiate the historical and physical findings. It is imprecise to rely upon any single or fixed combination of the above findings to accurately assess nutritional status or morbidity. Appreciation for the stresses and natural history of the disease process, in

Table 2-10. ELEMENTAL REQUIREMENTS FOR
DEPLETED ADULT SUBJECTS

Element	Daily infusion, per kg*
N	0.4 g
PO_4^{2-}	0.018 g
K^+	0.65 meq
Na^+	0.74 meq
Cl^-	0.56 meq
Ca^{2+}	0.13 meq

* Requirements listed are based on kilogram of ideal body
weight; appropriate adjustment to current body weight may be
necessary.
SOURCE: Adapted from Rudman D et al: *J Clin Invest* 55:94,
1975.

combination with nutritional assessment, remains the
basis for identifying patients in acute or anticipated need
of nutritional support.

Balance studies have documented the basal requirements for nonstressed, depleted patients who are undergoing nutritional support (Table 2-10). These guidelines
must be considered in relation to goals for gradual repletion of a malnourished patient or for maintenance of lean
tissue stores in an otherwise well-nourished subject.

The above basal requirements are inadequate for patients who have undergone major surgery or who have
suffered severe trauma or sepsis. The exact caloric and
nitrogen requirements necessary to maintain an individual in balance after severe injury are dependent upon the
extent of injury, the source and route of administered nutrients, and, to some extent, the degree of antecedent
malnutrition.

A fundamental goal of nutritional support is to meet the
energy requirements for metabolic processes, core temperature maintenance, and tissue repair. Failure to provide adequate nonprotein energy sources will lead to dissolution of lean tissue stores. The requirement for energy
may be measured by indirect calorimetry or estimated
from urinary nitrogen excretion which is proportional to
resting energy expenditure (REE) (Table 2-9). Basal energy expenditure (BEE) may also be estimated by the
equations of Harris and Benedict:

$$BEE \text{ (men)} = 66.47 + 13.75(W) + 5.0\,(H) - 6.76\,(A)$$
$$\text{kcal/day}$$
$$BEE \text{ (women)} = 655.1 + 9.56(W) + 1.85\,(H) - 4.68\,(A)$$
$$\text{kcal/day}$$

where W = weight, kg
H = height, cm
A = age, years

These equations are suitable for estimating energy requirements in 80 percent of hospitalized patients. A suitable correction for the degree of operative or traumatic
stress may then be applied as in Table 2-9 to determine
the resting energy expenditure. Nonprotein calories are
supplied in excess of energy expenditure because the uti-

lization of exogenous nutrients is decreased and energy
substrate demands are increased after traumatic or septic
insult. Appropriate nonprotein caloric needs are 1.2 to 1.5
times REE during enteral nutrition and 1.5 to 2.0 times
REE during intravenous nutrition.

The second objective of nutritional support is to meet
the substrate requirements for protein synthesis. Maintenance of protein synthesis is dependent upon many factors, including the nature and degree of insult, the source
and amount of exogenous protein, and prior nutritional
status. As a consequence, no single nutritional formulation is appropriate for all patients. An appropriate calorie-
nitrogen ratio (150 to 200:1) should be maintained, although recent evidence suggests that increased protein
intake (and a lower ratio) may be efficient in selected hypermetabolic patients. In the absence of severe renal or
hepatic dysfunction precluding the use of standard nutritional regimens, approximately 0.25 to 0.35 g of nitrogen/
kg of body weight should be provided daily.

Amino acid formulations designed to improve protein
kinetics in the posttraumatic or organ failure setting are
under investigation. Solutions enriched in branched-chain
amino acids are being used to preserve or enhance muscle
protein synthesis. Branched-chain amino acids are also
used in combination with reduced aromatic amino acid
concentrations to alleviate encephalopathy secondary to
hepatocellular dysfunction. Formulations designed to
improve nitrogen utilization by providing intact or keto
analogs of essential amino acids have gained wide acceptance in the management of acute renal failure.

The requirements for vitamins and essential trace minerals usually can be easily met in the average patient with
an uncomplicated postoperative course, and vitamins
usually are not given in the absence of preoperative deficiencies. Patients maintained on elemental diets or parenteral hyperalimentation require complete vitamin and
mineral supplementation. The commercial defined-
formula enteral diets contain varying amounts of essential
minerals and vitamins (Tables 2-11 and 2-12). It is necessary to ensure that adequate replacement is available in
the diet or by supplementation. Numerous commercial
vitamin preparations are available for intravenous or intramuscular use, although most do not contain vitamin K
and some do not contain vitamin B_{12} or folic acid. Supplemental trace minerals may now be given intravenously by
commercial preparations. Essential fatty acid supplementation may also be necessary, especially in patients with
depletion of adipose stores. Patients receiving intravenous feeding will require all of the above micronutrients
to prevent evolution of deficiencies.

Indications and Methods for Nutritional Support

The selection of patients who require partial or complete nutritional support has become increasingly important. The ability to provide complete nutritional support
in the starving patient and to counteract the nitrogen
losses in catabolic states with elemental diets or parenteral hyperalimentation represents a substantial contribu-

Table 2-11. CASEINATES AND WHOLE PROTEIN FORMULAS*

Formula	Criticare HN§	Ensure	Ensure HN	Ensure plus	Ensure plus HN	Entriton	Isotein HN	Isocal	Isocal HCN	Magnacal	NutriAid	Osmolite	Osmolite HN	Precision isotonic	Precision HN	Precision LR	Renu	Sustacal	Sustacal HC	TraumaCal	Travasorb MCT
NP. kcal/mL†	0.85	0.86	0.88	1.28	1.25	0.86	0.93	0.92	1.70	1.72	0.94	0.91	0.88	0.84	0.87	0.99	0.87	0.76	1.26	1.17	1.45
Nitrogen, g/L	6.00	5.92	7.10	8.80	10.0	5.60	10.8	5.44	12.0	11.2	6.29	5.92	7.10	4.64	7.04	4.16	5.60	9.60	9.76	13.20	5.92
Osmolality, mO/kg	650	450	470	600	650	300	300	300	740	590	350	300	310	300	557	525	330	625	650	550	312
Na, meq/L	27	32	40	46	50	61	27	23	34	43	33	23	40	34	42	30	21	40	36	52	32
K, meq/L	33	32	40	48	46	61	27	33	35	32	33	27	40	24	23	22	32	52	38	36	32
Cl, meq/L	30	30	40	46	45	56	27	30	34	26	30	23	40	28	33	31	18	44	36	45	30
Ca, meq/L	26	26	37	32	52	50	28	31	33	50	27	26	37	32	17	29	25	50	42	38	26
P, mmol/L	17	17	24	20	33	32	18	17	21	33	18	17	24	20	11	18	16	31	27	24	17
Mg, meq/L	17	17	25	26	34	33	19	17	22	15	17	17	25	21	11	19	16	14	28	17	17
Zn, mg/L	10	16	17	24	16	15	8.5	10	20		16	16	17	10	5	9	10		13	15	16
Cu, mg/L	1	1	1.5	1.6	1	2	1.1	1	2	2	1.1	1	1.5	1	0.7	1	2	2	2	1.5	1
Vitamins, 1/RDA/day‡	1.9	1.9	1.4	1.6	1.0	2.0	1.6	2.0	1.5	1.0	2.0	1.9	1.4	1.6	2.9	1.8	2.0	1.1	1.8	2.0	2.0

* Lactose-free.
† NP = nonprotein kilocalories per milliliters of solution.
‡ Volume in liters needed to meet the U.S. RDA per day.
§ This formula also contains synthetic amino acids.

SOURCE: Adapted from Legaspi A, Lowry SF: Agents affecting nutrition and homeostasis, in *Manual of Drug Therapy*. New York, Raven Press, 1985.

Table 2-12. ELEMENTAL AND PEPTIDE DIETS*

Formula	Vivonex	Vivonex HN	Vivonex TEN	Vital	Travasorb STD	Travasorb HN
NP, kcal/mL†	0.92	0.82	0.85	0.83	0.88	0.82
Nitrogen, g/L	3.36	6.72	6.08	6.72	4.80	7.20
Osmolality, mO/kg	550	810	630	460	560	560
Na, meq/L	20	23	20	16	40	40
K, meq/L	30	30	20	30	30	30
Cl, meq/L	20	23	23	19	42	38
Ca, meq/L	28	16	25	33	25	25
P, mmol/L	18	10	49	21	16	16
Mg, meq/L	18	10	17	22	16	16
Zn, mg/L	8	5	10	10	7.5	7.5
Cu, mg/L	1	0.7	1	1.3	1	1
Vitamins (1/RDA/day)‡	1.8	3.0	2.0	1.5	2.0	2.0

* Lactose-free.
† NP = Nonprotein kilocalories per milliliter of solution.
‡ Volume in liters needed to meet the U.S. RDA per day.
SOURCE: Adapted from Legaspi A, Lowry SF: Agents affecting nutrition and homeostasis, in *Manual of Drug Therapy*. New York, Raven Press, 1985.

tion. The need for nutritional support should be assessed during the preoperative and postoperative course of all but the most routine cases. However, it should be emphasized that the majority of surgical patients do not require special nutritional regimens. The reasonably well-nourished and otherwise healthy individual who undergoes an uncomplicated major surgical procedure has sufficient body fuel reserves to withstand the catabolic insult and partial starvation for at least 1 week. Adequate quantities of parenteral fluids with appropriate electrolyte composition and a minimum of 100 g of glucose daily to minimize protein catabolism will be all that is necessary in most patients. Assuming that the patient has a relatively uncomplicated postoperative course and resumes normal oral intake at the end of this period, defined-formula diets or parenteral hyperalimentation are probably unnecessary and inadvisable because of the associated risks. During the early anabolic phase, the patient must be provided with an adequate caloric intake of proper composition to meet the energy needs of the body and allow protein synthesis. A high calorie-nitrogen ratio (optimal ratio approximately 150 kcal/g nitrogen) and an adequate supply of vitamins and minerals are necessary for maximum anabolism during this period.

In contrast to this group, there are populations of surgical patients for whom an adequate nutritional regimen may be of critical importance for a successful outcome. These categories include preoperative patients who are chronically debilitated from their diseases or malnutrition and patients who have suffered trauma, sepsis, or surgical complications and cannot maintain an adequate caloric intake.

Specialized nutritional support can be given by enteral, enteral plus peripheral vein, and by central venous routes. The enteral route should be initially considered because it is simple, economical, and usually well toler-

ated in most patients. Nasopharyngeal, gastrostomy, and jejunostomy tube feedings may be considered for alimentation in patients who have a relatively normal gastrointestinal tract but cannot or will not eat. Elemental diets may be administered by similar routes when bulk and fat-free nutrients requiring minimal digestion are indicated. Finally, parenteral alimentation may be used for supplementation in the patient with limited oral intake or, more commonly, for complete nutritional management in the absence of oral intake.

Despite the failure to document clinical differences between the enteral and parenteral feeding routes with respect to the utilization of exogenous nutrients, the gastrointestinal tract serves a number of synthetic and immunologic functions that bear consideration in the design of nutritional support regimens. Toward this end, a number of approaches for preserving gastrointestinal mucosal integrity and gut mass, including luminal stimulation by digestible or nondigestible substrates, as well as infusion of critical intestinal fuel sources such as glutamine, are currently undergoing clinical trials.

The patient's ability to tolerate and absorb enteral feedings is determined by the rate of infusion, the osmolality, and the chemical nature of the product. Enteral feedings are often begun at a rate of 30 to 50 mL/h and are increased by 10 to 25 mL/h a day until the optimal volume is delivered. After full volume is attained, the concentration of the solution is increased slowly to the desired strength. If esophageal or gastric feedings are given, residual gastric volume should be monitored to reduce the risk of a major aspiration episode. If abdominal cramping or diarrhea occurs, the rate of administration or the concentration of the solution should be decreased. All feeding tubes should be thoroughly irrigated clear of solutions if feedings are interrupted or medications are given by this route.

NASOENTERIC TUBE FEEDING

The development of mercury-weighted silastic feeding tubes has improved the ability to provide safe and effective enteral nutrition. Use of such tubes represents a safer alternative to the practice of nasoesophageal or gastric feeding by large-bore red rubber or plastic tubes. Exceptions to this rule include patients with head and neck malignancies who will tolerate a blenderized diet that cannot easily be administered by smaller diameter tubes.

Nasoesophageal or gastric feedings should be used only in alert patients. The foremost contraindication for nasoesophageal or gastric tube feeding is unconsciousness or lack of protective laryngeal reflexes, which may result in life-threatening pulmonary complications due to aspiration. Even with a tracheostomy, it is inadvisable to feed mentally obtunded patients via such route, since feedings often can be recovered from tracheostomy suction, indicating continued aspiration of gastric contents. Pharyngeal tube feedings may be indicated for patients with oropharyngeal tumor; irritation may be prevented by inserting the tube into the pyriform sinus.

The nasojejunal tube may allow feeding beyond dysfunctional gastric stomas and high gastrointestinal fistulas. In such cases, it may be possible to maintain nutrition without a jejunostomy tube until stomal dysfunction relents or the fistula heals. Such tubes may be positioned in the upper small intestine by positioning the patient in a manner that promotes passage of the mercury-weighted tube into the desired intestinal segment. If this technique proves unsuccessful, placement may be effected by fluoroscopic guidance or by an experienced endoscopist. Proper position of the tube must be confirmed radiographically (with water-soluble opaque medium if necessary).

Whenever dietary preparations are administered into the gastrointestinal tract via tubes, it is advisable to employ bedside infusion pumps to ensure a constant rate of delivery over each 24-h period. The utilization of such pumps decreases the incidence of gastrointestinal side effects induced by too rapid delivery of hyperosmolar solutions, while at the same time allowing safer administration of larger daily volumes of nutrients, since gastric distention is minimized. Investigation is required for all abdominal complaints in such patients in view of reports of intussusception around feeding tubes placed more distally in the small intestine.

GASTROSTOMY TUBE FEEDING

The administration of blended food through a gastrostomy tube is a good method for feeding patients with a variety of chronic gastrointestinal lesions arising at or above the cardioesophageal junction. However, gastrostomy tube feedings are contraindicated for mentally obtunded patients with inadequate laryngeal reflexes. This feeding method should be used only in alert patients or in patients with total obstruction of the distal esophagus.

Generally, gastrostomies of the Stamm (serosa-lined, temporary) or modified Glassman (mucosa-lined, permanent) type are constructed. Percutaneous endoscopic gastrostomies (PEG) have proved to be a safe and effective method for pursuing enteral nutritional support. The feeding mixture may be ordinarily prepared food converted by a blender into a semiliquid. Hyperosmolarity of the feeding formula is not generally a problem as long as the pylorus is intact.

JEJUNOSTOMY TUBE FEEDING

Jejunostomy tube feedings are generally required for patients in whom nasoesophageal or gastrostomy tube feedings are contraindicated, e.g., comatose patients or patients with high gastrointestinal fistulas or obstructions, or in whom a nasojejunal feeding tube cannot be placed. The jejunostomy may be of the Roux en Y (permanent) or the Witzel (temporary) type. The latter is constructed by inserting a #18 French rubber catheter into the proximal jejunum approximately 12 in. distal to the ligament of Treitz. The wall of the jejunum is inverted over the tube for about 3 cm as it emerges from the bowel to create a serosa-lined tunnel that allows rapid sealing of the jejunal opening when the tube is removed. An alternative procedure is the placement of a smaller-bore polyethylene or silastic catheter. The tube is brought out through a stab wound in the left upper quadrant of the abdomen. The jejunum is sutured to the anterior abdominal wall at the point of tube entry to seal it from the peritoneal cavity.

Alternate methods that have gained wide acceptance include the needle catheter jejunostomy that is available in commercial kit form or may be constructed using subclavian catheter materials. In selected instances, jejunostomies may be placed endoscopically or converted from PEG catheters.

If the jejunostomy tube is inadvertently removed, blind attempts at reinsertion are contraindicated. If discovered within a few hours, the tube may be reinserted under fluoroscopic control to be sure it is in the bowel before feedings are resumed. The patient is observed for signs of peritonitis for 12 to 18 h after feedings are restarted. If there is any doubt about the position of the tube, it should be replaced surgically.

Feedings are safely begun 12 to 18 h after jejunostomy construction, even though peristalsis is not audible. Jejunostomy tube feedings are usually initiated with one of the many commercially available defined formula diets (Tables 2-11, 2-12). Such formulas, when provided by continuous infusion, are usually well tolerated.

With proper care, about 85 percent of jejunostomy patients tolerate their feedings. Diarrhea is usually controlled if the concentration and volume of formula are temporarily reduced. Failing this, feeding is halted for a day, then resumed from the beginning of the feeding regimen, progressing somewhat more slowly than before. If mild diarrhea or cramping persists, a pulverized Lomotil tablet or 8 to 10 drops of tincture of belladonna may be given through the tube 30 min prior to formula infusion. At times it may be necessary to give 5 mL paregoric 15 to 30 min before the formula to control cramping and diarrhea, but this should be employed sparingly and for as short a period as possible. In many cases, symptoms are relieved if the rate and volume of infusion are reduced and cold formula avoided. Failing control of diarrhea by the above means, or as an alternative method to opiates, the periodic administration of bulk-forming agents (Metamucil) may be helpful.

If the patient with a jejunostomy has a proximal bowel or biliary fistula draining more than 300 mL daily for prolonged periods, the fistular drainage may be collected by sump suction, cooled in an ice basin at bedside, and promptly refed in small increments throughout the day. To avoid jejunal overloading, the fistular fluid is refed between formula feedings. It is not advisable to refeed aspirated gastric juice, for this may cause jejunal irritation and profuse diarrhea. If the fistular drainage is profuse, it is usually not possible to refeed more than 2 L/day, and fluid and electrolyte losses must be replaced by appropriate intravenous supplements. Additional water may be given with the feedings or administered between the feedings as indicated. Occasionally, an elemental diet, as discussed below, may be indicated when other jejunostomy formulas are not tolerated.

ELEMENTAL DIETS

Commercial production of nutritionally complete liquid diets, derived in purified form either from natural foods or from foods prepared synthetically, has been given such designations as chemically defined or elemental diets.

Clinical experience with chemically formulated bulk-free elemental diets has been encouraging. These diets may be used for complete nutritional support or as dietary supplements for patients who are unable to eat or digest enough food to meet their energy requirements. They may be preferable to high-caloric parenteral feedings for patients who have at least part of the small bowel available for the absorption of simple sugars and amino acids. Elemental diets have been found useful for patients with depleted protein reserves secondary to gastrointestinal tract disease, such as ulcerative or granulomatous colitis and malabsorption syndrome, and for patients with only partial function of the gastrointestinal tract, such as the short bowel syndrome or gastric or small bowel fistulas with feeding distal to the fistula. The diets also have been used during preoperative bowel preparation.

As commercially prepared, these diets also contain base-line electrolytes, water- and fat-soluble vitamins (except vitamin K), and trace minerals. They contain no bulk and therefore produce a minimum of residue. Products such as Carnation Instant Breakfast and Meritene contain intact protein derived from milk products, eggs, or both and are designed for oral consumption in lactose tolerant patients. Other preparations contain intact protein from semipurified isolates of milk, soybean, or egg (Table 2-11). These do not contain lactose and are more readily tolerated in such lactase-deficiency states as gastroenteritis, intestinal resection, radiation, or genetic predisposition. Finally, there are several products whose protein content is either partially hydrolyzed or completely hydrolyzed to amino acids or dipeptides (Table

2-12). When digestion and absorption are normal, there appears to be little therapeutic advantage to the use of crystalline amino acid formulas. A listing of the basic constituents for several commercial preparations, as well as the volume necessary to achieve minimal daily requirements, is given in Table 2-11.

Special products designed for use in the presence of organ dysfunction are also available (Table 2-13). Amin-Aid provides essential amino acids and histidine with minimal electrolytes, vitamins, or bulk, but does yield 2 kcal/mL for use in the setting of renal failure. Hepatic Aid, which may be used in the presence of severe liver insufficiency, is enriched with branched-chain amino acids and is deficient in aromatic, ringed amino acids.

Fat may contribute less than 1 or as much as 47 percent of the calories in these commercial formulas. Most contain long-chain fats as corn oil, soy oil, or safflower oil. Some include medium-chain triglycerides, such as Precision-LR and Vital. Despite the high caloric density of fat, it does not increase the osmolality of the formula. When significant maldigestion or malabsorption is present, a diet low in fat or one supplemented with medium-chain triglycerides may be useful.

Specific products are limited in their overall clinical usefulness by virtue of the fixed content of nutrients. In recent years, there has been a trend in preparing enteral diets in modular form, where certain critical items, such as sodium, potassium, and fat, can be modified in concentration as dictated by clinical circumstances.

The amount of elemental diet required to maintain weight and nitrogen balance varies with the individual patient. In severe catabolic states the standard diet often fails to achieve positive nitrogen balance. Careful attention to water and electrolyte balance is mandatory, particularly when large quantities of fluid are being lost through fistulas or other routes. Additional sodium and potassium may be added to the mixture (not to exceed a total of 100 meq), although they should be given in intravenous fluids when larger quantities are needed. Water may be added to the mixture in the face of excessive pure water losses.

Complications include nausea, vomiting, and diarrhea which develop because of the high osmolarity of the diets. This generally can be controlled by decreasing the rate and or concentration of the mixture. Hypertonic nonketotic coma may occur in the presence of excessive water losses or if the diets are administered at concentrations above those recommended. Hyperglycemia and glycosuria may occur in any severely ill patient, particularly latent diabetics, and insulin may be indicated.

PARENTERAL ALIMENTATION

Dudrick et al. have demonstrated the clinical practicality of providing complete nutritional needs for an extended period of time using high-caloric parenteral feedings. Parenteral alimentation involves the continuous infusion of a hyperosmolar solution containing carbohydrates, proteins, fat, and other necessary nutrients through an indwelling catheter inserted into the superior

Table 2-13. SPECIALIZED FORMULATIONS FOR ENTERAL NUTRITION DURING ORGAN FAILURE*

Formula	Amin Aid	Hepatic Aid	Travasorb Hepatic	Travasorb Renal	TraumAid	Stresstein
NP, kcal/mL†	1.88	1.47	0.98	1.26	0.83	0.93
Nitrogen, g/L	2.35	6.47	4.4	4.4	7.58	11.2
Osmolality, mO/kg	1095	1150	690	590	675	910
EAA, g/L‡	18.6	22.15	20.0	13.8	26.2	89.6
BCAA, g/L§	7.5	15.3	14.5	6.67	15.0	61.6
Protein, g/L	19.4	42.6	29.0	23.0	43.0	70.0
Na, meq/L	<15	<15	19	0	23	28
K, meq/L	<6	<6	29	0	30	28
Cl, meq/L	0	0	19	0	23	29
Ca, meq/L	0	0	19	0	20	25
P, mmol/L	0	0	16	0	13	16
Mg, meq/L	0	0	15	0	11	17
Zn, mg/L	0	0	6.6	0	6.7	7.5
Cu, mg/L	0	0	0.8	0	0.7	1.0
Vitamins (1/RDA/day)‖	—	—	2.1	—	3.0	2.0

* Lactose-free.
† NP = nonprotein kilocalories per milliliter of solution.
‡ Essential amino acids, branched-chain amino acids included.
§ Branched-chain amino acids only; leucine, isoleucine, and valine.
‖ Volume in liters needed to meet the U.S. RDA per day.
SOURCE: Adapted from Legaspi A, Lowry SF: Agents affecting nutrition and homeostasis, in *Manual of Drug Therapy*. New York, Raven Press, 1985.

vena cava. In order to obtain the maximum benefit, the ratio of calories to nitrogen must be adequate (at least 100 to 150 kcal/g nitrogen) and the two materials must be infused simultaneously. When the sources of calories and nitrogen are given at different times, there is a significant decrease in nitrogen utilization. These nutrients can be given in quantities considerably greater than the basic caloric and nitrogen requirements, and this method has proved to be highly successful in achieving growth and development, positive nitrogen balance, and weight gain in a variety of clinical situations.

INDICATIONS FOR THE USE OF INTRAVENOUS HYPER-ALIMENTATION. The principal indications for parenteral alimentation are found in seriously ill patients suffering from malnutrition, sepsis, or surgical or accidental trauma when use of the gastrointestinal tract for feedings is not possible. It has been used in many instances either where it is not needed or where use of the gastrointestinal tract is more appropriate. In some instances, intravenous nutrition may be used to supplement inadequate oral intake. The safe and successful use of this regimen requires proper selection of patients with specific nutritional needs, experience with the technique, and an awareness of the associated complications. The fundamental goals are to provide sufficient calories and nitrogen substrate to promote tissue repair and to maintain the integrity or growth of the lean tissue mass. Listed below are situations in which parenteral nutrition has been used to successfully achieve these goals.

1. Newborn infants with catastrophic gastrointestinal anomalies, such as tracheoesophageal fistula, gastroschisis, omphalocele, or massive intestinal atresia

2. Infants who fail to thrive nonspecifically or secondarily to gastrointestinal insufficiency associated with the short bowel syndrome, malabsorption, enzyme deficiency, meconium ileus, or idiopathic diarrhea

3. Adult patients with short bowel syndrome secondary to massive small bowel resection or enteroenteric, enterocolic, enterovesical, or enterocutaneous fistulas

4. Patients with high alimentary tract obstructions without vascular compromise, secondary to achalasia, stricture, or neoplasia of the esophagus; gastric carcinoma; or pyloric obstruction

5. Surgical patients with prolonged paralytic ileus following major operations, multiple injuries, or blunt or open abdominal trauma, or patients with reflex ileus complicating various medical diseases

6. Patients with normal bowel length but with malabsorption secondary to sprue, hypoproteinemia, enzyme or pancreatic insufficiency, regional enteritis, or ulcerative colitis

7. Adult patients with functional gastrointestinal disorders such as esophageal dyskinesia following cerebral vascular accident, idiopathic diarrhea, psychogenic vomiting, or anorexia nervosa

8. Patients who cannot ingest food or who regurgitate and aspirate oral or tube feedings because of depressed or obtunded sensorium following severe metabolic derangements, neurologic disorders, intracranial surgery, or central nervous system trauma

9. Patients with excessive metabolic requirements secondary to severe trauma, such as extensive full-thickness burns, major fractures, or soft tissue injuries

10. Patients with granulomatous colitis, ulcerative colitis, and tuberculous enteritis, in which major portions of the absorptive mucosa are diseased

11. Paraplegics, quadriplegics, or debilitated patients with indolent decubitus ulcers in the pelvic areas, particularly when soilage and fecal contamination are a problem

12. Patients with malignancy, with or without cachexia, in

whom malnutrition might jeopardize successful delivery of a therapeutic option

13. Patients with potentially reversible acute renal failure, in whom marked catabolism results in the liberation of intracellular anions and cations, inducing hyperkalemia, hypermagnesemia, and hyperphosphatemia

Conditions *contraindicating* hyperalimentation include the following:

1. Lack of a specific goal for patient management, or where instead of extending a meaningful life, inevitable dying is prolonged
2. Periods of cardiovascular instability or severe metabolic derangement requiring control or correction before attempting hypertonic intravenous feeding
3. Feasible gastrointestinal tract feeding; in the vast majority of instances, this is the best route by which to provide nutrition
4. Patients in good nutritional status, in whom only short-term parenteral nutrition support is required or anticipated
5. Infants with less than 8 cm of small bowel, since virtually all have been unable to adapt sufficiently despite prolonged periods of parenteral nutrition
6. Patients who are irreversibly decerebrate or otherwise dehumanized

INSERTION OF CENTRAL VENOUS INFUSION CATHETER. The successful use of intravenous hyperalimentation generally depends upon the proper placement and management of the central venous feeding catheter. A 16-gauge, 8- or 12-in radiopaque catheter is introduced percutaneously through the subclavian or internal jugular vein and threaded into the superior vena cava. Although the technique for subclavian vein puncture (Fig. 2-5) has been quite popular, the internal jugular approach may be used (Fig. 2-6).

For insertion of the intravenous catheter through the subclavian vein, the patient is placed on his back in a 15° head-down position with a small pad placed between the shoulder blades to allow the shoulders to drop posteriorly. This allows expansion of the subclavian vein and easier penetration. The skin is scrubbed with ether or acetone to defat the surface and then with an iodophor compound. Drapes are carefully placed, and *scrupulous* aseptic precautions are observed. Local anesthetic is infiltrated into the skin, subcutaneous tissue, and periosteum at the inferior border of the midpoint of the clavicle. A 2-in-long, 14-gauge needle attached to a small syringe is

Fig. 2-5. Use of the subclavian vein for insertion of central venous catheter.

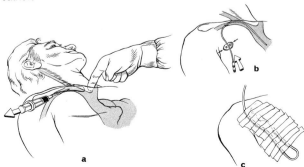

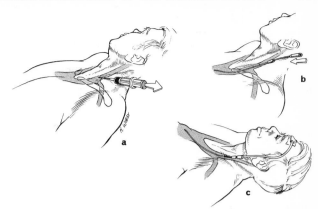

Fig. 2-6. Use of internal jugular vein for insertion of central venous catheter.

inserted, beveled down through the wheal, and advanced toward the tip of the operator's finger, which is pressed well into the patient's suprasternal notch. The needle should hug the inferior clavicular surface and go over the first rib into the subclavian vein. With slight negative pressure applied to the syringe, entrance into the vein will be noted by the appearance of blood. The needle is advanced a few millimeters further to be sure that it is entirely within the lumen of the vein. The patient is asked to perform a Valsalva maneuver, or the thumb is held over the needle hub as the syringe is removed to avoid air embolism. A 16-gauge, 8- or 12-in radiopaque catheter is then introduced through the needle and threaded into the superior vena cava. The needle is then withdrawn from the patient, and a small plastic splint is fitted over the junction of the catheter and needle to prevent catheter severance by the needle. The catheter is connected to a sterile intravenous administration tubing, and a slow infusion is begun while the catheter is sewn to the skin with a small synthetic suture. Antibiotic ointment is applied around the entrance of the catheter into the skin, and an occlusive dressing is applied over it including the junction of the intravenous tubing with the catheter. A chest film is immediately obtained to confirm the position of the radiopaque catheter in the vena cava and to check for a possible pneumothorax.

Every 2 or 3 days, the intravenous tubing is changed at the catheter entry site, the catheter site is scrubbed as for an operative procedure, and antibiotic ointment and a new occlusive dressing are applied. In general, withdrawal or administration of blood through the catheter or the use of the catheter for central venous pressure measurements should be avoided, since the risk of contamination and catheter occlusion are significantly increased.

The use of the internal jugular approach has also been quite satisfactory, especially for the pediatric age group. It is probably unwise, unless absolutely necessary, to place catheters into the inferior vena cava from the lower extremities because of the greater likelihood of sepsis and thromboembolic phenomena. Additionally, cutdown catheter insertions into the cephalic or basilic veins have not proved satisfactory.

Table 2-14. DEXTROSE–AMINO ACID FORMULAS DELIVERED VIA A CENTRAL LINE

Formula	Aminosyn			Freamine III		Novamine		Travasol	
	10%	8.5%	7%	10%	8.5%	11.4%	8.5%	10%	8.5%
Osmolality, mO/L	1000	850	700	950	810	1049	785	1000	1322
Total AA, g/100 mL*	9.86	8.53	6.97	9.70	8.25	11.41	8.50	10.00	8.50
Total EAA, g/100 mL†	4.70	4.06	3.32	4.63	3.94	5.11	3.80	4.05	3.34
PE, g/L‡	100	85	70	96	82	113	84	103	89
N§	15.7	13.4	11.0	15.3	13.0	18.0	13.4	16.5	14.3

Vitamins are usually supplemented with a multiple vitamin preparation containing: vitamin A, 10,000 units; ergocalciferol, 1000 units; vitamin E, 5 units; thiamine HCL, 50 mg; riboflavin, 10 mg; pyridoxine HCL, 15 mg; niacinamide, 100 mg; dexpanthenal, 25 mg; ascorbic acid, 500 mg.

* Total AA = total amino acids.
† Total EAA = total essential amino acids.
‡ PE = protein equivalent.
§ N = nitrogen.
SOURCE: Adapted from Legaspi A, Lowry SF: Agents affecting nutrition and homeostasis, in *Manual of Drug Therapy.* New York, Raven Press, 1985.

PREPARATION AND ADMINISTRATION OF SOLUTIONS. The basic solution contains a final concentration of 20 to 25% dextrose and 3 to 5% crystalline amino acids. The solutions are usually prepared in the pharmacy from commercially available kits containing the component solutions and transfer apparatus. Preparation in the pharmacy under laminar flow reduces the incidence of bacterial contamination of the solution. Proper preparation with suitable quality control is absolutely essential to avoid septic complications.

Since the formulation of commercially available alimentation solutions varies considerably with regard to amino acid and electrolyte concentration, it is imperative that the physician become thoroughly familiar with the levels of the components within the solution utilized (Table 2-14). Only in this manner may additives, in the form of additional electrolytes, be rationally planned to meet specific metabolic needs of the patient. One should recognize that the recommended concentrations of electrolytes are only estimates and that actual requirements may vary considerably (Table 2-10) between individual patients, dependent on routes of fluid and electrolyte loss, renal function, metabolic rate, cardiac function, and the underlying disease state.

Intravenous vitamin preparations should be added as recommended in Table 2-10. In addition, phytonadione (vitamin K_1) 10 mg and folic acid 5 mg should be administered intramuscularly once a week, since these are unstable in the hyperalimentation solution. Cyanocobalamin (vitamin B_{12}) 1 mg is given by intramuscular injection once a month. Intramuscular administration of iron may be required for patients with iron deficiency anemia although adequate mobilization of iron stores may occur once the patient is anabolic. During prolonged fat-free parenteral nutrition essential fatty acid deficiency may become clinically apparent, manifested by a dry, scaly dermatitis and loss of hair. The syndrome may be prevented by periodic infusion of a fat emulsion at a rate equal to 4 to 5% of total calories. Essential trace minerals may be required after prolonged total parenteral nutrition and may be supplied by direct addition of commercial preparations to dextrose amino acid solutions. The most frequent presentation of trace mineral deficiencies is the eczamatoid rash developing both diffusely and at intertriginous areas in zinc-deficient patients. Other rare trace mineral deficiencies include a microcytic anemia associated with copper deficiency and glucose intolerance presumably related to chromium deficiency. The latter complications are seldom seen except in patients receiving parenteral nutrition for extended periods of time. The daily administration of commercially available trace mineral supplements will obviate most such problems.

Depending upon fluid and nitrogen tolerance, parenteral nutrition solutions can generally be increased over 2 to 3 days to achieve the desired infusion rate. Insulin may be supplemented as necessary to ensure glucose tolerance. Wolfe and Elwyn have demonstrated that maximum efficiency of glucose utilization occurs at an infusion rate of 7 mg/(kg · min). Dextrose infusions above this level result in increased fat synthesis and provide no additional suppression of amino acid gluconeogenesis.

Rarely, additional intravenous fluids and electrolytes may be necessary with continued abnormal large losses of fluids. The patient should be carefully monitored for development of electrolyte, volume, acid-base, and septic complications. Vital signs and urinary output are regularly observed, and the patient should be weighed daily. Frequent adjustments of the volume and composition of the solutions are necessary during the course of therapy. Electrolytes are drawn daily until stable and every 2 or 3 days thereafter, and the hemogram, blood urea nitrogen, liver functions, phosphate, and magnesium are determined at least weekly.

The urine sugar level is checked every 6 h and blood sugar concentration at least once daily during the first few days of the infusion and at frequent intervals thereafter.

Relative glucose intolerance may occur following initiation of parenteral alimentation. Insulin may be supplemented as necessary to improve carbohydrate tolerance. The response of blood glucose to exogenous insulin is evaluated by frequent capillary blood determinations, rather than reliance upon glycosuria. If the blood sugar levels remain elevated or glycosuria persists, the dextrose concentration may be decreased, the infusion rate slowed, or regular insulin added to each bottle. The rise in blood glucose concentration observed after initiating an intravenous alimentation program may be temporary, as the normal pancreas increases its output of insulin in response to the continuous carbohydrate infusion. In patients with diabetes mellitus, additional crystalline or human insulin may be required.

The administration of adequate amounts of potassium is essential to achieve positive nitrogen balance and replace depleted intracellular stores. In addition, a significant shift of potassium ion from the extracellular to the intracellular space may take place because of the large glucose infusion, with resultant hypokalemia, metabolic alkalosis, and poor glucose utilization. In some cases as much as 240 meq of potassium ion daily may be required. Hypokalemia may cause glycosuria, which would be treated with potassium, not insulin. Thus, before giving insulin, the serum potassium level must be checked to avoid compounding the hypokalemia.

By virtue of the stress response following major trauma, sepsis, or burns, some patients may remain extremely insulin resistant.

Patients with insulin-dependent diabetes mellitus may exhibit wide fluctuations in blood glucose during parenteral nutrition. Partial replacement of lipid emulsions for dextrose calories may alleviate these problems in selected patients.

FAT EMULSIONS. Lipid emulsions derived from soybean or safflower oils are widely used as an adjunctive nutrient to prevent the development of essential fatty acid deficiency. Recent attention has also focused on their use as a major energy source in parenteral alimentation. Fat emulsion, dextrose, and amino acid combinations appear equally effective to carbohydrate and amino acid solutions in the repletion of nonstressed patients. The efficiency of fat as a caloric source in the traumatized, hypermetabolic patient is not well documented. There appears to be a theoretical advantage to the utilization of lipid emulsions in some septic and trauma patients where nonsuppressible fat oxidation and increased norepinephrine excretion accompany glucose infusion. Patients with abnormal fat transport or metabolism, lipoid nephrosis, coagulopathy, or serious pulmonary disease should not receive fat emulsions. Most investigators advise limitation of administered fat emulsions to between 2.0 and 2.5 g/kg of body weight per day.

SPECIAL FORMULATIONS. Numerous studies have documented the safety of parenteral alimentation in patients with renal failure. For this purpose, special formulations of essential amino acids may be indicated. Selection of the appropriate calorie and nitrogen concentrations must be judged by fluid tolerance, associated illnesses, and the frequency of dialysis. Appropriate use of dialysis is additive to nutritional support in improving survival of these patients. Solutions for patients with acute, oliguric renal failure contain a final dextrose concentration of 40 to 45% and only essential L-amino acids. In patients with nonoliguric renal failure, it may be possible to use both essential and nonessential amino acids to further promote protein synthesis.

Solutions designed for patients with hepatic failure contain increased levels of branched-chain amino acids and decreased concentrations of aromatic amino acids. Such solutions appear to improve encephalopathy but may not improve survival, which is dictated by the underlying hepatic pathology. Patients with moderate hepatic reserve and alcoholic hepatitis may also be treated with standard parenteral formulas to control encephalopathy and ascites.

Cachexia related to severe cardiac disease may be judiciously treated with highly concentrated dextrose and amino acid formulas that are low in sodium content.

COMPLICATIONS. Problems may arise either in the placement and maintenance of venous access or in the formulation and delivery of parenteral solutions. One of the more common and serious complications associated with long-term parenteral feeding is sepsis secondary to contamination of the central venous catheter. Contamination of solutions should be considered but is rare when proper pharmacy protocols have been followed. This problem occurs more frequently in patients with systemic sepsis and in many cases is due to hematogenous seeding of the catheter with bacteria. Usually, it is due to failure to observe strict aseptic precautions during preparation and administration of the solutions. One of the earliest signs of systemic sepsis may be the sudden development of glucose intolerance (with or without temperature increase) in a patient who previously has been maintained on parenteral alimentation without difficulty. When this occurs or if fever develops without obvious cause, a diligent search for a potential septic focus is indicated. Other causes of fever should also be investigated. If fever persists, the infusion catheter should be removed and cultured. Some centers are now replacing catheters considered at low risk for infection over a J-wire. Should evidence of infection persist over 24 to 48 h without a definable source, the catheter should be replaced in the opposite subclavian vein or into one of the internal jugular veins and the infusion restarted. It may be advisable to wait a short period of time before reinserting the catheter, especially if bacteremia or hemodynamic instability are present.

Other complications related to catheter placement include the development of pneumothorax, hemothorax, or hydrothorax; subclavian artery injury; cardiac arrhythmias if the catheter is placed into the atrium or the ventricle; air embolism or catheter embolism; and, rarely, cardiac perforation with tamponade. Clinically evident thrombophlebitis or thrombosis of the superior vena cava has been rare, but radiographically proved thrombophlebitis has been noted in up to 25 percent of selected patients. All these complications may be avoided by strict adherence to the techniques previously outlined.

Although there is a trend for increased utilization of

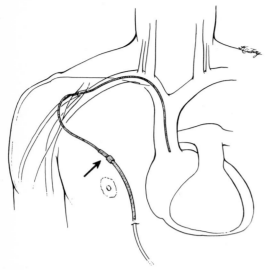

Fig. 2-7. A silastic catheter of the Hickman or Broviac type may be placed by percutaneous means into the superior vena cava or, as shown, by a venotomy in the cephalic, external, or internal jugular veins. The dacron cuff (arrow) may be positioned closer to the skin exit site than is demonstrated above. (Modified from: *Hickman RO et al: Surg Gynecol Obstet 148:871, 1979, with permission.*)

result in carbon dioxide retention and respiratory insufficiency. In addition, excess feeding has also been related to the development of hepatic steatosis or marked glycogen deposition in selected patients. Mild abnormalities of serum transaminases, alkaline phosphatase, and bilirubin may occur in many parenterally nourished patients. Failure of the tests to plateau or return toward normal over 7 to 14 days should suggest another etiology.

HOME PARENTERAL NUTRITION

Patients who do not require a hospital environment for management of their primary disease, yet cannot tolerate adequate enteral or oral feeding, *may* be candidates for home parenteral nutrition. Silastic catheters placed in the superior vena cava by the cephalic or internal jugular vein and tunneled over the chest wall to exit near the sternum have proved effective for this purpose (Fig. 2-7). Alternatives to this technique include the placement of subcutaneous infusion ports, which in preliminary trials have proved to be effective for long-term intravenous nutritional support. An absolute catheter-related infection rate of 0.3 per year per patient may be anticipated.

While home parenteral nutrition is generally more cost effective than similar inpatient methods, criteria for selection of patients must be more stringent than those listed above for hospitalized patients. Patients with terminal illnesses, lack of self-care ability, or a supportive home environment are *not* candidates for this method. The majority of patients will suffer from inflammatory bowel disease, motility disorders, or ischemic bowel infarction and resection.

An extended period of inpatient training is necessary to acquaint the patient and family with appropriate methods of solution preparation and delivery. This is best done in a multidisciplinary setting where professionals are thoroughly familiar with the acute and chronic complications of home parenteral nutrition. All patients on home parenteral nutrition should be placed on the registry maintained by Howard at the Oley Foundation (Albany Medical College). This will allow continued refinements in the clinical and technical management of these patients.

multiple lumen catheters for purposes of infusion therapy and monitoring critically ill patients, the risks, particularly of sepsis and of venous thrombosis, attending the prolonged use of such catheters may be increased. Efforts should be directed at replacing these catheters with standard single lumen intravenous feeding catheters at the earliest possible time. The acute nutritional management of surgical patients seldom requires the use of permanently implanted catheters (Fig. 2-7). Use of these catheters should be restricted to those nonseptic or high-risk patients requiring prolonged periods of nutritional and/or fluid therapy or for selected patients requiring frequent blood sampling.

Hyperosmolar nonketotic hyperglycemia may develop with normal rates of infusion in patients with impaired glucose tolerance or in any patient if the hypertonic solutions are administered too rapidly. This is a particularly common complication in latent diabetics and in patients following severe surgical stress or trauma. Treatment of the condition consists of volume replacement with correction of electrolyte abnormalities and the administration of insulin. This particularly serious complication can be avoided with careful attention to daily fluid balance and frequent determinations of urine and blood sugar levels and serum electrolyte content.

A number of volume, concentration, and compositional abnormalities may also develop, but these are largely avoided by careful attention to the details of patient management. This is particularly important for elderly patients and for patients with significant cardiovascular, renal, or hepatic disorders. Increasing experience has emphasized the importance of not "overfeeding" the parenterally nourished patient. This is particularly true of the depleted patient in whom excess calorie infusion may

Bibliography

Fluid and Electrolyte Therapy

Agus ZS, Wasserstein A, Goldfarb S: Disorders of calcium and magnesium homeostasis. *Am J Med* 72:473, 1982.

Arieff AI, Leach W, Park R, et al: Systemic effects of NaHCO$_3$ in experimental lactic acidosis in dogs. *Am J Physiol* 242:F586, 1982.

Astrup P, Jorgensen K, Andersen OS, et al: The acid-base metabolism: a new approach. *Lancet* 1:1035, 1960.

Baxter CR, Zedlitz WH, Shires GT: High-output acute renal failure complicating acute traumatic injury. *J Trauma* 4:467, 1964.

Bishop RL, Weisfeldt ML: Sodium bicarbonate administration during cardiac arrest: effect on arterial pH, pCO$_2$ and osmolality. *JAMA* 235:506, 1976.

Canizaro PC: Oxygen transport in shock, in Shires GT (ed.): *Shock and Related Problems*. New York, Churchill Livingstone, 1984, pp 95–110.

Canizaro PC, Prager MD, Shires GT: The infusion of Ringer's lactate solution during shock. *Am J Surg* 122:494, 1971.

Carrico CJ, Canizaro PC, Shires GT: Fluid resuscitation following injury. *Crit Care Med* 4:46, 1976.

Collins JA: Problems associated with the massive transfusion of stored blood. *Surgery* 75:274, 1974.

Gamble JL: Chemical anatomy, physiology and pathology of extracellular fluid. In lecture syllabus. Cambridge, MA, Harvard University Press, 1949.

Kwun BK, Boucherit T, Wong J, et al: Treatment of metabolic alkalosis with intravenous infusion of concentrated hydrochloric acid. *Am J Surg* 146:328, 1983.

Mattar JA, Weil MH, Shubin H, et al: Cardiac arrest in the critically ill. II. Hyperosmolal states following cardiac arrest. *Am J Med* 56:162, 1974.

Mengoli LR: Excerpts from the history of postoperative fluid therapy. *Am J Surg* 121:311, 1971.

Moore FD, Olesen KH, McMurrey JD, et al: *Body Cell Mass and Its Supporting Environment: Body Composition in Health and Disease*. Philadelphia, Saunders, 1963.

Moyer CA: *Fluid Balance*. Chicago, Year Book Medical Publishers, Inc, 1954.

Narins RG, Emmett M: Simple and mixed acid-base disorders: a practical approach. *Medicine* 59:161, 1980.

Roberts JP, Roberts JD, Skinner C, et al: Extracellular fluid deficit following operation and its correction with Ringer's lactate; a reassessment. *Ann Surg* 202:1, 1985.

Shires GT, Cunningham JN, Baker CRF, et al: Alterations in cellular membrane function during hemorrhagic shock in primates. *Ann Surg* 176:288, 1972.

Shires GT, Jackson DE: Postoperative salt tolerance. *Arch Surg* 84:703, 1962.

Shires GT III, Peitzman AB, Albert SA, et al: Response of extravascular lung water to intraoperative fluids. *Ann Surg* 197:515, 1983.

Stewart AF: Therapy of malignancy-associated hypercalcemia: 1983. *Am J Med* 74:475, 1983.

Thompson JE, Vollman RW, Austin DJ, et al: Prevention of hypotensive and renal complications of aortic surgery using balanced salt solution: thirteen year experience with 670 cases. *Ann Surg* 167:767, 1968.

Virgilio RW, Rice CL, Smith DE, et al: Crystalloid vs. colloid resuscitation: is one better? *Surgery* 85:129, 1979.

Wang C, Guyton SW: Hyperparathyroid crisis: clinical and pathologic studies of 14 patients. *Ann Surg* 190:782, 1979.

Wong ET, Rude RK, Singer FR, et al: A high prevalence of hypomagnesemia and hypermagnesemia in hospitalized patients. *Am J Clin Pathol* 79:348, 1983.

Wright HK, Gann DS: Correction of defect in free water excretion in postoperative patients by extracellular fluid volume expansion. *Ann Surg* 158:70, 1963.

Nutrition

Abel RM, Beck CH Jr, Abbott WM, et al: Improved survival from acute renal failure after treatment with intravenous essential l-amino acids and glucose. *N Engl J Med* 288:695, 1973.

Alexander JW, MacMillan BG, Stinnert JD, et al: Beneficial effects of aggressive protein feeding in severely burned children. *Ann Surg* 192:505, 1980.

Askanazi J, Rosenbaum SH, Hyman AI, et al: Respiratory changes induced by the large glucose loads of total parenteral nutrition. *JAMA* 243:1444, 1980.

Baker JP, Detsky AS, Stewart S, et al: Randomized trial of total parenteral nutrition in critically ill patients: metabolic effects of varying glucose-lipid ratios as the energy source. *Gastroenterology* 87:53, 1984.

Bartlett RH, Dechert RE, Mault JR, et al: Measurement of metabolism in multiple organ failure. *Surgery* 92:771, 1982.

Bessey PQ, Watters JM, Aoki TT, Wilmore DW: Combined hormonal infusion simulates the metabolic response to injury. *Ann Surg* 200:264, 1984.

Cahill GF Jr: Starvation in man. *N Engl J Med* 282:668, 1970.

Clague MB, Keir MJ, Wright PD, et al: The effects of nutrition and trauma on whole-body protein metabolism in man. *Clin Sci* 65:165, 1983.

Cuthbertson DP: The disturbance of metabolism produced by bony and non-bony injury, with notes on certain abnormal conditions of bone. *Biochem J* 24:1244, 1930.

Dahn MS, Lange P, Lobdell K, et al: Splanchnic and total body oxygen consumption differences in septic and injured patients. *Surgery* 101:69, 1987.

Dudrick SJ, Wilmore DW, Vars HM, et al: Long-term parenteral nutrition with growth, development, and positive nitrogen balance. *Surgery* 64:134, 1968.

Fischer JE (ed): *Surgical Nutrition*. Boston, Little, Brown, 1983.

Grant JP (ed): *Handbook of Total Parenteral Nutrition*. Philadelphia, Saunders, 1980.

Heymsfield SB, Bethel RA, Ansley JD, et al: Enteral hyperalimentation: an alternative to central venous hyperalimentation, *Ann Intern Med* 90:63, 1979.

Lindmark L, Bennegard K, Eden E, et al: Resting energy expenditure in malnourished patients with and without cancer. *Gastroenterology* 87:402, 1984.

Lowry SF: Host metabolic response to injury, in Shires GT, Davis JM (eds): *Host Defenses Advance in Trauma and Surgery*. New York, Raven Press, 1986.

Lowry SF, Brennan MF: Intravenous feeding of the cancer patient, in Caldwell MD, Rombeau JL (eds): *Clinical Nutrition*. Philadelphia, Saunders, 1985, vol II.

Mirtallo JM, Schneider PJ, Mavko K, et al: A comparison of essential and general amino acid infusions on the nutritional support of patients with compromised renal function, *J Parenter Enteral Nutr* 6:109, 1982.

Moore FD: *Metabolic Care of the Surgical Patient*. Philadelphia, Saunders, 1960.

Muggia-Sullam M, Bower RH, Murphy RF: Postoperative enteral versus parenteral nutritional support in gastrointestinal surgery: a matched prospective study. *Am J Surg* 149:106, 1985.

Mullen JL, Buzby GP, Matthews DC, et al: Reduction of operative morbidity and mortality by combined preoperative and postoperative nutritional support. *Ann Surg* 192:604, 1980.

Muller JM, Dienst C, Brenner V, et al: Pre-operative parenteral feeding in patients with gastrointestinal carcinoma. *Lancet* 1:68, 1982.

Rapp RP, Young B, Twyman D, et al: The favorable effect of early parenteral feeding on survival in head-injured patients. *J Neurosurg* 58:906, 1983.

Smith RC, Burkinshaw L, Hill GL: Optimal energy and nitrogen for gastroenterological patients requiring intravenous nutrition. *Gastroenterology* 82:445, 1982.

Twomey PL, Patching SC: Cost-effectiveness of nutritional support. *J Parenter Enteral Nutr* 9:3, 1985.

Wilmore WW (ed): *The Metabolic Management of the Critically Ill*. New York, Plenum Press, 1977.

Chapter 3

Hemostasis, Surgical Bleeding, and Transfusion

Seymour I. Schwartz

BIOLOGY OF HEMOSTASIS

Hemostasis is a complex process that prevents or terminates blood loss from the intravascular space, provides a fibrin network for tissue repair, and ultimately, removes the fibrin when it is no longer needed. Four major physiologic events participate, both in sequence and interdependently, in the hemostatic process. Vascular constriction, platelet plug formation, fibrin formation, and fibrinolysis occur in that general order, but the products of each of these four processes are interrelated in such a fashion that there is a continuum and multiple reinforcements (Fig. 3-1.).

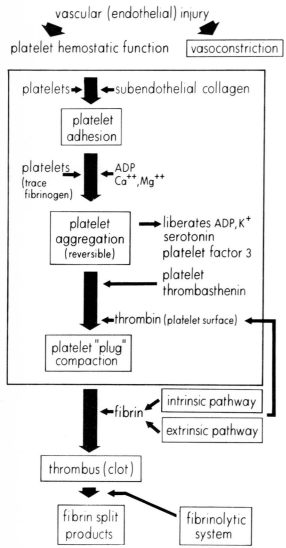

Fig. 3-1. Schematic representation of hemostasis.

tent vasodilator. Serotonin, 5-hydroxytryptamine (5-HT), released during platelet aggregation, is another vasoconstrictor, but it has been shown that when platelets have been depleted of serotonin in vivo, constriction is not inhibited. Bradykinin and fibrinopeptides in the coagulation schema are also capable of contracting smooth muscle. Some patients with mild bleeding disorders and a prolonged bleeding time have, as their only abnormality, capillary loops that fail to constrict in response to injury.

A lateral incision in a small artery may remain open because of physical forces, while complete transection of a similarly sized vessel contracts to the extent that bleeding may cease spontaneously. The vascular response factor should also include the contribution of pressure provided by surrounding tissues. Bleeding from a small venule ruptured by trauma, in the thigh of an athlete, may be negligible because of the compressive effect of surrounding muscle. In the same individual, bleeding from a similar vessel in the nasal mucosa may be significant. When there is low perivascular pressure, as seen in patients with muscle atrophy accompanying aging, prolonged steroid therapy, and in patients with the Ehlers-Danlos syndrome, bleeding tends to be more persistent.

Platelet Function

Platelets are 2-μm diameter fragments of megakaryocytes and number 200,000 to 400,000/mm^3 in circulating blood with a life span of 7 to 9 days. They play an integral role in hemostasis along two pathways. Platelets, which normally do not adhere to each other or to the normal vessel wall, form a plug that stops bleeding when vascular disruption occurs. Injury to the intima exposes subendothelial collagen to which platelets adhere within 15 s of the traumatic event. This requires von Willebrand factor (vWF), a protein that is lacking in patients with von Willebrand's disease. The platelets then expand and develop pseudopodal processes and also initiate a release reaction that recruits other platelets from the circulating blood. As a consequence, a loose platelet aggregate forms, sealing the disrupted blood vessel. The aggregation up to this point is reversible and is not associated with secretion. This process is known as *primary hemostasis*. The administration of heparin does not interfere with this reaction, and that fact explains why hemostasis can occur in the heparinized patient. Adenosine diphosphate (ADP) and serotonin are principal mediators in this process of adhesion and aggregation. Various prostaglandins have opposing activities. Arachidonic acid, released from platelet membranes, is converted by cyclooxygenase to PGG$_2$ and PGH$_2$, which, in turn, are converted to TXA$_2$, a potent platelet aggregator and vasoconstrictor. By contrast, PGE$_1$ (prostacycline) and PGE$_2$ inhibit aggregation and act as vasodilators.

ADP, released from damaged tissues and stimulated platelets, plus platelet factor 4 and trace thrombin on the platelet surface in the face of Ca^{2+} and Mg^{2+}, stimulate a platelet release reaction by which the content of the platelet and its granules is discharged. Fibrinogen is required for this process. The release reaction results in compac-

Vascular Constriction

Adherence of endothelial cells to adjacent endothelial cells may be sufficient to cause cessation of blood loss from the intravascular space. Vasoconstriction is the initial vascular response to injury even at the capillary level. It is dependent upon local contraction of smooth muscle that has a reflex response to various stimuli. The initial vascular constriction occurs prior to platelet adherence at the site of injury. Vasoconstriction is subsequently linked to platelet plug and fibrin formation. Thromboxane A$_2$ (TXA$_2$), that results from the release of arachidonic acid from platelet membranes during aggregation, is a powerful vasoconstrictor. By contrast, prostacycline, which is also secreted during the platelet release reaction, is a po-

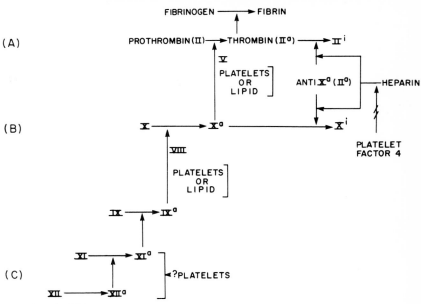

Fig. 3-2. Role of platelets in coagulation. Platelets or phospholipid accelerate reactions *A* and *B*. In addition, the role of platelets may be more complex in reaction *B* and may serve to protect factor X_a from inactivation by plasma inhibitors. Platelets may also play a part in activating the contact system *C*. Platelet factor 4 is the heparin-neutralizing substance (i = inactivated clotting factor). (From: *Weiss HJ: 1975, with permission.*)

tion of the platelets and the formation of an "amorphous" plug, wich is no longer reversible. This process is inhibited by cyclic AMP. As a consequence of the release reaction, platelet factor 3 is made available and contributes phospholipid to several stages of the coagulation cascade.

The lipoprotein surface provided by platelets catalyzes reactions that are involved in the conversion of prothrombin (factor II) into thrombin (Fig. 3-2). Platelet factor 3 is involved in the reaction by which activated factor IX (IXa), factor VIII, and calcium activate factor X. It is also involved in the reaction by which Xa, factor V, and Ca^{2+} activate factor II. Platelets may also play a role in the initial activation of factor XII and the activation of factor XI. Platelet factor 4 and β-thromboglobulin are also made available during the release reaction, and they may inhibit the activity of heparin and modify fibrin formation. The platelets also play a role in the fibrinolytic process by releasing an inhibitor of plasminogen activation.

Coagulation

Coagulation is the process by which prothrombin is converted into the proteolytic enzyme thrombin, which, in turn, cleaves the fibrinogen molecule to form insoluble fibrin in order to stabilize and add to the platelet plug. Coagulation consists of a series of zymogen activation stages in which circulating proenzymes are converted in sequence to activated proteases (Fig. 3-3). The traditional concept of the clotting system evolved from test tube

analysis and follows two pathways. The two pathways are the *intrinsic* pathway, which involves components normally present in blood, and the *extrinsic* pathway that is initiated by the tissue lipoprotein. In the intrinsic pathway factor XII is activated by binding to subendothelial collagen. Prekallikrein and high molecular weight kinogen amplify this contact phase. Activated factor XII (XIIa) proteolytically cleaves factor XI and also prekallikrein to form XIa and kallikrein. In the presence of Ca^{2+}, XIa activates factor IX (IXa). This, in turn, complexes with factor VIII, which can be activated to a more potent form by thrombin, and, in the presence of Ca^{2+} and the phospholipid platelet factor 3, activates factor X. In the extrinsic pathway, the tissue phospholipid, thromboplastin, reacts with factor VII and Ca^{2+} to activate factor X.

Activated factor X (Xa), produced by the two pathways, proteolyzes prothrombin (factor II) to form thrombin. This process is accelerated by factor V, tissue lipoproteins, platelet surface phospholipids, and Ca^{2+}. Thrombin activates the fibrin stabilizing factor (XIII) and cleaves fibrinopeptides A and B from fibrinogen (factor I) to form fibrin, a monomer that is cross-linked with XIIIa, to form a stable clot (Table 3-1).

All the coagulation factors except thromboplastin, Ca^{2+}, and most of factor VIII are synthesized in the liver. Factors II, VII, IX, and X require vitamin K for their production.

Fibrinolysis

Fibrinolysis is a natural process directed at maintaining the patency of blood vessels by lysis of fibrin deposits. Also involved in the maintenance of vascular patency is circulating ATIII which neutralizes the action of thrombin and other proteases in the coagulation cascade.

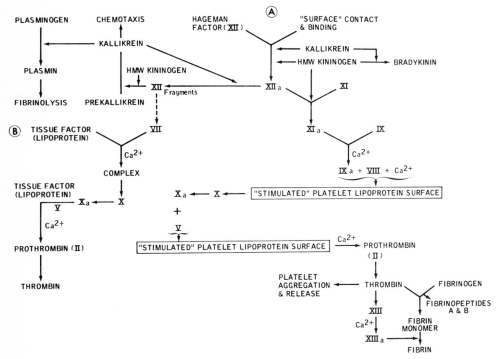

Fig. 3-3. Outline of the intrinsic (A) and extrinsic (B) pathways of fibrin formation. These interactions, which represent "secondary hemostasis," occur simultaneously with development of the hemostatic plug, i.e., primary hemostasis. The subendothelial blood vessel surface exposed by vascular damage or severance serves as a nidus for platelet adhesion and simulation. Factor XII (Hageman factor) also binds to the subendothelium and in so doing is converted from its precursor (zymogen) form to an activated molecule (XII$_a$). This interaction by itself (known as the contact phase) is relatively prolonged and inefficient. Amplification and enhancement occur by virtue of participation of prekalikrein and high-molecular-weight kininogen. The contact phase is also involved in initiation of fibrinolysis, kinin generation, and chemotaxis. Subsequent stages of intrinsic and extrinsic coagulation may be conceptualized as a biphasic catalytic system in which activated zymogens such as IX$_a$ form a complex with factor VIII. In the presence of calcium the complex catalyzes activation of factor X on the platelet lipoprotein surface. The X$_a$ receptor site on the platelet surface is known to be coagulation factor V (not phospholipid). Tissue factor lipoprotein (B) probably functions in a manner analogous to the stimulated platelet membrane. During activation of prothrombin by the X$_a$–V surface complex, prothrombin is bound via a calcium-mediated interaction. Three pairs of adjacent γ-carboxyglutamic acid residues are present on the prothrombin molecule, and each pair binds a calcium ion. In the absence of vitamin K an abnormal prothrombin molecule is synthesized containing glutamic but not γ-carboxyglutamic acid. Thus, calcium-mediated binding of prothrombin to the X$_a$–V-platelet lipoprotein complex is defective (these reactions have not yet been studied with platelets or platelet membranes, and the last statement is an assumption). Thrombin, a two-chain serine protease, cleaves arginine-glycine bonds of fibrinogen. One chain of thrombin (the B chain) closely resembles the serine proteases produced in the pancreas. Thrombin in concentrations that do not interact with fibrogen induces platelet aggregation and release. The stimulatory effect of the platelet surface may not be confined to coagulation proteins per se. It has been shown that tissue factor-type activity generated by leukocytes in the presence of endotoxin is enhanced by platelet membranes. (From: *Marcus AJ: 1978, with permission.*)

Fibrinolysis is initiated at the same time as the clotting mechanism under the influence of circulating kinases, tissue activators, and kallikrein present in many organs including venous endothelium. Fibrinolysis is dependent upon the enzyme, plasmin, which is derived from a precursor plasma protein (plasminogen) (Fig. 3-4). Plasminogen levels are known to rise as a consequence of exercise, venous occlusion, and anoxia. Plasminogen activation is also initiated by the activation of factor XII. The plasminogen is preferentially absorbed on fibrin deposits. The enzyme plasmin lyses fibrin and acts on other coagulant proteins, including fibrinogen, factor V, and factor VIII, as well. The smaller fragments of polypeptide products of fibrin that are produced interfere with normal platelet aggregation; the larger fragments are incorporated into the clot in lieu of normal fibrin monomers and result in an unstable clot. Human blood also contains an anti-plasmin that inhibits plasminogen activation, and platelets are believed to possess anti-fibrinolytic activity.

CONGENITAL HEMOSTATIC DEFECTS

Inheritance

The modes of inheritance of hemostatic disorders, with only rare exceptions, are three in type: (1) autosomal dominant, (2) autosomal recessive, and (3) sex-linked recessive. Since one chromosome of each of the 22 autosomal pairs normally is derived from each parent, any gene inherited as a part of an autosomal chromosome nor-

Table 3-1. NOMENCLATURE OF COAGULATION FACTORS

Factor I	Fibrinogen
Factor II	Prothrombin
Factor III	Thromboplastin (tissue or platelet factors)
Factor IV	Calcium
Factor V	Proaccelerin
Factor VI	(Same as factor V)
Factor VII	Proconvertin
Factor VIII	Antihemophilic factor A
Factor IX	Plasma thromboplastin component
Factor X	Stuart-Prower factor
Factor XI	Antihemophilic factor C
Factor XII	Hageman factor
Factor XIII	Fibrin stabilizing factor (Laki-Lorand)

mally will occur with equal frequency among males and females. Each child of a parent carrying an autosomal dominant gene has one chance in two of inheriting that trait. The most common hemostatic disorder transmitted by the autosomal dominant mode is von Willebrand's disease. Hereditary hemorrhagic telangiectasia and factor XI deficiency also appear to be transmitted in this fashion.

A normal individual should transmit no disease to his progeny. Occasionally, in a pedigree with an autosomal dominant gene, an *apparently* normal person may transmit disease to his or her child. The parent clearly carried the gene, which clinically expressed no defect. Explanation of this phenomenon is not at hand. The gene activity in the parent is referred to as "incompletely penetrant."

In inherited hemostatic disorders, the difference in clinical expression between dominant and recessive genes is a graded one rather than an "all-or-none" phenomenon. The heterozygous individual with an autosomal recessive trait may have a measurable deficiency of the factor governed by that gene, but no clinical disease. In order to demonstrate clinical expression of disease, the individual must be homozygous. This appears to be the case, for example, in factor X deficiency. The homozygote with clinical disease has less than 5 percent of factor X activity, while heterozygotes have levels ranging from 21 to 50 percent. Since the presumed heterozygotes within the same pedigree vary in factor X activity, it is convenient to suggest that the gene shows variable expression. Other hemostatic disorders probably inherited in this mode are factor V, factor VII, and factor I deficiencies.

Sex-linked recessive inheritance governs true hemophilia (factor VIII deficiency) and factor IX deficiency (Christmas disease). The genes for these diseases are recessive in expression and are carried on the female (X) chromosome. When paired with the normal X chromosome (the female carrier state), clinical disease is not present. When the affected X chromosome is paired with the normal male (Y) chromosome, clinical disease is expressed.

Theoretically, with the "graded" expression, the female carrier should be detectable in the laboratory. In fact, since the range of factor VIII activity normally is so broad, most female carriers *appear* to fall in the low-normal range. Estimates vary, but possibly as many as 50 percent of female carriers can be identified. Although the sex-linked recessive mode of inheritance has been confirmed repeatedly in true hemophilia, it seems likely that an *autosomal* gene also may influence factor VIII activity. This probability is emphasized by the autosomal dominant mode of inheritance of von Willebrand's disease, characterized by low factor VIII activity, and also by the patterns of variation in factor VIII activity among individuals within the same normal family and among different normal families.

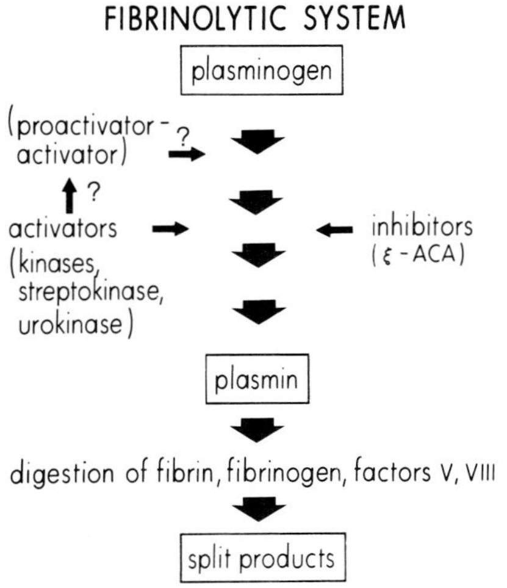

Platelet Deficiencies

The most common congenital platelet deficiency is an abnormality seen in *von Willebrand's disease* (see material below). In this disorder, the von Willebrand factor (vWF), which is missing, has been shown to be required for platelet adhesion to subendothelial collagen. Also, unlike platelets of normal patients that aggregate in vitro when ristocetin is added, platelets from patients with von Willebrand's disease fail to aggregate with the addition of ristocetin. Another inherited disorder affecting platelets is the rare *Bernard-Soulier syndrome*. Patients with Bernard-Soulier syndrome have normal levels of vWF and the addition of that factor does not affect aggregation of platelets in the presence of ristocetin. In Bernard-Soulier syndrome, the platelet membrane receptor for vWF, a portion of the glycoprotein I complex, is missing.

Glanzmann's thrombasthenia is a rare congenital disorder in which platelets fail to aggregate in the presence of ADP, and mediation of factors involved in clot retention is impaired also. Patients with *congenital afibrinogenemia* also have impairment of platelet aggregation because fibrinogen is required for this process to occur. Patients with congenital afibrinogenemia have disturbed platelet function, manifested by a prolonged bleeding time correctable by fibrinogen administration.

Fig. 3-4. Fibrinolytic system.

FIBRINOLYTIC SYSTEM

plasminogen

(proactivator → activator) → ?

↑ ?

activators → ← inhibitors (kinases, streptokinase, urokinase) (ε-ACA)

plasmin

digestion of fibrin, fibrinogen, factors V, VIII

split products

Congenital disorders of platelet secretion include *storage pool disease,* in which the platelets lack the storage capability of ADP required for aggregation. The Hermansky-Pudlak syndrome (occulocutaneous albinism, ceroidlike deposits in macrophages, and bleeding diathesis) is classified in this category. Congenital *primary release defects* have also been described and are responsible for prolonged bleeding time.

Congenital Defects of Coagulation Factors

FACTOR VIII DEFICIENCY (CLASSICAL HEMOPHILIA)

Classical hemophilia (hemophilia A) is a disease of males. The failure to synthesize normal factor VIII activity is inherited as a sex-linked recessive trait. Spontaneous mutations account for almost 20 percent of cases. The incidence of the disease is approximately 1:10,000 to 1:15,000 population, and the clinical manifestations can be extremely variable. The accuracy for detecting the carrier state now approaches 90 percent.

CLINICAL MANIFESTATIONS. Characteristically, the severity of clinical manifestations is related to the degree of deficiency of factor VIII. Spontaneous bleeding and severe complications are the rule when virtually no factor VIII can be detected in the plasma. When plasma factor VIII concentrations are in the range of 5 percent of normal, the patient may have no spontaneous bleeding yet may bleed severely with trauma or surgical treatment. Patients with levels greater than 5 percent of normal (greater than $0.05 \mu m/mL$) are considered mild hemophiliacs. Patients whose factor VIII levels fall between 1 and 5 percent of normal are considered moderately severe hemophiliacs. Typically, members of the same pedigree with true hemophilia will have approximately the same degree of clinical manifestations.

While the severely affected patient may bleed during early infancy, significant bleeding typically is noted first when the child is a toddler. At that time, in addition to the classic bleeding into joints, epistaxis and hematuria may be noted. Bleeding that is life-threatening may follow injury to the tongue or frenulum. Tracheal compression and retropharyngeal bleeding may follow tonsillar infection. Intracranial bleeding, associated with trauma in half the cases, accounts for 25 percent of deaths. Vascular and neural compromise may occur in relation to pressure secondary to bleeding into a soft tissue closed space. Equinus contracture deformity may be seen in severely hemophilic patients secondary to bleeding into the calf. Volkmann's contracture of the forearm and flexion contractures of the knees and elbows are also disabling sequelae of deep soft tissue bleeding.

Hemarthrosis is the most characteristic orthopaedic problem. Bleeding into the joint may cause few symptoms until distention of the joint capsule occurs. A large hemarthrosis generally is manifested by a tender, swollen, warm, and painful joint. Muscle spasm and pain around the joint arise from involvement of periarticular structures. These signs may mimic infection. The same ortho-

paedic problems are noted in association with severe factor IX deficiency (Christmas disease).

Retroperitoneal bleeding may follow lifting of a heavy object or strenuous exercise. Signs of posterior peritoneal irritation and spasm of the iliopsoas suggest the diagnosis. Hypovolemic shock may occur, since the amount of blood loss that can take place in this setting is enormous. The clinical manifestations of intramural intestinal hematoma are nausea and vomiting, crampy abdominal pain, and signs of peritoneal irritation mimic those of appendicitis. Fever and leukocytosis may be noted. Radiographs of the abdomen may fail to reveal an abnormality or may display a modest amount of ileus. Upper gastrointestinal examination may demonstrate a uniform thickening of mucosal folds which has been described as a "picket fence" or "stack of coins" appearance (Fig. 3-5). Intramural hematomas of the intestine occur with other hemostatic disorders and, therefore, should be considered

Fig. 3-5. Radiograph of patient with hemophilia. Note thickening of mucosal folds indicative of an intramural hematoma.

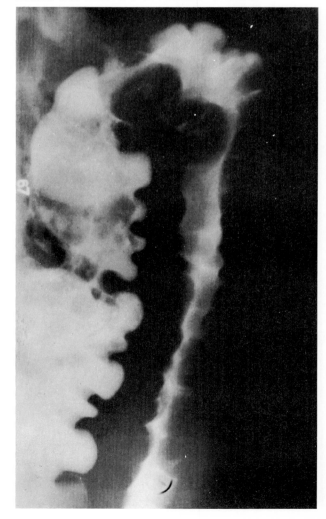

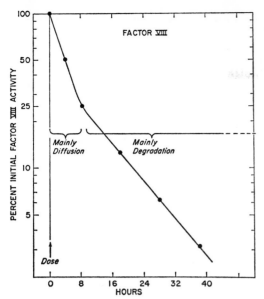

Fig. 3-6. Schematic representation of in vivo decay of a single dose of factor VIII. (From: *Shulman NR: 1968, with permission.*)

when any patient with a hemostatic problem presents with findings suggesting an acute intraabdominal process.

TREATMENT. Replacement Therapy. The plasma concentration of factor VIII necessary for maintenance of hemostatic integrity is normally quite small. Patients with as little as 2 to 3 percent of factor VIII activity usually do not bleed spontaneously. Once serious bleeding begins, however, a much higher level of factor VIII activity, probably approaching 30 percent, is necessary to achieve hemostasis.

The half-life of factor VIII is 8 to 12 h. Following administration of a given dose of factor VIII, approximately one-half of the initial posttransfusion activity disappears from the plasma in 4 h. This early disappearance is thought to be due, in large part, to diffusion from the intravascular space. The period of equilibration can extend for as long as 8 h, at which time only about one-quarter of the initial level remains in the circulating blood. From that time on, the slope of disappearance is less steep (Fig. 3-6). Twenty-four hours after a given dose, no more than 7 to 8 percent of administered factor VIII activity remains within the circulation.

One unit of factor VIII activity is considered that amount present in 1 mL of normal plasma. Actually, fresh frozen plasma contains 0.60 unit/mL. Theoretically, in a patient with 0 percent activity, to achieve an initial posttransfusion level of 60 percent of normal, using fresh plasma, a volume of plasma equal to 60 percent of the patient's estimated plasma volume would have to be administered. Table 3-2 shows approximate levels of factor VIII required for hemostasis in different lesions. The minimum hemostatic level of factor VIII for mild hemorrhages is 30 percent; for joint and muscle bleeding and major hemorrhages, it is 50 percent. For major surgery and life-threatening bleeding, levels of 80 to 100 percent

should be reached preoperatively and maintained above 30 percent for 2 weeks. Remembering the loss from the circulation, one-half the initial dose would need to be supplied every 12 h. The use of fresh plasma in such a circumstance would require a volume that is excessive. Factor VIII concentrates now available circumvent this problem. Cryoprecipitate concentrates of factor VIII can be regarded as containing 9.6 units/mL. The amount of material to be given can be computed from the formula

$$\frac{\text{Patient's weight (kg)} \times \text{desired rise of}}{\text{factor VIII (\% average normal)}} = R$$

where R is a factor that is fairly constant for any given type of material and represents the rise of factor VIII obtained in the patient's plasma for every unit of transfused factor VIII per kilogram of the patient's body weight. Half that amount is subsequently administered every 4 to 6 h to maintain a safe level. There is now a variety of factor VIII concentrates available. Regardless of the preparation employed, continued laboratory assessment of circulating factor VIII level is an important element in the control of these patients. Wet-frozen cryoprecipitate is preferred for replacement in patients with mild hemophilia since the risk of hepatitis is less than it is with factor VIII concentrates. The latter are preferred for major replacement problems. In mild hemophilia A and in mild von Willebrand's disease, DAVP (1-desamino-8-D-arginine vasopressin), a synthetic derivative of vasopressin, has been used to effect a dose-dependent increase of all factor VIII activities and to effect release of plasminogen activator. Patients undergoing orthopaedic or neurosurgical procedures should also receive a fibrinolytic inhibitor.

Following major surgical treatment of the hemophiliac, transfusion replacement of factor VIII should be continued for at least 10 days. Wounds should be well healed and all drains removed prior to the termination of therapy. If sutures remain, transfusion should be reinstituted prior to their removal. Many recent reports document the safety of major surgical procedures in hemophilic patients receiving replacement therapy. But in one large series, the incidence of postoperative hemorrhage did not improve over a 16-year period despite a threefold increase in dosage of factor VIII, suggesting that circulating factor VIII levels are not the sole determinant of bleeding in these patients.

The virus of homologous serum hepatitis is transmitted by the various concentrates of plasma. Other complications of replacement therapy include the appearance of inhibitors of factor VIII, which may arise in the hemophiliacs who have had transfusion. These inhibitors have been characterized as antibodies of the γ G variety. They tend to diminish in several weeks if further transfusion is not employed. Laboratory search for these factors should be carried out in every hemophilic patient who is considered a candidate for elective surgical treatment, as their presence complicates transfusion management. Paradoxical bleeding may occur in patients transfused to an appro-

Table 3-2. PRINCIPLES OF SUBSTITUTION THERAPY IN SURGERY IN PATIENTS WITH SEVERE BLEEDING DISORDERS

Type of operation and disease	Day of operation — Desirable level of (%)	Dosage — Initial units/kg	Dosage — Maintenance units/kg BW*	Interval (h)	Day 2–7 postoperatively — Desirable level of (%)	Dosage — Maintenance units/kg BW	Interval (h)	Day 8 postoperatively — Desirable level of (%)	Dosage — Maintenance units/kg BW	Interval (h)
Hemophilia A	VII:C	VIII:C			VIII:C			VIII:C		
Major surgery	50–150	50–60	25–30	4–6	40–60	20–40	4–8	15–25	10–15	12–24
Minor surgery	40–50	25–40	20–30	4–8	30–50	15–20	6–12			
Hemophilia B	IX:C	IX:C			IX:C			IX:C		
Major surgery	50–150	60–70	30–40	8–12	40–60	30–40	12–24	15–25	10–20	24–48
Minor surgery	40–50	40–40	20–30	8–12	30–50	15–20	24			
von Willebrand's disease	VIII:C	VIII:C			VIII:C			VIII:C		
Major surgery	50–70 BT† < 5 min	30–40	30–40	4–5	> 40 BT < 10 min	10–20	12	20–40	5–10	24–48
Minor surgery	VIII:C 20–50 BT < 5 min	10–20	10–20	4–5	VIII:C > 40 BT < 10 min	5–10	12			

* Body weight.

† Bleeding time according to Duke.

SOURCE: Nilsson IM, Larsson SA, Bergentz SE, 1987, with permission.

priate factor VIII level due to the development of abnormal platelet function.

Adjunctive Management. Treatment of soft tissue bleeding is directed at the prevention of airway obstruction and vascular and neural damage. These are accomplished best by the administration of sufficient factor VIII. Bed rest and cold packs can be of some assistance. In general, results of fasciotomy to relieve pressure have varied from disappointing to disastrous. The occasional development of large cysts has resulted in sufficient deformity and disability to require amputation.

The primary treatment of hemophilic hemarthrosis is directed at maintaining full range of motion and minimal destruction of the cartilage. Aspiration of blood from the hemophilic joint is not uniformly endorsed, and when regarded as necessary, it should be considered a major surgical event. Elevation of factor VIII level by transfusion is necessary. The procedure should be carried out in the operating room under strict sterile precautions. In most instances, aspiration is not required, and the combination of factor VIII replacement and local cold packing proves sufficient. Physiotherapy plays a critical role and should consist of *active* exercises, since the patient is unlikely to move the extremity to a point where bleeding will recur. Passive exercises often result in recurrence of bleeding. The reader is referred to the review by Curtiss for details of orthopaedic management.

The management of intramural intestinal hematoma and retroperitoneal bleeding is predicated on appropriate transfusion therapy and avoidance of surgical treatment. Even when a relatively minor procedure, such as trache-ostomy, is performed, the plasma level of factor VIII should be raised above 25 to 30 percent. Since dental hygiene usually is poor in hemophilic patients, dental and oral surgical treatment frequently are necessary. The same principles of transfusion therapy pertain, and the procedures should be delegated to well-trained personnel working where optimal care can be provided.

FACTOR IX DEFICIENCY (CHRISTMAS DISEASE)

Factor IX deficiency clinically is indistinguishable from factor VIII deficiency and also has an X-linked recessive mode of inheritance. These two entities were considered a single disease until 1952, when their unique deficiencies were documented. Factor IX deficiency accounts for 20 percent of hemophiliacs. Christmas disease, like classical hemophilia, can occur in severe, moderate, or mild forms according to the level of factor IX activity in the plasma. The severe form has a factor IX level of less than 1 percent; one-half of the patients belong to this group.

TREATMENT. Most patients with severe factor IX deficiency require substitution therapy on a regular basis. All patients require substitution therapy whenever minor or major surgery is performed. Currently, therapy is generally based on the administration of factor IX concentrates. Initially the rate of disappearance of factor IX from the circulation is more rapid than that of factor VIII; subsequently factor IX, with a half-life of 18 to 40 h, has a slower disappearance rate. A variety of factor IX concentrates is available. Good therapeutic results have been achieved with each of the concentrates and minimal side effects have been noted. Konyne, which contains 10 to 60 units of factor IX/mL, has produced good results, but thromboembolic complications had been reported. More recently, the preparations have had other activated clotting factors removed, and the incidence of thromboembolic complications has decreased. During severe hemorrhage, treatment should be directed at achieving plasma factor IX levels of 20 to 50 percent of normal for the first 3 to 5 days, and then maintaining the plasma level at 10 to 20 percent of normal for approximately 10 days. The usual daily dose is 30 to 50 μm/kg of body weight, followed by 20 μm/kg of body weight/24 h. When an operation is required, the plasma level of approximately 50 to 70 percent of normal should be achieved. Sixty microns per kilogram of body weight every 24 h is recommended during the operation and the first postoperative day, followed by 30 to 40 μm/kg every 24 h for the next 2 to 3 days, and 20 μm/kg every 24 h for the remainder of the week. In all instances, the levels should be monitored by laboratory determinations. The development of antibodies against factor IX represents a serious complication that is difficult to deal with. This occurs in about 10 percent of patients with Christmas disease. These patients are managed by withholding all infusion therapy with blood or plasma. High doses of factor IX concentrates combined with cyclophosphamide have been effective.

von WILLEBRAND'S DISEASE

von Willebrand's disease occurs as commonly as true hemophilia. The increasing recognition of this disease is related to more reliable factor VIII assays. This hereditary disorder of hemostasis is usually transmitted as an autosomally dominant trait but recessive inheritance may occur. The disease is characterized by a diminution of the level of factor VIII:C (procoagulant) activity that corrects the clotting abnormality in hemophilia A plasma. The reduction of factor VIII:C activity usually is not as great as that seen in classical hemophilia. Also unlike classical hemophilia, where factor VIII:C activity remains constant, in the patient with von Willebrand's disease variation in the level of circulating factor VIII:C activity may be noted. Characteristically, these patients also have a prolonged bleeding time, but this is less constant than the factor VIII:C reduction. A given patient may have an abnormal bleeding time on one occasion and a normal bleeding time on another. The level of factor VIII–related antigen (factor VIII:Ag) is disproportionately lower than that of factor VIII:C, and ristocetin fails to cause platelet aggregation in about 70 percent of patients with the disease.

CLINICAL MANIFESTATIONS. The manifestations of bleeding usually are mild and often overlooked until trauma or the stress of surgical treatment makes them apparent. A careful clinical history is, therefore, of great importance in these patients. Spontaneous manifestations often are limited to bleeding into the skin or mild mucous membrane bleeding. Epistaxis and menorrhagia have been relatively common in our personal experience. Serious bleeding following dental extractions and tonsillec-

tomy also are not uncommon. Fatal bleeding from the gastrointestinal tract has been described.

TREATMENT. Treatment is directed at correcting the bleeding time and factor VIII R:WF (the von Willebrand factor). Only cryoprecipitate is reliably effective. High-purity concentrates of factor VIII:C lack the required factor VIII R:WF. Ten to forty units per kilogram of cryoprecipitate are administered every 12 h to correct the bleeding time. Replacement therapy should be begun 1 day prior to a surgical procedure. Aspirin *must* be avoided for 10 days before an elective operation. Duration of treatment should be the same as that described for the patient with classical hemophilia.

FACTOR XI (PTA) DEFICIENCY (ROSENTHAL'S SYNDROME)

This uncommon and relatively mild disorder is inherited in an autosomally dominant fashion. Without careful laboratory testing, the affected males and females may be confused with von Willebrand's disease patients. A majority of patients are of Jewish ancestry.

Epistaxis is a common spontaneous clinical manifestation. The disease usually is recognized as a result of bleeding during and after operation. The bleeding usually is minor. Some patients have undergone major procedures without significant hemorrhage.

TREATMENT. Fresh frozen plasma is a suitable therapeutic medium. This factor disappears slowly from the circulation, and its biologic half-life may be as long as 80 h. An initial dose of 10 to 20 mL of plasma/kg of body weight can be given 6 or 8 h prior to anticipated surgical treatment, followed by a maintenance dose of 5 mL/kg administered every 24 h. Therapy usually can be discontinued several days earlier than with patients with more serious hemostatic disorders.

FACTOR V (PROACCELERIN) DEFICIENCY (PARAHEMOPHILIA)

This extremely rare deficiency usually is associated with mild bleeding, but serious bleeding may be encountered. The disease is transmitted as an autosomal recessive trait and is found in males and females alike. Only patients who presumably inherit the gene from both parents seem to be bleeders.

Factor V is synthesized in the liver but differs from prothrombin and factors VII, IX, and X in that factor V synthesis is not dependent upon vitamin K or inhibited by the administration of the coumarin drugs. Patients with severe parenchymal liver disease may be deficient in factor V. Both the prothrombin time (PT) and the partial-thromboplastin time (PTT) are prolonged, and the disorder is diagnosed by a specific assay. About one-third of patients have a prolonged bleeding time.

TREATMENT. Excessive bleeding may occur at the time of operation, usually in patients who have levels of less than 1 percent of normal factor V concentration. No more than 25 percent of normal activity is necessary for hemostasis during operative procedures. This level can be achieved by administering 15 mL of fresh frozen plasma per kilogram of body weight 12 h prior to operation. The administration of 7 to 10 mL/kg every 24 h will suffice to maintain hemostasis until healing has occurred. Once again, it is wise to administer the factor at the time of suture removal. Factor V, also known as labile factor, loses its activity during storage. Only plasma freshly frozen is applicable as therapy. Aspirin should be avoided in these patients.

FACTOR VII (PROCONVERTIN) DEFICIENCY

Factor VII (stable factor) deficiency is an uncommon but not rare disease. Mild clinical manifestations are the rule. The deficiency is inherited as an autosomal gene of "intermediate penetrance." The homozygous state results in significant deficiency and may be associated with serious bleeding. In these patients, spontaneous epistaxis, genitourinary and gastrointestinal bleeding, and even hemarthroses may be seen. The heterozygotes have minimal, if any, clinical manifestations. However, the correlation between factor VII level and bleeding is not good.

Factor VII, like factors II, IX, and X, requires vitamin K for synthesis. The synthesis is blocked by coumarin administration. Coumarin inhibition of synthesis is reversed by vitamin K administration. The administration of vitamin K to patients *congenitally* deficient in these activities will *not* result in synthesis and increased plasma levels.

As is also true for factor V–deficient patients and in patients with deficiencies of factors II and X, the one-stage prothrombin time is prolonged in patients with factor VII deficiency. Since factor VII is active only in the "extrinsic" blood-clotting system, deficient patients have a normal PTT and thrombin clotting time. A laboratory distinction between factor VII and factor X deficiency can be made by the use of the Stypven time test. Factor X is necessary for the effect of this viper venom in blood coagulation, while factor VII is not. Accordingly, the factor VII–deficient patient has a normal Stypven time.

TREATMENT. The biologic half-life of factor VII probably is the briefest of any of the blood-clotting factors— between 2 and 5 h. The initial half-life, thought to be due to equilibration between the intravascular and extravascular compartments, probably is no more than 30 min. The remainder of the disappearance time presumably represents catabolism and is estimated at between 5 and 6 h. Despite this relatively rapid disappearance, the transfusion management of patients with factor VII deficiency is not a great problem. Factor VII levels of less than 10 percent of normal are necessary before significant bleeding occurs. Even at these low levels of plasma activity, replacement transfusion is not always necessary for surgical procedures. Although the one-stage PT time recognizes deficiency of factor VII, this test is not an effective guide to the treatment of factor VII–deficient patients. The test is markedly abnormal at factor VII levels at which the deficient patient may not bleed. Transfusion of banked plasma, 10 mL/kg of body weight, on the day of

the operation, followed by half that amount daily for the next 5 or 6 days, provides adequate factor VII for hemostasis during major surgical treatment.

FACTOR X (STUART-PROWER) DEFICIENCY

This relatively rare deficiency is inherited as a highly penetrant incompletely recessive autosomal recessive trait and has been described in amyloidosis. An association between factor X deficiency and familial carotid body tumors has been reported. Clinically, affected patients are homozygotes, while the heterozygotes are clinically well and only minimally affected. The latter may demonstrate mild abnormalities with the one-stage PT and the PTT and the thromboplastin generation test. An assay is available.

TREATMENT. Little experience has been acquired in the surgical management of patients with factor X deficiency. Plasma levels of 10 to 40 percent of normal have proved sufficient to prevent significant bleeding following dental extractions. Plasma transfusion experiments in patients with factor X deficiency have demonstrated an 8- to 10-h first-phase disappearance time of half the administered activity, followed by a disappearance time estimated at 40 h. Applying these data, plasma levels of 15 percent or greater could be achieved by infusing 15 to 20 mL of frozen or normal plasma per kilogram of body weight initially, followed by half that amount per 24 h for 5 days. Prothrombin complex concentrates may be used. It is always prudent to give an additional infusion at the time of removal of the operative sutures.

INHERITED HYPOPROTHROMBINEMIA (FACTOR II DEFICIENCY)

This deficiency, inherited as an autosomal recessive trait, is perhaps the most rare of the inherited disorders of hemostasis. The prothrombin levels reported in affected patients have averaged about 10 percent of normal and are almost always less than 50 percent. Although the level of prothrombin activity required for hemostasis following surgical treatment is not precisely established, it seems likely that a level of 15 percent of normal is effective. The PTT is variably prolonged. An assay is available.

TREATMENT. The disappearance time of prothrombin from the intravascular compartment approximates that of factor X. An initial equilibration time of 9 h has been estimated, followed by a much slower disappearance of activity with another half-life of up to 3 days. Stored plasma contains factor II. Surgical treatment without faulty hemostasis should be possible in affected patients if an initial plasma infusion of 15 mL/kg of body weight is administered 12 to 24 h prior to the scheduled operation. This can be followed by an infusion of half this amount once daily until healing has occurred. Prothrombin complex concentrates may be used but are usually not warranted because they increase the risk of hepatitis and thromboembolic complications. Vitamin K is ineffective.

When the transfusion programs outlined above for deficiency of the prothrombin group of factors (factors II, V,

VII, and X) are employed, the one-stage prothrombin time does not return to normal. Rather, a one-stage prothrombin time slightly less than twice the control value is achieved. This is sufficient to result in normal hemostasis. Of the four "prothrombin" factors, only factor V must be provided as fresh or freshly frozen plasma. Stored plasma is equally effective as therapy for factors II, VII, and X.

INHERITED FIBRINOGEN ABNORMALITIES

Included in this category are patients with congenital afibrinogenemia, hypofibrinogenemia, and dysfibrinogenemia. Fewer than 200 cases of afibrinogenemia have been reported. This disorder is ascribed to an autosomal, recessive mode of inheritance. The affected individuals are presumably homozygous for the trait. Bleeding time may be markedly prolonged in some patients because fibrinogen is required for platelet aggregation. Conventional methods for measuring fibrinogen in the plasma give a zero value, but immunologic techniques may detect trace amounts of a fibrinogen-like protein. Patients have an indefinitely prolonged whole blood coagulation time, which can be corrected by the addition of fibrinogen. The deficiency, however, usually is less a clinical problem than is classical hemophilia. Bleeding usually begins early in life, and bleeding from the umbilical cord is a characteristic symptom. Bleeding may follow operations, dental extraction, and trauma but the most feared complication is intracranial bleeding following minor injury to the head.

Less profound inherited deficiencies of fibrinogen have been observed and categorized as congenital hypofibrinogenemia. Two groups of hypofibrinogenemic patients have been differentiated: those with fibrinogen values below 50 mg/dL and those with higher levels. The clinical manifestations depend on the fibrinogen concentration. Another congenital disorder is dysfibrinogenemia, in which there are structural defects in the fibrinogen molecule. Both the hypofibrinogenemia and the dysfibrinogenemia have a dominant mode of inheritance. Dysfibrinogenemic patients are frequently asymptomatic but may have moderate or severe bleeding associated with an operation. They have a propensity for thromboembolic disorders and have a higher incidence of wound dehiscence following operative intervention. The thrombin clotting time is diagnostic for this general category of abnormalities but definition of the precise abnormality requires a series of complex laboratory studies.

TREATMENT. Although the hemostatically optimal level of fibrinogen is not known, a level greater than 100 mg/dL is generally required during an operation. The patient's fibrinogen level should be raised above this prior to the procedure. Substitution therapy may be affected by the infusion of fresh frozen plasma or cryoprecipitate. In order to achieve a fibrinogen level near 100 mg/dL for 24 h, an initial dose of 20 to 25 mg fibrinogen/kg of body weight should be administered, followed by one-third the initial amount given on a daily basis throughout the postoperative period. But appropriate corrections must be based on actual fibrinogen measurements. Normal fibrinogen concentration should be maintained until wound healing is shown to be adequate.

CONGENITAL FACTOR XIII DEFICIENCY

This rare disorder is manifest by umbilical bleeding in the newborn and slow wound healing following an operation. In general, most of the bleeding manifestations are mild, but intracranial bleeding may result as a consequence of minor trauma. The mode of inheritance is an autosomal recessive trait. Immunologic assays have demonstrated deficiency of the protein. Therapy is accomplished with fresh frozen plasma, cryoprecipitate, or factor XIII concentrates. With major bleeding, or accompanying surgical intervention, the desired concentration of the recipient's plasma is 0.3 to 0.5 μm/mL. With minor bleeding or as prophylaxis, a level greater than 0.05 μm/mL is all that is required.

ACQUIRED HEMOSTATIC DEFECTS

Platelet Abnormalities

Thrombocytopenia is the most common abnormality of hemostasis that results in bleeding in the surgical patient. The patient may have a reduced platelet count due to a variety of disease processes such as idiopathic thrombocytopenic purpura, thrombotic thrombocytopenic purpura, and systemic lupus erythematosus, or secondary hypersplenism and splenomegaly of sarcoid, Gaucher's disease, lymphoma, and portal hypertension. In these circumstances the marrow usually demonstrates normal or increased number of megakaryocytes. By contrast, when thrombocytopenia occurs in patients with leukemia or uremia, and in those patients on cytotoxic therapy, there is generally a reduced number of megakaryocytes in the marrow.

Thrombocytopenia may occur acutely as the result of massive blood loss followed by replacement with stored blood. Exchange of one blood volume (11 units in a 75-kg man) decreases the platelet count from approximately 250,000/mm^3 to approximately 80,000/mm^3. Thrombocytopenia may be induced acutely by the administration of heparin and may be associated with thrombohemorrhagic complications. This situation, which is thought to have an immunologic basis, has been reported in 0.6 percent of patients receiving heparin. The lowest platelet counts occur after 4 to 15 days of treatment in patients given heparin for the first time and after 2 to 9 days in those given subsequent courses.

Thrombocytopenia is often accompanied by impaired platelet function. Impaired aggregation following the addition of ADP has been demonstrated in patients receiving a blood transfusion of more than 10 units. Uremia may be associated with increased bleeding time and an impaired aggregation, which can be corrected by hemodialysis or peritoneal dialysis. Defective aggregation and platelet secretion can occur in patients with thrombocythemia, polycythemia vera, or myelofibrosis. A variety of drugs interferes with platelet function. These include: aspirin, indomethacin, ibuprofen, dipyridamole, phenothiazides, penicillins, chelating agents, lidocaine, and cocaine.

The presence and extent of thrombocytopenia can be defined rapidly by a platelet count. In general, 60,000/mm^3 platelets are adequate for normal hemostasis, but if there is associated platelet dysfunction, there may be a poor circulation between the platelet count and the extent of bleeding. The template bleeding time is the most reliable in vivo test of platelet function.

When thrombocytopenia is present in a patient in whom an elective operation is entertained, it is managed based on the extent of the reduction of platelet count and the etiology. A count greater than 50,000/mm^3 requires no specific therapy. If thrombocytopenia is due to acute alcoholism, drug effect, or viral infection, the platelets will return to near normal levels within one to three weeks. Occasionally, severe thrombocytopenia may be secondary to vitamin B$_{12}$ or to folic acid deficiency, in which case it is associated with a megaloblastic bone marrow. This condition generally occurs 2 to 3 years after total gastrectomy or in association with severe intestinal malabsorption. In either case, supplying the appropriate nutrient will correct the thrombocytopenia in 2 to 3 days.

If the patient has idiopathic thrombocytopenia or lupus erythematosus, and a platelet count less than 50,000 per mm^3, an attempt to raise the platelet count with steroid therapy or plasmapheresis may prove successful (see Chap. 33). The administration of platelet transfusions in these patients with the spleen in place is generally ineffective. In an unusual circumstance, a preemptive splenectomy may be in order in a thrombocytopenic patient in whom a potentially bloody procedure is anticipated. Splenectomy alone should not be performed to correct the thrombocytopenia associated with splenomegaly secondary to portal hypertension.

Prophylactic platelet administration as a routine accompaniment to massive blood transfusion is not required or indicated to prevent a hemostatic defect. Platelet packs are administered preoperatively to rapidly increase the platelet count in surgical patients with thrombocytopenia due to marrow depression or in association with massive bleeding and replacement with banked blood. Special platelet transfusion sets are used to reduce the loss of platelets due to adherence. One unit of platelet concentrate contains approximately 5.5×10^{10} platelets and would be expected to increase the circulating platelet count by about 10×10^9/L in the average 70-kg man. Thus, a transfusion of 4 to 8 pool platelet concentrates should raise the count by 40 to 80×10^9/L and should provide adequate hemostasis, as documented by bleeding time and control of the hemorrhagic manifestations. Fever, infection, hepatosplenomegaly, and the presence of antiplatelet alloantibodies decrease the effectiveness of platelet transfusions. In patients refractory to standard platelet transfusions, the use of HLA-compatible platelets coupled with special processors has proved effective.

Platelet aggregometry has been applied to screening for potential donors.

Acquired Hypofibrinogenemia

DEFIBRINATION SYNDROME

The largest proportion of patients with fibrinogen-related problems of surgical concern are in this group. The fibrinogen deficiency rarely is an isolated defect because thrombocytopenia and factors II, V, and VIII deficiencies of variable severity usually accompany this state.

The majority of patients with acquired hypofibrinogenemia suffer from intravascular coagulation, more properly known as *defibrination syndrome* or *consumptive coagulopathy,* and it is to this group of patients that the term *disseminated intravascular coagulation* (DIC) has been applied. The syndrome, now recognized with increasing frequency, is caused by the introduction of thromboplastic materials into the circulation. Because this material is found in most tissues, many disease processes may activate the coagulation system. The hemorrhagic disasters of the perinatal period, e.g., retained dead fetus, premature separation of the placenta, and amniotic fluid embolus, primarily are due to this pathophysiologic mechanism. The hemorrhagic state following hemolytic transfusion reaction is also related to this process. Defibrination has been observed as a complication of extracorporeal circulation, disseminated carcinoma, lymphomas, thrombotic thrombocytopenia, rickettsial infection, snakebite, and shock. Release of thromboplastic material has long been a recognized complication of gram-negative sepsis and has been attributed to the effects of circulating endotoxin on platelets. Septicemia due to gram-positive organisms may also be associated with DIC.

The differentiation of DIC with secondary protective fibrinolysis from primary fibrinolytic states can be extremely difficult because the TT is prolonged in both cases, as is the PT and PTT. There is no laboratory test to confirm or exclude the diagnosis. The combination of a low platelet count, a positive plasma protamine test indicating the presence of fibrin monomer–fibrinogen complexes in the plasma, and reduced fibrinogen accompanied by increased fibrin degradation products viewed in the context of the patient's underlying disease is highly suggestive of the diagnosis.

TREATMENT. The most important facets of treatment are relieving the patient's causative, primary medical or surgical problem and maintaining adequate capillary flow. The use of intravenous fluids to maintain volume and, at times, vasodilators to open the arterioles is indicated. If blood flow deficiency is related to the inability of a damaged heart to pump, the use of drugs such as digitalis or Isuprel may be indicated. Viscosity may be affected by an increased hematocrit, and, therefore, a plasma expander may be beneficial.

If there is active bleeding, hemostatic factors should be replaced with fresh frozen plasma, cryoprecipitate, and

Certain surgical procedures should not be performed in the face of anticoagulation. In sites where even minor bleeding can cause great morbidity, e.g., the central nervous system and the eye, anticoagulants should be discontinued and, if necessary, reversed. Because of the added problem of local fibrinolysis, prostatic surgical treatment should not be carried out in a patient on anticoagulants. Procedures requiring blind needle introduction should be avoided. Deaths have been reported following sympathetic block for peripheral vascular disease in patients receiving anticoagulation.

Emergency operation occasionally is necessary in patients who have been heparinized as treatment for deep venous thrombosis. Reversal of heparinization may be desirable. The patient with repeated episodes of pulmonary embolization while fully heparinized is a potential candidate. Reversal of heparinization also can be a problem in cardiac and vascular surgical procedures. When the heparin has been given intravenously, its anticoagulant effect can be rapidly counteracted with protamine sulfate. Protamine sulfate also is administered intravenously. Theoretically, 1.28 mg should neutralize 1 mg of heparin. In fact, 1 mg of protamine may be given for each milligram of heparin given, provided the intravenous heparin was not given more than 2 h previously. Protamine sulfate in large doses also has an anticoagulant activity. The formation of both extrinsic and intrinsic prothrombinase can be retarded, prolonging the one-stage prothrombin time test and the partial thromboplastin time test. Some patients exhibit the phenomenon of "heparin rebound" following apparently adequate heparin neutralization with protamine. Prolongation of the clotting time again recurs after adequate postoperative antagonism of the heparin. This can contribute to postoperative bleeding. In our experience, this is the major cause of "unexplained" postoperative bleeding following cardiac and vascular surgical procedures. Activation of fibrinolysis and thrombocytopenia may also contribute to this problem.

Bleeding infrequently is related to hypoprothrombinemia if the prothrombin concentration is greater than 15 percent. In the elective surgical patient receiving coumarin therapy sufficient to effect anticoagulation, the drug can be discontinued several days prior to operation, and the prothrombin concentration then checked. A level greater than 50 percent is considered safe. If emergency surgical treatment is required, parenteral injection of vitamin K_1 can be used. Since the reversal effect may take 6 h, transfusion of whole blood or, preferably, freshly frozen plasma may be required. Parenteral administration of vitamin K also is indicated in elective surgical treatment of patients with biliary obstruction, malabsorption, and hypoprothrombinemia. The drug should result in a normal prothrombin time. In contrast, if the hypoprothrombinemia is related to hepatocellular dysfunction, vitamin K therapy is ineffective and should not be prolonged over a week if no response is noted. Vitamin K is an oxidant, and one must be aware that patients with red cell enzyme deficiencies may sustain hemolysis following its administration.

TESTS OF HEMOSTASIS AND BLOOD COAGULATION (Table 3-3)

The most important assessment of hemostasis is a careful history and physical examination. Only the history can indicate whether the patient has a hemorrhagic diathesis. Rather than asking a patient if he or she is a "bleeder," specific questions should be asked. These should include queries to determine if there was untoward bleeding during a major surgical procedure, or if there was *any* bleeding after a minor operation such as tonsillectomy, circumcision, or dental extraction, or if spontaneous bleeding was ever experienced. If there is a suggestion of bleeding diathesis, the age of onset and family history is helpful to determine whether a hereditary or acquired defect should be investigated. Questions should uncover a his-

Table 3-3. SCREENING TESTS IN ADULTS, HEALTHY TERM INFANTS, AND PREMATURE INFANTS

	Adults	*Term infants*	*Premature infants (32–35 weeks gestation)*
Platelet count (10^3/cm)*	300±50	259±35	239±50
Bleeding time (min)*	4±1.5	4±1.5	4±1.5
Prothrombin time (PT) (s)*	12–14	13–17	18
Partial thromboplastin time (PTT) (s)*	45	71	100
Thrombin time (TT) (s)*	10	14	14
Fibrinogen (mg/dL)†	200–350	117–225	—

* Values published by Hathaway and Bonnar.
† Values obtained in this laboratory.
Values for infants 35 to 39 weeks' gestation lie between those of term and 32 to 35 week infants.
Values for older children (>3 months) are the same as those for adults.
SOURCE: Karpatkin M, 1980, with permission.

tory of exposure to toxic agents, oral anticoagulants, and drugs that might interfere with hemostasis. Aspirin and ibuprofen are two of the more common medications in this category. A history of a recent regimen of broad spectrum antibiotics should alert the physician to the possibility of a deficiency of vitamin K–dependent clotting factors. Patients with malignancy may have a variety of abnormalities, such as compensated intravascular coagulation, and increased circulating fibrin complexes. Complex hemostatic disorders may accompany liver and renal failure.

PLATELET COUNT. Because thrombocytopenia is the most common abnormality of hemostasis in the surgical patient, determination of the level of circulating platelets is a critical screening test. Direct enumeration of blood platelets can be accomplished quite accurately. *Spontaneous* bleeding only rarely can be related to thrombocytopenia with platelet counts greater than 40,000/mm^3. Platelet counts of 60,000 to 70,000/mm^3 usually are sufficient to provide adequate hemostasis following trauma or surgical procedures if other hemostatic factors are normal. An abnormal count should be confirmed by inspection of the blood smear.

When an area where the red blood cells display their customary central pallor and where few of the red blood cells overlap one another is examined, 15 to 20 platelets per oil immersion field should be noted. If the blood is not anticoagulated before the smear is prepared, as many as half of these may be in clumps of three or four platelets. A well-stained blood smear that fails to display more than three or four platelets in at least every other oil immersion field can be considered significantly thrombocytopenic. In this situation, the patient's platelet count generally is less than 75,000/mm^3. Blood smears which must be searched because platelets appear in only every four or five oil immersion fields usually represent platelet counts of fewer than 40,000/mm^3. If cover slip smears have been prepared, the cover slips always should be mounted as matched pairs. Platelets occasionally stick to one of the cover slips, and examination of both will obviate a false impression of thrombocytopenia. Lightly stained blood smears may appear thrombocytopenic in that the platelets are not prominent enough to attract the examiner's attention.

Inspection of the blood smear has the other obvious advantage of permitting the examiner to identify additional pathologic features which may have meaning in the care of the patient. The presence of nucleated red blood cells or abnormal white cells can provide information important to the diagnosis. The presence of giant platelets or large fragments of megakaryocyte cytoplasm will also alert the examiner to possible pathologic platelet function.

BLEEDING TIME. This assesses both the interaction between platelets and a damaged blood vessel and the formation of the platelet plug. Bleeding time may be abnormal in thrombocytopenia, qualitative platelet disorders, von Willebrand's disease, and also in some patients with factor V deficiency, or hypofibrinogenemia. Aspirin ingested within one week will affect the results. The tests can be performed by a variety of techniques that do not have the same normal times or the same degree of accuracy. The Duke bleeding time, performed by incising the most dependent portion of the earlobe and measuring the time lapse until the bleeding ceases, normally should not exceed $3\frac{1}{2}$ min. The Ivy method is performed on the forearm after a blood pressure cuff has been inflated to 40 mmHg. It has an upper limit of normal of 5 min. The Mielke template technique, a modification of the Ivy method, provides more accurate results but may leave a scar.

OTHER TESTS OF PLATELET FUNCTION. Platelet aggregation can be assessed with a variety of induction agents to uncover specific abnormalities. The results may be affected by venipuncture, blood pH, temperature, duration of storage, and the equipment itself. The degree of abnormality detected by the test does not correlate with the extent of untoward bleeding. Aspirin is the most common cause of platelet aggregation abnormality. Failure of platelets to aggregate with the addition of arachidonate defines an aspirin effect. The failure of platelets to aggregate with ADP, epinephrine, and collagen is characteristic of Glanzmann's thrombasthenia. Abnormal platelet aggregation with ristocetin occurs in von Willebrand's disease and in Bernard-Soulier syndrome.

The ability of the platelets to liberate platelet factor 3 (phospholipid), essential in tiny amounts at several stages of the blood-clotting process (see Fig. 3-2), also can be measured. Impairment of platelet factor 3 release has been reported in conditions described as *thrombocytopathia*. This defect can represent a primary disease entity, but similar impairment has been described as a secondary phenomenon in uremia and liver disease. The inability of the platelet to make platelet factor 3 available for the clotting process may be a part of a more fundamental surface membrane abnormality. The ability of ADP, epinephrine, collagen, and arachidonic acid to liberate serotonin β-thromboglobulin, or platelet factor 4 can be measured.

PROTHROMBIN TIME (PT). This test measures the speed of the events described earlier as the extrinsic pathway of blood coagulation. A tissue source of procoagulant (thromboplastin), a lipoprotein, is added with calcium to an aliquot of citrated plasma and the clotting time determined. The laboratory should establish a normal dilution curve and normal values daily. The PT will be prolonged in the presence of even minute amounts of heparin. The presence of heparin, by its antithrombin action, will artificially prolong the clotting time of the mixture so that it appears that the prothrombin complex is low. Accordingly, an accurate prothrombin determination cannot be carried out in a patient receiving anticoagulation treatment with heparin until the heparin has disappeared from the plasma. This should be at least 5 h following the last intravenous dose. The amount of heparin used to maintain patency of an intravenous line is usually insufficient to alter the PT.

The use of tissue procoagulants in the test eliminates the roles of factors VIII, IX, XI, XII, and platelets. Properly done, the test will detect deficiencies of factors II, V, VII, X, and fibrinogen. The one-stage PT is the preferred method of controlling anticoagulation with the coumarin and indanedione drugs.

PARTIAL THROMBOPLASTIN TIME (PTT). The partial thromboplastin time is a screening test for the intrinsic clotting pathway. The in vitro clotting system now is sensitive to factors VIII, IX, XI, and XII, as well as the factors normally detected by the one-stage PT. The range of normal with this test varies with the product used. Each laboratory should establish a normal dilution curve daily, and the patient's plasma must be compared with a normal control.

The PTT, when used in conjunction with the one-stage prothrombin time, can help to place a clotting defect in the first or second stage of the clotting process. If the PTT is prolonged and the one-stage prothrombin time is normal, factors VIII, IX, XI, or XII may be deficient. If the PTT is normal and the one-stage PT is prolonged, a single or multiple deficiency of factors II, V, VII, or X or of fibrinogen may be present. The PTT is also abnormal in the presence of circulating anticoagulants or during heparin administration. It may be prolonged when heparin is used to maintain the patency of an intravenous line. The sensitivity of the test is such that only extremely mild cases of factor VIII or IX deficiency may be missed. In one study of over 600 patients with clotting abnormalities, only two mild abnormalities were not detected with this test.

THROMBIN TIME (TT). This test is of value in detecting qualitative abnormalities in fibrinogen and in detecting circulating anticoagulants and inhibitors of fibrin polymerization. The clotting time of the patient's plasma is measured following the addition of a standard amount of thrombin to a fixed volume of plasma. Controls of normal plasma must be run in parallel. Failure of the clot to form, in the absence of circulating inhibitors such as heparin or the fibrinolytic degradation products of fibrin and fibrinogen, is consistent with severe diminution of fibrinogen, usually well below 100 mg/dL. It is also prolonged when fibrinolysis is taking place.

OTHER TESTS OF COAGULATION. The fibrinogen level can be determined by clotting time measurements or gravimetrically. Specific assays of coagulation factors are performed by measuring clotting time of plasma congenitally lacking in one of these factors. Relatively simple tests permit identification of circulating anticoagulants. The simplest of these are based on the retardation of clotting of normal recalcified plasma by varying mixtures of the test plasma. The sensitivity of such tests usually can be increased by incubating the test plasma with the normal plasma for 30 min at body temperature prior to recalcification. Detection of factor XIII deficiency requires a special test.

TESTS OF FIBRINOLYSIS. Fibrin degradation products (FDP) can be measured by immunologic methods. The plasma protamine paracoagulation test (PPP) specifically detects fibrin monomers, but may be falsely positive in liver disease, thromboembolic disorders, renal disease, or pregnancy. Normally, dissolution of a recently formed blood clot will not occur for 48 h or more. When fibrinolysis is a significant factor in hemostatic failure, dissolu-

tion of the whole blood clot is observed in 2 h or less. The test has the disadvantage of being time consuming in a circumstance where time may be of the essence. In addition, a false impression of increased fibrinolytic activity may be gained from clots formed in patients with high hematocrits or in thrombocytopenia, where red cells may fall away from the clot. The euglobulin clot lysis time and dilute whole blood or plasma clot lysis time are more sensitive indices and permit more rapid evaluation of fibrinolysis.

The *thromboelastogram* is a graphic representation of clotting obtained by employing a special instrument, the thromboelastograph. The record obtained provides information about the clotting time, the speed of fibrin polymerization, and the strength and tendency toward dissolution of the clot. The instrument has provided information of research value but has not, in our experience, greatly aided the studies of clinical problems.

EVALUATION OF THE SURGICAL PATIENT AS A HEMOSTATIC RISK

Preoperative Evaluation of Hemostasis

The patient's history provides meaningful clues for the presence of a bleeding tendency. It is reasonable to use a questionnaire on which the patient indicates: (1) prolonged bleeding or swelling after biting the lip or tongue, (2) bruises without apparent injury, (3) prolonged bleeding after dental extraction, (4) excessive menstrual bleeding, (5) bleeding problems associated with major and minor operations, (6) medical problems receiving a physician's attention within the past 5 years, (7) medications including aspirin or remedies for headache taken within the past 10 days, and (8) a relative with a bleeding problem. Rapaport indicates that, based on the answers to these questions, one of the following conclusions can be reached: (1) hemostasis is apparently normal, (2) the history contains insufficient tests of hemostasis, or (3) there is a possibility or likelihood of a defect. He also proposes that this information, coupled with an appreciation of the planned operation, can be used to establish four levels of concern to determine the extent of preoperative testing.

In Level I, the history is negative and the procedure contemplated is relatively minor, e.g., breast biopsy or hernia repair: no screening tests are recommended. In Level II, the history is negative, screening tests may have been performed in the past, and a major operation is planned, but the procedure is usually not attended by significant bleeding: a platelet count and blood smear and PTT are recommended to detect thrombocytopenia, a circulating anticoagulant, or intravascular coagulation. Level III pertains to the patient whose history is suggestive of defective hemostasis and also to the patient who is to undergo an operative procedure in which hemostasis may be impaired, for example, operations using pump oxygenation or cell savers, or procedures in which a large, raw surface is anticipated. Level III also pertains to situations, such as intracranial operations, in which minimal postoperative bleeding could be injurious. In this level, a platelet count and bleeding time test should be performed to assess platelet function; a PT and PTT should be used to assess coagulation, and the fibrin clot should be incubated to screen for abnormal fibrinolysis. Level IV pertains to patients who present with a history highly suggestive of a hemostatic defect. A hematologist should be consulted, and, in addition to the tests prescribed for Level III patients, the bleeding time test should be repeated in 4 h following the ingestion of 600 mg of aspirin, provided that the operation is scheduled to take place 10 or more days after this study. In the case of an emergency procedure, platelet aggregation tests using ADP, collagen, epinephrine, and ristocetin should be performed, and a TT is indicated to detect dysfibrinogenemia or a circulating, weak, heparin-like anticoagulant. Patients with liver disease, renal failure, obstructive jaundice, and the possibility of a disseminated malignancy should have a platelet count, PT, and PTT performed preoperatively.

Evaluation of Excessive Intraoperative or Postoperative Bleeding

Excessive bleeding during or shortly after a surgical procedure may be due to one or more of the following factors: (1) ineffective local hemostasis, (2) complications of blood transfusion, (3) a previously undetected hemostatic defect, (4) consumptive coagulopathy and/or fibrinolysis. Excessive bleeding from the field of the procedure, unassociated with bleeding from other sites, e.g., central venous pressure or intravenous line or tracheostomy, usually suggests inadequate mechanical hemostasis rather than a defect in the biologic process. An exception to this rule applies to operations on the prostate, pancreas, and liver because operative trauma may stimulate local plasminogen activation and lead to increased fibrinolysis on the raw surface. In this circumstance 24 to 48 h interruption of plasminogen activation by the administration of EACA may prove effective.

Although one may be reasonably certain on clinical grounds that surgical bleeding is related to local problems, laboratory investigation must be confirmatory. Prompt examination should be made of the blood smear to determine the number of platelets, and an actual platelet count should be done if the smear is equivocal. A PTT, one-stage PT, and a TT all can be determined within minutes. Correct interpretation of the results should confirm the clinical impression or identify the problem.

As pointed out previously, massive blood transfusion is a well-documented cause of thrombocytopenia. Although most patients who receive 10 units or more of banked blood within a period of 24 h will be measurably thrombocytopenic, this is usually *not* associated with hemostatic failure. Therefore, prophylactic administration of platelets is not indicated, but if there is evidence of diffuse bleeding, 8 to 10 packs of fresh platelet concentrates should be given empirically, because no clear association has been documented between the platelet count, bleeding time, and the occurrence of profuse bleeding.

Another cause of hemostatic failure related to the administration of blood is a hemolytic transfusion reaction. The first hint of a transfusion reaction in an anesthetized patient may be diffuse bleeding in an operative field that had previously been dry. The pathogenesis of this bleeding is thought to be related to the release of ADP from hemolyzed red cells, resulting in diffuse platelet aggregation, following which the platelet clumps are swept out of the circulation. Release of procoagulants may result in progression of the clotting mechanism and intravascular defibrination. In addition, the fibrinolytic mechanism may be triggered.

Transfusion purpura is an uncommon cause of thrombocytopenia and associated bleeding following transfusion. In this circumstance, the donor platelets are of the uncommon Pl^{A1} group. These platelets sensitize the recipient, who makes antibody to the foreign platelet antigen. The foreign platelet antigen does not completely disappear from the recipient circulation but seems to attach to the recipient's own platelets. The antibody, which attains a sufficient titer within 6 or 7 days following the sensitizing transfusion, then destroys the recipient's own platelets. The resultant thrombocytopenia and bleeding may continue for several weeks. This uncommon cause of thrombocytopenia should be considered if bleeding follows transfusion by 5 or 6 days. Platelet transfusions are of little help in the management of this syndrome, since the new donor platelets usually are subject to the binding of antigen and damage from the antibody. Corticosteroids may be of some help in reducing the bleeding tendency. Posttransfusion purpura is self-limited, and the passage of several weeks inevitably leads to subsidence of the problem.

Disseminated intravascular coagulation (DIC) and disseminated fibrinolysis occur intraoperatively or postoperatively when control mechanisms fail to restrain the hemostatic process to the area of tissue damage. Either process can cause diffuse bleeding and can be caused by trauma, incompatible transfused blood, sepsis, necrotic tissue, fat emboli, retained products of conception. toxemia of pregnancy, large aneurysms, and liver diseases. It is important to distinguish between the two processes or the dominant element causing intraoperative or postoperative bleeding. No single test can confirm or exclude the diagnosis or distinguish between the two disorders. The combination of thrombocytopenia, defined by smear or platelet count, positive plasma protamine test for fibrin monomers, a low fibrinogen level and elevated fibrin degradation product (FDP) provides strong indications for DIC.

The simple single-tube clotting time test is helpful. Normally a clot forms within 10 min if there is periodic tilting of the test tube, and in 1 h the retraction begins. With DIC, formation occurs in a normal time and the clot promptly undergoes dissolution. The PT, PTT, and TT should be determined; this may be the most sensitive indicator of the three tests. Serial thrombin times, when used with the protamine sulfate test, have been used to differentiate the opposing mechanisms affecting hemostasis, i.e., DIC from fibrinolysis. The euglobulin lysis time provides a method of detecting diffuse fibrinolysis. The management of DIC and fibrinolysis has been presented previously.

A hemostatic defect may be imposed iatrogenically during surgical treatment employing extracorporeal bypass. Many etiologic factors may be involved, but the most commonly implicated is the introduction of heparin into the circulation. Bleeding after discontinuation of extracorporeal bypass may be due to inadequate neutralization of heparin with protamine sulfate. Since protamine sulfate is itself an anticoagulant when large doses are used, bleeding can be caused by these drugs. This is a rare occurrence. Rapid tests can be performed in vitro by adding small amounts of protamine sulfate to see if the clotting time is shortened. Other abnormalities attributed to extracorporeal circulation are defibrination and fibrinolysis. Fibrinolytic activity is often increased. These changes usually are related to the duration of pumping. Frequently there is a *lack* of clinical bleeding in the patients with laboratory evidence of fibrinolysis. Thrombocytopenia, hypofibrinogenemia, and reduction in factors V and VIII have been demonstrated. The thrombocytopenia usually is not severe, and the platelet count generally remains above $50,000/mm^3$. Evaluation of the patient with intraoperative or postoperative bleeding suspected of being due to hemostatic defect follows the same course previously outlined for preoperative evaluation of these patients.

Diffuse intraoperative and postoperative bleeding is a complication of biliary tract surgery in cirrhotic patients. This has been related to portal hypertension and coagulopathy associated with chronic liver disease. The tests used to distinguish DIC from fibrinolysis pertain. The therapeutic approach includes the intravenous administration of vasopressin to effect a temporary reduction in portal hypertension, and EACA to correct the increased fibrinolysis.

At times, an operation performed in a patient with sepsis is attended by continued bleeding. Severe hemorrhagic disorders due to thrombocytopenia have occurred consequent to gram-negative sepsis. The pathogenesis of endotoxin-induced thrombocytopenia has been studied in detail, and it has been suggested that a labile factor, possibly factor V, is necessary for this interaction. Defibrination and hemostatic failure also may occur with meningococcemia, *Clostridium welchii* sepsis, and staphylococcal sepsis. Hemolysis appears to be one mechanism in sepsis leading to defibrination. Evaluation of these patients includes platelet count, PT, PTT, and TT.

LOCAL HEMOSTASIS

Surgical bleeding, even when alarmingly excessive, is usually caused by ineffective local hemostasis. The goal of local hemostasis is to prevent the flow of blood from incised or transected blood vessels. This may be accomplished by interrupting the flow of blood to the involved area or by direct closure of the blood vessel wall defect. The techniques may be classified as mechanical, thermal, or chemical.

Mechanical Procedures

The oldest mechanical device to effect closure of a bleeding point or to prevent blood from entering the area of disruption is digital pressure. When pressure is applied to an artery proximal to an area of bleeding, profuse bleeding is reduced, permitting more definitive action. The Pringle maneuver of occluding the hepatic artery in the hepatoduodenal ligament as a method of controlling bleeding from a transected systic artery or from the surface of the liver is a classic example. Direct digital pressure over a bleeding site, such as a lateral rent in the inferior vena cava, is also effective. The finger has the advantage of being the least traumatic vascular hemostat. All clamps, including the so-called atraumatic vascular clamps, do result in damage to the intimal wall of the blood vessel. The obvious disadvantage of digital pressure is that it cannot be used permanently.

The hemostat also represents a temporary mechanical device to stem bleeding. In smaller and noncritical vessels, the trauma and adjacent tissue necrosis associated with the application of a hemostat are of little consequence. These minor disadvantages are outweighed by the mechanical advantage that the instrument offers to subsequent ligation. When bleeding occurs from a vessel that should be preserved, relatively atraumatic hemostats should be employed to limit the extent of intimal damage and subsequent thrombosis.

In general, a ligature replaces the hemostat as a permanent method of effecting hemostasis in a single vessel. When a vessel is transected, a simple ligature usually is sufficient. For large arteries with pulsation and longitudinal motion, transfixion suture to prevent slipping is indicated. When the bleeding site is from a lateral defect in the blood vessel wall, suture ligatures are required. The adventitia and media constitute the major holding forces within the walls of large vessels, and therefore multiple fine sutures are preferable to fewer larger sutures.

Historically, Aulus Cornelius Celsus devised the use of ligatures in the first century A.D. Because of the strong influence of Galen, who was inclined to cautery, this method did not gain popularity. Paré, in 1552, rediscovered the principle of ligature. In 1800, Physick used absorbable sutures of buckskin and parchment. In 1858, Simpson introduced the wire suture, and in 1881 Lister employed chromic catgut. Halsted, in the early 1900s, emphasized the importance of incorporating as little tissue as possible in the suture and indicated the advantages of silk. In 1911, Cushing reported on the use of silver clips to effect hemostasis in delicate vessels in critical areas. Recently, a wide variety of staples made of different metals, which are relatively inert in tissue, has been employed.

All sutures represent foreign material, and their selection is based on the characteristics of the material and the state of the wound. Nonabsorbable sutures, such as silk, polyethylene, and wire, evoke less tissue reaction than absorbable materials, such as catgut, polyglycolic acid (Dexon), and polygalactin (Vicryl). The latter are preferable, however, in the face of overt infection. The presence of nonabsorbable material in an infected wound can lead to extrusion or sinus tract formation. Wire is the least reactive of the nonabsorbable sutures but the most difficult to handle. Monofilament wire and coated sutures have an advantage over multifilament sutures in the presence of infection. The latter tend to fragment and permit sinus formation due to the interstices.

Diffuse bleeding from multiple transected vessels may be controlled by mechanical techniques which employ pressure directly over the bleeding area, pressure at a distance, or generalized pressure. These techniques are based on the premise that as pressure and flow are decreased in the area of vascular disruption, a clot will occur. As a standard procedure of military surgeons in the seventeenth century, pressure at a distance was effected by application of tourniquets and other pressure devices at pressure points proximal to bleeding sites. Now it is generally felt that direct pressure is preferable and is not attended by the danger of tissue necrosis associated with prolonged use of tourniquets. Gravitational suits have been employed to create generalized pressure and to decrease temporarily bleeding from ruptured major intraabdominal vessels.

Direct pressure applied by means of packs affords the best method of controlling diffuse bleeding from large areas. Rarely is it necessary to leave a pack at the bleeding site and remove it at a second sitting. If this is done, several days should elapse before removal, and the possibility of recurrent bleeding should be anticipated. The question as to whether hot wet packs or cold wet packs should be applied has been investigated. Unless the heat is so great as to denature protein, it may actually increase bleeding, whereas cold packs promote hemostasis by inducing vascular spasm and increasing endothelial adhesiveness. Bleeding from cut bone may be controlled by packing beeswax in the area. This material effects pressure and is relatively nonirritative to the body.

Thermal Agents

Galen's favoring of cautery influenced medicine for 1500 years, until the teachings of Paré were appreciated. The use of cautery was revitalized in 1928, when Cushing and Bovie applied this technique for effecting hemostasis of delicate vessels in recessed areas, such as the brain. Heat achieves hemostasis by denaturation of protein, which results in coagulation of large areas of tissue. With actual cautery, heat is transmitted from the instrument by conduction directly to the tissue; with electrocautery, heating occurs by induction from an alternating-current source.

When electrocautery is employed, the amplitude setting should be high enough to produce prompt coagulation but not so high as to set up an arc between the tissue and the cautery tip. This avoids burns outside the operative field and prevents exit of current through electrocardiographic leads or other monitoring devices. A negative plate should be placed beneath the patient whenever cautery is employed to avoid severe skin burns. The advantage of cautery is that it saves time; its disadvantage is that more tissue is necrosed than with precise ligature.

Certain anesthetic agents cannot be used with electrocautery because of the hazard of explosion.

A direct current can also result in electrical hemostasis. Since the protein moieties and cellular elements of blood have a negative surface charge, they are attracted to the positive pole, where a thrombus is formed. Direct currents in the 20- to 100-mA range have been applied to control diffuse bleeding from large serous surfaces. High-power argon-laser treatment has been applied successfully to the control of bleeding from superficial erosions.

At the other end of the thermal spectrum, cooling has been applied to control bleeding, particularly from the mucosa of the esophagus and stomach. Generalized hypothermia is of little avail, since, in order to reduce the blood flow to visceral organs, the systemic temperature must be brought down to the level of 35°C. At this point shivering and ventricular fibrillation may be encountered. Thrombocytopenia may also be a consequence of generalized cooling. Direct cooling with iced saline is effective and acts by increasing the local intravascular hematocrit and decreasing blood flow by vasoconstriction.

Extreme cooling, i.e., cryogenic surgery, has been applicable particularly in gynecology and neurosurgery. Temperatures ranging between −20 to −180°C are used, and freezing occurs around the tip of the cannula within 5 s. At temperatures of −20°C or below, the tissue, capillaries, small arterioles, and venules undergo cryogenic necrosis. This is caused by dehydration and denaturation of lipid molecules. The muscular walls of large arteries are an exception. Although the major arteries and blood may be frozen solid, the blood contained in these vessels does not clot. When thawing occurs, normal circulation is resumed.

Chemical Agents

Chemical agents vary in their hemostatic action. Some are vasoconstrictive, while others have coagulant properties. Still others are relatively inert but possess hygroscopic properties which increase their bulk and aid in plugging disrupted blood vessels.

Epinephrine, applied topically, induces vasoconstriction, but extensive application can result in considerable absorption and systemic effects. The drug generally is used on oozing sites in mucosal areas, during tonsillectomy, for example.

Historically, skeletal muscle was one of the first materials with locally hemostatic properties to be employed, its use having been introduced by Cushing in 1911. Shortly thereafter, hemostatic fibrin was manufactured. The properties required for local hemostatic materials include handling ease, rapid absorption, nonirritation, and hemostatic action independent of the general clotting mechanism. The most widely used of the commercially available materials are gelatin foam (Gelfoam), oxidized cellulose (Oxycel), oxidized regenerated cellulose (Surgicel), and micronized collagen (Avitene). All these materials act, in part, by transmitting pressure against the wound surface, and the interstices provide a scaffold on which the clot can organize (Table 3-4).

Gelfoam is made from animal skin gelatin which has

Table 3-4. ABSORBABLE HEMOSTATIC AGENTS

	Material	Time to hemostasis	Absorption time	Handling characteristics	Bactericidal property
Surgical,* absorbable hemostat	Oxidized regenerated cellulose	2–8 min	1–2 weeks	Flexible con-formable fabric does not adhere to wet gloves or instruments	Yes
Surgical Nu Knit,* absorbable hemostat	Oxidized regenerated cellulose	1–5 min	1–2 weeks	Dense, strong material pro-vides strong suture base. Does not adhere to wet instru-ments and gloves	Yes
Oxcel,[a] oxidized gauze	Oxidized gauze	2–8 min	3–4 weeks	Cotton fabric fibers may adhere to wet instruments and gloves	No
Gelfoam,[b] absorbable gelatin sponge	Purified gelatin	Not specified in labeling	4–6 weeks	Foam sponge softens when saturated with sodium chloride	No
Avitene,[c] microfibrillar collagen hemostat	Purified bovine corium collagen	1–5 min	12 weeks or less	Powder or non-woven-web may adhere to wet instruments or gloves	No
Thrombin,[d] thrombostat	Bovine origin	Dependent upon concentration, usually less than 1 min	N/A	Can be used in powder form or as a solution (sprayed on or applied with a sponge)	No
Instat,* collagen absorbable hemostat	Bovine dermal collagen	2–5 min	8–10 weeks	Sponge-like material maintains integrity when wet	No
Collastat,* absorbable collagen hemostatic sponge	Collagen from bovine deep flexor tendon (achilles tendon)	2–4 min	8 or more	Sponge-like material does not adhere to wet instruments or gloves	No
Helistat,[f] absorbable collagen hemostatic sponge	Collagen from bovine deep flexor tendon (achilles tendon)	2–4 min	8 or more weeks	Sponge-like material does not adhere to wet instru-ments or gloves	No

* Johnson & Johnson Products, Inc.
[a] Deseret
[b] Upjohn
[c] Alcon Laboratories
[d] Parke-Davis
[e] Kendall
[f] American Biomaterials Corp.

been denatured. In itself, Gelfoam has no intrinsic hemostatic action, but it can be used in combination with topical thrombin, for which it serves as an absorbable carrier. Its main hemostatic activity is related to the contact between blood and the large surface area of the sponge and to the pressure exerted by the weight of the sponge and absorbed blood. Prior to application of Gelfoam, the sponge should be moistened in saline or thrombin solution, and all the air should be removed from the interstices.

Oxycel and Surgicel are altered cellulose materials capable of reacting chemically with blood and producing a sticky mass which functions as an artificial clot. These substances are relatively inert and are removed by liquefaction in 1 week to 1 month. They should be dry when they are applied. Like Gelfoam, these materials are nontoxic and relatively nonirritating but are somewhat detrimental to wound healing and require phagocytosis to be removed. Surgicel has been shown to have an antibacterial effect. Microcrystalline collagen has been shown to be as effective as other materials as a topical hemostatic agent where a large surface is oozing.

TRANSFUSION

Background

In 1967, the tercentennial anniversary of the transfusion of blood into human beings was celebrated. In June of 1667, Jean-Baptiste Denis and a surgeon, Emmerez, transfused blood from a sheep into a fifteen-year-old boy who had been bled many times as treatment for fever. The patient apparently improved, and a successful experience was reported simultaneously in another patient. Because of two subsequent deaths associated with transfusion from animals to humans, criminal charges were brought against Denis. In April of 1668, further transfusions in humans were forbidden unless approved by the Faculty of Medicine in Paris. It was not until the nineteenth century that human blood was recognized as the only appropriate replacement. In 1900, Landsteiner and his associates introduced the concept of blood grouping and identified the major A, B and O groups. In 1939, the Rh group was recognized. Numerous other groups have been uncovered since that time. Development of sensitive cross-matching procedures took place in the 1940s, and with the impetus of World War II, blood transfusion became a common procedure. The introduction of various preservative solutions, such as acid citrate dextrose (ACD), citrate-phosphate-dextrose (CPD), and, recently, citrate-phosphate-double-dextrose adenine (CP2D-A), has been the major advance in blood banking.

As the scope of surgery has expanded, the requirement for larger amounts of blood for transfusion has increased. Approximately 14 percent of all patients operated upon, exclusive of procedures performed in the outpatient department or emergency area, are transfused. Of 604 adults who received blood at a university medical center in association with surgical treatment, 125 required over

5000 mL. The record administration in this hospital in a patient who survived was 100 units within a 36-h period. Preservation of blood and its constituents has been achieved by freezing, and emphasis has been placed on the use of plasma expanders and component therapy.

Characteristics of Blood and Replacement Therapy

BLOOD

Blood has been described as a vehicular organ that perfuses all other organs. It provides transportation of oxygen to satisfy the body's metabolic demands and removes the by-product carbon dioxide. Blood also transports chemical nutriments for, and waste products from, metabolic activity. Homeostatic governors, including hormones, coagulation factors, and antibodies, are carried to and from appropriate sites within the fluid portion of the blood. Red blood cells, with their oxygen-carrying capacity, white blood cells, which function in body defense processes, and platelets, which contribute to the hemostatic process, comprise the formed elements.

REPLACEMENT THERAPY

BANKED WHOLE BLOOD. Whole blood generally is collected in CPD or CP2D-adenine solution and stored at 4°C. Such blood is considered suitable for administration any time up to 35 days of storage. At least 70 percent of the transfused erythrocytes remain in the circulation 24 h posttransfusion and are viable. Normal survival of red blood cells is 110 to 120 days. Sixty days after transfusion, approximately 52 percent of the cells will survive if the transfusion uses fresh blood. The major loss occurs in the first 24 h after transfusion, and subsequent to that time the survival slope for red cells from fresh blood and stored blood is identical. Red cell changes include reduction of intracellular ATP and 2,3-diphosphoglycerate (2,3-DPG), which alters the curve of oxygen dissociation from hemoglobin, decreasing the oxygen transport function.

Banked blood is a poor source of platelets, since platelets lose their ability to survive transfusion after 24 h of storage, and those that survive are functionally defective. Among the clotting factors, factor II (prothrombin), factor VII, factor IX, and factor XI are stable in banked blood. Factor V levels are adequate for 1 to 2 weeks in banked blood, while factor VIII rapidly deteriorates during storage.

During the storage of whole blood, red cell metabolism and plasma protein degradation result in certain chemical changes in the plasma (Table 3-5). Lactic acid increases from 20 to 150 mg/dL, an amount which is insignificant. The pH decreases from 7 to 6.68 within 21 days. Little change in the sodium occurs, but the potassium concentration rises steadily to 32 meq at the end of 21 days. This must be considered when transfusing patients with anuria, oliguria, or hyperkalemia. In these cases, fresher blood or frozen red cells obviously are preferable. The ammonia concentration also rises steadily during storage,

Table 3-5. CHARACTERISTICS OF PLASMA STORED IN ACD SOLUTION
AT 4 ± 1°C

Constituents	Unit value	Days stored				
		0	7	14	21	28
Dextrose	mg/dL	350	300	245	210	190
Lactic acid	mg/dL	20	70	120	140	150
Inorganic phosphate	mg/dL	1.8	4.5	6.6	9.0	9.5
pH*		7.0	6.85	6.77	6.68	6.65
Hemoglobin	mg/dL	0–10	25	50	100	150
Sodium	meq/L	150	148	145	142	140
Potassium	meq/L	3–4	12	24	32	40
Ammonia	μg/dL	50	260	470	680	

* Determined with glass electrode.
SOURCE: Strumia MM, Crosby WH, et al: *Transfusion*. Philadelphia, Lippincott, 1963, with permission.)

from 50 to 680 μg at the end of 21 days. This may be of significance for the patient with hepatic disease. The high citrate content may reduce plasma ionized calcium if large volumes of stored blood are administered rapidly. This is most pertinent in children, in patients with hepatic dysfunction, and in patients undergoing cardiopulmonary bypass. The hemolysis that occurs during storage for 21 days is insignificant, since lysis of only about 1 percent of the red cells occurs and the free hemoglobin is rapidly cleared from the circulation following transfusion. Patients receiving large amounts of banked blood frequently have an elevation of the serum bilirubin for several days.

Typing and Cross Matching. In selecting blood for transfusion, serologic compatibility is established routinely for the recipients' and donors' A, B, O, and Rh groups. Cross matching between the donors' red cells and recipients' sera (the ''major'' cross match) is performed. As a rule, Rh-negative recipients should be transfused only with Rh-negative blood. Since this group represents 15 percent of the donor population, the supply may be limited. If the recipient is an elderly male who has not been transfused previously, the transfusion of Rh-positive blood is reasonable if Rh-negative blood is unavailable. Anti-Rh antibodies form within several weeks of transfusion. If further transfusions are needed within a few days, more Rh-positive blood can be used. Rh-positive blood should not be transfused to Rh-negative females who are capable of childbearing. Administration of hyperimmune anti-Rh globulin to Rh-negative women shortly after Rh sensitization largely eliminates Rh disease in subsequent offspring.

A variety of cell-serum interactions may be detected by careful cross matching. Incompatibility may be due to the fact that either the donor or recipient has been wrongly grouped.

In the patient who is receiving repeated transfusions, serum drawn not more than 48 h prior to cross matching should be utilized for matching with cells of the donor. Emergency blood transfusion can be performed with group O blood. If it is known that the prospective recipient is group AB, group A blood is preferable. The O donor blood should have low titers of anti-A and anti-B.

Such emergency cases are extremely rare, with the exception of battlefield casualties, and it should be possible to wait 10 min, during which time the patient's group can be determined and type-specific blood used. The use of plasma expanders in the meantime makes this delay particularly feasible.

When the blood of multiple donors is to be transfused, such as in the case of extracorporeal circulatory procedures, the question arises as to whether all samples should be cross-matched with each other. In determining compatibility, screening is performed in the usual fashion. Major cross matches are performed. In patients with malignant lymphoma and leukemia, cryoglobulins may be present, and the blood should be administered at room temperature. If these antibodies are present in high titer, hypothermia may be contraindicated.

In patients with thalassemia and, more particularly, with acquired hemolytic anemia, typing and cross matching may be difficult, and sufficient time should be allotted during the preoperative period to accumulate blood that may be required during the operation. Cross matching should always be carried out prior to the administration of dextran, since dextran interferes with the typing procedure.

Because banked blood may be stored for up to 35 days, the use of autologous predeposit transfusion is growing. In otherwise healthy, nonanemic patients, up to 5 to 6 units of blood may be collected for use in elective surgical procedures.

FRESH WHOLE BLOOD. This term refers to blood that is administered within 24 h of its donation. Due to the requirements for HB_sAg, HTLV-III, and syphilis testing, fresh blood is available only untested for such agents. Fresh whole blood is now believed an inadequate source of platelets and factor VIII.

PACKED RED CELLS AND FROZEN RED CELLS. Concentrated suspensions of red cells can be prepared by removing most of the supernatant plasma from the blood following settling of the cells or centrifugation. A small amount of plasma is left, so that the packed cell volume is approximately 70 percent.

Frozen red cells have an advantage in that their use

markedly reduces the risk of infusing antigens to which the patient has been previously sensitized. The red cell viability is improved and the ATP and 2,3-DPG concentrations are maintained. Either packed or frozen red cells are applicable in the treatment of anemia without hypovolemia. Their use reduces the danger of circulatory overload. Reactions secondary to allergens in plasma to which the recipient is sensitive also can be minimized.

LEUKOCYTE AND PLATELET-POOR RED CELLS. These are prepared by aspirating the buffy coat and supernatant plasma, following slow centrifugation or settling. The red cells then are washed with sterile isotonic solution. This should be done only for patients with demonstrated hypersensitivity to either leukocytes or platelets (buffy coat reactions). Usually this syndrome is manifest by fever, chilly sensations, and urticaria in the absence of hemolysis.

PLATELET CONCENTRATES. The indications for platelet transfusion are as follows: thrombocytopenia due to massive blood loss and replacement with stored blood, thrombocytopenia due to inadequate production, and qualitative platelet disorders. The preparations should be used within 120 h of blood donation. One unit of platelet concentrates has a volume of approximately 50 mL. The recovery of platelets in the recipient usually is no more than 60 percent of those present in the donor blood. The platelet concentrate consists of platelets prepared from a unit of platelet-rich plasma. These are resuspended in 30 mL of fluid and should be administered without a filter. The platelet concentrate has the advantage of obviating circulatory overload. Both preparations may harbor the hepatitis virus and account for allergic reactions similar to those due to whole blood. When treating thrombocytopenic bleeding or preparing some thrombocytopenic patients for surgery, it is advisable to elevate the platelet levels to the range of 50,000 to 100,000/mm^3 to provide continued protection. The development of isoimmunity remains one of the most important factors limiting usefulness of platelet transfusion. Isoantibodies are demonstrable in about 5 percent of patients after 1 to 10 transfusions, in 20 percent after 10 to 20 transfusions, and in 80 percent after more than 100 transfusions. The use of HL-A–compatible platelets addresses this problem.

FROZEN PLASMA AND VOLUME EXPANDERS. Frozen plasma prepared from freshly donated blood or fresh plamsa is necessary to provide factors V and VIII. The other plasma clotting factors are present in banked preparations. The use of plasma for therapy in patients with hypovolemia rarely is indicated. The risk of hepatitis is the same whether fresh frozen plasma or whole blood/red cells is administered. Ringer's lactate or buffered saline solution, administered in amounts two to three times the estimated blood loss, is effective in an emergency and is associated with fewer complications. Dextran or a combination of Ringer's lactate solution and normal human serum albumin are preferred for rapid plasma expansion. Commercially available dextran preparations probably should not be administered in amounts exceeding 1 L per day, since prolongation of bleeding time and hemorrhage can occur. Low-molecular-weight dextran, i.e., molecu-

lar weight of 30,000 to 40,000, has achieved recent popularity because it possesses a higher colloidal pressure than plasma and effects some reversal of erythrocyte agglutination.

CONCENTRATES. *Antihemophilic concentrates* are prepared from plasma and are available for the treatment of factor VIII deficiency. Some of these concentrates are twenty to thirty times as potent as an equal volume of fresh-frozen plasma. The simplest factor VIII concentrate is the plasma cryoprecipitate. *Albumin* also has been concentrated, so that 25 g may be administered and provide the osmotic equivalent of 500 mL of plasma. The advantage of albumin is that it is a hepatitis-free product.

Indications for Replacement of Blood or Its Elements

VOLUME REPLACEMENT. The most common indication for blood transfusion in diseases of surgical interest is the replenishment of the circulating blood volume. It is difficult to evaluate the volume deficit accurately.

A variety of techniques employing dyes or isotopically tagged colloids has been introduced to determine the blood volume more precisely. Values for "normal blood volume" are variable, and the techniques are relatively inaccurate when there is a rapidly changing situation, such as hemorrhage. Chronically ill and elderly patients may have a diminution of blood volume. In patients with cardiac decompensation, the blood volume may be greater than normal. Many patients with chronically reduced blood volume are well accommodated to that volume. Blood volume, in itself, does not serve as an absolute indication for transfusion. Measurement of hemoglobin or hematocrit is also used to interpret blood loss. This measurement is misleading in the face of acute blood loss, since the hematocrit may be normal in spite of a severely contracted blood volume. It has been shown that, after a healthy adult male lost approximately 1000 mL of blood rapidly, the venous hematocrit fell only 3 percent during the first hour, 5 percent at 24 h, 6 percent at 48 h, and 8 percent at 72 h, thus indicating the time required for the body to restore blood volume.

A healthy person can lose 450 mL in 15 min with only minor effects on the circulation and little change in blood pressure or pulse, as evidenced by the normal blood donor. The normal person may lose 1 L of blood rapidly without a fall in blood pressure as long as he remains supine. About 40 percent of blood volume, or 2 L of blood, usually is lost before significant hypotension develops. Loss of blood may be evaluated in the operating room by estimating the amount of blood in the wound and on the drapes and by weighing sponges. The loss determined by weighing sponges is only about 70 percent of true loss. In patients who have normal preoperative blood values, blood loss up to 20 percent of total blood volume (TBV) is replaced with crystalloid solutions. Blood loss up to 50 percent TBV is replaced with crystalloids and red blood cell concentrates. Blood loss above 50 percent TBV is replaced with crystalloids, red blood cells, and albumin or plasma. Continued bleeding above 50 percent TBV should receive the same components and fresh frozen plasma. If electrolyte solutions are used to replace blood volume, an amount three to four times the lost volume is required because of immediate diffusion into the interstitial space.

IMPROVEMENT IN OXYGEN-CARRYING CAPACITY. This is primarily a function of the red cell. When anemia can be treated by specific therapy, transfusion should be withheld. Acute anemias, such as hemolytic anemia, are more disabling physiologically than chronic anemia, since most patients with chronic anemia have undergone an adjustment to the situation. In pregnancy, there is a moderate drop in hematocrit, and transfusions are not indicated to correct the physiologic anemia of pregnancy prior to surgical treatment. The correction of chronic anemia prior to surgical treatment, though often performed, is difficult to justify, and there is no indication that anemia predisposes to wound dehiscence. Blood volume may be replaced with dextran solution or Ringer's lactate solution with a reduction of the hemoglobin to levels below 10 g and little demonstrable change in the effects of a reduction in oxygen-carrying capacity or the capacity to remove metabolic gaseous by-products. A stroma-free hemoglobin solution has been shown to have

ability to carry and exchange oxygen. Also, a whole blood substitute, Fluosol-DA, has been proposed as a solution with oxygen-handling capabilities.

REPLACEMENT OF CLOTTING FACTORS. Transfusion of platelets and/or proteins contributing to coagulation may be indicated in specific patients either prior to or during operation (Table 3-6). In the treatment of certain hemorrhagic conditions, it is to be appreciated that the clotting defects may be multiple and the injection of substitutes and extracts may be less effective than transfusion of fresh blood or fresh frozen plasma. Efficacy of fresh frozen plasma (FFP) in the management of coagulopathy in patients with liver disease and in patients receiving large amounts of stored blood is not well defined. There are insufficient data to specify criteria for transfusion of FFP. The initial volume of FFP needed for an effect on coagulation ranges between 600 to 2000 mL administered in 1 to 2 h. The rigid use of the PT and PTT to anticipate the effect of FFP is not justified.

When transfusion with fibrinogen is deemed necessary, a plasma level greater than 100 mg/dL should be maintained. The hypofibrinogenemia encountered during surgical treatment is frequently related to excessive consumption. Adequate levels of fibrinogen frequently will

Table 3-6. REPLACEMENT OF CLOTTING FACTORS

Factors	Normal level	Life span in vivo ($\frac{1}{2}$ life)	Fate during coagulation	Level required for safe hemostasis	Stability in ACD bank blood (4°)	Ideal agent for replacing deficit
I (fibrinogen)	200–400 mg/ 100 mL	72 h	Consumed	60–100 mg/ 100 mL	Very stable	Bank blood; concentrated fibrinogen
II (prothrombin)	20 mg/100 mL (100%)	72 h	Consumed	15–20%	Stable	Bank blood; concentrated preparation
V (proaccelerin, accelerator globulin labile factor)	100%	36 h	Consumed	5–20%	Labile (40% at 1 week)	Frozen fresh plasma; blood under 7 days
VII [proconvertin, serum prothrombin conversion accelerator (SPCA) stable factor]	100%	5 h	Survives	5–30%	Stable	Bank blood; concentrated preparation
VIII [antihemophilic factor (AHF), antihemophilic globulin (AHG)]	100% (50–150)	6–12 h	Consumed	30%	Labile (20–40% at 1 week)	Fresh frozen plasma; concentrated AHF; cryoprecipitate
IX [Christmas factor, plasma thromboplastin component (PTC), hemophilia B factor]	100%	24 h	Survives	20–30%	Stable	Fresh frozen plasma; bank blood concentrated preparation
X (Stuart-Prower factor)	100%	40 h	Survives	15–20%	Stable	Bank blood; concentrated preparation
XI [plasma thromboplasma antecedent (PTA)]	100%	Probably 40–80 h	Survives	10%	Probably stable	Bank blood
XII (Hageman factor)	100%	Unknown	Survives	Deficit produces no bleeding tendency	Stable	Replacement not required
XIII [fibrinase, fibrin-stabilizing factor (FSF)]	100%	4–7 days	Survives	Probably less than 1%	Stable	Bank blood
Platelets	150,000–400,000/ mm^3	8–11 days	Consumed	60,000–100,000/ mm^3	Very labile (40% at 20 h; 0 at 48 h)	Fresh blood or plasma; fresh platelet concentrate (not frozen plasma)

SOURCE: Salzman EW: Hemorrhagic disorders, in Kinney JM, Egdahl RH, Zuidema GD (eds): *Manual of Preoperative and Postoperative Care.* Philadelphia, Saunders, 1971, p 157, with permission.

return within hours without replacement therapy if the precipitating cause is corrected. Cryoprecipitate is a source of concentrated fibrinogen (250 mg/10 mL). Deficiency of factor V, per se, is relatively rare; although transfusion will increase the level, there is suggestion that the biologic half-life is short and may not exceed 12 h.

Hypoprothrombinemia and deficiency of factor VII in patients on anticoagulant therapy can be reversed with injection of vitamin K_1. In patients who are deficient in prothrombin, such as those with cirrhosis, and who require surgical treatment, transfusion with frozen plasma may effect immediate benefit.

Transfusion therapy for patients with hemophilia subjected to trauma or surgical procedure requires sufficient quantities to raise and maintain the level of factor VIII in the plasma to above 30 percent of normal. Transfusion of small amounts of factor VIII is not justified. If a life-threatening situation exists, large amounts must be used. The factor IX–deficient patient subjected to surgery or trauma also requires levels of 20 to 30 percent for secure hemostasis. Such levels are difficult to attain with plasma infusions despite the stability of factor IX in stored plasma. Factor IX concentrates are preferable. The biologic half-life of factor IX is appreciably longer than that of factor VIII.

Usually, the hemostatic mechanism is not markedly altered with platelet counts greater than 50,000/mm³. If thrombocytopenia is more pronounced, however, the transfusion of platelet concentrates may be indicated to prevent or treat active bleeding. The life span of freshly infused platelets is only about 10 days, and in some instances the recipient represents a hostile environment, and the survival is reduced to several hours. The usual dose is 1 unit/10 kg.

SPECIFIC INDICATIONS

SINGLE-UNIT TRANSFUSION. There has been a general trend toward condemning all single-unit transfusion on surgical services. As has been previously mentioned, they are usually uncalled for. The Committee on Blood of the American Medical Association found it necessary to oppose this trend, however, pointing out that it is a poor practice to order 2 units of blood to escape criticism for using a single unit, and an appropriate volume of blood should be given whenever transfusion is required.

MASSIVE TRANSFUSION. The term *massive transfusion* implies a single transfusion greater than 2500 mL, or 5000 mL transfused over a period of 24 h. The approximate percentages of *original* blood volume remaining after varying degrees of hemorrhage and transfusion are shown in Table 3-7. A variety of problems may attend the use of massive transfusion. Dilutional thrombocytopenia, impaired platelet function, and deficiencies of factors V, VIII, and XI may occur. The acid load present in stored blood may have an additive effect in a patient with preexisting acidosis. Routine alkalinization is not advisable, since this could have an adverse effect on the oxyhemoglobin dissociation curve and presents an additional so-

Table 3-7. PERCENTAGE OF ORIGINAL BLOOD VOLUME REMAINING IN A PATIENT WITH A 5-L BLOOD VOLUME TRANSFUSED WITH 500-ML UNITS

Situation*	Magnitude of hemorrhage and transfusion		
	1 Blood volume (10 units)	*2 Blood volumes (20 units)*	*3 Blood volumes (30 units)*
Best	37	14	5
Usual	25–30	10	2–4
Worst	18	3	0.4

* The "best" situation requires simultaneous and equal replacement during hemorrhage; the "worst" situation means initial loss of one-half blood volume not replaced until the hemorrhage has stopped.
SOURCE: After Collins, 1976.

dium load to a compromised patient. The increased potassium content of multiple units of stored blood does not provide clinical effects unless the patient is severely oliguric.

Citrate toxicity may be associated with massive transfusion, particularly in young children and patients with severe hypotension or liver disease. This is related to an excessive binding of ionized calcium and is usually corrected by spontaneous mobilization of calcium from bone. The physiologic consequences of citrate toxicity rarely have a significant effect. The function of hemoglobin is altered by storage in that the concentration of 2,3-DPG (diphosphoglyceric acid) falls to a negligible level by the third week. This results in an increased affinity of the red blood cells for oxygen and a less efficient oxygen delivery system. In itself, reduction of 2,3-DPG may not have a significant effect but when combined with acute anemia it may be an important factor.

When large transfusions are administered, a heat exchanger may be used to warm the blood, since hypothermia may cause a decrease in cardiac rate and output and a reduction in the blood pH. Warming the blood decreases significantly the frequency of intraoperative cardiac arrest.

The use of blood from many donors increases the possibility of hemolytic transfusion reaction due to incompatibility. This can be reduced by screening each potential donor in the pool and eliminating those who show possible incompatibility. Paradoxically, patients who survive a massive transfusion do not have a high probability of developing isoantibodies subsequently, and the risk is no greater than that from a single transfusion. The risk of posttransfusion hepatitis increases progressively with each succeeding unit. When administering massive transfusions, the pH, blood gases, and potassium should be measured regularly. Acidosis and abnormalities should be corrected. If diffuse bleeding occurs, coagulation screening tests and platelet counts should be performed, and deficits corrected with frozen plasma and platelet concentrates.

EXTRACORPOREAL CIRCULATION. The heparin used to prevent the blood from clotting is usually neutralized with protamine. A variety of physiologic compatible fluids, such as Ringer's lactate solution, buffered saline solution, and dextran, may be applied to prime the pump during extracorporeal circulation and reduce the need for blood. The platelet count falls progressively during the initial intraoperative and bypass period, in part due to dilution by non-blood-priming solutions. In general, the platelet count remains about half baseline but exceeds 100,000 per mm^3 during the postoperative period, and, therefore, platelet therapy is usually not required.

Methods of Administering Blood

ROUTINE ADMINISTRATION. The rate of transfusion depends upon the patient's status. Usually, 5 mL/min is administered for 1 min, following which 10 to 20 mL/min may be administered to complete routine transfusion. When marked oligemia is being treated, the first 500 mL may be given within 10 min, and the second 500 mL may be given equally rapidly in most cases. Cold blood may be used for this amount, but when larger amounts are administered, warm blood is desirable.

The gauge of the needle is a critical factor in the rate of flow. Flow also is determined by the height at which the bottle is suspended. In patients with peripheral circulatory failure, the veins may be constricted with resultant increased resistance to flow, necessitating raising the bottle. Positive pressure may be applied with an inflated blood pressure cuff surrounding the plastic bag.

When large transfusions are administered, it is important not to overload the circulation, and the use of central venous pressure monitoring is particularly pertinent. There is no practical advantage in the use of intraarterial transfusion over the intravenous route in the treatment of oligemia. It has been shown that coronary flow and systemic arterial pressure respond as rapidly and to the same extent whether the blood is administered intravenously or intraarterially. The theoretical advantage of intraarterial infusion for patients in whom the blood cannot pass from the venous to the arterial side of the circulation because of cardiac arrest or ineffective ventricular contraction is offset by the delay in setting up an intraarterial transfusion.

OTHER METHODS. Blood may be instilled intraperitoneally or into the medullary cavity of the sternum and long bones. Intrasternal and intramedullary transfusion may be painful, and the rate of administration is limited. Approximately 90 percent of red cells injected intraperitoneally enter the circulation, but uptake is not complete for at least a week, and therefore the method is not suitable when immediate transfusion is required.

Intraoperative autotransfusion has become increasingly popular; it is a potentially life-saving adjunct to the management of trauma and is useful in elective operations in which multiple transfusions are likely to be required, e.g., liver resection. A variety of devices is commercially available, but none satisfies all the requirements. The cell savers wash the blood and separate the cells and reinfuse washed red cells, but they are limited by the constraints of time and do not provide a rapid reinfusion. Others are directed toward retrieving blood and returning it directly in order to avoid the time lapse. A major disadvantage of autotransfusion is the associated hemolysis and accumulation of cellular debris; the red cell survival is normal. Blood suctioned gently from the peritoneal cavity and reinfused through a filter has been shown effective, and in one series of 123 transfusions using intraperitoneal blood in patients with ruptured ectopic gestation, there was only one death.

COMPLICATIONS

HEMOLYTIC REACTIONS. Hemolytic reactions due to incompatibility of A, B, O, and Rh groups or many other independent systems may result from errors in the laboratory of a clerical or technical nature or the administration of the wrong blood at the time of transfusion. Hemolytic reactions are characterized by intravascular destruction of red blood cells and consequent hemoglobinemia and hemoglobinuria. Circulating haptoglobin is capable of binding 100 mg of hemoglobin/dL of plasma, and the complex is cleared by the reticuloendothelial system. When the binding capacity is exceeded, free hemoglobin circulates, and the heme is released and combines with albumin to form methemalbumin. This is detected by a positive Schumm's test. When free hemoglobin exceeds 25 mg/dL of plasma, some is excreted in the urine, but in most subjects hemoglobinuria occurs when the total plasma level exceeds 150 mg/dL. The renal lesions that may occur consist of tubular necrosis and precipitation of hemoglobin within the tubules. Red cell stromal lipid is liberated, and this may initiate a disseminated intravascular coagulation. The kallikrein-bradykinin system may be activated and affect the circulatory system. Minor incompatibilities may occur, causing hemolysis within the reticuloendothelial system manifested by fever, a mild decrease in hemoglobin, and an increase in bilirubin. If the recipient has a low antibody titer at the time of transfusion, reaction may be delayed for several days.

Clinical Manifestations. There is an increased hazard in patients with a previous transfusion reaction. If the patient is awake, the most common symptoms are the sensation of heat and pain along the vein into which the blood is being transfused, flushing of the face, pain in the lumbar region, and constricting pain in the chest. The patient may experience chills, fever, and respiratory distress, hypotension, and tachycardia from amounts as small as 50 mL. In patients who are anesthetized and undergoing operation, the two signs which may call attention are abnormal bleeding and continued hypotension despite adequate replacement. The mortality and morbidity resulting from hemolytic reactions is high if the patient receives a full unit of incompatible blood. Acute hemorrhagic diatheses occur in 8 to 30 percent of patients. There is a sudden fall in the platelet count, an increase in fibrinolytic activity, and consumption of coagulation factors, especially V and VIII, due to disseminated intravascular clotting.

Rudowski reported the following incidences of clinical manifestations in a large series with hemolytic posttransfusion reactions: oliguria, 58 percent; hemoglobinuria, 56 percent; arterial hypotension, 50 percent; jaundice, 40 percent; nausea and vomiting, 30 percent; flank pain, 25 percent; cyanosis and hypothermia, 22 percent; dyspnea, 20 percent; chills, 18 percent; diffuse bleeding, 16 percent; neurologic signs, 10 percent; and allergic reaction, 6 percent. The laboratory criteria are hemoglobinuria with a concentration of free hemoglobin over 5 mg/dL, a serum haptoglobin level below 50 mg/dL, and serologic criteria to show antigen incompatibility of the donor and recipient blood. The simplest clinical diagnostic test is insertion of a bladder catheter and evaluation of the color and volume of the excreted urine, since hemoglobinuria and oliguria are the most characteristic signs. A positive Coombs' test indicating transfused cells coated with patient antibody also provides evidence.

Treatment. If a transfusion reaction is suspected, the transfusion should be stopped immediately, and a sample of the recipient's blood should be drawn and sent along with the suspected unit to the blood bank for comparison with the pretransfusion samples. The serum bilirubin should be determined in the recipient. Each gram of hemoglobin is converted to about 40 mg of bilirubin. The hemolytic reaction is characterized by an increase in the indirect reacting fraction.

A Foley catheter should be inserted and the hourly urine output recorded. Since renal toxicity is affected by the rate of urinary excretion and the pH and since alkalinizing the urine prevents precipitation of hemoglobin within the tubules, attempts are made to initiate diuresis and alkalinize the urine. This can be accomplished with 40 mg of furosemide plus 45 meq of bicarbonate. If marked oliguria or anuria occurs, the fluid intake and potassium intake are restricted, and the patient is treated as a case of renal shutdown. In some instances, dialysis is required. Following recovery from oliguria or anuria, diuresis is often copious and may be associated with significant losses of potassium and sodium that require replacement.

FEBRILE AND ALLERGIC REACTIONS. These are relatively frequent, occurring in about 1 percent of transfusions. Reactions are usually mild and are manifested by urticaria and fever and occur within 60 to 90 min of the start of transfusion. In rare instances, the reaction may be severe enough to cause anaphylactic shock. Allergic reactions are caused by transfusion of antibodies from hypersensitive donors or the transfusion of antigens to which the recipient is hypersensitive. Reactions may occur following the administration of whole blood, packed red cells, plasma, and antihemophilic factor. Treatment consists of antihistamines, epinephrine, and steroids, depending on the severity of the reaction. Re-

peated reactions can be prevented by use of leukocyte-depleted or washed red cells.

BACTERIAL SEPSIS. Bacterial contamination of infused blood is rare and may be acquired either from the contents of the container or the skin of the donor. Gram-negative organisms, especially coliform and *Pseudomonas* species, which are capable of growth at 4°C, are the most common cause. Clinical manifestations include fever, chills, abdominal cramps, vomiting, and diarrhea. There may be hemorrhagic manifestations and increased bleeding if the patient is undergoing surgical treatment. In some instances, bacterial toxins can produce profound shock. If the diagnosis is suspected, the transfusion should be discontinued and the blood cultured. Emergency treatment includes adrenergic blocking agents, oxygen, antibiotics, and, in some cases, judicious transfusion.

EMBOLISM. Although air embolism has been reported as a complication of intravenous transfusion, healthy animals tolerate large amounts of air injected intravenously at a rapid rate. In experimental animals, the minimum lethal dose averages 7.5 mL/kg, and the mortality rate accompanying this amount of air injection can be halved by placing the animal on the left side at the time of injection. This displaces the air away from the outflow tract in the right ventricle. It has been suggested that the normal adult generally will tolerate an embolism of 200 mL of air. Smaller amounts, however, can cause alarming signs and may be fatal. Manifestations of venous air embolism include a rise in venous pressure and cyanosis, a "mill wheel" murmur heard over the precordium, hypotension, tachycardia, and syncope. Death usually is related to primary respiratory failure. Treatment consists of placing the patient on the left side in a head-down position with the feet up. Arterial air embolism is manifested by dizziness and fainting, loss of consciousness, and convulsions. Air may be visible in the retinal arteries, and bubbles of air may flow from transected vessels.

Plastic tubes used for transfusion have also embolized after they have broken off within the vein. Plastic tubes have passed into the right atrium and the pulmonary artery, resulting in death. Embolized catheters have been removed successfully.

THROMBOPHLEBITIS. Prolonged infusions into peripheral veins using either needles, cannulae, or plastic tubes are associated with superficial venous thrombosis. Intravenous infusions which last more than 8 h are more likely to be followed by thrombophlebitis. There is an increased incidence in the lower limb as compared to upper limb infusions. Treatment consists of discontinuation of the infusion and local compressing. Embolism from superficial thrombophlebitis of this nature is extremely rare.

OVERTRANSFUSION AND PULMONARY EDEMA. Overloading the circulation is an avoidable complication. It may occur with rapid infusion of blood, plasma expanders, and other fluids, particularly in patients with heart disease. In order to prevent this complication, the central venous pressure should be monitored in these patients and whenever large amounts of fluid are administered.

Circulatory overloading is manifested by a rise in the venous pressure, dyspnea, and cough. Rales generally can be heard at the bases of the lungs. Treatment consists of stopping the infusion, placing the patient in a sitting position, and, occasionally, venous section for removal of blood.

Although acute pulmonary edema occurs more frequently following large transfusions, it has been reported in patients receiving small transfusions. A syndrome which can be confused with pulmonary edema consists of postoperative hypoxia seen in patients who have undergone cardiac surgical treatment and extracorporeal bypass procedures. A damaging factor apparently is carried by the perfusing blood, and immature plasma cells are found in the interalveolar tissue. The lesion represents an immune response to blood. The incidence is reduced by employing the hemodilution technique of pump priming.

TRANSMISSION OF DISEASE. Malaria, Chagas' disease, brucellosis, and syphilis are among the diseases that can be transmitted by blood transfusion. Syphilis has been reported following the transfusion of platelets. The storage temperature used for all other blood components (4°C or lower) kills the spirochete. The incubation period ranges from 4 weeks to 4 months. The first manifestation is the skin rash of secondary syphilis. Cure is readily achieved with brief penicillin therapy. Malaria can be transmitted by all blood components, including platelets, fresh frozen plasma, and frozen or deglycerolized red cells. The species most commonly implicated is *Plasmodium malariae*. The incubation period ranges between 8 to 100 days; the initial clinical manifestation is shaking chill and spiking fever. Cytomegalovirus (CMV) infection, causing a syndrome resembling infectious mononucleosis, was commonly observed following open heart surgery when large amounts of heparinized blood were used to prime the pump. The most significant morbidity and mortality occurs following transfusion of CMV-infected blood in low-birthweight infants born of mothers who were CMV antibody negative.

Posttransfusion viral hepatitis remains the most common fatal complication of blood transfusion. It is estimated that for every case of icteric posttransfusion viral hepatitis there are four anicteric cases, many of which are asymptomatic. Hepatitis is caused either by hepatitis B virus, or the non-A, non-B virus. The incubation period of the former is up to 6 months, the latter's may be as short as 2 weeks. A serologic marker for hepatitis B surface antigen (HB_sAg) is detectable, and since 1975, blood collecting agencies have been required to test all units of blood for this antigen. As a result, hepatitis B virus transmission has been reduced. Because there is no specific test for the non-A, non-B virus, careful screening of volunteer donors remains the only preventive measure.

The clinical manifestations of hepatitis include lethargy and anorexia as part of anicteric disease, icterus, and chronic liver disease. HB_sAg persists in about 35 percent of patients who develop serum hepatitis of type B. There is no risk from human serum albumin and other plasma protein fractions.

Immune serum globulin is effective in preventing type A hepatitis but is inconsistent in regard to type B. Accidental self-inoculation with material that is definitely known to contain HB_sAg, or transfusion of blood which is HB_sAg-positive, constitutes an indication for immediate use of human specific immunoglobulin (HSI) anti-HB_sAg. The presently recommended dose is 0.5 IgG given as an intramuscular injection. Recently, a vaccine has been developed against HB_sAg, and it is recommended that all surgeons undergo vaccination. Originally it was felt that a determination of the presence of antibody should be performed prior to undergoing the vaccination regimen, but this policy is no longer adhered to.

Acquired immunodeficiency syndrome (AIDS) is thought to be caused by a transmissible agent. One percent of all cases fall into none of the groups regarded as at high risk. This one percent had received a blood transfusion within 5 years of their illness. The risk of AIDS following blood transfusion has been estimated to be one case per million patients transfused and blood collecting agencies have taken measures to preclude donors to high-risk groups and to apply screening techniques. Blood donors are *not* at risk.

Bibliography

General

Colman RW, Hirsh J, Marder VJ, et al (eds): *Hemostasis and Thrombosis.* Philadelphia, Lippincott, 1982.

Rudowski WJ (ed): *Disorders of Hemostasis in Surgery.* Hanover, New Hampshire, The University Press of New England, 1977.

Biology of Hemostasis

Davie EW, Ratnoff OD: Waterfall sequence for intrinsic blood clotting. *Science* 145:1310, 1964.

Jackson CM, Nemerson Y: Blood coagulation. *Annu Rev Biochem* 49:765, 1980.

Macfarlane RG: Enzyme cascade in the blood clotting mechanism and its function as a biochemical amplifier. *Nature (Lond)* 202:498, 1964.

Marcus AJ: The role of lipids in platelet function: With particular reference to the arachidonic acid pathway. *J Lipid Res* 19:793, 1978.

Rodman NF: The morphologic basis of platelet function, in Brinkhous KM, Shermer RW, Mostofi FK (eds): *The Platelet.* Baltimore, Williams & Wilkins, 1971.

Shattil AJ, Bennett JS: Platelets and their membranes in hemostasis: Physiology and pathophysiology. *Ann Intern Med* 94:108, 1980.

Sherry S: Present concept of the fibrinolytic system. *Ser Haemat* 7:70, 1965.

Weiss HJ: Platelet physiology and abnormalities of platelet function. *N Engl J Med* 293:531, 1975.

Weiss HJ: Platelet physiology and abnormalities of platelet function. *N Engl J Med* 293:580, 1975.

Congenital Hemostatic Defects

Brown B, Steed DL, et al: General surgery in adult hemophiliacs. *Surgery* 99:154, 1986.

Curtiss PH Jr: Orthopedic management of patients with hereditary disorders of blood coagulation. *Mod Treat* 5:84, 1968.

Kasper CK, Bowlen AL, et al: Hematologic Management of hemophilia A for surgery. *JAMA* 253:1279, 1985.

Nilsson IM, Larsson SA, Bergentz S-E: The use of blood components in the treatment of congenital coagulation disorders. *World J Surg* 11:14, 1987.

Ratnoff OD: Hereditary disorders of hemostasis, in Stanbury JB, Wyngaarden JB, Fredrickson DS (eds): *The Metabolic Basis of Inherited Diseases,* 2d ed. New York, McGraw-Hill, 1966.

Rudowski WJ: Major surgery in haemophilia. *Annu Rev Coll Surg Engl.* 63:111, 1981.

Shulman NR: Surgical care of patients with hereditary disorders of blood coagulation. *Mod Treat* 5:61, 1968.

Acquired Hemostatic Defects

Bell WR: Disseminated intravascular coagulation. *Johns Hopkins Med J* 146:289, 1980.

Bennett B, Towler HMA: Haemostatic response to trauma. *Br Med Bull* 41:274, 1985.

Feinstein DI: Diagnosis and management of disseminated intravascular coagulation: The role of heparin therapy. *Blood* 60:284, 1982.

Griner PF: Drug effects on oral anticoagulants, in Weed RL (ed): *Hematology for Internists.* Boston, Little, Brown, 1971.

Hoak JC, Koepke JA: Platelet transfusions. *Clin Haematol* 5:69, 1976.

Klingensmith W: Surgical implications of hemorrhage during anticoagulant therapy. *Surg Gynecol Obstet* 125:1333, 1967.

Schwartz SI: Myeloproliferative disorders. *Ann Surg* 182:464, 1975.

Schwartz SI, Hoepp LM, Sachs S: Splenectomy for thrombocytopenia. *Surgery* 88:497, 1980.

Silver D, Kapsch DN, Tsoi EKM: Heparin-induced thrombocytopenia, thrombosis, and hemorrhage. *Ann Surg* 198:301, 1983.

Slichter SJ: Identification and management of defects in platelet hemostasis in massively transfused patients. *Prog Clin Biol Res* 108:225, 1982.

Tests of Hemostasis and Blood Coagulation

Bowie EJ, Owen CA Jr: The significance of abnormal preoperative hemostatic tests. *Prog Hemost Thromb* 5:179, 1980.

Karpatkin M: Screening tests in hemostasis. *Pediatr Clin North Am* 27:831, 1980.

Mielke CH, Kaneshiro MM, et al: The standardized normal ivy bleeding time and its prolongation by aspirin. *Blood* 34:204, 1969.

Nye SW, Graham JB, Brinkhous KM: The partial thromboplastin time as a screening test for the detection of latent bleeders. *Am J Med Sci* 243:279, 1962.

Quick AJ: Clinical interpretation of the one-stage prothrombin time. *Circulation* 24:1422, 1961.

Rapaport SI: Preoperative hemostatic evaluation: Which tests, if any? *Blood* 61:229, 1983.

Reid WO, Henry RL, et al: Hemostasis: The balance concept of procoagulant and inhibitor systems and use of the serial thrombin time (STT). *Medical Hypotheses* 15:169, 1984.

Evaluation of the Surgical Patient as a Hemostatic Risk

Biggs R, Macfarlane RG: *Human Blood Coagulation and Its Disorders,* 3d ed. Philadelphia, Davis, 1962.

Colman RW, Hirsh J, et al, (eds): *Hemostasis and Thrombosis.* Philadelphia, Lippincott, 1987.

Hougie C: *Fundamentals of Blood Coagulation in Clinical Medicine.* New York, McGraw-Hill, 1963.

Shulman NR, Aster RH, et al: Immunoreactions involving platelets. V. Posttransfusion purpura due to complement-fixing antibody against genetically controlled platelet antigen: Proposed mechanism for thrombocytopenia and its relevance. *Clin Invest* 40:1597, 1961.

Local Hemostasis

Abbott W, Austen WG: The effectiveness and mechanism of collagen-induced topical hemostasis. *Surgery* 78:723, 1975.

Cushing H: The control of bleeding in operations for brain tumor. *Ann Surg* 54:1, 1911.

Evans BE: Local hemostatic agents (and techniques). *Scand J Haematol* (suppl 40) 33:417, 1984.

Halsted WS: The employment of fine silk in preference to catgut and the advantages of transfixing tissues and vessels in controlling hemorrhage. *JAMA* 60:1119, 1913.

Jenkins HP, Clarke JS: Gelatin sponge: A new hemostatic substance. *Arch Surg* 51:253, 1945.

Sawyer PN, Wesolowski SA: Electrical hemostasis, in *Conference on Bleeding in the Surgical Patient. Ann NY Acad Sci* 115:455, 1964.

Schechter DS: History of the evolution of methods of hemostasis and the study of blood coagulation, in Ulin AW, Gollub SS (eds): *Surgical Bleeding: Handbook for Medicine, Surgery, and Specialties.* New York, McGraw-Hill, 1966.

Silverstein FE, Auth DC, et al: High power argon laser treatment via standard endoscope. I. A preliminary study of efficacy in control of experimental erosive bleeding. *Gastroenterology* 71:558, 1976.

Waltz JM, Cooper IS: Cryogenic surgery, in Ulin AW, Gollub SS (eds): *Surgical Bleeding: Handbook for Medicine, Surgery, and Specialties.* New York, McGraw-Hill, 1966.

Willman VL, Hanlon CR: The influence of temperature on surface bleeding: Favorable effects of local hypothermia. *Ann Surg* 143:660, 1956.

Transfusion

American Medical Association Committee on Blood: Single unit transfusions. *JAMA* 189:955, 1964.

Brzica SM, Pineda AA, Taswell HF: Autologous blood transfusion. *Mayo Clin Proc* 51:723, 1976.

Bunker JP, Stetson JB, et al: Citric acid intoxication. *JAMA* 157:1361, 1955.

Caceres E, Whittembury G: Evaluation of blood losses during surgical operations: Comparison of the gravimetric method with the blood volume determination. *Surgery* 45:681, 1959.

Case RB, Sarnoff SJ, et al: Intra-arterial and intravenous blood infusions in hemorrhagic shock: Comparison of effects on coronary blood flow and arterial pressure. *JAMA* 152:208, 1953.

Chaplin H Jr, Brittingham TE, Cassell M: Methods for preparation of suspensions of buffy coat–poor red blood cells for transfusion, including a report of 50 transfusions of suspensions of buffy coat-poor red blood cells prepared by a dextran sedimentation method. *Am J Clin Pathol* 31:373, 1959.

Collins JA: Massive blood transfusions, in *Clinics in Hematology.* Philadelphia, Saunders, 1976.

Glover JL, Broadie TA: Intraoperative autotransfusion. *World J Surg* 11:60, 1987.

Ham JM: Transfusion reactions, in Condon RE, DeCosse JJ (eds): *Surgical Care*. Philadelphia, Lea & Febiger, 1980, chap 12, pp 178–186.

Harrigan C, Lucas CE, et al: Serial changes in primary hemostasis after massive transfusion. *Surgery* 98:836, 1985.

Hoff HE, Guillemin R: The tercentenary of transfusion in man. *Cardiovasc Res Cent Bull* 6:47, 1967.

Hogman CF, Bagge L, Thoren L: The use of blood components in surgical transfusion therapy. *World J Surg* 11:2, 1987.

Ingram GIC: The bleeding complications of blood transfusion. *Transfusion* 5:1, 1965.

Katz R, Rodriguez J, Ward R: Posttransfusion hepatitis: Effect of modified gamma-globulin added to blood in vitro. *N Engl J Med* 285:925, 1971.

Keeling MM, Gray LA, et al: Intraoperative autotransfusion: Experience in 725 consecutive cases. *Ann Surg* 197:536, 1983.

Krevans JR, Jackson DP: Hemorrhagic disorder following massive whole blood transfusions. *JAMA* 159:171, 1955.

Krugman S, Giles JP, Hammond J: Viral hepatitis, type B (MS-2 strain): Prevention with specific hepatitis B immune serum globulin. *JAMA* 218:1665, 1971.

Lalich JJ, Schwartz SI: The role of aciduria in the development of hemoglobinuric nephrosis in dehydrated rabbits. *J Exp Med* 92:11, 1950.

Maloney JV Jr, Smythe CMcC, et al: Intra-arterial and intravenous transfusion. *Surg Gynecol Obstet* 97:529, 1953.

Messmer KFW: Acceptable hematocrit levels in surgical patients. *World J Surg* 11:41, 1987.

Peskin GW, O'Brien K, Rabiner SF: Stroma-free hemoglobin solution: The "ideal" blood substitute? *Surgery* 66:185, 1969.

Phillipps E, Fleischner FG: Pulmonary edema in the course of a blood transfusion without overloading the circulation. *Dis Chest* 50:619, 1966.

Pruitt BA Jr, Moncrief JA, Mason AD Jr: Efficacy of buffered saline as the sole replacement fluid following acute measured hemorrhage in man. *J Trauma* 7:767, 1967.

Reed RL, Ciavarella D, et al: Prophylactic platelet administration during massive transfusion. *Ann Surg* 203:40, 1986.

Rizza CR: Coagulation factor therapy. *Clin Haematol* 5:113, 1976.

Rudowski WJ: Complications associated with blood transfusion, in Allgower M, Bergentz SE, Calne RY, Gruber UF (eds): *Progress in Surgery*. New York, Karger, 1971.

Schwartz SI, Adams JT, Bauman AW: Splenectomy for hematologic disorders. *Curr Probl Surg,* May 1971.

Shires T, Coln D, et al: Fluid therapy in hemorrhagic shock. *Arch Surg* 88:688, 1964.

Snyder EL (ed): *Blood Transfusion Therapy: A Physician's Handbook*. Arlington, VA, American Association of Blood Banks, 1983.

Tocantis LM, O'Neill JF: Infusion of blood and other fluids into the general circulation via the bone marrow: Technique and results. *Surg Gynecol Obstet* 73:281, 1941.

Wallace J: Blood transfusion and transmissible disease. *Clin Haematol* 5:183, 1976.

Wilson RF, Bassett JS, Walt AJ: Five years experience with massive blood transfusions. *JAMA* 194:851, 1965.

Yankee RA: HL-A antigens and platelet therapy, in Baldini MG, Ebbe S (eds): *Platelets: Production, Function, Transfusion, and Storage*. New York, Grune and Stratton, 1974.

Chapter 4

Shock

G. Tom Shires III, Peter C. Canizaro, C. James Carrico, and G. Tom Shires

CLINICAL MANIFESTATIONS OF SHOCK

Classification; Clinical and Physiologic Manifestations of Shock

DEFINITION AND WORKING CLASSIFICATION

The scope of modern medicine is increasing steadily. As understanding of physiologic and biochemical derangements is broadened, so is the horizon of possibilities for the relief of illness. As more seriously ill patients are presented, the symptom complex of shock is more frequently encountered by the physician.

Although shock has been recognized for over 100 years, a clear definition and dissection of this complex and devastating state has emerged only slowly. Many attempts have been made over the years to define adequately the entity known as shock. In 1872, the elder Gross defined shock as a "manifestation of the rude unhinging of the machinery of life." Although the accuracy of this definition is unquestioned, it is obviously far from precise. In 1942, Wiggers, on the basis of an exhaustive examination of available evidence at that time, offered the definition: "Shock is a syndrome resulting from a depression of many functions, but in which reduction of the effective circulating blood volume is of basic importance, and in which impairment of the circulation steadily progresses until it eventuates in a state of irreversible circulatory failure." Blalock offered the definition in 1940: "Shock is a peripheral circulatory failure, resulting from a discrepancy in the size of the vascular bed and the volume of the intravascular fluid." A more modern definition has been devised by Simeone, who stated that shock may be defined as "a clinical condition characterized by signs and symptoms which arise when the cardiac output is insufficient to fill the arterial tree with blood under sufficient pressure to provide organs and tissues with adequate blood flow."

Shock of all forms appears to be invariably related to *inadequate tissue perfusion*. The low-flow state in vital organs seems to be the final common denominator in all forms of shock.

For purposes of a working clinical classification, the etiologic classification offered by Blalock in 1934 is still a useful and functional one. Blalock suggested four categories:

1. Hematogenic (oligemic)
2. Neurogenic (caused primarily by nervous influences)
3. Vasogenic (initially decreased vascular resistance and increased vascular capacity)
4. Cardiogenic
   a. Failure of the heart as a pump
   b. Unclassified category (including diminished cardiac output from various causes)

It is now clear that shock results from one or more of four separate but interrelated dysfunctions, involving (1) the pump (heart), (2) the fluid that is pumped (blood volume), (3) the arteriolar resistance vessels, and (4) the capacity of the venous vessels. These dysfunctions may be correlated as follows with Blalock's etiologic classification:

1. Cardiogenic shock implies failure of the heart as a pump and may be brought about by primary myocardial dysfunction from myocardial infarction, serious cardiac arrhythmias, or a variety of causes resulting in myocardial depression; or by miscellaneous causes, including mechanical restriction of cardiac function or venous obstruction such as occurs in the mediastinum with tension pneumothorax, vena cava obstruction, or cardiac tamponade.

2. Reduction in blood volume may take the form of loss of whole blood, of plasma, or of extracellular fluid in the extravascular space or a combination of these three.

3. Changes in arterial resistance or venous capacity may be brought about by specific disorders. A decrease in resistance may result from spinal anesthesia or from neurogenic reflexes, as in acute pain, or may accompany the end stages of hypovolemic shock. Septic shock may produce changes in peripheral arterial resistance and in venous capacity, as well as peripheral arteriovenous shunting.

Therapy of shock will obviously revolve around the etiologic type or combination of types of shock present in a given patient who has undergone trauma.

CLINICAL MANIFESTATIONS

The signs and symptoms of hypovolemic shock, when they are well established, are classic and usually easy to recognize. Most of the signs of clinical shock are characteristic of low peripheral blood flow and are contributed to by the effects of excess adrenosympathetic activity.

On first inspection the patient in shock presents an anxious, tired expression, which early is that of restlessness and anxiety and later becomes a picture of apathy or exhaustion. Typically, the skin feels cool and is pale and mottled, and there is evidence of decreased capillary flow exhibited by easy blanching of the skin, particularly the nail beds.

There are varying discrepancies in the classic picture of shock. In neurogenic shock, particularly that in response to spinal anesthesia, the pulse rate is normal or, more often, decreased; the pulse pressure is wide, and the pulse feels strong rather than weak. The rapid pulse characteristic of early hemorrhagic or wound shock may be absent, even if the patient has lost blood rapidly. This is also true if the position is supine or prone, in which case a rapid pulse may not appear until the patient is moved or elevated to a sitting position. The varying clinical picture in septic shock is discussed subsequently.

In observing a large number of patients in hemorrhagic hypovolemic shock, one sees remarkably varied but typical responses of the sensorium to the shock episode. Most young, healthy patients who sustain wound or hemorrhagic shock, when seen early after the wounding, will appear to be restless and anxious and give the appearance of great fear. Shortly after being seen by a physician and started on treatment, this restlessness frequently gives way to great apathy and the patient appears sleepy. When aroused, the patient may complain of weakness or of a chilly sensation, although not actually having a chill. If blood loss is unchecked, the patient's apathy and sleepiness will rapidly progress into coma. In treating a large number of accident victims, it has been our experience that patients who have bled into frank coma from which they cannot be aroused, resulting simply from blood loss alone (unassociated with other injuries such as brain damage), have usually sustained lethal blood loss. This sign usually indicates rapid massive hemorrhage for which compensations are inadequate to maintain sufficient cerebral blood flow to sustain consciousness.

Thirst seems to be a characteristic of the injured person and is found in most emergency room patients brought in acutely ill from trauma with or without shock. The studies carried out to elucidate the nature of the thirst are many and varied. Most of these patients have intense adrenal medullary stimulation from trauma, not necessarily accompanied by shock. Consequently caution must be used in allowing water intake, since dangerous water intoxication may be induced by this intense stimulus to imbibe liquids in the face of altered renal function.

Another characteristic of the patient in hemorrhagic shock is the low peripheral venous pressure, manifested on inspection by empty peripheral veins. Indeed, the starting of a simple intravenous infusion in a patient in hemorrhagic shock can be quite difficult. Obviously there are exceptions, such as shock due to cardiac tamponade, in which there is restriction to inflow of blood to the right side of the heart. In this instance the peripheral veins, including the neck veins, are distended.

Nausea and vomiting from hypovolemic shock are common. It is true that other causes should be sought, but shock alone may be first manifested in this manner.

Another classic finding in hemorrhagic hypovolemia is a fall in body "core" temperature. Whether this is due to a lowered metabolic rate or to lower perfusion in areas where body temperature is measured is unclear; recent animal studies suggest a protective effect of this hypothermia.

PHYSIOLOGIC CHANGES

BLOOD PRESSURE. Arterial blood pressure is normally maintained by the cardiac output and the peripheral vascular resistance. Thus, when the cardiac output is reduced because of loss of intravascular volume, the blood pressure may remain normal so long as the total peripheral vascular resistance can be increased to compensate for the reduction in cardiac output. The vascular resistance varies in different organs and in different parts of the same organ, depending on the local conditions that determine the state of vasoconstriction or vasodilatation at the time of the loss of intravascular volume. An example of the differential increase in peripheral resistance with reduction in cardiac output is seen in the change in distributional total blood flow to organs such as the heart and the brain, as opposed to that of most other organs that are not essential for immediate survival. In hemorrhagic shock the heart may receive 25 percent of the total cardiac output, as opposed to the normal 5 to 8 percent. The great increase in peripheral resistance in such organs as the skin and the kidney causes significant reduction in flow in these organs while providing a lifesaving diversion of the cardiac output to the brain and the heart. Consequently the blood pressure may not fall until the reduction in cardiac output or loss of blood volume is so great that the adaptive homeostatic mechanisms can no longer compensate for the reduced volume. As the deficit continues, however, there is a progressive hypotension.

PULSE RATE. Characteristically, reduction of the volume in the vascular tree is associated with tachycardia. A fall in pressure within the great vessels results in excitation of the sympathicoadrenal division of the autonomic nervous system and, simultaneously, inhibition of the medullovagal center (Marey's reflex). Consequently, with hemorrhage or loss of circulating blood volume, the resulting fall in arterial blood pressure should cause an increase in heart rate.

This compensatory mechanism is variable in its effectiveness. Obviously, the degree of loss of intravascular volume, the amount of reduction in venous return, and other variables such as ventricular function may markedly influence the ability of Marey's reflex to compensate for the reduction in blood volume. Work with slow hemorrhage in normal healthy volunteers by Shenkin et al. has shown that, as long as the supine position is maintained, as much as 1000 mL of blood may be lost without significant increase in pulse rate. Similarly, the pacemaker system of the heart within the sinoatrial node is obviously influenced by other stimuli, such as fear and anxiety, that may also accompany the trauma producing the loss of intravascular volume.

Consequently, during the course of observation and treatment of shock, changes in pulse rate are of value only when followed over an extended period. Change in pulse rate may indicate response to volume therapy once other external sources that may have changed cardiac rate are diminished or removed.

VASOCONSTRICTION. Increase in peripheral vascular resistance by production of peripheral vasoconstriction rapidly becomes maximal in an effort to compensate for the reduced cardiac output. Vascular resistance can be measured only indirectly in human beings and in animals. There is good evidence that early disproportionate reduction in vascular resistance in the heart occurs while there is still little change in vascular resistance in many organs. Subsequently, maximal vasoconstriction occurs in the skin, kidneys, liver, and finally, the brain. Concomitantly, there is generalized constriction of the veins in response to reduction in intravascular volume. Venoconstriction is a necessary homeostatic mechanism, since over half the total blood volume may be contained within the venous tree.

These vascular responses to hemorrhage are immediate and striking. Within seconds following the onset of hemorrhage there are unequivocal signs of sympathetic and adrenal activation. Serum catecholamine levels show prompt elevation, indicative of action of the adrenal medulla. The adrenocortical and pituitary hormones also show prompt increase in serum levels following shock. Many of the clinical signs associated with shock are simply signs of response of the sympathetic and adrenal medullary system to the insult sustained by the organism.

HEMODILUTION. All the responses to reduction of intravascular volume eventually result in decreased flow to tissues and initiation of compensatory mechanisms directed at correction of the low-flow state. One such compensation is movement of fluid into the circulation, resulting in hemodilution. This fluid, commonly known as extracellular fluid, has the composition of plasma but a lower protein content.

It is now clear, however, that the hematocrit or hemoglobin concentration in shock is simply an index of the balance between the amount of whole blood or plasma lost and the amount of extravascular extracellular fluid gained. For example, in hemorrhagic hypovolemia there is generally progressive hemodilution, which increases with the severity of the shock state. Obviously, in this circumstance there has been a greater movement of fluid from the extravascular to the intravascular space with progression of the shock. This is in contradistinction to shock associated with loss of intravascular volume due primarily to plasma loss. High-hematocrit shock may occur with massive losses of plasma and extravascular extracellular fluid, such as is associated with peritonitis, burns, large areas of soft tissue infection, and the crush syndrome.

The mechanism of hemodilution following hemorrhage is initially on the basis of the Starling hypothesis: that is, the reduction in hydrostatic pressure in the capillaries because of hypotension and arterial and arteriolar vasoconstriction results in a shift of the pressure gradient to favor the passage of fluid from the tissue extracellular space into the intravascular capillary bed. In addition,

Gann and others have shown a second phase of blood volume restitution via a hormonally mediated increase in extracellular osmolality.

BIOCHEMICAL CHANGES

The measurable biochemical changes that occur as a response to the stress invoked by shock fall into three fairly well-defined categories. These are (1) the changes invoked by the pituitary-adrenal response to stress, (2) the changes produced by a net reduction in organ perfusion imposed by a low rate of blood flow, and (3) the changes brought about by failing function within specific organs.

PITUITARY-ADRENAL. The immediate effects seen from adrenosympathetic activity are those associated with high circulating epinephrine levels. Characteristically, these include eosinopenia and lymphocytopenia along with thrombocytopenia. This doubtless represents the laboratory reflection of increased circulating epinephrine that can be measured and has been found to be elevated as an early response to shock. These changes are nonspecific and are found early in a patient with shock or severe trauma. The phenomena usually disappear rapidly. Other evidences of the pituitary and hormonal response to shock are seen in the well-known stress reaction or metabolic responses so well described by Moore. These include a striking negative nitrogen balance, retention of sodium and water, and an increase in the excretion of potassium.

LOW-FLOW STATE. Those changes incident to the low rate of blood flow during shock are now becoming better understood. More evidence is accumulating to support the observation that, as a result of a decreased blood flow or low rate of perfusion, there is a reduction in oxygen delivered to the vital organs and, consequently, a mandatory change from aerobic to anaerobic metabolism. In the switch from aerobic to anaerobic metabolism, energy made available by the oxidation of glucose is greatly reduced during shock. The most striking example of a shift in metabolism is the production of lactic acid as the end product instead of the normal aerobic end product, carbon dioxide. This is reflected in a metabolic acidosis with a reduction in the carbon dioxide–combining power of the blood. The available buffer base is progressively decreased by combining with the increased lactic acid, and the respiratory compensation that occurs early in the course of hemorrhagic shock is frequently inadequate. Consequently the progressive decline in pH toward a striking acidosis is hastened. Indeed, in several studies the ability of animals as well as human beings to recover from shock has been found to correlate with the degree of lactic acid production and the decrease in the alkali reserve and pH of the blood.

In some cases determination of blood pH may not accurately reflect changes in pH at the cellular level. After the induction of hemorrhagic shock in experimental animals, skeletal muscle surface pH changes precede those in blood, and minimal changes may be masked by the efficient blood buffer systems. Lactate and excess lactate levels correlate well with the clinical impression of the depth of shock, but the injuries producing the shock state have a much greater bearing on ultimate prognosis.

ORGAN FAILURE. The biochemical changes that appear incident to organ failure seem to be dependent in large part on the duration and severity of the shock. The changes in renal function induced by hypovolemia may vary from simple oliguria with a concentrated and acid urine to high-output renal failure with a urine of low specific gravity and high pH, or frank anuric renal failure. Similarly, the blood nonprotein nitrogen content depends on the degree of impairment in renal function. This may vary from slight or no retention of nitrogenous products to a steep and progressive rise that may require therapy.

Changes in ion concentration, including a rise of serum potassium, are dependent on many things, among them adrenal cortical response, the change in metabolism from aerobic to anaerobic with resultant release of potassium, and specific changes within tissues invoked by the shock. If renal function is maintained, the rise inevitably seen in serum potassium soon after the onset of shock is short-lived, in that the renal excretion of potassium is high during recovery from hemorrhagic shock. If renal function is impaired, the concentration of potassium and magnesium as well as creatinine can rise to high levels in the serum.

Although the kidney is quite sensitive to the physiologic alterations in shock, other organs vary in their response to various shock states. The lung is resistant to dysfunction induced by hemorrhage alone (see Pulmonary Responses). Concurrent direct lung injury or septic shock frequently lead to profound impairment in pulmonary function. Shock-induced changes in hepatocyte function may be reflected in early alterations in glucose metabolism and later alterations in bilirubin and protein metabolism. Loss of homeostasis in skeletal muscle, which represents a large proportion of body mass, produces major changes in fluid and electrolytes, as discussed below.

PATHOPHYSIOLOGIC RESPONSES TO SHOCK

Experimental Studies of the Response of Extracellular Fluid

EARLY RESULTS

Hypovolemic shock is the most common form seen clinically and is also the form that has been studied most intensively both clinically and in the laboratory. Most of our own studies have been carried out using hypovolemic shock produced by external blood loss as the model. A method has been developed that allows the simultaneous measurement of total-body red cell mass with the use of ^{51}Cr-tagged red blood cells and total-body plasma volume with the use of ^{131}I-tagged and, later, ^{125}I-tagged human serum albumin. In addition, total-body extracellular fluid can be measured simultaneously with the use of ^{35}S-tagged sodium sulfate. The three isotopes are simultaneously injected intravenously, and with the use of appropriate energy-differentiating counting instruments, all three isotopes can be traced after equilibration. Volumes are then determined by the dilution principle, using multiple sampling.

In an early study the three volumes were measured; splenectomized dogs were then bled a sublethal, sub-shock amount of 10 percent of the measured blood volume. After hemorrhage the three volumes were again measured. The loss of the amount of red blood cells and plasma removed during the hemorrhage could be detected by the method described. It was shown that the decrease in extracellular fluid volume was only the amount lost as plasma removed during the hemorrhage.

By use of the same model, volumes were measured before and after hemorrhage of 25 percent of the measured blood volume. This hemorrhage was again sublethal but produced hypotension. In this group of animals also the loss of the amount of red blood cells and plasma removed could be detected. In addition, however, the functional extracellular fluid volume as measured by the ^{35}S-tagged sodium sulfate was found to have decreased by 18 to 26 percent of the original volume. Since there was no measurable external loss of ^{35}S sulfate, this reduction was presumed to be an internal redistribution of extracellular fluid. Subsequent studies of external bleeding of 35, 45, and even over 50 percent hemorrhage always produced the same reduction in functional extracellular fluid as long as the animal was in shock.

In subsequent studies, splenectomized dogs were subjected to "irreversible" hemorrhagic shock according to a modified method of Wiggers, which utilizes a reservoir. Return of shed blood in this severe preparation resulted in the return of blood pressure to near control levels, followed by a fall in blood pressure within 1 to 16 h; death

resulted in 80 percent of the dogs, i.e., a standard mortality rate.

In one group of animals the three volumes were measured and the dogs were then subjected to shock by the Wiggers method. The three volumes were remeasured by reinjection during the period of shock; then shed blood was returned. The decrease in blood volume was the amount that had been removed. Concurrently, the functional extracellular fluid exhibited a decided reduction. Immediately after the return of the shed blood, the red cell mass returned to essentially normal levels, as did the plasma volume; however, there remained a deficit of functional extracellular fluid. In dogs treated with shed blood plus plasma (10 mL/kg), the losses during shock were again similar. After therapy with plasma, plus return of shed blood, there was a return of blood volume to normal. There remained, however, a decrease in functional extracellular fluid volume.

Dogs treated with an extracellular "mimic," such as a balanced salt solution plus shed blood, had comparable losses during shock. As in the previous groups, the blood volume returned essentially to normal after treatment. But dogs treated with salt solution plus shed blood exhibited return of functional extracellular fluid volume to control levels.

In this study only 20 percent of those dogs treated with shed blood alone survived longer than 24 h. When plasma was used in addition to whole blood as therapy, 30 percent of the dogs survived. Of the animals treated with lactated Ringer's solution plus shed blood, 70 percent survived (Fig. 4-1). The 80 percent mortality rate of a standard "irreversible" shock preparation was reduced to 30 percent by restoration of functional extracellular fluid volume in addition to return of shed blood.

Fig. 4-1. Acute hemorrhagic shock: survival study.

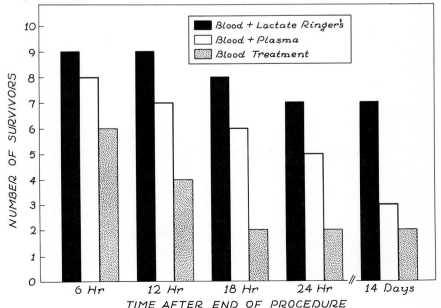

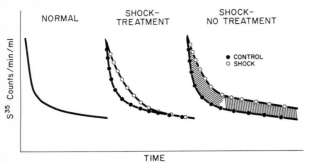

Fig. 4-2. Radiosulfate equilibration curve: semilogarithmic plot, summary model.

All these early studies of the measurement of the functional extracellular fluid were based on volume distribution curves of sulfate measured for approximately 1 h. At any point in the course of the curve there is a reduction in extracellular fluid in the untreated state of shock. Subsequent work has continued these volume distribution curves for many hours. In true untreated hemorrhagic shock there is a reduction in the total extracellular fluid, or final diluted volume of radiosulfate, when compared with preshock volumes (Fig. 4-2).

Even when a less severe shock preparation is used,

there is still a reduction in early equilibrating extracellular fluid or early available extracellular fluid, whereas the total anatomic extracellular fluid may remain normal. Subsequent studies have shown that if shock is not of sufficient duration to produce reduction in both functional and total extracellular fluid, the reduction may be only in functional extracellular fluid. Furthermore, if therapy is instituted quickly and blood pressure is returned to normal, a long sulfate equilibration curve may fail to reveal the acute reduction that was corrected early.

Consequently, the current status of sulfate as a measure of the functional extracellular fluid must be interpreted as indicating that early sulfate volume measurement reveals functional or available extracellular fluid and that prolonged measurement of the volume distribution curves gives total extracellular fluid values. If therapy has been instituted or has been completed, the reduction in total or even in the available extracellular fluid may not be measurable.

Unquestionably, some plasma, or transcapillary, refilling occurs in response to hemorrhage and to hemorrhagic shock. This response, however, is initially rather limited and, in severe hemorrhagic shock, is grossly inadequate to explain the reduction seen in interstitial fluid. Since there is no source for external loss, the question arose as to whether interstitial fluid might move into the cell mass in an isotonic fashion (Fig. 4-3).

Fig. 4-3. Interstitial fluid response to hemorrhagic shock.

NORMAL

VASCULAR TREE　　　**INTERSTITIAL FLUID**　　　**CELL FLUID**

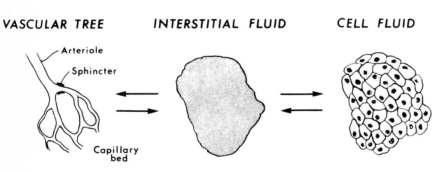

HEMORRHAGIC SHOCK

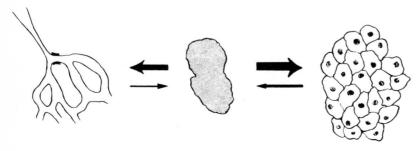

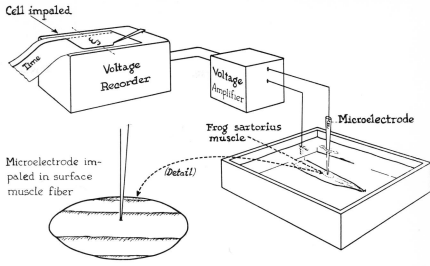

Fig. 4-4. Schematic of intracellular recording. [From: *Ruch and Fulton (eds): Medical Physiology and Biophysics, 18th ed, Philadelphia, Saunders, 1960, with permission.*]

CELLULAR STUDIES

Subsequently, studies of ion transport across the cell membrane were undertaken in order to determine the possibility of intracellular swelling in skeletal muscle in response to hemorrhagic shock. Using a Ling-Gerard ultramicroelectrode with glass tip diameter of less than 1 μm (Fig. 4-4), intracellular transmembrane potential recordings were made. The electrode was modified to record intracellular transmembrane potentials in vivo before, during, and after shock (Fig. 4-5).

Skeletal muscle measurements in acute hemorrhagic shock demonstrate a constant and sustained fall in the normally negative intracellular transmembrane potential. This may represent a reduction in efficiency of the sodium pump induced by tissue hypoxia; it is present only during shock-producing hypotension. Additional studies in splenectomized dogs showed that changes in variables such as pH, P_{CO_2}, and bicarbonate do not influence the transmembrane potential in shock. Even with progressive

Fig. 4-5. In vivo transmembrane potential measurement in rat skeletal muscle.

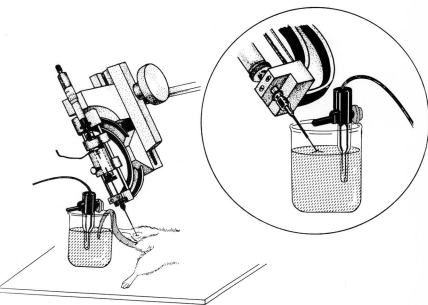

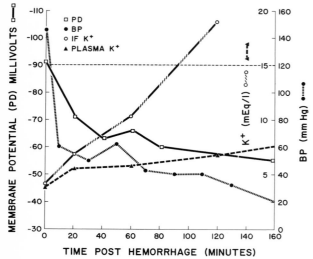

Fig. 4-6. Changes in membrane potential and interstitial K$^+$ in rats with hemorrhagic shock.

metabolic acidosis and its subsequent correction, the potential still follows the blood pressure and shock state.

Studies have been reported that utilized the ultramicroelectrode measurement of transmembrane potential combined with direct aspiration of skeletal muscle interstitial fluid by a modification of the technique of Hagberg. Using this technique, it was found that as blood pressure fell and transmembrane potential was reduced, plasma potassium rose slowly during the shock period (Fig. 4-6). The directly aspirated interstitial fluid potassium during the same period of time rose to a height of more than 15 meq/L of interstitial fluid. This explained where potassium, moving out of skeletal muscle cells,

was being sequestered as sodium chloride and water moved into muscle cells.

Additional studies have been performed in primates that show essentially the same phenomenon (Fig. 4-7). These studies also reveal that this cellular membrane transport is a reversible phenomenon; i.e., once the shock state is treated, transmembrane potential recovers. Concomitant muscle biopsies show clearly that muscle cells gain sodium, water, and chloride while losing potassium. Thus the data reveal an isotonic swelling of skeletal muscle cells in response to shock injury (Fig. 4-8).

Studies in human beings reveal the same response to shock injury. Interesting corroborative changes in action potentials of single cells in skeletal muscles have been revealed in primates (Fig. 4-9). One study shows a decrease in resting membrane potential, a decrease in amplitude of action potential, and prolongation of both repolarization and depolarization times. Resuscitation quickly reversed these changes, except for repolarization time, which remained prolonged for several days. This confirms in vitro the alterations in intracellular sodium and potassium concentrations that were measured by skeletal muscle biopsy and resting membrane potential measurements.

Maintenance of the transmembrane potential difference (PD) is an important cellular function of both excitable and nonexcitable tissues. The resting PD is generally agreed to depend upon an energy-dependent Na$^+$-K$^+$ transport mechanism. The specific energy substrate of this membrane-bound complex is adenosine triphosphate (ATP).

Changes in muscle and liver PD have been shown to be reliable indicators of cellular dysfunction in prolonged hemorrhagic shock. This cell membrane depolarization

Fig. 4-7. Changes in membrane potential and blood pressure in primates during hemorrhagic shock and after resuscitation.

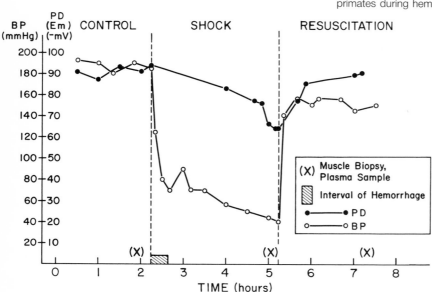

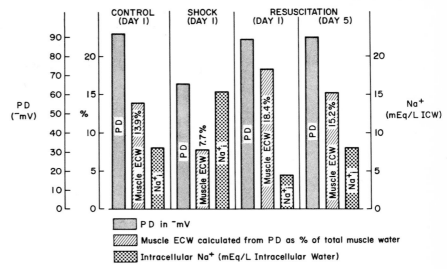

Fig. 4-8. Changes in membrane potential, extracellular water, and intracellular Na$^+$ in primates after resuscitation from hemorrhagic shock.

has been associated with cellular swelling, cellular uptake of sodium and chloride, and loss of potassium. Previous studies indicate that these abnormalities are due to failure of the active transport mechanism. The depletion of ATP in skeletal muscle, liver, and kidney in a hemorrhagic shock model in rats led to the proposal that the cellular dysfunction observed in hemorrhagic shock was secondary to inadequate energy stores. Subsequent studies reported markedly improved survival rates after hemorrhagic shock in animals that were administered ATP-MgCl$_2$ intramuscularly, intraperitoneally, or intravenously. In addition, restoration of tissue ATP levels was reported in the ATP-MgCl$_2$ resuscitated animals and was interpreted to be a result of entry into the cells of intact ATP molecules.

Our recent studies indicate that skeletal muscle ATP levels were maintained during prolonged hemorrhagic shock. Depletion of liver ATP or skeletal muscle creatine phosphate was not prevented by administration of intravenous ATP-MgCl$_2$. Cellular dysfunction in liver and muscle, indicated by depolarization of PD, was not ameliorated by infusion of ATP-MgCl$_2$.

Exogenously administered ATP is rapidly degraded in the plasma. In addition, several studies have demonstrated that ATP in the intact state does not cross the muscle cell membrane. Thus, late changes in cell energy contents appear to be the result of failing cellular function, rather than the primary cause of membrane failure in shock.

INTERPRETATION

Concisely stated, reduction in extracellular fluid in reversible hemorrhagic shock can consistently be shown (1) with extracellular fluid markers that enter cells slowly or not at all in the shock state when (2) reinjection of the extracellular fluid markers is utilized in the shock state, (3) extracellular fluid markers or tracers are allowed sufficient time for equilibration, (4) shock measurements are obtained while hemorrhagic shock is sustained, and (5) the shock preparation is sufficiently severe and is maintained until there is a change in cellular membrane transport.

Fig. 4-9. Action potentials in primates in hemorrhagic shock.

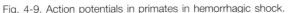

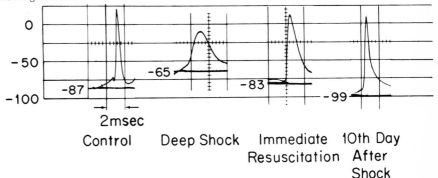

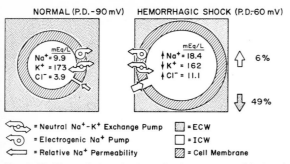

Fig. 4-10. Theoretic transport mechanisms responsible for alterations in potential difference *(PD)* and fluid-electrolyte distribution in hemorrhagic shock.

The data obtained from prior experiments support the use of transmembrane potential measurements as an accurate indicator of cellular alterations resulting from the low-flow state of hemorrhagic shock. Severe hypotension is associated with depression of transmembrane potential difference (PD) which is sustained in the presence of a continued shock state.

Transmembrane PD is generally agreed to be the result of either an electrogenic sodium pump (with active outward extrusion of sodium from muscle cells by a redox system) or a coupled sodium-potassium exchange pump with diffusion of sodium and potassium down their respective chemical gradients. In the latter theory the relative permeabilities of the membrane to the two ions must be considered and the potential interpreted on the basis of the Hodgkin-Katz-Goldman equation in which pNa^+ (relative permeability to sodium) is 0.01. Since permeability to potassium is assumed to be much greater than permeability to sodium in the cell membrane, the PD is essentially a potassium diffusion potential.

The present data thus suggest that skeletal muscle cells may be a principal site of fluid and electrolyte sequestration after severe, prolonged hemorrhagic shock. The exact mechanism for the production of electrolyte changes as well as for the notable diminution in extracellular water that occurs after hemorrhagic shock is not known. It appears that the changes may well represent a reduction in the efficiency of an active ionic pump mechanism or a selective increase in muscle cell membrane permeability to sodium, or both (Fig. 4-10). With a reset membrane potential, extracellular fluid electrolyte concentrations are unchanged. Consequently, from the Nernst equation, intracellular Cl^- must rise from 3.5 to 10 meq and intracellular Na^+ from 10 to 22 meq. Transposition of these data to the previously cited measurements in hemorrhagic shock is shown (Fig. 4-10). This model shows that only a 6 percent isotonic swelling of muscle cells will explain the major reduction in extracellular fluid measured in hemorrhagic shock. Studies are under way to determine the involvement of cell masses other than muscle during the course of hemorrhagic shock. One such study indicates that severe hemorrhagic shock of significant duration is associated with elevation of the internal sodium concentration of the red blood cells. The magnitude of these changes appears to be a function of both the severity and the duration of the shock process and seems to be well correlated with changes in clinical course when sequential sampling procedures are utilized.

There is a measurable reduction in extravascular extracellular fluid in response to sustained hemorrhagic shock. The cellular response to hypovolemic hypotension is characterized by a consistent change in active transport of ions. Evidence obtained directly from living cells indicates that sodium and water enter muscle cells, with resultant loss of cellular potassium to the extracellular fluid. The interstitial fluid holds the extruded potassium. Replenishment of the depleted extracellular fluid counteracts these changes at the cellular level and is an important feature of therapy in patients with hypovolemic shock.

Some interesting new data on the cellular transport mechanism indicate that the endorphins play an integral role in the pathophysiology of hemorrhagic shock. Blockade of these endogenous opiates by naloxone can significantly alter the course of this syndrome. While naloxone administration to normal rats had no effect on the circulation or cellular function, it improved the hemodynamic status of animals subjected to hemorrhagic shock, resulting in improved tissue perfusion. In addition, the administration of this drug prevented the cellular dysfunction normally seen in hemorrhagic shock.

Much current research in shock physiology addresses the role of not only endorphins but also other endogenous compounds that may exert effects on cardiovascular performance and membrane function. Thyrotropin-releasing hormone, arachidonic acid metabolites of both the cyclooxygenase and lipoxygenase pathways, and monochines, particularly cachectin, have all been implicated in the host response to shock. Further delineation of the complex actions of and interactions among these mediators should allow even more specific adjunctive therapies, in addition to fluid resuscitation, to be developed in the future.

Renal Responses

The observation was made long ago that during severe shock, from any cause, renal function essentially stops in human beings. The kidneys, like the skin and the liver, share in the relative oligemia which is a rapid compensatory mechanism in shock to divert blood flow to those organs, such as the brain and the heart, most vital for maintaining life. Consequently the relative oligemia suffered by the kidneys in response to shock is severe and immediate.

The development of oliguria and even anuria is apparently a direct function of the severity and duration of the renal ischemia during shock. In human beings, under normothermic conditions, normal kidneys will tolerate renal ischemia for periods varying from 15 min to a maximum of approximately 90 min. After this degree of ischemia, some functional and anatomic changes inevitably occur. With the use of hypothermia, the period of renal ischemia tolerated during hemorrhagic shock can be considerably prolonged.

SUBCLINICAL RENAL DAMAGE FOLLOWING INJURY AND SHOCK

In civilian and military practice, improved resuscitation with balanced electrolyte solution and blood and immediate corrective surgery have resulted in a great reduction in the incidence of primary oliguric renal failure. Recognition of nonoliguric renal failure as a less severe form of renal insufficiency suggested that graded renal damage might occur in association with systemic injury. Identification of patients with subclinical renal damage should be important in their postinjury care.

PATIENT STUDIES. A study was recently undertaken to determine the presence and degree of such renal damage during the early course of severely injured civilian patients. During the period of this study, 96,000 patients were treated in the emergency department, 988 of whom were admitted to the hospital for care of their injuries. Forty of the most severely injured were selected for continued care in a Trauma Research Unit after resuscitation and operative treatment of injuries. The criteria for inclusion in the study were hypotension following trauma and multiple long bone fractures.

All 40 patients showed generalized depression of renal function initially. Within 24 h of admission, 30 demonstrated return of clearances to normal ranges. The patients were divided into groups according to blood urea nitrogen (BUN) values (Fig. 4-11). Group I, considered to show a characteristic renal response to trauma, was selected on the basis of BUN values continuously below 20 g/dL after the first hospital day. This group included 30 of the 40 patients. Eight patients with renal dysfunction (Group II) showed persistent moderate elevation of BUN values above 20 g/dL. Two patients showed frank renal failure with rapidly progressing azotemia. One of these patients had sustained a gunshot wound of the renal

vein and vena cava and had had the renal pedicle on the involved side clamped for 1 h. The other patient, with a gunshot wound of the aortic bifurcation, represented failure of resuscitation. These two patients with renal failure are not considered in the subsequent comparisons between patients with the characteristic renal response (Group I) and those with renal dysfunction (Group II). Three patients with direct renal injury requiring suture or partial nephrectomy were included in Group I.

As would be expected on the basis of the selection criteria for the groups, glomerular filtration rate (GFR) was quite different for the two groups. Urea clearance (C_{urea}), another clearance primarily related to filtration, was depressed in both groups initially, with a rapid return to and above normal in the dysfunction group. Urine/plasma (U/P) urea ratio and osmolar clearances (C_{osm}) were different in the two groups only subsequent to 12 h after admission (Fig. 4-12).

Tubular resorption of water (TcH_2O) was significantly different in the two groups only at 18 and 24 h after admission. The trend in Group I was toward excretion of free water, while the trend in the dysfunction group was toward continued retention of free water. Cardiac output was not significantly different in the two groups.

Sodium clearances (C_{Na}) were similar in the two groups until after 12 h following admission. Subsequently C_{Na} fell in Group II. Postoperative sodium balance, represented as the difference between daily sodium intake and urinary sodium excretion, was different in the two groups. Group I showed positive sodium balance during day 1, balance during day 2, and negative balance during day 3. In Group II, the dysfunction group, increasing sodium retention occurred during each of the 3 days of the study.

There were no discernible differences between the two groups in age, type of injury, length of hypotensive episode, fluid administration, positive-pressure ventilation,

Fig. 4-11. Renal function after trauma: blood urea nitrogen values.

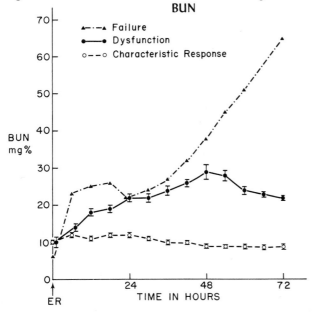

Fig. 4-12. Renal function after trauma: urine/plasma urea ratio.

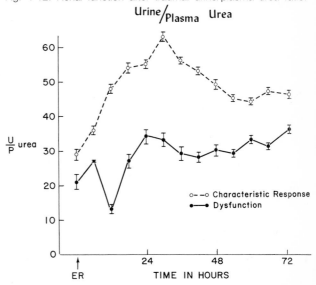

nephrotoxic antibiotics, minute urine volume, blood volume, or arterial P_{O_2} and pH.

Discussion

Classic renal clearance techniques have been used infrequently in surgical patients, partly because of errors inherent in the methods. All renal clearances are urine flow–sensitive. An increase in urine flow leads to a decrease in mean urine transit time. Consequently new filtrate washes out tubular and collecting system contents at a more rapid rate, yielding a factitiously high clearance. Conversely, a decrease in urine flow may lead to a factitiously low clearance. Errors in clearance measurements can be minimized by using constant mechanical infusion, long collection periods, and bladder washes. The long collection periods may obscure fluctuations during the period, but they provide accurate mean clearances.

In the normal human kidney, GFR may promptly increase 30 percent above basal level during diuresis. In the above-mentioned study, GFR was measured without fluid loading, and yet six of the patients in Group I showed a GFR above 150 mL/min, suggesting the presence of post-injury stimuli in the patients tending to increase GFR maximally. The patients with renal dysfunction (Group II) were presumably subject to similar stimuli but were unable to respond with any elevation in GFR because of renal damage or persistent neural or humoral influences affecting GFR.

Of interest is a study by Lucas et al. of the effects of albumin supplementation on renal function in 46 severely injured patients. Compared with a similar group of patients who received only crystalloid solutions and blood during resuscitation from hypovolemic shock, patients who received the additional albumin showed a decrease in GFR, C_{Na}, C_{osm}, and urine output. The authors postulated that these changes were due to increases in serum oncotic pressures in the glomerular tufts and peritubular vessels.

Endogenous creatinine clearance (C_{cr}) in both groups was always higher than GFR. Notable variation in C_{cr} in the injured patient was noted by Ladd, who concluded that endogenous C_{cr} was unsuitable for evaluation of GFR in battle casualties. Creatinine as determined by the Jaffe reaction overestimates the true creatinine in plasma, and since creatinine is secreted in human beings, the usual agreement of endogenous C_{cr} with inulin or iothalamate ^{125}I clearance is coincidental. Twofold and threefold increases in endogenous C_{cr} occur in association with the changes in muscle metabolism following severe trauma. Apparently normal values for C_{cr} may lead to a false sense of security when, in fact, the GFR may be reduced by a factor of 2 or 3 in the severely injured patient.

Muscle metabolism is profoundly altered in the injured patient, resulting in increased loads of creatinine and creatine presented to the kidney. In the early postinjury period, many patients had metabolic changes similar to those found in patients placed on a high protein diet. Even with increases in urea nitrogen load from tissue injury, multiple transfusions, and gluconeogenesis, these patients did not undergo azotemia and creatinemia. Azotemia and creatinemia are not inevitable consequences of severe tissue injury, and other factors are operative in the injured patient who exhibits such changes.

Small transient increases of GFR were apparent after administration of diuretics in some patients. In view of the demonstrated slow improvement in GFR that occurs after resuscitation and injury repair, it is difficult to ascribe increases in GFR during this early hospital period to furosemide. Further study of changes in GFR after administration of furosemide is indicated, however, in view of reports suggesting a beneficial effect of furosemide on renal function.

In a more recent study, Lucas et al. indicated that furosemide does not protect against renal failure by altering or increasing renal blood flow but may cause renal failure by producing hypovolemia. They were unable to demonstrate an increase in GFR, renal plasma flow, renal blood flow, or renal blood flow distribution in 54 critically ill surgical patients who received furosemide. Despite marked increases in urine output, C_{osm}, and C_{Na}, six of the patients developed renal failure, and five became hypotensive 2 to 10 h after administration of this diuretic.

C_{urea}, C_{cr}, C_{osm}, and U/P urea, U/P creatinine, and U/P osmolarity ratios have each been proposed as good clinical determinants of renal damage. Objections to the use of creatinine determinations alone have been noted above. Otherwise there is little to recommend any one of these tests over the others, since all relate filtration to some aspect of tubular function. Recognition of the need to measure at least one of the foregoing in urine and plasma simultaneously is important. U/P ratios approaching unity and clearances below 10 mL/min are diagnostic of some form of renal failure. Such determinations are of limited clinical use because many of the most difficult patients fall in an indeterminate group. Recently, Miller et al. have demonstrated the usefulness of comparing the fractional excretion of sodium with creatinine in oliguric patients. They demonstrated good separation of patients with prerenal oliguria from those with acute renal failure. There was very little overlap. The simplest such calculation comparing these two functions is the renal failure index $(U_{Na} \times PLCR)/U_{cr}$. An index of less than 1 usually indicates prerenal oliguria. An index of greater than 1 correlates well with acute renal failure.

A spectrum of secondary renal injury exists after severe trauma, varying from oliguric renal failure to transient depression of glomerular filtration and tubular function. Tissue trauma and multiple transfusions do not lead to azotemia in the injured patient with normal renal function. Conversely, even minimal persistent elevations of BUN are uniformly associated with significant renal dysfunction and sodium and water retention.

The more severely injured patient can be readily identified in the early postoperative phase by serial evaluation of the renal metabolism of urea or sodium. Identification of such patients should lead to meticulous supportive care, since the general metabolic reserve of the more severely injured patients is diminished and further insults are poorly tolerated.

HIGH-OUTPUT RENAL FAILURE

Posttraumatic acute renal insufficiency is well recognized as a highly lethal complication. The diagnosis is classically based on persistent oliguria and chemical evidence of uremia after stabilization of the circulation. The clinical course is characterized by oliguria of several days' to several weeks' duration, followed by a progressive rise in daily urine volume until both the excretory and concentrating functions of the kidney are gradually restored.

It is less well recognized that renal insufficiency may occur without an observed period of oliguria. This variant of renal insufficiency has been reported infrequently after burns, head injury, and soft tissue trauma. The reported cases are characterized by increasing azotemia, while the daily urine volume remains normal or increased. Many of these patients have an apparently inappropriate increase in urine volume, and the term *high-output renal failure* may best describe this entity, despite a theoretical objection. Until recently, this type of renal failure has not been noted frequently after trauma, nor has the clinical course been described in sufficient detail for recognition or management.

PATIENT STUDIES. This study describes the clinical course of acute renal failure without oliguria, emphasizing the problems encountered in management and suggesting renal ischemia as the basic causative mechanism (Fig. 4-13).

After severe abdominal trauma, the patients were in shock an average of 3.5 h, the individual times varying from 1 to 6 h. The average blood loss was 4.2 L and average blood replacement 3.6 L. The recorded blood loss was the amount measured at the time of operation. In most patients external bleeding was minimal. In addition to whole blood, they were given an average of 4 L of Ringer's lactate solution per patient prior to and during the operative procedure.

After operation the diagnosis of renal failure was not immediately suspected, since urine volumes were above 30 mL/h and few abnormalities were present in the initial values of blood urea nitrogen, potassium, sodium, carbon dioxide–combining power, and chlorides obtained on the first postoperative day.

In all cases not involving direct damage to the urinary tract, the urinalysis after operation showed specific gravities between 1.003 and 1.010, pH of 5.5 to 6.5, and urinary sediments containing at most a few red blood cells per high-power field and an occasional cast. The urine/plasma ratio of urea nitrogen was found to be slightly less than 20:1.

On the day of operation the minimum urinary output was 730 mL. This represented the output for less than 12 h in each case. There was a progressive increase in the mean urine volume for the first 6 to 8 days, reaching a peak of 2350 mL and returning gradually to normal between the sixteenth and seventeenth days. The continued high output of 3 L/day after the sixteenth day occurred in only one patient; the BUN in this patient did not return to normal for 37 days. Extremely high outputs were noted in some patients compared with the relatively normal values in others during the period of azotemia. The highest urine volumes were found in patients with the highest BUN values.

A progressive rise of the mean BUN during the 6 to 8 days after injury was followed by a gradual return to normal between the sixteenth and eighteenth days. The serum creatinine levels paralleled the azotemia, the highest value being 6.8 mg/dL. In all patients the increasing BUN level was paralleled by an increasing daily urinary volume. Similarly, the stepwise decline in blood urea was paralleled by a decreasing urinary volume.

In most instances the initial serum potassium values after operation were slightly below normal. In some the serum potassium levels were above 6 meq/L by the second or third postoperative day, while the remaining patients showed a slow but sustained rise. All the accelerated rises resulted from intravenous administration of potassium salts (not more than 60 meq/day). When the serum potassium reached 6 meq/L, treatment with cation exchange resins was instituted. This proved effective in preventing further rises in serum potassium. An increase in serum potassium from 5.5 to 9.2 meq/L was caused by the intravenous administration of 60 meq of KCl in a 12-h period. Extracorporeal hemodialysis was necessary to reduce the potassium intoxication that occurred.

Moderately low values for the carbon dioxide–combining power were present for the first 4 or 5 days after injury and represent a mild to moderate metabolic acidosis. All isotonic losses were replaced with lactated Ringer's solution when acidosis persisted. In most patients the acidosis was well controlled by the administration of isotonic lactate solutions, which occasionally resulted in a mild metabolic alkalosis, although two patients had carbon dioxide–combining power values between 15 and 18 meq/L despite lactate therapy and died on the tenth and twelfth postoperative days. After the eighth postoperative day carbon dioxide–combining powers were within a normal range without lactate administra-

Fig. 4-13. High-output renal failure.

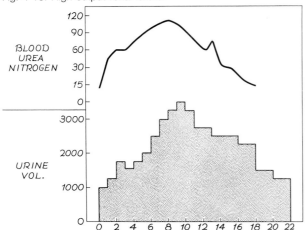

tion. The serum chlorides did not show a reciprocal relationship to the carbon dioxide–combining powers.

Serum sodium determinations were made throughout the period of renal failure. The highest values of 150 to 154 meq occurred during a trial of fluid restriction to determine whether the high urinary outputs were being induced by excessive administration of fluids. On these two occasions, hypernatremia was readily produced, indicating that the kidney was excreting a solute-poor urine.

Surviving patients were available for follow-up. Evaluation of renal function was carried out 1 to $1\frac{1}{2}$ years after injury. Determinations of blood urea nitrogen, creatinine, sodium, potassium, carbon dioxide, and chloride were normal. Intravenous pyelography was normal. The lowest urinary concentration obtained was 1.020, and excretion of phenolsulfonphthalein (PSP) exceeded 30 percent in 30 min in all patients studied. Within 3 months both tubular and glomerular functions had returned to normal.

Autopsy was performed on patients who died. Microscopic examination of the kidneys from these patients showed regenerating patchy tubular necrosis. The damage in each instance was principally to the distal nephron; less severe changes were seen in the proximal segments.

A typical course of high-output renal failure shows an increasing urea nitrogen that parallels the increasing urine volume, a mild metabolic acidosis, and an acute hyperkalemia produced by the administration of potassium salts. Recognition of the disease entity permits control of these abnormalities.

ANIMAL STUDIES. Animal experiments using dogs were carried out to determine the modifying effect of hypothermia on renal ischemia. After contralateral nephrectomy, the remaining renal pedicle was clamped for 2 h and released.

As seen in Fig. 4-14, Group A consists of normothermic controls. Group B dogs had regional renal hypothermia produced by irrigation of the peritoneal cavity with cold saline solution. Group C dogs had profound renal hypothermia to 25°C produced by circulating cold saline solution continuously around the kidney. This cooling technique has been previously described.

The results show progressive azotemia and death in untreated animals that are not cooled (Group A). There was only transient elevation of the BUN when the kidneys were cooled to 25°C (Group C). In Group B, regional hypothermia, the BUN rose to an average height of 60 mg/dL by the sixth to tenth day and gradually returned to normal between the twelfth and sixteenth days.

Utilizing this same model in six dogs with exteriorized ureters, minimum urine volumes of 400 mL/day were obtained without an observed period of oliguria. Usually the daily urine volume increased to between 600 and 900 mL/day before the BUN began to decline. Microscopic examination of these and six similarly treated animals, sacrificed between the fifth and tenth days, showed the tubular lesion to be confined principally to the distal tubules but with some proximal tubular involvement. These changes, both degenerative and regenerative, were scattered and irregular in distribution.

Consequently it can be seen that high-output renal failure in animals is an intermediate form of renal failure. With severe renal ischemia, unmodified oliguric renal failure inevitably resulted. When the kidney was protected with profound hypothermia, no significant renal failure resulted. On the other hand, with modest but practical protection to the kidney afforded by peritoneal sluicing with cold saline solution, moderate elevation of BUN associated with high urine volume was obtained. This protection resulted in recovery of the animal in each instance.

Discussion

Renal insufficiency without oliguria is important from the standpoint of recognition and clinical management of a variant of classic acute renal failure.

The clinical course of patients has been shown to be qualitatively the same as that occurring when oliguria is present. Quantitatively, however, these patients retain a limited ability to excrete acid products of metabolism, potassium, and urea. It is of primary importance that renal insufficiency of itself was not sufficient in terms of acidosis, uremia, potassium intoxication, or fluid volume control to cause death in this series.

The normal or high daily output of urine, although solute-poor, permits administration of fairly large quantities of water daily, in addition to replacement of isotonic salt losses such as those from gastrointestinal suction. The maintenance of normal extracellular fluid volume and normal serum sodium concentration is, therefore, easily accomplished when accurate daily outputs of each are obtained and losses are replaced accordingly. The quantity of fluids containing sodium may be administered as lactate to control the mild metabolic acidosis that occurs. The observations of Moore indicate that if the acidosis is not treated, it may become so severe as to become the outstanding abnormality in these cases.

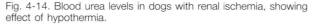

Fig. 4-14. Blood urea levels in dogs with renal ischemia, showing effect of hypothermia.

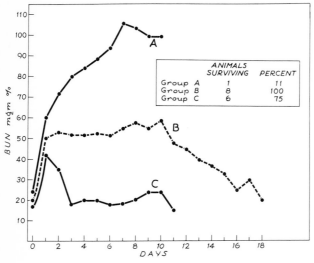

	ANIMALS SURVIVING	PERCENT
Group A	1	11
Group B	8	100
Group C	6	75

The chief dangers of high-output renal failure are (1) failure to recognize the existence of renal failure because of normal output and (2) the administration of potassium salts intravenously. Good urinary output and gastrointestinal involvement requiring suction would usually indicate the need for daily replacement of potassium. When this type of renal failure exists, however, potassium intoxication may be produced. In the early patients studied, five of nine required therapy for hyperkalemia. One required emergency hemodialysis for control of excessively high serum potassium levels. It is important that the serum level be determined daily and prior to the administration of any potassium-containing solutions.

The factors involved in the production of acute renal failure following trauma are incompletely understood, but renal ischemia is of unquestioned importance. This concept implies that the ischemia produces damage to the nephrons, which results in failure of the kidneys to excrete urine. Diuresis is felt to represent the recovery phase. Allowing for the physiologic variation between individuals and between given degrees of renal ischemia, a spectrum of the length of the oliguric phase should occur. This has been well documented by Teschan and Mason.

The frequency with which these cases occurred in relation to the small number of oliguric renal failures that were seen during the same period may represent differences in the therapy given during the ischemic episode. There are two outstanding differences in the therapy that we have routinely used. One is the administration of balanced salt solution along with whole blood in the resuscitation from hemorrhagic shock. It is well recognized that prolonged or severe extracellular fluid deficits are necessary for the production of renal failure in animals and may contribute to renal damage in human beings. The second difference in treatment is the use of renal hypothermia of a moderate degree to modify or prevent ischemic renal damage.

Clinical experience and laboratory experiments suggest that high-output renal failure represents the renal response to a less severe (or modified) episode of renal injury than that required to produce classic oliguric renal failure.

Pulmonary Responses

Acute respiratory failure following severe injury and critical illness has received increasing attention over the last two decades. With advances in the management of hemorrhagic shock and support of circulatory and renal function in injured patients, it has become apparent that 1 to 2 percent of significantly injured patients (with previously normal lungs) develop acute respiratory failure in the postinjury period. Initially this lung injury was thought to be specifically related to the shock state and its resuscitation. This is implied by such names as "shock lung" and "traumatic wet lung," which have been applied to acute respiratory insufficiency following injury. It is now recognized that there are many similarities in the pathophysiology and clinical presentation of acute lung injury following a variety of insults. This has resulted in the realization that the lung has a limited number of ways of reacting to injury and that several different causes of acute diffuse lung injury result in a similar pathophysiologic response. The common denominator of this response appears to be damage at the alveolar-capillary interface, with resulting leakage of proteinaceous fluid from the intravascular space into the interstitium and subsequently into alveolar spaces.

CLINICAL PRESENTATION. This injury with its resulting interstitial (and alveolar) edema produces a clinical picture ranging in severity from mild pulmonary dysfunction to progressive, eventually fatal, pulmonary failure. It differs from "classic" pulmonary failure in that the patients *are usually hypocarbic* rather than hypercarbic. The severe form has been labeled *adult respiratory distress* syndrome (ARDS) and is characterized by

1. Hypoxemia, which is relatively unresponsive to elevations of inspired oxygen concentration (indicating ventilation perfusion imbalance and shunting);
2. Decreased pulmonary compliance (progressively increased airway pressure required to achieve adequate tidal volume);
3. Chest x-ray changes, which are characteristically minimal in the early stages; with progression of the syndrome interstitial edema and diffuse bilateral infiltrates appear that may progress to widespread areas of consolidation;
4. Pulmonary edema due to cardiogenic causes or increased hydrostatic pressure, which should be ruled out, and this is generally done by the measurement of filling pressures.

The clinical criteria are summarized in Table 4-1.

Originally, four clinical stages were described. The first is quite subtle and is characterized by spontaneous hyperventilation with hypocarbia, diminished pulmonary compliance, and respiratory alkalosis. If the process continues, the patient progresses to the second stage, during which respiratory problems become more apparent. Persistent hyperventilation (with hypocarbia), progressive hypoxemia, decreased compliance, and an increase in pulmonary shunt fraction indicate that further pulmonary deterioration is occurring. Changes in chest roentgenograms are characteristically subtle during the early stages. As the syndrome advances to stage three (progressive pulmonary insufficiency) and stage four (terminal hypoxia with cardiac asystole), interstitial edema and diffuse infiltrates are observed on the roentgenograms.

Table 4-1. CLINICAL CRITERIA FOR POSTINJURY PULMONARY INSUFFICIENCY (ARDS)

Major
A. Hypoxemia (unresponsive)
B. Stiff lung (low compliance)
C. ↓ Resting volume (functional residual capacity)
D. X-ray (diffuse interstitial pattern)
E. ↑ Dead space ventilation

Minor
A. ↑ Cardiac output
B. Hyperventilation
C. R/O cardiogenic pulmonary edema

While these initial clinical descriptions are useful, several qualifying points are important. First, the early changes are nonspecific. Similar findings result from a variety of causes (e.g., early pneumonia, atelectasis, pulmonary edema). Second, the progression can be rapid and the stages are not clearly distinguishable. Studies of the incidence of ARDS have shown that >75 percent of patients developing "full-blown" ARDS do so within 24 h of the inciting cause and that 95 percent do so within 72 h. In these studies the diagnosis of ARDS required the following:

1. $Pa_{O_2} \leq 75$ mmHg while receiving $F_{I_{O_2}} \geq 0.5$
2. Diffuse pulmonary infiltrates
3. Pulmonary artery wedge pressure ≤ 18 mmHg
4. No alternate explanation for the above

Third, with currently available pulmonary support, progression to "stage four" is rare. While the mortality *associated with* ARDS remains high, death is rarely the result of respiratory failure alone.

PATHOPHYSIOLOGY. A review of basic terminology is shown in Table 4-2. The prominent derangements in pulmonary function associated with ARDS are (1) hypoxia that is unresponsive to increased inspired oxygen concentrations, (2) decreased pulmonary compliance (compliance defined as the amount of volume increase in the lungs obtained by a given increase in pressure), which clinically appears as "stiff lungs," and (3) a fall in resting lung volume, specifically a fall in the functional residual capacity. The functional residual capacity, as shown in Fig. 4-15, is the amount of air remaining in the lungs after a normal expiration.

The possible causes of hypoxia (decreased arterial P_{O_2}) are shown in Table 4-3. All clinicians are familiar with hypoventilation as a cause of hypoxia, as seen in the recovery room, but it is unlikely that hypoventilation is responsible for the hypoxia in this syndrome. Hypoventilation significant enough to produce hypoxia is associated with a rise in the P_{CO_2}. These patients, however, have an abnormally low P_{CO_2}.

Although diffusion defects can theoretically result from interstitial edema, they should respond to the administration of 100% oxygen. This is not the case in the patients in question, so diffusion defects alone appear to be unlikely causes of the clinical syndrome.

Ventilation/perfusion inequalities could explain the hypoxia seen in these patients, and shunting represents the ultimate ventilation/perfusion abnormality. This

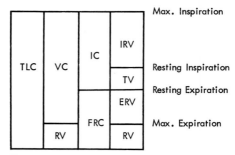

Fig. 4-15. Lung volumes and capacities: *TLC,* total lung capacity; *VC,* vital capacity; *IC,* inspiratory capacity; *FRC,* functional residual capacity; *RV,* residual volume; *ERV,* expiratory reserve volume; *TV,* tidal volume; *IRV,* inspiratory reserve volume.

statement deserves further explanation. Normally, there is autoregulation of ventilation and perfusion within the lung so that a balance exists between ventilation and perfusion of alveolar groups. When a group of alveoli become nonventilated or have decreased ventilation, compensatory mechanisms bring about a reflex decrease in blood supply to these alveoli. This, in its extreme, results in no ventilation and no perfusion to these alveolar units; thus no abnormality in terms of dead space ventilation or shunting occurs. The effects of loss of this normal balance or loss of compensatory mechanisms are shown in Fig. 4-16. On the left, alterations in blood flow are demonstrated. It can be seen that progressive decrease in blood flow with continued ventilation affects primarily carbon dioxide elimination. This can be defined as high ventilation/perfusion ratio and is usually reflected by increases in dead space ventilation. Such changes do not result in hypoxia. On the right side of Fig. 4-16 is shown the effect of reduction in ventilation while perfusion is maintained. It can be seen that progressive lowering of ventilation can result in hypoxia until the ultimate reduction, i.e., nonventilation, occurs. In theory, as long as any ventilation of the alveolus occurs, the hypoxia should be responsive to oxygen. This, then, is generally referred to as a ventilation/perfusion abnormality characterized by a low V/Q ratio. When alveolar collapse or nonventilation occurs for any reason, the hypoxia secondary to this is no longer responsive to oxygen; this is defined as a shunt.

Causes of pulmonary shunting are shown in Fig. 4-17. Shunting normally takes place, to the extent of about 3 percent of the cardiac output, through both intrapulmonary and extrapulmonary routes. Although pathologic shunts occur from extrapulmonary causes, intrapulmonary shunting appears to be the problem in ARDS. Basically, there is perfusion of alveoli that are collapsed or for

Table 4-2. BASIC TERMINOLOGY AND SYMBOLS

$\overline{V}_{O_2}$	Oxygen consumption
Q_T	Cardiac output
V_D/V_T	Physiologic dead space ventilation as fraction of tidal volume
Q_s/Q_t	Physiologic shunt as fraction of total cardiac output
AaD_{O_2}	Alveolar arterial gradient—oxygen
$F_{I_{O_2}}$	Fraction of inspired O_2
$V/\dot{Q}$	Ratio of ventilation to perfusion
Pa_{O_2}	Partial pressure, arterial, oxygen

Table 4-3. CAUSES OF HYPOXEMIA

1. Hypoventilation
2. Diffusion defects
3. V/Q abnormalities
4. Shunting

PULMONARY GAS EXCHANGE
CONTRIBUTING FACTORS

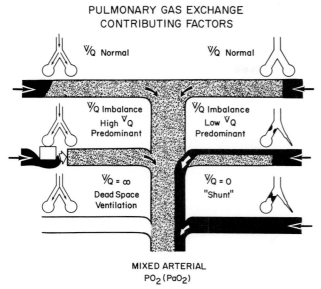

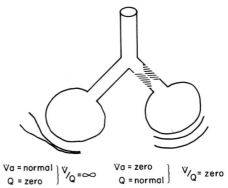

Fig. 4-18. Diagrammatic representation of mismatched ventilation and perfusion.

Fig. 4-16. Diagrammatic representation of ventilation/perfusion ratio (V/Q) abnormalities.

other reasons cannot be ventilated. The alveoli, for example, may be filled with secretions, exudate, blood, or edema.

Whatever the cause, the clinical picture appears to result from a distortion of the normal ventilation/perfusion balance. This concept is shown in Fig. 4-18. In some areas of the lung there is perfusion with poor ventilation; in other areas there is ventilation of nonperfused alveoli. This combination of abnormalities will produce decreased resting lung volume (functional residual capacity, or FRC), shunting, and increased dead space ventilation.

The common denominator producing the abnormalities in ventilation and perfusion and other abnormalities seen in ARDS is thought to be injury to the pulmonary capillary endothelium or alveolar epithelium. Injury to the capillary endothelium results in loss of integrity of the membrane, with increased permeability to albumin. The

consequent leak of protein-rich fluid leads to *interstitial pulmonary edema* and decreased pulmonary compliance. With continued leakage, the alveolar units become fluid-filled and hypoxia (shunting) ensues. Thus the entire clinical picture of ventilation of poorly perfused segments (capillary injury), decreased compliance (interstitial edema), perfusion of poorly ventilated segments, and loss of lung volume (partially and completely fluid-filled alveoli) appears to result from capillary injury with a "capillary leak."

ETIOLOGY. A variety of factors have been suggested as capable of producing ARDS (Table 4-4). Several of these are specific to, or frequently present in the trauma patient. Some of these have been clearly shown to predispose patients to the development of ARDS as shown in Table 4-5. The definition of these factors and possible mechanism of production are discussed below.

Blood-Borne Injury. Among individual conditions, *sepsis syndrome* is the most frequent single precipitant of ARDS. Sepsis syndrome has been defined as evidence of serious infection (temperature $\leq 35°C$ or $\geq 39°C$, white blood cell count <2000 or $>12,000$ cells/mm^3, positive blood cultures, or source of infection) accompanied by a deleterious systemic response (unexplained arterial hypotension with systolic blood pressure <90 mmHg for greater than 2 h, systemic vascular resistance less than 800 dyne · s/cm^5, or unexplained metabolic acidosis).

The risk of ARDS after bacteremia alone, on the other hand, is relatively low, increasing markedly if bacteremia is accompanied by a deleterious systemic response such as hypotension or thrombocytopenia. While sepsis can serve as an example of a number of factors that appear to produce ARDS as a result of blood-borne injury, the precise mechanism by which this occurs has not yet been elucidated and is the subject of extensive investigation. Some propose that the injury is a direct result of bacterial products on the capillary endothelium. Others present evidence for extensive injury resulting from products of activated leukocytes or platelets. This raises the challenging issue of host defense mechanisms activated and out of normal physiologic control. Several possibilities proposed are worthy of investigation (and are not mutually exclusive) and well may lead to enhanced understanding

Fig. 4-17. Mechanisms of arteriovenous admixture in pulmonary shunting.

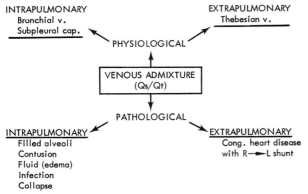

INTRAPULMONARY
Bronchial v.
Subpleural cap.

EXTRAPULMONARY
Thebesian v.

PHYSIOLOGICAL

VENOUS ADMIXTURE
(Qs/Qt)

PATHOLOGICAL

INTRAPULMONARY
Filled alveoli
Contusion
Fluid (edema)
Infection
Collapse

EXTRAPULMONARY
Cong. heart disease
with R→L shunt

Table 4-4. DISORDERS ASSOCIATED WITH (CAUSING) ADULT RESPIRATORY
DISTRESS SYNDROME

Blood-borne or vascular source of injury

Trauma (soft tissue or skeletal)*	Drug overdoses:
Sepsis*	Heroin, methadone, ethchlorvynol,
Fat embolism	acetylsalicylic acid, propoxyphene
Pancreatitis	Drug idiosyncratic reaction
Shock	Thrombotic thrombocytopenic purpura
Multiple transfusions:	Leukemia
Microemboli	Venous air embolism
Leukoagglutinin reaction	Head injury
Disseminated intravascular coagulation	Paraquat
Surface burns	Cardiopulmonary bypass/hemodialysis
Miliary tuberculosis	

Inhalation or airway source	*Direct or physical source*
Aspiration of gastric contents*	Lung contusion
Diffuse infectious pneumonia:* viral,	Radiation
mycoplasma, Legionnaires', pneumocystis	High altitude
Near-drowning*	Hanging
Irritant gas inhalation: NO_2, Cl_2, SO_2, NH_3	Reexpansion
Smoke inhalation	
O_2 toxicity	

* Common cause of ARDS.

of ARDS and of the multiple organ failure syndrome following injury and associated with sepsis. Whatever the precise mechanisms, it is becoming clearer that the end result of this blood-borne injury is massive disruption of the capillary endothelium and alveolar epithelium. The end result is loss of selectivity of the endothelium for albumin, interstitial edema, and eventual alveolar flooding and the clinical picture of ARDS.

Other predisposing factors for ARDS that probably operate in a similar fashion include massive soft tissue and skeletal trauma (with microemboli as a possible circulating agent); multiple blood transfusions (with particulate or activated humoral agents causing capillary injury); fat embolism; disseminated intervascular coagulation; and activation (or lack of metabolism) of other circulating agents as might occur in pancreatic injury, pancreatitis, and massive hepatic injury.

The role of hypotension (shock) alone as a precipitating factor continues to be questioned. It appears probable that the presence of severe hypotension may augment injury from other causes but that hypotension alone is rarely the sole cause.

Inhalation or Airway Injury. Aspiration of gastric contents is among the most common causes of ARDS in several series. The clinical picture and roentgenographic findings that we now call ARDS were described by Mendelson in a classic paper in which he also presented animal studies on the pathophysiology of lung injury, stressing the role of acid pH. As in sepsis, the precise mechanism remains under investigation. Although a pH of 2.5 or less was originally suggested as being necessary to produce lung injury in human beings, data now exist that suggest that aspiration of substances with pHs greater than 2.5 can also produce this clinical picture.

Table 4-5. INCIDENCE OF ARDS AFTER PREDISPOSING CLINICAL
CONDITIONS

	Single condition present			Multiple conditions present		
Clinical condition	Number	Number with ARDS	Incidence, %	Number*	Number with ARDS	Incidence, %
Sepsis syndrome	46	18	39	21	8	38
Aspiration	64	8	13	20	8	40
Multiple transfusions	31	8	26	37	12	32
Lung contusion	57	6	11	40	17	43
Multiple fractures	34	3	9	32	10	31
Near-drowning	5	2	40	6	4	67
Total	237	45	19	69	30	43

* Number with given condition as one of multiple risk conditions.

Despite the need to further define the mechanism, there is little question that aspiration of large amounts of gastric contents is a clear cause of ARDS. This has clinical significance, and in addition aspiration can serve as an example of other airway sources of injury. These include near-drowning, inhalation of toxic products (from burning wood, plastic, or chemical agents), oxygen toxicity, and diffuse infectious pneumonias.

Direct or Physical Lung Injury. Thoracic trauma with lung contusion is a well-established cause of ARDS. Here again, the mechanism requires continued investigation. ARDS can occur as a result of bilateral lung contusion due to chest trauma or blast injury. Lung contusion is usually localized and unilateral. Even a localized contusion can produce significant intrapulmonary shunting. The severe ARDS picture associated with bilateral contusions is more likely if the thoracic trauma is bilateral, although a severe unilateral blast injury can also result in ARDS involving both lungs. It has been suggested that significant increases in intrathoracic pressure occur with thoracic or abdominal injuries that produce much more extensive damage than initially appreciated on roentgenogram. There is little doubt that whatever the mechanism, "pulmonary contusions" are a predisposing factor in this devastating clinical picture. It is particularly important to recognize that this may not require evidence of extensive chest wall trauma. This is particularly true in children with their compliant chest walls.

Type and Amount of Resuscitative Fluid. The role of resuscitative fluids and the questions of the benefits of colloid versus crystalloid solutions have been a major area of controversy. Much of this concern has been based on knowledge of fluid exchange in the normal lung. This information is described mathematically in the following formula: $Q_f = K_w[(P_c - P_i) - \sigma_s(\pi_c - \pi_i)]$. A description of the symbols is as follows:

Q_f = net exchange of fluid across membrane
K_w = filtration coefficient of water
P_c = capillary hydrostatic pressure
P_i = interstitial hydrostatic pressure
σ_s = reflection coefficient of solute (factor by which ideal osmotic pressure is reduced owing to membrane permeability to solute; range of σ is 0 to 1.0)
π_c = capillary osmotic pressure
π_i = interstitial osmotic pressure

This concept is represented diagrammatically in Fig. 4-19.

If the pulmonary vasculature is normal, a fall in serum oncotic pressure renders the lungs more susceptible to pulmonary edema. Some authors reason that if crystalloid solutions are used in resuscitation, a fall in oncotic pressure might occur and cause or compound a pulmonary abnormality. If this were the case, the administration of colloid might be beneficial to the patient. The crucial flaw in the reasoning hinges upon the word "normal." Whether the injury leading to ARDS is to the endothelium or to the alveolar epithelium, the selectivity of the capillary for albumin and other large molecules is lost or impaired. Thus, the potential benefit of solutions containing high-molecular-weight compounds and the potential det-

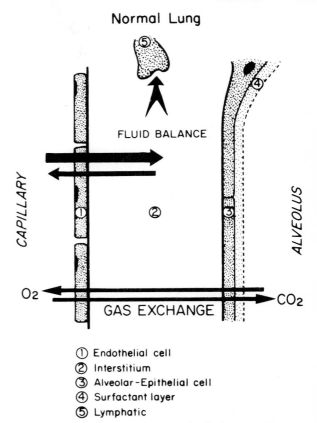

Fig. 4-19. Dynamic processes occurring in the normal lung.

riment of reasonable amounts of electrolyte-containing solutions become a nonissue. This will be discussed in more detail in the section on fluid therapy.

DIAGNOSIS. Rigid criteria for the diagnosis of ARDS have been previously outlined. It is generally agreed that if one waits until patients meet these criteria, any opportunity for preventive or early therapeutic measures is lost. The general approach to these patients is to attempt to identify high-risk patients, place them in an intensive care area, and carefully observe them for signs of ARDS. Particular emphasis is placed on changes in oxygenation, changes in respiratory rate or arterial P_{CO_2}, and changes in lung mechanics.

Assessment of the adequacy of pulmonary function should begin immediately after injury in those patients at risk for developing ARDS. Endotracheal tubes inserted for airway control during surgery should not be removed prematurely. In many patients an additional 4 to 6 h of intubation postoperatively will be sufficient to allow the physician to determine that ARDS is not a threat. Extubation should not be considered until adequate lung function has been demonstrated (described below). If several days of intubation are contemplated, a nasotracheal tube may be substituted for the endotracheal tube in the operating room. This will allow for greater patient comfort and acceptance.

Table 4-6. ASSESSMENT OF PULMONARY FUNCTION

Function	Acceptable	Consider institution of therapy*
Oxygenation:		
Partial pressure oxygen arterial blood	$Pa_{O_2} > 90$ mm or 40% $F_{I_{O_2}}$	<90 mmHg on 40% $F_{I_{O_2}}$ or decreasing
Partial pressure oxygen arterial blood to fraction inspired oxygen ratio ($Pa_{O_2}/F_{I_{O_2}}$)	$Pa_{O_2}/F_{I_{O_2}} > 250$	<250 or decreasing
Alveolar-arterial oxygen gradient (breathing 100% O_2 for 10 to 15 min)	50–200 mmHg	>200 mmHg or increasing
Ventilation:		
Partial pressure carbon dioxide arterial blood	35–40 mmHg	30 or decreasing
Minute volume	<12 L/min	Increasing
Mechanics:		
Rate	12–25/min	25 or increasing
Effective compliance	50 cm³/cmH₂O	50 or decreasing

* Trends over a period of time are useful in marginal situations.

A prerequisite for optimal lung function is normal cardiovascular status. Hemodynamic monitoring, therefore, should be instituted routinely. This includes recording of heart rate, arterial pressure, electrocardiogram, central venous pressure, and pulmonary artery pressure if indicated. Serial body weight, intake and output balance, bacteriologic studies, coagulation profile, and chest x-rays are important data.

Monitoring of pulmonary function can be conveniently divided into three general areas: evaluation of oxygenation, ventilation, and lung-thorax mechanics. Table 4-6 details the most easily obtained tests and includes normal values. As a general principle, isolated determinations are not as valuable as serial measurements obtained at regular intervals. Hypoxemia is often detected in apparently normal patients who appear to be doing well clinically.

The partial pressure of oxygen in the arterial blood (Pa_{O_2}) is the hallmark of adequacy of oxygenation. This must be considered in the light of the inspired oxygen concentration ($F_{I_{O_2}}$). A simple means of establishing a measurable relationship between Pa_{O_2} and $F_{I_{O_2}}$ is their ratio ($Pa_{O_2}/F_{I_{O_2}}$). Ratios between 250 and 500 are considered adequate, while a value of less than 250 is definitely abnormal. This ratio provides the clinician with a gross estimate of the efficacy of oxygenation at the bedside during rapid changes in therapy. It appears to be most reliable when the $F_{I_{O_2}}$ is between 0.3 and 0.7.

The alveolar-arterial oxygen difference (AaD_{O_2}) may allow rapid differentiation of the cause of hypoxemia. Of the four causes of hypoxemia (hypoventilation, diffusion defects, ventilation/perfusion abnormalities, and pulmonary shunt), only the intrapulmonary shunt should affect their index if the patient is breathing pure oxygen. The AaD_{O_2} is affected by cardiac output, O_2 consumption, the position of the hemoglobin/O_2 dissociation curve, and the magnitude of the pulmonary shunt. In particular, as the $F_{I_{O_2}}$ varies, the AaD_{O_2} varies widely. This greatly limits its value as an initial screening test.

The adequacy of ventilation is measured by the arterial partial pressure of carbon dioxide (Pa_{CO_2}). By definition, hypoventilation occurs when the Pa_{CO_2} is elevated. Postinjury pulmonary failure is usually associated with hypocapnia (hyperventilation). Therefore, the patient with a decrease in both Pa_{CO_2} and Pa_{O_2} probably has ARDS. Tidal volume (VT)—the amount of air breathed during one respiratory cycle—is another indication of the adequacy of ventilation. This is readily measured with a modestly priced respirometer. VT multiplied by the respiratory rate is called the *minute ventilation*. This value is easily derived but by itself is only a rough guide to adequate ventilation. In many postinjury patients, high minute ventilations are recorded. It is not established whether this is a compensatory response or an indicator of a pathologic condition.

The effective compliance (C_{eff}) may be quite valuable as an assessment of the ease of distensibility of lung and thoracic cage. This derived value is obtained by dividing the VT by the peak airway pressure. C_{eff} indicates the "stiffness" of the lungs, i.e., how difficult they are to ventilate (low C_{eff} means increased stiffness). A decreased C_{eff} may indicate increased extravascular lung water, airway constriction, or increased chest wall resistance (impaired bellows activity). Low values are usually found in patients with ARDS.

An adequate assessment of pulmonary function can be achieved by serial measurement of arterial blood gases, tidal volume, minute ventilation, and effective compliance. Several other monitoring devices have been advocated. The work of breathing is almost always increased in ARDS. This value is a measure of the mechanical cost of achieving adequate ventilation. The major disadvantage of this test is that it requires an intraesophageal balloon to measure transthoracic pressure and the availability of an analog computer for usable results. Although highly desirable, the measurement of the work of breathing is difficult in the critically ill patient.

Table 4-6 is intended as a guide for identifying patients who require increased attention. Careful investigation for causes of pulmonary deterioration (pneumothorax, fluid excess, lobar atelectasis, etc.) is indicated, and more extensive monitoring may be required prior to instituting therapy for ARDS.

MANAGEMENT. Support of Pulmonary Function, (Support of Oxygenation, and CO_2 Elimination). The most common indication for beginning ventilatory therapy is hypoxemia. Initial management should be to increase the $F_{I_{O_2}}$ both as a diagnostic test and to temporarily relieve hypoxemia if the Pa_{O_2} is less than 65 mmHg. For effective therapy, control of the airway must be achieved. The most rapid and reliable way to do this is the insertion of an endotracheal or nasotracheal tube. Mechanical ventilation may then be applied. Since a defect in the matching of ventilation to perfusion is present, therapy is directed at maintaining ventilation to marginally ventilated alveoli and recruiting collapsed or partially occluded alveoli. This will directly increase the FRC of the lungs.

Technique. The volume ventilator is the device most often chosen for the treatment of ARDS. The initial tidal volume setting may be 10 to 15 mL/kg body weight at a rate of 12 to 14 breaths per minute, with an inspiration: expiration ratio of 1:2. The ventilator is adjusted so that the patient can "trigger" additional ventilator breaths. This can be described as assisted mechanical ventilation (AMV). An $F_{I_{O_2}}$ of 0.4 should be applied initially and blood-gas determinations used to indicate the efficacy of this treatment. Humidification of the inspired air via a heated nebulizer is essential to avoid drying airway secretions.

Blood gases are checked within 10 to 20 min of beginning respiratory treatment to determine the patient's response. If hypoxemia persists on 40 percent oxygen, increasing the VT still further may be warranted in an effort to increase the FRC. The effect of this maneuver is best assessed by following serial compliance changes. If the C_{eff} is improving, benefit from increased VT may be expected. If C_{eff} decreases with an increase in VT, too much volume is being given to the patient. Lower tidal volume ventilation will then be required to minimize the risk of complications of ventilatory therapy. The compliance curve is shaped somewhat like the Starling curve of cardiac function, i.e., a plateau is reached, after which any increase in volume is achieved only at the expense of a marked increase in airway pressure.

Alternative methods of mechanical ventilatory support are available. One that is being used more frequently is intermittent mandatory ventilation (IMV). This is a technique of mechanical ventilation that allows the patient to breathe spontaneously and at the same time to receive periodic support from the ventilator.

Acceptable levels of Pa_{O_2} are between 65 and 80 mmHg. If this cannot be achieved with the treatment outlined above, there are two alternatives: manipulation $F_{I_{O_2}}$ and support of lung volume.

The $F_{I_{O_2}}$ may be increased to higher levels. Since pulmonary shunting is caused by continued perfusion of nonventilated alveoli, simply increasing the concentration of oxygen will have no significant effect on the shunt. In addition, washout of nitrogen from poorly ventilated alveoli will make them more susceptible to collapse, thus converting low V/Q areas to areas of shunt resulting in more atelectasis. Although there is still controversy over the role of O_2 toxicity in the genesis of ARDS (see above), the literature clearly indicates that prolonged use of high O_2 concentrations can produce a clinical picture similar to ARDS. A concentration of more than 50% O_2 is required to produce deleterious effects in patients with normal lungs, depending on the amount of time alveolar hyperoxia is maintained. The higher the O_2 concentrations, the less the time required to produce damage. Therefore every effort should be made to limit the $F_{I_{O_2}}$ to less than 0.5.

Since acceptable manipulation of the $F_{I_{O_2}}$ is limited, the second alternative is to recruit collapsed or partially collapsed alveoli with some modification of ventilatory therapy. This can be done by applying continuous positive end-expiratory pressure (PEEP) to the airway. PEEP may be achieved by either inserting an airflow resistance during expiration or using a ventilator with an end-expiratory plateau of positive pressure. Providing positive pressure throughout the respiratory cycle prevents alveolar and small airway collapse and may recruit lung units that were previously collapsed. The beneficial effects of this modality are (1) increased FRC, compliance, and Pa_{O_2}; (2) increased V/Q ratio (when initially low); (3) decreased pulmonary shunting; and (4) decreased mortality from ARDS.

Technique of PEEP. The commonly used volume ventilators have the capability of instituting PEEP without modifying the equipment. Although there is some controversy about the absolute level required, incremental increases in pressure are advocated. The usual beginning level is 5 cmH_2O of PEEP. Cardiorespiratory function is monitored after 10 to 15 min to assess the effects. If no beneficial effect is noted, further increases in PEEP follow in increments of 3 to 5 cmH_2O pressure.

There may be variable response to PEEP. While some patients respond with an immediate increase in Pa_{O_2}, others may not show improvement for $\frac{1}{2}$ to 1 h or longer. Therefore, absence of immediate response should not be interpreted as an absolute failure of PEEP. Each patient has a different but demonstrable optimal PEEP level that correlates well with the highest compliance. Thus a practical bedside monitor of the effectiveness of PEEP may be compliance.

Complications of PEEP. It has been shown that cardiac output may be decreased secondary to an increase in intrathoracic pressure and decreased venous return. This is usually significant only when the intravascular volume is decreased. Therefore, fluids should be given to assure a normal volume status before beginning PEEP therapy. Monitoring of the pulmonary wedge pressure is valuable in the assessment of volume prior to and during the administration of PEEP. Cardiac output may also be measured to assure normal values.

Excessive pressure applied to the terminal airways may overdistend and rupture normal alveoli, leading to pneumothorax. This complication of PEEP is uncommon below 20 cmH$_2$O pressure.

Close attention to the effective compliance can prevent excessive airway and alveolar pressure being applied during PEEP therapy. PEEP is most beneficial when FRC is low initially. In patients with a high FRC from preexisting lung disease (Chronic Obstructive Pulmonary Disease), any level of PEEP may be detrimental. This can be determined only by closely monitoring the patient's response to treatment, noting compliance especially.

Control of Pa$_{CO_2}$. Hyperventilation is a common problem in patients who are being artificially ventilated. Hypocarbia has been shown to be deleterious to the cerebral circulation (vasoconstriction) and the pulmonary circulation. Therefore, ventilatory therapy should be set to maintain normal levels of Pa$_{CO_2}$. With high tidal volume ventilation, a compensatory decrease in respiratory rate is necessary to maintain a normal Pa$_{CO_2}$. Increasing the inspired concentration of CO$_2$ or adding dead space have both been advocated as methods of increasing the Pa$_{CO_2}$ but are rarely effective in patients with ARDS. Effective control of the Pa$_{CO_2}$ requires heavy sedation or muscle relaxation and control of the patient's respiration. Decrease of the Pa$_{CO_2}$ below 30 is an indication for instituting respiratory control.

Oxygen-Carrying Capacity of Blood. Although the Pa$_{O_2}$ can be increased by higher levels of F$_{IO_2}$, it is the red blood cell that carries almost all the O$_2$ to the tissues. One unit of packed red cells carries more O$_2$ than plasma exposed to pure O$_2$ at hyperbaric pressure. Therefore, the hemoglobin (Hgb) concentration should be maintained between 12 and 14 g/dL. Attention should also be given to the acid-base status of the patient. Both acidosis and alkalosis produce shifts of the Hgb-O$_2$ dissociation curve that can affect the ability of Hgb to off-load O$_2$ at the tissue level.

Fluid Management. Fluid therapy can arbitrarily be divided into two phases when one is dealing with the acutely traumatized or critically ill patient. In the initial phase, or resuscitation phase, careful control of fluid volumes is important but may be difficult. Later, in the maintenance phase of fluid therapy, careful regulation of intake and output can be accomplished more easily. In both phases, the ideal would be the complete normalization of pulmonary vascular pressure. This can best be accomplished by invasive monitoring of pulmonary artery and central venous pressures. To avoid the complications of hydrostatic edema with resultant pulmonary dysfunction, continued monitoring of these parameters in acutely ill patients is essential. The values of these hemodynamic indices can guide the minute-by-minute volume replacement in the resuscitation phase and the hourly rates in the maintenance phase.

The type of fluid used for resuscitation and maintenance therapy is controversial. The two most common asanguinous fluids are isotonic balanced salt solutions and solutions containing albumin (colloid). Proponents of colloid therapy have stressed the sound physiologic principle of maintaining colloid osmotic pressure of the plasma (π_c) in the prevention of interstitial edema. Others

have argued that little or no change in plasma oncotic pressure occurs despite large volumes of balanced salt solutions. It is reasonable to assume that if the pulmonary membranes are injured the effect of oncotic pressure will be reduced, owing to the increased mobility of the protein species.

Randomized trials of crystalloid versus colloid therapy in acutely ill patients have been recently reported. Lowe and associates report no difference with regard to survival, incidence of pulmonary failure, or postresuscitation pulmonary function. Similarly, Virgilio and his colleagues have demonstrated the greater ease with which isotonic fluid therapy can be managed, despite its large volumes, as opposed to colloid therapy. On the other hand, others have suggested that the use of colloid solutions enhances the function of the myocardium and oxygen transport in patients with high cardiac indexes, whereas crystalloid tends to worsen pulmonary gas exchange.

Detrimental effects of albumin treatment have been proposed by several groups. It has been repeatedly demonstrated that albumin in the first several days of resuscitation has a negative inotropic effect and promotes fluid retention by limiting salt and water excretion. This same group has also suggested that albumin therapy may alter blood coagulation. Other investigators demonstrated an increased extravasation of albumin in the lungs after resuscitation with colloid solutions. This extravascular albumin may adversely affect fluid and protein movement in the lung.

Despite the conflict in the literature regarding the pros and cons of colloid therapy (albumin solutions), several points should be emphasized. Clinical and experimental studies generally find balanced salt solutions satisfactory for volume replacement. A second point is that massive volumes of isotonic salt solutions are necessary before severe changes in plasma osmotic pressure occur. A third point is that the changes that occur in colloid osmotic pressure may not be of importance in the injured lung because of the increased permeability of protein at the membrane level. Finally, the cost of albumin-containing solutions can be up to fifty times that of balanced salt solutions.

Based on the above, our approach is to treat the acutely ill or traumatized patient with blood and/or isotonic salt solutions, depending on the clinical status. Pulmonary vascular pressures are closely monitored to prevent the sequelae of overzealous therapy or hypovolemia.

Diuretics. Administration of diuretics has been proposed as a method for indirectly decreasing the amount of interstitial edema. Reports claiming a therapeutic role for diuretics in treating ARDS are not conclusive. There is no study that has randomly and prospectively shown that diuretics are as effective or more effective than ventilatory therapy alone. Our practice is to give small doses of furosemide *when hemodynamic studies indicate that fluid overload has occurred,* e.g., an elevated pulmonary artery wedge pressure. No attempt is made to "dry out" the patient by the long-term administration of diuretics. There is no solid evidence to suggest that lowering fluid volumes below normal will decrease the leak from injured capillaries. Such decreases in volume may have serious deleterious effects.

Corticosteroids and Anti-inflammatory Agents. Despite extensive interest in their use, there is no conclusive proof that pharmacologic doses of steroid should be part of the specific therapy of the ARDS syndrome. Data do exist to indicate that steroids may be effective in treating pulmonary fat embolism, and in selected patients with extensive acute fibrosis. Thus, we reserve steroid therapy for these clinical entities. Similarly, the use of other anti-inflammatory agents is unproved and should be confined to carefully constructed experimental trials.

Antibiotics. Phophylactic use of broad-spectrum antibiotics has no place in the primary therapy of ARDS. Indiscriminate use of these agents may allow the emergence of resistant strains of bacteria that are very difficult to treat. Many patients will already have been given antibiotics because of certain types of injury. Specific antibiotics are used to treat pulmonary sepsis. Their choice is determined by serial cultures of the sputum.

Ancillary Pulmonary Care. Patients treated in the intensive care unit tend to be bound to the bed by numerous tubes, wires, and catheters. Change in position then becomes a difficult problem. It has been shown, however, that significant improvement in oxygenation can result from frequent position changes. Maintenance of one position is likely to compound pulmonary abnormalities.

Routine pulmonary toilet, suctioning with sterile technique, and attempts to prevent pulmonary infection are very important. These must all be done on a routine basis.

PREVENTION. It has been suggested that early application of PEEP in high-risk patients could reduce the incidence of ARDS several-fold. This concept has been challenged by others. In a recent study we prospectively randomized 92 patients meeting entry criteria for ARDS risk factors to receive mechanical ventilation either without PEEP (control) or with 8 cm water PEEP (early PEEP). These therapies were continued for 72 h unless (1) ARDS developed or (2) the Pa_{O_2} was greater than 140 ($F_{I_{O_2}} = 0.5$) at 24 h and continued so following PEEP removal. This group included 65 trauma patients. The groups were comparable for age, severity of injury, number and types of ARDS risk factors, and additional oxygenation. Eleven of the 44 early PEEP patients (25 percent) and 13 of the 48 control patients (28 percent) developed ARDS. The incidence of atelectasis, pneumonia, and baro-trauma was the same in both groups as was mortality. Thus, we were unable to demonstrate any effect of early application of 8 cm of PEEP to high-risk patients on the incidence of ARDS. While this study does not rule out any potential benefit from early PEEP application, it effectively eliminates the possibility of a major reduction in the incidence of ARDS on a statistical basis. While there may be valid reasons for intubation and early mechanical support of injured patients, the probability that such treatment will significantly decrease the incidence of true ARDS is low. This is commensurate with the concept that a physical injury to the alveolar capillary interface has occurred. The impact of ventilatory support

Table 4-7. EARLY AND LATE MORTALITY IN ARDS PATIENTS BY IMMEDIATE CAUSE OF DEATH

	Early deaths (≤72 h)	Late deaths (>72 h)
Sepsis	3*	8
Respiratory	1	4†
Cardiac	1	5‡
Neurologic	3	4
Other	2	1

* Sepsis present prior to ARDS.
† All four with sepsis as a contributory cause.
‡ Three with sepsis as a contributory cause.

on the long-term progress of the disease remains debatable.

OUTCOME. Despite advances in ventilatory support and fluid management, the mortality associated with ARDS remains high. Most centers report mortalities of 50 percent or greater in patients who sustain rigidly defined ARDS. The causes of death, however, are rarely respiratory failure. In a recent review of ARDS patients at our institutions, we found that surprisingly few patients die as a direct consequence of respiratory failure (Table 4-7). Most of the early deaths (less than 72 h) are related to the underlying illness or injury. In contrast, sepsis was directly responsible for 38 percent of the late (greater than 72 h) ARDS deaths and was a contributing factor in 76 percent. This supports the intuitive impression that long-term survival in surgical patients with ARDS frequently depends on identification and elimination of the septic focus.

Summary. Acute pulmonary failure (ARDS) occurring in the injured patient has a variety of potential causes. Infection with systemic sepsis is the most common cause and the most amenable to definitive treatment. The chief functional defect, hypoxemia unresponsive to increased $F_{I_{O_2}}$, is treated with ventilatory therapy and support of lung volume (PEEP) on an empiric basis. Attempts at prevention with ventilatory means are of marginal value at best. Despite advances in ventilatory and fluid management, mortality has decreased little since the introduction of PEEP and long-term improvements in survival depend on identification and elimination of septic foci and on pharmacologic developments anticipated in the future.

Alterations in Oxygen Transport

Cell hypoxia and eventually cell death may result from the complex changes induced by shock, regardless of the type, and restoration of delivery of oxygen to the tissues at an adequate concentration and pressure forms the basis for treatment. In the past, attention was directed primarily toward the factors affecting oxygen transport capability, including the concentration and partial pressure of oxygen in the inspired air, alveolar ventilation, ventilation/perfusion relationships, cardiac output, blood volume, and hemoglobin concentration. The demonstration that the level of organic phosphates in the red blood cell has a significant effect on the position of the oxygen/hemoglobin dissociation curve has served to focus attention on the processes responsible for release of oxygen at the tissue level. Because of the clinical implication of these findings, a knowledge of factors regulating both uptake and release of oxygen has assumed increasing importance in the care of critically ill patients.

OXYGEN TRANSPORT

The oxygen transport system consists of several component processes that function collectively to extract oxygen from inspired air and deliver it at a partial pressure sufficient to allow rapid diffusion from blood into the body cells. Each of the component processes has its own internal controls, and failure of any one may be compensated for by adjustments in the remainder of the system. The functions of the oxygen transport system are summarized in the following formula:

$$\text{Oxygen consumption} = \text{arteriovenous oxygen difference} \times \frac{\text{cardiac output (L/min)}}{100}$$

The amount of oxygen in whole blood includes that bound to hemoglobin (1.38 mL O_2/g of hemoglobin) and a small amount dissolved in plasma (0.003 mL/mm of oxygen tension). The oxygen content of arterial (Ca_{O_2}) and venous blood (Cv_{O_2}) are calculated by the formula

$$\text{Oxygen content} = (1.38 \times \text{Hb}_{conc} \times \text{Hb}_{sat}) + (0.003 \times P_{O_2})$$

Consider a person with a hemoglobin of 15 g/dL, an arterial oxygen tension of 100 mmHg, a venous oxygen tension of 40 mmHg, arterial and venous hemoglobin saturations of 97 and 75 percent, respectively, and a cardiac output of 6 L/min. Substituting these values in the formulas above, arterial oxygen content is 20.4 vol%, venous oxygen content is 15.6 vol%, arteriovenous oxygen difference is 4.8 vol%, and oxygen consumption is 288 mL/min.

Changes in any one of these factors are of variable significance regarding oxygen delivery. For instance, pulmonary gas exchange with 20 percent inspired oxygen concentration (Fi_{O_2}) normally produces an arterial oxygen tension (Pa_{O_2}) of approximately 100 mmHg, slightly less than average alveolar oxygen tension. Increasing the Fi_{O_2} to 100 percent would raise Pa_{O_2} to approximately 650 mmHg. This would increase the amount of dissolved oxygen in the plasma from 0.3 to 2.0 vol% but would only increase the hemoglobin saturation from 97 to 100 percent. In contrast, even moderate changes in hemoglobin concentration or cardiac output have a strong influence on oxygen transport capability. A hemoglobin concentration of 10 g/dL (instead of 15) in the example above would reduce the oxygen-carrying capacity of the blood by one-third ($Ca_{O_2} = 13.7$ vol%). Coupled with a fall in cardiac output from 6 to 3 L/min, assuming that other variables remain unchanged, oxygen consumption theoretically would fall from 288 to 96 mL/min. This is a not infrequent

clinical occurrence, although oxygen consumption would be maintained at a higher level by adjustments in other parts of the system (e.g., increase of arteriovenous oxygen difference).

Therapy designed to improve tissue oxygenation, therefore, includes an evaluation of all factors affecting the oxygen transport system. Adjustment of inspired oxygen concentration and efforts to improve alveolar ventilation are of obvious importance; however, therapeutic attempts to maintain a normal hemoglobin concentration and cardiac output deserve special attention.

OXYGEN/HEMOGLOBIN DISSOCIATION CURVE

Another aspect of oxygen transport that deserves emphasis is the relationship between hemoglobin oxygen saturation and oxygen tension. The oxyhemoglobin dissociation curve describes hemoglobin affinity for oxygen, and its unusual sigmoid shape reflects the phenomenon of heme-heme interaction. Each of four heme groups in the hemoglobin molecule reacts with oxygen in a prescribed order, and uptake of an oxygen molecule by one heme group facilitates the oxygenation of the next heme group. The sigmoid configuration of this curve is particularly suitable for the uptake, transport, and subsequent release of oxygen. Since the upper portion of the dissociation curve is relatively flat, oxygen loading by hemoglobin may remain relatively normal despite wide variations in the alveolar oxygen tension. As oxygenated blood traverses the peripheral capillary, however, P_{O_2} drops from approximately 100 to 40 mmHg, hemoglobin saturation falls from 97 to 75 percent, and the blood releases just over 22 percent of its oxygen load (Fig. 4-20). Since P_{O_2} values at the peripheral capillary level fall on the steep portion of the curve, significant changes in oxygen release are produced by only small alterations in oxygen tension.

The position of the oxyhemoglobin dissociation curve along the horizontal axis is characteristically termed the P_{50} value. This reflects the oxygen tension necessary to saturate 50 percent of the hemoglobin with oxygen; the normal value is approximately 27 mmHg.

The importance of positional changes of the curve is also related to its sigmoid shape. Within limits, rightward or leftward shifts have little effect on arterial oxygen saturation if Pa_{O_2} is above 80 mmHg. At the peripheral capillary level, however, even small shifts of the curve may be important. A rightward shift of the dissociation curve (P_{50} above 27 mmHg) indicates decreased hemoglobin affinity for oxygen, while a leftward shift (P_{50} below 27 mmHg) is associated with an increase of hemoglobin/oxygen affinity. Compared with the normally positioned curve, more oxygen is released at any given P_{O_2} with a rightward-shifted curve and less is released with a leftward-shifted curve. Therefore, if arterial and venous oxygen tensions remain constant, arteriovenous oxygen difference increases with a rightward shift of the curve and decreases with a leftward shift (Fig. 4-21).

Changes in position of the oxygen/hemoglobin dissociation curve are significant in at least two respects. The

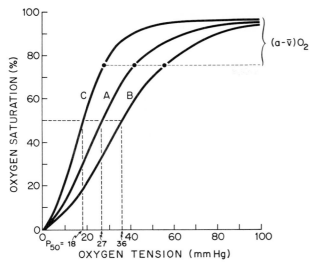

Fig. 4-20. Oxygen-hemoglobin dissociation curves in *(A)* normal, *(B)* rightward-shifted, and *(C)* leftward-shifted positions. The P_{50} value denotes the position of the curve along the horizontal axis and represents the oxygen tension (in mmHg) necessary to saturate 50 percent of available hemoglobin with oxygen. Note that as the curve moves toward the left, the arteriovenous oxygen difference, (a-v̄) O_2, can be maintained only by decreasing venous oxygen tension. (Adapted from: *Shappell SD, Lenfant CJM: Anesthesiology 37:127, 1972, with permission.*)

transfer of oxygen from the blood to the sites of intracellular utilization is directly related to the oxygen pressure differential. Thus a rightward shift of the curve is theoretically advantageous, since an equivalent amount of oxygen is released at a higher P_{O_2} than with a leftward-positioned curve. (Note that in curve *B* of Fig. 4-20, half of the oxygen would be released at a P_{O_2} of 36 mmHg; in curve

Fig. 4-21. Oxygen-hemoglobin dissociation curves similar to those in Fig. 4-20. Note that if arterial and venous oxygen tensions remain constant, arteriovenous oxygen difference decreases as the curve moves toward the left.

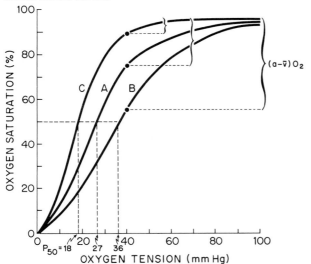

C, less than 10 percent of the oxygen would be released at the same P_{O_2}.) Second, the ability to maintain or enlarge the arteriovenous oxygen difference is dependent to some extent on the position of the curve. Normally, arterial hemoglobin saturation is near the upper limit and cannot be increased appreciably. Any enlargement of the arteriovenous oxygen difference necessitates reduction in venous hemoglobin saturation and venous oxygen tension Pv_{O_2}. As the curve moves to the left, maintenance of any given arteriovenous oxygen difference requires a progressive decrease in Pv_{O_2}. The fall in Pv_{O_2} is finally limited by the fact that a certain partial pressure is necessary for transfer of oxygen from the blood to the tissue cell. That level of oxygen pressure below which diffusion may be theoretically impaired and cellular function disturbed has been termed the "critical P_{O_2}."

Available data concerning the critical P_{O_2} are limited but suggest that it varies in individual organ systems and may depend on the level of activity of the tissues. Opitz and Schneider showed that oxygen uptake by the brain is impaired when venous oxygen tension falls below 20 to 25 mmHg, while Berne et al. indicated loss of myocardial function at oxygen tensions between 10 and 12 mmHg. With a leftward movement of the curve, therefore, maintaining or enlarging the arteriovenous oxygen difference is theoretically limited as the Pv_{O_2} approaches this critical level. Tissue oxygen delivery may be sustained in this instance by other mechanisms, principally by increasing cardiac output.

During hypovolemic shock, cardiac output is low and relatively fixed. Normally, enlargement of arteriovenous oxygen difference will partially compensate for the diminished blood flow; however, the response may be totally inadequate with a leftward shift of the dissociation curve. Continued survival and maintenance of essential organ function may be obtained only by shunting blood from tissues that tolerate a limited period of severe hypoxia (skin, skeletal muscle) to organs that require high oxygen flow rates (brain, heart).

FACTORS INFLUENCING THE POSITION OF THE OXYGEN/ HEMOGLOBIN DISSOCIATION CURVE

Attempts to ensure a normal or rightward-positioned dissociation curve may be essential during treatment of patients with low-flow states. Factors affecting the position of the curve have been summarized by Shappell and Lenfant and are outlined in Table 4-8. The main in vivo influences include changes in pH, temperature, partial pressure of carbon dioxide, and level of red blood cell organic phosphates. Changes in hydrogen ion concentration and temperature have predictable and instantaneous effects on the position of the curve, while P_{CO_2} exerts its influence both by changing pH and by a pH-independent effect. The quantitative effects of these influences on the dissociation curve have been reviewed in several excellent publications.

The position of the dissociation curve is also influenced by interaction of hemoglobin with organic phosphates in the red blood cell. Both ATP and 2,3-diphosphoglycerate

Table 4-8. FACTORS THAT ALTER HEMOGLOBIN/OXYGEN AFFINITY

Increase P_{50}	*Decrease P_{50}*
By direct effect:	By direct effect:
Increased [H$^+$]	Decreased [H$^+$]
temperature	temperature
P_{CO_2}	P_{CO_2}
DPG, ATP	DPG, ATP
Hb conc	Hb conc
Ionic strength	Ionic strength
Abnormal hemoglobin	Abnormal hemoglobin
Aldosterone	Carboxyhemoglobin
	Methemoglobin
By increasing DPG:	By decreasing DPG:
Decreased [H$^+$]	Increased [H$^+$]
Thyroid hormone	Decreased thyroid
Pyruvate kinase deficiency	hormone
Increased inorganic	Hexokinase deficiency
phosphate	Decreased inorganic
Cortisol	phosphate
Cell age (young)	Cell age (old)

SOURCE: Adapted from Shappell SD, Lenfant CJM: Adaptive, genetic and iatrogenic alterations of the oxyhemoglobin dissociation curve. *Anesthesiology* 37:127, 1971.

(DPG) bind to hemoglobin and lower the affinity of hemoglobin for oxygen, i.e., shift the dissociation curve to the right. In a quantitative sense, DPG is the more important of the two phosphates and exerts an additional influence in the intact red blood cell by lowering intracellular pH via Donnan equilibrium. Significant concentrations of DPG are found only in the red blood cell, and DPG is present in a concentration approximately equimolar with that of hemoglobin. DPG is a product of erythrocyte glycolysis, formed via a branch of the Embden-Myerhof pathway by conversion of 1,3-DPG to 2,3-DPG, catalyzed by diphosphoglycerate mutase.

Erythrocyte DPG undergoes considerable changes in response to several stimuli, with parallel changes in the position of the dissociation curve. Investigations have revealed that hypoxia increases erythrocyte DPG in conditions such as exercise, anemia, exposure to high altitude, cardiac failure, and various pulmonary diseases. The concomitant rightward shifts of the dissociation curve are thought to represent significant compensatory responses, allowing release of more oxygen at a higher P_{O_2}.

The regulation of DPG synthesis is complex and as yet not fully clarified. Although numerous factors influence the level of DPG (Table 4-8), the principal *mechanism* for increasing or decreasing its concentration appears to be related to the level of hydrogen ions in the red cell. DPG concentration increases as the red blood cell pH rises and decreases as the pH falls. These changes are due, in part, to the differential effects of pH on the activity of two red cell enzymes, DPG mutase and phosphatase. For instance, alkalosis stimulates DPG synthesis by increasing DPG-mutase activity and reducing the breakdown of DPG by DPG-phosphatase. The rise in red cell pH may be

secondary to elevation of whole blood pH or, as in hypoxic states, a relative increase in the amount of deoxyhemoglobin. The pH also influences DPG binding to hemoglobin and may affect other enzymes in the glycolytic cycle. The net effect of pH changes on DPG concentration, therefore, probably represents a combination of these (and other unknown) influences. It should be noted that the pH-induced changes in DPG concentration tend to counteract the direct pH effects on the curve via the Bohr effect. Therefore, the immediate rightward shift of the curve secondary to acute acidosis is eventually offset by a pH-induced reduction in DPG concentration.

DPG synthesis is also responsive to hormonal influences and the level of inorganic phosphate. The phosphate level is directly related to DPG concentration, and maintenance of a normal inorganic phosphate level during intravenous hyperalimentation is necessary to prevent a reduction in the level of erythrocyte 2,3-DPG. Thyroid hormone acts directly to increase DPG synthesis, a fact that probably explains the elevated levels of this compound in hyperthyroid patients. Cortisol and aldosterone both shift the dissociation curve to the right, thereby decreasing hemoglobin/oxygen affinity. The effects of cortisol are probably secondary to direct stimulation of DPG synthesis. Hemoglobin/oxygen affinity also increases as the erythrocyte ages, presumably owing to a decreasing DPG concentration.

BLOOD TRANSFUSIONS, ERYTHROCYTE DPG, AND OXYGEN DELIVERY

The acceptability for transfusion of blood that has been stored in ACD (acid citrate dextrose) solution for up to 3 weeks is based on survival of at least 70 percent of the cells in the recipient's circulation. During this 3-week period, however, there is a rapid decline in erythrocyte DPG and a progressive increase in hemoglobin/oxygen affinity. Following transfusion, several hours are required for the DPG levels to return to normal. These findings suggest that oxygen delivery may be impaired after the administration of large quantities of stored blood and have led to a reevaluation of transfusion practices.

Several studies in both experimental animals and human beings have failed to show significant impairment of tissue oxygenation with markedly reduced levels of erythrocyte DPG and leftward shifts of the oxygen dissociation curve. Similar findings were noted in our study of 45 injured patients who received more than 5 units of whole blood stored in ACD solution during resuscitation and the subsequent operative procedure. Erythrocyte DPG levels were below normal in a majority of these patients and correlated well with the amount and storage time of the transfused blood. There were no consistent correlations, however, between DPG concentration and the measured parameters of oxygen delivery. This lack of correlation may be explained by two observations. First, the position of the dissociation curve cannot be reliably predicted from a knowledge of the DPG concentration alone. DPG represents only one of several factors that affect the curve, and the final P_{50} represents a composite of these influences. Normal or elevated P_{50} values noted in several patients with low DPG concentrations were probably due to other factors (e.g., pH and temperature) that tended to counteract the influence of DPG. A second observation is the lack of a consistent relationship between the P_{50} value and oxygen consumption. The majority of patients with leftward shifts of the dissociation curve had reasonably normal arteriovenous oxygen difference and oxygen consumption. Additionally, several of the patients with narrowed arteriovenous oxygen differences maintained oxygen delivery simply by increasing the cardiac output.

These findings do not imply that the position of the dissociation curve and the factors that influence it are unimportant. They do suggest that a person with reasonably intact cardiovascular and pulmonary systems is able to tolerate rather significant leftward shifts of the oxygen dissociation curve. The consequences may be quite different, however, in a patient with limited compensatory mechanisms and in some therapeutic regimens followed without understanding of their effects on the position of the curve. An example of this is shown in Fig. 4-22. Despite the sharp reduction in cardiac output following hemorrhage to a mean blood pressure of 50 mmHg, the control dog with a normal P_{50} value was able to maintain normal oxygen delivery by increasing the arteriovenous oxygen difference from 4.5 to 10.6 mL. In contrast the DPG-depleted dog was unable to expand the arteriovenous oxygen difference sufficiently (P_{50} value 15 mmHg). The problem was compounded by attempts to correct pH to normal by infusion of sodium bicarbonate solution. The dissociation curve moved farther to the left (P_{50} value 8 mmHg), the hemoglobin concentration fell secondary to hemodilution, and oxygen consumption fell to near zero. Although extreme, the experimental conditions are not unlike those which may be found in the clinical setting.

Fig. 4-22. Effects of hemorrhagic shock and sodium bicarbonate infusion on oxygen consumption after exchange transfusion with fresh blood (dog *A*) and DPG-depleted blood (dog *B*). I, Control period; II, after exchange transfusion (DPG concentration 6.20 μM/mL RBC in dog *B*); III, after induction of hypotension; IV, continued hypotension and sodium bicarbonate infusion.

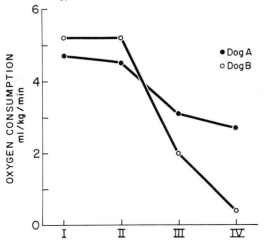

In summary, available evidence suggests that changes in hemoglobin/oxygen affinity, as reflected by the position of the oxygen dissociation curve, may be important in several circumstances. The elevated DPG concentrations and rightward shifts of the dissociation curve observed in hypoxic states (pulmonary disease, cardiac failure, anemia, exposure to high altitude, and so on) probably represent compensatory responses that facilitate oxygen unloading in the tissue capillaries. Oxygenation can be maintained in these instances by other mechanisms (e.g., increasing cardiac output) but at greater expense to body economy.

Leftward shifts of the dissociation curve observed following transfusions of stored blood, acute alkalosis, hypothermia, and so forth are, at best, undesirable phenomena and may significantly impair oxygen unloading. Although leftward shifts are tolerated in many circumstances, maintenance of a normally positioned dissociation curve may be of singular importance in patients with hypoxia, anemia, or hypotension when compensatory responses are limited.

THERAPEUTIC IMPLICATIONS

Obtaining a sufficient quantity of fresh blood for resuscitation of patients in hemorrhagic shock is difficult, and attempts are being made to find a suitable storage medium that will maintain the levels of organic phosphates (DPG, ATP) in red blood cells. In addition to DPG, maintenance of a sufficiently high ATP level is essential to maintain a flexible and highly deformable red cell membrane. The biconcave disc shape of a normal red blood cell is transformed toward a nondeformable spherocyte during storage. This loss of deformability hinders passage through the microcirculation and increases susceptibility of the cell to destruction. Although both DPG and ATP levels rapidly return to normal within 6 to 24 h, restoration may be delayed in the critically ill and massively transfused patient who is least able to tolerate increased microvascular resistance to flow and depression of tissue oxygenation. At the time of this writing, storage of blood in CPDA-1 (citrate phosphate dextrose adenine) solution seems to be the most practical alternative. Survival of red blood cells is similar after transfusion of blood stored in either ACD or CPDA-1 solution. Compared with blood stored in ACD solution, however, blood stored in CPDA-1 media has a higher pH, and DPG, ATP, and P_{50} are maintained at consistently higher levels. Additionally, use of CPDA-1 has increased the useful shelf storage life up to 35 days. Conversion from ACD to CPDA-1 solution for blood storage is a simple matter for blood banks and has been accomplished in most areas.

When large quantities of blood are administered, particularly in critically ill patients, some attention should be paid to the storage age of each unit of blood. If a significant portion of the blood administered has been stored for more than 7 to 10 days, every attempt should be made to obtain fresh blood for additional transfusion requirements. In our experience the institution of these simple changes, including conversion to CPDA-1 storage media, has been rewarding. The large reductions in DPG and P_{50} noted in the past are rarely seen today, even after massive transfusions.

Other factors that influence the position of the dissociation curve (Table 4-8) may also be important in the individual patient. For instance, the induction of respiratory alkalosis may produce an abrupt increase in hemoglobin/oxygen affinity. This is a common occurrence during operations and in patients requiring ventilatory assistance in the postoperative period; coupled with other factors that limit oxygen transport, the capacity to maintain tissue oxygenation may be sharply reduced. Similarly, the sudden correction of an acidosis, whether metabolic or respiratory, may have undesirable effects. In this regard the indiscriminate use of sodium bicarbonate during resuscitation of patients in hypovolemic shock is discouraged. The presence of a mild metabolic alkalosis is a common finding after resuscitation, owing in part to the alkalinizing effects of blood transfusions and the administration of lactated Ringer's solution. After infusion (and partial restoration of hepatic blood flow), the citrate and lactate contained in transfused blood and the lactate in lactated Ringer's solution are metabolized and bicarbonate is formed. If excessive quantities of sodium bicarbonate are administered simultaneously, a severe metabolic alkalosis may result. The alkaline pH may be highly undesirable, particularly in patients with hypoxia or low fixed cardiac output. Combined with other factors incident to blood replacement that increase hemoglobin/oxygen affinity (low DPG concentration and hypothermia), significant interference with oxygen unloading at the cellular level may occur.

The immediate and direct pH influences on the curve (via the Bohr effect) are eventually offset by reciprocal changes in DPG concentration. There is, however, a lag period of approximately 4 h before any change in DPG concentration is noted, and the final level is not reached until 48 h after induction of acidosis or alkalosis. The fact that the effects of sudden large changes in pH may persist for several hours should be considered during therapy. Correction of a metabolic acidosis, therefore, is properly directed toward correction of the underlying disorder. Bicarbonate therapy may be reserved for the treatment of severe metabolic acidosis, particularly following cardiac arrest, when *partial* correction of pH is essential to restore myocardial function. Similarly, pH correction in more protracted states of metabolic acidosis may be indicated but should be accomplished slowly.

Lowering body temperature also causes a leftward shift of the dissociation curve and an increase in hemoglobin/oxygen affinity, but any interference in oxygen delivery may be countered effectively by the hypothermia-induced reduction in metabolic requirements.

Rightward shifts of the curve are usually desirable and, unless extreme, rarely interfere with oxygen uptake in the lungs. Rightward shifts generally occur as a compensatory response to hypoxia, regardless of the cause. Nevertheless, in patients with severe arterial desaturation (exposure to high altitude, congestive failure, right-to-left cardiac shunts), any potential benefit from shifting the

curve farther to the right may be offset by interference with oxygen loading.

In a complex clinical setting, multiple factors that influence hemoglobin/oxygen affinity may be operative at any given time, and abrupt changes secondary to therapy or the disease process itself may occur. Evaluation of these multiple influences may be difficult, since few data concerning their cumulative effects are available. Nevertheless their *net* effect can be estimated by determining the position of the oxygen dissociation curve.

Techniques for constructing an oxygen dissociation curve are time-consuming and not readily available in most hospitals. For this reason we have developed a rapid, though less precise, method for estimating the position of the curve (the P_{50} value). Since the shape and slope of the curve do not change appreciably with changes in position, determination of a single point of the steep part of the slope should allow a rough estimate of the entire curve. To obviate the use of a tonometer, a single sample of venous blood is drawn anaerobically and the P_{O_2} and oxygen saturation is measured. (An arterial sample is unsuitable, since the values fall on the upper flat portion of the curve.) An estimated P_{50} value may then be obtained using the Severinghaus slide rule or a nomogram as depicted in Fig. 4-23. The nomogram represents a computer plot of a family of O_2 dissociation curves, using the correction factor for pH as suggested by Severinghaus. The point on the nomogram corresponding to the measured P_{O_2} and saturation values is found and traced to the

Fig. 4-23. Nomogram for estimation of P_{50} value (position of the oxygen-hemoglobin dissociation curve). The point on the nomogram corresponding to the measured P_{O_2} and saturation of a sample of venous blood is traced to the line representing 50 percent oxygen saturation. This intersect represents the estimated P_{50} (normal value approximately 27 mmHg). In the example shown, the venous blood sample P_{O_2} is 39 mmHg, the oxygen saturation 65 percent, and the P_{50} value 31 mmHg (a rightward-positioned dissociation curve).

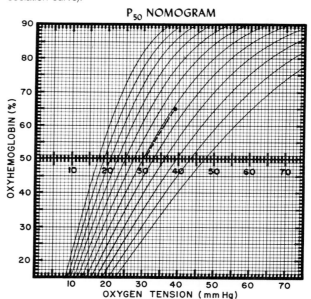

P_{50} NOMOGRAM

OXYHEMOGLOBIN (%)

OXYGEN TENSION (mmHg)

of cardiac output. Cardiac output can be estimated by using arteriovenous oxygen difference.

As with any patient who is at risk of developing serious cardiovascular complications, continuous monitoring of the crucial hemodynamic variables (heart rate, arterial pressure, central venous pressure, urinary output, electrolyte fluid balance) by using reliable equipment and accurate techniques will be required for the severely injured patient. In addition to the above "conventional" monitoring, the introduction into clinical practice of the thermodilution method for the determination of cardiac output at bedside by using the Swan-Ganz flow-directed catheter has made possible the continuous evaluation of cardiac function during various therapeutic interventions. Through the Swan-Ganz catheter, the pulmonary artery pressure and pulmonary capillary wedge pressure can be recorded concurrently with the injection of saline for the measurement of cardiac output. The diastolic pulmonary artery pressure or pulmonary capillary wedge pressure closely approximates the left atrial pressure, and either one can be taken as the left ventricular filling pressure. Stroke volume can be derived from cardiac output and heart rate. By plotting stroke volume versus left ventricular filling pressure, left ventricular curves can be constructed and myocardial performance can promptly be assessed under control conditions and during drug or fluid administration. With the above techniques, the main determinants of cardiac output (preload, blood pressure, and systemic arteriolar resistance) can instantaneously be monitored. Since generalized infection may adversely affect the outcome of the severely injured patient, care should be taken to introduce and maintain monitoring catheters under sterile conditions. For the same reason, pulmonary complications related to the Swan-Ganz catheter should be avoided, and the latter should not be introduced into the pulmonary circulation when contraindications exist (pulmonary rupture, pneumothorax, etc.).

With the use of these measurements the best method for treatment of a patient with hypotension and a complicated clinical picture can frequently be discerned. A depressed or normal central venous pressure that does not rise with rapid administration of a balanced salt solution usually indicates continuing hypovolemia. The diagnosis is supported by the presence of a measured decrease in cardiac output. If the hypovolemia is secondary to inadequate fluid replacement, a gradual and sustained rise in arterial pressure and cardiac output results from the administration of appropriate fluids. If continued fluid loss or acute bleeding is the cause, then fluid administration produces either a transient rise or no rise in the blood pressure and cardiac output.

The presence of an elevated central venous pressure or a central venous pressure that rises with the rapid administration of fluids (and produces either no change or a decrease in cardiac output) is indicative of impairment of the pumping mechanism. Usually this represents primary myocardial deficiency and must be treated accordingly; the defect in the pumping mechanism may occasionally be due to mechanical obstruction as with cardiac tamponade or mediastinal compression by intrapleural fluid or air. The possible presence of these surgically correctable lesions must be kept in mind, especially in the patient who has multiple injuries. Pulmonary embolism can produce a similar response but is rarely seen early in the course of the injured patient.

A normal or slightly increased central venous pressure with a normal or high cardiac output and disproportionate hypotension is usually due to a loss of peripheral vascular resistance. In this situation, the physician should suspect a "septic" component. Increased peripheral vascular resistance is the rule in oligemic shock. If accompanied by deficient myocardial function, the use of an inotropic agent (with minimal vasoconstrictor or preferably with vasodilator effects) may be beneficial. This should be done only after more direct therapy, such as volume replacement or digitalization, has been pursued. Hemodynamic measurements usually fail to show any indication for use of a vasoconstrictive agent in the treatment of hemorrhagic shock.

Several authors have questioned the value of central venous pressure measurements and pointed out that left ventricular overload and pulmonary edema can occur while right ventricular function (and the central venous pressure) remains adequate. This is particularly true after myocardial injury. In patients with normal cardiac reserve, however, *changes* in the central venous pressure with fluid infusion do indicate the ability of the myocardium to pump the volume presented to it. Properly applied, the central venous pressure remains a useful clinical tool in early resuscitation. Its interpretation can be augmented by measurement of pulmonary artery pressure and pulmonary wedge pressure, the latter approximating left atrial pressure. Such techniques are usually reserved for patients with more complicated problems, and the use of a balloon-tipped Swan-Ganz catheter is necessary.

A flow-directed pulmonary artery catheter is now available that provides continuous mixed venous oximetry. The potential benefits of this catheter in monitoring critically ill patients continue to be explored.

The ultimate hemodynamic criterion in the treatment of shock is the response of the patient. Adequate resuscitation is indicated when adequate cerebration and urine output are restored. Although diuresis by any means may be beneficial when a large pigment load is presented to the kidneys, the object of treatment in hypovolemic shock is to reestablish urine flow by adequate restoration of circulation and not to force urine flow in spite of inadequate resuscitation. The use of osmotic diuretics in uncorrected oligemic shock to produce "urine for urine's sake" would seem to have no physiologic basis and may, in fact, be detrimental by further depleting intravascular and extravascular extracellular fluid.

Cardiogenic Shock

In this form of shock the heart fails as a pump. Consequently primary therapy is directed toward the heart. Cardiac arrhythmias, whatever their origin, should be treated promptly. Cardiac tamponade, if this is the cause, should be relieved by pericardiocentesis. When the origin of the pump failure is myocardial infarction or myocarditis, the primary therapy again is directed toward the myocardial damage. If the myocardial damage is sufficiently severe to produce reduction in blood pressure, and indeed in organ perfusion, to the point that organ functions begin to fail, drugs with positive inotropic action may be efficacious.

HEMODYNAMIC MEASUREMENTS

Hemodynamic measurements play an important role in the management of postoperative patients with this type of hypotension. As previously described, the classic finding is a central venous or pulmonary artery pressure that is elevated or rises briskly with fluid administration. This is accompanied by a cardiac output that is depressed and fails to respond to fluid administration. In evaluating postoperative hypotension, as after an extensive procedure in the elderly or especially after cardiac surgery, the measurement of hemodynamic parameters may be of great benefit in differentiating hypovolemic hypotension from hypotension due to depressed myocardial function.

When hemodynamic measurements suggestive of deficient pumping action are found, myocardial insufficiency is usually at fault. It should be stressed again, however, that this can be due to mechanical obstruction (e.g., cardiac tamponade or mediastinal compression in the injured patient or pulmonary embolism in the postoperative patient), and treatment directed at primary myocardial insufficiency can lead to unnecessary delay and catastrophic results. Although identification of abnormalities causing mechanical obstruction to venous return or myocardial function must rest largely on clinical grounds, hemodynamic measurements may be of some benefit in that one may find a slow increase in cardiac output and arterial blood pressure accompanying the rising venous pressure produced by rapid fluid administration. This is in contrast to the picture usually seen in pure myocardial insufficiency, in which the cardiac output frequently falls in the face of a rising venous pressure. The rise in cardiac output probably occurs because the rising venous pressure is partially effective in overcoming the obstruction and maintaining a nearer to normal cardiac filling.

It has been demonstrated that with myocardial injury and after cardiac surgery, differences in functional reserve of the two ventricles occur and the central venous pressure alone loses a great deal of its reliability. Thus in these patients the use of pulmonary artery pressure, pulmonary wedge pressure, and, when feasible, left atrial pressure have their greatest value. Left atrial pressure (or left ventricular end-diastolic pressure) is not necessarily the same as right atrial pressure (or central venous pressure, or right ventricular end-diastolic pressure) under these circumstances.

In patients with low cardiac output from low blood volume who also have certain forms of heart disease, left atrial pressure may be considerably higher than right atrial pressure. Examples of such conditions are mitral stenosis and insufficiency, aortic stenosis and insufficiency, severe hypertension, and coronary artery dis-

ease. In such patients, unless one is actually measuring left atrial pressure, rapid infusion should probably be stopped when right atrial or central venous pressure reaches 12 mmHg (150 mm saline solution). The relation between changes in atrial pressure and changes in stroke volume or cardiac output at relatively high atrial pressures is not known. In most patients, however, when atrial pressures are about 15 mmHg (230 mm saline solution), further increases do not seem to increase cardiac output. Thus when central venous or right atrial pressure is less than 6 mmHg (80 mm saline solution), augmentation of blood volume is indicated. As the infusion proceeds, if central venous pressure rises rapidly and there is little evidence of increase in cardiac output, the infusion should probably be discontinued as being ineffective.

ABNORMALITIES IN CONTRACTILITY

In the condition in which there is low cardiac output and high atrial pressures and in which tamponade and ventricular outflow obstruction have been ruled out, there is probably an acute reduction of myocardial contractility. Treatment must therefore be directed toward improving contractility.

1. *Digitalis.* If time permits, digitalis is given, and digoxin is recommended. The estimated digitalizing dose given intravenously to a child or adult is 0.9 mg/m^2 of body surface area (1.5 mg for average adult). During digitalization, it is important to note that hypokalemia, hypercalcemia, and shock tend to increase the sensitivity of the heart to digitalis. Half or two-thirds of this may be given initially intravenously. An effect can be seen in 10 to 20 min, and the peak effect is reached in about 2 h. After 1 to 3 h, if no contraindication develops and further effect is desired, an additional one-sixth of the estimated digitalizing dose is given. This may be repeated after another 2 to 3 h. In less acute situations the same drug may be given orally; the digitalizing dose is then 1 mg/m^2. The estimated daily maintenance dose is one-quarter of the estimated digitalizing dose, usually given in divided doses.

2. *Inotropic Agents.* Dopamine in doses of 5 to 25 μg/(kg · min) intravenously may help restore the mean arterial blood pressure to a level of 70 to 80 mmHg to ensure adequate flow through cerebral and coronary vessels, particularly if they are partially occluded. The use of dopamine may result in an increase in cardiac output, without inducing an undesirable tachycardia. In doses less than 25 μg/(kg · min), there is either no change or a slight decrease in systemic vascular resistance and an increase in renal blood flow. At higher doses, alpha-adrenergic effects become predominant, resulting in systemic vasoconstriction and a decrease in renal blood flow.

Isoproterenol is rarely used today, particularly in patients with acute myocardial infarction, since it tends to increase myocardial oxygen consumption more than it increases coronary blood flow. In addition, it is not infrequently associated with tachyarrhythmias, particularly in a patient who has been digitalized.

The use of a vasopressor such as norepinephrine to

maintain a mean arterial blood pressure of approximately 70 to 75 mmHg may occasionally be indicated when other therapy has failed, including the use of dopamine.

Prior to treating patients with low cardiac output and high atrial pressures with these drugs on the basis that the cause is poor myocardial contractility, one must rule out pericardial tamponade. If high intrapericardial pressure exists in patients with high atrial and ventricular end-diastolic pressure, transmural pressure is low, and the poor output is due to end-diastolic ventricular volume and fiber length. The treatment is relief of the pericardial tamponade, which is about the only acute cause of high atrial pressures and small end-diastolic ventricular volume. A clinical analysis and chest x-ray are helpful in establishing the diagnosis. The presence of a paradoxic pulse should suggest strongly the presence of tamponade, and needle aspiration or open pericardiotomy is indicated.

3. *Ganglionic Blocking Agents.* Some patients with low cardiac output and high atrial pressures have relatively high arterial blood pressure. Systemic arteriolar resistance is high (*afterload-load* resisting shortening of myocardial sarcomeres). In these circumstances systolic left ventricular pressure is relatively high, as is systolic ventricular wall stress. Theoretically, reducing arterial blood pressure and systolic ventricular wall stress increases cardiac output. This can be done with an agent such as sodium nitroprusside. One should measure cardiac output before and during administration of this drug, and only if a significant increase in cardiac output has accompanied the decrease in arterial blood pressure should the drug be continued. Because of present uncertainties with the use of vasodilators (such as the effect on coronary, cerebral, liver, and renal blood flow) in this situation, it should be given only under special circumstances, and generally not in patients with hypovolemia.

In summary, attempts to diagnose and treat extramyocardial causes such as cardiac tamponade and pulmonary embolus should be made early in the course of cardiogenic shock. If the cause of shock is from primary failure of the myocardium as seen following acute myocardial infarction, the following modified guidelines suggested by Johnson and Gunnar seem reasonable.

After the diagnosis of cardiogenic shock has been made, an arterial line to measure direct arterial pressure and arterial blood gases, a Swan-Ganz catheter for measuring pulmonary artery and wedge pressures, and a Foley catheter should be inserted. Measurements of cardiac output by the thermal dilution technique can also be made using a specially constructed Swan-Ganz catheter. The response to treatment can then be effectively monitored by using these hemodynamic measurements.

1. If the patient is hypotensive and the wedge or pulmonary artery diastolic pressure is low, volume expansion with a suitable fluid is initiated.

2. If arterial pressure is low but pulmonary wedge pressure is 18 mmHg or above, an infusion of dopamine or dobutamine should be started. Dopamine is the preferable agent if arterial blood pressure can be maintained with low dosage levels without excessive tachycardia.

3. If the arterial systolic blood pressure is above 110 mmHg, the wedge pressure is above 18 mmHg, and there are signs of intense vasoconstriction with inadequate tissue perfusion, the cautious use of sodium nitroprusside may be indicated. It is emphasized that this form of therapy can be quite dangerous and careful monitoring of the effects of this agent is absolutely mandatory.

4. If the arterial pressure can be maintained with dopamine but wedge pressure remains elevated, the patient should be digitalized slowly and preload reduction considered.

5. If the patient's condition does not stabilize rapidly or if increasing amounts of pressor agents are necessary to maintain arterial pressure, and if the pulmonary wedge pressure remains elevated, the use of intraaortic balloon counterpulsation and cardiac catheterization should be considered.

Mechanical Assistance

The use of intraaortic balloon counterpulsation to maintain circulation in patients with severe cardiogenic shock due to failure of the myocardium is an established and effective form of therapy. The use of mechanical assistance should be considered early in the course of a patient with an acute myocardial infarction and pump failure who does not respond to the usual pharmacologic manipulations. Intraaortic balloon assistance can offer excellent temporary support of the circulation without increasing oxygen demands of the myocardium. While the patient is being supported in this manner, attempts should be made to find surgically correctable causes for the failure by evaluation of coronary artery anatomy and ventricular function. Patients not considered salvageable in the past may obtain excellent functional results with well-timed cardiac surgery following stabilization with the intraaortic balloon assistance device.

ABNORMALITIES IN RATE

Rapid ventricular rates (over 150 to 180 beats/min) are usually deleterious to cardiac output. Ventricular end-diastolic pressure is small because of the short period of ventricular filling with tachycardia, and ventricular extensibility is probably decreased because ventricular relaxation is not complete by the end of the extremely short diastolic period. Both tend to reduce stroke volume more than can be compensated for by the rapid heart rate, and cardiac output falls. If atrial fibrillation is the cardiac mechanism, digoxin is the drug of choice. Atrial flutter is more difficult to treat but should likewise be treated with digoxin. If no progress has been achieved with the drug after two-thirds of the digitalizing dose has been given, electroversion should be considered. Atrial tachycardia and premature atrial contractions as causes of excessively rapid heart rates are still more difficult to treat. Propranolol (Inderal) has been used with considerable success when the tachycardia was due to a resistant sinus tachycardia. Similarly, verapamil (Isoptin) has been used successfully for resistant tachyarrhythmias that are of atrial origin.

PVCs may on occasion cause fast ventricular rates.

Their tendency to cause ventricular fibrillation is of even greater concern. Lidocaine (Xylocaine) should be given intravenously in a single injection of 50 mg. If further lidocaine is needed, a solution containing 2 mg/mL of lidocaine can be given (1 to 4 mg/min) continuously. If it is used excessively, central nervous system irritability and depression of myocardial contractility may result. If protection against premature ventricular contractions is needed later, Pronestyl (procainamide hydrochloride) can be given orally in doses of 250 to 500 mg every 3 h. Bretylium tosylate has been useful in treating any resistant ventricular arrhythmias.

Low output associated with ventricular rates of less than 60 to 70 beats/min may occur in patients in whom cardiac performance is impaired. Because the myocardium is impaired, stroke volume cannot increase sufficiently to compensate for the slow rate. Regardless of whether the mechanism is sinus rhythm, atrial fibrillation with slow ventricular rate (too much digitalis or too little potassium), or complete atrioventricular dissociation, electrical pacing of the heart at a rate of 80 to 110 beats/min is advantageous. If there is a sinus mechanism, atrial pacing is preferred. Otherwise, direct ventricular pacing is indicated.

Neurogenic Shock

Neurogenic shock, or, by the older classification, "primary shock," is that form of shock which follows serious interference with the balance of vasodilator and vasoconstrictor influences to both arterioles and venules. This is the shock that is seen with clinical syncope, as with sudden exposure to unpleasant events such as the sight of blood, the hearing of bad tidings, or even the sudden onset of pain. Similarly, neurogenic shock is often observed with serious paralysis of vasomotor influences, as in high spinal anesthesia. The reflex interruption of nerve impulses also occurs with acute gastric dilatation.

The clinical picture of neurogenic shock is quite different from that classically seen in oligemic or hypovolemic shock. While the blood pressure may be extremely low, the pulse rate is usually slower than normal and is accompanied by dry, warm, and even flushed skin. Measurements made during neurogenic shock indicate a reduction in cardiac output, but this is accompanied by a decrease in resistance of arteriolar vessels as well as a decrease in the venous tone. Consequently there appears to be a normovolemic state with a greatly increased reservoir capacity in both arterioles and venules, thereby inducing a decreased venous return to the right side of the heart and subsequently a reduction in cardiac output.

If neurogenic shock is not corrected, a reduction of blood flow to the kidneys and damage to the brain result, and subsequently all the ravages of hypovolemic shock appear. Fortunately, treatment of neurogenic shock is usually obvious. Gastric dilatation can be rapidly treated with nasogastric suction. Shock in high spinal anesthesia can be treated effectively with a vasopressor such as ephedrine or phenylephrine (Neo-Synephrine), which will increase cardiac output as well as produce peripheral vasoconstriction. With the milder forms of neurogenic shock, such as fainting, simply removing the patient from the stimulus or relieving the pain will in itself be adequate therapy so that the vasoconstrictor nerves may regain the ability to maintain normal arteriolar and venous resistance.

There is rarely need for hemodynamic measurement in this usually benign and frequently self-limited form of hypotension. The exception to this occurs when this form of shock results from injury, as with spinal cord transection from trauma. In this instance there may be significant loss of blood and extracellular fluid into the area of injury surrounding the cord and vertebral column. Considerable confusion can arise as to the relative need for fluid replacement, as opposed to the need for vasopressor drugs, under these circumstances. Similarly, if surgical intervention for any reason becomes necessary, hemodynamic measurements may be of great value in the management of these patients. In uncomplicated neurogenic shock, central venous pressure should be normal or slightly low, with a normal or elevated cardiac output. If hypovolemia ensues, central venous pressure decreases, as does cardiac output. Thus, careful monitoring of central venous pressure may be necessary. Fluid administration without vasopressors in this form of hypotension may produce a gradually rising arterial pressure and cardiac output without elevation of central venous pressure, by gradually "filling" the expanded vascular pool; therefore, caution must be utilized during fluid administration.

In management of these patients balancing the two forms of therapy, slight volume overexpansion is much less deleterious than excessive vasopressor administration. The latter decreases organ perfusion in the presence of inadequate fluid replacement. Balance can best be obtained by maintaining a normal central venous pressure that rises slightly with rapid fluid administration (thus ensuring adequate volume) and using a vasopressor such as phenylephrine judiciously to support arterial pressure.

Septic Shock

During the past several years there has been a progressive increase in the incidence of shock secondary to sepsis, and the mortality rate remains in excess of 50 percent. This has occurred despite a better understanding of this entity, use of newer treatment regimens, and development of more potent antimicrobial agents. The most frequent causative organisms are gram-positive and gram-negative bacteria, although any agent capable of producing infection (including viruses, parasites, fungi, and rickettsiae) may initiate septic shock. Because of effective antibiotic control of most gram-positive infections, the majority of septic processes that result in shock are now caused by gram-negative bacteria. Among other causes, Altemeier and associates attribute this rising incidence of gram-negative sepsis to (1) the widespread use of antibiotics, with development of a reservoir of virulent and resistant organisms; (2) concentration in hospitals of large numbers of patients with established infections; (3) more extensive operations on elderly and poor-risk patients; (4) an increasing number of patients suffering from severe trauma; and (5) the use of steroids and immunosuppressive and anticancer agents.

GRAM-POSITIVE SEPSIS AND SHOCK

The shock state may be caused by gram-positive infections that produce massive fluid losses (necrotizing fasciitis) by dissemination of a potent exotoxin without evident bacteremia (*Clostridium perfringens, Clostridium tetani*) or, most often, by a fulminating infection from staphylococcus, streptococcus, or pneumococcus organisms. In the latter instance, shock is theoretically related to the release of exotoxins that many strains of staphylococcus and streptococcus (but not pneumococcus) are known to produce. The hemodynamic changes that occur are different from those seen in shock due to gram-negative organisms. Kwaan and Weil have noted hypotension of comparable severity in shock from both gram-positive and gram-negative infections, but their patients with gram-positive infections failed to show the other clinical manifestations of shock. Arterial resistance fell, but there was little or no reduction in cardiac output even with progressive hypotension. Urine flow was normal, sensorium clear, and perfusion of other organs was not grossly impaired, since neither acidosis nor a significant increase in serum lactic acid concentration appeared.

Treatment consists in the use of appropriate antibiotics, surgical drainage when indicated, and correction of any fluid volume deficit. A rapid and favorable response may be anticipated in many patients, and survival is substantially better than with gram-negative infections.

GRAM-NEGATIVE SEPSIS AND SHOCK

Gram-negative sepsis as a cause of shock is a more frequent and difficult problem. The highest incidence occurs during the seventh and eighth decades of life, and the response to treatment depends to a large extent on the age and previous health of the patient. There have been significant advances in the understanding of this entity, although much of the available information is still subject to controversy.

SOURCE. The most frequent source of gram-negative infections is the genitourinary system; almost half the patients have had an associated operation or instrumentation of the urinary tract. The second most frequent site of origin is the respiratory system, and many of the patients have an associated tracheostomy. Next in frequency is the alimentary system, with diseases such as peritonitis, intraabdominal abscess, and biliary tract infections; and then diseases of the integument, including burns and soft tissue infections. Indwelling venous catheters for monitoring and hyperalimentation are an increasing source of contamination, particularly with prolonged use. The reproductive system continues to be a significant source of infection (principally from septic abortions and postpartum infections), although the incidence is variable, depending on the hospital population.

The severity of septic shock varies considerably and appears to be a time-dose phenomenon, depending on the type and site of infection. For instance, mild hypotension following instrumentation of the genitourinary tract may represent nothing more than a transient bacteremia that is self-limited or responds to minimal therapy. In contrast, the patient with necrotizing pneumonia or multiple intraabdominal abscesses may have sepsis from an overwhelming number of organisms for a period of several days, and a much poorer prognosis. Similarly, the outlook is more favorable when the source of infection is accessible to surgical drainage, as in septic abortion, in which the infected products of conception can be removed readily. Variations in these factors must be considered when interpreting reported mortality rates and during the evaluation of new therapeutic regimens.

ASSOCIATED CONDITIONS. The presence of underlying disorders that limit cardiac, pulmonary, hepatic, or renal function increases the susceptibility to gram-negative infections and adversely affects the response to treatment. In Altemeier's reported series of 398 patients with gram-negative sepsis, almost half the patients had serious associated disease, including diabetes mellitus, malignant neoplasms, uremia, cirrhosis, burns, and malignant hematologic disorders. Of these conditions, cirrhosis of the liver appeared to have the most unfavorable prognosis. In addition, a small but significant number of patients were on corticosteroids or immunosuppressive agents, and corresponding mortality rates were 74 and 83 percent, respectively.

BACTERIOLOGY. The common causative organisms are similar to those found in the human gastrointestinal tract and include the coliform species and anaerobic bacilli. Recently the *Klebsiella*-Enterobacteriaceae-*Serratia* groups have been isolated with increasing frequency, and many are resistant to more conventional antibiotics. *Bacteroides* species are the predominant organisms in the fecal flora. These anaerobic organisms are difficult to culture and may account for a far greater number of infections than was previously reported. The majority of infections are caused by a single gram-negative organism, although in 10 to 20 percent of cases more than one organism may be isolated, particularly from intraabdominal sources. The isolates may be two or more gram-negative organisms or mixed cultures containing both gram-negative and gram-positive bacteria.

CLINICAL MANIFESTATIONS. Gram-negative infections are often recognized initially by the development of chills and elevated temperature above 101°F. The onset of shock may be abrupt and coincident with the signs and symptoms of sepsis or may occur several hours to days after recognition of an established infection. The complex hemodynamic abnormalities that follow are incompletely understood but are probably initiated by endotoxins from the cell walls of gram-negative bacteria. Intravenous injection of this lipopolysaccharide-protein complex into experimental animals will produce a shock state, but the hemodynamic responses vary in different animal species. The use of experimental animal models has contributed to our understanding of this entity, but direct extrapolation of the findings to human septic shock is difficult. A single injection of endotoxin into dogs causes pooling of blood in the splanchnic circulation, decreased venous return to the heart, reduction in cardiac output, and an abrupt fall in blood pressure. This initial response is transient and apparently due to hepatic venous outflow obstruction. Shortly thereafter the blood pressure rises toward normal but then slowly declines over the next several hours until death of the animal. This pattern is different from that seen in the subhuman primate and in human beings. Injection of *E. coli* endotoxin into human volunteers has been shown to produce (1) no response; (2) chills, fever, and vasoconstriction; or (3) peripheral vasodilation and a rise in cardiac output. These observations emphasize our lack of understanding of the effects of gram-negative infections and septicemia on the human circulation and the need for the development of more realistic experimental animal models.

Clinically, the shock state may be characterized by a primary adrenergic response, as seen in hypovolemic shock, with hypotension, peripheral vasoconstriction, and cold, clammy extremities. Earlier in the course, however, there may be an absence of adrenergic effects, with warm, dry extremities and decreased peripheral resistance. These diverse responses, presumably to the same stimulus, have led to a considerable amount of confusion over the clinical manifestations of septic shock, although a report by MacLean and associates tends to shed some light on this subject. They have noted two distinct hemodynamic patterns, depending on the volume status of the patient, and believe that the natural history of septic shock is one of progression from respiratory alkalosis to metabolic acidosis. A syndrome of early septic shock occurs in patients who are *normovolemic* prior to onset of sepsis and exhibit a hyperdynamic circulatory pattern characterized by (1) hypotension, (2) high cardiac output, (3) normal or increased blood volume, (4) normal or high central venous pressure, (5) low peripheral resistance, (6) warm, dry extremities, (7) hyperventilation, and (8) respiratory alkalosis. A typical patient with this pattern is the young, previously healthy person with a septic abortion. The high cardiac output is often associated with a decrease in oxygen utilization per unit flow, i.e., a narrowed arteriovenous oxygen difference. These findings can be explained by any of several mechanisms, but the two most likely possibilities are arteriovenous shunting and a primary cellular defect in the utilization of oxygen due to a direct effect of sepsis. In either case the presence of oliguria, altered sensorium, and blood lactate accumulation reflects the need for a further increase in flow despite the high cardiac output. MacLean suggests that treatment include measures to increase the cardiac output even more, combined with appropriate antibiotic therapy and early surgical drainage. In his series all but 4 of 28 patients with this hemodynamic pattern survived the episode of shock. If control of the infection is delayed or unsuccessful, the patient may pass into an acidotic phase with evidence of cellular damage (narrowing arteriovenous oxygen difference, decreasing oxygen consumption) and become refractory to further therapy.

In contrast, if septic shock develops in a patient who is *hypovolemic,* a hypodynamic pattern emerges characterized by (1) hypotension, (2) low cardiac output, (3) high peripheral resistance, (4) low central venous pressure, and (5) cold, cyanotic extremities. This response is typically seen in a patient with strangulation obstruction of the small bowel and a moderate to severe extracellular fluid and plasma volume deficit. If seen early, these patients are also alkalotic and will respond favorably to treatment. In the absence of overt cardiac failure, prompt volume replacement will often increase cardiac output, and a more favorable hyperdynamic circulation may develop. If therapy to combat sepsis is delayed or unsuccessful, the patient will inevitably have cardiac and circulatory failure, with a low fixed cardiac output and a resistant metabolic acidosis. At this point the patient may not be salvageable.

Our own experience in the treatment of septic shock tends to confirm MacLean's findings, although the presence of a metabolic acidosis has not necessarily been an ominous finding. We have seen several patients with hypodynamic and hyperdynamic circulatory patterns and metabolic acidosis in the early phase who have responded satisfactorily to therapy. The clinical picture may also be influenced by the patient's ability to meet the increased circulatory requirements imposed by sepsis. The elderly patient with limited cardiac reserve may be unable to increase cardiac output and enter the hyperdynamic phase, even with prompt volume replacement and measures designed to increase cardiac efficiency. In this instance the typical adrenergic response may persist, and the patient may rapidly succumb to the disease process.

The laboratory tests of value for diagnosis will depend to a large extent on the specific disease causing sepsis. Generally, the white blood cell count is appropriately elevated, but in debilitated and hypovolemic patients, those on immunosuppressive agents, and those with overwhelming sepsis, the white blood cell count may be normal or low. However, there is usually a noticeable left shift in the white blood cell differential, with many immature cell types. A falling platelet count may be an early and sensitive indicator of gram-negative septicemia, particularly in pediatric and burn patients. It has been suggested that endotoxin reacts with platelets, producing platelet aggregates that are subsequently trapped in the microcirculation. Patients at risk for sepsis should have serial platelet counts; a fall in the platelet count below 150,000 suggests the presence of gram-negative septicemia, and measures to find and eradicate the source should be undertaken. Rarely, a sudden fall in the platelet count may be a manifestation of disseminated intravascular coagulation (DIC), a syndrome known to be initiated by several stimuli, including endotoxin.

Progressive pulmonary insufficiency is characteristically seen in many patients with septic shock. Mild hypoxia with compensatory hyperventilation and respiratory alkalosis are commonly seen early in the course of shock in the absence of clinical or x-ray evidence of pulmonary disease. The arterial desaturation has been attributed to a variety of causes, including the presence of physiologic arteriovenous shunts in the pulmonary circulation secondary to perfusion of atelectatic or nonaerated alveoli. Regardless of the cause, the picture is frequently that of rapid deterioration of pulmonary function, development of patchy infiltrates that become confluent, superimposed bacterial infection, severe hypoxemia, and death.

Finally, it is worth emphasizing that development of mild hyperventilation, respiratory alkalosis, and an altered sensorium may be the earliest signs of gram-negative infection. This triad may precede the usual signs and symptoms of sepsis by several hours to several days. The exact cause is not known, although the condition is thought to represent a primary response to bacteremia. Early recognition of these findings, followed by a prompt search for the source of infection, may allow proper diagnosis prior to the onset of shock.

TREATMENT. The only effective way to reduce mortality in septic shock is by prompt recognition and treatment of the associated infection prior to the onset of shock. Once shock occurs, the control of infection by early surgical debridement or drainage and use of appropriate antibiotics represents *definitive* therapy. Other recommended measures, including fluid replacement, steroid administration, and the use of vasoactive drugs, represent *adjunctive* forms of therapy and are useful to prepare the patient prior to surgical intervention or to support the patient until the infectious process is controlled. This point deserves special emphasis, since death of the patient is inevitable if the infection cannot be adequately controlled.

As soon as gram-negative sepsis and shock are apparent, a prompt and thorough search for the source of infection is made while instituting other supportive measures. Because of the multiple complicating factors that may accompany endotoxemia, the patient is preferably treated in an intensive care unit. Careful monitoring of direct arterial pressure, central venous pressure (preferably pulmonary artery and pulmonary wedge pressures measured via a Swan-Ganz catheter), urine output, and arterial and central venous blood gases may be essential for proper management.

If the infectious process is amenable to drainage, operation is performed as soon as possible after initial stabilization of the patient's condition. In some cases surgical debridement or drainage of the infection must be accomplished before the patient will respond. These procedures may be performed under local or general anesthesia. For example, a patient with ascending cholangitis and shock secondary to sepsis may respond temporarily to supportive treatment. Improvement may be short-lived, however, unless prompt drainage of the biliary tract is instituted. The importance of surgical drainage is emphasized by the experience of MacLean et al. in their treatment of 53 patients. Forty-eight percent of their patients with infections amenable to surgical drainage survived, while only 23 percent of those not amenable to surgical treatment survived. More recently, Fry et al. emphasized the importance of surgical drainage and/or debridement in patients with infections caused by *Bacteroides* species. In a group of 98 consecutive adult patients with positive blood cultures for a *Bacteroides* organism, 77 had a mechanically treatable cause; most were due to intraabdominal abscess or an acutely perforated viscus.

Antibiotic Therapy. The use of specific antibiotics based on appropriate cultures and sensitivity tests is desirable when possible. The results may not be available for several days, but useful information may be gained from previous wound and blood cultures obtained during an earlier phase of the septic process and Gram's stain of appropriate material. Antibiotics must often be chosen, however, on the basis of the suspected organisms and their previous sensitivity patterns. These patterns are sufficiently diverse to preclude selection of a single antibiotic agent that will be effective against all the potential pathogens.

At present an effective combination of antibiotics in our hospital population when gastrointestinal tract organisms are suspected includes cefazolin or penicillin and gentamicin. This combination is effective against a majority of gram-negative organisms, with the notable exception of *Bacteroides* species. If presence of these organisms is suspected, an antibiotic of known effectiveness (e.g., cefoxitin or metronidazole) should be added to the regimen. Other antibiotics that are currently receiving extensive trials include a variety of third-generation cephalosporins, piperacillin, and imipenim.

When culture and sensitivity reports are available, more specific antibiotic coverage may be initiated if the infection is not under control. Altemeier and associates reported a mortality rate of 54 percent from sepsis in patients receiving inappropriate antibiotics and 28 percent when appropriate antibiotics were given.

Fluid Replacement. Prompt correction of preexisting fluid deficits is essential. A majority of patients will incur fluid losses from the disease processes that initiate sepsis and shock. "Third space losses," with massive sequestration of plasma and extracellular fluid, are characteristic of many surgical conditions, including peritonitis, burns, strangulation obstruction of the bowel, and extensive soft tissue infections.

The type of fluid used will vary, although most "third space losses" are properly replaced with a balanced salt solution such as Ringer's lactate. Any deficits in red blood cell mass should be corrected by the administration of packed cells or whole blood in order to maintain optimal oxygen-carrying capacity of the blood. Large quantities of replacement fluids are often needed in order to maintain an effective circulating volume. However, a fine balance exists between the need for volume replacement and the harmful effects that fluid overload may have on lungs already injured by the septic process. In this regard, attempts to increase pulmonary capillary osmotic pressure by the infusion of large volumes of plasma or albumin, in the absence of a specific need, may be detrimental. Because of the increase in pulmonary capillary permeability associated with severe sepsis, the use of large quantities of colloid solutions may result in an increase in extravascular pulmonary water. Careful replacement of "third space losses" with crystalloid solutions on the basis of patient response and continuous monitoring of the central venous or pulmonary artery and pulmonary wedge pressures are indicated.

Properly interpreted, the central venous pressure (CVP) will give a reliable estimate of the ability of the right side of the heart to pump the blood delivered to it. It is best used as an upper-limit guide; a rapid increase in central venous pressure, regardless of the initial level, may indicate that fluid is being administered too rapidly or that the heart is unable to handle additional volume. If central venous pressure is below 10 cm of water, fluids may be administered as rapidly as tolerated. If central venous pressure is above this level, fluids are still administered but at a slower rate of infusion. The central venous pressure may fall as blood pressure rises, owing to better perfusion of the coronary arteries and improved myocardial function. An abrupt rise in the central venous pressure or a fall in arterial pressure may indicate inability of the heart to respond, and the use of drugs that increase myocardial performance should be considered in conjunction with the use of a Swan-Ganz catheter.

In these instances, measurement of the CVP alone during fluid resuscitation is not sufficient, since it gives no direct information regarding function of the left side of the heart. Insertion of a Swan-Ganz catheter for measurements of *both* pulmonary artery (PA) and pulmonary capillary wedge (PW) pressure, the latter a reflection of left ventricular end-diastolic pressure, is necessary. This is particularly true in patients on mechanical ventilation and positive end-expiratory pressure.

Many patients will respond favorably to fluid administration combined with prompt control of the infection with a rise in blood pressure, an increase in urine output, warming of the extremities, and clearing of the sensorium. In these instances no additional therapy may be indicated.

Steroids. The use of pharmacologic doses of corticosteroids in the treatment of septic shock is controversial. There is no direct evidence that steroids are beneficial in these cases, although favorable responses, with improvement in cardiac, pulmonary, and renal functions and better survival rates, have been reported. Large doses of steroids are known to exert a modest inotropic effect on the heart and produce mild peripheral vasodilation. Although these salutary effects may be desirable, there are other, more potent drugs available with similar actions. Others have suggested that steroids protect the cell and its contents from the effects of endotoxin, for example, by stabilizing cellular and lysosomal membranes. In a prospective study of 172 consecutive patients in septic shock, Schumer noted a mortality rate of 10.4 percent in the steroid-treated patients, compared with a mortality rate of 38.4 percent in patients not receiving steroids. In a retrospective study of an additional 328 patients, the results were similar. Although impressive, evidence regarding the beneficial effects of steroids remains presumptive, because of many variables present in the clinical situation, including causes, associated conditions, and treatment.

Steroids may be administered concomitant with volume replacement or reserved for use if the response to fluid administration is only temporary or produces a rapid rise in central venous pressure. Many dosage schedules have been recommended, and most stress the need for a large initial dose and cessation of therapy within 48 to 72 h. One regimen is based on guidelines suggested by Lillehei. An initial dose of 15 to 30 mg/kg of body weight of methylprednisolone (or equivalent dose of dexametha-

sone) is given intravenously over a 5- to 10-min period. The same dose may be repeated within 2 to 4 h if the desired effects have not been achieved. If a beneficial response is obtained, additional injections are not given unless the effects are only short-lived. When the drug is used in this manner, there is rarely a need for more than two doses. It should be noted, however, that the current studies on immunosuppression by steroids may show that this effect outweighs other possible benefits from steroid therapy.

Vasoactive Drugs. Vasopressor drugs with prominent alpha-adrenergic effects are of limited value in treatment of this type of shock, since artificial attempts to maintain blood pressure without regard to flow are potentially harmful. Furthermore, they are probably contraindicated in hypovolemic patients with increased peripheral resistance, in view of the known deleterious effects of prolonged vasoconstriction. Beneficial effects attributed to these agents are probably due to their inotropic effects on the heart, although better drugs are available for this purpose. Rarely, use of vasoactive drugs with mixed alpha- and beta-adrenergic effects may be indicated in a patient with an elevated cardiac output and pronounced hypotension due to very low peripheral resistance. The increase in resistance (and slight increase in cardiac output) may produce a desired rise in blood pressure and improvement in flow.

Vasodilator drugs such as phenoxybenzamine have enjoyed some popularity, particularly when combined with additional fluid administration. Their use is based in part on improved survival of dogs when vasodilator drugs are given prior to the onset of endotoxic shock. These observations probably represent a specific canine response and cannot be directly extrapolated to human septic shock. Vasodilator agents have also been used in conjunction with adrenergic agents (for their inotropic effects), but data on their usefulness are limited.

Since the heart is frequently unable to meet the increased circulatory demands of sepsis, the use of an inotropic agent such as isoproterenol or dopamine would seem ideal when volume replacement and other measures have failed to restore adequate circulation. Dopamine, a naturally occurring catecholamine biochemical precursor of norepinephrine, is similar to isoproterenol in exerting positive inotropic and chronotropic effects on the heart by stimulation of beta-adrenergic receptors. Because of its lower potential for tachyarrhythmias and the ability to enhance renal blood flow when infused at a dose below $3 \ \mu\text{g/(kg} \cdot \text{min)}$, dopamine has virtually replaced isoproterenol as the agent of choice.

In summary, a "polypharmacy" approach is discouraged, although proper selection and use of vasoactive drugs may offer needed support until infection can be controlled or eradicated. If eradication is not possible, response to any of these drugs is only temporary. Determination of cardiac output, combined with arterial, pulmonary artery, and pulmonary wedge pressure measurements can be of great benefit in establishing the nature of the hemodynamic alterations and evaluating responses to therapy.

Digitalis. Although both Hinshaw and Greenfield have

shown that digitalis can prevent or reverse heart failure in animals following endotoxin injection, the clinical importance of this finding has yet to be established. We have not routinely administered digitalis to patients in septic shock in the absence of specific indications. Gram-negative sepsis and shock frequently occur in older patients with congestive failure or may precipitate cardiac failure in patients with limited cardiac reserve. In these instances digitalis can be administered cautiously in full doses, although toxicity may occur if the patient is hypokalemic or receiving isoproterenol.

Pulmonary Therapy. Many patients with sepsis and shock will develop significant pulmonary insufficiency and require maintenance of a controlled airway (via nasotracheal or endotracheal intubation) and assisted ventilation. (For a discussion of the adult respiratory distress syndrome as related to sepsis and the management of patients requiring ventilatory support, the reader is referred to the section Pulmonary Responses.)

Since inadequate tissue oxygenation is a consistent feature of shock, attention to all components of the oxygen transport system is essential (see the section Oxygen Transport). Efforts to maintain a normal or rightward-positioned oxygen/hemoglobin dissociation curve may be particularly important in view of reported reductions in red blood cell organic phosphates in late septic shock.

Bibliography

Clinical and Physiologic Manifestations of Shock

Baue AE, Wurth MS, Sayeed MM: The dynamics of altered ATP-dependent and ATP-yielding cell processes in shock. *Surgery* 72:94, 1972.

Bessey PQ, Brooks DC, Black PR: Epinephrine acutely mediates skeletal muscle insuline resistance. *Surgery* 94:172, 1983.

Blalock A: Shock: Further studies with particular reference to effects of hemorrhage. *Arch Surg* 29:837, 1937.

Blalock A: *Principles of Surgical Care, Shock and Other Problems.* St Louis, CV Mosby, 1940.

Canizaro PC, Prager MD, Shires GT: The infusion of Ringer's lactate solution during shock. *Am J Surg* 122:494, 1971.

Carey LC, Lowery BD, Cloutier CT: Treatment of acidosis. *Curr Probl Surg,* p 37, January 1971.

Gann DS, Carlson DE, et al: Impaired restitution of blood volume after large hemorrhage. *J Trauma* 21:598, 1981.

Gann DS, Dallman MF, Engelund WC: Reflex control and modulation of ACTH and corticosteroid. *Int Rev Physiol* 24:157, 1981.

Gross SG: *A System of Surgery: Pathological, Diagnostic, Therapeutic and Operative.* Philadelphia, Lea & Febiger, 1872.

Hiebert JM, McCormick JM, Egdahl RH: Direct measurement of insulin secretory rate: Studies of shocked primates and postoperative patients. *Ann Surg* 176:296, 1972.

Marey EJ: Loi qui preside a la frequence des battements du coeur. *CR Acad Sci* 52:95, 1861.

Mela LM, Miller LD, Nicholas GG: Influence of cellular acidosis and altered cation concentrations on shock-induced mitochondrian damage. *Surgery* 72:102, 1972.

Moore FD: *Metabolic Care of the Surgical Patient.* Philadelphia, Saunders, 1959.

Shamoon HM, Hendler R, Sherwin RS: Synergistic interactions among anti-insulin hormones in the pathogenesis of stress hyperglycemia in humans. *J Clin Endocrinol Metab* 52:1235, 1981.

Shenkin HS, et al: On the diagnosis of hemorrhage in man: A study of volunteers bled large amounts. *Am J Med Sci* 208:421, 1944.

Sherwin RS, Sacca L: Effect of epinephrine on glucose metabolism in humans: Contribution of the liver. *Am J Physiol* 247:E157, 1984.

Shires GT: Principles and management of hemorrhagic shock, in Shires GT: *Principles of Trauma Care,* 3d ed. New York, McGraw-Hill, 1985, pp 3–43.

Simeone FA: Shock, in *Christopher's Textbook of Surgery.* Philadelphia, Saunders, 1964, p 58.

Wiggers CJ: Present status of shock problem. *Physiol Rev* 22:74, 1942.

Wiggers HC, Ingraham RC, et al: Vasoconstriction and the development of irreversible hemorrhagic shock. *Am J Physiol* 153:511, 1948.

Response of Extracellular Fluid

Albert S, Shires GT III, et al: Effects of naloxone in hemorrhagic shock. *Surg Gynecol Obstet* 155:326, 1982.

Campion DS, et al: The effect of hemorrhagic shock on transmembrane potential. *Surgery* 66:1051, 1969.

Conway EJ: Nature and significance of concentration relations of potassium and sodium ions in skeletal muscle. *Physiol Rev* 37:84, 1957.

Cunningham JN Jr, Shires GT, Wagner Y: Cellular transport defects in hemorrhagic shock. *Surgery* 70:215, 1971.

Cunningham JN Jr, Shires GT, Wagner Y: Changes in intracellular sodium and potassium content of red blood cells in trauma and shock. *Am J Surg* 122:650, 1971.

Goldman DE: Potential, impedance and rectification in membranes. *J Physiol* 27:37, 1943.

Hagberg S, Haljamas H, Rockert H: Shock reactions in skeletal muscle: III. The electrolyte content of tissue fluid and blood plasma before and after induced hemorrhagic shock. *Ann Surg* 168:243, 1968.

Hodgkin AL, Katz B: The effect of sodium ions on the electrical activity of the giant axon of the squid. *J Physiol* 108:37, 1949.

Illner HP, Shires GT: The effect of hemorrhagic shock on potassium transport in skeletal muscle. *Surg Gynecol Obstet* 150:17, 1980.

Ling G, Gerard RW: The normal membrane potential of frog sartorius fibers. *J Cell Sci* 34:383, 1949.

Mela LM, Miller LD, Nicholas GG: Influence of cellular acidosis and altered cation concentrations on shock-induced mitochondrian damage. *Surgery* 72:102, 1972.

Middleton ES, Mathews R, Shires GT: Radiosulphate as a measure of the extracellular fluid in acute hemorrhagic shock. *Ann Surg* 170:174, 1969.

Peitzman AB, Shires GT III, et al: Effect of intravenous ATP-$MgCl_2$ on cellular function in liver and muscle in hemorrhagic shock. *Curr Surg* 300, September–October 1981.

Schloerb PR, Sieracki L, et al: Intravenous adenosine triphosphate (ATP) in hemorrhagic shock in rats. *Am J Physiol* 240:(1): R52, January 1981.

Shires GT, et al: Alterations in cellular membrane function during hemorrhagic shock in primates. *Ann Surg* 176:288, 1972.

Shires GT, Brown FT, et al: Distributional changes in extracellular fluid during acute hemorrhagic shock. *Surg Forum* 11:115, 1960.

Shires GT, Brown FT, Canizaro PC: *Shock*. Philadelphia, Saunders, 1973, chap 4.

Wilde WS: The chloride equilibrium in muscle. *Am J Physiol* 143:666, 1945.

Renal Responses

Baxter CR, Zedlitz WH, Shires GT: High output acute renal failure complicating traumatic injury. *J Trauma* 4:567, 1964.

Bush HL: Renal considerations in the injured patient. *Surg Clin North Am* 62:133, 1983.

Flear CTG, Clarke R: The influence of blood loss and blood transfusion upon changes in the metabolism of water, electrolytes and nitrogen following civilian trauma. *Clin Sci* 14:575, 1955.

Gerrick S, Ledgerwood AM, Lucas CE: Post-resuscitation hypertension: A reappraisal. *Arch Surg* 115:1486, 1980.

Hermreck AS: The pathophysiology of acute renal failure. *Surgery* 144:605, 1982.

Ladd M: *Battle Casualties in Korea*, vol 4. U.S. Army Medical Service Graduate School, Walter Reed Army Medical Center, 1956, p 193.

Lucas CE: Renal considerations in the injured patient. *Surg Clin North Am* 62:133, 1982.

Lucas CE, Ledgerwood AM, Higgins RF: Impaired salt and water excretion after albumin resuscitation for hypovolemic shock. *Surgery* 86:544, 1979.

Lucas CE, Weaver D, et al: Effects of albumin versus non-albumin resuscitation on plasma volume and renal excretory function. *J Trauma* 18:564, 1978.

Lucas CE, Zito JG, Carter KM: Questionable value of furosemide in preventing renal failure. *Surgery* 82:314, 1977.

Miller TR, Anderson RJ, et al: Urinary diagnostic indices in acute renal failure; a prospective study. *Ann Med* 89:47, 1978.

Stein JH, Lifschitz MD, Barnes LD: Current concepts on the pathophysiology of acute renal failure. *Am J Physiol* 234:171, 1982.

Teschan PE, et al: Post-traumatic renal insufficiency in military casualties: I Clinical characteristics. *Am J Med* 18:172, 1955.

Teschan PE, Mason AD: Reproducible experimental acute renal failure in rats. *Clin Res* 6:155, 1958.

Weissman C, Rosenbaum LM, et al: Massive perioperative polyuria. *J Trauma* 22:1028, 1982.

Wright HK, Gann DS: Correction of defect in free water excretion in postoperative patients by extracellular fluid volume expansion. *Ann Surg* 158:70, 1963.

Pulmonary Responses

Ashbaugh DG, Petty TL: Sepsis complicating the acute respiratory distress syndrome. *Surg Gynecol Obstet* 135:865, 1972.

Bell RC, Coalson JJ, et al: Multiple organ system failure and infection in adult respiratory distress syndrome. *Ann Intern Med* 99:293, 1983.

Burford TH, Burbank B: Traumatic wet lung: Observations on certain physiologic fundamentals of thoracic trauma. *J Thorac Surg* 14:415, 1945.

Clauss RH, et al: Effects of changing body position upon improved ventilation-perfusion relationships. *Circulation* (suppl II-37)38:214, 1968.

Dahn MS, Lucas CE, et al: Negative inotropic effects of albumin resuscitation for shock. *Surgery* 86:235, 1979.

Demling RH, Manohar M, et al: The effect of plasma oncotic pressure on the pulmonary microcirculation after hemorrhagic shock. *Surgery* 86:323, 1979.

Fowler AA, Hamman RF, et al: Adult respiratory distress syndrome: Risk with common predispositions. *Ann Intern Med* 98:593, 1983.

Fulton RL, Jones CE: The cause of post-traumatic pulmonary insufficiency in man. *Surg Gynecol Obstet* 140:179, 1975.

Greenfield S, Teres D, et al: Prevention of gram negative bacillary pneumonia using aerosol polymyxin as prophylaxis: I. Effect on the colonization pattern of the upper respiratory tract of seriously ill patients. *J Clin Invest* 52:2935, 1973.

Harken AH, Brennan MF, et al: The hemodynamic response to positive end-expiratory ventilation in hypovolemic patients. *Surgery* 76:786, 1974.

Herman CM: Detection and management of intraabdominal sepsis in ICU patients: Indications and outcomes. *Infect Surg* 2:737, 757, 1983.

Holcroft JW, Trunkey DD: Pulmonary extravasation of albumin during and after hemorrhagic shock in baboons. *J Surg Res* 18:91, 1975.

Horvitz JH, Carrico CJ, Shires GT: Pulmonary response to major injury. *Arch Surg* 108:349, 1974.

Liebman PR, Patten MT, et al: The mechanism of depressed cardiac output on positive end-expiratory pressure (PEEP). *Surgery* 83:594, 1978.

Lowe RJ, Moss GS, et al: Crystalloid vs. colloid in the etiology of pulmonary failure after trauma. A randomized trial in man. *Surgery* 81:676, 1977.

Lucas CE, Ledgerwood AM, Higgins RF: Impaired salt and water excretion after albumin resuscitation for hypovolemic shock. *Surgery* 86:544, 1979.

Mendelson CL: The aspiration of stomach content into the lungs during obstetric anesthesia. *Am J Obstet Gynecol* 52:191, 1946.

Montgomery AB, Stager MA, et al: Causes of mortality associated with the adult respiratory distress syndrome. *Am Rev Respir Dis* 132:485, 1985.

Moore FD, et al: *Post-traumatic Pulmonary Insufficiency*. Philadelphia, Saunders, 1969.

Pepe PE, Potkin RT, et al: Clinical predictors of the adult respiratory distress syndrome. *Am J Surg* 144:124, 1982.

Pepe PE, Hudson LD, Carrico CJ: Early application of positive end-expiratory pressure in patients at risk for the adult respiratory distress syndrome. *N Engl J Med* 311:281, 1984.

Peters RM, et al: Objective indications for respiratory therapy in post-trauma and post-operative patients. *Am J Surg* 124:262, 1972.

Pontoppidan H, et al: Acute respiratory failure in adults. *N Engl J Med* 287:690, 1972.

Robertson HT, Lakshminarayan S, Hudson LD: Lung injury following a 50 metre fall into water. *Thorax* 33:175, 1978.

Roscher R, Bittner R, et al: Pulmonary contusion: Clinical experience. *Arch Surg* 109:508, 1974.

Schwartz DJ, Wynne JW, et al: Pulmonary consequences of aspiration of gastric contents at pH values greater than 2.5. *Am Rev Respir Dis* 121:119, 1980.

Sinanan M, Maier RV, Carrico CJ: Laparotomy for intraabdominal sepsis in ICU patients: Indications and outcome. *Arch Surg* 119:652, 1984.

Staub NC: The forces regulating fluid filtration in the lung. *Microvas Res* 15:45, 1978.

Stothert JC, Weaver J, et al: Pulmonary vascular permeability after acid aspiration. *Surg Forum* 31:237, 1980.

Sturm JA, Carpenter MA, et al: Water and protein movement in the sheep lung after septic shock. Effect of colloid versus crystalloid resuscitation. *J Surg Res* 26:233, 1979.

Virgilio RW, Matildi LA, et al: Colloid vs. crystalloid volume resuscitation of patients with severe pulmonary insufficiency. *Surg Forum* 30:166, 1979.

Virgilio RW, Rice CL, et al: Crystalloid vs. colloid resuscitation. Is one better? *Surgery* 85:129, 1979.

Wahrenbrock ET: The effect of posture on pulmonary function and survival of anesthetized dogs. *J Surg Res* 10:13, 1970.

Weighelt JA, Mitchell RA, Snyder WH: Early positive end-expiratory pressure in the adult respiratory distress syndrome. *Arch Surg* 114:497, 1979.

Alterations in Oxygen Transport

Bellingham AJ, Detter JC, Lenfant C: Regulatory mechanisms of hemoglobin oxygen affinity in acidosis and alkalosis. *J Clin Invest* 50:700, 1971.

Benesch R, Benesch RE: The effect of organic phosphates from the human erythrocyte on the allosteric properties of hemoglobin. *Biochem Biophys Res Commun* 26:162, 1967.

Berne RM, Blackman JR, Gardner TH: Hypoxemia and coronary blood flow. *J Clin Invest* 36:1101, 1957.

Bowen JC, Fleming WH: Increased oxyhemoglobin affinity after transfusion of stored blood. *Ann Surg* 180:760, 1974.

Bunn HF, May MH, et al: Hemoglobin function in stored blood. *J Clin Invest* 48:311, 1969.

Canizaro, PC: Oxygen transport in shock, in Shires GT (ed): *Shock and Related Problems, Clinical Surgery International.* New York, Churchill Livingstone, 1984, vol 9, pp 127–147.

Canizaro PC, Nelson JL, et al: A technique for estimating the position of the oxygen-hemoglobin dissociation curve. *Ann Surg* 180:364, 1974.

Chaunutin A, Curnish RR: Effect of organic and inorganic phosphates on the oxygen equilibrium of human erythrocytes. *Arch Biochem Biophys* 121:96, 1967.

Collins JA: Problems associated with the massive transfusion of stored blood. *Surgery* 75:274, 1974.

Collins JA: Problems and perspectives in surgical hemotherapy. *Bibl Haematologica* 46:241, 1980.

Dennis RC, Vito L, et al: Improved myocardial performance following high 2-3 diphosphoglycerate red cell transfusions. *Surgery* 77:741, 1975.

Duvelleroy MA, Mehmel HC, Laver MB: Hemoglobin-oxygen equilibrium and coronary blood flow. *J Appl Physiol* 35:480, 1973.

Feola M, Gonzalez HF, et al: Development of a bovine stroma-free hemoglobin solution as a blood substitute. *Surg Gynecol Obstet* 157:399, 1983.

Fry DE, Woods M: The influence of oxyhemoglobin affinity on tissue oxygen consumption. *Ann Surg* 183:130, 1976.

Gould SA, Rosen AL, et al: Fluosol-DA as a red cell substitute in acute anemia. *N Engl J Med* 314(26):1653, 1986.

Harken AH: The surgical significance of the oxyhemoglobin dissociation curve. *Surg Gynecol Obstet* 144:935, 1977.

Holcroft JW, Trunkey DD: Extravascular lung water following hemorrhagic shock in the baboon; Comparison between resuscitation with Ringer's lactate and plasmanate. *Ann Surg* 180:408, 1974.

Hoyt DB, Greenburg AG, et al: Resuscitation with fluosol-DA 20%-tolerance to sepsis. *J Trauma* 26:8, 713, 1986.

Kalter ES, Carlson RW, Thijs LG: Effects of methylprednisolone on hemodynamics, arteriovenous oxygen difference, P_{50}, and 2,3-DPG in bacterial shock: A preliminary study. *Crit Care Med* 10:662, 1982.

Kovalik SG, Ledgerwood AM, et al: The cardiac effect of altered calcium homeostasis after albumin resuscitation. *J Trauma* 21:275, 1981.

Lenfant C, et al: Effects of altitude on oxygen binding by hemoglobin and on organic phosphate levels. *J Clin Invest* 47:2652, 1968.

Lenfant C, Ways P, Aucutt C: Effect of chronic hypoxic hypoxia on the O_2-Hb dissociation curve and respiratory gas transport in man. *Respir Physiol* 7:7, 1969.

Lucas CE, Ledgerwood AM, Huggins RF: Impaired salt and water excretion after albumin resuscitation for hypovolemic shock. *Surgery* 86:544, 1979.

Metsuno T, Ohyanagi H, Naito R: Clinical studies of a perfluorochemical whole blood substitute (Fluosol-DA). *Ann Surg* 195:60, 1982.

Opitz E, Schneider M: Über die Sauerstoffversorgung des Gehirns und den Mechanismus von Mangelverhungerung. *Ergeb Physiol* 46:126, 1950.

Oski FA, et al: The *in vitro* restoration of red cell 2,3-diphosphoglycerate levels in banked blood. *Blood* 37:52, 1971.

Oski FA, Marshal BE, et al: Exercise with anemia, the role of the left shifted or right shifted oxygen-hemoglobin equilibrium curve. *Ann Intern Med* 74:44, 1971.

Proctor HJ, Parker JC, et al: Treatment of severe hypoxia with red cells high in 2,3-diphosphoglycerate. *J Trauma* 13:340, 1973.

Severinghaus JW: Blood gas calculator. *J Appl Physiol* 21:1108, 1966.

Tremper KK, Friedman AE, et al: The preoperative treatment of severely anemic patients with a perfluorochemical oxygen-transport fluid, Fluosol-DA. *N Engl J Med* 307:277, 1982.

Valeri CR, Hirsch NM: Restoration *in vivo* of erythrocyte adenosine triphosphate, 2,3-diphosphoglycerate, potassium ion, and sodium ion concentrations following the transfusion of acid-citrate-dextrose-stored human red blood cells. *J Lab Clin Med* 73:722, 1969.

Valeri CR, Zaroulis CG: Rejuvenation and freezing of outdated stored human red cells. *N Engl J Med* 287:1307, 1972.

Woodson RD, Wranne B, Detter JC: Effect of increased blood oxygen affinity on work performance in rats. *J Clin Invest* 52:2717, 1973.

Therapy of Shock

Aeder MI, Crowe JP, et al: Technical limitations in the rapid infusion of intravenous fluids. *Ann Emerg Med* 14:307, 1985.

Altemeier WA, Todd JC, Inge WW: Gramnegative septicemia: A growing threat. *Ann Surg* 166:530, 1967.

Beecher HK: Preparation of battle casualties for surgery. *Ann Surg* 121:769, 1945.

Blaisdel FW: Controversy in shock research. Con: The role of steroids in septic shock. 8:673, 1981.

Canizaro PC, Praeger MD, Shires GT: The infusion of Ringer's lactate solution during shock. *Am J Surg* 122:494, 1971.

Civetta JM: A new look at the Starling equation. *Crit Care Med* 7(3):84, 1979.

Forrester JS, Diamond G, Chatterjee K: Medical therapy of acute myocardial infarction by application of hemodynamic subsets. *N Engl J Med* 295:1356, 1976.

Guntheroth WG, Abel FL, Mullins GL: The effect of Trendelenburg's position on blood pressure and carotid blood flow. *Surg Gynecol Obstet* 119:345, 1964.

Hagman CF, Bagge L, Thoren L: The use of blood components in surgical transfusion therapy. *World J Surg* 11, 2, 1987.

Holcroft JW: Impairment of venous return in hemorrhagic shock. *Surg Clin North Am* 62:25, 1982.

Holcroft JW, Trunkey DD: Further analysis of lung water in baboons resuscitated from hemorrhagic shock. *J Surg Res* 20:291, 1976.

Johnson SA, Gunnar RM: Treatment of shock in myocardial infarction. *JAMA* 237:2106, 1977.

Kolff J, Deeb GM: Artificial heart and left ventricular assist devices. *Surg Clin North Am* 65:3, 1985.

Krausz MM, Perel A, et al: Cardiopulmonary effects of volume loading in patients in septic shock. *Ann Surg* 185:429, 1977.

Loeb HS, Winslow EBJ, et al: Acute hemodynamic effects of dopamine in patients with shock. *Circulation* 44:163, 1971.

Lucas CE, Ledgerwood AM: The cardiopulmonary response to massive dose of steroids in patients with septic shock. *Arch Surg* 119:537, 1984.

Lucas CE, Ledgerwood AM, et al: Impaired pulmonary function after albumin resuscitation from shock. *J Trauma* 20:446, 1980.

MacLean LD, Mulligan WG, et al: Patterns of septic shock in man: A detailed study of 56 patients. *Ann Surg* 166:543, 1967.

Maier RV, Carrizo CJ: Development in the resuscitation of critically ill surgical patients, in Mannick JA, et al (eds): *Advances in Surgery*. Chicago, Year Book Medical Publishers, 1986, vol 19, pp 271–328.

Mason DT: Afterload reduction and cardiac performance: Physiological basis of systemic vasodilators as a new approach in treatment of congestive heart failure. *Am J Med* 65:106, 1978.

Messmer K: Blood substitutes in shock therapy, in Shires GT (ed): *Shock and Related Problems, Clinical Surgery International*. New York, Churchill Livingstone, 1984, vol 9, pp 192–205.

Myers ML, Austin TW, Sibbald WJ: Pulmonary artery catheter infections: A prospective study. *Ann Surg* 201:237, 1985.

Nelson LD: Continuous venous oximetry in surgical patients. *Ann Surg* 203:329, 1986.

Niarchos AP: Management of cardiovascular problems in the trauma patient, in Shires GT (ed): *Principles of Trauma Care*. New York, McGraw-Hill, 1985.

Schumer W: Controversy in shock research. Pro: The role of steroids in septic shock. *Circ Shock* 8:667, 1981.

Shatney CH, Deepika K, Militello PR: Efficacy of hetastarch in the resuscitation of patients with multisystem trauma and shock. *Arch Surg* 118:804, 1983.

Shires GT, Shires GT III: Hypovolemic shock, in Shires GT (ed): *Shock and Related Problems, Clinical Surgery International*. New York, Churchill Livingstone, 1984, vol 9, pp. 127–147.

Sprung CL, Caralis PV, Marcial EH: The effects of high dose corticosteroids in patients with septic shock. *N Engl J Med* 311:1137, 1984.

Swan HJC, et al: Catheterization of the heart in man with use of a flow-directed balloon-tipped catheter. *N Engl J Med* 283:447, 1970.

Trinkle JK, Rush BE, Eiseman B: Metabolism of lactate following major blood loss. *Surgery* 63:782, 1968.

Valeri CR: Optimal use of blood products in the treatment of hemorrhagic shock. *Surg Rounds* 4:38, 1981.

Wright CJ, Duff JH, et al: Regional capillary blood flow and oxygen uptake in severe sepsis. *Surg Gynecol Obstet* 132:637, 1971.

Chapter 5

Infections

Isidore Cohn, Jr., and George H. Bornside

INTRODUCTION

Infection is a dynamic process involving invasion of the body by pathogenic microorganisms and reaction of the tissues to organisms and their toxins. Soon after birth, a variety of microorganisms colonize the external and internal surfaces of the human body. This indigenous microflora usually does no harm; it produces no detectable pathologic effects in tissues and may be beneficial. Indeed, the normal intestinal flora functions as a barrier providing natural resistance against enteric infections with pathogens such as *Salmonella* and *Shigella* species.

Infection evolves into overt disease only when the equilibrium between host and parasite is upset. Of the thousands of species of microorganisms in nature, only a few hundred are known to be pathogenic for human beings.

Current thinking concerning clinical disease resulting from host and parasite interrelationships recognizes the role of the general health of the host, the previous contact with infectious microorganisms, the past clinical history, and various insults (toxic, traumatic, or therapeutic) of nonmicrobial origin. When the host's resistance is lowered, the indigenous microflora can become involved in infectious disease. This presents a dilemma to both the clinician and the microbiologist, as it must be decided which of the several microorganisms usually isolated from a clinical specimen are involved in the patient's disease. There are very few pathogenic species that cause disease at all times. Most organisms found in and on human beings often are harmless but are capable of causing disease in patients who are elderly, very young, or debilitated (Table 5-1).

Despite more than 80 years of aseptic surgery and more than 40 years of experience with antimicrobial agents, the surgeon finds that infections are as great a problem now as in the past. But the etiologic agents have changed. Streptococci and pneumococci are no longer the captains of death, because they can be controlled by antibiotics. Staphylococci *continue* to cause nosocomial (hospital-acquired) infections, but those gram-negative bacteria usually considered nonpathogens, opportunists, or secondary invaders have become a major problem. Nosocomial infection results from the transmission of pathogens to a previously uninfected patient from a source in the hospital environment (*cross infection*). Alternatively, the pathogens may come from patients themselves (*autoinfection*). They may be carriers of the pathogen or become colonized with virulent hospital strains during hospitalization. Many nosocomial infections have an iatrogenic basis (i.e., result from treatment by physicians and their professional collaborators). Frequent or prolonged use of supportive procedures such as indwelling vascular or urinary catheters, tracheostomies, and equipment for postoperative respiratory care are responsible for most iatrogenic infections. Nosocomial infection causes morbidity, mortality, expense to the patient, and increasing malpractice liability for the surgeon and hospital.

A *surgical infection* is an infection that requires surgical treatment and has developed before, or as a complication of, surgical treatment. Thus, a postoperative wound infection is also a specific nosocomial infection. Surgical infections may be analyzed in relation to procedures in clean or contaminated fields, the anatomic site or system involved, and the pathophysiologic activities of the causative microorganisms (Table 5-2). The microorganisms commonly encountered in surgical infections are the staphylococci, streptococci, clostridia, bacteroides, and the enteric bacteria. Most surgical incisions are contaminated but not infected with normal skin flora (bacteria such as coagulase-negative staphylococci and anaerobic diphtheroids). However, traumatic wounds are usually contaminated if not yet infected, and operations on infected or "contaminated" tissue usually result in infec-

Table 5-1. SOME INDIGENOUS MICROORGANISMS AND SOME INFECTIONS WITH WHICH THEY MAY BE INVOLVED

Microorganism	Infection
Aerobic or facultative:	
Achromobacter spp.	Bloodstream, burns, meningitis, urethritis
Acinetobacter spp.	Bloodstream, burns, meningitis, urethritis, pneumonia
Alkaligenes fecalis	Bloodstream, conjunctivitis, meningitis, respiratory tract, urinary tract
Candida albicans and other yeasts	Endocarditis, pneumonitis, septicemia, thrush, vulvovaginitis, candidosis
Corynebacterium spp.	Endocarditis, lung abscesses
Enterobacteriaceae (*Escherichia, Klebsiella, Enterobacter, Proteus,* etc.)	Abscesses, bloodstream, meningitis, peritonitis, pneumonia, wounds, urinary tract, endocarditis, pyelonephritis, cystitis
Haemophilus spp.	Bronchitis, conjunctivitis, meningitis, urinary tract
Moraxella spp.	Conjunctivitis
Nocardia spp.	Nocardiosis
Pseudomonas spp.	Bloodstream, burns, meningitis, urinary tract, wounds
Staphylococcus aureus	Abscesses, pneumonia, wounds, pseudomembranous enterocolitis
Staphylococcus epidermidis	Endocarditis, septicemia, thrombophlebitis
Streptococcus faecalis	Endocarditis, bloodstream, urinary tract, wounds, peritonitis, meningitis
Streptococcus viridans	Endocarditis
Anaerobic:	
Actinomyces spp.	Actinomycosis
Bacteroides spp.	Abscesses, endocarditis, peritonitis
Clostridium spp.	Cellulitis, myonecrosis, pseudomembranous enterocolitis
Fusobacterium spp.	Abscesses, myonecrosis, bacteremia
Lactobacillus spp.	Endocarditis
Peptostreptococcus spp.	Abscesses, myonecrosis
Veillonella spp.	Endocarditis

tion. Postoperative infections present a double hazard: First, the infection itself may result in toxemia or produce extensive tissue damage and perhaps septicemia. Second, the local effects of infection delay healing of the wound and may cause hemorrhage or disruption of the wound. In either case, the patient's hospitalization is extended.

GENERAL PRINCIPLES

Pathogenic species of bacteria have the capacity to invade and produce disease. However, disease is a biologic

Table 5-2. CLASSIFICATION OF SURGICAL INFECTIONS

I. Relative to final outcome
- A. Self-limiting infections: The patient recovers completely without medical or surgical treatment, or despite it (e.g., a boil).
- B. Serious infections requiring treatment: The outcome depends largely on the nature of treatment, the time after outset that it is administered, and clinical judgment (e.g., septicemia, pneumonia, empyema, primary peritonitis).
- C. Fulminating infections: These prove to be fatal or permanently disabling (e.g., retroperitoneal cellulitis).

II. Relative to time of onset
- A. Anteoperative surgical infections: These include all infections in which the microorganisms have gained entrance to the body before any operative procedure.
  1. Time and portal of entry are known—accidents.
  2. Time and portal of entry are not known—disease (infection) is established before the surgeon treats the patient.
- B. Operative surgical infections: These include all in which microorganisms gain entrance to the body during an operative procedure or as an immediate result of it (i.e., surgery may be considered either directly or indirectly responsible for the development of infection).
  1. Preventable operative surgical infections—failure of the surgeon or operating-room personnel to adhere to the principles of sterile procedure and all accepted and accredited practices
  2. Nonpreventable operative surgical infections
     - *a.* Pathogenic microorganisms already resident within body tissues (e.g., incision seeded with *Staphylococcus aureus* resident in ducts and glands of normal skin)
     - *b.* Microorganisms from a deep focus of infection (e.g., peritoneal abscess, lung abscess, etc.)
     - *c.* Microorganisms resident on the surface of normal mucous membranes (e.g., intestinal tract, respiratory tract, genitourinary tract)
     - *d.* Microorganisms on dust particles and borne by air currents
- C. Postoperative surgical infections: These are complications of the operation or the postoperative management of the patient.
  1. Surgical wound infection
  2. Respiratory tract infection
  3. Urinary tract infection

SOURCE: Modified from Meleney FL: *Treatise on Surgical Infections,* New York, Oxford University Press, 1948.

accident and represents a complex interaction between the microorganism and the host that occurs only under special circumstances. Healthy people may harbor pathogenic bacteria and yet be unaffected clinically. They are referred to as carriers of the particular pathogen. The healthy carrier of pathogenic microorganisms is the principal reservoir of most diseases. Although species such as *Staphylococcus aureus* and *Escherichia coli* are examples of pathogens, individual strains may be too feeble to cause infection. Feeble or noninvasive strains may cause infection if the resistance of the host is extremely low or if tremendous numbers of bacteria are introduced. Some bacteria that are nonpathogenic under ordinary conditions are opportunistic and may be pathogenic when the host-parasite equilibrium is upset, e.g., when normal flora is eliminated by antibiotics or when incision makes available a new area of the body. Antibiotic-resistant strains of *Staphylococcus aureus* of specific phage types, which cause nosocomial postoperative wound infections, may be endemic among carrier personnel of a particular hospital. Patients may become infected by direct contact with a carrier or may become infected with a hospital staphylococcus with which they have become colonized during hospitalization.

The term *virulence* refers to the tissue-invading powers of a specific strain of a pathogen and is used in two different ways: First, virulence describes quantitatively the smallest dose of a bacterial strain that will produce disease in a specified host. This assessment is usually conducted in experimental animals and may have no relation to human disease. Second, virulence describes an epidemiologic concept such as a given phage type of *Staphylococcus aureus* producing human disease more frequently than another. In this situation, virulence is based on ecologic advantage in the external environment but may not necessarily involve greater capacity to be virulent as measured by the critical dose of bacteria causing clinical infection.

A large infecting dose is favorable to the production of bacterial disease because only a small number of bacteria may actually reach a favorable site in the host. A sudden change to a different environment or to a new site may injure most of the inoculum. Moreover, the defense mechanisms of the host often destroy a large proportion of the invading organisms before they can become established. The greater the number of bacteria introduced into the host, the greater the amount of preformed toxins that will be carried along. Preformed toxins may protect bacteria from destruction during the period when they are adapting to the new environment and are incapable of producing additional toxin. The resistance of the host is shown in the ability to keep bacteria out of the body initially and, failing in this, to localize and destroy them. A healthy, unbroken skin is the first line of resistance. Although mucous membranes are less resistant, even here minute breaks usually provide for bacterial entry. It is then that active defensive measures come into play. Primary defenses include the system of fixed phagocytic cells (i.e., the histiocytes of the reticuloendothelial system) and mobile phagocytes. These are aided by antibacterial substances in blood plasma, lymph, and interstitial fluid, by physical barriers to the spread of bacteria (i.e., ground substances, serous and fibrous membranes), and by local and systemic reactions such as hyperemia, fever, and leukocytosis. Secondary defenses are dependent upon the presence of specific antigenic stimuli (bacteria and bacterial products). The antibodies formed in response to these antigens inhibit or destroy bacteria, or neutralize their toxins. In the presence of sufficient antibodies, the primary defenses are greatly accelerated, bacteria are phagocytized and digested more quickly than before, and the ability of serum to neutralize bacterial toxins is increased many thousandfold. The presence of other disease may greatly reduce resistance to microbial infection. For example, diabetes predisposes to infection of the skin and the genitourinary tract. Influenza, measles, and other viral infections markedly predispose to secondary bacterial infections of the respiratory tract. Malignant disease, malnutrition, chronic alcoholism, or metabolic disease may interfere seriously with an individual's resistance to infectious disease.

Bacteria cause disease by invading tissues and producing toxins. Bacterial invasion leads to demonstrable damage of host cells and tissues in the vicinity of the invasion, whereas bacterial toxins are transported by the blood and lymph to cause cytotoxic effects at sites removed from the initial lesion. Species such as *Streptococcus pyogenes* are both invasive and toxigenic. *Staphylococcus aureus* produces local damage but has little tendency to spread, although the local inflammatory response may be severe as in the case of carbuncles. *Clostridium tetani* is almost solely toxigenic. Generally, invasiveness and toxigenicity are not completely separable, since invasion involves some degree of toxin production and toxigenicity requires some degree of bacterial multiplication. *Exotoxins* are specific, soluble, diffusible proteins produced by certain bacteria as they multiply in a circumscribed area. Exotoxins lose their toxicity upon denaturation but retain much of their original antigenicity. Such modified exotoxins are called *toxoids*. Those prepared from *Clostridium tetani* are used to induce active immunity in man. The alpha toxin of *Clostridium perfringens* is a lecithinase that acts upon the membrane lipids of body cells and erythrocytes. *Endotoxins* are complex lipopolysaccharides of the bacterial cell wall produced by many gram-negative species. They are released only on partial or complete dissolution of the bacterial cell. Endotoxins are relatively heat-stable; many withstand temperatures of 60 to 100°C for 1 h. They do not form toxoids. Their toxicity is associated with the phospholipid moiety of the molecule, whereas their antigenic determinants are associated with the polysaccharide moiety.

Diagnosis

The classic signs and symptoms of infection are redness, swelling, heat, and pain. Redness of the skin is due to intense hyperemia. Swelling accompanies infection unless the infection is confined to bone that cannot swell. Heat results from hyperemia and may be detected even in the absence of redness. Pain is the most universal sign of infection. Along with pain goes tenderness, or pain to the touch, which is greatest over the area of maximal involvement. Loss of function is another sign of infection. It is brought about by reflex and by voluntary immobilization. The patient immobilizes the painful part in the most comfortable position. For example, a finger with an infected tendon sheath is kept flexed. In peritonitis, the abdominal muscles are maintained in a state of tonic contraction to keep the inflamed peritoneum beneath from moving. Fever and tachycardia are additional, albeit nonspecific, signs of infection. Fever and chills indicate septicemia, while an elevated pulse rate is a sign of a toxic state.

Leukocytosis accompanies an acute bacterial infection more often than a viral infection. The more severe the infection, the greater is the leukocytosis. In most surgical infections, the total leukocyte count is only slightly or moderately elevated. However, a high leukocyte count (35,000/mm³) occurs as a result of suppuration. The endotoxin released by gram-negative bacilli is thought to contribute to the production of high leukocyte counts. However, in the elderly, in the severely ill, and during therapy with antibiotic, some anticancer, and immunosuppressive drugs, white cell counts may be normal or low. The leukopenia of overwhelming sepsis is probably due to exhaustion of the supply of leukocytes and to bone marrow depression. Although the total number of leukocytes is normal in some infections, there is a preponderance of immature granulocytes, which may be increased above 85 percent compared with the normal below 75 percent ("shift to the left"). A chronic infection may be evident only by fatigue, low-grade fever, and perhaps anemia. Moreover, massive pyogenic abscesses may occur without leukocytosis, fever, or tenderness.

Exudate from the area of infection should be examined for color, odor, and consistency. The microorganisms causing a surgical infection often may be seen microscopically on gram-stained smears. For each bacterial cell observed under the oil-immersion lens, there are approximately 10⁵ similar organisms in each milliliter of exudate from which the smear was prepared. The staining and examination of slides are simple, rapid, inexpensive procedures that provide valuable and immediate information for the surgeon. Pus from deep-seated abscesses may be obtained by needle aspiration or at the time of definitive drainage. Exudate from surface infections may be examined directly. Specimens submitted to the bacteriologic laboratory should be collected before chemotherapy is begun and should be labeled adequately to identify the patient, the clinical diagnosis, and the nature and site of the specimen. The laboratory should be requested to do aerobic and anaerobic cultures and antibiotic-sensitivity tests. The surgeon must initiate treatment immediately upon clinical judgment, although the subsequent laboratory report will often make appropriate changes possible.

Biopsy is useful in establishing a diagnosis in granulomatous infections such as tuberculosis, syphilis, and mycoses. Additional sources of biopsy material are enlarged lymph nodes draining an area of infection or a sinus tract. Blood cultures are the single most definitive method of determining etiology in infectious disease and are often helpful in identifying the microorganisms causing surgical infection. Transient bacteremias accompany the early phase of many infections and may result from manipulation of infected or contaminated tissues (e.g., surgical incision of furuncles or abscesses, instrumentation of the genitourinary tract, and dental procedures). Bacteria usually enter the circulation via the lymphatic system. Consequently, when bacteria multiply at a site of local infection in tissues, the lymph drained from that area carries bacteria to the thoracic duct and eventually to the venous blood. However, a blood culture taken at the time of chill and fever may be negative for bacteria, as phagocytes promptly remove bacteria suddenly entering the bloodstream and chill and fever occur 30 to 90 min later. Thus, blood cultures should be taken at frequent intervals in a patient with febrile disease of unknown origin in an attempt to obtain blood before an expected chill and rise in temperature. A careful history and physical examination provide the basis for diagnosis and laboratory tests.

Surgical Therapy

It is necessary to distinguish between contamination and infection. Almost all wounds are contaminated with bacteria from the skin or from sources external to the patient. However, very few wounds become infected (i.e., exhibit disease manifested by inflammation, dehiscence, suppuration, and necrosis). The major clinical responses to wound infection are suppuration and invasion. Bacteria grow in the wound on substrates consisting of blood clots, lymph, leukocytes, and necrotic debris. Extension of the local inflammatory response to adjacent tissues is associated with a systemic reaction. The hazard of generalized infection is associated with all traumatic wounds. These and preoperative surgical infections are treated to overcome existing infection and to prevent postoperative infection. Local treatment consists of debridement of all necrotic or injured tissue, drainage of abscesses, removal of foreign bodies, and adjunctive therapy with antibiotics. Supportive measures governing the treatment of established surgical infections are bed rest, immobilization of the infected region, elevation to promote venous and lymphatic drainage, and relief of swelling and pain. Moist heat is applied to increase local blood supply, facilitate exudation, and hasten sloughing. The detailed management of wounds is discussed in Chap. 8 (Wound Healing and Wound Care).

Antibiotic Therapy

The adjunctive use of antibiotics in the treatment of infections is dependent upon an adequate blood supply and is most effective against acute infections such as cellulitis, septicemia, or peritonitis. Antibiotics have slight access to abscesses and penetrate by slow diffusion, if at all. In these situations, they should be used in conjunction with incision and drainage. Antibiotics are the primary treatment for acute spreading infections and should result in clinical improvement in 24 to 48 h. Change to a more effective antibiotic may be based on the culture and sensitivity report.

Although clinical judgment frequently must be used to select an antibiotic and although the causative microorganism often is revealed on microscopic examination of a gram-stained smear of exudate or pus, the infecting microorganisms should be identified and antibiotic sensitivities determined by the laboratory. Accordingly, the specimen for culture (pus, exudate, blood, or urine) should be obtained before chemotherapy is begun. In severe infections, exudate often can be inoculated on a blood agar plate and antibiotic sensitivity discs positioned so that rapid, presumptive sensitivity information can be obtained after incubation overnight or for several hours. This crude procedure does not replace the official pure culture studies of all microorganisms isolated from the specimen.

Hyperbaric Therapy

Brummelkamp and associates in Amsterdam introduced the hyperbaric oxygen chamber for operative procedures. In 1963 they reported the first use of hyperbaric oxygen for gas-producing infections. Both the patient and medical personnel were placed in a room-sized chamber in which the air pressure was raised to three times that of the normal atmosphere (i.e., 2280 mmHg, or 3 atm absolute). For seven periods of $1\frac{1}{2}$ h during 3 days, the pressurized patient inhaled 100 percent oxygen from a face mask. This increased the normal oxygen tension in plasma, lymph, and tissue fluids about fifteen to twenty times. Dramatic clinical improvement was described in most patients within the first day. Roding and colleagues advise that "operations be limited to opening the original wound and incising abscesses. Any further excision and removal of necrotic tissue can be done much later after clinical resolution. The advantage of postponement is that the operation can be performed in a dramatically improved patient who is no longer toxic." Large pressure chambers are available at only a few medical centers in the world and at special military and marine industrial facilities. In addition, much less expensive single-patient chambers are now available and are also used to treat patients. Therapy with hyperbaric oxygen, antibiotics, and surgical debridement has been effective for clostridial myonecrosis. Hyperbaric oxygenation appears to reduce toxemia and diminish the amount of tissue requiring excision. However, gas-producing infection due to anaerobic streptococci, *Escherichia coli,* and *Klebsiella* species showed no improvement after exposure to high-pressure oxygen. The use of hyperbaric oxygen is advocated as an adjunct to the surgical treatment of clostridial infections. In cases of clostridial myonecrosis, all conventional means of treatment should be employed, including early surgical debridement and administration of antibiotics. The reliability of immediate surgical treatment and adjunctive antibiotic therapy remains unquestioned.

SOME COMMON SURGICAL INFECTIONS

Cellulitis is a nonsuppurative inflammation of the subcutaneous tissues extending along connective tissue planes and across intercellular spaces. There is widespread swelling, redness, and pain without definite localization. Central necrosis and suppuration may occur at a later stage. In severe infections, blebs and bullae form on the skin. Although a variety of aerobic and anaerobic bacteria produce cellulitis, the hemolytic streptococci are the classic etiologic agents. Treatment consists of antibiotic therapy and rest. Failure of the inflammatory swelling to subside after 48 to 72 h of antibiotic therapy suggests that an abscess has developed, and that incision and drainage are needed.

Lymphangitis is an inflammation of lymphatic pathways that is usually visible as erythematous streaking of the skin. This is especially true in infections by hemolytic streptococci. Lymphangitis and the associated inflammatory swelling of lymph nodes *(lymphadenitis)* are a normal defense reaction against bacterial invasion and are frequently seen in the forearm of a patient with an infection of the hand or fingers. Most cases will respond to antibiotic therapy and rest.

Erysipelas is an acute spreading cellulitis and lymphangitis, usually caused by hemolytic streptococci that gain entrance through a break in the skin. There is a severe systemic as well as local reaction with abrupt onset, chills, fever, and prostration. The skin is red, swollen, and tender, and there is a distinct line of demarcation at the advancing margin of the infection. Erysipelas may develop on any cutaneous surface but commonly involves the face in a ''butterfly lesion'' over the nose and cheeks. Recurrent erysipelas in an extremity may lead to chronic lymphedema. Antibiotic therapy will usually halt the progress of the invasive infection, but the erythema disappears more slowly since it is a toxigenic consequence of bacterial invasion.

Infection in soft tissues is of paramount concern to the surgeon, and a variety of superficial infections will be discussed. An *abscess* is a localized collection of pus surrounded by an area of inflamed tissue in which hyperemia and infiltration of leukocytes is marked. A *furuncle,* or boil, is an abscess in a sweat gland or hair follicle. The inflammatory reaction is intense, leading to tissue necrosis and the formation of a central core. This is surrounded by a peripheral zone of cellulitis. An abscess beneath the corium of the skin is a *subepithelial abscess. Impetigo* is an acute contagious skin disease characterized by the formation of a series of intraepithelial abscesses. Gangrenous impetigo may occur as a complication in severe chronic debilitating diseases (e.g., chronic ulcerative colitis), and hemolytic streptococci and staphylococci can be cultured from the exudate. The lesions appear as multiple small pustules that extend and coalesce to form large areas of cutaneous gangrene and ulceration. Although management is similar to that of postoperative gangrene, favorable response is proportional to success in overcoming the primary disease.

A *carbuncle* is a multilocular suppurative extension of a furuncle into the subcutaneous tissues. The nape of the neck, dorsum of trunk, hands and digits, and hirsute portions of the chest and abdomen are apt to be involved. Individual compartments in a carbuncle are maintained through persistence of fascial attachments to the skin. As these numerous component locules rupture separately, individual fistulas appear. Most abscesses are caused by pyogenic cocci, usually *Staphylococcus aureus.* However, gram-negative bacilli and streptococci may be found coincidentally. Carbuncles may be more extensive than they appear and should be excised widely to prevent spread and to effect a cure. The wound contracts to a small scar, and a skin graft is not usually required.

The course of a furuncle is often self-limited and may require no specific therapy. However, furuncles can be serious and may become carbuncles. Large furuncles and abscesses should be incised and drained and the patient treated with antibiotics. Abscesses in the ''dangerous'' nasolabial area of the face bounded by the bridge of the nose and the angles of the mouth may become complicated by septic phlebitis with intracranial extension along the nasal veins to the cavernous sinus. The incidence of septic cavernous sinus thrombosis has declined since the introduction of antibiotics, and this lethal complication is now rare.

Bacteremia is defined as bacteria in the circulating blood with no indication of toxemia or other clinical manifestations. Bacteremia is usually transient and may last only a few moments, as the reticuloendothelial system localizes and destroys these organisms under favorable conditions. The normal individual probably experiences bacteremia, unknowingly, many times each year. This state follows dental procedures, major traumatic wounds, etc., and may be the means by which apparently isolated infections arise in internal organs, e.g., osteomyelitis, pyelonephritis (descending type), or subacute bacterial endocarditis.

Septicemia is a diffuse infection in which infectious bacteria and their toxins are present in the bloodstream. Septicemia may arise directly from the introduction of infecting organisms into the circulation but, as a rule, is secondary to a focus of infection within the body. The major routes by which bacteria reach the blood are (1) by direct extension and entrance into an open vessel, (2) by release of infected emboli following thrombosis of a blood vessel in an area of inflammation, (3) by discharge of infected lymph into the bloodstream following lymphangitis. Many specific diseases, e.g., typhoid fever and brucellosis, include a septicemic phase. In the absence of systemic disease, beta-hemolytic streptococci *(Streptococcus pyogenes)* are most frequently responsible. Septicemia caused by alpha-hemolytic streptococci *(Streptococcus viridans)* is usually a consequence of subacute bacterial endocarditis. The majority of bacteria that produce suppurative lesions may give rise to secondary septicemia. *Pyemia* is septicemia in which pyogenic microorganisms, most notably *Staphylococcus aureus,* and their toxins are carried in the bloodstream and sequentially initiate multiple focal abscesses in many parts of the body. Before the advent of chemotherapy, staphylococcic pyemia was almost always fatal; the mortality is still high. In *toxemia,* toxins are circulating in the blood, though the microorganism producing the toxin need not be. Toxemia is usually associated with infection by toxin-producing bacteria (e.g., the clostridia of gas gangrene and the diphtheria bacillus), but this is not always so. For example, botulinum toxin or staphylococcal enterotoxin may have been ingested directly to cause a profound toxemia without true infection.

PRINCIPLES OF ANTIBIOTIC THERAPY

Basic Considerations

Chemotherapeutic agents act primarily upon the parasite and not upon the host. They include antibiotics and metabolic antagonists such as the sulfonamides. An antibiotic is a chemical compound derived from, or produced by, living organisms and capable, at low concentrations, of inhibiting the life processes of microorganisms. *Bacteriostatic* agents prevent the growth of bacteria but do not destroy them. The defense mechanisms of the body then eliminate the bacteria which are unable to multiply. If the defenses are insufficient or if the bacteriostatic drug is withdrawn prematurely, then the bacterial population will resurge, and the patient will suffer a relapse. *Bactericidal* agents actively kill bacteria and must be employed in patients whose defense mechanisms are impaired or altered by disease or immunosuppressive therapy. The distinction between bactericidal and bacteriostatic effects is sometimes relative to duration of therapy and dosage. Some drugs are bacteriostatic at low concentrations and bactericidal at high concentrations. With most bactericidal drugs, the rate of killing increases with concentration. Antibiotic agents exert their effects in a variety of ways (Table 5-3). They may inhibit the synthesis of the bacterial cell wall and consequently interfere with the cell's osmotic defenses, or they may affect the barrier function of the cell membrane and cause loss of vital metabolites. An entirely different mode of action impairs the translation of genetic information and affects protein synthesis. Bacteriostatic drugs affect early stages of protein synthesis in the ribosome and result in an insufficiency, preventing growth and proliferation of bacteria without actually destroying them. However, bactericidal drugs cause the ribosome to miscode and consequently induce the manufacture of defective proteins or enzymes that poison the cell. Replication of deoxyribonucleic acid (DNA) in the chromosome at the level of the assembly of purine nucleotides may be affected by some antibiotics. Although their precise locus of action is not known, these drugs impede the replication of genetic information.

The addition of antibiotics to the armamentarium of the physician has revolutionized the practice of medicine but has been a double-edged sword. Antibiotics not only achieve a therapeutic effect but also alter the ecology of the patient's microflora. Excessive use of antibiotics may select for strains of bacteria whose resistance to antibiotics is transmitted by plasmids. It is pertinent to point out that the surgeon employs antibiotic drugs as adjunctive agents in the treatment of surgical infections, whereas the internist usually employs antibiotics as the primary treatment for medical infections. For the surgeon the aims of antibiotic therapy are much the same as those of surgical therapy, i.e., to control or eradicate bacterial infections acquired before or during hospitalization and to prevent infection from developing postoperatively. To obtain these goals, antibiotic agents are administered (1) systemically by either parenteral or oral routes, (2) preoperatively for preparation of the large intestine (intestinal antisepsis), or (3) locally by (a) topical irrigation, (b) topical application, (c) intraperitoneal, intrapleural, or intrathecal instillation or irrigation, and (d) intraluminal instillation into the large intestine or abscess cavity. Antibacterial drugs may be administered preoperatively, perioperatively, and postoperatively to prevent infection (prophylaxis) or to treat already established infection.

The fundamental principles governing the use of antibiotics are (1) administration of an agent active against the infecting microorganism, (2) adequate contact between the drug and the infecting microbe, (3) absence of (or minimal) toxic side effects or complications for the patient, and (4) utilization of host defenses to augment antibacterial effects of the antibiotic. The specificity of the antibiotic for the infecting microorganism is based upon laboratory identification and antibiotic-sensitivity studies. Clinical judgment is called upon in serious, rapidly developing infections, such as gram-negative shock. The surgeon must administer an antibiotic known to be effective against microorganisms that may be involved in the infection even though the specific microorganism is unknown. Many surgical infections are polymicrobic, and often it is necessary to choose a single antibiotic or a combination of antibiotics that will cover the broad range of probable pathogens. If possible, cultures should be taken before antibiotic therapy is initiated. The antibiotic is changed, if necessary, when culture and sensitivity reports become available from the laboratory.

The antibiotic must come in contact with the infecting microorganism. In an acute, diffuse infection, blood flow into the area of infection will usually deliver adequate levels of systemic antibiotic. A spreading cellulitis with lymphangitis and lymphadenitis often responds within 24 h to an appropriate antibiotic. However, since antibiotics cannot penetrate a thick-walled pyogenic abscess or an infected serous cavity, they should be used in conjunction with drainage of the abscess, debridement of necrotic tissue, and removal of any foreign bodies. These principles apply to every organ of the body. A spreading infection of the meninges responds to chemotherapy, but a brain abscess must be drained; a staphylococcal septicemia is treated by chemotherapy, but a pulp abscess of the fingertip must be drained.

The surgeon must be aware of toxic complications of antibiotics and should be prepared to treat them. Toxic effects range from minor skin rashes, drug fever, and gas-

Table 5-3. ANTIBIOTICS: MODES OF ACTION

Cellular site of inhibition	Bactericidal	Bacteriostatic
Cell wall synthesis	Penicillins Cephalosporins Vancomycin Bacitracin	
Barrier function of cell membrane	Polymyxin B Colistin Amphotericin B	Nystatin
Protein synthesis in ribosome	Streptomycin Aminoglycosides	Tetracyclines Chloramphenicol Erythromycin Clindamycin
DNA replication in chromosome	Griseofulvin	

trointestinal disturbances to renal tubular necrosis, loss of vision and hearing, irreversible blood dyscrasias, and anaphylactic shock. In addition, alterations in the normal flora of the body may occur in patients receiving prolonged antibiotic therapy. In most cases these changes produce no ill result, but in some the alterations of flora result in the rapid overgrowth of virulent, antibiotic-resistant bacteria that may have been present originally in small numbers (colonization). If the patient's general resistance to infection is depressed, a new infection may follow the antibiotic-induced alteration of flora (superinfection). The term *colonization* indicates an antibiotic-induced quantitative change in the resident microflora of the patient, a common consequence of antimicrobial therapy. There is no clinical evidence of secondary infection, and discontinuance of the antibiotic usually allows the normal flora to become reestablished. However, there is the risk that colonization will lead to superinfection, a clinical event that may be of great danger to the patient. The term *superinfection* usually refers to a new microbial disease induced by antibiotic therapy. Superinfection is most frequent with broad-spectrum antibiotics. Inhibition of the normal flora allows proliferation of species and strains of bacteria not inhibited by the antibiotic. Superinfection is often due to gram-negative bacilli and fungi that are more difficult to eradicate than are gram-positive streptococci and pneumococci. Superinfection may be fatal, usually occurs in elderly patients, and often follows therapy with aminoglycoside antibiotics (e.g., gentamicin and kanamycin) and other broad-spectrum drugs (either alone or in combination with penicillin). Clinical evidence of secondary infection (i.e., a rise in temperature, increased peripheral white blood cell count, and physical signs of a disease not present at the beginning of antibiotic therapy) indicates that colonization has progressed to superinfection. Serial superinfections with different antibiotic-resistant microbial species may occur in the same patient.

Secondary or opportunistic infections may also occur in patients with noninfectious diseases. For example, mycotic infections may develop in patients with lymphoma or leukemia. Deficiencies in host resistance as a result of disease (e.g., diabetes mellitus, hematopoietic disorders, renal failure, liver disease) or as a consequence of therapy with radiation, antimetabolites, or corticosteroids confer the potential for pathogenicity on many ordinary nonpathogenic microorganisms. Indwelling venous or urinary catheters also contribute to lowered host resistance. The term *suprainfection* designates a secondary infection unrelated to antibiotic therapy.

Chemoprophylaxis

A prophylactic antibiotic is administered to an uninfected patient who is in jeopardy of acquiring a surgical infection. There is controversy regarding prophylactic antibiotic therapy because prophylaxis has not always been as valuable as therapeutic use. In surgical patients, prophylactic antibiotics are administered to treat contaminated or potentially contaminated wounds before infec-

tion occurs. Bacterial contamination is a component of every surgical wound, and may arise exogenously from the operating team or the environment through a flaw in aseptic surgical technique, or endogenously from the patient's skin, respiratory, gastrointestinal, or genitourinary tracts. The administration of antibiotic agents to prevent infection cannot be substituted for either sound surgical judgment or strict aseptic technique. Prophylactic antimicrobial use has no place in clean operative procedures or in those carrying a minimal risk of sepsis, but should be considered for operations involving trauma or severe burns and for operations in infected tissues or those associated with heavy contamination (e.g., operations involving the large intestine). An equally beneficial role for chemoprophylaxis is prior to operations in patients especially prone to infection because of malnutrition, impoverished blood supply, or preexisting infection remote from the operative site. Other patient-risk factors are obesity, old age, immunodeficient states, and shock. The patient undergoing immunosuppressive therapy and/or requiring insertion of a permanent prosthetic device is particularly prone to surgical infections. Other treatment-specific factors include use of steroids and antineoplastic agents, radiotherapy, and operative procedures of long duration, such as cardiac and vascular procedures.

Surgical wounds may be designated as "clean," "contaminated," or "dirty" depending upon the presence or absence of prior infection and contact with the interior of the respiratory, urinary, or gastrointestinal tracts. Traumatic wounds are usually grossly contaminated, whereas elective clean surgical procedures may be slightly contaminated during the operative procedure. Infection does not necessarily follow contamination, since host factors as well as microbial factors are involved. However, the greater the contamination, the greater the possibility of consequent infection. Accordingly, in surgery of traumatic wounds or in elective "contaminated" or "dirty" surgery, antibiotic therapy should be started before the operation so that adequate levels of antibiotic may be obtained in tissue and body fluids during the operative procedure to prevent colonization during bacterial seeding of the operative field. In procedures of long duration it is necessary to maintain tissue levels of the antibiotic by intraoperative administration of the antibiotic agent.

Antibiotics also may be administered postoperatively, but should be limited to reduce the probability of adverse effects, the emergence of resistant microorganisms, and superinfection.

A prophylactic antibiotic regimen may not be successful if the drug is not effective against all potential pathogens or if the agent does not come in contact with susceptible pathogens at the site of infection. The antibiotic should be administered parenterally and in sufficient dosage to achieve high circulating blood levels.

Prophylactic antimicrobials are currently used in the following areas:

Cardiovascular (valve and open heart, coronary artery bypass)
Orthopaedic (hip-fracture repair involving implantation of foreign material, total hip replacement)

Obstetric and gynecologic (vaginal hysterectomy, cesarean section)

Biliary tract (acute cholecystitis, obstructive jaundice, or stones in common duct without jaundice, when the patient is more than seventy years of age)

Gastrointestinal (gastric ulcer or carcinoma, colonic procedures in patients with unobstructed gastrointestinal tract, resection of oropharyngeal or laryngeal carcinoma)

Urologic (bacteriuric patients prior to urologic procedures)

Neurosurgical procedures of long duration

Intestinal Antisepsis

Intestinal antisepsis is a form of antimicrobial prophylaxis employed by the surgeon to lower the high rate of infectious complications after colorectal surgery. Intestinal antisepsis reduces the patient's normal intestinal flora so that there will be fewer microorganisms present in the large intestine to gain access to sterile tissues during minor, inadvertent intraoperative spills. In addition, the reduction of the patient's normal microflora provides a measure of protection to anastomoses during the immediate postoperative period.

The protocol for preoperative preparation of the unobstructed large intestine includes the specific prophylactic use of oral antibiotics. Bacterial infection following elective colonic surgery results from unavoidable seeding of the wound with contents of the colon. This is manifested by intraabdominal abscesses and anastomotic disruption with resultant peritonitis and fistula formation. The ideal antibiotic agent for preoperative preparation of the colon has rapid bactericidal activity against pathogens in the gastrointestinal tract, minimal absorption, and the absence of undesirable or toxic side effects.

The traditional protocol for intestinal antisepsis is now of historical interest only. It involved a 3-day period of hospitalization during which the patient was placed on a low-residue (or clear liquid) diet, given a cathartic and daily enemas, and administered suitable oral antibiotics for 72 h prior to operation. Although mechanical cleansing alone diminishes the volume of bulk feces and, consequently, the total number of fecal bacteria, the remaining feces contain the usual large number of bacteria (on the order of 10^{11} bacteria per gram of feces). Thus, the potential for postoperative sepsis remains a major hazard. We believe that oral prophylactic antibiotics and mechanical cleansing are both essential for effective preoperative preparation of the large intestine. The Nichols-Condon method is currently the most widely used. It consists of a 2-day fluid diet, mechanical preparation, and oral neomycin and erythromycin base administered on the second day to diminish aerobic and anaerobic colonic microflora. One gram of each antibiotic is given at 1, 2, and 11 P.M.; the operation is scheduled for 8 A.M. the next day.

Alternate methods of mechanical preparation include whole-gut irrigation with a polyethylene-glycol-electrolyte lavage solution (Golytely) beginning on the day before surgery. The patient ingests 1 L of chilled solution per hour for a maximum of 5 h or until the rectal effluent is completely clear. Moreover, intravenous antibiotics are used by some surgeons preoperatively and/or postop-

eratively as an adjunct to (or even as an alternative to) the oral preoperative antimicrobial agents. Reduction of colonic microflora by oral antibiotic and the provision of high tissue levels of antibiotic during the perioperative period are worthwhile objectives in aiding the patient to avoid wound sepsis.

Intestinal antisepsis has been shown to reduce the incidence of postoperative complications related to bacteria but does not protect against errors of surgical skill or judgment. Collected studies show that the average incidence of wound infection is 20 percent in patients placed on intestinal antisepsis as compared with 48 percent or less in patients not on any form of preoperative intestinal antisepsis. As new antibiotics become available it is likely that the optimal regimen for preoperative preparation of the bowel for colorectal operations will change, but the benefit of appropriate intestinal antisepsis in operations on the colon and rectum is well established.

Intraperitoneal Antibiotic Therapy

The most frequent indications for the intraperitoneal instillation of antibiotics are perforated and gangrenous appendicitis, perforated peptic ulcer, gangrenous intestinal obstruction, traumatic perforation of the gastrointestinal tract at any level, intraabdominal abscess, and excessive spillage associated with elective colonic, gastric, or small bowel surgery. Intraperitoneally administered antibiotics may be useful in pelvic inflammatory disease, acute pancreatitis, major intraabdominal vascular procedures, closure of evisceration, and repair of large abdominal incisional hernias. To be effective for routine intraperitoneal instillation, the antibiotic must provide adequate control of endogenous enteric bacteria that may be expected in the peritoneal cavity, with minimal accompanying pain and local or systemic reaction. Clinical success and safety have been achieved with kanamycin and also with cephalothin.

In recent years povidone-iodine and other iodophors have been used as antiseptic solutions to irrigate wounds as well as the peritoneal cavity in diffuse peritonitis. Subsequent laboratory studies, however, have demonstrated that intraperitoneal instillation of nonlethal doses of povidone-iodine antiseptic solution into the peritoneal cavity caused a uniformly fatal outcome within the succeeding 24 h. When saline solution was instilled in place of povidone-iodine antiseptic solution, the experimental animals survived an average of 96 h. The more rapid death after treatment with povidone-iodine was not associated with differences in peritoneal microflora but with peritoneal absorption of excessive amounts of iodine. Iodophors cannot be recommended for use intraperitoneally and have been shown to offer no therapeutic benefit when used to irrigate experimental wounds.

ANTIMICROBIAL AGENTS

Antibiotics and chemotherapeutic agents that are useful currently in surgical practice are described briefly in this section. It is important to use an antibiotic agent for a sensitive microorganism and not to treat a particular disease. Precise antimicrobial therapy is based upon the laboratory culture and sensitivity report. Table 5-4 is a guide to the activities of antibiotics against microorganisms commonly involved in surgical infections. Table 5-5 summarizes the routes of administration and the doses commonly employed. The selection of antibiotic and dosage for a specific infection depends upon clinical judgment, bacterial sensitivity tests, and awareness of the toxicity of the drug. The white blood cell count is important in evaluating the response to antibiotic treatment and the appearance of adverse reactions in patients with infections.

Penicillins

The penicillins all share the 6-aminopenicillanic acid nucleus in which the beta-lactam ring is essential for antibacterial activity. Penicillins are bactericidal for susceptible bacteria by binding to receptors and blocking the synthesis of bacterial cell wall mucopeptide, producing osmotic instability and causing lysis. At adequate concentrations, penicillins are bactericidal against sensitive microorganisms, and are most effective during the stage of active bacterial multiplication. Inadequate concentrations may produce only bacteriostatic effects. Microorganisms that are resistant to penicillins produce beta-lactamases that hydrolyze the beta-lactam ring of some penicillins and inactivate the drug. Penicillins can be arranged in several groups:

1. Those with highest activity against gram-positive microorganisms, but susceptible to hydrolysis by beta-lactamases (e.g., penicillin G)
2. Those relatively resistant to beta-lactamases, but of lower activity against gram-positive microorganisms, and inactive against gram-negative microorganisms (e.g., methicillin, nafcillin)
3. Those with relatively high activity against both gram-positive and gram-negative microorganisms, but destroyed by beta-lactamases (e.g., ampicillin, carbenicillin, ticarcillin)
4. Those stable to gastric acid and suitable for oral administration (e.g., penicillin V, cloxacillin, ampicillin)

Penicillin G (benzyl penicillin) is active against almost all gram-positive pathogens. It is well absorbed but is not suitable for oral administration because it is destroyed by gastric acidity. Penicillin G is injected intramuscularly or intravenously and becomes distributed throughout the body in a few minutes. Hypersensitivity to penicillin is an important problem and is usually manifested as urticaria, but almost any type of allergic response may develop. Anaphylactic reactions may occur in the highly sensitized patient within minutes after an injection, and will require subcutaneous epinephrine. Penicillin G is the drug of choice (provided hypersensitivity does not exist) for severe infections produced by pneumococci, streptococci, non-beta-lactamase-producing staphylococci, meningococci, gonococci, clostridia, actinomycetes, treponemata, and bacteroides (except *Bacteroides fragilis*).

Semisynthetic penicillins are prepared by adding side chains to the 6-aminopenicillanic acid nucleus. They combine one or more of the following advantages: (1) they are acid-resistant and suitable for oral use; (2) they exert prolonged action in the body; (3) they are resistant to the beta-lactamases produced by *Staphylococcus aureus* and some gram-negative bacteria. Cloxacillin or dicloxacillin are preferred for oral use against lactamase-producing staphylococci. For severe infections, however, a parenteral formulation of methicillin, oxacillin, or nafcillin should be used.

Ampicillin, amoxicillin, carbenicillin, and ticarcillin are hydrolyzed by beta-lactamases but have greater activity than penicillin G against gram-negative bacteria. Ampicillin is slightly less active than penicillin G against most gram-positive bacteria. It is bacteriostatic in vitro against *Streptococcus faecalis* but is bactericidal in combination with an aminoglycoside. This combination is widely used to combat surgical sepsis. The ampicillin covers gram-positive species, particularly *Streptococcus faecalis;* the aminoglycoside covers facultative gram-negative species. Amoxicillin is similar to ampicillin. Carbenicillin resembles ampicillin but is more active against *Pseudomonas* and *Proteus* species; *Klebsiella* species are usually resistant. Ticarcillin resembles carbenicillin but is more active in vitro, requiring one-fourth to one-half the concentration of carbenicillin to kill *Pseudomonas aeruginosa.* Timentin is a parenteral combination of ticarcillin with clavulanic acid (as the potassium salt), a beta-lactamase inhibitor. The addition of clavulanate protects the ticarcillin from inactivation and extends its antibacterial spectrum, giving coverage of some *Enterobacteriaceae* (especially *Klebsiella*) and *Staphylococcus aureus* while retaining coverage against gram-positive cocci, including enterococci. The combination of amoxillin and clavulanate (Augmentin) provides an oral drug with activity against *S. aureus, Haemophilus influenzae,* and penicillinase-producing neisseriae. Despite the extended coverage provided by these combinations with clavulanate, older drugs and drug combinations may be equally effective.

Other new extended-spectrum penicillins include azlocillin, mezlocillin, and piperacillin. These are more active in vitro than carbenicillin or ticarcillin against gram-negatives such as *Klebsiella, Serratia,* and *Pseudomonas aeruginosa.* These newer agents are indicated in the treatment of infections caused by ticarcillin-resistant microorganisms.

Cephalosporins

The cephalosporins and cephamycins are related to the penicillins. In place of a 6-aminopenicillanic acid nucleus they have a nucleus of 7-aminocephalosporanic acid. They are bactericidal, and their mode of action is similar to that of penicillins, namely, inhibition of bacterial cell wall synthesis. A bewildering number of new semisynthetic cephalosporins have been developed and have entered into clinical practice since cephalothin was introduced in 1964. They are arranged into generations based on their expanding activity against gram-negative bacteria

Table 5-4. ANTIBIOTICS USEFUL AGAINST MICROORGANISMS IN SURGICAL INFECTIONS

Microorganism	First choice	Alternative agents
Gram-positive cocci:		
Staphylococcus aureus		
Lactamase-producing	Methicillin, nafcillin, oxacillin	A cephalosporin, clindamycin, vancomycin
Non-lactamase-producing	Penicillin G or V	A cephalosporin, clindamycin, vancomycin
Streptococcus pyogenes	Penicillin G or ampicillin	An erythromycin, a cephalosporin, vancomycin
Streptococcus pneumoniae	Penicillin G or V	An erythromycin, a cephalosporin, chloramphenicol
Streptococcus viridans	Penicillin G	An erythromycin, a cephalosporin, vancomycin
Streptococcus faecalis	Ampicillin or penicillin G with gentamicin or streptomycin	Vancomycin with gentamicin or streptomycin
Peptostreptococcus spp.	Penicillin G	Clindamycin, a tetracycline, chloramphenicol
Gram-negative cocci:		
Neisseria gonorrhoeae	Amoxicillin or ceftriaxone	Ampicillin, cefoxitin, chloramphenicol
Neisseria meningitidis	Penicillin G	Chloramphenicol
Gram-positive rods:		
Clostridium spp.	Penicillin G	Clindamycin, metronidazole, a tetracycline
Clostridium tetani	Penicillin G	A tetracycline
Clostridium difficile	Vancomycin	Metronidazole
Gram-negative rods:		
Acinetobacter spp.	Gentamicin	Amikacin, doxycycline
Bacteroides spp.		
Oropharyngeal strains	Penicillin G	Clindamycin, metronidazole, cefoxitin
Gastrointestinal strains	Clindamycin or metronidazole	Chloramphenicol, cefoxitin, ticarcillin
Campylobacter fetus	An erythromycin	A tetracycline, chloramphenicol
Enterobacter-Klebsiella-Serratia group	Ampicillin alone or with an aminoglycoside	Carbenicillin, ticarcillin, mezlocillin, or piperacillin alone or with an aminoglycoside, chloramphenicol
Escherichia coli	Ampicillin alone or with an aminoglycoside	Carbenicillin, ticarcillin, mezlocillin, or piperacillin alone or with an aminoglycoside, chloramphenicol
Fusobacterium spp.	Penicillin G	Clindamycin, metronidazole, chloramphenicol
Proteus mirabilis	Ampicillin	An aminoglycoside, carbenicillin, ticarcillin, mezlocillin, or piperacillin; a cephalosporin, chloramphenicol
Proteus spp. (indol-positive)	An aminoglycoside	Carbenicillin, ticarcillin, mezlocillin, or piperacillin; a cephalosporin, chloramphenicol
Providencia spp.	An aminoglycoside	Carbenicillin, ticarcillin, mezlocillin, or piperacillin; a cephalosporin, chloramphenicol
Pseudomonas aeruginosa	Gentamicin, tobramycin, or netlimicin, with carbenicillin, ticarcillin, mezlocillin, or piperacillin	Amikacin with carbenicillin, ticarcillin, mezlocillin, or piperacillin
Salmonella spp.	Ampicillin or amoxicillin	Chloramphenicol, trimethoprim-sulfamethoxazole
Actinomyces:		
Actinomyces israelii	Penicillin G	A tetracycline
Nocardia spp.	Sulfonamides	Trimethoprim-sulfamethoxazole, ampicillin
Fungi:		
Blastomyces dermatitidis	Amphotericin B	Ketoconazole
Candida albicans and other yeasts	Amphotericin B (± flucytosine)	Ketoconazole, miconazole (topical), nystatin (oral or topical)
Coccidioides immitis	Amphotericin B	Miconazole, ketoconazole
Cryptococcus neoformans	Amphotericin B (± flucytosine)	Ketoconazole, miconazole
Histoplasma capsulatum	Amphotericin B	Ketoconazole
Mucor spp.; *Rhizopus* spp.; *Aspergillus* spp.	Amphotericin B	
Paracoccidioides brasiliensis	Amphotericin B	Miconazole, ketoconazole
Sporotrichus schenckii	Potassium iodide	Amphotericin B

Table 5-5. ROUTES OF ADMINISTRATION AND DAILY DOSAGE OF ANTIBIOTICS COMMONLY USED IN ADULT SURGICAL PATIENTS HAVING NORMAL RENAL FUNCTION

Drug (trade name)	Oral	Intramuscular	Intravenous
Amikacin (Amiken)		15 mg/kg/day	15 mg/kg/day
Amoxicillin (Amoxil; others)	750–1500 mg/day		
Amphotericin (Fungizone)			0.25–1.5 mg/kg/day
Ampicillin (Polycillin; others)	1.2 g/day	150–200 mg/kg/day	150–200 mg/kg/day
Azlocillin (Azlin)			225–300 mg/kg/day
Carbenicillin (Geopen)		200–500 mg/kg/day	200–500mg/kg/day
Cefamandole (Mandol)		4–12 g/day	4–12 g/day
Cefazolin (Ancef, Kefzol)		1–10 g/day	1–10 g/day
Cefonicid (Monocid)		2–4 g/day	2–4 g/day
Cefoperazone (Cefobid)		2–4 g/day	2–4 g/day
Ceforanide (Precef)		1–2 g/day	1–2 g/day
Cefotaxime (Claforan)		2–12 g/day	2–12 g/day
Cefotetan (Apacef)		1–2 g/day	1–2 g/day
Cefoxitin (Mefoxin)		4–12 g/day	4–12 g/day
Ceftazidime (Fortaz)		2–6 g/day	2–6 g/day
Ceftizoxime (Cefizox)		2–12 g/day	2–12 g/day
Ceftriaxone (Rocephin)		1–2 g/day	1–2 g/day
Cefuroxime (Zinacef)		3–6 g/day	3–6 g/day
Cephalexin (Keflex)	1–4 g/day		
Chloramphenicol (Chloromycetin)	50–100 mg/kg/day		50–100 mg/kg/day
Clindamycin (Cleocin)	600–1800 mg/kg/day	600–2700 mg/kg/day	600–2700 mg/kg/day
Cloxacillin (Tegopen)	1–2 g/day		
Doxycycline (Vibramycin)	100–200 mg/day		100–200 mg/day
Erythromycin (Erythrocin; others)	1–2 g/day		1–2 g/day
Flucytosine (Ancobon)	50–150 mg/kg/day		
Gentamicin (Garamycin)		3–5 mg/kg/day	3–5 mg/kg/day
Kanamycin (Kantrex)		15 mg/kg/day	15 mg/kg/day
Ketoconazole (Nizoral)	200–1000 mg/day		
Methicillin (Staphcillin; others)		4–6 g/day	4–6 g/day
Metronidazole (Flagyl)	30 mg/kg/day		30 mg/kg/day
Mezlocillin (Mezlin)		16–18 g/day	16–18 g/day
Miconazole (Monistat)			600–3600 mg/day
Moxalactam (Moxam)		2–12 g/day	2–12 g/day
Nafcillin (Nafcil, Unipen)	Not recommended	2–6 g/day	2–6 g/day
Netlimicin (Netromycin)		3–6 mg/kg/day	3–6 mg/kg/day
Oxacillin (Prostaphlin)	2–6 g/day	2–6 g/day	2–6 g/day
Penicillin G		100,000–200,000 units/kg/day	100,000–300,000 units/kg/day
Piperacillin (Piperacil)		12–18 g/day	12–18 g/day
Streptomycin		2–4 g/day	Not recommended
Tetracycline (Achromycin; others)	1–2 g/day	Not recommended	1–2 g/day
Ticarcillin (Ticar)		200–300 mg/kg/day	200–300 mg/kg/day
Tobramycin (Nebcin)		3–5 mg/kg/day	3–5 mg/kg/day
Vancomycin (Vancocin)	1–2 g/day		2–3 g/day

(Table 5-6). All first-generation drugs have a similar spectrum, including activity against many gram-positive cocci (but not enterococci or methicillin-resistant *Staphylococcus aureus*), *Escherichia coli*, *Klebsiella pneumoniae*, and *Proteus mirabilis*. The presence of food in the stomach delays and reduces the peak serum level of the few oral cephalosporins by one-third. Most cephalosporins, however, are poorly absorbed from the gastrointestinal tract and must be given parenterally. Pain restricts intramuscular use for most of these drugs. The exception is cefazolin, which is best tolerated by this route. Cefazolin is as effective as cephalothin and is cheaper. Although all cephalosporins have activity against many gram-positive bacteria, the first-generation drugs are more active in this area than later drugs. On the other hand, the first-generation drugs have activity against only a few gram-negative

species, and of these many strains of *Escherichia coli*, *Klebsiella pneumoniae*, and *Proteus mirabilis* are now resistant to them. The first-generation cephalosporins are inactive against gram-negatives seen in nosocomial infections or against *Bacteroides fragilis*.

The second-generation cephalosporins have a wider spectrum against gram-negatives and are moderately active against many, including *E. coli*, *Klebsiella*, *Citrobacter*, *Enterobacter*, and *Proteus mirabilis*. Although cefamandole has been recommended for empiric therapy for patients having abdominal, pelvic, or cardiovascular surgery, other regimens provide better coverage and/or are less expensive. Cefamandole should not be used to treat intraabdominal infections caused by anaerobic bacteria. Cefoxitin can be used as a single agent in the treatment of most mixed aerobic-anaerobic infections of the skin and

Table 5-6. SOME CEPHALOSPORIN ANTIBIOTICS

Generic name	Trade name	Route of administration
First generation:		
Cephalothin	Keflin	I.M., I.V.
Cefazolin	Ancef, Kefzol	I.M., I.V.
Cephapirin	Cefadyl	I.M., I.V.
Cephadrine	Anspor, Velosef	P.O., I.M., I.V.
Cephalexin	Keflex	P.O.
Cefadroxil	Duricef, Ultracef	P.O.
Second generation:		
Cefamandole	Mandol	I.M., I.V.
Cefoxitin	Mefoxin	I.M., I.V.
Cefuroxime	Zinacef	I.M., I.V.
Ceforanide	Precef	I.M., I.V.
Cefonicid	Monocid	I.M., I.V.
Cefotetan	Apacef	I.M., I.V.
Cefaclor	Ceclor	P.O.
Third generation:		
Cefotaxime	Claforan	I.M., I.V.
Ceftizoxime	Cefizox	I.M., I.V.
Cefoperazone	Cefobid	I.M., I.V.
Moxalactam	Moxam	I.M., I.V.
Ceftazidime	Fortaz	I.M., I.V.
Ceftriaxone	Rocephin	I.M., I.V.

soft tissues, pelvic infections, and community-acquired abdominal sepsis. For nosocomial intraabdominal sepsis an aminoglycoside should be added to the regimen to expand the coverage for aerobic gram-negative bacilli. Neither cefamandole nor cefoxitin should be used to treat bacterial meningitis or infections caused by enterococci or methicillin-resistant *S. aureus*. Cefoxitin can be used in the prevention of infection after fecal soilage of the peritoneum due to trauma. It can be used to prevent infections in patients who cannot take oral neomycin-erythromycin bowel preparation owing to emergency operations or intestinal obstruction (Sanders et al.). The antibacterial spectrum of cefonicid is similar to that of cefamandole, but cefonicid has a half-life 6 to 10 times that of cefamandole. Accordingly, the typical dosing schedule with cefonicid is 1 to 2 g I.V. or I.M. q 24 h as contrasted to q 6 h for cefamandole.

The third-generation cephalosporins are newer and exhibit a wider spectrum against gram-negative bacilli than do the first- and second-generation drugs. For example, the third-generation drugs are a major therapeutic advance in the treatment of gram-negative meningitis, are very active against *Haemophilus influenzae* (including penicillinase-producing strains), and are more efficacious than the older cephalosporins in treating infection caused by gram-negative bacilli resistant to multiple antibiotics (i.e., nosocomial pathogens). This owes to their greater beta-lactamase stability and their high affinities for penicillin-binding proteins. These newer drugs, however, also display decreased activity against staphylococci, and their activity against gram-negative bacilli is often less predictable than that of the aminoglycosides. Their activity against anaerobes is inferior to that of cefoxitin, a

cheaper second-generation drug. Ceftizoxime, cefoperazone, and moxalactam have relatively long half-lives and may be administered on a q 8- to 12-h dosing schedule. Cefotaxime has a shorter half-life and should be administered on a q 4- to 6-h schedule. At our hospital ceftizoxime is restricted for use in treating infections due to gram-negative bacilli resistant to cefazolin and cefuroxime; cefoperazone may be used combined with an aminoglycoside in treating pseudomonal infections involving skin, soft tissues, and bones and joints in penicillin-allergic patients; cefotaxime is restricted for use in treating meningitis due to gram-negative bacilli; and ceftriaxone, which has a half-life of 6 to 9 h and may be administered once daily, is reserved for treating infections due to gram-negative bacilli resistant to cefazolin and cefuroxime. The third-generation cephalosporins have no place in the treatment of gram-positive or anaerobic infections, most community-acquired infections, or surgical prophylaxis. Based on their toxicities, moxalactam should be avoided and cefoperazone used with caution. The third-generation drugs are not cost-effective in most situations. Their economies in dosage because of long half-lives are offset by their high cost per gram and the frequent necessity of combining them with an aminoglycoside.

Erythromycins

Erythromycin is a macrocyclic lactone (i.e., a macrolide). It is active against pneumococci, beta-hemolytic streptococci, enterococci, many staphylococci, and clostridia. Erythromycin is bacteriostatic but may be bactericidal in higher concentrations, inhibiting bacterial protein synthesis. The antibiotic is uniformly distributed throughout the body and is excreted in the urine and bile. However, the major portion of the drug is metabolized in the body. Erythromycin base is generally well tolerated but may cause some gastrointestinal disturbance (nausea, vomiting, diarrhea, flatulence). Erythromycin is useful in pneumococcal and streptococcal infection, as a second choice in patients sensitive to penicillin, and for elimination of corynebacteria from the pharynx of carriers. Bacterial resistance to erythromycin is common during long-term treatment. Erythromycin is the agent of choice for treatment of mycoplasmal infections and Legionnaires' disease. It is useful in the treatment of actinomycosis.

Tetracyclines

The tetracyclines are a family of closely related antibiotics. Those now widely used are tetracycline, oxytetracycline, and doxycycline. There is no good evidence that tetracycline has any advantage over oxytetracycline in the treatment of disease or in the production of fewer side effects in the adult. Doxycycline possesses the advantage, because of its slower excretion, of requiring only one dose daily. Members of this group are broad-spectrum and active against those gram-positive species that are also sensitive to penicillin, against many gram-negative species that are not sensitive to penicillin, against *Treponema pallidum* and other treponemata, and against

Mycobacterium tuberculosis. They also inhibit the growth of actinomycetes, rickettsiae, mycoplasma, and agents of the psittacosis-lymphogranuloma venereum-trachoma group of *Chlamydia.* The tetracyclines are bacteriostatic. They interfere with protein synthesis by inhibiting amino acid transfer from RNA to microsomal protein. Resistance may be due to decreased permeability to the antibiotic. A microorganism resistant to one tetracycline is equally resistant to the others. Tetracyclines are usually administered orally; they become distributed throughout the body and appear to have affinity for fast-growing tissues, such as liver, tumors, and new bone. Tetracyclines (with the exception of doxycycline) are to be avoided in renal failure. Tetracyclines are deposited in teeth during early stages of calcification, causing a yellow to brownish discoloration that is undesirable cosmetically. Therefore, tetracycline treatment should be avoided in early childhood except for imperative reasons or when a short course will suffice. Liver damage has resulted from excessive doses. Replacement of suppressed normal flora by tetracycline-resistant microorganisms causes gastrointestinal disturbances such as nausea, vomiting, diarrhea, and flatulence. Superinfection with *Candida albicans* may produce soreness of the mouth and even thrush, which may spread to the pharynx and bronchi, or diarrhea and pruritus ani. Superinfection with *Proteus* and *Pseudomonas* species resistant to tetracycline commonly produces diarrhea. Superinfection with *Staphylococcus aureus* may produce a fatal staphylococcal enterocolitis. Activity against anaerobes is erratic. Tetracycline with penicillin is recommended for actinomycosis and, with sulfadiazine, for nocardiosis.

Chloramphenicol

Chloramphenicol is a broad-spectrum antibiotic; it is bacteriostatic and inhibits protein synthesis by interfering with messenger ribonucleic acid (mRNA). It is well absorbed orally and parenterally. About 90 percent can be detected in urine as an inactive conjugate with glucuronic acid; only about 10 percent appears as active antibiotic. Two different lethal toxic effects are known: First, a rare total aplasia of the bone marrow with aplastic anemia may occur during treatment or as long as 4 months afterward. Second, because of deficiency in detoxifying enzymes, premature infants may accumulate sufficient free chloramphenicol to cause an acute and usually fatal circulatory collapse (gray syndrome). Minor toxic effects include soreness of the mouth from overgrowth of *Candida albicans,* resulting from depression of normal flora due to antibiotic in the saliva, and optic neuritis in children with cystic fibrosis of the pancreas receiving treatment with chloramphenicol for pulmonary infection. Chloramphenicol should not be used for trivial infections or as a prophylactic agent to prevent bacterial infection. Chloramphenicol is the drug of choice for typhoid fever and other severe *Salmonella* infections, but since most *Salmonella* infections will respond to ampicillin, chloramphenicol should be used only if the patient does not respond to ampicillin or is allergic to it. Chloramphenicol is recommended for patients who cannot tolerate tetracyclines and for those who have rickettsial disease, psittacosis, or lymphopathia venereum. It can be a life-saving drug in the treatment of patients with meningitis when penicillin cannot be administered. Chloramphenicol is the drug of choice in the treatment of severe infections caused by such microorganisms as *Haemophilus influenzae* in patients allergic to penicillin. Prolonged usage and repeated exposure should be avoided. White cell count and differential should be taken daily, and therapy should be discontinued if leukopenia occurs.

Aminoglycosides

The aminoglycosides are bactericidal antibiotics having similar structural, antimicrobial, pharmacologic, and toxic characteristics, and include streptomycin, neomycin, kanamycin, gentamicin, tobramycin, amikacin, and netlimicin. These agents inhibit protein synthesis in bacteria by disorganizing the proper attachment of mRNA to the bacterial ribosome. Resistance to aminoglycosides is based upon either (1) a deficiency of ribosomal receptor; or (2) enzymatic destruction of the drug (plasmid mediated) by adenylylation (nucleotidylation) of hydroxyl groups, acetylation of amino groups, and phosphorylation of hydroxyl groups; or (3) impermeability to the drug or failure of active transport across cell membranes. The aminoglycosides possess a wide range of bactericidal activity against gram-negative and gram-positive bacteria and mycobacteria. There is little absorption from the alimentary tract and fairly slow renal excretion in unchanged form after intramuscular injection. This affords therapeutic levels for 6 to 8 h. Aminoglycosides exhibit a high degree of mutual cross resistance, a strong dose-related tendency to damage the auditory branch of the eighth nerve, and some possibility of damage to the kidney. This nephrotoxicity is indicated with rising serum creatinine levels or reduced creatinine clearance.

The use of streptomycin is now limited by its toxicity to the initial treatment of tuberculosis as a second or third drug, and is the drug of first choice in the treatment of infections due to *Pasteurella* species (i.e., tularemia, plague). Neomycin is used now only topically in ointments and orally (in conjunction with erythromycin base) for intestinal antisepsis to prepare the colon for elective surgery.

Kanamycin is closely related to neomycin but is less toxic. It is bactericidal for most gram-negative bacilli and has a spectrum of usefulness similar to amikacin or gentamicin, with the exception of *Pseudomonas aeruginosa,* against which kanamycin is ineffective. Kanamycin is completely absorbed following parenteral injection and is rapidly excreted in the urine.

Gentamicin is produced by a *Micromonospora.* This is designated by the suffix "micin," whereas the suffix "mycin" indicates derivation from a *Streptomyces.* Gentamicin is used in severe infections caused by gram-negative bacteria that are likely to be resistant to other, less toxic drugs. It is administered by intramuscular or intravenous injection and becomes well distributed. Gentamicin is almost quantitatively excreted unchanged in the urine, principally by glomerular filtration. The drug may be synergistic with beta-lactam antibiotics, such as cephalosporins or carbenicillin, against *Klebsiella* and *Pseudomonas,* respectively. Tobramycin is virtually identical with gentamicin in antibacterial activity but is less nephrotoxic. Netlimicin is similar in activity to gentamicin and to tobramycin. Amikacin is a semisynthetic derivative of kanamycin. It is relatively resistant to several of the enzymes that inactivate gentamicin, tobramycin and netlimicin, and can therefore be used against many strains of gram-negative bacilli to which these aminoglycosides are resistant. Parenteral aminoglycosides are among the most valuable agents available for the treatment of life-threatening infections by enteric gram-negative bacteria. Because of the emergence of resistant strains of *Pseudomonas, Proteus, Providencia,* and *Serratia,* hospitals usually designate a single aminoglycoside antibiotic, such as gentamicin, for primary use and hold the others in reserve for use against infections caused by resistant bacteria. Amikacin is preferred for nosocomial infections by gram-negative pathogens in severely ill, hospitalized patients.

Polypeptide Antibiotics

The polymyxins are basic polypeptides especially useful against *Pseudomonas aeruginosa.* They are bactericidal for most gram-negative bacteria, except *Proteus* species and *Neisseria* species. Fungi and all gram-positive bacteria are resistant. Polymyxin B and colistimethate (polymyxin E) have similar antibacterial activities. They are not absorbed from the alimentary tract but are well absorbed following intramuscular injection. The polymyxins are toxic, usually producing paresthesias, dizziness, and flushing, and nephrotoxicity and respiratory arrest following high dosages. The introduction of broad-spectrum penicillins, cephalosporins, and aminoglycosides has lessened the importance of polymyxins in the treatment of pseudomonal infections, and practically eliminated their need in clinical medicine.

Bacitracin is a bactericidal, polypeptide antibiotic active against gram-positive bacteria, including beta-lactamase-producing staphylococci, but inactive against common gram-negative bacilli. It is absorbed to only a slight extent from the alimentary tract, skin, wounds, or mucous membranes. Systemic administration of bacitracin is no longer used because of severe nephrotoxicity, but it is useful for irrigating wounds, infected joints, or abscess cavities. Bacitracin in ointment base is used topically, combined with neomycin or polymyxin, in treating infected wounds, suppurative conjunctivitis, and superficial infections.

Specialized Drugs

Lincomycin and clindamycin are lincosamides. They closely resemble erythromycin (although different in structure) in antibacterial activity against gram-positive microorganisms, become widely distributed in tissues, and are excreted through the bile. Because lincomycin is less active in vitro and has no clinical advantage over clindamycin, its use is not recommended. Clindamycin is useful primarily in the treatment of anaerobic infections, including those caused by *Bacteroides fragilis.* Mixed intraabdominal infections caused by anaerobes and aerobic gram-negative bacilli may be treated with clindamycin and an aminoglycoside. Infections such as aspiration pneumonia and anaerobic pleuropulmonary infections are best treated with penicillin, but the alternate agent of choice is clindamycin. Although clindamycin is active in vitro against streptococci, including pneumococci, alternative agents, such as erythromycin, are potentially less toxic. Bloody diarrhea with pseudomembranous colitis has been associated with clindamycin (as well as other antibiotics). This is due to a necrotizing toxin produced by *Clostridium difficile,* which is resistant to clindamycin and which becomes the predominant clostridial flora of the intestine during oral as well as parenteral administration of clindamycin.

Vancomycin is bactericidal for gram-positive microorganisms, including staphylococci, streptococci, and clostridia. It inhibits the synthesis of bacterial cell walls, but by a mechanism different from that of the penicillins. Vancomycin is regarded as a reserve antibiotic that is valuable in the treatment of life-threatening infections with multiresistant staphylococci and with streptococci (including *Streptococcus faecalis* endocarditis) in patients who are allergic to penicillin. The drug is administered intravenously. Since it is not absorbed from the gastrointestinal tract, oral administration is useful for the treatment of antibiotic-associated pseudomembranous colitis (caused by overgrowth of *Clostridium difficile*). Ototoxicity has been associated with prolonged serum concentrations greater than 60 to 80 μg/mL. Serum levels should be obtained. The serum half-life is prolonged in anuric patients.

Metronidazole (Flagyl) is a 5-nitroimidazole widely used in the treatment of trichomonal vaginitis, intestinal amebiasis, and giardiasis. It has become prominent because of its bactericidal action against all clinically important obligate anaerobic bacteria, such as *Bacteroides fragilis* and other species of bacteroides, fusobacteria, and clostridia. *Proprionibacterium, Actinomyces,* and microaerophilic streptococci are resistant. Metronidazole is the only drug exhibiting consistent bactericidal activity against *Bacteroides fragilis* at or close to the minimal inhibitory concentration. Its bactericidal activity depends on products resulting from the reduction of the 5-nitro group intracellularly at the low oxidation-reduction potential occurring within anaerobic microorganisms. This bactericidal metabolite is produced in both dividing and nondividing anaerobes.

Metronidazole has been used prophylactically in the perioperative period to prevent postoperative morbidity in patients undergoing elective colorectal and gynecologic operations. It has been given both intravenously and as a rectal suppository. Good results have been obtained in treating anaerobic and mixed aerobic-anaerobic infections, such as wound infections, abdominal abscesses, liver abscesses, perirectal abscesses, and decubitus ulcers. Metronidazole readily crosses the blood-brain barrier and has been effective in treating nontraumatic brain abscesses. Metronidazole may also be of value in dental surgery in decreasing the incidence of anaerobic infections. A combination of metronidazole and gentamicin is a relatively inexpensive, primary approach to treating intraabdominal and other polymicrobic infections. Metronidazole may cause peripheral neuropathy and convulsions in long-term therapy, and phlebitis if not buffered with sodium bicarbonate, but moderate reactions such as vomiting, diarrhea, and skin rash are more prevalent. Patients taking metronidazole should be warned against the use of alcohol because of the possibility of a disulfiram-like reaction. Although vancomycin is currently recommended for treating antibiotic-associated pseudomembranous colitis, metronidazole, which is much less expensive, may be used as an effective alternative treatment.

Imipenem is the first of a new class of beta-lactam antibiotics called carbapenems. It has the broadest antibacterial spectrum of any beta-lactam antibiotic now available (Barza). This includes gram-positive cocci (except methicillin-resistant staphylococci and some enterococci), gram-negative cocci, *Enterobacteriaceae, Pseudomonas aeruginosa,* and anaerobic bacilli including *Bacteroides fragilis.* Imipenem is administered intravenously in combination with an equal amount of cilastatin. The cilastatin inhibits renal tubular metabolism of imipenem, preventing the formation of potentially nephrotoxic compounds. Imipenem has been effective in treating mixed bacterial infections for which a combination of antibiotics, often including an aminoglycoside, are usually necessary—for example, pulmonary, gynecologic, and intraabdominal infections.

Antifungal Antibiotics

Antibiotics generally have no effect on pathogenic fungi, with the exception of the penicillins, which can be used to treat actinomycosis, and the sulfonamides, which can be used for nocardiosis. Pathogenic fungi are susceptible only to certain highly specialized drugs that usually have no antibacterial activity.

Amphotericin B is the only antifungal antibiotic effective in the treatment of systemic mycotic infections. It binds to sterols, specifically ergosterol, and interferes with the permeability of the fungal cell wall. Amphotericin B is the drug of choice for treatment of systemic candidosis, mucormycosis, disseminated active histoplasmosis, cryptococcosis, coccidioidomycosis, and pulmonary sporotrichosis. Amphotericin B is not appreciably absorbed from the gastrointestinal tract or the skin; it is administered intravenously or intrathecally, or instilled directly into the site of infection. Initial toxic effects commonly include fever, chills, nausea, vomiting, and headache. Toxic effects brought on by continued use may include anemia, thrombophlebitis at the site of injection, hypokalemia, rise of blood urea and serum creatinine levels, and permanent damage to the kidney.

Griseofulvin has its greatest activity against growing dermatophytes and is useful in treating superficial dermatomycoses of skin, hair, or nails due to species of *Mi-*crosporum, Epidermophyton, and Trichophyton. Griseofulvin is fungicidal, binds to RNA, impairs synthesis of nucleic acids and protein, and breaks down intracellular membranes of dermatophytes, but not of fungi causing systemic mycoses. This antifungal antibiotic is administered orally and is incorporated into liver, fat, keratin, and skeletal muscle. It is well tolerated even during long courses of treatment, and toxic effects (skin reactions, gastric discomfort, and neurologic reactions) are uncommon and rarely severe. Cultures are needed to determine that skin lesions are not due to *Candida* or bacteria, as these are not improved by griseofulvin and may be exacerbated by the antibiotic.

Nystatin is effective in the treatment of candidosis. It is fungistatic and damages the fungal cell membrane by binding to sterol sites in it. This antifungal antibiotic is not absorbed from the gastrointestinal tract, skin, or mucosal surfaces. It is used to treat gastrointestinal candidosis, which may result as a complication of therapy with broad-spectrum antibiotics. Such antibiotic-induced superinfection often disappears with discontinuance of the antibacterial therapy that provoked it. Nystatin is available in topical powders, creams, and ointments that may be useful in treating cutaneous and mucocutaneous aerueous candidosis. Nystatin tablets may be sucked for candida stomatitis; vaginal tablets are available for treatment of vaginal candidosis. Nystatin is harmless by local application. There have been rare cases of diarrhea, nausea, and vomiting after administration of large oral doses.

Flucytosine (5-fluorocytosine) is a halogenated pyrimidine inhibiting nucleic acid synthesis in yeastlike fungi. It is administered orally; there is good absorption and relatively low toxicity. Flucytosine may be effective for treatment of cryptococcosis and candidosis, but, when used alone, resistant organisms may emerge during therapy. However, the combination of amphotericin B plus flucytosine results in additive or even synergistic effects in systemic mycoses, reduces the dose requirement of amphotericin B alone, and may delay the emergence of resistance to flucytosine.

Miconazole and ketoconazole are imidazole derivatives having a broad spectrum of activity against dermatophytes, dimorphic fungi, yeast, and some bacteria. Miconazole is useful topically in the treatment of cutaneous and mucocutaneous candidal infections. Miconazole also can be given intravenously for the treatment of coccidioidomycosis, cryptococcosis, and candidosis when amphotericin B has failed or is contraindicated. Ketoconazole is clinically useful in the management of mucocutaneous candidosis, histoplasmosis, paracoccidioidomycosis, and dermatophytic infections. Therapeutic levels in blood are rapidly obtained after a single oral dose and are maintained for several hours.

Sulfonamides

Introduced in 1935, the sulfonamides initiated the modern antibacterial chemotherapeutic revolution in medicine. Their use antedates that of the antibiotics by several years, since penicillin did not become available until 1941. The sulfonamides are valuable agents in the management of some infections, particularly urinary tract infections due to *Escherichia coli,* and can be employed for the prophylaxis of recurrences of rheumatic fever. Although one of these compounds, mafenide acetate (Sulfamylon), has an important use in the topical therapy of severe burn wounds, the value of the sulfonamides in the treatment of surgical infections is severely limited by their inactivation by pus. The sulfonamides are bacteriostatic and active against both gram-positive and gram-negative bacteria. The drugs are strongly antagonized by *p*-aminobenzoic acid (PABA), an essential intermediate in the synthesis of folic acid by bacterial cells, and act as competitive inhibitors. Bacteria sensitive to the sulfonamides are unable to utilize preformed folic acid in the body and must synthesize it themselves. Folic acid acts as a coenzyme in the transfer of fragments containing one carbon atom, which are involved in the synthesis of amino acids (such as methionine and serine), purines, and thymine. These compounds also inhibit the activity of sulfonamides, but unlike PABA they are noncompetitive inhibitors, and their effect is not reversed by increasing the concentration of drugs. Accordingly, pus, which is rich in amino acids and purines made available by the breakdown of cellular protein and nucleic acids, inactivates the sulfonamides.

Some of the sulfonamides of use in surgical practice are sulfisoxazole (Gantrisin) and sulfamethoxazole (Gantanol), which are used for treating urinary tract infections, and mafenide (Sulfamylon), which is applied topically and used to treat burn wound infections. Mafenide is not inhibited by the products of tissue necrosis but causes pain. Of comparable value in the treatment of burns is the silver salt of sulfadiazine (Silvadene), which does not cause pain on application and is free of major toxicity.

Orally administered sulfonamides are rapidly absorbed in the stomach and duodenum and become distributed in all tissues and fluids. The sulfonamides are bound to either serum albumin or to tissue proteins, and they are detoxified in the liver. Both the drug and its less active metabolites are excreted by glomerular filtration. Sensitivity to one sulfonamide frequently confers sensitivity to others. Toxic reactions limiting sulfonamide therapy range from nausea, vomiting, and dermatitis to crystalluria, renal injury, hepatic damage, and hematologic disorders.

A fixed-dose combination of trimethoprim-sulfamethoxazole (Bactrim, Septra) is available in tablets for oral administration and also in a parenteral formulation. This combination is useful for the treatment of severe urinary tract infections, bronchitis in adults, pneumonia caused by *Pneumocystis carinii* (a presumed protozoan), and shigellosis. Trimethoprim-sulfamethoxazole is the drug of choice in typhoid fever with strains of *Salmonella typhi* resistant to both chloramphenicol and ampicillin.

STREPTOCOCCAL INFECTIONS

Streptococci form the dominant aerobic flora of the mouth and pharyngeal areas of human beings. They are gram-positive spherical or ovoid cells (rarely elongated into rods) arranged in pairs (short chains). Long chains are observed when the organism is cultured in fluid media. Although most species are aerobic or facultatively anaerobic, there are also species that are obligately anaerobic (e.g., *Peptostreptococcus putridus* and *Peptostreptococcus micros*) or microaerophilic. They may be divided into those which produce a soluble hemolysin and those which do not. Aerobes producing a clear zone of hemolysis on blood agar (beta hemolysis) include most of the species associated with primary streptococcal infections in human beings and can be subdivided into 15 broad groups (Lancefield groups) that are identified by precipitin tests with group-specific antisera against specific carbohydrate haptens (C antigens) of the streptococci. Strains belonging to Lancefield group A *(Streptococcus pyogenes)* are responsible for over 90 percent of human streptococcal infections. These group A strains can be further subdivided for epidemiologic studies into Griffith types according to their surface protein antigens (M, T, and R) by capillary precipitin or slide agglutination tests.

Another group of streptococci produce an ill-defined zone of partial hemolysis having a green or brownish-green color (alpha hemolysis). These are strains of *Streptococcus viridans*. Streptococci that are without effect on blood agar (nonhemolytic) include the fecal enterococci *(Streptococcus faecalis)*. Viridans and nonhemolytic streptococci are associated with chronic diseases or are nonpathogenic. *Streptococcus viridans* is part of the commensal flora of the mouth and throat and is dangerous in individuals with congenitally deformed or rheumatically damaged heart valves. It is the commonest cause of subacute bacterial endocarditis. *Streptococcus viridans* has been incriminated in apical tooth infections and is commonly found in carious teeth. Bacteremia frequently follows tooth extraction and even routine dental procedures. In otherwise healthy individuals the streptococci are rapidly removed from the circulation, but in those with heart lesions the organisms settle in or on the defective valves. Accordingly, patients with congenital or other valvular cardiac defects should be given penicillin prophylactically before and after any dental attention.

Nonhemolytic streptococci are always present in the colon and may be isolated from the terminal ileum and upper jejunum of 60 percent of surgical patients. These enterococci *(Streptococcus faecalis)* can cause suppurative lesions and urinary tract infections. Some strains of *Streptococcus faecalis* produce a true beta hemolysis; they belong to Lancefield group D.

Group A beta-hemolytic streptococci *(Streptococcus pyogenes)* are the principal causes of streptococcal pharyngitis, scarlet fever, and rheumatic fever. They also cause bacteremias following surgical procedures in patients with malignant disease. Groups B, C, D, F, and G are usually less virulent. Although group B streptococci are often isolated from patients with puerperal sepsis, with meningitis of the newborn, with diabetes mellitus, and/or with peripheral vascular insufficiency, they are also involved in pneumonias and infections of the male genitourinary tract. Since group C streptococci are part of the skin flora, they may be isolated from wounds and exudates more often than group B strains. The group G streptococci involved in infections usually originate in the genitourinary tract or skin, but they may also originate in the upper respiratory tract or gastrointestinal tract.

Streptococcus pyogenes is an invasive microorganism; it secretes two distinct hemolysins (streptolysins O and S) and several other products that aid in invasion. Streptolysin O is cardiotoxic and leukocidic and may be identical with leukocidin. Streptolysin S is a pure hemolysin responsible for beta hemolysis on blood agar plates. Hyaluronidase hydrolyzes hyaluronic acid and allows increased permeability of tissues. Streptokinase reduces fibrinolysis by activating the plasmin system. Streptodornase depolymerizes DNA. Erythrogenic toxin produces erythema when injected intradermally and is responsible for the punctate erythema of scarlet fever. The hyaluronidase and streptokinase produced by most strains of *Streptococcus pyogenes* are responsible for the spreading cellulitis (erysipelas) that is the typical streptococcal lesion. When abscess occurs, the pus is watery and often bloodstained due to the action of streptodornase and streptokinase, since the viscosity of pus is due to DNA and fibrin.

Erysipelas

Erysipelas is a spreading streptococcal cellulitis and lymphangitis with raised, sharply defined, irregular, reddish borders. Since erythrogenic toxin is produced in variable amounts by hemolytic streptococci, the development of cutaneous erythema is an inconstant manifestation of streptococcal infection. Minor skin abrasions and fissures predispose to these infections of the skin. The cutis is edematous and reddened, with a palpably raised border; the lesion is hot, tender, and painful. The classic lesion of erysipelas is a "butterfly" erythema centered around the nose and extending onto both cheeks. The systemic manifestations of erysipelas may be severe and suggest invasion via the lymphatics or bloodstream. Penicillin is usually effective against the invasive infection, but the erythema disappears more slowly.

Erysipeloid, a nonstreptococcal disease distinct from erysipelas, is a type of cutaneous cellulitis due to infection by *Erysipelothrix rhusopathiae,* a gram-positive, nonsporulating, facultative anaerobe in the family Corynebacteriaceae. The typical lesion is a violaceous nodule, often having a curved shape, which differs from that of erysipelas by its tendency to central clearing and the absence of suppuration. Human cases of erysipeloid may also occur as either a severe, generalized cutaneous disease or as septicemia with or without cutaneous involvement and often associated with endocarditis. Penicillin therapy is specific for most cases. Erysipelothrix infection is considered an occupational disease of abattoir workers, fish handlers, and others exposed to meat, poultry, and fish products.

Necrotizing Fasciitis

This is a life-threatening infection that may occur in only one or two patients a year in large city-county hospitals. The most significant manifestation of the infection is extensive necrosis of the superficial fascia with resultant widespread undermining of surrounding tissue and extreme systemic toxicity. The bacteria involved in about 90 percent of cases have usually been beta-hemolytic streptococci, or coagulase-positive staphylococci, or both. Gram-negative enteric pathogens alone have been associated with about 10 percent of cases of necrotizing fasciitis. The disease appears to be a clinical entity and not a specific bacterial infection. It has been described previously as hemolytic or acute streptococcal gangrene, gangrenous or necrotizing erysipelas, suppurative fasciitis, and hospital gangrene. Although necrotizing fasciitis may develop following surgical procedures such as appendectomy, the majority of cases have occurred outside the hospital following minor trauma such as abrasions, cuts, bruises, boils, injection of drugs, and insect bites on the extremities, particularly in individuals with diabetes and peripheral vascular disease. The chief diagnostic criterion for necrotizing fasciitis is superficial and widespread fascial necrosis. Cellulitis as well as edema (mild to massive) are present in most patients. The involved skin is pale red without distinct borders and with blisters or bullae. Pale red areas progress to a distinct purple. The diagnosis is confirmed by observation of (1) serosanguinous exudate; (2) swollen, stringy, dull gray, necrotic fascia with extensive undermining; and (3) a Gram-stained smear of the pus or fluid showing the types of bacteria involved and a substantial white blood cell response.

TREATMENT. This consists of multiple linear incisions over the affected area and debridement of all involved areas. In an open wound, the extent of undermining can be ascertained by passing a sterile hemostat along the plane just superficial to the deep fascia. In simple cellulitis or erysipelas, the hemostat cannot be passed. Before operation, the patient should be given a full dose of systemic antibiotic(s) effective against both hemolytic streptococci and penicillinase-producing staphylococci. The combination of an aminoglycoside and clindamycin and penicillin G or ampicillin covers the majority of pathogens involved. Therapy is continued postoperatively until the infection is controlled. Repeated debridement may be necessary if the patient continues to be febrile. With the appearance of clean granulation tissue after 5 to 10 days, the wound may be closed by skin graft or suture. Rea and Wyrick (1970) report a 30 percent mortality.

Peptostreptococci (anaerobic streptococci) are also pathogenic. They are normal inhabitants of the mouth, intestine, and vagina. They are abundant when oral hygiene is poor, and aspiration into the lungs and sinuses may lead to putrid lung abscess, empyema, and sinusitis. Brain abscesses often develop as complications of chronic or acute infections of the lungs, sinuses, or ears. *Peptostreptococcus putridus* has been isolated from cases of puerperal sepsis, brain abscess, and infected wounds. *Nonclostridial crepitant anaerobic cellulitis* is due to peptostreptococci, whereas *synergistic necrotizing cellulitis* with widespread involvement of deeper tissues is caused by the symbiotic activity of peptostreptococci, aerobic gram-negative rods, and frequently bacteroides.

Streptococcal Myonecrosis

Anaerobic streptococci can cause gas gangrene. Facultative streptococci and *Staphylococcus aureus* also may be isolated. *Streptococcal myonecrosis* resembles subacute clostridial gas gangrene and was not described until World War II. After an incubation period of 3 to 4 days, there is swelling, edema, and purulent wound exudate. These signs are followed by pain which rapidly becomes severe. Gas is present, and the infected muscle changes from pale and soft to bright red, striped with purple, and finally purple and gangrenous. The seropurulent discharge has a sour odor. In this disease, muscle is involved, in contrast to necrotizing fasciitis, in which the fascia is affected. Treatment consists of incision and drainage, antibiotic therapy, and supportive measures.

Progressive Synergistic Gangrene

As early as 1924, Meleney established the importance of microaerophilic and anaerobic streptococci in special wound infections known as progressive synergistic gangrene and chronic burrowing ulcer. *Meleney's progressive synergistic gangrene* characteristically develops in sutured, infected thoracic or abdominal incisions or around a colostomy, ileostomy, or simple abrasion. The initial lesion is a small, painful, superficial ulcer that gradually spreads. The central ulcerated area is surrounded by a rim of gangrenous skin, which in turn is encircled by a zone of purple erythema blending into a surrounding area of bright, painful erythema. There is seropurulent discharge. Cultures taken from the outer edematous part of the lesion yield microaerophilic or anaerobic nonhemolytic streptococci. Cultures taken from the central ulcerated area yield *Staphylococcus aureus* and sometimes gram-negative bacilli, such as *Proteus* species. However, clinical cases of progressive synergistic gangrene from which anaerobic or microaerophilic streptococci could not be isolated have been reported. Treatment involves wide excision and therapy with penicillin or chloramphenicol. Corticosteroids have been employed to aid healing. Ledingham and Tehrani find that the problem in acute dermal gangrene following surgery, such as necrotizing fasciitis and progressive synergistic gangrene, is no longer any apparent specificity of invading bacteria but rather a vicious cycle of infection, local ischemia, and diminished host defense mechanisms.

Meleney's Ulcer

Chronic burrowing or undermining ulcer, often designated as *Meleney's ulcer,* is caused by a nonhemolytic anaerobic or microaerophilic streptococcus. The lesion begins as a small, superficial ulcer following trauma or surgery and may also originate from an infected lymph node or subcutaneous abscess. The ulcer is only mildly painful, and systemic reaction is minimal. Slow, progressive enlargement of the lesion occurs over months or years. Infection of subcutaneous tissue is associated with ulceration of the overlying skin. Cutaneous gangrene is absent, and the edges of the undermined skin roll inward. The periphery of the lesion is erythematous, and the advancing edge of the lesion is characterized by pain and tenderness. Meleney's ulcer occurs most frequently after incision of a lymph node in the neck, axilla, or groin and after operations on the genital and intestinal tracts. As the lesion spreads, multiple ulcers and sinuses develop, producing epithelial strands and undermined bridges of skin. Treatment consists of debridement, drainage of sinuses, penicillin therapy, and split-thickness skin grafts over denuded areas as soon as the wound appears clean.

Peptostreptococci, either in pure culture or mixed with bacteroides, are frequently involved in appendiceal abscesses, peritonitis, abdominal wall sepsis, perirectal abscesses, and superficial abscesses related to infections of pilonidal and sebaceous cysts. Most abscesses are treated successfully by incision and drainage, and penicillin therapy. Peptostreptococcal infections, including septicemias, commonly occur in the female pelvic area following septic abortion and postpartum sepsis.

STAPHYLOCOCCAL INFECTIONS

Staphylococci form part of the permanent bacterial flora of the normal skin and nasopharynx and may cause a variety of infections, often characterized by suppuration, ranging from mild, localized pustules to lethal septicemias. Surgical and traumatic wounds are particularly susceptible to purulent infection. In stained preparations of pus, staphylococci appear as spherical cells occurring singly, in pairs, or in small clusters. They are gram-positive and nonmotile, and produce no spores. Staphylococci are aerobic or facultatively anaerobic and grow on ordinary unenriched bacteriologic media. They may produce pigmentation varying from white, orange, or yellow to golden. Blood agar is often hemolyzed (beta hemolysis). Two species are of medical importance: *Staphylococcus aureus* and *Staphylococcus epidermidis*. *Staphylococcus aureus* is usually associated with disease, and will be discussed subsequently. On the other hand, *Staphylococcus epidermidis* usually has not been considered a pathogen, but it has become recognized as an important cause of opportunistic infection following surgical procedures in which foreign materials and prostheses are placed in the patient. *Staphylococcus epidermidis* can cause endocarditis following open heart surgery and occasionally produces septicemia.

The criteria identifying staphylococci are colonial appearance on blood agar, gram stain reaction, microscopic morphologic features, production of coagulase, and fermentation of mannitol. *Staphylococcus aureus* is coagulase-positive and produces acid from mannitol. *Staphylococcus epidermidis* produces neither coagulase nor acid from mannitol. Filtrates of cultures of *Staphylococcus aureus* contain hemolysins, dermonecrotic and lethal factors, leukocidins, and enzymes. Strains of *Staphylococcus aureus* may be classified into groups on the basis of their susceptibility to various bacteriophages. Although phage typing of isolates is of value in epidemiologic investigations, it is not employed by the diagnostic laboratory for routine identification of clinical isolates.

Staphylococci are readily phagocytized by polymorphonuclear leukocytes, which may then be killed by the bacteria, presumably by their leukocidins. Although leukocidins, hemolysins, and coagulase are antigenic, antibodies to these antigens provide little or no protection. Since the antigenic components of staphylococci responsible for virulence are unknown, it has not been possible to make effective vaccines.

Staphylococcal infections in human beings depend upon many factors, including the type and number of staphylococci, the route of introduction, and the toxic substances produced by the staphylococci. Of equal importance are the susceptibility of the host, the previous exposure to specific strains, the general health and nutritional state, and the amount of trauma sustained. Factors such as toxemia, allergic reactions, starvation, and diabetes influence the onset and course of staphylococcal infections. Foreign body reaction as a consequence of sutures is an important factor in staphylococcal infection.

The skin is the most common site of staphylococcal infections. Lesions range from furuncles (boils) and carbuncles to surgical wound infections. Hospital-acquired staphylococcal infection by antibiotic-resistant strains reached epidemic proportion during the 1950s. The development and use of semisynthetic penicillinase-resistant penicillins has controlled these infections. However, the antibiotic-resistant staphylococci are now endemic in hospitals and pose a continual threat to the patient. A rapidly spreading cellulitis is sometimes seen with staphylococcal infections and should be treated vigorously with an appropriate antibiotic. Often there is pain, swelling, induration, patchy discoloration of the skin, and fever. Cellulitis may occur at the site of a venipuncture for intravenous cannulation. Staphylococcal abscesses characteristically begin in hair follicles or small sebaceous glands. An indurated area of cellulitis undergoes central necrosis and formation of an abscess having thick, odorless, and yellow or greenish pus. Staphylococci are a primary cause of acute wound sepsis and are involved in postoperative infections of "clean" incised wounds. The source of the infecting microorganisms is frequently exogenous. Virulent, antibiotic-resistant, hospital strains of *Staphylococcus aureus* may be carried in the nares and on the hands of physicians and hospital personnel, and these may be newly colonized on the skin of the patient. The air in the operating room may bear microorganisms from the nasopharynx, skin, hair, and clothing of the surgical staff and of the patient. Accordingly, it is essential to maintain strict, rigid rules for asepsis in the operating room.

Infected incisions should be opened widely and allowed to drain. Therapy with antistaphylococcal antibiotics should be initiated. Fulminating septicemias may arise from severe wound infections. The patient is ill with high fever, leukocytosis, toxemia, and evidence of irritation of the central nervous system. The mortality rate in fulminating untreated infections may be as high as 90 percent. If the infection persists, metastatic abscesses form in lungs, heart, kidneys, gallbladder, appendix, liver, peritoneum, and bone. Meningitis and brain abscesses hasten death. Endocarditis is a frequent complication of staphylococcal septicemia. Staphylococcal pneumonia is another nosocomial postoperative infection. It may be severe and is often associated with a tracheostomy. In fatal cases, the major finding at autopsy is marked pulmonary edema with little destruction of tissue.

Staphylococcal Enteritis

Enteritis with a drug-resistant staphylococcus following oral administration of a broad-spectrum antibiotic was first described by Kramer in 1948. Generally, this disease is benign with mild to moderate symptoms including nausea, vomiting, diarrhea, abdominal distention, fever, and weakness, but it may be fulminating and lead to septicemia and death. Discontinuance of the oral antibiotic usually leads to disappearance of symptoms. The prognosis is good so long as the intestinal mucosa remains intact.

Staphylococcal enterocolitis (pseudomembranous enterocolitis) is an acute inflammatory disease of the small and large intestine characterized by foci of epithelial necrosis and erosion of the mucosa. There is profuse, continuous diarrhea that soon becomes watery, contains desquamated, membranous patches, and often is greenish. The disease is a complication in debilitated surgical patients following therapy with broad-spectrum antibiotics. The use of neomycin in debilitated patients for preoperative intestinal antisepsis and for treatment of hepatic coma has resulted in staphylococcal enterocolitis. The major etiologic factors are suppression of normal gastrointestinal flora by a broad-spectrum antibiotic and acquisition of an enterotoxic strain of *Staphylococcus aureus* possessing multiple antibiotic resistance. Secondary factors are debilitation and an empty small bowel (as a result of preoperative starvation). Although stool cultures from some patients yield a pure culture of *Staphylococcus aureus,* pseudomembranous enterocolitis may exist without culturable *Staphylococcus aureus.* Conversely, *Staphylococcus aureus may exist in pure culture in the intestine of a patient with the symptoms of enteritis but in the absence of a pseudomembrane.* Discovery during the past decade of the role of toxin(s) of *Clostridium difficile* in antibiotic-associated pseudomembranous colitis explains some of these discrepancies. (Discussion is found under Clostridial Infections of the Gastrointestinal Tract.)

TREATMENT. Treatment consists of discontinuing previous antibiotics and employing a specific antistaphylococcal drug such as oral methicillin or oral vancomycin, hydration with intravenously administered fluids, replacement of electrolytes, intramuscular administration of corticosteroids, and attempts to reestablish a normal flora. The fulminating form of enterocolitis may be refractory to all forms of therapy and may result in death.

Peptococci and Disease?

Both obligately anaerobic staphylococci (peptococci) and facultatively anaerobic staphylococci grow in anaerobic cultures. However, the facultatives (e.g., *Staphylococcus aureus*) can be subcultured aerobically and separated from the peptococci that grow anaerobically only. In contrast to the role of pure cultures of staphylococci in disease, the peptococci may be found in wound infections, abscesses, and septicemias in association with bacteroides, clostridia, aerobic gram-negative bacilli, and aerobic cocci. These bacterial groups are major components of the normal flora of the skin and mucous membranes and can exert a role in mixed infections when these sites are disturbed. Peptococci (e.g., *Peptococcus magnus* and *Peptococcus asaccharolyticus*) account for approximately 20 percent of anaerobes found in clinical specimens from surgical patients (Holland et al.). Nevertheless, the peptococci have slight, if any, propensity to produce disease and seem unable to cause progressive infection in laboratory animals. This apparent nonpathogenicity is shared by many anaerobic species from normal flora found in anaerobic infections and has led to speculation that the unitarian theory of infection that has evolved from the monumental work of Koch and Ehrlich (one microbe, one disease, one drug) does not explain all infectious disease (Gorbach and Bartlett).

CLOSTRIDIAL INFECTIONS

The clostridia are large, gram-positive, rod-shaped microorganisms. They are ubiquitous. *Clostridium perfringens* is more widespread than any other pathogen. Its principal habitats are the soil and the intestinal tract of human beings and animals. The most characteristic feature of clostridia is the presence of an oval, central, or subterminal spore. In the case of *Clostridium tetani,* the spore is spherical and terminally located and produces a characteristic drumstick appearance. The clostridia are obligate anaerobes and can be cultured only on media having a low oxidation-reduction potential. This may be achieved by employing fresh media incubated in an anaerobic atmosphere in specially designed jars or with liquid media exposed to the atmosphere, but containing added reducing agents (such as sodium thioglycolate, powdered iron, or chopped meat).

The lesions produced by the pathogenic clostridia are due to their exotoxins. Gas gangrene is a necrosis of tissue along with putrefaction and is usually caused by clostridia derived from the intestine or soil. The infection is localized but its systemic effects are far-reaching. Gas gangrene is rarely a pure culture infection. It usually involves *Clostridium perfringens* along with other clostridial species, such as *Clostridium novyi, Clostridium septicum, Clostridium bifermentans (sordellii),* sometimes *Clostridium tetani* and *Clostridium botulinum,* and often nonpathogenic but proteolytic *Clostridium sporogenes* and *Clostridium histolyticum*. In addition, grampositive cocci and gram-negative enterobacteria are often present.

Clostridium perfringens is, nevertheless, the most important organism. Five types, A through F, have been described. They are differentiated on the basis of production of lethal toxins. All types produce alpha toxin, a lethal, necrotizing, hemolytic exotoxin, which is also a lecithinase. *Clostridium perfringens* type A produces the greatest amount of alpha toxin. In addition, some strains of type A produce variable amounts of hemolysin (theta toxin), collagenase (kappa toxin), hyaluronidase (mu toxin), and deoxyribonuclease (nu toxin).

Clostridial Wound Infection

MacLennan in 1962 described three types of anaerobic wound infection: simple contamination, clostridial cellulitis, and clostridial myonecrosis.

SIMPLE CONTAMINATION

Simple contamination of a wound by clostridia is common. It causes no discomfort to the patient and is of little concern to the surgeon. When anaerobes are digesting dead tissue, there may be a thin seropurulent exudate. If the necrotic material is removed, there will be no subsequent invasion of underlying tissues. The relatively common occurrence of clostridia in accidental wounds in the absence of anaerobic infection is probably due to the ubiquitous presence of these anaerobes and their spores. The absence of subsequent anaerobic infections is most likely due to unsuitable conditions for further multiplication of the contaminant and for toxin production. MacLennan estimated that between 10 and 30 percent of all severe civilian wounds were infected with spore-forming anaerobic bacilli. A high oxidation-reduction potential (Eh) due to the surrounding healthy tissues prevents colonization of the tissues. In the absence of treatment, however, cellulitis or myonecrosis may develop from the simple contamination, and the three types of anaerobic wound infection may be considered as ascending grades of severity.

CLOSTRIDIAL CELLULITIS

This is a gassy, crepitant infection involving necrotic tissue (killed by ischemia or trauma, but not by bacterial activity). Intact, healthy muscle is not invaded. The cellulitis is characterized as a foul-smelling, seropurulent infection of the depths and crevices of a wound. There is often local extension along fascial planes, but involvement of healthy muscle and marked toxemia are absent. Although *Clostridium perfringens* may be present, the predominant organisms are proteolytic and nontoxigenic clostridia, such as *Clostridium sporogenes* and *Clostridium tertium*. Clostridial cellulitis generally has a gradual onset; the incubation period is from 3 to 5 days; systemic effects are usually mild; there is no toxemia; the skin is rarely discolored; and there is little or no edema. This distinguishes the infection from gas gangrene. The spread of the cellulitis in the tissue spaces often has been rapid and extensive, necessitating immediate radical surgical drainage.

CLOSTRIDIAL MYONECROSIS (GAS GANGRENE)

This infection is rapid-spreading. It may be crepitant, or noncrepitant and edematous, mixed, or toxemic. The lesion also has been described as a "myositis," which is not as precise a term as is *myonecrosis*. The infection occurs in association with severe wounds of large muscle masses that have become contaminated with pathogenic clostridia, especially *Clostridium perfringens*. Such wounds are most commonly caused by the high-velocity missiles of modern warfare and by accidental trauma. Sometimes clostridial myonecrosis follows clean elective surgical procedures. Many patients with clostridial myonecrosis harbor a variety of anaerobic as well as aerobic bacteria. In fatal cases it is rare for only a single species to be present. Clostridial myonecrosis is most likely to develop in wounds in which there has been extensive laceration or devitalization of thick muscle masses, such as the buttock, thigh, and shoulder. Associated with such trauma is impaired arterial supply to the limb or muscle group and gross contamination of the wound by soil, clothing, and other foreign bodies. These conditions provide an ideal substrate for the development of clostridia. In anoxic muscle, glycolysis continues and the oxidation-reduction potential (Eh) of the muscle falls. With the accumulation of lactate, alkaline reservoirs become depleted, and the pH also falls. As a consequence of lowered Eh and pH, the proteinases present and the amino acids produced not only lower the pH further but provide substrate for the growth of clostridia. Once bacterial growth is established and toxins and other products of bacterial metabolism accumulate, the invasion of uninjured tissue is promoted, and the anaerobic infection is established. The infection is aided further by the fact that neither phagocytes nor antibodies can enter the necrotic lesion. Gas gangrene is considered to have begun when the infecting pathogenic anaerobes have produced sufficient toxins to overcome local defenses. Gas gangrene is relatively infrequent in clinical practice. The overall incidence is less than 2 percent, although from 4 to 40 percent of wounds may be contaminated with clostridia.

Clostridium septicum myonecrosis is related to malignancy. Debilitation and immunosuppression appear to underlie the resultant *Clostridium septicum* sepsis in patients with either hematologic or intestinal malignancy. Conversely, in a patient from whom *Clostridium septicum* is isolated, malignancy (e.g., hematologic or intestinal) should be suspected. In a patient with evidence of clostridial myonecrosis or sepsis and no external source, the cecum or distal ileum should be considered a likely site of malignancy.

TREATMENT. Early and adequate surgery is the most effective means of treating gas gangrene. Because of the rapid spread of the infection, a 24-h delay in treatment may be fatal. The diagnosis of gas gangrene is based on clinical evidence. Multiple longitudinal incisions for decompression and drainage and aggressive surgical debridement of all involved or devitalized tissues usually arrest the disease. If not or if early diagnosis was not made, then amputation is necessary. Antibiotic therapy with penicillin G and tetracycline has been most effective as an adjunct to operative treatment. Antitoxin is of no value therapeutically or prophylactically and should not be used. Adjunctive hyperbaric oxygenation has been used with success.

Infections of the Gastrointestinal Tract

Clostridia are usually present among the mixed flora in peritonitis, appendicitis, and strangulation intestinal obstruction. Quantitatively, the most numerous flora in peritoneal and loop fluids of dogs with experimental strangulation intestinal obstruction are clostridia, coliforms, bacterioides, and streptococci, in that order. Although it appears reasonable to assume that *Clostridium perfringens* actively participates in the pathophysiology of severe cases of appendicitis and acute cases of strangulated intestinal obstruction, direct clinical evidence is lacking. Experimental studies demonstrate that clostridial exotoxins contribute to the lethal activity of filter-sterilized strangulation fluids. However, this finding does not preclude a role for combinations of varying proportions of viable bacteria, bacterial endotoxins, and clostridial exotoxins. In biliary tract infections due to clostridia, acute emphysematous cholecystitis (gas gangrene of the gallbladder) and postcholecystectomy septicemia, it is generally believed that clostridia are transported to the liver from the gastrointestinal tract via the portal circulation and then excreted with the bile into the biliary tract. In postoperative gas gangrene of the abdominal wall, a rare complication of abdominal surgery, intestinal clostridia contaminate the abdominal wound at the time of operation. It occurs less often after operations on the stomach and duodenum than after those involving the lower intestinal tract. These infections are usually due to *Clostridium perfringens* and are fatal; they require awareness and early treatment. Gas gangrene of the abdominal wall must be distinguished from Meleney's progressive synergistic gangrene of the abdominal wall following drainage of appendiceal abscesses. Synergistic gangrene is a chronic, superficial progressive gangrene characterized by a slow, relentless progression, severe local symptoms, and absence of severe systemic symptoms. It is due to anaerobic cocci mixed with *Staphylococcus aureus, Streptococcus pyogenes, Pseudomonas aeruginosa,* or *Proteus* species.

ANTIBIOTIC-ASSOCIATED PSEUDOMEMBRANOUS COLITIS. In 1977 a toxin was first reported in the feces of patients with pseudomembranous colitis following antimicrobial therapy. Subsequent studies identified *Clostridium difficile* as the source of the toxin and suggested that antibiotic therapy altered the normal microflora of the colon and permitted overgrowth of *Clostridium difficile* in a previously colonized patient. The symptoms of antibiotic-associated colitis can appear during antimicrobial therapy or even as long as 2 or 3 weeks following its cessation. Watery diarrhea without gross blood is typical and may be accompanied by fever, abdominal pain, and leukocytosis. Sigmoidoscopy or colonoscopy reveals yellow-white, raised exudative plaques or pseudomembranes. The role of *Clostridium difficile* is demonstrated by isolating the microorganism from feces. Sterile filtrates of such feces produce cytotoxic effects when added to cell cultures. The cytotoxin(s) is neutralized by antitoxin produced from *Clostridium sordellii,* a closely related species.

Although almost all commonly used antibacterial agents have been implicated in antibiotic-associated colitis, those most frequently associated have been ampicillin, clindamycin, and cephalosporins. When diarrhea is not relieved by stopping the offending antibiotic, or when the diarrhea is severe, oral vancomycin is an effective treatment of *Clostridium difficile*-related colitis and diarrhea, and can be life-saving. Cholestyramime, an anion exchange resin that binds the toxins of *Clostridium difficile,* is an alternative for treatment of a patient who is not too seriously ill. However, if the drug fails or if the patient is seriously ill, oral vancomycin should be used. Oral metronidazole is also effective in treating *Clostridium difficile*-induced colitis.

Clostridium difficile is the most important cause of antibiotic-associated pseudomembranous colitis, which is most frequent in seriously ill, hospitalized patients. Only about 3 percent of healthy adults are reported to carry the microorganism in their stools, yet rates of antibiotic-associated colitis of 10 percent or higher have been found in some hospitals. This discrepancy suggests the possibility of nosocomial cross infection. Fekety et al. found that contamination with *Clostridium difficile* was common in the immediate environment of patients with the disease, and were able to isolate the microorganism from the hands and stools of asymptomatic hospital personnel. Therefore, such patients should be isolated.

Urogenital Infections

Postoperative infections due to *Clostridium perfringens* have occurred following procedures such as nephrectomy, lithotomy, and prostatectomy. Almost all uterine clostridial infections are due to *Clostridium perfringens.* They generally occur following criminal abortion and are rare following normal childbirth. Introduction of the organisms into the uterus is favored by instrumentation and manipulation. In modern obstetrics, the use of prophylactic antibiotic therapy and the wide use of cesarean section probably account for the decreasing frequency of this already rare form of uterine infection. In contrast, in cases of criminal abortion both endogenous and exogenous sources of contamination occur as the result of unskilled manipulations and the use of unsterile and unclean instruments and abortifacients. Once the interior of the puerperal or postabortal uterus has been contaminated, fragments of blood clot and necrotic tissue provide conditions favorable for multiplication of clostridia. Early diagnosis depends upon clinical recognition of such signs as jaundice, hypotension, tachycardia, shock, hemoglobinuria, uterine or perianal tenderness, and offensive vaginal discharge. The simplest method for the rapid detection of *Clostridium perfringens* is the demonstration of gram-positive rods with rounded ends in direct smears from the cervical os or canal. The treatment of uterine gas gangrene involves immediate chemotherapy, hyperbaric oxygenation, treatment of shock, hysterectomy, and management of renal failure. Penicillin is the antibiotic of choice.

Tetanus

This disease is a toxemia resulting from the growth of contaminating *Clostridium tetani* at a traumatized site and consequent production of exotoxin. In contrast to the clostridia of gas gangrene, *Clostridium tetani* is noninvasive, and neurotoxin is responsible for the symptoms of tetanus. The conditions necessary for the development of tetanus are the presence of the organisms or spores in the wound and favorable anaerobic conditions for bacterial growth and the elaboration of exotoxin. The presence of *Clostridium tetani* in soil and in the intestine of human beings and animals ensures that accidental wounds are exposed to the risk of contamination at the time of injury. However, as with other clostridial infections, the mere presence of *Clostridium tetani* or its spores in a wound is not followed always by tetanus, and the organism may be isolated from wounds in individuals who never develop tetanus. A low oxygen tension is necessary if *Clostridium tetani* is to grow. Currently, tetanus commonly follows mild injuries because the routine protective measures employed in severe cases may be omitted. The types of lesions leading to the development of tetanus are penetrating wounds due to splinters, thorns, rusty nails, and even dirty abrasions. In about 50 percent of cases, it is presumed that the wound was slight and healed before evidence of intoxication developed. Such mild injuries may not induce significant local anoxia, but they may be accompanied by other infections that lower the oxidation-reduction potential of the tissues to a point at which the spores of *Clostridium tetani* can germinate. For example, chronic ulcers of the leg, measles rash, boils, paronychia, and dental extractions have been implicated as modes of entry. In the United States, tetanus has become a disease primarily of unvaccinated adults. The median age of patients with nonneonatal tetanus varies from fifty-five to fifty-seven years; the median age for those dying from tetanus is from fifty-five to sixty years.

Currently, tetanus is seen in urban centers of the United States as a complication of narcotic addiction; *urban tetanus* has a mortality of 90 percent. *Tetanus neonatorum* results from contamination of the cut surface of the umbilical cord and is an important cause of infant mortality in developing countries where primitive unhygienic obstetric practices prevail. There is often continuous crying for hours followed by cessation of sucking and crying, convulsions, and fever. Severe spasm of the respiratory muscles is a common cause of death. *Postabortal tetanus* and *puerperal tetanus* result from unsterile manipulation or instrumentation of the genital tract. *Postoperative tetanus* sometimes follows elective surgical procedures, and is usually due to some breakdown in sterile technique, but it may also be caused by contamination from the patient's intestinal tract.

CLINICAL MANIFESTATIONS. The average incubation period for tetanus is from 7 to 10 days after injury, but it may range between 3 and 30 days. The incubation period is followed by the *period of onset,* that is, the time interval between the first symptom (usually trismus) and the onset of spasms. In severe cases reflex spasms may begin 12 h after onset, in moderately severe cases after 2 to 3 days, and in milder cases after 5 or more days. In general, the shorter the periods of incubation and onset, the worse the prognosis. Even with modern treatment, the mortality rate is rarely less than 30 percent.

Trismus is the most common early symptom. It often is combined with pain and stiffness in the neck, back, and abdomen. Occasionally dysphagia appears first. These symptoms increase according to the severity of the attack. Twenty-four hours after the onset, a patient with a moderately severe attack has a characteristically anxious expression (*risus sardonicus*) in which the eyebrows and the corners of the mouth are drawn up. The muscles of the neck and trunk are rigid to varying degrees, and the back is usually slightly arched. The patient is usually comfortable except for occasional pain in the neck or back, which tends to be made worse by movement. Manipulation of a limb or palpation of any part of the body tends to increase muscular rigidity and may bring on cramplike pain. Initially, reflex spasms are brought on by external stimuli, such as moving the patient or knocking the bed, but later they occur spontaneously at regular and increasingly shorter intervals until the height of the disease is reached. Spasms often begin with a sudden jerk. Every muscle in the body is thrown into intense tonic contraction, the jaws are tightly clenched, the head is retracted, the back is arched, the chest and abdomen are fixed, and the limbs are usually extended. A severe spasm may stop respiration. Spasms may last a few seconds or several minutes. When spasms occur frequently, they lead to rapid exhaustion and sometimes to death from asphyxiation. Without spasms, mortality is low; with severe spasms, few survive. Aspiration pneumonia is a common contributory cause of death.

Less common manifestations of the disease include local contracture of muscles in the neighborhood of the wound: *local tetanus*. This may precede the more generalized forms of involvement. *Cephalic tetanus* is a manifestation in which irritation or paralysis of cranial nerves appears early and dominates the picture. The facial nerve is affected most often, but ophthalmoplegia from involvement of the ocular nerves and spasm or paralysis of the tongue from involvement of the hypoglossal nerve may develop. Trismus and dysphagia may also be present. This condition, which is a type of local tetanus, follows wounds of the head and face, and the symptoms often appear first on the injured side.

Severe tetanus is terrible and often fatal, but those who recover do so completely. The patient who has survived tetanus is not immune and, unless immunized, is susceptible to a second attack. *Recurrent tetanus* in the same patient has been reported. Apparently a sublethal amount of tetanus toxin is not sufficient to provide an adequate antigenic stimulus for the production of active immunity.

The diagnosis of tetanus is a clinical one with bacteriologic confirmation sometimes possible. Frequently the presumed lesion has been so slight that it is not detectable at the time when clinical tetanus develops.

IMMUNIZATION. Prophylaxis with tetanus toxoid is the best means of preventing tetanus. For active immunization of individuals seven years old or over, the initial dose is 0.5 mL aluminum phosphate–adsorbed tetanus toxoid given intramuscularly, preferably in the left deltoid region, but it also may be given subcutaneously. This is repeated in 4 to 6 weeks, and a third injection is given in 6

to 12 months (or more). Only after this third injection is the basic series considered complete. For children six years old or under, diphtheria and tetanus toxoid combined with pertussis vaccine (DTP) is used. Delay in administering the second and third injections is not disadvantageous, and the series does not need to be restarted or repeated. Even after 25 years, a booster will rapidly recall complete active protection.

Following the initial dose of tetanus toxoid, nonimmunized individuals require approximately 30 days to acquire a safe antibody level (at least 0.01 I.U. of serum antitoxin per milliliter of blood). Patients are passively immunized in the interim by intramuscular administration of human hyperimmune globulin containing 250 units of tetanus antitoxin simultaneously with the toxoid. This protects for about 4 weeks. Passive immunization is not recommended for individuals who have received previous active immunization.

TREATMENT. Surgical care of wounds should be immediate. The most important features of surgical wound care are thorough cleansing and debridement. Foreign bodies and necrotic tissue can be contaminated massively with *Clostridium tetani* and establish wound conditions promoting growth and exotoxin production by *Clostridium tetani*. The wound should be left open until the patient has recovered from the convulsive stage of the disease. Antibiotic therapy with penicillin is effective against vegetative cells of *Clostridium tetani*. Tetracycline hydrochloride may be used if an allergy to penicillin exists. Antibiotics also are important as prophylaxis against respiratory infections, which are common in tetanus. Treatment of the patient with severe tetanus involves the use of muscle relaxants, sedation with Pentothal sodium, balance of fluid and electrolytes, control of respiratory secretions, and elimination of visceral stimuli such as distention of the urinary bladder and fecal impaction. A tracheostomy is performed if needed or when the period of onset is 1 day or less. Constant nursing care is required.

COMPLICATIONS. Tetanus is a particularly lethal disease, and death is generally due to respiratory arrest. Some complications of tetanus and its treatment are drug intoxication, especially from barbiturates; bronchopneumonia or other pulmonary infection; compression fracture of vertebrae, especially the thoracic vertebrae; anemia; and exhaustion, which may be so severe as a result of repeated convulsions that the patient lapses into coma and expires. Before human tetanus immune globulin was available, the risk of anaphylaxis complicated the use of bovine or equine tetanus antitoxin.

PROPHYLAXIS. The Committee on Trauma of the American College of Surgeons recommends the following guidelines (1979) for prophylaxis against tetanus in the management of wounds:

I. General principles
   A. The attending physician must determine for each patient with a wound, individually, what is required for adequate prophylaxis against tetanus.
   B. Regardless of the active immunization status of the patient, meticulous surgical care, including removal of all

devitalized tissue and foreign bodies, should be provided immediately for all wounds. Such care is essential as part of the prophylaxis against tetanus.

C. Passive immunization with Tetanus Immune Globulin-Human (called human T.I.G.) must be considered individually for each patient. The characteristics of the wound, conditions under which it was incurred, its treatment, its age, and the previous active immunization status of the patient must be considered. Passive immunization with human T.I.G. is not indicated, however, if the patient has ever received two or more injections of toxoid.

D. Every wounded patient should be given a written record of the immunization provided, with instructions to carry the record at all times, and if indicated, to complete active immunization. For precise tetanus prophylaxis, an accurate and immediately available history regarding previous active immunization against tetanus is required.

E. Immunization in adults requires at least three injections of toxoid. A routine booster of adsorbed toxoid is indicated every 10 years thereafter. In children under seven, immunization requires four injections of diphtheria and tetanus toxoids combined with pertussis vaccine. A fifth dose may be administered at four to six years of age. Thereafter, combined tetanus and diphtheria toxoid (adult type) is recommended for routine or wound boosters.

II. Specific measures for patients with wounds
  A. Previously immunized individuals
    1. When the attending physician has determined that the patient has been previously fully immunized and the last dose of toxoid was given within 10 years:
       a. For non-tetanus-prone wounds, no booster of toxoid is indicated.
       b. For tetanus-prone wounds and if more than 5 years has elapsed since the last dose, 0.5 mL adsorbed toxoid should be given. If excessive prior toxoid injections have been given, this booster may be omitted.
    2. When the patient has had two or more prior injections of toxoid and received the last dose more than 10 years previously, 0.5 mL adsorbed toxoid for both tetanus-prone and non-tetanus-prone wounds should be given. Passive immunization is not considered necessary.
  B. Individuals not adequately immunized, i.e., the patient has received only one or no prior injection of toxoid or the immunization history is unknown
    1. For non-tetanus-prone wounds, 0.5 mL adsorbed toxoid should be given.
    2. For tetanus-prone wounds:
       a. 0.5 mL adsorbed toxoid and 250 units (or more) of human T.I.G. (using different syringes, needles, and sites of injection) should be given.
       b. Administration of antibiotics should be considered, although the effectiveness of antibiotics for prophylaxis of tetanus remains unproved.

Medical students sometimes question on theoretical grounds the validity of administering toxoid and antitoxin (immune globulin) simultaneously to a previously unimmunized patient. The problem of interference during simultaneous active and passive immunization against tetanus has been studied quantitatively. There is some lowering of the antigenicity of toxoid, but the interference is not clinically significant if 250 units of tetanus immune globulin is injected. The antibody level in patients receiving immune globulin is protective for at least 4 weeks, and the second and third doses of toxoid produce an active antitoxin response. In addition, alum-adsorbed tetanus toxoid stimulates a quicker, higher, and more durable immunity than does plain toxoid because the aluminum in the preparation is an immunologic adjuvant. Use of the recommended adsorbed toxoid is, therefore, more reliable.

Wound Botulism

Botulism is an example of an intoxication resulting from the ingestion of exotoxin formed by *Clostridium botulinum* growing in improperly sterilized or inadequately preserved foods. Following gastrointestinal symptoms, botulism progresses to diplopia, blurred vision, and dysphagia and to a descending motor paralysis spreading to involve other cranial nerves and peripheral motor nerves. Although *C. botulinum* may be isolated from a wound as a simple contaminant, *wound botulism* is indicated by the presence of clinical signs of botulism. Wound botulism is a rare disease but should be suspected in any patient with a wound who presents with clinical signs of descending paralysis and a negative food history. Therapy of the wound is routine; therapy of the botulism is supportive, with respiratory care and assisted ventilation if required. Equine trivalent antitoxin should be given after testing for sensitivity to equine serum.

INFECTIONS CAUSED BY GRAM-NEGATIVE BACILLI

The gram-negative bacilli of importance to surgery are for the most part indigenous to human beings and often found in the intestinal tract. They are non-spore-forming rods, and they may be aerobes, facultative anaerobes, or obligate anaerobes. The role of some gram-negative bacilli as primary pathogens has long been known, e.g., *Pseudomonas aeruginosa* and *Salmonella typhi*. Others have been recognized only rarely as primary pathogens in human beings, e.g., *Serratia marcescens* and *Enterobacter aerogenes*. However, since the development of modern chemotherapy after World War II, the gram-negative bacilli have become increasingly important as causes of serious infection, particularly in hospitalized patients. Prior to the introduction of broad-spectrum antibiotics, the role of gram-negative bacilli as pathogens was usually overshadowed by the pneumococci, streptococci, and staphylococci. We now know that infection is most likely to occur when body defense mechanisms are either undeveloped or overtaxed, as in the case of infants and debilitated patients, and that therapeutic measures to combat one situation may provide an environment promoting the establishment of infection by almost any mixture of gram-negative bacilli. This situation prevails because of the great number of patients with impaired host defenses secondary to the use of multiple antibiotics, corticosteroids, immunosuppressive agents, antineoplastic drugs, and radiotherapy. Surgical procedures in which foreign bodies such as prosthetic valves or grafts are inserted appear to allow these less virulent species to become established

Table 5-7. TAXONOMY OF GRAM-NEGATIVE
BACILLI

Family	Tribe	Genus
Pseudomonaceae		*Pseudomonas*
Enterobacteriaceae	Eschericheae	*Escherichia (E. coli,* including *Alkalescens-Dispar* group)
		Shigella
	Edwardsielliae	*Edwardsiella*
	Salmonelleae	*Salmonella*
		Arizona
		Citrobacter (including Bethesda-Ballerup group)
	Klebsielleae	*Klebsiella*
		Enterobacter (including *Hafnia*)
		Pectobacterium
		Serratia
	Proteae	*Proteus*
		Providencia
Bacteroidaceae		*Bacteroides*
		Fusobacterium

and to produce infection. Indwelling venous and urethral catheters, endotracheal tubes and mechanical ventilators, peritoneal dialysis apparatus, and pump-oxygenators for extracorporeal circulation in cardiac surgery often serve as portals of entry for the gram-negative bacilli. The current taxonomic organization of gram-negative bacilli (aerobic, facultative, and anaerobic) is outlined in Table 5-7.

Aerobic and Facultative Bacteria

Pseudomonas aeruginosa is a strict aerobe; it is widely distributed and is frequently present in small numbers on healthy skin surfaces and in the normal intestinal flora of some individuals. *P. aeruginosa* is an opportunistic pathogen that can cause serious and lethal infections in debilitated or immunosuppressed patients, such as those with cancer, large burns, or cystic fibrosis, and is common in postoperative infections following the use of mechanical ventilators and indwelling urinary catheters. It is incriminated in primary infections such as meningitis resulting from lumbar puncture, traumatic injuries to the eye, and enteritis with associated bacteremia. Heroin addicts are subject to hematogenous pseudomonal osteomyelitis. Although *P. aeruginosa* is gram-negative and produces an endotoxin, its cell-wall lipopolysaccharides are not as toxic as those isolated from the enteric bacteria. It does, however, produce a variety of extracellular products that contribute to its pathogenicity, including hemolysins, proteases, an enterotoxin, and a heat-labile exotoxin. This exotoxin is more toxic than the other extracellular products or the endotoxin. *Pseudomonas* infections are treated with either tobramycin or gentamicin alone, or in

combination with carbenicillin or ticarcillin. Since resistant strains of *Pseudomonas* may be involved, antibiotic sensitivity tests should be performed.

Escherichia coli is found in the intestinal tract of human beings and animals and is the predominant facultative commensal in the normal intestinal flora. Although more than 145 different envelope capsular (K) antigens have been identified, the ability of a strain to be typed does not necessarily denote pathogenicity or virulence. Nevertheless, certain strains belonging to distinct antigenic types are *enteropathogenic,* others are *enterotoxigenic* by their capacity to produce toxins, and others are *enteroinvasive* by their ability to penetrate mucosal cells. These strains produce diarrheal disease, especially in infants. Stool isolates may have none, one, two, or all three of these pathogenic characteristics. *Escherichia coli* may produce meningitis, septicemia, endocarditis, appendiceal abscess, peritonitis, septic wounds, and pyogenic infections, chiefly urinary tract infections (pyelitis, cystitis, etc.) in pure culture or in association with fecal streptococci. *Escherichia coli* also has the capacity to produce a potent endotoxin that enters the circulation and induces shock. The antibiotic of choice in the treatment of the patient seriously ill with *Escherichia coli* sepsis is ampicillin alone or combined with gentamicin or tobramycin.

The *Salmonella* species are a large group of enteric pathogens transmitted via food and water. They cause enteric fevers (particularly typhoid fever), gastroenteritis, and septicemia. *Salmonella typhi* and *Salmonella enteritidis* pass from the small intestine by way of the lymphatics to the mesenteric glands. After multiplication there, they invade the bloodstream via the thoracic duct. Complications that may result from this hematogenous dissemination include thrombophlebitis, lymphadenitis, pneumonia, osteomyelitis, arthritis, endocarditis, and meningitis. Hemorrhage may occur from perforation of ulcers in lymphoid tissue of the intestine. The specific surgical treatment for perforation, i.e., simple closure or segmental resection, is determined by the pathologic findings encountered at operation. Chloramphenicol has long been advocated in the treatment of typhoid fever, but ampicillin is equally effective. Although postoperative wound infection due to *Salmonella typhi* is rare, recorded cases occur after gallbladder surgery in patients who are unsuspected typhoid carriers. Contaminated wound drainage and positive stools from such patients are distinct hazards to other hospitalized patients.

Before the introduction of modern chemotherapy, gram-negative bacilli of the tribe Klebsielleae were rarely noted as primary pathogens. However, along with other gram-negative bacilli, they have assumed increasing importance as causes of serious hospital-acquired infections. *Klebsiella pneumoniae* causes a severe pneumonia having a propensity for debilitated (frequently alcoholic) patients. *Klebsiella* has also been implicated in endocarditis, septic thrombophlebitis, septicemia, urinary tract infection, wound infection, crepitant cellulitis, and myonecrosis. *Enterobacter aerogenes* is a commensal in the intestinal tract of approximately 5 percent of healthy individuals. It has less pathogenic potential than strains of *Klebsiella* but is commonly involved in hospital-acquired sepsis. *Serratia marcescens* is another species formerly considered to be nonpathogenic for human beings. Although it too has low virulence for healthy individuals, it is now found primarily in hospitalized patients with some underlying disease. It may spread like other "hospital bacteria," and infection may not always produce clinical symptoms. Classically, *Serratia marcescens* has been recognized by its ability to produce a characteristic red pigment, and it has been thought to be an obligate pigment producer. However, the majority of strains of *Serratia marcescens* involved in hospital-acquired infections are nonpigmented and often have been mistaken for other enterobacteria. These nonchromogenic strains of *Serratia marcescens* now can be identified by appropriate biochemical tests. The *Klebsiella-Enterobacter-Serratia* species are often isolated in mixed culture from sputum, urine, blood, and wounds in which there are other potential pathogens such as streptococci, staphylococci, *Escherichia coli, Proteus* species, *Citrobacter* species, and *Pseudomonas aeruginosa*. Epidemiologic studies indicate that the particular strains and types of the gram-negative species producing infection are nosocomial and acquired in the intestinal tract of patients during hospitalization. They are often highly drug-resistant, and the overall mortality associated with bacteremia is approximately 50 percent. The risk of bacteremia appears to be related to the underlying disease of the patient and the nature of the infection (urinary tract, respiratory, wound infection, abscess, etc.). The antibiotic of choice in treatment of infections caused by the *Klebsiella-Enterobacter-Serratia* species is an aminoglycoside (gentamicin, tobramycin, netlimicin, or amikacin).

Gram-negative bacilli in the genera *Proteus* and *Providencia* also compete for prominence with the other aerobic gram-negatives in infections. Rapid and abundant urease production distinguishes *Proteus* from *Providencia*. These organisms often occur in abscesses, in infected wounds, and also in burns as one component of a mixed infection. They are resistant to most antibiotics, and what was originally a mixed infection may be converted into a pure proteus infection as a result of antibiotic therapy. Sepsis due to indol-negative *Proteus (Proteus mirabilis)* is treated with ampicillin, while that due to indol-positive species (*Proteus vulgaris, P. morganii,* and *P. rettgeri*) is treated with gentamicin, tobramycin, netlimicin, or amikacin. *Providencia* species are also sensitive to these aminoglycosides. The genus *Acinetobacter* includes gram-negative pleomorphic aerobes previously known by a wide variety of names. *Acinetobacter calcoaceticus* var. *anitratus* (formerly *Herellea vaginicola* and *Bacterium anitratum*) and *Acinetobacter calcoaceticus* var. *lwoffi* (formerly *Mima polymorpha*) are opportunists capable of causing therapy-potentiated infections in compromised patients. An aminoglycoside also constitutes appropriate therapy for these infections.

Anaerobic Bacteria

Obligately anaerobic bacteria, especially gram-negative bacilli, are found as normal flora on skin and all mucous membrane surfaces. They are by far the major component of the normal flora. In the normal oral cavity, anaerobes outnumber aerobes 10 to 1, and in the normal colon, 1000 to 1. When the mucous membrane barrier is disturbed by disease, trauma, or surgical procedures, these bacteria can invade adjacent tissue and may cause infection. In the upper respiratory tract and lungs, the major anaerobic pathogens are peptostreptococci, fusobacteria, and *Bacteroides melaninogenicus*. In intraabdominal infections, *Bacteroides fragilis* is the most frequent isolate; clostridia, peptostreptococci, and peptococci are also found. In infection of the female genital tract, the same anaerobes are also the principal pathogens. Although anaerobic infections often originate close to a mucosal surface, they may occur anywhere in the body as a result of direct or hematogenous spread. Clues to diagnosis include foul-smelling discharge, gas, necrotic tissue, abscess formation, and failure to obtain growth on aerobic culture despite the presence of organisms on Gram-stained direct smear. Anaerobes are associated with 90 percent of cases of intraabdominal abscess, 95 percent of appendiceal abscess, 90 percent of aspiration pneumonia, 95 percent of lung abscess, 85 percent of brain abscess, and 75 percent of upper tract female pelvic infections.

The bacteroides are obligately anaerobic, gram-negative, non-spore-forming bacilli. They are sometimes the only microorganisms found in clinical specimens but more often are found in association with other anaerobes and aerobes. Currently, human pathogens are assigned to the genus *Bacteroides* and the genus *Fusobacterium*. *Bacteroides* are rod-shaped cells with rounded ends and are sometimes coccobacillary; *Fusobacterium* may be bacilli with pointed ends or pleomorphic, filamentous forms with swellings and free, round bodies. Species causing infections in human beings are *Bacteroides fragilis, Bacteroides melaninogenicus, Fusobacterium fusiforme,* and *Fusobacterium necrophorus*.

In circumstances such as chronic illness, malignant disease, surgical treatment, and cystoscopy, the bacteroides may invade the bloodstream to cause septicemia and penetrate tissue and organs to produce abscesses. The clinical spectrum of infections varies from superficial infections to deep abscesses with overwhelming bacteremia and shock. The gastrointestinal tract, especially the colon and appendix, appears to be the most frequent source of bacteroides infection. Gynecologic infections involve the vagina, uterus, and contiguous structures, and are related to malignancy of pelvic organs, septic abortions, and postpartum complications. Upper respiratory tract infections and those of the nasopharynx, mouth, and jaw (tonsillar and peritonsillar abscesses, chronic otitis media, and dentoalveolar abscesses) have become relatively uncommon since the widespread use of antibiotics (penicillin or tetracycline) for the treatment of undiagnosed pharyngitis. Brain abscesses are a well-known complication of these upper respiratory tract infections in which bacteroides are involved along with other microorganisms, such as anaerobic streptococci.

Bacteroides bacteremia is characterized by a spiking fever, jaundice, and leukocytosis. In the patient more than forty years old, it is associated with chronic debilitating disease, hypotension, and a high mortality. Bacteremias have followed primary infection in the gastrointestinal, pelvic, and pharyngeal areas, and may originate from thrombophlebitis in these sites of infection. An indication of *Bacteroides* infection is the presence of a foul-smelling exudate from wounds or abscesses that contain gram-negative forms but produce no growth on aerobic culture. There appears to be a disposition toward *Bacteroides* infection in patients with underlying malignant disease. Often these patients have undergone elective intestinal surgery after preoperative intestinal antisepsis. This suggests that changes in the normal intestinal flora may predispose to *Bacteroides* infection. Therefore, the surgeon should be alert to the possibility of *Bacteroides* infection. A changing pattern of pyogenic abscesses of the liver has been characterized by an increased incidence of *Bacteroides* as the pathogen.

Treatment of anaerobic infections consists of surgical drainage of abscesses, excision of necrotic tissue, and appropriate antibiotic therapy. This should be based upon the results of sensitivity tests. Penicillin G is the drug of choice for most anaerobic infections, including those caused by oropharyngeal strains of *Bacteroides fragilis.* Infections caused by gastrointestinal strains of *Bacteroides fragilis,* however, require treatment with clindamycin. An alternative agent for either type of *Bacteroides* infection is metronidazole. (See Table 5-4 for other alternative agents.)

PSEUDOMYCOTIC INFECTIONS

Among the actinomycetes, *Actinomyces israelii* and *Nocardia asteroides* are isolated most frequently as human pathogens, although other species of each genus may also be implicated in human infections. Actinomycetes are true bacteria but traditionally have been studied and grouped with the fungi because of their resemblance to mycotic agents and their involvement in diseases resembling mycoses. Infections caused by these false fungi (pseudomyces) may be called pseudomycoses to separate them from true fungal infections. They will therefore be considered separately from the true mycoses.

Actinomycosis

Actinomyces israelii is a strict anaerobe present in normal oral flora. Actinomycosis is therefore an endogenous infection. There are three clinical types of actinomycosis: cervicofacial (the most common type), thoracic, and abdominal. A dense fibroblastic reaction is produced, and connective and granulation tissue tend to form a wall around the abscess. Wherever lesions occur, abscesses expand into contiguous tissue and form burrowing, tortuous sinuses to the outside, where they discharge pus and necrotic material. This pus contains dense clusters of organisms and hyphae appearing as macroscopic, yellow-brown "sulfur granules," which facilitate diagnosis when examined microscopically and cultured. Actinomycosis can be cured with massive doses of penicillin G or tetracycline. Surgical drainage of abscesses and aggressive

resection of damaged tissue are important adjuncts to long-term chemotherapy.

Nocardiosis

Nocardia, in contrast to actinomycetes, are aerobic inhabitants of soil and are not part of the normal flora of human beings. *Nocardia asteroides* and *Nocardia brasiliensis,* opportunistic pathogens for human beings, are less acid-fast than mycobacteria, and their filaments tend to branch. Nocardiosis tends to be progressive and fatal but is a rare disease. Pulmonary infection arises from inhalation of the organisms, while subcutaneous abscesses (mycetomas) result from contamination of skin wounds, usually of the hands and feet of laborers. Massive doses of sulfonamides, e.g., sulfadiazine 6 to 8 g/day orally for at least 4 to 6 months, is the preferred therapy; ampicillin is an alternate agent. Drainage of empyema and abscesses is an important surgical adjunct to chemotherapy.

MYCOTIC INFECTIONS

The relation of the surgeon to mycotic infection has changed in recent years. The need for surgical treatment has diminished because of more effective modern chemotherapy. However, the long-term use of cytotoxic agents, corticosteroids, and antibacterial drugs for patients with leukemia and neoplasms has increased the incidence of opportunistic mycotic infections. Among the pathogenic fungi to be discussed, *Blastomyces dermatitidis, Paracoccidioides brasiliensis, Histoplasma capsulatum, Cryptococcus neoformans,* and even *Coccidioides immitis* are frank pathogens but may be opportunistic to the extent that they cause progressive infections in debilitated patients more frequently than in healthy ones. Definite opportunistic infections are caused by species of *Mucor, Rhizopus, Aspergillus,* and *Candida.* Fungal infection threatens any compromised hosts, such as severely burned patients and those with implanted prosthetic devices and transplanted organs. Some of the symptoms of mycotic disease are chronic skin or mucous membrane lesions, low-grade fever, weight loss, chronic pulmonary or meningeal involvement, hepatosplenomegaly, and lymphadenopathy. Mycotic disease should be suspected unless another cause is clearly established. A mycosis may coexist with a lymphomatous disease, e.g., the association of histoplasmosis and cryptococcosis with Hodgkin's disease. A presumptive clinical diagnosis of a mycosis must be confirmed in the laboratory. Serologic tests are useful in reaching a presumptive diagnosis. The morphologic features of the fungus in tissue and culture are significant in identification.

The majority of patients with fungal infections seen by the physician have serious illness and present with typical symptoms of infection. Symptoms of pulmonary involvement frequently are present. Hematogenous dissemination of the disease produces manifestations such as tender swollen joints, draining subcutaneous abscesses, ulcerative lesions of the oropharynx, and meningitis. Many pa-

Table 5-8. MYCOSES IMPORTANT IN SURGICAL INFECTIONS

Type of disease	Mycosis	Representative fungus	Fungal morphology		
			Dimor-phism	Infected tissue	Laboratory culture
Systemic	Blastomycosis	*Blastomyces dermatidis*	Yes	Yeast	Mycelia
	Paracoccidioidomycosis	*Paracoccidioides brasiliensis*	Yes	Yeast	Mycelia
	Histoplasmosis	*Histoplasma capsulatum*	Yes	Yeast	Mycelia
	Coccidioidomycosis	*Coccidioides immitis*	Yes	Spherules	Mycelia
	Cryptococcosis	*Cryptococcus neoformans*	No	Yeast	Yeast
Subcutaneous	Sporotrichosis	*Sporotrichum schenckii*	Yes	Yeast	Mycelia
Systemic, particularly opportunistic	Phycomycosis	*Mucor corymbifera*	No	Mycelia	Mycelia
		Rhizopus oryzae	No	Mycelia	Mycelia
	Aspergillosis	*Aspergillus fumigatus*	No	Mycelia	Mycelia
	Candidosis	*Candida albicans*	Yes	Yeast and hyphae	Yeast and hyphae

tients with systemic mycoses, as well as those with dermatophytoses, have skin lesions that are painful, itching, weeping, crusting, malodorous, and disfiguring. Fungi of ever-increasing importance as agents of infection in surgical patients are grouped in Table 5-8 according to the type of disease they cause and will be discussed in the order shown.

Blastomycosis (North American Blastomycosis)

Blastomyces dermatitidis is a dimorphic fungus; it grows in tissues and in culture at 37°C as a spherical thick-walled, single-budding yeast and in culture at room temperature as a mold. Lateral, rounded conidia borne along hyphae are presumably the infectious spores. Demonstration of nonencapsulated, thick-walled, multinucleate yeast cells in pus, sputum, or tissue sections and their subsequent laboratory culture establish the diagnosis. Blastomycosis usually begins in the lungs as a subacute respiratory infection (pulmonary form) that gradually increases in severity over a period of weeks or months and sometimes resembles tuberculosis or carcinoma. Frequently, during the course of infection, patients develop skin lesions. These may be the only apparent signs of blastomycosis. Pulmonary blastomycosis spreads hematogenously to establish focal destructive lesions in other parts of the body. Spreading, ulcerated, crusted skin lesions in particular arise as metastases from the primary pulmonary lesions. Amphotericin B is indicated in treating all forms of blastomycosis. If surgery is indicated for diagnosis to rule out bronchogenic carcinoma, amphotericin is used both pre- and postoperatively to minimize operative spread.

Paracoccidioidomycosis (South American Blastomycosis)

Paracoccidioides brasiliensis is dimorphic and grows in tissue as a multiple-budding yeast, in contrast to the single-budding yeast in blastomycosis. Paracoccid-

ioidomycosis is characterized by primary pulmonary lesions with dissemination to visceral organs, by conspicuous ulcerative granulomas of the buccal and nasal mucosa, and by generalized lymphangitis. In blastomycosis, visceral organs are *not* involved. Treatment with amphotericin B is usually effective.

Histoplasmosis

Histoplasma capsulatum is dimorphic; it appears characteristically in infected tissues as many small, oval yeast cells packed within macrophages and reticuloendothelial cells; at room temperature it forms slowly growing mycelial colonies. This pathogen is present in soil, especially that enriched by feces of birds and bats, and is endemic in the Mississippi and Ohio valleys and along the Appalachian mountains of the United States. Inhalation of conidia leads to pulmonary infection. The initial infection is mild and may be inapparent or may occur as a primary acute disease. Symptoms may include fever, cough, chest pain, dyspnea, and pleurisy with effusion. Localized pulmonary histoplasmosis resembles tuberculosis in its histopathology. In a few individuals the infection becomes progressive and widely disseminated and may simulate miliary tuberculosis. Disseminated histoplasmosis primarily involves the reticuloendothelial system in various tissues and organs and often coexists in individuals who have tuberculosis, leukemia, or Hodgkin's disease. Histoplasmosis is treated with high doses of intravenous amphotericin B. In chronic cavitary disease surgical resection should be performed, with amphotericin therapy given before and after surgery to reduce postoperative complications and avoid relapse.

Coccidioidomycosis

Coccidioides immitis is a somewhat different dimorphic fungus; it varies in structure between a hyphal form found in soil and a spherule or sporangium form found in infected tissues. The sporangia are thick-walled structures filled with globular endospores or sporangiospores. At maturity the sporangium bursts and releases hundreds of endospores, each of which can form a new sporangium in tissue. When sporangia are plated on Sabouraud agar, growth of the mycelial form occurs. Barrel-shaped arthrospores are formed in the mycelium. These arthrospores are highly infectious and become airborne easily. The mycelial (saprophytic) form is readily converted into the sporangium (parasitic) form in human beings. *Coccidioides immitis* is endemic in the southwestern United States and adjacent Mexico, where it grows as a saprophyte in desert soils. Infection is established by inhalation of airborne arthrospores.

About 60 percent of infected individuals remain asymptomatic but become skin-sensitive to coccidioidin. The acute and most common form of coccidioidomycosis resembles influenza. When confined to the lungs, the disease is usually self-limited and heals with scarring. However, a chronic, progressive, granulomatous disease occurs in fewer than 1 percent of infected individuals. Years may elapse between primary infection and the more serious disseminated disease. Patients with disseminated coccidioidomycosis appear to have some defect in their immune response to the fungus. The symptoms are similar to those seen in advancing tuberculosis. Any organ or tissue of the body may be involved. However, the infection shows predilection for bone, skin, and subcutaneous tissue. This disease is not contagious, since it is spread only by saprophytic arthrospores. The majority of patients with primary infection recover without therapy or with only symptomatic care. Amphotericin B is used to treat disseminated coccidioidomycosis but is less effective than with blastomycosis, histoplasmosis, and cryptococcosis.

Cryptococcosis

Cryptococcus neoformans is *not dimorphic;* in both infected tissue and in culture it appears as encapsulated yeast cells. The yeast cells are thin-walled, but the large, clear polysaccharide capsules surrounding them are distinctive. *Cryptococcus neoformans* is found in dust and bird droppings. Inhalation of yeast cells is thought to initiate pulmonary infection, which may be inapparent or mild. There is little inflammatory response of invaded tissues. Cryptococcosis is a subacute or chronic mycotic infection most frequently involving tissues of the central nervous system but occasionally producing lesions in the lungs or skin. Cryptococcal meningitis is the most frequent form of disseminated disease and mimics tuberculous meningitis, brain abscess, or brain tumor. Pulmonary lesions are usually found at autopsy. Many patients with pulmonary or dermal cryptococcosis respond to therapy with flucytosine. Surgical resection is indicated for both cavitary and nodular pulmonary disease. When diagnosis is established by surgery, therapy with amphotericin B is begun postoperatively to avoid meningitis and recurrence. Amphotericin B is the drug of choice for cryptococcosis of the central nervous system. Cryptococcosis is an opportunistic mycosis in debilitated patients, particularly those with Hodgkin's disease or leukemia.

Sporotrichosis

Sporotrichum schenckii is dimorphic. When found in tissues or exudate stained by the periodic acid–Schiff technique, this fungus appears as fusiform bodies or round budding cells, but these are rarely seen. When these materials are cultured on Sabouraud agar at room temperature, the mycelial form grows. Microscopically, hyphae are slender and septate, and conidia are individually attached by sterigmata to a common conidiophore. Hyphae are converted to the yeast form by injection into mice and by cultivation at 37°C on an enriched medium. Human beings become infected by accidental subcutaneous inoculation from thorns and splinters. Sporotrichosis is a chronic progressive infection of the skin and subcutaneous tissue that frequently begins as a primary lesion of the skin of the hand or forearm and secondarily involves lymphatic channels and lymph nodes draining the area, which become cordlike, resulting in a chain of ulcers. Generalized infection occurs in the compromised host by way of the blood, and any organ or tissue can be the site of lesions. Symptoms are then related to the region involved. Orally administered potassium iodide is specific in sporotrichosis and must be continued for several weeks after recovery seems complete. Intravenous amphotericin B is indicated for disseminated sporotrichosis. *Sporotrichum schenckii* has caused suprainfection in patients with underlying hematologic malignant disease who have been treated with antitumor agents and steroids.

Phycomycosis

Species of *Mucor* and *Rhizopus* are saprophytes common in nature and are *not dimorphic*. They can produce rapidly fatal disease when they invade the brain, lungs, or other organs of a compromised host. These fungi may also produce a superficial infection of the skin with occasional ulceration and granuloma or abscess formation. *Mucor* and *Rhizopus* are opportunistic pathogens, and are held in check by normal serum factors that become diminished in individuals suffering from uncontrolled diabetes mellitus, blood dyscrasias, endocrine disturbances, malnutrition, and burns. Corticosteroid therapy and prolonged use of broad-spectrum antibiotics may also enhance susceptibility to phycomycosis. The local cutaneous lesions heal with proper hygiene and fungicides; extensive lesions may require debridement. Amphotericin B and correction of the underlying disease is the therapy for the acute form of phycomycosis. Amphotericin should be used to treat any patient not responding to other measures. Surgery should be considered for patients with pulmonary lesions not responsive to amphotericin.

Aspergillosis

Aspergillus has become an important pathogen in patients with impaired host defenses. These mycelial fungi are saprophytic and are not dimorphic but can cause local as well as disseminated disease. *Aspergillus fumigatus* is the most commonly reported species. Two forms of pulmonary aspergillosis are frequently seen: (1) pulmonary or bronchial aspergilloma (fungus ball), due to secondary invasion of a tuberculous or coccidioidal cavity, and (2) allergic bronchopulmonary aspergillosis. In the compromised host these may proceed to disseminated infection. Otomycosis is secondary to bacterial infection of the ear. The fungus grows on ear wax and macerated tissue. Systemic aspergillosis may complicate severe underlying diseases that are being treated with steroids, immunosuppressive drugs, or broad-spectrum antibiotics. Local superficial lesions often heal spontaneously with hygienic care. Localized abscesses and granulomas should be excised. Systemic infection requires treatment with amphotericin B. The prognosis in disseminated aspergillosis is poor; the patient often succumbs to the underlying disease.

Candidosis

Candida albicans is indigenous in human beings and is dimorphic; both yeast and mycelial forms are seen in infected tissue. *Candida albicans* affects mucous membranes and causes diseases ranging from thrush (oral candidosis) and vulvovaginal candidosis to systemic candidosis. The former are common medical problems, the latter an opportunistic infection of the compromised host. Patients with hemopoietic and lymphoreticular neoplasms, as well as those being treated with immunosuppressives, glucocorticoids, and broad-spectrum antibiotics, are particularly prone to systemic fungal infections. Patients with burns and those undergoing intravenous hyperalimentation are also prone to systemic candidosis. Candidal endocarditis, especially that due to *Candida parapsilosis,* is seen in drug addicts using intravenous heroin.

Thrush and other clinically distinctive candidal infections frequently result from antibacterial therapy, and discontinuance of the therapy will usually cause the antibiotic-induced superinfection to disappear. Topical nystatin is effective in treating candidal infections of the skin, mouth, and vagina. Amphotericin B is the mainstay in treating systemic candidosis. Oral flucytosine is considerably less toxic than amphotericin, but 50 percent of *Candida* strains are initially resistant. The use of combination therapy with amphotericin B and flucytosine produces an antifungal synergism using a lower and less toxic dose of amphotericin. Combination therapy has resulted in successful treatment of candidosis and also cryptococcosis.

SURGICAL ASEPSIS

Surgical asepsis, the prevention of the access of microorganisms to an operative wound, is achieved by methods designed to destroy bacteria or remove them from all objects coming in contact with the wound. Modern surgery is aseptic in the use of sterile instruments, sutures, and dressings and in the wearing of sterile gowns and rubber gloves by the operating personnel. Although this is pres-

ently the extent of routine sterility in surgical asepsis, the technology of germ-free research is able to provide sterile flexible plastic isolation chambers in which neonates or antibiotic-decontaminated patients may be maintained in a sterile environment. Operations may be performed in "surgical" isolators cemented to the operative site of the patient. The surgeon makes his incision through the site of attachment of the isolator, and the operation may be conducted in the absence of all microorganisms. There is considerable interest in unidirectional (laminar) airflow systems as a less absolute means of limiting the number of bacteria to which a patient is exposed. These systems recirculate air through high-efficiency particulate air filters that assure unidirectional flow in either a downward or horizontal direction. However, the advantages or necessity of such systems in operating rooms are controversial, since there has not been substantial evidence to demonstrate their effectiveness in reducing postoperative infections. The Committee on Control of Operating Room Environment of the American College of Surgeons does not recommend laminar airflow for general use in operating rooms.

It is necessary to resort to the use of antiseptics to degerm the site of the operation on the patient's skin. The surgeon and operating-room personnel usually use soaps or detergents containing antiseptics for scrubbing their hands before donning gloves or else rinse in an antiseptic after the scrub. An *antiseptic* is a chemical agent that either kills pathogenic microorganisms or inhibits their growth so long as there is contact between agent and microbe. By custom as well as by federal law, the term "antiseptic" is reserved for agents applied to the body. The antiseptic may actually be a disinfectant used in dilute solutions to avoid damage to tissues. A *disinfectant* is a germicidal, chemical substance used on inanimate objects to kill pathogenic microorganisms but not necessarily all others. These germicidal agents are used to disinfect instruments and other equipment that cannot be exposed to heat. They are essential for good housekeeping practices in hospitals, where they are used to disinfect floors, fabrics, and excreta. The first step in any process of biologic decontamination is thorough mechanical cleansing with soap or detergent and water to remove all traces of blood, pus, proteins, and mucus before the antiseptic or disinfectant is employed.

Sterilization

Sterilization is the process of killing all microorganisms (bacteria, spores, viruses, mycotic agents, and parasites). It is the ultimate in disinfection. The practical criterion of sterility is the failure of microbial growth to appear on tests in suitable bacteriologic media. Sterilization can be achieved by either physical or chemical agents. *Steam under pressure* is the most reliable means of sterilizing surgical supplies because of its power of penetration, microbiologic efficiency, ease of control, and economy of operation. Application of steam under a pressure of 15 psi (pounds per square inch) for 15 to 45 min will destroy all forms of life. Free-flowing steam, like boiling water, has a temperature of 100°C, but the same steam under pressure of 15 psi exerts a temperature of 121°C. Steam gives up heat by condensing into water. Thus when a bundle containing surgical pads or sponges is sterilized, the steam contacts the outer layer. There a portion of it condenses into water and releases heat. The steam then penetrates to a second layer, where another portion condenses and gives up heat. The steam thus approaches the center of the package, layer after layer, until the whole package is sterilized. The time of exposure depends upon the size of the parcel and its wrappings. Sterilization by steam under pressure is carried out in an autoclave. A major caution to be recognized when operating an autoclave is that a mixture of air and steam has a lower temperature than does pure steam. Therefore, when air is present in the chamber, the killing power of the process is diminished in proportion to the amount of air present. Most autoclaves depend upon gravity displacement of air from the chamber and from within articles being sterilized. Thus, improperly packed and positioned articles in the autoclave may fail to become sterile even though all physical conditions of the run may be correct. A new development in autoclaves is the high-vacuum sterilizer. A vacuum pump is incorporated into the system, and a vacuum is pulled in the chamber at the beginning and end of the sterilizing cycle. There is a considerable shortening of the time needed for sterilization, as only 3 min are needed to achieve sterility rather than the 20 min on the regular systems. In addition, there appears to be less damage to rubber, fabrics, and sharp instruments because of reduced exposure to moisture. There is less danger of creating air pockets and less chance of the steam's failing to penetrate to the center of bundles. Materials emerge dry, and much greater tolerances in packing the chamber are afforded.

Dry-heat sterilization is commonly used for glassware, for items that are injured by moisture, and for materials that resist penetration by steam, such as talc, vaseline, fats, and oils. The process consists of baking the material to be sterilized in a hot-air oven. At a temperature of 121°C (250°F) it takes about 6 h to sterilize glassware, but at 170°C (340°F) the time required is about 1 h. *Gas sterilization* is practical with ethylene oxide, a gas employed as a sterilizing agent in specially designed chambers in which temperatures and humidity can be controlled and from which air can be evacuated. The killing action is slow, and an exposure period from 3 to 6 h is needed. Sterilization employing ethylene oxide is used for delicate surgical instruments with optical lenses, for tubing and plastic parts of heart-lung machines and respirators, for prepacked commercial plastic products such as disposable syringes, and for blankets, pillows, and mattresses. Ethylene oxide is most reliable when applied to clean, dry surfaces that do not absorb the chemical. The gas dissolves in plastic, rubber, fabric, and leather, and chemical burns may occur when materials laden with ethylene oxide are applied to tissue. The dissolved chemical escapes from materials when they are exposed to air, and a minimum of 24 h of aeration is necessary to ensure removal of the gas from sterilized articles. However, solid metal or glass items may be used immediately after sterilization. *Radiation sterilization* refers to ionizing radiation by cobalt 60 sources (γ-radiation) and by electron accelerators (high-energy electrons). It is currently used commercially to sterilize disposable hospital supplies, such as plastic hypodermic syringes and sutures. Radiation sterilization of heat-sensitive pharmaceuticals has been recommended.

Chemical sterilization is currently achieved with a 2% aqueous solution of glutaraldehyde. This compound is an effective disinfectant for surgical, anesthetic, and dental equipment, rubber and plastic mouthpieces, catheters, and other heat-sensitive hospital equipment. Either a buffered alkaline solution (Cidex) or a potentiated acid solution (Sonacide) of glutaraldehyde may be used. They are equally bactericidal, sporicidal, and virucidal. Isopropyl alcohol may also be used for the chemical sterilization of instruments if they are first cleansed of all blood, pus, and body fluids. Only in the absence of spores is alcohol an effective sterilizing agent.

Degerming of Skin

Antiseptics incorporated into soaps are used for preoperative preparation of the skin at the operative site and for surgical hand scrubs by operating personnel. The bacteriologic content of normal skin consists of a resident flora, composed of coagulase-negative *Staphylococcus epidermidis* and anaerobic diphtheroides (e.g., *Propionibacterium acnes*), which reside on the surface of the skin, in hair follicles, and in the ducts of sebaceous glands. These bacteria can be diminished temporarily, but they cannot be permanently eradicated. They are not usually responsible for surgical infections. Superimposed upon the resident flora is a transient flora consisting of bacteria picked up as a result of temporary colonizing of the skin. In the hospital, this transient flora often consists of pathogens resistant to antibiotics and is likely to be composed of pathogenic strains of *Staphylococcus aureus* and gramnegative enterobacteria. Therefore, pathogenic bacteria on the hands of operating personnel at the time of operation must be removed by scrubbing and destroyed by an antiseptic agent. The patient's skin must be degermed in the area of operation prior to the incision. The most efficient method is a vigorous scrub with liquid soaps containing either hexachlorophene, an iodophor, or chlorhexidine.

Hexachlorophene is a bisphenol that disinfects the skin slowly. Commercial preparations containing 3% hexachlorophene, a detergent, and liquid soap are used for surgical scrubbing. Over a period of days, regular use of these surgical soaps brings about a progressive decrease in the number of bacteria on and in the skin. The hexachlorophene leaves an active film, which is renewed with each scrubbing. Consequently, its antibacterial activity persists so long as one continues to wash with soap containing hexachlorophene. A single washing with ordinary soap removes the antibacterial film. Hexachlorophene is effective against gram-positive pathogens such as *Staphy-*

lococcus aureus, but it is without activity against gram-negative bacteria, such as the pseudomonas and the enterobacteria. Significant blood levels have been found in frequent users, and vacuolar encephalopathy has been noted postmortem in premature infants bathed with hexachlorophene. It is also suspected of teratogenicity. Hexachlorophene preparations should be restricted for use only with specific indications, and removed from general use within a hospital.

Iodophors are organic complexes of iodine and a synthetic detergent. About 1% iodine is available in the formula, whose germicidal action results from the liberation of free iodine when the compound is diluted with water. The detergent in the complex enhances the bactericidal activity of the iodine. Advantages of iodophors are that they destroy both gram-positive and gram-negative bacterial cells, but not spores; they do not stain skin and clothing; and allergic reactions are reduced. However, they do not maintain adequate residual activity. Iodophors have been incorporated into surgical scrub soaps for hands and for the operative site, and are effective for this use, but they should not be used to lavage serous cavities. (Discussion is found under Intraperitoneal Antibiotic Therapy.)

Chlorhexidine gluconate is effective against gram-positive and gram-negative bacteria and fungi; it is sporicidal only at elevated temperatures. Chlorhexidine gluconate (4%) combined with 4% isopropanol in a sudsing base is used as a surgical hand scrub, a superficial skin wound cleanser, and a handwashing agent. Preoperative preparation of the skin is accomplished with a 0.5% solution of chlorhexidine in 70% isopropanol.

Other Surgical Antiseptics

No economical antiseptic or disinfectant is available to kill all microbial flora in a reasonable time at concentrations that will not irritate tissue or damage medical devices. However, there are several agents that have high reliability and low toxicity as surgical antiseptics. Among them are alcohol and iodine. The combination of inorganic iodine and alcohol, either as a tincture or as a mixture of 1 to 3% iodine with 70% ethyl or isopropyl alcohol, kills both gram-positive and gram-negative bacteria. Only a short contact time is needed, and the solution itself is not likely to be contaminated. Some patients, however, have adverse reactions to iodine, and most physicians hesitate to use this combination on mucous membranes or denuded skin. Aqueous iodophor solutions are available as an alternative. These also have a broad antimicrobic spectrum and are not likely to be contaminated, and they provoke adverse reaction less frequently than do inorganic tinctures of iodine. For patients sensitive to iodine, a thorough scrub with soap and water followed by a 2-min scrub with 70 to 90% ethyl or isopropyl alcohol is effective surgical antisepsis. Isopropyl alcohol is slightly more effective than ethyl alcohol when used as a 70% solution and is less expensive and more readily obtained because it is not potable. As a group, alcohols exhibit many desirable features. They are bactericidal, have a cleansing action, and evaporate readily. They do not, however, kill spores, and the best one can hope to accomplish with alcohol is to reduce the number of viable bacteria and destroy pathogens that may be on the skin as transients.

Aqueous quaternary ammonium compounds such as benzalkonium chloride (Zephiran chloride) are used diluted 1:750 for skin antisepsis for venipuncture and for disinfection of cystoscopes and bronchoscopes. They are less expensive than many other products and are nontoxic and nonallergenic but *must* be used with caution. Although they are potent bactericides in vitro and are particularly active against gram-positive cocci, benzalkonium antiseptics have been implicated in nosocomial infections by resistant *Pseudomonas capacia* and *Enterobacter* species that contaminate working solutions of these compounds. Accordingly, there are few applications for quaternary ammonium compounds in hospitals other than for environmental sanitation. Alternative surgical antiseptics such as iodine, iodophors, chlorhexidine, and alcohol have a broad antibacterial spectrum.

Bibliography

Introduction; General Principles; Surgical Infections

American College of Surgeons, Committee on Control of Surgical Infections: *Manual on Control of Surgical Infections,* 2d ed. Philadelphia, Lippincott, 1984.

Brummelkamp WH, Boerema I, et al: Treatment of clostridial infections with hyperbaric oxygen drenching: A report of 26 cases. *Lancet* 1:235–238, 1963.

Cruse PJE, Foord R: The epidemiology of wound infection: A 10-year prospective study of 62,939 wounds. *Surg Clin North Am* 60:27–40, 1980.

Hart GB, Lamb RC, et al: Gas gangrene: I. A collective review; II. A 15-year experience with hyperbaric oxygen. *J Trauma* 23:991–1000, 1983.

Holland JA, Hill GB, et al: Experimental and clinical experience with hyperbaric oxygen in the treatment of clostridial myonecrosis. *Surgery* 77:75–85, 1975.

Hunt TK: Surgical wound infections: An overview. *Am J Med* 70:712–718, 1981.

Meleney FL: *Treatise on Surgical Infections.* New York, Oxford University Press, 1948.

Meleney FL: *Clinical Aspects and Treatment of Surgical Infections.* Philadelphia, Saunders, 1949.

Polk HC Jr, Stone HH (eds): *Hospital-Acquired Infections in Surgery.* Baltimore, University Park Press, 1977.

Roding B, Groeneveld PHA, et al: Ten years of experience in the treatment of gas gangrene with hyperbaric oxygen. *Surg Gynecol Obstet* 134:579–585, 1972.

Basic Considerations of Antibiotic Therapy

Polk HC Jr, Ausobsky JR: The role of antibiotics in surgical infections. *Adv Surg* 16:225–275, 1983.

Pratt WB, Fekety R: *The Antimicrobial Drugs.* New York, Oxford University Press, 1986.

Yale CE, Peet WJ: Antibiotics in colon surgery. *Am J Surg* 122:787–791, 1971.

Chemoprophylaxis; Intestinal Antisepsis; Intraperitoneal Antibiotics

Bolton JS, Bornside GH, et al: Intraperitoneal povidone-iodine in experimental canine and murine peritonitis. *Am J Surg* 137:780–785, 1979.

Burke JF: Use of preventive antibiotics in clinical surgery. *Am Surg* 39:6–11, 1973.

Clarke JS, Condon RE, et al: Preoperative oral antibiotics reduce septic complications of colon operations: Results of prospective, randomized, double-blind clinical study. *Ann Surg* 186:251–259, 1977.

Cohn I Jr: *Intestinal Antisepsis*. Springfield, IL, Charles C Thomas, 1968.

Cohn I Jr: Intestinal antisepsis. *Surg Gynecol Obstet* 130:1006–1014, 1970.

Evans M, Pollock AV: Trials on trial: A review of trials of antibiotic prophylaxis. *Arch Surg* 119:109–113, 1984.

Fleites RA, Marshall JB, et al: The efficacy of polyethylene glycol-electrolyte lavage solution versus traditional mechanical bowel preparation for elective colonic surgery: a randomized, prospective, blinded clinical trial. *Surgery* 98:708–715, 1985.

Jagelman DG, Fazio VW, et al: A prospective randomized, double-blind study of 10% mannitol mechanical bowel preparation combined with oral neomycin and short-term, perioperative, intravenous flagyl as prophylaxis in elective colorectal resections. *Surgery* 98:861–865, 1985.

Nichols RL, Broido P, et al: Effect of preoperative neomycin-erythromycin intestinal preparation on the incidence of infectious complications following colon surgery. *Ann Surg* 178:453–462, 1973.

Nichols RL, Condon RE: Preoperative preparation of the colon. *Surg Gynecol Obstet* 132:323–337, 1971.

Rodeheaver G, Bellamy W, et al: Bactericidal activity and toxicity of iodine-containing solutions in wounds. *Arch Surg* 117:181–186, 1982.

Silverman SH, Ambrose NS, et al: The effect of peritoneal lavage with tetracycline solution in postoperative infection. *Dis Colon Rectum* 29:165–169, 1986.

Smith EB: A rationale for intraperitoneally administered antibiotic therapy. *Surg Gynecol Obstet* 143:561–564, 1976.

Antimicrobial Agents

Bartlett JG: Metronidazole. *Johns Hopkins Med J* 149:89–92, 1981.

Calderwood SB, Moellering RC Jr: Common adverse effects of antibacterial agents on major organ systems. *Surg Clin North Am* 60:65–81, 1980.

Conte JE Jr, Barriere SL: *Manual of Antibiotics and Infectious Diseases,* 5th ed. Philadelphia, Lea & Febiger, 1984.

Fry DE: Third generation cephalosporin antibiotics in surgical practice. *Am J Surg* 151:306–313, 1986.

Garrod LP, Lambert HP, et al: *Antibiotic and Chemotherapy,* 5th ed. Edinburgh, Churchill Livingstone, 1981.

Kagan BM (ed): *Antimicrobial Therapy,* 3d ed. Philadelphia, WB Saunders, 1980.

Sanders CV, Greenberg RN, et al: Cefamandole and cefoxitin. *Ann Intern Med* 103:70–78, 1985.

Streptococcal Infections

Aitken DR, Mackett MCT, et al: The changing pattern of hemolytic streptococcal gangrene. *Arch Surg* 117:561–567, 1982.

Altemeier WA, Culbertson WR: Acute non-clostridial crepitant cellulitis. *Surg Gynecol Obstet* 87:206–212, 1948.

Dellinger EP: Severe necrotizing soft-tissue infections: Multiple disease entities requiring a common approach. *JAMA* 246:1717–1721, 1981.

Dougherty SH: Role of enterococcus in intraabdominal sepsis. *Am J Surg* 148:308–312, 1984.

Giuliano A, Lewis R Jr, et al: Bacteriology of necrotizing fasciitis. *Am J Surg* 134:52–57, 1977.

Ledingham I McA, Tehrani MA: Diagnosis, clinical course and treatment of acute dermal gangrene. *Br J Surg* 62:364–372, 1975.

MacLennan JD: Streptococcal infection of muscle. *Lancet* 1:582–584, 1943.

Meleney FL, Friedman ST, et al: The treatment of progressive bacterial synergistic gangrene with penicillin. *Surgery* 18:423–435, 1945.

Rea WJ, Wyrick WJ Jr: Necrotizing fasciitis. *Ann Surg* 172:957–964, 1970.

Stone HH, Martin JD Jr: Synergistic necrotizing cellulitis. *Ann Surg* 175:702–711, 1972.

Staphylococcal Infections

Altemeier WA, Hummel RP, et al: Staphylococcal enterocolitis following antibiotic therapy, *Ann Surg* 157:847–858, 1963.

Elek SD: *Staphylococcus Pyogenes and Its Relation to Disease.* London, Livingstone Ltd., 1959.

Gorbach SL, Bartlett JG: Anaerobic infections: Old myths and new realities. *J Infect Dis* 130:307–310, 1974 (editorial).

Holland JW, Hill EO, et al: Numbers and types of anaerobic bacteria isolated from clinical specimens since 1960. *J Clin Microbiol* 5:20–25, 1977.

Kramer IRH: Fatal staphylococcal enteritis developing during streptomycin therapy by mouth. *Lancet* 2:646–647, 1948.

Clostridial Infections

Altemeier WA, Fullen WD: Prevention and treatment of gas gangrene. *JAMA* 217:806–813, 1971.

Altemeier WA, Hummel RP: Treatment of tetanus. *Surgery* 60:495–505, 1966.

Brooks GF, Buchanan TM, et al: Tetanus toxoid immunization of adults: A continuing need. *Ann Intern Med* 73:603–606, 1970.

Faust RA, Vickers OR, et al: Tetanus: 2,449 cases in 68 years at Charity Hospital. *J Trauma* 16:704–712, 1976.

Gerding DN, Olson MM, et al: *Clostridium difficile*-associated diarrhea and colitis in adults. A prospective case-controlled epidemiologic study. *Arch Intern Med* 146:95–100, 1986.

Kaiser CW, Milgram ML, et al: Distant nontraumatic clostridial myonecrosis and malignancy. *Cancer* 57:885–889, 1986.

Katlic MR, Derkac WM, et al: *Clostridium septicum* infection and malignancy. *Ann Surg* 193:361–364, 1982.

MacLennan JD: The histotoxic clostridial infections of man. *Bacteriol Rev* 26:177–276, 1962.

Matzkin H, Regen S: Naturally acquired immunity to tetanus toxin in an isolated community. *Infect Immun* 48:267–268, 1985.

Oakley CL: Gas gangrene. *Br Med Bull* 10:52–58, 1954.

Rubbo SD, Suri JC: Combined active-passive immunization against tetanus with human immune globlin. *Med J Aust* 2:109–113, 1965.

Willis AT: *Clostridia of Wound Infection.* London, Butterworth Scientific Publications, 1969.

Aerobic Infections

DiGioa RA, Kane JG, et al: Crepitant cellulitis and myonecrosis caused by Klebsiella. *JAMA* 237:2097–2098, 1977.

Doggett RG: *Pseudomonas Aeruginosa: Clinical Manifestations of Infection and Current Therapy.* New York, Academic Press, 1979.

Forkner CE Jr: *Pseudomonas Aeruginosa Infections.* New York, Grune & Stratton, 1960.

Reisig G, Schaffner W: Postoperative detection of *Salmonella typhi. Arch Surg* 104:349–350, 1972.

Steinhauer BW, Eickhoff TC, et al: The *Klebsiella-Enterobacter-Serratia* division: Chemical and epidemiologic characteristics. *Ann Intern Med* 65:1180–1194, 1966.

Sugerman HJ, Peyton JWR, et al: Gram-negative sepsis. *Curr Probl Surg* 18:405–475, 1981.

Wilkowske CJ, Washington JA II, et al: *Serratia marcescens:* Biochemical characteristics, antibiotic susceptibility patterns, and clinical significance. *JAMA* 214:2157–2162, 1970.

Anaerobic Infections

Anderson CB, Marr JJ, et al: Anaerobic infections in surgery: Clinical review. *Surgery* 79:313–324, 1976.

Finegold SM: *Anaerobic Bacteria in Human Disease.* New York, Academic Press, 1977.

Gorbach SL, Bartlett JG: Anaerobic infections. *N Engl J Med* 290:1177–1184; 1237–1245; 1289–1294, 1974.

Gorbach SL, Bartlett JG (eds): The role of clindamycin in anaerobic bacterial infections. *J Infect Dis* (suppl) 135: March 1977 (symposium).

Leigh DA: Wound infections due to *Bacteroides fragilis* following intestinal surgery. *Br J Surg* 62:375–378, 1975.

Sinkovics JG, Smith JP: Septicemia with bacteroides in patients with malignant disease. *Cancer* 25:663–671, 1970.

Stone HH, Kolb LD, et al: Incidence and significance of intraperitoneal anaerobic bacteria. *Ann Surg* 181:705–715, 1975.

Wilson SE, Finegold SM, et al: *Intra-abdominal Infection.* New York, McGraw-Hill, 1983.

Mycotic Infections

Bennett JE: Chemotherapy of systemic mycoses. *N Engl J Med* 290:30–32; 320–323, 1974.

Codish SD, Tobias JS, et al: Recent advances in the treatment of systemic mycotic infections. *Surg Gynecol Obstet* 148:435–447, 1979.

Emmons CW, Binford CH, et al: *Medical Mycology,* 3d ed. Philadelphia, Lea & Febiger, 1977.

Moss E, McQuown AL: *Atlas of Medical Mycology,* 3d ed. Baltimore, Williams & Wilkins, 1969.

Odds FC: *Candida and Candidosis,* Baltimore, University Park Press, 1979.

Schroter GPJ, Temple DR, et al: Crytococcosis after renal transplantation. *Surgery* 79:268–277, 1976.

Solomkin JS, Flohr A, et al: *Candida* infections in surgical patients: dose requirements and toxicity of amphotericin B. *Ann Surg* 195:177–185, 1982.

Stevens DA (ed): *Coccidioidomycosis: A Text.* New York, Plenum, 1980.

Surgical Asepsis

Block SS (ed): *Disinfection, Sterilization, and Preservation,* 3d ed. Philadelphia, Lea & Febiger, 1983.

Crowder VH Jr, Bornside GH, et al: Bacteriological comparison of hexachlorophene and polyvinylpyrrolidine-iodine surgical scrub soaps. *Am Surg* 33:906–911, 1967.

Kaul AF, Jewett JF: Agents and techniques for disinfection of the skin. *Surg Gynecol Obstet* 152:677–685, 1981.

Zamora JH: Chemical and microbiologic characteristics and toxicity of povidone-iodine solutions (review). *Am J Surg* 151:400–406, 1986.

Chapter 6

Trauma

G. Tom Shires, Erwin R. Thal, Ronald C. Jones, William H. Snyder, G. Tom Shires III, Robert N. McClelland, and Malcolm O. Perry

GENERAL CONSIDERATIONS

G. Tom Shires III and G. Tom Shires

The magnitude of the problem of trauma in the United States is probably not adequately appreciated. In this country trauma is the leading cause of death in the first four decades of life. It ranks overall as the fourth leading cause of death in the United States today; if arteriosclerosis is considered as a single entity, trauma is the third leading cause of death. Over 140,000 deaths occur each year from accidents. Automobile accidents alone kill more Americans annually than were lost during the entire Korean conflict. Unlike many serious disease entities in the United States, the incidence of and mortality from injuries is increasing each year.

Injury is the leading cause of physician contacts and leads to over 140 million bed days of annual disability. The Centers for Disease Control found that over 4 million years of future worklife are lost each year to injury versus 2.1 million to heart disease and 1.7 million to cancer.

Initial Resuscitation of the Severely Injured Patient

The patient with multiple injuries is best managed by one physician. When the responsibility is divided, evaluation of the patient's overall problems may be lacking and complications may not be recognized for several hours.

PRIORITY BY INJURY

There are three categories of patients, according to immediacy of injury. The first group includes injuries that interfere with vital physiologic function and therefore immediately threaten life, such as obstruction of an airway or bleeding from a gunshot wound. The primary treatment is to establish an airway and control the bleeding. This type of patient may require surgical treatment for massive internal bleeding within 5 to 10 min following arrival in the emergency room. The operating room should be alerted when the patient is admitted to the emergency room, and no time is wasted in getting the patient into "operative" condition. Often the control of hemorrhage is dependent on a rapid thoracotomy or laparotomy to occlude injured major vessels.

A second group of patients are those with injuries that offer no immediate threat to life. These include patients who have received gunshot wounds, stab wounds, or blunt trauma to the chest and abdomen but whose vital signs are stable. The majority of injured patients are in this category. Although they will require surgical procedures within 1 to 2 h, there is time for additional information to be obtained. Blood for typing and cross matching is drawn, and blood is made available if there is any possibility that the patient will require surgical intervention. If vital signs are stable, x-rays may be obtained to determine the course of the missile and the extent of possible associated injuries, such as fractures. Cystography and pyelography may be performed to assess hematuria. Since patients with penetrating and blunt abdominal injuries may develop shock at any moment, a physician must be in constant attendance during all evaluations. Patients who suddenly develop shock are immediately taken to the operating room without additional diagnostic procedures.

The third group of patients are those whose injuries produce occult damage. This group is composed primarily of patients who have sustained blunt trauma to the abdomen that may or may not require surgical intervention and in whom the exact nature of the injury is not apparent. These patients usually have time for extensive laboratory studies, x-rays, and more complete physical examination. Surgical intervention in this group may be delayed hours or days, as with delayed rupture of the spleen.

Patients who are severely injured are admitted to the emergency room in a trauma area equipped for emergency resuscitation. This room should contain such items as intravenous fluids, overhead operating-room light, oxygen, cardiac monitor and defibrillator, and a portable carriage that is suitable for an operating-room table in an emergency situation. A cabinet should be in the room containing equipment for endotracheal intubation, tracheostomy tray, closed drainage tray, venous section tray, central venous catheters, closed-chest drainage tubes, intravenous fluids with tubing, needles, and syringes for four-quadrant abdominal paracentesis, and pericardiocentesis and peritoneal lavage catheters. The cabinet shelf should have clearly visible labels under each tray or set of instruments. These trays and instruments should be kept in this trauma room and not in central supply, as a waiting period of even 5 min may prove fatal.

ADEQUATE AIRWAY. The first and most important emergency measure in the management of the severely injured patient is to establish an effective airway. A cabinet should be available at the head of the emergency room carriage in which a laryngoscope and cuffed endotracheal tubes of various sizes are available. Endotracheal intubation is the most rapid method of obtaining an adequate airway. Once an airway is established, a means of positive-pressure breathing such as an Ambu bag or anesthesia machine should be available, and a cuffed endotracheal tube is desirable, so that positive-pressure breathing may be accomplished if needed in the resuscitation or in the administration of anesthesia. Either wall suction or a portable suction machine must be available in the trauma room to remove pulmonary secretions, foreign bodies, and frequently, blood from the upper respiratory tract. In the presence of suspected cervical spine injuries, when an endotracheal tube cannot be readily inserted, a tracheostomy may be required.

SHOCK AND HEMORRHAGE. Shock is usually controlled while the patient's airway is being cleared by another person. Internal hemorrhage will require immediate surgical intervention. Hypovolemic shock is best prevented or controlled by starting intravenous infusions in at least two extremities, using 18-gauge or larger catheters. A balanced salt solution such as Ringer's lactate solution is usually started until blood is available. Blood for typing and cross matching is drawn at the time the intravenous fluid is started, and the balanced salt solution is given in addition to the blood. Shock resulting from a blood loss of 750 mL can usually be corrected by rapid administration of 2 L of Ringer's lactate solution over a 15- to 20-min period. Blood loss in excess of 750 mL usually requires the administration of whole blood in addition to balanced salt solution. Often, 2 L of balanced salt solution will replace the volume and correct hypotension so that no blood is necessary, reducing the possibility of blood transfusion reaction. When a patient initially responds to 1 to 2 L of balanced salt solution, as evidenced by a normal blood pressure and decrease in pulse rate, but subsequently becomes hypotensive, blood administration usually is indicated. However, by this time, type-specific blood usually is available and often crossmatched, which reduces the chances for a transfusion reaction. Should a patient not respond to the rapid administration of 2 L of balanced salt solution, uncrossmatched, type O, Rh-negative blood is administered without hesitation.

External bleeding is best controlled by direct finger pressure on the bleeding wound or vessel. Tourniquets are of little benefit in the control of major arterial bleeding and often injurious if they occlude collateral circulation. A frequent mistake is the placement of a tourniquet on an extremity tight enough to obstruct venous return but loose enough not to inhibit arterial flow; this only increases the blood loss and edema. The danger of tissue loss from tourniquet use is always present.

Superficial vessels may be ligated if they are readily seen; however, wounds are not probed in a blind attempt to place a hemostat on a vessel. As soon as bleeding is controlled, the wound is covered with a sterile dressing, and the patient is taken to the operating room, where the wound is more adequately visualized and proper instruments are available. The needless probing of wounds in the emergency room may lead to severe infection, which can be avoided by proper exploration including adequate irrigation and sterile surgical technique in the operating room.

NEUROLOGIC EVALUATION. After an adequate airway has been obtained and hemorrhage has been controlled, a gross neurologic evaluation of the patient is undertaken. Motor function in the four extremities should be verified. A progressing neurologic deficit following injury to the spinal cord may indicate the necessity for an emergency laminectomy. Decompression of a hematoma may result in return of function. Thoracoabdominal injuries usually take precedence over orthopaedic or neurologic injury.

CHEST INJURIES. Airway obstruction may be due to mucus, fragments of bone from facial fractures, dirt and debris, and, commonly, broken teeth or dentures. If the patient does not ventilate normally after an endotracheal tube is inserted, or a tracheostomy has been performed, several injuries should be considered. These include pneumothorax, hemothorax, cardiac tamponade, flail chest, and ruptured bronchus.

Pneumothorax. If a pneumothorax is questionable, an 18-gauge needle may be inserted into the chest in the anterior axillary line and aspiration done to reveal the presence of air. A chest x-ray is preferable, but often severe respiratory distress precludes time for x-ray confirmation. Tension pneumothorax with mediastinal shift is suggested by displacement of the trachea to the opposite side. Auscultation of the chest may reveal decreased breath sounds. The patient with a pneumothorax is treated with closed-chest drainage. As there is little danger from the insertion of a chest tube in the absence of a pneumothorax, an anterior chest tube should be inserted if there is doubt.

Hemothorax. Diagnosis of hemothorax is similar to that of pneumothorax. If the patient on the emergency-room cart is in distress, a needle may be inserted in the eighth interspace in the posterior axillary line and aspiration done to reveal a hemothorax. This is best drained with both anterior and posterior chest tubes. The anterior chest tube is placed in the second interspace in the midclavicular line and the posterior chest tube is placed in the eighth interspace in the posterior axillary line in the region between the midaxillary and posterior axillary line. Chest tubes are of large caliber so that adequate drainage may be maintained. Thoracotomy may be indicated, depending on the rate of bleeding or the presence of intrathoracic clots.

Cardiac Tamponade. During initial observation, an unsuspected cardiac tamponade may develop secondary to blunt or penetrating trauma. This is often not present on arrival in the emergency room but may develop after 1 to 2 h of observation. The clinical signs pathognomonic for cardiac tamponade are increased venous pressure, decreased pulse pressure, particularly with a paradoxical pulse and with or without cyanosis, and decreased heart sounds. The diagnosis may be subtle until the subsequent development of hypotension. Emergency treatment includes aspiration of the pericardial sac with an 18-gauge needle through the xiphocostal angle. Decompression of as little as 20 mL of aspirated blood may make a remarkable difference in the patient's vital signs. The high incidence of false-positive and false-negative findings on pericardiocentesis has led to the use of subxiphoid pericardial window in some centers. Depending on the cause of cardiac tamponade, immediate thoracotomy is usually required to repair the cardiac wound. When a patient arrives at the emergency room in shock without evidence of blood loss, this diagnosis should be suspected.

Flail Chest. Paradoxical chest wall motion from major blunt trauma has historically been managed by endotracheal intubation and mechanical ventilation or operative stabilization of the rib fractures. However, this approach has been replaced by ventilatory management based upon the physiologic derangement of the associated lung injury. Although this requires the careful assessment of arterial blood gases and clinical parameters of pulmonary function combined with vigorous pulmonary toilet, it allows many patients to overcome the morbidity associated with prolonged intubation and ventilation.

Ruptured Bronchus. After rupture of a bronchus, respiratory distress, hemoptysis, cyanosis, and a massive air leak with both mediastinal and subcutaneous emphysema and/or tension pneumothorax may be observed. Often the diagnosis is not obvious. There is a close relationship between fractures of the first and second ribs and rupture of a bronchus. If extrapleural hematoma is noted, special views of the first ribs are indicated. A ruptured bronchus is treated initially with closed-chest drainage. If this does not effectively keep the lung expanded, bronchoscopy and open thoracotomy with repair of the bronchus is indicated.

Open Chest Wounds. The patient with a chest injury resulting in a sucking chest wound is best managed by immediately covering the open wound with whatever material is available, such as a large vaseline gauze bandage or a thin sheet of plastic wrap. This prevents further shifting of the mediastinum and allows ventilation of the opposite lung. Chest tubes are usually inserted prior to operation, and immediate surgical intervention is indicated.

Ruptured Thoracic Aorta. The diagnosis may be suspected from chest x-ray showing a widened mediastinum and confirmed by arteriography. Immediate operation usually is indicated.

PENETRATING WOUNDS OF THE ABDOMINAL WALL. All penetrating injuries to the abdominal wall are explored locally in the emergency room to determine if the peritoneal cavity is penetrated. Exploration is usually accomplished by extending the stab wound and determining its depth. In the event that the extent of penetration cannot be determined or if the stab wound violates the peritoneal cavity, the abdominal cavity is lavaged. The mortality and morbidity from a negative abdominal exploration is negligible, but failure to discover such injuries as colon or liver injury for several hours may allow peritonitis and other complications to develop. All gunshot wounds of the abdomen should be explored whether penetration is evident or not. Shock waves from nonpenetrating gunshot wounds of the abdominal wall can easily transect bowel or lacerate the liver or spleen without entering the abdominal cavity. Most gunshot wounds that enter the peritoneal cavity damage a vessel, organ, or hollow viscus.

THE UNCONSCIOUS PATIENT. Patients with closed head injuries who are unconscious must have an airway established immediately. Hypotension rarely results from a closed head injury but is almost always caused by blood loss, usually in the thorax or abdomen. The cause of the blood loss is most rapidly determined by using an 18-gauge needle for immediate abdominal and chest taps, which may reveal nonclotting blood. The absence of blood does not rule out an intraabdominal or thoracic injury. Extreme care should be used in moving unconscious patients until injuries of the spine have been ruled out.

Immediate Nonoperative Surgical Care

Hematuria. A Foley catheter is routinely inserted, particularly following blunt trauma to the abdomen, to determine the presence of hematuria as well as to follow the urinary output during and immediately following the surgical procedure. Gross hematuria is evidence of urinary tract injury resulting from contusion, laceration, or rupture. If the patient's vital signs are stable and hematuria is present, a combined cystogram and intravenous pyelogram should be done. A single 15-min film is usually adequate to determine kidney function as well as indicate extravasation from the bladder, ureter, or kidneys. Failure to demonstrate extravasation does not rule out the possibility of a ruptured bladder or kidney. Should a nephrectomy be required during a laparotomy, functioning of the kidney on the opposite side should be proved. It is useless to attempt to visualize the kidneys by intravenous pyelogram when the patient is hypotensive. X-rays are delayed until the patient has been resuscitated and bleeding has been controlled in the operating room. If time is not available preoperatively for an intravenous pyelogram, a cassette may be placed under the patient prior to the start of surgical procedures and a pyelogram obtained intraoperatively.

FRACTURES. Fractures of the extremities are best managed immediately with splints for the extremities. Immobilization may prevent additional nerve and blood vessel injury and conversion of a closed fracture to an open one. The presence or absence of pulses in the fractured extremities should be noted on initial examination. Intravenous infusions should not be started in an injured extremity. Massive thoracoabdominal bleeding takes precedence over fractures, unless there is an accompanying arterial injury of such magnitude that there is danger of loss of limb. In such instances, it is often necessary to have two surgical teams working simultaneously.

Unstable pelvic ring fractures are best treated by early stabilization. The immediate application of external pelvic fixation not only allows early mobilization and pain relief but also may be lifesaving by controlling bleeding into the fracture hematoma.

ARTERIAL INJURIES. Any penetrating injury in the region of a major blood vessel or nerve deserves evaluation by arteriography. On initial examination, 18 percent of subsequently proved arterial injuries are noted to have a normal pulse distal to the arterial injury, and one-third of the patients have a palpable but diminished distal pulse. Vessel exploration in the region of the neck should be done under endotracheal anesthesia and may require resection of a portion of the clavicle for adequate visualization. Early recognition of an arterial injury is the most important factor in preserving a viable extremity or functioning distal organ.

Diagnosis and Management of Unapparent Injury

Blunt trauma to the abdomen may produce severe intraperitoneal or retroperitoneal injury with minimal physical findings. Bowel sounds may not be lost for several hours, and evidence of retroperitoneal or intraabdominal injury may not become apparent for as long as 18 h.

An abdominal paracentesis may be performed early in the observation period in patients with injuries from blunt trauma to the abdomen who have equivocal physical findings or altered consciousness. A 95 percent diagnostic accuracy is associated with the positive abdominal tap. A negative abdominal tap does not rule out intraabdominal injury and should be followed by peritoneal lavage or CT scan. Patients with signs of peritoneal irritation require exploratory laparotomy even in the absence of a positive abdominal tap or peritoneal lavage.

RADIOGRAPHS. These are taken when a patient's vital signs remain stable but are omitted for patients in severe shock. X-rays of the chest and abdomen are routinely performed to rule out foreign bodies such as knife blades within the depths of the wound. Patients sustaining gunshot wounds should have x-rays when possible in an attempt to trace the course of the missile. Patients sustaining blunt trauma often require multiple x-rays to rule out obscure fractures of the vertebral spine and retroperitoneal injuries. X-rays of extremities will be of value in determining whether or not the missile struck bone, fractured bone, or passed near vital structures.

NASOGASTRIC INTUBATION. A Levin tube is routinely inserted in most severely injured patients; exceptions include those patients with penetrating neck wounds, complex facial injuries, or suspected cervical spine fractures. Passage of the tube may provoke vomiting and empty the stomach of large particles, preventing subsequent aspiration during anesthesia. Esophageal or gastric injury from penetrating or blunt trauma may be diagnosed by finding bright red blood in the Levin tube drainage. Gastric intubation prevents gastric dilation during tracheal intubation and aids in the prevention of postoperative distention of the small bowel.

PROPHYLACTIC ANTIBIOTICS. Antibiotics are administered preoperatively to all patients sustaining penetrating wounds of the abdomen, beginning as soon as possible after the injured patient arrives in the emergency room. They may be discontinued if exploratory laparotomy is negative. Considerable experimental evidence indicates that prophylactic antibiotics in trauma are of benefit if administered within the first 3 h following injury. A retrospective review of a group of patients who sustained penetrating abdominal injuries showed that there was a decrease in the incidence of infections in those patients who received antibiotics preoperatively or intraoperatively as opposed to those who received antibiotics in the immediate postoperative period or therapeutically. This was significant for gunshot but not for stab wounds. A prospective study now being conducted indicates coverage should be against both aerobes and anaerobes.

Tetanus Prophylaxis. Following injury, immunized patients are administered a tetanus toxoid booster. In unimmunized patients the wound is debrided, and 250 units of tetanus human immune globulin is administered. Patients who were previously immunized but are now taking steroids, immunosuppressive therapy, or chemotherapy or who have had extensive irradiation should receive human immune globulin, since they may not have normal antibody response. Severely contaminated wounds should be left open or converted to open wounds when feasible.

PRINCIPLES IN THE MANAGEMENT OF WOUNDS

Ronald C. Jones and G. Tom Shires

Primary Wound Management

The most important single factor in the management of contaminated wounds is adequate debridement. This old surgical principle frequently has been forgotten since the advent of antibiotics. All tissue that is dead, has a poor blood supply, or is heavily contaminated should be removed if at all possible. This is particularly true of subcutaneous fat and muscle. Skin with impaired blood supply should be removed initially because of its tendency to become infected. Granulation tissue formation and later grafting procedures are preferable. Following sharp debridement and hemostasis, the wound is irrigated with copious quantities of saline solution, depending on the area and degree of soft tissue injury and contamination. That the incidence of wound infection is inversely proportional to the amount of irrigation and debridement at the time of injury has been demonstrated by Singleton and by Peterson and confirmed clinically many times.

LOCAL CARE OF WOUNDS

Glass or sharp instruments usually carry a minimal amount of foreign material into a wound and cause a minimal amount of tissue trauma. X-rays should be taken of any area in which the depth of the wound cannot clearly be seen. It is not uncommon for the deep portion of a stab wound to contain the tip of a knife blade or other foreign body. Stab wounds of soft tissues are explored in the emergency room with the gloved finger or under local anesthesia by extending the length of the laceration to determine the direction and extent of the wound and to rule out any major vessel, nerve, or organ injury. The wound is then irrigated with copious amounts of saline solution. If the wound is found not to penetrate the peritoneal cavity, a small soft-rubber Penrose drain is inserted and the wound is left open for drainage. The drain is removed in 24 h. Gunshot wounds are debrided externally and left open for drainage. Suturing these wounds leaves a closed contaminated space, and the infection can easily spread to surrounding soft tissue structures. Deep lacerations involving the extremity with damage to major vessels and tendons and massive muscle injury are managed by controlling major vessel bleeding and immediately wrapping the wound in sterile dressings. An x-ray is taken, if indicated, but a severe laceration is not explored until the patient is in the operating room. This procedure prevents undue contamination of the wound in the emergency room before the patient is adequately prepared. Minor lacerations can be managed in the emergency room.

Fascia usually can be approximated, and, depending on the type of wound, the skin and subcutaneous tissue may or may not be closed initially. These wounds are often left open and have delayed primary closure in 3 to 5 days. Damaged muscle due to gunshot wounds is debrided, hemostasis is obtained, and the wound is irrigated as outlined above. The wounds are packed open and closed with delayed closure. All patients with such wounds receive antibiotics and tetanus toxoid.

Antibacterial soaps or detergent materials are not used to irrigate wounds when muscle, tendon, or blood vessels are visible. Severe chemical irritation to these structures may occur, with resultant structure impairment and delayed wound healing.

Many factors, such as the number and virulence of organisms, blood supply of tissue, host resistance, shock, adequacy of surgical debridement, tissue tension, dead space, hemostasis, age, and associated diseases, are responsible for infection. Condie demonstrated in dogs that obliterating dead space reduced the occurrence of wound infection in the presence of contamination. Viable bacteria can be demonstrated in many surgical wounds at the time of closure; however, few incisions become infected.

Cosmetic appearance is a secondary consideration; the primary aim is to avoid infection and cover vital structures. No attempt at plastic repair is made at the initial closure of a potentially contaminated wound. Jagged edges of skin with poor blood supply are trimmed, and any resulting unpleasant scar can be cared for at a later date when no infection is present. Most lacerations, regardless of location, will never need revision if they meet the criteria previously outlined for the primary closure.

PUNCTURE WOUNDS. The most frequent puncture injury is that caused by a rusty nail in the foot. The patient is administered antibiotics both to prevent secondary infection and to aid in the prevention of tetanus, since this wound is not completely open to the air. Puncture wounds are debrided conservatively if they involve only the skin and subcutaneous tissue. Human tetanus immune globulin is given (250 mg) to the unimmunized patient. Debridement with conversion to an open wound and the administration of antibiotics and tetanus toxoid, whether or not the patient has been previously immunized, is also performed.

POWER MOWER INJURIES. Injuries resulting from the use of power mowers have increased in recent years. These include injuries from flying objects thrown from the power mower and from the mower itself to the hands and feet, particularly the fingers and toes. Treatment has consisted of covering exposed bones with muscle and leaving the entire wound open. These injuries almost uniformly become infected if an attempt is made to close the wound primarily. Patients are treated with systemic antibiotics and tetanus prophylaxis, and the wounds are packed with fine-mesh gauze. Skin grafting and reconstructive procedures should be delayed.

Emergency Laparotomy

INCISIONS. A midline incision is regularly used for exploratory laparotomy in patients with abdominal trauma and does not endanger the abdominal muscle, blood supply, or nerve supply, or damage aponeuroses. Minimal ligatures are used on bleeders that are contained in small bits of tissue, as each extra ligature is a foreign body and enhances the chance of a wound infection. Tissues should be kept moistened and gently handled. Surgical technique governs the development of wound infection as significantly as any single factor.

SUTURE. Number 0-Prolene is the suture material of choice for closing the uncomplicated midline abdominal incision, particularly in operations for traumatic lesions. It has not been the cause of draining sinuses following postoperative wound infections. Suture placement is probably the most important factor in the prevention of wound dehiscence. Sutures should not be placed at equal distances from the edge of the fascia, as they will fall in the same group of fibers; should one suture tear the fascia longitudinally, the tear may extend from suture to suture until dehiscence occurs. Sutures should be staggered or placed at varying intervals from the edge of the fascia. With such a closure, there should be no fear in having a patient cough vigorously for adequate postoperative pulmonary care. An occasional patient with minimal subcutaneous tissue will complain of pain in the incision when the suture is under a pressure point such as a belt. These sutures are easily removed under local anesthesia.

Simple interrupted suture is used to close the fascia and peritoneum in a single layer. This is felt to be superior to the figure-of-eight suture, because less tissue is gathered and the suture can be placed faster, thus reducing anesthesia time. Interrupted sutures are used instead of running sutures because a break in the suture material will not loosen the entire incision. Regardless of the type of suture or method of placement, the fascia should be loosely approximated and not strangulated. Tightening fascial sutures may lead to necrosis with the suture subsequently cutting through the tissue. Retention sutures have not been regularly used. Routine antibiotic irrigation of the wound for the prevention of infection has not been necessary.

Through-and-Through Closure Several local and systemic factors noted at the time of the original operation may make through-and-through closure the procedure of

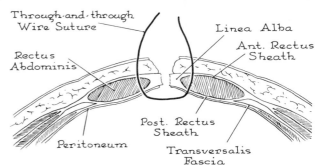

Fig. 6-1. Through-and-through wire closure. (From: *Shires GT: Care of the Trauma Patient. New York, McGraw-Hill, 1966, p 37, with permission.*)

choice (Fig. 6-1). This uses adjustable bridges and large braided nonabsorbable suture or German silver wire swaged on a large cutting needle. The bridges prevent cutting of skin by the wire and allow for swelling that occurs in the first 24 to 48 h postoperatively. The bridges can be adjusted to compensate for swelling of tissues. Wounds massively contaminated from shotgun wadding and fecal material, in patients with steroids, or associated with massive infection and peritonitis are best handled with through-and-through closure. Often a single patient may have several indications for this type of closure such as chronic pulmonary disease, obesity, and/or chronic debilitating disease. Occasionally through-and-through closure is used at the end of a lengthy operation with a long incision to shorten anesthesia time if the patient is not tolerating the procedure well. This type of closure is routinely used in the patient requiring reoperation in the early postoperative period because of gastrointestinal bleeding or intestinal obstruction. The wires are left in place for 3 weeks. This measure has proved to be sure, safe, timesaving, and often lifesaving.

INFECTION. Infection and severe abdominal distention are frequently mentioned as causative factors in dehiscence. Wound infection may be prevented in the markedly contaminated abdomen by leaving the skin and subcutaneous tissue open down to the fascia for delayed primary closure. This method is frequently used in long operations or with excessive contamination such as from feces. Abdominal wounds frequently harbor coliform organisms if bowel injury has been sustained. These wounds are packed open with fine-mesh gauze, changed daily for debridement, and either closed at 5 days or allowed to granulate until closure. This procedure will usually result in an excellent scar.

DRAINS. Subcutaneous drains will not substitute for good hemostasis. Failure to obtain hemostasis will give rise to a hematoma which is an excellent culture medium for an already contaminated wound. Drains from the abdominal cavity are usually brought out through a separate stab wound and by the most direct route. This is especially true for some liver and pancreatic injuries. Drainage of the free peritoneal cavity is not attempted.

Antibiotics

Following hemorrhage sepsis is the second most common cause of death in patients sustaining penetrating abdominal trauma and is a leading cause of postoperative mortality. Burke has demonstrated in animal models the relationship of time between contamination and implementation of antibiotic therapy. Experimentally, if antibiotics were delayed for greater than 3 h following contamination, the inflammatory response was unaltered, indicating antibiotics must be administered as soon after injury as possible. The incidence of infection following gunshot wounds is two or three times greater than following stab wounds.

Jones evaluated 257 patients sustaining penetrating abdominal trauma at Parkland Memorial Hospital in Dallas (PMH), 147 of whom had colon and small bowel injuries following penetrating abdominal trauma. Combination therapy using clindamycin/tobramycin was compared with single agents cefoxitin active against both aerobes and anaerobes and cefamandole active against aerobes but no anaerobes (Table 6-1). Cefoxitin was statistically more effective than cefamandole and comparable with clindamycin/tobramycin. Cefoxitin was also an effective agent in more serious infections including bacteremia, intraabdominal abscess, and severe operative soft tissue infections. Infection rate is higher in hypotensive patients than in normotensive patients (30 vs. 14 percent). Although Nichols could not correlate shock with infection, he did relate infection to number of units of blood transfused. In another report Gentry compared ticarcillin/tobramycin vs. cefamandole vs. cefoxitin and demonstrated cefoxitin to be comparable with combination therapy and superior to cefamandole. At PMH the usual dose of cefoxitin is 2 g q 6 h for 48 h following penetrating abdominal trauma. Nichols advocates 5 days of therapy in patients sustaining a colon injury. Oreskovich, administering penicillin and vibramycin or cefoxitin, was unable to demonstrate any difference in infection rate whether antibiotics were administered for 12 h or 5 days. However, these studies agree that it is important to cover *Bacteroides fragilis*.

Finegold and Gorbach have studied the microflora of the gastrointestinal tract, providing information regarding the bacteriology of intraabdominal injuries. They noted that the large intestine harbors predominantly anaerobic flora. These anaerobes have a total concentration of 10^{11} per gram and outnumber coliform organisms by 1000 to 10,000:1. Onderdonk using an animal model reported the concept of synergy between anaerobes and facultative bacteria as the mechanism for the abscess formation. Mortality related to coliform organisms injected into the peritoneal cavity, whereas abscess formation was associated with the combination of aerobes and anaerobes. Enterococcus strains alone did not produce mortality or abscess. Louie and Bartlett evaluated several single and combination antibiotics, and found that regimens most effective in reducing abscesses were those using clindamycin or cefoxitin, both of which are effective against anaerobes. They concluded in the animal model that the cefoxitin was superior to cefamandole.

Tally reported the sensitivities of 550 *Bacteroides fragilis* organisms and found none resistant to metronidazole. Approximately 7 or 8 percent were resistant to either clindamycin or piperacillin. Cefoxitin had 16 percent resistance. Over 40 percent of the *Bacteroides fragilis* were resistant to cefotaxime (Claforan) and cefoperazone (Cefobid).

Infection increases as the number of organ injuries increases and as the patient's age increases. Studies suggest that patients sustaining contamination of the peritoneal cavity with colonic contents probably benefit from antibiotic coverage effective against both aerobes and anaerobes. With colonic contamination the antibiotic is administered for a minimum of 48 h and, depending upon the condition of the patient and the number of associated injuries, may be administered for a longer period. Routine administration of an aminoglycoside is unnecessary following penetrating abdominal trauma and may contribute to renal damage.

Failure to debride nonviable tissue may result in infection and antibiotic failure. Surgical technique and appropriate surgical judgment such as whether or not to perform an intestinal anastomosis is just as important if not more so than the antibiotic chosen.

Following severe penetrating abdominal trauma, intraabdominal abscess formation remains common even with prophylactic antibiotic therapy. Jones retrospectively reviewed 50 patients who had sustained penetrating abdominal trauma and who subsequently developed intraabdominal abscess. Missile injuries were responsible for 92 percent of these injuries and 60 percent of these patients had associated colon injuries. The highest risk of infection follows missile injuries to the colon. The mortality in this review was 22 percent. The organisms recovered from these abscesses included *Escherichia coli*, *Klebsiella*, and *B. fragilis*. Gram-positive organisms included enterococcus, anaerobic streptococci, and *Clostridium*. Early diagnosis of intraabdominal abscess is usually easiest using a CT scan. Mortality from intraabdominal abscess has been reduced to 12 percent using the CT scan. With proper patient selection percutaneous drain-

Table 6-1. PENETRATING ABDOMINAL TRAUMA: COLON AND/OR SMALL BOWEL INJURIES AT PARKLAND MEMORIAL HOSPITAL (N = 147)

	Pt	Pt infections	Bacteremia abdominal abscess operative soft tissue
Cleocin/Tobra	51	15 (29%)	7 (14%)
Mandol	44	20 (45%)	11 (26%)
Cefoxitin	52	8 (15%)	5 (10%)
I vs. III		$p = 0.086$	$p = 0.515$
II vs. I and III		$p = 0.006$	$p = 0.048$

SOURCE: Jones RC, Thal ER, et al: *Ann Surg* 201:576, 1985, with permission.

age of intraabdominal abscess has had 80 percent satisfactory results. Following percutaneous drainage the patient may not respond as rapidly as with open surgical drainage and the drainage catheter may have to remain in place for several days, resulting in longer hospitalization. Gastrointestinal fistula and hemorrhage can occur with either approach.

INTRAPERITONEAL ANTIBIOTICS. Intraperitoneal antibiotic irrigation is not recommended. Toxic blood levels develop following intraperitoneal irrigation with kanamycin even with only 2 to 5 min of contact with the peritoneal cavity, and a significant amount of the irrigant cannot be recovered with suction. Patients with significant intraperitoneal contamination are given systemic antibiotics, the abdomen is irrigated with saline solution, which is of questionable value, and the fascia is closed. The skin and subcutaneous tissue may be left open for delayed primary closure, usually within 3 to 4 days following severe contamination. If the patient develops an infection following topical or intraperitoneal irrigation with antibiotics, the organisms isolated are often resistant to the antibiotic used.

BITES AND STINGS OF ANIMALS AND INSECTS
Ronald C. Jones and G. Tom Shires

Rabies

INCIDENCE. In the United States an estimated 2 million human beings are bitten by animals yearly, and one-half million are bitten by dogs. Any mammalian animal may carry rabies. In 1985 there were 5606 laboratory-confirmed cases of rabies. The animals most frequently reported infected and the percentage of the cases they accounted for were skunks (45 percent), raccoons (26 percent), bats (15 percent), foxes (3 percent), cattle (4 percent), dogs (2 percent), and cats (2 percent). Skunks, raccoons, and bats are the major hosts. Rabid skunks increased by 20 percent in 1985 to 2507. Raccoons represented 75 percent of all rabid animals in the mid-Atlantic states of Maryland, Pennsylvania, Virginia, West Virginia, and Washington, D.C. In 1981, for the first time, rabid cats outnumbered rabid dogs. Wildlife species accounted for 91 percent of the rabies in this country. Wildlife rabies has been reported in coyotes, opossum, otter, bobcats, bear, squirrel, deer, mink, woodchucks, coatis, ferrets, and a badger. Domestic rabies has been reported in cattle, dogs, cats, horses, mules, sheep, goats, swine, and guinea pigs. The Communicable Disease Center estimates that this represents less than 10 percent of the cases that actually exist. Mexico reported 10,756 cases of animal rabies of which 93 percent were in dogs. In the past 5 years, there has been an average of two cases of human rabies per year. Table 6-2 shows the incidence and frequency of reported rabies in the United States in various animals and in human beings by states or territory in 1985. Many of the cases of human rabies reported in the past 10 years have resulted from exposure outside the United States.

RABIES CONTROL. Saliva from a rabid animal contains large numbers of the rabies virus and is inoculated through a bite, any laceration, or a break in the skin. Animal experiments and at least two human infections indicate that animals and human beings can become infected by bats, without being bitten, by inhalation of rabies virus. Girard examined bats and demonstrated rabies virus in the brain, kidney, urine, salivary gland, adrenal gland, and liver, using the fluorescent antibody test.

The maintenance of wild and exotic animals such as skunks, raccoons, ocelots, and bobcats as household pets is discouraged since many of these animals are infected with rabies. If people insist on maintaining wild and exotic animals as household pets, the animals should be quarantined for a minimum of 90 days after capture and vaccinated at least 30 days prior to being released to an owner. Annual vaccination is recommended.

Dogs and cats bitten by a known rabid animal should be destroyed immediately. If the owner refuses to have this done, the unvaccinated animal should be placed in strict isolation for 6 months and vaccinated 1 month before being released. If the animal has been vaccinated within the previous 3 years, it should be revaccinated immediately and confined for 90 days. Since cat rabies cases now exceed the annually reported cases in dogs, immunization of cats should be required.

DIAGNOSIS. Circumstances of the Bite. Circumstances surrounding the attack frequently furnish vital information as to whether or not vaccine is indicated. Most domestic animal bites are provoked attacks; if this history is obtained, rabies vaccine can usually be withheld if the animal appears healthy. Children are frequently bitten while attempting to separate fighting animals or while teasing or accidentally hurting the animal. Bites during attempts to feed or handle an apparently healthy animal should generally be regarded as provoked. Frequently the patient has attempted to handle a sick animal. Although vaccination of the animal does not totally rule out the possibility of transmitting rabies, it is over 90 percent effective.

Bites from rodents, including squirrels, gerbils, chipmunks, guinea pigs, rats, and mice, seldom require specific rabies prophylaxis. Each case of possible exposure must be studied individually before a conclusion can be reached as to whether antirabies therapy is indicated. An unprovoked attack is more likely to indicate that the animal is rabid.

Extent and Location of Bite Wound. The likelihood that rabies will result from a bite varies with its extent and location. For convenience in approaching management, two categories of exposure are widely accepted:

Severe. Multiple or deep puncture wounds, or any bites on the head, face, neck, hands, or fingers.

Mild. Scratches, lacerations, or single bites on areas of the body other than the head, face, neck, hands, or fingers. Open wounds, such as abrasions, suspected of being contaminated with saliva also belong to this category.

Table 6-2. RABIES IN THE UNITED STATES BY STATE AND ANIMAL TYPE, 1985

	Dogs	Cats	Cattle	Domestic animal total*	Skunks	Bobcats	Raccoons	Bats	Wild animal total*	Total
Totals	116	127	213	503	2507	7	1487	830	5103	5606
Ala.	2	1		5	4		85	27	119	124
Alaska	2			2					41	43
Ariz.	1		1	3	86	1		29	120	123
Ark.	1	1	4	7	131			13	144	151
Calif.	5	2	5	13	421	2	2	136	573	586
Colo.		1		1				25	25	26
Conn.								7	7	7
Del.								1	1	1
D.C.	3			3			4	1	5	8
Fla.	1	1		2	4	2	111	21	144	146
Ga.	7	5		12	9		158	10	188	200
Hawaii										0
Idaho								10	10	10
Ill.	2	1	2	6	20			23	43	49
Ind.	1		1	2	11			11	22	24
Iowa	5	9	19	35	96			17	114	149
Kan.		2	3	6	50			4	55	61
Ky.	10		1	13	19			9	29	42
La.					14			10	24	24
Maine								1	1	1
Md.	1	11	3	17	6		672	34	743	760
Mass.								14	14	14
Mich.		2		2	6			17	24	26
Minn.	10	11	34	57	155		1	5	162	219
Miss.								10	10	10
Mo.	1		2	3	35			20	56	59
Mont.	2	5	15	26	207	1	2	12	224	250
Neb.	1	1	3	5	30			1	31	36
Nev.								15	15	15
N.H.								1	1	1
N.J.								38	38	38
N. Mex.		1		1	2			9	11	12
N.Y.		5	12	17	24		2	43	136	153
N.C.								12	12	12
N. Dak.	2	8	28	45	97		2	2	104	149
Ohio	1		2	4	9			15	26	30
Okla.	3	4	8	16	88			6	95	111
Oreg.								6	6	6
Pa.	3	10	4	20	81		285	44	429	449
R.I.										0
S.C.	3	7		11			40	11	51	62
S. Dak.	8	9	44	63	274		2	6	284	347
Tenn.	3			3	58			10	71	74
Tex.	28	22	13	74	404	1	3	99	514	588
Utah								4	4	4
Vt.								1	1	1
Va.	1	3	1	6	43		102	16	173	179
Wash.								5	5	5
W. Va.		1		2	8		15		27	29
Wis.	5	3	4	12	39		1	13	54	66
Wyo.	1	1	1	3	76			6	82	85
Guam										0
P.R.	3		3	6					35	41
V.I.										0

* Not shown in the table, but included in the totals are other domestic animals: horses and mules 38, sheep and goats 7, swine 2; other wild animals: coyotes 2, foxes 181, rodents and lagomorphs 23, other 66.

The only documented cases of rabies from human to human transmission occurred in four patients who received corneas transplanted from persons who died of rabies undiagnosed at the time of death.

Laboratory Diagnosis. The direct focus inhibition test of brain material is the recommended technique to diagnose rabies. The intracerebral inoculation of mice combined with the microscopic examination of brain tissue for Negri bodies is still one of the most useful tests in the laboratory diagnosis of rabies and should be used whenever human beings have been bitten by suspect animals and the direct focus inhibition test is negative.

MANAGEMENT OF BITING ANIMALS. Most animal bites of human beings are caused by dogs and cats, and in most instances it is possible to observe the biting animal for the development of rabies. Domestic animals that bite a person should be captured and observed for symptoms of rabies for 10 days. If none develop, the animals may be assumed to be nonrabid. If the animal dies or is killed, the head should not be damaged but should be sent promptly to a public health laboratory for examination. The tissue requires refrigeration, but not freezing, and transportation to the laboratory following death of the animal must be rapid. Clinical signs of rabies in wild animals cannot be interpreted reliably; therefore, any wild animal that bites or scratches a person should be killed at once (without unnecessary damage to the head) and the brain examined for evidence of rabies.

Information from the county health department regarding which animals, both domestic and wild, have been reported to be rabid within the past 10 years in the particular area may indicate a possible specific animal transmitting rabies.

PATIENT MANAGEMENT. Exposed Persons Previously Immunized. For mild exposure of a person who has demonstrated an antibody response to antirabies vaccination received in the past, two I.M. doses (1.0 mL each) of human diploid cell vaccine (HDCV), one immediately and one 3 days later, is recommended. RIG should not be given in these cases.

If it is not known whether an exposed person has had antibody previously demonstrated, the complete postexposure antirabies treatment (RIG plus five doses) may be necessary. Because of variation in vaccine potency and individual response, immunization should not be considered complete until antibody is demonstrated in the serum. If antibody can be demonstrated in a serum sample collected before vaccine is given, treatment can be discontinued after at least two doses of HDCV.

Preexposure Prophylaxis. Those whose vocations or avocations result in frequent contact with dogs, cats, foxes, skunks, or bats should also be considered for preexposure prophylaxis.

A significant number of citizens of the United States have been and, with increasing frequency, will continue to be exposed to rabies in other countries where rabies in dogs is a major problem. Because rabies in animals is widespread in large areas of Asia, Africa, and Latin America, the Foreign Quarantine Program of the U.S. Public Health Service has advised that preexposure immunization against rabies be suggested for Americans traveling in these areas. The dog remains the major source of human exposure.

Three 1-mL injections of HDCV given intradermally in the deltoid area on days 0, 7, and 21 or 28 are required. This series of three injections can be expected to have produced neutralizing antibody in all patients. Rabies has been reported to develop in a patient following four doses of HDCV when human rabies globulin was not also given. Serologic testing is not necessary after preexposure prophylaxis with HDCV administered by either the intradermal or intramuscular route. The intradermal route should not be used for postexposure prophylaxis. Chloroquine phosphate (administered for malaria) chemoprophylaxis may interfere with the antibody response to HDCV in persons traveling to the developing countries. In persons receiving preexposure prophylaxis in preparation for travel to a rabies endemic area, the intradermal dose route should be initiated early enough to allow the three-dose series to be completed 30 days or more before departure. If this is not possible, the intramuscular dose route should be used.

The intradermal human diploid cell rabies vaccine (HDCV) was licensed for preexposure use in the United States on May 30, 1986. Fishbein recently demonstrated that 95 percent of previously immunized persons who had inadequate titers at the time of booster responded with a fivefold increase in titer by day 7 after a single booster dose of HDCV. In contrast, persons receiving the primary rabies immunization do not begin to respond for 7 days and do not obtain significant titers from 10 to 14 days. For other persons, such as veterinarians and animal control officers in areas of low rabies endemicity, primary immunization may be all that is necessary until an exposure occurs. Routine 2-year boosters in the latter groups appear to be unnecessary and probably risky. Bernard demonstrated that intradermal boosters at 1 year following preexposure immunization resulted in generalized reaction, consisting primarily of headache, malaise, fever, muscle aches, joint pain, or generalized itching in 26 percent of patients.

Intradermal HDCV has not been approved for postexposure use. Should an exposure occur in any one who has had a recommended primary preexposure regimen of HDCV, the individual should receive two intramuscular (I.M.) booster doses of HDCV, one each on days 0 and 3.

Accidental Human Exposure to Vaccine. Accidental inoculation may occur in individuals during administration of animal rabies vaccine. Such exposures to inactivated vaccines constitute no known rabies hazard. There have been no cases of rabies resulting from needle or other exposure to a licensed modified live virus vaccine in the United States; however, the local or state health department can be contacted.

Postexposure Prophylaxis. *Incubation Period.* It is generally accepted that the incubation period for rabies in human beings ranges from 10 days to 1 year, most cases occurring 20 to 90 days from exposure. In cases of exposure of the head, neck, or upper extremities, the incubation period is potentially less than 30 days.

Immediate Local Care. Not all persons bitten by rabid animals contract the disease. Vigorous local treatment to remove possible rabies virus may be as important as specific antirabies therapy. Free bleeding from the wound is encouraged. Local care of an animal bite should consist of:

1. Thorough irrigation with copious amounts of saline solution;
2. Cleansing with a soap solution;
3. Debridement;
4. Administration of antibiotic when indicated to prevent bacterial infection;
5. Administration of tetanus toxoid;
6. Immediate suturing of the wound generally is not advised, since it may contribute to the development of rabies, but a severe laceration secondary to a dog bite may be sutured if exposure to rabies is unlikely.

Passive Immunization. Rabies immune globulin, human (RIG) (Cutter Laboratories, Hyperaperab and Merieux Institutes, IMOGAM) is antirabies gamma globulin prepared from hyperimmunized human donors. Human rabies immune globulin (HRIG) in combination with HDCV is considered the best postexposure prophylaxis. HRIG, 20 I.U./kg of body weight, is recommended for most exposures classified as severe, for all bites by rabid animals or those suspected of having rabies, for unprovoked bites by wild carnivores and bats, and for nonbite exposure to animals suspected of being rabid. A portion of the HRIG is used to infiltrate the wound, and the remainder is administered intramuscularly. HRIG is given only once, as early as possible following exposure and up to the eighth day. After the eighth day RIG is not indicated, since an antibody response to the vaccine is presumed to have occurred. The use of human immune antirabies globulin is accompanied by five intramuscular 1.0-mL doses of HDCV. If HRIG is not available, the recommended dose of equine antibodies serum is 40 I.U./kg of body weight (Table 6-3).

Table 6-3. POSTEXPOSURE ANTIRABIES TREATMENT GUIDE

Species of animal	Condition of animal at time of attack	Treatment of exposed person
Skunk Fox Coyote Raccoon Bat	Regard as rabid	HRIG + HDCV
Dog	Healthy	None
	Unknown (escaped)	HRIG + HDCV
Cat	Rabid or suspected rabid	HRIG + HDCV*
Other	Consider individually—see Circumstances of the Bite	

These recommendations are only a guide. They should be applied in conjunction with knowledge of the animal species involved, circumstances of the bite or other exposure, vaccination status of the animal, and presence of rabies in the region.

* Discontinue vaccine if tests of animal killed at time of attack are negative.

Active Immunization, Primary Immunization. Over 25,000 people per year undergo postexposure prophylaxis after bites by suspected or proved rabid animals. HDCV is an inactivated virus vaccine prepared from fixed rabies virus grown in human diploid cell culture. Five intramuscular 1.0-mL doses of HDCV on days 0, 3, 7, 14, and 28 are administered. The WHO currently recommends a sixth dose 90 days after the first dose. All injections are given in the deltoid area. The routine serologic testing of persons who receive recommended preexposure or postexposure treatment regimens of HDCV is not necessary, nor is it necessary to perform routine serologic testing following booster doses of HDCV for persons given the recommended primary HDCV vaccination or those shown to have had an adequate antibody response to primary vaccination with duck embryo vaccine or other rabies vaccination. The vaccine may be stopped if the animal is proved nonrabid.

Evidence from laboratory and field experience in many areas of the world indicates that postexposure prophylaxis combined with local wound treatment, vaccine, and rabies immune globulin is uniformly effective when appropriately used. However, rabies has occasionally developed in human beings who have received postexposure rabies prophylaxis with the vaccine alone.

Booster Doses. In persons continuously exposed to the risk of rabies, booster doses of HDCV should be given at 2-year intervals. A previously immunized person who is exposed to rabies should receive two doses I.M. of 1 mL of HDCV, one immediately and one 3 days later. Laboratory workers in rabies biologic exposure areas should be tested for rabies antibody every 6 months and vaccinated when antibody as measured with the rapid fluorescent-focus inhibition test is low. HRIG is not indicated.

Side Reaction to Vaccine. Following vaccination with HDCV, reactions have included warmth, redness, pain, swelling, and itching at the infection site in approximately 15 to 25 percent of patients. Other side effects have included fever, nausea, vomiting and diarrhea, lymphadenopathy, headache, and dizziness. Rarely have systemic reactions including hives and anaphylaxis occurred. Two cases of illness resembling Guillain-Barré syndrome have been reported.

Precautions and Contraindications. *Immunosuppression.* Corticosteroids and other immunosuppressive agents and immunosuppressive illnesses can interfere with the active immunity in predisposed patients developing rabies. Immunosuppressive agents should not be administered during postexposure therapy, unless essential for the treatment of other conditions. When rabies and postexposure prophylaxis are administered to persons receiving steroids or other immunosuppressive therapy, it is especially important that serum be tested for serum antibody to ensure that an adequate response has developed.

Pregnancy. Because of the potential consequences of inadequately treated rabies exposure and limited data to indicate that fetal abnormalities have not been associated with rabies vaccination, pregnancy is not considered a contraindication to postexposure prophylaxis.

Allergies. Persons with histories of hypersensitivities should be given rabies vaccines with caution. When a patient with a history suggesting hypersensitivity to HDCV must be given that vaccine, antihistamines can be given; epinephrine should be readily available to counteract antiphylactic reactions, and the person should be carefully observed.

Manifestations and Treatment of Disease. Rabid dogs are noted to have purposeless movements with snapping, drooling, and vocal cord paralysis. Death usually occurs in 2 to 5 days. Human beings die essentially the same way. There are 2 to 4 days of prodromal symptoms before the patient reaches the excited stage. Paresthesia in the region of the bite is an important early symptom. Symptoms noted with the onset of clinical rabies include headaches, vertigo, stiff neck, malaise, lethargy, and severe pulmonary symptoms including wheezing, hyperventilation, and dyspnea. The patient may have spasm of the throat muscles with dysphagia. The outstanding clinical symptom of rabies is related to swallowing. Drooling, maniacal behavior, and convulsions ensue and are followed by coma, paralysis, and death.

Instead of sedation and symptomatic treatment only, it is now recognized that intensive respiratory supportive care may be beneficial, in view of a case of human rabies in which the patient survived. Strict attention was given to the management of airway, pulmonary care, cardiac arrhythmias, and seizures. This included tracheostomy, vigorous suctioning, Dilantin for seizures, close monitoring of blood gases, electrocardiograms, electroencephalograms, and a ventricular shunt. Nursing care is extremely important.

At least one case of human rabies has been treated with interferon in the United States. In animal studies interferon has been shown to offer protection against challenge by rabies virus only when it is administered before or shortly after virus challenge. Once clinical disease develops, the use of interferon is justified because clinical rabies is almost uniformly fatal despite active or passive immunization.

Snakebites

INCIDENCE. In North America all the poisonous snakes of medical importance are members of the family Crotalidae, or pit vipers, with the exception of the coral snake, of the Elapidae family. Coral snakes are scattered from Florida to southern Arizona, are biologically related to the Indian cobra, and produce a different envenomation syndrome from the crotalids. The pit vipers include the rattlesnake, cottonmouth moccasin, and copperhead.

Approximately 8000 persons are bitten each year by poisonous snakes. Over 98 percent of snakebites occur on the extremities. Thirty-five percent of snakebites occur in children less than ten years of age, usually in an area around their homes. Since 1960, an average of 14 victims have died annually as a result of snakebites. Five states account for 70 percent of these deaths: Texas, Georgia, Florida, Alabama, and southern California. Rattlesnakes are responsible for approximately 70 percent of all deaths

due to snakebites. Death from the bite of a copperhead is extremely rare.

POISONOUS VERSUS NONPOISONOUS SNAKES. Pit vipers are named for the characteristic pit, a heat-sensitive organ, that is located between the eye and the nostril on each side of the head. As a rule, these snakes may be identified by their elliptical pupils, as opposed to the round pupil of harmless snakes. Nonpoisonous snakes do not have pits. However, the coral snake does have a round pupil and lacks the facial pit. Pit vipers have two well-developed fangs that protrude from the maxillae, whereas nonpoisonous snakes have rows of teeth without fangs. Pit vipers also may be identified by turning the snake's belly upward and noting the single row of subcaudal plates. Nonpoisonous snakes have a double row of subcaudal plates (Fig. 6-2). The coral snake is a brightly colored small snake with red, yellow, and black rings. This color combination occurs also in nonpoisonous snakes, but the alternating colors are different. Only the coral snake has a red ring next to a yellow ring; when red touches yellow, it is a coral snake. The nose of the coral snake is black.

The venoms of poisonous snakes consist of enzymatic, complex proteins that affect all soft tissues. Venoms have been shown to have neurotoxic, hemorrhagic, thrombogenic, hemolytic, cytotoxic, antifribin, and anticoagulant effects. Phospholipase A is probably responsible for hemolysis. Most venoms contain hyaluronidase, which enhances the rapid spread of venom by way of the superficial lymphatics. There may be considerable variation in the venom effect. Either neurotoxic features such as muscle cramping, fasciculation, weakness, and respiratory paralysis or hemolytic characteristics may predominate depending on the snake and the patient.

CLINICAL MANIFESTATIONS. Pain from the bite of a poisonous snake is excruciating and probably the symptom that most easily differentiates poisonous from nonpoisonous snakebites. Poisonous snakes characteristically produce one or two fang marks, whereas nonpoisonous snakes may produce rows of punctures. Local signs and symptoms may include swelling, tenderness, pain, and ecchymosis and may appear within minutes at the site of the venom injection. If no edema or pain is present within 30 min following the injury, the pit viper probably did not inject any venom. Swelling may continue to increase for 24 h. Hemorrhagic vesiculations, bullae, and petechiae may appear between 8 and 36 h, with thrombosis of superficial vessels and eventual sloughing of tissues. Systemic symptoms include paresthesias and muscle fasciculations. Muscle fasciculations are most common following a rattlesnake bite and often are in the perioral region. Fasciculations almost never follow a copperhead bite and rarely follow a cottonmouth bite. They are often seen in the face muscles and over the neck, back, and the involved extremity, and may occur within 10 min. Hypotension, weakness, sweating and chills, dizziness, nausea, and vomiting are other systemic symptoms.

Rattlesnake. Most rattlesnakes probably eject less than 50 percent of their venom during a single biting act. Following a rattlesnake bite, ecchymosis, hemorrhagic

CHARACTERISTICS OF SNAKES

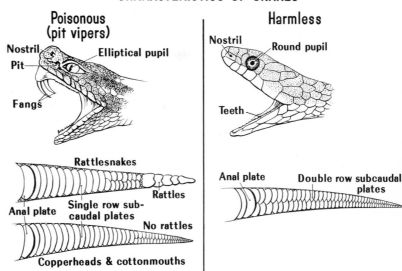

Fig. 6-2. Characteristics of poisonous and nonpoisonous snakes. (From: *Parrish HM: Texas State J Med 60:592, 1964, with permission.*)

vesiculations, swelling of the regional lymph nodes, weakness, fainting, and sweating commonly are reported. The venom produces deleterious changes in the blood cells, defects in blood coagulation, injuries to the intimal linings of vessels, damage to the heart muscles, alterations in respiration, and, to a lesser extent, changes in neuromuscular conduction. Pulmonary edema is common in severe poisoning, and hemorrhage into the lungs, kidneys, heart, and peritoneum may occur. Hematemesis, melena, changes in salivation, and muscle fasciculations may be seen. Urinalysis may reveal hematuria, glycosuria, and proteinuria. Red blood cells and platelets may decrease, and bleeding and clotting times are usually prolonged.

Coral Snakes. The coral snake contributes to only 3 percent of all bites and 1.5 percent of all deaths from poisonous snakes. Bites by the coral snake occasionally provoke blurred vision, ptosis, drowsiness, increased salivation, and sweating. The patient may notice paresthesia about the mouth and throat, sometimes slurring of speech, and nausea and vomiting. Pain is not a constant complaint, nor is edema a constant finding. Thus coral snake venom causes more extensive changes in the nervous system, but death may occur from cardiovascular collapse.

LABORATORY EVALUATION. Blood should be immediately drawn for typing and cross matching, because hemolysis may later make this difficult. Since hemolysis and injury to kidneys and liver may occur, it is important to follow alterations in clotting mechanism and renal and liver function as well as electrolyte status. Routine tests include a complete blood count, platelet count, prothrombin time, partial thromboplastin time, urinalysis, blood sugar, BUN, and electrolytes. Additional tests depending on the severity of the bite include fibrinogen, red cell fragility, clotting time, and clot retraction time.

LOCAL TREATMENT. The treatment of the bite of a poisonous snake varies considerably but is related to the length of time from the bite until treatment is instituted. Application of a tourniquet, incision, and suction are appropriate if employed within 1 h from the time of the bite. The Committee on Trauma of the American College of Surgeons in consultation with many experts in this field developed a poster for emergency department use entitled "Management of Poisonous Snakebites."

Immobilization. Patients are kept quiet, and the extremity is immobilized. Splinting the limb may inhibit the local diffusion of venom by stopping the movement of muscle bellies within their sheaths. Snyder and Knowles have shown in animals that exercise greatly enhances the absorption of venom and as much as 30 percent may be absorbed within 30 min following vigorous exercise.

Tourniquet. The snake injects venom into the subcutaneous tissue, and this is absorbed by the lymphatics. As almost none of the venom is absorbed through the bloodstream, the tourniquet is applied loosely to obstruct only venous and lymphatic flow. The index finger should be easily inserted beneath the tourniquet after its application. The distal pulse is checked and should be palpable after tourniquet application. The tourniquet is not released once applied and may be left in place during the 30 min that suction is being applied. Snyder and Knowles have injected ^{131}I-tagged venom into dogs and have demonstrated that if the tourniquet is applied promptly, less than 10 percent of the venom leaves the leg of the dog in 2 h. The tourniquet may be removed (1) as soon as an intravenous infusion is started, (2) when antivenin is ready for administration, and (3) if the patient is not in shock.

EMERGENCY DEPARTMENT MANAGEMENT OF POISONOUS SNAKEBITES

Clinical evaluation of the victim

1. Assess respiratory status.
2. Assess circulatory status.
3. Determine the extent of systemic reaction from the presence of hypotension; nausea; vomiting; sweating; weakness; or neurotoxic symptoms such as dizziness, perioral paresthesia, ptosis, paralysis, or muscle fasciculations.
4. Inspect the area of the bite, noting one or more fang marks (although a coral snake may leave none), swelling, pain, or ecchymoses.
5. Identify the snake if possible. Most bites are from nonpoisonous snakes.

Laboratory evaluation

1. Routine tests:
    a. Complete blood count
    b. Type and cross match
    c. Prothrombin time
    d. Partial thromboplastin time
    e. Platelet count
    f. Urinalysis
    g. Blood sugar; blood urea nitrogen (BUN); electrolytes
2. Additional tests, depending on the severity of the bite:
    a. Fibrinogen
    b. Red cell fragility
    c. Clotting time
    d. Clot retraction time

Grade of envenomation

The grade of envenomation will vary with time after the bite. (If the victim is seen early, severe envenomation may be underassessed.) Observe at least 6 h after the bite.

1. Indications of minimal envenomation:
    a. Local symptoms and signs
    b. Few systemic symptoms and signs
    c. Minimal laboratory abnormalities
2. Indications of moderate envenomation:
    a. Swelling that progresses beyond the area of the bite
    b. Some systemic symptoms and signs
    c. Abnormal laboratory findings—i.e., abnormal clotting factors; a fall in hematocrit or platelets
3. Indication of severe envenomation:
    a. Marked local symptoms and signs
    b. Severe systemic symptoms and signs
    c. Significant abnormalities in laboratory findings

Treatment

1. Start intravenous infusion of balanced salt solution if any evidence of envenomation exists.
2. Oxygen and appropriate vasopressors should be available.
3. Keep the bitten part level with the heart.
4. Release compression band (if one has been applied) only if:
    a. The patient is not in shock
    b. An intravenous line has been established
    c. Antivenin is available
5. Local care of the area of the bite:
    a. If the victim is treated within 30 min of the bite, incise at least full-thickness skin to the depth of the bite. Apply suction for 20 min.
    b. Some consultants with extensive experience and good results recommend early exploration of the snakebite area under local or general anesthesia as primary therapy, to diagnose the status of envenomation and to determine the depth and amount of tissue destruction.
    c. Cryotherapy is not indicated in the emergency department.
6. Update tetanus immunization.
7. Antivenin (see Grade of Envenomation):
    a. Withhold antivenin from patients without symptoms or signs of envenomation.
    b. Withhold antivenin from patients exhibiting local but not systemic symptoms or signs. Many patients will not require antivenin. (Copperhead venom is not usually very toxic, and rarely necessitates antivenin.)
    c. Admit all patients who receive antivenin.
    d. Administer antivenin intravenously in a continuous saline drip on the basis of grade of envenomation:
        • Minimal: 0 to 4 vials
        • Moderate: 5 to 9 vials, especially in children and the elderly
        • Severe: 10 to 15 or more vials
    Administer antivenin only after a skin test. Read product information carefully.

EMERGENCY DEPARTMENT MANAGEMENT OF POISONOUS SNAKEBITES (continued)

e. Epinephrine 1/1000 in a syringe should be available before antivenin is given.

f. Judge the amount of antivenin by improvement in symptoms and signs, not by the patient's weight. Children may need more antivenin than adults.

g. If systemic manifestations are severe, antivenin should be given rapidly, by intravenous drip, in large doses.

8. Watch for vascular insufficiency or compartment syndrome. Fasciotomy may be required if distal vascularity is impaired by swelling.

Additional antivenin considerations:

- Polyvalent antivenin (Wyeth Laboratories) is the current antivenin of choice for all North American rattlesnake, water moccasin (cottonmouth), and copperhead bites.
- North American coral snake antivenin (Wyeth Laboratories) should be used for eastern coral snakebites only—not for western or Arizona coral snakebites.

Incision and Suction. Incision and suction may be of benefit if accomplished within 30 min after snakebite. Approximately 50 percent of subcutaneously injected venom can be removed when the suction is started within 3 min. Treatment in the first 5 min is important, since half the value of suction is lost after 15 min and almost all after 30 min. A 30-min period of suction extracts about 90 percent of the venom that can be removed by this procedure. The incision should be ¼ in. long and ⅛ to ¼ in. deep, longitudinal and not cruciate. When two fang marks are seen, the depth of the venom injection is generally considered to be one-third of the distance between the fang marks. A good rule of thumb has been to incise the skin and subcutaneous tissue in length the same distance as between the fang marks to ensure adequate drainage. A superficial incision may be easily accomplished by raising the skin with a pinch between two fingers. Severe bites may result in envenomations between the fascia, and surgical exploration may be indicated. Incisions made proximal to the bite do not usually recover enough venom to make the procedure worthwhile and thus are contraindicated.

When a suction cup is not available after incisions have been made, mouth suction may be used if the mucosa of the mouth is intact. Snake venom is not absorbed through an intact oral mucosa but may be absorbed when there is any denuded area or minor laceration of the mucosa. The digestive juices neutralize poisonous snake venom if it is swallowed.

Russell has demonstrated that the serosanguinous fluid removed during suction contains substances that when injected into animals produce a fall in systemic blood pressure and changes in respiratory rates and alterations in the electrocardiogram and electroencephalogram similar to those observed following injection of crude Crotalus venom. If exudate removed during suction contains venom, its removal should increase the chances of survival.

Excision. Snyder and Knowles showed that wide excision of the entire area around the snakebite within 1 h from the time of injection can remove most of the venom. Excision of the fang marks including skin and subcutaneous tissue should be considered in severe bites and in patients known to be allergic to horse serum who are seen within 1 h following the bite. However, the average snakebite does not require surgical excision. This procedure is reserved for the most severe envenomations. Most fatalities from snakebites do not occur for 6 to 48 h following the bite, giving time to institute other first aid measures. Excision often causes severe scarring and possible skin graft.

Cryotherapy. This form of therapy has been used but is not recommended, as it only increases the local area of necrosis. McCollough and Gennard analyzed cryotherapy in relation to amputation and noted that 75 percent of children requiring amputation following snakebite had received cryotherapy. Cooling or refrigeration experimentally produces intense vasoconstriction and thus decreases the amount of antivenin getting into the area of the bite. Gill found that dogs developed edema and ecchymosis just as rapidly and extensively with cryotherapy as without it. There was no evidence to suggest inactivation of venom by tissue temperature of 15°C and below.

SYSTEMIC TREATMENT. The most important treatment for a snakebite is antivenin, although many patients will not require it. Copperhead venom is not usually very toxic and rarely necessitates antivenin. In 1954 polyvalent Crotalidae antivenin became commercially available. Most snakebite fatalities in the United States during the past 20 years have involved either delay in obtaining treatment, no antivenin treatment, or inadequate dosage. Because antivenin contains horse serum, its administration requires prior skin testing. Epinephrine 1/1000 in a syringe should be available before antivenin is given.

Information concerning identification of a snake or proper antivenin frequently can be obtained from the nearest zoo herpetarium. A major problem with bites by exotic poisonous snakes is the choice and availability of suitable antiserum. Physicians confronted with this situation may obtain advice from the local poison control center or from the Antivenin Index Center of the Oklahoma Poison Information Center, Oklahoma City, Oklahoma (405-271-5454).

Because the rattlesnake, cottonmouth moccasin, and copperhead belong to the same biologic family, their bites can be treated by the same antivenin (antivenin Crotalidae polyvalent).

The coral snakebite is rare, and the antivenin is different from that for the pit vipers. A North American coral snake (*Micrurus fulvius*) antivenin has been developed. It effectively treats Micrurus coral snakebites but is not effective in treating bites of Micruroides, the genus native to Arizona and New Mexico. Coral snake antivenin can be obtained from many state health departments. Also, a large supply has been stocked at the U.S. Public Health Service National Communicable Disease Center in Atlanta, Georgia.

The time of antivenin administration depends upon the snake involved. If the bite is from a snake with a quick-acting venom, such as a king cobra or mamba, an initial dose of antivenin may be required as part of the first-aid treatment. However, for bites by most snakes, such as rattlesnakes and others with less virulent venom, antivenin should be withheld until a physician can determine if it is indicated. Approximately 30 percent of all poisonous snakebites in the United States result in no envenomation.

The indication for antivenin is governed by the degree of envenomation, as outlined by Wood et al. and modified by Parrish and by McCollough and Gennard:

Grade 0—no envenomation: One or more fang marks; minimal pain; less than 1 in. of surrounding edema and erythema at 12 h; no systemic involvement.

Grade 1—minimal envenomation: Fang marks; moderate to severe pain; 1 to 5 in. of surrounding edema and erythema in the first 12 h after bite; systemic involvement usually not present.

Grade II—moderate envenomation: Fang marks; severe pain; 6 to 12 in. of surrounding edema and erythema in the first 12 h after bite; possible systemic involvement including nausea, vomiting, giddiness, shock, or neurotoxic symptoms.

Grade III—severe envenomation: Fang marks; severe pain; more than 12 in. of surrounding edema and erythema in first 12 h after bite; grade II symptoms of systemic involvement usually present and may include generalized petechiae and ecchymosis.

Grade IV—very severe envenomation: Systemic involvement is always present, and symptoms may include renal failure, blood-tinged secretions, coma, and death; local edema may extend beyond the involved extremity to the ipsilateral trunk.

With frequent observations using this classification, the severity of the bite will be found to increase with time, and thus a change in grade is observed. Most bites will have reached a final staging within 12 h.

Antivenin usually is not required for grades 0 or 1 envenomation. Grade II may require 3 or 4 ampules, and grade III usually requires 5 to 15 ampules. If symptoms increase, several ampules may be required during the first 2 h. Because children are smaller, they receive relatively larger doses of venom, which places them in a higher-risk group. Thus, the smaller the patient, the relatively larger the required dose of antivenin. Proper dosage can be estimated by observing the clinical signs and symptoms. If systemic manifestations are severe, antivenin should be given rapidly, by intravenous drip, in large doses.

The injection of antivenin locally around the bite is not advised, as massive edema usually occurs in that area. Absorption from this area is poor, and additional anti-

venin fluid will further decrease perfusion and perhaps increase tissue anoxia.

If any antivenin is indicated, 3 to 5 vials are given by intravenous drip in 500 mL of normal saline solution or 5 percent glucose solution. If severe systemic symptoms are already present, 6 to 8 vials are added. McCollough and Gennard have demonstrated in studies with radioisotopes that antivenin accumulates at the site of the bite more rapidly after intravenous than after intramuscular administration. The dose of intravenously administered antivenin can be more easily titrated with response to treatment, and the amount administered is based on improvement in signs and symptoms, not on weight of the patient. Antivenin is administered until severe local or systemic symptoms improve. When it is obvious that antivenin therapy will be instituted, the tourniquet should be left in place until antivenin is started intravenously. All patients who receive antivenin are admitted to the hospital.

If too much time has elapsed for excision to be effective and the patient is allergic to horse serum, a slow infusion of 1 ampule of antivenin in 250 mL of 5% glucose solution may be given in a 90-min period with constant monitoring of the blood pressure and electrocardiogram depending on the seriousness of the bite. This is accomplished in an active emergency department or an intensive care unit where resuscitation equipment and personnel trained in resuscitation are available. If an immediate reaction occurs, the antivenin is stopped, and a vasopressor, epinephrine, and perhaps an antihistamine may be required, depending on the severity of the reaction.

The incidence of serum sickness is directly related to the volume of horse serum injected. Of patients receiving 100 to 200 mL of horse serum, 85 percent will have some degree of sensitivity in 8 to 12 days following injection. This complication will have to be dealt with at a later time, since some patients may require from 1 to 5 ampules of antiserum every 4 to 6 h.

Steroids have been used but are of questionable benefit. Russell experimentally used doses of methylprednisolone up to 100 mg/kg in mice and noted that steroids neither affected survival nor prevented tissue damage and inflammation. When used in association with the antivenin, there is a decreased incidence of serum sickness. According to Parrish, cortisone and ACTH do not affect the survival rate of animals poisoned with pit viper venom. Tracheal intubation and prolonged ventilation may be required for respiratory failure. Acute renal failure may require renal dialysis.

Intravenous fluids are frequently required to replace the decreased extracellular fluid volume resulting from edema formation. Fascial planes may become very tense, with obstruction of venous and later arterial flow, requiring fasciotomy. Adequate antivenin treatment usually makes surgical intervention unnecessary. Roberts has advocated intracompartment pressure monitoring and found it to be elevated in two cases. However, careful monitoring of skin color, distal pulses, and capillary refill of the nail bed may prove helpful in determining if fasciotomy is indicated.

These patients may need blood, since anemia can develop from the hematologic effects. As afibrinogenemia has been reported, fibrinogen may be required. Vitamin K may also be required. Bleeding and clotting abnormalities are treated with antivenin in addition to blood components. Antibiotics are started immediately to prevent secondary infection, and tetanus toxoid is administered. The most common species of organisms isolated from rattlesnake venom are *P. aeruginosa*, *Proteus* species, *Clostridium* species, and *B. fragilis*.

Stinging Insects and Animals

HYMENOPTERA

The most important insects that produce serious and possibly fatal anaphylactic reactions are the arthropods of the order Hymenoptera. This group includes the honeybee, bumblebee, wasp, yellow and black hornet, and the fire ant. The venom of these stinging insects is just as potent as that of snakes and causes more deaths in the United States yearly than are caused by snakebites. Drop for drop, the venom of the bee is just as potent as that of the rattlesnake. Parrish noted that, of 460 deaths between 1950 and 1959, 50 percent were due to Hymenoptera, 30 percent due to poisonous snakes, and 14 percent due to spiders. Scorpions accounted for eight deaths. No other poisonous creature killed more than 5 persons.

Insects of the Hymenoptera group, except the bee, retain their stinger and are in a position to sting repeatedly, each time injecting some portion of the venom sac contents. The worker honeybee sinks its barbed sting into the skin, and it cannot be withdrawn. As the bee attempts to escape, it is disemboweled. The stinger with the bowel, muscles, and venom sac attached are left behind. The muscles controlling the venom sac, although separated from the bee, rhythmically contract for as long as 20 min, driving the stinger deeper and deeper into the skin, and continuing to inject venom.

Bee venoms contain histamine, serotonin, acetylcholine, formic acid, phospholipase A, hyaluronidase, and other proteins. Once the proteins of these insects are injected, the patient may become sensitized and be a candidate for anaphylactic response with the next sting.

CLINICAL MANIFESTATIONS. Symptoms consist of one or more of the following: localized pain, swelling, generalized erythema, a feeling of intense heat throughout the body, headache, blurred vision, injected conjunctivae, swollen and tender joints, itching, apprehension, urticaria, petechial hemorrhages of skin and mucous membranes, dizziness, weakness, sweating, severe nausea, abdominal cramps, dyspnea, constriction of the chest, asthma, angioneurotic edema, vascular collapse, and possible death from anaphylaxis. Fatal cases may manifest glottal and laryngeal edema, pulmonary and cerebral edema, visceral congestion, meningeal hyperemia, and intraventricular hemorrhage. Death apparently results from a combination of shock, respiratory failure, and central nervous system changes. Most deaths from insect stings occur within 15 to 30 min following the bite or sting.

TREATMENT. Early application of a tourniquet may prevent rapid spread of the venom. Affected persons should be taught to remove the venom sac if present, being careful not to squeeze the sac. It may be necessary for some patients to carry an emergency kit, which is commercially available, supplied with a tourniquet, sublingual isoproterenol in 10-mg tablets, epinephrine hydrochloride aerosol for inhalation to reduce bronchospasm and laryngeal edema, and tweezers to remove the sting and venom sac until a physician is available. Patients should be taught to give themselves an epinephrine injection. Patients having severe reactions should first receive 0.3 to 0.5 mL of a 1:1000 solution of epinephrine intravenously. Antihistamines also may be intravenously administered, and oxygen may be given. If wheezing continues, aminophylline may be given slowly intravenously. Occasionally, the patient may require a tracheostomy.

DESENSITIZATION. The Insect Allergy Committee of the American Academy of Allergy noted that 50 percent of people who had a severe generalized reaction to stings had no previous history of a severe reaction. A sharp rise was noted in the proportion of serious reaction after the age of thirty, suggesting increasing sensitivity as the total number of stings increase. Patients with a history of severe local or systemic involvement following insect stings should be desensitized. Venom immunotherapy is safe and is highly effective within a few weeks. Venom immunotherapy is the recommended form of prophylaxis for insect sting allergy.

It has been suspected that a refractory period of 10 to 14 days persists following an insect sting during which skin tests may be negative. Therefore, skin tests should be delayed several weeks after stinging and be performed with extreme caution. Cross reactions to the wasp, bee, and yellow jacket may occur.

STINGRAYS

Approximately 750 persons each year are stung by stingrays. However, during the past 60 years, only two deaths in this country have been attributed to the venom of the stingray.

As the spine, which is curved and has serrated edges, enters the flesh, the sheath surrounding the spine ruptures, and venom is released. As the spine is withdrawn, fragments of the sheath may remain in the wound. The wound edges are often jagged and bleed freely. Pain is usually immediate and severe, increasing to maximum intensity in 1 to 2 h and lasting for 12 to 48 h.

TREATMENT. This consists of copious irrigation with water to wash out any toxin and fragments of the spine's integumentary sheath. Russell noted that the venom is inactivated when exposed to heat. Therefore, the area of the bite should be placed in water as hot as the patient can stand without injury for 30 min to 1 h. After soaking, the wound may be further debrided and treated appropriately. Patients treated in this manner were shown to have rapid and uncomplicated healing of the wound. Patients not treated with heat had tissue necrosis with prolonged drainage and chronically infected wounds.

PORTUGUESE MAN-OF-WAR

This coelenterate is commonly found along our southern Atlantic coast. Its tentacles are covered with thousands of stinging cells, the nematocytes, capable of emitting microscopic organelles, the nematocysts, each of which consists of a small sphere containing a coiled hollow thread. When activated by touch, the thread is uncoiled with such force that it can penetrate skin and even rubber gloves. On contact, venom in the cyst is injected into the victim through the thread. This sting produces extreme pain and often signs of clinical shock; however, no deaths have been reported due to this sting alone.

Following a severe sting there may be almost immediate severe nausea, gastric cramping, and constriction and tightness of throat and chest with severe muscle spasm. There is intense burning pain with weakness and perhaps cyanosis with respiratory distress.

TREATMENT. The most important emergency treatment is to inactivate the nematocysts immediately, to prevent their continuous firing of toxins. This is accomplished by application to the involved area of a substance of high alcohol content, such as rubbing alcohol. This is followed by application of a drying agent, such as flour, baking soda, talc, or shaving cream. The tentacles may then be removed by shaving. Alkaline agents, such as baking soda, are then applied to the involved area in order to neutralize the toxins, which are acidic. Antihistamines may be helpful in controlling the inflammatory response after these emergency treatments. Demerol and Benadryl may dramatically relieve the pain and symptoms. Aerosol corticosteroid-analgesic balm is helpful.

Spider Bites

BLACK WIDOW SPIDER

The most common biting spider in the United States is the black widow *(Latrodectus mactans)* (Fig. 6-3). The spider is black and globular, with a red hourglass mark on the abdomen. Latrodectism is a syndrome characterized

by severe muscular pain and stiffness, nausea, vomiting, and headache. The female spider has a reddish orange hourglass on its ventral surface. *Latrodectus* venom is primarily neurotoxic in action and appears to center on the spinal cord. Following a bite by the black widow spider, the majority of patients experience pain within 30 min and a small wheal with an area of erythema appears. Nausea and vomiting occurs in approximately one-third of patients, headache in one-fourth, and dyspnea may occur.

The time of onset of symptoms following the bite is from 30 min to 6 h. The severe symptoms last from 24 to 48 h. Generalized muscle spasm is the most prominent physical finding. Cramping muscle spasms occur in the thighs, lumbar region, abdomen, or thorax. Priapism and ejaculation have been reported.

Even if the bite is on an extremity, the spasm may involve the abdomen and chest. Although the abdomen is rigid, it is nontender and patients do not demonstrate signs and symptoms of generalized peritonitis. Less commonly the patient may have hypertension, hyperreflexia, and urinary retention. Most patients recover within 24 h.

TREATMENT. Treatment has consisted of narcotics for the relief of pain and a muscle relaxant for relief of spasm. Either methocarbamol (Robaxin) or 10 mL of a 10% solution of calcium gluconate relieves symptoms. It is believed that calcium acts by depressing the threshold for depolarization at the neuromuscular junctions. Calcium gluconate may give instant relief of muscular pain as well as relieving muscular spasm. Methocarbamol can be administered intravenously, 10 mL over a 5-min period with a second ampule started in a saline solution drip. Although antivenin *(Lactrodectus mactans)* is available, it is rarely required. The manufacturer recommends its use for patients younger than sixteen years or older than sixty years and for patients with underlying cardiovascular diseases. The antivenin is prepared from horse serum and is administered intramuscularly after appropriate skin tests. Hospitalization may be required for the young, elderly, and patients with significant chronic diseases or with severe signs and symptoms of envenomation.

NORTH AMERICAN LOXOSCELISM

The distinguishing mark of the *Loxosceles reclusa* is the darker violin-shaped band over the dorsal cephalothorax (Fig. 6-4). The spider is native to the south central United States and is found both indoors and outdoors. They are frequently found in attics, closets, old clothes, wood piles, boat docks, and in infrequently worn shoes. The first recognized and documented case in the United States by a *Loxosceles reclusa* was published in 1957.

CLINICAL MANIFESTATIONS. The body ranges from 7 mm to 1.2 cm and including the legs ranges from 2 to 3 cm. The initial bite may go unnoticed or be accompanied by a mild stinging sensation. Pain may recur 6 to 8 h afterward. A mild envenomation is associated with local urticaria and erythema. This usually resolves spontaneously. More severe bites result in progression to necrosis and sloughing of skin with residual ulcer formation. A generalized macular and erythematous rash may appear in 12 to

Fig. 6-3. Abdominal view of a female black widow spider showing the hourglass marking. (From: *Paton BC: Surg Clin North Am 43:*537, 1963, with permission.)

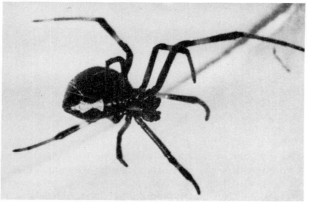

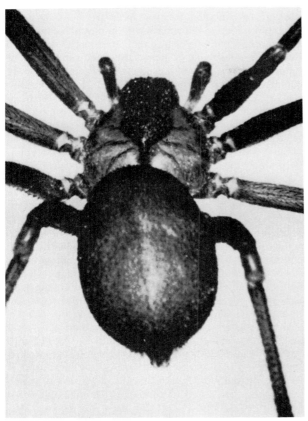

Fig. 6-4. The distinguishing mark of the *Loxosceles reclusa* is the darker violin-shaped band over the dorsal cephalothorax. (From: *Dillaha CJ, Jansen GT, et al: JAMA 188:33, 1964, with permission.*)

24 h. Erythema develops, with bleb or blister formation surrounded by an irregular area of ischemia. A zone of hemorrhage and induration and a surrounding halo of erythema may develop peripherally. The central ischemia turns dark, an eschar forms by the seventh day, and by the fourteenth day the area sloughs, leaving an open ulcer. Approximately 3 weeks is required for the lesion to heal. The pain may be out of proportion for the size of the area involved. The progression from blue to black gives the bite a necrotic appearance, and the more severe ones develop within a few hours to 2 days. Lesions found in areas of fatty tissue such as thigh, buttocks, and abdomen tend to be more extensive and result in severe scar formation. The necrotic lesions usually do not involve tendons or muscles.

Systemically, the patient may have fever, nausea, vomiting, arthralgia, and malaise. Severe systemic manifestations may occur in 24 to 48 h in small children, with fever, chills, malaise, weakness, nausea, vomiting, joint pain, and even petechial eruption. The two principal systemic effects, hemolysis and thrombocytopenia, have been responsible for deaths. Hemoglobinemia, hemoglobinuria, leukocytosis, and proteinuria may also occur. Renal failure can develop secondary to hemoglobinuria. *Loxosceles* venom is chiefly cytotoxic in action.

Laboratory studies are obtained in patients with severe envenomation including prothrombin time, PTT, platelet count, and urinalysis.

The current understanding of the pathophysiology of the bite is that intravascular coagulation and the formation of microthrombi within the capillary occur, leading to capillary occlusion, hemorrhage, and necrosis.

TREATMENT. Immediate excision with primary closure has been advocated as the treatment of choice. This usually is not possible since patients rarely can be certain that they were bitten by a brown recluse spider. Likewise, the excision may be inadequate, allowing venom to migrate in the residual tissue, resulting in ulcer formation requiring reexcision and often grafting. Treatment of loxoscelism seems to be conservative, because of the difficulty in predicting the severity of the bite. Various treatments have been advocated in addition to early excision such as corticosteroids, heparin, regitine, dextran, and infusion, but clinical studies have failed to identify the benefit of these agents. The dose for steroids has varied from 30 to 80 mg of methylprednisolone daily tapered over a period of several days. Excision of the necrotic area with skin grafting may be required at a later date.

Rees has recently reported using a leukocyte inhibitor, dapsone, used in leprosy, to be effective in reducing inflammation at the site of the brown recluse venom injection. Many of the patients were treated 48 h or more following the bite. Some received surgical excision and others were treated conservatively with dapsone 100 mg daily for 14 days before surgical excision, if required. They concluded that the incidence of scarring and deformity was much less in the dapsone treated group than with observation and subsequent surgical excision. Only one patient required hospitalization while on dapsone therapy compared with 50 percent in the observed group. These data imply that the high incidence of delayed wound healing, abscess formation, and objectionable scarring may be avoided if surgical therapy is delayed until the eschar has matured. The mechanism of action of dapsone is unclear. There are significant side effects associated with dapsone treatment including dose-dependent hemolytic anemia, methemoglobinemia, and rash. Rees suggests obtaining blood for G6PD levels and hematocrit before dapsone therapy. Complete blood counts are recommended weekly since reduction in leukocytes, platelets, or severe anemia due to hemolysis may develop. Hemolysis may be exaggerated in individuals with glucose-6-phosphate-dehydrogenate (G6PD) deficiency. Whether or not dapsone improves morbidity following brown spider bites awaits further clinical evaluation. Conservative therapy seems to be the preferred treatment. Excision of the necrotic area with skin grafting may be required at a later date.

PENETRATING WOUNDS OF THE NECK AND THORACIC INLET

Although penetrating injuries of the neck are uncommon in civilian surgical practice, the concentration of deep vital structures makes any cutaneous wound a potentially serious injury. Life-threatening consequences of unrepaired injuries of the larynx, trachea, pharynx, esophagus, and blood vessels of the neck and thoracic inlet mandate early diagnosis and operative correction. There is general agreement that penetrating wounds with overt evidence of deep injuries require urgent operations. A difference of opinion exists regarding the necessity for operative exploration of patients without evidence of such injuries. Numerous reports document similar results in patients treated by routine operative explorations and those observed, with or without adjunctive diagnostic studies, and operated upon for positive tests or evolving clinical findings.

GENERAL CONSIDERATIONS. Before World War II, the treatment of penetrating wounds of the neck was largely nonsurgical unless major bleeding or deep injuries were obvious. Reported mortality rates were 18 percent of 188 cases in the Spanish-American War and 11 percent of 594 cases in World War I. During World War II the mortality rate fell to 7 percent, probably because of a variety of factors, including earlier tracheostomy, more frequent and expedient surgical exploration, antibiotics, and improvements in surgical and anesthetic techniques.

Since 1960, numerous civilian series have been reported and mortality rates approximate 5 percent. Most deaths are due to spinal cord and blood vessel injuries, although tracheal and esophageal wounds account for some. Fogelman and Stewart pointed out that the mortality rate for their cases that were promptly explored was 6 percent, whereas for those in which surgical intervention was omitted or postponed the mortality rate was 35 percent.

Mandatory (Routine) Exploration. Based on the improved results of operative care of penetrating neck injuries, the policy evolved in many major trauma centers of "treating the platysma like the peritoneum" and exploring virtually all neck wounds that penetrated the platysma. In 1967, Jones et al. reviewed 274 penetrating neck wounds treated in this manner at Parkland Memorial Hospital. There were 11 deaths, for a mortality rate of 3.6 percent. Of the fatalities, four were due to complications from spinal cord injuries, three from massive hemorrhage, and the remainder from cerebral complications of vascular or laryngotracheal injuries. Of the 274 cases, 103 (38 percent) explorations were negative, i.e., with no hematoma, no significant bleeding, and no damage to any named structure in the neck, although the tract of the injury frequently was within millimeters of vital structures. In the negative explorations there were no deaths and the only complication was a superficial wound infection that cleared promptly with drainage. These patients usually were discharged within 72 h to clinic follow-up if there were no associated injuries. Similar results have been documented more recently in the series reported by Saletta et al. and Roon and Christensen. These three series represent 700 patients, 327 (47 percent) of whom had major structural injuries. Thirty-one (4.4 percent) of these patients with important injuries were considered preoperatively to be "clinically negative." Most of these silent injuries were not life-threatening, but many patients with serious injuries had soft signs indicating their presence.

Selective Exploration. Because of the frequency of negative explorations resulting from the policy of mandatory exploration, a number of trauma centers have begun the selective management of penetrating neck injuries. Patients with overt signs of vascular or visceral injuries are promptly operated upon and those with "clinically negative" penetrating wounds are monitored by repeated physical examinations, with or without radiographic and endoscopic diagnostic procedures. Reports summarizing the results of selective management of more than 1200 patients with penetrating neck trauma have been published since 1983. About half the patients in most series underwent explorations because of clinical or radiographic evidence of deep injuries, and the rate of negative explorations was in the range of 20 to 30 percent. Subsequent explorations were infrequently required and minimal morbidity occurred in observed patients. No significant differences in mortality or morbidity were demonstrated between series managed by mandatory or selective exploration, including the randomized single-institution study by Golueke. Variable cost saving may result from a selective management policy, depending on the extent to which diagnostic studies are used.

Clinical evidence of an underlying vascular or visceral injury mandates operative exploration in any patient with penetrating cervical trauma. Acute symptoms and signs suggesting cervical vascular injuries include arterial bleeding, hematoma, diminished distal pulsation, bruit, unexplained shock, and cerebral changes indicative of an ischemic or embolic event. Findings suggesting aerodigestive tract injuries include stridor, dysphonia, aphonia, hemoptysis, hematemesis, dysphagia, odynophagia, and subcutaneous emphysema. Most laryngotracheal injuries acutely cause symptoms and physical findings, while vascular and pharyngoesophageal injuries are more often initially occult.

In hemodynamically stable and "clinically negative" patients with penetrating neck trauma, careful examination of the wound is an important aspect of estimating the potential for morbid injuries. If the extent of the injury is not apparent, the wound is very gently probed with a small hemostat, only to the depth of the platysma muscle. If the platysma has been penetrated, the probing is discontinued. Neck wounds should not be probed beneath the platysma muscle because hemostasis may be disrupted. A valid appraisal of the likelihood of deep injury requires knowledge of the anatomic relationships of the visceral and vascular structures of the neck. Wounds in the posterior triangle are less often associated with serious visceral and vascular injuries than those in the anterior and lateral aspects of the neck. Directly anterior wounds infrequently injure the esophagus without an intervening tracheal injury that is usually manifest by subcutaneous emphysema or air escaping from the wound. Plain films of the neck may be useful diagnostically by demonstrating subfascial air or, in the case of missile wounds, may assist in defining the trajectory by revealing a retained bullet or metallic fragments in bone.

Because a penetrating wound may be the only sign indicating the presence of a major vascular injury, arteriography has become an important modality in the manage-

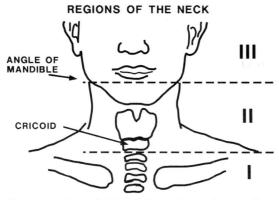

REGIONS OF THE NECK

ANGLE OF
MANDIBLE

CRICOID

III

II

I

Fig. 6-5. Arbitrary division of the cervical region into three zones. Management of penetrating wounds of the neck is based on the area involved. (From: *Monson DO et al: 1969, with permission.*)

ment of neck injuries. The validity of biplane multifilm arteriography in the evaluation of peripheral arterial injuries was documented by Snyder et al. These studies may be useful in precisely defining the site of an arterial injury, as well as for the purpose of confirming arterial integrity. Monson's division of the neck into three zones is useful in considering the arteriographic evaluation of penetrating neck trauma (Fig. 6-5): Zone I—below a horizontal line 1 cm above the claviculomanubrial junction or inferior to the cricoid cartilage; Zone II—between Zone I and the angle of the mandible; and Zone III—between the angle of the mandible and the base of the skull. Zones II and III are considered the neck proper and Zone I is the base of the neck or thoracic inlet. Arteriography has been used extensively and successfully to exclude arterial injuries in the selective management of cervical trauma. Many authors recommend its routine use in stable patients with overt signs of arterial injury, especially in Zones I and III because of the potential technical problems with exposure and vascular control in these regions. This will be considered more thoroughly in the section on specific injuries.

The possibility of underlying pharyngoesophageal injury has remained a problem in the management of "clinically negative" penetrating neck trauma. Important laryngotracheal injuries are essentially always overt, arterial injuries can be accurately diagnosed arteriographically, and occult venous injuries are unlikely to have much morbid potential. The validity of nonoperative exclusion of pharyngoesophageal injuries has not been thoroughly addressed. In an attempt to resolve this issue, 118 patients with penetrating neck trauma in Zones II or III treated at Parkland Memorial Hospital were prospectively studied. Essentially all patients had cervical arteriography, barium esophagrams, and flexible and rigid endoscopies, followed by operative neck explorations. Esophageal injuries were found at exploration in 10 patients; barium swallows and rigid esophagoscopies detected the injuries in eight of the nine patients so studied. Flexible endoscopy was inaccurate, yielding falsely negative results in five of the eight patients with esophageal perforations having this examination. Of 108 patients in whom esophageal injuries were operatively excluded, false-positive studies occurred in none of the 103 patients having barium swallows, one of the 98 patients having flexible esophagoscopies, and five of the 107 patients undergoing rigid endoscopies. The patient with a falsely negative barium swallow had a positive rigid endoscopy, and the esophogram demonstrated the injury in the single patient with a negative rigid endoscopic examination. Therefore, all patients with esophageal injuries had at least one positive study preoperatively. The sensitivity (ability of a test to detect an injury if present) for barium swallow and rigid esophagoscopy was 89 percent. The specificity (ability of a test to exclude an injury if absent) was 100 and 95 percent for barium swallow and rigid esophagoscopy, respectively.

Summary. Patients with clinical findings of vascular or visceral injuries are operatively explored in the operating room under general anesthesia. Patients with altered sensoriums in whom appropriate information, examinations, and diagnostic studies are impossible are also explored. Based on the above data, our current recommendations for stable patients with penetrating injuries in Zones II and III, without clinical evidence of vascular or aerodigestive tract injuries, include biplane four-vessel cervical angiography, barium esophagography in two projections with cineradiography, and rigid esophagoscopy. If arteriography reveals an injury requiring operation, no further studies are performed and the patient is operatively explored. If arteriography is negative, barium esophagography is performed. If esophagography is normal, important injury is considered unlikely and the patient is admitted for observation. If esophagography is positive, operative exploration is recommended, preceded by rigid esophagoscopy under general anesthesia. If esophagoscopy is negative, the judgment regarding proceeding with operative exploration is based on the certainty of the abnormality seen on esophagram. If any of the aforementioned studies cannot be adequately completed or are equivocal, operative exploration is recommended. Patients with injuries in Zone I are more liberally explored, despite the absence of objective clinical findings, because the site of injury is less amenable to observation, unexpected bleeding is difficult to control nonoperatively, and the validity of arteriographic exclusion is questionable.

Success with selective management of penetrating neck trauma requires surgeons and radiologists experienced in evaluating such injuries and the 24-h availability of precise radiologic studies. In addition, the necessary commitment of time and personnel for careful and repeated patient observation is substantially greater than is required for a cervical exploration. Routine exploration probably remains the safest approach to the management of penetrating neck injuries for surgeons working in hospitals caring for a limited number of traumatized patients.

The cost of observation without radiologic studies is clearly less than for an operative procedure and a brief postoperative stay. The expense of several radiologic studies makes the cost of the two modes of treatment more similar. Additional expenses mount related to the number of patients requiring operative procedures after the diagnostic studies. It seems that the total expense of a policy of mandatory exploration is likely to be at least equal to if not less than for selective management.

TREATMENT. Initial Evaluation and Management. On admission to the emergency room, all patients with neck injuries are immediately evaluated regarding their systemic condition, i.e., airway patency and adequacy of ventilation, blood pressure, pulse, and mental state. Peripheral signs of shock such as sweating, cold skin, and collapsed veins should be recorded. If there is external bleeding, pressure is applied for temporary hemostasis. Adequate ventilation may require endotracheal intubation in obtunded patients or tracheostomy if a laryngotracheal injury or a cervical hematoma has caused upper airway obstruction. One or two large-bore intravenous cannulas are inserted in peripheral veins and an infusion of Ringer's lactate solution is started while blood is drawn for typing and cross matching. If shock is present, the fluid is given rapidly; if there is no evidence of blood loss, the intravenous solutions are kept going by slow drip. When indicated, whole blood is administered as soon as it is available. Usually the salt solution will temporarily reverse the shock state until cross-matched blood is available. If shock is severe and is not improved promptly by the Ringer's lactate solution, type O, Rh-negative low-titer unmatched blood is infused rapidly until matched blood is available. Plasma has also been used but has no advantage over salt solutions; i.e., both are quite helpful temporarily, although neither is a substitute for whole blood. Tube thoracostomy is often necessary for intrathoracic bleeding or pneumothorax from the commonly associated pulmonary injuries. If there is no clinical evidence of pneumothorax or hemothorax and the patient's condition is stable, an upright chest film is obtained with a physician in constant attendance. No attempt is made to pass a nasogastric tube in the emergency room because of the danger of recurrent hemorrhage as a result of coughing or gagging.

The major initial risk is airway compromise for patients with injuries of the neck proper and exsanguinating hemorrhage for those with penetrating trauma entering the mediastinum. The clinical presentation of patients with superior mediastinal vascular injuries varies from innocuous-appearing cutaneous wounds to terminal hemorrhagic shock. Hemostasis may be transient and spontaneously break down, or it may be disrupted by changes in intravascular or intrathoracic pressure. Acute hemorrhage from these injuries can sometimes be controlled by external pressure, but occasionally control requires an anterolateral thoracotomy in the emergency room. The innominate and right subclavian vessels can be controlled through a right thoracotomy and the left subclavian artery controlled through a left chest incision.

Special x-ray studies such as contrast esophagography and arteriography may be useful but are considered only in hemodynamically stable patients. The use of these studies was previously summarized from the standpoint of diagnostic maneuvers, but arteriography as a preoperative study will be considered in more detail in this section. The potential benefits from preoperative arteriography can be related, in part, to the location of the wound. The neck proper extends from the base of the skull to about the level of the cricoid cartilage. This area corresponds to Zones II and III described by Monson (Fig. 6-5) or to the middle and upper neck. Penetrating wounds coursing inferior to the cricoid are considered wounds of the thoracic inlet or base of the neck (Zone I). An upper neck wound whose course extends above the angle of the mandible (Zone III) often presents dangerous intraoperative problems. Arteriographic definition of the site and extent of arterial injury may importantly alter operative plans. Internal carotid injuries near the base of the skull are difficult to expose and cephalad control may be essentially impossible. Initial extracranial-intracranial arterial bypass (EC-IC) is a reasonable consideration in patients with such injuries. Cerebral protection, with an initial EC-IC, may occasionally be important in cephalad injuries with continued flow because intraluminal shunt insertion is often not possible. In addition, reconstruction of the internal carotid artery may not be technically feasible and ligation may be required. Operative control of mid-neck carotid wounds (between the mandible and the level of the cricoid cartilage—Zone II) is usually simple and arteriographic definition is less important. Vertebral artery injuries that may otherwise go undetected may be demonstrated if arteriography is performed on patients with injuries in this region.

Penetrating wounds in the low neck (Zone I) may involve vessels of the superior mediastinum and require thoracic incisions for adequate exposure. Arteriography is potentially helpful in such wounds, but the necessary delay poses substantial risk. In most anatomic sites, exacting arteriography accurately defines specific arterial lesions and confirms arterial integrity. In the superior mediastinum there are many important structures, and risk of occult hemorrhage argues against substituting arteriography for operative exploration. The concentration of major arteries increases the likelihood of missing minor arteriographic defects that indicate the presence of major injuries. Such inaccuracies result because of the superimposition of dye columns caused by the spatial orientation of these vessels. The validity of "exclusion" arteriography, established for extremity injuries, cannot be transposed to the diagnostic evaluation of mediastinal wounds. For these reasons, operative exploration is indicated for most penetrating injuries suspected of entering the mediastinum.

Although arteriography may not reliably exclude mediastinal vascular injuries, it can be helpful in defining the site of arterial wounds. The decision to use arteriography for planning the operation must take into account delay and the risk of cardiovascular deterioration. The bleeding may be tamponaded by soft tissues, but this is tenuous, as emphasized in a report by Flint of 146 patients with base-of-the-neck vascular injuries. Of the 90 patients initially normotensive, six (7 percent) became profoundly hypotensive en route to or shortly after arrival in the operating room. Rapid hemostasis was obtained operatively in all six patients and all survived, but the personnel and facilities available in the operating room played a major role. If these unanticipated events had occurred in the radiology suite, the outcome would most likely have been different. In summary, preoperative arteriography is frequently helpful in evaluating patients with potential arterial injuries of the neck and thoracic inlet, but it should not be used to obviate the need for operative exploration in patients with intrathoracic bleeding, and arteriograms should be considered only in stable patients.

The frequent absence of overt signs of vascular trauma and the minimal morbidity imposed by operative exploration was documented in the review by Flint et al. of 146 patients with base-of-the-neck vascular injuries. Thirty-two percent of these patients had no diagnostic signs of vascular injuries. Even innominate and subclavian vessel wounds had no overt manifestations in 29 percent of these patients with such injuries. Most of the injuries in these patients were adequately managed with cervical or transverse clavicular incisions, and very few of those without overt injury manifestations required thoracic incisions.

Anesthesia. Exploration is performed under general anesthesia, using an orotracheal airway with an inflatable cuff. The anesthetic agent varies considerably according to the specific problem, necessity for rapid induction, circulatory status, and preexisting disease. There are no specific contraindications in patients with neck injuries to any of the commonly used anesthetic agents or relaxants.

Anesthetic induction requires attention to different problems in patients with superior mediastinal injuries as compared with those with wounds of the neck proper. Intubation while awake is preferred in patients with wounds of the neck proper because difficulties imposed by cervical hematomas or upper airway edema may delay adequate oxygenation in paralyzed patients. In these wounds, disruption of existing hemostasis by retching or struggling with intubation is usually amenable to control by external pressure. On the other hand, intubation in patients with superior mediastinal wounds may produce major hemorrhage that cannot be controlled by local pressure. These patients less often have structural alterations of the upper airway, and intubation can more safely follow the infusion of muscle relaxants. Because gastric decompression is omitted to avoid sudden alterations in intrathoracic pressure, precautions are necessary in the technique of induction to minimize the aspiration risk. In either instance, preinduction preparation for emergency tracheostomy is essential.

The chest is again examined just before induction, because pneumothorax may develop slowly following a neck wound, appearing an hour or longer after an initially negative chest x-ray. Wounds in the base of the neck following a downward path may cause minimal apical pulmonary injuries so that a pneumothorax is not apparent initially and may not be manifest until after the patient is intubated. This should be kept in mind as a cause for hypotension or hypoxia during anesthesia.

Technique of Operation. With adequate control of the ventilatory and cardiovascular systems, the surgeon can now safely and adequately explore the structures that may be injured. Patient positioning and preparation of the sterile field require foresight concerning operative exposure and the need for venous autografts. The supine position with some cervical extension is used. The prepared operative field includes the neck, chest, anterior shoulders, and a separate site for harvesting saphenous vein.

The incision is planned to allow full exposure of the tract of injury. Proximal and distal control of the major blood vessels must also be considered in the length and position of the incision. Incisions commonly used are the oblique incision along the anterior border of the sternocleidomastoid muscle, the horizontal clavicular incision with resection of the medial portion of the clavicle, median sternotomy, and anterolateral thoracotomy. A collar incision is occasionally useful for bilateral injuries or those primarily involving the larynx or proximal trachea.

The tract of injury is followed to its depth, with systematic examination of each adjacent structure. Blast injury, especially from high-velocity missiles, may not be immediately apparent and requires careful evaluation. If injuries to the major blood vessels are suspected, tapes are passed around the vessels proximal and distal to the point of suspected injury before local clots are removed. Injured structures are repaired as outlined in the following paragraphs and muscles are anatomically approximated.

Most soft tissue neck wounds are drained for 24 to 48 h using Penrose drains or Silastic suction catheters to prevent the accumulation of blood and serum. If the pharynx or esophagus is injured, drainage is continued for 4 to 8 days. In the case of a massive gunshot wound, such as close-range shotgun injury, the wound is left open initially and, if possible, a delayed primary closure is performed 3 to 4 days later.

Specific Injuries

VASCULAR INJURIES. Clinical problems posed by acute vascular injuries are best considered by dividing the discussion into injuries of the neck proper (Zones II and III) and those of the base of the neck or thoracic inlet (Zone I). Cerebral ischemia and tracheal compression from contained bleeding are the major concerns with injuries of the middle and upper neck. External hemorrhage can usually be controlled by pressure, and the diagnosis is signaled by an adjacent penetrating wound, a bruit, or a neurologic deficit. The major problems of vascular injuries of the thoracic inlet are exsanguinating hemorrhage, early diagnosis, and operative exposure. Operative techniques of vessel repair are straightforward and infrequently pose important management problems. Although the specific vessel injured is sometimes defined by preoperative arteriography, the surgical management of potential vascular injuries must often proceed without this information.

Cervical Blood Vessels. Major vascular injuries in this region include the common carotid artery and its extracranial branches, the vertebral artery, and the internal jugular vein. Special attention is directed to preoperative neurologic evaluation because cerebral infarction may affect the intraoperative decision regarding flow restoration. Transient hypotension may exaggerate cerebral ischemia, but it does not appear to have a predictably deleterious effect on eventual neurologic status. Rapid fluid volume restitution and restoration of normal blood pressure is important for physiologic reasons and also allows a more accurate evaluation of the neurologic consequences of the injury. Thal and associates described the relationship between preoperative neurologic status, vascular procedure, and results in 60 patients with carotid injuries. Forty-one (68 percent) patients were neurologically intact preoperatively and 19 (32 percent) had deficits of varying severity. It was concluded from this review that vascular reconstruction was advisable in patients with mild deficits and in those with severe deficits in whom prograde flow was present preoperatively. Ligation was recommended in patients with severe neurologic deficits and no preoperative prograde flow. Ligation may occasionally be appropriate for patients with neurologic deficits and persistent prograde flow in whom thrombus exists in the cephalad vessel. If thrombectomy cannot be performed without risk of cerebral embolization, ligation may be the best choice. Arterial reconstruction, if feasible, was recommended in essentially all neurologically intact patients. The only exception is the patient with obstructed prograde flow and intraluminal thrombus in the cephalad vessel. If reconstruction risked cerebral embolization, ligation was suggested. Controversy continues regarding the therapeutic implications of preoperative neurologic deficits. Recent reviews by Unger et al. and by Liekweg and Greenfield support the recommendation that injured carotid arteries should be reconstructed, if technically feasible, in all except comatose patients with prograde flow. In these authors' opinion, flow should also be restored in patients without prograde flow, except those with severe or rapidly progressing deficits and seriously depressed sensoriums.

Operative Technique. Before the induction of anesthesia, preparations are made for the performance of emergency tracheostomy in the event of intubation difficulties. Stability of the cervical spine should be confirmed before intubation, particularly in high-velocity missile trauma. If an internal carotid injury near the base of the skull has been demonstrated arteriographically, exposure may be difficult and an additional 1 to 2 cm can be obtained by jaw dislocation or subluxation. The mandible is pulled inferiorly and anteriorly and held in place with dental wires.

Patients with potential or proved carotid injuries should be handled with consideration given to the tenuous hemostasis provided by soft tissue tamponade and the likelihood of intraluminal thrombus. A vigorous antiseptic scrub may dislodge a clot and cause either bleeding or embolization. Preparation of the operative field preferably includes the shoulder and anterior chest in case further exposure is required, as well as a site for harvesting a venous autograft.

Incision extensions that may be necessary are described with vascular injuries of the thoracic inlet. Shunts are rarely needed for repairs of common carotid injuries if the cephalad clamp does not occlude communication between the external and internal carotid arteries. Adequate collateral flow from the external carotid is easily verified by momentarily releasing the cephalad clamp. Following proximal and distal occlusion, with or without an intraluminal shunt, repair is carried out by standard vascular techniques. Injuries of the internal jugular vein are primarily repaired if this can be readily accomplished by lateral venorrhaphy, patch venoplasty, or end-to-end anastomosis. Unilateral ligation is well tolerated and the use of interposition grafts to restore venous continuity is not justified.

The common use of preoperative arteriography in recent years has uncovered an increasing number of vertebral artery injuries. In the past these injuries have been recognized infrequently, apparently because vertebral flow is not essential, and the size and course of the vessel make overt manifestations uncommon. Acute complications of vertebral artery injury are rare, but massive hemorrhage may be lethal. An AV fistula is the most common late complication, usually diagnosed months or years after injury. The incidence of these sequelae is unknown. Meier et al. described a series of 13 patients with acute vertebral artery trauma treated at Parkland Hospital during a 3-year period. During this time period 54 carotid injuries were treated, yielding a comparative incidence of about 20 percent for vertebral artery injuries.

Forty-one patients with penetrating vertebral artery injuries treated at the same institution during an 11-year period have recently been reviewed by Reid and Weigelt. Five of these patients were in shock on arrival but no patient presented with or developed neurologic signs attributable to the vertebral-basilar system. Three-quarters of these patients had no clinical findings of arterial injuries other than the penetrating wound or a stable hematoma. The remaining patients had expanding hematomas and four had overt arterial hemorrhage. The diagnosis was made arteriographically in 35 patients and during urgent operative explorations in the remainder. Proximal and distal vertebral artery ligations were performed in 28 patients; 13 had only proximal ligations and two were treated nonoperatively. Several complications developed in the patients having only proximal ligations and the authors recommend both proximal and distal ligations when feasible. Because the frequency of untoward sequelae of vertebral artery injuries is unknown, the indications for operations in asymptomatic patients are not clear. Reid and Weigelt recommended ligation of injured vertebral arteries in all patients with normal contralateral arteries if no spinal cord branches arise from the injured vessels but state that nonoperative management may be reasonable in asymptomatic patients with arteriographically minimal injuries. The site of proximal ligation is immediately distal to the subclavian origin of the vertebral artery. The site of distal ligation depends on the location of injury and can be performed as high as the C1-C2 interspace, when the artery is free of the bony canal.

Base of the Neck (Thoracic Inlet). Thoracic inlet injuries involve the vessels of the superior mediastinum that are proximate to the pleural spaces and separated from the surgeon by the claviculosternal "shield." The specific vessels include the innominate, the subclavian, and the proximal common carotid arteries and adjacent veins. Anatomic characteristics make the diagnosis of injured vessels difficult and impede rapid hemostasis and operative exposure for vascular control and repair. Exsanguinating hemorrhage is the predominant risk; bleeding may not be easily recognized because of free decompression into the pleural spaces. Abundant collateral blood supply generally protects against cerebral or upper extremity ischemia but also disguises the injury by maintaining distal perfusion and exaggerates blood loss during operative exposure. The major clinical differences between these injuries and those in the neck proper are obscure hemorrhage, difficulty obtaining immediate hemostasis, the extensive incisions that may be required for exposure, and the infrequency of cerebral ischemia.

Rapid resuscitation, liberal surgical exploration, and a thorough knowledge of the operative approach are the necessary ingredients of success. Indications to consider early surgical exploration are listed in Table 6-4. Diagnostic errors and subsequent inappropriately conservative management rarely occur with overt signs of major vascular injury. Unfortunately, many of these injuries appear innocuous at the time of presentation, and a high index of suspicion is necessary. In this circumstance platysmal penetration and proximity of the wound to a major vascular structure are used as indications for surgical exploration. As previously discussed, arteriography to modify the principle of proximity and penetration exploration remains controversial. It may prove useful if immediately available, but valuable time should not be wasted with studies if objective evidence of major vascular injury exists.

Important factors in the management of these injuries are emphasized by the series of Flint et al. During an 11-year period, 146 patients with 206 injuries of major vascular structures at the base of the neck were treated. Arterial injuries accounted for 49 percent, including 36 injuries to the subclavian artery, 29 to the common carotid, and 7 to the innominate artery. Of the 74 venous injuries, there were 31 to the subclavian vein, 32 to the internal jugular, and 11 to the innominate vein. Signs and symptoms of major vascular injury were equivocal in many patients and totally absent in 32 percent of the patients. These patients were explored on the basis of platysmal penetra-

Table 6-4. FINDINGS SUGGESTING MAJOR VASCULAR INJURY

Obvious or direct evidence of injury:
1. Circulatory instability
2. Excessive external bleeding
3. A large or progressing hematoma
4. Distal pulse deficit
5. Neurologic deficit involving nerves anatomically adjacent to major vascular structures
6. Massive or continued intrathoracic bleeding

Indirect evidence indicating injury:
1. A wound above the clavicle or manubrium that penetrates the platysma muscle
2. Thoracic wounds whose trajectory traverses the superior mediastinum or thoracic inlet.
3. Mediastinal widening demonstrated radiographically

---

tion and the proximity of the wound to a major vascular structure. The overall mortality was 7.8 percent and was generally related to the magnitude of associated injuries or the extent of blood loss before operation. Thirteen percent of the patients with arterial trauma died, compared with 3 percent of those with venous injuries. Early and liberal surgical exploration with emphasis on adequate exposure resulted in low mortality and morbidity rates in this large series.

Operative Technique. Vessel exposure and control of hemorrhage are the major problems in the operative management of thoracic inlet injuries. The varied vessels and adjacent structures that may be involved and the overlying bony shield are the basis of these problems. The inaccuracy of preoperative wound localization and the wide exposure often required for vascular control make a flexible operative approach essential. A variety of incisions may be needed, often involving the mobilization of overlying bony structures, as illustrated in Fig. 6-6. The initial incision may not provide adequate exposure and may require extension or another separate incision. Such extensions or additional incisions were required in 25 percent of 146 patients with these injuries reported by Flint et al. The supine position and a wide operative field including the entire neck, chest, and upper arms offers the most operative flexibility.

The approaches used to expose these injuries are the oblique cervical and horizontal clavicular incisions, median sternotomy, left anterolateral thoracotomy, and a musculoskeletal chest wall flap (Fig. 6-6). The right oblique cervical incision generally is adequate to expose the entire right common carotid artery. The horizontal clavicular incision with subperiosteal resection of the medial half of the clavicle adequately exposes the right subclavian vessels. Extension to a median sternotomy is necessary to expose the innominate artery. The distal left common carotid artery is easily exposed through a left oblique neck incision, but the proximal vessel requires a sternal extension. The distal left subclavian artery can be reached through a horizontal clavicular incision, but its proximal portion requires a sternotomy or, more appropriately, a left anterolateral thoracotomy. A musculoskeletal flap, or "trapdoor," may be used to expose the proximal left carotid and the entire left subclavian arteries and the left innominate vein. This is formed by combining horizontal clavicular, superior median sternotomy, and anterolateral thoracotomy incisions. Most base-of-the-neck injuries can be exposed through the oblique cervical and/or horizontal clavicular incisions. Major extensions should be made without hesitation when these incisions provide inadequate exposure. The vascular repair seldom is difficult and most often can be accomplished by lateral arteriorrhaphy or end-to-end anastomosis. When graft interposition is required, autogenous material is preferred.

The operative approach to penetrating injuries of the base of the neck is appropriately based on the presenting clinical picture, supplemented when possible by arteriography. The factors considered in choosing the primary incision are hemodynamic status, predicted wound course, site of the injury, and evidence of intrathoracic

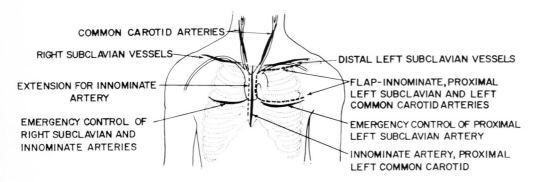

COMMON CAROTID ARTERIES

RIGHT SUBCLAVIAN VESSELS

DISTAL LEFT SUBCLAVIAN VESSELS

EXTENSION FOR INNOMINATE ARTERY

FLAP-INNOMINATE, PROXIMAL LEFT SUBCLAVIAN AND LEFT COMMON CAROTID ARTERIES

EMERGENCY CONTROL OF RIGHT SUBCLAVIAN AND INNOMINATE ARTERIES

EMERGENCY CONTROL OF PROXIMAL LEFT SUBCLAVIAN ARTERY

INNOMINATE ARTERY, PROXIMAL LEFT COMMON CAROTID

Fig. 6-6. Incisions and extensions for base-of-the-neck vascular injuries.

bleeding. Sound judgment and the flexibility to widely extend incisions result in maximal required exposure and minimal incisional complications and morbidity.

In unstable patients with suspected major mediastinal injuries, especially in the presence of large or continuing intrathoracic bleeding, initial thoracic incisions are advisable. This usually implies a median sternotomy, but if the wound is on the left and a proximal left subclavian injury is suspected, an anterolateral thoracotomy is performed. Anterolateral thoracotomy is performed on the side of injury in patients with massive intrathoracic bleeding if sternal splitting instruments are not immediately available.

Oblique cervical and horizontal clavicular incisions often provide adequate exposure without the added risk and morbidity of thoracotomy. One of these incisions is appropriate in stable patients with cervical, periclavicular, or supramanubrial wounds without evidence of deep mediastinal penetration or intrathoracic hemorrhage. A wide operative field is essential, however, and extension to a thoracic incision is made without hesitation.

The oblique cervical incision provides adequate exposure for most cervical wounds without evidence of mediastinal penetration. In the series of Flint et al., this incision provided adequate exposure for the control and repair of 84 percent of internal jugular vein and 76 percent of common carotid injuries. Lateral extension with resection of the medial half of the clavicle is sometimes necessary for additional exposure. Using this extension, satisfactory access was obtained in more than 90 percent of patients with common carotid and internal jugular injuries. If difficulty with proximal exposure is encountered during the dissection of either common carotid artery, a midsternal extension is made.

The horizontal clavicular incision is initially used in stable patients with periclavicular or supramanubrial wounds and suspected mediastinal penetration but without notable intrathoracic bleeding. Eighty-seven percent of subclavian vein injuries, 75 percent of innominate vein injuries, and 60 percent of subclavian artery injuries were

successfully repaired by Flint and associates using this incision.

If possible, complete proximal and distal vascular control should precede dissection into the immediate area of suspected injury and the tamponading hematoma. If exposure is inadequate during the dissection of either proximal common carotid artery or the right subclavian artery, a midsternal extension should be made without hesitation. If proximal exposure is inadequate during the transclavicular dissection of the left subclavian artery, a left anterolateral thoracotomy is performed and, if additional exposure is required, midsternal extension forms a musculoskeletal flap.

The repair of the vascular injury, once isolated, seldom presents a major problem and can usually be accomplished by lateral arteriorrhaphy or end-to-end anastomosis. When graft interposition is required, autogenous material is preferred. The use of shunts or extracorporeal circulation to maintain cerebral flow should be considered if flow is reduced in more than one of the vessels supplying the brain. Vascular reconstruction is desirable, but because of the rich collateral circulation, single arterial ligations can usually be safely performed, especially when survival depends on early completion of the operation. Measurement of "stump" pressures may be helpful in predicting the consequences of major arterial ligations. Venous ligation usually results in minimal morbidity and may be indicated when optimal repair is not possible, although both innominate veins should not be ligated.

LARYNX AND TRACHEA. The signs and symptoms of laryngeal and tracheal injuries include respiratory distress, hoarseness, hemoptysis, and subcutaneous emphysema. As emphasized earlier, essentially all penetrating laryngotracheal injuries are clinically obvious and this fact may be useful in predicting the course of a missile. Subcutaneous air is not diagnostic of such an injury since air may enter through the skin wound or be due to an injury of the esophagus, bronchus, or lung.

Whenever laryngeal or tracheal injury produces difficulty breathing in the emergency room, a tracheostomy is performed before transfer of the patient to the operating suite. If the patient is hoarse or the wound is near the thyroid or larynx, laryngoscopy is performed preoperatively, when feasible, to evaluate the larynx and function of the recurrent laryngeal nerves. Direct laryngoscopy, using a small-diameter flexible endoscope, is more often successful and less cumbersome than indirect laryngoscopy in the acutely traumatized patient.

Tracheal wounds are usually obvious during operative exploration, but if the injury cannot be identified the endotracheal tube cuff should be deflated to increase intratracheal pressure and enhance the air leak. Clean lacerations of the trachea or larynx are closed using synthetic absorbable suture such as Dexon or Vicryl. These materials result in less frequent problems with chronic granulation tissue postoperatively. Tracheal wounds can more often be primarily repaired than was previously thought. If a tracheostomy is not also performed, an endotracheal tube may be indicated for several days postoperatively to ensure an adequate airway. A tracheostomy may be required instead of or in addition to primary repair, depending on the site and size of the defect and the magnitude of associated injuries. Patients with laryngeal injuries should have normal anatomy reconstructed as accurately as possible to lessen subsequent airway and speech difficulties. If a tracheostomy is required, it is maintained until healing is complete and laryngeal or tracheal edema has subsided, usually in 4 to 8 days.

PHARYNX AND ESOPHAGUS. The clinical findings suggesting pharyngeal or esophageal injury are hematemesis, dysphagia, and subcutaneous emphysema. Carefully performed barium esophagography with cineradiography in two projections may be used to exclude esophageal injury in the asymptomatic patient with platysmal penetration. False-negative examinations occasionally occur, and all patients are closely observed in the hospital and without oral intake for at least 24 h. Pharyngoesophageal injuries are notoriously silent, and a high index of suspicion and a liberal attitude regarding operative exploration result in the lowest incidence of missed esophageal perforations.

After adequate debridement, injuries of the pharynx and esophagus usually may be primarily repaired using an inner layer of absorbable suture such as Vicryl or Dexon and an outer layer of silk, cotton, or Prolene. If a small esophageal injury is suspected but cannot be demonstrated during exploration, an anesthetic mask may be applied to the nose and mouth and positive pressure exerted while the wound is filled with saline solution. Bubbles may disclose the point of injury. It is vital to drain all such wounds, because infections and salivary leaks are potential complications. If there is massive loss of esophageal tissue, as with a close-range shotgun blast, it may be necessary to perform a cutaneous esophagostomy for feeding purposes and a cutaneous pharyngostomy for salivary drainage. A secondary reconstruction will be required after initial healing is complete. A small plastic nasogastric tube is used for feeding for 8 to 10 days following major esophageal injuries, unless a gastrostomy is deemed preferable.

NERVE INJURIES. A preoperative neurologic examination is performed, whenever possible, to identify injured nerves. The brachial plexus, deep cervical plexus, phrenic nerves, and the cranial nerves are systematically tested. The vagus and recurrent laryngeal nerves can be evaluated by examining the vocal cords. A hypoglossal or spinal accessory nerve injury is particularly easy to miss unless a preoperative neurologic examination is performed. An associated head injury or alcoholic intoxication often impedes an adequate neurologic examination. Whenever possible, severed or lacerated nerves are debrided and repaired primarily using interrupted fine silk sutures on the perineurium.

SALIVARY GLANDS. The diagnosis of salivary gland injury is usually made during operative exploration but, if suspected preoperatively, may be made with sialography. Debridement, hemostasis, and simple drainage provide effective treatment. In the absence of ductal obstruction, a salivary fistula rarely occurs after injury to the gland substance. When the major duct is injured, it may be repaired with fine silk over a ureteral catheter stent. The catheter should be removed after repair is completed. When repair is not feasible because of the patient's condition or for some other compelling reason, the duct may be ligated and the gland allowed to atrophy, or the duct may be reimplanted in the mucosa at a later time. If a salivary fistula does occur postoperatively and fails to close spontaneously, irradiation usually arrests salivary flow, but it is not advisable in children or young adults.

MISCELLANEOUS INJURIES. Thyroid injuries require only debridement of devitalized tissue, hemostasis, and adequate drainage. The thoracic duct may be injured with wounds near the left innominate-jugular venous bifurcation. Repair of the duct is not feasible because of its friability, but simple ligation is adequate. The duct may divide immediately before entering the vein or there may be tributaries from the head and arm and multiple ligations may be required for lymphostasis. The area should be thoroughly dried and inspected before closing, because a large collection of lymph may occur postoperatively from even a small leak. If lymph does accumulate, incision and drainage with the application of a bulky pressure dressing for a few days will usually effect closure of the lymphatic fistula. Injured right thoracic ducts, though less frequent, are treated similarly.

ABDOMINAL TRAUMA

Erwin R. Thal, Robert N. McClelland, Ronald C. Jones, Malcolm O. Perry, and G. Tom Shires

The incidence of abdominal trauma continues to increase. Each year about 3.5 million persons in the United States are injured in automobile accidents, and many of these injuries involve the abdominal contents. Mortality rates are generally higher in patients sustaining blunt trauma than in those with penetrating wounds. Although newer and better diagnostic techniques such as computed tomography are now available, blunt trauma still presents a difficult challenge to the clinician. The spleen, liver, kidneys, and bowel are the most frequently injured abdominal organs. In a review of several series of blunt ab-

Table 6-5. FREQUENCY OF INJURY IN
ABDOMINAL TRAUMA

Viscera injured	Frequency, %
Spleen	26.2
Kidneys	24.2
Intestines	16.2
Liver	15.6
Abdominal wall	3.6
Retroperitoneal hematoma	2.7
Mesentery	2.5
Pancreas	1.4
Diaphragm	1.1

dominal trauma the frequency of injury has been determined (see Table 6-5).

Early diagnosis facilitates optimal management. Initial evaluation serves as a baseline but is frequently difficult because of the masking of abdominal injury by other associated injuries. Often the patient is unconscious because of alcoholism, drug abuse, shock, or associated head injury. Chest trauma, orthopedic problems, and retroperitoneal injuries may further complicate the diagnostic process. Another misleading factor in diagnosis, often not recognized, is that relatively trivial injuries may rupture abdominal viscera. The index of suspicion must be high, even in cases of supposedly minor abdominal trauma, if diagnostic errors are to be avoided.

CLINICAL MANIFESTATIONS. The evaluation of the patient with blunt abdominal trauma begins with a careful history and physical examination. Knowing the mechanism of injury is essential in discerning the likelihood of abdominal injury. Information about the patient and the accident scene can be obtained from the paramedics, witnesses, family, police, and the patient as well. Factors such as rapid deceleration, impaling forces, and seat belt restraints make abdominal viscera prone to injury. Physical examination in the alert patient remains the most reliable predictor of injury, yet this will be misleading as either a false-positive or false-negative examination in 10 to 20 percent of patients. The entire patient must be examined as well as the abdomen because of the high incidence of associated trauma. Fitzgerald et al. reported extraabdominal injuries were present in 97 percent of patients with abdominal injuries who were dead upon arrival at the hospital and in 70 percent of those admitted alive. In spite of the explosion of diagnostic technology, if the diagnosis is unclear, one must depend on repeated physical examinations done at frequent intervals by the same examiner. One cannot overemphasize the importance of the bedside clinical evaluation in determining which patients will benefit from operative management of their injuries.

Abdominal pain and tenderness when present are very reliable findings. Abdominal rigidity, and/or involuntary guarding, are indicative of intraperitoneal injury, and even when present alone, warrant exploratory celiotomy without further diagnostic procedures. It is important to note that blood in the peritoneal cavity may or may not cause irritation; hence hemoperitoneum may or may not produce significant physical findings. Patients with an altered state of consciousness resulting from closed head injuries, alcoholism, or drug abuse also may demonstrate evidence of abdominal discomfort. Injuries to organs in the retroperitoneal space such as pancreas, duodenum, kidney, and blood vessels, by virtue of their anatomic location, frequently do not produce signs of peritoneal irritation such as rebound tenderness, referred pain, and abdominal wall rigidity.

Newer diagnostic studies and better imaging techniques such as computed tomography have increased the clinician's ability to rapidly identify abdominal injuries. These studies have significantly helped to reduce the number of negative celiotomies. In a small number of cases it will be difficult to determine the extent of injury and occasional negative procedures will be performed. It is still preferable to perform a negative celiotomy on occasion with virtually no mortality and very little morbidity than to suffer the consequences of a missed injury.

In patients with blunt abdominal trauma, determinations of alterations in blood pressure are often useful. A valuable sign of continuing intraabdominal hemorrhage is transient elevation of the blood pressure to normal levels for a few minutes followed by return to hypotensive levels with the rapid infusion of 500 to 1000 mL of Ringer's lactate solution. Patients who are hypotensive from minimal blood loss or from neurogenic shock usually do not behave in this manner. The Ringer's lactate solution generally is infused over a period of 15 to 20 min while other measures, such as blood typing and cross matching, are being carried out. Postural hypotension, when the patient assumes the erect position, is another useful sign of continuing intraabdominal bleeding. Often subtle signs of hemorrhage such as mild to moderate tachycardia, tachypnea, narrowing of the pulse pressure, and cool skin temperature will be early manifestations of intraabdominal hemorrhage. Blood loss in the range of 30 to 40 percent of the blood volume will be necessary to produce sustained marked hypotension with a systolic blood pressure consistently below 60 to 70 mmHg.

DIAGNOSTIC PROCEDURES. Whereas history and physical examination remain the most reliable diagnostic modalities, other diagnostic aids will frequently confirm clinical suspicions. In general, laboratory determinations do not offer much help in the young, previously healthy traumatized patient.

Sudden acute blood loss may not be adequately reflected by early hemograms; hence, a normal hemoglobin and hematocrit shortly after injury may be misleading. Serum glucose and creatinine determinations may be helpful in elderly patients suspected of having diabetes or renal insufficiency. Whereas serum electrolytes are rarely abnormal, the serum potassium level is extremely important if operation is contemplated. Unrecognized hypokalemia may lead to disastrous consequences. A serum amylase level, when elevated, is a relatively reliable predictor of intraabdominal injury although not always an indication for operative intervention. In addition to being elevated with pancreatic injury, abnormal amylase levels are also seen in injuries to the duodenum and upper small bowel. Leakage of the amylase-containing fluid is rapidly absorbed into the blood from the peritoneal cavity.

Serum isoenzyme amylase analysis has been advocated by some authors to be more specific than total amylase for pancreatic injury; however, other reports refute this hypothesis.

Studies of urinary sediment are useful, since hematuria may indicate injury to the genitourinary tract. Recent studies indicate that dipstick urinalysis is very accurate in determining hematuria in addition to being very cost-effective. If the patient with abdominal injury cannot void, catheterization should be done to obtain urine for examination. Catheterization is contraindicated prior to obtaining an urethrogram, if there is a scrotal hematoma, perineal hematoma, blood at the tip of the male meatus, or a high-riding or floating prostate on rectal examination. In these instances injury to the urethra is suspected and additional damage may be done if a catheter is blindly inserted.

Levin tubes are inserted in all patients sustaining blunt abdominal trauma. The stomach contents are aspirated and the aspirate is examined for the presence of blood. In addition, a Levin tube provides decompression of the stomach, prevents gastric dilatation, and prevents aspiration with the induction of anesthesia. The instillation of 30 to 60 mL of an antacid in the Levin tube will neutralize the stomach contents and further minimize the ravages of aspiration, should it occur.

Blood-gas determinations should be obtained in all multiply injured patients and, in particular, those patients with a history of chronic pulmonary disease, chest injuries, or possible aspiration.

Radiologic Findings. For patients who have sustained severe abdominal injury and in whom other clinical signs obviously point to such injury, radiography, for diagnosis, may dangerously delay surgical intervention. For some patients with stable vital signs and questionable diagnoses of intraabdominal injury, x-ray studies may occasionally be helpful. When a patient is suspected of having intraabdominal injuries, upright films of the chest should be made, in addition to supine films of the abdomen. Occasionally additional information may be obtained from lateral and left lateral decubitus films. The skeletal system is surveyed for fractures or dislocations. Examination of the soft tissues may give information about changes in size, shape, or position of many viscera. Pneumoperitoneum may be diagnosed with the patient in the erect or lateral decubitus positions. Indirect evidence of solid viscera rupture with secondary hemorrhage may be presumed by an increase in density in the region, by displacement of neighboring viscera, or by accumulation of fluid between the gas shadows of bowel loops. If a gastric, duodenal, or upper jejunal rupture is suspected, the appearance of pneumoperitoneum may be facilitated by injecting 750 to 1000 mL of air into the nasogastric tube, after which the patient sits in a semierect position for 10 min before an upright chest film or left lateral decubitus film of the abdomen is made. Films should also be made prior to the air injection for purposes of comparison if the patient's condition permits.

Examination of the upper gastrointestinal tract by contrast radiography using a water-soluble opaque medium may identify an injury of the stomach, duodenum, or upper small bowel. Although rarely needed or used, it may be helpful in identifying an intramural duodenal hematoma. Contrast material is frequently used in conjunction with computed tomography. The use of barium mixtures for this is dangerous, since a severe peritoneal reaction may be caused by barium if it leaks through a gastrointestinal perforation. This is especially true if there is fecal contamination in the peritoneal cavity from a concomitant colon injury.

Intravenous pyelograms should be done if feasible for patients with hematuria or other evidence of genitourinary injury, not only to establish the nature of the injury but also to determine if both kidneys are functioning prior to surgical intervention in case an injured kidney must be removed. It is important to note that occasional renal injuries are not detected by intravenous pyelography and, if clinically suspected, may be better confirmed by arteriography or computed tomography. If arteriography is contemplated, the intravenous pyelogram and cystogram can be obtained at the conclusion of the angiogram, thereby eliminating one study and conserving time. If necessary, intravenous pyelograms may be done during the surgical procedure to determine the presence of a functional kidney on one side before removing the other kidney.

Cystograms using a minimum of 300 mL of contrast material to adequately distend the bladder may also be useful for diagnosing bladder injury or perforation from blunt abdominal trauma, but normal cystograms do not necessarily rule out bladder injury.

Computed tomography. As experience is gained, the CT scan and perhaps later the MRI will provide excellent images of intraabdominal viscera. Resolution is excellent for solid organs such as the liver and spleen as seen in Fig. 6-7. Whereas lavage is unreliable for retroperitoneal

Fig. 6-7. Markedly disrupted spleen with blood seen surrounding the splenic remnant.

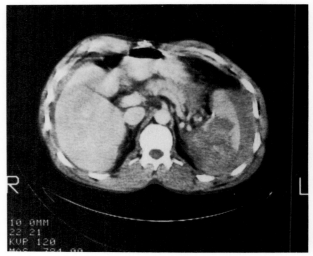

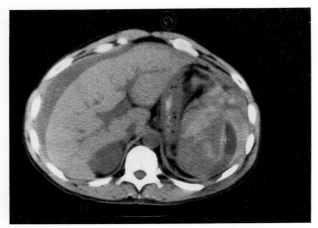

Fig. 6-8. Large spleen with inhomogeneous density representing blood in and around the spleen. Small fluid level seen within the spleen. Free fluid (blood) in the abdomen and surrounding liver. There are areas of high density (clotted blood) within lower-density fluid.

injuries the CT scan has a distinct advantage in this area. Pancreatic injuries are frequently identified with clarity.

Hollow organs are harder to evaluate unless contrast material is used. This is recommended and given both orally and intravenously. Intravenous contrast will permit assessment of the genitourinary system and possibly obviate the need for an intravenous pyelogram.

Fluid collections, usually blood, may be seen surrounding organs or in dependent places such as the pelvis (Fig. 6-8). Contained hematomas can be seen within solid organs that would be missed with lavage if there is no free blood in the peritoneal cavity (Fig. 6-9).

It must be emphasized that unstable patients are not candidates for computed tomography. The length of the procedure will vary according to whether contrast is used, experience with the technology, and the availability

Fig. 6-9. Patient fell two stories. Large intraparenchymal hematoma seen in right lobe of liver.

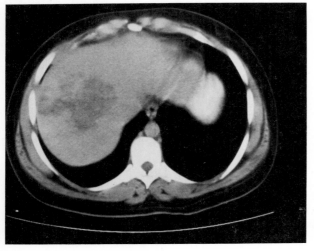

of the scanner. Again, valuable time should not be wasted if hemodynamic stability is in question.

Early reports are very enthusiastic, but caution must be given to the fact that significant injuries have been missed with CT scans and hence continued clinical evaluation is essential for optimal care in spite of a negative procedure.

The emergence of the CT scan has led to consideration of nonoperative management of some selected injuries. Until the natural history of these injuries is better defined, specific recommendations regarding nonoperative therapy should be withheld.

Arteriography. Selective arteriography is another available study occasionally used in diagnosis of blunt abdominal trauma. Selective catheterization of the celiac, mesenteric, or renal vessels may be performed. A film taken several minutes after injection can be used as an excretory urogram.

Arteriography is useful in assessing renal artery injury and is routinely employed if a kidney is not promptly visualized with intravenous pyelography. Intimal tears, aortic occlusion, and traumatic aneurysms are often seen in conjunction with seat belt injuries and are occasionally associated with serious lumbosacral trauma.

When continued pelvic bleeding occurs with extension into the retroperitoneal space secondary to pelvic fractures, arteriography may be beneficial in localizing the site of bleeding. Additionally, vasospastic agents or hemostatic agents such as autologous clot may be embolized to control bleeding. Again, it must be emphasized that time should not be wasted on adjunctive procedures when surgical intervention is indicated.

Scintiscanning. Both liver and splenic scanning have been described in conjunction with blunt abdominal trauma. This technique primarily is limited to those patients whose diagnoses are uncertain and whose conditions remain stable. The radionuclide most frequently used is ^{99mm}Tc sulfur colloid. Most series reporting results of this technique are small and emphasize the relative inaccuracy of the examination.

Paracentesis. Needle abdominal paracentesis is a useful diagnostic aid only for those cases of abdominal trauma in which, after physical examination, the examiner continues to suspect intraabdominal hemorrhage. The abdominal tap has been particularly useful as a diagnostic adjunct for comatose patients with head injury in whom adequate physical examination of the abdomen is not possible. A review of this procedure shows a diagnostic accuracy of 95 percent if blood is aspirated. A negative tap is extremely unreliable and should be followed by another diagnostic study such as peritoneal lavage. In female patients with suspected intraabdominal hemorrhage, culdocentesis may be positive for blood when abdominal taps are negative.

The technique was well described by Drapanas and McDonald and is illustrated in Fig. 6-10. The abdomen is prepped with an iodinated compound or other standard solutions. An 18-gauge short-bevel spinal needle is attached to a syringe and inserted through the abdominal wall after prior infiltration with a local anesthetic agent. Suction is applied to the syringe as the needle is slowly

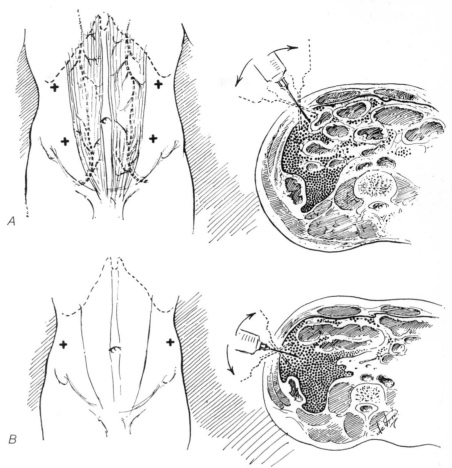

Fig. 6-10. *A*. Technique for four-quadrant peritoneal taps. Preferred location for aspiration of each quadrant is shown. Note that puncture through the rectus abdominis sheath is avoided. *B*. Technique for bilateral flank taps. Aspiration is performed in each flank midway between the costal margin and iliac spine. In our experience, bilateral flank taps are equally reliable as, and more easily performed than, four-quadrant taps in cases of abdominal trauma. (From: *Drapanas T, McDonald J: Surgery 50:742, 1961, with permission.*)

advanced into the abdomen at the sites illustrated. Return of a minimum of 0.1 mL of nonclotting blood constitutes a positive tap. Occasionally, an intraabdominal blood vessel may be entered, but this blood will clot and differentiate it from blood obtained from the free peritoneal cavity. Bilateral flank taps are as reliable as four-quadrant taps and may be more reliable if only small amounts of blood are present. Puncture of the rectus abdominis sheath anteriorly should be avoided. This will prevent a rectus abdominis sheath hematoma resulting from injury to the epigastric vessel and diminish the chance of penetrating the intestine, since gas-filled loops of bowel tend to float anteriorly in an abdomen containing fluid or blood. Actually, the danger of penetrating the intestine is slight; several studies have shown that penetration with an 18-gauge needle is harmless, as a hole in the bowel seals off quite rapidly with no leakage. Other technical considerations include the following: (1) Areas of abdominal scars or other points of possible bowel fixation to the abdominal wall should be avoided. (2) The direction of the needle inside the abdominal cavity should be changed only by withdrawing the point of the needle superficial to the peritoneum, redirecting the needle, and reintroducing it into the peritoneal cavity. (3) Peritoneal taps should be avoided in the presence of markedly distended bowel, since abnormally elevated intraluminal pressure may cause continued leakage.

Paracentesis is simple, quick, and safe with relatively few complications. A positive needle tap is quite accurate, but the major drawback is the high percentage of false-negative results.

Peritoneal Lavage. Because of the poor reliability of paracentesis, if nonclotting blood is not aspirated, other procedures have been developed to detect intraabdominal injury. Canizaro et al. described the use of intraperitoneal saline infusions in animals. Root et al. first described the technique of peritoneal lavage in human beings in 1965 and subsequently reported a series of 304 patients with a 96 percent accuracy. Numerous reviews of this procedure have proved peritoneal lavage to be a safe and reliable adjunctive procedure for evaluating patients with blunt abdominal trauma. The indications for this technique are patients with closed head injuries, altered consciousness, spinal cord injuries, equivocal abdominal findings, and negative needle paracentesis. It is not recommended for patients with gunshot wounds to the lower chest or abdomen, stab wounds to the back, previous abdominal procedures, presence of dilated bowel, late pregnancy, or positive needle paracentesis.

Several techniques have been described. The Lazarus-Nelson approach utilizes a small Teflon catheter inserted over a previously placed flexible guide wire. The technique popularized by Perry selects a point in the lower midline below the umbilicus approximately one-third of the distance between that and the pubic symphysis. After decompression of the urinary bladder and the stomach by the use of a Levin tube, the skin is cleansed and prepared with an iodinated antiseptic solution. A wheal is raised with 1% lidocaine with epinephrine and the skin incised with a #11 scalpel. At this point a standard peritoneal dialysis catheter can be inserted, and the trocar advanced carefully until it just penetrates the peritoneum (Fig. 6-11). An alternative and perhaps safer method is to incise the abdominal wall to the peritoneum and insert the trocar under direct vision. Once the peritoneum is penetrated, the trocar is removed and the dialysis catheter advanced toward the pelvis. A syringe is then attached to the catheter and the peritoneal cavity is aspirated.

Nonclotting blood will often be aspirated through the larger catheter in spite of a negative needle paracentesis. If no blood is aspirated, a liter of balanced salt solution (Ringer's lactate) is rapidly infused into the peritoneal cavity over 5 to 10 min. For children and small adults 10 to 15 mL/kg is used. The patient is then turned from side to side in order to further mix the blood and fluid. If other injuries such as pelvic or long bone fractures are present, this step is eliminated.

The empty intravenous-fluid bottle is lowered and the fluid siphoned out of the peritoneal cavity. A sample is sent to the laboratory for quantitative analysis. In addition to obtaining red cell and white cell counts, it is important to determine the presence or absence of amylase,

Fig. 6-11. Insertion of catheter for peritoneal lavage in the lower midline below the umbilicus.

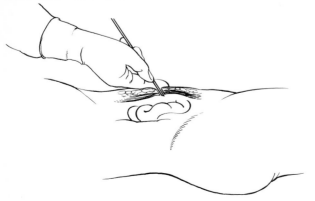

bile, or bacteria. Greater than 100,000 RBC/mm^3, 500 WBC/mm^3, or detection of bile, bacteria, food fibers, or amylase in excess of normal serum values is considered a positive study. Some have recommended colorimetric methods, but these do not appear to be as accurate as quantitative analysis of the fluid. Controversy exists regarding the number of red cells that constitute a positive study. Most authors agree with 100,000 for blunt trauma but figures as low as 1000 have been reported for penetrating trauma.

It must be emphasized that peritoneal lavage is very inaccurate in predicting retroperitoneal injuries. Unless the posterior peritoneum has been torn or considerable time has elapsed between the injury and lavage, most pancreatic injuries are not detected. The same is true for duodenal, urologic, and major vessel injuries that are retroperitoneal. Diaphragmatic injuries likewise are rarely detected by peritoneal lavage. Complications, although very rare (1 to 2 percent), occur frequently enough that lavage is not recommended for every patient suspected of abdominal injury. A negative lavage, however, may spare the patient an exploratory celiotomy. The role of peritoneal lavage is now being reassessed and its use redefined since the emergence of computed tomography. There clearly is a place for both diagnostic tests.

Other Procedures. Sonography has been used in the evaluation of blunt abdominal injury but is not nearly as accurate as computed tomography. Although some advocate laparoscopy, this technique as well as needleoscopy provides a less than complete examination and cannot be recommended at this time for the multiply injured patient.

Penetrating Trauma

STAB WOUNDS

Diagnosis of penetrating injuries of the abdomen does not usually present the difficult problem often posed by blunt abdominal trauma. Three methods of management have evolved: (1) routine exploration of all patients with abdominal stab wounds, (2) selective management, or (3) exploration following demonstration of peritoneal cavity and/or visceral injury.

Before 1960 there was little controversy, since essentially all surgeons agreed that penetrating trauma to the abdomen required exploratory celiotomy to rule out visceral injury. This agreement was first challenged by Shaftan in 1960, who recommended exploratory celiotomy only for patients with physical evidence of injury due to penetrating abdominal trauma and observation in the hospital for those without evidence of visceral injury. The major controversy now revolves around the following issues, which assume paramount importance: (1) How reliable are the various diagnostic criteria for visceral injury? (2) What is the effect of delayed celiotomy on the complication and mortality rate in patients who have no clinical manifestations of visceral injury after penetrating trauma, but who subsequently develop such manifestations? (3) Does negative celiotomy cause significant morbidity and mortality?

Some clinicians favor mandatory celiotomy for all patients who have sustained penetrating abdominal trauma. This point of view was supported by Bull and Mathewson, who found that 23 percent of 78 patients with significant intraabdominal injury confirmed at celiotomy and due to penetrating abdominal wounds had had no physical signs preoperatively. In contrast, 18 percent of 100 patients with possible penetrating injuries in whom the peritoneal cavity was not entered did have physical findings suggestive of visceral injury.

In spite of the fact that there is virtually no mortality associated with a negative celiotomy, most series report postoperative complications in the range of 10 to 20 percent. A recent review of 247 patients with negative celiotomies at Parkland Hospital revealed a 2 percent incidence of small bowel obstruction. Seventy-five percent of the patients had an average follow-up of 57 months. Because of the high incidence of negative celiotomy following routine exploration, most trauma centers have abandoned this approach.

Selective management of abdominal stab wounds is now recommended by many authors. Following clinical assessment, the decision to perform exploratory celiotomy is based on the following factors: (1) physical signs of peritoneal injury; (2) unexplained shock; (3) loss of bowel sounds; (4) evisceration of omentum or a viscus; (5) evidence of blood in the stomach, bladder, or rectum; and (6) evidence of visceral injury such as pneumoperitoneum or visceral displacement on x-ray films. Occasionally, other diagnostic studies are employed, including intravenous pyelography, cystography, arteriography, needle paracentesis, peritoneal lavage, or computed tomography (CT). In the absence of any indication of visceral injury, these patients are admitted to the hospital for a 24- to 48-h period of observation and are reevaluated frequently, preferably by the same observer. If the patient's condition deteriorates or changes significantly, exploratory celiotomy is performed. Nance and Cohn reported a reduction in the percentage of negative celiotomies following selective management from 53 to 11 percent; 4.8 percent of 210 patients initially observed subsequently required an operation when manifestations of visceral injury developed. This delay in surgical treatment caused no mortality or significant morbidity.

An alternative approach to either routine exploration or selective management involves the use of adjunctive methods to help determine whether penetration of the peritoneal cavity has occurred. The decision to operate is based upon confirmation of peritoneal penetration and/or visceral injury. Cornell et al. have described the diagnostic injection of radiopaque contrast material. Following aseptic preparation of the wound site, a small catheter is inserted into the wound and held tightly by a purse-string suture; 50 to 100 mL of contrast media is injected; and anteroposterior, lateral, and oblique films of the abdomen are obtained. Contrast media seen within the peritoneal cavity is an indication of peritoneal penetration. Objections to this technique are the following: (1) some patients are hypersensitive to the contrast material; (2) injection of this material may be quite painful, thereby masking further evaluation; (3) the incidence of false-positive and false-negative results is as high as 15 to 25 percent in some series; (4) the technique is impractical for multiple stab wounds.

Local exploration is another modality that may provide useful information. The abdominal wall is prepared with an antiseptic agent. Using local anesthesia, the wound is opened sufficiently to visualize the complete course and depth of the tract. Often with adequate light, instruments, assistance, and exposure, it is obvious that a wound thought to have penetrated the peritoneal cavity is actually superficial and not damaging to the viscera. These patients are managed by simple drainage and outpatient follow-up if other injuries do not require hospitalization. Local wound exploration must involve more than simple instrument probing to determine penetration. This blind probing may be misleading, since a tortuous wound tract may allow passage of the probe for only a short distance, creating a false impression of nonpenetration. If the end of the tract cannot be visualized or the peritoneum is penetrated, local exploration is considered positive. This technique is equally useful for stab wounds of the back, although the thickness of the paraspinous muscles may prevent visualization of the end of the wound tract. Frequently, innocuous small stab wounds of the back significantly damage such retroperitoneal structures as the inferior vena cava, ureter, pancreas, or duodenum. A recent review of over 300 abdominal stab wounds by the authors indicated that nearly 20 percent of the patients could be discharged from the emergency room without hospital admission based on a negative local exploration that clearly demonstrated the end of the tract.

The abdominal viscera are at risk to injury with stab wounds of the lower chest as well as the abdomen. Figure 6-12 indicates the diaphragmatic excursion with maximal inspiration and expiration and clearly demonstrates elevation of the diaphragm as high as the fourth to fifth intercostal space anteriorly. Wounds at or below this level are therefore evaluated for abdominal injury as well.

If the stab wound to the chest is located below the fifth intercostal space and medial to the anterior axillary line and there is no obvious indication for operation, peritoneal lavage is performed. If lavage is negative, the patient is admitted to the hospital and observed for 24 to 48 h. If lavage is positive, operation is performed.

Patients with stab wounds of the abdomen located medial to the anterior axillary line are evaluated clinically. If there is no indication for operation, local exploration is performed. If the end of the tract is not visualized or the peritoneum has been penetrated but the abdominal physical findings are considered negative, lavage is similarly performed. Since lavage is unpredictable in determining retroperitoneal injuries, this method of management is limited to lower chest and abdominal wounds that are located between the two anterior axillary lines. Whereas these wounds have previously been treated by routine celiotomy, a review of 123 patients treated in this manner successfully reduced the incidence of negative celiotomies from 25.6 to 4.1 percent; 70 percent of the patients in this series were spared operative procedures,

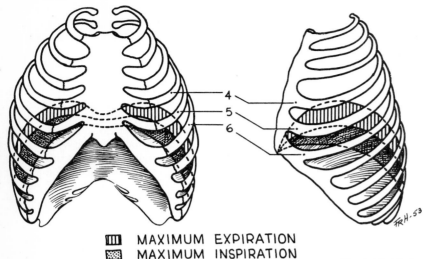

■ MAXIMUM EXPIRATION
▨ MAXIMUM INSPIRATION

Fig. 6-12. Maximum diaphragmatic respiratory excursion. (From: *Shefts LM: Surg Clin North Am 38:1577, 1958, with permission.*)

while 2.3 percent of the 88 patients initially observed were subsequently operated upon but did not suffer any ill effects from delayed surgical treatment.

Patients with posterior wounds lateral to the anterior axillary line are not lavaged because of this method's unreliability with retroperitoneal injuries. In many centers these wounds are treated according to the criteria for selective management; other institutions recommend operative intervention to rule out visceral injury.

Since lower chest wounds may penetrate the diaphragm, it is important to evacuate air and blood from the pleural space with chest tubes prior to celiotomy. Although a pneumothorax may not be indicated by x-ray or physical examination, prophylactic insertion of an anterior chest tube will decrease the danger of a tension pneumothorax developing during induction of anesthesia and subsequent abdominal exploration.

GUNSHOT WOUNDS

The incidence of visceral injury in patients with abdominal gunshot wounds is at least 90 percent, as compared with 30 to 40 percent in patients with abdominal stab wounds. There is an eightfold to tenfold difference in mortality rates associated with gunshot wounds when compared with stab wounds.

It is not possible to predict the path of a missile by merely observing the entrance and exit wounds or connecting a line between an entrance wound and the appearance of a bullet on the x-ray film. These missiles may bounce, tumble, ricochet, and embolize.

Extraperitoneal gunshot wounds may produce intraabdominal injury by blast effect. In a report by Edwards and Gaspard, 14 percent of 35 patients sustaining gunshot wounds to the abdomen without penetration of the peritoneal cavity sustained at least one visceral injury.

Any bullet passing in proximity to the peritoneal cavity requires exploratory celiotomy. This includes all wounds of the lower chest and abdomen, flank, and back. Approximately 25 percent of lower chest wounds will produce intraabdominal injury. Celiotomy is recommended for patients with entrance wounds below the fifth intercostal space. If the patient's condition permits, anterior-posterior and lateral films of the abdomen should be made to locate the missile. Selective management, the use of radiopaque material, local exploration, or peritoneal lavage are not recommended for patients sustaining gunshot wounds in proximity to the abdomen. A review of 59 gunshot wound patients all of whom were taken to the operating room in spite of a negative physical examination and negative periotoneal lavage had a 25 percent incidence of visceral injury. Injuries not detected by either modality included the colon, diaphragm, kidney, pancreas, and aorta.

Once the diagnosis of intraabdominal injury is established and resuscitation is instituted, the abdomen is explored. A long midline incision is preferred for the following reasons: (1) It may be made much more rapidly than other incisions, a matter of vital importance when attempting rapid control of exsanguinating hemorrhage. (2) It gives wide access to all parts of the abdomen, which transverse incisions do not. (3) It may be readily extended into either side of the thorax or continued superiorly as a median sternotomy in case of combined thoracoabdominal injury or when better abdominal exposure is required. (4) It may be rapidly closed, which is or great importance in decreasing the anesthesia and operative time in gravely injured patients.

MANAGEMENT OF PATIENTS WITH EXSANGUINATING ABDOMINAL HEMORRHAGE. With improvement of prehospital care, more patients are arriving at the hospital in extremis. Frequently this condition is due to massive intraabdominal hemorrhage that is refractory to standard resuscitative measures. Ledgerwood and associates have advocated performing preliminary left thoracotomy and temporary thoracic aortic occlusion prior to opening the abdomen in patients with massive hemoperitoneum, tense abdominal distention, and persistent hypotension. The descending thoracic aorta is quickly and bluntly dissected circumferentially and occluded by a straight vascular clamp just above the diaphragm. Although this procedure may have occasional applicability, caution is expressed because it requires opening another major cavity, it increases afterload on the heart, the blood supply to the spinal cord may be interrupted, renal circulation is diminished, and it is ineffective in controlling major venous bleeding.

Once the abdomen is opened, the aortic clamp can be slowly released following stabilization of the patient, and proximal control gained at a lower level. A medium or large Richardson retractor may be used to obtain rapid temporary occlusion of the abdominal aorta just below the diaphragm. The lesser curvature of the stomach is pulled inferiorly, and the flat surface of the retractor blade is compressed firmly against the abdominal aorta, thus occluding it against the vertebra just beneath the diaphragm.

With effective control of massive hemorrhage, resuscitation can be successfully completed, ensuring continuous perfusion to the heart and brain and minimizing the possibility of sudden cardiac arrest.

Stomach

Injuries to the stomach from blunt trauma are infrequent, perhaps because of a relative lack of fixation of the stomach and its protected position; but penetrating injuries of the stomach from gunshot wounds occur frequently.

DIAGNOSIS. The diagnosis of gastric injury is generally suspected from the course of the penetrating object, and, at times, additional suspicion of gastric injury arises from the presence of bloody fluid aspirated from the Levin tube. Generally, wounds of the anterior stomach wall are easily seen at celiotomy. Because of the possibility of missing posterior stomach wall wounds, it is important in all cases of proved or possible gastric injury to open the lesser sac through the gastrocolic omentum. This permits the entire posterior aspect of the stomach to be searched for injury. The points of attachment of the greater and lesser omenta on the greater and lesser curvatures of the stomach, respectively, should also be carefully inspected. If a hematoma is noted at the mesenteric attachment, it should be evacuated and the stomach wall at that site carefully inspected for injury.

TREATMENT. Gastric wounds are repaired by first placing a continuous locked 2-0 suture through all layers of the gastric wall (Vicryl or Dexon suture material may be preferable to chromic catgut); a purse-string suture in the stomach does not provide adequate hemostasis. This hemostatic stitch is very important to control extensive bleeding that may occur from the rich submucosal network of blood vessels in the stomach. After this inner layer closure, an outer inverting row of interrupted nonabsorbable mattress sutures of the Lembert or Halsted type is placed. The outer row of sutures provides adequate serosal approximation of the stomach wall, seals off

readily, and prevents leaks. These sutures in the outer layer should not be through-and-through, as is the first row of sutures, but should extend through the seromuscular coat and the submucosal layer of the stomach. Wounds of the stomach are not drained externally, since they are unlikely to leak, as duodenal wounds may. However, it is very important to suction the peritoneal cavity, with special attention to the subhepatic and subphrenic spaces and the lesser sac, so that all food particles and gastric juice spilled into these areas are removed.

After operation for a gastric wound, nasogastric tube suction should be maintained for several days until active peristalsis resumes and the danger of postoperative gastric dilatation passes. The gastric aspirate should be observed for excessive bleeding, which may occur if the hemostatic suture line is inadequate. If bleeding is brisk or persists, the patient should be immediately reexplored to control the gastric bleeding point. After peristalsis resumes, gastric aspiration is discontinued and the patient is initially started on clear liquids and rapidly advanced to a normal diet.

COMPLICATIONS Complications that may develop after stomach injury are hemorrhage from, or leakage of, the suture line and development of subhepatic, subphrenic, or lesser sac abscesses secondary to spilling of contaminated gastric contents. Development of such abscesses is suspected after gastric wounds in patients who fail to do well postoperatively and who have unexplainable fever for more than a few days. If contamination seems heavy, the skin and subcutaneous tissue should be left open until the wound appears clean.

Duodenum

Injuries to the duodenum and small bowel comprise about one-quarter of blunt and penetrating abdominal trauma. In 1947, Lauritzen reported the mortality rate of retroperitoneal duodenal perforation as approximately 60 percent and related it to the difficulty in establishing an early diagnosis. Burrus et al., in 1961, reported a series of 86 duodenal injuries with an overall mortality of 26 percent.

Mortality rates for duodenal injuries have steadily decreased and are directly proportional to the number and severity of associated injuries as well as the time between injury and treatment. Lucas and Ledgerwood reported a mortality rate of 40 percent in patients who were not operated upon in the first 24 h after injury, in contrast to a mortality of only 11 percent among those operated upon within less than 24 h. The improving mortality rate among patients with duodenal injuries is indicated by four series of duodenal wounds reported since 1978. The total number of patients in these series was 677 and the mortality rates ranged from 10.5 to 14 percent. The mortality rate for simple stab wounds involving only the duodenum should be significantly less than 5 percent, while the mortality for severe blunt trauma or shotgun wounds to the duodenum ranges from about 35 to more than 50 percent, especially when such trauma is combined with serious pancreatic injuries.

DIAGNOSIS. The diagnosis of blunt trauma to the duodenum and small bowel is considerably more difficult than that of penetrating trauma to these organs. With duodenal or small bowel trauma, all the characteristic signs of injury to abdominal viscera may be minimal or absent for several reasons: (1) The injury of the duodenum following blunt trauma is frequently retroperitoneal, so that duodenal contents leak into the retroperitoneal area rather than into the free perioteoneal cavity. (2) Duodenal and small bowel fluid may cause minimal contamination and may not lead to early signs of bacterial peritonitis. This is not true of injuries of the intraperitoneal duodenum, in which duodenal fluid freely flows into the peritoneal cavity. The highly alkaline pH of this fluid causes immediate chemical irritation of the peritoneum and physical signs of such irritation.

Injuries of the duodenum or upper small bowel should be suspected in any patient who receives a blow to the upper abdomen or lower chest, such as from a steering wheel. Testicular pain should raise suspicion of retroperitoneal duodenal rupture. Also, pain referred to the shoulders, chest, and back may be associated with perforation of the duodenum and small intestine.

Several diagnostic aids may be helpful in determining rupture of the duodenum or small bowel. First, needle paracentesis of the abdomen, especially in the right gutter region or in the upper quadrants, may be helpful if blood, bile, or abnormal amounts of small bowel contents are aspirated. Plain radiographs of the abdomen are helpful and may be diagnostic, but absence of free intraperitoneal air does not rule out bowel perforation. Retroperitoneal rupture of the duodenum is not often diagnosed by x-ray. However, the diagnosis may be based on detection of a large accumulation of air about the right kidney or along the psoas muscle margins. After x-ray films of the abdomen and upright chest films are made to search for intraabdominal air collections, it is helpful to inject air through the nasogastric tube to produce or enlarge these air collections so they are more readily detectable. The accuracy of radiographic studies may also be increased by giving the patient a water-soluble radiopaque contrast medium orally and making abdominal x-ray films to detect leakage of the medium from the duodenum or small bowel. Such diagnostic procedures are unnecessary if other clinical signs indicate the need for exploratory celiotomy. Federle et al. have shown that computerized tomography may be useful in the diagnosis of intraabdominal trauma, especially in the retroperitoneal area, where ruptures of the third and fourth portions of the duodenum are likely to occur.

When a celiotomy is done for suspected intraabdominal injury, duodenal lesions are often missed, especially retroperitoneal lesions of the third or fourth portions. This is due to superficial observation, inadequate exposure, and lack of persistence on the part of the surgeon. It has been reported that duodenal perforations have been missed initially in 33 to 50 percent of the various reported series of retroperitoneal duodenal injuries. To avoid overlooking duodenal trauma and contributing to the high mortality from duodenal wounds, it is important to inspect the entire duodenum during abdominal exploration

for trauma. This is especially true if a retroperitoneal hematoma is noted near the duodenum or if there is crepitation or bile-stained fluid along the lateral margins of the duodenum retroperitoneally. If these signs are noted or if the duodenum is contused, it should be widely mobilized by the Kocher maneuver, incising the peritoneum along its lateral margin, so that the duodenum can be completely mobilized along with the head of the pancreas. Thus, small areas of perforation in the retroperitoneal aspect of the duodenum may be identified. Often retroperitoneal wounds of the duodenum that were missed at initial exploration are not recognized until several days later when bile-stained fluid drains from the abdominal wound of a patient who has continued to do poorly postoperatively. The following signs, in addition to those mentioned previously, require careful exploration of the duodenum and the retroduodenal area: elevation of the posterior peritoneum with glassy-appearing edema; petechiae or fat necrosis over the ascending and transverse colon or mesocolon; retroperitoneal phlegmon; hematoma over the head of the pancreas extending into the base of the mesocolon; fat necrosis of the retroperitoneal tissues; and/or discoloration of retroperitoneal tissues—dark from hemorrhage, grayish from suppuration, or yellowish from bile.

The third and fourth portions of the duodenum may be exposed by mobilizing the cecum, right colon, hepatic flexure of the colon, and mesenteries of these organs up to and including the ligament of Treitz, carrying the dissection of the mesocolon along the attachment at the root of the small bowel mesentery, as shown in Fig. 6-13.

TREATMENT. The local treatment of the duodenal perforation itself depends more on the size of the perforation than on any other single factor. In general, an attempt is made to close the duodenal perforation if this can be done without decreasing the lumen of the duodenum. This closure is carried out with a continuous locking 3-0 suture through all layers of the duodenal wall (preferably using Vicryl or Dexon suture material) followed by an outer layer of nonabsorbable interrupted mattress sutures in the seromuscular layer of the duodenum. After this, the duodenum is carefully palpated to exclude stenosis. If the perforation is so large that simple closure will cause a stricture of the duodenum, consideration should be given to (1) complete division of the duodenum and an end-to-end anastomosis or (2) division of the duodenum, closure of both ends, and a gastroenterostomy.

Kobold and Thal first reported a method of managing large duodenal defects that previously might have required one of the above techniques of duodenal division. Their method consisted of using a retrocolic loop of proximal jejunum that is sutured over a large defect in the duodenum, with an inner row of absorbable sutures taken between the torn edge of the duodenum and the seromuscular layer of the jejunum and an outer layer of nonabsorbable mattress sutures taken between the seromuscular coats of the duodenum and the jejunum. Animal studies, as well as clinical usage, have shown the feasibility of this ''patching'' technique in managing large duodenal defects (Fig. 6-14). Large duodenal wounds and duodenal wounds that have dehisced also have been managed

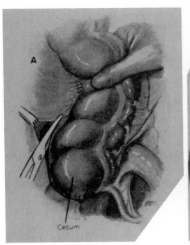
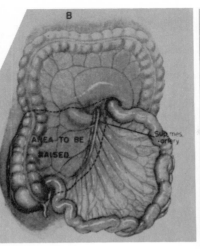
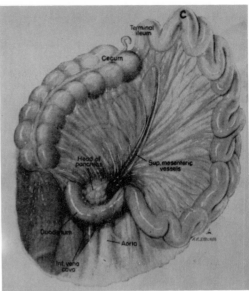

Fig. 6-13. A technique for the exposure of the third and fourth portions of the duodenum. *A* and *B*. Initial dissection for mobilization of the right side of the colon, small intestine, and mesentery. *C*. Exposure obtained of the third and fourth portions of the duodenum. (From: *Cattell RB, Braasch JW: Surg Gynecol Obstet 111:379, 1960, with permission.*)

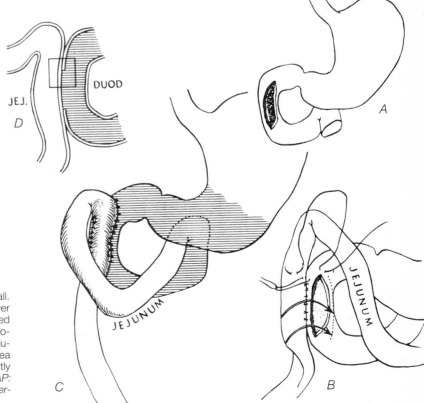

Fig. 6-14. *A*. Area of excision of duodenal wall. *B*. Technique of placement of intact jejunum over the wound to form a patch. *C*. The completed closure. *D*. Cross section of the completed closure showing the relationship of the intact jejunum to the duodenal perforation. The boxed area is the site from which tissue was subsequently removed for study. (From: *Kobold EE, Thal AP: Surg Gynecol Obstet 116:340, 1963, with permission.*)

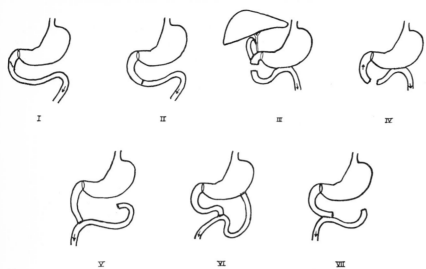

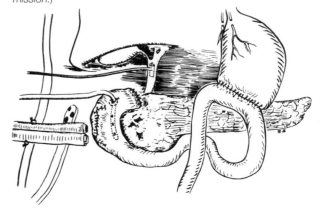

Fig. 6-15. Diagrammatic representation of various operative procedures in a series of cases. I, Simple closure; II, end-to-end duodenoduodenostomy; III and IV, closure of both ends of duodenum and gastroenterostomy; V, closure of distal duodenum and duodenojejunostomy; VI, duodenojejunostomy and gastroduodenostomy; VII, resection of fourth part of duodenum and duodenojejunostomy. (From: *Cleveland HC, Waddell WR: Surg Clin North Am 43:413, 1963, with permission.*)

by anastomosis of the open end or the side of a defunctionalized Roux en Y loop of proximal jejunum over the duodenal defect.

If the region of the ampulla is involved in a duodenal injury, the common bile duct should be identified by insertion of a T tube, since reimplantation of the common duct sometimes may be necessary. Approximately 75 to 80 percent of all duodenal injuries can be closed by debridement of the wound edges and simple suture. However, for the other 20 to 25 percent, one of the reparative procedures described above recommended by Cleveland and Waddell is used (Fig. 6-15). Rarely, even a pancreaticoduodenectomy may be necessary to manage extensive devitalizing trauma to the duodenum and periampullar region, especially when such injuries are combined with severe pancreatic trauma and it is difficult to control bleeding (see the section Combined Duodenum and Pancreatic Injuries).

Very severe injuries of the duodenum or combined severe injuries of the pancreas and duodenum may be treated by a Berne duodenal "diverticulization" procedure instead of by pancreatoduodenal resection unless the destruction and devitalization of the pancreas and duodenum is too extensive. The duodenal diverticulization procedure was first described by Berne and associates in 1960. This operation is illustrated in Fig. 6-16. This operation consists of diversion of the alimentary stream away from the injured duodenum and pancreatic head. This is achieved by removing the gastric antrum, closing the duodenal stump, and performing a Billroth II gastrojejunostomy and vagotomy. The duodenal laceration is closed with interrupted monofilament nonabsorbable sutures, and the duodenum is decompressed with a tube duodenostomy to reduce the possibility of disruption of the duodenal suture line from increased pressure within the duodenal stump. The tube duodenostomy is performed by inserting a #12 or #14 French straight rubber

catheter into the lateral duodenal wall through a stab wound, securing the tube with a purse-string suture. The area of the combined pancreatic and duodenal injuries is then extensively drained with several large Penrose drains and a soft suction drain. Closed suction drains may be preferable to Penrose drains if the area of tissue de-

Fig. 6-16. The essential components of duodenal diverticulization including gastric antrectomy, tube duodenostomy, gastrojejunostomy, and drainage of the biliary tract may be advisable. (From: *Berne CJ, Donovan AJ, et al: Am J Surg 127:503, 1974, with permission.*)

struction is not too extensive. The biliary tract is drained by inserting a T tube into the common duct or by performing a tube cholecystostomy. In 1974, Berne and associates reported the use of this operation in the treatment of 50 patients with severe pancreatic and duodenal injuries with a mortality rate of only 16 percent, which is gratifyingly low for patients with such grave injuries. Even though duodenal and pancreatic fistulae may develop in patients undergoing the Berne duodenal diverticulization procedure, these lesions are generally well tolerated since they are, in effect, end rather than lateral fistulae because the gastric contents are diverted from the duodenum and pancreas. In the experience reported by Berne and associates, there were seven duodenal fistulae and five pancreatic fistulae among their 50 patients, but all closed spontaneously.

An alternative method for diverting the gastric contents from severe duodenal injuries was reported by Vaughn and associates. This procedure consists of repair of the duodenal wound, followed by a gastrotomy on the greater curvature of the antrum of the stomach in a site selected for gastrojejunostomy. Through this opening, the pylorus is closed with sutures of chromic catgut (or Vicryl suture). Gastrojejunostomy, side-to-side, is then accomplished (Fig. 6-17). These surgeons used this procedure in 75 patients selected from 175 consecutive patients who had duodenal trauma. The mortality was 19 percent and the rate of fistula formation was 5 percent among the patients treated by pyloric exclusion and gastrojejunostomy, in contrast to a 14 percent mortality rate and a 2 percent fistulization rate in the entire series of 175 patients. The mortality and fistulization rates were somewhat higher in the pyloric exclusion group, probably because these patients had more severe duodenal injuries. Two of the three patients who developed duodenal fistulae after pyloric exclusion had spontaneous closure of the fistula, and the remaining patient required surgical closure. Vaughan and associates note that in other series of duodenal injuries the rate of lateral duodenal fistula formation has ranged between 6 and 14 percent regardless of the type of closure. This compares very favorably with

the 2 percent overall fistulization rate in their series of 175 patients with duodenal injuries. Kelly and associates have performed the same type of pyloric exclusion with gastrojejunostomy but have used staples instead of sutures as employed by Vaughan and associates to close the pylorus.

Prevention of Duodenal Fistulization after Duodenal Trauma. Various surgeons suggest that duodenal fistulas can be prevented by prolonged decompression of the duodenum after closure of the wound. This may be especially indicated in more severe injuries of the duodenum and can be accomplished in several ways. Snyder and associates performed duodenal tube decompression in 53 percent of the 190 of their patients with duodenal injuries who had duodenorrhaphies. The reasons for duodenal decompression in their series were difficult to determine retrospectively but were probably related to the surgeon's subjective impression of the severity of the duodenal wound. In this series, duodenal fistulae developed in 9 percent and caused death in 4 percent of those who had duodenal decompression. A review of their patients did not allow comment on the efficacy of tube duodenostomy in the prevention of fistulae. However, they did state that the morbidity and mortality might have been greater if tube decompression had not been used. These results suggest that decompression is not a complete safeguard against fistula formation. Stone and Fabian reported a series of 321 patients with duodenal wounds and the most recent 237 were all managed with duodenal decompression via a gastrostomy tube and twin jejunostomy tubes (one passing retrograde into the duodenum). Only one duodenal fistula (0.5 percent) occurred in 210 surviving patients. In contrast, failure to decompress the duodenum was associated with an 8 percent leak rate. Thus, tube decompression of the duodenum is a reasonable and probably effective adjunct in the management of selected duodenal wounds. However, decompression is not an effective substitute for careful reconstructions of severe duodenal injuries.

Reliance on an abdominal drain in the management of duodenal trauma has varied considerably, although several reports suggest that routine drainage of the duodenal suture line may favor fistula formation. However, other clinical analyses have reached the opposite conclusion and use of a drain has been urged to provide a tract for discharge of intestinal contents if a duodenal leak occurs. Objective data about drainage of duodenal wounds are lacking, and the argument remains unsettled about whether a soft rubber drain should or should not be used. Probably, in the opinion of most surgeons, drainage is considered advisable.

Postoperative Care. After repair of duodenal injuries, decompression with a nasogastric or gastrostomy tube is usually continued for about 5 to 7 days to protect the suture lines. If fistulae form, gastroduodenal decompression should be continued for prolonged periods and a sump drain should be inserted into the drain site for continuous active suction of the fistulous tract. This is done to prevent the possible spread of duodenal fluid throughout the peritoneal cavity, to prevent collapse and healing of the

Fig. 6-17. Duodenal injury and method of excluding the pylorus. (From: *Vaughan GD, Frazier OH, et al: Am J Surg 134:785, 1977, with permission.*)

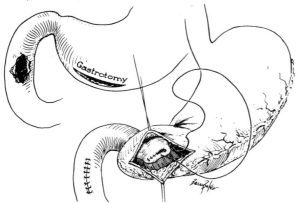

fistulous tract, to prevent digestion of the skin by duodenal fluid draining onto the skin, and to aid calculation and replacement of fluid and electrolyte losses from the fistula. Also, when a duodenal fistula develops, the patient is placed on central intravenous hyperalimentation according to the principles of Dudrick and associates, which are discussed in Chap. 2. This regimen maintains excellent nutrition and may reduce the volume of gastrointestinal secretions. Occasionally, the duodenal fistula does not spontaneously close despite adequate nonoperative treatment with intravenous hyperalimentation and sump drainage. In such cases, when a reasonable trial of conservative treatment has been made and the patient is in optimal condition for reoperation, the abdomen is opened and completely explored to rule out distal bowel obstruction that may be causing the fistula to persist. The fistula is exposed at its origin from the duodenum, and a Roux en Y defunctionalized limb of proximal jejunum is brought up to the fistula and anastomosed to it. This anastomosis may use either the end or the side (after closing the end of the jejunal limb) of the defunctionalized jejunum. This procedure permanently diverts the fistula drainage internally and is very effective.

INTRAMURAL HEMATOMA

Intramural hematoma of the duodenum is usually due to blunt abdominal trauma, including child abuse, which causes rupture of intramural duodenal blood vessels with formation of a dark, sausage-shaped mass in the submucosal layer of the duodenal wall. The hematoma may cause partial or complete duodenal obstruction, but the obstruction is usually partial. The patient has signs of a high small bowel obstruction, with nausea and vomiting associated with upper abdominal pain and tenderness, and sometimes a suggestion of a right upper quadrant mass on palpation of the abdomen. Plain films of the abdomen may show an ill-defined right upper quadrant mass and obliteration of the right psoas shadow. Felson and Levin have shown that an upper gastrointestinal tract series is generally diagnostic, showing dilation of the duodenal lumen with the appearance of a "coiled spring" in the second and third portions of the duodenum due to the crowding of the valvulae conniventes by the hematoma. The serum amylase level may be elevated. An intramural duodenal hematoma may also occur spontaneously in patients on anticoagulants.

Wooley and associates state that traditionally the recommended treatment for intramural duodenal hematoma has been surgical. The most common operation has been simple evacuation of the hematoma; however, gastroenterostomy as well as duodenal resection has been performed. Izant and Drucker in 1964 suggested that most infants and children with intramural duodenal hematomas could be successfully treated without surgical intervention. Nonsurgical treatment of these patients consists of cessation of oral intake, nasogastric suction, and intravenous replacement of fluids and electrolytes. Holgerson and Bishop in 1977 reported on nine patients with intramural duodenal hematomas, only one of whom was operated on. It is now increasingly evident that when there is no indication of bowel perforation, most patients with this condition will respond to the conservative treatment noted above.

Small Bowel

Injuries to the small bowel are more common than injuries to the duodenum or colon. Eighty percent of bowel injuries occur between the duodenojejunal junction and the terminal ileum, with approximately 10 percent each in the duodenum and the large intestine. The usual mechanism of small bowel injury from blunt trauma is crushing of the small bowel against the vertebral column. Rupture of the small bowel is also caused by shearing and tearing forces applied to the abdomen, and rarely by sudden elevation of the intraluminal pressure of the bowel with bursting from such sudden high pressure. Williams and Sargent have experimentally shown that rupture due to sudden elevation of pressure within the bowel is quite unusual.

In exploring the abdomen for injuries to the small bowel, it is important to inspect minutely the entire circumference of the small bowel and its attached mesentery from the ligament of Treitz to the ileocecal valve. The bowel may be completely transected in one or more places in blunt trauma with or without severe injury to the mesentery and its blood supply; at times, the mesentery may be torn from a segment of bowel, thus depriving the bowel of its blood supply. Penetrating trauma to the small bowel from a gunshot wound or stab wound is common, although, surprisingly, it has been noted at the time that in patients with a stab wound of the abdomen, the small bowel has been spared. This is probably because the great mobility of the small bowel allows it to slide away from the knife, a much less likely occurrence with gunshot wounds than with stab wounds.

TREATMENT. Small, single perforations of the small bowel may be closed safely with a single layer of interrupted nonabsorbable mattress sutures that include and invert the seromuscular and submucosal coats of the bowel. A hemostatic stitch, as required for stomach wounds, is not necessary for small bowel injuries, because the small bowel does not tend to continue bleeding from the submucosal plexus, as does the stomach. However, individual bleeders should be ligated with fine suture material. An advantage of a single-layer closure is its rapidity of performance, which is important in patients in precarious condition after multiple trauma.

Two small perforations of the bowel that are very close together may often be repaired by converting the wounds into one and closing the resulting defect as a single linear wound. This type of repair does not constrict the lumen of the bowel as much as two separate lines of suture placed close together and is more secure. Multiple perforations of the small bowel may occur after injury from shotgun pellets. Each one of these injuries should be carefully sought out and closed with interrupted rows of nonabsorbable mattress sutures.

Long linear lacerations of the small bowel lumen also should be closed with a single row of nonabsorbable sutures after ligating any persistent bleeders with small nonabsorbable sutures. Longitudinal lacerations may be closed in a longitudinal direction or transversely according to the Heineke-Mikulicz principle.

Small bowel injuries produced by high-velocity missiles cause severe contusions of tissue surrounding the actual perforation. Because the contusion is a site of potential tissue necrosis and bowel leakage caused by thrombosis of vessels in the area of blast injury, it should be debrided. The debridement should extend into viable bowel where active bleeding is obtained. If the wound is too large or is long and longitudinal, the bowel may not be adequately closed without compromising the lumen, and the damaged segment should be resected. Also, if there are multiple wounds in a short segment of bowel, it is much safer and easier to resect the injured segment than to attempt to suture each of the closely spaced wounds, with resulting impairment of the bowel lumen and blood supply and subsequent obstruction and/or necrosis and leakage. Perforations or lacerations to the mesenteric border, unless they are quite small, are difficult to repair and frequently are associated with vascular impairment. They also should be managed by resection of the involved bowel if an adequate closure cannot be obtained without impairment of the blood supply. Following transection the bowel should be reanastomosed after debriding contused and damaged areas on either side of the wound back to normal intestine that has a good blood supply. Careful attention should be given to leaving uninjured mesentery adjacent to the suture line of the reanastomosis.

Extensive segments of bowel may be avulsed from the mesentery, so that the bowel loses its blood supply. All the necrotic or potentially necrotic bowel and injured mesentery must be resected and an end-to-end anastomosis made between uninjured bowel attached to uninjured mesentery.

Contusions of the small bowel should be assumed to be larger than is apparent. Such injuries are dangerous, since they may lead to subsequent necrosis and perforation. Contusions up to 1 cm in diameter may be turned in with a row of fine nonabsorbable mattress sutures. Larger contusions should be resected.

Temporary control of bowel spillage can be quickly obtained by stapling either the perforation or both ends of a transection while attention is directed toward managing more serious problems. After stabilization has been accomplished the bowel can be repaired more leisurely as described above. Postoperative care of patients with wounds of the small bowel includes maintenance of nasogastric suction and low oral intake until adequate bowel activity returns. Leakage from suture lines and intestinal obstruction rarely occur if small bowel wounds are properly managed.

Colon Injuries

The morbidity and mortality from acute injuries to the colon and rectum have been significantly reduced by an aggressive surgical approach. This has been largely influenced by the experiences of military surgeons during World War II, the Korean conflict, and the Vietnam War.

In World War II, an impressive improvement in the mortality from wounds of the colon was noted. This was due to several factors including improved methods of triage and transportation, effective replacement of blood and fluid, and early surgical intervention combined with ancillary use of antibiotics.

The mortality rate for wounds of the colon of 37 percent in World War II was reduced to approximately 15 percent during the action in Korea. The majority of military surgeons treating acute injuries of the colon tended to exteriorize the wound as an artificial anus to prevent further soilage of the peritoneal cavity. This approach to these particular wounds was duly carried over into civilian practice and reflected in the subsequent reduction in mortality and morbidity. In the later phase of the Korean conflict, however, some modification of the aggressive technique was noted in that small, primary wounds treated early were handled by primary closure without exteriorization.

Acute wounds of the colon that occur in a civilian environment exhibit features that may modify the indications for exteriorization of the wound. The types of injury usually noted in a military situation resulted from either high-velocity missiles or fragmentation missiles in which there was massive destruction of tissue and usually gross soilage of the peritoneal cavity. In the civilian environment, the wounds more often are caused by low-velocity missiles and usually are unassociated with massive destruction of surrounding organs and tissue. The time from wounding to initial treatment in the civilian situation is generally somewhat less than that noted during military conflict. Similarly, associated injuries occurring in civilian accidents do not tend to be so numerous or so massive as those in a military environment, and this has a definite influence on morbidity and mortality.

ETIOLOGY. Acute injuries of the colon and rectum may be divided into penetrating wounds and wounds resulting from blunt trauma. In the former group, accidental colon injuries may be the result of industrial accidents involving explosions resulting in impalement, penetrating injuries from flying objects, or blast injuries.

These injuries may be either the direct result of explosives or the result of accidents involving sources of greatly compressed air. External acts of violence constitute an important source of injuries to the colon, and these are generally penetrating injuries caused by guns or knives or, on rarer occasions, blunt abdominal trauma. Wounds of the rectum, particularly, may be the result of instrumentation during the process of sigmoidoscopy, the administration of enemas, or unnatural sexual behavior. There may also be perforations of the colorectum by foreign bodies that pass through the alimentary canal into the colon. Inadvertent penetration of the colon or rectum may occur during difficult operations; this is especially true of pelvic operations for neoplastic or severe inflammatory disease. Falls resulting in impalement upon sharp objects may produce wounds of the rectum. Automobile accidents and other forms of blunt trauma may also produce acute injuries to the colon and rectum.

DIAGNOSIS. A systematic diagnostic approach to problems of abdominal trauma is necessary, but specific examinations of the colon and rectum may be necessary to delineate an injury. This is particularly pertinent in those instances in which instrumentation is the cause of suspected perforation. Rectal examination and sigmoidoscopy should occupy a prominent place in the examination of these patients. Diagnostic abdominal x-ray studies should be employed to determine if there is a perforation with leakage of air into the free peritoneal cavity. Anteroposterior and lateral decubitus views are particularly helpful in these instances. Contrast studies of the colon should be employed rarely and cautiously in view of the high morbidity and mortality associated with leakage of barium and feces into the free peritoneal cavity. Aqueous opaque media, such as Gastrografin, are preferable when penetration of the colon is suspected.

TREATMENT. The general principles of management of patients with abdominal trauma apply to those patients who have acute injuries of the colon. It is important that the time from wounding to definitive operation be as short as possible, and aggressive replacement of fluid and blood losses should be undertaken at once. Patients with penetrating abdominal trauma or suspected colon or rectal injury should have a broad-spectrum antibiotic with aerobic and anaerobic coverage begun prior to surgery.

A thorough and complete exploration of all abdominal viscera is made, for the morbidity and mortality vary directly with the number of associated injuries. Bleeding should be controlled as rapidly as possible and immediate efforts made to reduce peritoneal soilage from any penetrating wound of an abdominal viscus. The specific care of the wound of the colon should be approached by noting the anatomic differences between the intraperitoneal and extraperitoneal large intestine. Particular attention must be paid to the type of wound, its location, the amount of tissue destruction, the presence of associated injuries, and the time from wounding to definitive care.

Small primary wounds located on the antimesenteric border that are seen quite early, in which there is minimal tissue destruction, and minimal or no peritoneal soiling including those of the left colon, in the absence of associated injuries of other abdominal viscera, may often be adequately managed by a primary two-layer closure.

The mucosa is approximated with a running lock suture of 3-0 absorbable suture and the seromuscular layers are closed with interrupted permanent sutures using the Lembert technique. High-velocity missile wounds associated with shock, large fecal contamination, and significant associated injuries should rarely if ever be closed primarily. Tissue destruction in these cases is often excessive and may not be readily apparent.

A less well-accepted modification of primary closure in which the repaired colon wound is exteriorized and then returned to the abdominal cavity, usually about 10 to 14 days later, has been reported by several groups of surgeons. If the repaired colon wound fails to heal after exteriorization, it is converted to a colostomy and managed in the usual manner; otherwise the patient is returned to the operating room and, under general anesthesia, the repaired and well-healed segment of bowel is freed up and dropped back into the peritoneal cavity. In general, the colon wounds managed by exteriorization-repair are somewhat more severe than those managed by simple primary closure. Flint and associates have classified colon injuries into three grades. His classification has been used to determine the type of repair that is most appropriate. It includes: Grade 1—isolated colonic injuries with minimal fecal contamination, no shock and minimal delay (these injuries are most suitable for primary repair). Grade 2—through and through perforation, lacerations, moderate contamination, and associated injuries. Grade 3—severe tissue loss, devascularization of the colon, heavy contamination, prolonged hypotension, or significant delay in treatment (these wounds should routinely be managed by exteriorization as a colostomy, by primary repair and a proximal colostomy, resection and colostomy with mucous fistula, or a Hartmann closure of the distal colonic segment).

Favorable experiences with selective use of exteriorization-repair have been reported by Lou and associates and by Dang and associates. In 65 to 75 percent of the patients in these series the colon wound healed and could be returned to the peritoneal cavity after several days. The mortality rates were zero and the colon-related morbidity rates were 18 percent in both of these experiences. These two series consisted of a total of 88 patients who had exteriorization-repairs. Probably less than 15 percent of patients with colon injuries can be treated in this manner. It is important to emphasize that if exteriorization-repair is used, a generous opening must be made in the abdominal wall to permit exteriorization of the repaired wound without obstruction of the colon.

Burch and associates recently reported a series of 727 patients with colon injuries. Primary repair was accomplished in 52 percent, the majority of which were simple closure. Seventy-eight percent of right colon injuries, 62 percent of transverse colon injuries, and 32 percent of left colon injuries were closed primarily. The late mortality rate (>48 h) was 1.2 percent for primary repair compared with 9.2 percent for patients treated with a colostomy. It should be noted that more seriously injured patients had a colostomy, hence the higher mortality rate, but with careful selection primary repair can be safely accomplished.

Acute injuries of the intraperitoneal colon resulting from high-velocity missiles that are associated with extensive destruction of tissues or that are large and ragged in nature and are located near or involve the mesenteric border should not be closed primarily. If located in the ascending, transverse, or descending colon, the wound may be exteriorized as a colostomy. Similarly, if the time from wounding to definitive care is relatively long, allowing seeding of the peritoneal cavity with a large number of bacteria, some type of colostomy should be performed either as a wound exteriorization or as a proximal diverting colostomy. Primary closure of the distal wounds is then permissible. Although a loop colostomy may be done for expediency, a completely diverting double-barrel colostomy is favored. It is preferable to open the loop colostomy immediately, usually with the cautery in order to secure early, complete fecal diversion. This is performed in the operating room after all the wounds are closed and dressed. When there are associated massive injuries to other viscera, although the colon wound itself might fulfill the indications for primary closure, a colostomy is indicated. In some instances, there may be massive injury of the cecum or of the ileocecal area, in which case it will be necessary to resect the injured bowel and do an ileotransverse colostomy.

Recent enthusiasm for primary repair in part has been predicated on a feeling that there is an excessive morbidity associated with colostomy closure. Thal and Yeary reported their experience with 137 patients who had colostomy closures following trauma. The morbidity in their series was 10.2 percent, including wound infection 5.1 percent, bowel obstruction 2.9 percent, and fistula formation 1.5 percent. There was no mortality in their series. They concluded that the morbidity following colostomy closure was low enough so as not to be a factor in the consideration of primary repair versus colostomy as an initial operative procedure.

Localized minor wounds of the right colon and cecum that do not produce extensive destruction of the large bowel and are not associated with massive soilage or serious injuries to other viscera may often be managed by primary closure and appendicostomy. In these instances, after debridement and careful closure of the laceration of the cecum, tube appendicostomy is performed to decompress this segment. Seromuscular sutures are placed about the base of the appendix and secured to the lateral parietal peritoneum in order to prevent intraperitoneal leakage about the area of the tube insertion. By this technique, suitable decompression of the cecum and right colon may be obtained, and removal of the tube appendicostomy permits the vent to close spontaneously.

The extraperitoneal perforations of the rectum must be evaluated under the same principles employed for colon injuries within the peritoneal cavity. If clean lacerations with minimal spillage are seen early, primary bowel repair may be indicated if the wound is accessible. Presacral drains should then be inserted. Associated perineal wounds should be debrided and, if grossly contaminated, left open. If debridement is adequate and these wounds are clean, they may be closed with drainage. Any damage to the anal sphincter may be repaired at this time. When a perineal wound is present but not penetrating the colon, it should be debrided widely and if not grossly contaminated then may be closed with drainage. Where there is no perineal wound but there is significant tissue destruction about the extraperitoneal rectum, presacral drainage should be instituted.

For all injuries of the rectum, complete diversion of the fecal stream is mandatory and can be accomplished by constructing a proximal double-barrel colostomy. Even in those instances where the rectal wound has been closed and diverting colostomy performed, presacral drainage is necessary.

Drainage of the retrorectal area is extremely important. This can be established by making a curvilinear incision in the posterior perianal area, incising the anococcygeal ligament, and bluntly dissecting into the presacral space. Two Penrose drains will usually suffice, but with extensive injuries, it may be necessary to utilize sump drainage for a few days.

Lavenson and Cohen, on the basis of their experience in the Vietnam conflict, strongly recommended removal of all feces from the distal rectum. This is accomplished by irrigating copious amounts of saline solution through the defunctionalized segment until the return is clear. They report a significant decrease in mortality and complication rates when utilizing this technique. Military injuries are generally associated with higher-velocity missiles and cause more fecal contamination and blast injury to surrounding pelvic tissue. In civilian injuries, distal irrigation may not be as important, as evidenced by Trunkey and Shires, who report a lower morbidity and mortality rate in their series, in which distal irrigation was not employed but adequate drainage and diversion were used.

Serious perineal injuries are treated in a similar manner. Even in the absence of rectal injury, sepsis can be avoided by early fecal diversion. Failure to recognize this potential problem may lead to extensive soft tissue infections extending from the knee to the axilla, with potential involvement of the anterior and posterior abdominal wall.

Early closure of the colostomy is indicated in patients who have completely recovered and have no distal colon injury. It is desirable to close the simple colostomy in 2 or 3 weeks. Prior to closure, both limbs of the colon should be visualized radiographically to assure that no lesion persists. Mechanical and bacterial cleansing of the colon is effected preoperatively.

Liver

Injury to the liver is suspected in all patients with penetrating or blunt trauma that involves the lower chest and upper abdomen. Among patients with penetrating abdominal trauma, the liver is second only to the small bowel as the organ most commonly injured; among those with blunt trauma, the liver is second only to the spleen as the most commonly injured organ. About 80 percent of liver injuries occur as a result of penetrating trauma from stab wounds or gunshot wounds; only 15 to 20 percent occur from blunt trauma. In recent years, the incidence of stab wounds has diminished while the incidence of gunshot wounds, especially those caused by higher-velocity and larger-caliber missiles, and blunt trauma has increased. These changes in the types of liver injuries, the more rapid transport of patients with hepatic trauma to treatment facilities, and better resuscitation methods have caused an increase in the severity of liver injuries that are likely to confront the surgeon.

Early exploration, prompt replacement of blood and use of balanced electrolyte solution, antibiotics, proper choice of surgical treatment, and adequate drainage are all factors that have led to increased survival rates. The average overall mortality rate of patients with hepatic trauma is about 10 to 15 percent. However, this rate is directly related to the severity of the liver injury and the presence of associated visceral trauma. The mortality rate of stab wounds to the liver without associated organ injury is only about 1 percent. When significant liver trauma is associated with injuries of more than five other intraabdominal organs, or when major hepatic resection is required to control the bleeding, the mortality rate rises to about 45 to 50 percent.

TREATMENT. After initial resuscitation and diagnostic maneuvers, patients with suspected hepatic injuries are rapidly moved to the operating room. The entire abdomen and chest are "prepped" and draped, and a long upper midline abdominal incision is made. Sources of bleeding from the liver and abdomen are quickly appraised, and temporary control of the bleeding is obtained by manual compression or packs placed over the bleeding sites and by temporary occlusion of appropriate major vessels. Digital compression of the hepatic artery and portal vein to occlude temporarily the blood flow to the liver (the Pringle maneuver) may control or slow hepatic hemorrhage in some patients, but more often it is necessary to combine the Pringle maneuver with compression packs placed over the liver injury to control hemorrhage effectively. There is general agreement that, in the normothermic liver, blood flow to the liver can be completely occluded with safety for at least 15 min and probably longer without causing any hepatocellular damage. If it is necessary to occlude the hepatic blood supply for more than 15 min, the vascular occlusion can be briefly interrupted every 10 or 15 min to allow short periods of uninterrupted hepatic blood flow. In a small, uncontrolled clinical experience with 22 patients who had complex hepatic injuries, Pachter and Spencer gave an intravenous bolus of methylprednisolone (30 to 40 mg/kg) before hepatic inflow occlusion.

This use of steroids may have been responsible for increasing tolerance to inflow occlusion beyond 20 min in 82 percent; however, it is emphasized that this was an uncontrolled observation. In addition, Pachter and Spencer used 2 L of iced Ringer's lactate solution intraperitoneally to induce some degree of hepatic hypothermia. Again, this method of protection against warm ischemia was not adequately evaluated, since an intrahepatic temperature probe was not used to confirm the achievement of local hepatic hypothermia. Induced hypothermia may have adverse cardiac effects and should be used cautiously if used at all.

Definitive treatment of liver injuries may be accomplished by drainage alone, suture or hemostatic maneuvers and drainage, or variations of hepatic resection or resectional debridement.

Drainage Alone. Hepatic hemorrhage ceases spontaneously by the time the abdomen is opened or stops soon after compression of the bleeding site in about half of patients with liver injuries. In such patients, the only treatment necessary is adequate drainage of the injury. Suturing of nonbleeding liver injuries is unnecessary. This is emphasized by Trunkey, Shires, McClelland and by Lucas and Ledgerwood who reported no rebleeding among several hundred patients with liver injuries that stopped bleeding spontaneously or soon after temporary pack compression. Suturing of nonbleeding liver wounds may cause bleeding and needlessly traumatizes hepatic tissue.

In the opinion of most surgeons who manage large numbers of hepatic injuries, these injuries should be drained externally. A combination of Penrose drains and sump suction drains is often used when treating massive injuries. Large, 1-in.-wide Penrose drains should be brought out posterolaterally, as dependently as possible, through an abdominal stab wound to achieve the best drainage by gravity. It is important to make an adequate opening in the abdominal wall, sufficient to admit at least two fingers, to assure optimal function of the Penrose drains; otherwise, the drains act as plugs rather than drains. Adequate drainage of the perihepatic space in patients with liver injuries greatly reduces the formation of infected collections of bile, blood, and tissue fluid in the subphrenic and subhepatic spaces. The Silastic suction drains now available are generally very effective in providing aspiration drainage for most patients with liver injuries. It is preferable to bring suction drains out through small stab wounds in the abdominal wall that are separate from the Penrose drains if both types are used. In large patients with more extensive liver wounds, it may be preferable to resect the lateral half or two-thirds of the right twelfth rib to achieve more effective gravity drainage. The Penrose drains are left in place 5 to 10 days, thereafter being slowly removed over a 3-day period. Only at this time is a firm, fibrinous tract formed about the drains that ensures adequate external drainage of the material that accumulates in the abdomen after the drain is removed. Suction drains generally should remain in place until drainage is less than 25 to 30 mL of fluid daily. Some authors have suggested that minor injuries may be managed without drainage; however, the evidence is inconclusive at this time.

Suture, Hemostatic Techniques, and Drainage. Bleeding persists despite temporary compression packing of the injury site in approximately half of patients with liver injuries. Definitive hemostasis of persistently bleeding liver injuries usually can be achieved by liver sutures. Simple interrupted sutures are placed 2 cm from the wound margins, using 2-0 or 0 chromic sutures swaged onto a 2-in. blunt-tipped "liver needle." This allows gentle but firm approximation of the wound edges, thereby stopping most bleeding that originates from the outer 2 cm of the liver parenchyma immediately beneath the hepatic capsule. Passage of the suture through buttressing material such as Surgicel, Gelfoam, or omentum is seldom needed if the sutures are placed 2 cm from the margin of the injury and tied gently. However, if a bolster is needed, it is preferable to use a vascularized pedicle of omentum instead of foreign material. Trunkey, Shires, and McClelland have abandoned the technique previously described using interlocking mattress sutures for hemostasis. These authors now recommend direct suture ligation of the bleeding vessel as an attempt to reduce the chance of strangulation and subsequent necrosis by mattress sutures.

Microcrystalline collagen powder (Avitene) may be used in selected patients to control bleeding from minor liver wounds. Unlike other material such as Gelfoam, Avitene can be left in liver wounds without inciting significant foreign body reaction.

The use of liver sutures to obtain hemostasis from both the entrance and exit sites of long gunshot tracts in the liver is controversial. However, Lucas and Ledgerwood state that this technique was successfully used in several of their patients who otherwise would have required extensive surgery. Placement of the liver sutures at both ends of the bullet tract stops bleeding arising from the subcapsular area, which is the usual source. During their 5-year prospective review, Lucas and Ledgerwood found that only one patient developed an intrahepatic abscess following use of this technique, and no patients developed hemobilia after closure of both ends of a long gunshot tract. They noted that continued bleeding that persists after closure of both ends of a tract is usually identified at the initial operation by blood oozing between the liver sutures or by an increase in the size of the liver within 10 min after placement of the sutures. If there is persistent bleeding from the tract, hemostasis is best achieved by opening the tract and individually ligating the bleeding vessels.

Ligation of an appropriate major branch of the hepatic artery (i.e., the right or left branch) while reported in the past is now rarely advocated. Lucas and Ledgerwood did not find ligation of major branches of the hepatic artery as effective in arresting hemorrhage, possibly because some of these patients were bleeding from major venous injuries. It is suggested that the right or left hepatic artery should not be ligated if a simple temporary compression pack or suturing of a bleeding injury controls the hemorrhage.

Flint and Polk reviewed their large experience with hepatic artery ligation in the management of liver trauma. Critical reanalysis of their results showed that hepatic artery ligation was actually required in only 12.4 percent of their 540 patients with liver trauma rather than in the 17 percent who actually had this procedure. They also pointed out that the unrealistic expectation that hepatic artery ligation would control venous bleeding undoubtedly led to late recognition of hepatic and portal vein injuries in patients who continued to bleed after hepatic artery ligation. In their present approach to bleeding liver lacerations, Flint and Polk initially pack the liver wound and manually compress the liver while restoring blood volume and controlling other bleeding sites. Preparations are made and the packs are removed. If bleeding recurs, the porta is occluded temporarily with a vascular clamp. If hemorrhage continues after the Pringle maneuver, the wound is repacked and a search is made for hepatic venous injury. When porta compression controls hemorrhage, the laceration is gently explored for specific bleeding sites amenable to suture ligation. After this, devitalized liver tissue is debrided and the area is drained.

The use of a pedicle of omentum as an autogenous pack to control hemorrhage in major hepatic injuries has been recommended by Stone and Lamb and by Pachter and Spencer. The omental pedicle provides the necessary bulk to fill a traumatic crevice in the liver so as to obstruct further hemorrhage without causing pressure necrosis of the surrounding hepatic parenchyma. In large liver wounds, this viable pack of omentum may eliminate dead space as well as tamponading venous oozing from the liver.

Resection. Resectional debridement or limited wedge resection is recommended to control bleeding from ragged liver injuries that may be caused by shotgun wounds, high-velocity rifle wounds, and severe blunt injuries. Limited resectional debridement of shattered liver tissue usually achieves hemostasis from such injuries effectively and safely. The margins of resectional debridement should be 2 or 3 cm beyond the point of injury, and bleeding during debridement is controlled by digital parenchymal compression and/or temporary occlusion of the inflow of blood to the liver at the porta hepatis. The liver parenchyma is separated bluntly by finger fracture, a suction tip, or a scalpel handle. Vessels and bile ducts are secured by individual suture ligation or by metal hemoclips as these structures are encountered. It is not necessary to oppose the margins of the resection with interrupted liver sutures if bleeding from the resected surface is controlled. If such hemostasis is not achieved, the omental pack referred to above may be employed.

Anatomic hepatic lobectomy to control bleeding, especially from the right lobe, is preferably reserved for patients in whom (1) hepatic suturing is unsuccessful; (2) resectional debridement or hepatotomy with intraparenchymal hemostasis is precluded by the anatomic location of the injury; (3) occlusion of the hepatic artery fails to control hemorrhage. Although resectional debridement or sublobar hepatic resection may be required in about 4 or 5 percent of all patients with liver injuries, no more than 2 or 3 percent require anatomic, lobar resection to control hemorrhage. Most of the few patients with liver injuries who require major hepatic lobectomies to control bleeding have massive, shattering injuries to the major hepatic veins at or near the junction with the vena cava (Fig. 6-18). If it becomes apparent that major lobar resection is necessary, the hepatic bleeding is temporarily controlled by manual compression of packs placed over the liver wound and by a Pringle maneuver while the midline abdominal incision is extended by performing a median sternotomy.

A median sternotomy is much more quickly and easily made and closed than a right thoracoabdominal incision, causes considerably less diaphragmatic injury, provides much easier access to the vena cava and hepatic veins, permits easier insertion of a retrohepatic vena caval shunt if this is required, and causes less postoperative pain and pulmonary morbidity than a right thoracoabdominal incision.

After wide exposure is obtained by the median sternotomy extension of the midline abdominal incision, Rumel tourniquets are placed about the vena cava superior and inferior to the liver. The superior tape is placed about the vena cava superior to the central tendon of the diaphragm after this portion of the vena cava is exposed by opening the pericardium. These tapes permit temporary occlusion of the vena cava for insertion of an intracaval shunt if vascular isolation of the liver is required during hepatic lobectomy because of major retrohepatic vena cava or major hepatic vein injury near where these veins enter the vena cava. The hepatic artery, portal vein, and bile ducts supplying the lobe to be resected are then suture-ligated and divided. After this, hepatic resection can be done by

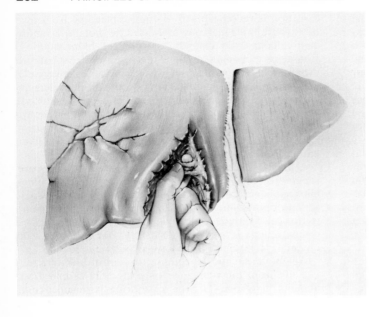

Fig. 6-18. Typical liver injury requiring hepatic resection.

dividing Glisson's capsule with a cautery along the line appropriate for the lobe being removed. The lobe is removed by fracturing through the liver substance along the line of resection with the thumb and forefinger or with the top of an abdominal suction tube from which the guard has been removed. As the blood vessels and bile ducts are encountered within the liver, they are isolated by passing a right-angle clamp around them and are then ligated and divided. After the larger vessels and ducts are suture-ligated, the smaller ones are secured with metal hemoclips. No attempt is made to secure the hepatic veins at their junction with the retrohepatic vena cava before beginning the resection; instead, it is much easier and safer to isolate and suture-ligate or oversew the appropriate major hepatic veins as they are encountered posteriorly during the liver resection. The resection begins anteriorly and progresses posteriorly toward the right or left side of the vena cava, keeping to the right or left of the middle hepatic vein (depending upon whether a right or left lobectomy is being done). The middle hepatic vein demarcates the right from the left lobe of the liver and passes in a line from the middle of the gallbladder bed posteriorly to the midportion of the retrohepatic vena cava. The hepatic veins and other large vascular structures must be oversewn, since simple ligatures on these large structures often slip off and cause catastrophic bleeding.

The Lin hepatic compression clamp may be helpful in performing resections. With the use of this clamp, there is considerable reduction in blood loss and operating time, but its availability should not cause a broadening of the strict indications for liver resection for trauma. The clamp can be used for resecting the liver only when the liver has been severely shattered and devitalized without injury to the retrohepatic vena cava or the major hepatic veins near the junction of the vena cava.

Vascular Isolation. Vascular isolation may be required in a highly selective group of patients with liver injuries.

This technique allows the surgeon to control bleeding from and to repair retrohepatic vena caval or major hepatic venous injuries. Vascular isolation of the liver is attained by using one of two techniques. The first of these techniques employs occlusive vascular clamps placed across the aorta just below the diaphragm, on the porta hepatis, and across the inferior vena cava above and below the liver. This technique may be associated with cardiac dysrhythmias and renal insufficiency. The second technique for obtaining vascular isolation of the liver was first described and reported by Schrock and associates and further successful experience with this reported by Yellin and associates. When this technique is used, retrohepatic vena caval and hepatic venous isolation is attained by inserting a #36 endotracheal tube with an inflatable balloon near the caudal end via the right atrial appendage of the heart. The tube is then passed down the retrohepatic cava and shunts blood around the liver from the lower portion of the body to the right heart. Control of vascular inflow to the liver is obtained by placing a Rumel tourniquet or vascular clamp on the porta hepatis. The introduction of the intracaval shunt via the right atrial appendage is most expeditiously done through a median sternotomy. Also, it is suggested that three equidistant "guy" sutures should be placed in the right atrial wall somewhat outside the atrial purse-string suture before making the atrial opening in the center of the purse-string suture to insert the shunt tube. These "guy" sutures are then spread apart and held up by assistants as the atrium is opened; this greatly facilitates insertion of the shunt by stabilization of the atrial wall. Defore and associates reported survival of 7 of 15 patients with major vena caval or hepatic vein injuries following vascular isolation and introduction of an intracaval shunt as described. Nevertheless, this technique is difficult and somewhat dangerous to perform and should be used only when it is certain that the vena caval and/or hepatic vein injuries are severe enough that bleeding can be controlled in no other way. In the latter instance, the shunt may be lifesaving. It is also emphasized that the results with the shunt probably can be improved if it is used promptly as soon as it becomes apparent that no other method will achieve hemostasis. In some experiences reporting poor results with the shunt, its use may have been delayed too long and the massive transfusions required in the interim may have led to an intractable coagulopathy. In reviewing 60 patients from several institutions in whom the shunt was used, Walt found a survival rate of 20 percent and very probably most of these patients would not have survived without the shunt.

Another method for controlling hemorrhage from the retrohepatic vena cava or major hepatic veins has been described by the authors. If the major venous laceration is in such a position in the suprahepatic vena cava or the extrahepatic portion of the hepatic veins, a Foley catheter may be quickly inserted into the exposed laceration. The balloon of the Foley catheter is then inflated and gently pulled up against the wall of the vena cava or hepatic vein to occlude the laceration, arrest the hemorrhage, and thus permit repair of the venous laceration with relatively good exposure and little blood loss.

It is again emphasized that these methods should not be used except by a skillful and experienced surgeon in whose judgment exsanguination will occur unless vascular isolation is carried out. If such is not the case, the temporary use of gauze packing to control intractable hemorrhage may still be indicated. A recent experience with the use of packs to control hemorrhage in patients with hepatic trauma was reported by Feliciano and associates. These surgeons recommend intraabdominal gauze packing for hepatic tamponade in patients with continued or uncontrollable hepatic parenchymal oozing despite all attempts at surgical control of extensive injuries. The packing can be removed at relaparotomy or on rare occasions through the abdominal drain site. Nine of the ten patients initially reported survived and there were no cases of rebleeding after removal of the packing. The packs were removed when their hemodynamic status was satisfactory, bleeding seemed to be under control, and other systemic problems did not preclude another general anesthetic to remove the packs. The packs are generally removed 3 to 4 days after the original operation. Feliciano and associates note that reoperation to remove the packs is not necessary, but a "second-look" operation is valuable since it permits further debridement of nonviable tissue, irrigation of the subphrenic and subhepatic spaces, and insertion of clean perihepatic drains. A warning must be given against indiscriminate packing as a primary treatment for liver injuries, as was often done with catastrophic results many years ago. In this regard, Feliciano and associates state that packing is a valuable adjunct for controlling hepatic hemorrhage in highly selected patients and should be performed early if indicated. Appropriate use of this packing technique will often preclude massive transfusions and subsequent fatal coagulopathy problems. Placing a steridrape between the liver surface and the pack has been recommended. This technical point will facilitate the removal of the pack without disturbing the hemostasis or clot formation that has been achieved at the injury site.

SUBCAPSULAR HEMATOMA. The treatment of subcapsular hematomas of the liver is somewhat controversial. Left alone, these may (1) resolve spontaneously, (2) expand and burst with delayed intraperitoneal bleeding, (3) cause a hepatic abscess, or (4) decompress into the biliary tree and cause hematobilia. The risk of inducing massive hemorrhage, at times uncontrollable, accompanies attempts at incision and evacuation.

Richie and Fonkalsrud reported a series of subcapsular hematoma patients who were treated nonoperatively. They emphasize that severe bleeding may result in some patients in whom hematomas of the liver are unroofed, and they further noted that since some hematomas are centrally located within the liver, they often do not lend themselves to resection or control by hepatic artery ligation. These authors recommended performing an emergency liver scan, although CT scans would be preferable now, on patients with probable blunt hepatic trauma who do not have persistent hemorrhage or shock and who do not have other indications for immediate laparotomy, such as positive needle paracentesis of the abdomen or positive peritoneal lavage. If the patient's condition remains stable, and a subcapsular hematoma is seen on liver scan, they recommend close observation in the hospital by means of frequent physical examinations, serial hematocrit determinations, and performance of liver function tests. The status of the hematoma is apprised by serial CT scans to be certain it is resolving and not increasing in size. Geis and associates have also reported a successful experience with the treatment of subcapsular and intrahepatic hematomas. These authors emphasize that serious sequelae of these lesions may occur approximately 1 to 28 days after injury. They also pointed out that one-quarter of their 16 patients with intrahepatic hematomas had palpable livers and all of these had large hematomas visualized by hepatic scan. Furthermore, three of the four with large hematomas had complications. Thus, they caution that a palpable liver is an ominous sign that indicates a large hematoma and a very high incidence of serious complications. Other recent favorable experiences with the nonoperative management of subcapsular hematomas of the liver have been reported by Cheatham and associates and by Lambeth and Rubin.

Emergency hepatic arteriography for patients in stable condition with probable subcapsular or intrahepatic hematomas due to blunt trauma may be used on rare occasions.

An advantage of hepatic arteriography in some stable patients with intrahepatic hematomas is that this technique can be used therapeutically as well as diagnostically. If a site of arterial hemorrhage is visualized arteriographically, the hemorrhage may be controlled nonoperatively and atraumatically by embolizing several 2-mm^2 pieces of Gelfoam through the hepatic arterial catheter. These emboli obstruct the bleeding site and prevent further bleeding.

Hematobilia. Hematobilia is caused by arterial hemorrhage into the biliary tract after liver trauma; classically it presents with a triad of findings consisting of upper or lower gastrointestinal hemorrhage, obstructing jaundice, and colicky abdominal pain. In the past, the standard treatment for this condition consisted of hepatic resection or hepatotomy with direct exposure and suture ligation of the bleeding artery. Such treatment is often associated with considerable blood loss and high operative mortality and morbidity. There are now several reports of successful management of traumatic hematobilia by ligation of the hepatic arteries supplying the involved lobe of the liver. Also, in 1976, Walter and associates first reported successful control of hematobilia by hepatic artery catheter embolization. Since that time, Heimbach and his colleagues and Perlberger have also successfully treated traumatic hematobilia with angiographic embolization.

COMPLICATIONS. Major nonfatal complications occur in approximately 20 percent of patients with liver injuries. Since the thorax is involved in many hepatic injuries, there is a high incidence of pulmonary complications. Also, the incidence of intraabdominal and perihepatic abscesses ranges from 4.5 to 20 percent. The probability of such abscess formation increases with more complex injuries of the liver and with the presence of associated colon injuries.

Patients with major lobar resections may be expected to have some postoperative bilirubin elevation, probably secondary to transient biliary obstruction by blood clots and temporary hepatic insufficiency (due to shock, loss of hepatic mass, operative trauma, and occasionally, postoperative sepsis). Hyperbilirubinemia usually disappears within about 3 weeks, with no further surgical treatment required for the relief of jaundice. Liver function studies generally show hepatic impairment but usually return to normal after several weeks. Glucose metabolism is altered after resection, and in the early postoperative period it may be necessary to give the patient supplemental glucose solutions. Studies indicate that survival is possible with only 20 percent of the normal hepatic mass, and that within 1 to 2 years, most of the resected hepatic tissue is replaced by hepatic regeneration.

Although Merendino and associates and Perry and LaFave suggested that T-tube drainage of the common bile duct should be carried out after hepatic resections, reports by Lucas and Walt and by Pinkerton and associates suggest that septic complications and bleeding from gastroduodenal stress ulcers are significantly increased by T-tube drainage. Lucas and Walt, in a well-controlled prospective study, supported the position that effective biliary decompression is not achieved by the T tube and that drainage of the common duct may increase the incidence of complications in patients with hepatic trauma, especially those due to infection and bile duct obstruction (i.e., jaundice, cholangitis, and bile duct stricture). T-tube drainage of the uninjured bile duct associated with hepatic injuries is no longer advocated.

Gallbladder

Although perforations of the gallbladder due to blunt trauma are very unusual, penetrating abdominal trauma frequently causes gallbladder injuries. Penetrating or avulsion injuries of the gallbladder are best managed by cholecystectomy, but in unstable patients with other severe injuries, when, in the surgeon's judgment, cholecystectomy is inadvisable, a tube cholecystostomy should be done, with placement of drains around the gallbladder and the subhepatic space. In general, simple suture of a gallbladder perforation is not recommended because of the probability of bile leakage. After about 4 weeks, if a patient who has had a tube cholecystostomy is doing well, a cholangiogram is performed through the cholecystostomy tube, and if this shows that the gallbladder and biliary ducts are normal, with free flow of contrast material into the duodenum, the cholecystostomy tube can be removed. Routine cholecystectomy after removal of the cholecystostomy tube in patients who have sustained gallbladder trauma is unnecessary, but it is probably advisable to perform an oral cholecystogram or sonogram several months after injury to determine the status of the gallbladder.

Extrahepatic Biliary Tree

PENETRATING INJURIES

The diagnosis of penetrating injuries of the extrahepatic biliary tree usually presents no problem as compared with the diagnosis of blunt trauma of the biliary tree, which may be difficult unless intraabdominal hemorrhage occurs. When the hepatic artery and portal vein are involved, the mortality rate is inordinately high because of massive hemorrhage that may be virtually impossible to control before irreversible hypoxic damage occurs to the brain and myocardium. Probably most patients with injuries to the extrahepatic biliary tree and one of the major vessels in the hepatoduodenal ligament do not survive to come to surgical exploration. This is especially true when the wounding agent is a large-caliber, high-velocity missile. In contrast, wounds of the gallbladder, which are seen frequently after penetrating abdominal trauma, have a low mortality rate and are not so commonly associated with injuries to the major vessels in the hepatoduodenal ligament.

While opening the abdomen, blood and bile seen issuing from the subhepatic region indicate possible injury to the biliary tree. At times, the amount of bile, blood, or contusion may be minimal, and the gallbladder, cystic duct, and hepatoduodenal structures must be carefully inspected to evaluate the significance of any subserosal hematoma or bile staining. If the patient has survived to be surgically explored, generally no massive bleeding from the subhepatic region will be noted initially. However, many times in obtaining exposure of the hepatoduodenal ligament structures, clots that have formed and tamponaded major bleeding sites may be dislodged, with recurrence of vigorous bleeding from the portal vein, hepatic artery, or their branches, which are so frequently injured when the bile ducts are injured.

Generally, the hemorrhage may be immediately arrested by lacing the fingers in the foramen of Winslow and compressing the hepatoduodenal ligament (the Pringle maneuver). Following this, after removing the free blood and obtaining good exposure while maintaining finger tamponade as above, more definitive control of the hemorrhage may be obtained by placing vascular or rubbershod clamps across all the structures in the hepatoduodenal ligament. One clamp should be placed as far distal as possible on the hepatoduodenal ligament, and this maneuver is aided by dividing the lateral serosal reflection of the duodenum and reflecting the duodenum and head of the pancreas medially. Another clamp is then placed on the hepatoduodenal ligament through the foramen of Winslow as near the liver hilus as possible.

After hemorrhage is controlled, the serosa of the hepatoduodenal ligament at the site of the hematoma formation is incised, and the disruption of the portal vein or hepatic artery is visualized by rapidly dissecting out these structures. When the defects in the major vessels are located, repair is carried out with 5-0 arterial sutures using the general principles and techniques of vascular surgery. The vascular repair should be done only after careful exposure of the defect, but also with dispatch, since the known safe occlusion period of hepatic vascular inflow is limited. As noted in the section on liver trauma, it may be possible to extend this period by giving an intravenous bolus of methylprednisolone according to Pachter and Spencer.

The management of blunt and penetrating injuries of the extrahepatic biliary tree was reviewed by Busuttil and associates who treated 21 patients with severe injuries to the porta hepatis over a 10-year period. Fourteen of these patients had bile duct injuries, eight had complete transection of the common duct, and five had a tangential or incomplete disruption with a portion of the duct wall remaining intact. Five of the eight patients who had complete transection had primary end-to-end repair with T-tube stenting, while three underwent primary Roux en Y choledochojejunostomy. All patients with incomplete disruptions had primary repairs with or without T-tube stenting. Of the five patients with complete disruptions who had primary end-to-end anastomosis of the bile duct with T-tube stenting, all required secondary biliary tract reconstruction by some type because of subsequent bile duct stricture. In contrast, no patient with complete transection treated by means of a primary Roux en Y choledochojejunostomy or choledochoduodenostomy required reoperation.

Busuttil and associates state that the most important factor in determining how to manage the bile duct injury is whether or not the duct is completely or incompletely transected. From their experience, complete transection almost always ends with stricture if the duct is primarily repaired end-to-end but has a favorable outcome if some type of duct-enteric anastomosis is done. These findings were reported by Belzer some years ago when he showed that an incomplete ductal injury could be successfully repaired by duct anastomosis or patch (vein or gallbladder graft); however, a complete division, when mobilized for primary anastomosis or patch, almost always ends in stricture Also, Longmire recommended duct-enteric anastomosis as the best method for the early treatment of injuries to the extrahepatic bile ducts.

Busuttil and his colleagues further state that if the duct has been perforated or incompletely divided, primary repair can be successfully performed. There seems to be no definitive evidence that the presence or absence of a T-tube stent makes any difference in the rate of success in these cases. However, Busuttil and associates believe that a T-tube stent should not be used if the duct is of small caliber.

If the patient is in poor condition and cannot tolerate a prolonged procedure for definitive repair of the bile duct, then the defects of the biliary duct may be repaired by simple bridging with a T tube fixed in place with a suture at either end of the ductal defect; secondary repair can then be done as soon as the patient can tolerate it. If possible, however, definitive repair should be done, since recurrent strictures are more likely after the more difficult secondary repairs of the bile ducts.

If the gallbladder and cystic duct are intact, the biliary-enteric bypass to repair a ductal injury also may be done between the gallbladder and jejunum with ligation of the distal and proximal limbs of the damaged common duct. Also, it may be more expedient at times to use a simple loop of jejunum instead of a Roux en Y limb to perform the bypass procedure.

BLUNT TRAUMA

Blunt trauma to the biliary tree deserves separate discussion, not because the surgical management differs, but because of its relative rarity and difficulty of diagnosis. Soderstrom and associates reported that through December 1979, there were 101 patients with gallbladder injuries due to blunt abdominal trauma reported in the English literature. This included 31 patients from their own experience; these 31 patients represented 2.1 percent of 1349 patients who had blunt intraabdominal injuries from 1973 through 1979 at the Maryland Institute for Emergency Medical Services System. The usual mechanism of closed injury to the extrahepatic biliary tree is a shearing force applied to the common duct.

When blunt trauma to the biliary tree is severe enough to result in a free flow of bile into the peritoneal cavity, the characteristic picture of bile peritonitis occurs. According to Sturmer and Wilt, the usual history involves a crushing injury to the right upper quadrant, the epigastrium, or the lower part of the chest, which results in severe pain and may be followed by shock. Bile or nonclotting blood may be found on peritoneal tap or lavage.

Shock is usually secondary to the marked outpouring of extracellular fluid into the peritoneal cavity due to the chemical irritation of the peritoneum by bile. The initial chemical peritonitis caused by bile may be followed shortly after by bacterial peritonitis. If biliary leakage is minimal, shock may be of relatively short duration or may be absent, and abdominal signs initially may be slight. This may be followed by the recovery and well-being of the patient, which may last for periods up to 5 or 10 days. However, the onset of jaundice on about the third day is a fairly constant sign. The appearance of clay-colored stools and the presence of bile in the urine may be noticed from the second to the fifth day after injury of the duct.

Carmichael reported that of 12 deaths due to common duct avulsion, delay in surgical treatment of the 22 survivors following common bile duct avulsion averaged 9 days.

A gradual increase in abdominal size may occur during the first 10 days that may be unattended by the usual signs of peritonitis in patients with bile duct rupture. This increasing abdominal girth is accompanied by progressive signs of extracellular fluid volume deficit and by evidence of infection manifest by fever and leukocytosis. In the reported cases of transection of the common duct, the site of transection was uniformly in the retroduodenal area of the superior margin of the pancreas. This serves to emphasize the importance of extensive medial reflection of the duodenum to explore the retroperitoneal duodenum as well as the distal common duct and pancreas in patients undergoing celiotomy for blunt abdominal trauma.

In reviewing the surgical treatment of the 34 patients reported to have blunt injuries of the common bile duct, Carmichael notes that 9 of the earlier patients were treated by simple external drainage and 7 of these 9 patients died. Of the two survivors of simple drainage, choledochoduodenostomy was required for stricture 2½ months after injury in one and a primary repair of a stricture was done later in the other. Thus, simple drainage is unwise because of the high mortality and high stricture rate associated with this method of treatment. Although many surgeons recommend primary end-to-end repair, three developed strictures and one of these died with cholangitis and cirrhosis. Moreover, T-tube stents were used in the initial repair of the duct in all three of the patients who developed strictures after end-to-end reconstruction. Longmire has stated that primary repair of the common duct should be attempted only if there is an adequate lumen, no inflammation, and a short injured segment of the duct. Carmichael advocates choledochoduodenostomy when the distal duct is unsuitable for primary repair or is missing. Of eight choledochoduodenostomies in his review, all did well except one, who required a cholecystojejunostomy to reestablish bile flow. No duodenal fistulae occurred. Choledochojejunostomy with or without a Roux en Y jejunal limb was done in six patients, and all of these did well. Finally, Carmichael reported that cholecystoenterostomy was done in seven cases, with ligation of the distal bile duct. This operation was associated with one death and two revisions.

Thus, Carmichael concluded that the most successful procedures in reconstruction of the avulsed common bile duct are Roux en Y choledochojejunostomy or choledochoduodenostomy. Choledochojejunostomy offers a better exposure if a future operation is required, a tension-free anastomosis, and a technically easier mucosa-to-mucosa anastomosis. Also, this procedure avoids the lateral duodenal fistula that may occur after choledochoduodenostomy.

The postoperative therapy of biliary tract injuries, in which bile peritonitis is an important complicating feature, should include adequate replacement of extracellular fluid volume deficits, which may require intravenous infusion of several liters of balanced salt solutions in 24 h.

These solutions should be given as soon as possible preoperatively and continued throughout the surgical procedure and postoperatively to avoid extracellular fluid volume deficit. Broad-spectrum antibiotics should be given before the surgical procedure and continued during the operation and postoperatively until the chances of sepsis diminish.

The overall mortality in the collected series of common duct injuries reported by Carmichael was 35 percent; however, the mortality from biliary tract injuries probably should be below 5 to 10 percent if they are discovered early and treated appropriately.

Portal Vein

Approximately 90 percent of portal vein injuries occur because of penetrating trauma. They are frequently associated with other visceral injuries, most commonly to the inferior vena cava, liver, pancreas, and stomach. Mattox and associates reported a survival rate of 50 percent in their series of 22 patients with portal vein injuries. Lateral venorrhaphy, if possible, is the preferred method of treatment. Mattox suggests performing a portacaval or mesocaval shunt as an alternative treatment of portal vein injury if suture repair is impossible and patient's general condition is stable. In contrast, Fish reported that four of five patients who had portacaval shunts for portal vein reconstruction after trauma developed hepatic decompensation or encephalopathy, whereas those complications were not observed in patients undergoing portal vein ligation.

The insertion of an autogenous vein graft to bridge the defect in the portal vein (using the left common iliac vein, left renal vein, or a paneled saphenous vein graft) may be preferable to a portacaval shunt if the patient's condition is stable and the proximal and distal ends of the injured vein are suitable for the insertion of a graft. This procedure should prevent portal hypertension or hepatic deterioration that may occur if the vein is ligated. However, if associated injuries are severe, ligation of the portal vein may make it possible to save the patient. Even though portal vein ligation may cause portal hypertension, interruption of the vein is compatible with patient's survival in about 80 percent of the cases. It should, of course, be emphasized that in those with associated hepatic arterial injuries, a good repair of the hepatic artery must be achieved before accepting treatment of portal vein injuries by ligation. It has been reported recently that 80 percent of 20 patients survived portal vein ligation when lateral venorrhaphy was not possible. However, because of obstruction to portal outflow, acute splanchnic hypervolemia develops simultaneously with peripheral hypovolemia. Patients have died of such splanchnic pooling after portal vein ligation. Since this problem has been appreciated, these patients have been followed closely with either central venous or pulmonary artery pressure measurements to maintain a functionally normal peripheral blood volume. This may require overtransfusions of a volume of blood almost equal to the patient's own normal blood volume.

Pancreas

Ronald C. Jones and G. Tom Shires

Travers described the first pancreatic injury found in an intoxicated woman who was struck by a stage coach wheel in England in 1827. Approximately 70 percent of pancreatic injuries are caused by penetrating and 30 percent result from blunt trauma. Between 1950 and 1985, 500 patients were initially treated for penetrating and blunt pancreatic trauma at Parkland Memorial Hospital (PMH) in Dallas.

DIAGNOSIS. Diagnosis of pancreatic injuries is based upon a complete history, including the mechanism of injury, thorough physical examination, serum amylase level, and adequate visualization of the pancreas at surgical exploration.

Following isolated blunt pancreatic trauma, symptoms are often mild and delayed and physical signs may be absent or minimal. Usually, however, there is at least mild upper abdominal tenderness, but in the absence of a history of significant trauma or severe symptoms, this sign may be overlooked. Injuries to retroperitoneal organs such as the pancreas may not produce clinical findings of loss of bowel sounds, tenderness, guarding, or spasm for several hours.

Computed tomography of the abdomen may become the most specific method of diagnosing organ injury preoperatively, particularly following blunt trauma. It should not take the place of a good physical examination or close follow-up observation.

Serum Amylase Determination. Over 25 years ago, Matthewson and Halter advocated routine serum amylase determinations in patients sustaining blunt trauma and emphasized that pancreatic injury was more common than had been previously appreciated. Serum amylase elevation alone is not an indication for exploratory celiotomy. If signs of peritonitis are present (such as spasm, tenderness, and absent bowel sounds), then a celiotomy is performed. Unrecognized severe pancreatic injury can be a fatal lesion, particularly when it is accompanied by disruption of pancreatic tissue and leakage of pancreatic juice.

Many patients have been found to have an elevated serum amylase level but negative abdominal findings. These patients are closely observed for evidence of peritonitis or until the amylase level returns to normal. An amylase determination is performed on peritoneal lavage fluid, but the elevation is more often due to small bowel injury than to pancreatic injury.

Sometimes the serum amylase is elevated in less than 2 h following injury, but the longer the delay from injury to surgery, the more likely an elevation. A preoperative serum amylase determination was performed in 270 patients in the PMH study. Only 16 percent of the patients had preoperative elevations of serum amylase following penetrating trauma and 61 percent of patients had an elevation following blunt trauma. Even with complete transection of pancreas only 65 percent of the patients had elevated serum amylase levels. Berni noted that the serum amylase level was elevated in two-thirds of their patients with blunt trauma compared with 10 percent of those with penetrating pancreatic injury. Amylase determinations may be misleading. Olsen stated that 33 percent of patients with hyperamylasemia had no significant intraabdominal trauma, and no patient in his series with hyperamylasemia had significant intraabdominal injury without other evidence of trauma. He reemphasized that hyperamylasemia alone without any other evidence of visceral injury is not an indication for exploratory celiotomy. Serum amylase is not a reliable indicator of pancreatic injury. The serum amylase is indicated as a diagnostic test following blunt trauma but is of no benefit following penetrating trauma and thus is not cost-effective. Though these various reports show that it is unwise to perform exploratory celiotomy on the basis of elevated amylase levels alone, the detection of hyperamylasemia in asymptomatic patients who have sustained abdominal trauma cannot simply be dismissed. These patients are admitted to the hospital and closely observed. Plain abdominal x-ray films may show evidence of retroperitoneal trauma. This is suspected when there is obliteration of the psoas margin, retroperitoneal air along a psoas margin or around the upper pole of the right kidney, or displacement of the stomach.

Since pancreatic injury is relatively uncommon it has been difficult to assess the true value of CT scan in preoperative diagnosis of transection of the pancreatic duct. Cook reported CT findings in 20 patients who subsequently underwent laparotomy or autopsy. In three patients a CT diagnosis of pancreatic contusion or traumatic pseudocyst was surgically proved; in four other patients the CT diagnosis was pancreatic contusion; however, at surgery the pancreas was normal. The CT can document gross pancreatic injury demonstrating parenchymal disruption, focal or diffuse enlargement, and peripancreatic fluid collection. The majority of missed diagnoses is due to unopacified bowel loops adjacent to the pancreas that may be mistaken for focal pancreatic swelling. Peripancreatic hematoma from trauma to the spleen, left kidney, and streak artifacts are other causes for diagnostic errors. Nasogastric tubes should be retracted to the gastroesophageal junction to more readily visualize the pancreas. Jeffrey correctly diagnosed 11 of 13 pancreatic injuries. However, three represented delayed diagnosis with pseudocysts formation. There were two false-negative results in the remaining 10 patients who had pancreatic fractures. Thus, 20 percent of acute pancreatic injuries were missed.

As more experience is gained with endoscopic retrograde pancreatography, it is possible that this technique may have a role in the diagnosis of pancreatic injury. Gougeon advocated transduodenal pancreatography using the fiberoptic duodenoscope intraoperatively to determine ductal injury. Taxier utilized endoscopic retrograde pancreatography to evaluate the pancreas after trauma, but primarily in patients with delayed diagnosis of pancreas injury. Emergency endoscopic retrograde cholangiopancreatography would require expertise and rapid availability to be of value in the critically ill patient.

Surgical Exploration. When preoperative diagnostic

studies indicate a probability of pancreatic injury, it is necessary to visualize the entire pancreas. The head of the pancreas and the duodenum are completely mobilized to the midline by performing a Kocher maneuver. The gastrocolic omentum is also divided in order to enter the lesser sac and view the entire body of the pancreas.

Any retroperitoneal hematoma in the upper part of the abdomen or a peripancreatic hematoma should be considered presumptive evidence of pancreatic injury and should be explored. Over 60 percent of patients sustaining penetrating trauma have an associated retroperitoneal injury, but pancreatic injury occurs in only 20 percent of patients following blunt trauma.

ASSOCIATED INJURIES. Isolated pancreatic injury is rare following penetrating trauma but occurs in 20 percent of blunt injuries. Associated injuries are usually more obvious indications for surgical exploration than suspected pancreatic injury. Death and serious complications are frequent in pancreatic trauma but are rarely caused by the pancreatic injury. Although the pancreas is a vascular organ, it is not often responsible for uncontrollable hemorrhage. When profuse bleeding occurs from the pancreatic area, the pancreas is mobilized and the superior mesenteric and the splenic vessels, the aorta, and the vena cava are inspected, since they are often the source of severe hemorrhage. Because of the location of the pancreas, injuries to the liver and the stomach are frequent following penetrating trauma whereas liver and spleen are more commonly injured following blunt trauma.

MANAGEMENT. Drainage. After bleeding from the pancreas or from adjacent major blood vessels is controlled, the extent of the pancreatic injury is determined. Simple pancreatic contusions without capsular or ductal disruption and without persistent hemorrhage require no suturing or debridement. These injuries are drained with a sump drain placed directly at the site of the pancreatic contusion and brought out along a short, direct tract at the tip of the twelfth rib. The drains are left in place for 10 days, since several patients have been observed to have minimal pancreatic drainage for up to 7 days and then have significant increase in drainage. Lack of drainage to such areas of unrecognized capsular injury may lead to complications associated with intraabdominal collections of pancreatic secretions such as pseudocysts, pancreatic abscesses, and lesser-sac abscesses. Simple drainage is a satisfactory method of management in 75 percent of patients sustaining either stab or gunshot wounds. In the last 100 patients evaluated for septic complications, 9 percent had an associated infection of the drain tract. As a result of this septic complication and intraabdominal abscess formation, closed sump drainage is now utilized in favor of combined Penrose and sump drainage. However, there are few data to support this conclusion.

Fistulae may develop following pancreatic contusion and 4 of the 10 fistulae that drained for greater than 1 month in the PMH series followed contusion injuries.

Distal Pancreatectomy. The most effective method of treatment for pancreatic injuries with obvious disruption of the pancreatic duct in the body or tail of the gland is distal pancreatectomy. This is performed at the point where the main duct is injured, and allows removal of the traumatized and devitalized tissue.

When performing a distal pancreatectomy, sutures are placed in the superior and inferior borders of the pancreas approximately 1.5 to 2 cm from the edge. This, along with isolation of the splenic vessels during distal pancreatectomy, prevents unnecessary blood loss and probably provides better visualization. In resecting the distal pancreas, the cut edge is beveled in a fish-mouth fashion. This enables a better closure of the proximal end of the pancreas. The transected duct of Wirsung in the remaining proximal gland is ligated with a transfixion suture of fine monofilament, nonabsorbable material such as Prolene, to discourage fistula formation. The cut surface of the transected proximal pancreas is oversewn with interrupted, interlocking mattress sutures, which facilitates hemostasis. The auto stapler has been used with excellent results. This method of management provides hemostasis and prevents fistula formation. The stump of the pancreas is extensively drained with a sump drain.

Most patients sustaining a stab or gunshot wound do not require surgical resection. A conservative approach in the absence of proved ductal injury results in a low mortality. Liberal use of resective debridement for only possible ductal injury contributes to a higher mortality. Simple drainage of the pancreas is the treatment of choice for most penetrating injuries, particularly in the unstable patient.

During the past 5 years less than 10 percent of patients at PMH have undergone distal pancreatectomy for penetrating and blunt trauma. Approximately 25 percent of patients undergoing a distal pancreatectomy develop an intraabdominal abscess.

Pseudocysts almost never develop following distal pancreatectomy and sump drainage. Approximately 10 percent of patients managed by distal pancreatectomy die usually secondary to sepsis and associated injuries. One disadvantage to distal pancreatectomy is the frequent iatrogenic associated splenic injury necessitating splenectomy. Patients who are extremely unstable and who have pancreatic injury can always be managed conservatively with drainage alone and if they survive the pancreatic injury can be managed at a later date. Four patients in the PMH series died intraoperatively while undergoing distal pancreatectomy, two of whom could have been managed with drainage. Some patients who initially appear to have pancreatic duct damage may do well with drainage alone, and obviously the suspected ductal injury has not occurred.

The integrity of the pancreatic duct can be determined by opening the duodenum and performing a pancreatogram or performing a distal pancreatectomy with pancreatogram. These diagnostic procedures are rarely indicated, particularly if the duodenum is intact and if the spleen is uninjured. Iatrogenic splenic injury associated with distal pancreatectomy is common. If pancreatic ductal injury is doubtful, simple drainage is performed. In an unstable patient with questionable ductal injury, drainage is the treatment of choice.

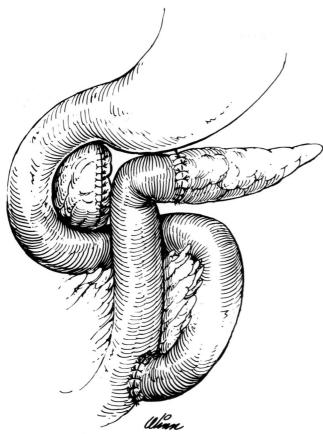

Fig. 6-19. Technique of Roux en Y anastomosis to the transected body of the pancreas.

Roux en Y Pancreaticojejunostomy. Several methods of treating pancreatic transection have been described. For the pancreas completely transected over the superior mesenteric vessels and to the right of these vessels, a Roux en Y anastomosis to the distal pancreas with oversew of the end of the proximal segment may be used, particularly if the spleen is not injured (Fig. 6-19). This treatment has been recommended by Jones and Shires for treatment of injuries that require removal of 80 percent or more of the pancreas. Transections of less magnitude are treated by simple distal pancreatectomy. This method leaves all functioning pancreatic tissue, thereby avoiding the possibility of pancreatic insufficiency or diabetes. The risk of injury to the underlying splenic vessels is less with this mode of treatment than with resection. The possibility of fistula and pseudocyst formation is also minimized.

The Roux en Y anastomosis is accomplished using permanent sutures placed approximately 1 cm apart in a single-layer anastomosis. Once this anastomosis is accomplished, drainage is established with sump drains. Unless the completely severed pancreatic duct is managed with definitive surgery, a pseudocyst or fistula will almost always result. A Roux en Y anastomosis to one fragment of the severed pancreas is little more time-consuming than resection of the distal fragment, which often requires a splenectomy.

PANCREATIC INSUFFICIENCY. The normal pancreas is approximately 12 to 15 cm in length. Eleven patients in the Parkland Memorial Hospital series required 80 percent or more resection; three of these patients required from 35 to 100 units of insulin per day and an additional three patients had elevated blood sugar levels and abnormal glucose tolerance tests. A twelfth patient underwent a pancreaticoduodenectomy and developed pancreatic insufficiency and blood glucose elevations in excess of 500 mg/dL. Roux en Y drainage is considered only for patients who would otherwise require 80 percent or more resection of the distal pancreas which fortunately is an uncommon injury. Although implantation of both ends of the pancreas is no longer used at PMH, a modification described by Letton and Wilson remains an alternative; pancreaticojejunostomy may not be indicated when there is associated colonic contamination. Several authors have reported pancreatic insufficiency and diabetes as complications of extensive pancreatic resection.

Complete Transection. Approximately two-thirds of the patients with complete transection of the pancreas will have a preoperative elevation of serum amylase. The majority of patients are managed with distal pancreatectomy; however, the occasional patient without splenic trauma can be managed with a Roux en Y anastomosis to the distal portion of the pancreas. This anastomosis is not performed in the presence of colonic contamination or if the pancreas has poor consistency and will not securely hold sutures. If the surgeon is not accustomed to pancreatic anastomosis, a distal pancreatectomy may be a wiser choice.

Isolated Pancreatic Injuries. Isolated pancreatic injuries occurred in over 20 percent of patients sustaining blunt trauma in the PMH series and none died, although six had complete transections. There were eight penetrating injuries and none of these patients died. This supports the conclusion that pancreatic injury is rarely the cause of death.

Combined Duodenum and Pancreatic Injuries. Over 20 percent of penetrating pancreatic injuries are associated with duodenal trauma, but less than 10 percent of blunt injuries have duodenal trauma. The mortality for combined pancreaticoduodenal trauma is 20 percent, mostly from associated injuries, but excluding intraoperative deaths the mortality is only 15 percent.

These injuries are usually managed by drainage of the pancreas and suture of the duodenum. A duodenostomy tube may be inserted, but it is difficult to demonstrate that this decreases morbidity or mortality. Duodenal fistula following duodenostomy tube insertion was higher than without duodenostomy, but more severe injuries were treated with a duodenostomy tube.

Pyloric exclusion has been used by Vaughan resulting in only a 5 percent duodenal fistula rate. Berne diverticulization has been advocated for moderately severe injuries and pancreaticoduodenectomy for the most extensive injuries. Most patients in the PMH series with combined pancreaticoduodenal injuries treated with

Berne diverticularization have had major complications, such as duodenal, biliary, and pancreatic fistula with sepsis and death. Indications for Berne diverticulization have not been clearly delineated. Pyloric exclusion is a simpler and less time-consuming operation and prevents duodenal fistula formation.

Pancreaticoduodenectomy. Pancreaticoduodenectomy has been reported as a method of management in approximately 120 patients in over 30 series in the literature with a mortality rate of 30 percent following penetrating injuries and over 20 percent following blunt trauma for a combined mortality rate of 25 percent. Strict indications for pancreaticoduodenectomy include combined pancreaticoduodenal injuries in which the duodenum cannot be repaired or is not viable or there is uncontrollable hemorrhage from the pancreas. In the presence of colonic injuries, intraabdominal abscess is frequent. Prior to performing a pancreaticoduodenectomy the presence of a pancreatic ductal injury should be verified. With duodenal rupture cannulation of the pancreatic duct with pancreatogram is easily performed. An alternative method of determining ductal injury is by mobilizing the tail of the pancreas and performing a pancreatogram through the distal pancreatic duct. Hemostatic sutures are placed 2 cm into the superior and inferior portions of the pancreas prior to incising the tail. The common duct is identified and proved to be intact by operative cholangiogram or by passing a catheter through the common duct and into the duodenum. If the common bile duct and major duct system are intact and the duodenal injury can be closed, a pancreaticoduodenectomy is not indicated. Avulsion of the common duct from the duodenum with avascular duodenal wall, and stellate fracture with bleeding from a crushing injury of the head of the pancreas may be indications for pancreaticoduodenectomy. The overall condition of the patient and associated injuries must be considered prior to submitting the patient to several more hours of surgery. There are times when this procedure is necessary, but they are rare, particularly if the duodenum is intact. Complications following pancreaticoduodenectomy are common. Thus mortality rate of this procedure must be low to justify its use if any other form of management can be employed.

In addition to fistula formation and abscesses, marginal ulceration with upper gastrointestinal bleeding has occurred following pancreaticoduodenectomy in which a vagotomy or subtotal gastric resection was not performed. Symptoms of dumping, diabetes, and weight loss with diarrhea have occurred following pancreaticoduodenectomy for trauma. Postoperative bleeding into the intestinal tract from the pancreaticojejunostomy requiring reoperation has been reported.

COMPLICATIONS. Complications following pancreatic trauma include fistula, pancreatic abscesses, vascular necrosis with hemorrhage from the drain site, pseudocyst formation, and intestinal fistula secondary to suture line breakdown from pancreatic juice activation.

Fistula. Most pancreatic fistulae are minor and close within a period of 1 month. Major pancreatic fistulae have been arbitrarily defined as those which drain longer than 1 month. The frequency of pancreatic fistulae depends on definition, and the rate is higher if defined as drainage for 1 week rather than 1 month. The serum amylase level is frequently elevated while the fistula is present, probably because of transperitoneal absorption. Almost all pancreatic fistulae will eventually spontaneously close; therefore, treatment is conservative. Attention must be given to preventing autodigestion of the surrounding skin.

Many patients with pancreatic fistulae can continue oral intake of food, especially if the fistula drains less than 500 mL each day and the volume does not increase significantly when the patient eats. In the presence of large-volume pancreatic fistulae, it is preferable to institute intravenous hyperalimentation. Intravenous hyperalimentation has two beneficial effects on such patients: (1) It maintains excellent nutrition and nitrogen balance without stimulating the pancreas, as do oral feedings; and (2) intravenous hyperalimentation can significantly reduce the volume of pancreatic exocrine secretion by one-half or more.

Pseudocyst. A pancreatic pseudocyst is a false cyst the wall of which is inflammatory fibrous tissue that does not contain epithelium but is made of those structures surrounding the region of the pancreas in the retroperitoneum. The most frequent symptoms associated with a pancreatic pseudocyst are an abdominal mass, pain, nausea, and vomiting. The serum amylase level may be elevated for a long time prior to this diagnosis. Diagnosis is by sonography or computed tomography. The pseudocyst rarely spontaneously resolves. Pancreatic pseudocyst is now a rare complication following pancreatic trauma if the pancreas has been explored and managed appropriately, such management including adequate drainage. The preferred method of draining pancreatic pseudocysts is internally by either cyst gastrostomy or Roux en Y cyst jejunostomy.

Sepsis. Intraabdominal abscess is a common complication following multiple abdominal trauma and is the second most common cause of death. Although pancreatic fistulae rarely cause death, they occasionally give rise to lesser-sac abscesses and subphrenic abscess. Subphrenic abscess is frequently associated with injuries to the liver, spleen, and colon. The location of a right or left subdiaphragmatic abscess is predictable in most patients depending on whether the associated injury was to the spleen or to the liver. A lesser-sac abscess may contribute to either sepsis or retroperitoneal bleeding and death. In almost all patients in whom the pancreatic injury contributes to death, there is association with severe sepsis. Sepsis usually is associated with duodenal and colonic fistula, renal failure, and occasionally pulmonary embolus. Cultures of the abscess grow a predominance of mixed gram-negative organisms; however, staphylococci and enterococci may be present. The serum amylase level is not consistently elevated in patients with a pancreatic or lesser-sac abscess. The method of management of pancreatic abscess consists of adequate debridement and drainage, frequently with gastrostomy and feeding jejunostomy.

Hemorrhagic pancreatitis may present with massive

Table 6-6. PANCREATIC TRAUMA, 1950–1984

	Pt	*Died*	*Mortality, %*
Penetrating			
Stab	76	4	5
Gunshot	252	55	22
Shotgun	34	19	56
Blunt	138	26	19
Total	500	104	21

SOURCE: Jones RC: Management of pancreatic trauma. *Am J Surg* 150:698, 1985, with permission.

bleeding from the drain tract, probably from erosion of ligated retroperitoneal vessels.

Mortality. The mortality rate caused by pancreatic injury is variable and is chiefly related to hemorrhage from major blood vessels. The mortality following stab wounds is 5 percent, gunshot wounds 22 percent, and blunt trauma 19 percent (Table 6-6).

Recognition of pancreatic injury at the time of initial surgical exploration is the key to decreasing the morbidity rate of pancreatic injury. It is best accomplished by opening the lesser sac through the gastrocolic ligament and directly visualizing the pancreas. There are several reasons why the pancreatic injury appears not to be the cause of death. The mortality for isolated pancreatic injury is less than 1 percent. Patients developing shock following injury have a 40 percent mortality in association with pancreatic trauma whereas the normotensive patient with pancreatic injury had a 4 percent mortality, and no patient with an isolated pancreatic injury in the PMH series died. The mortality rate due to the pancreatic injury in the multiply injured patient is less than 3 percent.

SUMMARY. The majority of patients who sustain pancreatic injury can be managed with sump drainage including most with gunshot wounds to the head of the pancreas. Pancreaticoduodenectomy may be indicated in 2 to 3 percent. Patients who require resection of 80 percent or more of the pancreas and do not have splenic injuries should be considered for a Roux en Y anastomosis to the distal pancreas after ductal injury has been proved. The severity of injury often dictates the appropriate treatment. A conservative approach is indicated for most pancreatic injuries, resulting in shorter operating time and less blood loss in the unstable patient with multiple injuries. Most important is identification of ductal injury at the initial operation and institution of surgical drainage.

Spleen

The spleen is the abdominal organ most frequently injured by blunt trauma: such injuries to the spleen represent approximately one-quarter of all blunt injuries of the abdominal viscera. The spleen also is often injured by penetrating abdominal trauma and is frequently associated with blunt and penetrating thoracoabdominal injuries.

DIAGNOSIS. The diagnosis of splenic injury is usually easily made with penetrating trauma but is often more difficult in patients sustaining blunt trauma. The clinical manifestations are the systemic symptoms and signs of hemorrhage and local evidence of peritoneal irritation in the region of the spleen. Only about 30 to 40 percent of patients with splenic injury present with a systolic blood pressure below 100 mmHg. However, many patients with splenic trauma may develop hypotension and tachycardia when assuming the sitting position. A tender abdomen with guarding and distention is apparent in only about 50 to 60 percent of those patients with splenic rupture.

A history of injury, which may be seemingly slight, followed by abdominal pain, predominantly in the left upper quadrant, left shoulder pain, and syncope is very significant. Often the left shoulder pain, or Kehr's sign, occurs only when the patient is in a supine or head-down position. This is caused by irritation of the inferior surface of the left side of the diaphragm by free blood or blood clots. Elevation of the foot of the bed or pressure in the left subcostal region may occasionally reproduce pain at the top of the left shoulder. Ballance's sign, which refers to fixed dullness to percussion in the left flank and dullness in the right flank that disappears on change of position of the patient, thus indicating large quantities of clot in the perisplenic region and free blood in the remainder of the peritoneal cavity, may be helpful in establishing the diagnosis. Whereas a decreased or falling hematocrit, leukocytosis of more than 15,000, x-ray findings such as fractures of the left lower ribs, gastric displacement, loss of splenic outline, and splinting or elevation of the left diaphragm are useful diagnostic findings, they are frequently absent.

Abdominal paracentesis and diagnostic peritoneal lavage are extremely helpful in establishing the diagnosis in doubtful cases, particularly in patients whose sensibility is obtunded by other injuries. In patients with splenic trauma the incidence of false-negative diagnostic peritoneal lavage is reported, in repeated series, to be less than 1 percent.

Radionuclide scans are occasionally used to detect splenic injury and to follow patients who are treated by either nonoperative therapy or one of the many splenic preservation procedures. Computerized tomography is now a preferable procedure and has essentially replaced the nuclear scans for this purpose as a diagnostic aid. It is an accurate, simple way to diagnose subcapsular hematomas and more extensive transcapsular lacerations. Jeffrey et al. reported correct interpretation in 49 of the first 50 patients studied with 28 true-negatives and 21 of 22 true-positives being identified.

Delayed rupture of the spleen was first described by Baudet in 1902, and the asymptomatic interval between abdominal injury and rupture of the spleen is known as the latent period of Baudet. It was postulated that bleeding appeared several days after injury because (1) a subcapsular splenic hematoma gradually increased in size until it caused a delayed rupture of the splenic capsule and intraperitoneal hemorrhage or (2) there was initial bleeding from a splenic laceration that ceased spontaneously but began again in several days or weeks when the perisplenic hematoma became dislodged. This concept has been challenged by Olsen and Polley and by Benjamin and associates. These authors report a rate of delayed rupture of the spleen of less than 1 percent in over 600 patients. They suggest that delayed splenic rupture is an unusual occurrence and that the 15 percent incidence reported in older papers actually represents a delay in diagnosis rather than a delayed rupture in those patients.

TREATMENT. King and Shumacker in 1952 reported that all five patients under six months who had splenectomies developed meningitis or overwhelming septicemia. Two of these five patients died. This observation stimulated further investigation followed by considerable confusion and contradictory remarks into the relationship between splenectomy and what was later termed overwhelming postsplenectomy infection (OPSI). This syndrome is characterized by an abrupt onset of overwhelming sepsis, massive bacteremia, usually pneumococcal, followed by early death.

Eraklis and Filler reported a mortality rate of 0.8 percent in 342 patients under age sixteen who had splenectomy for trauma. Singer reviewed 23 series from the literature including 2795 patients. The risk of sepsis was 1.45 percent in the 688 patients (300 adults) who had splenectomy for trauma. Only four of these patients died for a mortality rate of 0.58 percent. This has been compared with the general population where a death rate due to sepsis is estimated at 0.01 percent. This comparison is not accurate as the two groups are dissimilar by virtue of the fact the former group have all sustained some type of trauma and undergone an operative procedure that is not accounted for in the control group.

O'Neal and McDonald reported a mortality rate of 2.7 percent in a series of 356 adult patients. There were no fatalities in the 115 patients with splenectomy for trauma. All of the deaths in the series occurred in patients whose spleen was removed in conjunction with other nontraumatic elective procedures or patients with proved malignancies.

The literature supporting this syndrome in the adult trauma patient is increasing but still is not as convincing as for pediatric and nontrauma patients. Nevertheless, stimulated by these and many other reports describing the immunologic abnormalities and pathophysiology of the overwhelming sepsis syndrome, a more conservative approach has evolved concerning the management of splenic trauma. Nonoperative therapy in the pediatric age group has been advocated by Aronson et al., Ein et al., and others. This approach has several distressing aspects. In assessing the patient with multiple trauma one cannot assume the spleen is the only injured organ; hence other injuries may be missed in as many as 30 percent of patients. Nonoperative therapy requires a prolonged hospitalization that is generally accomplished in an intensive care unit. Other drawbacks include a prolonged convalescence, increased hospital cost, and risk and complications associated with repeated blood transfusions, such as delayed autoimmune disease.

Based upon an extensive review of the literature, Luna

and Dellinger concluded that the 1 to 2 percent incidence figures for postsplenectomy infection represented a 10- to 20-fold overestimation of the true incidence. These authors quoted a 60 percent success rate in three series of nonoperative observation in adults who were initially stable without evidence of blood loss. Ninety-three percent of the patients who failed nonoperative management required a splenectomy, suggesting that splenic salvage rates were not improved by nonoperative observation when the initial injury was felt to be relatively minor.

Luna further states it has been estimated that 35 to 40 percent of patients who are successfully observed will require a blood transfusion that averages 40 to 50 percent of their blood volume. Although symptoms may occur in only 50 percent of patients with non-A non-B hepatitis and only 20 percent become icteric, it is estimated that the per unit risk for a single unit transfusion may approach 3 percent. The posttransfusion hepatitis death rate per unit of blood transfused is 0.14 percent.

Proper management of patients with splenic injuries is still controversial, and continued reevaluation of data is necessary. It is possible that failure of nonoperative therapy frequently results in splenectomy rather than splenorraphy (the preferable procedure) and the increased incidence of blood transfusion with its attendant disease transmission problems may outweigh any theoretic advantages of avoiding surgery. Luna and Dellinger also concluded that in adults 0.26 percent of the observed patients die (0.17 percent for pediatric patients) compared with 0.06 percent for those operated upon initially.

A more rational approach to the problem is splenic preservation in carefully selected patients at the time of operation. The procedures include (1) no therapy for nonbleeding capsular lacerations, (2) application of microfibrillar collagen or other hemostatic agents to minor lacerations with minimal bleeding, (3) suture repair of more extensive injuries, (4) partial splenectomy for splenic injuries that do not involve the hilus. Contraindications to splenic salvage procedures as recommended by Traub include (1) patient instability secondary to major associated injuries, (2) splenic avulsion or extensive fragmentation, (3) extensive hilar vascular injury, (4) failure to attain splenic hemostasis. Relative contraindications include significant peritoneal contamination from concomitant bowel injury and rupture of a diseased spleen.

Increasing experimental data and clinical evidence indicate that an intact spleen is required to produce important opsonic antibodies that are necessary for optimal function of the macrophage system and production of immunoglobulins. Sepsis is a rather frequent occurrence following splenectomy for certain hematologic disorders, many of which have diffuse reticuloendothelial abnormalities. Many of these patients, however, receive various forms of therapy that alter immunity and response to infection. Splenectomy is still a safe procedure and the indicated procedure of choice in many patients.

OPERATIVE TECHNIQUE (See Chap. 33). Although drainage of the splenic bed following elective splenectomy is controversial, there is little question that drainage should be employed when splenectomy is performed under most emergency conditions. The incidence of drain tract infections and subphrenic abscess has been reported to be as high as 25 to 50 percent when drains were used, in contrast to 5 to 12 percent when drains were not employed. Many of these infections, however, were related to the presence of associated injuries, usually in the gastrointestinal tract, or to the immunologic defects often present in patients requiring splenectomies for conditions other than trauma, and not to the drains per se. The routine use of drains following splenectomy for trauma is supported by the series reported by Naylor and Shires. These authors reported an incidence of subphrenic abscess of only 3.4 percent in 408 patients undergoing splenectomy for trauma. Among the 72 patients who had splenectomy for trauma involving the spleen alone, there were no subphrenic abscesses and an incidence of drain tract infection of only 1.3 percent. Thus, while it cannot be proved that drainage of the splenic bed after splenectomy for trauma reduces the incidence of subphrenic collections, it is most probable that drainage in such cases does not increase the incidence of subphrenic abscess. Also in those instances of splenic injury in which there is any question of associated pancreatic or gastric trauma, drainage of the splenic bed may prevent complications that could arise if such unrecognized injuries were not drained. Even those authors who incriminate the usage of splenic bed drains report no higher incidence of subphrenic abscess or other infections if the drains are removed before the sixth postsplenectomy day.

Another area of controversy is the issue of prophylactic antibiotics in the postsplenectomized patient, particularly in the pediatric age group. Most authors advocate prophylactic penicillin therapy until at least age five years, but it has been recommended that protection be extended into the teenage years, and isolated reports suggest indefinite protection. The use of long-term antibiotics is not without untoward effects, such as drug sensitivity, bacterial resistance, and suppression of natural immunologic defenses. Patient compliance over a long period of time is very poor. Patients who have undergone splenectomy are advised to contact their physician at the first sign of any febrile illness.

Pneumococcal vaccination is recommended following splenectomy. This should protect against 80 to 85 percent of the pneumococcal strains leading to sepsis. It must be stressed, however, that although pneumococcus is the most prevalent offending organism, the syndrome can be caused by other organisms such as meningococcus and *Haemophilus influenzae*. Currently there are no recommendations for a second or booster dose of pneumococcal vaccine. Asplenic patients should be considered immunocompromised, receive close follow-up, and be instructed about the potential risks of the asplenic state.

MORTALITY. Factors contributing to mortality following splenic injury include (1) associated injury, (2) mechanism of injury, (3) presence of shock on admission to hospital, and (4) advanced age. Naylor and associates reported an overall mortality rate of 11.2 percent in their series of 408 patients, which compares favorably with that in other reports.

Retroperitoneal Hematoma

The management of traumatic retroperitoneal hematoma is a controversial problem. The most common cause of retroperitoneal hemorrhage, according to Baylis et al. and according to the experience at Parkland Memorial Hospital, is pelvic fracture, which accounts for about 60 percent of all traumatic retroperitoneal hematomas. The diagnosis of retroperitoneal hematoma is most difficult following blunt, nonpenetrating trauma to the abdomen, and should be suspected in any patient following trauma who has signs and symptoms of hemorrhagic shock but no obvious source of hemorrhage. Hemorrhage within the retroperitoneal area may be massive and may exceed 2000 mL of blood. Experimental data have shown that as much as 4000 mL of fluid can extravasate into the retroperitoneal space under pressure equal to that in the pelvic vessels.

DIAGNOSIS. Abdominal pain occurs in approximately 60 percent of patients, and back pain in about 25 percent. The abdominal pain is usually vague and generalized but is occasionally localized over the hematoma. Local or generalized tenderness is present in about two-thirds of the patients, and shock occurs in approximately 40 percent. Occasionally, a tender mass is palpable through the abdomen or in the flanks, and in some cases, rectal examination will reveal a boggy mass anterior or posterior to the rectum. Dullness to percussion over the flanks or the abdomen that does not vary with changing positions of the patient has been recorded in some instances. At times, discoloration of the flanks from retroperitoneal hemorrhage has been noted after the lapse of a few hours (Grey Turner's sign). Progressive decreases in the hemoglobin and hematocrit is a consistent finding, and hematuria is found in 80 percent of patients. Hematuria may represent the first clue to the development of a retroperitoneal hematoma.

Somewhat more than half the patients produce free, nonclotting blood on diagnostic paracentesis or lavage of the abdomen; this blood is generally related to the presence of both retroperitoneal and intraabdominal hemorrhage. However, if the retroperitoneal hematoma that occurs without intraperitoneal hemorrhage is large enough to yield a so-called false-positive peritoneal tap or lavage from retroperitoneal hemorrhage alone, then the hematoma itself may require abdominal exploration to search for the persistent source of the retroperitoneal bleeding. If a large pelvic hematoma is suspected, special care should be taken when performing lavage so as not to inadvertently enter the hematoma, which may cause significant and difficult to control hemorrhage.

Radiography, according to Baylis et al., has been valuable in several respects; approximately two-thirds of the patients with peritoneal hematoma have had fractures of the pelvis, and other x-ray findings have included obliteration of the psoas shadow in 30 percent, abdominal mass in 5 percent, and paralytic ileus in 8 percent. Also, displaced bowel-gas shadows and fractured vertebrae have been noted. Intravenous pyelograms and/or retrograde cystograms are generally obtained in patients with sus-

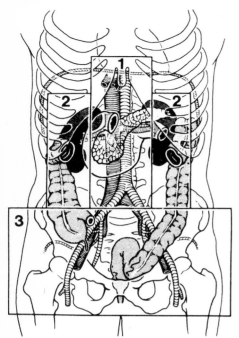

Fig. 6-20. Retroperitoneal classification. Zone 1 = central-medial retroperitoneal hematomas. Zone 2 = flank retroperitoneal hematomas. Zone 3 = pelvic retroperitoneal hematomas. [From: *Sheldon GF: Retroperitoneal hematoma, in Blaisdell WF, Trunkey DD (eds): Abdominal Trauma. New York, Thieme-Stratton, 1982, p 281, with permission.*]

pected retroperitoneal hematomas, if the patient's condition is stable. Arteriography and CT scan may be helpful in establishing the diagnosis of retroperitoneal injury. In the patient whose condition is deteriorating, however, immediate exploration is performed without obtaining such studies, in order to attempt rapid control of progressive bleeding. Many retroperitoneal hematomas from pelvic fractures will tamponade themselves within a short time, and the patient's condition will remain stable.

TREATMENT. One of the most frequently debated areas of abdominal surgery is that of the proper management of retroperitoneal injuries. The major controversy centers around the question of whether to open and explore retroperitoneal hematomas depending upon the anatomic location. The retroperitoneum has been divided into three areas in an attempt to clarify the various problems encountered (Fig. 6-20). Area 1 is the upper central area and extends from the diaphragmatic hiatus to the sacral promontory. Area 2 consists of the right and left flank, and area 3 consists of the pelvis.

The decision to open the hematoma is dependent upon several considerations. These include the wounding mechanism, the location, and the intraoperative evaluation of the size of the hematoma. There is general agreement that all penetrating injuries should be explored as well as all hematomas in the central medial area from the hiatus to the sacrum (area 1).

Injuries located in the flanks (area 2) are frequently individualized. The most common injury in this area is the

kidney, renovascular pedicle, and posterior colon. Once again, penetrating injuries in this area should be explored. Patients with blunt trauma are often managed selectively. If the evaluation of the kidney has been unremarkable, including an arteriogram, and the hematoma is lateral or contained in Gerota's fascia and not expanding, many authors recommend nonexploration. If, however, the hematoma is expanding or large and the preoperative evaluation is incomplete or inconclusive, it is best to investigate this area of potential injury. Prior to opening Gerota's fascia, it is extremely important to gain control of the renal artery and vein so that if massive hemorrhage is encountered the surgeon will be in a position to control it. If there is any question of a hematoma around the large bowel, it must be completely explored.

Large retroperitoneal hematomas that are located deep in the pelvis (area 3) and associated with pelvis fractures are best not explored. It is important to be certain there is no injury to the distal aorta, iliac vessels, or takeoff of the internal iliac vessels. If major vessels are not explored at the time that hematomas occur near them, major and sometimes fatal postoperative bleeding may occur. Present-day vascular surgical techniques obviate the fear of incurring massive hemorrhage as a contraindication to exploring retroperitoneal hematomas.

Ligation of one or both hypogastric arteries may, at times, control persistent bleeding in the pelvic retroperitoneal space from pelvic fractures that cannot be controlled by any other means. Certainly it is preferable to locate a single vessel that is bleeding and either ligate or repair it. Selective arteriography, either intraoperatively or in the x-ray department, and infusion of vasospastic drugs or the embolization of autologous clots or hemostatic agents may be beneficial in controlling this type of hemorrhage. On rare occasions it may be necessary to pack the pelvis with large lap packs for 24 to 48 h in order to achieve hemostasis.

Inferior Vena Cava

Inferior vena caval injuries associated with penetrating abdominal wounds are being seen with increasing frequency. It has been reported that 1 in every 50 gunshot wounds and 1 in every 300 knife wounds of the abdomen will injure the vena cava. These are serious injuries: one-third of the patients die before reaching the hospital, and up to half the remaining persons will die during hospitalization. Most deaths occur from bleeding because of the inherent difficulties in controlling injuries of large veins, but significant wounds of other structures, especially in the retroperitoneum, are common and often adversely affect therapeutic efforts.

ETIOLOGY AND DISTRIBUTION. Most injuries of the inferior vena cava are caused by gunshot wounds, but stab wounds or blunt trauma may also be involved (Table 6-7). Simple penetrating wounds produced by knives and low-velocity missiles are less lethal than those wounds caused by shotguns, high-velocity bullets, and especially blunt trauma. Widespread serious damage to other structures, particularly liver and major arteries and veins, are likely

Table 6-7. CAUSES OF INFERIOR VENA CAVAL
INJURIES

	Total	Died	Mortality, %
Bullet	69	23	33
Shotgun	8	6	75
Stab	12	2	17
Blunt	12	11	92
Total	101	42	42

to result from shotgun wounds and blunt trauma to the abdomen and lower part of the chest.

The infrarenal vena cava is most susceptible and most often injured (Table 6-8). The level of injury is a major determinant of survival, and injuries of the suprarenal, intrahepatic vena cava are extremely dangerous, especially when accompanied by wounds of hepatic and renal veins. Difficulties in exposure and control are invariably encountered, and adjunctive measures are often necessary.

DIAGNOSIS. Injuries of the inferior vena cava should be considered in all cases of penetrating wounds of the abdomen and lower part of the chest. Because of the vagaries of the trajectory of bullets, innocent-appearing small-caliber wounds may produce serious damage to retroperitoneal structures, without intraabdominal organ injury. Patients who have suffered stab wounds of the back or lower part of the chest may also harbor unsuspected caval injuries.

One of the major determinants of survival of these patients is the presence of hemorrhagic shock on admission. This is often a clue that despite the absence of identifying physical findings, major vascular injuries are present. Hemoperitoneum, hemothorax, subcutaneous blood staining from retroperitoneal bleeding, and evidence of distal vena caval obstruction may be helpful in diagnosis.

Except for direct venous studies with contrast media, radiographic examination is rarely specific. Routine x-ray studies, including anteroposterior and lateral films of the chest and abdomen, are useful and are recommended, but in a patient in unstable condition these should be obtained in the operating room as preparations for surgery are in progress. It is usually best not to delay surgery for elaborate studies if firm indications for exploration exist.

TREATMENT. As alluded to in the discussion of other vascular injuries, associated injuries are common and are a major factor in survival of these patients (Table 6-9).

Table 6-8. LOCATION OF INFERIOR VENA
CAVAL INJURY

	Total	Died	Mortality, %
Above renal veins	19	11	58
At renal vein level	21	13	62
Below renal veins	47	14	30
Bifurcation	14	4	29

Table 6-9. INJURIES ASSOCIATED WITH
INFERIOR VENA CAVAL INJURY

Aorta, iliac artery	13	Kidney	21
Major splanchnic vessel	26	Pancreas	18
Renal artery or vein	20	Spleen	10
Liver	46	Colon	27
Duodenum	27	Other	21

Prior to exploration, resuscitation and attention to other problems often are important. An adequate airway must be obtained, volume and blood deficits repaired, and fractures stabilized. Vena caval injuries that require clamping may reduce the effectiveness of using lower-extremity veins for fluid administration, and at least one large-bore catheter should be placed into the upper-extremity venous system. This line is best reserved for blood and fluid administration and should not be used for primary anesthetic manipulations.

Thoracotomy may be required, especially in patients with suprarenal caval injuries. If transatrial intracaval shunts are needed, a median sternotomy offers good exposure for this maneuver as well as for control of associated hepatic injuries.

Abdominal exploration is performed through a midline incision that can be extended as required, and median sternotomy can be added if necessary. Rapid abdominal exploration will usually expose major injuries and establish priorities of repair. It is usually wise to control the bleeding, pause, and complete volume and blood restoration before definitive repairs are begun. Attempts to complete bowel repairs while bleeding persists from other injuries often extend the hypotensive episode and increase blood loss.

Centrally located retroperitoneal hematomas above the pelvis often harbor significant injuries, and usually are explored. Damage to other retroperitoneal structures is common (79 percent) and not always evident without formal exploration. The size or stability of the hematoma does not offer reliable evidence as to the presence or absence of significant injuries. Continued bleeding from the vena caval injury, however, is ominous. Patients actively bleeding at the time of operation have a very high mortality rate, especially if the vena caval injury is at or above the renal arteries and veins (Table 6-10).

Initial control of bleeding can usually be obtained with pressure and packs. Occasionally temporary occlusion of the abdominal aorta at the diaphragmatic hiatus is useful in reducing blood loss from high caval injuries. Exposure

Table 6-10. RELATIONSHIP OF BLEEDING AND
MORTALITY FROM INFERIOR VENA CAVAL
INJURIES

	Total	Died	Mortality, %
Active bleeding	41	32	78
Tamponade	57	9	16
Not specified	3	0	0

Simple Anterior Repair

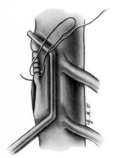

Fig. 6-21. Repair of anterior laceration of the inferior vena cava. Note the use of a partially occlusive clamp.

Anterior and Posterior Rotation Repair Repair

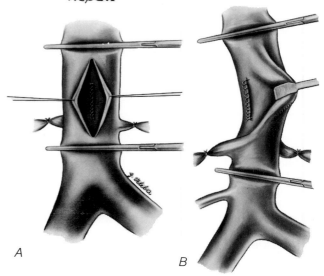

A

B

Fig. 6-22. Repair of through-and-through injury to the inferior vena cava. *A.* Anterior laceration is enlarged to permit closure of the posterior wall from within the lumen. *B.* Rotation of the posteroinferior vena cava.

of the inferior vena cava is obtained by reflecting medially the right colon, duodenum, and pancreas. Direct tamponade, manually or with sponge sticks, is usually effective in controlling bleeding. Simple lacerations or punctures are most common, but transections, avulsion, or multiple lacerations may be encountered, and control may be very difficult in the last group.

Simple lacerations can be controlled with gentle digital pressure and sutured by simply passing the needle under the occluding finger. In some cases the edge of the wound can be held gently in apposition with vascular forceps or blunt Allis clamps while repair is effected. Balloon catheter tamponade has also been employed for control of these wounds. Partial occlusion with vascular clamps is a useful technique and can be instituted after the initial use of other maneuvers (Fig. 6-21). These simple tangential wounds usually can be repaired without injury to lumbar veins, but occasionally ligation of gonadal and lumbar tributaries is required (Fig. 6-22).

Transections may be repaired by end-to-end vascular surgical techniques after mobilizing the vena cava. If there are multiple caval wounds requiring complicated repairs, or if repair poses an undue risk in a patient with multiple injuries, infrarenal ligation is preferable. In most cases construction of venous grafts is not required, and the time and effort necessary to perform these repairs may increase the operative morbidity and mortality.

Wounds at or above the renal veins are difficult to expose and repair. If bleeding from behind the liver is encountered and is not easily identified as coming from a laceration of the anterior cava wall below the caudate lobe, an intracaval shunt may be needed. The liver can be rotated medially after division of supporting ligaments, and if intrahepatic vena cava or combined hepatic vein lacerations are present, the shunt can be inserted as described by Schrock et al. The transatrial approach is easier than inserting the shunt from the intrarenal vena cava, and is very useful in managing these extremely dangerous wounds. A large chest tube (34 to 38 F tube) with a proximal side hole is inserted through the atrial appendage, and the tip is placed near the orifices of the renal veins. Umbilical tapes encircling the inferior vena cava within the

pericardium and above the renal veins secure the catheter. The side hole in the catheter is placed at a level to permit the return of blood via the tube into the right atrium. This shunt, occasionally combined with temporary occlusion of the portal triad, will usually allow sufficient control of bleeding to effect repairs. This technique is rarely required.

Unlike injuries of the infrarenal cava, most wounds above the renal veins should be repaired. Ligation of the inferior vena cava at this level produces serious complications. Some survivors have been reported, and those were usually in operations uncomplicated by hypotension, shock, or multiple injuries.

Those vascular procedures used in other areas are effective in repairing the suprarenal vena cava. Simple venorrhaphy often may suffice, but patch graft angioplasty or anastomosis may be needed (Fig. 6-23). If graft interposition is required, autogenous venous grafts obtained from the infrarenal cava or iliac vein are preferred (Fig. 6-24). Concomitant repair of hepatic vein injuries can be effected, but in some cases ligation may be preferable.

These repairs can usually be completed within 30 min, a period of ischemia well tolerated by the normothermic liver. Regional hypothermia may be induced with iced saline solution by irrigation techniques, thus conferring further protection of the liver during more prolonged ischemia.

COMPLICATIONS. In patients with isolated wounds of the inferior vena cava, repair is usually effective and complications are few. In these patients, two episodes of ileofemoral venous thrombosis have been encountered,

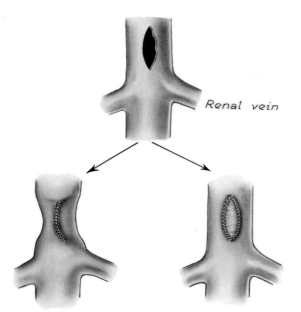

Renal vein

Fig. 6-23. Repair of the inferior vena cava using a patch graft to prevent stenosis.

and an additional patient had a pulmonary embolus. Pancreatitis has also been encountered, and recurrent retroperitoneal bleeding occurred in one patient.

The mortality in patients with isolated inferior vena caval injuries was 11 percent in the present series, but 67 percent of the patients with one or more major vessel injuries died. All the patients with inferior vena caval wounds at or above the renal veins had significant associated injuries, usually liver and bowel, occasionally pancreas, stomach, and lung. The mortality is high in this group of patients, especially if the inferior vena cava is actively bleeding at surgery.

Female Reproductive Organs

Injuries to the female reproductive organs are infrequently seen following either blunt or penetrating trauma

Fig. 6-24. Interposition of an excised segment of the infrarenal inferior vena cava to establish continuity of the suprarenal inferior vena cava.

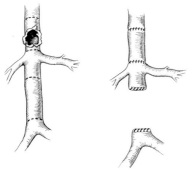

to the abdomen. A series reported by Quast and Jordan revealed only 27 patients with gynecologic injuries in a 16-year period at their hospital. Two of those injuries resulted from blunt trauma with rupture of the uterus in patients who were in the immediate postpartum period. These are apparently the only cases recorded of rupture of the nonpregnant uterus. The remaining injuries were penetrating wounds. An enlarged uterus was present in 10 of their patients. Six patients were pregnant, two had large uterine myomas, and two were in the postpartum period. No cases of rupture of an unenlarged uterus by blunt trauma have been recorded, however. Rupture of the pregnant uterus due to blunt trauma is rare but has occurred in a number of instances. The major threat to the fetus in blunt trauma is placental abruption, which if complete, will result in fetal demise. Of blunt and penetrating wounds to the female reproductive tract, 90 percent involve the uterine corpus and 10 percent involve the remaining adnexa.

In the past serious questions have been raised about the efficacy of pregnant patients wearing seat belts in automobiles. Crosby et al, have shown rather conclusively that more maternal and fetal lives have been saved by the use of lap belts, with or without shoulder harnesses, than by not using them.

The diagnostic evaluation of the pregnant patient sustaining traumatic injury should be undertaken with careful consideration for radiation exposure. Many procedures can be condensed to give maximum information with minimal exposure. On the contrary, no necessary procedure should be withheld because of a known or suspected pregnancy.

The most common cause of fetal death in automobile accidents is maternal death; therefore, important diagnostic and therapeutic measures designed to save the mother should be performed. In general, intrauterine exposure to diagnostic radiation is not an indication to terminate a pregnancy.

Pregnant patients sustaining penetrating trauma are managed the same as nonpregnant patients. It may be difficult to perform lavage in the late second and third trimester for stab wounds, but patients sustaining gunshot wounds should be formally explored in the operating room. In spite of the fact the gravid uterus may afford considerable protection to abdominal viscera, these organs are still at risk.

TREATMENT. The signs and symptoms from a ruptured pregnant uterus are those of abrupt and massive intraperitoneal hemorrhage. Associated with these findings are generalized abdominal pain and tenderness, abdominal distention, ileus, and the absence of fetal heart sounds and movements. If the patient arrives at the hospital alive (which is not often the case), immediate blood volume and extracellular fluid replacement must be instituted through several large-bore intravenous catheters, preferably placed in the upper extremities, since there may be an interference with venous return from lower extremities of those patients. Urgent celiotomy is necessary to control hemorrhage, even though the patient may still be in shock at the time. Probably the only anesthesia that will be required is assisted respiration with 100% oxygen administered through an endotracheal tube. Other agents may be added if and when shock abates. The treatment of choice is evacuation of the uterus, closure of the disruption with large chromic catgut sutures, and thorough peritoneal toilet with removal of all blood and foreign tissue.

Wounds of the uterus and adnexa are repaired by figure-of-eight chromic catgut sutures without drainage in most instances, although in occasional patients hysterectomy is indicated, as in injury of the lower uterine segment and major uterine vessels caused by high-velocity missiles. In these instances, hysterectomy is preferable to an attempted suture repair, since repair may cause stenosis of the cervical canal with resultant hematometra and dystocia. Also, hysterectomy for lower-uterine-segment injuries is indicated to obtain proper control of bleeding vessels and to help rule out uretheral injury at the point where the ureter and uterine artery are in juxtaposition.

It is best to leave the vaginal cuff partially open following hysterectomy for trauma, because of the likelihood of vaginal cuff or cul-de-sac abscess formation, especially if there is appreciable blast injury or concomitant colon injury. If abscesses occur and the vaginal cuff has been left open, it is usually a relatively simple matter to drain the abscess with a finger inserted through the vagina into the open cuff. If gross fecal contamination is present from colon injury, the cuff should be left open and a Penrose drain led out of the vagina from the cul-de-sac. This drain may be secured to the vaginal cuff by a single small chromic catgut suture.

If massive uncontrollable or recurrent bleeding occurs following trauma to the female pelvic organs, it may be rapidly and adequately controlled by bilateral in-continuity ligations of the hypogastric arteries with nonabsorbable suture material. This will not often be required but should be borne in mind as a very helpful and possibly lifesaving procedure.

Following injury to the pregnant uterus, the loss of the fetus is quite high. Quast and Jordan reported a salvage of only 1 of 10 pregnancies. One patient who was pregnant at the time of a tangential knife injury of the uterus had a uterine repair for penetrating trauma and subsequently delivered the child uneventfully per vagina.

Other instances have been reported in which penetrating uterine injury during pregnancy has been repaired with ensuing normal delivery. Quast and Jordan found that 81 percent of their patients with uterine injuries during pregnancy delivered subsequently per vagina with no difficulty. The cesarean section rate was 19 percent. Of the patients they followed after uterine injury, all who were in the childbearing age subsequently were able to conceive children. In this group, the abortion rate for these later pregnancies was 16 percent, with no apparent cause found.

By far the majority of pregnant patients with uterine injuries will abort shortly after the injury, frequently requiring curettage to control bleeding after spontaneous abortion. Others will require elective emptying of the uterine contents at the time of celiotomy in order to secure adequate hemostasis and uterine repair. Intravenous oxytocin should be given in such instances to aid in uterine contraction and hemostasis after hysterotomy.

Abdominal Wall

Injury to the abdominal wall without peritoneal injury is often difficult to diagnose. Muscular guarding and rigidity are frequently present, and it may be impossible to rule out intraabdominal injury from a hematoma of the abdominal wall. Such hematomas are usually due to rupture of the rectus abdominis or the epigastric artery by direct trauma or severe muscular exertion. The epigastric artery may also be injured by penetrating trauma, resulting in a hemoperitoneum. The patient may become hypotensive from such an injury because of the severe intraperitoneal bleeding that sometimes occurs.

The mass from the rectus abdominis hematoma is below the umbilicus in over 80 percent of the cases. To distinguish this mass from intraperitoneal masses, patients should be requested to raise their heads against resistance; the mass should disappear if it is intraperitoneal and remain the same if it is in the abdominal wall. This sign is not completely reliable, and if adjunctive diagnostic aids such as paracentesis and lavage are equivocal, then abdominal celiotomy should be performed.

On occasion missile injuries will appear to be limited to the abdominal wall. Depending upon the bullet caliber, distance at which it was shot, and body habitus blast effect may injure hollow and solid abdominal viscera without actual penetration of the peritoneum. Local wound exploration, peritoneal lavage, and computed tomography are unreliable in these cases. As stated above, these patients are best treated by celiotomy.

Bibliography

General Considerations

Shires GT: *Principles of Trauma Care.* New York, McGraw-Hill, 1985.

Principles in Wound Management and Antibiotics

Alexander JW, Kaplan JZ, Altemeier WA: Role of suture materials in the development of wound infection. *Ann Surg* 165:192, 1967.

Burke JF: The effective period of antibiotic action in experimental incisions and dermal lesions. *Surgery* 50:161, 1961.

Condie JP, Ferguson DJ: Experimental wound infections: Contamination versus surgical technique. *Surgery* 50:367, 1961.

Dunphy JE, Jackson DS: Practical applications of experimental studies in the care of the primarily closed wound. *Am J Surg* 104:273, 1962.

Finegold SM: Intestinal bacteria. *Calif Med* 110:455, 1969.

Gentry LO, Feliciano DD, Lea AS: Perioperative antibiotic therapy for penetrating injuries to the abdomen. *Ann Surg* 200:561, 1984.

Gorbach SL: Intestinal microflora. *Gastroenterology* 60:1110, 1971.

Jones RC: in Shires G Thomas (ed): *Care of the Trauma Patient,* 2d ed. New York, McGraw-Hill, 1978.

Jones RC, Thal ER, et al: Evaluation of antibiotic therapy following penetrating abdominal trauma 201:576, 1985.

Jones RC: Newer antibiotics for the surgeon. *Am J Surg* 152:577, 1986.

Louie TJ, Onderdonk AB, et al: Therapy for experimental intraabdominal sepsis: Comparison of four cephalosporins with clindomycin plus gentamicin. *J Infect Dis* 135:5, 1977.

Mann LS, Spinazzola AJ, et al: Disruption of abdominal wounds. *JAMA* 180:99, 1962.

Nichols RL, Smith JW, Klein DB: Risk of infection after penetrating abdominal trauma. *N Engl J Med* 311:1065, 1984.

Onderdonk AD, Bartlett JG, Louie T: Microbial synergy in experimental abdominal abscess. *Infect Immun* 13:22, 1976.

Oreskovitch MD, Dellinger EP, Lennard S: Duration of preventive antibiotic administration for penetrating abdominal trauma. *Arch Surg* 117:200, 1982.

Thadepalli H, Gorbach SL, et al: Abdominal trauma, anaerobes and antibiotics. *Surg Gynecol Obstet* 137:270, 1973.

Thorngate S, Ferguson DJ: Effect of tension on healing of aponeurotic wounds. *Surgery* 44:619, 1958.

Wagner DH: Errors in the choice of abdominal wall incisions and in their closure. *Surg Clin North Am* 38:175, 1958.

Bites and Stings of Animals and Insects

Anderson LJ, Baer GM, Smith JS: Rapid antibody response to human diploid rabies vaccine. *Am J Epidemiol* 113:270, 1981.

Auer AI, Hershey FB: Surgery for necrotic bites of the brown spider. *Arch Surg* 108:612, 1974.

Berger RS, Addelstein GH, Anderson PC: Intravascular coagulation: The cause of necrotic arachnoidism. *Invest Dermatol* 61:142, 1973.

Bernard KW, Mallonie J, Wright JC: Preexposure immunization with intradermal human diploid cell rabies vaccine—Risks and benefits of primary and booster vaccinations. *JAMA* 257:1059, 1987.

Bernstein B, Erhlich F: Brown recluse spider bites. *J Emerg Med* 4:457, 1986.

Bitseff EL, Garoni WJ, et al: The management of stingray injuries of the extremities. *South Med J* 63:417, 1970.

CDC Rabies Surveillance Annual Summary 1985, U.S. Department of Health and Human Services, issued 1986.

Christopher DG, Rodning CB: Crotalidae Envenomation. *South Med J* 79:159, 1986.

Compendium of Animal Rabies Control. *Mortality and Morbidity Weekly Report* 35:53, 1987.

Davidson T: Inside world of the honeybee. *Natl Geograph* 154:188, 1959.

Dillaha CJ, Jansen GT, et al: North American loxoscelism. *JAMA* 188:33, 1964.

Emergency Department Management of Poisonous Snake Bites, American College of Surgeons Committee on Trauma, February 1981.

Fardon DW, Wingo CW, et al: The treatment of brown spider bites. *Plast Reconstr Surg* 40:482, 1967.

Fishbein DB, Bernard KW, Miller KD: Early kinetics of the antibody response after booster immunizations after human diploid cell vaccine. *Am J Trop Med Hyg* 35:663, 1986.

Golden DBK, Langlois J, et al: Treatment failures with whole-body extract therapy of insect sting allergy. *JAMA* 246(21):2460, 1981.

Golden DBK, Valentine MD, et al: Regimens of hymenoptera venom immunotherapy. *Ann Intern Med* 92:620, 1980.

Goldstein EJC, Citron DM, et al: Bacteriology of rattlesnake venom and implications for therapy. *J Infect Dis* 140(5):818, 1979.

Huang TT, Blackwell SJ, Lewis SR: Tissue necrosis in snakebite. *Tex Med* 77:53, 1981.

Huang TT, Lynch JB, et al: The use of excisional therapy in the management of snakebite. *Ann Surg* 179:598, 1974.

Human diploid cell rabies vaccine. *Med Let* 22(22):93, 1980.

Hunt KJ, Valentine MD, et al: A controlled trial of immunotherapy in insect hypersensitivity. *N Engl J Med* 299:157, 1978.

Ledbetter EO: What's new in the management of snakebite. *Tex Med* 77:41, 1981.

Levine MI: Insect stings. *JAMA* 217:964, 1971.

Marr JJ: Portuguese man-of-war envenomization. *JAMA* 199:115, 1967.

Marteic Z: Lactrodectism: Variations in clinical manifestations produced by Lactrodectus species of spiders. *Toxicon* 21:457, 1983.

Parrish HM: Incidence of treated snakebites in the United States. *Public Health Rept (US)* 31:269,1966.

Parrish HM, Carr CA: Bites by copperheads in the United States. *JAMA* 201:927, 1967.

Portuguese man-of-war. *JAMA* 192:994, 1965 (editorial).

Rabies prevention in the United States. Recommendations of the Public Health Service, Immunization Advisory Committee. *Mortality and Morbidity Weekly Report* 33(28):393, July 1984.

Rabies prevention: Supplementary statement on the preexposure use of human diploid cells rabies vaccine by the intradermal route. *JAMA* 257:1037, 1987.

Rees R, Shack RB, Withers E: Management of brown recluse spider bites. *Plast Reconstr Surg* 68:768, 1981.

Rees RS, Altenbern DP, et al: Brown recluse spider bites: A comparison of early surgical excision vs. dapsone and delayed surgical excision. *Ann Surg* 202:659, 1985.

Reisman RE, Arbesman CE, Lazell M: Clinical and immunological studies of venom immunotherapy. *Clin Allergy* 9:167, 1979.

Roberts RS, Csenscsitz TA, Heard CW: Upper extremity compartment syndromes following pit viper envenomation. *Clin Orthop* 193:184, 1985.

Russell FE: *Snake Venom Poisoning.* Philadelphia, Lippincott, 1980.

Russell FE, Carlson RW, et al: Snake venom poisoning in the United States—Experiences with 550 cases. *JAMA* 233:341, 1975.

Schwartz HJ, Lockey RF, et al: A multicenter study on skin test reactivity of human volunteers to venom as compared to whole-body hymenoptera antigens. *J Allergy Clin Immunol* 67:81, 1981.

Snyder CC, Knowles RP: Snake bite! *Consultant (SKF)* 3:44, 1963.

Sprenger TR, Bailey WJ: Snakebite treatment in the United States—Review. *Int J Dermatol* 25:479, 1986.

Strauss MB, Orris WL: Injuries to divers by marine animals: A simplified approach to recognition and management. *Milit Med* February 1974.

Timms PK, Gibbons RB: Lactrodectism—Effects of the black widow spider bites. *West J Med* 144:315, 1986.

Van Mierop LHS: Poisonous snakebite: A review. II. Symptomatology and treatment. *J Fla Med Assoc* 63(3):201, 1976.

Van Mierop LHS, Kitchesn CS: Defibrination syndrome following bites by the eastern diamondback rattlesnake. *J Fla Med Assoc* 67:31, 1980.

Wasserman GS, Anderson PC: Loxoscelism and necrotic arachnoidism. *J Toxicol Clin Toxicol* 21:451, 1984.

Penetrating Wounds of the Neck and Thoracic Inlet

Ayuyao AM, Kaledzi YL, et al: Penetrating neck wounds: Mandatory versus selective exploration. *Ann Surg* 202:563, 1985.

Dunbar LL, Adkins RB, Waterhouse G: Penetrating injuries to the neck: Selective management. *Am Surg* 50:198, 1984.

Flint LM, Snyder WH, et al: Management of major vascular injuries in the base of the neck: An 11-year experience with 146 cases. *Arch Surg* 106:407, 1973.

Fogelman MJ, Stewart RD: Penetrating wounds of the neck. *Am J Surg* 91:581, 1956.

Gewertz BL, Samson DS, et al: Management of penetrating injuries of the internal carotid artery at the base of the skull utilizing extracranial-intracranial bypass. *J Trauma* 20:365, 1980.

Golueke PJ, Goldstein AS, et al: Routine versus selective exploration of penetrating neck injuries: A randomized prospective study. *J Trauma* 24:1010, 1984.

Graham JM, Feliciano DV, et al: Management of subclavian vascular injuries. *J Trauma* 20:537, 1980.

Hiatt JR, Busuttil RW, Wilson SE: Impact of routine arteriography on management of penetrating neck injuries. *J Vasc Surg* 1:860, 1984.

Jones RF, Terrell JC, Salyer KE: Penetrating wounds of the neck: An analysis of 274 cases. *J Trauma* 7:228, 1967.

Jurkovich GJ, Zingarelli W, et al: Penetrating neck trauma: Diagnostic studies in the asymptomatic patient. *J Trauma* 25:819, 1985.

Larson DL, Cohn AM: Management of acute laryngeal injury: A critical review. *J Trauma* 16:858, 1976.

Liekweg WG, Greenfield LJ: Management of penetrating carotid artery injury. *Ann Surg* 188:587, 1978.

Meier DE, Brink BE, Fry WJ: Vertebral artery trauma: Acute recognition and treatment. *Arch Surg* 116:236, 1981.

Metzdorff MT, Lowe DK: Operation or observation for penetrating neck wounds? A retrospective analysis. *Am J Surg* 147:646, 1984.

Monson DO, Saletta JD, Freeark RJ: Carotid-vertebral trauma. *J Trauma* 9:987, 1969.

Narrod JA, Moore EE: Selective management of penetrating neck injuries. *Arch Surg* 119:574, 1984.

Noyes LD, McSwain NE Jr, Markowitz IP: Panendoscopy with arteriography versus mandatory exploration of penetrating wounds of the neck. *Ann Surg* 204:21, 1986.

Obeid FN, Haddad GS, et al: A critical reappraisal of a mandatory exploration policy for penetrating wounds of the neck. *Surg Gynecol Obstet* 160:517, 1985.

Ordog GJ, Albin D, et al: 110 bullet wounds to the neck. *J Trauma* 25:238, 1985.

Prakashchandra MR, Bhatti MFK, et al: Penetrating injuries of the neck: Criteria for exploration. *J Trauma* 23:47, 1983.

Reid JDS, Weigelt JA: Forty-three cases of vertebral artery trauma. Presented at the 47th Annual Meeting of The American Association for the Surgery of Trauma, Montreal, Quebec, Canada, September 1987.

Roon AJ, Christensen N: Evaluation and treatment of penetrating cervical injuries. *J Trauma* 19:391, 1979.

Rosoff L Sr, White EJ: Perforation of the esophagus. *Am J Surg* 128:207, 1974.

Saletta JD, Lowe RJ, et al: Penetrating trauma of the neck. *J Trauma* 16:579, 1976.

Snyder WH III, Thal ER, et al: The validity of normal arteriography in penetrating trauma. *Arch Surg* 113:424, 1978.

Symbas PN, Hatcher CR Jr, Boehm GAW: Acute penetrating tracheal trauma. *Ann Thorac Surg* 22:473, 1976.

Thal ER, Snyder WH III, et al: Management of carotid artery injuries. *Surgery* 76:955, 1974.

Thomas AN, Goodman PC, Roon AJ: Role of angiography in cervicothoracic trauma. *J Thorac Cardiovasc Surg* 76:633, 1978.

Unger WS, Tucker WS Jr, et al: Carotid arterial trauma. *Surgery* 87:477, 1980.

Weigelt JA, Thal ER, et al: Diagnosis of penetrating cervical esophageal injuries. Presented at the 39th Annual Meeting of the Southwestern Surgical Congress, San Diego, California, April 1987.

Abdominal Trauma

Ahmad W, Polk HC Jr: Blunt abdominal trauma. A prospective study with selective peritoneal lavage. *Arch Surg* 111:489, 1976.

Arango A, Baxter CR, Shires GT: Surgical management of traumatic injuries of the right colon; 20 years civilian experience. *Arch Surg* 114:703, 1979.

Aronson DZ, Scherz AW, Einhorn AH: Nonoperative management of splenic trauma in children: A report of six consecutive cases. *Pediatrics* 60:482, 1977.

Bach RD, Frey CF: Diagnosis and treatment of pancreatic trauma. *Am J Surg* 121:20, 1971.

Backwinkel K: Rupture of the rectus abdominis muscle. *Arch Surg* 90:35, 1965.

Balfanz JR, Nesbit ME, Jarvis C: Overwhelming sepsis following splenectomy for trauma. *J Pediatr* 88:458, 1976.

Barnes JP, Diamonon JS: Traumatic rupture of the gallbladder due to nonpenetrating injury. *Tex State J Med* 59:785, 1963.

Bartizal JF, Boyd DR, et al: A critical review of management of 392 colonic and rectal injuries. *Dis Colon Rectum* 17(3):313, 1974.

Bass EM, Crosier JH: Percutaneous control of posttraumatic hepatic hemorrhage by gelfoam embolization. *J Trauma* 17(1):61, 1977.

Baudet quoted by Terry JH, Self MM, Howard JM: A discussion of injuries of the spleen. *Surgery* 40:615, 1956.

Baylis SM, Lansing EH, Glas WW: Traumatic retroperitoneal hematoma. *Am J Surg* 103:477, 1962.

Beall AC, Bricker DL, et al: Surgical considerations in the management of civilian colon injuries. *Ann Surg* 173:971, 1971.

Benjamin CI, Engrav LH, Perry JF Jr: Delayed rupture or delayed diagnosis of rupture of the spleen. *Surg Gynecol Obstet* 142:171, 1976.

Berne CJ, Donovan AJ, et al: Duodenal "diverticulization" for duodenal and pancreatic injury. *Am J Surg* 127:503, 1974.

Bull JC Jr, Mathewson C Jr: Exploratory laparotomy in patients with penetrating wounds of the abdomen. *Am J Surg* 116:223, 1968.

Buntain WL, Lynn HB: Splenorrhaphy: Changing concepts for the traumatized spleen. *Surgery* 86:784, 1977.

Burch JM, Brock JC, et al: The injured colon. *Surg* 203(6):701, 1986.

Burrington JD: Surgical repair of a ruptured spleen in children: Report of eight cases. *Arch Surg* 112:417, 1977.

Burrington JD: Preservation of the traumatized spleen in children. *Contemp Surg* 15:11, 1979.

Busuttil RW, Kitahama A, et al: Management of injuries to the porta hepatis. *Ann Surg* 191(5):641, 1980.

Canizaro PC, Fitts CT, Sawyer RB: Diagnostic abdominal paracentesis: A proposed adjunctive measure. *US Army Surg Res Unit Annl Rept* June 1964.

Carmichael DH: Avulsion of the common bile duct by blunt trauma. *South Med J* 72(2):166, 1980.

Cassebaum WH, Bukanz SL, et al: Ligation of the inferior vena cava above the renal vein of a sole kidney with recovery. *Am J Surg* 113:667, 1967.

Cattell RB, Braasch JW: A technique for the exposure of the third and fourth portions of the duodenum. *Surg Gynecol Obstet* 111:379, 1960.

Cerise EJ, Scully JH Jr: Blunt trauma to the small intestine. *J Trauma* 10(1):46, 1970.

Cheatham JE Jr, Smith EI, et al: Nonoperative management of subcapsular hematomas of the liver. *Am J Surg* 140:851, 1980.

Cobb LM, Vinocur CD, et al: Intestinal perforation due to blunt trauma in children in an era of increased nonoperative treatment. *J Trauma* 26(5):461, 1986.

Cook A, Levine BA, et al: Traditional treatment of colon injuries. *Arch Surg* 119:591, 1984.

Cook DE, Walsh JW, et al: Upper abdominal trauma: Pitfalls in CT diagnosis. *Radiology* 159:65, 1986.

Cornell WP, Ebert PA, et al: A new nonoperative technique for the diagnosis of penetrating injuries to the abdomen. *J Trauma* 7:307, 1967.

Crosby W: Safety of lap belt restraints for pregnant victims of automobile collisions. *N Engl J Med* 248:632, 1971.

Crosby W: Committee on medical aspects of automobile safety belts during pregnancy. *JAMA* 221:20, 1972.

Curtis LE, Simonian S, et al: Evaluation of the effectiveness of controlled pH in management of massive upper gastrointestinal bleeding. *Am J Surg* 125:474, 1973.

Dang CV, Peter ET, et al: Trauma of the colon. Early drop-back of exteriorized repair. *Arch Surg* 117:652, 1982.

Dauterive AH, Flancbaum L, Cox EF: Blunt intestinal trauma. A modern-day review. *Ann Surg* 201(2):198, 1985.

Dawes LG, Aprahamian C, et al: The risk of infection after colon injury. *Surgery* 100(4):796, 1986.

Defore WW Jr, Mattox KL, et al: Management of 1,590 consecutive cases of liver trauma. *Arch Surg* 111:493, 1976.

Dickerman JD: Bacterial infection and the asplenic host: A review. *J Trauma* 16(8):662, 1976.

Dickerman JD: Splenectomy and sepsis: A warning. *Pediatrics* 63:938, 1979.

Dixon JA, Miller F, McCloskey D: Anatomy and techniques in segmental splenectomy. *Surg Gynecol Obstet* 150:516, 1980.

Donohue JH, Crass RA, Trunkey DD: The management of duodenal and other small intestinal trauma. *World J Surg* 9(6):904, 1985.

Douglas GJ, Simpson JS: The conservative management of splenic trauma. *J Pediatr Surg* 6:565, 1971.

Drapanas T, McDonald J: Peritoneal tap in abdominal trauma. *Surgery* 100:22, 1960.

Dudrick SJ, Wilmore DW, et al: Spontaneous closure of traumatic pancreatoduodenal fistulas with total intravenous nutrition. *J Trauma* 10(7):542, 1970.

Duke JH, Jones RC, Shires GT: Management of injuries to the inferior vena cava. *Am J Surg* 110:759, 1965.

Edwards J, Gaspard DJ: Visceral injury due to extraperitoneal gunshot wounds. *Arch Surg* 108:865, 1974.

Ein SH, Shandling B, Simpson JS: Nonoperative management of traumatized spleen in children: How and why. *J Pediatr Surg* 13:117, 1978.

Eraklis AJ, Filler RM: Splenectomy in childhood: A review of 1413 cases. *J Pediatr Surg* 4:382, 1972.

Fabian TC, Mangiante EC, et al: A prospective study of 91 patients undergoing both computed tomography and peritoneal lavage following blunt abdominal trauma. *J Trauma* 26(7):602, 1986.

Federle MP, Richard AC, et al: Computed tomography in blunt abdominal trauma. *Arch Surg* 117:645, 1982.

Feliciano DV, Jordan GL, et al: Management of 1000 consecutive cases of hepatic trauma (1979–1984). *Ann Surg* 204(4):438, 1986.

Feliciano DV, Mattox KL, Jordan GL Jr: Intra-abdominal packing for control of hepatic hemorrhage: A reappraisal. *J Trauma* 21(4):285, 1981.

Feliciano DV, Mattox KL, et al: Packing for control of hepatic hemorrhage. *J Trauma* 26(8):738, 1986.

Felson B, Levin EJ: Intramural hematoma of the duodenum: Diagnostic roentgen sign. *Radiology* 63:828, 1954.

Fischer RP, Beverlin BC, et al: Diagnostic peritoneal lavage: Fourteen years and 2586 patients later. *Am J Surg* 136:701, 1978.

Fish JC: Reconstruction of the portal vein: Case reports and literature review. *Am Surg* 32:472, 1966.

Fitzgerald JB, Crawford E, DeBakey ME: Surgical considerations of abdominal injuries: Analysis of 200 cases. *Am J Surg* 100:22, 1960.

Flint LM, Vitale GC, et al: The injured colon. Relationships of management to complications. *Ann Surg* 193:619, 1981.

Flint LM Jr, McCoy M, et al: Duodenal injury. Analysis of common misconceptions in diagnosis and treatment. *Ann Surg* 191:697, 1980.

Flint LM, Polk HC Jr: Selective hepatic artery ligation: Limitations and failures. *J Trauma* 19(5):319, 1979.

Foley WJ, Gaines RD, Fry WJ: Pancreaticoduodenectomy for severe trauma to the head of the pancreas and the associated structures: Report of three cases. *Ann Surg* 170:759, 1969.

Forde KA, Ganepola AP: Is mandatory exploration for penetrating abdominal trauma extinct? The morbidity and mortality of negative exploration in a large municipal hospital. *J Trauma* 14(9):764, 1974.

Freeark RJ, Corley RD, et al: Unusual aspects of pancreatoduodenal trauma. *J Trauma* 6:482, 1966.

Fullen WD, McDonough JJ, et al: Sternal splitting approach for major hepatic or retrohepatic vena cava injury. *J Trauma* 14(11):903, 1974.

Fullen WD, Selle JG, et al: Intramural duodenal hematoma. *Ann Surg* 179:549, 1974.

Geis WP, Schulz KA, et al: The fate of unruptured intrahepatic hematomas. *Surgery* 90(4):689, 1981.

Giddings WP, Wolff LH: Penetrating wounds of the stomach, duodenum, and small intestine. *Surg Clin North Am* 38:1605, 1958.

Giuliano A: Is splenic salvage safe in the traumatized patient? *Arch Surg* 116:651, 1981.

Gougon FW, Legros G, Archambaul TA: Pancreatic trauma, new diagnostic approach. *Surgery* 132:400, 1976.

Graham JM, Mattox KL, et al: Traumatic injuries of the inferior vena cava. *Arch Surg* 113:413, 1978.

Graham JM, Mattox KL, Jordan GL: Traumatic injuries of the pancreas. *Am J Surg* 136:744, 1978.

Green JB, Shackford SR, et al: Late septic complications in adults following splenectomy for trauma: A prospective analysis in 144 patients. *J Trauma* 26(11):999, 1986.

Haddad GH, Pizzi WF, et al: Abdominal signs and sinograms as dependable criteria for the selective management of stab-wounds of the abdomen. *Ann Surg* 172:61, 1970.

Heimbach DM, Ferguson GS, Harley JD: Treatment of traumatic hemobilia with angiographic embolization. *J Trauma* 18(3):221, 1978.

Holgerson LO, Bishop HC: Nonoperative treatment of duodenal hematoma. *J Pediatr Surg* 12:11, 1976.

Howman-Giles R, Gilday DL, et al: Splenic trauma—nonoperative management and long term follow-up by scintiscan, *J Pediat Surg* 13:121, 1978.

Ivatury RR, Nallathambi M, et al: Liver packing for uncontrolled hemorrhage. *J Trauma* 26(8):744, 1986.

Izant RJ, Drucker WR: Duodenal obstruction due to intramural hematoma in children. *J Trauma* 4:797, 1964.

Jackson GL, Thal ER: Management of stabwounds of the back and flank. *J Trauma* 19(9):660, 1979.

Jeffrey RB, Federle MP, Goodman PC: CT of splenic trauma. *Radiology* 141:729, 1981.

Jeffrey RB Jr, Federle MP, Crass RA: Computed tomography of pancreatic trauma. *Radiology* 147:491, 1983.

Jones RC: Management of pancreatic trauma. *Ann Surg* 187(5):555, May 1978.

Jones RC: Management of pancreatic trauma. *Am J Surg* 150:698, 1985.

Jones RC, Shires GT: The management of pancreatic injuries. *Arch Surg* 90:502, 1965.

Jones RC, McClelland RN, et al: Difficult closures of the duodenal stump. *Arch Surg* 94:696, 1967.

Jones RC, Thal ER, et al: Evaluation of antibiotic therapy following penetrating abdominal trauma. *Ann Surg* 120(5):576, 1985.

Kelly G, Norton L, et al: The continuing challenge of duodenal injuries. *J Trauma* 18(3):160, 1978.

King H, Shumacker HB Jr: Splenic studies: I. Susceptibility to infection after splenectomy performed in infancy. *Ann Surg* 136:239, 1952.

Kobold EE, Thal AP: A simple method for the management of experimental wounds of the duodenum. *Surg Gynecol Obstet* 116:340, 1963.

Kudsk KA, Sheldon GF, Lim RC Jr: Atrial-caval shunting (ACS) after trauma. *J Trauma* 22(2):81, 1982.

Lambeth W, Rubin BR: Nonoperative management of intrahepatic hemorrhage and hematoma following blunt trauma. *Surg Gynecol Obstet* 148:507, 1979.

Lavenson GS, Cohen A: Management of rectal injuries. *Am J Surg* 122:226, 1971.

Ledgerwood AM, Kazmers M, Lucas CE: The role of thoracic aortic occlusion for massive hemoperitoneum. *J Trauma* 16(8):610, 1976.

Letton AH, Wilson JP: Traumatic severance of pancreas treated by Roux-y anastomosis. *Surg Gynecol Obstet* 109:473, 1959.

Lim RC, Glickman MG, Hunt TK: Angiography in patients with blunt trauma to the chest and abdomen. *Surg Clin North Am* 52(3):551, 1972.

LoCicero J III, Tajima T, Drapanas T: A half-century of experience in the management of colon injuries: Changing concepts. *J Trauma* 15(7):575, 1975.

Longmore WP: Early management of injury to the extrahepatic biliary tract. *JAMA* 165:822, 1966.

Lou Sister MA, Johnson AP, et al: Exteriorized repair in the management of colon injuries. *Arch Surg* 116:926, 1981.

Lucas CE: What is the role of biliary drainage in liver trauma? *Am J Surg* 120:509, 1970.

Lucas CE, Ledgerwood AM: Factors influencing outcome after blunt duodenal injury. *J Trauma* 15(10):839, 1975.

Lucas CE, Ledgerwood AM: Prospective evaluation of hemostatic techniques for liver injuries. *J Trauma* 16(6):442, 1976.

Lucas CE, Walt AJ: Analysis of randomized biliary drainage for liver trauma in 189 patients. *J Trauma* 12(11):925, 1972.

Lucas CE, Canizaro PC, Shires GT: Repair of hepatic venous intrahepatic vena caval, and portal venous injuries, in Madding GF, Kennedy PA: *Trauma to the Liver,* 2d ed. Philadelphia, Saunders, 1971, chap 10, p 146.

Luna G, Dellinger EP: Nonoperative observation therapy for splenic injuries. *Am J Surg* 153:462, 1987.

McLelland BA, Hanna SS, et al: Analysis of peritoneal lavage parameters in blunt abdominal trauma. *J Trauma* 25(5):393, 1985.

McClelland RN, Shires T: Management of liver trauma in 259 consecutive patients. *Ann Surg* 161:248, 1965.

McClelland RN, Shires T, Poulos E: Hepatic resection for massive trauma. *J Trauma* 4:282, 1964.

McInnis WD, Aust JB, et al: Traumatic injuries of the duodenum: A comparison of 1° closure and the jejunal patch. *J Trauma* 15(10):847, 1975.

Mahon PA, Sutton JE Jr: Nonoperative management of adult splenic injury due to blunt trauma: A warning. *Am J Surg* 149:716, 1985.

Malangoni MA, Levine AW, et al: Management of injury to the spleen in adults. Results of early operation and observation. *Ann Surg* 200(6):702, 1984.

Martin TD, Feliciano DV, et al: Severe duodenal injuries. Treatment with pyloric exclusion and gastrojejunostomy. *Arch Surg* 118(17):631, 1983.

Mattox KL, Espada R, Beall AC Jr: Traumatic injury to the portal vein. *Ann Surg* 181:519, 1975.

Maynard AL, Oropeza G: Mandatory operation for penetrating wounds of the abdomen. *Am J Surg* 115:307, 1968.

Mays ET: Lobar dearterialization for exsanguinating wounds of the liver. *J Trauma* 12(5):397, 1972.

Miller DR: Median sternotomy extension of abdominal incision for hepatic lobectomy. *Ann Surg* 175:193, 1972.

Moore FA, Moore EE, et al: Risk of splenic salvage after trauma. *Am J Surg* 148:800, 1984.

Moretz JA III, Campbell DP, et al: Significance of serum amylase level in evaluating pancreatic trauma. *Am J Surg* 130:739, 1975.

Morgenstern L: Microcrystalline collagen used in experimental splenic injury: A new surface hemostatic agent. *Arch Surg* 109:44, 1974.

Morgenstern L, Shapiro SJ: Techniques of splenic conservation. *Arch Surg* 114:449, 1979.

Morton JR, Jordan GL: Traumatic duodenal injuries: Review of 131 cases. *J Trauma* 8(2):127, 1968.

Mucha P Jr, Daly RC, Farnell MB: Selective management of blunt splenic trauma. *J Trauma* 26(11):970, 1986.

Nance FC, Cohn I Jr: Surgical judgment in the management of stab wounds of the abdomen: A retrospective and prospective analysis based on a study of 600 stabbed patients. *Ann Surg* 170:569, 1969.

Nance FC, Wennar MH, et al: Surgical judgment in the management of penetrating wounds of the abdomen: Experience with 2212 patients. *Ann Surg* 179:639, 1974.

Naylor R, Coln D, Shires GT: Morbidity and mortality from injuries to the spleen. *J Trauma* 14(9):773, 1974.

Nichols RL, Smith JW, et al: Risk of infection after penetrating abdominal trauma. *N Engl J Med* 311(17):1065, 1984.

Oakes DD: Splenic trauma. *Curr Probl Surg* 17:342, 1981.

Olsen WR: The serum amylase in blunt abdominal trauma. *J Trauma* 13(3):200, 1973.

Olsen WR, Polley TZ Jr: A second look at delayed splenic rupture. *Arch Surg* 112:422, 1977.

Olsen WR, Redman HC, Hildreth DH: Quantitative peritoneal lavage in blunt abdominal trauma. *Arch Surg* 104:536, 1972.

O'Neal BJ, McDonald JC: The risk of sepsis in the asplenic adult. *Ann Surg* 194:775, 1981.

Oreskovich MR, Carrico CJ: Stab wounds of the anterior abdomen. Analysis of management plan using local wound exploration and quantitative peritoneal lavage. *Ann Surg* 198(4):411, 1983.

Pachter HL, Pennington R, et al: Simplified distal pancreatectomy with the auto suture stapler: Preliminary clinical observations. *Surgery* 85:166, 1979.

Pachter HL, Spencer FC: Recent concepts in the treatment of hepatic trauma. Facts and fallacies. *Ann Surg* 190(4):423, 1979.

Pachter HL, Spencer FC, et al: The management of juxtahepatic venous injuries without an atriocaval shunt: Preliminary clinical observations. *Surgery* 99(5):569, 1986.

Parvin S, Smith DE, et al: Effectiveness of peritoneal lavage in blunt abdominal trauma. *Ann Surg* 181:255, 1975.

Peitzman AB, Makaroun MS, et al: Prospective study of computed tomography in initial management of blunt abdominal trauma, *J Trauma* 26(7):585, 1986.

Perlberger RR: Control of hemobilia by angiographic embolization. *AJR* 128:672, 1977.

Perry JF Jr, DeMeules JE, Root HD: Diagnostic peritoneal lavage in blunt abdominal trauma. *Surg Gynecol Obstet* 131:742, 1970.

Perry JF Jr, LaFave JW: Biliary decompression without other external drainage in treatment of liver injuries. *Surgery* 55:351, 1964.

Perry MO: *The Management of Acute Vascular Injuries*. Baltimore, Williams & Wilkins, 1981, p 105.

Perry MO, Thal ER, Shires GT: Management of arterial injuries. *Ann Surg* 173:403, 1971.

Printen KJ, Freeark RJ, Shoemaker WC: Conservative management of penetrating abdominal wounds. *Arch Surg* 96:899, 1968.

Quast DC, Jordan GL: Traumatic wounds of the female reproductive organs. *J Trauma* 4:839, 1964.

Reinhardt GF, Hubay CA: Surgical management of traumatic hemobilia. *Am J Surg* 121:328, 1971.

Reinhoff WF, Donahoo JS: Isolated complete rupture of the pancreas from non-penetrating abdominal trauma treated by distal resection. *Am Surg* 33:148, 1967.

Richie JP, Fonkalsrud EW: Subcapsular hematoma of the liver. *Arch Surg* 104:781, 1972.

Root HD, Hauser CW, et al: Diagnostic peritoneal lavage. *Surgery* 57:633, 1965.

Rosoff L, Cohen JL, et al: Injuries of the spleen. *Surg Clin North Am* 52(3):667, 1972.

Rydell WB Jr: Complete transection of the common bile duct due to blunt abdominal trauma. *Arch Surg* 100:724, 1970.

Ryzoff RI, Shaftan GW, Herbsman H: Selective conservatism in abdominal trauma. *Surgery* 59:650, 1966.

Salyer K, McClelland RN: Pancreaticoduodenectomy for trauma. *Arch Surg* 95:636, 1967.

Schrock T, Blaisdell FW, Mathewson C: Management of blunt trauma to the liver and hepatic veins. *Arch Surg* 96:698, 1968.

Schrock T, Christensen N: Management of perforating injuries of the colon. *Surg Gynecol Obstet* 135:65, 1972.

Seaver R, Lynch J, et al: Hypogastric artery ligation for uncontrollable hemorrhage in acute pelvic trauma. *Surgery* 55:516, 1964.

Shackford SR, Sise MJ, et al: Evaluation of splenorrhaphy: A grading system for splenic trauma. *J Trauma* 21(7):538, 1981.

Shaftan GW: Indications for operation in abdominal trauma. *Am J Surg* 99:657, 1960.

Shannon FL, Moore EE: Primary repair of the colon: When is it a safe alternative? *Surg* 98(4):851, 1985.

Sheldon GF, Cohn L, Blaisdell W: Surgical treatment of pancreatic trauma. *J Trauma* 10:795, 1970.

Sheldon GF, Lim RC Jr, et al: *Ann Surg* 202(5):539, 1985.

Shires GT, Jackson D, Williams J: Temporary duodenal decompression as an adjunct to gastric resection for duodenal ulcer. *Am Surg* 28:709, 1962.

Singer DB: Postsplenectomy sepsis, in Rosenberg HS, Bolande RP (eds): *Perspectives in Pediatric Pathology*. Chicago, Year Book Medical, 1973, vol 1, p 285.

Smiley K, Perry MO: Balloon catheter tamponade of major vascular wounds. *Am J Surg* 121:326, 1971.

Smithwick W III, Gertner HR Jr, Zuidema GD: Injection of hypaque (sodium diatrizoate) in the management of abdominal stab wounds. *Surg Gynecol Obstet* 127:1215, 1968.

Snyder WH III, Weigelt JA, et al: The surgical management of duodenal trauma. *Arch Surg* 115:422, 1980.

Soderstrom CA, Maekawa K, et al: Gallbladder injuries resulting from blunt abdominal trauma. An experience and review. *Ann Surg* 193(1):60, 1981.

Sparkman RS: Massive hemobilia following traumatic rupture of the liver. *Ann Surg* 138:899, 1953.

Starzl TE, Kaupp HA, et al: Penetrating injuries of the inferior vena cava. *Surg Clin North Am* 43:387, 1963.

Steele M, Lim RC: Advances in management of splenic injuries. *Am J Surg* 130:159, 1975.

Stone HH, Fabian TC: Management of duodenal wounds. *J Trauma* 19(5):334, 1979.

Stone HH, Lamb JM: Use of pedicled omentum as an autogenous pack for control of hemorrhage in major injuries of the liver. *Surg Gynecol Obstet* 141:92, 1975.

Strate RG, Grieco JC: Blunt injury to the colon and rectum. *J Trauma* 23(5):384, 1983.

Strauch GO: Preservation of splenic function in adults and children with injured spleens. *Am J Surg* 137:478, 1979.

Sturmer FC, Wilt KE: Complete division of the common duct from external blunt trauma. *Am J Surg* 105:781, 1963.

Taxier M, Sivak MV, et al: Endoscopic retrograde pancreatography in the evaluation of trauma to the pancreas. *Surg Gynecol Obstet* 150:65, 1980.

Thal ER: Evaluation of peritoneal lavage and local exploration in lower chest and abdominal stabwounds. *J Trauma* 17:642, 1977.

Thal ER: Peritoneal lavage. Reliability of RBC count in patients with stab wounds to the chest. *Arch Surg* 119:579, 1984.

Thal ER, May RA, Beesinger D: Peritoneal lavage: Its unreliability in gunshot wounds of the lower chest and abdomen. *Arch Surg* 115:430, 1980.

Thal ER, Shires GT: Peritoneal lavage in blunt abdominal trauma. *Am J Surg* 125:64, 1973.

Thal ER, Yeary EC: Morbidity of colostomy closure following colon trauma. *J Trauma* 20(4):287, 1980.

Thompson JS, Moore EE, Moore JB: Comparison of penetrating injuries of the right and left colon. *Ann Surg* 193:414, 1981.

Traub AC, Perry JF: Splenic preservation following splenic trauma. *J Trauma* 22(6):496, 1982.

Trunkey D, Hays RJ, Shires GT: Management of rectal trauma. *J Trauma* 13(5):411, 1973.

Trunkey D, Shires GT, McClelland RN: Management of liver trauma in 811 consecutive patients. *Ann Surg* 179(5):522, 1974.

Tuggle D, Huber PJ Jr: Management of rectal trauma. *Am J Surg* 148:806, 1984.

Turpin I, State D, Schwartz A: Injuries to the inferior vena cava and their management. *Am J Surg* 134:25, 1977.

Vannix RS, Carter R, et al: Surgical management of colon trauma in civilian practice. *Am J Surg* 106:364, 1963.

Van Stiegmann G, Moore EE, Moore GE: Failure of spleen repair. *J Trauma* 19:698, 1979.

Vaughan GD III, Frazier OH, et al: The use of pyloric exclusion in the management of severe duodenal injuries. *Am J Surg* 134:785, 1977.

Walt AJ: The mythology of hepatic trauma—or Babel revisited. *Am J Surg* 135:12, 1978.

Walter JF, Baaso BT, Cannon WB: Successful transcatheter embolic control of massive hematobilia secondary to liver biopsy. *AJR* 127:847, 1976.

Weichert RF III, Hewitt RL, Drapanas T: Blunt injuries to intrahepatic vena cava and hepatic veins with survival. *Am J Surg* 121:322, 1971.

Weinstein ME, Govin GG, Rice CL: Splenorrhaphy for splenic trauma. *J Trauma* 19:692, 1979.

Wilder JR, Habermann ET, Schachner SJ: Selective surgical intervention for stab wounds of the abdomen. *Surgery* 61:231, 1967.

Wilder JR, Lotfi MW, Jurani P: Comparative study of mandatory and selective surgical intervention in stab wounds of the abdomen. *Surgery* 69:546, 1971.

Witek JT, Spencer RP, et al: Diagnostic spleen scans in occult splenic injury. *J Trauma* 14:197, 1974.

Woolley MM, Mahour GH, Sloan T: Duodenal hematoma in infancy and childhood. Changing etiology and changing treatment. *Am J Surg* 136:8, 1978.

Yajko RD, Seydel F, Trimble C: Rupture of the stomach from blunt abdominal trauma. *J Trauma* 15(3):177, 1975.

Yellin AE, Chaffee CB, Donovan AJ: Vascular isolation in treatment of juxtahepatic venous injuries. *Arch Surg* 102:566, 1971.

Yasugi H, Mizumoto R, et al: Changes in carbohydrate metabolism and endocrine function of remnant pancreas after major pancreatic resection. *Am J Surg* 132:577, 1976.

Yasugi H, Rosoff L Sr: Pancreatoduodenectomy for combined pancreatoduodenal injuries. *Arch Surg* 110:1177, 1975.

Burns

P. William Curreri and Arnold Luterman

The complex pathophysiologic alterations that accompany major thermal injury present the surgeon with an extraordinary therapeutic challenge. During the past two decades, few areas of medical science have experienced more rapid development of new treatment modalities. As a result, marked improvement in the care of patients with major burn injury has been noted. Comprehensive treatment centers now utilize sophisticated, multidisciplinary teams to aid in the diagnosis of rapidly changing physiologic responses to the injury and to assist in providing the vast array of specialized therapeutic services that are necessary to minimize morbidity and mortality.

Burn injury constitutes a major national health problem. More than 2 million persons suffer thermal injury annually, of whom 100,000 must be hospitalized. Burn injuries are now exceeded only by motor vehicle accidents as a cause of accidental death. As in other types of trauma, thermal injury frequently afflicts children and young adults. Prolonged morbidity, as well as temporary or permanent disability, associated with thermal injury results in a staggering economic drain on social resources. Hospital and medical costs for the treatment of burn injuries are now estimated at greater than one billion dollars a year. Financial support is often required to defray expenses associated with prolonged hospitalization, loss of family income sources, and replacement of lost labor within the working force.

ETIOLOGY OF BURNS

Burns are caused by the application of heat to the body. The depth of the resulting burn injury will be dependent on the intensity and duration of heat application and the conductivity of the tissues involved. The most common heat sources are an open flame and hot liquid. In addition, thermal injury is frequently observed in patients who have been exposed to direct contact with hot metal, toxic chemicals, or high-voltage electric current. Damage as a result of heat rarely occurs below 45°C. Between 45 and 50°C, gradations of cell injury may occur; and above 50°C, denaturation of protein elements of the cell becomes apparent.

Laboratory accidents, civilian assaults, industrial mishaps, and inexpert application of agents used for medical purposes account for most of the chemical burns in the civilian population. At least 25,000 products capable of producing chemical burns are available for use in industry, agriculture, military science, and the home. The number of patients with chemical burns requiring professional medical care is estimated to exceed 60,000 per year. At least 3000 deaths annually in the United States can be attributed to cutaneous and gastrointestinal chemical injuries. A principal difference between thermal and chemical injury is the length of time during which tissue destruction continues, since the chemical agent causes progressive damage until inactivated by reaction with tissue, while thermal injury ceases shortly after removal of the heat source. Tissue destruction associated with exposure to chemicals may be limited by application of large volumes of water to dilute the offending agent and reduce its contact time. Compared with thermal injury, the severe, full-thickness chemical burn may appear deceptively superficial, with only mild bronze discoloration of intact skin during the first few postburn days.

Electrical injuries cause 2400 admissions to emergency rooms annually, accounting for 3 percent of all admissions to major burn centers and resulting in 1500 deaths per year. The number of accidents is steadily increasing. One-third of all major electrical accidents occur in electrical workers, one-third in construction workers, and the remainder in non-work-related settings such as home accidents. The extremities are the most common sites of contact with electric current, with the upper limbs involved more frequently than the lower limbs.

In contrast to both thermal and chemical burns, electrical injury usually results in minimal destruction of skin. The magnitude of the injury is directly related to the amount of current passing through tissue between the point of contact with the electrical source and the exit site at which the patient is grounded. The magnitude of current passing through various organs is indirectly related to the resistance of the tissue. Nerve, blood, and muscle offer the least resistance to electric current and thus sustain the maximum amount of tissue damage. As a result, cutaneous injury may be apparent only at the entrance and exit sites, although considerable deep tissue destruction of upper and lower extremity musculature may be present.

The cross-sectional area of different portions of the body will also determine the extent of damage produced. In those portions of the body with small cross-sectional areas (e.g., a distal limb), current density and the temperatures generated will be higher than in those areas of greater cross-sectional area.

The electrical resistance of skin can vary dramatically depending on its moisture, cleanliness, and thickness. The average resistance measurement for skin is 40,000 ohms. Calloused skin may have a resistance as high as 1 million ohms, while the resistance of moist skin may be as low as 300 ohms.

Small, deep burns in the antecubital space or in the axilla are often observed in the patient with severe electrical injury of the upper extremity. These burns result from the arcing of current across the joint via the path of least resistance, the skin moistened with perspiration. When arc burns are present, they are nearly always accompanied by extensive, deep muscular destruction. This type of injury is frequently associated with release of hemochromagens into the bloodstream that are excreted via the urinary tract. Thus, "port-wine" colored urine containing myoglobin is not unusual following major electrical injury.

IMMEDIATE THERAPY

Initial therapy of the patient with a major burn should be directed toward restoration of normal physiologic parameters and prevention of life-threatening complications. With the exception of chemical burns, in which the toxic agent must be diluted with water and physically removed as rapidly as possible to prevent further tissue destruction, the burn wound is of secondary importance during the first few hours after the injury.

Maintenance of Airway

Immediate pulmonary complications may become manifest in the thermally injured patient. Excessive exposure to smoke may result in carbon monoxide poisoning. Carbon monoxide is a colorless, odorless gas with an affinity for hemoglobin approximately 210 times greater than that of oxygen. Patients with carbon monoxide poisoning exhibit the signs and symptoms of hypoxia, which may range from pronounced tachypnea and agitation to respiratory arrest and coma.

The diagnosis may be quickly confirmed by analyzing the concentration of carboxyhemoglobin in the blood. Treatment includes the administration of 100% oxygen, with ventilatory support if necessary, in order to displace the tightly bound carbon monoxide from the hemoglobin molecule. Since carbon monoxide is not toxic to lungs per se, the syndrome is entirely reversible, provided anoxic damage to distant tissues (e.g., the central nervous system) has not occurred. Although several decades ago few patients with severe carbon monoxide poisoning survived long enough to reach the emergency room, the development of sophisticated paramedical teams trained to insert endotracheal tubes and administer ventilatory support in the field has allowed greater salvage of such patients in the last several years.

Upper airway obstruction in patients with burns of the head and neck may occur during the first 48 hours after injury. The obstruction is related to soft tissue edema of the oral pharynx and vocal cords following exposure to hot gases. Direct thermal injury to the lower respiratory tract is exceedingly unusual, since the nose and oral pharynx are extremely efficient heat exchangers, allowing cooling of inhaled hot gas prior to its entrance into the trachea. Since it is more difficult to extract heat from liquid, direct thermal injury of the lower respiratory tract is occasionally noted in patients injured by superheated steam.

Upper airway obstruction is usually heralded by an increase in the respiratory rate and progressive hoarseness. In addition, a patient may exhibit increased difficulty in clearing bronchial secretions as the vocal cords become more edematous. Confirmation of impending obstruction is made by direct visualization of the posterior oral phar-

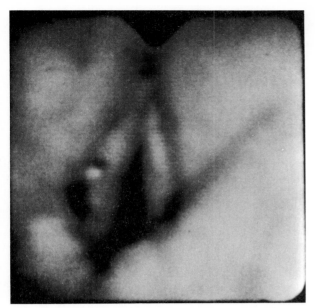

Fig. 7-1. Vocal cords seen through a fiberoptic bronchoscope shows swelling, vesicles, and carbonaceous deposits.

ynx and cords, utilizing either direct laryngoscopy or fiberoptic endoscopy (Fig. 7-1). The latter is usually preferred, since at the same time, assessment of smoke inhalation may be accomplished by visualizing the lower respiratory tract.

Impending upper airway obstruction is treated by the immediate insertion of an endotracheal tube. Tracheos-

tomy is performed only when nasotracheal or endotracheal intubation is impossible. Soft tissue edema is maximal at between 24 and 48 h. Therefore, the endotracheal tube is usually not removed until the third postburn day. Direct visualization of the posterior pharynx and larynx is performed prior to extubation to determine if swelling has decreased. Reintubation, if required, often is technically difficult to perform.

Intravenous Resuscitation

Cardiovascular alterations occur almost immediately following burn injury. There is a massive shift of fluid and electrolytes from the intravascular and extracellular fluid space into the cells. Reversion of water and sodium from the intracellular fluid back into the extracellular fluid begins between 24 and 48 h but is not complete until the tenth postburn day. In general, these changes are directly proportional to the extent and depth of burn. Therefore, any consideration of fluid resuscitation to prevent hypovolemic shock requires an accurate estimation of the magnitude of burn injury. The burned wound is three-dimensional; therefore, not only the depth but the surface area involved must be estimated.

Burns are classified as first, second, or third degree (Table 7-1). First-degree burns are characterized by simple erythema of the skin, with only microscopic destruction of superficial layers of the epidermis. A mild sunburn is characteristic of a first-degree injury. The first-degree injury is of little clinical significance, since the water barrier of the skin is not disturbed. Systemic cardiovascular disturbances are rarely observed following first-degree

Table 7-1. CLASSIFICATION OF BURNS

Classification	Morphology	Clinical appearance	Cause
First degree	Only superficial layers of epidermis devitalized; dilatation and congestion of intradermal vessels	Erythema only—blanches on pressure	Ultraviolet exposure (ultraviolet light, sunburn), very short flash
Second degree	Destruction of varying depths of epidermis with coagulation necrosis; clefting of epidermis with fluid collection (blister formation); congestion and coagulation in subdermal plexus. Some skin elements remain viable (often only skin appendages), from which epithelial regeneration can occur*	Erythematous, weeping, painful. Blisters and bullae often present. Superficial layers of skin can be readily wiped away. Remaining skin elements waxy white, soft, dry, insensitive	Short flash, spill scald
Third degree	Destruction of all skin elements; coagulation of subdermal plexus	Dry, hard, inelastic, translucent, with thrombosed vein visible	Flame, immersion scald, chemical contact, electric current

* Initial injury may be partial-thickness, with only dermal appendages (hair follicles and glands) remaining, but these skin elements are readily destroyed by infection, with resulting conversion to full-thickness (third-degree) burn.

burn injury. The burns rapidly heal if the patient avoids further exposure to a heat source. First-degree burns are *not* considered when estimating the magnitude of burn injury for purposes of planning intravenous fluid replacement.

Second- and third-degree burns are of equal physiologic significance and may be summated in the estimate of total body surface burn injury. Second-degree burns extend through the epidermis into the dermis. By definition, viable epithelial elements from which epithelial regeneration can occur are retained in second-degree burn injury; thus the burn is often described as *partial-thickness*. Even when most of the epithelium is destroyed, regeneration may occur from epithelial cells surrounding hair follicles or sweat glands. On the other hand, third-degree burns are characterized by total irreversible destruction of all the skin, dermal appendages, and epithelial elements. Spontaneous regeneration of epithelium is not possible, and the burns are described as *full-thickness*. Such burns require the application of skin grafts if the development of scar tissue is to be avoided.

Since skin varies in thickness in different parts of the body, application of the same intensity of heat for a given period of time will result in a burn that will vary in depth, depending on the thickness of the skin itself in the local area, as well as the existence and degree of development of the dermal appendages (sweat glands and hair follicles) and dermal papillae. In the very old person, in whom dermal papillae and appendages are atrophic, and in the very young, in whom they have not yet fully developed, deep burns result from the same heat intensity that produces a moderate second-degree burn in the middle-aged adult. Since the skin of the back is thicker than that on any other part of the body, full-thickness burns are less common in this area. On the other hand, skin covering the inner arm is extraordinarily thin, thus full-thickness injury is frequently observed in this area.

The length and width of the burn wound is expressed as a percentage of the total body surface area displaying either second- or third-degree burns. The extent of the body surface involved is most commonly estimated by the "rule of nines" (Table 7-2). The major anatomic portions of the adult may be divided into multiples of 9 percent of the body surface area. The proportion of each of these areas with second- or third-degree burns is esti-

mated, and the summation of these estimates represents the percentage of the total body surface area burn. Because the surface area of the head and neck in childhood is significantly larger than 9 percent of the total body surface area and the surface area associated with the lower extremities is smaller, the rule of nines may not be used to estimate total body surface area burns in children. For example, a one-year-old child has 19 percent of the total body surface area associated with the head, as compared with only 7 percent in the adult patient. In contrast, each lower extremity represents only 13 percent of the total body surface area in the year-old infant. Thus the total body surface area burn in children is best estimated by the utilization of charts that relate regional body surface to age (Figure 7-2). A useful rule of thumb for estimating the amount of body surface area involved by a scattered burn injury is the *palm of hand rule*. The surface area of the patient's palm is roughly 1 percent of the total body surface area.

Over the past 20 years, many resuscitation formulas have been developed as guides to initial resuscitation in hypovolemic shock following thermal injury. Most utilize various combinations of crystalloid and colloid solutions but differ widely in the ratio of colloid to crystalloid, as well as the rate of fluid administration. The ideal resuscitation formula would rapidly restore normal hemodynamic stability. Such a response is dependent on the rate at which fluid is lost from the extracellular fluid compartment, the composition of the fluid lost, and the ability of various solutions to restore an effective circulating extracellular volume. Unfortunately, most formulas have been derived empirically from clinical experience, in which the amount of fluid required to restore renal function was accepted as optimal replacement therapy.

Although controversy still remains over "the solution" for resuscitation in burn shock, scientific investigation supports the need for both crystalloid and colloid solutions. *It is of relatively little consequence which formula is utilized to begin such therapy, as long as this is modified according to the patient's changing requirements.* The formula shown in Table 7-3 has been popularized by Baxter and is known as the *Parkland formula*. This formula has been adopted in most burn centers and is currently the standard against which new formulas must be compared. Data from numerous studies now suggest that both volume and the sodium ion are critical to providing adequate resuscitation in hypovolemic burn shock. Administration of crystalloid solution results in early expansion of depleted plasma and extracellular fluid volumes and return of the cardiac output toward normal. After 24 h, colloid remains the most effective solution to maintain plasma volume without further increasing edema formation. The Parkland formula was derived to provide specific replacement of known deficits measured by simultaneous determinations of red cell volume, plasma volume, extracellular fluid volume, and cardiac output during burn shock. The formula calls for the administration of 4 mL of lactated Ringer's solution/kg of body weight/percent of body surface area burn during the first 24 h postinjury. Fluid therapy during the second 24 h,

Table 7-2. "RULE OF NINES" FOR ESTIMATING PERCENTAGE OF BODY SURFACE INVOLVED IN BURNS

Anatomic area	Percent of body surface
Head	9
Right upper extremity	9
Left upper extremity	9
Right lower extremity	18
Left lower extremity	18
Anterior trunk	18
Posterior trunk	18
Neck	1

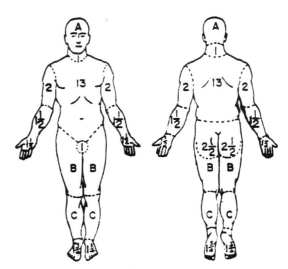

UNIVERSITY OF SOUTH ALABAMA MEDICAL CENTER
HOSPITAL AND CLINICS

BURN CHART

Relative Percentage of Areas Affected by Growth

Age	Age in Years					
	0	1	5	10	15	ADULT
A − $\frac{1}{2}$ of head	$9\frac{1}{2}$	$8\frac{1}{2}$	$6\frac{1}{2}$	$5\frac{1}{2}$	$4\frac{1}{2}$	$3\frac{1}{2}$
B − $\frac{1}{2}$ of one thigh	$2\frac{3}{4}$	$3\frac{1}{4}$	4	$4\frac{1}{4}$	$4\frac{1}{2}$	$4\frac{3}{4}$
C − $\frac{1}{2}$ of one leg	$2\frac{1}{2}$	$2\frac{1}{2}$	$2\frac{3}{4}$	3	$3\frac{1}{4}$	$3\frac{1}{2}$

Total Percent Burned_____ 2° +_____ 3° =_____

Fig. 7-2. Burn charts are used to determine exactly what percent of the total body surface area is involved.

Table 7-3. FLUID RESUSCITATION OF BURNED PATIENTS: PARKLAND FORMULA

First 24 h:
 Electrolyte solution (lactated Ringer's): 4 mL/kg body wt./% second- and third-degree burn
 Administration rate: $\frac{1}{2}$ first 8 h, $\frac{1}{4}$ second 8 h, $\frac{1}{4}$ third 8 h
 Urine output: 30–70 mL/h

Second 24 h:
 Glucose in water (D_5W): To replace evaporative water loss, maintaining serum sodium concentration of 140 meq/L
 Colloid solution (plasma): To maintain plasma volume in patients with more than 40% second- and third-degree burns
 Urine output: 30–100 mL/h

according to this formula, consists in the administration of free water (5% dextrose in water) in quantities sufficient to maintain the serum sodium concentration at 140 meq/L (approximately 4 to 5 L in a 70-kg patient with a 50 percent burn) and plasma sufficient to return the plasma volume to normal and sustain adequate perfusion of peripheral organs and tissues (approximately 250 mL for each 10 percent total body surface area burn over 20 percent). Supplemental potassium replacement is usually not required during the first few days of management. The catabolic state caused by the burn injury results in increased urine levels of potassium with a decrease in total body potassium. The serum level of potassium remains normal or slightly elevated. When nutritional support is instituted and an anabolic state created, large amounts of potassium may be required to replenish this deficit and avoid acute decrease in serum potassium concentration.

During the first 24 h, the rate of fluid administration is adjusted to correspond as closely as possible with the rate of extracellular fluid loss. Baxter's studies have confirmed that extracellular deficits occur rapidly within the first 6 to 12 h postinjury. Therefore, one-half of the total calculated fluid volume is delivered during the first 8 h *from the time of injury* and the remaining fluids more slowly over the next 16 h.

The adequacy of resuscitation can best be judged by frequent measurements of vital signs, central venous pressure, hourly urine output, and observation of general mental and physical response. Urine output (normal, 30 to 100 mL/h in the adult) still remains one of the most reliable guides to adequacy of fluid therapy. Acute tubular necrosis, with resultant renal failure, is extremely rare in an adequately resuscitated patient, with the possible exception of a patient in whom there is extensive muscle damage (electrical burns) resulting in hemachromogen release and intratubular protein precipitation. Therefore, oliguria during the early postburn period is most often an indication of inadequate resuscitation, and increased fluid administration is the treatment of choice. Restriction of fluid is almost never indicated, and the administration of diuretics should be reserved for those cases in which tubular damage from circulating pigments appears likely, and then only after a sufficient amount of resuscitation fluids has been administered.

Urinary outputs of 30 to 100 mL/h should be maintained during the first 24 h in the adult patient. In the absence of hypoxia related to respiratory dysfunction, the patient's sensorium accurately reflects cerebral circulation. Well-resuscitated patients with major thermal injury rarely display hysteria, acute anxiety, or hostility.

The indications to use central venous catheters, Swan-Ganz catheters, and arterial lines in burn patients are identical to those for any trauma victim. The burn injury does not contraindicate their use (when needed) even if entrance through a burned site is necessary. Nonburned areas are preferred because of the difficulty in securing a catheter to eschar. All intravenous lines should be changed every 72 h whether or not they traverse burned tissue to lower the risk of septic thrombophlebitis and its sequelae.

Sedation

One of the most frequent therapeutic errors in the treatment of patients with major burns is the overuse of sedation. An insignificant burn of a minute area incurred during a common household mishap may be quite painful. Projection of such an experience by medical and paramedical personnel has resulted in marked overestimation of the pain associated with a major burn. If there is full-thickness skin destruction, the intrinsic sensory nerve endings have also been destroyed and the wound itself is painless. In contrast, the second-degree burn can be quite painful initially. Pain from a burn injury is markedly increased when the wound is roughly handled, or by exposing the wound to a cold environment. It is essential to completely examine the burn patient to determine if other injuries have occurred. When the physical examination is over, however, the wounds should be covered and the patient kept warm. This usually minimizes the pain from the burn sites, thereby decreasing the need for analgesics.

Sedative and analgesic medications must never be administered before hypoxia, hypovolemia, or both have been excluded, both states commonly producing an anxious, thrashing, disoriented patient. When given they should be kept at an *absolute minimum* to prevent depression of cardiopulmonary function and to allow evaluation of the sensorium, an important indicator of the adequacy of fluid resuscitation. Decreased peripheral circulation to muscle and skin is often associated with the hypovolemic state, so any narcotics administered intramuscularly or subcutaneously are subject to erratic uptake. Therefore, narcotics should always be administered in small doses by the intravenous route during the first 4 to 5 days. Administration by this route ensures rapid and predictable concentrations of the drug in the central nervous system and prevents the narcosis that may result following fluid resuscitation if repeated doses of narcotics have been administered by the intramuscular route.

Antibiotics

Subsequent to thermal injury, microorganisms contaminating the surfaces of the wound and persisting in the depth of the hair follicles and sweat glands begin to proliferate rapidly if topical chemotherapeutic agents are not applied. In the absence of topical chemotherapy, the superficial areas of the burn wound contain up to 100 million organisms per gram of tissue within 48 h following injury.

Characteristically, gram-positive organisms are responsible for this initial proliferation and colonization of the burn wound. At one time, most experienced clinicians prophylactically administered penicillin to patients with major burn injuries for a period of 3 to 4 days. Routine prophylactic administration of penicillin in the immediate postburn period is no longer recommended. Recent studies have demonstrated that the routine administration of prophylactic penicillin fails to lower the incidence of early gram-positive cellulitis, increases the incidence of yeast colonization of the gastrointestinal tract, and is associated with more rapid emergence of resistant gram-negative organisms in the burn wound. Penicillin prophylaxis, as a routine, has now been discontinued in most burn centers, and the incidence of early streptococcal cellulitis has not increased.

The full-thickness burn wound is relatively avascular. When it becomes infected, the avascular tissue may prevent the ingress of host defense factors and systemically administered antibiotics. The burn wound, once infected, may behave like an undrained abscess. Despite the current availability of newer antibiotic agents, some of which may penetrate to the eschar, one cannot rely totally on systemic agents as the sole mechanism of controlling microorganism proliferation in the burn wound. Other modalities such as topical antibiotics must be employed.

Systemic antibiotic agents are most useful in treating specific distant bacterial infections (e.g., pneumonia) that may complicate the burn victim's hospital course.

Tetanus Prophylaxis

All burn injuries must be considered contaminated, and tetanus prophylaxis is mandatory except in those patients actively immunized within the preceding 12 months. If a booster was received within the preceding 10 years, the intramuscular administration of 0.5 mL of absorbed tetanus toxoid will usually provide adequate prophylaxis. In the absence of active immunization within 10 years prior to the burn injury, 250 to 500 units of tetanus immunoglobulin (human) should be simultaneously administered at another site, utilizing a different syringe and needle so as to prevent inactivation of the immune globulin by toxoid.

Escharotomy

A principal characteristic of human skin is a remarkable degree of elasticity, which allows the skin to stretch with only minimum applied force. The elasticity of skin allows considerable edema of underlying soft tissues without increasing central limb pressure, which might impede either venous outflow or arterial inflow. If the skin were unyielding, a patient with a severely sprained ankle might lose blood flow to the distal foot as soft tissue edema occurred. Skin with second-degree injury retains its elastic properties. Full-thickness injury (third degree) is characterized by almost complete loss of elasticity. Thus circumferential third-degree burns are frequently associated with decreased peripheral blood flow as fluid resuscitation, accompanied by soft tissue edema, progresses. Failure to recognize this situation may result in unnecessary loss of distal extremities.

The usual clinical signs associated with poor peripheral blood flow in the nonburned patient, that is, diminished peripheral pulses and decreased skin temperature, are unreliable in patients with severe thermal injury. Hypovolemia with peripheral vasoconstriction usually results in decreased temperature of distal extremities in all patients with major second- and third-degree burns, and distal pulses often may not be felt as a result of overlying soft tissue edema preventing palpation of the underlying artery. More reliable signs of decreased peripheral flow in patients with circumferential third-degree burns are slow capillary refill (observed in the nail beds) and the onset of neurologic deficits. The most accurate monitoring device for assessing distal blood flow to extremities is the ultrasonic Doppler, which allows repetitive evaluation of both venous and arterial flow in the digital arteries and veins.

Patients with burns involving the extremities should have the affected limb elevated to minimize soft tissue edema. Should vascular impairment become apparent, however, escharotomies should immediately be performed. An escharotomy is simply an incision through the full depth of the eschar, thus relieving underlying pressure on the central arteries and veins. These incisions may be performed without anesthesia, since third-degree burns are anesthetic. Blood loss is minimal because of the extensive intracapillary coagulation that has occurred as a result of the thermal injury. The escharotomies are usually performed on the lateral and medial aspects of the extremity and must be carried across the joints, since the skin is most tightly adherent to the underlying fascia at these points and vascular obstruction is most likely to occur in these areas. In the upper extremity, the escharotomy should extend through all areas of third-degree burn down to and including the thenar and hypothenar spaces, in order to preserve the intrinsic muscles of the hand. Similarly, in the lower extremities, escharotomies should extend to the base of the large and small toes if the foot exhibits extensive third-degree burns. Escharotomies should only be performed once resuscitation is in progress and an adequate intravascular volume has been achieved. Once escharotomies have been performed, signs of adequate peripheral perfusion are to be expected. Persistent impairment of peripheral blood flow requires reassessment of intravascular volume status, and the extent and depth of the escharotomies. Fasciotomies may be considered at this stage.

Fasciotomy, a linear excision of the deep fascia surrounding the muscles, is rarely indicated in patients with severe burns. In rare instances of extensive incineration when burns involve not only the skin but the underlying fat and muscle, fasciotomy becomes necessary as a result of swelling within the muscle compartments. More frequently, fasciotomy is required in the treatment of electrical burns where there has been extensive muscle injury that appears potentially reversible.

Gastric Decompression

Most patients with more than 20 percent total body surface area burns will develop a reflex paralytic ileus some time during the first 24 h. Although bowel sounds are usually active for 6 to 10 h following the injury, intestinal motility is gradually lost for a short period of time during the latter half of the first 24 h. Unfortunately, the development of ileus frequently occurs at the time when medical and nursing surveillance has relaxed and the patient is asleep following sedation and restoration of fluid volume. Vomiting in such a patient carries a high risk of pulmonary aspiration, a complication associated with severe morbidity and high mortality. For this reason, patients with major burns require a nasogastric tube, so that the stomach may be effectively decompressed until normal gastrointestinal motility has been demonstrated.

The insertion of a nasogastric tube will also allow inspection of the gastric contents at periodic intervals. Patients with major burns are at risk of hemorrhagic gastritis as a result of increased stress. For this reason, gastric aspirates should be monitored frequently for the presence of frank blood or guaiac-positive material, and antacid should be instilled through the nasogastric tube at hourly intervals to prevent superficial erosions of the gastric mucosa.

Histamine H_2 receptor antagonists that suppress gastric acid secretion may also be used to prevent or treat stress gastritis. In elderly patients and at high doses, certain of these compounds may produce central nervous system changes such as confusion, slurred speech, delirium, and hallucinations. Fever, serum creatinine changes, leukopenia, bradycardia, and diarrhea have been reported to occur infrequently. Therefore, these compounds are usually used if stress gastritis develops despite adequate antacid administration.

Medical Evacuation

Although most hospitals are equipped to provide emergency therapy of the patient with a major burn, the majority of community hospitals have neither the nursing nor the paramedical expertise to comfortably care for a patient with massive burn injury. Furthermore, because of the special physical requirements necessary for optimal treatment of such patients, personnel in community hospitals often transfer such patients to special facilities as soon as appropriate arrangements can be made. Guidelines for hospitalization or transfer to a burn treatment facility are outlined in Table 7-4.

Extensive experience with medical evacuation of severely burned soldiers during the Korean and Vietnam wars has yielded valuable information that may assist in ensuring safe transfer of burned patients. In general, such patients tolerate evacuation best if they are moved within the first 24 to 48 h. Prior to transfer, a fluid resuscitation program should be started. Patients with a larger than 20 percent burn should have a Foley catheter inserted into the bladder, so that urinary output can be monitored during the evacuation and fluid administration appropriately adjusted. Pulmonary function should be assessed, and if impending upper airway obstruction or severe smoke inhalation is suspected, an endotracheal tube should be inserted prior to transfer. Extensive debridement or treatment of the burn wounds is unnecessary and is generally to be avoided, since it interferes with evaluation of the burn wound by the receiving hospital. Rather, the

Table 7-4. TRIAGE CRITERIA

Burn size	Admit to hospital	Transfer to burn treatment facility
Total	>15%	>20%
Third degree	>2%	>10%
Age	<5 or >60	<5 or >60
Airway or inhalation injury	Present	Severe
Electric injury	Present	Severe
Significant associated injury or preexisting disease	Present	Present
Deep burns of face, hands, feet, or perineum	Present	Present
Suspected child abuse	Present	Present

SOURCE: American College of Surgeons, *Bulletin,* October 1979.

wounds should be temporarily wrapped in sterile dressings to provide maximal comfort during the transfer. If air evacuation is to be utilized, it is especially important to insert a nasogastric tube, since air within the stomach will expand at increased altitude, often inducing acute gastric distention and vomiting. This, in turn, could result in aspiration pneumonitis, which would be particularly compromising in a patient with the smoke inhalation syndrome.

THERAPY OF THE BURN WOUND

Debridement and Excision

Second-degree wounds (partial-thickness burn injury) usually present as vesicular lesions. Unless very small, the overlying blister should be punctured and the nonviable skin removed. This permits the direct application of topical chemotherapeutic agents to the underlying viable dermal remnants. Failure to prevent secondary bacterial infection of deep second-degree burn wounds may result in conversion of the partial-thickness injury to a full-thickness injury. Debridement can usually be accomplished without anesthesia, utilizing careful surgical technique and modest amounts of sedation prior to removing the nonviable superficial epithelium.

The nonviable skin of the third-degree burn is referred to as the *eschar.* Usually the eschar remains tightly adherent to the underlying subcutaneous tissues and cannot be sharply debrided without severe hemorrhage and significant pain. Therefore, except in special circumstances, only loose eschar, which may be debrided without anesthesia or excessive blood loss, is removed initially. The remaining eschar is left intact, and efforts are made to prevent bacterial colonization and invasion by the use of topical chemotherapeutic agents. Topical chemotherapeutic agents do not sterilize the third-degree burn eschar, and eventually bacterial growth will occur. The topical agents are employed to control the rate of proliferation of bacteria within the burn wound, so as to prevent invasion of underlying viable tissue, with entrance of bacteria into the bloodstream. At about 18 to 24 days following burn injury, the third-degree burn eschar will separate from the underlying viable tissue as a result of the liberation of bacterial proteases. At this time, it is extraordinarily important that the eschar be promptly debrided, in order to prevent systemic sepsis as a result of localized abscess formation beneath the eschar. Normally, the patients are taken to a hydrotherapy area once or twice a day during the first 3 weeks in order to cleanse the surface of the eschar and to inspect the wound. Each day, the physician debrides any loose areas of eschar and carefully inspects the wound and unroofs any localized abscess pockets.

Modern surgical principles dictate the surgical debridement of nonviable tissue in the treatment of major injury. In the case of burn injury, however, immediate total debridement of nonviable eschar is not always possible. Some investigators have advocated the use of topical enzyme preparations to more rapidly remove the eschar. The advantages of such an approach include debridement without anesthesia and limitation of associated hemorrhage. The efficacy of currently available enzymes has not been conclusively demonstrated. Furthermore, most enzyme preparations require the use of overlying wet dressings to maintain the activity of the enzyme. Such dressings promote wound infection, since they provide a warm, moist environment. In addition, some of the enzyme preparations inhibit the effectiveness of topical chemotherapeutic agents in controlling the rate of proliferation of bacterial growth. Therefore, other authors have condemned the use of enzymatic debridement, maintaining that the risks of sepsis far outweigh the benefits of early debridement. In addition, some enzyme preparations do not effectively differentiate nonviable eschar from underlying normal tissues, and erosion of vessels in viable tissue occasionally induces unexpected bleeding from the wound.

Tangential excision of deep second- and third-degree wounds has become increasingly more popular in major burn centers in the past decade. The eschar is tangentially excised utilizing a specially designed knife or an air-driven dermatome to sequentially remove layers of the eschar in sheets approximately 0.010 in. in thickness until viable tissue, as evidenced by capillary bleeding, is encountered. Primary closure is achieved by immediate grafting with autograft (if adequate donor sites are available) or temporary closure with heterograft, homograft, or synthetic barrier dressings. The procedure, although technically easy to perform, requires experience in determining an adequate level of excision. This is especially true when full-thickness injury has occurred and the level of excision is into the subcutaneous fat. Viability of this relatively avascular layer is often difficult to appreciate. The decision to perform early tangential excision (within 72 h of admission) must depend on analysis of both potential risks and benefits of this technique. The major advantage is a shortened hospital stay and potentially improved function when wounds extend across joints. The major disadvantage is the risk of performing a major surgical procedure (with significant blood loss) requiring general anesthesia in an already critically injured patient. Most centers now employ tangential excision for deep second- or third-degree burns of functionally critical areas, such as hands and face, and to shorten the hospital course in relatively good risk patients.

Several investigators have utilized the carbon dioxide laser to excise third-degree burn eschar. The CO_2 laser allows removal of tissue with relatively little blood loss, and the level of excision can be readily selected by the surgeon. The procedure is very slow, because of the limited power that can be generated by the CO_2 laser with safety for both the patient and the operating room personnel. Thus the procedure results in prolonged operating time. Furthermore, the required equipment is expensive and somewhat cumbersome to use. Since the laser beam may cause serious damage to the retina following exposure, operating room personnel must wear protective glasses. Finally, the laser energy is partially dissipated in the underlying viable tissue (the graft recipient site), and the resulting injury to superficial cells may prevent acceptance of heterograft, homograft, and autograft.

When third-degree burns are relatively limited in size (less than 5 percent), as may occur following contact with a hot piece of metal, the full-thickness eschar may be excised primarily under anesthesia without excessive hemorrhage. The wound should be covered immediately with autograft. This approach markedly decreases postburn morbidity and often results in a better cosmetic appearance.

Children with massive injuries (greater than 70 percent of total body surface area being third degree) have been successfully treated with staged, extensive excision to fascia of all burned areas. The open wounds are immediately covered with viable homograft that is allowed to "take." Immunosuppression with antithymocytic globulin (ATG) has been utilized by at least two investigators. Immunosuppression has not been proved efficacious, however, and can only be recommended for use in specialized burn facilities actively involved in clinical investigation of skin transplant immunology. This approach has not proved to be of value in treating the massively burned adult.

Adult patients with massive burn injuries of more than 70 percent total body surface burns, of which at least 60 percent is third-degree, should undergo early, deep burn wound excision. Such procedures should be attempted only in major centers, since this approach requires enormous medical, paramedical, and nursing support. Prior to excision, the burn wound must be sterile or contain only a relatively low concentration of bacteria (less than 10^4 organisms per gram of tissue). Some authors advocate the preoperative infusion of antibiotics by subeschar clysis into the eschar that is to be excised. In this manner, maximum antibiotic concentration is achieved in the relatively avascular eschar, and the chances of seeding the bloodstream during the procedure are presumably reduced. Both the eschar and the underlying subcutaneous fat are excised. The exposed deep fascia must be immediately covered with homograft. Failure to provide immediate physiologic coverage results in desiccation of the fascia and subsequent secondary infection. Thus an unlimited bank of homograft, obtained from cadavers, must be maintained. Furthermore, excision of 20 percent of the total body surface is frequently associated with loss of the patient's complete blood volume. Centers using this approach must have blood banks capable of providing significant quantities of both stored and fresh blood. In some cases, the blood loss has been reduced by utilizing deliberate hypotensive anesthesia during the procedure. Obviously, the operative procedure inflicts great stress on the patient, who already will have evidenced marked pathophysiologic alterations. Extraordinary intensive care support by both physicians and specialized nursing personnel is therefore required postoperatively in the intensive care area.

Patients with electrical injuries often have injury to the muscle compartments of the extremity. Early surgical exploration, fasciotomy, and removal of nonviable muscle should be performed when motor dysfunction or massive edema of the extremity occurs. Repeat exploration within a few days may be required to further debride necrotic tissue. In the interim, the wounds can temporarily be closed with heterografts.

Cutaneous burns resulting from contact with hot tar or asphalt are not infrequently encountered. By the time the physician sees the patient, the tar has solidified on the burn wound as it has cooled. It may be removed by applying generous quantities of Neopolycin ointment to the burn wound, over which a large occlusive dressing is applied. The dressing may be removed 18 to 24 h later. At this time most or all of the tar will be dissolved, and a water-soluble topical chemotherapeutic agent may be applied.

Topical Chemotherapy

Modern antibacterial topical therapy was advocated by Monafo and Moyer in the early 1960s. These investigators used aqueous silver nitrate (0.5%) solution as a continuous wet soak, in combination with large, bulky dressings. The mode of action of silver nitrate is not specifically known but probably depends on the free silver ion, which is active at relatively low concentrations. Silver nitrate is effective against most gram-positive organisms and most strains of *Pseudomonas,* although it has limited effectiveness against other gram-negative bacteria such as *Enterobacter* and *Klebsiella.* The agent sterilizes the surface of the wound but has limited penetration of deeper tissues. Therefore, the eschar must be removed rapidly when deep bacterial colonization occurs, in order to prevent invasion of underlying viable tissue. The major complication associated with the use of silver nitrate solution is severe electrolyte depletion (primarily sodium and chloride), necessitating frequent monitoring of serum electrolytes, since specific replacement therapy is required. Silver nitrate therapy has been acclaimed as the most economical topical agent. The drug itself is inexpensive and available in most hospital pharmacies. The large quantities of dressings required, the increased nursing personnel requirements to effect the dressing changes, and the major housekeeping problems associated with discoloration caused on contact by precipitation of silver salts significantly increase the cost of this form of treatment. In addition, the necessity for bulky dressings inhibits the early active movement of extremities and therefore encourages less than optimum joint function.

In the mid-1960s, Lindberg, Moncrief, and Mason introduced mafenide acetate (Sulfamylon), a topically applied cream that allowed open treatment of burn wounds. Mafenide acetate has proved effective against a wide range of gram-positive and gram-negative organisms, as well as most anaerobes. This drug actively diffuses through the eschar, thus providing protection in the depth of the eschar at the interface between the viable and nonviable tissue. Since the burns remain exposed, wounds can be more readily examined. In addition, the treatment does not interfere with intensive physical therapy and allows uninhibited treatment of associated soft tissue inju-

ries. Unfortunately, the drug is a potent inhibitor of carbonic anhydrase and therefore may induce acid-base derangements. Acidosis may develop rapidly in the presence of pulmonary dysfunction. The use of the drug is associated with a pronounced reduction of the buffering capacity of the blood, as a result of increased bicarbonate excretion by the kidney, and simultaneous hypocapnea secondary to hyperventilation. Other disadvantages associated with the use of this drug include pain on application, an occasional hypersensitivity reaction (5 to 7 percent), delayed eschar separation due to improved bacterial control, and the emergence of opportunistic infections, including *Providencia, Serratia,* fungal, yeast, and viral infections.

Silver sulfadiazine (Silvadene), developed by Fox in the late 1960s, has essentially the same bacterial spectrum as mafenide acetate but is associated with fewer disadvantages. The major side effects are hypersensitivity reaction to sulfa (5 to 7 percent), delayed eschar separation, and emergence of opportunistic infections. The agent appears to desiccate the wound less than other topical drugs and consequently keeps the eschar soft, allowing for greater joint mobility. It does not inhibit carbonic anhydrase activity, and its application is soothing rather than painful.

Betadine, a water-soluble topical antiseptic complex of polyvinylpyrrolidone (povidone) iodine, is effective against a wide range of gram-positive and gram-negative organisms, as well as some fungi. The drug is manufactured as an ointment and as an aerosol cream. The drug readily diffuses through the eschar and is absorbed and excreted rapidly. Systemic toxicity is apparently rare. One major disadvantage of this agent is its propensity to cause rapid desiccation of the eschar, resulting in interference with progressive active physical therapy programs. In addition, its application to partial-thickness burns may be associated with mild to moderate pain. This agent has only recently been extensively used for the topical therapy of burns and, as in the case of other topical agents, emergence of opportunistic infections may be expected after more extensive experience.

The properties of each of the currently utilized topical chemotherapeutic agents are summarized in Table 7-5. Newer and even more effective topical agents are currently in clinical trial and may be expected to be marketed in the near future. It is important to emphasize that burn wounds treated with these topical agents are not sterilized; rather, the bacterial population is effectively suppressed and remains at levels below that associated with the development of invasive burn wound sepsis. Furthermore, the agents are effective in preventing bacterial conversion of second-degree burns to full-thickness injury, thus reducing the amount of skin that might be required had the agents not been employed.

Bacteriologic Monitoring

Despite the use of topical chemotherapeutic agents, some patients, particularly those with burns of more than 60 percent of the total body surface, will evidence pro-

Table 7-5. PROPERTIES OF TOPICAL CHEMOTHERAPEUTIC AGENTS

Agent	Antibacterial spectrum	Dressings required?	Disadvantages
Sodium mafenide (Sulfamylon)	Gram-positive and gram-negative organisms and most anaerobes	No	Pain on application; skin allergy; carbonic anhydrase inhibition; resistant organisms
Silver nitrate 0.5%	Most gram-positive organisms and some strains of *Pseudomonas*	Yes	Hyponatremia; hypochloremia; failure to penetrate eschar; methemoglobinemia
Silver sulfadiazine (Silvadene)	Gram-positive and gram-negative organisms and *Candida albicans*	No	Skin allergy; resistant organisms
Povidone-iodine (Betadine)	Gram-positive organisms and fungi; possibly less effective vs. some gram-negative organisms	Yes (cream) No (aerosol)	Pain on application; excessive drying of eschar

gressive colonization of the burn wound, with subsequent invasion of viable tissue and bloodstream dissemination of the bacteria. Therefore, clinical bacteriologic monitoring of the burn wound is imperative in order to diagnose incipient burn wound sepsis and effect immediate treatment.

In general, cultures of the burn wound surface have failed to accurately predict progressive bacterial colonization or incipient burn wound sepsis. Qualitative and quantitative correlation is poor between flora on the surface of the burn wound and bacterial colonization of the deep layers of the eschar. Blood cultures, although helpful if bacteral growth is demonstrated, have not proved particularly useful, since life-threatening sepsis may occur in the absence of bacteremia, and the presence of bacteria in the bloodstream is a relatively late phenomenon, often just preceding death. Bacterial growth in burn wounds is best monitored by semiquantitative burn wound biopsy cultures. Multiple full-thickness wound biopsies are obtained serially from representative areas of the burn wound. The tissue is weighed, homogenized, serially diluted, and inoculated on blood agar and eosin–methylene blue plates. In this manner, the precise number of viable organisms per gram of tissue can be calculated. When wound biopsy cultures reveal more than 10^5 organisms per gram of tissue or a hundredfold increase in the concentration of organisms per gram of tissue is observed within a 48-h period, it may be assumed that the organisms have escaped effective control by the topical chemotherapeutic agent and that burn wound sepsis is incipient.

Heterograft and Homograft

All terrestrial mammals require an intact epithelial covering in order to maintain water, electrolyte, and thermal homeostasis. Following spontaneous separation of eschar or after surgical removal by tangential or fascial excision, the wound can be temporarily covered with a biologic dressing. Either porcine heterograft or homograft obtained from cadavers is most commonly utilized. The application of these materials, providing early temporary wound closure, can contribute to the prevention and con-

trol of infection, the preservation of healthy granulation tissue, and maintenance of joint function. Specifically, the physiologic dressings decrease evaporative water loss and diminish heat loss secondary to evaporation; they cover exposed sensory nerves and therefore decrease pain associated with the open wound; and they protect neurovascular tissue and tendons that would otherwise be exposed. When the physiologic dressing adheres to the underlying granulation tissue, bacterial proliferation is readily inhibited, since the heterograft or homograft provides an acceptable surface against which neutrophils may entrap bacteria. Until the wound is ready for definitive autograft, deeper tissues are protected from desiccation. The physiologic dressings prevent the development of hypermature granulation tissue and promote a well-nourished recipient bed, and they act as an excellent test material to determine the optimal time for subsequent autograft. When adherence is observed, the bed may be assumed to be in optimal condition for autograft, and postoperative loss of split-thickness skin grafts (autografts) will rarely occur.

Heterograft and homograft are most commonly used for temporary coverage of open wounds, as described above. The grafts are removed within 5 days and replaced with new physiologic dressing until autografting has been accomplished. These physiologic dressings may also be utilized to debride untidy wounds immediately after eschar separation. The heterograft or homograft hastens separation of very tiny pieces of eschar left behind at the time of debridement. It should be emphasized, however, that physiologic dressings may be used for this purpose with safety only if more than 95 percent of the eschar has been mechanically removed in the course of daily debridement or by surgical excision.

Either heterograft or homograft may be used electively over reepithelializing deep second-degree burns, once superficial necrotic debris has been entirely removed (usually 5 to 7 days). Adherent physiologic dressings at this time will promote the rate of reepithelialization and decrease pain in the wound, allowing decreased hospitalization time. Some clinicians utilize heterograft or homograft to immediately cover very superficial second-degree burns. The advantages of such treatment include marked decrease in pain, decreased hospitalization, earlier return of joint function, and more rapid reepithelialization of the burn. Utilization of physiologic dressings in this manner must be undertaken with caution. One must be certain that the wound is indeed extremely superficial in depth with minimal necrotic tissue, since coverage of a deeper wound essentially closes an open abscess and may precipitate burn wound sepsis. In addition, the homograft or heterograft must be applied within hours after the burn injury, before colonization with microbial organisms occurs.

It is important that the physiologic dressing and burn wound be inspected within 24 h to ensure continued adherence to the dermal remnants. Should the physiologic dressing become dislodged or should fluid accumulate beneath it, the material should be removed immediately and the wound treated with topical chemotherapeutic agents in the conventional manner. If the heterograft or homograft remains adherent, it is important that it not be removed but rather be allowed to separate spontaneously as reepithelialization occurs. Frequent changing of physiologic dressings applied to second-degree burns results in sequential removal of epithelial cells at the time of removal and may convert them to full-thickness burn wounds.

Autograft

Definitive closure of burn wounds as soon as possible after injury is the ultimate objective of all burn wound care. There are, however, priorities of coverage dictated by functional and cosmetic considerations. In general, the hands, feet, joints, and face should be covered prior to nonfunctional surfaces. Autografts may be applied as sheets of skin without the need of suture fixation or ''pie crusting'' incisions to allow release of plasma. Fixation with bandaging is not required unless accidental dislodgment is likely, e.g., on circumferentially burned limbs or on burns of patients with uncontrollable motion. Exposure of the freshly applied autograft allows continuous graft inspection and early evacuation of any collections of blood or serum that may occur beneath the graft. When dressings are used, they should be removed 72 h following grafting. If the grafts are adherent, active motion of the burned area may be begun.

Patients with extensive burns often present a serious disproportion between the area requiring autografting and available donor sites. Mesh or expanded grafts may be utilized to cover large areas from limited donor sites. After harvest of the skin grafts, the grafts are placed on plastic carriers and passed through a Tanner-Vanderput mesh dermatome. A series of parallel incisions is made in the sheet graft, allowing expansion of up to six times the area of the original donor site. The small interstices are rapidly filled by epithelialization (4 to 8 days), resulting in a somewhat thinner but physiologically functional skin cover. When mesh grafts are used, moist protective dressings or dressings with material that will maintain a moisture barrier (semipermeable or impermeable) prevent the deeper tissues (exposed through the interstices

of the mesh graft) from desiccating. Once the epithelium has extended from the edges of the mesh across the interstices, the grafts may be exposed to room air and humidity. In general, mesh grafts are not used on the face, hands, feet, and flexion creases, since the healed grafts are not as cosmetically acceptable as intact autografts. In addition, mesh grafts are less able to withstand recurrent localized trauma.

Synthetics

Synthetic skin substitutes possess many theoretical advantages over their biologic counterparts (heterograft, homograft). Synthetic materials can be mass-produced, have an indefinite shelf life, are relatively inert, and are comparatively inexpensive. Numerous products are now available for very specific types of wounds; results are equal to those produced by biologic materials.

''Spray-on'' polymeric dressings have, in general, been abandoned. In extensive testing they were found safe in treating superficial second-degree burns and donor sites. When used, however, they required daily inspection of the wound for purulence or nonadherence of the dressing, and their use on deeper second- or third-degree burns was contraindicated.

A variety of synthetic sheet dressings with varying water permeability and adherence properties are now available. These have proved useful in the treatment of donor sites and superficial second-degree burns and as temporary dressings after surgical excision of the eschar. Poor adherence remains a major problem with these materials, so their use for extended periods of time following major burn wound excision is not recommended.

Recently a bilayer artificial skin composed of a temporary silastic epidermis and a porous collagen chondroitin 6-sulfate fibrillar dermis has been developed. Following grafting, the dermal component is populated with fibroblasts and vessels from the wound bed. The silastic epidermis remains firmly adherent but can be removed weeks or even months later when autograft tissue is available for transplantation. When the silastic is removed, extremely thin (0.003 to 0.004 in. thick) epidermal grafts are placed on the newly formed dermal bed. The extremely thin donor sites heal rapidly, allowing earlier recropping if required.

The neodermis produced with the use of artificial skin microscopically resembles normal dermis. The gross feel and texture of the neodermis is more analogous to normal dermis than to scar tissue. Artificial skin currently is being tested in a number of centers in this country, and preliminary results are excellent.

GENERAL THERAPEUTIC CONSIDERATIONS

Metabolism and Nutrition

Hypermetabolism characterizes the human response to major injury. Several investigators have now shown a direct relationship between the magnitude and duration of the hypermetabolic response and the severity of the sustained trauma. Wilmore has demonstrated a curvilinear relationship between the resting metabolic expenditure and the magnitude of total body surface burn in human patients. Resting metabolic rate approached a maximum response of approximately twice normal in patients with burns of more than 60 percent of the total body surface. Both Reiss and Wilmore have documented caloric expenditure in excess of 60 kcal/($m^2 \cdot$ h) in patients with major thermal injury. Total daily energy consumption during the nonresting state in severely burned patients approached 40 kcal for each percent of body surface burned, plus 25 kcal/kg of body weight.

Previously, the hypermetabolic response was attributed in part to obligatory energy losses in the form of heat associated with a marked increase in evaporative water loss. The increase in evaporative water loss results from destruction of the water barrier within the skin. If water evaporation is mechanically prevented, however, there is no significant decrease in the metabolic rate observed in the burn patient. Furthermore, one cannot reduce oxygen consumption in thermally injured patients to normal levels by manipulation of environmental temperature and humidity. This suggests that the hypermetabolic response is non-temperature-dependent. A close correlation has been demonstrated between oxygen consumption and urinary catecholamine excretion. In addition, hypermetabolic response has been partially blocked by the administration of alpha- and beta-adrenergic blocking agents. The hypermetabolic response in human beings is associated with increased rectal and skin temperatures, and animal experiments have demonstrated that burn injury is associated with a true increase in critical temperature. These studies suggest that the hypermetabolic response to burn injury is mediated through the hypothalamic temperature center, which emits an efferent signal expressed via catecholamine excretion.

In addition to elevated energy requirements, a marked catabolic response accompanies severe burn injury. The postburn catabolism is associated with weight loss, retarded wound healing, and negative nitrogen, potassium, sulfur, and phosphorus balance. Again, the magnitude and duration of the catabolic response roughly parallels the severity of the burn injury. Up to 30 g of nitrogen/day may be recovered from the urine of severely burned patients. If extraordinary means to provide excessive dietary nitrogen are not pursued, negative nitrogen balance may be observed for up to 2 months following the thermal accident. However, protein catabolism does not proceed uniformly in all tissues. Structural and functional integrity of vital organs such as the heart and liver is maintained at the expense of muscle protein.

Posttraumatic negative nitrogen balance can be ameliorated if sufficient caloric and nitrogen intake is provided. More than 20 g of nitrogen/m^2 of body surface per day is required in patients with major burns during the first postburn month in order to maintain positive nitrogen balance. During the second postburn month, nitrogen intake of 13 to 16 g/($m^2 \cdot$ day) will maintain nitrogen equilibrium. The catabolic response in burn patients is associated with increased levels of glucagon and catecholamine (catabolic hormones) in the plasma and depressed levels of insulin (anabolic hormone).

Total oxidation of a normal 70-kg male would yield approximately 166,000 endogenous kcal. It is estimated that healthy persons can tolerate acute losses of up to one-third of lean body weight before death ensues. Thus an extensively burned adult, with energy requirements of 5000 kcal/day, becomes a severe nutritional risk within 2 weeks, assuming no oral or parenteral caloric intake. Since most of the kinetic energy requirements of the supine, bedridden patient are associated with maintenance of normal respiratory function, the most common cause of death in these patients is pulmonary sepsis. An ineffective respiratory effort results in progressive atelectasis and subsequent lung infection by opportunistic pathogens.

The clinical consequences of inadequate nutritional replacement include profound weight loss, development of superior mesenteric artery syndrome, decreased immunologic response, diminished leukocyte function (host resistance), impaired wound healing, and severe inhibition of cellular active transport, resulting in cellular dysfunction.

Current knowledge of the hypermetabolic response following injury allows more rational therapy aimed at preventing morbid consequences of acute malnutrition. Control of the environment by maintaining an externally warm temperature (31°C) will alleviate patient discomfort and shivering associated with a cold environment and prevent further increases in the metabolic rate subsequent to cold stress (Fig. 7-3). Furthermore, apprehension and pain may be treated appropriately with narcotics and tranquilizers, since both these stresses are known to potentiate the release of catecholamines.

Effective prohylaxis against infection and timely closure of the burn wound will ameliorate both the catabolic and the hypermetabolic response to burn injury. A progressive physical therapy program will also enhance the deposition of protein into lean muscle mass, which allows performance of kinetic work required for maintenance of normal function.

The cornerstone of nutritional management of the burn patient is the provision of adequate exogenous calories and nitrogen to prevent prolonged catabolism. Whenever possible, the gastrointestinal tract should be used for the various dietary regimens designed to supply the nutritional needs of the patient. Maintenance of adequate nutrition is best monitored by accurate daily measurements of body weight. Postburn weight loss of less than 10 percent is usually well tolerated, provided the patient was not nutritionally depleted prior to the burn injury. Weight loss that exceeds 10 percent of the preburn weight is often associated with an increased incidence of morbidity.

When the voluntary food intake of the burned patient is insufficient to provide for positive energy balance, the physician must intervene with forced feedings, by either the parenteral or the enteral route. Enteral feedings may be accomplished by insertion of a small silastic nasogastric feeding tube through which nutrients are delivered

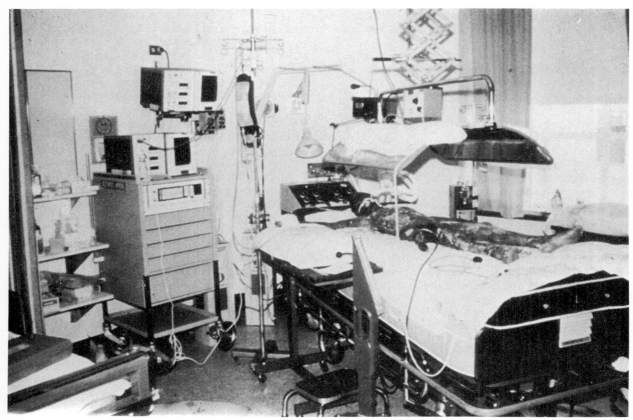

Fig. 7-3. Burn patients require well-equipped facilities for optimum care. The patient is maintained in a warm environment under a heat shield to minimize cold stress.

24 h a day via a constant delivery pump. Usually patients with major burns tolerate a complete homogenized diet. Partially digested or elemental diets are usually contraindicated, since the higher osmolality associated with these diets often results in gastric distention, profuse diarrhea, or dehydration when large caloric intakes are administered. When positive energy balance is unobtainable by utilization of the gastrointestinal route alone, intravenous hyperalimentation should be employed simultaneously in order to avoid prolonged periods of malnutrition. The intravenous administration of fat emulsions and amino acid solutions by peripheral vein may also be used to supplement enteral caloric intake, if necessary.

Physical Therapy, Splinting, and Rehabilitation

Contractures associated with serious loss of joint function may complicate severe thermal injury. It has now been documented that a progressive physical therapy program implemented immediately after hospital admission is associated with preservation of range of motion in joints with overlying burn injury. It should be emphasized that the program must begin on the day of admission and be continued until the burn wounds are healed and normal range of joint motion can be maintained by the patient. Major burn centers have found it necessary to employ full-time physical therapists to supervise active physical therapy at the bedside during waking hours. Repetitive exercises are conducted in the direction opposite that of any anticipated deformity.

Prolonged immobilization must be avoided, and early motion following skin grafting should be encouraged. In addition, proper positioning during bed rest must be monitored, and splints must be manufactured to maintain anticontracture positions during sleep. When a carefully supervised program of physical therapy is an integral part of burn wound care, 85 percent of the joints underlying surface burns should have a normal range of motion at the completion of therapy. The upper extremities are more susceptible to the deleterious effects of prolonged immobilization than the lower extremities. The ideal position for the lower extremities (knees extended, feet in neutral position) is comfortable to the patient and relatively easy to maintain in either the prone or supine position. The shoulders, however, are difficult to position or splint in patients with extensive burns. Elevation and abduction of the arm at the shoulder joint are often uncomfortable, and a patient with burns at the shoulder invariably assumes and maintains a position of adduction and extension if not carefully monitored by nursing personnel and therapists.

Many factors influence the success of a physical therapy program, including patient motivation, but no factor

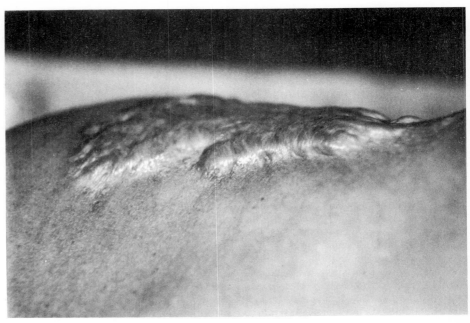

Fig. 7-4. Hypertrophic scarring usually develops in areas of second-degree burns that have spontaneously healed.

is more deleterious to the preservation of motion than delay of treatment. Daily range-of-motion evaluation and appropriate daily exercises to achieve maximum potential range of motion in joints underlying both second- and third-degree surface burns are of paramount importance. Goals should be established during the early postburn period, which must be rapidly achieved and thereafter maintained. The patient should be encouraged to pursue daily self-care activities as soon as possible. By the time of discharge, the patient should be as independent as possible and should have mastered a home physical therapy program to maintain function.

The development of hypertrophic scars may occur after hospital discharge (Fig. 7-4). The resultant scar overgrowth may inhibit function and often causes severe disfigurement. Larson and his associates have reported reduction of hypertrophic scar formation following the application of conforming isoprene splints and/or elastic garments during the convalescent period (Fig. 7-5). A variety of new materials are now available that can be placed deep to the pressure garments or splints to concentrate pressure on critical contoured areas (bridge of nose, chin, neck, web spaces of the hand). A new technique using clear high-temperature plastic is also available to control scarring about the face. An exact casting of the face is first made using plaster, over which the high-temperature plastic is molded. The resultant face mask is applied to the face as soon as the burns have healed.

All these devices exert pressure on the scar, causing better alignment of collagen fibrils and reduction of local interstitial edema. Splints and pressure devices are started when the patient is in the burn center, and the

Fig. 7-5. Form-fitted elastic compression garments may help to minimize hypertrophic scarring.

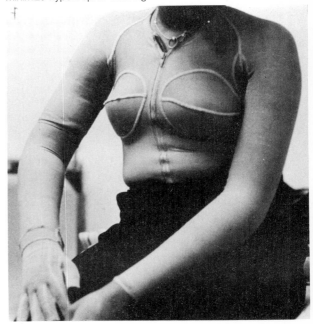

devices are continued for at least 6 months after discharge to discourage the delayed development of a hypertrophic scar.

COMPLICATIONS

Smoke Inhalation Syndrome

Smoke inhalation syndrome is an acute pulmonary dysfunction related to lower respiratory tract pathophysiology occurring within 72 h after exposure to gaseous products of incomplete combustion (primarily aldehydes). The severity of this syndrome is a function of the type of smoke inhaled, its amount, and the magnitude of the accompanying thermal injury. Patients with smoke inhalation syndrome frequently exhibit *no* physical signs or symptoms of injury during the first 24 h after sustaining a major burn. Smoke inhalation should be highly suspected in patients burned within an enclosed space, patients injured while under the influence of alcohol or drugs, and patients who lost consciousness at the time of the accident. Such patients are most likely to have inhaled large amounts of smoke prior to being evacuated from the scene of the fire.

Diagnosis is dependent on a high index of suspicion and careful physical and laboratory examination (Table 7-6). At the time of initial examination, sputum should be obtained from the lower respiratory tract and examined for the presence of carbon. When carbonaceous sputum is noted, the patient should be hospitalized and observed for the development of severe respiratory dysfunction within 18 to 36 h. Carboxyhemoglobin concentration should be measured as soon as the patient reaches the hospital. Normal carboxyhemoglobin levels are of relatively little value, since the patient may have been exposed to smoke containing low concentrations of carbon monoxide or may have been treated effectively with oxygen by paramedical personnel prior to arrival at the hospital. The presence of increased concentrations of carboxyhemoglobin suggests the inhalation of a significant amount of smoke, and the patient should be retained in the hospital for observation, since most such patients will later develop a pathophysiologic condition of the lower respiratory tract following recovery from carbon monoxide poisoning. Within 6 to 12 h after injury, the hospitalized patient should be subjected to fiberoptic bronchoscopy to assess the lower respiratory tract. Direct visualization of the trachea and bronchus provides approximately 86 percent accuracy in indicating significant smoke inhalation. Objective findings include the extramucosal appearance of carbonaceous material, bronchorrhea, mucosal edema, vesicles, erythema, hemorrhage, and ulceration.

The Pa_{O_2} while the patient is breathing 100 percent oxygen may also be utilized to monitor for the development of smoke inhalation syndrome. Patients with an initial Pa_{O_2} of less than 300 should be suspected of significant smoke inhalation. This test also has an accuracy of approximately 86 percent.

Other authors have utilized a ^{133}Xe scan to diagnose lower respiratory tract injury. An abnormal scan following the injection of ^{133}Xe into a peripheral vein is indicated by incomplete washout from the lungs within 90 s or the presence of local radioisotopic trapping. The test is 87 percent accurate but has been infrequently utilized, since it requires the movement of severely ill patients to special radioactivity-counting facilities.

Between 24 and 48 h after injury, the patient exhibits progressive bronchospasm with expiratory wheezes, rales, tachypnea, and progressive respiratory failure. The subsequent development of bronchopneumonia secondary to bacterial growth distal to occluding plugs (consisting of inspissated mucus and sloughed bronchial epithelium) is a fairly constant feature. Radiographic changes are usually not noted until 72 h after the injury (Fig. 7-6).

The treatment of smoke inhalation syndrome can be divided into nonspecific and specific therapy. Nonspecific modalities include rapid fluid resuscitation of burn shock, performance of escharotomies of the chest and the abdomen, the provision of external dry heat, and frequent monitoring of respiratory function. Prompt intravenous fluid resuscitation and restoration of normal intravascular volume prevents exacerbation of central nervous system hypoxia. When circumferential third-degree burns of the chest and abdomen are present, chest wall and diaphragmatic excursion are inhibited unless escharotomies are performed. The provision of an externally warm environment minimizes oxygen demand associated with an increased metabolic rate. Most important, however, is the frequent assessment of respiratory function by repetitive

Table 7-6. SMOKE INHALATION SYNDROME

History: Enclosed space, alcohol/drugs, unconsciousness
Physical Exam.: Altered mental status, carbon in sputum, delayed symptoms

Diagnostic tests	Advantages	Disadvantages
Carboxyhemoglobin	Simple, rapid	Nonspecific, rapid disappearance
Fiberoptic bronchoscopy	Simple, rapid, objective	
^{133}Xe scan	Objective	Complicated, expensive
AaD$_{O_2}$ gradient	Simple, rapid, ? objective	Unproved

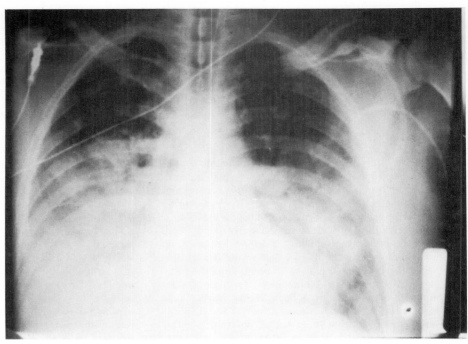

Fig. 7-6. Chest x-ray changes secondary to smoke inhalation may not be evident for 72 h. The clinical syndrome that develops is similar to the adult respiratory distress syndrome.

physical examination, serial determinations of arterial P_{O_2}, and pulmonary compliance, which often decreases prior to a significant fall in the arterial P_{O_2}.

Specific treatment includes the provision of humidified air and oxygen as required. If respiratory failure is incipient, endotracheal intubation should be performed and the patient supported with mechanical ventilation. Often it is necessary to institute positive end-expiratory pressure (PEEP) to prevent progressive respiratory failure. Intravenous administration of bronchodilators often alleviates the severe bronchospasm. Routine use of steroids should be avoided. Administration to patients with smoke inhalation may lead to up to three times higher incidence of infectious complications and increased mortality. When smoke inhalation syndrome is complicated by pneumonia, appropriate antibiotics should be administered by a parenteral route. Prophylactic antibiotics either parenterally or by aerosolization are contraindicated. They do not lower the incidence of subsequent infection and may result in the emergence of highly resistant strains of bacteria.

Burn Wound Sepsis

One of the principal causes of death following massive thermal injury is burn wound sepsis. Burn wound sepsis is characterized by the active invasion of microorganisms into viable subeschar tissue, with subsequent bacteremia. Third-degree burn wounds are essentially avascular, so systemic delivery of antibiotics via the bloodstream does not reliably suppress microbiological growth within the burn wound. Moreover, host resistance to infection is now known to be markedly diminished in patients with major thermal injury. Complement abnormalities, hypo-gammaglobulinemia, cell-mediated immunity, decreased neutrophil intracellular bacterial killing, and abnormalities in the inflammatory response within the burn wound have all been described. In addition, there is a marked decrease in neutrophil and monocyte chemotactic responsiveness. These two factors, markedly decreased perfusion of the eschar and severely compromised host resistance to infection, may result in rapid bacterial colonization if topical chemotherapeutic agents are not utilized. Although the topical agents have reduced the incidence of bacterial invasion of the viable subeschar tissue, bacterial proliferation may still escape the control of all currently used chemotherapeutic preparations particularly if they are used for prolonged periods. Early excision of eschar with closure obviates this problem. This technique may not always be feasible, however, necessitating a nonsurgical approach, i.e., spontaneous separation of eschar with delayed autografting. When bacterial escape is proved by quantitative wound biopsy, administration of antibiotics by needle clysis beneath the eschar has been employed with success. This therapy is most effective when initiated at the time wound colonization reaches 10^4 organisms per gram of tissue. Antibiotics administered by subeschar clysis should be selected after review of in vitro sensitivity of the offending organism. The entire daily "systemic" dose of the selected antibiotic should be dissolved in a solution of isotonic saline solution or half-strength saline solution of sufficient quantity to infuse each 44-cm² area of burn eschar with 25 mL of solution once daily.

Utilization of antibiotics administered by subeschar clysis has allowed recovery of children with documented *Pseudomonas* burn wound sepsis accompanied by ecthyma gangrenosum. Prior to the utilization of subeschar antibiotics, the complication of *Pseudomonas* septicemia was uniformly fatal in burn patients. Up to 50 percent survival was reported in such patients in 1974 by Loebl and his colleagues.

Distant Septic Complications

Because of decreased host resistance, distant septic complications are not unusual in patients with severe burn injury. Bronchopneumonia is the most common complicating infection. Sputum cultures from such patients usually reveal the same microorganism that has colonized the burn wound. Bacteria may be aerosolized from the burn wound and inhaled in large doses as the patient is manipulated during the course of daily wound care. In about one-third of burn patients with pneumonia the bacteria are seeded via the bloodstream (hematogenous pneumonia) as a complication of burn wound sepsis. Conventional treatment with systemic antibiotics and respiratory support is indicated when septic pulmonary infiltrates are diagnosed by physical examination or chest radiography.

Suppurative thrombophlebitis occurs more frequently in patients with massive thermal injury than in other hospitalized patients with severe illness. This complication follows prolonged venous cannulation with polyethylene catheters utilized for the delivery of intravenous fluid. In contrast to bland thrombophlebitis, this type often exhibits no abnormal physical signs. Calf tenderness and edema are only infrequently present. More commonly, the patient presents with bacteremia of unknown origin. Blood cultures often yield staphylococci. The diagnosis may be confirmed by surgical exploration of all peripheral veins that have been cannulated during hospitalization. The vein is opened and milked in a retrograde manner, and any effluent is observed. If pus can be identified, the diagnosis is confirmed. In the absence of liquefied suppurative material, the vein should be biopsied and subjected to frozen section. Bacterial colonization of the intima of the vein also strongly suggests the presence of suppurative thrombophlebitis. The incidence of suppurative thrombophlebitis may be markedly reduced in the burn population by limiting the duration of any single intravenous catheter to periods of 72 h or less. Should the complication occur, the offending vein must be excised in its entirety. Failure to employ prompt surgical treatment usually results in fatal bacteremia.

Thermally injured cartilage is another common site of bacterial infection. Cartilage is relatively avascular, and local host resistance to established infection is diminished as a result. The cartilage of the external ear is covered only by cutaneous tissue and thus frequently is injured when full-thickness burns of the ear are sustained. The development of suppurative chondritis often may be prevented in patients with severe ear burns by minimizing external pressure upon the ear. Such patients should sleep without bed pillows and be prevented from assuming a lateral position with the burned ear down. When suppurative chondritis occurs, either in the cartilage of the external ear or in other cartilaginous structures, surgical excision of the involved cartilage is necessary to arrest progressive septic destruction.

Gastrointestinal Complications

Gastric and duodenal ulcers have been reported previously as a common complication of major thermal injury. These ulcers were first described by Curling in 1842 and have been reported to occur in as many as 25 percent of hospitalized burn cases. The incidence of Curling's ulcers has been markedly reduced during recent years, and operative intervention for upper gastrointestinal bleeding following burn injury is only rarely necessary today. In the past, 85 percent of upper gastrointestinal hemorrhage was associated with bacteremia. The decreased incidence of Curling's ulcer is associated with the reduced frequency of major septic complications, the prophylactic introduction of antacids into the stomach via a gastrointestinal tube (maintenance of a neutral pH in gastric aspirates), and the improved provision of nutritional supplements, allowing more rapid healing of small acute mucosal erosions.

If major upper gastrointestinal hemorrhage should occur, the patient should be promptly treated with iced saline solution lavage and blood volume replacement begun. When hemorrhage cannot be controlled by conservative means, prompt surgical intervention is indicated, since these critically ill patients do not tolerate prolonged periods of hypovolemic shock. The abdominal cavity can be, and often must be, opened through the burn wound. At closure, the subcutaneous tissue and skin are left open to prevent soft tissue infection. Once the bleeding source is identified by gastrotomy or duodenotomy, hemostasis is obtained by oversewing the base of the ulcer. Blood volume replacement is continued until the patient's condition is stable, and then a vagotomy and hemigastrectomy should be performed. Lesser procedures are associated with an unacceptable incidence of rebleeding, and reoperation carries a prohibitive surgical risk.

SPECIAL PROBLEMS

Long Bone Fractures

Often physicians are confronted with a patient who has sustained a long bone fracture with overlying cutaneous burns. Such a patient cannot be treated with closed cylinder casts, since second-degree burns will rapidly convert to full-thickness injuries as a result of bacterial growth. Furthermore, bacterial growth will be unchecked in third-degree burns, resulting in subsequent burn wound sepsis. Open repair of the fracture is generally contraindicated unless simultaneous excision of all burn tissue and autograft closure is possible. The fracture should be immobilized by insertion of Steinman pins or Kirschner wires in order to effect suspension of the extremity in balanced skeletal traction. The burn wounds can then be left exposed and treatment with topical chemotherapeutic agents initiated. The wounds must be cleansed and inspected daily and the chemotherapeutic agent reapplied.

Following electrical burn, bone may be thermally injured at the entrance and exit sites. This is most likely to occur when the entrance or exit site is on the scalp, the sternum, or the anterior leg. In these locations the underlying bone is in close approximation to the overlying skin. The burn wound is debrided of nonviable soft tissue, and topical chemotherapeutic agents are applied to remaining soft tissue defects and the exposed nonviable bone. When granulation tissue has developed over the soft tissue, temporary coverage with physiologic dressings is instituted until the soft tissue is definitively grafted. After soft tissue wounds are closed, the devitalized bone is decorticated until bleeding bone is encountered. Granulation tissue will develop from the endothelium of the vessels and eventually cover the remaining viable bone. Split-thickness skin graft can then be successfully applied.

Burn Injury of Joints

Occasionally burn injury may extend down to and include the joint capsules. Such injuries are most likely to occur where the overlying skin and soft tissue are relatively thin. The interphalangeal joints of the dorsal surfaces of the fingers and toes are most commonly involved. When it is apparent that the joint capsule has been devitalized and the joint is open, the cartilage should be surgically removed and a formal arthrodesis performed to allow ankylosis of the joint in an optimal position. Interphalangeal joints should be fixed in the extended position or with just a few degrees of flexion. Crossed Kirschner wires are utilized to hold joint position until healing of adjacent bony surfaces has occurred at about 6 weeks. When arthrodesis of joints is necessary, it is particularly important to maintain maximal function of adjoining joints. Ankylosis of the interphalangeal joints results in little long-term disability as long as metacarpophalangeal and metatarsophalangeal joint function is maintained.

Occasionally patients with burns of the hand cannot be maintained in appropriate position by splints during the acute postburn period. This problem most frequently occurs in infants and young children, in whom the fingers are not long enough to allow application of appropriate pressure dressings to maintain optimal extremity position within the splint. In such patients the temporal insertion of a single axial wire through both interphalangeal joints of each finger prevents interphalangeal flexion contractures. The wires are removed at 3 weeks and aggressive active physical therapy is employed to regain finger flexion.

Burns of the Face

Because of its exposed position, the head, with its appendages and orifices, is an anatomic area frequently burned. The protective action of the lids and the constant moisture that surrounds the ocular structures prevents the eyes from being directly involved by thermal injury, except in cases of contact, chemical, or electrical burns. Injury due to these agents often results in perforation of the cornea or opacification of the cornea, which may require later correction with a corneal graft. Moreover, third-degree burn injury of the lids may cause retraction of the lids, allowing the cornea to be constantly exposed to the drying action of air. Thus extreme care must be directed toward protecting the cornea of the eye. The instillation of artificial tears (methyl cellulose) and the use of antibiotic ointments are often required to prevent corneal desiccation. When such third-degree burn injuries are present, it is often beneficial to perform tarsorrhaphies shortly after the burn injury, limiting subsequent lid contraction deformity. The upper and lower tarsal plates are sewn together in such a fashion as to allow union of the two cartilaginous structures. The patient is able to see through a small peephole in the center of the eye, where the upper and lower lids are not joined. The tarsorrhaphies are not released until long after autografting has been accomplished and further lid contraction is not expected. Skin should be grafted over the lids as soon as eschar separation is complete. If subsequent lid retraction still occurs, reconstruction of the eyelids is accomplished by blepharorrhaphy.

Patients with second- or third-degree burn injury of the face may develop microstomia as a result of gradual fibrosis of the circumoral tissues. Prophylactic treatment to prevent this complication is particularly cumbersome and of only limited success. Surgical reconstruction of the mouth may be carried out 1 year after the burn injury.

Frequently patients become very self-conscious about major or minor postburn scarring on the face. Most scars should be treated initially by conservative management, utilizing elastic pressure masks for a period of 1 to 2 years. Attempts at early surgical reconstruction are often unsuccessful, since the tissue remains extraordinarily hyperactive for a year or more. Scar revision for cosmetic purposes should generally not be attempted for an interval of 1.5 to 2 years following the burn injury.

MORBIDITY AND MORTALITY

Whereas survival after burns of 30 percent of the total body surface area was infrequent 25 years ago, today very few patients with injuries of this magnitude die. The size of a burn injury capable of producing a 50 percent mortality has steadily risen over the past 30 years. Currently the LD_{50} by age group is in the range of 62, 63, and 38 percent total body surface area for patients with ages from 0 to 14, 15 to 40, and 40 to 65 years, respectively. Patients over the age of 65 years have a 50 percent mortality with burns of only 25 percent total body surface area. Chronic disease states in this group frequently interfere with appropriate physiologic response to major thermal injury.

More importantly, the development of multidisciplinary teams to ensure total care of the burn patient has markedly reduced the morbidity associated with this severe injury. At several centers, more than 90 percent of surviving patients have been able to return to an occupation as remunerative as their preinjury employment. Self-respect and independence are preserved, and the quality of life experienced by the patient usually approaches, or in some cases exceeds, the preinjury level.

Bibliography

General

Artz CP, Moncrief JA, Pruitt BA Jr: *Burns: A Team Approach.* Philadelphia, Saunders, 1978.

Curreri PW, Luterman A, et al: Burn injury, analysis of survival and hospitalization time for 937 patients. *Ann Surg* 192:472, 1980.

Curreri PW, Marvin JA: Advances in clinical care of burn patients. *West J Med* 123:275, 1975.

Monofo WW: *The Treatment of Burns: Principles and Practice.* St. Louis, WA Green, 1971.

Pruitt BA Jr: The burn patient: I. Initial care. II. Later care and complications of thermal injury. *Curr Probl Surg* April–May 1979.

Shuck JM, Moncrief JA: The management of burns. *Curr Probl Surg* (monograph), February 1969.

Etiology of Burns

Baxter CR: Present concepts in the management of major electrical injury. *Surg Clin North Am* 50:1401, 1970.

Curreri PW, Asch MJ, Pruitt BA Jr: The treatment of chemical burns: Specialized diagnostic, therapeutic, and prognostic considerations. *J Trauma* 10:634, 1970.

Gruber RP, Laub DR, Vistnes LM: The effect of hydrotherapy on the clinical course and pH of experimental cutaneous chemical burns. *Plast Reconstr Surg* 55:200, 1975.

Jelenko C: Chemicals that burn. *J Trauma* 14:65, 1974.

Immediate Therapy

Baxter CR: Crystalloid resuscitation of burn shock, in Polk HC, Stone HH (eds): *Contemporary Burn Management.* Boston, Little, Brown and Company, 1971, p 7.

Baxter CR, Marvin JA, Curreri PW: Fluid and electrolyte therapy of burn shock. *Heart and Lung* 2:707, 1973.

Baxter CR, Marvin JA, Curreri PW: Early management of thermal burns. *Postgrad Med* 55:131, 1974.

Curreri PW, Marvin JA: Advances in the clinical care of burn patients. *West J Med* 123:275, 1975.

Hummel RP, MacMillan GB, Altemeier WA: Topical and systemic antibacterial agents in the treatment of burns. *Ann Surg* 172:370, 1970.

Loebl EC, Baxter CR, Curreri PW: The mechanism of erythrocyte destruction in the early post-burn period. *Ann Surg* 178:681, 1973.

Loebl EC, Marvin JA, et al: Erythrocyte survival following thermal injury. *J Surg Res* 16:96, 1974.

Salisbury RE, McKeel DW, Mason AD Jr: Ischemic necrosis of the intrinsic muscles of the hand after thermal injury. *J Bone Joint Surg [Am]* 56-A:1701, 1974.

Simon TL, Curreri PW, Harker LA: Kinetic characterization of hemostasis in thermal injury. *J Lab Clin Med* 89:702, 1977.

Therapy of the Burn Wound

Bromberg BE, Song IC, Mohn MP: The use of pig skin as a temporary biological dressing. *Plast Reconstr Surg* 36:80, 1965.

Burke JF, Quinby WC, et al: Immunosuppression and temporary skin transplantation in the treatment of massive third degree burns. *Ann Surg* 182:183, 1975.

Burke JF, Yannas IV, et al: Successful use of physiologically acceptable artificial skin in the treatment of extensive burn injury. *Ann Surg* 194:413, 1981.

Curreri PW, Desai MH, et al: Safety and efficacy of a new synthetic burn dressing. *Arch Surg* 115:925, 1980.

DiVincenti FC, Curreri PW, Pruitt BA Jr: Use of mesh skin autografts in the burn patient. *Plast Reconstr Surg* 44:464, 1969.

Durthschi MB, Orgain C, Counts CW, et al: A prospective study of prophylactic penicillin in acutely burned hospitalized patients. *J Trauma* 22:11, 1982.

Fox CL, Roppole BW, Stanford W: Control of *Pseudomonas* infection in burns by silver sulfadiazine. *Surg Gynecol Obstet* 128:1021, 1969.

Hummel RP, Kautz PD, et al: The continuing problem of sepsis following enzymatic debridement of burns. *J Trauma* 14:572, 1974.

James JH, Watson ACH: The use of OPSITE, a vapour permeable dressing on skin graft donor sites. *Br J Plast Surg* 28:107, 1975.

Lindberg RB, Moncrief JA, Mason AD Jr: Control of experimental and clinical burn wound sepsis by topical application of sulfamylon compounds. *Ann NY Acad Sci* 150:950, 1968.

Luterman A, Kraft E, Kookless S: Biologic dressings, an appraisal of current practices. *J Burn Care Rehab* 1:18, 1980.

MacMillan BB: Deep excision and early grafting, in Polk HC, Stone HH (eds): *Contemporary Burn Management.* Boston, Little, Brown and Company, 1971, p 357.

Monafo WW, Aulenbacher CE, Pappalardo E: Early tangential excision of the eschars of major burns. *Arch Surg* 104:503, 1972.

Monafo WW, Moyer CA: Effectiveness of dilute aqueous silver nitrate in the treatment of major burns. *Arch Surg* 91:200, 1965.

Pruitt BA Jr, Curreri PW: The burn wound and its care. *Arch Surg* 103:461, 1971.

Pruitt BA Jr, Curreri PW: The use of homograft and heterograft skin, in Polk HC, Stone HH (eds): *Contemporary Burn Management.* Boston, Little, Brown and Company, 1971, p 397.

Salisbury RE, Hunt JL, et al: Management of electrical burns of the upper extremities. *Plast Reconstr Surg* 51:648, 1973.

Snyder WH, Bowles BM, MacMillan GB: The use of expansion meshed grafts in the acute and reconstructive management of thermal injury: A clinical evaluation. *J Trauma* 10:740, 1970.

Travis MJ, Thornton J, et al: Current status of skin substitutes. *Surg Clin North Am* 50:1233, 1978.

General Therapeutic Considerations

Curreri PW: Long-term supranormal dietary programs in extensively burned patients, in Sheets WL, Cowan GSM Jr (eds): *Intravenous Hyperalimentation.* Philadelphia, Lea & Febiger, 1972, p 136.

Curreri PW: Metabolic and nutritional aspects of thermal injury. *Burns* 2:16, 1975.

Curreri PW, Hicks JE, et al: Inhibition of active sodium transport in erythrocytes from burn patients. *Surg Gynecol Obstet* 139:538, 1974.

Curreri PW, Richmond D, et al: Dietary requirements of patients with major burns. *J Am Diet Assoc* 65:415, 1974.

Curreri PW, Wilmore DW, et al: Intracellular cation alterations following major trauma: Effect of supranormal caloric intake. *J Trauma* 11:390, 1971.

Dobbs ER, Curreri PW: Burns: Analysis of results of physical therapy in 681 patients. *J Trauma* 12:242, 1972.

Larson DL, Abston S, Evans EB: Splints and traction, in Polk HC, Stone HH (eds): *Contemporary Burn Management*. Boston, Little, Brown and Company, 1971, p 419.

Larson DL, Abston S, et al: Techniques for decreasing scar formation and contractures in the burn patient. *J Trauma* 11:807, 1971.

Reiss E, Pearson E, Artz CP: The metabolic response to burns. *J Clin Invest* 35:62, 1956.

Rickler JM, Bruck HM, et al: Superior mesenteric artery syndrome as a consequence of burn injury. *J Trauma* 12:979, 1972.

Salisbury RE, Palm L: Dynamic splinting for dorsal burns of the hand. *Plast Reconstr Surg* 51:226, 1973.

Sawchuk RJ, Zaske DE: Drug kinetics in burn patients. *Clin Pharmakokinet* 5:548, 1980.

Wilmore DW: Hormonal responses and their effect on metabolism. *Surg Clin North Am* 56:999, 1976.

Wilmore DW, Curreri PW, et al: Supranormal dietary intake in thermally injured metabolic patients. *Surg Gynecol Obstet* 132:881, 1971.

Wilmore DW, Mason AD Jr, et al: Effect of ambient temperature on heat production and heat loss in burn patients. *J Appl Physiol* 38:593, 1975.

Wilmore DW, Mason AD Jr, Pruitt BA Jr: Insulin response to glucose in hypermetabolic burn patients. *Ann Surg* 183:314, 1976.

Wilmore DW, Orcutt TW, et al: Alterations in hypothalamic function following thermal injury. *J Trauma* 15:697, 1975.

Zawacki BC, Spitzer KW, et al: Does increased evaporative water loss cause hypermetabolism in burn patients? *Ann Surg* 171:236, 1970.

Special Problems

Achauer BM, Allyn PA, et al: Pulmonary complications of burns: The major threat to the burn patient. *Ann Surg* 177:311, 1972.

Achauer BM, Bartlett RH, et al: Internal fixation in the management of the burned hand. *Arch Surg* 108:814, 1974.

Alston DW, Kozerefski P, et al: Materials for pressure inserts in the control of hypertrophic scar tissue. *J Burn Care Rehab* January–February 1981.

Altman LC, Klebanoff SJ, Curreri PW: Abnormalities of monocyte hemotaxis following thermal injury. *J Surg Res* 22:616, 1977.

Asch MJ, Curreri PW, Pruitt BA Jr: Thermal injury involving bone: A report of 32 cases. *J Trauma* 12:135, 1972.

Asch MJ, Moylan JA Jr, et al: Ocular complications associated with burns: Review of a five-year experience including 104 patients. *J Trauma* 11:857, 1971.

Bartlett RH, Allyn PA: Pulmonary management of the burned patient. *Heart and Lung* 2:714, 1973.

Bruck HM, Pruitt BA Jr: Curling's ulcer in children: A 12-year review of 63 cases. *J Trauma* 12:490, 1972.

Curreri PW, Bruck HM, et al: *Providencia stuartii* sepsis: A new challenge in treatment of thermal injury. *Ann Surg* 177:133, 1973.

Curreri PW, Heck EL, et al: Stimulated nitroblue tetrazolium test to assess neutrophil antibacterial function: Prediction of wound sepsis in burned patients. *Surgery* 74:6, 1973.

Heck EL, Browne L, et al: Evaluation of leukocyte function in burned individuals by *in vitro* oxygen consumption. *J Trauma* 15:486, 1975.

Heimbach DM: Smoke inhalation. *Top Emer Med* 3:75, 1981.

Loebl EC, Marvin JA, et al: The method of quantitative burn-wound biopsy cultures and its routine use in the care of the burned patient. *Am J Clin Pathol* 61:20, 1974.

Loebl EC, Marvin JA, et al: Survival with ecthyma gangrenosum, a previously fatal complication of burns. *J Trauma*. 14:370, 1974.

Loebl EC, Marvin JA, et al: The use of quantitative biopsy cultures in bacteriologic monitoring of burn patients. *J Surg Res* 16:1, 1974.

Marvin JA, Heck EL, et al: Usefulness of blood cultures in confirming septic complications in burn patients: Evaluation of a new culture method. *J Trauma* 15:657, 1975.

Moncrief JA: Burns of specific areas. *J Trauma* 5:278, 1965.

Moylan JA: Inhalation injury—a primary determinant of survival following major burns. *J Burn Care Rehab* March–April 1981.

Moylan JA: Smoke inhalation and burn injuries. *Surg Clin North Am* 60:1533, 1980.

Pruitt BA Jr, Erickson DR, Morris A: Progressive pulmonary insufficiency and other pulmonary complications of thermal injury. *J Trauma* 15:369, 1975.

Pruitt BA Jr, Foley FD: The use of biopsies in burn patient care. *Surgery* 73:887, 1973.

Pruitt BA Jr, Goodwin CW: Stress ulcer disease in the burned patient. *World J Surg* 5:209, 1981.

Quan PE, Rau SB, et al: Control of scar tissue in the finger web spaces by use of graded pressure inserts. *J Burn Care Rehab* January–February 1981.

Reckler JM, Flemma RJ, Pruitt BA Jr: Costal chondritis: An unusual complication in the burned patient. *J Trauma* 13:76, 1973.

Rosenthal A, Czaja AJ, Pruitt BA Jr: Gastrin levels and gastric acidity in the pathogenesis of acute gastroduodenal disease after burns. *Surg Gynecol Obstet* 144:232, 1977.

Silverstein P, Peterson HD: Treatment of eyelid deformities due to burns. *Plast Reconstr Surg* 51:38, 1973.

Voorhis CC, Law EJ, MacMillan BG: Operative treatment of Curling's ulcer in children: Report of 4 cases with 3 survivors. *J Trauma* 14:175, 1974.

Wanner A, Cutchavaree A: Early recognition of upper airway obstruction following smoke inhalation. *Am Rev Respir Dis* 180:1421, 1973.

Warden JD, Mason AD, Pruitt BA Jr: Suppression of leukocyte chemotaxis *in vitro* by chemotherapeutic agents used in management of thermal injuries. *Ann Surg* 181:363, 1975.

Chapter 8

Wound Healing and Wound Care

Erle E. Peacock, Jr.

INTRODUCTION

During the course of human evolution a valuable defense mechanism—the ability to regenerate compound tissues—was replaced by a much less complicated and far less valuable process—the phenomenon of healing. Although ability to heal has been of enormous importance in natural selection, restoration of physical integrity by synthesis of scar tissue can be regarded, at best, as only a method of preserving homeostasis and cannot be compared with the more pristine function of multi-germ-layer regeneration. Moreover, the fibrous tissue synthesis stage of healing can be detrimental even to the extent of destroying the organism that it sought to preserve. Examples are the potentially fatal deformity of valve leaflets incurred during healing of rheumatic fever valvulitis, development of posthepatitic cirrhosis, and development of esophageal stenosis after swallowing a corrosive agent. The patient may survive the initial disease or injury only to succumb months or years later from complications of fibrous tissue synthesis during healing.

Posthepatitic cirrhosis is of special interest to students of biology of wound healing, because the liver is probably the only example of a compound organ in human beings in which almost embryonic propensity for secondary regeneration appears to be retained. Under most circum-stances, the liver can be counted upon to regenerate most, if not all, of preinjury mass; in fact, the failure of regeneration to occur with normal rapidity and effectiveness in severe nodular cirrhosis gives the impression that only overgrowth of fibrous tissue may have prevented hepatic regeneration. The significance of this hypothesis reflects the possibility that fibrous protein synthesis anywhere in the body chokes or overpowers cellular regeneration; from an evolutionary standpoint, such a hypothesis has some factual basis. The hydrozoan *Tubularia* will sometimes regenerate an amputated hydranth without forming a connective tissue scar; at other times the organism will merely heal the wound by formation of scar tissue. When scar tissue is found, only an abortive attempt at regeneration can be identified. Another example can be found during development of newts when the ability to regenerate is disappearing. If during this time connective tissue synthesis is blocked by pharmacologic agents, the ability to regenerate a new limb will be prolonged.

With the possible exception of the liver, regeneration in human beings is essentially limited to simple tissue such as epithelium; compound structures such as skin, deep organs, and nervous system can heal only by sealing the wound in a manner to be described. The sealing process varies, depending upon whether structural integrity is interrupted or tissue substance is removed. In both types of wounds, epithelization is the fundamental process that seals the wound, and fibrous tissue synthesis and remodeling is the process that provides structural strength. When tissue is missing, an additional process—contraction—moves tissue edges into closer approximation so that epithelization and fibrous protein synthesis can accomplish their objectives. Simple as this description may sound, most of the mistakes made by physicians in treating wounds are attributable to failure to realize and understand the limitations and end results of these fundamental processes and how they differ from pristine regeneration. Thus optimal wound management requires detailed knowledge of epithelization, fibrous protein synthesis, and the biology of wound contraction. Study of these processes requires, in addition, some knowledge of the milieu in which they occur—the ground substance.

WOUND CONTRACTION

In 1793, John Hunter wrote, "In the amputation of the thick thigh (which is naturally 7, 8, or more inches in diameter) . . . the cicatrix shall be no broader than a crown piece." The essence of this quotation is that full-thickness wounds of organs (including skin) do not heal by synthesis of fibrous scar with the exact dimensions of the original defect. A crown piece in Hunter's time was 1½ in. in diameter, thus over 90 percent of the amputation wound was closed by centripetal movement of skin edges. This process is called *contraction*—a dynamic term denoting action, which should not be used interchangeably with "contracture," the correct term for the end result (Fig. 8-1*A* and *B*). Just as loss of brain or stomach produces a permanent defect in human beings, loss of skin also is permanent, and when a defect in the integument occurs, restoration of integrity is dependent largely upon stretching surrounding skin to cover exposed subcutaneous tissue. Obviously, stretching skin will distort movable features such as lips, eyelids, breasts, or digits. The fundamental process in contraction can be illustrated perfectly and the end result predicted positively by simply grasping the edges of a gaping wound and manually coapting them. Such replication of the contraction process produces the exact deformity that will result from natural wound contraction over a longer period of time. If it is not physically possible to coapt the edges of a wound

by reasonable external force, one can be certain that natural processes also will not be effective, as the amount of skin present is all that will be available to be stretched over the wound. Unnatural stretching by an implanted expansion device, of course, is an exception to this statement. The area that remains uncovered will either remain as an open granulating wound or, if it is small, be covered by epithelium, which is a poor substitute for normal skin and establishes a potentially dangerous area for the development of epidermoid carcinoma.

Thus the effectiveness of the contraction process in producing complete wound closure and the cosmetic and functional deformity that closure by contraction produces are related to the amount of skin available in a given area of the body. Because the hands and face of a young person do not contain excess skin, closure of a defect by contraction causes distortion of facial features or restriction of joint motion. In areas where there is redundancy of skin, such as the cervical region or face of old people, wound contraction can be extremely effective in closing defects without producing cosmetic or functional abnormalities. Where an excess of skin is not present but flex-

Fig. 8-1. *A.* Severe contracture produced by full-thickness skin loss in burn wound of neck and face. Note ectropion of lower lip. *B.* Release of contracture in same patient shown in Fig. 8-1*A.* Contracture was released by excising scar tissue and resurfacing the defect with several split-thickness skin grafts. Note absence of wrinkling of graft and restoration of cervical profile. Facial scars ultimately excised and resurfaced.

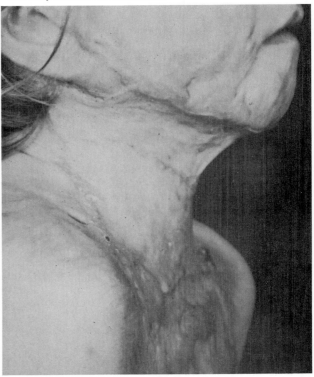

A   B

ion or extension of a joint will move wound edges together, wound contraction inexorably results in movement of the joint into an extreme position. After healing has occurred, the joint will be fixed because of lack of a satisfactory envelope. When loss of skin occurs over an area such as the malleolar surface of the lower leg and ankle, wound contraction simply cannot occur because there is not enough skin to stretch over the defect. In this instance the wound either becomes covered by a thin, almost gelatinous film of epithelium or remains open for an indefinite length of time.

Three questions immediately arise about the contraction process: What starts it? What stops it? What is the mechanism by which it occurs? On first consideration, the answer to the first question appears obvious, in that interruption of the integrity of skin always seems to be the initiating stimulus. Close examination of the series of events that occur following removal of a piece of full-thickness skin, however, reveals that wound contraction does not begin immediately; about 4 days elapse before movement of the edges is measurable. This so-called lag phase of healing seems to include the contraction phenomenon, and it can only be surmised that a set of conditions must be established or an assembly of cells or energy source completed before the actual work of mobilizing skin edges begins. One might surmise also that reestablishment of physical integrity is the stimulus that stops contraction; but again, measurement of the timing of other events reveals that contraction of a wound does not stop immediately with closure; indeed, wounds that were not caused by a loss of tissue and that have their edges approximated immediately will sometimes undergo considerable contraction. Even closure of a wound by the application of a free skin graft or pedicle flap does not stop the contracting process once movement of wound edges has begun (Fig. 8-2). An interesting observation is that the rate of wound contraction is not the same for all points on the circumference of a wound unless the wound is a perfect circle. The ultimate configuration of the scar produced by a contracting wound is the result of variations in the rate of movement of different segments as well as the firmness of attachment of different areas of the skin to both movable and immovable structures. From a practical standpoint, the surgeon may use such information to reduce the final extent of wound contraction. For example, a wound created by bringing ileum through the abdominal wall to form a permanent ileostomy can produce ileal obstruction if the skin opening undergoes contraction. One way to minimize skin wound contraction is to make the skin incision a perfect circle.

The first step in studying the mechanism of wound contraction is to try to define precisely where the fundamental process is located. In the crudest analysis it must be determined whether centripetal movement occurs because an energy or power source located outside the defect is pushing the skin edges in or whether a centrally located power source is pulling the skin edges to the center of the defect. Curiously, even after 35 years of intensive study, the answer is not entirely clear. There is good evidence that energy is being expended in both areas, and

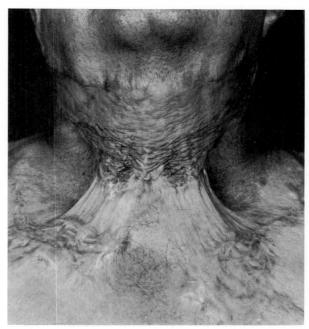

Fig. 8-2. Appearance of split-thickness skin graft applied to granulating wound while undergoing contraction. Note wrinkled appearance of graft and effect of continued contraction on surrounding skin.

the question becomes whether both processes are effective or whether only one is effective and the other either is reacting to wound contraction or is insufficient to produce effective tissue movement.

Over the years most investigators have assumed either that central granulation tissue in a contracting wound was retracting and pulling the normal skin over the granulating base or that contents of the wound were being absorbed as the skin edges moved toward the center. In 1958, Grillo et al. awakened interest in this question by reporting some experiments designed to determine whether changes in the central mass of wound tissue were pulling the skin edges together or whether central wound tissue was merely adjusting to movement of wound edges propelled by peripheral force. The commonly held opinion that dehydration of wound tissue was responsible for contraction was destroyed by Grillo's measurements, which showed that water content of central wound tissue at the beginning of wound contraction had not changed significantly at the end of contraction. The assumption that collagen synthesis and contraction might be responsible for drawing wound edges together also was disproved by direct measurement of collagen content of wound tissue during contraction. Although collagen content increases significantly between the fifth and eighth day of healing, total collagen in the wound falls significantly after 4 weeks and cannot be correlated with rate of wound contraction. Moreover, rate of wound contraction is not affected by suppressing collagen synthesis or interfering with cross linking.

The result of such studies was that attention became

focused upon living cells as the motor units in the contraction process. Wound contraction occurs only in living organisms, and the force that produces migration of wound edges is generated by living cells. As might be expected, a cytochrome poison, such as potassium cyanide, can be shown to impair wound contraction although it does not abolish the process completely. Migration of mesodermal cells in tissue culture also has been shown to be restricted by a cytochrome poison. These observations are readily reversible, which suggests an inverse relationship between inhibition of aerobic respiration and cell migration.

In an attempt to determine if cells responsible for wound contraction were located in granulation tissue, Grillo excised all central wound tissue from wounds in guinea pigs every day during the contracting process. Curiously, excision of central tissue did not affect rate of wound contraction. Such data are not conclusive in localizing the mechanism of wound contracture, however, because they cannot be correlated with results produced by other manipulations of the central mass of wound tissue. For instance, if a square of granulation tissue in the center of a healing wound is outlined by tattoo marks and then separated from the rest of the wound tissue by circumferential incision during wound contraction, two interesting observations can be made: The centrally migrating wound edge will retract peripherally, and the centrally circumcised area of granulation tissue will contract centrally. This finding leads one to the inescapable conclusion that granulation tissue between two wound edges was not being compressed by peripheral skin moving inward but was under considerable tension produced by the advancing wound edges. Moreover, in other experiments, wounds that were splinted for several days and then released did not show marked acceleration of wound contraction following removal of the splint if central granulation tissue was incised. Additional evidence that tension in granulation tissue is causally related to wound contraction is found in the ingenious experiments of James and Newcombe, who measured the contraction force of granulation tissue and plotted it against the length of tissue elements and the cross-sectional area of granulation tissue. No significant correlation between wound tension and overall wound area could be shown, but a highly significant correlation was found between cross-sectional area of granulation tissue and the tension that was developed during wound contraction. Such studies suggest that granulation tissue under tension resembles stretched elastic tissue, in that the amount of tension produced is related to cross-sectional area and not to overall length or surface area. These data, plus the demonstration that granulation tissue contains cells of a type that can exert migratory force of a magnitude necessary to mobilize skin edges, strongly suggest that the machinery for wound contraction is located in the central granulating mass. A recent discovery by Majno et al. of highly specialized cells (termed *myofibroblasts*) with smooth-muscle-like contracting powers lends additional support to this concept.

Grillo found that although wound contraction was not inhibited by excising the entire central mass of granulation tissue, it could be stopped decisively by excising a very limited zone of tissue just beneath the advancing dermal edge. The term "picture frame area" was developed to describe the strategic location of cells that appear to constitute the machinery for wound contraction. Histologic examination of the "picture frame area" reveals a collection of large, stellate, pale-staining cells that have been thought to be the cells responsible for moving the overlying dermis.

Presently it can be said only that recent investigations have eliminated changes in nonliving materials as the cause of wound contraction and have established that the movement of wound edges requires a high order of energy transfer performed by living cells. No unifying hypothesis exists by which all the available data can be explained or the exact site or mechanism of action of wound contraction identified. The apparently incompatible findings of Grillo and of Abercrombie and James concerning the importance of the central granulation tissue can probably best be resolved by hypothesizing that the wound margin makes its way over the surface of movable granulation tissue, and as it does so, it forces it by counteraction in a centrifugal direction, thus putting central granulation tissue under enough tension to cause retraction when it is excised or divided. Regardless of the exact location, however, the phenomenon of wound contraction is one of the most predictable and powerful of all biologic reactions and must be positively reckoned with in the management of wounds where tissue has been lost. The process is carried out by myofibroblasts. Under the microscope, myofibroblasts show characteristics of fibroblasts and smooth muscle cells including a rough endoplasmic reticulum, microfilament bundles similar to smooth muscle, and abundant microtubules that apparently perform a bracing function. In contrast to normal fibroblasts, myofibroblasts often are joined by hemidesmosomes, allowing the cells to "pull on each other." Histochemical studies indicate that the common contractile protein in smooth muscle cells and myofibroblasts is actin. Wound contraction can be controlled by topical application of smooth muscle inhibitors such as Trocinate. Inhibitors of microtubule formation such as colchicine and vinblastine also inhibit wound contracture under experimental conditions. Colchicine has been found to be too toxic to utilize clinically in the control of wound contraction in human beings.

EPITHELIZATION

An attempt to cover by regenerating epidermis any area of the body denuded of skin is the first irrefutable sign of wound repair and occurs long before any evidence of connective tissue synthesis. Factors that control movement of epidermal cells and the mechanism by which cells cover a denuded area are important to students of wound healing for two reasons. The first is that epithelization is necessary in the repair of all types of wounds if a watertight seal is to occur. Protection from fluid and particulate-matter contamination and maintenance of an internal milieu are dependent upon the physical characteristics of keratin. It should be pointed out, however, that just as the plastic liner of a home swimming pool contributes only a watertight seal while structural stability is maintained by concrete blocks, the epidermis, although essential to maintain a watertight seal, provides very little structural strength. It is the surrounding fibrous protein framework that gives strength to a scar (Fig. 8-3). Actually, no cellular structure or globular protein can impart much strength in the repair of a wound. When structural strength is needed, fibrous protein must be utilized. Thus highly cellular organs, such as liver, spleen, kidney, or brain, have almost no structural strength and cannot be sutured as effectively as fibrous tissue organs, such as dura, dermis, fascia, or peritoneum. A wound healed only by epithelium will stop "weeping" and be safe from bacterial invasion as long as the epithelium is intact, but the slightest trauma literally will wipe off what is hardly more than a gelatinous film; thus no degree of permanent protection has been achieved.

Second, epithelization is of great importance in the study of wound healing, because when certain variations in the control of cell division and cell movement occur, normal epithelization becomes uncontrolled growth, with awesome invasive potential. The recognized potential for development of cancer in certain types of wound scars (radiant-energy-induced wounds particularly) and in all wounds that are prevented from healing over a long period of time emphasizes the close similarity between cancer and the healing process (Fig. 8-4*A* and *B*). Actually, a histologic section from a 5-day-old healing wound can be interpreted as fibrosarcoma if none of the historical details are available. Healing is dependent upon what may be thought of as a return to embryonic status; at certain times in the healing process the overall picture—characterized by mitosis, pleomorphism, disorganization, and loss of polarity—resembles uncontrolled growth of a malignant neoplasm. A major difference exists, however: the factor of control. In a healing wound, the embryonic state is temporary and some controlling influence brings order out of disorder, a resting state to rapidly multiplying cells, and a remodeling of recently synthesized fibrous tissue to produce purposeful structural patterns. In a neoplasm, however, the situation is similar to a healing wound in which the factor of control never reappears, so that healing continues without purpose or control until the entire organism is consumed by direct extension or metastasis of the products of regeneration. Considered in this way, there may be only a fine distinction between healing and malignant growth; it may be that when we understand all the factors that influence cells to return to embryonic activity during healing, and even more important, the factors that control their growth and movement after healing has been accomplished, an important step will have been taken in solving the riddle of cancer. For now, however, it is important to remember that the stimulus following injury to overcome entropy and develop embryonic kinetics is one of the most powerful and predictable phenomena in biology.

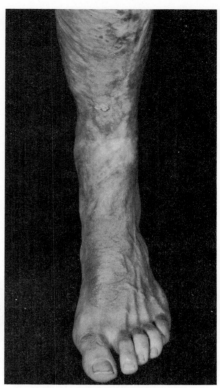

Fig. 8-3. Third-degree burn of lower leg following healing by epithelization. Absence of dermis accounts for shiny appearance and relative fragility of the surface.

Apparently cell division and ameboid movement cease only when cells are surrounded by other cells of their own type; this characteristic of cells has something to do with determining the direction in which a mass of cells will move. Weiss observed that when epithelial and mesenchymal cells are mixed and suspended in a proper medium, random movement of cells occurs, causing numerous collisions. Collisions of dissimilar cells (i.e., epidermal and mesenchymal) result in repulsion, whereas collision of similar cells results in two cells sticking together and developing protoplasmic bridges and protofibrils. Thus random movements and collisions over a sufficient period of time invariably result in cells of similar type becoming agglutinated on one side of the medium and the remainder becoming agglutinated on the other side. As increasing portions of the circumference of a cell membrane become satisfied by attaching to cells of similar lineage, the remaining unsatisfied sides become the exploring or searching surface; thus some degree of polarity for the whole mass is established. Failure to achieve complete surface contact with other cells results in a continued state of embryonic activity. One does not have to use much imagination to predict that as cells continue to be driven by an insatiable desire to contact cells of similar type, the risk of loss of control over replication and locomotion increases. Until more is known about the factors involved in control of cell growth and movement,

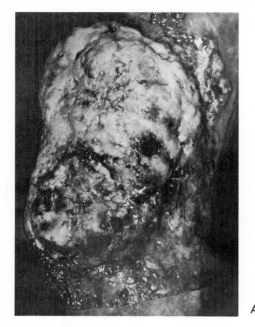

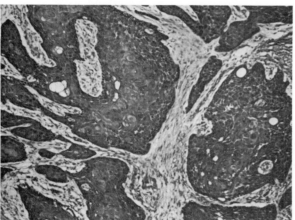

Fig. 8-4. *A.* Epidermoid carcinoma in open third-degree burn wound of thigh. Burn is 15 years old. *B.* Microscopic appearance. Carcinoma developing in burn wounds metastasizes by vascular routes more frequently than other carcinomas.

however, one can only take cognizance of the fact that any wound that is prevented from healing is potentially a malignant neoplasm.

Wounds caused by certain agents such as radiant energy or specific chemicals have unusual propensity for developing cancer in scars or chronic ulcers. In wounds induced by radiant energy, the length of time before cancer develops appears to be directly proportional to the wavelength of the damaging ray. Thus thermal burn wounds and scars may require 20 years for invasive cancer to develop, while in gamma- or x-ray-induced wounds cancer may develop in a few months. Solar and cosmic radiation, a causative agent in most human skin cancer, is short-wavelength radiation, but because it is filtered by

atmosphere and melanin, human development of epidermoid cancer from this source usually does not occur until late in life.

The development of cancer is more rare in surgical or traumatic wounds than in radiant-energy or chemical-induced wounds. No type of wound is exempt, however, when healing has been prevented by constant reinjury or inadequate skin replacement. Even in postphlebitic leg ulcer (a common chronic ulcer) cancer may develop over a long period of time.

The mechanism by which epithelium attempts to close a wound has caused considerable speculation. Previous descriptions of the process, based on the assumption that mitosis was not a prominent occurrence, are not correct. Although it is difficult to find mitotic figures in the advancing margin of epithelium, the works of Bullough and of Gillman and Penn have shown conclusively that mitosis does occur in several layers of epithelium and that it is a recognizable part of epithelization. Theoretically, it should be possible for a wound of any size to be epithelized, although there is a practical limit in clinical practice to the size of the area that will become epithelialized naturally.

Two important gross and histologic differences between normal epithelization in a healing wound and abnormal epithelial growth in epidermoid cancer are size and shape of the peripheral cell mass. A striking feature in a normally healing wound is diminishing thickness to monolayer proportions of the advancing cell front (Fig. 8-5*A* and *B*). In carcinoma, cells pile up and tumble over one another to produce a grossly umbilicated appearance (Fig. 8-6*A* and *B*). Loss of surface protein appears to be a key factor in changes in cell adhesiveness. Thus in normal epithelial regeneration, even though mitosis does occur, the most fundamental process is dedifferentiation and cell movement by development of ruffled membranes and pseudopods. The process begins early (within hours) and results in flat, thin, resting cells at the margin of the wound. These cells develop ruffled membranes and move across the center of the wound. When this occurs, the cell seems to adopt the characteristics of a typical basal cell; if it comes to rest in a more superficial position, it becomes a typical prickle cell.

In incised and sutured wounds, epithelization produces a watertight seal in 24 hours even though there is a dip where the cells have migrated into the crevice. Although the area of regeneration thickens with addition of more cells, the center of the wound remains somewhat inverted until underlying connective tissue synthesis pushes the epithelium into an everted position. Gillman and Penn have pointed out that the cutaneous tract of a skin suture on either side of the scar is also a wound of the epithelium, and that the inverted contour of epithelium over the wound also occurs along the path of a suture to the extent that a completely epithelized tract may be produced or a small cyst formed after a suture is removed.

Epithelization of a surface wound (whether partial thickness of skin such as an abrasion, or split-thickness skin-graft donor site, or full-thickness wound such as postphlebitic ulcer of the ankle) involves similar movement of epithelial cells but over a much more hazardous terrain and greater distance than incised and sutured wounds. The early escape of blood and serum in open wounds produces a scab, and the regenerating epithelium moves beneath the scab, literally detaching it from the underlying surface as it seals the wound. Actually, epithelium does not move along the interface between dermis or fat and the scab but seems to prefer to infiltrate or actually cut through the fibrous tissue substrate by elaborating an enzyme that renders collagen soluble. This phenomenon is the result of tissue collagenase elaborated at the interface between epithelium and mesenchymal tissue. Confirmation of the observation that epithelium literally cuts its own path through fibrous and fibrinous tissue may be extremely important in understanding the remodeling of deep fibrous tissue to produce a new dermal-epithelial interface. A significant problem in recent attempts to grow epithelium on artificial collagen substrate for replacement of burned skin has been difficulty in reproducing rete pegs to provide stable adherence of cells to fibrous protein.

The protective influence of a scab or other cover (eschar, surgical dressing, etc.) to prevent physical trauma, drying, hemorrhage, contact with caustic materials, and the like is the basis for medical care of secondarily healing wounds. In the final analysis, successful epithelization occurs only if the cumulative effect of physical manipulation, drying, bacterial enzymes, wound area, etc., does not exceed the finite capacity of available cells to divide, dedifferentiate, and move across the surface. Considered in the simplest analysis, it may be that interruption of epidermis merely allows the epidermis to do what it normally would do if it had room, since cell movement and cell division are to a large extent prevented in the intact epidermis by the compression effect of surrounding cells.

Epidermal growth factor (EGF), a single polypeptide chain of 53 amino acid residues that contains three intramolecular disulfide bonds, has been identified and extracted from a number of tissues. EGF enhances a number of cellular events that are part of the mitogenic response during wound healing. Local application of EGF enhances the accumulation of cells and ground substances in experimental wounds. EGF has not been shown to be of any clinical value in the treatment of healing wounds in human beings.

GROUND SUBSTANCE

Even as late as 1952, some treatises on wound healing made no mention of the role of ground substance. The mystery surrounding ground substance is nowhere better exemplified than in the name itself, a mistranslation of the German *grundsubstance,* which referred to a mysterious matrix from which all the formed elements of connective tissue were believed to originate. A similar connotation was expressed by the French *substance fondamentale.* Modern definitions have done little to clarify the true nature of this amorphous material, and the best that can be said, even now, is that the term ''ground substance'' usu-

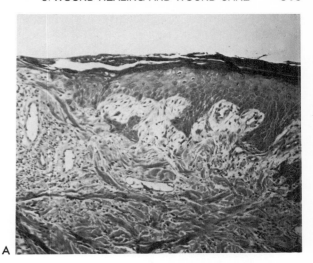

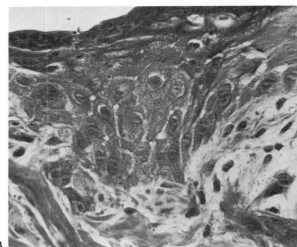

Fig. 8-5. *A.* Low-power view of epithelium advancing over granulating surface in a human wound. Note decreased thickness of advancing margin. *B.* High-power view of advancing epithelium in granulating human wound. Note dedifferentiation of cells, deep migratory activity suggesting subsurface enzyme activity at epithelial-mesenchymal tissue interface, and absence of visible mitotic activity.

ally refers to a continuous nonfibrillar matrix including water and electrolytes through which metabolites diffuse between blood vessels and cells. Recent investigations on the function of one component, fibronectin, have failed to reveal anything more specific than a general structural frame. Histologically, ground substance is identified by a remarkable propensity to absorb certain dyes such as toluidine blue and to undergo characteristic reactions with periodic acid. By such staining reactions it can be seen that ground substance is relatively organized in some areas, such as basement membrane, and undergoes, during inflammation and healing, characteristic changes in staining reaction called *metachromasia.* Such histochemical reactions seem to be due to reactions with mucopolysaccharides, many of which contain hexosamine. Be-

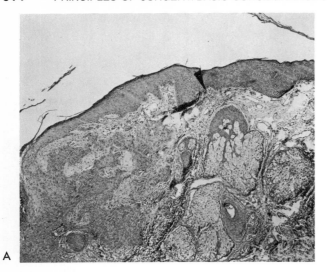

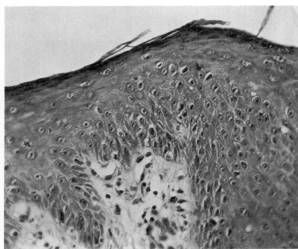

Fig. 8-6. *A.* Low-power view of epidermoid carcinoma of skin. Note accumulation of cells producing increased thickness of epithelium without purposeful migratory activity. *B.* High-power view of epidermoid carcinoma. Note numerous mitotic figures.

most closely associated with the fibrillar elements of connective tissue. Thus changes in sulfated acid mucopolysaccharides are most likely to be of significance during the healing process, and, indeed, such substances are found to be increased during early stages of wound healing. Determination of actual amounts of any of the components of ground substance may be misleading, however, as synthesis and deposition involve polymerizing reactions and formation of giant molecules with molecular weight varying between 10,000 and 10,000,000.

Because the healing process is characterized by polymerizing aggregating reactions, it is interesting to speculate upon the role of mucopolysaccharides. Discovery that acid-sulfated mucopolysaccharides accumulate during healing raises the question of whether linkages between fibrillar proteins and ground substance occur. The same question has been raised about normal tissues such as tendons, where chondroitin C is a prominent portion of the ground substance; stabilization of tendon by cross linkages between collagen fibrils and chondroitin C has not been demonstrated conclusively. Chondroitin A protein complex seems important in stabilization of cartilage, and destruction of this complex by local injection of papain in a rabbit's ear will produce a lop-ear deformity that will return to normal as soon as the complex is reconstituted. It seems likely that ground substance is most important in the phenomenon of healing because of its relation to collagen synthesis and remodeling. Although chemical linkages between mucopolysaccharides and collagen have been extremely difficult to identify, chemical bonds are present that may be important in the development of strength or orientation of collagen fibers and fibrils. Certainly the assembly of collagen subunits into fibrils and fibers is dependent upon many environmental conditions, including a purely physical template or lattice. Variations in the relative amounts of sulfated fractions are believed by some to be instrumental in determining the configurations of collagen fibrils, but how much this complicated substance actually participates in the healing process is not clear.

COLLAGEN

As far as the questions that patients ask their physicians following repair of wounds are concerned, fibrous protein synthesis is the essence of healing. Accurate answers to such questions as "When do the stitches come out?" "When can I go back to work?" "How bad will the scar be?" and others are dependent upon a thorough knowledge of collagen synthesis, collagen degradation, and the factors that influence equilibrium between the two. Unfortunately, there are gaps in our knowledge about collagen metabolism; but enough is known so that the care of wounds does not have to be a mixture of craft and religion, as Paré expressed it, but can be, in most instances, a scientific exercise with a predictable outcome. Even such seeming trivia as the selection of a suture or dressing material can be the result of logical reasoning based upon factual knowledge.

cause of characteristic staining reactions, attention has been focused on the acid mucopolysaccharides, even though it must be remembered that they account for only a small portion of ground substance. As a result, errors have been made by measuring hexosamine in connective tissues and drawing conclusions about the relative amount and importance of ground substance.

Meyer's division of the acid mucopolysaccharides into two major groups has been useful in the study of wound healing. These groups are nonsulfated mucopolysaccharides, of which hyaluronic acid and chondroitin can be easily identified, and sulfated mucopolysaccharides, of which chondroitin sulfate A, chondroitin sulfate B, chondroitin sulfate C, heparitin sulfate, and keratosulfate have been identified. Presently it seems that the nonsulfated group is the main component of the structureless gel fraction of ground substance and that the sulfated group is

Collagen is an extracellular secretion from specialized fibroblasts, and the monomeric particles or basic molecules that fibroblasts synthesize are frequently called *tropocollagen*. The tropocollagen molecule is one of the largest biologic macromolecules, with a molecular weight of about 300,000 and dimensions of 15 Å in width and 2800 Å in length. It is a stiff, elongated rod that can be visualized by an electron microscope and is soluble in cold salt solution. Thus tropocollagen is sometimes referred to as saline-extractable, or salt-soluble, collagen.

Recently it has become evident that genetic pleomorphism is expressed in subtypes of collagen molecules. Three types of collagens can be recognized by analyzing the composition of α1 and α2 chains. Type I collagen is the most prevalent type in the mature vertebrate organism. Type II collagen appears limited to cartilage and is found primarily in human articular and costal cartilages and in chick embryo bones. Type III collagen is found in association with Type I collagen and is most prevalent in tissue undergoing remodeling or fetal organogenesis. Type III collagen also appears to be an important component of tissues with an unusual degree of elasticity, such as those of the aorta, esophagus, and uterus. Other types and subtypes of collagen appear only in highly specialized tissue and do not appear important in wound healing biology.

The amino acids found only in collagen, and used to identify it in analytical procedures, are hydroxyproline and hydroxylysine. The amount of collagen in a specimen of tissue is determined by measuring the amount of hydroxyproline and multiplying the result by a factor of 7.8. Other fibrous tissues such as elastin do not contain significant amounts of hydroxyproline. Formerly it was believed that hydroxyproline in collagen had much to do with the formation of various intra- and intermolecular cross links that give collagen molecules, fibers, and fibrils their characteristic rigidity. The three-plane fixation of the triple-helix structure results, teleologically speaking, in being able to rely on collagen to transmit energy accurately in tendons or to support nonfibrous structures such as muscle. The supporting nonelastic properties of collagen can be destroyed by rupturing cross links within and between molecules, but fortunately, the destruction of cross links to this extent requires rather harsh treatment for mature collagen, such as temperatures over 70°C or exposure to strong acids or alkalies. Under these circumstances, what is produced is gelatin, which, of course, has no structural strength even though the essential amino acids are present. Hydroxylation of proline and lysine also are important in transport of collagen molecules across cell membranes.

Synthesis of collagen is an intracellular phenomenon that occurs on polysomes; a critical stage in construction of the molecule is the hydroxylation of proline to produce hydroxyproline. Externally administered hydroxyproline is excreted rapidly in the urine and apparently cannot be utilized by fibroblasts to synthesize collagen. Among other things, one of the metabolic defects that can be identified in collagen-deficiency diseases such as scurvy is accumulation of proline-rich precursors and deficiency of hydroxy-proline-containing polypeptides. During active collagen synthesis, rough endoplasmic reticulum in fibroblasts forms characteristic parallel lines, or canaliculi, and it appears that monomeric molecules are excreted into the extracellular milieu through these canaliculi. In ascorbic acid deficiency, the microsomes do not form parallel lines of canaliculi but are arranged, instead, in large cystic spaces. It is from these areas that proline-rich and hydroxy-proline-poor amorphous material is found.

Before aggregation and normal assembly can occur, a specific extracellular enzyme, procollagen peptidase, is needed to remove nonhelical terminal extensions from both the N-terminal and C-terminal ends of collagen molecules. The terminal peptide extensions of the collagen molecule are registration peptides facilitating triple-helix formation. These terminal peptides interfere with subsequent fibril aggregation and failure to remove them because of congenital absence of procollagen peptidase results in poorly assembled collagen with marked structural abnormalities. A type of Ehlers-Danlos syndrome has been found to be the result of persistent pro-α chains. A similar condition appears to be responsible for the structural malformations called dermatosparaxis in a disease first observed in Belgian cattle.

Monomeric collagen particles exposed to proper pH, temperature, osmotic conditions, etc., in the intercellular milieu aggregate or polymerize rapidly by the formation of cross links of various types. The most important such cross links are covalent ester bonds such as a Schiff's base between an amino group of one molecule and an aldehyde group of another. Oxidative deamination of lysine by an important enzyme, lysyl oxidase, is a necessary first step in formation of covalent ester cross links. In addition, other types of cross links, such as oppositely charged electrostatic groups and Van der Waals interactions, are involved in assembling monomeric particles into polymerized aggregates.

The rodlike collagen molecules appear to lie in staggered, overlapping, parallel formation, with one-quarter-length overlap. It is this staggered one-quarter-overlap arrangement of tightly packed units that gives collagen a typical repeating axial periodicity of 640 Å. Whenever collagen molecules are assembled under physiologic conditions such as those provided by the extracellular ground substance, typical fibrils with 640-Å repeating periods are produced. In certain laboratory preparations, however, it is possible to alter the characteristic 640-Å periodicity by forcing the monomeric particles to line up exactly parallel or end-on. This can be accomplished by adding glycoprotein to the milieu or by charging the preparation with a high-energy system such as adenosine triphosphate. Under these conditions, fibrils with band widths of 2000 Å can be produced; such atypical fibers are called *segment long-spacing fibers,* or *fibrous long-spacing fibrils.* These preparations have been extremely valuable in the laboratory, as they have revealed much about the size and method of polymerization of collagen molecules; they are not of any physiologic importance, however, as far as is known.

Although the collagen molecule basically is a triple

helix with a spiral configuration, heat-sensitive intramolecular cross links prevent it from having elastic or recoil properties. However, if a collagen fiber or fibril is placed in a water bath with a small weight suspended from one end and the temperature of the bath is elevated, a point will be reached when the heat-sensitive intramolecular cross links will be destroyed and recoil of the spiral polypeptide chain will occur. The temperature at which this phenomenon occurs is called the *thermal shrinkage temperature,* and the magnitude of this reaction is such that a fiber or fibril will shrink to one-third physiologic length. The thermal shrinkage temperature of collagen, therefore, is an excellent indicator of the strength and degree of inter- and intramolecular bonding. By measuring the thermal shrinkage temperature of various types of collagen, it has been possible to learn about variations in bonding under physiologic conditions and, in some instances, to correlate the development of physical properties of collagen with the extent of cross linking. From such studies it has become clear that cross linking, among other factors, is a function of aging; the older a specimen of collagen becomes, the firmer and more numerous the cross links are. Thus, collagen gel that is only a few minutes old has relatively few cross links, has low thermal shrinkage temperature, and is so flimsy that cold salt solution solubilizes it. If the gel is allowed to mature for 24 h, the number and strength of the cross links increase to the extent that a weak acid may be needed to depolymerize even a portion of it and a higher temperature will be required to cause it to undergo thermal shrinkage. If the aggregate is allowed to polymerize for several weeks, the maximum number and firmness of cross links will be realized, with the result that a strong acid may be needed to get even a portion of the collagen into monomeric units and the thermal shrinkage temperature will be the highest yet. In summary, therefore, both solubility and thermal shrinkage temperatures can be used to measure the age of collagen as represented by the effectiveness of the cross-linking process.

In addition to naturally occurring cross links such as ester bonds, artificial cross links can be added to change the physical properties of collagen. Just as adding an agent that shares electrons easily, such as a sulfur molecule, will increase the strength of rubber (vulcanization) sevenfold, addition of a similar agent such as the methyl group in formaldehyde will increase the number and kinds of cross links in collagen. Just how much the addition and destruction of cross links has to do with physical properties of wound-repair collagen in scar tissue is not known. It has been shown, however, that addition of methyl or amide cross links will increase the tensile strength of scar tissue in incised and sutured wounds in rats as much as threefold on the eighth postwound day. That variations in cross linking are partially responsible, however, for the final appearance, texture, or elasticity of human scars is becoming more certain.

At this point, other factors involved in tensile strength must be considered, for cross linking may have very little to do with tensile strength after fibrils and fibers have been formed. It is highly unlikely, in the opinion of the author, that fibrils and fibers are cross-linked very efficiently, because the average distance between fibrils is of the order of 1 μm. Chemical cross links are approximately 2.8 Å, which means that the distance is roughly 500 times too great for the usual types of cross links to span the distance between fibrils. However, because addition of cross links such as methyl or amide bonds definitely increases tensile strength in wet scar tissue, the inescapable conclusion seems to be that rupture of scar tissue must occur, to some extent, along inter- and intramolecular planes. There is no uniform agreement on this point, and the question of the importance of cross linking in the development of strength in scar tissue must be investigated further.

After a certain amount of collagen has been synthesized, the most important factor in gain of strength may be the physical weave of fibrils and fibers. Certainly it is possible to vary the physical properties of other fibrous materials by varying the weave of the small components exclusive of any chemical bonds. A good example of this principle is to be found in the physical weave of a nylon stocking. Nylon thread is nonelastic, yet a nylon stocking can be made elastic by properly weaving the fibers. Transposed to a biologic system, nonelastic tendon or fascia shows physical characteristics similar to nylon thread, while elasticity of the wall of the aorta is similar to that of a nylon stocking.

The old concept of collagen as a static, adynamic substance—the excelsior of the body—is erroneous. Actually, as will be shown later, collagen in wound scar is a relatively dynamic structure that, like other tissues, is undergoing constant remodeling and replacement. After the forty-second day of wound healing there is no measurable increase in the amount of collagen in a healing wound, and yet the scar continues to gain strength for at least 2 years. Thus changes in collagen, such as increased cross linking and rearrangement of fibers and fibrils, must be occurring. Turnover of collagen in a healing wound is extensive. Most newly synthesized collagen is replaced as the scar matures and literally all of the collagen in a fibrous transplant, such as a skin graft, will be removed and replaced ultimately.

Before we leave the subject of remodeling, it is important to mention a disease, lathyrism, which has been useful in the study of collagen metabolism and which is beginning to have far-reaching implications for control of human scar tissue. The disease, recognized by Hippocrates, is caused by excessive ingestion of certain peas of the genus *Lathyrus*. Considerable differences exist between the human form of the disease, which is manifested by spastic paralysis, and the disease in laboratory animals, which is characterized by skeletal and cardiovascular abnormalities secondary to altered collagen metabolism. The active and highly potent fraction that produces altered collagen metabolism is beta-aminopropionitrile. Considerable data are available on the effect of this substance on both developing and mature tissues. Most such data support the hypothesis that the primary effect of beta-aminopropionitrile is to block the formation of inter- and intramolecular cross links during all stages of collagen aggregation. Thus beta-aminopropionitrile affects growing tissue more than adult tissue. Characteristically, beta-aminopropionitrile produces a significant increase in saline-extractable collagen, as it prevents the assembly of monomeric collagen units into stable fibrils and fibers. There is evidence that fibril formation is not stopped during lathyrism but that cross linking in fibrils is so unstable that cold saline will solubilize much of the collagen that was assembled during beta-aminopropionitrile poisoning. Growing embryos literally become saline-soluble under the effect of beta-aminopropionitrile, and mature animals will develop hernias or die suddenly of dissecting aneurysms. Wound healing, as might be predicted, is affected by beta-aminopropionitrile; there is cessation of gain in tensile strength within hours after the agent is administered; saline-extractable collagen increases approximately ten times. Clinical implications of the beta-aminopropionitrile effect are exciting, for it is a clear-cut demonstration that it is possible to alter the physical properties of collagen in dramatic fashion. Because some of the effects of fibrous tissue healing in specialized organs, such as the liver or heart, can be more ruinous to health than the disease or injury that preceded healing, the demonstration that some control over deep scar formation is possible is an exciting one. If, in addition, mature recently synthesized collagen also could be solubilized selectively, a major breakthrough in many disease processes could evolve. Highly purified beta-aminopropionitrile has been administered to human beings with scleroderma, urethral stricture, and keloid. It can be given safely to human beings, but is not available for treatment of human diseases. At this time, penicillamine, a lathyrogenic agent as well as a copper chelater previously utilized to treat Wilson's disease, is being used to treat arthritis in human beings and also is being studied as a treatment for undesirable scar tissue.

Several times in this chapter the term "remodeling" of scar tissue has been used. The thoughtful student is likely to be concerned over such a term, as it connotes not just synthesis of collagen but collagen breakdown as well. Because no enzyme able to lyse collagen had been identified in human beings until approximately 25 years ago, collagen turnover in either normal tissue or wound scar was suspect. Even though no such mechanism could be demonstrated, however, indirect evidence has been abundant that some enzyme or mechanism for solubilizing collagen must exist. There is always some extractable collagen in the skin of even the oldest and most depleted individuals. Obviously, if all tropocollagen were going into the skin, the dermis would soon be as thick as elephant hide. Some collagen must be coming out of dermis, and the relatively constant thickness of skin only attests to an equilibrium that exists between collagen synthesis and degradation. Cutaneous scars are raised above the surface 2 to 4 weeks after injury; yet they usually soften, become pliable, and decrease considerably in size with passage of time. The loss of 50 percent of collagen from the gravid uterus 36 hours after parturition and the rapid disappearance of dermis when tetraplegic patients are allowed to lie unattended attest that human beings possess

an effective enzyme capable of degrading mature collagen. Search for such an enzyme was unsuccessful for a long time because it was assumed that the enzyme could be extracted from tissue. In 1963, Gross, Lapiere, and Tanzer hypothesized that collagenolytic enzyme was the product of living cells and that contact with a living cell was necessary in order for collagenolysis to occur. In one of the most important experiments performed in the wound-healing field during that era, the hypothesis was tested by preparing culture plates of reconstituted collagen and amphibian Tyrode culture medium. Specimens of tissue from the rapidly absorbing tail of a metamorphosing tadpole (a structure containing mostly collagen that is absorbed and not broken off during metamorphosis) were placed on the collagen-Tyrode substrate, and the culture plates were incubated under tissue culture conditions. After several days a clear zone appeared around each implant, and if the tissues were kept alive long enough, the entire substrate became lysed by collagenolytic activity. Failure of the cells to survive stops collagenolytic activity immediately; even after lysis has begun, it can be stopped by killing the cells. Thus Gross and Lapiere demonstrated that collagenolytic enzyme is a product of living cells and that cells that produce enzyme need to be in close contact with collagen fibers for lysis to occur. Riley and Peacock cultured a variety of normal and pathologic human tissues and found collagenolytic enzyme to be widely distributed, particularly in epithelium-containing structures.

The most uniformly positive tissue for collagenolytic enzyme in human beings is cutaneous scar. Scar tissue reveals positive lytic activity approximately 10 days after closure of a cutaneous laceration, and a high level of activity has been found in dermal scars as long as 30 years after injury. Granulation tissue is only slightly active; burn eschar does not show any activity for about 2 weeks. Between 2 and 3 weeks after a third-degree burn, however, cultures of separating dermal eschar are strongly positive for collagenolytic activity. These findings suggest that invasion of dead eschar by underlying connective tissue cells or undermining epidermal cells is necessary for contact between cells and heat-tanned collagen. Retarded wound healing may be the result of excessive collagenolysis. Serum, cysteine, and progesterone have been shown to inhibit tissue collagenase acting at neutral pH. Progesterone in ophthalmic concentrations is the agent of choice in treating corneal injury, particularly alkali burns in which delayed tissue collagenase activity is the cause of rupture of the globe.

By measuring collagen synthesis and collagen breakdown, it is possible to study healing from the standpoint of variations in metabolic equilibrium. Considered as such, scar tissue is a product of opposing forces of collagen synthesis and collagen destruction, and the result of such forces will vary according to the relative rate and effectiveness of each. The maximum amount of total collagen in a healing wound is found by the forty-second day. Although increased amounts of saline-extractable collagen (compared with nonwounded resting dermis) can be extracted from scar tissue for as long as 18 months, there is no further gain in insoluble (or mature) collagen. The conclusion would seem to be that, even though remodeling of the collagen continues, equilibrium has been established between collagen synthesis and collagen destruction. Demonstration by Cohen of accelerated collagen synthesis and deposition and collagenolytic activity in human keloids probably represents an abnormality of such an equilibrium.

The concept that all collagen to some extent, and healing wound collagen particularly, is undergoing simultaneous construction and destruction can serve as a basis for speculation concerning some of the previously unexplainable findings in the healing process. One such enigma is the behavior of wounds during ascorbic acid depletion. In the classic descriptions of scurvy it is important to remember that sailors' wounds did not just fail to heal; they actually disrupted months after thay had healed perfectly. This observation has been verified in animals and raises the question of whether collagen is dependent upon ascorbic acid for structural integrity. It is known that collagen can be repeatedly depolymerized and reconstituted in the laboratory without contact with ascorbic acid, and artificially reconstituted collagen does not lose tensile strength. Therefore, the notion that vitamin C has anything to do with strength of mature scar tissue is untenable. Because synthesis of new collagen is blocked during ascorbic acid deficiency, and because collagenolytic activity probably proceeds normally, a possible explanation for old scar dehiscence would seem to be that tissue previously in equilibrium becomes unbalanced by having synthesis knocked out and lysis continue. Inexorably, the scar will become weaker until a point is reached where normal tissue tension produces disruption.

Although to some extent hypothetical (actual quantitative measurements of lysis and synthesis are not sensitive enough now to prove or disprove the equilibrium hypothesis), the theory is important as it relates to the whole field of conditions erroneously referred to in the past as "collagen diseases." The collagen in such diseases is precipitated under physiologic conditions and, as might be predicted, is normal as far as can be determined by electron or light microscopy, x-ray defraction, or amino acid analysis. Thus all the evidence supports the idea that so-called collagen diseases represent abnormal amounts of collagen in abnormal places but are not specific diseases of the collagen molecule or fibril. Such an explanation is entirely logical, as one cannot have a disease of a nonliving structure. Collagen is a crystalline protein in which the nearest thing that could be classified as a disease process is the abnormal construction of collagen during lathyrism. The collagen in such diseases as rheumatic fever, dermatomyositis, and scleroderma is more accurately considered as the ash or scar from a burnt-out primary wound or inflammatory process. In the other direction, destruction of collagen in diseases such as rheumatoid arthritis is, at least partially, the result of excessive tissue collagenase activity. The concept of the collagen system as a dynamic, constantly remodeling one opens the door for investigation of a large number of diseases of unknown cause that are characterized by deficient or excessive collagen formation.

SEQUENCE OF EVENTS: SUMMARY

Once the basic processes in the healing phenomenon have been mastered, the student has only to relate them to one another in proper sequence to be ready to start the study of what physicians can do to aid healing. The most important concept in this regard is the understanding that healing is not a series of events but is a concert of simultaneously occurring processes, some of which continue for many years after physical integrity of wounded tissue has been reestablished. The most dramatic events, such as sealing the wound, regaining tensile strength sufficient to permit normal stress, and acquiring a scar that is cosmetically and functionally acceptable, occur in a relatively short period of time. Long-term processes, such as remodeling of collagen and development of cancer in scar tissue, fortunately are not processes that cause patients much concern. Although the basic processes are much the same in an incised and sutured wound properly coapted (healing by primary intention) and a wound in which tissue has been lost so that healing must occur by contraction and epithelization (secondary healing, or healing by secondary intention), the time required for secondary healing is so much longer and the area involved usually so much greater that it is convenient to study the secondary healing process to see how the basic steps in wound healing relate to one another.

The first thing that happens after full-thickness skin loss is that normal elasticity of the skin and external tension produced in some areas by muscle pull enlarge the defect according to the amount of force exerted and the direction over which it acts. Thus the shape of a skin defect may have little relation to the size or shape of the fragment of tissue that was removed. If hemorrhage is not too severe, a clot forms quickly, then contracts and dehydrates to form a scab. Because a scab is essentially a dehydrated, fully contracted blood clot, it is less durable and effective in closing the wound than collagenous eschar. Nevertheless, a scab serves a useful purpose in providing limited protection from external contamination, satisfactory maintenance of internal hemostasis, and a surface beneath which cell migration and movement of wound edges can occur. Classically, the beginning of wound healing is described as the "lag" phase—an inaccurate term that carries the connotation that there is a period when nothing of importance is happening. Actually, a great number of important things are happening even though they usually are not considered part of the healing process. One soon recognizes, however, that almost instantly following infliction of an injury the stage for healing is set, and the props and background for the events that are to follow are essentially those of controlled inflammation. Study of the biology of repair has emphasized that the most successful reparative processes occur against a background of inflammation and that, up to the point of necrosis, how well the wound heals is related to the amount of inflammation present. Specifically, the release of various amines from connective tissue mast cells, perfusion of capillaries surrounding the defect, change in permeability of capillary walls, release of enzymes, fluid, and protein into extracellular spaces, accumulation of white blood cells and connective tissue cells, and formation of thrombi in peripheral lymphatic channels are well-known changes in general inflammation that are important in providing the best milieu for repair to proceed. It is only when bacteria, foreign bodies, medications, or accumulation of destructive enzymes cause necrosis of tissue that inflammation becomes a deterrent to healing. Therefore, the author prefers to see the term ''lag'' phase replaced by strong emphasis on inflammation as an active part of the reparative process.

Approximately 12 h after injury has occurred, and at a time when inflammation has been established, epithelial migration—the first clear-cut sign of rebuilding—occurs. In a primary wound, epithelization is complete in a few hours; in a secondary healing wound, migration of cells is rapid at first, but as the line of cells from the wound margin becomes extended and the epithelial probe dwindles to a monolayer, progress becomes slower, so that days or even weeks elapse before epithelization is complete. After 4 or 5 days, however, epithelization is assisted as the machinery of wound contraction begins, and the wound margins start central movement.

A great amount of activity takes place in the center of the wound after a scar or eschar has been removed and before epithelium has covered the surface. Grossly, the surface that was once gray or yellow-brown and smooth becomes bright red and granular. The reason for this is an extravagant proliferation of richly perfused capillary loops. The knuckles or loops of blood vessels impart a granular appearance to the surface, and it is because of them that the wound is often described as granulating or showing granulation tissue. Granulation tissue provides a good defense against invasion by surface contaminants, but it is fragile and produces a difficult terrain for advancing epithelial cells. This is particularly true if surface infection, edema, or deep fibrous tissue interfere with return circulation. When this happens, the fiery red granular dots will change to a purple, soggy, gray-black cluster that may fill the entire wound cavity and spill over the wound edge, thus eliminating the possibility of epithelization.

Although no visible signs of collagen synthesis can be found until the fourth to sixth day, biochemical evidence of collagen synthesis can be found between the second and fourth days. The level of hydroxyproline in wound tissue rises rapidly, and the saline-extractable-collagen level becomes elevated shortly thereafter. Before signs of collagen synthesis occur, the ground substance changes, as evidenced by accumulation of sulfated mucopolysaccharides and development of metachromasia. On or about the seventh day wounds will show a delicate fine reticulum of young collagen fibrils. Actually, the gelation that is occurring at this time is so random that polymerization of new collagen fibrils is much like that of a new gel in a laboratory beaker—without purposeful orientation or polarity. There is a short period when young fibrils and fibers take silver stains selectively, and it is thought that this property reflects the presence of large numbers of unsatisfied bonding sites; mature collagen fibers do not stain selectively with silver. As fibrogenesis proceeds, purposefully oriented fibers seem to become thicker, presumably because they are accruing more collagen particles; nonpurposefully oriented fibers disappear. The overall effect appears to be one of lacing the wound edges together by a three-dimensional weave. In secondary wounds the mass of scar tissue becomes dense, compact, and smaller in circumference but shows little in the way of purposeful organization. The overall direction is one of replacing granulation tissue, allowing the surface to become covered with epithelium, and filling in the remaining skin defect with scar tissue after contraction is complete. As far as filling the defect is concerned, contraction is the major influence; it exerts full potential before scar-tissue synthesis is complete. The central scar seems to remodel itself to fill the defect after contraction is over. Thus wounds surrounded by mobile and redundant skin will have a small central scar, while wounds surrounded with tight nonmovable skin will have relatively large central scars regardless of the size of the defect.

Development of tensile strength (strength per unit of scar tissue) and burst strength (strength of the entire wound) is the result initially of blood vessels growing across the wound, epithelization, and aggregation of globular protein. Later, collagen synthesis is important. The effect of vascularization and epithelization, although relatively small, is adequate on the fifth day to hold wound edges, if not under excessive tension, coapted without sutures. The really significant gain in tensile strength begins about the fifth day, however, when collagen synthesis becomes apparent; tensile strength measurements in laboratory animals usually are recorded from that day. Increase in strength is rapid for 17 days and slow for an additional 10 days; there is an almost imperceptible gain in tensile strength for at least 2 years. In spite of the measurable increase in tensile strength for such a long period, strength of scar in rat skin never quite reaches that of unwounded skin.

Collagen content of the wound tissue rises rapidly between the sixth and the seventeenth days but increases very little after the seventeenth day and none at all after the forty-second day. Gain in strength after the seventeenth day, therefore, is due primarily to remodeling of collagen and, hence, is not correlated with total collagen content except for a very short portion of the healing curve.

When a normally healing wound is disrupted mechanically after the fifth day and immediately resutured, the return of tensile strength is so rapid that within 2 days the burst strength is nearly what it would have been had the secondary wound not occurred. This phenomenon, commonly called the *secondary healing effect,* has been studied intensely to determine the exact mechanism of rapid gain of tensile strength following repair of a secondary wound. Curiously, it is neither more rapid collagen synthesis nor more rapid assembly of collagen subunits; secondary wounds contain slightly less collagen than primary wounds of the same age. Because the thermal shrinkage temperature of secondary wound collagen is significantly higher than that of primary wounds of the same age, it has been suggested that more effective cross linking or better physical weave of collagen subunits is responsible for the rapid gain in strength of secondary wounds. The demonstration by Madden and Smith that secondary healing is really nothing more than continued primary healing (without a lag phase) invalidates previous cross-linking theories of secondary wound healing. Whatever the explanation, however, the machinery for producing rapid gain in tensile strength in secondary wounds is limited to an area of 7 mm around the first wound. Excision of skin edges more than 7 mm circumferential to the primary wound results in secondary wound healing at the same rate as in a primary wound.

WOUND CARE

From a treatment standpoint, there are essentially two types of wounds: those which are characterized by loss of tissue and those in which no tissue has been lost. Lacerations are an example of wounds without tissue loss, and avulsions or burns are examples of wounds that, in addition to interruption of surface continuity, result in loss of tissue. A question that must be answered for both is whether immediate closure can be performed safely. Whether the wound can be closed by suturing the edges together or a graft of some sort is required, a decision must be reached about whether closure can be immediate or should be delayed until the danger of infection is past.

The key to deciding when a wound should be closed is an understanding of the difference between contamination and infection; the trick to determining when one has become the other is the ability to recognize and interpret signs of inflammation. A contaminated wound can be converted by skillfully performed surgery into a clean wound that can then be closed safely; an infected wound cannot be surgically debrided without high risk of failure, including the potentially lethal complications of interfering with natural localizing processes. The history and physical examination contribute valuable information, because the length of time needed for contamination to become infection reflects, among other things, the strength of the bacterial inoculum and the ability of the substrate to combat invasion. A clean razor slice of highly vascular skin of the face might be closed safely 48 h after injury, whereas a stable-floor-nail penetration of the foot of an elderly person might not be closed safely 1 min after injury. Laboratory data also are helpful, particularly when considering the time to close a secondary healing wound. Quantitative measurements of the number of bacteria in tissue samples have shown that concentrations greater than 10^5 organisms per gram of tissue are likely to cause abscess and wound breakdown following second-

ary closure. If the concentration of bacteria in tissue is significantly less than 10^5 organisms per gram of tissue, the chances of successful wound closure are much improved. Because contaminated wounds have bacteria only on the surface and ideally the surface will be mechanically or hydrodynamically cleansed, quantitative bacteriology is reserved primarily for diagnosis of granulating previously infected wounds.

Once the decision has been made to close a laceration, the surrounding skin should be prepared with suitable antiseptic and local anesthetic injected. A guide to application of antiseptic is never to put anything in a wound that could not be tolerated comfortably in the conjunctival sac. Any caustic solution that is capable of sterilizing the surface of the skin will also destroy delicate cells on the surface of the wound. Therefore, harsh antiseptics should be applied only to the edge of a wound, never within it. Recent popular use of povidone iodine solution to irrigate or soak wound tissues may offer some advantages over saline irrigation, but data presently are not convincing. Moreover, absorption following prolonged use in large wounds such as burns or in wounds containing serous membranes such as peritoneum or pleura has caused significant complications. Debridement of a wound can be done either hydrodynamically or mechanically. When the wound contains only surface contaminants not attached to wound tissues, a copious stream of saline will flush foreign bodies and undesirable organisms out of the wound cavity. When devitalized or contused tissue fragments are still attached to the wound tissues and external contaminants are partially driven into the tissues, however, surgical excision of affected tissues must be performed. When there is a redundancy of tissue and there are no important structures in the depth of the wound, such as nerve or tendon, the best type of debridement is excision of the entire wound to produce a new wound that is surgically clean. When there is a shortage of tissue or when a wound involves important structures that cannot be sacrificed without producing disability, damaged tissue must be carefully dissected until all dead tissue and extraneous material have been removed. In a wound of the hand involving numerous tendons and nerves, this type of debridement may be tedious and require several hours to perform.

After the wound has been debrided, proper suture materials must be selected for closure. There are two major types of sutures, absorbable and nonabsorbable, and selection of the proper suture should be based on what has been learned about the biology of the healing process. For the most part, absorbable sutures, which are made of sheep intestines or synthetic polymers, are used when infection is known to be present or when debridement has been difficult and thoroughness is in doubt.

Plain gut sutures will be solubilized by tissue collagenase in less than 10 days, while gut that has been tanned lightly with chromium salts will remain structurally intact for approximately 3 weeks. Gut sutures are usually not used when they can be avoided because the reaction to a foreign animal protein is considerably greater than the reaction to such substances as cotton, silk, and nylon.

Synthetic absorbable sutures are not as locally irritating as animal proteins but because the collagen-synthesis stage of wound healing is barely under way at 10 days and scar tissue is far from mature even at 3 weeks, a more permanent material may be needed.

Nonabsorbable sutures are usually preferable because they produce less tissue reaction and can remain permanently below the surface of the integument. The major disadvantage of permanent sutures is that if they are placed in areas where infection develops, the suture material can harbor organisms; hence infection will not subside until the sutures are removed. A nonabsorbable suture of steel or some alloy may be mechanically irritating, and sometimes an inflammatory reaction develops around nonabsorbable sutures that resembles a local allergic phenomenon. Sutures are placed in different types of tissue for different reasons; before a suture is selected and placed in a wound, the questions should be asked: What is the suture required to do? and How long does it need to do it? Sutures that are placed in tissues to hold wound edges together under tension should be placed in fibrous tissue. Sutures placed in cellular tissues such as fat, epidermis, liver, or kidney provide little structural strength, as they tend to cut through tissues, having no appreciable strength. Sutures in weak tissues usually are used to obliterate a potential cavity (dead space), provide hemostasis, or act as a fine-adjustment leveling device on the surface of the skin. Objectives for such sutures are met in a few hours; thus absorbable sutures can be used satisfactorily if they are desirable.

A typical facial wound involving skin, subcutaneous fat, fascia, and superficial muscle might be repaired in the following way: After local anesthesia has been administered, the skin prepared, contaminants flushed out with saline solution, and any dead fragments of tissue excised, closure is performed. The muscle, being primarily cellular, does not hold sutures well. Muscle is closed primarily to stop hemorrhage and to obliterate dead space. A synthetic absorbable suture is satisfactory for these purposes. Fibrous tissue surrounding muscle has significant strength, however, and should be closed with a permanent suture of silk or some synthetic substance. If the skin is closed in a single layer, the retracted subcutaneous fat might not come together completely, thus producing a cavity that would become filled with blood and possibly infected. A loosely tied suture in subcutaneous fat, although it contributes almost nothing to tensile strength because it does not pass through fibrous tissue, may be utilized to obliterate a subcutaneous cavity and discourage hemorrhage. After the subcutaneous tissue has been closed, a decision should be made about the desired final appearane of the surface scar. The width of the wound following closure of the subcutaneous tissue will be an accurate indicator of how wide the final cutaneous scar will be if the next sutures merely approximate skin edges and are tied on the outside. The reason is that, if suture marks are to be avoided, skin sutures should be removed in 6 to 8 days because of development of inflammatory reaction, epithelial lined tracts, or small stitch abscesses. Although the wound edges may be accurately coapted

with only a hairline scar at the time that cutaneous sutures are removed, the wound is held together only by epithelium, blood vessels, and globular protein. Even though it usually will not dehisce before collagen production takes over, the scar will stretch and widen during the ensuing 21 days while collagen formation and remodeling occur. The result usually is that a 7-day-old 1-mm-wide scar may become a 1-cm-wide scar 3 weeks after the sutures have been removed. One way to reduce widening of a scar after skin sutures are removed is to place permanent sutures in the fibrous protein layers of the skin to bring the edges together. This is accomplished by a subcuticular or intradermal suture of fine silk or synthetic material. The overlying epidermis is gently retracted, and sutures are placed in the lower part of the dermis. The knot is sometimes placed deep in subcutaneous tissue but can be tied superficially provided that the ends of the suture are cut close and the knot and suture ends are covered by overlying epithelium. It is important to use a very fine suture that will not be palpable beneath the epithelium and a clear or light-colored suture material that will not show through translucent epithelium. It has been shown recently that permanent subcuticular sutures will not eliminate completely secondary widening of a scar; such sutures will reduce the extent of transverse remodeling in many wounds, however.

After subcuticular sutures have been placed, the skin edges will be as close together as it is possible to bring them; yet the overlying epithelial edges may be vertically uneven. A final row of sutures of fine silk or synthetic material that serve as a fine adjustment or leveler of the epithelial edges is frequently utilized to produce an even surface. Because these sutures are in cellular tissue, they contribute little to the strength of the wound and should not be placed more than 1 mm from the wound edge. They should be tied loosely and removed before any epithelial reaction develops. Actually, external sutures in a wound closed in this manner probably can be removed in a few hours or as soon as the plasma clot seals the epithelial edges. For practical purposes, however, they are not removed until the first dressing, whenever that may be. In recent years the use of external cutaneous sutures has been partially eliminated by the development of various types of adhesive strips that can be used to hold skin edges together without producing epithelial sinuses or reaction.

When should sutures be removed? is a question frequently asked of surgeons. The answer is simple: when they have done the job they were put in to do, namely, hold the wound edges together until adequate tensile strength has developed. To set a finite period of time for removal of sutures is to imply that wounds heal at a standard rate; but the rate of healing is variable even in different parts of the body and under different conditions in a single individual. Instead of counting days until sutures can be removed, the wound must be examined; sometimes one or two sutures must be removed to see if the skin edges are sufficiently adherent to permit removal of all sutures. In wounds where a narrow scar is important and where some tension is unavoidable, it is advisable to splint the immature scar with adhesive strips for 2 or 3 weeks or until new collagen has attained sufficient strength and reliability.

The appearance of a linear scar frequently is worse between the third and fifth weeks after wound closure than it is at the time sutures are removed. The irregular, raised, purplish appearance of immature scar tissue can be a cause of great concern to young patients. Resorption of excess collagen, development of pliability, and the fading of undesirable color are called *maturation* of the scar, and maturation occurs more rapidly in older people than in the young. Children and teen-age patients, particularly, may have a distressing amount of red color in scars for several years. This condition is temporary, however, and redness should not be an indication for secondary surgical revision.

Scars should be revised secondarily only after they have undergone maximum maturation. Beefy, red, hypertrophic, immature scars usually recur after excision, and it is often amazing how much natural improvement will occur if sufficient time is allowed. It is seldom wise to attempt surgical improvement of a scar in less than 6 months; often natural improvement will continue for as long as 12 months.

Secondary revision should not be performed with the idea of changing the color of a scar or with the idea that a scar can be eliminated completely. All that secondary revision can accomplish is to take out a scar that resulted from unskilled closure or closure under unsatisfactory conditions and to close the defect as skillfully as possible under optimal conditions. Leveling uneven edges, changing the direction so that the scar does not cross lines of changing dimensions, and supporting a wide scar by the use of meticulously placed subcuticular sutures are the main improvements that can be accomplished. If scar tissue is elevated slightly above the level of surrounding skin, abrasion of that area with sandpaper or rotating brush will produce a smooth denuded surface over which new epithelium will spread in a more even plane.

Wounds characterized by a loss of skin can be allowed to heal by contraction and epithelization if there is sufficient skin to be stretched across the defect. This is usually permitted only when infection prevents primary closure and when contraction does not produce a contracture that would interfere with function or produce a cosmetically unacceptable scar. In all other wounds, a skin graft should be performed to replace the skin that has been lost.

At the moment, there is no known catalyst to accelerate normal wound healing; about all that a physician can do to aid normal healing is to protect the wound from physical, chemical, or bacteriologic complications that retard or prevent healing. Abnormal healing sometimes can be corrected as in the utilization of topical vitamin A to correct inhibition of epithelization caused by cortisone therapy. Vitamin A does not accelerate epithelization over normal expectation; it only corrects inhibition of epithelization caused by a specific drug effect. Platelet-derived growth factor, activated wound macrophages, *Staphylococcus aureus* bacterial strains, epidermal

growth factor, and cartilage-derived growth factor are some of the biological substances that presently are being evaluated as wound-healing stimulants because of theoretical considerations or the early results of animal experiments. Protection usually means the use of an artificial dressing unless a natural dressing material, such as an eschar or scab, can serve the same purpose. Once the scab or eschar deteriorates, however, it, like any other dressing material, must be changed (debrided), and either definitive coverage provided or an artificial dressing applied. As in the selection of suture materials, choosing dressing materials involves a clear understanding of the objectives of each component of the dressing and the fundamental biologic processes that the dressing is supposed to protect. The first layer of a dressing is usually made of fine-mesh gauze, so that granulation tissue will not penetrate the interstices and cause hemorrhage when the dressing is removed. A long search for a pharmacologic substance to incorporate in the gauze to stimulate epithelial growth has been unsuccessful so far. Because certain by-products of the azo dye industry are carcinogenic, it was hoped that related dyes such as scarlet red might offer epithelial stimulation without being carcinogenic. All such substances have been disappointing, however, although most surgeons do use a gauze impregnated with some bland substance such as petroleum jelly or topical antibiotic in a water-soluble base. The main value of such medicated dressings is that there is less adherence of epithelium and vascular tissue to the dressing, hence less interference with wound healing when the dressing is changed. Dry gauze is a perfectly satisfactory dressing for most wound surfaces, however, and when carefully applied and removed, it can be as atraumatic as any other material. The usual coarse 4×4 hospital gauze sponge with cotton-filled center is not a good material to place against open wounds; the interstices permit permeation by vascular tissue, and the cotton lint that is included becomes embedded in the wound. Sponges, mechanics' waste, cotton, and the like are used to give bulk to a dressing after the fine-mesh gauze has been applied to make the dressing conform to a desired shape and immobilize the wounded part. Nonstretchable, firm, roller gauze bandage and adhesive tape are used to complete the dressing in a typical occlusive (erroneously called "pressure") dressing. The nonstretchable gauze and adhesive tape provide a compact and stable immobilizing influence. A clean wound has very little drainage and no odor, and does not have to be dressed very often.

Infected wounds have considerable drainage and odor and, therefore, must be dressed often to provide suitable drainage and tolerable appearance. It is common practice to use a wet dressing on infected wounds, which means that the inside layers of the dressing are intentionally moistened with saline solution or some other substance. The realization that there is no catalytic effect upon healing or any control of infection from water and that maceration of skin or eschar produces favorable conditions for bacterial or fungus growth throws doubt upon the beneficial effects to be obtained by applying a wet dressing. The usual answer is that drainage is increased by capillary action or that debridement is accomplished as detritus sticks to the dressing. Such reasoning has never seemed logical to the author; a dry dressing will absorb more wound drainage than a wet one, and debridement can usually be accomplished more efficiently by surgical means. It often appears that wounds become clean more quickly with the use of wet dressings, but in the author's experience this is partly because wet dressings are changed more often. Of course, less pain may be associated with wet-dressing changes than with dry-dressing changes. However, when dry dressings are changed frequently and skillfully, surface detritus may be removed more effectively by dry dressings than by wet ones. One sound reason for using a wet dressing, however, is that wet heat is more penetrating than dry heat, and when additional warmth is desirable to increase the local inflammatory response, a warm moist dressing is effective. Failure to keep a moist dressing warm by the addition of external heat, however, results in a cold soggy dressing that has no particular virtue and is definitely inferior to a frequently changed dry one. The objective is to keep wound secretions from accumulating and retarding repair by enzyme activity. Fibrinolysins, particularly, inhibit healing.

SKIN GRAFTS

Skin grafts are classified as free grafts (meaning that they are separated completely from their donor sites before being transferred to recipient areas) and pedicle grafts (which maintain a vascular connection with the general circulation). Free grafts are full-thickness (which means that the entire thickness of the skin, including epidermis and dermis, is transferred) and split-thickness (which means that the entire epidermis and only a portion of the dermis are transferred). The remainder of the dermis after split-thickness skin grafting remains at the donor site.

The "take" of a free graft refers to a pink appearance that occurs between the third and fifth days after transfer, signifying that vascular connections have developed between the recipient bed and the transplant. Before this time, free grafts are white (unless microvascular surgery has provided instantaneous restoration of circulation) and do not show any change in color when pressed upon and released. It is a matter of considerable conjecture whether there is diffusion of gases and nutrients between cells of the graft and underlying capillaries prior to development of actual vascular connections, and it has been assumed in the past that diffusion was necessary to keep cells nourished during the first few days. When grafts that include more than full thickness of the skin do not survive as free transplants, or when split-thickness grafts with pus or blood interposed between graft and capillary bed do not survive, it has been considered that diffusion could not occur through fat, pus, blood, etc. It seems more likely now, however, that diffusion is not important in the take of a graft and that mechanical barriers such as pus, blood, or fat prevent the take of a free graft by preventing

vascular connections from developing. Whatever the reason, the thicker the graft, the more likely will be the failure of take if mechanical or inflammatory conditions at the graft-wound interface are less than optimal. For this reason, thin grafts are used to cover less than ideally prepared wounds; full-thickness grafts are reserved for surgically produced wounds under optimal conditions.

In taking a full-thickness skin graft the surgeon produces a wound that will have to be closed by suturing the edges together or by applying a split-thickness skin graft from another donor site. If this is not done, closing a wound in one area with a graft will leave a wound of the same size and shape at the donor site. Full-thickness grafts are usually small grafts that can be taken from a place where there is an excess of thin skin, such as the inframammary fold or the groin, where the donor site can be closed by suturing the skin edges together.

It was once thought that split-thickness skin grafts must be taken through the level of the dermal-epidermal undulating interface so that small islands of stratum germinativum cells would remain to reepithelialize the denuded surface. Because of this notion, surgeons were careful to take grafts as thin as possible, and the taking of a split-thickness skin graft was relegated to only a few highly skilled individuals (Fig. 8-7). It seems obvious now that if it were possible to take a graft through only the epithelium, a satisfactory take would be unlikely. Most of the cells would be dead, and the covered wound would be resurfaced by cells that would provide no better coverage than that which would have occurred from normal epithelization. The qualities of skin other than waterproofing (strength, flexibility, appearance, etc.) that are desired in a graft are qualities provided by dermis. The final appearance of both recipient and donor sites, therefore, reflects the amount of dermis that has been transferred and the amount of dermis that is left behind. Epithelial cells migrate out of deep glands and hair follicles, and donor sites

Fig. 8-7. Removal of thick split-thickness skin graft with a freehand knife. The largest possible grafts can be taken by this method. Most grafts are taken with a dermatome.

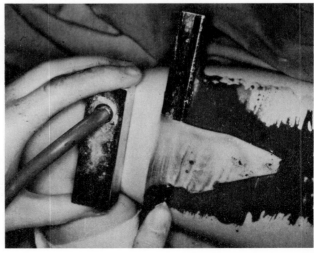

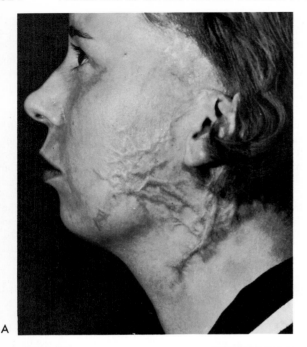

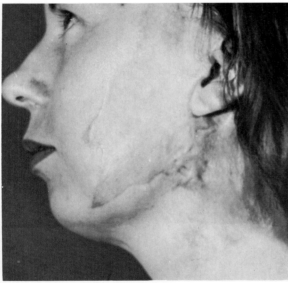

Fig. 8-8. *A.* Hypertrophic scar produced by deep second-degree burn. Although a significant amount of full-thickness skin has not been lost, overproduction of collagen has produced an unsightly scar. *B.* Patient shown in Fig. 8-8*A* following excision of facial portion of scar and application of a thick split-thickness skin graft. Cervical portion of scar resurfaced later. A single graft covering facial and cervical areas would obliterate submandibular groove. Note that scar at junction of graft and skin is most prominent near angle of mouth where motion and tension are unavoidable. Although different in texture, hue, and thickness from normal skin, the graft provides a smooth surface over which cosmetics can be applied more effectively than over previous scar.

that do not extend through the entire depth of the dermis will be reepithelialized from these sources. Dermis, being a complex organ and not a simple tissue, does not regenerate, however, and if all the properties of normal dermis are desired in the recipient area, full-thickness dermis must be transferred; if less than the full thickness is transferred, the resulting graft will be abnormal in appearance and function.

In choosing the thickness of a free skin graft, qualities that are desired in the recipient area must be balanced against cost incurred in the donor site. How such factors influence selection of graft thickness can be illustrated by comparing two extremes in wound and donor-site conditions. In a large thermal burn, the recipient area is not optimal in that usually it is infected, edematous, and involves a large area. The take of a graft therefore is uncertain, and revascularization is problematic. From the standpoint of the donor site, it may be necessary to procure several grafts from the same area to obtain enough skin for the entire wound; thus rapid healing, with remaining dermis thick enough for subsequent grafts to be taken, is mandatory. In this case, both donor-site and recipient conditions require thin grafts. In contrast, a 2-cm-diameter wound caused by loss of skin from the cheek of a young person presents an entirely different set of requirements for an optimal graft. The recipient bed should be optimal if excised immediately; the need for full-thickness dermis is mandatory so that normal texture, color, and thickness will produce the most cosmetically acceptable result. The graft usually is small, and so a variety of areas with a 2-cm redundancy of skin can be found for a donor site. Thus all factors point to the selection of a full-thickness graft. In other wounds the choice may not be quite so clear, but the principles involved in these two cases are the factors that must be considered in selection of any free graft (Fig. 8-8*A* and *B*).

Split-thickness skin grafts have a tendency to develop deep pigmentation after transfer. It is important to warn patients who recently have had split-thickness skin grafts placed on exposed areas of the body that protection from solar radiation is advisable for at least 6 months. Thick grafts have less tendency to develop undesirable pigment, and usually will blend into new surroundings more quickly than thin ones.

Finally, a word should be said about the concept of a "dressing graft." Split-thickness skin is the best possible dressing material for an open wound, and failure of surgeons to take advantage of this fact usually is based on the mistaken notion that placing a split-thickness skin graft on a wound is tantamount to closing the wound. Although the possibility that some portion or all of the graft may take and thus close the wound is the main advantage in using split-thickness skin grafts as a dressing material, placing the graft on a wound of questionable suitability for closure does not in itself produce a closed wound in the same manner as suturing two full-thickness skin edges together. Actually, a skin dressing does not close the wound any more than a petroleum jelly gauze dressing. If the wound has been inadequately debrided or infection is not yet controlled, the graft will slough in a few days and may disappear by the time of the first dressing. In such instances nothing will have been lost except a few square centimeters of split-thickness skin from the donor area. Dressing a questionable wound of relatively small size with split-thickness skin, therefore, is a sort of biologic test to determine suitability for closure, as well as providing some benefit if even a part of the graft survives. Xenografts of porcine skin, human allografts of split-thickness skin, and human amnion also are used as biologic dressings to test the suitability of the wound for definitive closure and to prevent metabolic and infectious complications of large wounds remaining open for protracted periods. Such grafts should be removed before take occurs and often are changed several times before optimum conditions for autograft application are obtained. In the judgment of the author, a porcine xenograft is a poor choice for a biologic dressing. Availability through a commercial source makes it easy for a surgeon to obtain porcine grafts, but expense and theoretical considerations of crossing major histocompatibility loci augur strongly for using human skin obtained from autopsy specimens or amnion obtained from the delivery room instead.

When more than the skin has been lost, and the skin plus some other tissue such as fat, tendon, muscle, or nerve must be replaced to restore function and appearance, transfer of skin by pedicle flap or direct vascular anastomosis is required (Fig. 8-9). As the name implies, pedicle transfers maintain vascular connection with the host, so that interruption of the capillary circulation never occurs. The vessels that are most important during transfer of tissue are the vessels in the subdermal plexus. These vessels are relatively large, frequently longitudinally oriented, and are located on the undersurface of the dermis superficial to subcutaneous fat. One frequently hears that a pedicle flap has been made thicker than actually needed for cosmetic or functional purposes in order to provide a safe blood supply. Fat on the undersurface of a flap does not add any appreciable blood supply, and it may be removed safely to produce as thin a pedicle as needed, provided the important vessels lying on the undersurface of the dermis are not injured. The problem in transplanting tissue by the pedicle method is to design a pedicle so that the base is as narrow as possible in relation to the length needed to cover the deficient area. It becomes a matter of considerable judgment, therefore, to gauge the shape and dimensions of a flap so that blood supply through the intact pedicle will be adequate to nourish the distal end of the flap. A great deal depends upon the natural profuseness of vascular beds; thus it is possible to move a pedicle flap on the face or cervical region that is three times as long as it is wide, while it may not be possible (without performing preliminary procedures to increase the blood supply) to transfer a flap on the leg that is no longer than it is wide. The blood supply in the base of a contemplated flap can be improved by performing a procedure commonly referred to as delay of the flap. The principle of delay is to reduce blood supply gradually to small segments of the circumference of the flap and thus improve the remaining blood supply to the point where a pedicle that was of insufficient width before

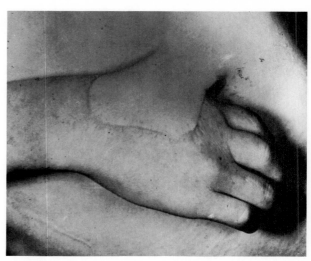

Fig. 8-9. Abdominal pedicle flap applied to dorsum of hand. Scar on hand has been turned back to resurface the raw side of pedicle and a portion of the donor site. Flap will be separated from the abdominal wall in 18 days.

the flap was delayed becomes adequate to nourish the flap. The mechanism by which delay (gradual interruption of a portion of the blood supply to a flap) improves circulation in the base is not completely clear. It seems doubtful that new blood vessels actually grow into the area, although casual observation of changes in the vessels at the base suggests that this is what may happen. The rapidity with which delay improves the circulation strongly suggests, however, that the release of various amines, probably in response to changes in pH secondary to increased anaerobic metabolism, causes a closure of normally open shunts that prevent perfusion of the entire capillary network. The effect is a substantial hyperemia at the base of the flap; over a period of several weeks and after several delaying procedures, the vessels in the pedicle base become racemose in appearance, and the amount of blood flow is increased to the extent that a relatively long flap can be transferred on a narrow pedicle. Following transfer of a flap, circulation must be observed carefully for the first 48 h, as signs of impending circulatory embarrassment occur before irreversible thrombosis and cell death. It is not unusual for the distal end of a flap to be dusky following transfer; venous spasm secondary to the trauma of rotation may be all that is involved. Improvement usually occurs in a few hours, but during this time the danger of venous thrombosis is increased; if there is progression of cyanosis and edema, the possibility that tension on veins is interfering with return circulation must be investigated by removing a few sutures. Perhaps the most serious, but still reversible, sign of impending venous thrombosis is development of a sharp line of color differentiation. A gradual change from normal pink to slight cyanosis is not so significant as a clearcut line demarcating the area of circulatory deficiency. Even if all sutures have to be removed and the flap returned to its original bed, the sign must be attended to, or

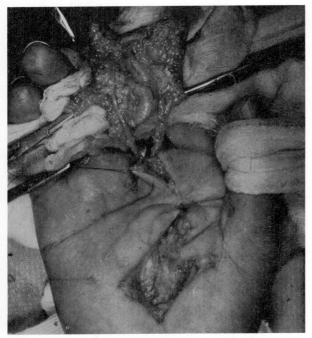

Fig. 8-10. Island pedicle flap developed during amputation of long finger. The flap is nourished by a single digital artery and nerve. Sensation is preserved by including a digital nerve in the vascular pedicle.

an irreversible demarcation will soon develop, signifying complete thrombosis and certain distal necrosis. In sensibly planned and adequately prepared flaps, one does not have to be particularly concerned about arterial insufficiency; venous drainage is the function that develops complications. Complications usually are the result of too much tension, poor dressing, hematoma, or infection.

The use of heparin and low-molecular-weight dextran has seemed to be beneficial in dangerously compromised circulation. Recently smoking has been shown to affect adversely circulation in face flaps. Hyperbaric oxygenation has been reported instrumental in saving flaps of laboratory animals, but is not practical for managing human flaps.

Advancement flaps and rotation flaps are the simplest pedicle transfers. They are dependent upon redundancy of soft tissue adjacent to a defect so that the donor defect can be closed by approximating the skin edges or applying split-thickness skin grafts. More complicated flaps require the use of an arm as a carrier to provide circulation during the period that skin is detached from the original donor site, such as abdominal wall, and transferred to a distant site, such as the lower leg. Because of similarity of tissue characteristics, safety in transfer, and expense and time involved, it is desirable to design flaps as close to the point where they are needed as possible.

One of the most sophisticated rotation flaps is an island pedicle flap (Fig. 8-10), which combines the pedicle principle of intact blood and nerve supply with some of the advantages of a free graft. The principle of the island pedicle is that careful dissection of the artery and vein (and sometimes the nerve) to a piece of skin can be performed so that the skin is detached from surrounding skin and remains attached to the body only by essentials for survival—an artery, a vein, and sometimes a nerve. Depending on the length of these structures, it is possible to move a full-thickness skin and fat graft, or an intact finger, or a portion of a finger or toe, a long distance. Transfer of hair-bearing portions of the scalp on a temporal artery-and-vein supported flap to the supraorbital region for eyebrow reconstruction and transfer of a finger to replace a missing thumb are examples of island pedicle transfers.

Fig. 8-11. Elevation of tensor fascia lata fascia, muscle, and overlying skin without delay.

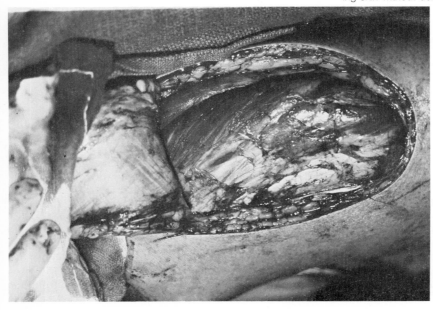

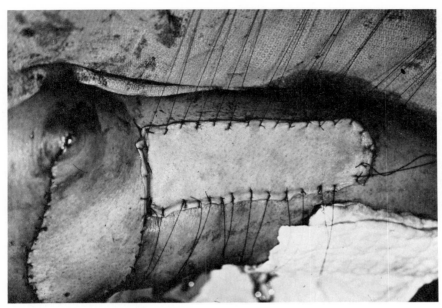

Fig. 8-12. Rotation of tensor fascia lata myocutaneous flap to cover debrided trochanteric decubitus ulcer.

The need to perform time-consuming and costly delay procedures has been reduced significantly by the development of myocutaneous and free microvascular transfer flaps. Discovery that muscle under skin supplies blood vessels sufficient to nourish skin is the basis for composite flaps, called myocutaneous, that transfer intact muscle, subcutaneous tissue, and overlying skin as a single unit rotated on the relatively narrow vascular supply of the muscle. Pectoralis major, latissimus dorsi, gracilis, and tensor fascia lata myocutaneous flaps are used fre-

quently to transfer skin and subcutaneous tissue without delay procedures. An example of a tensor fascia lata myocutaneous flap rotated 180° to a trochanteric defect on the single artery and vein nourishing the muscle is shown in Figs. 8-11 and 8-12. Perhaps the most elegant such transfer is a free flap in which muscle, muscle and skin, or skin alone is transferred to a distant site. After transfer, the blood vessels are sutured by microvascular technique to vessels in the recipient area, thus reestablishing active circulation. Latissimus dorsi, gracilis,

Fig. 8-13. Outline of latissimus dorsi muscle and skin flap.

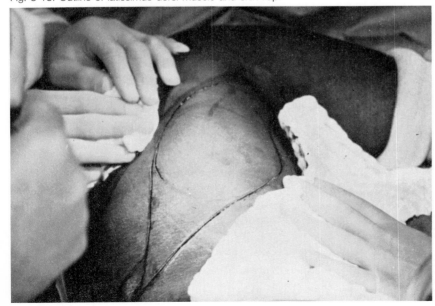

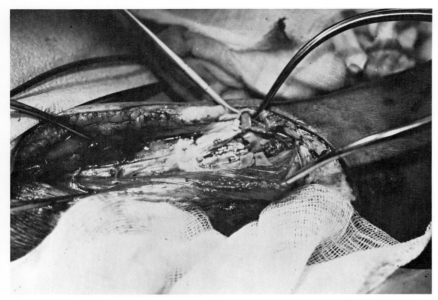

Fig. 8-14. Preparation of anterior tibial artery and veins to receive thoracodorsal vessels of latissimus free flap.

groin, and scapular skin flaps have been very successful in restoring surface defects in the lower leg and foot. Free jejunal and omental grafts have been utilized in the head and neck. Transfer of rib, subcutaneous tissue, and overlying skin by microvascular anastomosis of intercostal vessels to facial vessels has been useful in reconstructing composite defects of the face and lower jaw. An example of free-flap transfer of a latissimus dorsi and overlying back skin flap to the lower leg with anastomosis of the thoracodorsal vessels to the anterior tibial (end-to-side) artery and vein is shown in Figs. 8-13 to 8-15.

Finally, in the opinion of many, maturity in restorative surgery can be measured, in part, by how often one thinks

Fig. 8-15. Latissimus free flap on leg following microvascular anastomosis of thoracodorsal vessels to anterior tibial artery and vein.

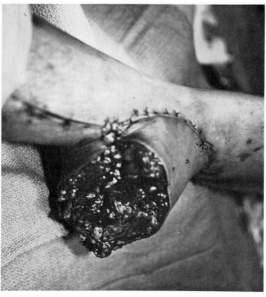

of a pedicle flap as the only means of rebuilding a damaged area and then devises a way to make a free graft suffice. Pedicles are dramatic, particularly as used by military surgeons to rebuild enormous tissue defects caused by high-explosive wounds; fortunately, however, civilian injuries are not often so devastating, and the practical points of expense, length of time away from work, utilization of hospital facilities, and the like have to be considered in each case where a pedicle could be used. In addition, although areas such as the face may appear in photographs to have been superbly restored by massive flaps, yet it must be remembered that flaps have no dynamic function; they are expressionless, and often look better in photographs than they do as part of the constantly moving facial features. A recent development that has reduced the need for distant pedicle flaps is local tissue expansion with an implanted inflatable device. Gradual stretching of skin for 4 to 6 weeks can be accomplished with such a device so that local rotation advancement flaps become possible in areas where local skin was not sufficient to resurface the defect before expansion. When a pedicle flap is needed, nothing else will suffice, and pedicles are an extremely valuable part of restorative surgery. The high cost of donor-site mutilation, length of time required for transfer, and adynamic features, however, make the pedicle flap definitely second choice to a free graft if a free graft can be used.

Bibliography

Wound Contraction

Abercrombie M, James DW, Newcombe JF: Wound contraction in rabbit skin, studied by splinting the wound margins. *J Anat* 94:170, 1960.

Ariyan S, Enriquez R, Krizek T: Wound contraction and fibrocontractive disorders. *Arch Surg* 113:1034, 1978.

Danes B, Leinfelder PJ: Cytological and respiratory effects of cyanide on tissue cultures. *J Cell Comp Physiol* 37:427, 1951.

Ehrlich HP, Grislis G, Hunt TK: Evidence for the involvement of microtubules in wound contraction. *Ann Surg* 133:706, 1977.

Grillo HC, Gross J: Studies in wound healing. III. Contraction in vitamin C deficiency. *Proc Soc Exp Biol Med* 101:268, 1959.

Grillo HC, Watts GT, Gross J: Studies in wound healing. I. Contraction and wound contents. *Ann Surg* 148:145, 1958.

Madden JW, Carlson EE, Hines J: Presence of modified fibroblasts in ischemic contracture of the intrinsic musculature of the hand. *Surg Gynecol Obstet* 140:509, 1975.

Madden JW, Morton D Jr, Peacock EE Jr: Contraction of experimental wounds. I. Inhibiting wound contraction by using a topical smooth muscle antagonist. *Surgery* 76:18, 1974.

Majno G, Babbiani G, et al: Contraction of granulation tissue *in vitro:* Similarity with smooth muscle. *Science* 173:548, 1971.

Phillips JL, Peacock EE: Importance of horizontal plane cell mass integrity in wound contraction. *Proc Soc Exp Biol Med* 117:539, 1964.

Rudolph R: Contraction and the control of contraction. *World J Surg* 4:288, 1980.

Rudolph R, Guber S, Woodward M: Inhibition of myofibroblasts by skin grafts. *Plast Reconstr Surg* 63:173, 1979.

Ryan GB, Cliff WJ, et al: Myofibroblasts in human granulation tissue. *Hum Pathol* 5:55, 1974.

Watts GT, Grillo HC, Gross J: Studies in wound healing. II. The role of granulation tissue in contraction. *Ann Surg* 148:153, 1958.

Epithelization

Alexander SA: Patterns of epidermal cell polarity in healing open wounds. *J Surg Res* 31:456, 1981.

Alexander SA, Gonoff RB: The glycosaminoglycans of open wounds. *J Surg Res* 29:499, 1980.

Alvarez OM, Mertz PM, Eaglstein WH: The effect of occlusive dressings on collagen synthesis and re-epithelialization in superficial wounds. *J Surg Res* 35:142, 1983.

Argyris TS: The regulation of epidermal hyperplastic growth, CRC critical review. *Toxicology* 9:151, 1981.

Franklin JD, Lynch JB: Effects of topical applications of epidermal growth factor on wound healing. *Plast Reconstr Surg* 64:766, 1979.

Gillman T, Penn J: Studies on the repair of cutaneous wounds. *Med Proc* 2(suppl 3): 121, 1956.

Laato M, Niinikoski J, et al: Stimulation of wound healing by epidermal growth factor. *Ann Surg* 203:379, 1986.

Sullivan DJ, Epstein WS: Mitotic activity of wounded human epidermis. *J Invest Dermatol* 41:39, 1963.

Collagen

Baur PS, Parks DH: The myofibroblast anchoring strand—the fibronectin connection in wound healing and the possible loci of collagen fibril assembly. *J Trauma* 23:853, 1983.

Bornstein P: Disorders of connective tissue function and the aging process: a synthesis and review of current concepts and findings. *Mech Ageing Dev* 5:305, 1976.

Cohen IK, Keiser HR, Sjoerdsma A: Collagen synthesis in human keloid and hypertrophic scar. *Surg Forum* 22:488, 1971.

Dayer J, Russell RG, Krane SM: Collagenase production by rheumatoid synovial cells: stimulation by a human lymphocyte factor. *Science* 195:181, 1977.

Diegelmann RF, Cohen IK, Kaplan AM: The role of macrophages in wound repair: a review. *Plast Reconstr Surg* 68:107, 1981.

Duskin D, Bornstein P: Impaired conversion of procollagen to collagen by fibroblasts and bone treated with tunicamycin, an inhibitor of protein glycosylation. *J Biol Chem* 252:955, 1977.

Ellis H: Internal overhealing: The problem of intraperitoneal adhesions. *World J Surg* 4:303, 1980.

Ellis H, Lapiere CM: Collagenolytic activity in amphibian tissues: A tissue culture assay. *Proc Natl Acad Sci USA* 48:1014, 1962.

Fleischmajer R, Olsen BR, Kühn K (eds): Biology, chemistry, and pathology of collagen. *Ann NY Acad Sci* 460, 1985.

Hoffmann H, Olsen B, et al: Segment-long-spacing aggregates and isolation of COOH-terminal peptides from type I procollagen. *Proc Natl Acad Sci USA* 73:4304, 1976.

Madden JW: Some aspects of fibrogenesis during the healing of primary and secondary wounds. *Surg Gynecol Obstet* 115:408, 1962.

Miller ES: Biochemical characteristics and biological significance of the genetically-distinct collagens. *Mol Cell Biochem* 13:165, 1976.

Olsen B, Hoffmann H, Prockop DJ: Interchain disulfide bonds at the COOH-terminal end of procollagen synthesized by matrix-free cells from chick embryonic tendon and cartilage. *Arch Biochem Biophys* 175:341, 1976.

Peacock EE Jr: Collagenolysis: The other side of the equation. *World J Surg* 4:297, 1980.

Prockop DJ, Kivirikko KI, et al: The biosynthesis of collagen and its disorders. *N Engl J Med* (3001):13, 1979.

Raju DR, Jindrak K, et al: A study of the critical bacterial inoculum to cause a stimulus to wound healing. *Surg Gynecol Obstet* 144:347, 1977.

Riley WB Jr, Peacock EE Jr.: Identification, distribution, and significance of a collagenolytic enzyme in human tissue. *Proc Soc Biol Med* 214:207, 1967.

Wound Care

Ariyan S, Cuono CB: Use of the pectoralis major myocutaneous flap for reconstruction of large cervical, facial or cranial defects. *Am J Surg* 140:503, 1980.

Bucknall TE, Ellis H: *Wound Healing for Surgeons.* Philadelphia, WB Saunders, 1984.

Cutting CB, Bardach J, Finseth F: Hemodynamics of the delayed skin flap: A total blood flow study. *Br J Plast Surg.* 34:133, 1981.

Faulk WP, Stevens PJ, et al: Human amnion as an adjunct in wound healing. *Lancet* 1(8179): 1156, May 31, 1980.

Harii K: Myocutaneous flaps—clinical applications and refinements. *Ann Plast Surg* 40:440, 1980.

Hunt TK, Dunphy JE: *Fundamentals of Wound Management.* New York, Appleton-Century-Crofts, 1979.

Leighton WD, Johnson ML, Friedland JA: Use of the temporary soft tissue expander in post traumatic alopecia. *Plast Reconstr Surg* 77:737, 1986.

McGregor JC, Buchan AC: Clinical experience with the tensor fasciae latae myocutaneous flap. *Br J Surg* 33:270, 1980.

Mulliken JB, Healey NA: Pathogenesis of skin flap necrosis from an underlying hematoma. *Plast Reconstr Surg* 64:540, 1979.

Olivari N: Use of thirty latissimus dorsi flaps. *Plast Reconstr Surg* 64:654, 1979.

Peacock EE Jr: *Wound Repair,* 3d ed. Philadelphia, Saunders, 1984.

Peacock EE Jr: Wound healing, in *The Scientific Management of Surgical Patients*. Boston, Little, Brown, 1983, chap 2.

Serafin D, Riefohl R, et al: Vascularized rib-periosteal and osteocutaneous reconstruction of the maxilla and mandible: An assessment. *Plast Reconstr Surg* 66:718, 1980.

Sindelar WF, Mason GR: Intraperitoneal irrigation with povidone-iodine solution for the prevention of intraabdominal abscesses in the bacterially contaminated abdomen. *Surg Gynecol Obstet* 148:409, 1979.

Teh BT: Why do skin grafts fail? *Plast Reconstr Surg* 63:323, 1979.

Chapter 9

Oncology

Donald L. Morton, James S. Economou, Charles M. Haskell, and Robert G. Parker

INTRODUCTION

Oncology (from the Greek *onkos,* mass, or tumor, and *logos,* study) is the study of neoplastic diseases. Neoplasms are an altered cell population characterized by an excessive, nonuseful proliferation of cells that have be- come unresponsive to normal control mechanisms and to the organizing influences of adjacent tissues. Malignant neoplasms are composed of cancer cells that exhibit un- controlled proliferation and impair the function of normal organs by local tissue invasion and metastatic spread to distant anatomic sites. Benign neoplasms are composed of normal-appearing cells that do not invade locally or metastasize to other sites.

Cancer has plagued human beings since antiquity, and many of its clinical manifestations were described by Hippocrates (460–375 B.C.). Neoplasms have been identi- fied in all species of animals including the lower verte- brates, such as amphibia and fish. The wide distribution of neoplasia in natural and human history suggests that cancer may be common to all multicellular organisms.

Neoplastic disease is the second most frequent cause of death in the United States. The magnitude of the cancer problem is exemplified by the fact that three of every ten persons living today has or will develop cancer. An esti- mated 73 million Americans, 30 percent of those pres- ently alive, will develop cancer sometime during their lifetime. Approximately 40 percent of those who get cancer will survive for at least 5 years after treatment. Until recently such facts caused many physicians and sur- geons to approach the cancer patient with feelings of pessi- mism and despair that frequently interfered with adequate therapy.

Fortunately, exciting developments in tumor immunol- ogy, viral oncology, and molecular biology and advances in the therapy of some neoplasms led to a rebirth of inter- est in the basic biologic and clinical problems posed by cancer. Specialty boards have been established in medi- cal oncology and gynecologic oncology. A wide variety of scientists from many disciplines have been attracted to cancer research. As a result, more advances have been made in cancer therapy in the past 10 years than in all previous times. This chapter is designed to introduce the student to general principles that can be used as the basis for acquiring further knowledge in this rapidly growing field.

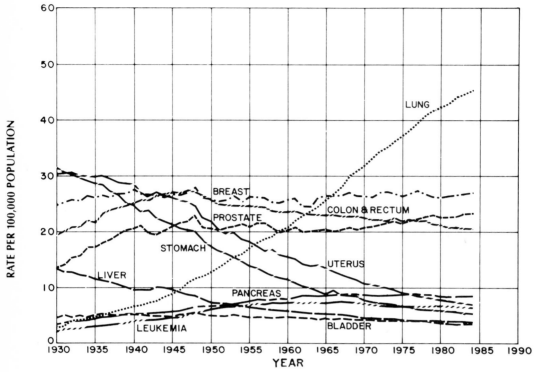

Fig. 9-1. Cancer death rates by site, United States, 1930–1984. (From: *National Vital Statistics Division and Bureau of the Census, United States.*)

EPIDEMIOLOGY

The changes in death rates from cancer by body site for males and females in the United States during the past 45 years are summarized in Fig. 9-1. Although there has been a decrease in mortality from certain neoplasms, the overall cancer death rates continue to show a slow, steady increase.

The mortality rates from lung cancer have increased steadily and probably represent the most dramatic change for any cancer site. There will be about 150,000 new cases of lung cancer in the United States in 1987, and the incidence in black males and females continues to rise. Thirteen percent of all lung cancer patients are alive 5 years after diagnosis. Compared with 40 years ago, the mortality has risen from 18.3 to 67.5 per 100,000 for men and from 4.6 to 16.6 for women. Lung cancer represents the leading cause of cancer death when both sexes are considered.

Pancreatic cancer death rates also have steadily increased through the years. Today, the rates are twice what they were in women and three times that in men when compared with 1930.

There has been a striking reduction during the past 50 years in death rates caused by cancers of the stomach and uterus. The stomach cancer death rate is now less than one-fourth the 1930 rate in men and less than one-fifth the 1930 rate in women, although there has been little improvement in the survival rates of stomach cancer. The reason for this declining incidence is unknown.

Death rates due to uterine cancer are only one-half what they were 40 years ago. In this case, the causes of the reduction are known to be earlier detection and improved treatment for cancer of the uterine cervix and corpus.

The incidence of cancer in different sites and the mortality rate in each sex are compared in Fig. 9-2. The sites most frequently causing death in males, in order of decreasing frequency, are (1) lung, (2) colon and rectum, and (3) prostate. The sites, in order of decreasing frequency in females, are (1) lung, (2) breast, and (3) colon and rectum.

The incidence of various types of neoplasms differs from the death rates for the same neoplasms (Fig. 9-2) because different forms of cancer are not equally lethal. The most significant 5-year survival rates are achieved in patients with cancer of the skin, cervix, uterus, and bladder; the lowest survival occurs in patients with pancreatic cancer. Lung cancer is the leading cause of cancer death even though skin cancer occurs more commonly.

Females tend to have a greater number of 5-year survivals with cancers of any given primary site than males, although the reasons are unknown at this time. The overall 5-year survival for women with cancer is 50 percent,

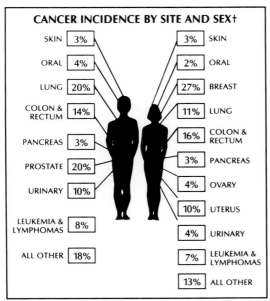

Fig. 9-2. Estimated cancer incidence by site and sex, 1987 estimates. *(American Cancer Society, Cancer Facts and Figures, 1987.)*

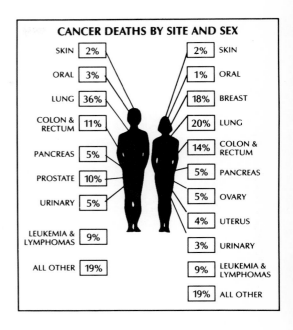

compared with only 31 percent for men. The overall 5-year cancer survival rates for common malignant tumors of selected sites are shown in Fig. 9-3.

ETIOLOGY

While many etiologic agents for cancer have been recognized, some for centuries, the underlying molecular mechanisms have only recently been better understood. A discussion of current thinking about oncogenes and growth factors will be preceded by a review of classical etiologic agents and epidemiological factors.

CHEMICAL CARCINOGENS. The first cause-and-effect relation between a carcinogenic stimulus and the development of cancer in human beings was described by Percival Pott, an English surgeon, in 1775, when he described a cancer of the scrotum frequently occurring in chimney sweeps. Yamagiwa and Ichikawa, working from 1915 to 1918, identified the carcinogen when they experimentally produced cancers by painting the ears of rabbits with coal tar. Kennaway and Cook, in studies from 1924 to 1932, demonstrated that pure hydrocarbons, such as 1,2-dibenzanthracene and similar compounds isolated from coal tar, were carcinogenic agents. Subsequently, a variety of chemical agents have been found that are capable of inducing neoplasms in experimental animals and in human beings. These chemicals are called *carcinogens.* There may be many years separating the time of exposure to a carcinogen and subsequent development of a neoplasm. Consequently, the present-day evaluation of the safety of food additives or other products for human consumption that are chronically ingested over long periods of time is a most difficult task.

A variety of chemicals associated with different types of human neoplasms are shown in Table 9-1. Aromatic amines are known to cause tumors of the urinary tract; workers in the dye industry have a higher incidence of this type of cancer. Benzene has been associated with acute leukemia in shoe repairmen in Italy, solvent manufacturers, painters, and printers who use it as a solvent. Coal tar, pitch, creosote, and anthracene have been associated with cancer of the skin, larynx, and bronchus. A variety of paraffin oils, waxes, and tars are associated with cancer of the skin. Isopropyl oil has been associated with cancer of the sinuses, larynx, and bronchus in workers exposed to it. Mesotheliomas occur very frequently in miners and ship workers who have been exposed to asbestos. Certain metals have been associated with tumors, including chromium, nickel, and arsenic.

PHYSICAL CARCINOGENS. Ionizing radiation was found to be carcinogenic in the 1920s when subcutaneous sarcomas were induced by radium implants in experimental animals. The carcinogenic effects of radiation in human beings were recognized when radium dial painters who commonly licked brushes containing radioactive materials developed bone cancers. Since then, many examples of the carcinogenic effects of radiation have been recognized. Physicians and dentists exposed to multiple x-ray exposures develop recurrent skin cancer. Cancer of the thyroid in adults is frequently associated with neck irradiation in early childhood. The survivors of the atomic bomb detonations show an increased incidence of leukemia. Ultraviolet light on exposed areas may foster the

FIVE YEAR CANCER SURVIVAL RATES* FOR SELECTED SITES

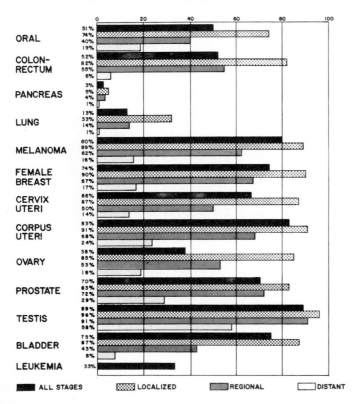

*Adjusted for normal life expectancy
This chart is based on cases diagnosed in 1974-1982

Source: Surveillance and Operations Research Branch,
National Cancer Institute

Fig. 9-3. Five-year cancer survival rates for selected sites. *(American Cancer Society, Cancer Facts and Figures, 1987.)*

development of skin cancer. Farmers and sailors have an increased incidence of skin cancers from excessive exposure to sunlight, as do fair-skinned people living in tropical regions.

Mechanical Irritation. Chronic mechanical irritation may be associated with the development of cancer, although the exact mechanisms are unknown. Examples include the malignant degeneration in old burn scars (the chronic ulcer of Marjolin), and cancer of the liver and bladder subsequent to parasitic infestation by schistosomes.

Tumor viruses have become increasingly implicated as primary etiologic agents for a small number of human tumors. That viruses could cause cancers in animals and induce cell transformation in vitro was demonstrated many years ago. The study of retroviruses in particular has led to the discovery of oncogenes (see below) and provided the first clear insight into the molecular mechanisms of neoplasia.

Epidemiologic and molecular biologic evidence has circumstantially implicated a number of viruses with human malignancies: Hepatitis B and hepatocellular carcinoma, human T-cell leukemia virus and adult T-cell leukemia/lymphoma, Epstein-Barr virus with both Burkitt's lymphoma and nasopharyngeal carcinoma, and herpes simplex virus-2 and cervical cancer.

HEREDITARY FACTORS. Genetic factors are of major importance in determining the effectiveness of chemical, physical, and viral carcinogens in animals.

Clear-cut examples in human cancer development are demonstrated when the same type of cancer occurs in identical twins, when colon cancer develops in family members with familial polyposis, and with the familial patterns associated with breast cancer. Cancer of the breast is about three times more common in the daughters of women with premenopausal breast cancer and in women whose blood relatives have had at least two incidences of breast cancer. Furthermore, the daughters develop breast cancers at a younger age than did their mothers.

A more indirect genetic role is found in certain families who seem to have an increased incidence of neoplastic diseases. A clearly defined pattern of inheritance has been established for some of these tumors. It is often difficult to assess the importance of environmental factors in these cases. Substantiated examples include a pattern of dominant inheritance in some families for diseases such as retinoblastoma, lipomatosis, and colonic polyposis. In other families, there may be an association of multiple diseases that may include one or more neoplasms. An

Table 9-1. CHEMICAL AND PHYSICAL CARCINOGENS IN HUMAN BEINGS

Carcinogen	*Site of neoplasm*	*Site exposed*	*Persons at risk*
Chemical agents:			
Aromatic amines, especially β-naphthylamine	Urinary tract	Cutaneous and respiratory	Chemical workers producing dye stuffs, rodenticides, laboratory reagents
Benzol or benzene	Blood, lymphatic organs	Cutaneous and respiratory	Coal-tar refiners, solvent manufacturers, painters, printers, mechanics
Coal tar, pitch, creosote, anthracene, tobacco	Skin, larynx, bronchus	Cutaneous and respiratory	Coke-oven workers, coal-tar distillers, lumber industry workers, chemical workers, smokers
Petroleum, shale and paraffin oils, waxes, tars	Skin	Cutaneous	Workers in oil refineries, wax and asphalt producers, mechanics
Isopropyl oils	Sinus, larynx, bronchus	Respiratory	Producers of isopropyl alcohol
Asbestos	Bronchus, mesothelioma of pleura	Respiratory, generally >2 years	Asbestos miners, shippers, millers
Chromium	Bronchus	Respiratory and cutaneous	Workers engaged in chromate ore reduction
Nickel	Nasal cavity, sinus, bronchus	Respiratory	Nickel miners, shippers, and refiners
Arsenic	Skin, bronchus, bladder	Respiratory	Smelters, pesticide manufacturers
Physical agents:			
Ionizing radiation	Skin, thyroid, tongue, tonsil, sinus, bone, blood	Local or systemic, therapeutic (e.g., treatment of spondylitic polycythemia)	Radium dial workers
	Bronchus	Respiratory	Pitchblende miners
Ultraviolet radiation	Skin	Cutaneous	Farmers, other outdoor workers, sailors, fishermen, and fair-skinned people in tropical climates

example of this is the association of pheochromocytoma with medullary (amyloid-producing) carcinoma of the thyroid, cerebellocortical hemangioblastoma, or neurofibromatosis. Other examples include some cases of polyendocrine adenomas (pituitary, parathyroid, pancreas), including the Zollinger-Ellison syndrome and hereditary adenocarcinomatosis (adenocarcinoma of the colon, stomach, uterus, and ovary occurring in different members of the same family). There are also several relatively rare heritable nonneoplastic diseases that have been associated with malignant tumors with great frequency. An example is the high incidence of skin cancer in patients with xeroderma pigmentosa. There also is an association between dermal inclusion cysts and multiple carcinomas of the colon, polyposis, multiple bony exostoses, and benign connective tissue tumors (Gardner's syndrome).

There are marked differences in the frequency of certain neoplastic diseases with respect to age, sex, and other constitutional factors suggesting that additional host determinants may be important. Acute lymphocytic leukemia is essentially a disease of childhood, whereas malignant melanoma is essentially a postpubertal disease. Testicular tumors and Hodgkin's disease are more frequent in young adults, and breast cancer is far more common in women than in men. In many other tumors, the frequency in both sexes increases markedly with increasing age.

GEOGRAPHIC FACTORS. Neoplasms may be found in all human populations, but there are some striking racial and regional differences in the occurrence of specific types of cancer. Although it is difficult to separate the genetic from the environmental factors, such as diet or habits, it is important to be aware of certain particularly strong differences. In a comparison study with the Caucasian population of the United States, Shimkin noted the following differences in cancer incidence:

1. High incidence of cancer of the stomach in Scandinavia, Iceland, and Japan
2. High incidence of primary cancer of the liver in South and West Africa
3. High incidence of cancer of the nasopharynx in China
4. High incidence of cancer of the urinary bladder in Egypt
5. Low rate of colorectal cancer in black Africa
6. Low incidence of cancer of the prostate and breast in Japan
7. Low incidence of cancer of the uterine cervix in Israel and in Jewish women in general
8. Low incidence of cancer of the skin in blacks

Custom and environment obviously play an important role in the development of cancer. Migration of populations usually causes a shift toward the patterns of cancer incidence of the host country. For example, in Japan there is a very high incidence of stomach cancer and a relatively low incidence of lung cancer. However, a second generation Japanese-American has a low risk of stomach cancer, and if a heavy smoker, he has as high a risk of lung cancer as his American counterpart.

For unknown reasons, socioeconomic factors may also influence cancer incidence. Cancer of the stomach and of the cervix are three to four times more frequent in lower economic groups than in middle and higher economic groups. On the other hand, cancer of the breast, leukemia, and multiple myeloma are more frequent in higher socioeconomic groups.

PRECANCEROUS CONDITIONS. Some clinical disorders, such as leukoplakia, actinic keratosis, polyps of the colon or rectum, neurofibromas, dysplasia of the cervix or bronchial mucosa, and chronic ulcerative colitis, are described as precancerous because they are so frequently followed by the development of cancer. It is particularly important that the physician be aware of these conditions in order to conduct careful follow-up of these patients.

ONCOGENES AND GROWTH FACTORS. Many lines of research in the molecular mechanisms of cancer have led to the discovery of oncogenes, which, when improperly regulated, cause the cell to enhance or decrease essential products associated with growth and differentiation and to exhibit the unrestricted growth and dissemination characteristic of cancer.

Much of our insight into oncogenes comes from the study of retroviruses. These are RNA tumor viruses found in avian and mammalian systems that can cause carcinomas, sarcomas, leukemias, and lymphomas. Retroviruses have an enzyme, reverse transcriptase, which permits the single-stranded viral genomic RNA to be transcribed into complementary DNA (cDNA). This cDNA may then integrate very efficiently into the cellular genome (Fig. 9-4). There are two major subgroups of oncogenic retroviruses—acute and chronic. Acute transforming retroviruses induce tumors in experimental animals within a few weeks while chronic transforming viruses do so after many months.

The Rous sarcoma virus (RSV) is a classic acute transforming virus whose genome is depicted in Fig. 9-4. The GAG gene codes for a structural protein found in the viral core, the POL gene codes for reverse transcriptase, and ENV is the viral envelope glycoprotein. The RSV genome also contains a V-*Src* gene that is known as the viral oncogene. The V-*Src* gene is responsible for the in vitro and in vivo oncogenic potential of RSV.

Current evidence has shown that all viral oncogenes are derived from normal cellular genomes called proto-oncogenes or cellular oncogenes (C-onc). About 20 different cellular oncogenes have been characterized, and these genes are highly conserved in evolution. Homologous oncogene sequences can be found in the genomic DNA of mammals, fish, birds, yeast, invertebrates, and *Drosophila*. However, viral oncogenes are not exact copies of cellular oncogenes, and the difference may range from a single amino acid substitution, to deletions, insertions, or major truncations. These observations have led to the general theory that cellular oncogenes are normal and perhaps important genes that regulate growth and differentiation. Molecular alterations of the oncogene itself or of its regulation may result in abnormal growth and differentiation of the cell.

Our understanding of cellular oncogenes makes the behavior of chronic transforming retroviruses easier to understand. These viruses do not contain oncogenes. These viruses, however, may integrate near cellular oncogenes, placing these under the potent viral transcriptional control.

For several oncogene families (V-*abl*, V-*erb* B, V-*ets*, V-*mos*, V-*myb*, V-H-*ras*, V-k-*ras*, and V-*sis*) there is circumstantial evidence of their association with human malignancies, most of which belong to the *ras* family.

During evolution, families of cellular oncogenes with

Fig. 9-4. The genome organization of Rous sarcoma virus, the reverse transcription of viral genome into cDNA, and subsequent integration into the chromosome.

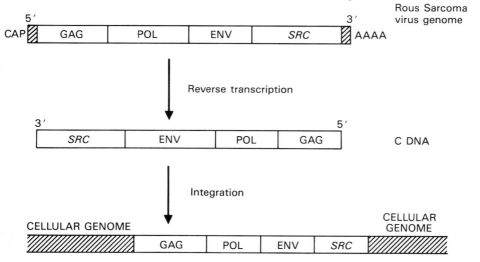

similar structures seem to have arisen. The *ras* genes (Ha, K-, and N-*ras*) is one such family. The Ha-*ras* cellular oncogene is homologous to the Harvey murine sarcoma virus and has been circumstantially associated with human bladder, lung, and kidney cancers. Other *ras* oncogenes have been associated with other human cancers. *Ras* oncogenes code for a highly homologous series of proteins of 21,000 daltons called p21 proteins. Normal p21 proteins are located on the cytoplasmic surface of the cell membrane, have GTPase activity, and are thought to be intimately involved in some way with the regulation of cell proliferation. Malignant transformation by *ras* oncogenes is caused by a single point mutation in the amino terminal region of the *ras* gene. These mutations are confined to two "hot spots," codons 12 and 61, which result in a mutant p21 protein that lacks GTPase activity. Our understanding of the mechanism of transformation in a setting of a mutated *ras* gene product is still incomplete, but the mutational loss of GTPase activity gives the cell a growth-promoting signal in some way. It is interesting that such mutations can be caused by known carcinogens such as nitroso-methyl-urea and dimethyl nitrosamine.

Another major oncogene family specifies gene products that have tyrosine kinase activity. This oncogene family includes the *src* oncogene of the previously described RSV. Tyrosine kinases are capable of phosphorylating tyrosine residues on various proteins, and those oncogenes possessing this activity all share extensive homology around the kinase domains of their various gene products. Perhaps less than 0.1 percent of all protein phosphorylation occurs at tyrosine residues, but this enzymatic activity must be relevant to cell proliferation and oncogenesis. A number of receptors for normal growth factors—platelet-derived growth factor (PDGF), epidermal growth factor (EGF), and insulin-like growth factor (IGF 1)—have intrinsic tyrosine kinase activity when activated by an appropriate ligand. PDGF is a small glycoprotein stored in platelet alpha granules that can signal fibroblasts in the G0 phase to enter the cell-division cycle (G1-S-G2-M-G1). Progression through G1 to S (DNA replication) requires EGF and IGF. PDGF is highly homologous to the *sis* viral oncogene product, the oncogene of the simian sarcoma virus (Fig. 9-5). While normal fibroblasts do not have detectable c-*sis* messenger RNA, many human sarcomas do, and some release PDGF-like growth factors that may stimulate these tumors in an autocrine fashion. Normal fibroblast division appears to be regulated by the interaction of several cellular oncogenes (which code for normal growth factors and their receptors). These results provide a basis for understanding how mutations in any of these oncogenes could result in unrestricted proliferation. The V-*erb* B oncogene codes for a truncated form of the EGF receptor, a gene product that has the tyrosine kinase and transmembrane domains but lacks the normal ligand receptor. This mutant growth factor receptor may act as if it is persistently activated.

Myc-like oncogenes are associated with Burkitt's lymphoma, neuroblastoma, retinoblastomas, and other human tumors. The study of N-*myc* oncogene in neuroblastomas provides an example of another form of aberrant oncogene expression–oncogene amplification. In oncogene amplification, the cell increases the number of copies of the oncogene, and its expression may be greatly enhanced. N-*myc* amplification correlates closely with tumor progression. The absence of N-*myc* gene amplification (namely, one copy per tumor cell) was associated with a favorable response to conventional therapy, regardless of stage at diagnosis. The generally favorable

Fig. 9-5. *A.* Homology between V-*erb* B gene product and epidermal growth factor receptor. *B.* Homology between V-*sis* gene product and platelet-derived growth factor (PDGF).

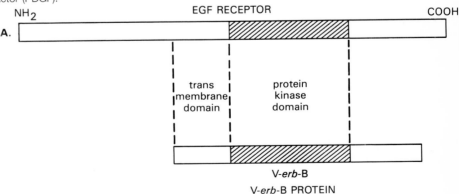

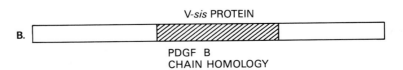

stage IV S, characterized by skin and liver metastases, also had single oncogene copies. Neuroblastomas with N-*myc* amplification (3 to 10 or > 10 copies) had a higher incidence of progression after conventional therapy. The N-*myc* oncogene appears to play a key role in determining the aggressiveness of neuroblastomas and is being used as an important intrastage prognostic factor. Early studies suggest that HER-2/*neu* oncogene amplification in breast cancer may also be correlated with prognosis.

Chromosomal abnormalities frequently occur in human cancers. Such gene rearrangements may activate or suppress important regulatory genes. A well-studied example is the gene translocation in Burkitt's lymphoma in which the long arm of chromosome 8 is translocated to number 14 (or occasionally 2 or 22). The long arm of 8 has the C-*myc* oncogene while 14, 2, and 22 have loci for various immunoglobulin genes. The result is an abnormal regulation and timing of C-*myc* expression. Also, the classic translocation involving chromosomes 9 and 22 producing the Philadelphia chromosome of chronic myelogenous leukemia involves repositioning the C-*abl* oncogene.

The clinical applications of oncogene research are only just being realized. The greatest benefit will be a molecular understanding of the mechanism of oncogenesis. Examining the oncogene activity of individual tumors even now permits intrastage prognostic assessment. Recently, a monoclonal antibody to the gene product of the N-*myc* oncogene is being used to histochemically stain neuroblastoma cells. A *ras*-specific monoclonal antibody has been found to intensely stain cells from areas of carcinoma in situ and invasive carcinoma in colon and breast cancer. Therapeutic strategies in the future may involve the creation of drugs that suppress oncogene expression or their products.

MULTIFACTORIAL ETIOLOGY. It is likely that all individual cancers are the result of multiple factors, such as an interaction of an oncogenic virus with a chemical or physical carcinogen. It is also possible that two chemical carcinogens may act synergistically to increase the incidence of cancer. A chemical may be a carcinogen only in a host with a hereditary susceptibility. When condensations of smog or cigarette smoke are applied separately to the cheek pouch of the golden hamster, there is a low but definite incidence of tumor. However, when they are applied together, there is a markedly increased incidence of tumors. Similarly, viruses have enhanced the oncogenic effects of smog and cigarette smoke in tissue culture. It is very possible that such synergistic interactions occur in human beings.

The possibility that multiple factors may be involved in the etiology of human neoplasia, rather than any one, may increase the chances of ultimate cancer prevention. For example, in carcinoma of the lung, it may be that in addition to heavy cigarette smoking (perhaps only chronic irritation), one requires a specific genetic background (since not all heavy smokers develop cancer of the lung), suitable male hormonal factors (since males are more frequently affected), and a virus. In addition, the latent period between start of smoking and high incidence of lung cancer is roughly 35 years. Although cigarette smoking may not be the only cause of lung cancer, it is the only factor that can be controlled. On the basis of present knowledge, lung cancer could be prevented by eliminating cigarette smoking altogether or by limiting cigarette smoking to a shorter period of time.

Custom and environment obviously are involved in the etiology of this cancer. Although cigarette smoking has been strongly implicated as a cause of squamous cell carcinoma of the lung, the habit is sufficiently ingrained in people in the United States to make its total elimination extremely difficult. Habits and customs in other parts of the world may be equally difficult to eliminate. The inhalation of snuff and the mastication of betel nuts have been associated with nasal and oral pharynx tumors, but the use of such materials continues despite their known carcinogenic effects. Nevertheless, efforts to identify the causative factors and to educate people regarding these factors must be continued.

BIOLOGY

Regardless of the etiologic agent, the cancer cell is a progeny of a normal cell that has lost its cellular mechanisms for controlling proliferation. The cancer cell differs from a normal cell in a variety of ways, but none of its new characteristics are absolutely indicative of malignancy. Cytogenetic studies of some cancer cells have revealed various abnormalities in chromosome number and appearance. However, these changes have not been shared by all cancer cells, and many cancer cells have normal chromosomal profiles.

Almost all malignant neoplasms seem to arise from a single cell that has undergone malignant transformation to form a malignant clone (group of cells); however, other human neoplasms such as the neurofibromas occurring in von Recklinghausen's disease may develop from multiple clones of cells. Simultaneously multifocal origins of carcinoma of the breast, oral pharynx, colon, and other organs also have been observed. Studies of patients with breast carcinoma have demonstrated that at least 30 percent have other areas involved with in situ carcinoma. Nevertheless, the primary tumor mass that was the cause for clinical presentation arises from a single cell alone.

Cancer cells generally proliferate faster than normal cells, except for leukocytes or cells of the intestinal mucosa. However, the proliferative rate decreases as the tumor mass grows; the proportion of cells undergoing mitosis is much greater when there are only a few cancer cells present than when there are many cells present in a large tumor mass. There are many rapid changes in the mitotic fraction of neoplasms during the initial growth phase, but after the tumor mass is 1 cm in diameter, the rate of division usually follows a predictable pattern.

After neoplastic transformation has occurred, the cancer cell differs from the normal cell not only in proliferative index but also in morphology, biochemistry, antigenic expression, and many other aspects.

MORPHOLOGIC CHANGES. Malignant cells tend to revert to more primitive cell types, that is, to dedifferentiate. The normal orderly tissue patterns are lost or replaced by the random piling up of malignant cells without definite pattern. Other histologic changes may include cellular pleomorphism, a high index of mitoses, and hyperchromatism in the nucleus and nucleoli. Invasion of adjacent normal structures also may be seen microscopically. These morphologic changes are the basis for histopathologic or cytologic diagnoses of cancer and usually allow very accurate diagnosis of neoplastic diseases.

BIOCHEMICAL CHANGES. The biochemical activity of cancer cells is similar, though not identical, to that of normal cells. A great diversity exists in the biochemical characteristics of different tumor cells, usually correlating with rate of proliferation. Changes in DNA, RNA, and the chemical architecture of the cellular membrane of malignant cells are associated with the loss of contact inhibition to proliferation and intercellular adhesiveness. However, no single biochemical alteration has yet been defined that is absolutely characteristic of malignant transformation.

Reversion of the normal cellular biochemistry to that of the embryonal cells produces distinctive embryonal substances whose presence in the adult may be used to diagnose cancer. The carcinoembryonic antigen associated with gastrointestinal cancers, and α-fetoglobulin associated with hepatoma and embryonal cancers are thought to be examples of this type. The synthesis of these substances may be due to depression of fetal gene function that occurs during oncogenesis.

Malignant cells may also produce biologically active substances that are normally produced by the cells from which the neoplasm originated. The release of these substances may cause symptoms similar to hyperfunction of that particular organ, for example, hyperparathyroidism produced by parathyroid carcinomas. Neoplasms may also produce biologically active substances that are not normally produced by the cells of origin. Some bronchogenic carcinomas may produce parathyroidlike hormones, ACTH, antidiuretic hormones, and other hormones.

The mechanism of this ectopic hormone secretion is based upon the hypothesis of variable genetic activity or *selective derepression* of a specific gene. All cells contain the same genes; however, only about 10 percent of these genes are expressed in any one cell type; the remainder are repressed. Cancer cells are primitive cells; with dedifferentiation, they acquire the ability to express some of these previously repressed genes. This new genetic expression is responsible for the production of a new specific-messenger RNA and the production of new polypeptides and hormones.

GROWTH RATES OF NEOPLASMS. Approximately two-thirds of the growth of human neoplasms occurs before they are clinically detectable. If one assumes that a cancer begins from a single cell, then it takes about 30 exponential divisions to produce a 1-cm nodule (1 billion cells). At 45 exponential divisions the patient is apt to be dead from the sheer bulk of the malignant tumor.

The growth rate of tumors can be expressed by the *tumor doubling time*, i.e., the time it takes for a tumor to double in volume. Tumor doubling times appear to be an accurate and precise method for comparing the biologic aggressiveness of neoplasms in different patients. This measurement is particularly applicable to metastatic pulmonary lesions, since these are usually peripheral in location and are discretely delineated on chest radiographs, so that accurate serial measurements are easily obtainable.

The method used in the measurement of the tumor doubling time is illustrated in Fig. 9-6. Briefly, the average of the greater and the lesser diameters of each metastatic nodule is determined from successive chest radiographs. The averages are plotted on semilogarithmic paper against the time in days between these points; the slope of this line represents the rate of tumor growth. Where this line crosses any two doubling lines, the horizontal distance between them represents the tumor doubling time in days. This measurement has been shown to be an accurate and reproducible method for the quantitation of the rate and pattern of tumor growth in individual patients.

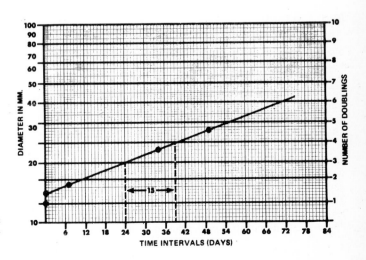

Fig. 9-6. Method of plotting tumor doubling time, based upon the direct measurement of the changing diameters of metastatic pulmonary nodules. (From: *Joseph WL et al: J Thorac Cardiovasc Surg 61:23, 1971, with permission.*)

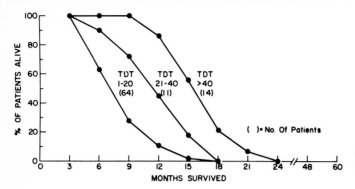

Fig. 9-7. Survival curves in 89 untreated patients following the onset of pulmonary metastases, showing three groups based upon tumor doubling time. (From: *Joseph WL et al: J Thorac Cardiovasc Surg 61:23, 1971, with permission.*)

The tumor doubling time varies from 8 to 600 days; most tumors double in 20 to 100 days. The measurement of tumor doubling times can be extremely helpful in determining prognosis, in evaluating response to chemotherapeutic agents, and in comparing responses to different therapeutic regimens.

In one study the tumor doubling times of a large series of patients with pulmonary metastases from tumors of different histologic types were measured. Wide variations within particular types of neoplasms were found. The tumor doubling time correlated closely with the length of survival in three distinct groups of patients. This is illustrated in Fig. 9-7. This correlation might be expected, because the tumor doubling time represents the balance between the intrinsic proliferative rate of the tumor cell and the patient's inhibiting defense mechanisms.

On the basis of growth dynamics, most human tumors have been present in the body for at least 1 year and many for as long as 10 years prior to their clinical detection. Thus, it appears that there is a long period of time between the inception of neoplastic transformation and the development of clinical cancer. During this time, detection may be possible and surgical treatment might result in cure. Tests must be perfected to detect cancer earlier, to shorten this preclinical interval and make surgical treatment more successful.

Immunobiology

The concept that cancer patients may develop an immune response against their neoplasms is not new. This view became very popular at the turn of the century when it was found that strong immunity could be induced against transplantable neoplasms in randomly bred laboratory rodents. A period of intense laboratory and clinical investigation followed, in anticipation that tumor immunity might lead to control of malignant disease. However, it soon became evident that the immunity was not directed against tumor-specific antigens (TSA), but instead was against normal tissue antigens in the neoplasm due to genetic differences between tumor donor and recipient. Thereafter, interest in tumor immunology declined because no antigens other than the transplantation antigens could be demonstrated in neoplasms.

Interest in the immunology of neoplastic diseases was reawakened in the 1950s when tumor-specific antigens were conclusively demonstrated in methylcholanthrene-induced sarcomas in mice. In order to eliminate any histocompatibility factors the investigators used inbred strains of rodents that, after many years of inbreeding, had the genetic homogeneity of monozygotic twins. Specific tumor transplantation resistance was induced by presensitization with a transplant of tumor tissue that was allowed to grow for a time and then was excised. The immunized rodents were then resistant to challenge with further transplants of the same neoplasm (Fig. 9-8). However, the immunity induced in these animals was relative, not absolute. Whereas a challenge with 100,000 tumor cells produced a growing tumor in control mice, it did not in the immune mice. Challenge with larger numbers of

Fig. 9-8. Mouse A, immunized with benzpyrene-induced tumor t, resists subsequent challenge with t tumor cells. Challenge with cells from another benzpyrene-induced tumor, t_2, leads to progressive tumor growth and death of the mouse.

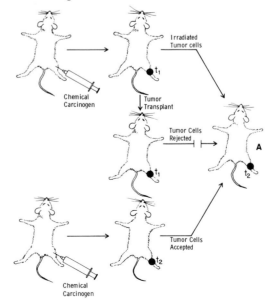

cells (1 to 10 million), however, usually overwhelmed the immunologic defense, and progressive tumor growth was observed.

Tumor-specific antigens have been demonstrated in most viral, chemical, and physical-carcinogen-induced neoplasms and possibly in some spontaneous tumors. During the past 25 years there has been tremendous progress in tumor immunology. Because tumor antigens were first identified by their ability to elicit rejection when transplanted from one animal to another, they became known as "tumor-specific transplantation antigens." Other assays have been developed, and these antigens are rarely referred to by this term. However, fundamental questions concerning the expression of tumor-specific antigens by human tumors, the host response to these antigens, and the ability to manipulate the response to achieve tumor regression continue to be the goals of human tumor immunology.

ANTIGENIC SPECIFICITY OF ANIMAL NEOPLASMS. The wide variety of viral-, chemical-, and physical-carcinogen-induced neoplasms for which tumor-specific transplantation antigens were originally demonstrated are summarized in Table 9-2. The antigenic specificities of these major types of carcinogenic agents have been found to be quite different.

Table 9-2. TUMOR-SPECIFIC ANTIGENS CAPABLE OF INDUCING REJECTION RESPONSES IN SYNGENEIC HOSTS

Inducing agent	*Antigenic specificity*

Chemical carcinogens:
  3-Methylcholanthrene
  1,2,5,6-Dibenzanthracene
  9,10-Dimethylbenzanthracene
  3,4,9,10-Dibenzpyrene
  3,4-Benzpyrene-dimethylam-
    inoazobenzene
Physical agents:
  Films
    Millipore filter
    Cellophane film
  Radiation
    Ultraviolet
    ^{90}Sr
	Antigens distinct for each individual neoplasm

Virus:
  DNA
    Polyoma
    SV-40
    Adenovirus 12,18
    Shope papilloma
  RNA:
    Mammary tumor agent
    Leukemia
      Gross
      Moloney ⎫
      Rauscher ⎬ Shared common
      Friend   ⎭ antigens
      Graffi
      Rich
      Rous (Schmidt-Ruppin)
	Common antigens in each neoplasm induced by the same virus

Tumor-Specific Antigens of Neoplasms Induced by Chemical and Physical Carcinogens. These are individually distinct for each tumor, even if induced by the same carcinogen, in the same strain, and of the identical histologic type (Fig. 9-9). For example, injection of a chemical carcinogen such as benzpyrene in two inbred mice of the same strain will result in two antigenically different tumors, t_1 and t_2. If mouse *A* is immunized with irradiated tumor cells from t_1, it will subsequently reject tumor cells from the same tumor transplanted into an intermediate host. However, the same animal, immune to t_1, will develop a tumor when injected with the same number of tumor cells from t_2.

Tumor-Specific Antigens of Neoplasms Induced by Viral Carcinogens. In contrast to the unique tumor-specific antigens of chemical-carcinogen-induced tumors, the tumor-specific antigens of viral-induced neoplasms are common to all neoplasms induced by the same virus, but differ from those induced by other viruses (Fig. 9-9). For example, with inbred mice of the same strain, mouse *A* is immunized with SV-40 virus alone, mouse *B* is immunized with *irradiated* tumor cells from an SV-40 virus-induced mouse tumor, and mouse *C* is immunized with tumor cells from an SV-40 virus-induced rat tumor. All will reject challenge of tumor cells from SV-40 virus-induced tumor t. However, challenge with the same tumor cells in mice *D* and *E*, immunized with either polyoma virus alone or polyoma virus-induced tumor cells, leads to progressive tumor growth and death.

Although the generalization that virus-induced neoplasms contain common antigens and chemical-carcinogen-induced neoplasms contain individually distinct antigens is usually correct, more recent studies have demonstrated that this distinction is not as absolute as originally believed. Common antigens related to leukemia viral antigens have been found in chemical-carcinogen-induced sarcomas, and some carcinogen-induced neoplasms arising in the bladder have contained common antigens. Furthermore, spontaneous mouse mammary carcinomas induced by the mammary tumor virus contain individually distinct antigens in addition to the common antigens of the mammary tumor virus.

EFFECTOR MECHANISMS IN TUMOR IMMUNITY. The host provides a number of effector mechanisms with theoretical and proved effectiveness in the immune destruction of tumors. The important effectors include tumor-antigen-specific antibodies, mononuclear phagocytes, natural killer cells, and cytotoxic T lymphocytes, neutrophils, and K cells.

Antitumor Antibodies. There are five classes of immunoglobulin molecules (IgG, A, M, D, E) in human beings. The major antibody classes associated with tumor immunity are IgM and IgG. The antigen-binding region of the antibody molecule is located in the aminoterminal or Fab portion. Binding of antibody to the tumor target cell does not by itself result in growth suppression or destruction. It serves only as a recognition signal for cytolytic effectors such as complement, macrophages, or K cells to perform the cytotoxic event. Antitumor antibodies of the

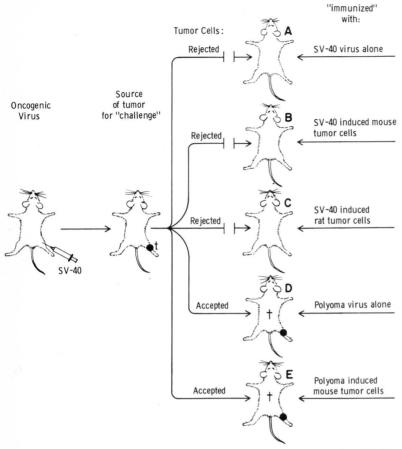

Fig. 9-9. Mice A, B, and C, immunized with SV-40 virus or SV-40 virus-induced tumor cells, reject challenge of tumor cells from SV-40 virus-induced tumor t. Challenge with the same tumor cells in mice D and E, immunized with polyoma virus or polyoma virus-induced tumor cells, leads to progressive tumor growth and death of the mouse.

appropriate subclass are effective in suppressing small numbers of tumor cells in certain experimental settings. Recently, the administration of human monoclonal antibodies specific for tumor-associated antigens to tumor-bearing patients has shown promising results.

Complement. The classical complement system is composed of a group of serum proteins (Cl-9), most of which are β-globulins. The binding of the C1 to the appropriate immunoglobulin subclass (IgG1, IgG3, IgM in human beings) initiates a cascade of component activation and macromolecular aggregation that results in (1) release of the anaphylatoxins C3a and C5a, which causes neutrophil chemotaxis, neutrophil activation, increased vascular permeability, release of histamine from mast cells, and smooth muscle contraction; and (2) assembly of the C5-9 membrane attack complex, which inserts in the lipid bilayer of the target cell membrane, forming a "doughnut" and thus providing for the free exchange of water and electrolytes and the consequent osmotic lysis of the cell. The alternative complement pathway provides for the assembly and activation of complement on target membranes without antibody or C1 fixation and appears to be more important in microbial immunity.

Antibody-Dependent Cell-Mediated Cytotoxicity (ADCC). Antibody-coated tumor cells may be killed by a variety of cellular effectors that are able to engage via Fc receptors on the effector cell surface. Thus, the antibody molecule provides the specific recognition signal while the otherwise quiescent and nonspecific effector cell is directed to the target cells to provide the cytotoxic event. Monocytes and macrophages are very efficient cytotoxic effectors in the ADCC system. The so-called K cell, a poorly defined lymphocyte of uncertain lineage that closely resembles the NK cell, is quite active. In addition, neutrophils and perhaps eosinophils and platelets are active in certain settings. The mechanisms of killing by these ADCC effectors are not fully defined.

Mononuclear Phagocytes. Cells of the mononuclear phagocytic system play a central role in immunity. They are composed of circulating monocytes, macrophages in the alveolus, spleen, and lymph node, Kupffer cells in the liver, and brain microglial cells. Circulating monocytes are the best studied of these cells and are of greater interest to the tumor immunologist because of their ability to migrate to sites of inflammation and tumor.

Macrophages have a number of important immunoregulatory and cytotoxic functions. They help to initiate immune response by serving as antigen-presenting cells. Such cells are especially abundant in germinal centers of lymph nodes and as Langerhans cells in the skin. In addition, macrophages have a wide range of regulatory, tumoricidal, and bactericidal properties. Elaboration of such lymphokines as interleukin-1 (IL-1) is important in T and B lymphocyte activation and the generation of fever. Macrophages also produce monocytotoxins that include tumor necrosis factor (TNF) which has a broad range of cytocidal and regulatory properties (see lymphokine section). Many other macrophage products—prostaglandins, complement components, proteolytic enzymes and hydrolases, hydrogen peroxide, superoxides—mediate other regulatory and cytotoxic functions. Macrophage function is initiated and enhanced by the process of "activation." Activation is a complex multistep process characterized by morphologic changes (maturation, spreading, pinocytosis, synthesis of lysosomal granules), elaboration of monokines and cytotoxins, and enhanced bactericidal activity. Macrophages may be activated by lymphokines (IFNY), bacterial products (endotoxin), and antibody-coated targets.

Natural Killer Cells. NK cells comprise about 5 percent of peripheral blood leukocytes and morphologically are large granular lymphocytes. NK cells, freshly isolated from the peripheral blood leukocytes and morphologically large granular lymphocytes, are capable of killing certain tumor target cells in short-term in vitro assays. This killing does not require immunologic memory or specificity and is not restricted by the major histocompatibility complex (as with cytolytic T lymphocytes). NK cells may be found in the peripheral blood, spleen, and bone marrow but are found infrequently in the thymus, lymph nodes, or lymph. NK cells can kill a selected repertoire of cultured and freshly isolated human tumor cells, but many appear to be resistant. The mechanism of NK lysis is not fully understood but requires cell contact and may be mediated by cytotoxins contained in their cytoplasmic azurophilic granules. The target structure recognized by NK cells as well as the lineage of NK cells is still being debated. A number of biologic response modifiers such as interleukin-2 (IL-2) and interferon (IFN) will augment NK activity in vitro and in vivo. Prostaglandin E2, which can be produced by macrophages and tumor cells, suppresses NK activity. There is much convincing circumstantial evidence to suggest that NK cells are important in immunologic surveillance and eradication of small numbers of tumor cells. It is unlikely that they play an effective role in the immune response against established tumors, and NK cells found within tumors have defective function. A current area of interest is the use of biologic response modifiers such as IL-2 to augment NK function in cancer patients.

Lymphokine-Activated Killer Cells. See below, section on Immunotherapy.

Cytolytic T Lymphocytes. The classic cytotoxic cell of cellular immunity is the cytotoxic T lymphocyte (Tc), the only one with intrinsic immunological specificity by virtue of its antigen-specific receptor. The T cell receptor is composed of two disulfide linked peptides (α and β) which recognize foreign antigens only in association with Class I major histocompatibility complex (MHC) antigens (HLA-A,B,C). Class I MHC antigens are glycoproteins with molecular weight of 44,000, are associated with β2-microglobulin, and are present on all cells except erythrocytes. This is an important concept since T cells sensitized to viral or tumor antigens of one MHC haplotype are unable to recognize and kill cells bearing the same foreign antigen in association with a different haplotype. Other MHC antigens such as Class II or D region antigens are important in cooperation and interaction between cells in the immune system.

Cytolytic T cells (Tc) induce ultrastructural lesions in the membrane lipid bilayer of nucleated target cells. As with the complement (C9) membrane lesion, these Tc-mediated lesions appear to be caused by polymerization of 18 to 20 precursor molecules (termed "perforins") into tubular complexes that perforate the cell membrane. These molecules and lymphotoxin, a cytotoxin similar in action to and sharing some homology with TNF, are under intense scrutiny as the effector molecules for Tc and other cytotoxic cells. Cytotoxic T lymphocytes may be clonally expanded in the presence of IL-2, and such cytotoxic T cell clones are valuable research tools and potential therapeutic agents.

Suppressor T cells can be induced by tumor antigen, products other than antigens (e.g., prostaglandins), and direct interactions with immune cells. There are also suggestions that there are natural suppressor cells that control immune reactions. Suppressor T cells are themselves regulated by countersuppressor T cells. It is logical that immunotherapy should consist of modulators of suppressor cells along with appropriate stimulation. In recent years emphasis in immunotherapy has been on biologic response modifiers. These agents include cyclophosphamide, cimetidine, and indomethacin which are used primarily to inhibit immune suppression and to augment tumor immunity.

BIOLOGIC RESPONSE MODIFIERS. Genetic engineering technology has permitted large-scale production of purified, homogeneous lymphokines. Some of these factors can be used in supraphysiologic doses to modify host tumor immunity in vivo or immune effectors in vitro.

Interleukin-1. Interleukin-1 (IL-1) is a lymphokine originally defined as a thymocyte mitogen produced by activated macrophages. It is now known that many different types of cells produce IL-1 (including monocytes, macrophages, dendritic cells, Langerhans cells, endothelial cells, neutrophils, NK cells, microglial cells), and that two IL-1 molecules exist that have broad ranges of immunologic, biologic, and inflammatory properties.

There are two IL-1 genes whose gene products—IL-1α

and IL-1β—both have molecular weights of 17,000. These two molecules have only a 20 percent amino acid sequence homology, although there are a number of regions of close homology between the α and the β forms that may represent common functional domains. Both IL-1α and IL-1β bind to the same surface membrane receptor on target cells to effect their hormonal action.

IL-1 has many biologic effects, and it has not yet been fully determined which, if any, of these properties segregate to the α or β species. IL-1 induces some T cells to produce IL-2 and others to express IL-2 receptors, which is important in the clonal expansion of T cell subsets. IL-1 may also have a maturation effect on pre-B cells and participate in the proliferation of mature B cells by inducing the production of interferon β₂. Thus, IL-1 has a vital and integral role in cellular and humoral immunity. In addition, IL-1 initiates the febrile response, directly acts on the bone marrow to cause release of neutrophils into the circulation, induces hepatic synthesis of acute-phase proteins, induces skeletal muscle catabolism, and promotes the degradation of cartilage matrix. IL-1 can cause the production and release of IL-2 and tumor necrosis factor (TNF) by appropriate target cells and is thereby able to initiate a cascade of important inflammatory and immunoregulatory functions, many of which remain to be fully defined.

Interleukin-2. Interleukin-2 (IL-2) is a glycoprotein with a molecular weight of 15,000 that is produced by helper T lymphocytes. Originally called "T-cell growth factor," IL-2 can support the long-term proliferation of T cells in culture. IL-2 has been cloned in *Escherichia coli* and the recombinant nonglycosylated form and is fully active and available in large quantities for experimental and clinical studies.

IL-2 augments the generation of cytolytic T lymphocytes, natural killer (NK) cells, lymphokine activated killer (LAK) cells, and alloantigen responsiveness. This lymphokine may help in restoring immunocompetence from certain immunodeficiency states. Human recombinant IL-2 is currently being used in clinical immunotherapy trials.

TUMOR NECROSIS FACTOR. Tumor necrosis factor (TNF) was originally described as a protein found in the sera of mice sensitized with *Corynebacterium parvum* or *Bacillus* Calmette-Guérin and then challenged with bacterial endotoxin. TNF causes hemorrhagic necrosis of certain experimental tumors in mice. It is likely that TNF was responsible for the occasional necrosis of human tumors induced by "Coley's toxins" when these bacterial toxins were used in the 1930s. It is now known that TNF has a broad range of biologic activities.

TNF is a peptide hormone whose subunit molecular weight is 17,000. TNF is produced by monocytes, macrophages, endothelial cells, large granular lymphocytes, and neutrophils. The TNF gene is closely linked to the lymphotoxin gene with which it shares 30 percent amino acid sequence homology. Properties of TNF include (1) direct cytotoxicity for certain cells, (2) stimulation of procoagulant activity by vascular endothelial cells (which may contribute to the phenomenon of in vivo hemorrhage

necrosis of tumors), (3) activation of neutrophil adherence and phagocytosis, and (4) induction of fever by direct effect on the hypothalamic thermoregulatory center. Shires has demonstrated that this protein can cause many of the effects of endotoxin shock. TNF is one of the major effector molecules of macrophage-mediated cytotoxicity of tumor cells, plays a central role in the pathogenesis of endotoxin-induced shock, and may account for the wasting and catabolic state associated with chronic illness and cancer. Some investigators who feel that the term "tumor necrosis factor" is misleadingly narrow have coined the term "cachectin" instead.

Interferons. Interferons (IFN) were discovered about 30 years ago as antiviral agents. There are three major classes of IFNs, α, β, γ, all of which have now been fully characterized and cloned using recombinant DNA technology. There are over a dozen physicochemically related IFN subtypes, all with a molecular weight of about 20,000. IFNα used to be called leukocyte IFN and is produced by monocytes. IFNβ (fibroblast IFN) has the same molecular weight as IFNβ. Only one species of IFNγ has been identified, and it is produced by immune T cells. IFNγ has also been called immune IFN and macrophage activating factor (MAF). IFNγ has a molecular weight of 25,000 and shares only 12 percent amino acid sequence homology with other IFNs.

IFNs have diverse effect on many different cell types. IFNs have a wide range of direct antitumor effects whose sensitivity may be related to IFN receptor expression. IFNs may augment expression of MHC antigens and alter membrane lipids and cytoskeleton. IFNs also may augment the activity of cytotoxic T lymphocytes, NK cells, K cells, and tumoricidal macrophages.

IFNs have been used in clinical trials since the early 1970s, but only recently have purified, recombinant IFNs become available for clinical use. IFNα A as a single agent can cause partial and occasionally complete responses in leukemia, Kaposi's sarcoma, breast carcinoma, renal cell carcinoma, lymphomas, malignant melanoma, and others. IFNβ may have some activity with multiple myeloma and lymphoma. Less is known about the therapeutic efficacy of IFNγ.

IFNs may act synergistically with other biologic response modifiers (other IFN classes, IL-2, etc.), and it may be in this setting that they will find more effective clinical applications.

IMMUNE SURVEILLANCE. The concept of immunologic surveillance is based upon the premise that carcinogenesis occurs frequently as a spontaneous mutation, from chemical carcinogens or from oncogenic viruses. Burnet postulated that the teleology of the immune system was to recognize the foreignness of tumor-specific antigens on the neoplastic cells and to mount an immune response capable of eliminating them. In this context, clinical cancer would represent a failure of the mechanisms for immunologic destruction, although it may be the exception rather than the rule. The NK cells may be the basis of the surveillance system because they can recognize new antigens, whereas the T cells do not seem to have this capability.

Mechanisms for Evasion of Immune Surveillance. If neoplastic cells are capable of eliciting a host immune response that leads to their specific destruction, it is pertinent to ask why or how cancer develops. A variety of possible ways by which cancer cells evade the immune surveillance mechanisms have been described:

Insufficient antigenicity to evoke an immune response may account for the growth of some neoplasms. Tumor antigens and tumor-associated antigens are usually weaker immunogens than transplantation antigens. Some neoplastic cells may have either an extremely weak tumor antigen or an extremely low density of tumor antigens on the cell surface. Thus, the tumor cell with the stronger tumor antigen may be recognized and eliminated, whereas those cells with weak tumor antigens may escape detection and destruction.

Antigenic modulation of a thymus leukemia (TL) antigen has been observed on a murine lymphoma cell. The TL antigen disappears when the cell is transplanted in immunized hosts or carried in tissue culture containing specific antibody, but it will reappear when the tumor cells are passed in tissue culture without antibody or transplanted in unimmunized hosts. Furthermore, antigenic shift may be another form of antigenic modulation whereby tumor cells escape control immunologic surveillance. This phenomenon has been described with certain animal neoplasms in which the lung metastases are antigenically different from the primary tumor.

Immunologic indifference may explain the observation by Old and associates that small numbers of tumor cells having tumor-specific antigens develop into progressively growing tumors although larger numbers of cells are rejected. In this instance the small number of cells may not be immunogenic enough and can "sneak through" the host immune response.

Immunosuppression by irradiation, neonatal thymectomy, chemotherapy, or steroid or antilymphocyte globulin administration usually increases the frequency and growth rate, and shortens the latency period, for both virus- and carcinogen-induced neoplasms in experimental animals. The incidence of cancer in human beings increases significantly with advancing years as the immune response to a variety of antigens decreases. Furthermore, in human beings with congenital immunodeficiency diseases, the incidence of spontaneous cancer is 10,000 times that of the general age-matched population. In human organ transplant recipients on immunosuppressive drugs, the incidence of spontaneous cancer is more than seventy times that of the general age-matched population. NK function may be depressed in patients who develop cancer. Renal transplant patients and patients with Chédiak-Higashi disease who have a high incidence of lymphoproliferative disorders appear to have abnormal NK cell function.

Immunologic tolerance that develops during the fetal or neonatal periods owing to exposure to tumor-specific antigens or an oncogenic virus may account for tumor growth in some animals when the immunologic surveillance system would otherwise afford protection. Bittner discovered in 1936 that C3H female mice transmitted mammary tumor virus (MTV) through the milk to their nursing young that later induced mammary tumors in a high percentage of their adult female progeny. Morton demonstrated that mice infected as neonates subsequently became tolerant to the tumor-specific antigens of the MTV-induced neoplasms and consequently could not be immunized against them as adults. Newborn mice foster-nursed on non-MTV-carrying mothers from another strain were not tolerant to the virus and, when adult, could be effectively immunized against the MTV-induced mammary tumors. The incidence of mammary tumors in these foster-nursed mice was much lower than in those nursed on MTV-infected mothers.

Low-dose immunologic tolerance similar to that seen with transplantation systems, but secondary to prolonged exposure to small amounts of weak tumor-specific antigens may account for the growth of some tumors. Low-dose tolerance may explain the development of metastases from breast cancer in immunocompetent patients many years after radical mastectomy.

CLINICAL EVIDENCE FOR TUMOR IMMUNITY IN HUMAN BEINGS

For obvious reasons the tumor transplantation techniques used to demonstrate these tumor-specific antigens of animal neoplasms were not applicable to the study of human tumors. Nevertheless, there are a number of well-documented clinical observations that suggest human host immune defenses against cancer. Although other physiologic, endocrinologic, and biologic explanations can be given for these observations, they are most easily explained on an immunologic basis:

1. Spontaneous regression of established tumors is a rare but well-documented phenomenon. Sometimes these regressions have followed a minor viral or bacterial infection. Although spontaneous regression has been observed in many different tumor types, it is most frequently seen in neuroblastomas of children, malignant melanoma, choriocarcinoma, adenocarcinoma of the kidney, and soft tissue sarcomas. However, spontaneous regression occurs less frequently than 0.5 percent in all types, except for neuroblastomas.

   Spontaneous regression of small pulmonary metastases following the surgical removal of the primary tumor has been observed and occurs most frequently in hypernephromas. Spontaneous regression also may account for the prolonged survival or cure of patients after incomplete surgical excision of the cancer.

2. Recurrence of tumor 10 years after successful treatment of the primary is often manifested by rapid tumor growth and death. Although endocrinologic changes may account for some of these observations in breast cancer, in other tumors this course suggests a host defense that inhibits the tumor growth during the disease-free interval.

3. Microscopic evidence of the histiocytic, plasmocytic, lymphocytic, and eosinophilic infiltration, which resembles that seen in an organ transplant or tumor transplant that is undergoing rejection in a human being, is associated with an improved prognosis. For example, in stomach cancer, these findings correlate better with survival than does adequate surgical removal of the tumor.

4. The presence of many tumor cells in the peripheral blood, lymphatics, pleural cavity, and operative wounds of patients

who subsequently never develop metastases suggests host immune defense.

5. There is a low incidence of successful growth of tumor tissue, or autotransplants in patients with advanced disease. The resistance against tumor growth was relative rather than absolute, since challenge with greater numbers of cancer cells usually resulted in tumor growth. The immune nature of this resistance was suggested when autologous leukocytes or plasma was mixed with these tumor cells, and cancer growth decreased in approximately half the patients studied.

IMMUNOLOGIC EVIDENCE FOR TUMOR-ASSOCIATED ANTIGENS IN HUMAN NEOPLASMS. During the past 20 years, a variety of sensitive immunologic techniques has demonstrated that many human neoplasms contained antigens that appear to be at least tumor-related if not uniquely specific. These antigens are capable of eliciting an immune response in human beings.

Humoral antibodies have been shown by the immunofluorescence, complement fixation, immunocytolosis, and immunodiffusion techniques. Cellular immunity has been demonstrated by lymphocyte-mediated cytotoxicity (the ability of lymphocytes to kill tumor cells in tissue culture), lymphocyte blastogenesis tests (the ability of lymphocytes to be stimulated to proliferate by tumor antigens), and migration inhibition tests (macrophages or other blood leukocytes inhibited in their migration by tumor-specific antigens). Finally, it has been found that cancer patients develop delayed cutaneous hypersensitivity reactions to tumor antigens. Thus, it has become increasingly apparent that some tumor antigens are capable of eliciting an immune response that can be monitored by the immunologic techniques used to study other types of immune reactions. The wide variety of human neoplasms in which tumor antigens have been detected are listed in Table 9-3. The precise specificity of these antigens remains controversial.

Various classes of antigens may be expressed by a malignant cell. For example, the fetal or differentiation antigens that are normal on the cells of the developing fetus, but not on adult normal cells, are expressed on many types of tumor cells. Group-specific antigens have been found on tumor cells of the same histologic type, on tumor cells of various histologic types, and on some normal cells. Individual-specific antigens appear to be like the highly restricted specific antigens on chemically in-

Table 9-3. HUMAN NEOPLASMS WITH DEMONSTRATED TUMOR-ASSOCIATED ANTIGENS

Burkitt's lymphoma
Malignant melanoma
Neuroblastoma
Osteosarcoma
Soft tissue sarcomas
Colon carcinoma
Breast carcinoma
Leukemia
Lung carcinoma
Bladder carcinoma
Renal carcinoma

duced sarcomas in animals. At issue is whether there are antigens on human tumors that are never expressed by the normal fetal or adult cells. These antigens would be truly tumor-specific. Most authorities agree that at the present time there is insufficient evidence for the existence of such tumor-specific antigens. Nevertheless, many types of *tumor-associated* antigens have been demonstrated whose specificity is restricted to human tumor and fetal tissues.

Differentiation, or Fetal, Antigens. Most tumor-associated antigens are located on the cell surface, where they are susceptible to immune attack by antibodies or lymphocytes. Thus, they are probably of considerable importance in the tumor-host relationship. However, there are other types of antigens that may not be located at the cell surface, although they are more or less specific for the neoplastic state. One such group is composed of the fetal, or carcinoembryonic, antigens.

Fetal antigens are produced by normal fetal organs during embryonic development. Their production is repressed shortly after birth, and they are not produced in significant quantities in normal adult organs. However, during neoplastic transformation, reversion of the cell to the embryonic state is accompanied by a renewed production of these fetal antigens. The fetal antigens are thought to represent the phenotypic expression of genes active during fetal life but not expressed during normal adult life. Their occurrence in tumors is thought to be secondary to alterations in the pattern of gene regulation as the result of the dedifferentiation and reversion of the cell to a primitive embryonic state.

The carcinoembryonic, or fetal, antigens initially were thought to be a useful means of detecting malignant disease before other clinical evidence of disease is apparent or as a detector of recurrence following therapy to provide a basis for further treatment. Fetal antigens that are common to many different histologic types of human neoplasms have been described, as have those that are restricted to the organ of origin.

α-Fetoglobulin. The α-fetoglobulin circulating in approximately 70 percent of patients with primary hepatomas is found in normal human fetal serum up to 1 year after birth. The fetal antigen also has been found occasionally in patients with gastric cancer, prostatic cancer, and primitive testicular tumors such as teratomas, although it appears to be relatively specific for hepatomas. The specificity of the test was demonstrated when adult monkeys were given hepatic carcinogens; α-fetoglobulin appeared in the serum of a high percentage of these monkeys prior to any histologic evidence of neoplastic change.

The α-fetoglobulin test has been clinically evaluated and found to be useful in the diagnosis of hepatomas. It is not positive in patients with rapidly dividing cells due to hepatic regeneration following liver resection or in those with cirrhosis.

Carcinoembryonic Antigen. The carcinoembryonic antigen (CEA) reported in 1965 by Gold and Freedman is another tumor-associated antigen occurring in fetal gut, liver, and pancreas during the first two trimesters of gestation. This antigen was originally thought to be specific for adenocarcinomas arising in the gastrointestinal tract and pancreas, but more recently it has been found in a variety of carcinomas, sarcomas, and lymphomas of many different histologic types.

Since the CEA appears in the bloodstream, it was initially thought to be of great importance as a diagnostic tool for malignant disease prior to other clinical evidence of cancer. A radioimmunoassay capable of detecting nanogram quantities of CEA in the blood was developed. However, elevated CEA levels were found in patients with a variety of nonmalignant conditions including alcoholic cirrhosis, pancreatitis, cholecystitis, colonic diverticulitis, and ulcerative colitis. This test has not been useful as a serologic method for the diagnosis of malignant tumor.

The serum levels of CEA do appear to correlate with the extent of known carcinomas of the colon. Metastasis to the liver is frequently associated with the highest levels. It has been shown that the CEA level drops during the postoperative period in those patients who have successful resection of the tumor. Patients who develop tumor recurrence often show a rise in CEA titer to the preoperative levels. Thus, CEA may be of some value for following the clinical course of patients with known malignant disease in order to detect evidence of recurrence prior to its becoming clinically detectable.

GENERAL IMMUNE COMPETENCE OF CANCER PATIENTS. A number of studies have tested the general functional capacity of the cancer patient's immunologic system. Such studies can be grouped into two categories— those concerned with humoral antibody production and those dealing with cell-mediated immune reactions.

Formation of humoral antibody to known antigenic substances has been studied by many investigators, who have found most cancer patients have the ability to form humoral antibodies against a variety of antigenic substances, even in the presence of advanced disease. There is no evidence to implicate a defect in humoral antibody production in most cancer patients.

The cell-mediated immune reactions have been measured by the cancer patient's ability to manifest delayed cutaneous hypersensitivity to a variety of common skin test antigens to which most normal persons are reactive by virtue of previous exposure such as to mumps, tuberculin, streptokinase, or streptodornase. In addition, a primary immune response was tested against a new antigen by studying the survival of skin allografts and by sensitizing patients to an antigen, such as the contact sensitizer dinitrochlorobenzene (DNCB). DNCB reacts with proteins in the skin and forms a hapten that sensitizes the immunocompetent patient (Fig. 9-10). Cell-mediated immunity can be studied with an in vitro test that requires lymphocyte recognition and proliferation in response to foreign tissue antigens or mitogens such as phytohemagglutinin.

These immunologic studies revealed that cell-mediated immune reactions are significantly impaired in patients with lymphoreticular neoplasia. Since these diseases usually diffusely involve the immune effector system, this

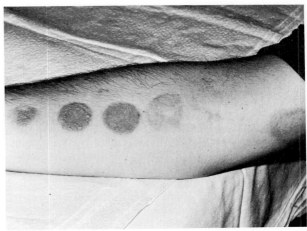

Fig. 9-10. Positive reaction to dinitrochlorobenzene (DNCB), showing initial exposure and subsequent challenges.

might be expected. In patients with solid tumors, the degree of immunologic impairment seems to vary with the extent of disease. Patients with localized tumors rarely have detectable defects in immunocompetence, whereas patients with advanced disease are often anergic.

The etiology of immunosuppression in cancer patients remains obscure. It is possible that immunosuppression could be the result of a humoral factor elaborated by the cancer cell or a complex physiologic response against the cancer cell that can depress normal cell-mediated immunity.

HYBRIDOMAS AND MONOCLONAL ANTIBODIES. Kohler and Milstein developed a method for producing large amounts of antibody with specificity against only one set of antigenic determinants. With this technique, plasma cells are fused to myeloma cells in such a way that a single clone of antibody-producing cells can be selected and grown in tissue culture indefinitely. This ability to produce a single clone of cells making huge quantities of a single antibody molecule has revolutionized immunology and, perhaps, tumor biology.

Much of the uncertainty and disagreement concerning tumor-specific antigens may be related to the assay systems used in their demonstration. The creation of hybridomas that produce antibodies against a single antigen makes the study of tumor immunology and tumor-specific antigens more precise.

Hybridomas have produced monoclonal antibody that appears to react with the tumor-specific antigens of target cells. Such antibody could be used to develop immunodiagnostic techniques. Radioimmunoassays for serum-borne tumor antigens and scans using labeled antibody have been reported. Specific monoclonal antibody has been used for immunotherapy of cancer patients with observed regressions in a significant proportion of treated patients. Attempts are being made to link specific monoclonal antibody to cytoxic agents such as Adriamycin or ricins in order to deliver lethal drugs to a tumor without affecting the normal tissues.

It is too early to assess the impact of hybridomas and monoclonal antibodies on human cancers. However, it is easy to envision a new age for immunodiagnosis and immunotherapy based on this technological advance.

POSSIBLE APPLICATIONS OF IMMUNOBIOLOGY TO CANCER THERAPY. There are many possible applications of cancer immunobiology to cancer therapy besides those of the immunotherapy. Immunoprevention by vaccine prepared from the common tumor antigens or tumor viral antigens is theoretically possible. However, because of the long latency period of most human neoplasms, it would require several decades to evaluate such a vaccine even if it were already in hand.

Immunobiology has great potential as a guide to standard cancer therapy. Immunologic monitoring of cancer patients undergoing therapy for malignant disease could be extremely useful in determining choice of therapy, as well as determining the patient's response to the therapy. Immunologic testing also may be useful in following the patient's response to certain therapeutic modalities that are known to be immunosuppressive, such as chemotherapy or radiation therapy, so that therapeutic regimens that are nonimmunosuppressive may be devised. Furthermore, with multiphase immune monitoring, it may become possible to carry out immunologic engineering in patients with defective immune responses. The deficiencies then might be corrected by appropriate adjunctive therapy once the site of the defect has been diagnosed.

PATHOLOGY

When confronted with a mass, the clinician must first determine whether it is neoplastic or inflammatory. If the mass is suspect for neoplasia, a biopsy is necessary before a specific diagnosis can be made.

In general, biopsy of a tumor must be obtained before therapy is instituted since the histology of the tumor will determine the mode of treatment. The pathologist's interpretation of materials submitted for microscopic examination depends not only upon experience and the quality of the material submitted but also upon the clinical history and findings on the patient and a review of any previous biopsy material. The features to which pathologists must direct their attention are partly histologic, that is, the arrangement of the tumor cells and their relation to the surrounding tissue, and partly cytologic, namely, the nature of the tumor cells and, in particular, the appearance of the nucleus and nucleoli.

The characteristics of benign and malignant neoplasms are listed in Table 9-4. *Anaplasia* means lack of differentiation. *Polarity* is the normal orderly alignment of epithelial cells, which are arranged in sheets. One of the early signs of malignant change is the loss of this normal polarity, so that the cells may present as a disorderly arrangement in relation to the surface and to each other. *Nuclear changes* of the malignant cells are often seen as enlarged and hyperchromic nuclei. These three features may all be seen before invasion of the deeper tissues has occurred. *Preinvasive carcinoma,* or *carcinoma in situ,* will demonstrate this change with no evidence of invasion of deeper histologic layers.

One of the most characteristic features of malignant disease is the ability to infiltrate and destroy deeper cellular layers and adjacent tissues, e.g., malignant colonic epithelial cells invading the muscular or serosal layers of the colon. In contrast, a benign tumor grows by expansion, compressing the surrounding tissues to form a capsule, but does not infiltrate these tissues.

On the basis of these microscopic criteria, the pathologist usually has no difficulty in determining whether the neoplasm is malignant or benign. Sometimes the microscopic diagnosis is difficult and opinions are divided among the different pathologists examining the tissue. When this happens, several options are open to the clinician: If the biopsy is not adequate, more material should be obtained. Special stains are sometimes helpful, such as oil red O, to show fat globules as in liposarcoma. Biopsy material may be examined by electron microscopy or even with immunologic stains to detect surface antigens such as those seen on subtypes of malignant lymphomas. Outside expert opinion may be useful, such as from the Armed Forces Institute of Pathology or the National Can-

Table 9-4. GENERAL CHARACTERISTICS OF BENIGN AND MALIGNANT NEOPLASMS

Characteristic	Benign neoplasms	Malignant neoplasms
Nuclear structure	Normal size, staining, and shape	Large, hyperchromatic with variation in size and shape
Mitotic figures	Usually rare	Frequent and perhaps atypical
Anaplasia	Absent	Varying degree
Polarity	Orderly arrangement	Disorderly arrangement
Local invasion or infiltration	Absent (except angioma)	Usually present
Capsule	Present	Absent or a pseudocapsule
Recurrence	Absent or rare	Frequent
Metastases	Absent	Frequent
Growth	Slow, self-limited	Often rapid
Systemic effects	Rare, except for neoplasms	Frequent

cer Institute, which act as referral centers for patients with unusual malignant neoplasms.

The electron microscope has been helpful in diagnosing some undifferentiated tumors, such as malignant melanoma and soft tissue sarcomas. Hormonal assay may be helpful, as in diagnosing a glucagon-producing alpha cell cancer of the pancreas. However, it is well to remember that sometimes tumors produce biologic substances that are not normally produced by the tissue from which they originated. For example, estrogen receptors have been found in neoplasms other than breast cancer.

It may not be possible, in certain situations, to differentiate histologically between a benign and a malignant neoplasm, as with the parathyroid carcinomas, giant cell sarcomas of bone, and thymomas. In these cases, clinical characteristics of the lesions in terms of the development of recurrence, metastases, and progressive growth may be the only differentiating criteria available to the clinician.

CLASSIFICATION OF NEOPLASMS. Many different classifications of tumors exist, but the most useful one is based upon the cell type of tissue of origin. When the neoplasm is undifferentiated, the special methods discussed above may help to classify it.

Neoplasms arising from epithelial cells regardless of whether in the ectoderm or the entoderm are known as carcinomas. Sarcomas arise from connective tissue and cells of mesenchymal origin and include tumors of fibrous, muscular, fatty, vascular, and skeletal origin. Teratoma signifies a neoplasm in which anaplastic, immature somatic cells, comparable with blastoderm, are usually dominant; it exhibits varying degrees of differentiation into mature somatic cells of ectodermal, mesodermal, and entodermal types. Teratomas occur in the testis, ovary, and mediastinum. A simplified classification of benign and malignant neoplasms arising from different sites is given in Table 9-5.

GRADING OF MALIGNANCY. Broders classified carcinomas into four grades according to their degree of differentiation, the appearance of cells, their nuclei, and the number of mitotic figures. On this basis, the least malignant are classified as grade 1, and the most malignant are grade 4. In general, the lower-grade, more differentiated neoplasms are less malignant and tend to metastasize less frequently than the higher-grade, more anaplastic ones.

CARCINOMA IN SITU AND PREMALIGNANT LESIONS. Carcinoma in situ is a lesion with the cytologic characteristics of malignant tumors but with no detectable invasion into the surrounding tissue or infiltration into deeper cell layers. Most likely these in situ lesions develop into invasive cancer after variable delay periods. The interval between the detection of carcinoma in situ of the cervix and invasive carcinoma may be 10 to 15 years. Carcinoma in situ also occurs in the skin, bronchus, stomach, and pharynx. When these lesions are adequately treated, a cure is assured.

ROUTES FOR SPREAD OF NEOPLASMS. There are few subjects of greater importance to the oncologist than the spread of cancer. Much is known about the routes of spread but little about the conditions that determine that spread. Some cancers are metastatic at the time of their clinical discovery, while others of the same type and in the same organ tissue may remain localized for years.

Metastases may entirely dominate the clinical picture, while the primary tumor remains latent and asymptomatic. Some patients present with metastatic cancer and no evidence of a primary site. For example, metastases to the brain secondary to silent cancers in the bronchus or the gastrointestinal tract are often mistaken for primary brain tumors.

Knowledge of the particular manner in which different types of cancer spread is important in planning therapy. In general, a malignant tumor may spread by four routes: directly by infiltrating surrounding tissue; via lymphatics;

Table 9-5. SIMPLE CLASSIFICATION OF NEOPLASMS

Tissue of origin	Site of origin	Benign	Malignant
Epithelial origin (ectoderm or entoderm)	Skin, mouth, larynx, lung, esophagus, urinary tract, cervix	Papilloma	Squamous cell carcinoma
	Breast, stomach, colon, pancreas, liver	Adenoma	Adenocarcinoma
Mesodermal origin	Fibrous tissue	Fibroma	Fibrosarcoma
	Muscular tissue	Leiomyoma, rhabdomyoma	Leiomyosarcoma, rhabdomyosarcoma
	Fatty tissue	Lipoma	Liposarcoma
	Vascular tissue	Angioma	Angiosarcoma
	Hemopoietic tissue		Leukemia, multiple myeloma, lymphoma
	Bone	Osteoma, chondroma	Osteogenic sarcoma, chondrosarcoma
Special types:			
Melanocytes	Skin, eye	Nevus	Malignant melanoma
Neural tissue	Brain, spinal cord nerve	Astrocytoma Ganglioneuroma	Glioblastoma multiforme Neuroblastoma
Trophoblast	Placenta, testis	Chorioepithelioma	Choriocarcinoma
Notochord	Spine	Chordoma	Chordoma
Blastoderm	Mediastinum, ovary, testis	Teratoma	Teratoma

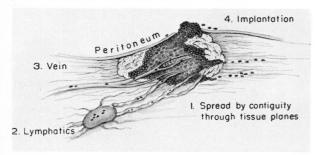

Fig. 9-11. Four mechanisms of the dissemination of cancer cells. This is a diagrammatic illustration; the original tumor could be one of many organs with cells disseminating by the four mechanisms. (From: *Cole WH et al: Dissemination of Cancer. New York, Appleton-Century-Crofts, 1961, with permission.*)

by vascular invasion; or by implantation in serous cavities (Fig. 9-11). Knowledge of the patterns of neoplastic spread in different types of cancer is important in planning definitive therapy. However, many cancers will spread by more than one route, and an orderly course of metastases cannot be relied upon. For example, many patients with breast cancer or melanoma may manifest distant metastatic disease in lungs or liver but will never develop evidence of lymph node metastases. Metastatic patterns of various types of human tumors are summarized in Table 9-6.

Direct Extension. Cancer cells may spread by direct extension through tissue spaces. Some neoplasms, such as soft tissue sarcomas and adenocarcinomas of the stomach or esophagus, may extend for considerable distances (10 to 15 cm) along tissue planes beyond the palpable tumor mass. Other neoplasms, such as basal cell carcinoma of

skin, rarely extend for more than a few millimeters beyond the visible margin. Even though some of the central nervous system tumors rarely spread, their location can cause death by interfering with vital CNS functions.

Lymphatic Spread. Tumor cells can readily enter lymphatics and extend along these channels by permeation or embolism through the regional lymphatics to lymph nodes. Permeation is the growth of a colony of tumor cells along the course of the lymph vessel. This occurs commonly in the skin lymphatics in carcinoma of the breast and in the perineural lymphatics in carcinoma of the prostate.

Spread along the lymphatics of embolism to the regional nodes or distant lymph nodes is of much greater importance. Lymph node metastases are first confined to the subcapsular space; at this stage the node is not enlarged and may appear normal to the naked eye. Gradually the tumor cells permeate the sinusoids and replace the parenchyma. There is little direct spread from node to node, because the capsule is not penetrated until a late stage. The tumor cells travel by anastomosing lymphatics, and the spread occurs in other nodes by way of collateral lymph channels. When a lymph node containing tumor is more than 3 cm in diameter, tumor has usually extended beyond the capsule into the perinodal fat.

The lymph from the abdominal organs and lower extremities drains into the cisterna chyli and then into the thoracic duct, which finally opens into the left jugular vein. Tumor cells probably freely pass from the lymph to the bloodstream. Originally, oncologists believed that solid neoplasms involved regional lymph nodes and then spread into the bloodstream by drainage through the lymphatics into the thoracic duct and to other parts of the body. An alternative explanation favored by many oncol-

Table 9-6. ESTIMATED FREQUENCY* OF PATTERNS OF NEOPLASTIC SPREAD FOR COMMON HUMAN NEOPLASMS

Neoplasm	Hematogenous	Lymphatic	Local infiltration (expressed as local recurrence)
Adenocarcinoma			
Breast	4	3	2
Colon	3	3	1
Stomach	4	4	3
Pancreas	4	4	3
Epidermoid carcinoma			
Lung	4	3	2
Oral pharynx	1	3	3
Larynx	1	3	2
Cutaneous neoplasm			
Squamous cell carcinoma	1	2	1
Melanomas	3	3	2
Basal cell carcinomas	0	0	1
Sarcomas			
Bones	4	1	1
Soft tissue	4	1	3
Brain neoplasms	0	0	4

* 0—Does not occur, 1—1 to 15 percent, 2—15 to 30 percent, 3— > 30 percent, and 4— > 50 percent.

ogists assumes that the presence of cancer cells in regional lymph nodes indicates an unfavorable host-tumor relationship and the likelihood of distant metastases.

Lymphatic involvement is extremely common in epithelial neoplasms of all types, except basal cell carcinoma of the skin, which does not metastasize to regional lymphatics. Sarcomas metastasize to lymph nodes only 2 to 5 percent of the time.

VASCULAR SPREAD. Cancer cells may reach the bloodstream either through the thoracic duct or by invasion of blood vessels. Capillaries are almost always invaded. The veins are invaded frequently, the arteries rarely. The chief reason for the striking differences in invasion characteristics between arteries and veins appears to be that lymphatics frequently penetrate the walls of the large veins from without and form a plexus reaching to the subendothelial region, thus providing a portal of entry for tumor cells through the vein wall. When the vascular endothelium is destroyed, a thrombus forms that is quickly invaded by tumor. This combination of thrombus and tumor may detach to form large tumor emboli. Vascular invasion is commonly seen in both carcinomas and sarcomas and is associated with a poor prognosis. Some types of neoplasms have a remarkable tendency to grow as a solid column along the course of veins, for example, renal carcinomas and sarcomas. Renal carcinomas have been known to grow out of the renal vein into the inferior vena cava and up the inferior vena cava to the right atrium.

Spread through Serous Cavities. Tumor cells occasionally gain entrance to serous cavities via direct growth of tumor through the wall of an organ. Many tumor cells are capable of growth in suspension without a supporting matrix and may grow and spread within the peritoneal cavity or attach to serous surfaces. In either case, it is common for tumor cells to spread widely when they encounter a space lined with a serous surface. Thus, widespread peritoneal seeding is commonly seen with gastrointestinal neoplasms and tumors of ovarian origin. A similar mechanism appears to operate in the case of malignant gliomas, which may spread widely within the central nervous system via cerebral spinal fluid.

CLINICAL MANIFESTATIONS OF CANCER

The clinical presentation of cancer is varied and inconstant. Cancer may appear as an asymptomatic lesion too small to be seen without magnification or special studies such as a mammogram. It may appear as an asymptomatic lump, or the patient may complain of symptoms that are subsequently found to be caused by an underlying malignancy. Often, symptoms are nonspecific and resemble those of nonmalignant diseases.

The clinical abnormalities produced by advancing neoplastic diseases may be grouped into two categories—those abnormalities which stem directly from the presence of a tumor mass and those physiologic derangements which are produced indirectly. By teaching patients those key symptoms of cancer which require medical evaluation, earlier diagnosis and treatment may be achieved.

Table 9-7. CANCER'S SEVEN WARNING SIGNALS

Change in bowel or bladder habits
A sore that does not heal
Unusual bleeding or discharge
Thickening or lump in breast or elsewhere
Indigestion or difficulty in swallowing
Obvious change in wart or mole
Nagging cough or hoarseness

The onset of the neoplastic state is difficult to date in human beings. As previously discussed, a prolonged latent or induction period is likely before clinically detectable disease evolves. Therefore, the use of the word "early" in describing a cancer may lead to confusion. To avoid this, we will use the terms "early" and "late" in relation to the clinical stage of a neoplasm rather than to indicate its duration in the body. When viewed in this manner, the curable cancer may have been present a long time prior to its diagnosis and therapy. The term *early* usually means a neoplasm that can be effectively treated. These neoplasms are small rather than large, do not extend into essential organs, and have not metastasized. Some lesions that have been present for years still may be early, whereas other lesions with more rapid growth rates may be *late* even if present for only a few months.

The "Seven Danger Signals of Cancer," as formulated by the American Cancer Society, are listed in Table 9-7. These may be helpful in the ongoing effort to educate people and increase the frequency of early diagnosis for certain major tumors. The more common patterns of clinical presentation, and some of the more common syndromes related to cancer will be discussed in detail in the paragraphs that follow.

Carcinoma in situ and other premalignant lesions were discussed earlier under pathology and will not be discussed further here.

SIGNS OF EXPANSILE GROWTH. The signs attributable to the expansile growth of a tumor depend upon its location. When the neoplasm is either on or near the surface of the body, it may present simply as a visible or palpable mass. In the gastrointestinal, biliary, respiratory, and urinary tracts, signs are frequently related to obstruction. Examples are vomiting, jaundice, cough, or urinary retention. Within the central nervous system, expansile growth may cause pain, paralysis, or sensory loss.

Expansile growth of a tumor may also result in destruction of host tissues. Examples are pathologic fractures, hepatic insufficiency, and Addison's disease.

SIGNS OF INFILTRATIVE GROWTH. Pain, numbness, and paralysis may result when tumor infiltrates nerves. Frequently, signs of nerve invasion are also signs of incurability. Examples are lumbosacral plexus pain in cancer of the cervix and rectum, dorsal and lumbar spine pain in cancer of the pancreas, and the shoulder and arm pain and palsy when carcinoma of the lung infiltrates the brachial plexus. Other signs of infiltration generally denoting incurability are thickening of the uterine ligaments

Table 9-8. UNKNOWN PRIMARY TUMORS PRESENTING AS METASTASES

Site of metastasis	Primary neoplasm
Lymph nodes:	
Cervical nodes	Nasopharynx, pharynx, oral cavity, thyroid, larynx, lymphomas
Supraclavicular nodes	Bronchus, breast, stomach, esophagus, pancreas, colon, testis, ovary, cervix
Axillary nodes	Breast, melanoma, lymphoma
Inguinal nodes	Genitalia, anus, melanoma
Skin and subcutaneous tissues	Melanoma, breast, bronchus, stomach, kidney
Lung	Breast, colon, kidney, stomach, testis, melanoma, thyroid, sarcomas
Liver	Stomach, colon, breast, pancreas, bronchus
Ovary	Stomach, colon
Bones	Breast, bronchus, prostate, thyroid
Central nervous system	Breast, bronchus, kidney, colon
Serous cavities	Bronchus, breast, ovary, lymphoma

in cancer of the cervix and fixation to the chest wall in breast cancer.

SIGNS OF TUMOR NECROSIS: BLEEDING AND INFECTION. Tumors may become necrotic, ulcerate, and bleed. Fatigue and weakness may be the only symptoms or signs in cancer of the stomach or right colon, because the tumor ulceration and bleeding have resulted in anemia. If a cancer becomes ulcerated and infected, the signs of inflammation include edema, pain, tenderness, and fever. The inflammation caused by cecal cancer can mimic the clinical symptoms of acute appendicitis or cholecystitis. Therefore, response of such inflammation to antibiotics or the healing of an ulcer does *not* necessarily indicate a nonneoplastic lesion.

Tumor necrosis at any site may produce fever, leukocytosis, elevation of sedimentation rate, anorexia, and malaise. Such necrosis constitutes one of the causes of the "fever of unknown origin." Keller and Williams, in studies of 46 patients with unexplained fever, found that in 19 who underwent exploratory laparotomy the cause of the fever was intraabdominal malignant disease.

UNKNOWN PRIMARY TUMORS PRESENTING AS METASTASES. Usually the site of origin of a metastasis is known. However, the initial presentation of a tumor may be at a distance from its origin. In fact, the primary neoplasm giving rise to the metastases may have regressed completely and may never be detected in some neoplasms, such as malignant melanoma and carcinomas of the oral pharynx. Surgical resection of the metastatic lesions may result in long-term cure without the site of the primary ever being detected.

The most frequent sites of presentation of metastatic neoplasms are the cervical and supraclavicular lymph nodes, lungs, liver, bones, and brain. The most common metastatic sites for unknown primary neoplasms are listed in Table 9-8.

SYSTEMIC MANIFESTATION OF MALIGNANT DISEASE. Tumors may have a variety of remote and systemic effects that contribute to morbidity. Cancer patients frequently develop unusual symptoms and physiologic derangements that cannot be attributed to the mechanical presence of primary or metastatic disease, or to physiologic changes resulting from hormones normally secreted by the tissue of origin.

Some symptoms, such as the cachexia of carcinomatosis, may result from competition between the tumor and the host for basic components of the same metabolic pool. However, the pathogenesis of many of these disorders is unknown. Some of these nonmetastatic, systemic manifestations of malignant tumors are thought to result from (1) the ectopic production of known hormones; (2) the secretion of unidentified, physiologically active substances that do not resemble known hormones but that have hormonelike effects; (3) autoimmune phenomena in which the host is sensitized to an antigen from the tumor; and/or (4) toxic substances secreted from the tumor.

The nonmetastatic clinical manifestations of malignant disease and the neoplasms with which they are associated are presented in Table 9-9. Sometimes palliative surgery is indicated to treat these systemic manifestations, for example, resection of metastases that are producing hormones that induce hypercalcemia, or hypoglycemia.

CANCER DIAGNOSIS AND STAGING EXTENT OF CANCER

Diagnosis

Diagnosis of cancer should proceed in an orderly fashion: careful history, thorough physical examination with examination of the blood and urine, and investigation of suspicious findings by appropriate radiologic examinations and radioisotope scans.

A *history* of any of the following is suspicious and should prompt a search for cancer: weight loss; loss of appetite; bleeding or a discharge from any body orifice or nipple; a sore that is slow to heal; changing color or size of a mole; persistent cough or wheeze; change in voice; difficulty in swallowing; growing lump either in or under the skin, in the breast, in the abdomen, or in the muscles; and/or change of bowel habits.

Physical examination includes a thorough search of the entire skin surface for squamous cell and basal cell carcinomas, indurated lesions, ulcers, suspicious or irritated nevi, nodules, and other signs of malignant disease. Lymph nodes should be palpated for enlargement. Breasts should be carefully examined. All body orifices should be examined. A Papanicolaou smear from the cervix should be obtained prior to a bimanual pelvic exami-

Table 9-9. SYSTEMIC MANIFESTATIONS OF MALIGNANT DISEASE

Clinical manifestations	Associated neoplasms	Clinical manifestations	Associated neoplasms
Cutaneous		Hormonal and metabolic effects of nonendocrine tumors	
Acanthosis nigricans	Cancer of stomach, lung, and breast		
Dermatomyositis	Cancer of stomach, breast, lung, and ovary	Hypoglycemia (mechanism unknown)	Retroperitoneal or mediastinal mesenchymal tumors, hepatic tumors
Erythema multiforme, exfoliative dermatitis, bullous pemphigoid	Allergic response to a variety of neoplasms, lymphoma, myeloma	Cushing's syndrome (increased ACTH)	Cancer of the lung, malignant thymoma, pancreatic cancer
Peutz-Jeghers syndrome	Intestinal polyposis	Hypercalcemia (increased PTH, vitamin D-like substances or bone destruction)	Cancer of lung, kidney, breast, uterus, sarcomas, hemopoietic neoplasms
Hematologic			
Abdominal red cell mass			
Erythrocytosis (increased erythropoietin)	Renal cell carcinoma, hepatoma, uterine myoma, cerebellar tumors, pheochromocytoma	Hyponatremia (increased ADH)	Cancer of lung, intracranial tumors
Anemia:		Hyperthyroidism (increased TSH)	Choriocarcinoma, testicular embryonal carcinoma
Myelophthisic	All tumors	Precocious puberty and/or gynecomastia (increased gonadotropin)	Hepatoma, lung, adrenal cancer, testicular tumors
Hypoproliferative	Thymoma, renal cell carcinoma		
Hemolytic	Hemopoietic neoplasm	Zollinger-Ellison syndrome (increased gastrin secretion)	Pancreatic nonbeta islet cell adenomas
Miscellaneous causes (infection, bleeding, radiation effects, uremia, etc.)		Elevated liver enzymes	Renal cell carcinoma
		Anorexia and weight loss	Most neoplasms
Abnormal leukocyte or platelet mass		Hyperuricemia	Hemopoietic neoplasms
Leukemoid reactions	Miscellaneous neoplasms	Atypical carcinoid syndrome	Pancreatic duct, islet cell, gastric, thyroid, and oat cell cancer of lung
Leukopenia	Hemopoietic neoplasms, lung, pancreas		
Thrombocytosis		Nonmetastatic neuromuscular	
Coagulation and bleeding disorder		Multifocal leukoencephalopathy	Hemopoietic neoplasms
Disseminated intravascular coagulation (DIC)	Mucin-secreting adenocarcinoma	Subacute cerebellar degeneration	Multiple neoplasms, especially of lung, ovary, and breast
Vascular			
Thrombophlebitis	Cancer of lung, reproductive tract, pancreas, and breast	Polyneuropathy and/or myopathy	Multiple neoplasms, especially of lung, ovary, and breast
Fibrinogen deficiency (increased fibrinolysis)	Cancer of prostate and lung	Myasthenia gravis	Thymoma
Flushing, vasodilatation, violaceous skin, asthma	Carcinoid tumor		

SOURCE: Modified from Owens AH Jr: Neoplastic diseases, in Harvey AM et al: *The Principles and Practice of Medicine.* New York, Appleton-Century-Crofts, 1972, with permission.

nation. Rectal examination should include proctoscopic examination of patients who have hemorrhoids or rectal symptoms. The oral pharynx should be examined with special attention to the floor of the mouth. Indirect laryngoscopy should be performed if the patient is hoarse, has a neck mass, or is suspected of having an intrathoracic neoplasm or cancer of the thyroid gland.

Laboratory examination should include complete blood cell count, urinalysis, examination of stool for occult blood, and chest radiograph. Other tests should be ordered where indicated by symptoms. Before operating on a patient for cure or palliation, a metastatic work-up should be done, directed by symptoms and the most likely site of metastases. Prior to extensive disfiguring or disabling procedures, tomograms of the lungs, bone marrow biopsy, scalene node biopsy, isotope scans, or arteri-

ography may be useful in determining whether the neoplasm is still localized. Cytologic examination should be performed if a pleural effusion or ascites is present.

Diagnosis of solid tumors rests upon locating and performing a biopsy of the lesion. This goal is most easily fulfilled when the tumor is near the body surface or involves one of the orifices of the body that can be examined with appropriate visual instruments, such as a bronchoscope, proctoscope, or cystoscope. Carcinomas of the breast, tongue, or rectum can be seen or palpated, and a portion can be excised for definitive diagnosis.

The most difficult cancers to diagnose, and unfortunately the most lethal ones, occur in the internal organs. Space-occupying lesions in the internal organs may grow quite large before causing symptoms. Techniques that may be useful in localizing such lesions include barium examinations of the gastrointestinal tract; examination of the bronchial tree by endoscopy media; selective arteriography of major vessels supplying internal organs; radioisotopes and radiopaque dyes that concentrate in various organs such as the liver, gallbladder, kidney, and lymph nodes; and ultrasonography and abdominal computer-assisted tomography (CT scans are rapidly becoming the most useful investigative studies for intraabdominal tumors). Exploratory surgery is often required to confirm the diagnosis and to obtain biopsy.

CANCER DETECTION EXAMINATION. Any given individual stands approximately 1 chance in 4 of developing cancer during his or her lifetime. Therefore, in screening 1000 persons for an entire life span, we will find cancer in 250 of them. Since a person can harbor more than one primary cancer and a second lesion will develop with increasing frequency as the number of people who have survived the first one increases, we might count on a very crude estimate of 350 cancers in our population of 1000. Since we expect people to live an average of 72 years, we must carry out 72,000 annual examinations to discover 350 cancers, or less than 5 cancers per 1000 examinations. By directing our search to the middle and late adult years when the incidence is highest, we might conceivably double the yield to 10 per 1000. Thus, the chances of detecting cancer in a given annual examination are no more than 1 in 100 even under the most optimal circumstances.

The problem of cancer detection is further complicated by the relative insensitivity of our methods for clinical cancer detection. The earliest neoplasms must be at least 1 cm in size before they are detectable by physical examination, and often tumor masses up to 10 cm in diameter will go undetected if in the liver, retroperitoneum, or other "silent" areas.

Both physicians and patients have been rather slow to adopt the habit of periodic examinations to detect asymptomatic tumors. Although approximately 1 in 4 Americans will develop cancer in a lifetime, it is difficult to determine whether mass screening will have an impact on the cure rate for cancer. The problem most likely will be solved by selecting certain high-risk groups and screening those periodically. For example, Papanicolaou smears yearly in women over thirty have markedly decreased the death rate from carcinoma of the cervix. The use of mammography to screen postmenopausal women may also have an impact on reducing the death rate from breast cancer. However, periodic chest x-rays or proctoscopy may not affect the cure rate for carcinoma of the lung or colon. Much research remains to be done in the field of cancer detection and screening before routine screening examinations can be expected to improve survival.

Perhaps as more sensitive methods are developed for detection of cancers at an earlier stage, screening can be done more effectively. One hope for such a screening test has been the development of immunologic assays for detection of tumor antigens or antibodies in the patient's serum. Examples of these assays include those for α-fetoprotein and carcinoembryonic antigen.

BIOPSY. It is imperative that microscopic proof of malignant disease be obtained prior to institution of treatment, since significant morbidity and mortality may result from all forms of cancer therapy. The specific type of antitumor therapy will depend upon the histologic type of tumor which must be established by biopsy. Significant errors have been made when biopsies were not obtained; examples are radical mastectomies for fat necrosis and radiation therapy for renal cysts.

Even when biopsy reports from another hospital are available, the slides of the previous biopsy must be obtained and reviewed prior to the institution of therapy. This is essential because, not infrequently and particularly in rare neoplasms, an erroneous interpretation may have been made. *Definitive therapy cannot be planned rationally without knowing the nature of the neoplastic lesion.*

Three methods for biopsy of suspicious tissue are commonly used. They are the *needle,* the *incisional,* and the *excisional,* or open, biopsy; each has its advantages and disadvantages. Regardless of method used, the pathologic interpretation of the tumor mass can be valid only if a representative section of tumor is obtained. A problem of "sampling error" can occur with the needle and the incisional biopsies when only a small portion of the total tumor mass is submitted for pathologic examination.

Needle biopsy is the simplest method and may be used for biopsy of subcutaneous masses, muscular masses, and some internal organs, such as liver, kidney, and pancreas. Further, this method is inexpensive and causes minimal disturbance of the surrounding tissue. The danger of implanting tumor cells in a needle track during aspiration biopsy is extremely small and can be avoided if the location of the needle track is such that it can be excised easily at the time of the definitive surgical procedure. Needle biopsy may be disadvantageous when the specimen is quite small and not representative of the total tumor, or the needle may miss the space-occupying lesion. Hence, a needle or aspiration biopsy does require experience to interpret. A negative report for malignant disease is always viewed with skepticism and should be followed by incisional or excisional biopsy if there is any doubt. Some centers have used fine-needle aspiration cytology. In this procedure, a fine needle is inserted into the tumor, and strands of single cells are obtained for cytologic diagnosis. This procedure is extremely useful for a number of tumors but requires considerable skill to interpret and should only be done by an experienced pathologist.

Incisional biopsy involves removal of only a portion of a tumor mass for pathologic examination. It is best performed under circumstances where, if tumor cells are spilled at the time of biopsy, the incisional wound can be encompassed and totally excised at the time of the definitive surgical procedure. Incisional biopsy includes removal of portions of tumor with forceps during endoscopic examination of the bronchus, esophagus, rectum, and bladder. Incisional biopsy is indicated for deeper subcutaneous or muscular tumor masses when needle biopsy fails to establish a diagnosis.

The incisional biopsy is also used when a tumor is so large that total local excision would prejudice any subsequent adequate, wide, locally curative resection because of the wide tissue planes that are necessarily exposed by biopsy. Such biopsy should take a deep section of tumor, as well as a margin of normal tissue, if possible. Incisional biopsy does suffer from the same hazard as the needle biopsy in that the removed portion may not be representative of all the involved tissue; hence, a negative biopsy does not preclude the presence of cancer in the remaining mass. Another theoretic objection to the incisional method is the possibility that the surgeon may seed cancer cells into the operative wound or that exposed open lymphatics may transport the cells to distant sites. Despite these dangers, one must keep in mind that definitive surgical procedures cannot be planned rationally without knowing the nature of the neoplastic lesion.

Excisional biopsy is total local removal of the tumor mass. This is used for small, discrete masses, 2 to 3 cm in diameter, when local removal will not interfere with the wider excision required for permanent local control. A major advantage of an excisional biopsy is that it gives the entire lesion to the pathologist. However, this method is contraindicated in large tumor masses because, again, the biopsy procedure often scatters tumor cells throughout a large biopsy incision that must be widely and totally encompassed by subsequent definitive surgical procedures. Therefore, excisional biopsy is usually contraindicated for skeletal and soft tissue sarcomas, although it is ideally suitable for superficial squamous or basal cell carcinomas and malignant melanomas. Surgeons should always mark the excisional biopsy margins with sutures so that if removal is incomplete, they will know where tumor margin was positive should further excision be indicated.

Biopsy incisions should be closed with meticulous hemostasis, since it may be possible for a collecting hematoma to extend tumor cell contamination by widespread infiltration of tissue planes. Contaminated instruments, gloves, gowns, and drapes should be discarded and replaced with noncontaminated substitutes when the definitive procedure is to follow immediately after the biopsy procedure.

The excisional method is principally used for polypoid lesions of the colon, for thyroid and breast nodules, for small skin lesions, and when the pathologist cannot make a definitive diagnosis from tissue removed by incisional biopsy. An unbiopsied lump is surgically removed when the suspicious character of the lesion, the need for its removal whatever the diagnosis, and the nonmutilating nature of the operation make such an approach reasonably definitive. Examples of such procedures include hemithyroidectomy for thyroid nodules, partial colectomy for lesions at any point beyond the reach of the sigmoidoscope, or a right colectomy for a cecal mass that might be inflammatory or neoplastic.

Lymph nodes should be carefully selected for biopsy. Cervical lymph nodes should not be biopsied until a careful search for a primary tumor has been made. Indirect laryngoscopy, pharyngoscopy, esophagoscopy, bronchoscopy, and thyroid scan may be included in the workup. Enlargement of the upper cervical nodes is usually due to metastases from laryngeal, oropharyngeal, and nasopharyngeal neoplasms. Supraclavicular nodes are more frequently enlarged from metastases originating in the thoracic or abdominal cavity.

The specimen may be prepared for pathologic examination by either frozen or permanent sections. Frozen sections are made immediately, and pathologic diagnosis can be obtained within 10 to 20 min. Although frozen sections may be as adequate as permanent sections for diagnosis of some neoplasms, most pathologists would prefer to make a definitive diagnosis in questionable cases on permanent sections. Although such sections require 1 to 2 days for processing, it is usually best to have a definite diagnosis before discussing the therapeutic options. Therefore, frozen sections are used when the diagnosis is required at the time of major surgery and when it is in the patient's best interests to have the definitive resectional surgery carried out at that time.

Occasionally, an exploratory thoracotomy or laparotomy will be necessary to obtain tissue for microscopic examination and confirmation of diagnosis. As a general rule, regardless of the clinical picture, the neoplastic nature of the disease process must be confirmed by frozen section examination prior to closure of the wound. This is critical because the permanent sections may fail to confirm the neoplastic nature of the pathologic process, and the patient will have experienced the morbidity of operation without obtaining a diagnosis.

Exfoliative cytology constitutes one possible method for the early diagnosis of certain types of neoplasms. This technique is based upon the fact that cancer cells are shed from the surfaces of neoplasms arising in epithelial-lined body cavities and orifices, such as the vagina, bronchus, and stomach. These cells can be collected, stained, and recognized as malignant because of their individual morphologic changes.

Staging Extent of Cancer

The extent of the patient's tumor by clinical evaluation at the time of initial presentation is called the *clinical stage*. In addition to making an exact histologic diagnosis of cancer, it is essential that the clinical stage of the disease be determined prior to making a decision regarding therapy. This is especially important when the patient initially presents for treatment, but also it is often desirable to repeat some of the diagnostic procedures periodically during the patient's course in order to assess his or her true status. The recognized importance of this staging has led to a variety of international and national attempts to standardize the staging of the patient with cancer. To date, no single system has been universally accepted (Table 9-10). Stage I usually indicates a neoplasm confined to its primary site of origin, Stage II indicates metastases to the regional lymph nodes, and Stages III and IV indicate distant metastatic spread.

The Union Internationale Contre Cancrum (UICC) has attempted to standardize one system for all nations. This has been called the TNM system because it relies on a statement of tumor extent in terms of the primary tumor (T), presence or absence of node metastases (N), and the

Table 9-10. CHRONOLOGY AND TYPES OF
STAGING RECOGNIZED BY THE AMERICAN
JOINT COMMITTEE ON CANCER*

Stage	Comment
cTNM	*Clinical-diagnostic staging:* The extent of disease using all information available prior to first definitive treatment, including pathologic confirmation of extent of disease by biopsy or invasive techniques
pTNM	*Postsurgical resection-pathologic staging:* The extent of disease using all data available at the time of surgery and on examination of a completely resected specimen
sTNM	*Surgical-evaluative staging:* The extent of disease using all clinical information available plus that obtained on surgical exploration; usually done for a few inaccessible tumors that are not amenable to definitive resection
rTNM	*Retreatment staging:* The classification when restaging is necessary for additional or secondary definitive treatment after a (disease-free) interval following first treatment
aTNM	*Autopsy staging:* Used only when the cancer is first diagnosed at autopsy

* From Beahrs OH, Myers MH (eds): *Manual for Staging of Cancer,* 2d ed., published for the American Joint Committee on Cancer by Philadelphia, Lippincott, 1983, p 6, with permission.

presence or absence of distant metastases (M). The system was developed following careful analysis of the results of treatment in patients with various constellations of clinical findings. It was found that patients with larger tumors did less well than those with smaller tumors; hence, the separation of various stages on the basis of tumor size. For different tumors size criteria vary, but in this system decreasing prognosis is indicated by increasing numbers after the T, such as T_1, T_2, T_3, or T_4 for lesions of increasing sizes. The presence or absence of regional spread is usually indicated by variations in the secondary category, under N for nodes. The absence of nodal metastasis is designated as N_0; the presence of nodal metastasis is N_1; for more extensive nodal involvement, additional numbers may be used. Finally, distant metastases are indicated by adding a subscript 1 following M for metastases, or a subscript 0 for their absence. Thus, a small lesion that has neither spread to regional nodes nor metastasized would be designated as a $T_1N_0M_0$ lesion. A lesion that was larger and involved regional nodes but without distant metastases might be identified as a $T_2N_1M_0$ lesion. A larger neoplasm with both regional and distant metastases would be designated a $T_3N_1M_1$ lesion. For some tumor types such as soft tissue sarcoma a G for grade of malignancy is added. High-grade tumors are more anaplastic and tend to metastasize sooner.

The American Joint Committee on Cancer recognizes several types of cancer staging schemas (Table 9-10). The clinical-diagnostic staging (cTNM) represents the extent of disease prior to first definitive treatment. Postsurgical resection-pathologic staging (pTNM) provides additional information after operation, and is especially useful in planning adjuvant therapy for many types of tumors. Other staging types include surgical-evaluative staging (sTNM) usually for tumors that cannot be resected, retreatment staging (rTNM) usually after a disease-free interval, and autopsy staging (aTNM).

The importance of accurate staging when designating a therapeutic program for a patient with cancer cannot be overemphasized. It is an important consideration when comparing the results of therapy in different centers, and as therapeutic methods for cancer improve, it is only by careful staging that new forms of therapy can be appropriately evaluated. For example, only accurate staging can identify patients, such as those with Stage II breast cancer, whose more advanced disease is still potentially curable by adjuvant therapy. These patients probably have subclinical metastases at the time of operation.

Unfortunately, one of the great deficiencies of the present staging methods is their inability to detect subclinical microscopic metastatic lesions. Many patients who are treated for apparently localized cancers already have disseminated metastases. For example, about one-half of those patients who have cancer of the breast and who undergo mastectomy have subclinical distant metastasis at the time of the operation.

THERAPY

General Considerations

At present, approximately 55 percent of all cancer patients are treated by surgical resection (40 percent by surgery alone); 34 percent by radiation therapy (16 percent by radiation therapy alone); and 22 percent by chemotherapy alone or in combination with the other modalities. As the use of chemotherapy as an adjuvant to surgery increases, it is likely that a much larger percentage of patients will have chemotherapy as part of their cancer treatment. At the present time, most patients with potentially curable solid tumors are treated with surgery. In an effort to improve overall cure rates, radiation and chemotherapy can be added to the surgical procedure.

Surgery and radiation therapy today represent the most successful means of dealing with cancer as long as it remains localized to the primary site and regional lymph nodes. Since these forms of therapy exert their effect locally, neither can be considered curative once the disease has metastasized beyond the local region, although both methods of therapy may be useful as palliative treatment. Chemotherapy and immunotherapy, unlike surgery and radiation therapy, represent systemic forms of treatment effective against tumor cells already metastatic to distant organ sites. These systemic therapeutic modalities have a greater chance of curing patients with a minimum number of tumor cells than those with clinically evident disease. Thus, though surgery and radiation therapy cannot be curative unless the tumor is confined locally or regionally, they can decrease the patient's tumor burden so that chemotherapy or immunotherapy may become more effective. During the past several years, enough evidence has accumulated to suggest that treatment combining surgery, radiation therapy, chemotherapy, and, possibly, immunotherapy will significantly improve cure rates above those achieved with any single therapeutic modality.

Cancer treatment, therefore, should be approached in an interdisciplinary manner. Just as oncology should be approached as a unique field of study, so cancer should be regarded as a single but complex disease requiring a multidisciplinary approach. The practice of assigning certain types of neoplasms to surgery, radiation therapy, or medicine with a further division into various anatomically oriented specialties should be discontinued.

GOALS OF THERAPY—CURE OR PALLIATION. Once the diagnosis of malignant disease has been made and the extent of disease determined, a decision must be made about the specific therapy. *Is the patient curable?* This is the foremost question that must be answered before the physician recommends aggressive therapy with its attendant complications. The goals of therapy vary with the extent of the cancer. If the cancer is localized without evidence of spread, the goal is to eradicate the cancer and cure the patient. When the cancer is spread beyond local cure, the goal is to control the patient's symptoms and to maintain maximum activity for the longest possible period of time. Palliation should be measured in terms of useful life. Diabetes is not cured, but the manifestations of the disease are controlled so that a patient has many years of activity and useful life. Goals for the palliation of patients living with cancer are similar.

Patients are generally judged as incurable if they have distant metastases or evidence of extensive local infiltration of adjacent organs or structures. The most common criterion for incurability is distant metastases. However, some patients are potentially curable even if they have distant metastases. For example, patients with solitary pulmonary metastases may be curable by resection, and even those with widespread metastases who have choriocarcinoma may be curable with chemotherapy. Histologic proof of distant metastases should be obtained before the patient is assessed as incurable. Occasionally, an exploratory celiotomy or thoracotomy may be necessary to determine the nature of equivocal lesions in the lungs or liver. In some situations, e.g., multiple pulmonary metastases, the clinical situation may point so overwhelmingly to distant metastases that the patient may safely be considered incurable without biopsy.

Local extension may be a criterion of incurability. For each anatomic site, there are certain local criteria that place the patient unequivocally in an incurable status, while others imply a poor prognosis but are not absolutely indicative of incurability. In equivocal situations after extensive studies have failed to demonstrate metastatic or incurable local extension, the patient deserves the benefit of doubt and should be treated for cure.

CHOICE OF THERAPY. Surgery, radiation therapy, and chemotherapy are the most frequently used therapeutic modalities in the fight against cancer. Each may play a role in both curative and palliative therapy. Immunotherapy is a new modality that has a limited role in cancer therapy at the present time, but one that may become increasingly useful in the future. In choosing therapy, a variety of factors must be considered regardless of whether the aim is cure or palliation. The natural history of the disease and the results obtained from each type of therapy must be known prior to choosing a modality or combination of modalities.

The patient's general condition and the presence of any coexisting disease must be considered in planning therapy. Surgery may be contraindicated in a patient who has recently experienced a myocardial infarction. A patient with preexisting diabetes will be much more susceptible to the toxic effects of hormonal therapy with corticosteroids. Renal disease may increase the toxicity of some of the chemotherapeutic drugs, such as methotrexate. In addition, any evidence of infection or bleeding in a patient may make any form of cancer therapy dangerous, requiring vigorous treatment prior to the initiation of definitive therapy.

The psychologic makeup of the patient and the patient's life situation must be considered. A patient who is unable to accept the realities of a given treatment should be offered an alternative approach when possible. This is particularly true of any surgical procedures that significantly alter appearance or that involve change of organ function requiring the patient's daily care, such as colostomy. Experimental forms of therapy, such as intraarterial infusion of drugs, should also be avoided in some patients. Obviously, a patient who is going to be unwilling to tolerate the inconvenience of an intraarterial catheter and who might remove it without medical approval should not undergo such treatment.

Adjuvant Therapy

Even though extensive staging procedures indicate that a tumor localized to the primary site and regional lymph nodes is potentially curable by local therapy (either surgery or radiation), about 60 percent of malignant tumors will ultimately recur. Obviously, patients whose tumors fall into this category have subclinical metastases at the time of diagnosis. The probability for cure may be improved if systemic therapy is coupled to the local treatment. This adjuvant treatment can consist of chemotherapeutic agents or, in some instances, immunotherapy using vaccines or nonspecific stimulants.

The rationale for chemotherapy under these circumstances relates to the principles of the log cell kill hypothesis—a given dose of drug kills a constant fraction of cells, the so-called first-order cell kill. However, the drugs must be given when the number of tumor cells is low enough to permit destruction but at doses that can be tolerated by the patient. The opportunity for cure probably occurs during the early stage of the disease or immediately after surgery when tumor burden is minimal. At the present time, most trials of adjuvant chemotherapy are experimental; however, the results of extensive breast cancer trials have convinced most clinicians that adjuvant chemotherapy for premenopausal patients with Stage II carcinoma of the breast can improve disease-free survival. Other subsets of breast cancer patients also may respond to adjuvant chemotherapy, although these results are less clear-cut. Other tumors that seem to respond to adjuvant chemotherapy are Wilms' tumor, osteosarcoma, Ewing's sarcoma, and ovarian carcinomas.

Surgical Therapy

Surgical treatment represents the most frequently used and the most successful single method of cancer therapy currently available. More patients are cured of cancer by surgery than by any other therapeutic modality. However, only about one-third of cancer patients are cured by surgery alone, since surgical therapy, with few exceptions, is curative only in those patients in whom the disease is localized to the primary site and regional nodes.

Cancer surgery has been based upon the concept that cancer begins as a local disease and spreads in an orderly fashion from the primary site to adjacent tissues by direct extension to the regional lymph nodes by lymphatics and through the blood vessels. The surgical procedure was designed to remove the primary neoplasms and the usual contiguous routes of spread with the aim of removing *every* cancer cell from the body. New evidence suggests that many malignancies have a relatively long latency period and probably shed cells throughout the body as they grow. Surgery, in these instances, would be considered as a means for local control of the disease. This decrease in tumor burden could alter the host-tumor balance to favor the patient with minimal metastases.

Advances in surgical techniques, anesthesia, and supportive care (blood transfusion, antibiotics, and fluid and electrolyte management) have permitted the development of more radical and extensive operative procedures. These advances have resulted in significant improvements in the cure rates for certain human neoplasms. Ultraradical operations have been extended to their anatomic limits, permitting the surgical removal of nearly all organs. Unfortunately, these more radical procedures have often failed to significantly increase cure rates.

There have been few significant improvements in the management of most human neoplasms by surgery alone during the past two decades. Furthermore, advances in cancer surgery techniques beyond those presently practiced are unlikely to significantly change the cure rates of most human neoplasms. It would appear, then, that any therapeutic advances must come from the combination of other modalities with cancer surgery.

PREOPERATIVE PREPARATION. Often, the patient's physical condition is relatively poor. Many malignant tumors seem to have a toxic effect on the host disproportionate to the size of the lesion. Patients may have a poor nutritional status because of interference with normal alimentary function as with cancers of the oral pharynx, esophagus, and intestinal tract. Pain may contribute to anorexia and severe electrolyte disorder. Anemia, vitamin defi-

ciencies, and defects in the coagulation mechanisms must be corrected before an operation can be safely performed.

Every effort should be made to correct nutritional deficiencies, restore depleted blood volumes, and correct hypoproteinemia prior to extensive surgical procedures. Total parenteral nutrition can be used to prepare the malnourished patient for a major operation. Otherwise the operative morbidity and mortality following extensive cancer operations will be excessive.

CANCER SURGERY

Once the decision has been made to proceed with surgical therapy, the operative procedure should be planned carefully. It is essential to realize that the best, and often the only, opportunity for cure is at the time of the first operation. If the neoplasm is incompletely excised at that time, tissue planes, lymphatics, and blood vessels are violated and tumor cells are seeded throughout the wound. Any recurrence that follows may be difficult to separate from the inflammatory reaction and scarring that can distort tissue planes to a point where tumor margins are indistinct. Therefore, enucleation or incomplete excision of tumor masses is *never* indicated as a therapeutic measure.

PREVENTION OF CANCER CELL IMPLANTATION DURING SURGERY. Local recurrence of cancer following surgery may be due to incomplete removal or spillage of cancer cells into the operative area (Fig. 9-12). The cancer surgeon constantly must be aware of the possible danger of transferring cancer cells by inoculation into the surrounding tissues during the course of an operation. As soon as the incision is made, all edges of the wound should be protected with a plastic drape to prevent tumor cell contamination. This precaution is exemplified best when laparotomy or thoracotomy is performed for malignant disease within the abdomen or thorax.

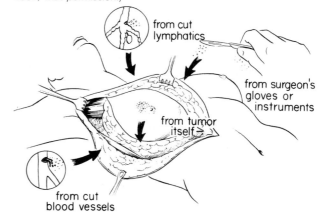

Fig. 9-12. During the operative procedure, cancer cells may be seeded in the wound by direct contact with the primary tumor, with lymph nodes containing metastatic tumor, or with contaminated gloves and instruments. Cancer cells may also enter the wound via cut lymphatics and divided blood vessels. (From: *Cole WH et al: Dissemination of Cancer. New York, Appleton-Century-Crofts, 1961, with permission.*)

from cut lymphatics

from surgeon's gloves or instruments

from tumor itself →

from cut blood vessels

Tumor cells may be inadvertently transplanted from the primary site to other sites during the surgical procedure. When preliminary biopsy has been done, the entire operative field should be reprepared after the biopsy incision is closed. The instruments and gloves used during the biopsy are not used again, because they may have been contaminated. Even the basin of saline solution in which the surgeon's gloved hand is dipped may be contaminated with cancer cells. The importance of this is illustrated by a patient with breast cancer who had a skin graft taken from the thigh to close a skin defect after a mastectomy. Later tumor nodules having the same histologic characteristics as the primary neoplasm developed on the thigh at the skin graft donor site.

If the tumor is entered during the operative procedure, the risk of implanting cancer cells into the wound is greatly increased. Should this happen, the operative field must be isolated; the cut surface of the tumor must be cauterized with the electrocautery and isolated from the remainder of the wound; and the contaminated knife, instruments, and gloves must be discarded. Then, and then only, can the operation continue through a new plane of dissection allowing a much wider margin around the tumor.

Many different cytotoxic solutions have been used to irrigate the wound following cancer surgery in an effort to sterilize the operative site. None have been very effective in decreasing the local recurrence rate, with the exception of 0.5% formaldehyde used to prevent local recurrence from carcinoma of the cervix. Sodium hypochlorite solution, nitrogen mustard, and thiotepa have all been tried, with little success.

The rate of local recurrence in the suture line following resection for carcinoma of the colon is about 10 percent. There has been some success with various techniques to prevent this local recurrence. Ligation of the bowel with umbilical tape proximal and distal to the tumor, or anastomosis, or irrigation of the cut ends of the colon with bichloride of mercury solution and then excision of the edge of each end of the bowel have been used and have decreased the recurrence rate to less than 2 percent. The use of closed anastomosis and iodized sutures has decreased the anastomotic recurrence rate in the laboratory. Local recurrence can occur despite every effort to isolate the tumor or avoid spilling cancer cells into the operative field. For example, tumor in local lymphatics may be unrecognized at the time of the initial operation, or blood-borne cells may implant the fresh wound. Usually a local recurrence is associated with systemic disease and is an unfavorable prognostic factor.

PREVENTION OF VASCULAR DISSEMINATION AT SURGERY. Blood-borne metastases are a major factor in the death of patients with most tumors. Although cancer cells have been identified in the blood of many cancer patients, only a small number of these circulating cancer cells survive because of host resistance and other factors. Thus, tumor embolism and metastases are not synonymous. In fact, there appears to be little difference in the prognosis of patients with or without tumor cells in their blood preoperatively. However, there is a correlation between the presence of tumor cells seen in the blood during the operative procedure and prognosis. Furthermore, manipulation of the tumor at any time in the surgical procedure can greatly increase the number of cancer cells recovered from the blood.

Definite measures should be taken to prevent the dissemination of tumor cells during the operation. These can include (1) avoiding manipulation of the tumor ("no-touch" technique), (2) early ligation of the vascular pedicle, (3) the use of tourniquets on all extremity tumors.

Since any manipulation of the tumor mass may result in exfoliation of tumor cells into the lymphatics and blood, such manipulation must be kept to a minimum prior to the operative procedure, during preparation of the skin with antiseptic agents as well as during the operative procedure. Furthermore, it is imperative to use an incision of proper size to minimize unnecessary manipulation of the tumor. One that is too small will not permit the necessary wide excision without excessive handling. Turnbull and associates have reported a significant higher survival in left colon cancer using the no-touch technique, which combines minimal manipulation, early ligation of the vascular pedicle, and wide excision. However, the importance of early ligation of the vascular pedicle has been questioned by Stearns, who reported similar results without the early ligation.

TYPES OF CANCER OPERATIONS. Local Resection. Wide local resection in which an adequate margin of normal tissue is removed with the tumor mass may be adequate treatment for certain low-grade neoplasms that do not metastasize to regional nodes or widely infiltrate adjacent tissues. Basal cell carcinomas and the mixed tumors of the parotid gland are examples of such neoplasms. However, it is essential that at least some normal tissue surrounding the tumor is excised in order to prevent local recurrence.

Radical Local Resection. Some neoplasms may spread widely by infiltration into adjacent tissues. This is especially true for soft tissue sarcomas and esophageal and gastric carcinomas. For this reason, it is necessary to remove a wide margin of normal tissue with the neoplasm in these cases. The wide normal-tissue margin between the line of excision and the tumor mass also acts as a protective barrier against tumor cell spill into the severed lymphatics and vessels. The greater the thickness of normal tissue between the plane of dissection and the tumor, the greater likelihood of a complete local excision.

If the tumor was previously explored but not removed or if an incisional biopsy was performed, it is extremely important that a wide segment of skin and the underlying muscles, fat, and fascia be removed far beyond the limits of the original incision, because tumor cells may have been implanted in the incision at the time of this initial operation.

It must be constantly emphasized that malignant neoplasms are not well encapsulated. A pseudocapsule composed of a compression zone of neoplastic cells usually covers the tumor. This apparent encapsulation offers a great temptation for simple enucleation, because the tumor may be dislodged from its bed so easily. This temptation must be resisted. The surgeon must cut through normal tissue at all times and should never encounter the neoplasm during its removal. Dissection should proceed with meticulous care to avoid tumor cell spill. Retraction always should be away from, rather than toward, the tumor. It is important for the surgeon to remember to be as far as possible from the gross extent of the tumor on all sides including the deep aspect. Skin, subcutaneous fat, and muscle usually can be sacrificed with impunity and little functional loss. Involvement of major vessels, nerves, joints, or bones may require sacrifice of these structures and even amputation in order to obtain a curative result. During the surgical procedure, the extent of operation should be determined not only by the concern for cure, but also by functional considerations.

All deeply situated sarcomas lying between or within muscle groups require the removal of all muscle bundles from their origin to insertion within that particular fascial compartment; all surrounding or adjacent fascia, periosteum, vessels, nerves, and connective tissues; and all skin adjacent to the lesions. These procedures are imperative when surgery alone is used to treat sarcomas, because these lesions tend to infiltrate along fascial and muscle planes far beyond the palpable limits of the tumor. As surgeons proceed with the operation, they may be forced to alter their initial operative plan as they visualize the extent of tumor and as the pathology reports of frozen section examinations of surgical margins are made available. These decisions as to extent of resection are difficult and require experienced judgment. In borderline situations, it is usually better to proceed with a potentially curative resection of the tumor mass unless there is histologic confirmation that the lesion has extended beyond the boundaries of possible surgical resection. Advances in the use of combined modality therapy for skeletal and soft tissue sarcomas have permitted the salvage rather than amputation of extremities for selected patients (see the section on Combined Modality Therapy).

Radical Resection with en Bloc Excision of Lymphatics. Since many neoplasms commonly metastasize by way of the lymphatics, operations have been designed to remove the primary neoplasm and the regional lymph nodes draining that area in continuity with all the intervening tissues. Conditions are best for this type of operation when the collecting nodes of the lymphatic channels draining the neoplasm lie adjacent to the primary site or if there is a single avenue of lymphatic drainage that can be removed without sacrificing vital structures. It is important to avoid cutting across involved lymphatic channels because such action greatly increases the possibility of local disease recurrence.

This principle was applied to breast cancer by Meyer and by Halsted at the turn of the century and has formed the foundation of cancer surgery for many years. At the present time, it is generally agreed that such en bloc regional lymph node dissections should be performed in patients having clinical involvement of nodes by metastatic tumor. In many cases, the tumor has already spread beyond the regional nodes, and the cure rates following such procedures may be quite low. En bloc removal of the involved nodes offers the only chance for cure and provides significant palliation and local control. Therefore, the defeatist attitude toward metastatically involved regional nodes must be discouraged.

The high rate of local cancer recurrence following surgical resection when lymph nodes are grossly involved and the high error rate when palpation is used to assess the extent of the involvement have led to routine dissection of regional nodes close to the primary tumor even though they are not clinically involved. Microscopic examination of the excised lymph nodes in these patients who have no clinical evidence of palpable enlargement reveals evidence of tumor spread in 20 to 40 percent of carcinomas and melanomas. This concept is supported by comparison of the higher 5-year survival rate of patients showing microscopic involvement of lymph nodes with that of patients in whom lymph node involvement was clinically recognizable.

Recently some surgeons have challenged the concept of elective, or prophylactic, lymph node dissection in cases where the regional nodes are not obviously involved, because it is not clear whether cure rates are improved if the nodes are removed before they are palpable. However, in many types of cancer the foreknowledge of tumor in regional nodes does affect the staging of the patient and can alter the treatment modality. For example, patients with breast cancer who have metastases to regional nodes may benefit considerably from adjuvant chemotherapy as would some patients with deep melanomas. Furthermore, a comparison of experimental results from one institution with another depends upon accurate staging of each patient at the time of the initiation of therapy. For these reasons, the decision to recommend a prophylactic lymph node dissection must be based on the likelihood of benefit to the patient.

Randomized prospective studies will be necessary to answer the question of which patients do best after prophylactic dissection. Until then, the surgeon must weigh benefit against risk for each patient. Certainly, the argument against lymphadenectomy because it diminishes the host's immune system has not been proved by experimental studies, and should not be a consideration when planning therapy.

Extensive Surgical Procedures. Some slow-growing primary tumors may reach enormous size and may locally infiltrate widely without developing distant metastasis. Supraradical operative procedures can be undertaken for these extensive, nearly inoperable tumors, with cure of occasional patients. Although surgical care, anesthesia, blood replacement, and physiologic monitoring are much improved over the past, these operations should not be undertaken except by experienced surgeons who can select those patients most likely to benefit. Furthermore, these extensive surgical procedures sometimes offer a chance for a cure that is not possible by other means, and are justified in selected situations when extensive laboratory work-up shows no evidence of distant metastases. However, the surgeon must be willing to accept the responsibility for the postoperative emotional rehabilitation of the patient before undertaking such extensive procedures as the pelvic exenteration, hemipelvectomy, forequarter amputation, or mutilating operations for head and neck carcinomas.

Pelvic exenteration is a well-conceived operation capable of curing patients with radiation-treated recurrent cancer of the cervix and certain well-differentiated and locally extensive adenocarcinomas of the rectum. This operation removes the pelvic organs (bladder, uterus, and rectum) and all soft tissues within the pelvis. Bowel function is restored with colostomy. Urinary tract drainage is established by anastomosis of ureters into a segment of bowel (ileum or sigmoid colon). The 5-year relapse-free survival from pelvic exenteration is 25 percent in this situation.

Hemipelvectomy (resection of the lower extremity and iliac bone) can sometimes be curative for skeletal sarcomas limited to the head of the femur or acetabulum or to one-half of the pelvic structures, and in some slowly growing soft tissue sarcomas of the upper thigh and buttock that recur locally but metastasize slowly. Forequarter amputation (resection of the upper extremity and scapula) can offer similar results when the neoplasm is limited to the bones of the scapula and upper humerus or to the soft tissues of the shoulder girdle.

SURGERY OF RECURRENT CANCER. There is a definite role for surgical resection of localized recurrent neoplasms of low-grade malignancy and slow growth where further resection may produce a long period of remission. Additional surgical procedures are frequently successful in controlling recurrent soft tissue sarcomas, anastomotic recurrences of colon cancer, certain basal and squamous carcinomas of skin, and recurrent breast cancer.

Routine "second-look" operations to detect early recurrence of colon cancer were advocated by Gilbertsen and Wangensteen. The results of this second-look procedure have not been impressive and do not appear to justify its routine use. However, various tumor markers, such as CEA, have been extremely useful for selecting patients likely to benefit from reoperation. In general, a local recurrence can be treated surgically or with radiation. The surgeon must decide which form of treatment will achieve local control with the lowest morbidity.

RESECTION OF METASTASES. Although logic would suggest that once a neoplasm has metastasized to a distant site it should no longer be curable by surgical resection, removal of metastatic lesions in the lung, liver, or brain has occasionally produced a clinical cure. Therefore, in selected patients with slowly growing neoplasms, resections of the metastatic lesions may be indicated, especially if the metastasis is solitary. Prior to undertaking resection, an extensive laboratory work-up should rule out metastatic spread to other body areas.

Some patients with isolated liver metastases may benefit from surgical resection. Those patients with a solitary metastasis, or metastases located in one lobe, are often successfully treated with resection. Approximately 25 percent of these patients will survive for 5 years. However, less than 5 percent with colon cancer metastatic to the liver are candidates for this type of treatment. Most of these patients have diffuse disease and are best treated with systemic or intraarterial chemotherapy. Occasionally, resection is recommended for the patient whose primary tumor is controlled and who has no evidence of other metastases. As can be seen in Fig. 9-13, the result can be very gratifying.

The results of resection of pulmonary metastatic lesions have been much more satisfactory. In fact, resection of a solitary pulmonary metastasis provides a higher rate of 5-year survival than resection of primary bronchogenic carcinoma of the lung. Resection of pulmonary metastases may be indicated even when more than one metastatic lesion is present. Many patients die from their pulmonary metastases; resection could provide cure. Our experience has shown that patients with tumor doubling times greater than 40 days received significant palliation from their pulmonary resections and remained free of disease for as long as 5 years. In contrast, patients with tumor doubling times of less than 20 days did not significantly benefit from resection of their metastatic lesions (Fig. 9-14).

ADMINISTRATION OF CHEMOTHERAPY BY ARTERIAL INFUSION OR ISOLATED PERFUSION. The concentration of chemotherapeutic drugs can be greatly increased when the drug is administered directly into the artery supplying the neoplastic lesion. Continuous infusion of chemotherapeutic drugs over a period of weeks can be carried out

Fig. 9-13. Resected liver and smiling patient at 10-year anniversary of operation for hepatic metastases.

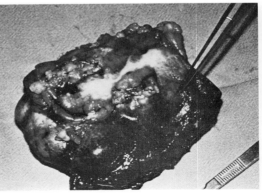
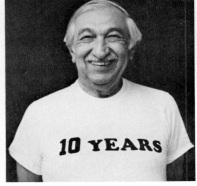

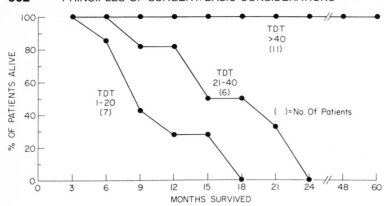

Fig. 9-14. Survival curves of 24 untreated patients following onset of pulmonary metastases. (From: *Joseph WL et al: J Thorac Cardiovasc Surg 61:23, 1971, with permission.*)

with portable infusion pumps attached to a catheter placed in the artery. Some striking remissions using this technique have been observed, although they usually have been of short duration. It appears logical to assume that this manner of administering chemotherapeutic agents would increase their effectiveness because of the greater concentrations obtainable. Patients with hepatoma have responded well to the intraarterial infusion of 5-FU. Hepatic artery ligation and 5-FU infusion have been combined with some success in treating patients with metastatic colon carcinoma.

Hepatic artery ligation itself may be of benefit in the management of hepatic metastases. Because metastases derive their blood supply predominantly from the hepatic artery whereas normal liver tissue receives blood from both the arterial and portal system, the ligation may induce tumor necrosis. In the absence of hypotension or sepsis, it is surprisingly well tolerated.

One ingenious method of administering increased concentrations of chemotherapeutic drugs involves the isolated perfusion technique. The artery and veins supplying the tumor-bearing extremity are cannulated and isolated from the systemic circulation by connection to a pump-oxygenator. The tumor is then perfused for up to 90 min with oxygenated blood containing cancerocidal drugs in amounts that would be prohibitively poisonous if infused through the general circulation.

Heating the blood with a heat exchanger similar to that used for cardiopulmonary bypass appears to increase the effectiveness of the chemotherapeutic drugs. Hyperthermic perfusion with chemotherapeutic agents may be worthwhile in treating satellite or intransient metastasis from malignant melanoma and primary or recurrent sarcomas of the extremities. Some long-term survivors with malignant melanoma treated by this technique have been reported. Furthermore, Stehlin reports that hyperthermic perfusion of chemotherapeutic drugs, when combined with radiation therapy, may decrease the necessity of amputation in some primary or recurrent sarcomas that are bordering on vital structures of the extremity.

Despite long experience with intraarterial infusion and regional perfusion for the administration of chemotherapeutic drugs, there is still no general agreement about their usefulness. Many chemotherapists believe systemic

administration of drugs would be equally effective. We have observed more dramatic responses from the infusion/perfusion techniques than from systemic administration of chemotherapeutic drugs.

Heat itself may be an effective agent against some types of tumor (see section on Hyperthermia), and when combined with chemotherapy, may be an important tool for the treatment of metastatic or recurrent cancers. Hyperthermia is currently being evaluated in several centers in the United States, and has been reported to prolong survival when combined with intraarterial chemotherapy for treatment of hepatic metastases.

PALLIATIVE SURGERY. Surgical procedures are sometimes indicated to relieve symptoms, to reduce the severity of the patient's illness, or to prolong a useful comfortable life without attempting to cure the patient. Such an operation is justified to relieve pain, hemorrhage, obstruction, or infection when it can be done without great risk to the patient, and when it improves the quality of life even if it does not prolong it. Surgery that only prolongs a miserable existence certainly does not benefit the patient.

Some examples of palliative surgical procedures are (1) colostomy, enteroenterostomy, or gastrojejunostomy to relieve obstruction; (2) chordotomy to control pain; (3) cystectomy for infected, bleeding tumors of the bladder; (4) amputation for painful infected tumors in the extremities; (5) simple mastectomy for carcinoma of the breast, even in the presence of distant metastases, when the primary tumor is infected, large, ulcerated, and locally resectable; and (6) colon resection in the presence of hepatic metastases.

Radiation Therapy

Radiation therapy, like surgical therapy, must be judged by the frequency of local and regional control of tumor in proportion to treatment-induced morbidity. Ionizing radiations are effective in controlling a variety of malignant tumors and, consequently, are used in the management of 50 to 60 percent of all patients with cancer. Proper use of the method requires that the radiation oncologist be directly involved in the selection of patients and evaluation of these patients before, during, and after treatment, as well as be responsible for the treatment application.

Ionizing radiations can be accurately delivered to a body part without anatomic restrictions. This enables the destruction of tumors with preservation of the anatomy and, consequently, of function and cosmesis, if the anatomy is intact prior to treatment. Thus, radiation treatment is biologically and functionally most effective for small tumors, which have not destroyed adjacent normal tissues.

Radiation therapy is less influenced than surgical therapy or chemotherapy by concurrent medical problems, although treatment-related sequelae may be more frequent and/or severe in patients with certain systemic illnesses, such as diabetes or hypertension. Disadvantages of the method include the increase of some sequelae with time, and the long overall treatment period, although treatment usually is on an outpatient basis and daily contact allows the opportunity to provide continued support of the patient.

The appearance of late sequelae today may be the unfortunate consequence of treatment techniques long abandoned. Thus, it is important that the selection of radiation therapy be based on today's potential for accomplishment and limitation of undesired side effects.

PHYSICAL BASIS. Ionizing radiations are characterized by their capacity to ionize (and excite) atoms and molecules in an absorber such as tissue. They may be electromagnetic (x-rays, gamma rays) or corpuscular (electrons, protons, neutrons) and of natural origin (gamma rays from radium) or artificial origin (x-rays or gamma rays from cobalt 60). Inasmuch as the basic physical mechanisms of action of all ionizing radiations are the same, the different observed effects of equal physical doses are the result of differences in spatial and/or temporal distributions.

Current conventional clinical radiation therapy includes the use of x-rays, high-energy electrons, gamma rays from cobalt 60 and cesium 137, and beta rays. Protons, heavy ions, and neutrons are being clinically investigated.

For decades, doses at the point of interest, such as in the tumor or spinal cord, were grossly extrapolated from skin reactions or doses measured in air (the roentgen). Currently, radiation doses used clinically are actually absorbed doses measured in the patient, such as by placement of thermoluminescent dosimeters, or in a phantom, which stimulates the human being. The actual measurements then are adapted for precise clinical application through the use of computer programs. Based on the 1980 I.C.R.U. recommendations, doses are preferably quantified in units of grays (Gy), with 1 Gy equal to 1 joule per kilogram of the absorber. Thus, 1 Gy equals 100 rad and 1 cGy equals 1 rad.

For proper clinical use, these accurately measured physical doses must correlate total dose, overall time of application, number and size of increments, dose rate, and pattern of application. For example, a single increment of 1000 cGy produces far different results than does 1000 cGy divided into 10 daily increments of 100 cGy. The biologic results can be further changed by reducing the dose rate of 150 to 250 cGy/min conventionally used in photon teletherapy to 5 cGy/min, as used for total body irradiation.

Today's availability of modern radiation therapy was initially facilitated by the widespread distribution of cobalt 60 teletherapy units, dating to 1949, and their later replacement or augmentation by versatile 4- to 6-MeV linear accelerators. Such modern equipment provides short treatment times and isocentric patient setups, as well as relative "skin sparing," decreased absorption in bone, and sharp beam margins with less side scatter. The relative depth doses (point of interest as a percent of the surface or maximum dose) and the cost increase as the energy of the particle striking the target to produce the x-rays increases. Unfortunately, the terms supervoltage and megavoltage have been used imprecisely, but it is proper to consider units above 2 MV peak energy as megavoltage generators.

An interest in delivering doses throughout tumors that are higher than achievable with external beam therapy has resulted in a renewed interest in the direct placement of a range of newly developed radioactive isotopes (^{192}Ir, ^{137}Cs, ^{125}I) into selected cancers. Such treatment of cancers of the breast, prostate, brain, lung, oral cavity, pharynx, and eye has led the radiation oncologist into the operating room and into closer cooperation with many surgeons.

Although technological and engineering developments have enabled modern radiation therapy, future advances are likely to be based on the better understanding of the biology of tumors.

RADIOCHEMICAL BASIS. The initial physical absorption of energy requires only about 10^{-12} s. Radiochemical events, which are initiated by this absorption, require another 10^{-10} s in mammalian cells and tissues. These nearly instantaneous reactions may initiate biologic processes not detected for years (carcinogenesis) or even generations (changes in offspring). Sixty to seventy percent of radiation-induced damage is considered secondary to the ionization of water (indirect effect). The remaining changes are the result of the ionization and excitation of intracellular targets (direct effect). The free radicals produced have a short lifetime (10^{-5} to 10^{-10} s) prior to recombining and so have a short range of action. However, orderly recombination of ionization products can be modified by the presence of substances such as oxygen and sulfhydril compounds.

BIOLOGIC BASIS. Most clinical radiation therapy to the current time has been empirical. However, radiobiology studies now are providing a scientific basis for clinical applications and will provide a basis for future developments.

Modern cellular radiobiology dates to the development of tumor cell culture by Puck and Marcus in the mid-1950s. Mammalian cell dose-survival curves quantitatively correlate reproductive cell death with total radiation dose. The inherent radiosensitivity of most mammalian normal or tumor cells is remarkably similar, with doses of 110 to 240 cGy consistently reducing reproductive cell survival to 37 percent (D_0 dose). Therefore, differences in the rapidity and completeness of response of human tumors and normal tissues must be based on other factors such as the capacity to repair sublethal damage, cell cycle time, distribution of cells in the replication cycle, and repopulation.

The difference between radiosensitivity and radiocurability is important. Radiosensitivity is the measure of susceptibility of cells to injury by ionizing radiations. This injury may be lethal to the cell through interruption of the capacity to replicate indefinitely (reproductive death) or through metabolic incapacitation or structural degeneration independent of progression of the cell through the reproductive cycle (interphase death).

Radioresistance is the reciprocal of radiosensitivity and so both terms are relative. All mammalian cells are radiosensitive through a narrow range (D_{37} or D_0 = 110 to 240 cGy) when measured by reproductive death.

Radiocurability, which is permanent tumor control allowing survival of the host, is related primarily to tumor size, site, and type, and less to radiosensitivity. Most radiocurable tumors are only moderately responsive when measured by rate of gross decrease in size (epidermoid carcinomas of the oral cavity, pharynx, larynx, skin, cervic, and adenocarcinomas of the breast, prostate, and uterus). Indeed, except for seminoma, many of the rapidly responding tumors (non-Hodgkin's lymphomas, undifferentiated carcinomas) are not radiocurable, usually because of widespread extent.

Radiation-instigated cell killing can be modified in several ways. Inasmuch as molecular oxygen must be present for maximal cell killing by ionizing radiations, tumor cellular hypoxia can decrease the effectiveness of radiation therapy by as much as a factor of 3. This may explain the postirradiation persistence of tumor cells when there is necrosis or fibrosis.

Heat directly kills cells and alters radiosensitivity. Hyperthermia is an attractive adjuvant to radiation therapy because it is effective during the S-phase of the cell cycle and is not adversely influenced by hypoxia, and it blocks repair of sublethal damage (see section on Hyperthermia).

The intrinsic radiosensitivity of cells can be increased by altering the target DNA, such as by replacing thymidine with halogenated pyrimidine analogs (BUdR, IUdR) during cell replication. Cell killing can be increased by inhibiting the postirradiation repair processes. For example, the repair of DNA strand breaks can be inhibited by actinomycin D and Adriamycin, and by heat (42 to 45°C). Unfortunately, current methods of altering the target DNA and inhibiting postirradiation repair are not selective for tumor cells and so do not favorably alter the therapeutic ratio.

Cell killing can be modified by changes of the dose rate. As the dose rate decreases, cell killing, per unit of dose, decreases. Low dose rates, i.e., less than 10 cGy/min, may favor repair in normal cells. This is exploited clinically in improving lung tolerance in total body irradiation

and allowing very large total doses in interstitial and intracavitary treatments.

Inherent cellular radiosensitivity to photons varies by a factor of approximately 2, depending on position in the cell cycle. Thus, frequent doses of photons may decrease the radiosensitivity of a homogeneous population of cells by selectively killing cells in the most vulnerable phase of the cycle.

Such variations in radiosensitivity to photons related to cell age, repair of sublethal damage, and hypoxia are minimized by the use of high-energy particles (fast neutrons, heavy ions, pi mesons), thus providing a basis for investigation of these radiations.

CLINICAL BASIS. Like surgery and chemotherapy, radiation therapy has definite indications and contraindications. Irradiation may be the only anticipated treatment or it may be combined with surgery and/or chemotherapy.

Whether radiation therapy may be useful is based on factors related to both the tumor (type, primary site, extent) and the host (general condition, local and regional tissue status). Inasmuch as all forms of cancer treatment may cause serious morbidity and once used may enforce an initial diagnosis, it is essential that a diagnosis be positively established, if possible. This usually means identification of tumor by biopsy. An unfortunate historic activity, a trial of radiation therapy to determine "sensitivity," not only was biologically meaningless but was detrimental because of destruction of evidence necessary to identify the tumor properly. On a rare occasion, when biopsy may pose an unreasonable risk to the patient (brain stem, optic tract), treatment may be licensed by strong diagnostic evidence. The introduction of computerized tomography (CT) and magnetic resonance imaging (MRI) should reduce unfortunate diagnostic errors. Once the tumor identity has been established, reappearance after treatment, particularly in palliative situations, may require less potentially morbid diagnostic efforts.

Histologic tumor type and grade may be useful pretherapeutic predictors of biologic behavior and radiosensitivity (Table 9-11). However, this evidence is much less useful in predicting radiocurability.

The potential for tumor control by radiation therapy is more closely related to tumor size and primary site. Generally, as tumors increase in size, the likelihood of radiocurability decreases, presumably related to a direct correlation of tumor cell number and radiation dose required to kill all the tumor cells. The primary tumor site predicts biologic behavior and dictates which adjacent normal tissues must tolerate the incidental irradiation. For example, small epidermoid carcinomas of the uterine cervix and vocal cords are localized and can be eradicated by radiation doses tolerated by the surrounding normal tissues. Larger tumors at the same sites are less frequently controlled by similar doses and, in addition, are more likely to spread regionally, thus requiring treatment of a larger volume with consequent reduction of normal tissue tolerance.

After initial evaluation of the patient, the objective of radiation therapy must be defined. If the cancer is radio-

Table 9-11. RELATIVE RADIOSENSITIVITY OF
MALIGNANT TUMORS

(Listed in order of decreasing radiosensitivity)

Malignant tumors arising from hemopoietic organs
(lymphosarcoma, myeloma)
Hodgkin's disease
Seminomas and dysgerminomas
Ewing's sarcoma of the bone
Basal cell carcinomas of the skin
Epidermoid carcinomas arising by metaplasia from columnar
epithelium
Epidermoid carcinomas of the mucous membranes,
mucocutaneous junctions, and skin
Adenocarcinomas of the endometrium, breast, gastrointestinal
system, and endocrine glands
Soft tissue sarcomas
Chondrosarcomas
Neurogenic sarcomas
Osteosarcomas
Malignant melanomas

SOURCE: From Ackerman LV, del Regato JA: *Cancer: Diagnosis, Treatment, and Prognosis,* 4th ed. St Louis, Mosby, 1970, with permission.

curable, patient inconvenience, relatively high cost, and a moderate risk of serious treatment-related morbidity should be considered in that fortunate perspective. If the objective is palliation of bothersome cancer-related symptoms or signs, these consequences of treatment usually are not acceptable.

Radiation treatment planning and delivery have become highly complicated. In most patients, the primary tumor and its regional spread are graphically displayed in three dimensions and incorporated in a planned treatment volume. The best method of delivery of the radiations is selected from a range of options including multiple beams of photons and/or electrons, sometimes augmented by interstitial and/or intracavitary applications. The dosimetry data are incorporated in computer-assisted programs, which allow rapid, accurate calculations of the desired options.

Repetitive treatment delivery can be accurate to within a few millimeters, if required (proton or heavy ion beam treatment of choroidal melanoma or linear accelerator treatment of retinoblastoma).

Doses to different sites in the same patient may vary according to need. The treatment plan may include the integration of different types of radiations. For example, a primary squamous cell cancer of the oral tongue or cervix may receive a high local dose from an isotope source, while regional lymph nodes, which may harbor metastases, may receive lower doses from a photon teletherapy source. The integration of all the components of such a comprehensive plan for radiation therapy is possible only when directed by a single, trained, responsible physician.

Even when seemingly indicated, radiation therapy may be inappropriate because of host factors. These may include general debility, making the tolerance to vigorous irradiation unlikely; or there may be local tissue changes

precluding high-dose local treatment; or the patient may fear the treatment, making its proper use impossible.

Radiation therapy is increasingly being used in planned combination with surgery and/or chemotherapy. Multidisciplinary treatment implies continuous cooperation of all physicians involved in planning, delivering, and monitoring a treatment program. The objective of combined surgery and radiation therapy is improved local and regional control of tumor. Both methods may be directed to the same site, as when resection of a cancer of the hypopharynx is followed by irradiation, or when irradiation of a soft tissue sarcoma in an extremity is followed by surgery; or each method may be directed to a different site, as when orchiectomy is followed by irradiation of the retroperitoneal lymph nodes, or when a neck dissection follows interstitial irradiation of a cancer of the oral tongue.

When surgery and radiation therapy are directed to the same site, the interval between their use depends on a range of facors, which should be decided by mutual agreement. Thus, low-dose irradiation of a soft tissue sarcoma may be followed by resection in 10 to 14 days, while rectosigmoid resection should be delayed 4 to 6 weeks after high-dose pelvic irradiation to allow for regression of edema and hyperemia. Most postoperative radiation therapy is with high doses directed to sites at high risk for persistent tumor and so should be delayed until wound healing is as complete as possible.

Such planned combined treatment is in stark contrast to the use of one method to rescue the failure of the other. In these circumstances, the effectiveness of the second method is reduced. Surgery in tissues heavily irradiated in a curative attempt many months before is difficult because of fibrosis, loss of tissue planes, and decreased vascularity, and the frequency and severity of complications are consequently increased. Irradiation of tumor regrowing in tissues altered by surgery is likely to be less effective, often because of decreased vascularity, and more morbid, as when bowel is fixed by adhesions, resulting in high doses to small segments.

Every effective anticancer therapy may produce undesirable and, occasionally, dangerous side effects. It is important to recognize that the potential to cause and avoid serious sequelae is much different today from in the past. Also, the incidence of treatment-related side effects varies with the philosophy of the radiation oncologist, who must answer whether the risks of frequent serious sequelae are worth slightly more frequent tumor control.

Early radiation-induced reactions, although undesirable, are self-limited. These include anorexia and even nausea, fatigue, diarrhea, esophagitis, skin and mucosal reactions, epilation, and hematopoietic suppression.

The clinically important severe sequelae of radiation therapy, such as bowel stenosis and bone necrosis, become evident months or years after treatment (Table 9-12). Often these are predictable and can be minimized by good modern treatment. Such developments, if the result of well-considered risks, can be correlated with unavoidable sequelae of other treatments. For example, is a colostomy, made necessary because of radiation-induced stenosis of bowel occurring during curative irra-

Table 9-12. LOCAL EFFECTS OF RADIATION

Organ	Acute changes	Chronic changes
Skin	Wet or dry epidermitis	Ruunning
	Radiodermatitis	Ulceration
	Epilation	
Gastrointestinal tract	Edema, ulceration, infection, diarrhea, hepatitis	Stricture, ulceration, and perforation
Kidney		Nephritis, renal insufficiency
Bladder	Dysuria	Ulceration
Gonads	Sterility	Atrophy, menopause
Hemopoietic tissue	Lymphopenia	Pancytopenia
Bone	Cessation of epiphyseal growth	Necrosis
Lung	Pneumonitis	Pulmonary fibrosis
Heart	Acute pericarditis, myocarditis	Chronic pericarditis, myocarditis
Eye	Conjunctivitis	Cataracts
Nervous system	Cerebral edema	Radiation myelitis

diation of advanced cancer of the cervix, less acceptable than a planned colostomy that is part of an abdominal perineal resection?

The risks of radiation carcinogenesis occasionally are considered to be contraindications to radiation therapy. While ionizing radiations are weak co-carcinogens in the laboratory and have caused cancers in humans, the risk under today's clinical conditions should receive no more consideration than death related to anesthetics or drug sensitivities. In recent studies of over 2000 patients with head and neck cancer, and 2000 patients with cancer of

Table 9-13. RADIATION THERAPY AS AN ADJUNCT TO SURGERY (LOCALLY ADVANCED CANCERS)

Preoperative radiation therapy
  Cure rate increased with these locally advanced
    carcinomas:
      Larynx
      Laryngopharynx
      Esophagus
      Bladder
      Uterus
      Retinoblastoma
      Paranasal sinuses
      Superior pulmonary sulcus
      Soft tissue sarcomas (liposarcomas)
      Bulky cervical node metastases from epidermoid
        carcinoma of the head and neck
  Local recurrence decreased with these locally advanced
    carcinomas:
      Rectum
      Endometrium
      Head and neck (epidermoid) with clinically positive
        lymph nodes
Postoperative radiation therapy
  Carcinoma of the lung for mediastinal node metastases
  Seminoma (periaortic and iliac node areas)
  Medulloblastoma (after biopsy)
  Wilms' tumor
  Bladder
  Ovary (dysgerminoma, granulosa cell, and
    cystadenocarcinoma)

the breast; the therapeutic use of ionizing radiations caused no detectable increase in second cancers. The development of leukemia in patients irradiated for Hodgkin's disease is correlated with the use of alkylating agents. No such increase in leukemia was noted in 29,493 patients irradiated for carcinoma of the cervix and observed for 60,000 person-years.

SUMMARY. Modern radiation therapy is a full-fledged partner of surgery and chemotherapy in the treatment of the patient with cancer (Table 9-13). The widespread availability of adequately trained physicians and support personnel, versatile megavoltage generators, sophisticated dosimetry, and computer-assisted treatment planning, and even elementary radiobiologic understanding, dates but a few years. Consequently, today's potential for accomplishment should not be judged on historical performance.

The necessity of correlating cancer biology in the human being, basic radiobiology and physics, radiation responses in tumors and normal tissues, and continuing evaluation of performance to facilitate the selection and treatment of patients dictates that the use of radiation therapy be decided by a trained physician, the radiation oncologist, just as the use of surgery must be decided by the trained surgeon.

Chemotherapy

The treatment of cancer with drugs was initiated in 1941 by Huggins and Hodges, with the discovery that estrogens palliated prostatic cancer. Polyfunctional alkylating agents were developed in the later 1940s, as a result of experimental work performed during World War II. Since then there has been a tremendous increase in the number of chemotherapeutic drugs available; at present at least five major classes of drugs, plus an additional group of miscellaneous drugs, are available (Table 9-14). Although full elucidation of this complex field is beyond the scope of this chapter, certain general principles will be described regarding the use of chemotherapy. This section will consider the mechanisms of action of the major

Table 9-14. DRUGS USED IN TREATMENT OF NONHEMATOLOGIC NEOPLASMS

Drugs	Route of administration	Cell cycle phase specificity*	Acute toxicity†	Principal delayed or cumulative toxicity†
Alkylating agents:		Nonspecific	N & V§	BM§, cyclophosphamide may cause alopecia, hemorrhagic cystitis
Nitrogen mustard	I.V.		N & V	
Chlorambucil	P.O.§		None	
Phenylalanine mustard	P.O., I.V.‡, I.A.‡		None	
Cyclophosphamide	P.O., I.V.		N & V	
Thiotepa	I.V.		None	
Antimetabolites:				
Methotrexate	P.O., I.M., I.V.	Specific	None	BM, stomatitis, hepatitis
5-Fluorouracil	I.V.	Nonspecific	N & V	BM, stomatitis, diarrhea, nausea, alopecia
Hydroxyurea	P.O., I.V.‡	Specific	None	BM
Antibiotics:				
Actinomycin D	I.V.		N & V	BM, alopecia, stomatitis
Mithramycin	I.V.		None	BM and hemorrhagic diathesis
Doxorubicin	I.V.		N & V, fever	BM, cardiac toxicity, stomatitis, alopecia
Bleomycin	I.V., S.C., I.M.		Fever	Skin changes, pulmonary fibrosis
Vinca alkaloids:				
Vincristine	I.V.	Specific	N & V, rare	Constipation, BM, peripheral neuropathy, alopecia
Vinblastine				
Steroid hormones:				
Adrenal corticoids	P.O., I.V., I.M.	(?) Nonspecific	None	Hypertension, peptic ulcer, diabetes, increased susceptibility to infection
Androgens	P.O., I.M.	Unknown	None	Fluid retention, masculinization; may cause hypercalcemia in breast cancer
Estrogens	P.O.	Unknown	N & V, occasional	Fluid retention, uterine bleeding; may cause hypercalcemia in breast cancer
Progestins	P.O., I.M.	Unknown	None	May cause hypercalcemia in breast cancer
Antiestrogens	P.O.	Unknown	None	Transient bone marrow suppression; may cause hypercalcemia in breast cancer
Miscellaneous:				
Nitrosoureas‡ BCNU CCNU	I.V., P.O.	Nonspecific	N & V	BM (may be delayed 4–6 weeks), liver dysfunction
Imidazole carboxamide	I.V., I.A.‡	Nonspecific	N & V	BM, hepatotoxicity, fever
Mitotane (o, p-DDD)	P.O.	Unknown	N & V	Skin eruptions, mental depression, muscle tremors
Cisplatin	I.V.	Nonspecific	N & V	Hearing loss, renal dysfunction
Etoposide	I.V.	Nonspecific	N & V	BM; neurotoxicity

* The distinction between a phase-specific and non-phase-specific drug may not be absolute. Some authorities distinguish additional categories or use different names for these categories, but these are not considered in this chapter since their clinical relevance remains to be defined.

† See manufacturer's package inserts for usual doses and for additional toxicity data.

‡ Experimental drug or route of administration; not yet approved by the Food and Drug Administration or Division of Biological Standards; it may be available from the Cancer Chemotherapy National Service Center, Bethesda, Maryland.

§ N & V = nausea and vomiting; BM = bone marrow depression; P.O. = orally (per os); I.A. = intraarterial.

classes of chemotherapeutic drugs, the biologic and pharmacologic factors that are important in understanding drug therapy, and guidelines for the use of chemotherapy in patients with nonhematologic malignant conditions.

MECHANISMS OF ACTION. The majority of antineoplastic drugs appear to affect either enzymes, directly, or substrates of enzyme systems. In most cases the effects on enzymes or substrates relate to DNA synthesis or function, apparently by inhibiting cells that are undergoing DNA synthesis. Drugs that act by inhibiting the enzymes of nucleic acid synthesis are called *antimetabolites.*

Methotrexate, a structural analog of folinic acid, appears to act as a nearly irreversible inhibitor of the active site of the enzyme dihydrofolate reductase, which is necessary for DNA synthesis. Another commonly used antimetabolite is 5-FU, which appears to act as a reversible inhibitor of the enzyme thymidylate synthetase, which is necessary for the synthesis of thymidine, which is then used in DNA synthesis. This class of compounds acts directly on enzymes as either reversible or irreversible inhibitors, leading to the synthesis of abnormal DNA due to the incorporation of an abnormal building block or to disrup-

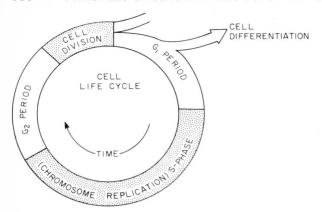

Fig. 9-15. Schematic diagram of the cell life cycle. G_1 is the first "gap" period, and G_2 is the second "gap" period. [From: *Baserga R (ed): The Cell Cycle and Cancer. New York, Marcel Dekker, 1971,* with permission.]

tion of DNA synthesis due to the lack of an essential building block.

Other major drugs appear to work primarily by affecting substrates. The usual substrate affected is the DNA macromolecule, although some of these agents will interfere with other substrates, such as proteins, and may have other diverse effects. Three major chemical classes of drugs appear to act by affecting specific substrates. The alkylating agents are extremely reactive compounds that can substitute an alkyl group (for example, $R—CH_2—CH_2^+$) for the hydrogen atoms of many organic compounds. The primary compounds affected appear to be the nucleic acids, especially DNA. Such alkylation produces breaks in the DNA molecule and cross linking of the twin strands of DNA, thus interfering with DNA replication and the transcription of RNA. Since these effects are somewhat similar to that seen with ionizing radiation, alkylating agents are sometimes called "radiomimetic." Another group of compounds that appear to work primarily on substrates are the *antibiotics*. These are natural products derived from certain soil fungi. They produce their antineoplastic effect by forming relatively stable complexes with DNA, thereby inhibiting the synthesis of DNA and RNA. The final class of drugs acting primarily on substrates is the *vinca alkaloids*. Although their total mechanism of action may not be completely defined, it is apparent that they can bind to microtubular proteins necessary for cell division. These proteins form the spindle apparatus that allows the chromosomes to separate to either end of the dividing cell; the vinca alkaloids appear to be able to dissolve this protein, leading to death of the cell during mitosis.

Table 9-14 lists representative examples of each group along with selected characteristics considered to be of clinical importance.

BIOLOGIC AND PHARMACOLOGIC FACTORS IN CANCER THERAPY. A major theme in pharmacology has been the study of variations in drug absorption, distribution, metabolism, and excretion as related to a stable, invariant biologic receptor. In cancer chemotherapy, however, the

biologic receptor, the cancer cell, is a variable and fluctuating target. Thus, the kinetics of tumor growth must be given as much attention as the kinetics of drug absorption or metabolism when considering cancer chemotherapy. Specifically, five general principles of tumor biology relevant to treatment appear to be extremely important. These include an understanding of (1) antineoplastic drug action as a function of the cell cycle, (2) tumor cell population growth, (3) tumor cell heterogeneity and drug resistance, (4) the log–cell kill hypothesis, and (5) the critical role of drug scheduling in optimizing therapy. These biologic factors will be reviewed first, followed by a brief discussion of clinical pharmacologic factors that are especially important in cancer chemotherapy.

Drug Action and the Cell Cycle. The life cycle of all cells, both normal and neoplastic, starts with mitosis, or cell division. This is followed either by differentiation or a series of biochemically distinct phases known, in sequence, as G_1 (the first "gap" phase), S phase (DNA synthesis), G_2 (second "gap" phase), and mitosis (Fig. 9-15). Although these events are similar in neoplastic and normal cells, there appear to be some quantitative differences in the duration of the cycle and the sensitivity of cells to drugs during various phases of the cell cycle. Because of these differences, one must differentiate between drugs that kill cells only during specific phases of the cycle *(phase-specific)*, and drugs that kill cells during all or most phases of the cell cycle *(phase-nonspecific)*. The distinction between a phase-specific and phase-nonspecific drug may not be absolute. Some authorities distinguish additional categories or use different names for these categories. In particular, some workers separate the phase-nonspecific drugs into an additional two categories: *cycle-specific* and *non-cycle-specific*. For this discussion, drugs that can affect multiple phases of the cell cycle or that appear to be effective against nondividing cells are grouped together under the term *phase-nonspecific*, since the clinical usefulness of this group appears to be correlated with their lack of phase specificity.

Gompertz and Cell Population Growth. The human organism consists of communities of cells, many of which are capable of self-renewal through cell division. Generally these renewable populations grow rapidly when they are small in number and slowly when they are large. Thus, the fetus grows rapidly, but the adult organism remains constant in size, thanks to a balance between cell production and cell loss. This relation between size and growth rate may be expressed quantitatively in either of two ways: (1) as a function of volume doubling times (time for any given number of cells to double in number) or (2) as a function of the growth fraction (that fraction of cells undergoing division at any one time). Figure 9-16 presents a logarithmic plot of human fetal and childhood growth against time and includes specific data on the volume doubling times during growth. Growth in the early years is clearly exponential with a high growth fraction and very short volume doubling times. As time passes, the doubling time lengthens and the growth fraction decreases. The general slope of this curve can be expressed mathematically as an exponentially decreasing function.

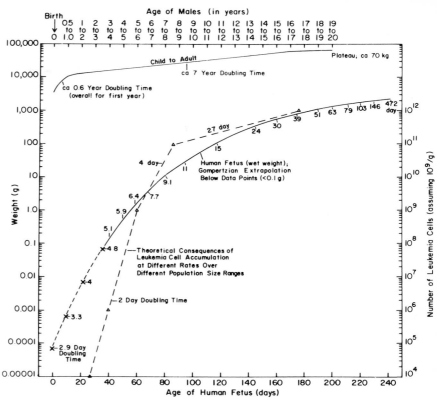

Fig. 9-16. Human fetal and childhood growth as a Gompertzian process, and the theoretic consequences of accumulation of leukemic cells at different rates over varying population ranges. (From: *Skipper HE, Perry S: Cancer Res 30:1883, 1970, with permission.*)

The specific equation describing this relationship was originally derived by the eighteenth century mathematician Gompertz; therefore, biologic growth that conforms to this pattern is referred to as *Gompertzian growth*. Interestingly, evidence that not only normal cell growth but neoplastic cell growth follows a Gompertzian pattern is increasing. At least 18 different animal tumors conform to a Gompertzian growth curve, and Sullivan and Salmon have shown that human myeloma follows a Gompertzian growth pattern.

Tumor Cell Heterogeneity and Drug Resistance. Tumor cells appear to be intrinsically unstable and highly susceptible to mutation. For some tumors, multiple clones of cells may arise through the process of mutation, leading to a highly heterogeneous population of cells with differing sensitivity patterns to various chemotherapeutic agents. This phenomenon, known as tumor cell heterogeneity, has important implications for cancer treatment. It implies that the larger the size of the tumor, the more likely there will be resistance to multiple chemotherapeutic agents. Since drug resistance is the most important reason for the failure of cancer chemotherapy, it implies that chemotherapy should be used as early as possible in the natural history of the cancer in order to assure the highest probability that the tumor will be sensitive to treatment.

The Clonogenic Assay. The search for an in vitro sensitivity test for malignant tumors, analogous to the culture and sensitivity tests in use for bacteria, continues to command the attention of oncologists. Most currently used chemosensitivity tests are based on the human tumor stem cell—or clonogenic—assay developed by Hamburger and Salmon. In this system, single-cell suspensions derived from a biopsied tumor are plated in vitro on a soft agar medium and exposed to various chemotherapeutic agents. Malignant cells alone possess the capability of sustained growth in the semisolid agar medium. The growth of the cultured malignant cells is measured either by the number of colonies formed (usually defined as 30 or more cells per colony as counted by an automated optical scanner) or by the incorporation of radioactive substrates such as tritiated thymidine. The two techniques have been shown to give equivalent results, with the latter technique having the advantages of shorter turnaround time (5 days versus 2 to 3 weeks) and elimination of clumping artifacts (clumps of nonviable tumor cells incorrectly scored as viable colonies). In either method, the in vitro growth of drug-treated tumor cells is compared with untreated "control" cells to determine in vitro sensitivity.

Numerous studies have demonstrated that clonogenic assays, regardless of the exact method employed, have similar predictive accuracies for sensitivity and resistance. Predictive accuracy for sensitivity, defined as the percent probability that a tumor that is sensitive in vitro will be responsive clinically, has consistently ranged from 50 to 65 percent in these studies. Predictive accuracy for resistance, the probability that a tumor that is resistant in vitro will not respond clinically, has been much higher— 85 to 95 percent—suggesting that these assays may be particularly useful for determining which tumors will fail to respond to chemotherapy. Prospective trials have been carried out that confirm the ability of the clonogenic assay to direct chemotherapy. A prospective, randomized trial of the assay has recently been completed in which patients treated with single-agent chemotherapy selected by the assay had a significantly higher clinical response rate than those treated with the physicians's choice of drug.

Despite these favorable results, problems remain. Low in vitro growth rates are common for some tumor types, such as sarcomas and primary breast cancers. Heterogeneity of the chemosensitivity of a tumor, either in the same tumor deposit over time or between two different deposits of the same tumor (e.g., a primary and a metastasis) is a significant theoretical concern and probably a real factor in limiting the predictive accuracy of these assays. Chemotherapeutic combinations—clinically used far more than single-drug therapy—have not been tested as rigorously as single agents. More than any other factor, however, the lack of available active antineoplastic drugs limits the clinical usefulness of predictive testing for most common tumor types. For this reason, attempts have been made to use the clonogenic assay for screening potential new anticancer drugs, with some success.

At present, routine use of in vitro sensitivity testing cannot be advocated for all tumors. Such tests represent a potent research tool and a potential aid in the ongoing search for new antitumor agents. In selected cases, assay-directed chemotherapy can yield a higher likelihood of success than the clinician's best choice. As technical and methodological advances continue to improve in vitro growth rates, it is anticipated that the number of patients who can benefit from in vitro sensitivity testing will increase.

The Log–Cell Kill Hypothesis. Antineoplastic drugs are incapable of killing all cancer cells at any given exposure; rather, they will kill a variable fraction of cells from a very few up to a maximum of 99.99 percent. The fractional cell kill observed can usually be graphed on semilog paper as a line with a negative exponential slope, and so experimental chemotherapeutic data are usually expressed in logarithmic terms. Since the body burden of tumor cells in a human being with an advanced malignant tumor may be greater than 10^{12} cells, and since the best one can hope for with a single maximal exposure of tumor cells to a drug is 2 log–cell kill, it is apparent that treatment must be repeated many times in order to achieve even partial control. Theoretically, this hypothesis also suggests that chemotherapeutic drugs may not be capable of totally eradicating any given population of tumor cells. There is good evidence that immunotherapy does not face this restriction, since it can completely eradicate small numbers of tumor cells; however, it may be totally inef-

fective against larger tumor cell masses (greater than 0.1 mg of tumor in most model systems).

Drug Scheduling and Combination Therapy. Studies with experimental animal tumors have conclusively demonstrated the critical importance of drug scheduling in therapy. Cytosine arabinoside, an antimetabolite that kills only cells in S phase, must be given frequently in order to assure contact with cancer cells during this critical period. When this drug is so employed, it is possible to "cure" some forms of murine leukemia, whereas maximally tolerated doses of the drug given at less frequent intervals fail to prolong survival. On the other hand, cyclophosphamide (Cytoxan), which is phase-nonspecific, achieves optimal suppression of most experimental neoplasms when given on an intermittent schedule.

A second factor related to drug scheduling is the growth status of any given tumor. In general, solid tumors with a large tumor mass will be growing slowly, and will have a small growth fraction (less than 10 percent) and a prolonged tumor volume doubling time. Since relatively few of these cells are dividing, these tumors are generally resistant to phase-specific drugs. Thus, the usual treatment for advanced nonhematologic tumors has been with phase-nonspecific drugs, such as the alkylating agents or 5-FU. However, successful treatment with such phase-nonspecific drugs may render the tumor more susceptible to phase-specific drugs, by converting the tumor from one with a low growth fraction with few of the cells in S phase to one with a higher growth fraction with many cells in S phase.

It is clear that the optimal way to use chemotherapy against most forms of human cancer is by using combinations of drugs. Since cancer chemotherapy usually involves the use of toxic drugs, one must design programs of combination chemotherapy with care in order to minimize dangerous toxicity. In general, the successful programs of combination chemotherapy have been designed with the following criteria in mind: (1) only drugs active against the tumor in question are included; (2) drugs included have different mechanisms of action, in order to minimize the possibility of drug resistance; and (3) drugs chosen generally have different spectra of clinical toxicity, thus allowing the administration of full or nearly full doses of each of the active agents.

Clinical Pharmacology. In addition to the principles relating to tumor biology described above, numerous pharmacologic principles must be considered in cancer chemotherapy. The first such consideration relates to the route of administration of a drug or a combination of drugs. A variety of routes can be chosen, such as oral, intravenous, intramuscular, intraarterial, or local application. By using a carefully selected parenteral route of administration, difficulties related to absorption of drugs are avoided. It also may be possible to improve the antitumor effect of a given drug. Particularly promising in this regard has been the use of drugs by the intraarterial route, such as when the primary tumor is in the liver or on an extremity. Using a portable infusion pump, drugs can be continuously infused over weeks or months. An extension of this approach has been with isolation-perfusion of an extremity with high doses of chemotherapy. As newer drugs are developed, particularly drugs with very short half-life periods, it is likely that the choice of the route of administration will become increasingly important.

A second consideration relates to transport mechanisms for the drug in question. If the drug is transported on serum proteins, it is possible that other drugs may alter significantly the proportion of the bound and free anticancer drug. An example of this is the ability of salicylates to displace methotrexate from its binding site on albumin. In this setting, high doses of salicylates may result in augmented host toxicity from methotrexate.

Another consideration is the possible effect of drug interactions when drugs are given in combinations. One well-established drug interaction involves allopurinol, a xanthine oxidase inhibitor, when it is used with 6-mercaptopurine (6-MP). Since degradation of 6-MP is catalyzed by xanthine oxidase, the use of allopurinol along with full doses of 6-MP has been shown in the past to be dangerous. Normal function of organs important in drug metabolism or degradation may be critical to the biologic fate of a drug. For example, serious liver disease may increase the toxicity of drugs that are cleared by that route, such as vincristine or Adriamycin. Severe neurotoxicity has been observed in patients with concomitant liver disease when given otherwise clinically well-tolerated doses of vincristine.

The route of excretion of a drug may be critical. Methotrexate is primarily excreted by the kidney, and even modest elevation of the BUN (blood urea nitrogen) may be associated with major hematologic toxicity from the use of relatively low doses of methotrexate. For this reason the status of the kidneys must be observed very closely in all patients receiving methotrexate therapy. In fact, it is wise to observe renal function in all patients receiving cancer chemotherapeutic drugs, since nearly all of them have some extent of excretion by the renal route. In addition, it is not unusual for a brisk response to chemotherapy to result in elaboration of large amounts of uric acid, from the breakdown of the nucleic acids of the destroyed cancer cells. Uric acid nephropathy may result. Pretreatment with allopurinol may prevent this complication.

A final factor relates to the ability of a given drug to enter the cancer cell: many drugs require direct access to a specific biochemical pathway within the cell, and failure to gain entry will be associated with drug resistance. To some extent this effect may be overcome by giving very large doses of the drug; however, this is usually associated with unacceptable drug toxicity. An exception to this limitation may be the experimental use of large doses of methotrexate and its antidote, citrovorum factor. Cancer cells appear to lack this transport system. When normal and cancer cells are exposed to massive doses of methotrexate, a high intracellular drug concentration results. When the antidote is subsequently given in lower doses, the normal cells are "rescued" by virtue of the cell membrane transport system. Future work with this treatment

and with others that rely on the transport of drugs across cell membranes may result in further improvements in drug therapy.

The most common cause of treatment failure is the development of drug resistance by tumor cells. Recent studies with human tumors grown in short-term tissue culture suggest that clinical tests for such drug resistance may be possible. Salmon and coworkers have successfully used such "clonogenic assays" to predict drug resistance, and there is widespread interest in the use of such tests clinically. Further work with these assays is needed, but they are very promising as a useful clinical tool.

Ultimately, all factors that might alter either the concentration of the critical drug at its primary site of action or the duration of time available for such activity should be considered in the use of drugs. This may be expressed as a function of concentration times time, and because of its importance it is commonly referred to as the $C \times T$ function.

CHEMOTHERAPY AS AN ADJUVANT TO CANCER SURGERY. The proved ineffectiveness of surgical resection alone for many types of neoplasms has led many investigators to the use of cancer chemotherapeutic agents as adjunctive treatment. It was postulated that these agents might control microscopic foci of cancer already disseminated in the body. Controlled clinical trials have been carried out to determine the effectiveness of single chemotherapeutic agents when combined with surgical resection for carcinomas of the breast, lung, stomach, and colon. Very few significant benefits have been demonstrated thus far using single agents. However, the chemotherapeutic agents chosen for these studies, their dosage, and the duration of administration may not have been optimal for the desired result. It is likely that future applications of this concept using newer chemotherapeutic agents in combination for prolonged periods of time may well result in improved survival for these patients. This approach may be further enhanced by advances in immunotherapy and radiation therapy. An example of one approach to adjuvant chemotherapy as applied to breast cancer appears later in this chapter.

GUIDELINES FOR CHEMOTHERAPY IN PATIENTS WITH NONHEMATOLOGIC MALIGNANT TUMORS. The initial major question a physician must ask when considering chemotherapy for any patient with a neoplasm is whether benefit will result with tolerable toxicity. The physician must have all the facts regarding the patient, including the type, extent, and grade of the malignant tumor, its expected natural history, the results of current therapy, and the psychologic makeup of the patient. In addition, one must consider the following three principles:

1. The patient should have a histologic diagnosis of a malignant disease that is known to respond in a reasonable percentage of cases in a manner beneficial to the patient. Table 9-15 outlines the current status of cancer chemotherapy for a variety of nonhematologic neoplasms. Brief comment on specific drug-sensitive neoplasms will be presented subsequently. In general, patients in whom disease usually or often responds to chemotherapy should receive drug treatment, unless there is a specific contraindication. In addition, patients suspected of

Table 9-15. CURRENT STATUS OF CANCER
CHEMOTHERAPY FOR
NONHEMATOLOGIC NEOPLASMS

Disease	Major drugs used
Chemotherapy used alone with curative intent	
Gestational trophoblastic neoplasia	Methotrexate, actinomycin C, vinca alkaloids, alkylating agents, cisplatin
Testicular tumors	Cisplatin, vinblastine or etoposide, bleomycin
Chemotherapy used with curative intent as part of combined modality therapy	
Wilms' tumor	Actinomycin D, vincristine
Ewing's sarcoma	Cyclophosphamide, vincristine, actinomycin D, doxorubicin
Osteosarcoma	Doxorubicin, methotrexate, cisplatin
Breast cancer	Cyclophosphamide, methotrexate, 5-fluorouracil, doxorubicin
Ovarian cancer	Cisplatin, doxorubicin, cyclophosphamide
Medulloblastoma	Methotrexate
Chemotherapy used with major palliative intent	
Small-cell lung cancer	Cyclophosphamide, vincristine, doxorubicin, etoposide
Prostatic carcinoma	Estrogens
Endometrial carcinoma	Progestins
Adrenal carcinoma	o, p'-DDD
Islet cell carcinoma	Streptozocin
Soft tissue sarcomas	Doxorubicin, cyclophosphamide, cisplatin
Advanced poorly differentiated carcinoma of unknown primary origin	Cisplatin, bleomycin, vinblastine

**Chemotherapy is experimental or is given
with minimal hope of palliation**

Epidermoid carcinomas of the head and neck, cervix, lung,
and from an unknown primary site
Adenocarcinomas of the gastrointestinal tract, pancreas, liver,
bile ducts, lung, and from an unknown primary site
Carcinomas of the bladder or kidney
Melanoma
Neuroblastoma
Brain tumors
Carcinoid tumors

having minimal residual disease (micrometastases) after local
therapy also may be candidates for adjuvant chemotherapy.
Such therapy would be questionable for those patients with a
tumor known to be minimally inhibited by commercially
available drugs. Experimental therapy may be warranted for
these patients.

2. It is absolutely essential that there be adequate facilities to
monitor the potential toxicity outlined in Table 9-14, and physicians should not initiate therapy unless they are adequately
trained in the use of drugs and committed to monitoring the
patient for drug therapy. Chemotherapy is generally contraindicated for patients with nonhematologic malignant condi-

tions if they have major bleeding or infection, although patients with leukemia and, in some cases, lymphomas may
require treatment even during such episodes in order to control life-threatening bleeding or infection. Patients with major
dysfunction of an organ system particularly susceptible to the
toxicity of a cancer chemotherapeutic drug must be followed
carefully and may be more suitably treated with an alternative
drug. An example of this latter situation would be a patient
with a severe neuromyopathy, who might be better treated
with drugs other than vinca alkaloids, as these may exacer-
bate the condition. Patients in whom a rapid response to therapy is possible or who have preexisting renal disease should
be treated with allopurinol to prevent the complication of uric
acid nephropathy. Finally, patients who are under active
chemotherapy and develop severe toxicity may require aggressive support with platelets, red blood cells, antibiotics, or
in some cases, white blood cells for control of infection.

3. Cancer chemotherapeutic drugs are toxic. In order to minimize unwarranted toxicity, the physician should conduct a
diligent search for disease markers to assist in monitoring
treatment. Ideally, several parameters of tumor response
should be followed in order to objectively assess the response
to therapy. Some factors that can be considered in assessing
response to treatment are described in more detail in Table
9-16. As a general rule, tumor size is of particular importance.
Most oncologists require a 50 percent reduction in the product
of the greater and lesser diameters of any given tumor to accept the change as a "partial response."

The specific choice of a drug or drugs for a given patient
with cancer and the precise choice of a dose and schedule for
such single agent or combination therapy are best decided in
the light of current therapeutic research. To some extent such
choices can be determined by referring to Table 9-16 and the
following section. Other useful sources of information include
the *Medical Letter on Drugs and Therapeutics,* which period-

Table 9-16. CRITERIA FOR RESPONSES IN
PATIENTS WITH SOLID TUMORS

Tumor size	Palpation and measurement with calipers
	Radiologic measurement
	Radioisotope scans
	Ultrasound
	CAT scan
	Magnetic resonance imaging (MRI)
Tumor products	Quantitative level of chorionic gonadotropin (choriocarcinoma and certain testicular tumors)
	Quantitative level of carcinoembryonic antigen (CEA) in bowel cancer
	Quantitative level of α-fetoprotein in hepatoma or testicular tumors
	Serum or urine paraproteins in myeloma
	Urinary adrenal hormone (adrenal carcinoma treated with o,p'-DDD)
Improvement in symptoms or sign of tumor	Improvement in hypercalcemia (particularly with carcinoma involving bone)
	Improvement in obstruction due to tumor (such as bowel obstruction or obstructed ureter)
	Disappearance of effusions from tumors involving pleura, peritoneum, or obstructing lymphatics
	Subjective symptoms are important to patient but are generally poor indicators of antitumor response

ically publishes information on the choice of therapy in the treatment of cancer; books on the treatment of cancer (such as that edited by Haskell); and the specialty journals of cancer (*Cancer; Cancer Treatment Reports; The Journal of Clinical Oncology; Seminars in Oncology*).

ILLUSTRATIVE NEOPLASMS HIGHLY RESPONSIVE TO CHEMOTHERAPY. Trophoblastic Tumors of the Uterus. Metastatic gestational choriocarcinoma is curable in 80 to 90 percent of women using chemotherapeutic drugs alone. The discovery by Li et al. in 1956 that methotrexate could control metastatic disease in women with choriocarcinoma represents a landmark in the history of cancer chemotherapy. Subsequent systematic study of this disease has markedly increased our understanding about cancer and its treatment. Certain points are worthy of special mention.

1. Methotrexate must be started as soon as possible after the diagnosis has been made. This relates to the finding that the best prognosis, with cure rates of 95 to 100 percent, is seen in patients whose disease is treated within 4 months of onset, in whom metastases do not include the brain or liver, and in whom 24-h urine quantities of human chorionic gonadotropins (HCG) are less than 100,000 I.U.
2. Combination chemotherapy should be used if the initial response to chemotherapy is suboptimal or if the patient presents with high titers of HCG, with liver or brain involvement, or with symptoms present longer than 4 months. Second-line drugs for this disease include actinomycin D, vincristine, alkylating agents, and doxorubicin.
3. Therapy should be continued for 6 months after the chorionic gonadotropin titer has returned to normal. This is even more important than eliminating radiographic evidence of disease, since residual pulmonary lesions may be present despite cure of clinical growths. This is analogous to the residual changes of many nonneoplastic diseases, such as tuberculosis.

Germ-Cell Tumors of the Testis. All forms of testicular cancer are now considered to be highly responsive to chemotherapy. This was initially proved in patients with advanced embryonal cell carcinomas, yolk sac tumors, and choriocarcinoma using various combinations of cisplatin, bleomycin, and vinblastine. Subsequently, the same has been shown for patients with bulky or advanced seminoma. Currently, the major difference between the treatment of advanced seminoma and the various forms of "nonseminomatous germ-cell tumors" of the testis is how one utilizes combined modality therapy. Both groups of patients with advanced, bulky disease now receive immediate combination agent chemotherapy for at least 4 months. Patients with nonseminomatous tumors with persistently elevated levels of the tumor markers alphafetoprotein or beta-chorionic gonadotropin may be treated even longer. After the completion of chemotherapy, patients with seminoma may receive additional radiation therapy to areas of previously known disease or to residual masses. Masses that persist after this therapy are almost always scar tissue or necrotic tumor, so surgery plays no role in these patients. They are considered potentially cured with chemotherapy alone, or with the combination of chemotherapy and radiation therapy. The situation is very different, however, for the various forms of nonseminomatous tumor. These tumors tend to consist of a heterogeneous population of tumor cells, and it is not unusual for chemotherapy to eradicate the drug-sensitive population, leaving histologically benign teratomas. These "benign" tumors are resistant to radiation therapy, and they can be locally aggressive, so they must be surgically removed. Thus, patients with nonseminomatous tumors usually undergo surgical exploration rather than radiation therapy following the completion of combination chemotherapy.

Carcinoma of the Prostate. The mainstays of therapy for disseminated cancer of the prostate are orchiectomy and estrogen therapy. These modalities have increased survival of these patients modestly, and they are of major palliative value in controlling pain. Many different doses of the most commonly used estrogenic hormone have been employed. However, data from the Veterans Administration Cooperative Research Group have shown up to a 25 percent increased mortality from cardiovascular diseases in a group of patients treated with moderately high doses (5 mg daily) of diethylstilbestrol. A prospective study has since proved that a low dose of 1 mg daily results in good antitumor effects without significant cardiovascular toxicity.

Wilms' Tumor. Improvements in survival for patients with Wilms' tumor have developed steadily in recent years. Whereas this was once considered a hopeless tumor to treat, it is now possible to control the disease for substantial periods of time in 80 percent of children with the disease. This improvement involves the sequential use of optimal surgery, radiation therapy, and chemotherapy with actinomycin D and/or vincristine. A national study group is currently trying to resolve the optimal combination of these modalities; however, it is clear that the addition of effective chemotherapy has substantially improved the care of these patients.

Carcinoma of the Breast. Recent developments involving a combination chemotherapy, estradiol receptor protein, competitive inhibitors of estrogen, medical adrenalectomy, and adjuvant chemotherapy have substantially changed the contemporary treatment of this disease.

Most physicians are currently treating advanced breast cancer with multiple combinations of drugs. One such combination includes 5-FU, cyclophosphamide, vincristine, methotrexate, and sometimes prednisone (CMFVP). Another combination includes Adriamycin and cyclophosphamide (AC) or 5-FU, Adriamycin, and cyclophosphamide (FAC). Response rates for these combinations have been generally 50 percent or greater, compared with 20 to 35 percent for the same drugs used as single agents. The median duration of response with combination chemotherapy has been in the range of 9 months.

Changing concepts of the biology of breast cancer have stimulated a number of clinical trials of adjuvant chemotherapy using single or multiple agents given intermittently over prolonged periods after operation. Many such studies are currently in progress, and most have demonstrated a reduced early recurrence rate for patients treated with adjuvant chemotherapy. One study has also shown an improved 10-year survival rate for patients

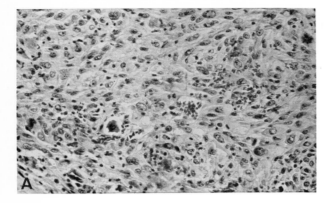

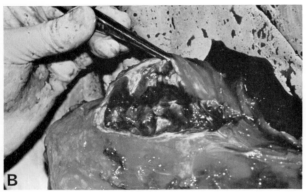

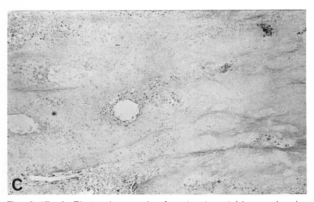

Fig. 9-17. *A.* Photomicrograph of pretreatment biopsy showing osteosarcoma with minimal necrosis (×250). *B.* Resected surgical specimen following preoperative treatment with intraarterial Adriamycin and radiation therapy. Note gross tumor liquefaction and necrosis. *C.* Photomicrograph of posttreatment specimen showing 99 percent tumor necrosis with loss of nuclei (×40). (From: *Morton DL et al: Ann Surg 184:268, 1976, with permission.*)

treated after operation with cyclophosphamide, methotrexate, and 5-fluorouracil (CMF). If these exciting preliminary results are confirmed, they will mark the first real impact on the natural history of breast cancer since the Halsted radical mastectomy.

A number of interesting therapeutic options in breast cancer are being evaluated by studies currently in progress. These include investigations to determine (1) the optimal combination and sequence of drugs and/or hormonal agents; (2) the efficacy of adjuvant chemoimmunotherapy, chemohormonal therapy, or hormonal manipulation used alone in women with estradiol receptor–positive tumors; (3) whether surgical adrenalectomy and medical adrenalectomy using aminoglutethimide are comparable; and (4) the usefulness of the estrogen antagonist tamoxifen in different patient groups.

COMBINED MODALITY THERAPY. Pediatric oncologists pioneered the use of combined modality therapy—radiation in combination with chemotherapy and surgical therapy—to overcome childhood neoplasms. The cure rate for localized retinoblastoma and other sarcomas in children has been increased dramatically with combined therapy. Wilms' tumor can be cured 75 percent of the time if surgical therapy is followed by radiation and chemotherapy, an increase of 40 percent over operation alone. Embryonal rhabdomyosarcoma responds best to combinations of radiation, chemotherapy, and operation.

Until recently, the effectiveness of multimodality therapy had been demonstrated only occasionally for adult neoplasms. An example illustrates the complexity of such combined therapy for skeletal and soft tissue sarcomas.

Surgical therapy, the accepted method for management of most skeletal and soft tisue sarcomas of the extremity, has been associated with frequent treatment failure. Even with amputation, approximately 50 percent of patients with soft tissue sarcoma and 80 percent of those with sarcomas of bone eventually developed and died from their distant metastases. In an attempt to improve results of treatment for the sarcomas, a regimen of combined pre- and postoperative therapy was developed. Preoperative continuous intraarterial infusion of doxorubicin and radiation therapy followed by surgical resection achieved preservation of a functional extremity in most patients with no decrease in survival.

The preoperative therapy with intraarterial Adriamycin followed by radiation was found to produce extensive tumor cell necrosis as high as 88 percent (Fig. 9-17*A, B, C*). The effectiveness of this preoperative therapy permitted local resection of the sarcoma and salvage of a viable, functional extremity. Local recurrence rates are as low as with amputation, and long-term results are functionally and psychologically superior.

Early data suggest that multimodality therapy may be effective for small localized breast cancers. In several studies, radiation and minimal surgery were as effective as mastectomy for control of small breast cancers. Survival and local recurrence rates were the same for both groups, and patients treated with multimodality therapy were spared the physical deformity and the psychological problems of mastectomy.

Immunotherapy

One of the basic problems associated with all forms of cancer therapy is caused by the similarities in the biochemical and subcellular constituents of the cancer and normal cells. Although some cancer cells may have a rapid rate of cell division when compared with normal cells of the same organ, there are other normal cells in the body (e.g., those in the bone marrow and intestinal epithelium) that may grow even more rapidly. Hence, any therapy designed to inhibit the proliferation rate of cancer cells may also inhibit the function of these normal cells. Radiation and chemotherapy can injure the normal tissue as well as tumor cells. Similarly, cancer surgery often requires the sacrifice of normal tissues and organs to ensure an adequate margin around the cancer cells. In contrast, immunotherapy depends upon basic antigenic differences between neoplastic and normal cells for its therapeutic effect.

In contrast, immunotherapy is a logical adjunct for the treatment of subclinical microscopic disease following definitive cancer surgery, radiation therapy, or chemotherapy, for the following reasons: (1) Patients who have only small foci of cancer cells remaining after destruction of the major tumor bulk are the most likely to benefit from immunotherapy, because the tumor mass that must be destroyed is smallest at that time. (2) The specificity of the immune response provides a possible therapeutic tool that has selectivity for small numbers of cancer cells not possible with any other therapeutic modality. (3) Patients with disease in earlier stages are more likely to respond to immunotherapeutic maneuvers, since the cancer patient's general immune competence is greatest when the disease is localized and is often impaired after metastasis. (4) Immunotherapy should complement rather than interfere with currently available methods of cancer therapy. However, since both irradiation and chemotherapy are immunosuppressive, the use of immunotherapy in combination with these therapeutic modalities must be carefully controlled.

Numerous attempts at immunotherapy of cancer have been undertaken since the turn of the century. Although an occasional striking regression was obtained, in most cases the results were neither impressive nor consistent, and interest in this treatment modality declined until recently. With the availability of large quantities of purified biological response modifiers (such as interleukin-1 and -2, interferon, tumor necrosis factor) made available by recombinant DNA technology, a patient's immune defenses may be dramatically manipulated in a number of ways. These scientific advances, coupled with a clearer understanding of the regulation of tumor immunity, have ushered in a new era for the clinical immunotherapy of human cancer.

ACTIVE SPECIFIC IMMUNOTHERAPY. This form of immunotherapy is an effort to stimulate the host to generate a specific immune response to its tumor, generally with the use of tumor cell or tumor antigen vaccines. In this method of treatment, efforts are made to increase the patient's tumor immunity by altering the tumor antigen in such a way that it becomes more antigenic before immunizing the patient.

Most attempts at immunotherapy in human beings have involved vaccines composed of whole tumor cells inactivated by a variety of different methods to render the cells incapable of proliferation. These methods have included radiation, mitomycin C treatment, freezing and thawing,

or heat treatment. Although such techniques have prevented progressive tumor growth, they may have inactivated the tumor-specific antigens as well. For example, the same freezing and thawing technique frequently used to prepare human tumor vaccines has often inactivated tumor-specific antigens of carcinogen-induced animal neoplasms.

Studies with animal neoplasms demonstrate that living tumor cells administered intradermally in numbers insufficient for progressive tumor growth generally are the most effective immunogens. The possibility that living tumor cells might result in tumor growth at the inoculation site has inhibited the use of such vaccines in human beings. However, it would seem that with certain tumors that share common tumor-specific antigens, such as skeletal and soft tissue sarcomas, one patient could be immunized with an allogenic vaccine of living tumor cells from another patient. An immune response could be induced against the foreign HLA transplantation antigens on the tumor cells, causing their rejection. Theoretically this immunization should induce a strong immune response against a common cross-reacting tumor-specific antigen as well.

Repeated attempts have been made to increase the antigenicity of tumor vaccines by modifying the tumor cells in a variety of ways. These have included coupling highly antigenic carrier proteins such as rabbit γ-globulin to the tumor cells, and chemical treatment by agents such as iodoacetate and, more recently, with neuraminidase and concanavalin A. Regression of established tumors has been observed in animals following active immunotherapy with such vaccines (Fig. 9-18).

Many of these experiments have used immunological adjuvants as well, such as bacillus Calmette-Guérin

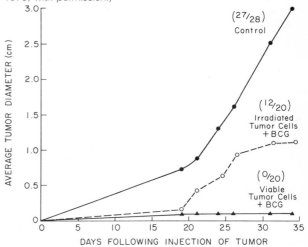

Fig. 9-18. Immunotherapy experiments with a transplantable liposarcoma in syngeneic strain 2 guinea pigs: 1×10^5 liposarcoma tumor cells were inoculated intramuscularly into the leg, and immunotherapy was initiated intradermally in four sites on the back with 1×10^6 living or 1×10^7 irradiated tumor cells mixed with bacillus Calmette-Guérin (BCG). (From: *Morton DL et al: Ann Surg 172:740, 1970, with permission.*)

(BCG) vaccine, *Corynebacterium parvum,* and Freund's adjuvant, in an attempt to enhance the host's immune response to the native or modified tumor antigens.

The ideal tumor vaccine in many respects, however, would be one composed of the isolated and purified tumor-specific transplantation antigens from the cell surface. Such vaccines would have the advantages of safety, stability, and ease of administration. Previous experience gained with guinea pig sarcomas from which isolated and partially purified tumor-specific antigen preparations induced good immunity to tumor challenge suggests that success can be anticipated for this approach. However, to date, there has been little progress along these lines with the human tumor-associated transplantation antigen.

In summary, active immunotherapy using vaccines prepared in a variety of ways combined with many different types of immunoadjuvants has been used in clinical trials. It can be demonstrated clearly that such autoimmunization procedures do enhance patients' immune responses to their own tumors. Results to date, however, have not been impressive, although newer knowledge about lymphokines that modulate the immune response suggests that active immunotherapy may become more effective in the future.

PASSIVE IMMUNOTHERAPY. In passive immunotherapy, tumor-specific antiserum is used systemically in an effort to suppress tumor. This approach is fraught with a number of theoretic and practical problems. Passive immunotherapy, for a number of reasons, is only effective in suppressing small numbers of tumor cells and must work in concert with host effectors (complement, macrophages, K cells, etc.) to effect a cytotoxic action on target cells. Moreover, only antibodies of certain classes and subclasses can interact effectively with certain cellular effectors. Finally, most of the better characterized human tumor-specific antisera are murine monoclonal antibodies that, because of their antigenicity, have limited applications in human beings. Recently, Irie and Morton have successfully used a human monoclonal IgM antibody specific for ganglioside GD2 to successfully treat human melanoma satellite lesions. The emerging field of human monoclonal antibodies will likely make these immunotherapy modalities more practical and effective.

IMMUNOTOXINS. Immunotoxins are tumor-specific antibodies to which are attached toxic molecules. This intuitively appealing concept, first proposed by Paul Ehrlich one century ago, employs the antibody molecule to preferentially localize anticancer agents in the vicinity of tumors. It obviates the need for the host to supply effector cells or complement to mediate tumor destruction. Monoclonal antibodies are preferred to heterologous antiserum since they permit the use of homogeneous, purified antibodies of defined specificity. A wide range of toxic molecules has been tested in vitro and includes radioactive isotopes, traditional cancer drugs, and plant and bacterial toxins. Recombinant DNA technology now permits the creation of hybrid or chimeric immunotoxin molecules in which the Fc portion of the immunoglobulin molecule has been replaced by a polypeptide toxin sequence. Immunotoxins are currently undergoing clinical trials, although their overall therapeutic efficiency in clinical oncology is unproved.

ADOPTIVE IMMUNOTHERAPY. In adoptive immunotherapy, immune lymphoid cells are transferred to a recipient to mediate tumor destruction. In many experimental murine tumors, in vivo transfer of lymphocytes from an immune mouse to a tumor-bearing mouse can cause dramatic tumor regression (Fig. 9-19). These immune lymphocytes are tumor-antigen-specific, display major histocompatibility complex restriction, and have classical T cell markers; thus, they are classical cytolytic T lymphocytes. In these animal models, it is necessary to use large numbers of cells from immunized, syngeneic (genetically identical) donor mice. This effective immunotherapeutic modality is unfortunately technically impractical in human beings.

Rosenberg and colleagues have pioneered the study of adoptive immunotherapy using so-called lymphokine-activated killer (LAK) cells. LAK cells are cytolytic lymphocytes that are generated in the presence of interleukin-2 (IL-2). Treatment of human lymphocytes from almost any source (peripheral blood, lymph nodes, spleen, thymus, bone marrow) results in the creation of cytolytic cells capable of killing a wide range of fresh and cultured human cancer cells but not normal cells. The biochemical nature of this tumor-specific recognition and killing is not fully defined. Human LAK cells do not have T cell markers and are not MHC or antigen-specific in their killing. It is not yet certain whether they represent a novel cell type or are expanded and modified from an NK precursor pool.

Extensive animal experiments demonstrate the ability of systemically administered LAK cells and IL-2 to cause dramatic regression of many different types of primary and metastatic tumors. Clinical trials using autologous LAK cells (obtained by repeated leukopheresis and in vitro IL-2 expansion) and systemically administered IL-2 have resulted in clear, objective responses in some patients with bulky metastatic cancer. Administration of high doses of IL-2 alone have some clinical efficacy but considerable toxicity. Even greater toxicity is seen with combined administration of LAK cells and IL-2 and includes fluid retention and renal dysfunction. Nevertheless, these impressive studies, in patients with large tumor burdens, are an exciting glimpse of the potential of properly manipulated immune systems.

NONSPECIFIC IMMUNOTHERAPY

The theoretic basis for nonspecific immunotherapy depends upon the observation that certain substances, such as mixed bacterial toxins and fractions of the tubercle bacillus, have the ability to nonspecifically enhance host resistance to most viral, fungal, and bacterial agents. Although the exact mechanism is unknown, these agents do appear to stimulate immune response to a wide variety of antigens, including tumor antigens.

Historically, a type of nonspecific immunotherapy was described by Bradford Coley at the turn of the century in one of the first reports of a tumor regression possibly in-

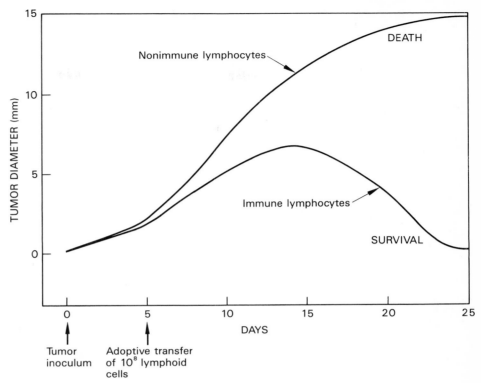

Fig. 9-19. Regression of experimental tumor upon adoptive transfers of immune lymphocytes.

duced by immunologic means. Coley's interest in the possible value of such therapy was stimulated when he observed a recurrent inoperable sarcoma of the neck regress completely for 7 years after the patient had had attacks of erysipelas. This observation led to the development of Coley's toxins, a mixture of killed bacterial vaccines. Coley injected this admixture directly into tumor lesions or gave it intravenously. Some impressive regressions of tumors and long-term cures resulted from these agents. Because the responses were inconsistent, Coley's toxins never received widespread use, and interest in them died out. Recent interest in a nonspecific immunotherapy of a similar type has been revived using attenuated bovine tuberculosis bacillus (BCG).

Our work with BCG began more than 20 years ago, when we injected BCG into metastatic nodules in the skin and subcutaneous tissues in patients with malignant melanoma. We observed that the intratumor injection of BCG caused 90 percent of the intradermal metastases to regress in patients who were immunologically competent. In addition, in about 20 percent of these patients, uninjected nodules were observed to regress. Satellite, in-transit metastases, and local recurrence often can be controlled in the extremity by this technique; however, many of these patients still develop systemic metastases. Although the intratumor injection of BCG may not control systemic disease, it is nonetheless a very useful method to control local disease that avoids the side effects of chemotherapy and can result in long-term survival.

There are several possible mechanisms to explain tumor regression following BCG injection; both specific and nonspecific immune reactions were probably involved. The tumor cells may be killed as "innocent bystanders" during the delayed cutaneous hypersensitivity reaction that occurs when lymphocytes and macrophages attack BCG dispersed throughout the tumor nodule. This is supported by the observation that the intratumor injection of BCG works only in patients who can be sensitized to BCG, as shown by their delayed cutaneous hypersensitivity reaction to PPD.

In addition to the nonspecific effect, a specific immune response to melanoma-associated tumor antigens also occurs in some patients because an associated rising titer of antimelanoma antibody is observed following BCG immunotherapy. Sequential biopsies of tumor nodules following BCG inoculation reveals that the regression of these nodules is associated with a granulomatous infiltration of lymphocytes, monocytes, and fibroblasts surrounding and infiltrating the melanoma cells. Furthermore, the regression of melanoma nodules not given injection with BCG is accompanied by the appearance of lymphocyte infiltrates within the regressing melanoma tumor nodules (Fig. 9-20). The specific antitumor effect may result from more lymphocytes and macrophages coming into contact with the tumor cells so that the afferent limb of the immune response is increased. Conversely, it may work via the effector limb of the immune response by bringing greater numbers of both stimulated and unstimulated lymphocytes to the tumor.

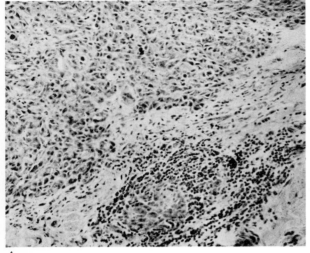

A

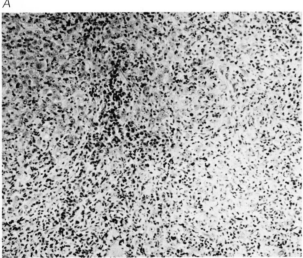

B

Fig. 9-20. *A.* Subcutaneous metastasis of malignant melanoma prior to immunotherapy with BCG. Note the absence of lymphocytic and monocytic infiltration among the tumor cells. *B.* Subcutaneous metastasis that has decreased in size from 10 to 5 mm during the 6-week period following immunotherapy with BCG injections into other melanoma nodules. BCG was *not* injected into this nodule. Note the marked lymphocytic and monocytic infiltration among the melanoma cells. (From: *Morton DL et al: Ann Surg 172:740, 1970, with permission.*)

Our results have now been confirmed by a number of investigators. The observation that the intratumor injection of BCG occasionally led to the regression of uninjected nodules suggested that BCG might be useful as an adjuvant to operation to control micrometastatic disease in human beings. BCG has been shown to prevent growth of spontaneous metastases in some animal tumor models where variables of tumor load and time of BCG vaccination can be carefully controlled. In human beings, a number of preliminary reports have suggested that intradermal BCG delays recurrence in patients with melanoma

who are at high risk because of metastases to regional nodes. However, in our prospective randomized trial of adjuvant immunotherapy, BCG did not diminish the recurrence rate, but did significantly extend survival once the disease recurred.

BCG is only one of a wide variety of agents that can nonspecifically stimulate the immune system's response to a variety of different types of antigens. Examples of other agents include *Corynebacterium parvum,* MER (methanol-extractable residue of BCG), bacterial antitoxins, and polynucleotides.

Other impressive results with nonspecific immunotherapy come from the studies of Klein in patients with basal and squamous cell carcinomas of the skin. Here the induction of delayed hypersensitivity reactions to DNCB resulted in the resolution of more than 90 percent of superficial basal or squamous cell carcinomas. Klein observed that the mixture of multiple antigens such as PPD, mumps, and *Candida* increased the delayed hypersensitivity and effectiveness of this form of immunotherapy.

Another form of nonspecific immunotherapy involves the use of agents capable of restoring depressed immune responses. Several agents have been proposed in such a context, including thymic hormones such as thymosin and the antihelminthic drug levamisole.

The rational application of immunotherapy to human cancer will depend, to a large extent, on a better knowledge of tumor-associated antigens in human neoplasms and methods for increasing the immune response against these antigens. Specificity for cancer cells cannot be achieved by any other known therapeutic means, but the potency of immunotherapy is limited.

Expectations of dramatic benefits from immunotherapy for malignant disease have been high; however, the results of many clinical trials have fallen short of these expectations. The theoretical advantages of a specific systemic antitumor adjuvant with minimal toxicity continues to make immunotherapy a promising avenue of future investigation. At the present time, its use should be limited to cancer facilities where the effects of this form of treatment can be scientifically evaluated.

SURGERY AS IMMUNOTHERAPY

A tumor may promote its own growth by a number of immune mechanisms. The cancer cell may act as a "factory" that is constantly producing both immunosuppressive factors and tumor-associated antigens (Fig. 9-21). The specific and nonspecific immunosuppression decreases the patient's immune defenses and facilitates growth of the tumor. In numerous studies, this immunosuppression appears to be related to the presence of the tumor.

The key to recovery of the balance in the host-tumor relationship depends on destruction or removal of the tumor cell "factory." Surgery appears to be the most efficient means of removing the factory. Once the mass of tumor is gone, the patient with cancer is more likely to be able to mount an immune response that may destroy any subclinical foci of tumor cells scattered through the body.

CANCER SURGERY AS IMMUNOTHERAPY

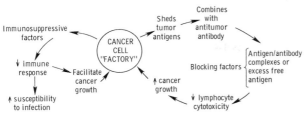

Fig. 9-21. Schematic of cancer cell factory as it might function to enhance its growth by producing immunosuppression in the host. Theoretically, cancer surgery removes the cancer factory and its associated immunosuppressants, which allows the host immune responses to return to normal. (From: *Morton DL et al: Chest 71:640, 1977, with permission.*)

However, if the recovery of the immune response is inadequate or if the number of tumor cells in any distant metastatic focus is too large, the patient may fail to regain control of the disease. Nonetheless, surgery for cancer becomes the first step in immunotherapy.

If this thesis is correct, it would follow that the approach to the surgical treatment for solid neoplasms must change dramatically. The future lies not in treating every patient with a solid neoplasm as one with localized disease but in assuming that the local disease is merely a manifestation of a systemic illness, whether or not the patient has overt metastatic disease. Not until we accept surgery as merely the first step in the treatment of cancer can we significantly improve our rates of cure. Therapeutic advances eventually must come from a multimethod combination of immunotherapy and chemotherapy with surgical therapy or radiotherapy. Unlike surgery and radiotherapy, both local treatments, the triple combinations represent a systemic treatment effective against tumor cells already metastatic to distant sites. However, at present, systemic therapeutic techniques have greater potential for curing those patients with a minimal number of tumor cells, rather than those with clinically evident disease. Surgery for apparently localized tumors can favorably affect the host-tumor relationship and may even cure the patient with subclinical distant metastases. However, debulking the unresectable or recurrent tumors in the patient with metastatic disease is usually unsuccessful and rarely indicated.

Hyperthermia*

National efforts are under way to establish additional safe and reliable forms of therapy. Results in laboratory models, animals, and initial human clinical trials have been very encouraging and suggest that thermal therapy—hyperthermia—may have a substantive role in future cancer treatment. In 1967, Cavaliere and his colleagues in Rome announced that tumor cells were apparently selectively thermosensitive compared with normal cells at

---

* Storm FK (ed): *Hyperthermia in Cancer Therapy*. Chicago, Year Book Medical Publishers, 1985.

temperatures from 42 to 45°C (108 to 113°F). During the late 1960s and early 1970s, evidence continued to suggest that at 42 to 45°C tumor cells were slightly more sensitive to heat than normal cells. When a cell subline derived from a non-tumor-producing line acquired high tumor-producing ability, it also acquired reduced thermotolerance. These and other investigations both in vitro and in vivo suggested that the acquisition of malignant potential was associated with increased thermosensitivity.

Investigators have found that a major factor in cell killing at 42°C is the irreversible damage to cancer cell respiration. Coincident alterations appear to take place in nucleic acid and protein synthesis that include a reduction of activity in many vital enzyme systems. These factors, associated with an increase in cell-wall membrane permeability and the liberation of lysozymes, probably account for the autolytic cell destruction after hyperthermia. The efficacy of thermocytotoxicity increased rapidly as temperatures were increased from 42 to 45°C, the threshold of thermal pain in human beings. At such temperatures, the differential thermosensitivity between malignant and normal cells is reduced and replaced by a linear cell kill from progressive protein denaturation. Thus, at 45°C, host tissue tolerance becomes a prime concern in the design of clinical trials.

It is well known from experiments on exposed tumors that energy concentrated within a tumor, from interstitial implants, focused ultrasound, or microwaves potentially provides enough local heat for tumor destruction. Less well known is the fact that nonfocused microwaves and capacitive, inductive, and magnetic-loop radio-frequency applicators can heat a region of the host that contains the tumor, providing "selective tumor heating," this having remarkable implications for the treatment of deep-seated tumors. Extensive temperature measurements during hyperthermia therapy in spontaneous animal and human tumors demonstrate that many tumors selectively retain more heat than normal tissues because their neovascularity is physiologically unresponsive to thermal stress and is incapable of regulating and augmenting blood flow. Thus effective independent tumor heating is possible deep within the body, even without the ability to focus such energy.

Interstitial hyperthermia has been achieved by passing a low-frequency current between electrodes implanted directly into tumors. While invasive, this technique has been useful for small accessible tumors where the full extent of the lesion was known (for example, oropharynx, vagina, and rectum). Liquid silicone impregnated with finely powdered iron particles has been used to occlude the vascular beds of tumors. The potential for selectively heating the metallic material that remains in the tumor in the vulcanized silicone offers promise. Ultrasound, a well-defined and spatially manipulative source of acoustic energy when focused, has potential for noninvasive selective heating of a target volume at depth. However, unlike electromagnetic energy, ultrasound does not propagate effectively through air and is ineffective near air-containing spaces (for example, oral-nasal cavity and respiratory and gastrointestinal tracts). Most clinical trials have been limited to superficial tumors heated to 43 to 45°C. Microwaves have produced effective noninvasive localized hyperthermia to large areas of surface tissues and have been quite useful for treatment of superficial tumors. Radio frequency (RF) has provided a means for both local and regional in-depth noninvasive hyperthermia, particularly when magnetic-loop applicators are employed. These create a strong electromagnetic field into which the body or limb is immersed. This approach permits safe and effective heating of visceral human tumors and has provided most of the available knowledge about the effects of localized heat therapy on deep internal human cancers.

Effective hyperthermia can be achieved in most superficial and visceral solid human tumors regardless of histopathologic type, although it is most effective for large tumors. Some tumors cannot be safely heated to 42°C and seem to retain their ability to regulate blood flow and dissipate heat. Distinct histologic changes occur in effectively heated tumor cells but not in stromal or vascular cells within the tumor, or in adjacent normal tissues. Rapid autolytic disintegration of heat-damaged tumor cells is observed, followed by a marked increase in connective stroma associated with progressive scar formation. Progressive coagulation necrosis occurs at 45°C, although its results appear to differ depending on the location of the tumor. Superficial tumors generally slough off, whereas visceral tumors may not significantly change in size after a transient increase in size during treatment. Therefore, biopsy or careful assessment of tumor doubling time (for example, stabilization of a previously progressive tumor) is necessary to determine the effects of high-temperature internal tumor therapy.

At temperatures greater than 45°C, tumors display extensive vascular thrombosis. Subsequent resection has been facilitated in some instances by the avascular nature of the tumor. Heat also sensitizes tissues to ionizing radiation. Hyperthermia has been combined with radiation therapy, both external beam and interstitial, in an effort to produce a synergistic or additive response. Several investigators have concluded that hypoxic cells may be at least as sensitive to hyperthermia as oxygenated cells, forming one rationale for combination therapy. Others have suggested that the primary effect of hyperthermia is to inhibit cellular recovery from sublethal radiation injury. As previously noted, heat seems to alter tumor cell membrane permeability. This finding suggested that enhanced intracellular drug uptake might occur at elevated temperatures, which has since been documented in in vitro studies. A recent review of laboratory investigations has shown an additional 2- to 3-log kill at 43 to 45°C over that at 37°C for thiotepa, bleomycin, phenylalanine mustard (L-PAM), amphotericin B, methyl-CCNU, CCNU, cisplatin, methotrexate, and Adriamycin. The best-known clinical example of this synergism can be found in regional hyperthermic chemotherapeutic limb perfusion for in-transit metastatic melanoma. Once hyperthermia therapy is optimized, it may be possible to achieve responses at lower drug doses, which, in turn, may reduce drug toxicity and prolong the duration of therapy. It also may be possible to reinstitute use of previously less effective drugs with the expectation of enhanced activity due to hyperthermia.

PROGNOSIS

Predicting the future course of a patient's malignant disease is one of the most difficult problems an oncologist faces. At the present time, it is impossible to predict the future course of a given patient except in general terms. However, a number of known factors are important in determining prognosis.

The *site of origin* of the primary tumor is one of the most important factors influencing prognosis. The propensity of a neoplasm to metastasize to distant sites varies according to its tissue of origin. Over 90 percent of carcinomas of the lung, pancreas, and esophagus spread beyond their primary site and cause death, whereas carcinomas of the skin, breast, and thyroid glands are frequently localized and curable, even when metastatic in some patients.

The *stage of disease* at the time of initial treatment is of considerable importance in determining survival for all types of neoplasms. The chance for cure is best when the neoplasm is confined to the organ of origin. The smaller the primary neoplasm, the better the prognosis, as well. Thus, in situ carcinoma of the cervix, carcinomas of the breast less than 1 cm in diameter, and small polypoid carcinomas of the colon are generally curable; larger neoplasms may not be curable. Direct extension into adjacent organs or metastases to regional nodes suggest a more guarded prognosis, although many patients are still curable at this stage of the disease. The spread of cancer by the bloodstream with metastases to distant sites portends a grave prognosis, and few patients are curable at this stage. As a general rule, lymph node involvement sharply reduces survival probability by about one-half that of patients without involved nodes. The total number of involved nodes is an important prognostic guide.

The *histopathologic features* of the neoplasm correlate in a general way to prognosis. The more undifferentiated, highly malignant-appearing neoplasms with frequent mitosis are more likely to develop early distant spread and local recurrence. However, some very malignant neoplasms still can be cured with adequate treatment. Venous invasion is a grave prognostic factor in all types of neoplasia.

Host immune factors, as previously discussed, may be an important factor in determining prognosis. Immunologic methods for monitoring immune responses are currently under development. It is already apparent that those patients who have spontaneous depression of their immune responses have a uniformly poor prognosis following therapy.

The *age of the patient* may be an important factor affecting prognosis. Some oncologists believe that neoplasms in younger patients carry a poorer prognosis than the same tumors in middle-aged or elderly patients, although elderly patients may have associated medical problems that do not permit adequate treatment of the cancer. While there may be some validity in this concept, it should not be overemphasized, because many young patients have a good prognosis. In fact, some have a much better prognosis than adults with the same neoplasms. Those neoplasms which occur prior to one year of age generally have a better prognosis than those which occur later in childhood. This can be determined in the following manner: The child is usually cured of the neoplasm if free of disease for 9 months after treatment, plus double the age at the time treatment was begun. This concept is based upon the supposition that if the earliest cancer cell started with conception and if the cancer grew at a constant rate, then it would reach a certain size at the time treatment was initiated. If treatment was successful in eliminating all cancer cells except one, then in a period equal to 9 months plus double the age of the child, the cancer size would again be equivalent to the original tumor mass. Therefore, if there is no recurrence after this time span, it can be assumed that the patient is cured.

The *adequacy of treatment* is most relevant to prognosis for certain types of neoplasms. The cure rate for some neoplasms, such as soft tissue sarcomas and certain childhood neoplasms, may be twice as high in sophisticated cancer centers when compared with cure rates in small community hospitals where experience and supportive systems are less extensive.

PSYCHOLOGIC MANAGEMENT OF THE CANCER PATIENT

The physician can ease the cancer patient's fear of the disease by free and open communication. Psychologic support and education are necessary in order for the patient to deal with any disability that may result from therapy. Examples include training in the care of a stoma following curative surgery for colonic and rectal cancer or referral to lay groups associated with the American Cancer Society for counseling the anxious patient with an altered body image resulting from mastectomy.

Despite the prognostic factors discussed previously, it is still impossible to predict the exact course of any malignant tumor. Patients with the most grim prognoses are occasionally cured by aggressive therapy, and spontaneous regressions are sometimes observed even in patients with metastases. In contrast, some patients with apparently localized disease may be dead of disseminated cancer in a few months. This uncertainty about the future is one of the most difficult adjustments faced by cancer patients and their families. Most reassuring in this regard is to emphasize that for each month that passes following successful treatment of the primary neoplasm, the chances for cure improve. This is particularly correct for tumors such as squamous cell carcinoma of the lung or oral pharynx. Although other, more slowly growing neoplasms, such as carcinoma of the breast and malignant melanoma, may recur after disease-free intervals of 10 or 20 years, the chances of recurrence also decrease with

time. Recognition that cancer is a chronic disease is an important aspect of management. Long-term, consistent follow-up provides opportunities for reassurance and usually can ensure detection of recurrence at an early stage.

Some patients do not want to know about their illness for fear of having their suspicions verified. Never lie to a patient, even if requested by the family. In general, gentle and optimistic truth is best. Untruths often create barriers between patients and their families that can lead to psychologic isolation of patients who are unable to discuss their fears and anxieties with those they need most.

With the patient for whom primary cancer therapy has failed, one of the most difficult problems faced by the physician is "What should the patient be told?" Most oncologists who deal exclusively with cancer patients agree that the incurable patient also must be told the truth as gently and optimistically as possible. Hope and reassurance as to the physician's continuing concern are best sustained by continuing active treatment until it is certain that the patient can no longer benefit. Realistic and consistent support is actually more important to the patient and the family at this stage of the disease than earlier. There is increasing evidence that patients tolerate the process of dying much better when cared for in this manner.

Some incurable patients are unable to accept the realities of the situation. In this case, it is essential that a responsible family member be informed. The life duration of the incurable patient is so uncertain that predictions should be avoided. If, as frequently happens, the relatives insist upon some estimate, a combined minimum-maximum prognosis, such as from 6 months to 2 years, will help the family accept this uncertainty.

The basic aim in caring for the patient with advanced cancer is to prolong useful life, but not useless suffering. The patient should be permitted to die with dignity when active therapy can no longer be of benefit.

Bibliography

Etiology

American Cancer Society: *Cancer Facts and Figures*. New York, 1987.

Barbocid M: Human oncogenes, in DeVita VY, Hellmen S, Rosenberg SA (eds): *Important Advances in Oncology*. Philadelphia, Lippincott, 1986, p 3.

Barratt RW, Tatum EL: Carcinogenic mutagens. *Ann NY Acad Sci* 71:1072, 1958.

Bishop JM: The molecular genetics of cancer. *Science* 235:305, 1987.

Bishop JM: Retroviruses and cancer genes. *Cancer* 55:2329, 1985.

Bister K, Jansen HW: Oncogenes in retroviruses and cells; biochemistry and molecular genetics. *Adv Cancer Res* 47:99, 1986.

Boice JD Jr, Fraumeni JF Jr (eds): *Radiation Carcinogenesis: Epidemiology and Biological Significance*. New York, Raven, 1984.

Boyland E: The history and future of chemical carcinogenesis. *Br Med Bull* 36:5, 1980.

Butlin HT: Cancer of the scrotum in chimney-sweeps and others: I. Secondary cancer without primary cancer. II. Why foreign sweeps do not suffer from scrotal cancer. III. Tar and paraffin cancer. *Br Med J* 1:1341; 2:1; 3:66, 1892.

Campisi J, Fingert HJ, Pardee AB: Basic biology and biochemistry of cancer, in Knapp RC, Berkowitz RS (eds): *Gynecologic Oncology.* New York, Macmillan, 1984, chap 2.

Doll R: The epidemiology of cancer. *Cancer* 45:2475, 1980.

Elson LE, Betts TE: Death rates from cancer of the respiratory and oral tracts in different countries in relation to the types of tobacco smoked. *Eur J Cancer* 17:109, 1981.

Garfinkel MA: Cancer mortality in nonsmokers; prospective study by the American Cancer Society. *J Natl Cancer Inst* 65:1169, 1981.

Heuper WC: Environmental cancer, in Homburger F (ed): *The Physiopathology of Cancer.* New York, Harper & Row, 1959, p 919.

Kennaway EC: The formation of a cancer producing substance from isoprene (2-methyl-butadiene). *J Pathol Bacteriol* 27:233, 1924.

Kindt TJ, Robinson MA: Major histocompatibility complex antigens, in Paul WE (ed): *Fundamental Immunology.* New York, Raven, 1984, pp 347–378.

Land H, Parada LF, Weinberg RA: Cellular oncogenes and multistep carcinogenesis. *Science* 222:771, 1983.

Lee Y-T (Margaret): Cancer statistics of Chinese versus Americans. *J Surg Oncol* 27:355, 1981.

Locke FB, King H: Cancer mortality risk among Japanese in the United States. *J Natl Cancer Inst* 65:1149, 1980.

Lorenz E: Radioactivity and lung cancer: a critical review of lung cancer in the miners of Schneeburg and Joachimstall. *Cancer Res* 5:1, 1944.

Martland HS: Occupational poisoning in manufacture of luminous watch dials: General review of hazard caused by ingestion of luminous paint with special reference to the New Jersey cases. *JAMA* 92:466, 1929.

Minz B, Fleischman RA: Teratocarcinomas and other neoplasms as developmental defects in gene expression. *Adv Cancer Res* 34:211, 1981.

Porter CD, White CJ: Multiple carcinomata following chronic x-ray dermatitis. *Ann Surg* 46:649, 1970.

Pott P: *Chirurgical Observations Relative to the Cataract, the Polypus of the Nose, the Cancer of the Scrotum, the Different Kinds of Ruptures, and the Mortification of the Toes and Feet.* London, Hawkes, Clarke and Collins, 1775.

Prehn RT: Specific isoantigenicities among chemically induced tumors. *Ann NY Acad Sci* 101:107, 1962.

Rous P: Transmission of a malignant new growth by means of a cell-free filtrate. *JAMA* 56:198, 1911.

Schottenfeld D: The epidemiology of cancer: an overview. *Cancer* 47:1095, 1981.

Schreiber MM, Bozzo PD, et al: Malignant melanoma in Southern Arizona: Increasing incidence and sunlight as an etiologic factor. *Arch Dermatol* 117:6, 1981.

Seeger RG, Brodeur GM, et al: Association of multiple copies of the V-mvc oncogene with rapid progression of neuroblastomas. *N Engl J Med* 313:1111, 1985.

Shimkin MB: Research on the causes and nature of cancer, in del Regato JA, Spjut HJ (eds): *Cancer.* St. Louis, Mosby, 1977, p 3.

Storer JB: Radiation carcinogenesis, in Becker FF (ed): *Cancer: A Comprehensive Treatise,* 2d ed. New York, Plenum, 1982, vol 1, pp 629–659.

Varmus HE: The discovery of cellular oncogenes and their role in neoplasia. *Cancer* 55:2324, 1985.

VanBeveren C, Vermal M: Homology among oncogenes. *Curr Top Microbiol Immunol* 123:73, 1986.

Waterfield MD, Scrace GT, Whittle N, et al: Platelet-derived growth factor is structurally related to the putative transforming protein p28 in sarcoma virus. *Nature* 304:35, 1983.

Wigle DT, Mae Y, et al: Relative importance of smoking as a risk factor for selected cancers. *Can J Publ Health* 71:269, 1980.

Biology and Immunobiology

Black PH: Shedding from the cell surface of normal and cancer cells. *Adv Cancer Res* 32:75, 1980.

Burnet FM: *Immunological Surveillance.* New York, Pergamon, 1970.

Drysdale BE, Zacharcheck CM, Shin HS: Mechanisms of macrophage mediated cytotoxicity: Production of a soluble cytotoxic factor. *J Immunol* 131:2362, 1983.

Eilber FR, Morton DL: Impaired immunologic reactivity and recurrence following cancer surgery. *Cancer* 25:362, 1970.

Eilber FR, Nizze A, Morton DL: Sequential evaluation of general immune competence in cancer patients: correlation with clinical course. *Cancer* 35:660, 1975.

Everson TC, Cole WH: *Spontaneous Regression of Cancer.* Philadelphia, Saunders, 1966.

Fidler IJ, Hart IR: Biological diversity in metastatic neoplasms: Origins and implications. *Science* 217:998–1003, 1982.

Foley EJ: Antigenic properties of methylcholanthrene-induced tumors in mice of the strain or origin. *Cancer Res* 13:835, 1953.

Gatti RA, Good RA: Occurrence of malignancy in immunodeficiency diseases: A literature review. *Cancer* 28:89, 1971.

Giuliano AE, Rangel DM, et al: Serum-mediated immunosuppression in lung cancer. *Cancer* 43:917, 1979.

Gold P, Freedman SO: Specific carcinoembryonic antigens of the human digestive system. *J Exp Med* 122:467, 1965.

Golightly MG, D'Amore P, et al: Studies on cytotoxicity generated in human mixed lymphocyte cultures. III. Natural killerlike cytotoxicity mediated by human lymphocytes with receptors for IgM. *Cell Immunol* 70:219, 1982.

Golub SH, D'Amore P, et al: Systemic administration of human leukocyte interferon to melanoma patients. II. Cellular events associated with changes in NK cytotoxicity. *J Natl Cancer Inst* 68:711, 1982.

Golub SH, Dorey F, et al: Systemic administration of human leukocyte interferon to melanoma patients. I. Effects of NK function and cell populations. *J Natl Cancer Inst* 68:703, 1982.

Goodwin WE: Regression of hypernephromas. *JAMA* 20:609, 1968.

Gupta RK, Morton DL: Clinical significance of tumor-associated antigens and anti-tumor antibodies in human malignant melanoma, in Reisfeld RA, Ferrone S (eds): *Melanoma Antibodies and Antigens.* New York, Plenum, 1982, p. 139.

Henney CS, Gillis S: Cell-mediated cytotoxicity, in Paul WE (ed): *Fundamental Immunology.* New York, Raven, 1984, pp 669–684.

Klein G: Tumor antigens. *Ann Rev Microbiol* 20:223, 1966.

Kohler PF: Human complement system, in Samter M (ed): *Immunologic Diseases,* 3d ed. Boston, Little, Brown, 1979, pp 244–280.

Morton DL: Acquired immunological tolerance and carcinogenesis by the mammary tumor virus. I. Influence of neonatal infection with the mammary tumor virus on the growth of spontaneous mammary adenocarcinomas. *J Natl Cancer Inst* 42:311, 1969.

Morton DL, Eilber FR, et al: Immunological factors in human sarcomas and melanomas: A rational basis for immunotherapy. *Ann Surg* 172:740, 1970.

Morton DL, Holmes EC, et al: Immunological aspects of neoplasia: a rational basis for immunotherapy. *Ann Intern Med* 74:587, 1971.

Old LJ, Boyse EA: Antigens of tumors and leukemias induced by virus. *Fed Proc* 24:1009, 1965.

Old LJ, Boyse EA, Stockert E: Antigenic properties of experimental leukemias: I. Serological studies in vitro with spontaneous and radiation-induced leukemias. *J Natl Cancer Inst* 31:977, 1963.

Old LJ, Stockert E, et al: Antigenic modulation: loss of TL antigen from cells exposed to TL antibody: Study of the phenomenon in vitro. *J Exp Med* 127:523, 1968.

Paul WE: *Fundmental Immunology.* New York, Raven, 1984.

Piessens WF: Evidence of human cancer immunity. *Cancer* 26:1212, 1970.

Pilch YH, Meyers GH, et al: Prospects for the immunotherapy of cancer: Part I, Basic concepts of tumor immunology. *Curr Probl Surg* January 1975, p 1.

Pitot HC: The natural history of neoplastic development: the relation of experimental models to human cancer. *Cancer* 49:1206, 1982.

Prehn RT, Main JM: Immunity to methylcholanthrene-induced sarcomas. *J Natl Cancer Inst* 18:769, 1957.

Reinherz EL, Meuner SC, Schlossman SF: The human T cell receptor: Analysis with cytotoxic T cell clones. *Immunol Rev* 74:83, 1983.

Skipper HE: In *The Proliferation and Spread of Neoplastic Cells.* Baltimore, Williams & Wilkins, 1968.

Southam CM, Brunschwig W, et al: The effect of leukocytes on transplantability of human cancer. *Cancer* 19:1743, 1966.

Stutman O: The immunological surveillance hypothesis, in Herberman RB (ed): *Basic and Clinical Tumor Immunology.* Boston, Martinus Nijhoff, 1983, pp 1–81.

Sugarbaker EV: *Cancer Metastasis: A Product of Tumor-Host Interactions.* Chicago, Year Book Medical Publishers, 1979, no 7, vol 3, pp 1–59.

Watson JD, Mochizuki DY, Gillis S: Molecular characterization of interleukin-2. *Fed Proc* 42:2747, 1983.

Watson JD, Tooze J, Kurtz DT: *Recombinant DNA.* Scientific American, New York, 1983.

Pathology

Anderson W: The general pathology of tumors, in *Boyd's Pathology for the Surgeon.* Philadelphia, Saunders, 1967, p 92.

Bloom HJG, Richardson WW, Harries EJ: Natural history of untreated breast cancer (1805–1933): Comparison of untreated and treated cases according to histological grade of malignancy. *Br Med J* 2:213, 1962.

Boyd W: *An Introduction to the Study of Disease.* Philadelphia, Lea & Febiger, 1971, p 210.

Cole WH, McDonald GO, et al: *Dissemination of Cancer.* New York, Appleton-Century-Crofts, 1961.

Collins VP, Leoffler RK, Tivey H: Observations on growth rates of human tumors. *Am J Roentgenol Radium Ther Nucl Med* 76:988, 1956.

Everson TC: Spontaneous regression of cancer. *Ann NY Acad Sci* 114:721, 1964.

Garland LH, Coulson W, Wollin E: The rate of growth and apparent duration of untreated primary bronchial carcinoma. *Cancer* 16:694, 1963.

Hawkins RS, Roberts MM, et al: Oestrogen receptors and breast cancer: Current status. *Br J Surg* 67:153, 1980.

MacMahon B, Feng MA: Prenatal origin of childhood leukemia: Evidence from twins. *N Engl J Med* 270:1082, 1964.

Moertel CG: Incidence and significance of multiple primary malignant neoplasms. *Ann NY Acad Sci* 114:886, 1964.

Pearson HA, Grello FW, Cane EC Jr: Leukemia in identical twins. *N Engl J Med* 268:1151, 1963.

Pund ER, Nettles TB, et al: Preinvasive and invasive carcinoma of the cervix uteri: Pathogenesis, detection, differential diagnosis, and pathologic basis for management. *Am J Obstet Gynecol* 55:831, 1948.

Rigler LB: Natural history of untreated lung cancer. *Ann NY Acad Sci* 114:755, 1964.

Russell WO, Ibanex ML, et al: Thyroid carcinoma: Classification, intraglandular dissemination, and clinicopathologic study based upon whole organ sections of 80 glands. *Cancer* 16:1425, 1963.

Slaughter DP: Multicentric origin of intraoral carcinoma. *Surgery* 20:133, 1946.

Viadana E, Kwai-Lung A: Patterns of metastases in adenocarcinomas of man. *J Med* 6:1. 1975.

Clinical Manifestations

Barrie JG, Knapper WH, Strong EW: Cervical nodal metastases of unknown origin. *Am J Surg* 120:466, 1970.

Bhattacharya SK, Sealy WC: Paraneoplastic syndromes resulting from elaboration of ectopic hormones, antigens, and bizarre toxins. *Curr Probl Surg* May 1972.

Giuliano AE, Moseley AS, et al: Clinical aspects of unknown primary melanoma. *Ann Surg* 191:98, 1981.

Greenberg BE: Cervical lymph node metastases from unknown primary sites. *Cancer* 19:1091, 1966.

Jesse RH, Neff LF: Metastatic carcinoma in cervical nodes with an unknown primary lesion. *Am J Surg* 112:547, 1966.

Keller JW, Williams RD: Laparotomy for unexplained fever. *Arch Surg* 90:494, 1965.

Myers WPL, Tashima CK, Rothschild EO: Endocrine syndromes associated with non-endocrine neoplasms. *Med Clin North Am* 50:763, 1966.

Diagnosis and Staging

Commission on Clinical Oncology of the Union Internationale Contre Cancrum: *TNM Classification of Malignant Tumors.* International Clinics against Cancer, Geneva, 1968.

Copeland MM: American Joint Committee on Cancer Staging and End Results Reporting: Objectives and progress. *Cancer* 18:1637, 1965.

Eilber FR, Holmes EC, Morton DL: Immunotherapy as an adjunct to surgery in treatment of cancer. *World J Surg* 1:547, 1977.

Finck ST, Giuliano AE, et al: Results of ilioinguinal dissection for stage II melanoma, *Ann Surg* 196:180, 1982.

Jones SE: Importance of staging in Hodgkin's disease. *Semin Oncol* 7:126, 1980.

Russell WO, Cohen J, et al: A clinical and pathological staging system for soft tissue sarcomas. *Cancer* 40:1562, 1977.

Williams PA: A productive history and physical examination in the prevention and early detection of cancer. *Cancer* 47:1146, 1981.

Surgery

Barnes JP: Physiologic resection of the right colon. *Surg Gynecol Obstet* 94:722, 1952.

Cole WH, Packard D, Southwich HW: Carcinoma of the colon with special reference to prevention of recurrence. *JAMA* 155:1549, 1954.

Deckers PJ, Ketcham AS, et al: Pelvic exenteration for primary carcinoma of the uterine cervix. *Obstet Gynecol* 37:647, 1971.

Eilber FR, Grant TT, et al: Internal hemipelvectomy—excision of the hemipelvis with limb preservation: an alternative to hemipelvectomy. *Cancer* 43:806, 1979.

Eilber FR, Mirra JJ, et al: Is amputation necessary for sarcomas? A 7-year experience with limb salvage. *Am J Surg* 192:431, 1980.

Flanagan L, Foster JH: Hepatic resection for metastatic cancer. *Am J Surg* 113:551, 1967.

Gilbertsen VA, Wangensteen OH: A summary of thirteen years' experience with the second look program. *Surg Gynecol Obstet* 114:438, 1962.

Giuliano AE, Eilber FR, et al: The management of locally recurrent soft tissue sarcoma. *Ann Surg* 196:87, 1982.

Halsted WS: The results of operations for the cure of cancer of the breast performed at the Johns Hopkins Hospital from June 1889 to January 1894. *Ann Surg* 20:297, 1894.

Huggins C, Bergenstal DM: Inhibition of human mammary and prostatic cancer by adrenalectomy. *Cancer Res* 12:134, 1952.

Kiselow M, Butcher HR, Bricker EM: Results of the radical surgical treatment of advanced pelvic cancer: A fifteen-year study. *Ann Surg* 166:436, 1967.

Miles WE: A method of performing abdomino-perineal excision for carcinoma of the rectum and the terminal portion of the pelvic colon. *Lancet* 2:1812, 1908.

Miller DR, Albritten FF Jr: Principles of surgery for cancer, in Nealon TF Jr (ed): *Management of the Patient with Cancer.* Philadelphia, Saunders, 1966, p 154.

Mockman S, Curreri AR, Ansfield FJ: Second-look operation for colon carcinoma after fluorouracil therapy. *Arch Surg* 100:527, 1970.

Mueller CB, Jeffries W: Cancer of the breast: Its outcome as measured by the rate of dying and causes of death. *Ann Surg* 182:334, 1975.

Patt YZ, Chuang VP, et al: The palliative role of hepatic arterial infusion and arterial occlusion in colorectal carcinoma metastatic to the liver. *Lancet* 1:349, 1981.

Pierce EH, Clagett OT, et al: Biopsy of the breast followed by delayed radical mastectomy. *Surg Gynecol Obstet* 103:559, 1956.

Ramming KP: Is partial hepatectomy, intrahepatic artery infusion of 5-FU, or systemic chemotherapy the best form of treatment for colon carcinoma metastatic to the liver? in O'Connell TX (ed): *Controversies in Surgical Oncology.* Philadelphia, Saunders, 1981, p. 246.

Ramming KP, Sparks FC, et al: Hepatic artery ligation and 5-fluorouracil infusion for metastatic colon carcinoma and primary hepatoma. *Am J Surg* 132:236, 1976.

Ramming KP, Sparks FC, et al: Management of hepatic metastases. *Semin Oncol* 4:71, 1977.

Roberts SS, Hengesh JW, et al: Prognostic significance of cancer cells in the circulating blood: A ten year evaluation. *Am J Surg* 113:757, 1967.

Stearns MW, Schottenfeld D: Techniques for the surgical management of colon cancer. *Cancer* 28:165, 1971.

Stehlin JS: Hyperthermic perfusion with chemotherapy for cancer of the extremities. *Surg Gynecol Obstet* 129:305, 1969.

Stehlin JS Jr, Giovanella BC, et al: Results of hyperthermic perfusion for melanoma of the extremities. *Surg Gynecol Obstet* 140:339, 1975.

Storm FK, Kaiser L, et al: Thermo-chemotherapy for melanoma metastases in liver. *Cancer* 49:1243, 1982.

Turnbull RB, Kyle K, et al: Cancer of the colon: the influence of the no-touch isolation technic on survival rates. *Ann Surg* 166:420, 1967.

Veronesi U, Saccozzi R, et al: Comparing radical mastectomy and quadrectomy, axillary dissection, and radiotherapy in patients with small cancers of the breast. *N Engl J Med* 305:6, 1981.

Watkins E, Khazei AM, Nabra KS: Surgical basis for arterial infusion chemotherapy of disseminated carcinoma of the liver. *Surg Gynecol Obstet* 130:581, 1970.

Wilkens EW Jr: The surgical management of metastatic neoplasms of the lung. *J Thorac Cardiovasc Surg* 42:298, 1961.

Radiation Therapy

Baker AR: Local procedure in the management of rectal cancer. *Semin Oncol* 7:385, 1980.

Harris JR, Recht A, et al: Time course and prognosis of local recurrence following primary radiation therapy for early breast cancer. *J Clin Oncol* 2:37, 1984.

Harris JR, Beadle GF, Hellam S: Clinical studies on the use of radiation therapy as primary treatment of early breast cancer. *Cancer* 53:705, 1984.

Higgens GS Jr, Conn JH, et al: Preoperative radiotherapy for colo-rectal cancer. *Ann Surg* 181:624, 1974.

Johns HE, Cunningham JR: In *The Physics of Radiology.* Springfield, Ill., Charles C Thomas, 1977.

Kaplan HS: Historic milestones in radiobiology and radiation therapy. *Semin Oncol* 6:479, 1979.

Kotalik JF: Multiple daily fractions in radiotherapy. *Cancer Treat Rev* 8:127, 1981.

Moss WT, Brand WN: *Therapeutic Radiology; Rationale, Technique, Results,* 3d ed. St. Louis, C. V. Mosby, 1969.

Paulson DL, Shaw RR, et al: Combined preoperative irradiation and resection for bronchogenic carcinoma. *J Thorac Cardiovasc Surg* 44:281, 1962.

Powers WE, Tolmach LJ: Preoperative radiation therapy: Biologic basis and experimental investigation. *Nature* 201:272, 1964.

Stevens KR: A review of the value of radiation therapy for adenocarcinoma of the rectum and sigmoid. *Fron Gastrointest Res* 5:93, 1979.

Till JE, McCulloch EA: A direct measurement of the radiation sensitivity of normal mouse bone marrow cells. *Radiat Res* 14:213, 1961.

Chemotherapy

Bailor JC, Byar DP: Estrogen treatment for cancer of the prostate. *Cancer* 26:257, 1970.

Baserga R: Molecular biology of the cell cycle. *Int J Radiat Biol* 49:219, 1986.

Bonadonna G, Brusamolino E, et al: Combination chemotherapy as an adjuvant treatment in operable breast cancer. *N Engl J Med* 294:405, 1976.

Bruce WR: The action of chemotherapeutic agents at the cellular level and effects of these agents on hematopoietic and lymphomatous tissue. *Can Cancer Conf* 7:53, 1966.

Calabresi P, Schein PS, Rosenberg SA: *Medical Oncology: Basic Principles and Clinical Management of Cancer.* New York, Macmillan, 1985.

Chabner B (ed): *Pharmacologic Principles of Cancer Treatment.* Philadelphia, Saunders, 1982.

Chabner BA: The oncologic end game (Karnofsky Memorial Lecture). *J Clin Oncol* 4:625, 1986.

De Vita VT, Hellman S, Rosenberg SA (eds): *Cancer Principles and Practice of Oncology,* 2d ed. Philadelphia, Lippincott, 1985.

Einhorn LH: Testicular cancer as a model for a curable neoplasm: The Richard and Hinda Rosenthal Foundation Award Lecture. *Cancer Res* 41:3275, 1981.

Erlichman C: Potential applications of therapeutic drug monitoring in treatment of neoplastic disease by antineoplastic agents. *Clin Biochem* 19:101, 1986.

Gilman A: The initial clinical trial of nitrogen mustard. *Am J Surg* 105:574, 1963.

Greco FA, Vaughn WK, Hainsworth JD: Advanced poorly differentiated carcinoma of unknown primary site: Recognition of a treatable syndrome. *Ann Intern Med* 104:547, 1986.

Haskell CM (ed): *Cancer Treatment.* 2d ed. Philadelphia, Saunders, 1985.

Huggins C, Hodges CV: Studies on prostatic cancer. I. The effect of castration, of estrogen and androgen injection on serum phosphatases in metastatic carcinoma of the prostate. *Cancer Res* 1:293, 1941.

Lewis JL: Chemotherapy of gestational choriocarcinoma. *Cancer* 30:1517, 1972.

Li MC, Hertz R, Spencer DB: Effect of methotrexate therapy upon choriocarcinoma and chorioadenoma. *Proc Soc Exp Biol Med* 93:361, 1956.

Salmon SE: Cloning of human tumor stem cells, in *Progress in Clinical and Biologic Research.* New York, A.R. Liss, 1980.

Schabel FM Jr: The use of tumor growth kinetics in planning "curative" chemotherapy of advanced solid tumors. *Cancer Res* 29:2384, 1969.

Schnipper LE: Clinical implications of tumor-cell heterogeneity. *N Engl J Med* 314:1423, 1986.

Skipper HE: Cancer chemotherapy is many things: GHA Clowes Memorial Lecture. *Cancer Res* 31: 1173, 1971.

Skipper HE, Perry S: Kinetics of normal and leukemic leukocyte populations and relevance to chemotherapy. *Cancer Res* 30:1883, 1970.

Strawitz JG: Cancer chemotherapy using isolation perfusion, in Brodsky I, Kahn SB, Moyer JH (eds): *Cancer Chemotherapy II.* New York, Grune & Stratton, 1972, p 443.

Sullivan PW, Salmon SE: Kinetics of tumor growth and regression in IgG multiple myeloma. *J Clin Invest* 51:1697, 1972.

Tannock IF: Experimental chemotherapy and concepts related to the cell cycle. *Int J Radiat Biol* 49:335, 1986.

Combined Therapy

Burk MW, Morton DL: Adjuvant cancer therapy: Rationale for its use. *Surg Clin North Am* 61:1245, 1981.

Eilber FR, Morton DL, et al: Limb salvage for skeletal and soft tissue sarcomas: Multidisciplinary preoperative therapy. *Proc Int Colloquium Cancer* 1981/2001, 1981.

Gilbert HA, Kagan RA, Winkley J: Soft tissue sarcomas of the extremities: Their natural history, treatment and radiation sensitivity. *J Surg Oncol* 7:303, 1975.

Haskell CM, Eilber FR, Morton DL: Adriamycin (NSC-12317) by arterial infusion. *Cancer Chemother Rep* 6:187, 1974.

Haskell CM, Silverstein MJ, et al: Multimodality cancer therapy in man: A pilot study of adriamycin by arterial infusion. *Cancer* 33:1485, 1974.

Jaffe N, Frei E, III, et al: Adjuvant methotrexate and citrovorum factor treatment of osteogenic sarcoma. *N Engl J Med* 291:994, 1974.

Lindberg RD: The role of radiation therapy in the treatment of soft tissue sarcoma in adults, in *Proceedings of 7th National Cancer Congress.* Philadelphia, Lippincott, 1972.

McNeer GD, Cantin J, et al: Effectiveness of radiation therapy in the management of sarcoma of the soft somatic tissues. *Cancer* 22:391, 1968.

Martin RG, Butler JJ, Albores SS: Soft tissue tumors: Surgical treatment and results, in *Tumors of Bone and Soft Tissue.* Chicago, Year Book Medical Publishers, 1965, p 333.

Morton DL, Eilber FR: Soft tissue sarcomas, in Holland JF, Frei E III (eds): *Cancer Medicine.* Philadelphia, Lea & Febiger, 1982, p 2141.

Morton DL, Eilber FR, Sondak VK, Economou JS (eds): *The Soft Tissue Sarcomas.* Orlando, Grune & Stratton, 1987.

Morton DL, Eilber FR, et al: Limb salvage from a multidisciplinary treatment approach for skeletal and soft tissue sarcomas of the extremity. *Ann Surg,* 184:268, 1976.

Murphy WT: The role of radiation therapy in the management of soft somatic tissue sarcoma. *Proc. 6th Natl. Cancer Congress* 1968, p 775.

Rosen G, Murphy ML, et al: Chemotherapy, en bloc resection and prosthetic bone replacement in the treatment of osteogenic sarcoma. *Cancer* 37:1, 1976.

Rosen G, Suwansirikal S, et al: High dose methotrexate with citrovorum factor rescue and Adriamycin in childhood osteosarcoma. *Cancer* 33:1151, 1974.

Rossi A, Bonodonna G: Current impact of adjuvant chemotherapy on resectable cancer. *Cancer Chemother Pharmacol* 3:17, 1979.

Storm FK (ed): *Hyperthermia in Cancer Therapy.* Chicago, Year Book Medical Publishers, 1985.

Suit HD, Russell WO: Radiation therapy of soft tissue sarcomas. *Cancer* 36:759, 1975.

Suit HD, Russell WO, Martin RG: Sarcoma of soft tissue: Clinical and histopathological parameters and response to treatment. *Cancer* 35:1478, 1974.

Townsend CM Jr, Eilber FR, Morton DL: Skeletal and soft tissue sarcomas: Results of treatment with adjuvant immunotherapy. *JAMA* 236:2187, 1976.

Immunotherapy

Bordon EC: Interferons and cancer: How the promise is being kept, in Gresser I (ed): *Interferon.* London, Academic, 1984, pp 43–83.

Buick RN, Salmon SE: Variables in the demonstration of human tumor clonogenicity: Cell interactions and semi-solid support, in Salmon SE (ed): *Cloning of Human Tumor Stem Cells.* New York, Alan R Liss, 1980, p 199.

Cobbald SP, Waldmann H: Therapeutic potential of monovalent monoclonal antibodies. *Nature* 308:460, 1984.

Deckers PJ, Pilch YH: RNA-mediated transfer of tumor immunity: A new model for immunotherapy of cancer. *Cancer* 28:1219, 1971.

Economou JS: The role of antibody in tumor immunity. *Surg Gynecol Obstet* 153:417, 1981.

Eilber FR, Morton DL, et al: Adjuvant immunotherapy with BCG in treatment of regional lymph node metastases from malignant melanoma. *N Engl J Med* 294:237, 1976.

Grimm EA, Ramsey KM, et al: Lymphokine-activated killer cell phenomenon II. Precursor phenotype is serologically distinct from peripheral I lymphocytes, memory cytotoxic thymus-derived lymphocytes, and natural killer cells. *J Exp Med* 157:884, 1983.

Gutterman JU, Mavligit GM, Hersh EM: Chemoimmunotherapy of human solid tumors. *Med Clin North Am* 60:441, 1976.

Halpern BN, Biozzi G, et al: Correlation entre l'activitie phagocytaire du système reticulo-endothelial et la production d'anticorps antibacteriens. *C R Soc Biol (Paris)* 152:758, 1958.

Holland JF, Bekesi JG: Immunotherapy of human leukemia with neuraminidase-modified cells. *Med Clin North Am* 60:539, 1976.

Irie RF, Morton DC: Regression of cutaneous metastatic melanoma by intralesional injection with human monoclonal antibody to ganglioside GD2. *Proc Natl Acad Sci* 83:8694, 1986.

Israel L, Edelstein RL: *Nonspecific Immunostimulation with Corynebacterium parvum in Human Cancer.* Baltimore, Williams & Wilkins, 1974.

Jansen FK, Blythman HE, et al: Immunotoxins: Hybrid molecules combining high specificity and potent cytotoxicity. *Immunol Rev* 62:185, 1982.

Klein E: Hypersensitivity reactions at tumor site. *Cancer Res* 29:2351, 1969.

Klein E, Holterman O, et al: Immunotherapy for accessible tumors utilizing delayed hypersensitivity reactions and separated components of the immune system. *Med Clin North Am* 60:389, 1976.

Lotze MT, Matory YL, et al: Clinical effects and toxicity of interleukin-2 in patients with cancer. *Cancer* 58:2764, 1986.

Lloyd KO: Human tumor antigens: Detection and characterization with monoclonal antibodies, in Herberman RB (ed): *Basic and Clinical Tumor Immunology.* Boston, Martinus Nijhoff, 1983, pp 159–214.

McKneally MF, Maver C, Kausel H: Regional immunotherapy of lung cancer with intrapleural BCG. *Lancet* 1:377, 1976.

Magnani JL, Steplewski Z, et al: Identification of the gastrointestinal and pancreatic cancer-associated antigen detected by monoclonal antibody 19-9 in the sera of patients as a mucin. *Cancer Res* 43:5489, 1983.

Moertel CG, Ritts RE Jr, et al: Clinical studies of methanol extraction residue fraction of bacillus Calmette-Guérin as an immunostimulant in patients with advanced cancer. *Cancer* 35:3075, 1975.

Morton DL: Cancer immunotherapy: An overview. *Semin Oncol* 1:297, 1974.

Morton DL: Changing concepts of cancer surgery: Surgery as immunotherapy. *Am J Surg* 135:367, 1978.

Morton DL, Eilber FR, et al: Multimodality therapy of malignant melanoma, skeletal and soft tissue sarcomas using immunotherapy, chemotherapy and radiation therapy, in Salmon S and Jones S (eds): *Adjuvant Therapy of Cancer III.* New York, Grune & Stratton, 1981, p 241.

Morton DL, Eilber FR, et al: BCG immunotherapy of malignant melanoma: Summary of a seven-year experience. *Ann Surg* 180:635, 1974.

Morton DL, Holmes EC, Golub SH: Immunologic aspects of lung cancer. *Chest* 71:640, 1977.

Nathanson L: Use of BCG in treatment of human neoplasms: A review. *Semin Oncol* 1:337, 1974.

Oettgen HF, Pinsky CM, Delmonte L: Treatment of cancer with immunomodulators: *Corynebacterium parvum* and Levamisole. *Med Clin North Am* 60:463, 1976.

Rojas AF, Feierstein JM, et al: Levamisole in advanced human breast cancer. *Lancet* 1:211, 1976.

Rosenberg SA: Adoptive immunotherapy of cancer: Accomplishments and prospects. *Cancer Treat Rep* 68:233, 1984.

Rosenberg SA: Lymphokine-activated killer cells: A new approach to immunotherapy of cancer. *J Natl Cancer Inst* 75:595, 1985.

Rosenberg SA, Lotze MT, et al: Observations on the systemic administration of autologous lymphokine-activated killer cells and recombinant interleukin-2 to patients with metastatic cancer. *N Engl J Med* 313:1485, 1985.

Sparks FC: Hazards and complications of BCG immunotherapy. *Med Clin North Am* 60:499, 1976.

Vitetta ES, Drolick KA, et al: Immunotoxins: A new approach to cancer therapy. *Science* 219:644, 1983.

Prognosis

Dunphy JE: On caring for the patient with cancer. *N Engl J Med* 295:313, 1976.

Sutherland AM: Psychological impact of cancer and its therapy. *CA* 32:159, 1981.

Wangensteen OH: Should patients be told they have cancer? *Surgery* 27:944, 1950.

Psychologic Management

Hodgson TA: Social and economic implications of cancer in the United States. *Ann NY Acad Sci* 363:189, 1981.

Meyerowitz BE, Sparks FC, et al: Psychosocial impact of adjuvant chemo-immunotherapy for breast cancer. *Cancer* 43:1613, 1979.

Chapter 10

Transplantation

Richard L. Simmons, Richard J. Migliori, Craig R. Smith, Keith Reemtsma, and John S. Najarian

Human beings do not burst like balloons—they fall apart, piece by piece. Clinical organ transplantation is designed to replace the exhausted parts as they fall. Because the immunologic barrier of allograft rejection stands in the way of attaining chimerism between host and graft, immunologists and surgeons have been working together since World War II to circumvent the rejection reaction. Unfortunately, the problems remain unsolved. Despite the clinical success of kidney, liver, pancreas, heart, and bone marrow transplantation, organs are still rejected, and the attempts to prevent rejection can be fatal. The field of clinical transplantation, though no longer experimental, remains in flux.

The first part of this chapter discusses the immunobiology of the allograft, the rejection reaction, and the means for achieving immunosuppression. The current and incipient clinical applications of these biologic principles and techniques to the human patient are discussed in the second section.

IMMUNOBIOLOGY OF THE ALLOGRAFT

Tissue or organ grafts between individuals of the same species (*allografts,* or *homografts*) are rejected with a vigor proportional to the degree of the genetic disparity between the individuals. Grafts between individuals of different species (*xenografts,* or *heterografts*) are rejected even more rapidly. Grafts between identical twins (*isografts, isogeneic grafts,* or *syngeneic grafts*) or from individuals to themselves (*autografts,* or *autogenous grafts*) survive indefinitely after the vascular supply has been reestablished.

Allografts normally survive the transplant operation as well as isografts. If the recipient has not previously encountered the antigens present on the donor graft, the allograft is not morphologically or physiologically distinguishable from the isograft in the early posttransplant period—the rejection process normally takes several days. Medawar first noted that skin grafts between unrelated rabbits appeared normal until the fourth or fifth day. At that time inflammation appeared within the graft bed in the form of a dense leukocyte infiltrate that led to necrosis of the entire graft by about the tenth day. He further demonstrated that the rejection process is the result of immunologic mechanisms. Whereas the "first-set rejection" takes place in 10 or 11 days, a second graft from the same rabbit resulted in an accelerated "second-set rejection." The process of first-set and second-set rejection of an allogeneic graft takes place whether or not the graft is *orthotopic* (a graft placed in the anatomic position normally occupied by such tissue) or *heterotopic* (placed in other than the original location). The reaction is immunologically specific for the antigens involved, and the second-set rejections occur only when the recipient has been sensitized to antigens shared with the first graft.

Transplantation (Histocompatibility) Antigens

The rejection of an allograft is elicited by foreign histocompatibility antigens on the grafted tissue. Many antigens can serve as histocompatibility antigens. For example, the ABO blood group antigens will elicit rapid graft rejections in hosts with natural isoantibody. Similarly, xenografts between distant species are rejected rapidly because tissue incompatibilities are so profound between most species that preformed antibodies may exist in the recipient of the graft. Alloantigeneic incompatibilities between members of a species vary, however, and strong antigens can lead to graft rejection within 8 days, while weaker differences will permit graft survival of well over 100 days.

THE IMMUNOGENETICS OF HISTOCOMPATIBILITY

The strongest of the transplantation antigens is the expression of a single chromosomal region called the *major histocompatibility complex* (MHC) (Fig. 10-1). In human beings the MHC is located on chromosome 6. All mammals have a similar MHC, but the nomenclature varies among species. In human beings, the gene products of the MHC were first investigated on leukocytes and were named *human leukocyte antigens* (HLA). Naturally, the first-discovered antigens would be likely to be the major determinants.

The presence of HLA antigens on a cell surface can be detected in one of two ways. The serologic method uses antigen-specific antisera, which binds to cells carrying the antigen. A second method measures the reactivity of host lymphocytes to lymphocytes from potential graft donors. The responding lymphocytes are reacting to other cellular

Fig. 10-1. Gene map of chromosome 6 in human beings. This segment of the chromosome between the locus coding for the enzyme glyoxylase (GLO) and HLA-A is usually referred to as the HLA complex. The loci of HLA can be divided into two classes: Class I loci include HLA-A, HLA-B, and HLA-C, whereas the Class II loci include HLA-DR, HLA-DP, and HLA-DQ. Gene products of the Class I molecules are glycoproteins consisting of a heavy chain that penetrates the cell membrane. The heavy chain is folded into three immunoglobulin-like domains (α_1, α_2, and α_3). A B_2 microglobulin unit completes the structure. The Class II molecules consist of two polypeptide chains, both of which penetrate the cell membrane. The extracellular part of each chain is folded into two domains. The domains adjacent to the cell membrane are homologous with the α_3 and B_2M domains of the Class I antigens and the constant domain of the immunoglobulin molecule. [From: *deVries RRP, Van Rood JJ (eds): Immunobiology of HLA Class I and Class II Molecules. Basel (Switzerland), Karger, 1985, with permission.*]

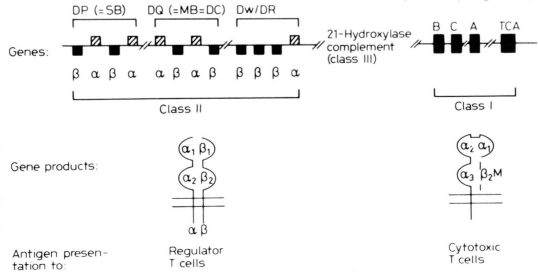

transplantation antigens. The antigens that can best trigger the proliferation of allogeneic lymphocytes were designated *Class II antigens*. The antigens that trigger allogeneic lymphocyte proliferation poorly were designated *Class I antigens*. Both Class I and Class II antigens can now be detected by specific antisera. The Class I antigens are expressions of those portions of the MHC supergene called HLA-A, HLA-B, and HLA-C. The Class II antigens are expressions of HLA-D, D, DQ, and DW/DR subloci.

HLA Class I molecules can be detected on the cell surfaces of almost all nucleated cells. In contrast HLA Class II molecules are found only on cells of the immune system—macrophages, dendritic cells, B cells, and activated T cells. Resting T lymphocytes do not express Class II antigens. Both Class I and Class II antigens each are composed of two polypeptide chains with variable and constant regions. The polymorphism is expressed in the variable regions of each molecule distant from the cell membrane. The portion of molecule closest to the cell membrane shows considerable homology between Class I and Class II molecules and also with the constant part of immunoglobulin molecules. This fact suggests that a common evolutionary origin exists between these three molecules (Fig. 10-1).

The HLA antigens have formed the basis for transplantation tissue typing for many years. Because of extreme polymorphism, only rarely do two unrelated individuals share all the antigens expressed. Relatives, on the other hand, often share some antigens because each person inherits one chromosome and, hence, one set of HLA antigens from each parent (Fig. 10-2), and because all the HLA antigens are expressed (codominant) on the cell surface.

The MHC subloci have been found to be closely linked but separable, and therefore genetic crossover between them, though unusual, can occur. As shown in Fig. 10-2, the parental HLA-A, -B, and -D pairs are usually inherited together, and the antigens originating from one chromosome are called *HLA haplotype*. Almost always the haplotype the child receives from each parent corresponds to the haplotype of one of the parental chromosomes. When crossover occurs during meiosis, however, the child receives a recombinant haplotype from a parent. (In the example shown, recombination occurred between A and B antigens. Recombination can occur between B and D also.)

Detection of the A, B, and D alleles for tissue typing requires banks of monospecific antisera. Typing was thought to be clinically useful because it seemed clear that survival of transplanted organs between family members correlated with the closeness of the HLA antigen match. The clinical results of organ transplantation have not, however, clearly demonstrated the importance of HLA-A and -B identity in organ transplantation between unrelated (cadaver) donor–recipient pairs. This apparent paradox seems caused by the fact that inheritance of the MHC in its entirety is important for graft survival rather than simple sharing of several HLA antigens.

It is important to recognize that there are genes on

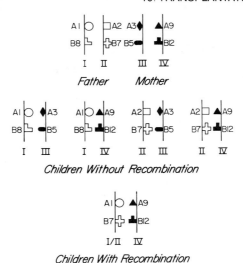

Children Without Recombination

Children With Recombination Between Subloci

Fig. 10-2. Hypothetic examples of inheritance of serologically detectable HLA antigens of the A and B series. Four offspring of mating between parents with chromosomes labeled I-II and III-IV are shown, as well as one possible result of recombination within the HLA region and subsequent inheritance. The parental chromosomes are usually transmitted intact, and the offspring receive one chromosome containing an A and B pair from each parent. Occasionally, however, crossover occurs and the child receives a recombinant antigen pair from a parent. For simplicity, genes coding for the C and D series of antigens within the HLA complex are not shown. See Fig. 10-1 for the presumed location of the genes within the HLA complex.

other chromosomes outside the MHC that code for weaker histocompatibility loci. In human beings, such antigens are not well understood, but a graft from a sibling identical at the HLA locus will be rejected if immunosuppressive drugs are not utilized. Such rejections are the natural consequence of these minor histocompatibility loci.

NORMAL ROLE FOR THE MHC. The functions of histocompatibility antigens are not totally understood, but clearly they do not exist merely to thwart the efforts of transplant surgeons. Most likely they are important to the recognition phenomena during cell-cell interactions within the same organism. For example, the T lymphocyte can recognize certain microbial antigens and initiate immune responses against them most efficiently when those antigens are associated with certain of its own HLA determinants. Thus HLA polymorphism is useful to the host in antimicrobial immunity.

DISTRIBUTION OF HLA ANTIGENS. Not all cells and tissues express equivalent amounts of HLA antigens. Some cells even express greater or lesser quantities at different phases of the cell cycle. Most adult parenchymal cells express Class I antigens, but only passenger leukocytes have a full complement of Class II antigens. For this reason, it is possible to deplete experimental grafts of their passenger leukocytes and diminish the strength of the rejection response. In clinical practice, however, these techniques are not yet possible. Almost all transplanted organs contain enough HLA antigens to elicit prompt rejection by a normal host, and there is evidence that the expression of HLA Class II antigens can be induced on parenchymal cells in the presence of an immune response. This reaction seems to be the result of the action of interferon-gamma on parenchymal cells.

Histocompatibility Matching

It is obvious that, other things being equal, the less antigenic the graft, the less the host will react against it. In human transplantation, when the donor and recipient are identical twins, there is no antigenic difference, and the tissues are accepted. When the donor and recipient are siblings or when a parent donor is used for offspring, there is a greater statistical likelihood of antigen sharing between donor and recipient than when a cadaver or other unrelated donor is used.

Several methods have been developed for the purpose of demonstrating antigenic similarities between donor and recipient prior to transplantation, so that donor and recipient pairs that are relatively histocompatible may be selected.

The best current method is called leukocyte typing.

HLA antigens on circulating lymphocytes can be detected with antisera derived originally from multiply transfused patients or from women with multiple pregnancies. Some of the antisera seem to recognize groups of antigens, and others recognize single antigens (*monospecific antisera*). Using the patient's leukocytes and a group of standard antisera, it is thus possible to characterize most of the strong HLA antigens in both donor and host. Only HLA antigens can be routinely determined in this way. Weaker histocompatibility antigens at other loci have not been detected by serologic techniques in human beings.

Antigens are currently detected by isolating lymphocytes from the peripheral blood of potential donors or recipients. The cells are incubated with antisera of various specificities and rabbit serum as a source of complement. Cells that react with antibodies in the serum die in the presence of complement and can be stained with vital dyes. Typing sera is becoming increasingly standardized. A typical set of results from the University of Minnesota typing laboratories is illustrated in Table 10-1.

Histocompatibility typing is useful in determining the best match between donor and recipient when family donors are utilized. Siblings who share all HLA antigens

Table 10-1. LYMPHOCYTE ANTIGEN TYPING REPORT OF THEORETICAL FAMILY*

Family member	ABO	*HLA-A locus*												*HLA-DR locus*									
		A1	A2	A3	A9	A10	A11	A28	Aw19	Aw34	Aw36	Aw43	DR1	DR2	DR3	DR4	DR5	DRw6	DR7	DRw8	DRw9	DRw10
Father AB	A	+	−	+	−	−	−	−	−	−	−	−	−	−	+	+	−	−	−	−	−	−
Mother CD	A	−	+	−	−	−	−	+	−	−	−	−	−	+	−	−	−	−	+	−	−	−
Son AC (patient)	O	+	−	−	−	−	−	+	−	−	−	−	−	+	−	+	−	−	−	−	−	−
Son AD	A	+	+	−	−	−	−	−	−	−	−	−	−	+	−	−	−	−	+	−	−	−
Daughter BC	O	−	−	+	−	−	−	+	−	−	−	−	−	+	−	+	−	−	−	−	−	−
Daughter BD	A	−	+	+	−	−	−	−	−	−	−	−	−	+	−	+	−	−	+	−	−	−
Daughter AC	O	+	−	−	−	−	−	+	−	−	−	−	−	+	−	+	−	−	−	−	−	−

Family member	ABO	*HLB-B locus*																		
		B5	B7	B8	B12	B13	B14	B15	Bw16	B17	B18	Bw21	Bw22	B27	Bw35	B37	B40	Bw41	Bw42	Bw47
Father AB	A	−	−	+	−	−	−	−	−	−	−	−	−	−	+	−	−	−	−	−
Mother CD	A	−	−	−	−	−	−	−	−	−	−	+	−	−	+	−	−	−	−	−
Son AC (patient)	O	−	−	+	−	−	−	−	−	−	−	−	−	−	+	−	−	−	−	−
Son AD	A	−	−	+	−	−	−	−	−	−	−	+	−	−	−	−	−	−	−	−
Daughter BC	O	−	−	−	−	−	−	−	−	−	−	−	−	−	+	+	−	−	−	−
Daughter BD	A	−	−	−	−	−	−	−	−	−	−	+	−	−	+	−	−	−	−	−
Daughter AC	O	−	−	+	−	−	−	−	−	−	−	−	−	−	+	−	−	−	−	−

* The specifications for the A, B, C, and DR loci are those currently used at the University of Minnesota.

Son AC is the prospective transplant recipient. Daughter AC is a perfect match for all four antigens; she shares the inheritance of both HLA haplotypes and is the ideal donor. Both parents, son AD, and daughter BC share only one haplotype with the potential recipient and are theoretically not as good donors. Daughter BD shares no HLA haplotypes with the recipient and is the poorest donor in the family.

More important than the HLA type are the ABO blood types. The father, mother, son AD, and daughter BD *cannot* donate, because they are all blood group A and the recipient is blood group O and possesses anti-A antibodies in his serum.

are the best possible donor-recipient pair. But several points about histocompatibility matching deserve emphasis:

1. Recipients receiving grafts, even from donors who are HLA identical matches with them, will still reject the graft (although more slowly) unless immunosuppressive drugs are utilized. Only an identical twin is truly a perfect match.
2. Even with poor histocompatibility matches between relatives, the results are frequently good, which probably indicates it is sometimes possible to suppress even great degrees of antigenic incompatibility.
3. Even with a good histocompatibility match, the graft may fail if the host happens to have preformed antibodies against a donor's tissue. These antibodies can be recognized if recipient serum is allowed to react with donor lymphocytes in a cytotoxicity test. This test, called *cross matching,* should be performed with fresh serum as a final test of compatibility prior to transplant. Preformed cytotoxic antibodies to donor tissue cannot be detected by the usual typing procedure itself.
4. The presence of ABH isohemagglutinins will most often lead to the prompt rejection of tissue bearing incompatible blood group substances.
5. Despite the results of tissue typing, a related donor has generally produced better transplant results than an unrelated (cadaver) donor.
6. Tissue typing for unrelated cadaver donors has not been successful, with one exception: HLA-identity of all detectable antigens correlates with a higher incidence of graft success. But such identity is rare.

MIXED LYMPHOCYTE CULTURE (MLC). The other method capable of detecting degrees of histocompatibility between donor and recipient is the MLC test, which detects differences principally at the Class II locus. Lymphocytes of the recipient are mixed with lymphocytes of the donor in tissue culture. If significant antigenic differences exist between the two, they will respond by transformation into blast cells, DNA synthesis, and mitosis. The incorporation of tritiated thymidine into DNA can be quantified to assess the degree of stimulation. As the test was originally devised, it was a two-way test—cells of the donor were capable of reacting against cells of the recipient and vice versa. In order to isolate the response of the recipient cells to the donor antigens, the donor lymphocytes can be inactivated by irradiation. The test is not useful as a screening test for cadaver organ transplantation but retains usefulness in related bone-marrow transplantation.

The Immune Apparatus

The immune response to the histocompatibility antigens on the cells of transplanted organs triggers the rejection reaction. At birth, human beings are already immunologically competent and have undergone a complex developmental process. It is now agreed that there is a single hemopoietic stem cell, found in the extraembryonic yolk sac. The daughter stem cells migrate to various centers for further differentiation. Within these centers, progenitor cells for erythrocytes, eosinophils, basophils, neutrophils, and lymphoid cells arise, depending on the local microchemical environment. It is likely that further proliferation of these progenitor stem cells depends on the action of "poietins," which tend to expand the populations of specialized cells in the way that erythropoietin acts on the erythrocyte line (Fig. 10-3).

The lymphoid cell line first appears within two primary (or central) lymphoid tissues. The thymus governs the development of cellular immunity. In birds, the bursa of Fabricius governs the development of humoral immunity. The bursa exists as a clearly defined central lymphoid structure only in birds. The equivalent of the bursa of Fabricius has not been defined in mammals, but there is evidence that it exists—perhaps within the fetal liver or bone marrow. In human beings the characteristics of sex-linked agammaglobulinemia of the Bruton type—very low levels of immunoglobulins, with normal cellular immunity and thymus-derived lymphocytes—suggest that the bursa equivalent has failed to develop.

Both the thymus and the bursa (or its equivalent) are responsible for the further development of the peripheral lymphoid tissues, i.e., spleen, lymph nodes, Peyer's patches. Certain areas of the lymph node are dependent on the functional presence of the thymus and the bursa (Fig. 10-4). The paracortical regions between the cortical germinal centers and the medulla are dependent on the thymus, while the germinal centers themselves and the medullary cord lymphoid tissue are under the developmental control of the bursal equivalent. Therefore, thymectomy early in the neonatal period or congenital thymic deficiency results in failure of development of the paracortical regions of the lymph nodes. In chickens, bursectomy leads to failure of development of germinal centers and medullary cord lymphoid tissues.

All cells that were once dependent on the thymus for their development are called *T cells.* T cells represent the immunocompetent cell population responsible for the development of cellular rather than humoral immunity. These reactions include delayed hypersensitivity reactions, as well as many of the early reactions responsible for allograft rejection.

The *B cells* descend from stem cells in the bone marrow and become responsible for the manufacture of circulating immunoglobulins and thus for humoral immunity (Fig. 10-3). The B cells appear to be relatively sessile, but their end products, immunoglobulin antibodies, can interact with foreign antigens at distant sites. The T cells responsible for cell-mediated immunity are of necessity more peripatetic and must migrate to the periphery in order to neutralize foreign antigens.

The lymphoid system is the seat of the body's immunologic response and the small mature lymphocytes and the plasma cells are the immunocompetent cells. Once the lymphocytes (T or B cells) have migrated to the peripheral lymphoid tissue, they are fully immunocompetent. It is likely that Burnet's clonal selection theory holds true—i.e., a state of preparedness for a certain antigen or group of related antigens exists within a lymphoid cell so that it is only capable of responding to a narrow range of genetically determined antigenic specificities. For this reason only a small percentage of the lymphocytes in the body will respond to a specific antigen.

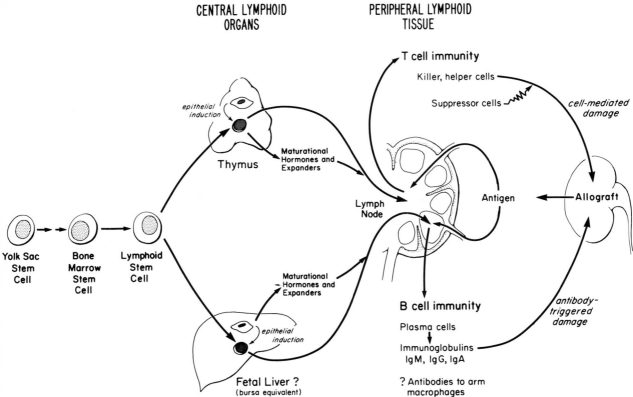

CENTRAL LYMPHOID ORGANS

PERIPHERAL LYMPHOID TISSUE

Fig. 10-3. Encapsulation of the extraordinarily complex developmental sequences of the immune system. Certain of the known inducers, expanders, growth factors, and sites of maturation needed to establish the T and B cell lines are presented. Much of this takes place before birth, so transplant recipients are fully competent with established peripheral lymphoid populations in the lymph nodes, Peyer's patches, and spleen. Therefore, clinical immunosuppression consists principally of lymphocyte depletion and inhibition of the activation of antigen-stimulated lymphocytes. [From: *Foker JE, Simmons RL, Najarian JS: Principles of immunosuppression, in Sabiston DC Jr (ed): Davis-Christopher Textbook of Surgery. Philadelphia, Saunders, 1977, p 506, with permission.*]

In order for a lymphocyte to respond to its predetermined antigen, it must have a specific chemical receptor for that antigen on its cell surface (Fig. 10-5). B cells possess a receptor very similar to an immunoglobulin. T cells have receptor molecules whose structures share many structural similarities with immunoglobulin and also with both Class I and Class II histocompatibility antigens (see Figs. 10-1 and 10-5). Attached to these shared constant (c) regions close to the cell membrane are variable (v) por-

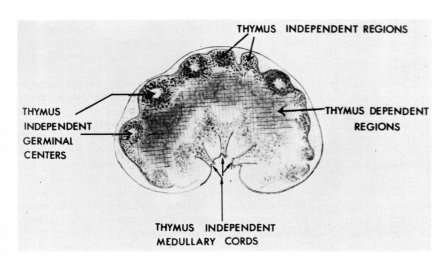

Fig. 10-4. The thymus-dependent and thymus-independent areas are illustrated in this schematic representation of a lymph node. [From: *Good RA, Finstad J: Structure and development of the immune system, in Najarian JS, Simmons RL (eds): Transplantation. Philadelphia, Lea & Febiger, 1972, p 26, with permission.*]

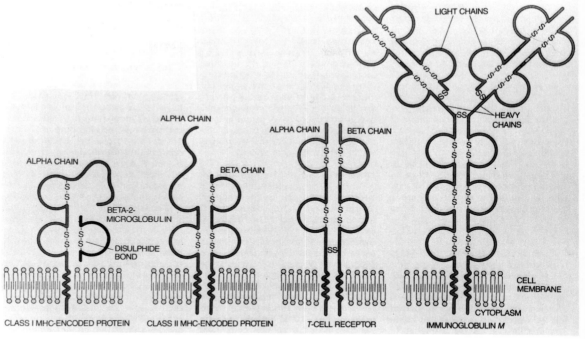

Fig. 10-5. Homology between HLA antigens and antigen binding molecules on the surfaces of lymphocytes. The molecular structures are similar and the molecules share similar amino acid sequences. (From: *Mannack P, Kappler J: The T cell and its receptor. Sci Am 254:36, 1986, with permission.*)

tions of the receptor molecule that permit it to bind and be activated by specific antigens. The variable portion of the T receptor molecule does not resemble an immunoglobulin, however.

Immunologic Events in Allograft Rejection

INDUCTION OF IMMUNITY

ROLE OF THE SMALL LYMPHOCYTE. Mature lymphocytes appear to sit in a state of immunologic readiness. The small lymphocyte can react to its bound antigen by proliferation, differentiation, maturation, and the production of molecules (antibodies, protein markers on the cell surface, lymphokines) that can react with the antigen and recruit other mediators of the immune response. After proliferation some of these cells have a life span of many years so that a much larger pool of antigen-reactive cells (memory cells) remains. Such cells also may be capable of a more rapid response.

THE AFFERENT ARC. The small lymphocyte thus recognizes the immunogenic determinants and translates that recognition into an immunologic response. The first phase of the immunologic response has been called afferent arc. It involves the grafting process itself, the release of the immunogenic histocompatibility antigens from the graft, the processing and recognition of the immunogens,

and the stimulation of the responsive lymphoid cell population. After organ allografting, this process takes place principally within the graft, and to a lesser degree in the lymphoid depots.

The immunogens of a grafted organ, being surface components of the cell membrane, are readily available to the recipient's T lymphocytes that percolate through the transplanted organ. In order for the lymphocyte to become sensitized, however, an accessory cell of the monocyte-macrophage lineage is necessary. In the case of protein antigens, the macrophage efficiently traps an antigen, processes it, and presents it in a form more easily recognized by the T cell receptor. For this to occur, the responding lymphocyte and the macrophage must share identical Class II antigens on their cell surfaces. This is strong evidence for the importance of self-recognition of cooperating cells in the immune response.

The accessory cell has a second function as well, namely, to provide a second signal by means of a secreted (monokine) molecule that enhances T cell responses in its immediate vicinity. The most important monokine in the activation of T cell responses is called interleukin-1 (IL-1) (Fig. 10-6). But interleukin-1 has many other functions including mediating the production of fever and metabolic change during inflammatory responses.

Within the microenvironment of the immune cellular response, however, IL-1 has well-defined functions. In cooperation with antigen binding by the T cell, IL-1 fosters the appearance of receptors for a second lymphokine on the cell surface of the antigen-reactive cell, namely, IL-2 receptors. Interleukin-2 (IL-2) is simultaneously secreted by antigen-responsive helper cells. Interaction of

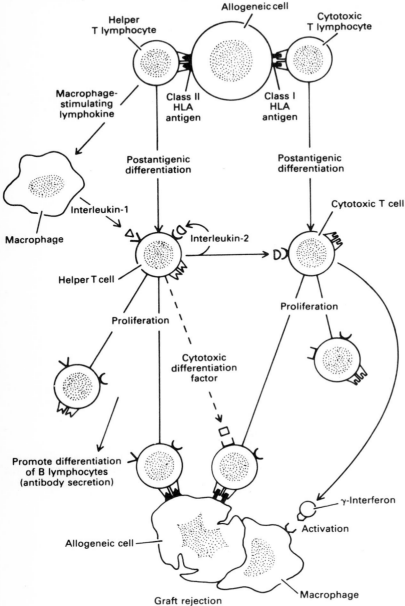

Fig. 10-6. Cellular immune response of T cells to transplantation antigens. The sequence leading to the proliferation of alloreactive T cells includes antigen, interleukin-1, and interleukin-2. (Adapted from: *Strom TB: Kidney Int 26:353, 1984, with permission.*)

IL-2 with its receptor allows the cell to proliferate and mature (Fig. 10-6).

CELL-CELL INTERACTIONS. During graft rejection, antigen-responsive clones of lymphocytes do not act alone. They not only require accessory cells plus interleukin, they also interact with other lymphocytes. Extensive lymphocyte-lymphocyte interaction is needed for the development of maximum lymphocyte proliferative and cytotoxic activity. The cooperation occurs both between T and B cells and between defined subpopulations of T cells.

The requirement for cooperation between T and B cells was established by showing that neither cell population

alone could mount an immune response to certain antigens, whereas mixtures of the two cell types resulted in the production of high levels of antibody. Because B cells are the precursors of antibody-forming cells and T cells do not synthesize readily detectable amounts of immunoglobulin, certain T cells must serve as "helper cells" that assist B cells to differentiate into producers of antibody. An antibody response to the major histocompatibility antigens requires this cooperation, and suspensions of B cells alone in tissue culture will not effectively produce antibodies to these antigens unless T cells are added. Therefore, T-cell recognition of the antigen is necessary for the production of specific antibody by the B cell. Not all T cells can function in this role, only the subgroup of helper T cells (T_H). A full antibody response to most antigens seems to require aid from T_H cells.

Just as T_H cells are necessary for B-cell antibody response, T_H cells are needed for the development of lymphocyte-mediated cytotoxicity. The lymphocytes that produce direct cytotoxicity are also T cells: effector (T_E), or killer cells. The T_H cell is required for the T_E cell to develop fully the capacity to inflict cell damage. Cell-associated histocompatibility antigens are prominent among the antigens that require T_H-T_E cell cooperation for induction of maximum cytotoxicity.

There is evidence that yet another T-cell subgroup can inhibit either the development of antibody-producing B cells or the generation of T_E cells. These regulatory lymphocytes have been called suppressor T (T_S) cells.

The elucidation of these interactions has occupied many cellular immunologists during the past decade. Convincing experimental demonstration of lymphocyte-lymphocyte interaction required the various cells to be identified and separated from the bulk populations of lymphocytes in vitro. This was facilitated by the discovery of distinct antigenic proteins on the surfaces of the various subsets of lymphocytes. Antibodies to these surface marker proteins could then be used to deplete or enrich the bulk populations of a specific cell type and thereby clarify the function of each cell type. Table 10-2 lists the functional lymphocyte subtypes and the markers they possess.

Once the lymphocyte subpopulations were identified, the mechanisms of their interaction could be elucidated.

Table 10-2. FUNCTIONAL SUBPOPULATIONS OF LYMPHOCYTES

A. T lymphocytes
 1. Regulatory T lymphocytes
  a. Helper cells
  b. Suppressor cells
 2. Effector T lymphocytes
  a. Delayed hypersensitivity (DHT)
  b. Mixed lymphocyte reactivity
  c. Cytotoxic T lymphocyte (CTL or "killer" cells)
B. B lymphocytes
 1. Precursors of antibody-forming cells Bμ, Bγ, Bα, Bϵ
 2. Memory cells
 3. ? Regulatory B lymphocytes

SOURCE: From Katz DH: The immune system: An overview, in Fudenberg HH, Stites DP, Caldwell JL, Wells JV (eds): *Basic and Clinical Immunology,* 3d ed. Los Altos, CA, Lange Medical Publications, 1980, p 1.

Most interactions seem to involve the manufacture and release of soluble substances *(lymphokines)* by stimulated cells that trigger responder cells that bear receptors for these lymphokines. Table 10-3 lists some of the lymphokines that have been studied and their putative function.

The most powerful of the lymphokines secreted by activated T_H cells is called interleukin-2. T_E cells cannot secrete interleukin-2, but T_E cells require it in order to proliferate and mature. The interaction of the antigen-responsive T_H cell with the antigen plus interleukin-1 permits it to secrete interleukin-2, which acts on both T_H and T_E cells to permit expansion of the antigen-sensitive clones. A second set of lymphokines that act on antigen-stimulated B cells is necessary for B cells expansion (Fig. 10-6, Table 10-3).

Table 10-3. LYMPHOKINES RELEASED BY ANTIGEN-ACTIVATED T CELLS

Lymphokine		Target cell and function
		Other lymphocytes
Interleukin-2	IL-2	Maintains growth of activated T cells
B cell growth factor	BCGF	Maintains B cell growth
B cell differentiation factor	BCDF	Induces B cell differentiation
Suppressor factor		Suppresses T and B cell functions, not well characterized
		Macrophages
Macrophage activating factor	MAF	Activates macrophages, may be same as gamma-IFN
Migration inhibition factor	MIF	Inhibits macrophage mobility
Macrophage chemotactic factor	MCF	Attracts macrophages
Procoagulant induction		An activation activity, affects coagulation
Fc receptor induction		Induces elevated number of Fc receptors
		Polymorphonuclear leukocytes
Eosinophil chemotactic factor	ECF	Attracts eosinophils
Eosinophil stimulator		Induces eosinophilia
Chemotactic factor		Attracts PMN
		Donor tissue
Gamma-interferon	IFN	Induces elevated MHC expression and has antiviral activity, may be the same as MAF
Lymphotoxin	LT	May be involved in cell damage mediated by LC
		Bone marrow
Interleukin-3	IL-3	Promotes the growth and differentiation of stem cells
Colony stimulating factor	CSF	As above, may include IL-3

Most evidence supports the idea that B lymphoid differentiation to antibody-producing cells is accompanied by cellular proliferation. When the B cell proliferates, morphologic differentiation accompanies the proliferation, and the result is a plasma cell busily engaged in making specific antibody. Conversion from a transformed cell to a plasma cell is seen within a few days of grafting, in both organ allografts and the lymphoid tissue stimulated by these transplants.

The situation for T cells responding to Class I and Class II alloantigens during allograft rejection has proved to be a fascinating variation on the standard immunologic response. Class II alloantigens stimulate T_H cells preferentially and Class I alloantigens stimulate T_E cells preferentially (Fig. 10-6). The T_E cells, after proliferation under the influence of interleukin-2 from helper cells responding to Class II antigens, mature into cells that interact with cells bearing Class I antigens. Such an interaction leads to donor cell death. The T_E and T_H precursors respond to different alloantigens within the closely linked HLA complex, and different T-cell types appear to accomplish differentiation and proliferation. Differentiation requires proliferation, but quite unexpectedly they occur in different cells.

EXPRESSION OF IMMUNITY: GRAFT DESTRUCTION

Specifically sensitized T_E cells are present within most rejecting allografts and are capable of inflicting damage. Alloantigenically stimulated T_H cells are there as well, and can secrete lymphokines (Table 10-3) capable of mediating delayed hypersensitivity reactions. But specifically sensitized cells are in the minority and it is likely that a small number of specifically sensitized lymphoid cells initiate a rejection reaction but that the completion of reaction requires many nonsensitized cells as well. Polymorphonuclear eosinophils, leukocytes (PMNs), plasma cells, and unsensitized mononuclear cells are all part of the rejection process. Furthermore, there is convincing evidence that antibody can initiate graft destruction in the relative absence of a cellular reaction under appropriate circumstances.

In Vitro Lysis of Target Cells by Cytotoxic Lymphocytes. The specifically sensitized lymphoid cells that collect at the site of an allograft have long been known to damage the donor tissues directly in the absence of humoral antibody or complement. Direct contact between the sensitized lymphocyte and the target cell appears to be important. The mechanism of cell membrane damage has not been identified. Several cytotoxic agents have been found that may be released by the lymphocytes, but the specificity of the reaction in vitro favors the idea that interaction of cell surfaces is important to direct the damage of the target cell.

EFFECTOR MOLECULES (LYMPHOKINES) RELEASED BY ACTIVATED LYMPHOCYTES. The release of cytotoxic factors by lymphocytes infiltrating an allograft would be the most direct way to damage foreign cells, but probably not the most efficient, since nonspecific cell killing would result. Several other kinds of molecules are released by specifically sensitized T cells, and these products or lymphokines serve to activate and enlist macrophages, polymorphonuclear leukocytes (PMNs), lymphocytes, etc., so that the initial cellular response is amplified. Several lymphokines have been identified, but it is not yet clear whether there is a small number of molecules with multiple functions or whether a different molecule is specific for each function (Table 10-3).

Macrophages seem to be very active participants in graft rejection; their role does not end with antigen processing. Two of the most investigated lymphokines, migration inhibitory factor (MIF) and chemotactic factor (CF), may serve to attract macrophages and then inhibit their escape. Other lymphokines function to activate the macrophage. Macrophages resemble lymphocytes in that they have resting and activated states. In the later phase, the cytoplasm has the appearance of great activity, both morphologically and enzymatically. Phagocytosis, pinocytosis, and bacteriostatic and tumoricidal activities are increased. The levels of many intracellular enzymes, including the digestive enzymes found in lysosomes, are markedly elevated. Macrophages found at the site of graft rejection appear to be in the activated state and thus better able to participate in tissue destruction.

A host of other activities has been ascribed to the lymphokines. Neutrophils, basophils, and eosinophils are attracted by them (Table 10-3). Growth inhibitory and cytotoxic activities against target cells have been described in vitro. Several apparent lymphokines affect lymphocytes themselves and can be shown under suitable experimental conditions to stimulate mitoses and increase antibody production. Transformed lymphocytes also release a vascular permeability factor in addition to the cytotoxic lymphokines. Little is known about the permeability factor(s) and its possible effect on an allograft rejection. Tissue edema is, however, a prominent feature of graft rejection, and it may join the vascular permeability factors released by the complement activation and neutrophil and platelet participation in the efferent arc of rejection.

ROLE OF ANTIBODY IN ALLOGRAFT REJECTION. Circulating antibody is not an obligatory participant in the rejection of solid tissue allografts. In fact, the inability to make immunoglobulin does not preclude graft rejection. There is now no doubt, however, that rejection can be mediated by alloantibodies—especially the rejection of vascularized organ allografts.

Humoral antibody provides only the recognition portion of graft rejection. Unlike cell-mediated immunity, where the recognition system is intimately associated with the destruction of the target, humoral antibody must activate other systems in order to effect cell death.

Although antibodies bind to allografts, such binding is of no consequence by itself, and the antibody would probably be cleared during the course of normal cell membrane repair. The combination of antibody with the antigen produces an active complex, which triggers a number of nonspecific effector pathways (Fig. 10-7). Each effector pathway typically consists of a sequential activation of enzymes that attract and hold active cells, produce vascular permeability, release enzymes capable

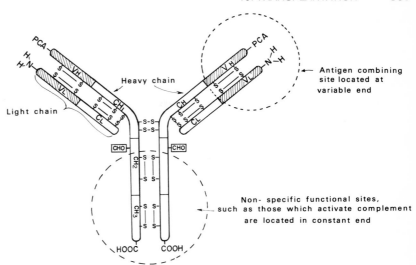

Fig. 10-7. Structure of the IgG antibody molecule. V_H and V_L are the variable portions of the heavy and light chains, respectively, and together they form the antigen-combining site. C_L is the constant portion of the light chain. CH_1, CH_2, and CH_3 are the subunits forming the invariable area of the heavy chain. The approximate positions of the inter- and intrachain disulfide bridges are shown. [From: *Foker JE, Simmons RL, Najarian JS: Allograft rejection: I. The induction of immunity: The afferent arc, in Najarian JS, Simmons RL (eds): Transplantation. Philadelphia, Lea & Febiger, 1972, p 63, with permission.*]

of degrading cell surfaces and other proteins, release factors causing smooth muscle contraction, and precipitate the formation of fibrin clots.

The immunologic response, therefore, can be both efficient and discriminatory. Relatively few specifically differentiated cells can produce molecules that will perform the recognition function. Since few cells are committed to each antigen, many more antigens can be discriminated. The antibodies in turn initiate a relatively general effector mechanism that can destroy the graft.

THE COMPLEMENT SYSTEM. The most important of the several effector molecular cascade systems triggered by antigen binding by antibody is the complement system. The combination of antibody (of IgG_1, IgG_2, IgG_3, or IgM classes) with antigen changes the conformation of the antibody molecule. Included in this change is the activation of a site on the constant (Fc) end of the antibody molecule, which then triggers the complement pathway. The alternate (properdin) pathway can be set off by the immunologically nonspecific serum proteins of the properdin system reacting with sugar structures found on bacterial surfaces and conceivably mammalian cells; its role in graft rejection, however, is unknown. The components of both pathways are circulating protein molecules that, when activated, react in a sequential fashion. At present, the system is known to be made up of a number of distinct molecules that are capable of interacting with one another, with antibody, and with cell membranes. Once activated they can act enzymatically on the next molecule in the sequence, which serves as the inactive substrate. Components C6 and C9 are nonenzymatic and bind to the previous components, resulting in conformational and activity changes.

Most of the biologically significant activities of the complement system arise during activation of the last six reacting complement components, C3 and C5 through C9 (Fig. 10-8). The two parallel but entirely independent initial pathways—the classic and the alternate pathways—both lead to activation of the terminal, biologically important portion of the sequence, involving the reactions of C5 through C9. The terminal portion of the complement sequence may also be directly activated by certain noncomplement serum and cellular enzymes without participation of the early reaction factors. For example, fibrinolytic enzymes in plasma and certain lysosomal enzymes will activate the C3 and C5 stages.

The classic complement pathway (Fig. 10-8) appears to be the most important for immune reactions. Three biologic consequences of complement activation are most important in transplantation rejection.

1. Complement has been shown to be capable of mediating lytic destruction of many kinds of cells to which antibodies have bound. The active components are in the C8 and C9 complexes, but the mechanism of lysis is not clear; perhaps enzymatic activity of the complex damages the membrane directly.
2. Many kinds of cells possess receptors for the C3b or C4b (activated) components, including B lymphocytes, neutrophils, monocytes, and macrophages. If C3b or C4b attach to a damaged cell they may act as opsonins, bringing the target cells in contact with the phagocytic macrophages and monocytes or exposing the surface antigens of these cells to B lymphocytes.
3. Many of the complement cleavage products have biologic actions of their own. For example, C4a and C2b act as kinins. C3a has chemotactic activity for polymorphonuclear leukocytes, causes the release of histamine from mast cells (anaphylatoxin activity), has a kinin activity, and causes immune adherence. C5a is a very potent chemotactic factor, stimulates histamine release from mast cells, and attracts neutrophils and liberates lysosomes from them.

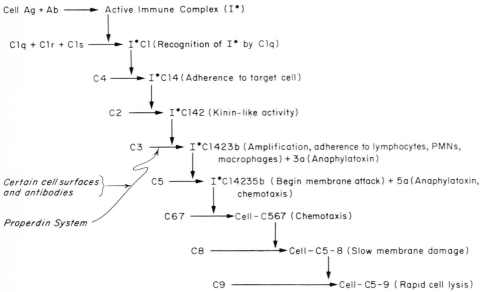

```
Cell Ag + Ab ─────────▶ Active Immune Complex (I*)
                                    │
                                    ▼
C1q + C1r + C1s ─────────▶ I*C1 (Recognition of I* by C1q)
                                    │
                                    ▼
C4 ─────────▶ I*C14 (Adherence to target cell)
                                    │
                                    ▼
C2 ─────────▶ I*C142 (Kinin-like activity)
                                    │
                                    ▼
C3 ─────────▶ I*C1423b (Amplification, adherence to lymphocytes, PMNs,
                          macrophages) + 3a (Anaphylatoxin)
                                    │
                                    ▼
Certain cell surfaces }          C5 ─────────▶ I*C14235b (Begin membrane attack) + 5a (Anaphylatoxin,
and antibodies        }                          chemotaxis)
                                    │
Properdin System                    ▼
                        C67 ─────────▶ Cell-C567 (Chemotaxis)
                                    │
                                    ▼
                        C8 ─────────▶ Cell-C5-8 (Slow membrane damage)
                                    │
                                    ▼
                        C9 ─────────▶ Cell-C5-9 (Rapid cell lysis)
```

Fig. 10-8. The complement pathways and the biologic activity released at each step. The classic pathway begins with a specific antigen-antibody reaction. The properdin pathway is triggered by a more nonspecific interaction between cell surfaces and the molecules that make up the properdin systems. Both pathways, however, converge at the C3 step, where most of the biologic activity associated with complement activation begins. Amplification also occurs at several steps, but it is greatest at C3. The subsequent steps lead to the molecular condensation on the target cell surface, which ultimately results in membrane damage and lysis. There are several other important consequences of complement activation. The presence of these molecules on the target cell surface makes them adherent to other cells. Macrophages, platelets, polymorphonuclear leukocytes, and lymphocytes adhere and increase the damage to the graft cells. The steps through C5 are largely enzymatic in nature; the C3 and C5 components, for example, are split during activation, releasing chemotactic and vasoactive (anaphylatoxins) molecules. Attachment of the C5b molecule to the cell begins the condensation ending in membrane damage; this seems to occur away from the immune complex. Interaction of the C6,C7 components results, additionally, in the release of another chemotactic factor. The activation of the complement pathway, therefore, contributes to many of the features seen in allograft rejection; cellular infiltrates, adherent PMNs and platelets, thrombosed vessels, interstitial edema, and cellular damage.

Therefore, complement activation releases kinins that increase vascular permeability, leading to edema; attracts polymorphonuclear leukocytes that release other vasoactive compounds and lysosomal enzymes; encourages phagocytosis of damaged tissue; releases lysosomal enzymes from macrophages; opsonizes cells; binds cells to damaged cell surfaces (immune adherence); and leads to cell death.

An important biologic characteristic of the complement system as well as the other cascade systems discussed in this section is that they are capable of self-amplification. Thus, in one study 450 C4 molecules were found fixed to each sensitized sheep red blood cell, but each erythrocyte had approximately 100,000 C3 components on its surface. In addition, the C3 components were distributed over the cell membrane surface, rather than confined to the site of the antigen-antibody combination, thus enlarging the area of effect. Although this step produces the greatest numerical amplification, other steps in the complement pathway also expand the number of active molecules.

THE CLOTTING SYSTEM. Theoretically the deposition of fibrin in the allografted organ may arise in two ways: The first, the so-called *extrinsic pathway* of thrombin formation, requires tissue thromboplastin to initiate the sequence of events. The release of this cellular substance may follow damage to the endothelial cell membranes either by antibody and complement or through the direct cytotoxic effect of lymphocytes. The activation of complement through C3 would also promote the adherence of platelets, which, in turn, would stimulate platelet retraction and release of platelet phospholipids. These phospholipids have been shown to promote clotting.

The second method of inducing clot formation, the *intrinsic pathway,* has the potential to be activated directly by immunologic reaction. In the intrinsic pathway, Hageman factor (factor XII) begins a sequence that proceeds through factors XI, IX, VII, and V to the activation

of prothrombin factor to form thrombin with the eventual polymerization of fibrin. Antigen-antibody complexes will activate Hageman factor to trigger this cascade and produce clotting in vitro in the absence of platelets. Thus, an entry into the intrinsic pathway is present within the interactions of antigens and antibodies (Fig. 10-9).

As the reaction proceeds and tissue damage is produced, tissue thromboplastin is released, collagen fibers are exposed, and clotting is facilitated. It is now generally hypothesized that the progressive obliterative vascular reaction of a chronically rejecting allograft is a by-product of fibrin laid down along endothelium that has been damaged by immune mechanisms.

THE KININ SYSTEM. The kinin, or kallikrein, system is initiated by activation of coagulation factor XII, leading

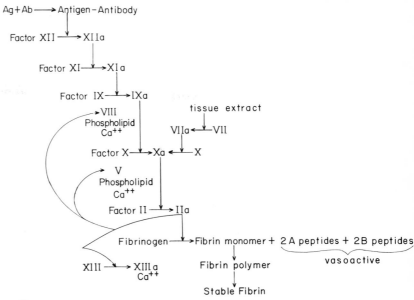

Fig. 10-9. The coagulation cascade system. Fibrin and two vasoactive peptides are the final products of the cascade. The two modes of activation of the system are diagrammed. Factor XII (Hageman factor) can be activated by immune complexes initiating the intrinsic pathway. Tissue damage (presumably produced by immunologic damage) could precipitate the extrinsic system. In both systems, the factors shown, with the probable exceptions of V and VIII, are enzymes. Activation of the pathways involves the sequential conversions of these enzymes to active forms (represented by XIIa, XIa, etc.). [From: *Najarian JS, Foker JE: Allograft rejection: II. The expression of immunity: The efferent arc, in Najarian JS, Simmons RL (eds): Transplantation. Philadelphia, Lea & Febiger, 1972, p 94, with permission.*]

eventually to the formation of kallikrein, which acts on kininogen, an α-globulin substrate in the plasma, and results in bradykinin. Bradykinin is one of the kinins, a group of active peptides that are rather rapidly inactivated, after formation, by kininases present in plasma. The kinins possess a variety of biologic activities, including chemotaxis of PMNs, smooth muscle contraction, dilatation of peripheral arterioles, and increase of capillary permeability. The involvement of the kinin system in graft rejection is likely but is as yet unproved.

INTERRELATIONSHIPS OF THE MOLECULAR CASCADE SYSTEMS (Fig. 10-10). Antigen-antibody complexes activate complement and Hageman factor. Hageman factor in turn produces clotting, activates plasmin, and perhaps directly activates complement. Plasmin in turn can activate C3 to produce, among other effects, chemotactic factors, immune adherence, and opsonization. Activation of Hageman factor also leads to kinin production. Activation of the complement system produces aggregation of platelets and, consequently, initiation of the clotting mechanism. Thrombin formation, in turn, stimulates the production of plasmin from plasminogen. Prostaglandin activity is released following complement activation, and may contribute to vascular permeability, although the significance of this in allograft rejection remains unclear.

Not only are the activators of these systems interrelated, but also the inhibitors are intertwined. The C1 esterase inhibitor also decreases the activity of the kinin and plasmin systems. Neither activation nor inhibition of one system can occur without affecting the other pathways.

The complexity of the allograft reaction is just beginning to be understood. Not only does it involve a variety of recognition molecules (antibodies) and presumably a similar variety of specifically sensitized cells; there is much recent evidence that unsensitized lymphocytes can be specifically directed and actively lyse target allogenic cells by a coating with antibody. In addition, the main force of the reaction may be produced by a bewildering array of amplifying chain reactions that include both molecular amplification schemes and cellular amplifiers. The activation of complement, the clotting system, kinin formation, and the stimulation of PMN, macrophages, and platelet assault produce a variety of damage to the transplanted organ. Included are occlusive phenomena within the graft vessels, induced permeability of these same vessels with interstitial edema accumulation, disruption of cellular basement membranes, and the infiltration of the graft with a profusion of cell types (Fig. 10-10).

AN INTEGRATED VIEW OF THE REJECTION OF ORGAN ALLOGRAFTS. Rejection morphology has two main components: The first component is the host response, and it is composed of effector cells and molecules, both immunologically specific and nonspecific. In rapid rejections these comprise most, if not all, of the pathologic picture so that the speed of the reaction virtually precludes response by the organ cells. The second component becomes prominent only with longer survival of the transplanted organ and encompasses morphologic alterations peculiar to the injured organ.

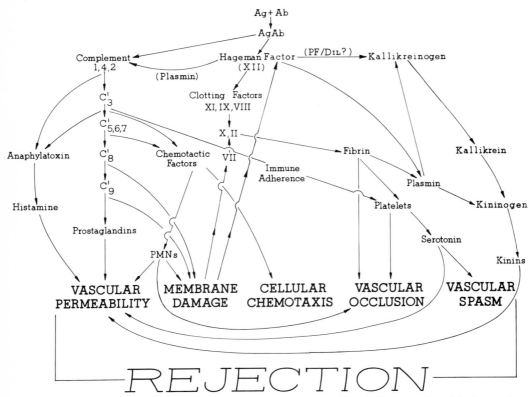

Fig. 10-10. Integration of the humoral amplification system in graft rejection. This diagram suggests the complexity of allograft rejection. The three main cascade pathways—complement, clotting, and kinin—generate many active molecules, including the kinins, chemotactic factors, anaphylatoxins, histamine, and serotonin. These molecules, together with platelets and polymorphonuclear leukocytes (PMNs), produce the destructive effects on the graft. The most prominent consequences include increased vascular permeability (edema), spasm, and occlusion, as well as cell and basement membrane damage and cellular chemotaxis (infiltration). It is clear that these systems do not operate singly but tend to activate each other. Not shown are the many interlocking inhibitory factors that keep these systems in check once they are activated. [From: *Najarian JS, Foker JE: Allograft rejection: II. The expression of immunity: The efferent arc, in Najarian JS, Simmons RL (eds): Transplantation. Philadelphia, Lea & Febiger, 1972, p 94, with permission.*]

A predictable series of events ensues when an unsensitized patient is allografted. The first visible change is a perivascular infiltration of round cells (Fig. 10-11). The accumulation of cells is not significant for several hours after transplantation but can reach considerable numbers within 48 h. The original enclaves around small vessels spread, and the interstitial space is further infiltrated. A potpourri of cells accumulates: cells resembling small lymphocytes are seen, as well as large transformed lymphocytes with basophilic cytoplasm. Large histiocytes or macrophages are just beginning to arrive in numbers. Plasma cells are still relatively scarce; as a terminal product of cellular differentiation, they may require several cell divisions before they appear in the organ (Fig. 10-12).

Antibody and complement are deposited in the area of the capillaries, and some of the infiltrating lymphoid cells are producing immunoglobulins by the third day. Recognition molecules (antibody) as well as sensitized cells are therefore present early in the allograft reaction.

Sensitized lymphoid cells, upon recognizing the foreign tissue, release several mediators of inflammation and cell damage. The release of cytotoxic factors directly injures membranes of adjacent cells. Mitogenic products stimulate division of lymphoid cells, perhaps expanding the immunocompetent population. Activated, phagocytic macrophages are effectively concentrated in the area by migration inhibitory factor and other chemotactic factors. In addition, vascular permeability agents are released.

Meanwhile, complement is fixed, thereby producing chemotactic factors, anaphylatoxins, and finally cellular damage when the terminal components are activated. Capillary permeability is increased by anaphylatoxins from the complement chain and probably by kinins. Interstitial edema becomes prominent. At the same time there are several additional inducements to cellular infiltration. The complement cascade generates molecules that produce immune adherence and others that have chemotactic activity. Damaged cells release additional compounds that contribute to infiltration by PMNs as well as other cells. PMNs in turn release vasoactive amines (including histamine or serotonin, depending on the species) and

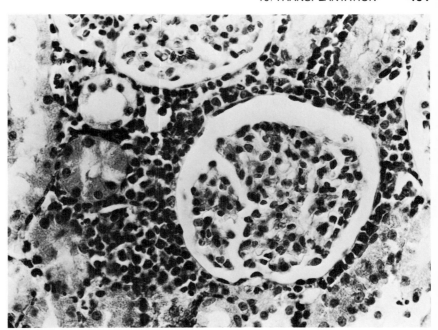

Fig. 10-11. Canine renal allograft 48 h after transplantation into unmodified recipient. Round cell infiltration, usually the first overt sign of host activity against the allograft, is apparent within 6 to 12 h after transplantation. By 48 h the number of invading cells is substantial. The original perivascular infiltrate has surrounded a glomerulus and adjacent tubules. [From: *Foker JE, Najarian JS: Allograft rejection: III. The pathobiology of organ rejection, in Najarian JS, Simmons RL (eds): Transplantation. Philadelphia, Lea & Febiger, 1972, p 122, with permission.*]

additional vascular permeability-promoting factors. The PMNs squeeze through the enlarged endothelial cell junctions and release proteolytic cathepsins D and E, causing basement membrane damage.

Fibrin and α-macroglobulins, whose contribution is not understood, are deposited by 7 days. During this time, lymphoid cells have continued to accumulate and, joined by significant numbers of plasma cells and PMNs, obscure the normal architecture. The round cell population presumably contains many macrophages and other immunologic nonspecific cells at this point. Increasingly frequent mitoses may indicate the production of immunocompetent cells within the graft.

The small vessels become plugged with fibrin and platelets, diminishing the perfusion and preventing function. In this relatively rapid sequence of events the organ has little chance to respond, and the pathologic process is dominated by the host effector pathways.

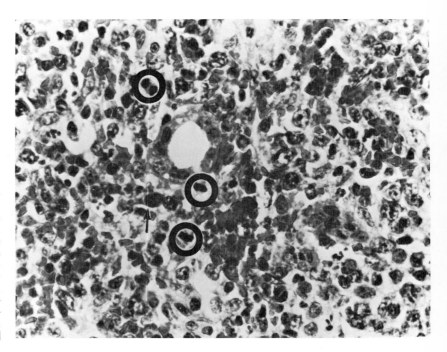

Fig. 10-12. Canine renal allograft 4 days after transplantation into an unmodified recipient. Invading cells all but obscure the architecture of the kidney. Numerous mitoses (circles) can be found, and this cellular proliferation may be producing immunologically competent cells within the graft. A plasma cell (arrow) is present, but most of the cells resemble lymphocytes and macrophages. [From: *Foker JE, Najarian JS: Allograft rejection: III. The pathobiology of organ rejection, in Najarian JS, Simmons RL (eds): Transplantation. Philadelphia, Lea & Febiger, 1972, p 122, with permission.*]

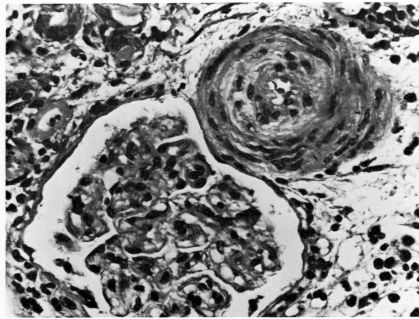

Fig. 10-13. A rejected human allograft removed 18 months post-transplant. The lumen of the arteriole has all but disappeared as a consequence of hyperplasia of the cells of the vessel. Most of the thickening of the wall is probably due to proliferation of smooth muscle cells, with spindle-shaped nuclei. Endothelial cells, with rounder nuclei, almost fill the lumen. [From: *Foker JE, Najarian JS: Allograft rejection: III. The pathobiology of organ rejection, in Najarian JS, Simmons RL (eds): Transplantation. Philadelphia, Lea & Febiger, 1972, p 122, with permission.*]

Obviously, rejection modified by immunosuppressive agents is not a distinct morphologic classification. The morphologic features associated with this more chronic rejection become dominated by the response of the organ tissue itself. Here the normal response of tissue to injury predominates in the pathologic picture. A good deal of endothelial cell damage occurs in the allograft, and the responses of cellular repair, hypertrophy and hyperplasia, follow.

Endothelial cell damage also elicits repair processes. Aggregations of platelets within the intimal layer are resolved, and the dissolution of the thrombi is accompanied by the infiltration of macrophages and foam cells. The result is a thickened intimal layer with the loss of smooth endothelial lining and the presence of vacuolated cells. The lumen narrows as a result. Narrowing of the vessel lumen is also a consequence of the medial thickening. Studies using nonimmunologic disease models have shown that most of the cells proliferating in response to the stimulus of injury are smooth muscle cells. A reasonable extrapolation is that hyperplasia of these cells produces much of the lumenal narrowing in the allograft (Fig. 10-13).

Although the exposed position of the endothelial cells and the striking proliferation of the smooth muscle cells argue for their being an important target of the immune reaction, there is evidence that the basement and elastic membranes of the vessel absorb a major portion of immune-mediated damage. Either immune complexes or antibodies to the vascular basement membrane activate complement and attract polymorphonuclear cells. These nonspecific effector cells release at least four protein factors that increase the permeability of the vessel and in addition produce cathepsins D and E, which digest base-

ment membranes. The PMNs are active in reaching the basement membrane and will lift the endothelial cells to gain this access.

Platelets may be of greater significance than PMNs in mediating damage. Immune complexes (which activate complement) will result in platelet adherence and the release of vasoactive substances. Platelet aggregation leads to the release of histamine, serotonin, and other capillary permeability factors that expose more basement membrane; the exposed collagen fibers of the basement membrane further enhance platelet aggregation. Platelets and PMNs drawn to these sites release cathepsins, elastases, and phosphatases that increase destruction and attract other nonspecific cellular effectors including macrophages.

The myocardial cell is the characteristic cell of the heart, the tubular cell of the kidney, the acinar and islet cell of the pancreas, etc. The differentiation and function of these cells demand an ample oxygen supply, and if destroyed, they cannot be replaced by further cellular division. Therefore, compromise of respiration by vascular endothelial and medial hypertrophy, intravascular aggregations of platelets, and interstitial accumulations of edema and mononuclear cells will have predictable consequences for these cells. They will atrophy, and death may be followed by replacement fibrosis (Fig. 10-14).

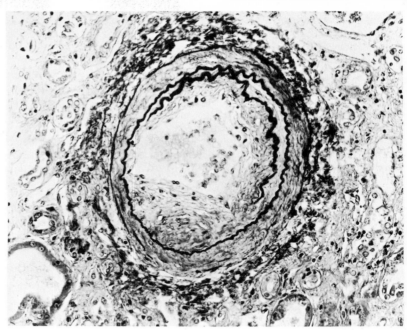

Fig. 10-14. Extensive damage to the small artery in a human renal allograft removed 14 months posttransplant is apparent. The elastic membranes are badly frayed, and the elastica interna has been destroyed entirely along half the circumference of the vessel. The intimal layer shows extensive disruption and loss of cells. The cells remaining are often vacuolated. The lumen is narrowed by tissue from several origins: proliferation of smooth muscle cells in the media, endothelial cell swelling and hyperplasia, and the presence of an organized thrombus. The adventitial area shows damage and edema formation. Note also that severe tubular atrophy and interstitial fibrosis are present. [From: *Foker JE, Najarian JS: Allograft rejection: III. The pathobiology of organ rejection, in Najarian JS, Simmons RL (eds): Transplantation. Philadelphia, Lea & Febiger, 1972, p 122, with permission.*]

The interstitial area concomitantly increases in size. The interstitial area, however, has much activity in its own right. Repair of immunologic damage stimulates many fibroblastic cells to proliferate, and it attracts macrophages. The persisting immunogenic capacity of the allograft is indicated by the inevitable presence of infiltrating plasma cells and lymphoid cells.

It is impossible to determine what proportions of these effects result from ischemia produced by vascular occlusion, interstitial edema, or cellular infiltrates. Similarly, the contribution made by the direct cytotoxic action of specific and nonspecific effector cells and molecules is unknown.

CIRCUMVENTING REJECTION

Clinical Immunosuppression

Theoretically, there are a number of methods by which the allograft rejection response can be suppressed including (1) destroying the immunocompetent cells prior to transplantation, (2) making the antigen unrecognizable or even toxic to the reactive lymphocyte clones, (3) interfering with antigen processing by the recipient cells, (4) inhibiting lymphocyte transformation and proliferation, (5) limiting lymphocyte differentiation into killer or antibody-synthesizing cells, (6) activating sufficient numbers of suppressor lymphocytes, (7) inhibiting destruction of graft cells by killer lymphocytes, (8) interfering with the combination of immunoglobulins with target antigens, or (9) preventing tissue damage by the nonspecific cells or antigen-antibody complexes.

In practice, a clinically useful immunosuppression largely depends on the destruction of the immunocompetent cells and on inhibiting the differentiation and proliferation of these cells. Methods of inducing specific immune tolerance by various antigen preparations prior to grafting, or by inhibiting sensitized cells and antibodies after they have produced, have not been clinically successful. It is more difficult to inhibit the immune response after it is underway, so less can be gained clinically after sensitization has occurred. To be most effective, immunosuppression must be present at the time of transplantation, or even before. Nevertheless, some success can be achieved in reversing the exacerbations of the rejection reaction seen in clinical transplantation.

ANTIPROLIFERATIVE AGENTS

Most traditional immunosuppressive agents act to impair the proliferation of lymphocytes. Such agents include the antimetabolites, alkylating agents, toxic antibiotics, and x-ray. They inhibit the full expression of the immune response by preventing the differentiation and division of the immunocompetent lymphocyte after it encounters the antigen. All of them, however, fall into one of two broad mechanistic categories. Either they structurally resemble needed metabolites or they combine with certain cellular components, such as DNA, and thereby interfere with cell function.

The former group, the antimetabolites, have a structural similarity to cell metabolites and either inhibit enzymes of that metabolic pathway or are incorporated during synthesis to produce faulty molecules. The antimetabolites include purine, pyrimidine, and folic acid analogs, which are most effective against proliferating and differentiating cells. They are given at the time of transplantation when the immunocompetent cells are first stimulated, and then for the life of the graft to interfere with the continuing stimulus to the immune system.

Alkylating agents and certain antibiotics include those compounds that combine with DNA and other cellular components. Although these agents would be useful in the pretransplant period to reduce the number of effective immunocompetent cells in the recipients, and thereafter to prevent proliferation, they are so toxic that their use has been limited to bone marrow transplantation and as occasional substitutes for azathioprine.

PURINE ANALOGS. The purine analog azathioprine (AZ) (Imuran) has been the most widely used immunosuppressive drug in clinical organ transplantation. Azathioprine is 6-mercaptopurine (6-MP) plus a side chain to protect the labile sulfhydryl group. In the liver, the side chain is split off to form the active compound, 6-MP. The mechanism of action would seem to be similar for these two compounds; however, azathioprine seems to enjoy the advantage of slightly lower toxicity.

Full metabolic activity comes in the cell with the addition of ribose 5-phosphate from phosphoribosyl pyrophosphate to form 6-MP ribonucleotide. The structural resemblance of this molecule to inosine monophosphate is obvious, and 6-MP ribonucleotide inhibits the enzymes that begin to convert inosine nucleotide to adenosine and guanosine monophosphate (Fig. 10-15). In addition, the presence of 6-MP ribonucleotides slows the entire purine biosynthetic pathway by fraudulent feedback inhibition of an early step. The steric similarity to either adenosine or guanine nucleotides is not great enough to allow significant incorporation into DNA or RNA and synthesis of

faulty molecules. The result of inhibiting these several enzymes, however, is to block the synthesis of cellular RNA, DNA, certain cofactors, and other active nucleotides.

The toxicity of azathioprine results from the same mechanisms. Its primary toxic effect is bone marrow suppression, leading to leukopenia. Liver toxicity can also result, possibly because of the high rate of RNA synthesis by these cells. The mechanism is unclear, however, because hepatic dysfunction does not seem to be dose-related.

Although pyrimidine analogs have been studied extensively as immunosuppressants in the laboratory, they have only limited clinical use.

FOLIC ACID ANTAGONISTS. The folic acid antagonists, aminopterin and methotrexate, inhibit the enzyme dihydrofolate reductase, and prevent the conversion of folic acid to tetrahydrofolic acid. This step is necessary for the synthesis of DNA, RNA, and certain coenzymes; again, proliferating cell systems are most affected.

Some of the toxicity of aminopterin and methotrexate can be abrogated by the administration of folinic acid some hours or even days after the use of the antagonist. Nevertheless, the ratio of immunosuppression to toxicity has not justified their use in clinical kidney transplantation. The immune reactions that accompany bone marrow transplantation are more difficult to control, and methotrexate is used to both prevent and reverse the severe graft-versus-host reactions that occur. Since methotrexate is usually used with one or more other drugs, its toxic effects can be difficult to identify. Megaloblastic hemopoiesis, mucosal breakdown with severe gastrointestinal bleeding, and liver damage seem to be related to methotrexate therapy. These effects, even with high dosages of

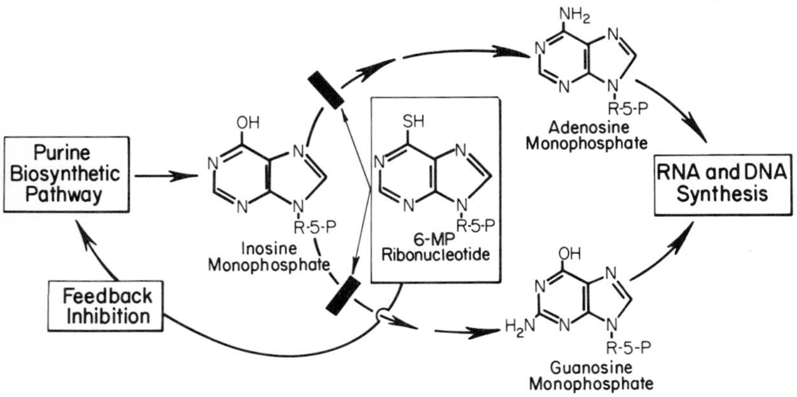

Fig. 10-15. Mechanism of antimetabolite action. 6-Mercaptopurine (6-MP) ribonucleotide resembles inosine monophosphate in its steric configuration. It thereby competes with inosine in its transformation into adenosine monophosphate and guanosine monophosphate and their subsequent incorporation into RNA and DNA. In addition, 6-MP inhibits the purine biosynthetic pathway, since it resembles a product of that biosynthetic pathway (feedback inhibition). [From: *Simmons RL, Foker JE, Najarian JS: Principles of immunosuppression, in Sabiston DC Jr (ed): Davis-Christopher Textbook of Surgery. Philadelphia, Saunders, 1972, p 471, with permission.*]

methotrexate, can usually be prevented by folinic acid (citrovorum rescue). Obviously, depression of the transplanted marrow may also result from the activity of methotrexate, although assigning the cause may be difficult in the complex clinical situation.

ALKYLATING AGENTS. The alkylating agents have highly reactive rings as part of the molecular structure. These unstable rings have electron-seeking points that combine with electron-rich nucleophilic groups such as the tertiary nitrogens in purines and pyrimidines, or with —NH$_2$, —COOH, —SH, and —PO$_3$H$_2$ groups on a variety of molecules. The high-energy rings of alkylating agents break and combine with these constituents to form stable covalent bonds. Obviously, many cell components have such groups, including DNA, RNA, and the enzymatic and structural proteins. Alkylation of DNA is probably the most detrimental. If the DNA strands are not repaired, chromosomal replication will be faulty in proliferating cells. Both DNA and RNA can be alkylated at several points, but a common site appears to be N-7 of the guanine ring (Fig. 10-16). Mispairing of DNA during replication may result from the presence of the alkylating agent itself, the clipping out of the alkylated guanine residue, or the cleavage of an alkylated guanine ring. Also chain breaks and cross-linkages frequently interfere with chain replication.

Since the damage to DNA can be repaired, these effects are apparently time-dependent. Consequently, the administration of alkylating agents just before and during stimulation by the antigen would most interfere with the ability of the immunocompetent cells to respond to that antigen. Continued use of the alkylating agents would also muffle the proliferative response of these cells in the face of a persistent stimulus. There are differences, however, in the response of T and B cells. The B cell seems to be more susceptible to cyclophosphamide than the T cell. This drug is a potent inhibitor of antibody formation, but its effect on skin or kidney rejection is much less spectacular. The reason for this apparent difference is unknown.

The usefulness of alkylating agents, which include nitrogen mustard, phenylalanine mustard, busulfan, and cyclophosphamide, is limited by their toxicity. Even so, cyclophosphamide has been used with good results in renal transplantation when liver toxicity prohibited the use of azathioprine. Cyclophosphamide is frequently used in clinical bone marrow transplantation, where it potentiates the effects of radiation and enhances the disruption of DNA. When cyclophosphamide is used, lower doses of radiation are required to deplete the recipient bone marrow population and provide space for donor cells. When leukemia is the indication for bone marrow transplantation, cyclophosphamide will aid in the destruction of these cells.

Toxicity is high, however, and predictable reactions occur, principally to rapidly replicating cell populations. Stomatitis, nausea, vomiting, diarrhea, skin rash, anemia, and alopecia are all common reactions. The more specific effects of cyclophosphamide administration are prompt fluid retention, occasionally severe hemorrhagic cystitis, and cardiac toxicity. The cardiac and edema problems suggest that even nonreplicating cell populations are adversely affected by this drug.

ANTIBIOTICS. The immunosuppressive antibiotics include the inhibitors of nucleic acid synthesis, and chloramphenicol and puromycin, which interfere with cellular protein synthesis. Actinomycin D binds to the guanine residue of DNA, thereby sterically interfering with RNA polymerase and, consequently, with DNA-directed RNA

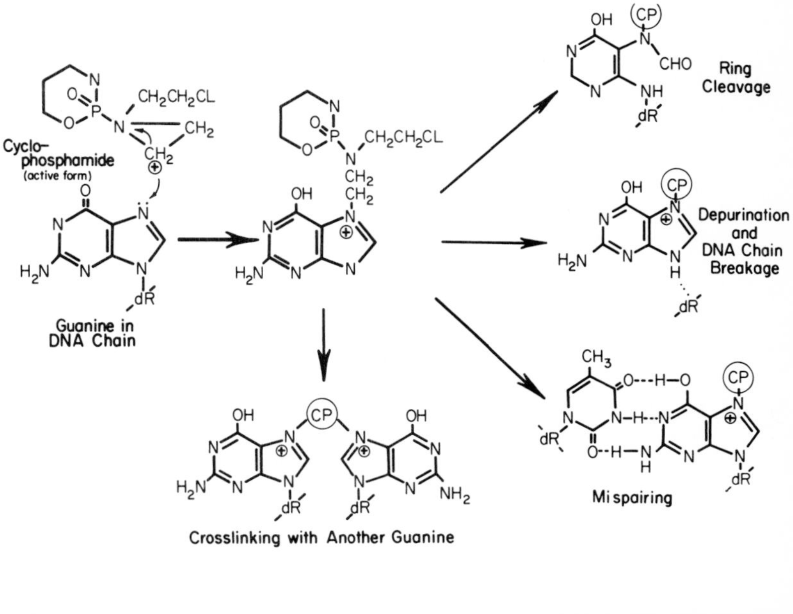

Fig. 10-16. Mechanism of the action of the alkylating agent cyclophosphamide (CP). CP binds to the guanine molecule within the DNA chain. The guanine-CP complex leads to further damage to the DNA molecule. Four examples of the damage to DNA are shown. [From: *Simmons RL, Foker JE, Najarian JS: Principles of immunosuppression, in Sabiston DC Jr (ed): Davis-Christopher Textbook of Surgery. Philadelphia, Saunders, 1972, p 471, with permission.*]

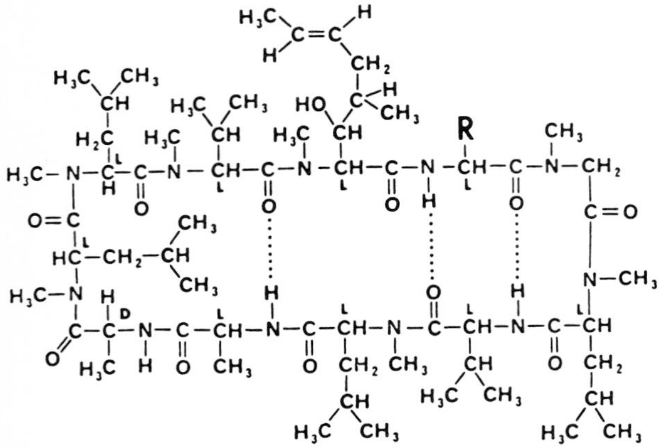

Fig. 10-17. Structure of cyclosporine. CyA,R = —CH₂CH₃; CyD,R = —CH(CH₃)₂.

synthesis. Mitomycin C combines with cellular DNA and hinders replication. None of these agents is clinically useful as an immunosuppressive agent for transplantation.

CYCLOSPORINE. Cyclosporine is a fungal cyclic peptide (Fig. 10-17) which represents an entire new class of clinically important immunosuppressive agents. It is not an alkylating, antimitotic, or lympholytic agent. Its action at the molecular level seems highly specific, not just for lymphoid cells, but rather for certain subpopulations of T cells.

Cyclosporine strongly inhibits the formation of cytotoxic T cells in mixed lymphocyte culture, and prophylactic administration is strongly suppressive of allograft rejection. Indeed, rejection or graft-versus-host disease can sometimes be overcome or reversed. Stopping the drug permits rejection to resume so that cyclosporine plus antigen does not lead to permanent tolerance.

Cyclosporine does not appear to affect precursor hematopoietic cells, resting or dividing lymphocytes, or macrophage functions. It acts by interfering with the production of the lymphokine interleukin II, which is normally essential for lymphocyte proliferation. Thus the expansion of antigen-responsive clones of T lymphocytes is suppressed. T suppressor cells, however, are not inhibited. Additive immunosuppressive effects can be achieved in combination with ALG, azathioprine, prednisone, irradiation, and other anti-inflammatory drugs.

Cyclosporine has virtually revolutionized clinical transplantation. In combination with modest doses of prednisone, it appears to be of equal clinical utility, or superior, to ALG-azathioprine and prednisone. Its renal toxicity is a serious disadvantage but can usually be controlled by reducing the dose or combining it with conventional immunosuppressive drugs. A minor disadvantage is that it can only be administered by mouth in a lipid-soluble medium (milk, oil), and its absorption is unpredictable. An intravenous formulation is also available but nephrotoxicity is a problem. In clinically useful doses, cyclosporine is no more likely to induce lymphoma formation than the older immunosuppressive agents.

IMMUNOSUPPRESSION BY LYMPHOCYTE DEPLETION

ADRENAL CORTICOSTEROIDS. Despite uncertainty about their mechanism of action, steroids are necessary for successful human organ transplantation and are commonly used to produce immunosuppression in other types of patients.

Many effects of steroids are known (Fig. 10-18). The problem is deciding which are primary and which are secondary actions. Steroids cross the cell membrane and bind to specific receptors in the cytoplasm of most cells, lymphocytes included. The steroid-receptor complex then enters the nucleus and interacts with DNA in an unknown way. In lymphocytes, DNA, RNA, and protein synthesis is inhibited, as is glucose and amino acid transport. At a sufficient dosage, lymphocyte degeneration and lysis occur. Cytolysis can readily be produced in vivo, and T cells appear to be most susceptible. The primary antilymphocyte action of steroids may be to deplete small lymphocytes before they are activated by antigen. Steroids also suppress most of the accessory functions of macrophages including the ability to secrete interleukin-1.

The functional effects of steroids are predictable, and all T-cell responses are depressed. Paradoxically, the steroid-resistant thymocytes that remain after an injection of steroids have increased activity, but the net immunologic capability of the treated animal is reduced.

Although B-cell activity and antibody production are relatively unaffected by steroids, many other cell types that participate in graft rejection are damaged. Both macrophage and neutrophil chemotaxis and phagocytosis are inhibited. The accumulation of neutrophils, macrophages, and monocytes at sites of immune and inflammatory activity is reduced. Steroids also increase the membrane stability of digestive lysosomal particles in these cells, which reduces their inflammatory activity. Inflammation is so intertwined with any substantial immune reaction that the various effects are inseparable. The variety of immunologic activities that steroids will suppress means that their effectiveness against the rejection reaction is probably the sum of many influences. Steroids alone cannot prevent clinical allograft rejection, but, together with other compounds, they are potent in both preventing and reversing rejection reactions.

Steroid toxicity of some degree is frequent and commonly includes a cushingoid appearance. Other characteristic problems from steroid therapy are hypertension; weight gain; peptic ulcers and gastrointestinal bleeding; euphoric personality changes; cataract formation; hyperglycemia, which may progress to steroid diabetes; and osteoporosis with avascular necrosis of bone. The appearance and severity of these complications vary considerably, but all too frequently they are life-threatening or disabling. Clinical transplantation will be improved tremendously when more specific means of immunosuppression are developed and present steroid dosages can be reduced.

ANTILYMPHOCYTE GLOBULIN. A variety of antibody preparations designed to react with immunoresponsive

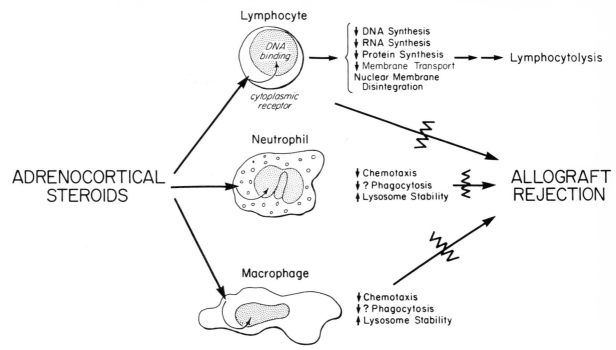

Fig. 10-18. Adrenocortical steroids play an important role in clinical allograft immunosuppression. Many apparent sites of action have been located experimentally. These compounds bind to cytoplasmic receptors, and this complex combines with DNA. How this relates to the many functional consequences of steroids presented in this diagram is unclear. In the complex clinical transplantation setting it is not possible to determine if the primary suppression of lymphocytes is more important than the anti-inflammatory effects on neutrophils and macrophages in the suppression of allograft rejection reactions. The suppression of interleukin-1 production by macrophages is probably a most important mechanism.

lymphocytes are available, and their number and variety will increase in the next few years. They are designed to prevent and to treat graft rejection.

Heterologous polyclonal antilymphocyte globulins (ALG) are produced when thoracic duct, peripheral blood, lymph nodes, thymus, or spleen lymphocytes are injected into animals of a different species. Cell membranes or cultured lymphocytes serve equally well to provide the antigenic stimulation. The addition of adjuvants, usually Freund's complete adjuvant, is used to enhance the immunogenicity of the foreign lymphocytes and produce sera that are consistently more immunosuppressive. The rabbit and the horse are commonly used to produce antisera for clinical transplantation.

The antibodies produced in this crude way are reactive with a number of different epitopes on the many subsets of lymphocytes injected. As a consequence, the immunosuppressive effect is the net result of the destruction of many lymphocyte subsets.

The action of heterologous polyclonal ALG seems to be directed mainly against the T cell. ALG therefore interferes most with the cell-mediated reactions-allograft rejection, tuberculin sensitivity, and the graft-versus-host reaction. ALG can abolish preexisting delayed hypersensitivity reactions, and larger doses will prolong the survival of some xenografts. ALG has a definite, but lesser, effect on antibody production to T-cell-dependent antigens.

Although these preparations, purified and administered intravenously, have been widely used in clinical transplantation with beneficial results in both the prevention and treatment of organ allograft rejection, monoclonal reagents with more predictable reactivity are becoming available. Such antibodies are the products of cell fusions between antilymphocyte antibody-producing clones of mouse B cells and laboratory myeloma cells. The resulting hybridomas have become rendered immortal and each cell line produces a single antibody directed to a single antigen on a human lymphocyte. If the target cell is a cell type essential for the immune response, such as a T cell, severe degrees of immunosuppression can be induced in the recipient of the monoclonal antibody. Mouse monoclonal antibody directed against T cells is now available for clinical use in the treatment of rejection.

The toxicity of any heterologous antibody prepared against human tissue depends in part on its cross reactivity with other tissue antigens, and the ability of the patient to make antibodies against the protein itself. Polyclonal ALG can produce anemia and thrombocytopenia despite prior absorption with human platelets and red cell stroma. Monoclonal antibodies have few cross reactions, but fever, chills, nausea, diarrhea, and aseptic meningitis are frequently seen during the intravenous administration of the first few doses. All heterologous globulins can elicit allergic reactions against themselves. These are generally mild and infrequent, but monoclonal antibodies are strongly antigenic so that they are less effective after 1 or 2 weeks of use. Polyclonal antibody preparations seem to be repeatedly effective.

RADIATION. Radiation was probably the first agent used to produce immunosuppression. Ionizing radiation (x-rays, alpha rays, beta rays) affects both cellular proteins and nucleic acids. Despite the fact that relatively small dosages of irradiation may disrupt the secondary protein structure formed by hydrogen bonding and the tertiary conformation that results, biologically significant alterations of protein function seem to require very high dosages. Consequently, most of the immunosuppressive effects of x-radiation are caused by changes produced in nucleic acids. DNA is particularly vulnerable, and therefore so is cellular replication. The most important of the several modes of damage is the production of scattered breaks in the deoxyribose-phosphate backbone of DNA (Fig. 10-19). Disruption of either the carbon-carbon bonds of the deoxyribotides or the bonds involving the phosphate groups produces breaks in one of the DNA strands. Occasionally both strands are broken at the same point. Other sites of damage, such as the bases themselves, are even less frequent.

Repair mechanisms exist to mend the breaks, but insuf-

Fig. 10-19. X-ray-induced damage of DNA molecule. Irradiation frequently induces single breaks in the deoxyribotide backbone of the DNA double helix. More rarely, irradiation induces double breaks within the backbone. [From: Simmons RL, Foker JE, Najarian JS: Principles of immunosuppression, in Sabiston DC Jr (ed): Davis-Christopher Textbook of Surgery. Philadelphia, Saunders, 1972, p 471, with permission.]

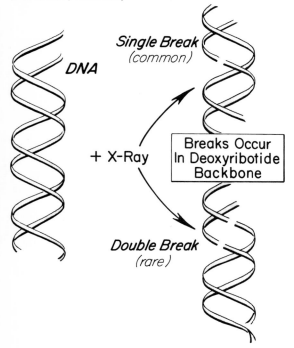

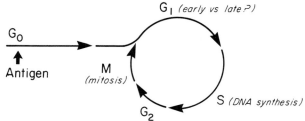

Fig. 10-20. The phases of the cell cycle. Following stimulation by an antigen, or other type of mitogen, small lymphocytes are activated. They are converted from the resting G_0 phase to the active G_1 phase. The G_1 phase lasts 10 h or longer before DNA synthesis (S phase) begins. The S phase lasts about 10 h and is followed by a short (2 to 4 h) G_2 phase before mitosis (M phase). M phase is relatively brief, usually less than 2 to 3 h, after which the cells are returned to the G_1 phase. The susceptibility of the cell to the immunosuppressive agents used in transplantation varies with the phase of the cycle. Periods of most intense nucleic acid synthesis, particularly S phase, are most vulnerable to the antimetabolites. As discussed in the text, the resting G_0 lymphocyte is also susceptible to several of the clinically used immunosuppressive agents. [From: Foker JE, Simmons RL, Najarian JS: Principles of immunosuppression, in Sabiston DC Jr (ed): Davis-Christopher Textbook of Surgery. Philadelphia, Saunders, 1977, p 509, with permission.]

ficient time may be available in the dividing cell. Therefore, the effectiveness of radiation is dependent upon the phase of the cell cycle in which the cell is found (Fig. 10-20). Cells in the M or G_2 phase are most sensitive to irradiation. Presumably, DNA breaks that occur during these phases cannot be repaired quickly enough, and the synthetic events and precise apportionment of cellular components that occur during mitosis may become scrambled. Conversely, the early G_1 phase and the latter part of the S phase are the most resistant portions of the cell cycle. Although irradiation is, in general, most effective just prior to or during mitosis, lymphocytes are a special case. For reasons that are not known, these cells are also sensitive in their resting, or G_0, phase.

The effect of irradiation on the immune response depends greatly on its timing with relation to antigen exposure. When an antigen is given soon after irradiation, the immune response will be inhibited because there is insufficient time for the immunocompetent cell population to recover before the antigen is encountered. If radiation is given during the time of maximal proliferation of the immunocompetent population to an antigen (soon after antigen administration), the immune response will be strongly inhibited. On the other hand, if antigenic stimulation is delayed long enough for the precursor cells to recover from the radiation, there will even be a slight augmentation of the response. Radiation is ineffective if given long after the antigen, when a mature population of effector cells has been formed.

Total body irradiation has limited use in clinical transplantation because the toxicity is too great. Fractionated doses of radiation to the lymphoid tissues (total lymphoid irradiation), similar to that used in the treatment of Hodgkin's disease, is under investigation. Profound immunosuppression is produced, and low dosages of azathioprine and prednisone can maintain the effect. Local irradiation of the graft may also provide some immunosuppressive effects by damaging invading lymphocytes as well as producing nonspecific anti-inflammatory effects.

Both total body radiation and total lymphoid irradiation have been used to eliminate the immune reactivity of patients in preparation for bone marrow transplantation. Cytotoxic chemotherapy is used in combination. The toxicity is predictable. The rapidly replicating skin and gastrointestinal tract are universally affected, and nausea, vomiting, diarrhea, and skin changes occur.

THYMECTOMY. The atrophic adult mammalian thymus continues to play a small role in maintaining immunologic responsiveness. Its extirpation can enhance the effects of immunosuppressive agents or irradiation. Unfortunately, thymectomy has not been useful in clinical transplantation.

LYMPHOID EXTIRPATION AND SPLENECTOMY. Immunity becomes rapidly systemic. It is not confined for long to the regional lymph nodes or to a single major lymphoid organ like the spleen. Splenectomy, however, appears to be beneficial in combination with ALG, azathioprine, and prednisone in prolonging human organ allograft survival. Its effect may simply be to reduce the toxicity of the myelosuppressive drugs so that greater doses of azathioprine can be tolerated in splenectomized transplant recipients. Because splenectomy also increases the risk of subsequent infection, it is used less often in organ transplantation.

THORACIC DUCT DRAINAGE. Cannulation and drainage of the thoracic duct will deplete the body of a large proportion of its circulating T lymphocytes, and such depletion will lead to prolongation of allograft survival and to lesser decreases in the capacity for antibody synthesis. Thoracic duct cannulation and drainage have been used for clinical immunosuppression with great success, but the procedure is cumbersome. The indwelling cannula can become plugged or infected and protein depletion may result if the cell-free lymph is not reinfused. It is doubtful whether this complicated technique, which requires prolonged hospitalization, is superior to drug therapy.

ADVERSE CONSEQUENCES OF IMMUNOSUPPRESSIVE THERAPY

The complications of immunosuppressive therapy in recipients of organ allografts are difficult to distinguish from the complications of recurrent rejection. Patients who do not have rejection episodes generally do not suffer major complications of immunosuppressive therapy. Conversely, the patient who requires repeated large doses of prednisone to avoid further rejection episodes or who suffers diminished renal function in the presence of high doses of azathioprine will have potentially lethal complications. The major complications all relate to a relative inability to respond effectively to a large variety of pathogenic, and even to normally saprophytic, organisms. There may be, moreover, a decrease in the normal capacity to destroy mutant, potentially neoplastic cells.

PARAMETERS OF IMMUNOSUPPRESSION. Can immunosuppression be measured in any other way than by graft function? All methods of clinical immunologic monitoring are restricted to measuring the specific or nonspecific responses of peripheral blood lymphocytes—the spleen, thymus, and lymph nodes not being readily available. With this restriction in mind, an immunosuppressive effect can be detected during the first 2 weeks after kidney transplantation. The response of the patient's circulating lymphocyte to either the mitogen phytohemagglutinin (PHA) or to foreign leukocytes is depressed. In recipients of ALG, azathioprine, and prednisone, the loss of reactivity is proportional to the decrease in number of circulating T cells. The T-cell number in cyclosporine recipients is not diminished, but there may be some alteration in the relative proportions of helper and suppressor T cells. In some recipients of long-surviving grafts, peripheral blood lymphocytes may not respond to graft antigens in vitro. There is no other reliable way to monitor the level of immunosuppression achieved. Nor is it possible to predict incipient rejection accurately. Because the degree of immunosuppression cannot yet be measured, the dosages of immunosuppressive agents are regulated instead by toxicity produced.

BACTERIAL AND FUNGAL INFECTION. Immunosuppression understandably increases the risk of infection. The routine posttransplant immunosuppression regimen does not necessarily result in a higher bacterial infection rate. With suitable aseptic precautions and antibiotic perioperative prophylaxis, the postoperative wound infection incidence is very low. When there are no severe rejection reactions and the graft maintains good function, the day-to-day bacterial challenge to the recipient is handled. Although urinary tract infections are frequent, they are usually mild and easily controlled by antibiotics.

We do not mean to imply that bacterial infection is an insignificant problem for transplantation patients. On the contrary, infection is still the most common complication of immunosuppression, and overall it is the most common cause of death in transplant recipients (Fig. 10-21). Infections are the natural consequence of impaired healing of visceral anastomoses after renal, liver, or pancreatic transplantation. Increasing experience has reduced the incidence of perigraft infections, however, and the most common infections are now caused by organisms that are normally weakly pathogenic. Antibiotics will eradicate the more aggressive bacteria, but they leave opportunistic organisms free to colonize the susceptible transplant patient. The opportunistic organisms, which are normally eliminated by cellular mechanisms, can now blossom in the face of the relative T-cell depression. Fungi are prominent opportunists, and they can cause cutaneous, mucosal, pulmonary, and central nervous system infections, as well as generalized sepsis. *Candida* infections are probably the most common. The inevitable mucosal candidiasis can be satisfactorily prevented by oral mycostatin.

Aspergillus species are probably the second most common cause of fungal infection and typically produce upper lobe pulmonary cavities and brain abscesses. There have been many reports of hospital epidemics traceable to con-

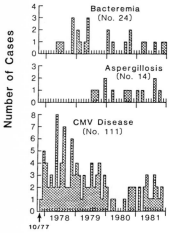

Fig. 10-21. Incidence of infections in 535 consecutive transplants performed between October 1977 and September 1981, at the University of Minnesota hospital, and followed until January 1982. The incidence varied widely, even though the rate of transplantation was the same, i.e., 10 to 15 transplants per month. The reasons for this variation are not clear. (From: *Peterson PK, Ferguson R, et al: Infectious diseases in hospitalized renal transplant recipients: A prospective study of a complex and evolving problem. Medicine, 61:360, 1982, with permission.*)

struction or ventilation problems. *Rhizopus oryzae, Histoplasma capsulatum,* and *Cryptococcus neoformans* also invade the lung, and the latter is the most common cause of meningitis. The indolent bacterium *Nocardia asteroides* occasionally infects, producing nodular pulmonary lesions. The protozoan *Pneumocystis carinii,* more commonly seen in patients undergoing cancer chemotherapy, usually causes a diffuse alveolar infiltrate.

Standard patient isolation precautions are of little use against these organisms, and prophylactic antibiotics are not available for most of them. Prevention is dependent upon avoiding excessive dosages of immunosuppressive agents in a futile attempt to prolong the function of a rejected graft. Some protection against *P. carinii, Nocardia,* the pneumococcus, *Listeria, Legionella,* and other susceptible organisms may be provided by the prophylactic trimethoprim and sulfamethoxazole. The pneumococcal vaccine may ultimately be useful.

VIRAL INFECTIONS. Viral infections seem to be almost ubiquitous among kidney transplant recipients. The herpes group of DNA viruses are most common etiologic agents. Infection or antibody response to cytomegalovirus (CMV) is found in 50 to 90 percent of patients after renal transplantation (Fig. 10-21). Herpes simplex infection occurs in about 25 percent and zoster in 10 percent of graft recipients; both can be prevented or treated with the antiviral agent acyclovir. Epstein–Barr virus (EBV) commonly infects transplant patients, but most infections are mild. EBV is associated with posttransplant malignancy in rare patients, however.

Antigenic evidence for hepatitis B virus infection can be detected in many transplant patients and non-A, non-B hepatitis is probably a cause of liver failure in some long-term survivors. Immunosuppressed patients have both typical and atypical patterns of infection. Hepatitis is particularly illustrative. Transplantation and hemodialysis patients may have no symptoms of acute hepatitis, but antibody responses and viral elimination are unusual. For this reason, persistent active hepatitis is a common finding in long-term survivors and a common underlying cause of death years after the transplant.

Cytomegalovirus (CMV) is the most important infectious illness that afflicts immunosuppressed transplant patients. CMV infection can produce a spectrum of illness typically characterized by fever, neutropenia, arthralgias, malaise, myocarditis, pancreatitis, or gastrointestinal ulceration. The most severe illnesses are acquired as primary infections from latent virus residing in the grafted tissue. Less often blood transfusions are the vector. Some cases of apparently new infection represent reactivation of latent intracellular viruses. Transplant recipients who do not have antibodies to CMV and who receive grafts from donors who do are at highest risk. The use of antilymphocyte antibody preparations for immunosuppression increases the risk. Recipients of cyclosporine appear to be at lower risk.

The typical CMV infection is a mild febrile illness, followed by an antibody response and regression of viral symptoms. A rejection episode sometimes accompanies the viral infection and raises the controversy of whether the virus triggers the rejection episode. These patients usually recover but may continue to excrete CMV in urine or saliva despite the presence of antibodies to CMV. In certain patients, however, there is no effective immune response, and the infection can be lethal. The virus itself induces a profound state of immunosuppression rendering these patients exquisitely susceptible to bacterial or fungal opportunists. Many serious infections are superinfections in patients already suffering CMV infections.

PREVENTION OF INFECTION. The incidence of severe, near-fatal infections has been reduced through a number of precautions. (1) The most important precaution is to eliminate all sources of infection prior to transplantation, especially those in the urinary tract and dialysis access site. Other sources of infection should be sought by routine preoperative cultures and careful examination. If any source is found, it should be eliminated by the appropriate use of surgical drainage or antibiotic therapy. (2) When technical problems are avoided, wound sepsis is uncommon. Urinary, biliary, or pancreatic anastomotic breakdown especially predisposes to wound infection. (3) Organs from related and well-matched cadavers elicit less frequent and less vigorous rejection reactions. If repeated rejection can be avoided, the doses of immunosuppressive drugs can be minimized and the rate and severity of infection will diminish. (4) Many patients who die of infection develop leukopenia (especially neutropenia) at some time. Some bouts of leukopenia can be attributed to cytomegalovirus infections. Leukopenia can be prevented by careful reduction in azathioprine doses when the leukocyte count or platelet count falls. The use of other bone marrow depressants (chloramphenicol) should be avoided in patients already on azathioprine therapy. Cyclosporine A is not myelosuppressive and should reduce the incidence of neutropenia. (5) Protective isolation protocols were formerly used to minimize infections in the initial postoperative care. Most transplant units have discontinued their use because they restrict access to the patients, impose psychologic stress, and are probably ineffective against viral, fungal, or endogenous bacteria.

MALIGNANCY. Cancer has been an unexpectedly frequent companion of clinical transplantation. The incidence of cancer is not high enough, however, to contraindicate the transplant procedure. Tumors in transplant recipients have come from two general sources. A rare cause is the inadvertent transplantation of a cancer from a cadaver donor in whom the cancer was unsuspected. These tumors can sometimes be treated simply by halting immunosuppression therapy and allowing rejection of the tumor tissue, as well as the transplant, to occur.

The more common cancers are the primary tumors that appear in the immunosuppressed recipient. Only certain tumors grow more readily in immunodepressed patients. Seventy-five percent of the spontaneous cancers are either epithelial or lymphoid in origin. Carcinoma in situ of the cervix, carcinoma of the lip, and squamous or basal cell carcinomas of the skin account for about half of this group, while B-cell lymphomas make up the remainder. It has been estimated that the risks to the transplant recipient of developing cervical cancer, skin cancer, or lymphoma are increased by 4, 40, and 350 times, respectively. The lymphomas are unusual both in their frequency and in their behavior. Almost 50 percent of the immunosuppressed patients with lymphomas have brain involvement, which occurs in only 1 percent of nontransplanted related cases of lymphoma. These lymphomas, although initially responsive to radiation therapy, are usually fatal.

Recent evidence suggests that all lymphomas are not true neoplasms. Immunologic analysis has indicated that these tumors secrete several different types of immunoglobulins, i.e., they do not have the monoclonal characteristics of cancer. Most evidence suggests that some may represent uncontrolled B-cell proliferative responses to EBV. At this stage, antiviral chemotherapy with acyclovir appears promising. Subsequently true lymphoid neoplasms seem to evolve from chromosomal abnormalities; such true monoclonal malignancies have not responded well to conventional cancer chemotherapy.

We do not know why transplant patients have an increased risk for these cancers. It has been postulated that the surveillance and elimination of tumor cells as they arise by lymphocytes is an important natural defense of human beings against cancer. Certainly this function might be abnormal in immunodepressed patients. Another possibility is the use of mutagens like azathioprine as immunosuppressive drugs. There is also growing evidence that herpes viruses, to which the immunosuppressed patient is manifestly susceptible, can induce these neoplasms. EBV is almost certainly the cause of the polyclonal B-cell lymphoproliferative disorder that evolves into a monoclonal lymphoma. All these lesions contain the EBV genome as part of the cellular DNA.

Less certain is the possibility that cancers of the epithelium may be a consequence of herpes virus transformation. This group of viruses is carcinogenic in animals and infects epithelial cells of lip, skin, and genital tissue. Circumstantial evidence exists for a role in human cervical cancer. Herpes viruses are usually dormant, but the stress of transplantation or the action of antimetabolite may activate them. The viruses might then either proliferate and cause a clinical viral illness or produce cellular transformation into cancer cells. Similarly, the Papova viruses are probably the cause of skin cancer in immunosuppressed patients.

CUSHING'S DISEASE. Most transplant patients who receive steroid therapy develop Cushing's syndrome. The appearance of the face is altered by rounding, puffiness, and plethora; fat tends to be redistributed from the extremities to the trunk and face. There is also an increased growth of fine hair over the thighs and trunk and sometimes over the face. Acne may appear or increase, and insomnia and increased appetite are noted. The underlying metabolic changes can be even more serious: The continuing breakdown of protein and diversion of amino acids to glucose increase the need for insulin and result in weight gain, fat deposition, muscle wasting, thinning of the skin with striae, and sometimes the development of steroid diabetes, cataracts, and osteoporosis. In some patients a myopathy develops, the nature of which is unknown. The cushingoid changes may represent such a problem that transplant nephrectomy will be necessary on that basis alone.

GASTROINTESTINAL BLEEDING. Gastrointestinal bleeding due to reactivation of a preexisting ulcer or diffuse ulceration of the gastrointestinal tract can be a fatal complication. The relative pathogenetic contribution of progressive uremia and steroid administration is unknown, but when bleeding appears, it can be difficult to control by nonoperative means. Occasionally the use of cimetidine or the intramesenteric arterial infusion of vasopressin is effective.

During moderate doses of steroid therapy, episodes of gastrointestinal bleeding can be almost totally prevented by the use of antacids between meals. In patients with rejection who require high steroid dosage, antacid therapy must be intensified with each increase in steroid administration. Pretransplant antiulcer operations have been used in patients with peptic disease.

OTHER INTESTINAL COMPLICATIONS. A number of colonic complications, including diverticulitis, bleeding, and ulceration, are associated with immunosuppressive treatment. A syndrome of acute cecal ulceration with gastrointestinal bleeding is due to cytomegalovirus. Cytomegalovirus underlies sporadic ulcer disease in other enteric locations as well.

CATARACTS. Cataracts are common in patients who require steroids. The cataracts, which develop slowly, appear to be independent of the absolute prednisone dosage.

THROMBOSIS AND THROMBOEMBOLIC PHENOMENA. Thrombophlebitis may occur in the renal transplant recipient, particularly on the side of the graft where the venous anastomosis may become partially or completely thrombosed. The diagnosis is difficult because swelling of the leg on the side of the transplant site is an occasional sign of rejection, associated with increases in weight, pulmonary infiltrates, and slight increases in serum creatinine level. When the differential diagnosis is difficult, a femoral venogram is indicated. The diagnosis of pulmonary embolism may also be difficult because clinical thrombophlebitis seldom precedes the embolus.

HYPERTENSION. Many of the patients who come to renal transplantation are already hypertensive. Hypertension can usually be controlled with dialysis or, in rare refractory cases, with nephrectomy. Hypertension in most patients will develop soon after transplantation, but posttransplant hypertension can be easily controlled with dietary salt restriction and drugs. The hypertension seems to be due not only to prednisone but also to failure to regulate the normal salt and water balance in the early posttransplant period and secretion of renin by the kidney. Hypertension may be aggravated by rejection. It should be remembered, however, that significant hypertension may be due to renal arterial stenosis, and arteriography may be necessary for the differentiation.

DISORDERS OF CALCIUM METABOLISM. Patients frequently come to renal transplantation with renal osteodystrophy. Alterations in vitamin D metabolism and secondary hyperparathyroidism are prominent factors in the pathogenesis of skeletal disease. Long-standing acidosis may likewise be contributory. The resulting osteoporosis, osteomalacia, and osteitis fibrosa cystica in the child can lead to growth restriction, epiphysiolysis, skeletal deformities, and pathologic fractures. The bone disease in some cases can be arrested with pharmacologic dosages of vitamin D or aluminum hydroxide.

Hemodialysis can correct the uremic state, but the bone disease may actually progress if the stimulus to parathyroid hormone secretion is not effectively eliminated. Great attention should be directed toward keeping the dialysate calcium concentration at a level (6 to 7 mg/dL) that does not promote calcium loss from the blood. Parathyroidectomy is sometimes required to help arrest progressive bone disease but is not indicated for hypercalcemia alone after transplant. Parathyroidectomy seems primarily indicated for patients on chronic hemodialysis in whom transplantation is not planned.

MUSCULOSKELETAL COMPLICATIONS. A disturbing complication of successful renal transplantation is avascular necrosis of the femoral heads and other bones. Its occurrence is most closely correlated with the dosage of steroid used. Transient rheumatoid symptoms precede changes visible by radiography by several months. The bone changes apparently occur secondarily to steroid osteopenia or osteonecrosis with resulting microfractures. Alterations in lipid metabolism caused by fluctuating high levels of steroids likewise appear to be important in the pathogenesis. The treatment is for the most part symptomatic. It is doubtful that bone lesions can revascularize sufficiently to restore normal architecture in the presence of maintenance steroids. Should symptoms increase, replacement arthroplasty is usually successful.

Migratory arthralgia, myalgia, and tendonitis are common, but persistent joint pain and swelling are most often signs of intraarticular infection. Occasionally, an unexplained septic arthritis crops up in these patients; mycobacterial infections are most commonly reported.

PANCREATITIS. Pancreatitis may appear suddenly and unexpectedly in renal allograft recipients, and recurrent bouts may prove to be fatal. It has been attributed variously to corticosteroid therapy, azathioprine, cytomegalovirus, or hepatitis virus. Steroids are known to thicken pancreatic secretions.

ERYTHREMIA AND ANEMIA. The transplanted kidney is apparently fully capable of manufacturing erythropoietin. During rejection, the serum level may be increased. Erythremia also may appear, but apparently it is not related to elevated erythropoietin levels. Phlebotomy has been advised for hemoglobin levels greater than 16 g/dL.

Anemia usually is not present except in association with uremia or immunodepression secondary to azathioprine toxicity. A microangiopathic hemolytic anemia has also been thought to be induced by the vascular changes within the chronically rejecting kidney.

GROWTH. Since chronic renal failure itself is inhibitory to development, uremic children are usually far behind their peers in size. After successful transplantation their growth response is highly variable and may depend on age, previous growth rate, renal function, and immunosuppressive drug regimen. Many children return to a normal growth rate; unfortunately the growth that was lost during their original illness is not made up, so these children will always be smaller than their peers.

PREGNANCY. Many normal children have been born to renal transplanted women despite their use of mutagenic immunosuppressive drugs. The pregnancies of renal transplanted recipients are frequently complicated, however, by toxemia and bacterial and viral infections, particularly of the urinary tract. Both toxemia and infection may contribute to a higher incidence of premature labor and small neonates. Another important problem that must be faced is the decreased life expectancy of the transplant recipient. Parenthood is a long-term obligation, and counseling of these patients should include a discussion of these considerations.

CLINICAL TISSUE AND TRANSPLANTATION

Clinical allotransplants may be of several types: (1) temporary free grafts, such as skin allografts and blood transfusions; (2) partially inert struts that provide a framework for the ingrowth of host tissue, such as bone, cartilage, nerve, tendon, and fascial grafts; (3) permanent, partially privileged, structurally free grafts, such as cornea, blood vessels, and heart valves; (4) partially privileged functional free grafts such as parathyroid, ovary, and testes; (5) whole organ grafts, such as pancreas, kidney, liver, lung, and heart; and (6) bone marrow that acts as a functional replacement of the entire hemopoietic and lymphopoietic systems. Immunosuppression is warranted only for grafts essential for life. Tooth bud and thyroid grafts, which would require immunosuppression for any success, are trivial grafts and are easily replaced by prostheses or medication.

Clinical autotransplants have been carried out with hair, skin, teeth, kidney, legs, arms, veins, arteries, pericardium, valves, bone, cartilage, fascia, fat, tendons, nerves, stomach, bowel, parathyroid, thyroid, ovary, testis, adrenal, and hemopoietic tissue. Allotransplants have been carried out employing cornea, teeth, thyroid, parathyroid, adrenal, ovary, testis, pituitary, spleen, lymph node, bone marrow, skin, bone, cartilage, fascia, tendons, nerves, arteries, valves, veins, hemopoietic tissue, pancreas, duodenum, intestine, kidney, liver, lung, and heart. Xenografts of skin, heart valves, heart, kidney, testis, bone, and cartilage have been tried in the past.

Skin

Autotransplants of skin containing hair are used to reconstruct eyebrows or to replace the scalp after traumatic avulsion. Autotransplants of individual hair roots are sometimes used as a treatment for baldness. Skin autotransplants have been used to reconstruct the esophagus, urinary tract, vagina, and hernial weaknesses as well as the usual surface defects. The main use of skin autografts is to cover and replace areas destroyed by trauma, burn, or operation.

Skin allotransplants are also used quite extensively in burned patients when autochthonous skin is not available. The theory behind this is that the skin allograft provides a better coverage than any other material, and during the period of time when it is taking, it prevents the continued spread of sepsis. Skin allografts are commonly used in three different ways: In the first they are applied as a dressing to the freshly excised burned area and are removed after 10 to 14 days. At this time additional allografts are reapplied if the area does not appear to be clean enough to accept autografts. The second method is to place pinch grafts of autografted skin within defects created in a sheet allograft covering large defects. As the allografted skin is gradually rejected, it is replaced by epithelial cells that grow in from the autografts. In a modification of these techniques widely meshed autografts are covered with a sheet allograft to protect both the ungrafted areas and the fragile autograft. The allografts are eventually lifted off by the regenerating autograft.

Xenografts of skin are commonly used as temporary biologic dressings and are replaced at 1- to 5-day intervals. Fresh porcine skin is more physiologic and bacteriostatic but should be removed before it becomes vascularized. Commercial preparations of porcine skin are nonviable and do not become vascularized. A vast array of synthetic substitutes as well as animal collagenous materials are being developed, but their value must be compared with the present optimum temporary dressing, allograft.

Vascular Grafts

AUTOGRAFTS

Vein autografts have been used for over 50 years to replace segments of damaged arteries. This is still the best bypass graft for occluded vessels in the lower extremity.

After a period of time in the arterial circuit the vein wall thickens, and the vein becomes somewhat arterialized. Although there are occasional instances in which vein grafts weaken and rupture, by and large they make very satisfactory arterial substitutes. The two most common usages at the present time are in femoropopliteal artery–saphenous vein bypass grafts and coronary artery bypass grafts. Pieces of autologous vein are also used as patch grafts. It is possible too to carry out successful autologous vein grafts to bridge defects in veins, although veins are less likely to stay open than arteries.

Autografted arteries are also sometimes used as vascular replacements; most often the hypogastric artery is utilized. Pieces of pericardium are sometimes used to patch defects or divert flow in the repair of intracardiac defects.

ALLOGRAFTS

Allografted arteries are seldom used now. There are three reasons for this: (1) aneurysms sometimes occur, with rupture and a fatal outcome; (2) plastic prostheses have proved so suitable for the larger blood vessels; (3) for smaller blood vessels the use of the autologous saphenous vein has proved to be better than either prostheses or allografts. Arterial allografts, even if viable, do not survive but in part are replaced by host tissue and in part persist as semi-inert material.

When organs are transplanted, the artery supplying the organ becomes an arterial allograft. It has been shown that the epithelium of smaller blood vessels is antigenic and some degree of allograft rejection occurs.

Fresh, sterile aortic valve allografts have been used quite extensively. They appear to elicit a minimal antigenic response when compared with arterial allografts. Even so, gradual thickening, immobility, and calcification of these valves occur; their functional life expectancy is short. Preserved porcine valve xenografts are more useful, but loss of mobility sometimes indicates their replacement.

Vein allografts have been used for a number of years in sporadic fashion, and umbilical vein allografts have become commercially available for arterial bypass. Allografts have always been inferior to fresh autografts because of the rejection reaction that these grafts elicit. For some reason there has been a great reluctance among surgeons and others to accept the fact that arterial and venous allografts are antigenic. It is true that the antigenicity is relatively mild and that the graft can provide structural function even in the face of the immunologic response, but it eventually limits the life of the graft.

Fascia

Fascial autografts, either free or attached at one end, are used as living sutures for the repair of inguinal hernias; for the repair of chest wall defects, torn ligaments and tendons, abdominal wall hernias, and defects in the pleura, dura, diaphragm, trachea, and esophagus; for wrapping aneurysms; in arthroplasty; for fascial slings to correct paralysis of the facial muscles; in the stabilization of fractures and joints; in the construction of flexor sheaths; and to correct urinary incontinence. Fascial autografts have been used most commonly because of their convenience and ready availability. Some freeze-dried, preserved (nonviable) allografts have been used, however, and these dead grafts have united with muscle nearly as quickly as living fascia. Such allografts lose much of their histoincompatibility and serve as strong lattice for the ingrowth of autologous tissue.

Tendon

Free tendon autografts are used every day in standard surgical procedures. By far the most common use is that of repairing severed flexor tendons to the fingers. Usually the palmaris longus, plantaris, or extensor tendons of the toes are used, and the graft is inserted from the level of the midpalm of the hand to the distal phalanx. Tendon allografts are rarely of clinical use.

Nerve

Nerve autotransplants are used to bridge defects in important motor nerves or sometimes to transfer the function of one nerve into the distal end of another, to repair a severed facial or recurrent laryngeal nerve, for instance. The autografts undergo Wallerian degeneration with proliferation of Schwann cells and are penetrated by regenerating fibers of the host's nerve after a few weeks. When the nerve graft is thick, the center of the graft may develop a zone of avascular necrosis through which regeneration fails to occur. This does not happen with thin grafts. As a consequence of this, some investigators have advocated the use of cable grafts consisting of several strands of smaller nerves to bridge defects in nerves of larger caliber. Experimental work is being done to evaluate the function of vascularized nerve grafts transferred with microsurgical techniques. Motor recovery can occur as well as sensory recovery.

When allografts are used, the rate and intensity of nerve fiber penetration are less, and the outcome is far inferior to that obtained with autografts. In general they should probably be used only when autografts cannot be obtained. Xenografts have been tried but appear to be of no value to human beings. It is likely that the inflammatory rejection response interferes with the passage of autologous nerve endings down the transplanted nerve sheath.

Cornea

Perhaps the most common clinical allotransplant is that of the cornea. The eye should be harvested from cadavers within 6 h after death. Eyes removed more than 36 h after death are unsuitable for corneal transplantation. The whole eye is generally preserved in a sterile container at a temperature of 3 to 5°C, and the graft is cut from it at the time of use. The eye is suspended from a suture passed through the severed optic nerve to keep it from coming in contact with the sides of the vessel. Eye banks store the cornea in nutrient media at 4 or 34°C as long as 1 month.

Two types of corneal transplants are utilized: the full-thickness graft and the lamellar, or partial-thickness, graft. The full-thickness graft gives the best results, but infrequently complications such as secondary glaucoma, anterior synechiae, and a partial lifting off of the graft, causing astigmatism or opacification, occur. These complications are avoided in lamellar keratoplasty, which is the operation of choice when the corneal opacity does not involve the full thickness of the cornea. In order to achieve a successful graft there must be good apposition between the graft and the host, the graft must be in contact with healthy cornea at some point in the circumference if it is to remain transparent, and blood vessels must not invade the graft to any appreciable extent.

The best patients for grafting are those with central corneal scars and healthy surrounding cornea with no vascularization, keratoconus, especially if the apex of the cone is beginning to break down, and corneal dystrophy. Indolent corneal abscesses, perforating ulcers of the cornea, and descemetocele have less positive outcomes. The results are also somewhat less good in acne rosacea and herpetic keratitis because of the danger of recurrence of the disease.

Corneal grafts are apparently so successful because they remain effectively isolated from the host's cells so long as the graft itself and the cornea directly around it remain avascular. Systemic immunosuppression is used only on rare occasions. Many corneal grafts remain clear indefinitely, although occasionally a graft that has remained clear for several weeks becomes opaque. Apparently the fibrous barrier that is formed at the junction between the host and the graft is almost impervious to blood vessels and helps to maintain the isolation of the graft even when vessels have entered the host's cornea. The clouding over of a previously clear graft is due to the allograft reaction, usually because of vascularization.

Bone

Bone implants are used for the following indications: (1) to hasten the healing of defects and cavities, e.g., the use of cancellous bone chips in the residual defect after curettage of a unicameral bone cyst; (2) to supplement bony union in cases of delayed healing or pseudarthrosis arising after fracture, e.g., sliding or barrel stave grafts for nonunion of tibial shaft fractures, or to supplement the healing of certain fresh acquired or surgical fractures where skeletal continuity is problematic, e.g., cancellous autogenous implants for fractures of both bones of the forearm in an adult, (3) to reconstruct contour or major skeletal defects arising as a result of surgery trauma, disease, or congenital malformation, e.g., replacement of calvarial defects after surgery for trauma by compact bone implants.

Bone grafts are used to provide one or more of the following: (1) a source of viable osteoblasts (bone production); (2) a source of replacement for lost skeletal architecture (bone conduction); or (3) new bone formation (bone induction). Autografts of cancellous bone may provide all three: a source of living bone cells when harvested in thin strips where diffusion will provide cell nourishment, conduction of new bone formation along the cancellous surfaces, and bone induction from the matrix component diffusion that induces the differentiation of mesenchymal cells to form new bone. Autografts of cortical bone, such as fibular struts, may provide some small amount of living cells but primarily serve to reconstruct skeletal defects without the problems of antigenicity encountered in allografts. Allografts are generally reserved for large defects that cannot be filled or bridged by autografts without major disability at the donor site. Allografts will only provide for conduction and induction of a new bone. Combinations of autogenous cancellous grafts with cortical autografts or allografts are frequently used to hasten incorporation of these grafts to the recipient sites.

A variety of grafting techniques have been devised to meet the differing clinical requirements. The most frequent types of bone grafts are autogenous grafts with or without internal fixation. These may be applied as barrel stave grafts, sliding grafts, or cancellous chips. In addition, there are vascularized pedicle grafts of two types, those with a bony base, and muscle pedicle grafts. Microvascular anastomosis to provide free viable bone grafts or composite bone and soft tissue grafts has been useful in major defects of the limbs from trauma or neoplasia. Similarly, in some locations, vascularized grafts may be mobilized and rotated on their vascular pedicle to provide a viable graft without the requirement of anastomosis.

Autografts are preferred for clinical use, since the cellular elements of bone allografts usually elicit a rejection response. Bone allografts do elicit new bone formation (osteoinduction) and serve as struts for the ingrowth of autologous bone (osteoconduction). When properly prepared, the immune response to the allograft can be substantially reduced. As such, allografts are of great clinical use.

For the most part stored or processed bone allografts are used in clinical situations. Preservation methods include (1) refrigeration, (2) freezing, (3) freeze-drying, (4) decalcification, or (5) any one of the above plus irradiation for sterilization. Such nonviable grafts mainly serve to stimulate and conduct new autologous bone formation.

Cartilage

It has been long known that cartilage can be successfully transferred between individuals of different genetic backgrounds without the need for immunosuppression therapy. This immunologic privilege is attributable in adult articular cartilage to the absence of a blood supply. Under normal circumstances the fluid-nutritional needs are met via the synovial fluid. Thus, the absence of direct vascular contact and the presence of a dense proteoglycan-collagen matrix will insulate the chondrocytes from the host immune response.

Free autografts of cartilage have been used most extensively in plastic reconstructive surgery (1) to rebuild the contours of the nose after congenital or posttraumatic deformity, (2) to reconstruct the pinna, and (3) to fill out defects in the facial bones and the skull.

The fresh cartilage autograft comes closest to fulfilling the description of an ideal cartilage graft: it should maintain its structure, have the potential for growth and repair, provoke no untoward reaction, and form a firm union with host tissues, persisting without loss of viability or absorption. Recent experimental and clinical application of rib perichondrial grafts as a source of new cartilage growth remains promising as an autograft technique for small joints.

The fresh cartilage allograft, however, has been reported to be a reasonable substitute for the autograft in particular circumstances because of its greater ease of procurement. The major drawback of such grafts is that despite the immunologic privilege of cartilage, the bulk of experimental and clinical evidence suggests that the tendency for late deterioration and absorption is somewhat greater than that of autografts. Furthermore, the potential for infection or transmission of viral-induced disease is similar to other living tissue transplants that are not proved sterile by culture or donor serology.

The preserved cartilaginous allograft has been used as a substitute for the fresh implant primarily because of the convenience that storage of such implants in cartilage banks provides. Refrigerated and chemically preserved frozen sections of cartilage have all been used with variable success.

COMPOSITE GRAFTS OF BONE AND CARTILAGE

Composite grafts involve the surgical transfer of entire functional units rather than the implantation of bits and pieces of cartilage or bone.

EPIPHYSEAL GROWTH PLATES. The object of the transplantation of epiphyseal growth plates is to restore longitudinal growth in hypoplastic limbs, whether congenital or acquired. This type of procedure has been used in efforts to improve the function of children with congenital deficiency of the radius. In these cases, autotransplantation of the proximal fibula has been used as a substitute for the radial deficiency. Although, in some cases, enlargement of the transplant could be demonstrated, this was always inferior to the natural growth potential and has not been sufficient to justify incorporation of this procedure into the surgical armamentarium. Microvascular transfer of epiphyseal growth plates shows continued growth and hypertrophy. This technique is now under clinical trial for restoring growth in damaged limbs.

OSTEOCHONDRAL GRAFTS. The diseases that destroy the articular cartilage are common. The osteochondral or osteoarticular graft might be a useful substitute. Transplants of articular cartilage, in conjunction with a very thin shell of subchondral supporting bone, are still in the experimental stage. Both allogenic and autogenous composites are now being applied in clinical trials in selected centers.

TRANSPLANT OF HEMIJOINTS OR WHOLE JOINTS. The experimental transplantation of joints was initiated by Judet in 1908. Autografts tend to heal their osteosynthesis sites, revascularize the bony component, and in general maintain the articular surfaces in a fair state of preservation. On the other hand, both fresh and preserved allogenic transplants give unpredictable results, sometimes healing well with good function, and other times showing progressive deterioration. The latter changes in the allogeneic groups are associated with delayed revascularization of the bony component, subchondral fracture and collapse, and synovial invasion of the joint surfaces. (Animal work suggests that immunosuppressive techniques can abort this phenomenon.) Artificial hemijoints or whole joints have superseded transplantation, at least for the present, but are more commonly used as composite replacements in major segmental defects. These composites generally use an allogeneic bone segment with an artificial joint implant to allow soft tissue reattachment around the joint for better function; host tendons and ligaments will generally reattach to the allograft and do not grow into a metal implant.

Extremity Replantation

Autotransplants or replantation of extremities have been carried out with increasing frequency in recent years. These procedures have usually involved the upper extremity, because the chances for good functional recovery are far greater in the arm than in the leg. Excellent prostheses exist for the lower extremity, but they are much less satisfactory for the upper. The major advantage of replantation is the development of useful sensation in the replanted extremity.

Shortening of the reimplanted extremity usually is necessary, and this produces much more incapacity in the leg than in the arm. Replantation of the leg might be considered when the opposite leg has been extensively damaged or lost or when the amputation has been so high that good prostheses are not available. Advances in microsurgery have made replantation of digits routine for the experienced microsurgeon.

The technique of limb replantation initially requires a general evaluation of the patient to assess other associated injuries. This should include radiography of the proximal stump as well as the amputated extremity itself, and particularly of the spine to be certain that the spinal roots to the extremity have not been avulsed. After securing hemostasis with pressure and being certain that no serious injury has been overlooked, the replantation can begin. During this initial phase the severed limb should be placed in a plastic container and packed in ice. The extremity should not be frozen, however, and for that reason, dry ice should be avoided. The limb may be replanted even though several hours have elapsed between its severance and the start of replantation. The exact critical period of ischemia has not definitely been established, but it appears that at least 12 h for a limb and up to 36 h for a finger can elapse with successful results after replantation. The more distal the amputation, the less ischemia-sensitive muscle tissue is in the extremity and prolonged cold ischemia is tolerated.

Prior to replantation a thorough debridement of grossly devitalized tissue is carried out. The bone is fixed first so that the limb will be stabilized before beginning the repairs of the vessels and nerve supply. Bones may require slight shortening to freshen up the ends and to gain additional length for relaxation of the arteries and nerves, and closure of soft tissue. Intramedullary fixation is used whenever possible.

After proper fixation of the bones, and repair of the tendons, the blood vessels are joined. In a distal amputation, a microsurgical team is required. The precise sequence of repair varies from surgeon to surgeon, but often the largest vein is joined first, so that there will be outflow available at the moment when the blood is ready to flow through the artery. It is important to join normal vessels beyond the zone of injury using vein grafts as necessary. If a nerve gap exists, nerve repair is delayed until healing is complete and a nerve graft can be done. If the nerve has been cleanly severed, immediate primary repair is carried out. A better result is obtained in distal nerve transections than in proximal ones, and in young people as compared with older ones. Distal sensory nerves give the most favorable results. Motor recovery in the median nerve is much more successful than in the ulnar nerve.

After completing the arterial and venous anastomoses and after either joining the ends of the nerves or deciding to perform a nerve graft as a secondary procedure, attention is turned to the soft tissues. With the blood supply restored, viability of tissues is easier to ascertain, and debridement can be completed. The shortening of the bone makes it possible to join several muscles together with a view to covering the blood vessels with living tissues. If soft tissue loss is minimal, the coverage can be achieved with the skin of the extremity, and other defects can be covered with split-thickness skin grafts. If the soft tissue defect is great and no covering is available, the defect must be covered by a pedicle flap. The newer microsurgical techniques permit the use of free revascularized myocutaneous flaps, usually as a secondary procedure.

In the postoperative period the patient's limb must be kept in an elevated position to minimize edema. It is important to do a fasciotomy, including carpel tunnel release, at the end of the replantation to avoid compartment swelling from ischemic damage to the arm musculature. Heparin and dextran are not generally used postoperatively. Some degree of hypotension may occur as a consequence of leakage of plasma into the replanted extremity and acute blood loss. This is particularly true of proximal extremity injuries. The hypotension is counteracted by the administration of plasma.

In a major limb amputation there is a period of acute acidosis as a consequence of absorption of metabolic products from the ischemic extremity and venous return begins. This acidosis is aggressively treated with the administration of bicarbonate. Both bicarbonate and mannitol are administered to protect against myoglobin renal damage and prophylactic antibiotics are also administered. If early severe sepsis supervenes, the extremity may have to be amputated. Low-grade late infection, usually consisting of osteomyelitis, is treated by drainage and irrigation. The fixation materials are left in place until the bone heals, even in the face of sepsis—because fixation must be achieved if possible.

Passive movement of all joints is begun immediately and continued throughout the course of treatment. Galvanic stimulation of the intrinsic muscles of the hand or foot can be utilized to maintain the tone of muscles. Extensive physical therapy is instituted as soon as wound healing is complete. If primary nerve suture has not been carried out, the nerves are reexplored 6 weeks or more after the injury, and grafting is carried out then. The long-term functional results have been good.

Muscle and Musculocutaneous Grafts

Occasionally, following a severe trauma or extirpative surgery, vital structures such as brain, bone periosteum, tendon, nerve, and major vascular structures become exposed in a wound. Such wounds require full-thickness flap coverage to preserve the viability of these important structures and promote functional recovery. In situations where no local or regional flaps are available for transfer, autogenous muscle or musculocutaneous flaps must be grafted using microsurgical techniques. The most commonly used muscles and musculocutaneous flaps are the rectus abdominis perfused on the inferior epigastric arterial pedicle, and the latissimus dorsi, perfused by the thoracodorsal artery and vein. Microsurgical transfer of these muscles results in minimal donor site functional morbidity, and provides a large volume of tissue for reconstruction of the wound.

Following harvest, the muscles are revascularized using appropriate recipient vessels in the region of wound. Care must be taken to perform the microsurgical anastomosis outside the zone of injury so that normal vessels are used to revascularize the flap. Utilization of an end-to-side anastomosis has a theoretically increased patency rate and does not jeopardize distal perfusion of an already injured extremity. These free flap transfers are commonly done by organized microsurgical teams where technical skills are maintained by a high volume of replantation and reconstructive surgery.

Other free flaps are occasionally employed for specialized situations. The skin and soft tissue of dorsum of the foot, perfused by the dorsalis pedis artery and thin skin of the volar forearm perfused by the radial artery are occasionally used for reconstructions in the head, neck, and face where their thinness and malleability are an asset. The great toe or the second toe perfused on the dorsalis pedis axis can be transferred to reconstruct the thumb or hand where no digits are available for opposition. These transfers are extremely complex, and require reconnection of tendons, nerves, and bone, as well as successful microvascular anastomosis.

Microsurgical techniques have significantly increased the reconstructive surgeon's armamentarium. Using microsurgery, a wide variety of autogenous transplants are possible and can provide functioning tissue where it is needed. Successful methods of immunosuppression are being developed and will ultimately allow microsurgeons to transfer functioning heterografts for reconstructive purposes.

Hemopoietic and Lymphoid Tissues

BONE MARROW

Bone marrow is easily destroyed by whole-body ionizing irradiation, drugs, or chemicals. In contrast, the mature peripheral blood cells are in most instances not sensitive to injury by irradiation or by chemical substances, but these cells have a relatively short life span, and a regular supply of new cells is needed. In leukemia, the bone marrow is replaced by tumor cells, a situation effectively the same as that existing when marrow is destroyed by other means.

Injury to bone marrow by drugs, chemicals, and diseases poses several clinical problems. Bone marrow transplants between identical twins have been successfully carried out in many cases of irradiation exposure, aplastic anemia, and leukemia. Autologous marrow transplantation has also been found useful after planned treatment with toxic levels of alkylating agents.

Marrow allotransplants are far less successful. Marrow is highly immunogenic and will be readily rejected by the immunologically normal host. If, however, the marrow is allotransplanted into an immunologically crippled (irradiated, immunosuppressed) host, a chimera is produced. The problem then becomes, not destruction of the marrow by the host, but the maturation of donor marrow stem cells that results in total immunological competence and rejection of the host by the graft. This graft-versus-host (GVH) phenomenon is not seen with skin, kidney, heart, and liver grafts, but it is a major unsolved problem in the transplantation of foreign bone marrow, white blood cells, and lymphoid tissues. GVH disease does not occur in bone marrow transplants between identical human twins, and the GVH reaction is less severe if the donor and recipient are identical at the entire HLA locus.

The major sites of injury in GVH reactions are the lymphatic tissues, the skin, the intestine, and the liver of the host. Dermatitis, diarrhea, loss of weight, poor liver function, and infection associated with immunoincompetence are intrinsic parts of the reaction. The GVH reactions in bone marrow transplantation in human beings have been of overwhelming importance and are the major problem in this growing clinical area. Some of the experimental and clinical approaches to the problem of the control of GVH disease are listed in Table 10-4. A combination of tissue typing and immunologic suppression is now used to control the GVH reaction in human beings, but selective deletion from the transplanted marrow of T-cell precursors responsible for GVH may soon be practical. Monoclonal antibodies directed against potentially immunoreactive cells in the mixed population of bone marrow cells are promising.

A long-range goal in marrow transplantation is the use of these grafts as a means of promoting acceptance of other organs, such as liver, heart, and kidney. Once the

Table 10-4. SOME APPROACHES TO THE CONTROL OF GRAFT-VERSUS-HOST DISEASE

A. Immunologic compatibility:* histocompatibility typing and matching of donor and recipient
B. Immunologic suppression
  1. Treatment of marrow recipient
     a. Methotrexate*
     b. Cyclophosphamide*
     c. Antilymphocyte serum*
     d. Cyclosporine*
  2. Treatment of marrow donor: antilymphocyte serum
C. Removal of immunologically active cells
  1. Treatment of the marrow in vitro with ALG or monoclonal antibodies against selected T-cell subpopulations
  2. Cell separation.
D. Innate absence of immunocompetent cells; use of fetal and newborn blood-forming tissue as the donor source

* Currently in clinical use.

Table 10-5. INDICATIONS FOR PARATHYROID TRANSPLANTATION

1. Autotransplantation
   a. Severe secondary hyperparathyroidism
   b. Primary generalized parathyroid hyperplasia
   c. Inadvertent removal of parathyroid tissue
2. Allotransplantation
   a. Congenital absence of parathyroid glands—DiGeorge's syndrome
   b. Iatrogenic aparathyroidism that is not controllable with a medical regimen

foreign marrow is established, a state of relative or complete specific nonreactivity against donor antigens is conferred, and other tissues taken from the same donor as the marrow can be successfully transplanted without further immunosuppression.

In practice, human bone marrow allotransplantation has enjoyed increasing success. More than 2000 transplants are carried out yearly in the United States. HLA-identical marrow transplants (from matched siblings) are commonly used to treat aplastic anemias, combined immunodeficiency disease, and thalassemia major. The majority of patients enjoy long-term disease-free survival. Marrow transplantation is now used to treat other acquired and congenital disorders of hemapoietic stem cells and congenital enzymatic defects. Transplantation for leukemia is less successful. The best results are achieved in the treatment of chronic myelogenous leukemia in the chronic phase, and for acute nonlymphoblastic leukemia in first remission.

Aside from transplants between identical twins, transplantation with HLA-matched but nonidentical twin marrow is very successful with the best record of successful engraftment and the least severe GVH disease. The use of non-HLA-matched donors is far less successful. In these patients, marrow allotransplantation requires much larger doses of immunosuppressive cytotoxic drugs than those used to gain acceptance of kidney grafts. Furthermore, the GVH disease in these HLA-mismatched recipients has been difficult to control. Matching unrelated donors at the HLA locus is better than using mismatched relatives as donors.

THYMUS

The congenital absence of thymic tissue prevents the maturation of the entire T-cell system. Such patients are deficient in cell-mediated immune responses and those B-cell responses requiring T-cell interaction. Transplantation of an embryonic fresh or cultured thymus into such patients has resulted in considerable improvement in these normal defense mechanisms. The exact indications

and success rates have not been fully defined, but this is a promising field of investigation.

Endocrine Grafts (Other than the Pancreas)

The placement of endocrine fragments as autografts into intramuscular pockets has been successful in several clinical situations. The indications for parathyroid autotransplantation are listed in Table 10-5. When it appears possible that a patient may have insufficient parathyroid tissue following removal of the thyroid gland, or of all four parathyroid glands for chief cell hyperplasia, the glands should be diced and implanted into intramuscular pockets. The volar forearm muscle is a useful site for autotransplantation because the parathyroids are readily available for subsequent excision if hyperparathyroidism recurs. Their function can be easily assessed by hormone assay of antecubital vein blood.

Similar indications for other endocrine organs have been suggested. None of these indications has been well defined, however, because hormonal replacement (parathyroids excepted) is simpler. The prognosis for endocrine allotransplants is in doubt for the same reason. Replacement therapy for endocrine deficiency (aside from insulin deficiencies) is generally adequate, and there is seldom an indication for the use of systemic immunosuppressive drugs to eliminate the need for endocrine replacement therapy. In the case of parathyroid allotransplants, there has been an insistent and recurrently hopeful effort. Parathyroid deficiency is not treated with specific hormone replacement, but rather with calcium and vitamin D, which give inadequate results. An occasionally successful parathyroid allotransplant in a patient with a functioning renal allograft already receiving immunosuppressive drugs has been reported.

ORGAN TRANSPLANTATION

Pancreas

The discovery of insulin in 1921 was hailed as the cure of diabetes; it prevented death from diabetic coma, controlled the overt symptoms of diabetes, and provided an increased life expectancy. As diabetic patients lived longer, however, previously unseen complications developed. Diabetes was responsible for at least 30,000 deaths in 1974, and it is the leading cause of new cases of blindness in adults. Diabetics are seventeen times more liable to kidney disease, five times more liable to gangrene of the extremities, and twice as likely to develop heart diseases. Obviously, new approaches to treatment are required. Pancreas and islet transplantation offer the possibility that the development and progression of diabetic lesions will be prevented by precise regulation of carbohydrate metabolism—control not yet achieved by injected insulin.

An unresolved question is whether juvenile-onset diabetics suffer only from a lack of insulin or whether the absence of insulin reflects other subcellular derangements. Whether normalization of carbohydrate metabolism in these patients will prevent the development of systemic lesions is still unanswered. Several observations, however, support the hypothesis that angiopathic lesions associated with diabetes are secondary to abnormal metabolism:

1. Nephropathy and retinopathy occur in patients who develop diabetes as a result of other disease states (e.g., hemochromatosis) or after total pancreatectomy.
2. Numerous longitudinal clinical studies have shown a relationship between duration of the disease, control of plasma glucose, and development of lesions.
3. Nephropathy and retinopathy occur in animals with induced diabetes.
4. Studies in animals have demonstrated that reduction of hyperglycemia by insulin therapy or by transplantation of whole pancreas or islets prevents or minimizes formation of diabetic lesions in the eye, kidney, and nerve.
5. Kidneys transplanted from normal to diabetic rats develop histologic lesions characteristic of diabetes in the rat, whereas kidneys transplanted from diabetic to normal rats showed disappearance or lack of progression of these lesions.

These observations suggest that it may be possible to prevent the systemic complications of diabetes by insulin released from transplanted pancreatic islets. Alternative methods to provide precise glucose homeostasis, such as an implantable glucose sensor coupled to an insulin pump, are also possible, however.

WHOLE ORGAN

Either whole organ or distal segmental pancreatic transplants will ameliorate experimental diabetes. In addition to the expected problems associated with the control of immunologic rejection and the need for immunosuppressive drugs, there are special technical concerns. Of these, the major problem is difficulty in establishing drainage of the pancreatic duct. Theoretically, ligation of the pancreatic duct should result in atrophy of exocrine tissue without affecting endocrine tissue. But in practice a severe inflammatory reaction occurs and leads to a constricting fibrosis that damages even the islets. Filling the ductal system with plastic is an alternative approach to the prevention of exocrine secretion. Unfortunately pancreatic fibrosis remains a problem with this technique as well.

All alternative approaches are less successful. Initial attempts used a combined pancreaticoduodenal approach, with the duodenum serving as a conduit for drainage of exocrine enzymes. When a generous segment of transplanted duodenum was used, however, it was particularly susceptible to rejection and to anastomotic leakage. These complications can be eliminated by direct anastomosis of the pancreatic duct to an enteric drainage site, but fistulas are common. Permitting the duct to drain freely into the peritoneal cavity for absorption has been successful in animals, but some patients develop ascites. The use of a short segment of duodenum anastomosed to the bladder seems to be the most successful solution. Graft thrombosis and other complications associated with graft pancreatitis continue to plague progress in this field. Despite these problems, more than 1000 clinical transplants have been performed. Usually cadaver organs are used, and most recipients already have diabetic end-stage renal disease; both kidney and pancreas are transplanted at a single operation. Increasingly, however, as success grows, pancreas transplantation will be carried out in patients before advanced renal disease occurs.

Successful whole-organ or segmental pancreatic transplants produce circulating insulin and normal plasma glucose levels. When the venous drainage of the pancreatic graft is hooked up to the systemic circulation, the circulating insulin levels are higher than when the venous anastomosis is made to the portal system, although the plasma glucose levels are similar. Rejection episodes are as difficult to reverse as they are to detect. By the time glucose levels become abnormal, rejection is usually too far advanced, and serum enzyme levels do not become elevated. When the pancreatic duct is anastomosed to the bladder, however, the urine amylase level falls early in the rejection response. Thus, the most successful technical solution seems to permit better immunologic monitoring of the rejection response.

Experience in human beings has shown that functioning vascularized pancreatic allograft will correct the metabolic deficiency in diabetes. The techniques (Figs. 10-22 and 10-23) are now safer and more successful. The results of transplant carried out between 1983 and 1986 are illustrated in Fig. 10-24. Most current clinical research continues to focus on methods of controlling pancreatic exocrine secretion without inducing pancreatitis in the transplant. Rejection, thrombosis, and fibrosis remain serious barriers to widespread clinical application, even though fistula formation is now an unusual problem.

ISLET TISSUE

It is not necessary to transplant the pancreas in order to cure diabetes; transplantation of the pancreatic islets will suffice. The current technique for isolation of islets from the pancreas involves mechanical disruption, enzymatic digestion, and density-gradient separation. Isolated adult islets infused into the portal vein will produce long-lasting control of diabetes in rats. This technique has also been successfully applied to the autotransplantation of islets in people who require total pancreatectomy for chronic painful pancreatitis.

Clinical islet allotransplantation has been frustrated by

A.
Duct Injection

B.
Enteric Drainage

C.
Urinary Drainage

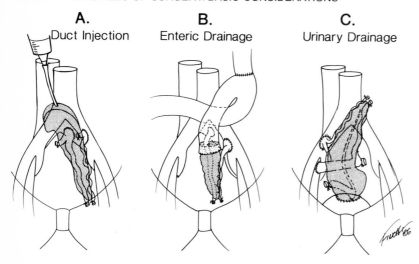

Fig. 10-22. Technique of pancreas transplantation. The body and tail can be transplanted with anastomoses of splenic vessels of donor pancreas to iliac vessels of recipient. The duct can be injected with a polymer to occlude it, or the duct can be anastomosed to a loop of bowel or the bladder. These techniques are still in use in some centers. (Adapted from: *Sutherland DER, Kendall D, et al: Surg Clin North Am 66:557, 1986, with permission.*)

the apparent increased susceptibility of islets to allograft rejection. Survival is difficult to achieve even when immunosuppression that will prolong skin, kidney, or heart allografts is used. The clinical application of islet transplantation will also require techniques such as cold storage or culture to preserve the cells.

The experimental evidence that islet tissue graft can prevent, halt, and even improve the vascular and neurological lesions of diabetes provides a tremendous impetus to continue research, despite these formidable difficulties.

Gastrointestinal Tract

Various segments of intestine can be autotransplanted by removal from the body and reimplantation. Stomach, small bowel, and colon can be used to replace esophagus, with reimplantation of the vascular supply. Allotransplantation of the small bowel and stomach has been carried out experimentally. These grafts are rejected in the usual fashion, and within the same general period as kidneys and other organs. There is some evidence that the lymphoid tissue within the intestinal wall can initiate a graft-versus-host reaction.

Although there is little apparent clinical use for a gastric transplant, there is a definite need for transplantation of the small bowel. Infarction of the bowel sometimes requires excision of the entire small bowel, and this leads to a nutritional deficiency that requires expensive and cumbersome parenteral alimentation. Patients with various nutritional and motility problems, as well as certain patients with Crohn's disease, might benefit from safe

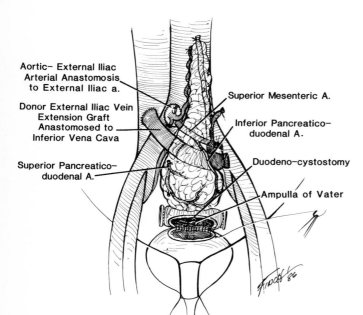

Aortic– External Iliac
Arterial Anastomosis
to External Iliac a.

Donor External Iliac Vein
Extension Graft
Anastomosed to
Inferior Vena Cava

Superior Pancreatico-
duodenal A.

Superior Mesenteric A.

Inferior Pancreatico-
duodenal A.

Duodeno–cystostomy

Ampulla of Vater

Fig. 10-23. Preferred method of pancreatic-duodenal transplantation. The whole pancreas is used. The celiac axis and superior mesenteric arteries are anastomosed to the iliac artery. The portal vein provides venous drainage. The duodenum is anastomosed to the bladder. [From: *Sutherland DER, Najarian JS, in Simmons RL, Finch M, et al (eds): Manual of Vascular Access, Organ Donation, and Transplantation. New York, Springer-Verlag, 1984, with permission.*]

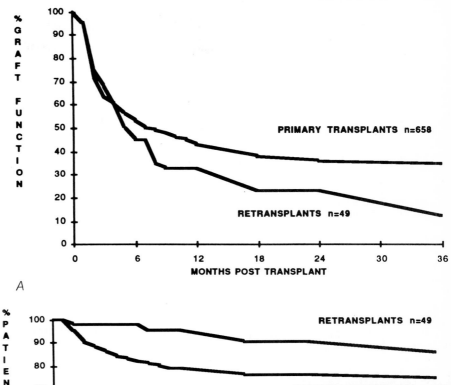

Fig. 10-24. Results from the World Pancreas Registry. *A*. Insulin-independent graft function. *B*. Recipient survival rate for primary transplants and retransplants reported between January 1, 1983, and August 31, 1986.

and successful bowel transplantation. A few attempts in human beings have been successful for several months, but no long-term survival has been achieved.

Liver

Liver transplantation has become a highly successful solution to a variety of congenital and acquired hepatic disorders in thousands of patients. A liver transplant may be positioned in the normal anatomic location (orthotopic transplantation) following a total hepatectomy of the recipient. Alternatively, the donor organ can be placed in an ectopic site (heterotopic transplantation), generally with retention of the host's liver (auxiliary transplantation). Orthotopic grafts are universally preferred by clinicians because experimental heterotopic grafts have been so unsuccessful.

INDICATIONS FOR LIVER TRANSPLANTATION. In theory, liver transplantation is appropriate for any disease that will cause total liver failure (Table 10-6). Chronic active hepatitis is the most common indication for liver transplantation in adults, followed by alcoholic cirrhosis, primary biliary cirrhosis, and secondary biliary cirrhosis.

Table 10-6. COMMON INDICATIONS FOR HEPATIC TRANSPLANTATION

Adult	*Children*
Chronic active hepatitis	Biliary atresia
Alcoholic cirrhosis	Chronic active hepatitis
Primary biliary cirrhosis	Hepatoma
Secondary biliary cirrhosis	Neonatal hepatitis
Secondary cholangitis	General hepatic fibrosis
α-1-Anti-trypsin deficiency	Secondary biliary cirrhosis
Hemachromatosis	Inborn errors of metabolism
Budd–Chiari syndrome	
Acute hepatitis B	

Modified from Ascher NL, Simmons RL, Najarian JS: Host hepatectomy and liver transplantation, in Simmons RL, Finch ME, Ascher NL, Najarian JS (eds): *Manual of Vascular Access, Organ Donation, and Transplantation.* New York, Springer-Verlag, 1984, pp 255–284.

Also, certain patients with rare types of malignancy confined to the liver may benefit from a liver graft.

In children the most common indication for transplantation is extrahepatic biliary atresia. Virtually all these patients previously have had one or more Kasai procedures. Transplantation is technically feasible in infants weighing as little as 5 kg; in patients smaller than this, the portal vein is usually too small to remain patent.

Naturally transplantation is contraindicated in any patient with (1) irreversible infection, (2) widespread malignancy, (3) concurrent disease (e.g., myocardial failure, old age) that would seriously impair survival, or (4) a high risk for recurrent disease in the transplant organ. Because active hepatitis also usually recurs, the presence of HBsAg or HBeAg antigenemia is a relative contraindication. The risk of recurrent alcoholism also makes alcoholic cirrhosis a relative contraindication unless the patient has abstained from alcohol for at least 2 years. In patients with sclerosing cholangitis, active ulcerative colitis also rules out liver transplantation. Patients with portal vein thrombosis cannot be successfully revascularized with orthotopic grafts.

PREOPERATIVE EVALUATION OF THE RECIPIENT. Intensive preoperative evaluation is designed to (1) characterize those physiologic defects in hepatic, pulmonary, renal, or cardiac function that will influence the patient's chance of survival, (2) determine whether the transplant is technically feasible for that particular patient, and (3) search out sites of occult infection and malignancy (Table 10-7).

During the complete history and physical examination, special attention is given to specific extrahepatic organ systems. For example, fluid overload and congestive heart failure are frequently present and must be treated with fluid restriction, diuretics, and lanoxin. In adults, roentgenograms of the chest and electrocardiograms are obtained, and a stress exercise test is done if recommended after a formal cardiology consultation.

Attention to respiratory reserve is important. Because all patients are respirator-dependent in the early post-transplant period, knowledge of their prior pulmonary

Table 10-7. WORK-UP OF POTENTIAL RECIPIENTS FOR LIVER TRANSPLANTATION

1. General
   a. History and physical examination
   b. Chest roentgenogram
   c. Electrocardiogram (ECG)
   d. Serum electrolytes
   e. Fasting blood sugar
2. Hematology
   a. Hemoglobin, leukocyte count, and differential count
   b. Platelet count, bleeding-clotting time, prothrombin time, partial thromboplastin time, thrombin time (factor analysis)
3. Hepatic
   a. Bilirubin, alkaline phosphatase, serum glutamic–pyruvic transaminase (SGPT), aspartate aminotransferase (AST)
   b. Protein electrophoresis
   c. Serum amino acid analysis
   d. α-Fetoprotein
   e. Ultrasound
   f. Ascitic cytology and culture
4. Nutritional evaluation
   a. Transferrin, prealbumin, serum amino acid analysis
5. Renal
   a. Urinalysis
   b. Blood urea nitrogen (BUN), serum creatinine
   c. 24-h creatinine clearance
6. Calcium metabolism (primary biliary cirrhosis)
   a. (Bone roentgenograms: hands, skull, clavical, lamina dura)
   b. (Ca, PO$_4$, Mg, alkaline phosphatase)
   c. (Parathormone)
7. Gastrointestinal
   a. Upper GI series
   b. Upper GI endoscopy
   c. (Variceal sclerotherapy)
8. Immunologic studies
   a. Blood type (ABO)
   b. Tissue typing including serial cytotoxic antibody determinations
9. Pulmonary function studies
   a. Chest roentgenogram
   b. Blood gases
   c. Pulmonary function tests
10. Infectious work-up
    a. Chest roentgenogram
    b. Blood, urine, throat, feces, ascites cultures
    c. Hepatitis screen
    d. Dental consult
11. Financial-social rehabilitation

The tests enclosed within parentheses are not administered routinely during the potential recipient work-up, but only when the circumstances indicate.

Modified from Ascher NL, Simmons RL, Najarian JS: Host hepatectomy and liver transplantation, in Simmons RL, Finch ME, Ascher NL, Najarian JS (eds): *Manual of Vascular Access, Organ Donation, and Transplantation.* New York, Springer-Verlag, 1984, pp 255–284.

function will help during the process of weaning from the respirator. Therefore, pulmonary function tests are obtained on all adult patients but only arterial blood gases and chest roentgenograms are necessary for pediatric patients. Postoperative ascites or a marginally oversized donor liver can further compromise respiratory function.

A variety of preoperative tests are obtained to assess hepatocellular function (Table 10-7). Hepatitis screening results will determine the need for hyperimmune globulin to prevent recurrent hepatitis, and unsuspected tumors are sought using a-fetoprotein, hepatic ultrasound, and computerized axial tomography (CAT). A coagulation profile is obtained to document functional capacity of the liver and predict the need for correction. An uncorrectible prothrombin time abnormality is a poor prognostic sign. A radionuclide hepatic excretion scan will reveal unsuspected biliary calculi that must be removed from the common bile duct at the time of recipient hepatectomy. An upper gastrointestinal series and upper gastrointestinal endoscopy will reveal the presence of gastric or esophageal varices. Sclerotherapy is used to treat bleeding esophageal varices while the patient is awaiting transplantation. Oral nystatin antifungal prophylaxis must be used to prevent invasive candidosis at the sclerotherapy site.

Patency of the portal vein system must be determined before transplantation because occlusion of the portal vein contraindicates liver transplant. CAT scans used to detect silent malignancy may also show portal vein patency. If either CAT scan or ultrasonography fails to visualize the portal vein, celiac angiography, with special attention to the venous phase, may be required.

The value of immunologic testing has not been determined, but most centers prefer that liver donors and recipients are ABO compatible. Liver donor organs are far too scarce, and the time before transplantation is too short for the time-consuming HLA matching tests to be performed.

While awaiting transplant a program of pretransplant management is set up to optimize the patient's general condition and to improve the suboptimal function of the multiple organ systems. Nutritional and respiratory functions receive special attention. All patients, especially those with pulmonary insufficiency, are begun on an intensive program of pulmonary toilet and exercise. For example, smokers must stop smoking, and postural drainage and short courses of broad-spectrum antibiotics may be necessary to treat bacterial infection.

The judicious use of furosemide and aldactone diuretic treatment of ascites is weighed against the possibility of exacerbating renal insufficiency. Blood volume is maximized using colloid to treat the prerenal component of the hepatorenal syndrome.

The patient's preoperative nutritional status may be enhanced by cautiously increasing dietary protein while monitoring the serum ammonia and serial amino acid profiles. Sclerotherapy is implemented as needed for bleeding varices.

IMMEDIATE PRETRANSPLANT MANAGEMENT. A rigidly defined protocol must be set up for the recipient as soon as a potential cadaver donor is located. Most of the procedures simply reassess the patient's condition while others are designed to prevent infection, replace blood loss, correct coagulation defects, and institute immunosuppression. Prophylactic antibiotics are begun to reduce colonization of the gastrointestinal tract, to minimize wound infection, or to provide protection against herpes virus infection.

Immediate preoperative exchange transfusion is indicated in all patients with impaired coagulation parameters, even though an effective exchange often results from the replacement of lost blood during the early stages of the operation. To effect rapid replacement of blood loss or perform exchange transfusion, central venous cannulation must be carried out. Systemic arterial and pulmonary artery pressure measurements should be monitored during the administration of fresh frozen plasma and load-reducing agents. This requires both arterial and pulmonary artery cannulation (Swan–Ganz catheter).

TECHNIQUE. Liver transplantation is a relatively straightforward procedure, although excessive bleeding, brought on by the extensive collateral venous system caused by the patient's portal hypertension, makes the native hepatectomy the most difficult part of the transplant process. Complications can occur if there is a septic focus, or if residual scars exist from prior operations (portosystemic shunts; attempts at biliary decompression). If technical difficulties prohibit the completion of the liver transplant, the patient will die.

The following eight precautions should be followed: (1) Do not remove the spleen (bleeding is excessive, removal obviates an important portosystemic collateral pathway, and splenic vein flow may be essential to maintain a patent portal vein); (2) minimize retroperitoneal dissection; (3) do not interfere with collateral vessels; (4) avoid thoracic incisions; (5) preserve the blood supply to the distal common duct by minimizing dissection in this region; (6) preserve as much length of suprahepatic vena cava, portal vein, hepatic artery, and infrahepatic vena cava as possible; (7) avoid clamp injury to the renal vessels; and (8) match the weights of donor and recipient ±20 percent. In children the donor can be smaller by as much as 20 percent but only minimally larger.

The most common incision for an orthotopic liver graft is a transverse abdominal incision. The diseased liver is dissected free and clamps are applied to the suprahepatic and intrahepatic vena cavas, the portal vein, and the hepatic artery. The liver can then be removed and replaced by the cadaver liver. Many surgeons perform a portal vein–to–superior vena cava temporary shunt so that the splanchnic venous bed does not become excessively congested during clamping of the vein. A concurrent temporary inferior vena cava–to–superior vena cava shunt minimizes renal venous congestion and permits the return of blood to the heart during the anhepatic phase.

The allograft anastomoses are shown in Fig. 10-25. The suprahepatic caval anastomosis is the most difficult to perform. The second anastomosis is usually the portal vein to minimize venous congestion of the intestine. After the portal vein anastomosis is completed, the inferior hepatic caval clamps should be briefly removed, leaving the suprahepatic vena cava clamped. The portal vein inflow should be opened to allow the liver to be perfused with warm blood. This sequence is useful to remove the cold perfusate from the liver and prevent systemic hypothermia and heparinization. As soon as the perfusate is

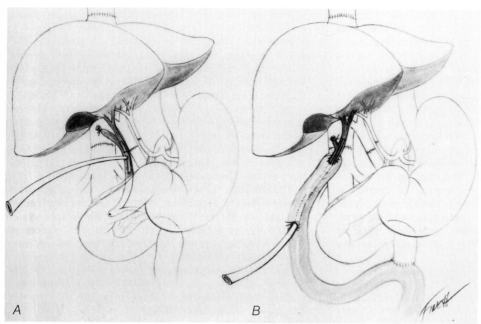

Fig. 10-25. Completed orthotopic liver transplant in *(A)* adults and *(B)* children. The two preferred methods of biliary reconstruction are illustrated. [From: *Ascher NL, Najarian JS, et al, in Simmons RL, Finch M, et al (eds): Manual of Vascular Access, Organ Donation, and Transplantation. New York, Springer-Verlag, 1984, with permission.*]

washed from the liver and it becomes firm and pink, the intrahepatic vena cava is clamped, and the suprahepatic vena cava clamp is removed. The remaining vascular anastomoses (hepatic artery, inferior vena cava) can then be accomplished.

Following the vascular anastomoses, biliary drainage must be obtained. A direct bile duct–to–bile duct anastomosis is preferred in adults. A choledochojejunostomy is preferred in children.

As many as 30 to 40 percent of patients have double hepatic arteries, and one of them may arise from the superior mesenteric artery. Care must be taken during the donor operation to preserve this arterial supply to the transplanted liver.

A common complication is paralysis of the right side of the diaphragm, which apparently results from crushing of the right phrenic nerve by the vascular clamp applied to the suprahepatic inferior vena cava. Enough length must be preserved during total hepatectomy for the clamp to be applied without impinging on the diaphragm.

POSTOPERATIVE MANAGEMENT. The early posttransplant management of liver recipients is so complex that protocols have been designed to guarantee that crucial details are not omitted. If renal function is satisfactory, cyclosporine and prednisone are preferred for immunosuppression. If renal function is poor, cyclosporine is omitted and antilymphoblast serum and azathioprine are used.

Some degree of acute tubular necrosis is common in the immediate postoperative period, probably because of poor perfusion due to blood loss and the clamping of the inferior vena cava with renal venous hypertension. If renal function is already compromised, the nephrotoxic effect of cyclosporine can be minimized by delaying its

use until 12 h after transplantation. Constant monitoring of renal function and cyclosporine levels will ensure the precise adjustment of the dosage.

Respiratory support is usually required for at least 24 to 48 h after extubation. Most patients can then be transferred to a regular nursing ward. Nasogastric suction is maintained until bowel function returns, and intravenous hyperalimentation is used until they can eat. Levels of BUN, creatinine, electrolytes, calcium, phosphate, white blood cell count, and hemoglobin are determined daily. Chest roentgenograms are taken daily for 5 days, and whenever the patient becomes febrile, to seek evidence for atelectasis, pneumonia, diaphragmatic paralysis, and pleural effusion. Culture samples are taken as indicated.

Monitoring liver transplant function with frequent chemical determination of coagulation parameters (especially prothrombin time, factor V levels, the serum bilirubin, transaminase, and alkaline phosphatase levels) is mandatory. Changes in these levels can signal rejection, ischemia, viral infection, cholangitis, or mechanical obstruction.

A radionuclide excretory cholangiogram is performed on postoperative day 3 and at weekly intervals; excretion of the radioisotope by the liver into the small bowel by 45 min is considered to be normal. A delay can reflect hepatocellular damage during death of the donor, complications of the donor operation, prolonged cold storage, vascular compromise, or rejection. Also, delayed excretion into the biliary tree can reflect rejection, hepatocellular damage from ischemia, or viral infection. Delayed passage into the small bowel can indicate mechanical obstruction or breakdown. A T-tube cholangiogram (performed with gravity) will diagnose breakdown at the site of biliary drainage, or if a T tube has not been used (e.g., with a cholecystojejunostomy), transhepatic cholangiography may be necessary to evaluate the biliary system.

During rejection lymphocytes infiltrate portal tracts and central veins, with varying degrees of bile duct epithelial damage; therefore, a percutaneous liver transplant biopsy and culture is the only way to differentiate among rejection, ischemia, viral infection, and cholangitis. Rejection is treated initially with intravenous steroids or with antilymphoblast globulin. The presence of polymorphonuclear leukocytes within the portal tracts indicates cholangitis. The patient is treated with antibiotics and a search is made for a mechanical obstruction as an underlying cause. Cytomegalovirus hepatitis is treated with ganciclovir.

Postoperative Complications. The most serious complication is primary nonfunction, in which the liver fails to function sufficiently well to support life. This may be a result of ischemia, technical factors, or accelerated rejection. Primary nonfunction is first suspected when factor V levels in the plasma fail to return to normal.

Intraoperative bleeding results from many causes: Extensive portasystemic shunts are almost always present and global coagulation defects always exist. Even when hemostasis appears adequate during operation, bleeding is a special hazard in the immediate postoperative period. Coagulation parameters, including platelet levels and serum calcium levels, must be measured during closure of the abdomen so that they can be corrected. Blood loss may continue into the postoperative period, although immediate normal transplant function will minimize these complications. A normal prothrombin time and factor V level are early signs that normal function has returned.

Thrombotic occlusion of either the hepatic artery or portal vein will cause sudden deterioration of hepatic function. The bilirubin and transaminase values rise rapidly, coagulopathy, hyperkalemia, and hypoglycemia appear, and the liver fails to extract radionuclides during liver scan. In many centers, these catastrophes are indications for retransplantation.

Vena caval stenosis (most often the suprahepatic anastomosis) leads to edema in the lower trunk and renal insufficiency. An angiogram of the vena cava will confirm the diagnosis. Operative repair must be undertaken. Milder degrees of stenosis of the suprahepatic vena cava anastomosis in children declare themselves by nonspecific alterations in hepatic function: persistent ascites, elevated bilirubin, and hepatic enzymes. Balloon angioplasty can be used for vena cava stenosis in the late postoperative period.

Respiratory complications are common. Liver transplant recipients have ascites, pleural effusion, paralyzed diaphragms, and a new edematous liver. The operative pain and spasms of the abdominal wall add to the high risk of pulmonary complications. The atelectasis can easily become complicated by pneumonia. Prophylaxis includes both training the prospective recipients to use their accessory respiratory muscles, and vigorous pulmonary toilet in the postoperative period. The liberal use of bronchoscopy to reexpand atelectatic lung segments and to remove (and culture) purulent material is also helpful. Function usually returns to a paralyzed diaphragm within 3 to 4 weeks. The ascites can be drained via peritoneal dialysis catheters if care is taken to maintain asepsis. Provided that liver function is good and infection does not supervene, almost all patients can be weaned from their often lengthy respirator dependence.

Renal malfunction is common both before and after transplantation, but the posttransplant problems can be minimized by attention to a number of details: (1) maintain renal perfusion in the preoperative period by maintenance of blood volume; (2) do not compromise the renal veins or the right renal artery as it courses behind the vena cava; (3) use a portasystemic shunt during the operation to reduce renal vein pressure during the anhepatic phase; (4) intravenous cyclosporine should be infused slowly in low doses during the initial periods of recovery so that peak blood cyclosporine levels remain below nephrotoxic levels; (5) stop the use of cyclosporine therapy with the first sign of renal compromise, and temporarily use conventional immunotherapy (ALG, azathioprine); (6) avoid nephrotoxic agents (aminoglycosides, amphotericin B); and (7) remove ascites to reduce intraabdominal pressure.

Although infectious complications are no longer the most common causes of death after liver transplantation, they continue to be a major problem. For example, the incidence of bacterial sepsis has diminished with the use of cyclosporine and newer methods of biliary drainage. Cholangitis and biliary anastomotic breakdown are now rare. Even so, perioperative antibiotics should be used in repeated doses during operation because the blood loss is great and the operation is long. Topical antibiotics (0.1% cephapirin) used repeatedly during the operation will obviate the need for repeated systemic doses. Postoperative antibiotics should be based on intraoperative culture results of contaminated material.

Oral trimethoprim sulfamethoxazole will reduce the postoperative incidence of *Pneumocystis carinii* and *Nocardia* infections, as it does in renal transplant patients.

Fungal infections remain a major problem in liver recipients but can be controlled by the preoperative and postoperative use of high-dose oral, esophageal, and gastric nystatin. Also, prompt institution of systemic amphotericin B for candidosis without fungemia will minimize the adverse consequences.

Central venous pressure lines should be removed as soon as possible to decrease the chance of their colonization.

Viral infections are a major problem the most serious of which is cytomegalovirus (CMV). CMV can be treated with ganciclovir, a new antiviral drug. Acyclovir will not prevent or cure CMV, but it will prevent herpes simplex.

Cholangitis in the absence of discernible biliary obstruction is more common than previously described. Only by biopsy of the transplant can it be diagnosed. Cul-

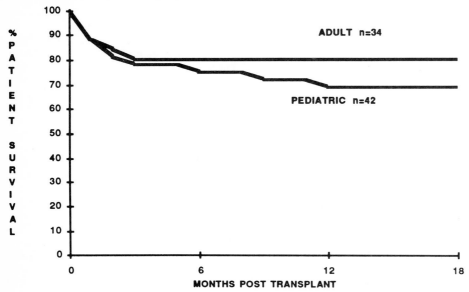

Fig. 10-26. Results of adult and pediatric liver transplants performed at the University of Minnesota between April 1984 and March 1987.

ture of the specimen permits rational antimicrobial therapy.

Subclinical and reversible rejection episodes are commonly detected if liver biopsies are carried out at weekly intervals. Rejection may occur at any time in the postoperative period including the first 24 h, but most cases occur at least several weeks after transplantation.

RESULTS. Although the first liver transplant in a human being was performed in 1963, the procedure was not successful until 1967. From then until 1978 the results were generally poor, with 1-year survival figures ranging from 25 to 30 percent. The longest-living survivor is well 12 years after transplantation. Since 1979, Starzl's group has enjoyed markedly improved survival, in the range of 70 to 80 percent for 1 year. The results of hepatic transplantation have improved with the use of cyclosporine. Currently, a combination of steroids, azathioprine, and cyclosporine are used for the prophylaxis of rejection following liver transplantation at the University of Minnesota. The results using this regimen are shown in Fig. 10-26.

Heart, Heart-Lung, and Single Lung

Craig R. Smith and Keith Reemtsma

HEART

HISTORICAL DEVELOPMENT. Cardiac transplantation is a young field that has progressed dramatically in the 1980s. Christiaan Barnard performed the first human heart transplant in 1967; this stimulated a flurry of imitation throughout the world. Disappointing results led to a backlash of public disparagement, and early eclipse into disfavor by 1970. More cardiac transplants were performed in 1968 (54) than were performed in any subsequent year until 1981.

Public discouragement with early clinical results tended to overshadow the substantial experimental foundations of the procedure. Heterotopic transplants, in which the heart is placed in parallel in the circulation, were done as early as 1905 by Carrel and Guthrie. Orthotopic transplants, in which the donor heart replaces the recipient heart, were first done successfully in dogs by Lower and Shumway in 1959. By 1967 the operative technique was well refined, and the procedure was reproducible in animals. Operative technique has changed remarkably little in 20 years. Because he was so actively involved in the experimental development of the field, Shumway persevered clinically, and nurtured the field through the 1970s. By 1982 the series at Stanford enjoyed 50 percent survival at 5 years.

With the clinical introduction of cyclosporine in 1982, cardiac transplantation entered a phase of exponential growth. More transplants were done in 1985 (984) than were done from 1967 to 1984. At the beginning of the 1980s, fewer than 10 centers were performing cardiac transplants, a number that has grown to more than 80.

SPECTRUM OF DISEASE. Patients requiring cardiac transplantation can be combined under a diagnosis of congestive cardiomyopathy, a broad category of diverse pathogenesis, defined by histopathology and functional characteristics. The "idiopathic" cardiomyopathies are a heterogeneous group of conditions sharing common end-stage pathology characterized by dilated cardiac chambers, myocardial degeneration, and fibrosis. Viral cardiomyopathy is thought to account for the majority of "idiopathic" cases. Specific diagnoses such as familial cardiomyopathy, alcoholic cardiomyopathy, or postpartum cardiomyopathy account for a small fraction of the group, since most are ultimately idiopathic. Idiopathic cardiomyopathy primarily attacks young and otherwise healthy patients.

Ischemic cardiomyopathy is loosely defined as an end-stage manifestation of coronary atherosclerosis. Compared with patients with idiopathic cardiomyopathy, patients with ischemic cardiomyopathy are generally older and have a higher frequency of associated problems such as diabetes and peripheral vascular disease. Patients with end-stage ventricular failure associated with valvular disease are infrequently transplanted and are difficult to classify. Congenital heart disease presents similar problems, and transplantation in childhood is elected for a combination of idiopathic cardiomyopathies and primary congenital lesions, such as hypoplastic left heart syndrome. However defined, such cases account for a small percentage of cardiac transplants.

The age range for all patients transplanted from 1967 through early 1986 is 4 days to 66 years, with a mean age of 40 plus or minus 12 years. The broad distribution of age over the middle decades reflects overlap between the differing age distributions of idiopathic and ischemic cardiomyopathy. If eligibility for transplant were not influenced by age, the distribution of diagnoses would shift toward those of coronary atherosclerosis, with all its associated problems, and the mean age would increase accordingly. At present, 57 percent of all patients transplanted have had idiopathic cardiomyopathy, 40 percent have had ischemic cardiomyopathy, and 3 percent have had congenital heart disease or other diagnoses. Eighty percent of patients transplanted have been men. It is not clear whether this is due to differences in the expression of cardiomyopathies by gender or to differences in selection criteria favoring men.

RECIPIENT SELECTION. Recipients are selected from among patients with end-stage ventricular failure, clinically NYHA Class III–IV, who are unlikely to survive more than 1 year, and for whom there is no alternative therapy. Selection criteria (Table 10-8) continue to be quite strict because of the belief that heart donors are a scarce resource that must be distributed preferentially to those with the greatest chance of benefit. The proper psychosocial profile includes evidence of ability to comply with an elaborate regimen of postoperative care. Until recently patients older than 55 years were excluded, but at present carefully selected older patients are being transplanted when the other essential criteria are met.

Contraindications include systemic diseases likely to compromise long-term survival, such as malignancy, severe peripheral vascular disease or autoimmune vasculitis, and renal or hepatic dysfunction not likely to respond to an improvement in cardiac output. Diabetes and peptic ulcer disease have been considered relative contraindications.

The level of pulmonary vascular resistance in a potential recipient is given particular attention. In all patients with left ventricular failure, regardless of etiology, pulmonary artery pressure (PAP) increases as left atrial pressure rises. Pulmonary vascular resistance (PVR) increases variably but can become extremely elevated and fixed. A normal donor heart, accustomed to low pulmonary artery pressure and resistance, will fail immediately if placed in a recipient with sufficiently elevated PVR. Therefore, right heart catheterization provides essential information regarding operative risk. PVR index equals mean PAP minus wedge pressure divided by cardiac index and is assigned dimensionless units called Wood's units (WU). The normal range is 0 to 3 WU. Cardiac output is frequently used for the denominator, but some accuracy in prediction is lost when the patient's body surface area is significantly greater or less than 1.0 m^2. At the time of catheterization, patients with elevated PAP and PVR receive a trial infusion of nitroprusside or prostaglandin E-1, observing the effect on PVR as the infusion rate is increased up to the point at which systemic pressure falls below an acceptable level. If the PVR can be reduced to less than 5 WU, the patient is considered an acceptable risk. At the same time, pulmonary artery systolic pressure that remains greater than 50 mmHg is reason for concern but not necessarily for exclusion.

DONOR EVALUATION. Estimates based on current recipient acceptance criteria suggest that about 14,000 people per year in the United States could benefit from cardiac transplant. Estimates of the number of potential heart donors suggest that a maximum of 2000 are available each year. Under such conditions the cornerstone of any cardiac transplant program is an effective system for identifying and managing potential donors.

Table 10-9 summarizes the process of donor evaluation. It must be emphasized that such listings are guidelines and not requirements, and a balance must be reached between the desire to use only ideal donors and the need to minimize the mortality on the recipient waiting list. Many of the exclusions made are not meant to imply that the heart is not functioning perfectly well in the donor but are based on concern about the ability of the donor heart to tolerate ischemia during the cold preservation period. The limits of an acceptable donor heart are still being defined, and extending the limits would be one way to increase the number of potential donors.

The donor heart is ischemic from the time the aortic cross clamp is applied in the donor until the cross clamp is

Table 10-8. SELECTION OF RECIPIENTS FOR CARDIAC TRANSPLANTATION

Indications:	End-stage ventricular failure
	NYHA Class III–IV existence
	Poor 6- to 12-month prognosis for survival
	Medically compliant psychosocial profile
	No alternative treatment
Contraindications:	Systemic disease (vascular, autoimmune)
	Irreversible renal/hepatic insufficiency
	Neoplasia
	High, fixed pulmonary vascular resistance
	Active infection
Relative contraindications:	Age > 55 years
	Diabetes mellitus
	Active peptic ulcer disease

Table 10-9. ELEMENTS OF DONOR EVALUATION

Travel time (major variable in ischemic time)
Age (male < 40, female < 50)
Size (approximately recipient weight ±20%)
ABO blood group
Lymphocyte cross match (controversial)
Etiology of brain death
   Blunt trauma: rule out myocardial contusion
   Penetrating trauma and primary neurologic:
     look carefully at medical history
Medical history
   Cardiac history
   Hypertension
   I.V. drug abuse
   Smoking
   Alcoholism
Hemodynamic history since admission
   Cardiac arrest or prolonged hypotension
   Cardioactive and vasoactive drug requirements
   Central venous pressure
Cardiac
   ECG: ST-T waves can be misleading in brain death
   Echocardiogram: contractility, regional wall motion
   Evaluation by cardiologist
Pulmonary
   Oxygenation
   Chest x-ray: contusion, pneumothorax, infiltrates, edema
Serology
   Hepatitis B
   HTLV-III
   Cytomegalovirus

removed from the recipient, and ideally this ischemic period is kept under 4 h. Travel time between the donor and recipient hospitals is usually the main determinant of ischemic time; so expedient transportation is arranged accordingly. Age criteria are set to minimize the risk of using a heart with silent coronary atherosclerosis. Size matching is designed to avoid extreme discrepancies in the atrial and great vessel anastomoses, and to avoid any predictable mismatch in hemodynamics, as might occur if a small female heart is placed in a man with borderline acceptable PVR.

Major blood group compatibility is essential. The importance of a prospective lymphocyte cross match remains controversial in the transplantation of solid organs other than the kidney. As a practical matter, time constraints usually prohibit prospective cross matching.

Victims of blunt trauma must be assessed carefully for myocardial contusion, which can be present with few objective findings. On the other hand many normal hearts will be thrown away if indirect evidence such as thoracic fractions and pulmonary contusions is overemphasized. Victims of penetrating trauma frequently have a social profile that makes attention to certain features of medical history such as I.V. drug abuse important. Patients with primary neurologic brain death (i.e., subarachnoid hemorrhage) require close scrutiny for evidence of major hypertension and its cardiac sequelae.

Features of the hemodynamic course that might be alarming in isolation, such as cardiac arrest or a high-dose dopamine infusion, need to be considered in context or good donors will be wasted. A common scenario is a patient on high-dose dopamine with diabetes insipidus and a low CVP, who can be taken off dopamine after volume replacement.

The ECG should be normal, but striking ST-T changes can be associated with cerebrovascular accidents, hypothermia and electrolyte abnormalities. Echocardiography is extremely helpful under such circumstances, as it is in the evaluation of blunt trauma, to assess contractility and search for focal wall motion abnormalities.

A fairly broad spectrum of pulmonary pathology can be tolerated as long as oxygenation is adequate and sepsis is avoided. Extensive traumatic injury should raise the index of suspicion for myocardial contusion but is not an independent exclusion.

Positive serology for HTLV-III or hepatitis B excludes a potential donor. The information can be difficult to obtain quickly but should be insisted upon if the donor's medical and social history suggests increased risk. Knowledge of the potential recipient's cytomegalovirus (CMV) titer is required to interpret a positive CMV titer in the donor. Acute CMV infection in an immunosuppressed seronegative recipient is very serious and appears to be transmissible with the heart. Although many CMV positive recipients will experience CMV reactivation infection after transplant, it is far less serious. Of course, use of a seronegative donor for a seronegative recipient does not guarantee safety, since the disease can be transmitted equally well through blood transfusion.

DONOR OPERATION. The procedure is timed in coordination with teams removing liver and kidneys, and with the team preparing for implantation in the recipient. The heart is exposed through a median sternotomy, and a final assessment is made by visual inspection. Heparin is given. Removal begins with ligation of the superior vena cava and division of the inferior vena cava and pulmonary veins (Fig. 10-27). This is done as the first step in order to decompress the heart and avoid any ventricular distention with the aorta occluded. An aortic cross clamp is applied just proximal to the innominate artery. Preservation is begun by infusing hyperkalemic cardioplegia solution at 4°C into the aortic root to produce a prompt arrest in diastole. The cooling provided by coronary perfusion is augmented by immersion in saline solution at 4°C. The heart is observed closely for distention, which can be relieved if necessary by passing a finger across the mitral valve from the opening in the pulmonary veins. Finally the aorta and pulmonary artery are divided distally (Fig. 10-28); the heart is removed from the pericardium and wrapped in ice for transport.

RECIPIENT OPERATION. The recipient operation begins with median sternotomy and cannulation for cardiopulmonary bypass, using two separate venous cannulae that can be snared in the cavae. The cannulae are inserted well away from the atrioventricular groove, where the right atrial anastomosis will eventually be made. To minimize ischemic time, close communication is maintained with the donor team so that implantation can proceed as soon as the donor heart arrives in the recipient operating room. The patient is placed on total cardiopulmonary bypass

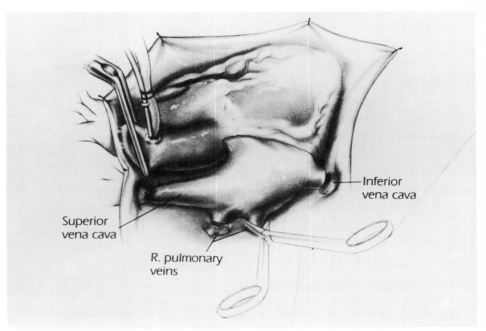

Fig. 10-27. Donor cardiectomy. The aortic cross clamp has been applied, and cardioplegia is being infused through a cannula in the aortic root. The superior vena cava has been ligated. The inferior vena cava and right superior pulmonary vein have been divided, and the scissors are about to divide the right inferior pulmonary vein. For the next few minutes attention is directed toward achieving a rapid arrest without ventricular distention, and beginning topical hypothermia with iced saline irrigation.

with moderate systemic hypothermia. The recipient aorta is cross-clamped just proximal to the innominate artery, and the heart is removed by dividing the great vessels at their commissures and separating the atria from the ventricles at the atrioventricular groove. Both atrial appendages are excised. The posterior aspects of both atria are left intact and connected by the interatrial septum. The donor heart is brought onto the field, trimmed appropriately, and carefully inspected, looking particularly for a

patent foramen ovale. If a patent foramen is left open, a significant right-to-left shunt can occur in patients with residual pulmonary hypertension. Implantation proceeds with anastomosis of the left atria, followed by the right atria, pulmonary arteries, and aortae (Fig. 10-29). Size discrepancies are easily accommodated in the atrial suture lines. Significant aortic size discrepancy is quite common, especially when there is a large age difference between donor and recipient. Remarkably large mis-

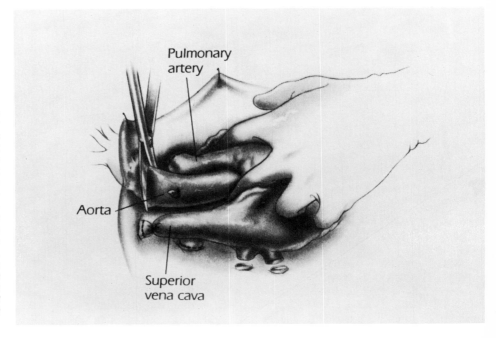

Fig. 10-28. Donor cardiectomy. The scissors are about to divide the aorta. The pulmonary artery and superior vena cava will be divided next and the donor heart removed for transport. The pulmonary artery is usually divided at or beyond the bifurcation to preserve all possible length. It is convenient to divide the right pulmonary artery just to the right of the superior vena cava (dotted line) and divide the left pulmonary artery at the pericardial reflection. (From: *Doty DB: Cardiac surgery: A looseleaf workbook and update service. "TRANSPL" section in Update 3. Chicago, Year Book Medical Publishers, 1986, with permission.*)

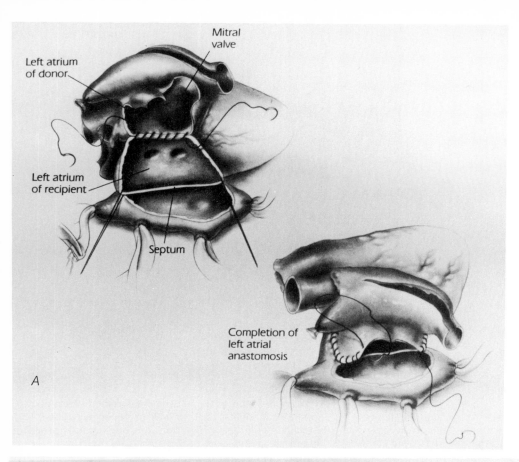

Left atrium
of donor

Mitral
valve

Left atrium
of recipient

Septum

Completion of
left atrial
anastomosis

A

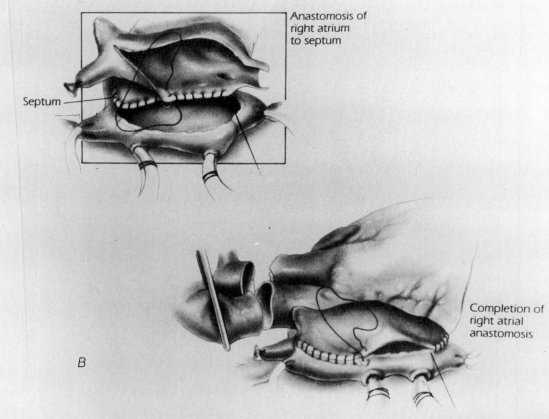

Anastomosis of
right atrium
to septum

Septum

Completion of
right atrial
anastomosis

B

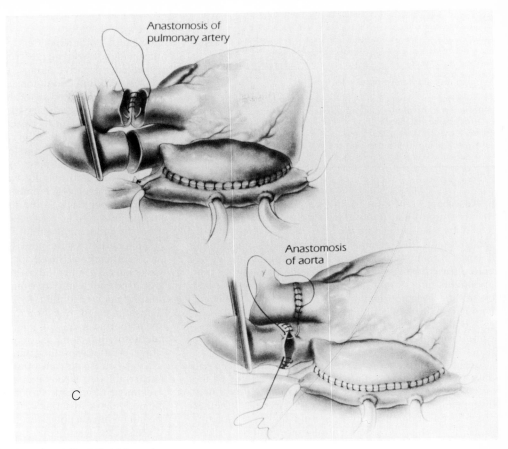

Anastomosis of
pulmonary artery

Anastomosis
of aorta

C

Fig. 10-29. *A*. Implantation of the donor heart. The left atrial anasto-mosis is begun adjacent to the left atrial appendage of the donor and the confluence of the left pulmonary veins in the recipient (upper figure). It is completed by joining the right edge of the donor left atrium to the interatrial septum (lower figure). Note the opening in the right atrium, which is directed from the inferior vena caval orifice toward the middle of the right atrial appendage. *B*. Implanta-tion of the donor heart. The right atrial anastomosis is begun by rolling the posterior edge of the right atriotomy over to the interatrial septum, where the suture line overlaps the septal segment of the left atrial suture line just completed (upper figure). The closure di-verges from the left atrium at the inferior and superior ends of the septum and continues anteriorly (lower figure). *C*. Implantation of the donor heart. The pulmonary artery (upper figure) and aorta (lower figure) are trimmed and joined with a continuous suture, be-ginning posteriorly. Discrepancies in circumference are taken up with careful suture spacing. (From: *Doty DB: Cardiac surgery: A looseleaf workbook and update service. "TRANSPL" section in Update 3. Chicago, Year Book Medical Publishers, 1986, with per-mission.*)

matches can be accommodated with a careful anastomo-sis, in part because of the elasticity of youthful aortic tis-sue. The cross clamp is removed, and a spontaneous rhythm is restored. The sinus node of the donor heart becomes the dominant pacemaker. The recipient's intrin-sic rhythm frequently persists, producing regular noncon-ducted contractions of the native atrial tissue and a sec-ond independent P-wave on the posttransplant ECG.

Early postoperative care is identical in most respects to that given any patient following open heart surgery, ex-

cept that strict reverse isolation is observed. The dener-vated heart often requires a period of chronotropic sup-port, which is usually provided by isoproteronol infusion or epicardial pacing to maintain a heart rate of 90 to 110. Virtually all patients demonstrate a degree of right ven-tricular decompensation as the donor right ventricle tries to adapt to the residual elevated PVR in the recipient. Clinical manifestations include a rising central venous pressure, a right ventricular gallop, and edema. Echocar-diography done during this period typically shows de-creased right ventricular contractility with chamber dila-tion, and may show tricuspid insufficiency. In correctly selected patients these findings will return to normal as the PVR gradually falls, but inotropic and vasodilator support may be required for many days.

IMMUNOSUPPRESSION. Maintenance immunosuppres-sion (Table 10-10) consists primarily of oral cyclosporine and prednisone, usually given twice daily. Cyclosporine dosage is adjusted to maintain an appropriate blood or serum level. Complex interactions with other medications are frequently seen, especially with drugs metabolized in the liver. Dilantin is a common example.

Unfortunately, in spite of its miraculous immunosup-pressive effects, cyclosporine has significant renal and other toxicity. A decrease in renal function and a rise in systemic blood pressure are seen over time in a high per-centage of patients, and appear to be dose-related. There

Table 10-10. IMMUNOSUPPRESSION FOLLOWING CARDIAC TRANSPLANT

Maintenance immunosuppression:

1. Cyclosporine: Usually 4–8 mg/kg P.O. b.i.d., adjust to maintain serum level 100–300 ng/mL
2. Prednisone: 0.2 mg/kg P.O. b.i.d., taper after 3–6 months to ≤0.1 mg/kg P.O. b.i.d.
3. Azathioprine (optional—protocols vary): 1–2 mg/kg P.O. q.d.

has also been some concern that chronic low-grade rejection not controlled by cyclosporine and not easily detected by routine endomyocardial biopsy might be responsible for the gradual development of myocardial fibrosis in many patients, and for the appearance of severe diffuse coronary artery disease in about 10 percent of patients after 1 year. Many programs have responded by adding azathioprine to their maintenance regimen, hoping to gain a reduction in cyclosporine dosage as well as a boost in the level of maintenance immunosuppression. It is not yet clear that this approach will produce any benefits.

Beginning 3 to 6 months posttransplant the prednisone dose is tapered slowly to a level about one-third of the initial dose. Most features of a cushingoid habitus slowly disappear as the prednisone dose is tapered. Whether other chronic complications of steroid administration (arthopathy, myopathy, glucose intolerance) will be avoided remains to be seen.

REJECTION. Rejection is monitored by right ventricular endomyocardial biopsy, done at least weekly in the first month, then less frequently on a tapering schedule. At the time of each biopsy a right heart catheterization is performed. Most rejection episodes have normal hemodynamics, but a low cardiac output, low mixed venous oxygen saturation, and elevated right atrial or wedge pressures raise suspicion of rejection. The biopsy is performed through the same venipuncture with a flexible biopsy forceps passed into the right ventricle. Adequate sampling is important, since the false negative rate only drops below 5 percent when three or more pieces of muscle can be examined on the slide. The biopsy material can be fixed, stained, and examined microscopically within 24 h.

Histologic evidence of myocyte necrosis is considered diagnostic of significant rejection. Inflammatory cell infiltrates are considered abnormal but are usually not treated as rejection in the absence of myocyte necrosis in patients on cyclosporine. All suspected rejection episodes are considered in clinical context, especially if the histological diagnosis is ambiguous. Subjective signs are frequently subtle but may include malaise, fatigue, and frank dyspnea or orthopnea. Physical findings are usually absent but can include tachycardia, a ventricular gallop, rales, and edema. Diminution in ECG voltage is correlated with rejection in patients maintained on azathioprine and steroids but is without value in patients on cyclosporine. Echocardiography can add suggestive findings but is not independently diagnostic. Occasionally all the evidence will suggest rejection in the presence of a repeatedly negative biopsy. In such cases, once bacterial sepsis, viral infection, constrictive pericarditis, and tamponade are excluded, a left heart catheterization is likely to show diffuse coronary disease.

About 95 percent of rejection episodes can be treated initially with steroids. Many institutions prefer to give intravenous methylprednisolone (usually 1 g/day for 3 days) as initial treatment. At Columbia Presbyterian rejection is treated initially with an increase in oral prednisone to 50 mg twice daily for 3 days, followed by a 10 mg/day taper back to the maintenance dose, a protocol designed to reduce the incidence of infectious complications by reducing the total steroid dose (Fig. 10-30). Rejection episodes unresponsive to the oral pulse are treated with intravenous methylprednisolone, unless they are associated with hemodynamic instability or a low serum cyclosporine level, in which case intramuscular rabbit antithymocyte globulin (R-ATG) is added simultaneously. Uncomplicated rejection associated with an adequate cyclosporine level but failing to respond to intravenous methylprednisolone is treated with R-ATG as a third stage. The oral prednisone protocol described has been effective in 91 percent of all rejection episodes, and half the remainder have been salvaged with the adjunctive treatment described. Patients who present initially with hemodynamic instability are at high risk and are promptly begun on intravenous steroid and antithymocyte globulin.

RESULTS. Results are being carefully tabulated in the Registry of the International Society for Heart Transplantation, which presently includes just over 3500 cases (January 1987). With early (30-day) mortality included, 1-year survival expectancy is 79 percent (Fig. 10-31). Survival remains high thereafter, with 77 percent actuarial survival at 5 years. Improvement in results since the introduction of cyclosporine is evident when the curve for patients treated with cyclosporine is compared with that for noncyclosporine patients. One-year survival with cyclosporine is 79 versus 66 percent without cyclosporine, and at 5 years the difference is 77 versus 55 percent. The curves are significantly different ($p < 0.01$).

Although long-term survival appears to be excellent, perioperative mortality remains high. During 1985 there was 12 percent mortality during the first 30 days. In cyclosporine-treated patients, 30-day mortality was attributed to rejection in 22 percent, infection in 20 percent, and "cardiac" and other causes in the majority (58 percent). The most common cardiac causes of early mortality are poor donor selection, poor donor preservation, and prohibitive pulmonary hypertension in the recipient. In comparison with patients treated with azathioprine and steroids, cyclosporine has significantly reduced the frequency of early death due to rejection, from 32 to 22 percent, but has had no significant impact of deaths due to other causes.

For all patients risk falls dramatically during the first year. Three-quarters of the first-year mortality occurs during the first quarter of the year. Although the period of high risk coincides with the period having the greatest

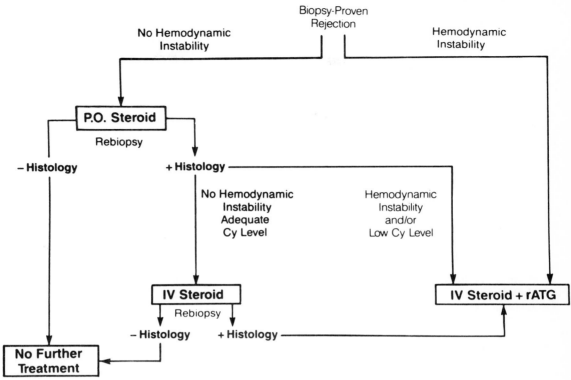

Fig. 10-30. Treatment algorithm for biopsy-proved rejection used at Columbia Presbyterian Medical Center. Ninety-five percent of all rejection episodes are treated initially with oral steroid. "Cy level" is the cyclosporine level. (From: *Michler, Smith, et al, with permission.*)

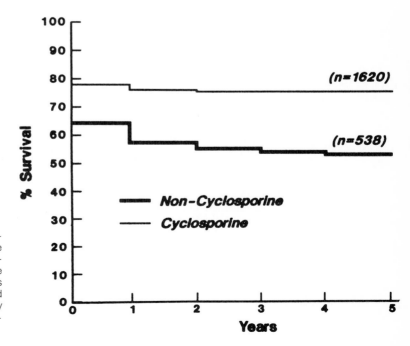

Fig. 10-31. Overall actuarial survival of patients transplanted from 1978 through 1985, compiled for the most recent Official Report of the Registry of the International Society for Heart Transplantation in June 1986. Early (30-day) mortality (about 10 percent) is included. The curves for cyclosporine-treated and non-cyclosporine-treated patients are significantly different (p < 0.01). (From: *Solis and Kaye, with permission.*)

frequency of rejection episodes, it is complications of immunosuppression, infection in particular, that accounts for the highest mortality. In patients treated with cyclosporine, the percentage of mortality due to infection increases from 20 percent at 30 days to 29 percent at 60 days, and eventually accounts for about 40 percent of the mortality in the registry. Death due to rejection remains relatively stable throughout at 20 to 25 percent.

Infectious complications in cardiac transplant recipients are most often pulmonary. Opportunistic pathogens predominate, and include *Pneumocystis carinii, Cytomegalovirus, Legionella,* and fungi. Antibacterial and antifungal agents will control most infections if the level of immunosuppression can be tightly controlled.

Most chronic complications can also be viewed as consequences of immunosuppression. Slowly progressive renal insufficiency and hypertension are still common in patients on long-term cyclosporine, although it appears that tighter control of dosage will arrest the problem. Malignancies occur in 2 to 5 percent of patients, and have a spectrum of pathology characteristic of immunosuppressed patients.

Lymphoma, especially non-Hodgkin's lymphoma, Kaposi's sarcoma, and other relatively unusual neoplasms predominate. Problems related to regulatory physiology in a denervated heart, which were the subject of much speculation and experimental modeling in the early years, do not appear to be major. The adaptive mechanisms are incompletely understood, and probably involve a combination of humoral control and receptor regulation. By whatever mechanism, the autoregulation of cardiac output is remarkably well preserved after cardiac transplantation.

One unfortunate consequence of denervation is that angina cannot occur as a premonitory symptom in patients developing graft atherosclerosis, so that these patients tend to present with sudden death or congestive heart failure. The coronary atherosclerosis seen in cardiac transplants is characteristically diffuse and progressive, frequently occurring in the first 1 to 2 years, with an incidence of about 10 percent. The leading suspicion regarding etiology is that the phenomenon reflects chronic low-grade rejection that is poorly detected by conventional means, and raises concern that the incidence may continue to increase. Every large series by now contains several patients who have required retransplantation for this problem.

The most impressive results are those measured by functional status. In Stanford's first 106 patients, 97 percent were restored to NYHA Class I existence. Assessments of employment status are complicated by the fact that many patients were originally students or housewives, but if return to a previous life-style is used as the criterion, 82 percent of the Stanford series did so. At Columbia Presbyterian, 62 percent of patients have returned to their previous life-style after 6 months, a figure that rises to 100 percent after 2 years.

Cardiac transplantation is now a well-established therapy for end-stage heart failure, but progress is needed in several areas. Age limits are being stretched in both directions. As yet there is no evidence to substantiate the intuitive notion that results in older patients will be less satisfactory, but only small numbers are available for analysis at present. At the other end of the spectrum, results in infants and children have been disappointing, with 1-year survival of only 49 percent in the 0- to 10-year age group recorded in the registry. Although the management of immunosuppression in infants and small children has proved to be very difficult, progress is anticipated with experience.

Endomyocardial biopsy is a reliable method for monitoring rejection, but it remains an invasive procedure with measurable risks. Noninvasive methods for the diagnosis of rejection are the focus of intensive research activity in echocardiography, nuclear scanning, magnetic resonance imaging, and labeled antimyosin monoclonal antibody, to name a few.

The most imposing problem of all is the rapid increase in demand for the procedure in the face of a limited inventory of replacement parts. The efficiency of human donor procurement efforts is increasing steadily but will inevitably lag behind, especially if age criteria are relaxed substantially. Use of the artificial heart as permanent replacement may regain popularity if the trend continues, and if use of the artificial heart as a temporary bridge to transplant continues to have encouraging results. Another alternative is the use of nonhuman donors (xenografts), which has received scant attention in the past but gained sudden notoriety recently when Bailey transplanted a baboon heart into a human infant with hypoplastic left heart syndrome. The child survived 20 days. In a heterotopic primate model recently developed at Columbia Presbyterian, 12-fold improvement in survival over controls was obtained with conventional (cyclosporine and steroid) immunosuppression. If success is achieved in the orthotopic position, it is hoped that chimpanzees and other species could be used to expand the donor pool.

Heterotopic Transplantation

In heterotopic transplantation, the donor heart is placed in parallel in the circulation. Experimentally this has been done in both sides of the thorax, in the abdomen, the neck, and the inguinal region. Clinically, it is placed in the right chest, with separate left atrial, right atrial, aortic, and pulmonary arterial anastomoses (Fig. 10-32). Advocates of the procedure have cited the advantage of having the native heart in place during severe rejection episodes, and the advantage of using donors smaller than could be used in the orthotopic position. Results obtained to date in the heterotopic position do not support wide application of this approach. The largest series in the world is at the Groote Schuur Hospital in South Africa, and a recent report (May 1986) documented a disappointing 55 percent 1-year survival and 22 percent 5-year survival in 49 patients. The authors currently recommend heterotopic transplantation only for certain conditions: patients with pulmonary vascular resistance too

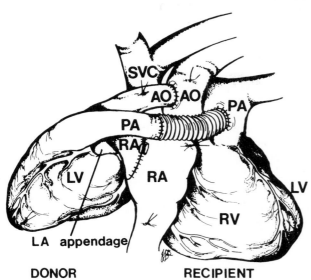

DONOR   **RECIPIENT**

Fig. 10-32. A completed heterotopic cardiac transplant. The donor aorta (AO) crosses over the superior vena cava (SVC) and is anastomosed end-to-side to the recipient aorta. The donor pulmonary artery (PA) reaches the recipient PA by adding a segment of Dacron tube graft. The right atrial (RA) anastomosis lies partially obscured by the PA. The left atrial anastomosis, performed first because it is most posterior, is not visible, although the left atrial appendage can be seen (LA appendage). The procedure is performed on total cardiopulmonary bypass with aortic and bicaval cannulation. (From: *Novitzky D, Cooper DKC, et al: The surgical technique of heterotopic heart transplantation. Ann Thor Surg 36:476–482, 1983, with permission.*)

high for orthotopic transplantation, and patients whose critical condition demands use of a donor heart too small to be used orthotopically.

HEART-LUNG

The first successful human heart-lung transplant was performed by Reitz in 1981, following several years of work in the laboratory at Stanford spent developing the method in a primate model. Three previous attempts in human beings, in 1968 (Cooley), 1969 (Lillihei), and 1971 (Barnard) were all early failures. Reitz's first patient was a woman with primary pulmonary hypertension who was leading a virtually normal life until her death due to unrelated causes.

SPECTRUM OF DISEASE. Patients who might benefit from heart-lung transplant have suffered irreversible damage to both the heart and lungs. Such patients can be divided into two groups—those with pulmonary vascular disease and those with respiratory disease. In pulmonary vascular diseases the high-resistance circulatory disorder is primary, while in respiratory diseases chronic disturbance in gas exchange and alveolar mechanics leads to a secondary increase in pulmonary vascular resistance. Even though both pathways end in right ventricular failure, there is therapeutic relevance in this distinction. Pulmonary vascular diseases reach end stage with no signifi-

cant tracheobronchial or alveolar abnormalities, and with no effect on chest wall mechanics, so that the entire disease process is removed at transplant. By contrast, respiratory diseases reach a cardiac end stage after years of worsening ventilatory mechanics, so that heart-lung transplant still leaves behind an older, nutritionally depleted patient with chronically infected secretions and distorted thoracic anatomy, with attenuated diaphragmatic and intercostal musculature. The results of heart-lung transplant have been very poor when performed for respiratory disease, although the total numbers are still small.

RECIPIENT SELECTION. The cardinal fact guiding selection of candidates for heart-lung transplant is the rarity of suitable donors, which makes it mandatory to select only patients with the greatest probability of a good outcome. Results have been best in young patients with end-stage primary pulmonary hypertension (PPH) or Eisenmenger's syndrome. In patients thought to have PPH it is important to exclude chronic pulmonary thromboembolism, both because of concern about recurrence after transplant, and because certain patients with thromboembolic occlusion of both pulmonary arteries can benefit from pulmonary thromboendarterectomy. In such cases there is no reliable substitute for pulmonary angiography, although magnetic resonance imaging is promising.

In patients with Eisenmenger's syndrome correctable lesions that may have been overlooked should be excluded, and any previous history of cardiothoracic operation carefully reviewed. Based on the limited experience accumulated to date, patients who have had previous operations have had nearly insurmountable bleeding problems, with operative mortality greater than 50 percent. The problem tends to be particularly severe in Eisenmenger's patients with primary cyanotic lesions, who usually have large systemic-pulmonary collaterals throughout the mediastinum, and form highly vascular adhesions. History of a previous cardiothoracic operation is very nearly an absolute contraindication to heart-lung transplant in 1987.

DONOR SELECTION. In addition to the familiar criteria for a satisfactory cardiac donor, heart-lung donors must have a clear chest x-ray, normal gas exchange, and clean tracheobronchial secretions (Table 10-11). The lungs tend to deteriorate quickly in most patients with brain death. Even if neurogenic pulmonary edema or contusion from blunt trauma are absent, the lungs remain susceptible to the insults of mechanical ventilation and airway colonization with nosocomial pathogens. It is also important to

Table 10-11. CRITERIA FOR A SATISFACTORY HEART-LUNG DONOR

1. Satisfactory heart donor
2. Clear chest x-ray
3. Normal gas exchange ($P_{O_2} > 90$ torr with $F_{I_{O_2}} \geq 40\%$, PEEP ≥ 5 cm)
4. Clean secretions (no more than a few colonizing organisms)
5. Close size match

have a close size match between the donor lungs and the recipient thorax, to avoid chronic basal atelectasis and infection when the lungs are too large, and to avoid large pleural effusions when the lungs are too small. After using height and weight as a rough guide, thoracic dimensions are carefully compared by overlapping comparable donor and recipient chest x-rays. Ideally, the overlap should be a centimeter or less in all dimensions.

DONOR OPERATION. Techniques for preservation of the heart and lungs have been very slow to develop, and dependence on the cumbersome transfer of an intact donor from another hospital to an adjacent operating room has greatly retarded the growth rate of the procedure. Methods for preservation that would allow distant procurement remain somewhat controversial. Cooling on cardiopulmonary bypass, cooling with pulmonary artery perfusion, topical hypothermia alone, and preservation in an autoperfusion apparatus all have advocates. A method developed at Stanford, attractive in its relative simplicity, has been used very recently and successfully for distant procurement in two patients at Stanford, two patients at the University of Pittsburgh, and one patient at Columbia Presbyterian, with ischemic times ranging up to 4 h and 45 min. The technique consists of high-volume pulmonary artery flush with modified Collin's solution at 4°C, preceded by pulmonary vasodilation with a prostaglandin E-1 infusion, and standard cardioplegic arrest of the

heart. The technique seems to offer great hope for the future.

The heart and lungs can be removed from the donor through a median sternotomy or a bilateral anterior thoracotomy, which is preferred by Hardesty and Griffith. The anterior contents of the mediastinum are removed, and the major structures isolated. Heparin is given. Whatever method of lung preservation is to be used is begun, the aorta is clamped just proximal to the innominate artery, and the heart is arrested with cardioplegia. The trachea is divided several rings above the carina after clamping distally with the lungs partially inflated, and the organs are dissected free of their posterior mediastinal attachments, taking care to achieve hemostasis on the organ block. The organs are immersed in cold saline for transport.

RECIPIENT OPERATION. The recipient operation is performed through a median sternotomy. Both pleural cavities are entered. Both phrenic nerves are dissected free on pedicles of pericardium from the diaphragms to a point just above the pulmonary arteries. The trachea is exposed deep to the aorta and just superior to the pulmonary artery bifurcation, where it will later be divided just above the carina. The patient is placed on cardiopulmonary bypass with moderate systemic hypothermia, using aortic and bicaval cannulation, the heart is excised, leaving the posterior aspects of both atria, and the great vessels are divided at their commissures (Figs. 10-33 and 10-34).

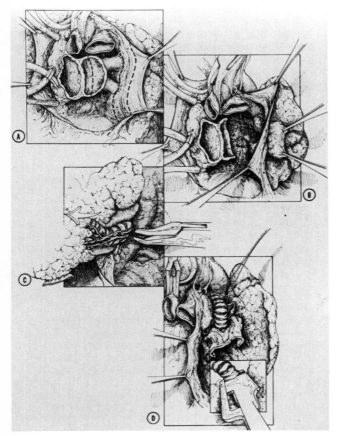

Fig. 10-33. *A.* The recipient atria after removal of the heart. Incisions are made so as to preserve the phrenic nerve in a "ribbon" of pericardium. The left and right pulmonary veins are separated by a longitudinal incision in the posterior left atrial wall and thus into the oblique sinus. *B.* The left pulmonary veins are withdrawn beneath the phrenic nerve. The vagus nerve is immediately posterior. *C.* The left lung is progressively mobilized, and the bronchial arteries are secured. *D.* The left pulmonary artery is divided and the bronchus is stapled and cut. (Copyright B. Hyams.) (From: *Jamieson, Stinson, et al, with permission.*)

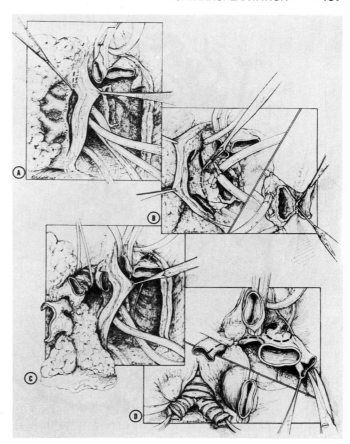

Fig. 10-34. *A.* The right phrenic nerve is separated from the hilum. *B.* The right pulmonary veins are separated from the right atrium. *C.* The right pulmonary ligament is divided, the lung is mobilized, and the pulmonary artery and bronchus are cut. *D.* The remnants of the pulmonary artery are removed, leaving the area around the ductus ligament and recurrent nerve. The trachea and bronchial remnants are exposed to the right of the aorta. The trachea is cut just above the carina. (Copyright B. Hyams.) (From: *Jamieson, Stinson, et al, with permission.*)

Removing the heart improves exposure for the difficult posterior hilar and mediastinal dissection that follows. The two lungs are excised separately along with the left atrium. Both cavae are mobilized to provide room for the new right lung to pass under the right atrium. The atrial septum becomes the posterior free wall of the new atrium; so a patent foramen or ASD must be closed securely. Any remaining pulmonary artery is removed, leaving a small patch containing the ligamentum arteriosum so that injury to the recurrent nerve can be avoided. The recipient trachea is divided just above the carina, the new organ block is brought onto the field, and the donor trachea is divided just above the carina. Implantation begins with anastomosis of the trachea, usually with a simple continuous suture, followed by right atrial and aortic anastomoses. The lungs are passed under each phrenic pedicle, with the right lung passing under the right atrium as well (Fig. 10-35).

The technical keys to operation are hemostasis in the middle mediastinum and protection of both phrenic nerves, both vagus nerves, and the recurrent nerve. Hemostasis can be very difficult to achieve, especially in patients with large bronchial collateral vessels. Postoperative bleeding has been a major problem, one that can begin a vicious cycle of massive transfusion and deteriorating pulmonary function. Paralyzed diaphragms and gastric dilatation can contribute to difficulties maintaining lung expansion. Pyloroplasty has been required in at least two patients.

POSTOPERATIVE CARE. The early postoperative challenge is to maintain full lung expansion and good gas exchange. Before and after extubation tracheobronchial secretions are managed with bronchoscopy and vigorous pulmonary toilet. Pleural effusions are common and can interfere with lung expansion; they are managed with thoracentesis or tube thoracostomy. During the first 2 weeks, before lymphatic drainage is reestablished and ischemic injury has healed, the lungs are kept as dry as possible with vigorous diuresis.

Immunosuppression is modified by problems unique to the lungs. Because steroid administration is known to impair bronchial healing, tracheal healing is carefully protected by withholding maintenance steroids for 2 to 3 weeks. Maintenance cyclosporine treatment is augmented during that period with azathioprine, and frequently with antithymocyte globulin as well. Steroid treatment for rejection is not withheld if indicated.

A greater problem is that diagnosis of rejection in the lungs is very difficult, and surveillance for cardiac rejection with endomyocardial biopsies cannot be relied upon to faithfully mirror activity in the lungs. Diagnosis of lung rejection is still a complex clinical judgment in most

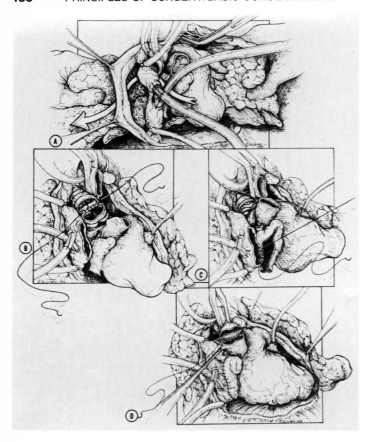

Fig. 10-35. Reimplantation: *A.* The right lung passes beneath the right atrial remnant and the phrenic nerve. *B.* The tracheal anastomosis is performed first, commencing with the posterior wall. *C.* The right atrial anastomosis. *D.* The aortic anastomosis. (Copyright B. Hyams.) (From: *Jamieson, Stinson, et al, with permission.*)

cases, based on an intuitive synthesis of evidence provided by arterial blood gases, chest x-rays, bronchoscopy, and airway cultures. At present, the more sophisticated methods brought to bear, such as bronchoalveolar lavage and labeled leukocyte scanning, can differentiate normal from abnormal but fail to make the crucial distinction between infection and rejection.

If fever, tachycardia, diffuse pulmonary infiltrates, and worsening oxygenation occur, the tracheobronchial tree is aggressively cultured, and an endomyocardial biopsy is obtained. If the cardiac biopsy and the cultures are negative, a trial course of intravenous methylprednisolone (1 g/day for 3 days) may be given, anticipating prompt improvement if the presumptive diagnosis of isolated pulmonary rejection is correct. If the response is inadequate and infection is still securely excluded, a course of antithymocyte globulin can be given. The most difficult distinction to make is between viral pneumonia and rejection, which can be clinically indistinguishable. Because viral pneumonia will become rapidly progressive when treated as rejection, it is necessary on occasion to resort to open lung biopsy in ambiguous situations. In the first few postoperative weeks it can be equally difficult to distinguish rejection from early ischemic/edematous changes, although the consequence of error is not quite as great.

Routine surveillance for cardiac rejection is carried out with endomyocardial biopsy on a regular basis, and cardiac rejection is treated with steroids and/or antithymocyte globulin. A curious feature of heart-lung transplantation is that cardiac rejection is seen with much lower frequency than in cardiac transplantation ($p < 0.01$).

RESULTS. In early 1986, with just 91 cases recorded in the Registry of the International Society for Heart Transplantation, 1-year survival was a rather disappointing 54 percent. On the other hand, the 3-year actuarial survival of 51 percent provides some reason for optimism, implying that the survival curve will remain quite flat. As with cardiac transplantation, the mortality is skewed heavily toward the early postoperative period, and survival in the first year should improve with experience. Patients who have done well have shown remarkable functional improvement comparable with that seen in cardiac transplant patients. The first 10 survivors in the Stanford series were restudied at an average of almost 2 years postoperatively, and were found to have essentially normal pulmonary function.

Some caution is still warranted because of the frequency with which bronchiolitis obliterans is being observed in late survivors. Obliterative bronchiolitis was detectable in half of Stanford's first 20 long-term survivors at a mean of 11 months, with similar experience beginning to emerge from other series. Mortality has been 30 to 50 percent with at least half the remainder demonstrating significant functional impairment. Retransplant has been successfully performed once at Stanford and once in England. The cause of bronchiolitis obliterans is not known. Opinion divides between those who believe the cause to be chronic inadequately treated rejection, and those who suspect a relationship to chronic infection, especially with *Pneumocystis*. The latter theory is supported by the high frequency of *Pneumocystis* colonization in survivors.

It is fair to conclude that heart-lung transplant offers an excellent therapeutic alternative in certain diseases for which no other treatment exists, but long-term durability remains uncertain, and the procedure is likely to remain a therapeutic frontier for the rest of the decade.

SINGLE LUNG

The first human lung transplant was performed in 1963, and was followed by more than 45 attempts around the world during the next 20 years, without a single long-term success. Average survival was less than 10 days. Bronchial healing seemed to pose an insolvable problem, since dehiscence of the bronchial anastomosis was a lethal complication seen in almost every patient surviving more than 7 days. The focus of effort shifted to the laboratory, where Cooper and other members of the Toronto Lung Transplant Group confirmed that steroids markedly inhibited bronchial healing, while cyclosporine and azathioprine did not. Directing their attention to the tenuous vascularity of bronchial anastomoses, the group found that placement of a pedicled omental wrap around the anastomosis restored systemic blood supply to the site within 4 days. Patient selection criteria also underwent refinement as it was recognized that single lung transplantation in patients with emphysema set the stage for major ventilation/perfusion mismatch, because of preferential ventilation and air trapping in the highly compliant native lung at the same time that perfusion was directed almost exclusively to the low compliance vascular bed of the transplanted lung.

Applying the lessons learned in their laboratory, the group in Toronto performed a successful single lung transplant in 1983 in a fifty-eight-year-old man with idiopathic pulmonary fibrosis. That patient returned to work in 3 months, and in 1986 had no difficulty tolerating emergency resection of a leaking abdominal aortic aneurysm. By the end of 1986 seven single lung transplants had been performed in Toronto with five long-term survivors, all demonstrating similar outstanding improvement in their quality of life. The criteria used to select recipients were highly restrictive, and their initial experience focused entirely on patients with pulmonary fibrosis, avoiding patients with emphysema and cystic fibrosis. All patients had to be weaned from steroids before transplant, and all had reasonably well preserved right ventricular function.

The procedures were done through a posterolateral thoracotomy, with a pulmonary artery anastomosis, a broad left atrial cuff anastomosis for pulmonary venous drainage, and a bronchial anastomosis reinforced with a pedicled omental wrap (Fig. 10-36). Heparinization and

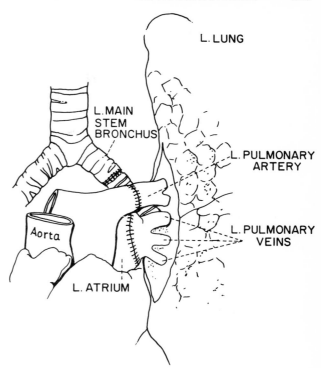

Fig. 10-36. Technique for single lung transplantation, left lung. A cuff of left atrium remains at the confluence of the donor pulmonary veins, so that the anastomosis can be made through the wall of the left atrial cuff rather than through each individual pulmonary vein. After completion of the anastomoses, omentum is brought into the pleural space and circumferentially wrapped around the bronchial anastomosis (not shown).

cardiopulmonary bypass were required in only one case. The left lung was transplanted in most cases, because the mobility of the left diaphragm allowed implantation of an oversized lung. Maintenance steroids were withheld for 3 weeks, although numerous intravenous doses of methylprednisolone were given in each case when a clinical diagnosis of rejection was made. Cyclosporine, azathioprine, and antilymphocyte globulin (ALG) were used initially for immunosuppression, discontinuing the ALG after 5 to 7 days. Perfusion lung scans appeared to be useful in the diagnosis of rejection, demonstrating a shift in perfusion away from the transplanted lung, presumably a reflection of increased pulmonary vascular resistance during rejection.

The results in Toronto are being followed internationally with great interest, and it is likely that the latter half of the 1980s will see a burst of activity in clinical single lung transplantation. It is not clear that the procedure can be extended to patients falling outside the highly selective criteria applied successfully in Toronto. It still appears that patients with end-stage pulmonary disease who have significant right ventricular failure will be operable only with combined heart-lung transplant, which requires extension of that procedure into a patient group in which results to date have been uniformly disappointing. Patients with preserved right ventricular function but with obstructive or septic bilateral pulmonary disease present additional problems. This category is potentially quite large, containing many patients with emphysema and cystic fibrosis, but single lung transplant would appear to be unsuitable because of the potential for ventilation-perfusion mismatching, and the risk of septic contamination of the transplanted lung. Double lung transplantation may prove suitable for such patients. During 1986 one such procedure was performed at Toronto, and three were performed in England, with encouraging early results.

Transplantation for pulmonary disease is still in an exciting embryonic stage that can be expected to demonstrate considerable differentiation during the next several years. The procedure will need to be tailored specifically to the underlying disease process. At present it appears that patients with preserved right ventricular function should receive a single lung transplant for pulmonary fibrosis, and double lung transplant for obstructive and septic diseases. Heart-lung transplant should be reserved for patients with pulmonary vascular disease, and possibly for selected patients with nonvascular pulmonary disease and significant right ventricular failure.

Kidney

The technical knowledge necessary to perform kidney transplants has been available since the turn of the century, when Carrel and Guthrie developed the techniques of vascular suture. Renal transplantation is now the treatment of choice for many patients with renal failure, although hemodialysis and peritoneal dialysis serve as an adequate substitute for most patients.

INDICATIONS AND CONTRAINDICATIONS. The precise indications for the selection of recipients of renal allotransplants have never been defined. In general, irreversible renal failure is the only indication necessary for the patient with a normal urinary outflow tract and without active infection, severe malnutrition, disseminated malignancy, or life-limiting systemic disease. Lower tract abnormalities can usually be corrected. The only absolute contraindications are active infection or malignant disease that cannot be brought under control. A partial list of diseases for which transplantation has been carried out is included in Table 10-12.

Transplantation, when successful, offers a greater degree of rehabilitation to the uremic patient than does either hemodialysis or peritoneal dialysis. The risks are also slightly greater because immunosuppression is required for the duration of graft function. Rigid guidelines that dictate certain therapies for individual patients have not been established. In general, however, children should be transplanted because growth is better after transplantation. Diabetics seem to have fewer problems after transplantation than during dialysis. Older patients without related donors, however, may survive longer on hemodialysis. All patients with HLA-identical sibling donors should certainly be transplanted. In other groups of patients, the indications are less clear, and the preference of the individual is the dominant factor. Most patients who have had a transplant—even one that has

Table 10-12. INDICATIONS FOR RENAL TRANSPLANTATION

Irreversible chronic renal failure	Irreversible acute failure
Chronic pyelonephritis	Cortical necrosis
Chronic glomerulonephritis	Hemolytic uremic syndrome
Diabetic nephropathy	Acute and subacute glomerulonephritis
Goodpasture's disease	Anaphylactoid purpura (Henoch–Schönlein)
Hypocomplementemic nephritis	Acute tubular necrosis
Steroid-resistant nephrotic syndrome	Trauma requiring nephrectomy
Hypertensive nephrosclerosis	Renal vascular diseases
Obstructive uropathy	Renal artery occlusion
Acquired	Renal vein thrombosis
Congenital	Tumors requiring nephrectomy
Congenital disorders	Renal carcinoma
Aplasia	Wilms' tumor
Hypoplasia	Tuberous sclerosis
Horseshoe kidney	Other
Hereditary nephropathies	Multiple myeloma
Alport's syndrome	Macroglobulinemia
Polycystic kidney disease	Wegner's disease
Medullary cystic disease	Scleroderma
Metabolic disorders	Lupus erythematosus
Hyperoxaluria	Polyarteritis (periarteritis nodosa)
Nephrocalcinosis	
Gout	
Oxalosis	
Amyloidosis	
Cystinosis	

Modified from Simmons RL, Ascher NL, Najarian JS: Host hepatectomy and liver transplantation, in Simmons RL, Finch ME, Ascher NL, Najarian JS (eds): *Manual of Vascular Access, Organ Donation, and Transplantation.* New York, Springer-Verlag, 1984, pp 255–284.

failed—prefer life with a kidney transplantation to life on dialysis.

A few renal diseases will recur in transplants but such diseases are only relative contraindications; foral glomerulosclerosis, hemolytic uremia syndrome, membranoproliferative glomerulonephritis of the dense-deposit type, and diabetes are among them.

A number of metabolic diseases (gout, oxalosis, cystinosis, hyperoxaluria, nephrocalcinosis, and amyloidosis) have very little in common except for the accumulation within the kidney of abnormal deposits associated with renal failure. Transplants in most of these diseases can be successful, although recurrence after oxalosis is common.

The psychologic disturbances exhibited by some patients with chronic renal failure are not contraindications to selection. It is extremely difficult to judge the psychologic and social stability of a patient with chronic illness. Similarly, one cannot exclude, out of hand, patients with coronary disease or cerebrovascular accidents. Patients with severe liver disease, however, are more susceptible to cyclosporine or azathioprine toxicity and sepsis. Liver disease, therefore, remains a relative contraindication.

More important than the actual selection technique of the potential recipient is the choice of time for the institution of treatment by dialysis or transplantation. Treatment by either technique should always be instituted prior to the development of uremic complications. Once hypertension, pericarditis, cardiac failure, severe anemia, and neuropathy appear, management is markedly complicated and rehabilitation compromised. Ideally, the conservative management of patients treated for progressive renal functional deterioration should be carried out in conjunction with nephrologists associated with both dialysis and transplant centers. In this way, the complication of severe uremia can be rapidly prevented by treatment without the delays inherent in the referral process.

The traditional indication for the institution of dialysis has been a serum creatinine level greater than 15 mg/dL or a creatinine clearance less than 3 mL/min despite meticulous conservative care. It is obvious that there are exceptions to this rule. Some patients, particularly patients with polycystic kidney disease, with serum creatinine levels greater than 15 mg/dL can be maintained well for months on dietary management. In other patients, especially diabetic patients, severe complications of uremia will develop long before the serum creatinine reaches that level. The most pernicious of these complications is peripheral neuropathy. If there are signs of motor involvement, the patient should have dialysis and transplantation without delay, since very rapid progression of the disease can make it impossible ever to rehabilitate such a patient. Another indication for early dialysis-transplantation is uncontrollable hypertension, or hypertension that can be controlled only at the expense of severe orthostatic hypotension and other side effects. Severe anemia with anemic symptoms (dyspnea at the mildest exertion), severe bone disease (especially in children), and the failure of the patient to maintain a diet or carry on social and family obligations all should lead to early dialysis and transplantation. There is little to be gained by a delay of 3 to 6 months, and lives may be lost in futile attempts at conservative management.

Since some of the complications of uremia may appear suddenly during conservative management, it is extremely important that the patient be fully evaluated as early in the course of progressive uremia as possible. In addition to the medical evaluation, this preparation should include interviews with the hospital, the rehabilitation clinic, and social service in order to ameliorate the financial and social difficulties that may accompany dialysis and transplantation. Rehabilitation of the patient can be actively pursued even prior to the institution of definitive treatment.

Although most patients with end-stage renal disease will undergo a period of dialysis prior to transplant, many patients who are carefully followed for progressive uremia can be transplanted without dialysis. In this way, the number of vascular or peritoneal access procedures necessary for dialysis can be reduced and care can be rendered more economically.

PREPARATION FOR TRANSPLANTATION. The pretransplantation studies are listed in Table 10-13. Most of these studies are used by many transplant groups and for patients on dialysis. A few deserve elaboration.

The urinary tract should be evaluated for patency of its outflow and absence of ureterovesical reflux. In general, a voiding cystogram suffices. That test makes it possible to determine that the urethra is unobstructed, that the bladder empties, that there are no abnormalities of the bladder wall, and that there is no ureteral reflux. It is almost impossible to evaluate bladder emptying in the presence of ureterovesical reflux. Contraction of the bladder wall leads to reflux of the urine into the ureters, which then empty back into the bladder when the bladder wall is relaxed. It may be necessary to remove both ureters at the ureterovesical junction prior to evaluation of the bladder for competence.

The upper gastrointestinal tract should be evaluated for the possibility of a preexisting peptic ulceration. Pretransplant treatment regimens have almost completely eliminated upper gastrointestinal tract bleeding as a complication of steroid administration after transplant.

Because so many patients with uremia also have hearing deficits, periodic audiograms should be carried out.

Tissue Typing and Cross Matching. The principles of transplantation immunogenetics have been presented in detail above. Prior to transplantation, tissue typing to match donor and recipient should be carried out—both for the selection for the most appropriate donor and for the determination of the prognostic implications of tissue matching. It is possible at present to type most patients completely at the HLA-A, -B, and -D/DR loci (Table 10-1). This is extremely valuable in family donor selection because HLA identity between siblings occurs 25 percent of the time. Transplants between such perfectly matched siblings have long-term success rates of 95 percent. There is controversy whether matching unrelated cadaver donors with recipients will have beneficial consequences for the outcome of renal transplantation. Whatever the con-

Table 10-13. WORK-UP OF POTENTIAL
RECIPIENTS OF RENAL TRANSPLANTATION

1. General
   a. History and physical examination
   b. Chest x-ray
   c. ECG
   d. Electrophoresis
   e. Fasting blood sugar
2. Hematologic
   a. Hemoglobin
   b. Leukocyte count and differential count
   c. Platelet count
   d. Bleeding-clotting time
   e. Prothrombin time, partial thromboplastin time, thrombin time
3. Renal
   a. Flat plate of abdomen (kidney size) (tomography)
   b. Creatinine clearance
   c. 24-H protein excretion
   d. (Electrophoresis/urine, protein excretion selectivity)
   e. Electrolyte status in blood
   f. (Electrolyte status in urine)
   g. Urinalysis ×3
   h. Urine culture ×3
   i. (Renal biopsy)
4. Signs of hyperparathyroidism
   a. Bone x-ray (hands, skull, clavicle, lamina dura)
   b. Ca, PO_4, Mg, alkaline phosphatase
5. Hypertensive work-up
   a. Chest x-ray (heart size)
   b. ECG
   c. Ophthalmic examination
   d. Serial blood pressure
6. Urologic evaluation
   a. Voiding cystogram
   b. (Retrograde pyelography)
   c. (Cystometrography)
   d. (Bladder biopsy)
   e. (Bladder stimulation)
7. Upper gastrointestinal x-ray, cholecystogram (colon x-ray in older patients)
8. Pap smear
9. Dental consultation and correction of any infectious problem
10. Typing
    a. ABO
    b. Blood pedigree
    c. Tissue typing including serial cytotoxic antibody determinations
11. (Pulmonary function studies)
12. Infectious work-up
    a. Chest x-ray
    b. Urine culture
    c. Blood culture
    d. (Sinus-teeth x-ray; ear, nose, and throat consultation)
13. Financial-social rehabilitation
    a. (Psychologic-psychiatric)

NOTE: The tests listed within parentheses are not administered routinely during the potential recipient work-up, but only when the circumstances so indicate.

troversies about matching, it is important to determine whether a putative recipient has antibodies against antigens on donor tissue. Patients who have been presensitized by blood transfusion, pregnancy, or previous transplantation can then be identified by serum reactivity against a panel of normal leukocytes bearing known HLA specificities.

Because many patients have preformed antibodies against a potential renal allograft donor, cross matching of the patient's serum to detect antibodies against donor leukocytes must be carried out immediately prior to the transplant. If these preformed antibody barriers are crossed, immediate (hyperacute) or accelerated rejection frequently ensues. Varying cross-matching techniques have varying degrees of sensitivity, and the most sensitive method should be utilized. Organ preservation techniques currently permit prolonged storage of kidneys (up to 48 and frequently 72 h) so that cross-matching techniques that take several hours can always precede transplantation.

Most transplant units draw serum samples monthly on all patients awaiting transplantation in order to detect the formation of antidonor antibodies. The use of several of these sera for final cross matching should always be performed, since antibodies appear and disappear without apparent reason in recipients. Nevertheless, if a patient has previously made antibodies against the putative donor, it is likely that an accelerated rejection will occur and that that donor should not be utilized.

Transfusion. For many years blood transfusions to prospective transplant recipients were avoided as much as possible. Physicians recognized that sensitization to the histocompatibility antigens of the blood donor would occur and that cross matching of the donor kidney to the transfused recipient would be more difficult. Paradoxically, most data now agree that transplants to transfused patients are much more successful than transplants to the untransfused. The reason is not clear, but much data support the idea that a degree of specific immunologic nonreactivity may be induced to the transfused histocompatibility antigens. Whatever the reason, most transplant centers permit transfusions as needed for the uremic patient awaiting transplantation. Some centers perform deliberate transfusions from either the prospective related donor or from random donors. In practice, an immunosuppressive drug (azathioprine or cyclosporine) is often administered during pretransplant transfusions to minimize sensitization and maximize the development of tolerance.

Dialysis. Dialysis is not an essential preparation for all transplant patients, but most patients do require a period of dialysis because of preexistent uremia. Dialysis removes toxic products of small molecular size from the blood and reinstitutes acid-base balance and electrolyte homeostasis. Although such treatment will not relieve all the complications of uremia, it will prevent death in most cases. In hemodialysis, blood is passed through a tubing composed of a semipermeable membrane, so that dialyzable substances within the blood pass into the dialysis bath and dialyzable materials within the bath pass into the blood. Peritoneal dialysis uses the peritoneum as the semipermeable membrane, and the peritoneal cavity as the container of the dialysis bath.

Vascular Access for Hemodialysis. The Quinton–Scribner cannula was the instrument first widely used for access to

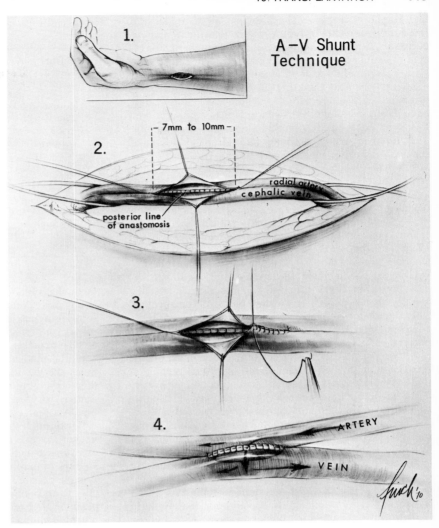

1.

A–V Shunt Technique

2.

– 7mm to 10mm –

radial artery
cephalic vein

posterior line of anastomosis

3.

4.

ARTERY

VEIN

Fig. 10-37. Technique for constructing an arteriovenous anastomosis between radial artery and cephalic vein at the wrist. [From: *Kjellstrand CM, Simmons RL, et al: Kidney: I. Recipient selection, medical management, and dialysis, in Najarian JS, Simmons RL (eds): Transplantation. Philadelphia, Lea & Febiger, 1972, p 148, with permission.*]

blood in dialysis. This technique used cannulation of an artery and a vein with an external arteriovenous shunt. The persistence of the cannulae within the vessels and the subsequent passage through the skin had predictable consequences—the cannulae clotted, the cutaneous fistulas became infected, and the shunt was in danger of bleeding. Similar problems occur when long-term subclavian vein cannulation is used for vascular access, but such external systems using intravascular cannulation are still very useful for short-term hemodialysis.

For prolonged vascular access without prosthetic implants the best technique uses a subcutaneous arteriovenous fistula, usually constructed between the radial artery and the cephalic vein at the wrist (Fig. 10-37). The superficial veins become dilated, and blood can be ob-

tained for passage through the dialyzer by the use of two large-bore needles inserted into the dilated venous system.

Many modifications of these fistulas have been devised that utilize vascular or prosthetic grafts to bridge gaps between artery and vein, but all provide a dilated subcutaneous vessel for repeated puncture with large-bore needles.

Peritoneal dialysis is a useful but less efficient alternative. The dialysis fluid is alternately infused into the peritoneal cavity and drained off. This technique requires the permanent implantation of a catheter through the abdominal wall. The catheter is capped when not in use. Peritoneal dialysis is most useful for children, and its principal disadvantage is a high incidence of bacterial peritonitis. Although even repeated peritoneal infections are rarely fatal, they render the dialysis treatment increasingly inefficient.

Dialysis as a definitive treatment for end-stage renal failure is a lifesaving, effective treatment for both short-

and long-term therapy. The principal disadvantages are the energy-consuming nature of the treatment that requires a continuous commitment of the patient and physician to details of daily care. For this reason, transplantation, if successful, is preferable for younger patients.

SELECTION AND EVALUATION OF LIVING DONOR. The principles of histocompatibility typing and matching have been described above. From the recipient's point of view it is generally preferable that the donor be a biologic relative. Even mismatched sibling and parent kidneys may survive with better function and for more prolonged periods than do closely matched cadaver kidneys. Before the advent of histocompatibility typing, it was shown that kidneys from sibling donors functioned better than kidneys from parental donors. Because the genes governing the expression of histocompatibility antigens are situated at one (complex) locus, there will always be one major allelic difference between the parent and the offspring, whereas one-fourth of siblings will be identical, one-half will have a one haplotype difference, and one-fourth will have both haplotypes different. Tissue typing can usually identify that sibling (if any) who shares all the serologically detectable antigens at the major histocompatibility complex (MHC). Such sibling grafts have a better than 95 percent chance for long-term success.

A living related donor offers other advantages to the recipient: the delay between renal failure and rehabilitation is shorter, posttransplant renal function is usually immediate, and there are fewer rejection episodes, so that smaller doses of immunosuppressive drugs are required.

The major blood group antigens (ABO) are strong transplantation antigens. Although a number of successful allotransplants have been carried out across isoantibody barriers, it is generally unwise to perform transplants into patients with known preformed isohemagglutinins against the donor blood type. The same rules apply to clinical transplantation that apply to transfusion, i.e., AB is the universal recipient and O the universal donor. When such blood type barriers are crossed, the most violent type of hyperacute rejection reaction may occur. There is some evidence to suggest that Lewis blood group factors (but not Rh, Duffy, Kell) act as histocompatibility antigens.

The living related donor should be in perfect health to minimize any risks inherent in an operation of this magnitude. Rare deaths following renal donation from a healthy person have been reported, and the utmost caution must be exerted not to harm or diminish the renal reserve of a healthy volunteer. Table 10-14 lists the examinations routinely carried out on volunteer related donors.

Ethical Problems. Selection of a related donor is made on the basis of histocompatibility testing when possible; often, however, there is only one volunteer. The ethical and social problems of donor selection have been extensively discussed elsewhere, but brief consideration is pertinent here.

In practice, the recipient should be informed of the risks and benefits of receiving a kidney from a related donor. The recipient knows best which relatives can be approached and which cannot. When a volunteer appears

Table 10-14. PROTOCOL FOR LIVING RELATED DONOR WORK-UP

1. History and physical examination.
2. Hematology: hematocrit, leukocyte count, differential count, platelet count
3. Coagulation: prothrombin time, partial thromboplastin time, thrombin time
4. Chemistry: serum Na^+, K^+, Cl^-, CO^{2-}, SGOT, bilirubin, uric acid, Ca^{2+}, P, BUN, creatinine, fasting blood sugar, glucose tolerance test
5. Urine: urinalysis, 24-h urine for creatinine clearance
6. Microbiology: clean-catch urine culture $\times 2$
7. Immunology: blood type (major and minor), tissue typing, leukocyte cross match for recipient antidonor and leukocyte antibodies; VDRL; screen for hepatitis
8. X-ray: chest x-ray, intravenous pyelogram (IVP), renal arteriograms
9. Isotope: bilateral renogram
10. Electrocardiogram

he or she is blood-typed and tissue-typed. If the volunteer is acceptable on these grounds, the risk of donor nephrectomy is explained to him or her. The risk to life in an otherwise perfectly healthy patient has been estimated to be 0.05 percent. The long-term risk has been estimated by actuarial statistics to that incurred by driving a car 16 miles every working day. Much evidence suggests that no long-term harm results from life with a single kidney. Although risks are small, the pain, anxiety, and loss of work time are real.

It is difficult to conceive of a living related donor who is not subject to some family pressure to donate. That such pressures exist, however, is evidence that people have feelings of family and role obligations within the society. When a person freely volunteers to donate, both the benefits to the recipient and the risks to the donor are explained. No pressure is exerted to persuade or dissuade potential donors. They are not subjected to extensive psychologic interviews or testing. Careful studies of actual donors indicate a remarkably favorable psychologic response in most donors, but some ambivalence and conflict within the family occur in a minority. On occasion, when the potential donor expresses anxiety concerning the donation, it is necessary to fabricate a medical excuse not to donate that can be used by the otherwise medically and immunologically compatible donor.

Sometimes it is necessary or advisable to use donors under the age of eighteen. This has frequently been necessary for identical-twin transplants. The use of such donors, however, should be restricted to those circumstances in which other donors are not available. A court of law will find it difficult to decide whether an adolescent should donate to parents or siblings when family pressure may exist. Teen-aged donors have been used when they have insisted on donation and the court has agreed to it.

Unrelated persons are not generally encouraged to donate, since the results are no better than those achieved with cadaver donors.

SELECTION OF CADAVER DONOR. The ideal cadaver kidney donor (1) is young, (2) has remained normotensive until a short time before death, (3) is free of transmissible infection and malignant disease, and (4) has died in the hospital after observation for a number of hours, during which time blood group and tissue type have been determined and urinary function has been assessed. Under these ideal conditions the donor kidneys can be removed within minutes to minimize the warm ischemia time. It is often necessary, however, to compromise with these ideal principles. The age of the donor is not of crucial importance but kidneys from young children have decreased survival. A donated kidney can recover from long periods of shock and anuria that occur while it is still in the donor. But not more than 1 h of warm ischemia time should elapse during donation.

Criteria of Brain Death. The procurement of cadaver organs for transplantation has raised some serious moral, ethical, legal, and psychologic problems. The first problem is to establish when death occurs. Since the decision is a clinical one, made by the physician in the interest of the patient (potential donor), it should be based primarily on clinical criteria of irreversible brainstem damage—fixed, dilated pupils; absent reflexes; unresponsiveness to external stimuli; and the inability to maintain vital functions such as respiration, heartbeat, and blood pressure without artificial means. The decision should be made by physicians who are not associated with the potential recipient in any way, either as the referring physician or as a member of the transplant team. The exact criteria vary among institutions. Table 10-15 lists the guidelines for the determination of death reported to the President's Commission for the Study of Ethical Problems in Medicine and Biomedical and Behavioral Research by a panel of medical consultants.

In the past, a falling blood pressure has been used as a criterion of brain death, but this sign is frequently the result of dehydration due to diabetes insipidus. This is aggravated by loss of vasomotor tone, which produces hypotension. Almost all patients with brain death can be maintained for prolonged periods with normal vital signs using plasma and vasopressors; cardiac stimulants are rarely required. Urinary output can likewise be maintained with hydration and diuretics. Even the head-injury patient who has been anuric and in shock for many hours can be restored to hemodynamic stability by restoration of a normal blood volume.

The principles of organ preservation are described in a subsequent section. The advances in organ preservation have alleviated the urgency of cadaver transplantation. It is possible to harvest kidneys at the moment of death and preserve them in iced solutions for more than 24 h until the transplant recipients are ready. Kidneys can now be routinely preserved by hypothermic perfusion for more than 48 h (see subsequent section). The use of machines for this purpose has increased the availability of cadaver kidneys because the kidneys can be transported for long distances. The development of preservation also allows for more careful typing, matching, shipping, and sharing of organs between various centers.

ORGAN HARVEST. Related Living Donor. The actual technique of the donor operation is not as crucial as those

Table 10-15. CRITERIA FOR DETERMINATION OF DEATH

An individual with the findings in either section A (cardiopulmonary) or B (neurologic) is dead.

A. Cardiopulmonary
An individual with irreversible cessation of circulatory and respiratory functions is dead.
  1. Cessation is recognized by an appropriate clinical examination . . . absence of responsiveness, heartbeat, respiratory effort.
  2. Irreversibility is recognized by persistent cessation of functions during an appropriate period of observation and/or trial of therapy.
B. Neurologic
An individual with irreversible cessation of all functions of the entire brain, including the brainstem, is dead.
  1. Cessation is recognized when evaluation discloses findings of *a* and *b*:
     a. Cerebral functions are absent.
     b. Brainstem functions are absent.
  2. Irreversibility is recognized when evaluation discloses findings of *a* and *b* and *c*:
     a. The cause of coma is established and is sufficient to account for the loss of brain functions.
     b. The possibility of recovery of any brain functions is excluded.
     c. The cessation of all brain function persists for an appropriate period of observation and/or trial of therapy.

SOURCE: From Report of the medical consultants on the diagnosis of death to the President's Commission for the Study of Ethical Problems in Medicine and Biomedical and Behavioral Research, Guidelines for the determination of death. *JAMA* 246:2184, 1981.

factors that maintain urinary output in the donated kidney and in the remaining donor kidney. An active diuresis in the donor at the moment of renal artery occlusion favors prompt function in the recipient. For these reasons, the urine output is monitored throughout the donor operation and should not fall below 1 mL/min per kidney. The patient is hydrated several hours prior to operation, and both colloid [5 mL/(kg · h)] and crystalloid [5 mL/(kg · h)] solutions are administered during the operation, with constant attention to the central venous pressure and the urine output. Mannitol and furosemide are given shortly before the kidney is removed. In addition, systemic heparinization is carried out a few minutes before the renal artery is occluded. The heparin is then counteracted with protamine.

The donor operation is carried out through a flank incision and a retroperitoneal approach. The peritoneum is retracted, the ureter identified, and a length of ureter is dissected free. The ureter is then transected (preserving its blood supply from the renal pelvis) so that the urinary output of the donor kidney can be observed throughout the operation. The remainder of the ureter is dissected free up to the renal vein. A large lumbar vein, the ovarian or testicular vein, and the adrenal branch of the renal vein are doubly ligated on the left side. There are no major branches of the renal vein on the right side. Dissection on the renal vein is carried down to the vena cava. The artery is not dissected free until the dissection of the renal vein is complete. The kidney is not removed until urinary output from the donor kidney itself is excellent. At that time the renal artery and vein are sequentially clamped and divided.

Minor complications of nephrectomy in healthy related donors are common, but serious complications are quite rare. The function of the remaining kidney increases to about 70 percent of the preoperative value. Prolonged follow-ups indicate that the health and life expectancy of the donor are not adversely affected by donation.

Cadaver Donor. The technique of kidney harvest from a cadaver donor depends to a large degree on the status of the donor's circulation. If the cadaver is brain-dead but with intact circulation and urine output, nephrectomy can be performed at leisure via the transperitoneal route.

If the donor has a sudden irreversible circulatory collapse, the kidneys must be removed more rapidly to minimize ischemia time. Heparin is administered, and both kidneys are removed together by clamping the aorta and vena cava above the origin of the renal arteries and veins and pulling the kidneys up together, prior to transection of the aorta and vena cava below the origin of the renal vessels and the ureters in the pelvis. Prompt cooling of the organs is required, and both kidneys can be perfused with iced crystalloid solution prior to storing them in the cold or perfusing them on preservation machines.

TECHNIQUE. Preparation. It is probably not necessary to remove the kidneys from most patients. Removal of the patient's diseased kidneys may be considered to control hypertension to eliminate a source of infection or eliminate the nephrotic syndrome. Recurrence of the glomerulonephritis in the transplanted kidney is not known to be aggravated by the presence of the diseased kidneys. Asymptomatic polycystic kidneys rarely present a problem.

When indicated, most transplantation centers perform the nephrectomy sometime prior to transplantation in order to minimize the surgical stress at transplantation when immunosuppressant drugs are utilized and optimal transplant function desired, or to completely eliminate urinary tract infection before immunosuppression is begun.

When two-stage transplantation is carried out (i.e., nephrectomy preceding the transplantation by a week or 10 days), the postnephrectomy management is simple. Hyperkalemia is a recurrent postnephrectomy problem, but it can usually be prevented if a 20 percent glucose solution is administered prophylactically (with insulin if the patient has diabetes). Rectal ion-exchange resins may be required to control hyperkalemia. Dialysis can usually be postponed 2 or 3 days with these techniques. Delay in reinstituting dialysis is preferred if heparinization is required. Peritoneal dialysis can be resumed immediately to avoid clotting of the catheter.

Splenectomy or thymectomy, or both, have also been performed in kidney recipients prior to transplantation but both have fallen into disuse.

During preparation for transplantation, sepsis from any source must be scrupulously removed. Frequent sources of sepsis are (1) the hemodialysis cannulae, if present, (2) the bladder in patients with preexisting urinary tract infections, (3) the skin of patients with uremic dermatitis, and (4) dental caries. The bladder of the totally anuric patient frequently becomes infected and should be irrigated with appropriate antimicrobial agents several times weekly prior to grafting.

Dialysis should be frequent and intense in the immediate pretransplantation period. Recipients of cadaver kidneys will have little preparation time prior to transplantation. Many patients will be maintained on systemic anticoagulants because of clotting problems in hemodialysis shunts; the anticoagulants must be discontinued, and vitamin K must be administered.

Transplantation. The operative technique of renal transplantation has become standardized. A retroperitoneal approach is used to the iliac vessels, and the renal artery and vein are anastomosed to the iliac vessels as shown in Figs. 10-38 and 10-39.

There must be no deficit in blood volume following the vascular anastomoses. Hypovolemia interferes with the rapid resumption of renal function. Urine usually appears within a few minutes of completion of the vascular anastomoses in related living donor kidneys; mannitol and furosemide may be helpful in hastening the appearance of urine, a useful sign that there are no serious technical deficiencies.

Fig. 10-38. Sites of anastomoses of renal vein to the side of the iliac vein. [From: *Simmons RL, Kjellstrand CM, Najarian JS: Kidney: II. Technique, complications, and results, in Najarian JS, Simmons RL (eds): Transplantation. Philadelphia, Lea & Febiger, 1972, p 445, with permission.*]

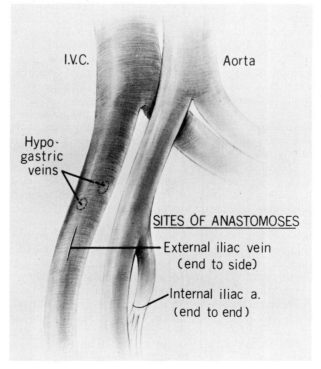

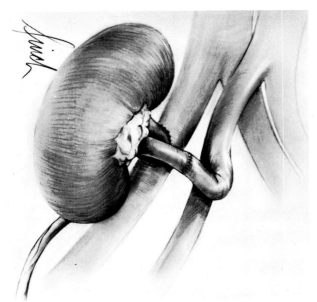

Fig. 10-39. Completed anastomosis of hypogastric artery to renal artery, and of renal vein to common iliac vein. [From: *Simmons RL, Kjellstrand CM, Najarian JS: Kidney: II. Technique, complications, and results, in Najarian JS, Simmons RL (eds): Transplantation. Philadelphia, Lea & Febiger, 1972, p 445, with permission.*]

Three methods are generally available for establishing urinary tract continuity. The preferred method involves ureteroneocystostomy. Pyeloureterostomy and ureteroureterostomy have also been used. Systemic or topical perioperative antibodies will help prevent wound infections.

Anesthesia in the Anephric Patient. Certain precautions are necessary during any operation on an anephric patient. In particular, certain anesthetics are excreted almost exclusively by the kidney and should not be used. These include the muscle relaxant gallamine triethiodide. Both curare and succinylcholine are metabolized by the liver, but both may also be accompanied by prolonged paralysis in the postoperative period. In the case of succinylcholine, a number of investigators have found that serum cholinesterase is broken down during hemodialysis. In such patients, succinylcholine would be expected to have prolonged action. Conduction anesthesia has been used, but most anesthesiologists prefer general anesthesia.

In the administration of anesthetics and fluids, it should always be assumed that the kidney will not function immediately after transplantation, even if dialysis is rarely required after transplantation. Similar thinking should be employed with regard to hyperkalemia in the uremic patient. Other concerns of the anesthesiologist are the loss of the hypertensive state after induction of anesthesia to normal levels, and the low hematocrit in patients with chronic uremia. The hematocrit should be raised to 30 prior to transplantation, and hypovolemia due to excessive ultrafiltration during hemodialysis should be avoided.

POSTTRANSPLANTATION CARE. The management of kidney allograft patients in the early posttransplant period does not differ radically from the management of other postoperative patients. Vital signs are monitored frequently for the first day, and the central venous pressure is utilized as a guide to blood volume. A Foley catheter is left in the bladder, which is not irrigated unless clots are thought to be occluding the catheter. The urine output is measured at least every hour. The volume of urine should be replaced with intravenous fluids. A convenient replacement solution consists of one-half normal saline solution with 5% dextrose and water and 10 meq of sodium bicarbonate per liter. Potassium need not be added to the intravenous fluids except in small children, whose urinary electrolytes should be replaced milliequivalent for milliequivalent. Diabetic patients should receive continuous insulin infusion intravenously to maintain blood sugars in the slightly hyperglycemic range (150 to 200 mg/dL).

The urinary output in the early postoperative period may be enormous, partly because of tubular dysfunction but primarily because of the overhydrated state of even the best-dialyzed patient. A creatinine clearance obtained on the evening of transplantation will be helpful in assessing renal function.

The Foley catheter can be removed almost any time after the first day. The tip of the catheter should be cultured at that time. Moderate hypertension is frequently seen in the early posttransplant period, and a low-sodium diet and low doses of antihypertensive medication (α-methyldopa, hydrochlorothiazide, or hydralazine) are useful to counteract this tendency. Antacids are useful in preventing the appearance of gastrointestinal ulceration of patients on immunosuppressive drugs. The patient is allowed out of bed and oral fluids are begun on the first postoperative day.

The 2-h creatinine clearance determination can be useful in interpreting early oliguria, but the test is not routine. The hematocrit should be followed at 4-h intervals, since rebleeding is a rare but severe complication that can produce oliguria and the onset of acute tubular necrosis (ATN).

A base-line sonogram and ^{131}I Hippuran renogram are usually performed soon after transplantation. Intravenous pyelography (IVP) is rarely necessary. Determinations of blood urea nitrogen (BUN), serum creatinine, and creatinine clearance suffice to estimate daily renal functions. Serum electrolyte determinations can usually be discontinued after good renal function is established. Periodic leukocyte and platelet counts are necessary to assay the state of the bone marrow during immunosuppression. Rarely, hyperglycemia and hypercalcemia are complications, and therefore blood sugar and calcium levels should be determined from time to time. The diabetic patient will require frequent blood sugar determinations and adjustments of insulin dosage.

Prophylactic Immunosuppression. Standard immunosuppressive management at most clinical transplant centers now consists of cyclosporine and prednisone. Because of cyclosporine's nephrotoxic properties, ALG or azathioprine, or both are sometimes employed until renal

Table 10-16. PROPHYLACTIC IMMUNOSUPPRESSION FOR RENAL TRANSPLANTATION AT THE UNIVERSITY OF MINNESOTA

A. Antilymphoblast globulin (ALG)
 1. 20 mg/kg intravenously daily
B. Azathioprine (evening dose after checking leukocyte count)
 1. Preoperative dose is 5 mg/kg per day
 2. First and second postoperative days: 5 mg/kg
 3. Third through sixth postoperative days: 4 mg/kg
 4. Seventh postoperative day: 3 mg/kg; maintain at 2 to 3 mg/kg
 5. Adjust at all times with respect to WBC, platelet count, and renal function
 6. Caution: Reduce dosage to 1.5 mg/kg for severe renal functional impairment
C. Prednisone
 1. 0.25 mg/kg every 6 h for 1st week
 2. 0.25 mg/kg per day for 2d week
 3. 0.5 mg/kg per day for 3d week
 4. Reduce dose slowly to achieve a maintenance dose of 0.5 mg/kg per day
D. Cyclosporine
 1. Start at 8 mg/kg per day on day 5. Adjust dose to achieve whole blood levels approximating 200 mg/mL

function approaches more normal levels Table 10-16). Then ALG is stopped and cyclosporine started. Most centers are currently individualizing the concurrent use of all four of these drugs, but cyclosporine has replaced azathioprine as the backbone of the regimen. A higher dose of prednisone or methylprednisone is used for rejection episodes. Some centers reserve the use of ALG or monoclonal antilymphocyte antibodies to treat steroid-resistant rejection epidoses.

COMPLICATIONS. **Renal Failure.** The most serious complication of renal transplantation is the failure of the graft to initiate or maintain function. Although the causes of failure can easily be defined, the differential diagnosis may, at the time, be impossible. The functional failure of the kidney is best examined in relation to the time after transplantation. The kidney may (1) never function, (2) have delayed onset of functions, (3) fail to function after a brief or prolonged time, or (4) gradually lose its function over a period of months or years. In each phase, four general diagnoses should be considered: (1) ischemic damage to the kidney; (2) rejection of the kidney by reactions directed against histocompatibility antigens on the kidney; (3) technical complications; and (4) the development of renal disease, either a new disease or recurrence of the original.

The simplest and best assay for decreased renal function is the frequent determination of BUN and serum creatinine, and the determination of creatinine clearance. Sonograms and renograms are also useful. The differential diagnosis of renal malfunction, however, may require percutaneous pyelography, arteriography, and renal biopsy.

Early Anuria and Oliguria

Early anuria or oliguria is a major diagnostic problem. The possibilities include (1) hypovolemia, (2) thrombosis of the renal artery or renal vein, (3) hyperacute rejection of the kidney, (4) ischemic renal damage (ATN), (5) compression of the kidney (by hematoma, seroma, or lymph), and (6) obstruction of the urinary flow.

The investigation of early posttransplant anuria should be rapidly performed in a strict sequence. The Foley catheter should first be irrigated and/or changed to remove any question of catheter obstruction. Unfortunately, whatever the cause of anuria, a clot can be obtained by bladder irrigation in the first posttransplant day. The clot may not be the primary cause of anuria, however, because blood will clot within the bladder if the urine is not copious enough to wash it out prior to coagulation. Therefore, even if a clot is present within the urinary catheter, the urine output should be monitored for the first 10 to 15 min after emptying the bladder to determine urine output adequacy.

If the obstructed catheter has not caused the oliguria, one must rule out hemorrhage and hypovolemia combined with compression or displacement of the kidney by the hematoma. If hypotension and tachycardia are present and the central venous pressure is low, hypovolemia is very likely. A radiograph of the abdomen will reveal displacement of the intraperitoneal contents by a massive hematoma. Echography and repeated hematocrit determinations will confirm the diagnosis. The normal degree of ischemic damage to the transplanted kidney plus hypovolemia and compression of the kidney and vessels by a hematoma all conspire to impair renal function. If anuria or severe oliguria is present, restoration of the blood volume will seldom suffice to restore renal function, even if furosemide or other diuretics are used. Many patients will require reexploration to control the bleeding point. After exploration, if the period of hypovolemia and renal compression has been relatively brief and diuretics have been used during ischemia, prompt restoration of renal function usually occurs.

The diagnosis of bleeding is frequently apparent and obviates the need for the next step in the investigation sequence—an [131]I Hippuran renogram (Fig. 10-40). The renogram permits assessment of the blood flow to the kidney and the ability of the kidney to concentrate and excrete the Hippuran. The results are never diagnostic. If the vascular phase and concentration are near normal, however, the renal arterial and venous anastomoses are patent. If the Hippuran uptake by the kidney is severely depressed, a renal arteriogram should be done. Arteriography will assess the renal arterial anastomosis, and if it reveals the presence of intravascular thrombosis of the kidney the diagnosis of hyperacute rejection will be suggested.

Technical Complications. Thrombosis of the renal arterial anastomosis is rare. Partial obstruction due to torsion or kinking of the vessels is more common and should be promptly repaired. When the renogram demonstrated poor concentration of the [131]I Hippuran, an arteriogram should be performed to detect correctable technical complications (Fig. 10-41). Thrombosis of the renal vein occurs even more rarely than thrombosis of the renal artery. When it does occur, thrombosis of the artery ensues because the collateral venous circulation of the kidney has

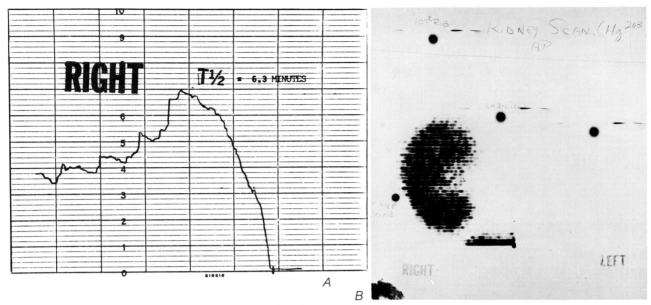

Fig. 10-40. Function of a homotransplanted kidney. *A.* A radiograph showing a half-life of 6.3 min and a completely normal-appearing curve. *B.* A scan of the same transplant showing excellent uptake in the kidney and the appearance of the radioactive material in the bladder. This transplant continued to have excellent function 5½ years later. (From: *Hume DM: Advances in Surgery, vol II. Chicago, Year Book Medical Publishers, 1966, with permission.*)

Fig. 10-41. Correctable arterial complications in the early posttransplant period. Oliguria was present in both patients. [131]I Hippuran revealed poor vascular phase. The arteriograms revealed torsion distal to the renal arterial anastomosis, which was corrected by a reanastomosis. [From: *Simmons RL, Kjellstrand CM, Najarian JS: Kidney: II. Technique, complications, and results, in Najarian JS, Simmons RL (eds): Transplantation. Philadelphia, Lea & Febiger, 1972, with permission.*]

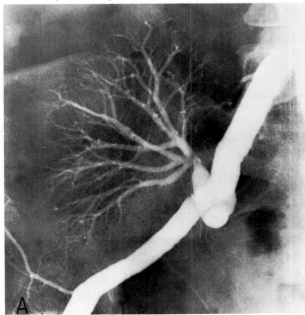

been interrupted by the transplant procedure. Partial thrombosis of the renal and iliac veins has occurred. Usually, this is accompanied by swelling of the ipsilateral lower extremity, fever, and evidence of pulmonary embolism.

Formerly, one of the most common, and most frequently fatal, complications following renal transplantation was urinary extravasation due to distal ureteral necrosis. Rejection was seldom at fault. The problem can generally be avoided by (1) using the ureter as short as possible; (2) avoiding tension at the ureteroneocystostomy site; (3) avoiding hematomas within the wound, which put tension on the ureter and also interfere with the developing collateral blood supply to the distal ureter; (4) avoiding transperitoneal "clotheslining" of the ureter by always placing the ureter in the retroperitoneal position where tension will be minimal and the collateral blood supply can develop.

Urinary extravasation is a serious complication that can lead to infection. It demands urgent reexploration with reimplantation of the ureter into the bladder, nephrostomy, or performance of a pyeloureterostomy to the host ureter. On occasion, the pelvis of the transplanted kidney may be involved, and nephrectomy may be required. Delay in definitive repair will frequently lead to infection, loss of the kidney, and death.

Technical errors can become manifest long after the immediate posttransplant period. Arterial stenosis, venous thrombosis, and late ureteral leaks and strictures are frequently confused with rejection (see below). Prior to any antirejection treatment, technical problems should be ruled out by echography, arteriography, renography, or percutaneous nephrostograms.

Hyperacute Rejection. Hyperacute rejection of the kidney is almost always mediated by humoral antibody, with the subsequent participation of the complement, coagulation, and kinin cascade systems. Platelets, PMNs, and

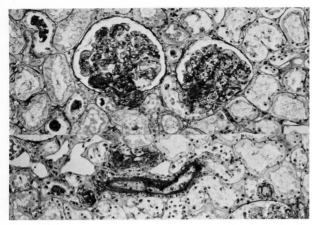

Fig. 10-42. Hyperacute renal rejection 20 h posttransplantation in a twenty-five-year-old male. Hyperacute rejection is characterized initially by fibrin and platelet thrombosis and fibrinoid necrosis of glomerular tufts, renal arterioles, and small arteries. A massive polymorphonuclear leukocyte reaction, interstitial hemorrhage, and tubular necrosis occur with subsequent cortical infarction 24 to 36 h posttransplantation. (×160.) (From: *Richard K. Sibley, personal communication.*)

vasospasm may also play a role. Classical hyperacute rejection is now rare because laboratory techniques can demonstrate cytotoxic antibody directed against donor histocompatibility antigens positive cross match. A rare patient will have a hyperacute rejection in the absence of demonstrable cytotoxic antibody. Indeed, detectable cytotoxic antibody will appear and disappear at intervals in patients awaiting transplantation. In the classic hyperacute rejection, the kidney will fail to regain its normal turgor and healthy pink color after anastomoses are established. Biopsy and histologic study at this time may reveal leukocytes in the glomerular capillaries, and intravascular renal thrombosis follows (Fig. 10-42). Definite evidence of a hyperacute rejection should be treated by immediate nephrectomy. A less acute rejection may occur, however, and renal function may not fail until a day or two following transplantation. Such rapid rejection has been differentiated by the term *accelerated rejection.*

Acute Tubular Necrosis. The diagnosis of ischemic renal injury is one of exclusion. If all other causes of renal functional failure in the early posttransplant period have been ruled out, one must assume that the diagnosis is ATN. "Acute tubular necrosis" in clinical parlance refers to kidneys whose function is impaired from ischemia or a variety of other causes. If kidneys from this clinical spectrum are biopsied, they most frequently show only hydropic changes. The more severe the insult, the more likely will be the presence of tubular necrosis. The correlation between tubule pathology and function, however, is not always good and suggests the interplay with other mechanisms, including prolonged vasoconstriction and vascular endothelial cell swelling. Most kidneys will recover, but sometimes disruption is so severe that cellular repair is not possible.

ATN occurs most commonly in cadaver recipients when the donor had undergone long periods of stress and hypotensive insult to the kidney to be transplanted. Another cause of recipient ATN is a long period of warm ischemia preceding transplantation. Kidneys with warm ischemic intervals greater than 1 h should not be utilized for transplantation, because function will seldom return to normal. Cold ischemia is much better tolerated, and preservation up to 48 h is now very satisfactory.

Almost all transplanted kidneys have undergone some degree of damage secondary to trauma and ischemia. A second trauma (hypovolemia, hypoxemia, renal compression, bacteremia, allergic reactions to ALG) that normally might not result in ATN in normal kidneys may cause oliguria in transplanted kidneys. One must not diagnose rejection and institute massive steroid therapy in the early posttransplant period without ruling out the possibility that an additional insult to an already damaged kidney has occurred and that the diagnosis is not acute rejection but ATN. Renal biopsy may be necessary to make this differentiation.

The management of the patient with ATN is simple. Urinary flow will resume in almost all cases within 2 or 3 weeks, but anuria for as long as 6 weeks with total recovery has been observed. ^{131}I Hippuran renograms are useful in following improvement prior to resumption of urinary flow. Dialysis is maintained intermittently during the period of oliguria. A number of studies have shown that the long-term function of renal transplants is independent of the presence or absence of oliguria in the early posttransplant period.

Rejection

Technical errors may not become evident for several weeks post grafting, and any trauma can aggravate the degree of ATN in a previously damaged kidney. Nevertheless most renal failure appearing after the first posttransplant week can be attributed to rejection.

With better immunosuppression, the acute rejection episodes that formerly appeared in the first month following transplantation are seen less and less frequently. The majority of patients, however, will sustain at least one acute rejection episode during the first 3 to 4 months following transplantation. Clinical rejection is rarely an all-or-nothing reaction, and the first episode seldom progresses to complete renal destruction. The functional changes induced by rejection appear to be in large part reversible; therefore, the recognition and treatment of the rejection episode prior to the development of severe renal damage is of extreme importance. Usually the rejection reaction responds to increased prednisone doses and local irradiation. Even with prompt treatment the creatinine clearance may be permanently impaired, however slightly, following each clinical rejection episode.

Differential Diagnosis. The clinical picture of a rejection reaction may be distressingly similar to several other problems: ureter leak or obstruction, hemorrhage with consequent ATN, infection, or stenosis or twist in the renal artery or vein. Classic renal rejection is characterized by oliguria, enlargement and tenderness of the graft, malaise, fever, leukocytosis, hypertension, weight gain,

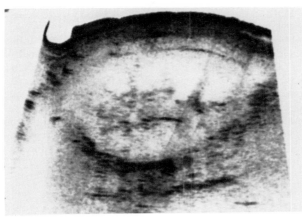

Fig. 10-43. Longitudinal sonogram of a renal transplant during episode of acute rejection (characterized clinically by anuria, fever, weight increase, and elevated creatinine levels to 0.079 mg/mL). Note enlarged pyramids of decreased echogenicity anteriorly. Interpyramidal cortex (septa of Bertin) shown as echogenic bands between pyramids. The kidney appears enlarged and more globular in shape compared with a base-line study 4 weeks earlier. Biopsy confirmed severe acute rejection requiring transplant nephrectomy 3 days after the sonogram. (From: *Frick MP, Feinberg SB, et al: Ultrasound in acute renal transplant rejection. Radiology 138:659, 1981, with permission.*)

Table 10-17. STANDARD ANTIREJECTION THERAPY AT THE UNIVERSITY OF MINNESOTA

1. Therapy
   a. Prednisone: 2 mg/kg × 3 days; then 1.5 mg/kg × 3 days; then 1.0 mg/kg × 3 days; thereafter reduce prednisone slowly to a maintenance dose.
   b. Azathioprine: Regulate dose to prevent leukopenia; do not increase.
   c. Irradiate kidney transplant: 150 rad every other day for three doses.
2. Adjuncts
   a. Reinstitute antacid therapy.
   b. Reinstitute oral nystatin (100,000 units twice daily) to prevent mucosal candidiasis.
   c. Reduce protein and fluid intake if renal function is significantly impaired.

and peripheral edema. Laboratory studies have shown lymphocyturia, red cell casts, proteinuria, immunoglobulin fragments, fibrin fragments in the urine, complementuria, lysozymuria, decreased urine sodium excretion, renal tubular acidosis, and increased lactic dehydrogenase in the urine. The level of the blood urea nitrogen increases, as does serum creatinine. Creatinine clearance is obviously decreased; renograms will show slow uptake of the Hippuran and slow urinary excretion. Echography can show edema of the renal papillae (Fig. 10-43).

The most important parameter to follow is the serum creatinine level. Unlike the BUN, which is sensitive to a number of changes (steroid administration, fever, and high-protein diet), serum creatinine levels are relatively stable for each patient. The creatinine clearance is more sensitive, but it depends on a carefully timed collection of urine.

The most reliable clinical signs of renal functional deterioration are a slight decrease in urinary output, slow weight gain, small increases in diastolic blood pressure, and edema of the lower extremity on the side of the graft. A peripheral leukocyte count and a serum creatinine level should be determined to confirm renal functional deterioration. A renogram and echogram should be promptly performed and compared with those obtained at the peak of renal function (usually prior to discharge from the hospital) to rule out urinary extravasation, urinary obstruction, or ureteral stenosis. Arteriography is seldom necessary but may reveal (1) characteristic changes of decreased concentration of dye flowing into the kidney, (2) decreased nephrogram effect, (3) an irregularity of the cortical vasculature and intralobar vasculature character-

istic of rejection, and (4) normal renal artery and anastomosis, eliminating the possibility of a technical problem.

Renal biopsy should be a definitive diagnostic tool. Both open biopsy and needle biopsy techniques have been described, and the histologic changes of rejection are characteristic (Figs. 10-11 through 10-14). A normal kidney biopsy is diagnostic, but a biopsy that reveals renal damage may merely reflect acute rejection, a chronic ongoing process, exacerbation of the pre-existing renal disease, or damage due to infection or radiation. With experience, however, needle biopsy of transplanted kidneys is a safe procedure and usually provides the diagnosis. Aspiration of the kidney to obtain cells for cytologic analysis can also be used to diagnose rejection.

Treatment. Most institutions have developed a standard rejection regimen for allografted kidneys (Table 10-17). This standard regimen can be repeated as many as three times within a 2-month period in patients for whom rejection appears to be unremitting. If it is repeated more often than that, infection may appear and be lethal. The decision to stop immunosuppression and sacrifice the transplant frequently depends on subtle factors and is difficult to make, particularly in patients who have deterioration of renal function over a period of months and years.

Renal Failure due to Recurrent Disease

Certain diseases are known to recur in the transplanted kidney. These are listed in Table 10-18. Transplantation is not necessarily contraindicated in these diseases since the recurrence is unpredictable and the transplant may provide long-term palliation that is superior in the individual case to dialysis. The best example is diabetes, in which the histologic features of diabetes often recur with only gradual deterioration of function.

RESULTS. Figure 10-44 shows the results of renal transplantation in adults at the University of Minnesota for the years since 1984 when a combination ALG, azathioprine, cyclosporine, and prednisone therapy was initiated.

TRANSPLANTATION IN CHILDREN. Renal failure in children is a common cause of death. Traditionally, young children have not been considered ideal candidates for renal transplantation, although excellent results have

Table 10-18. RISK OF RECURRENCE OF
PRIMARY RENAL DISEASE
FOLLOWING TRANSPLANTATION

High risk
  Focal sclerosis (proliferative type)
  IgA disease
  Membrano-proliferative glomerulonephritis
    (dense-deposit disease type)
  Hemolytic uremic syndrome
  Diabetes mellitus
  Oxalosis
Moderate risk
  Antiglomerular basement membrane disease
  Scleroderma
Low risk
  Membranous glomerulonephritis
  Amyloidosis
  Rapidly progressive crescentic
    AP nephritis
  Lupus
  Wegner's
No risk
  Congenital nephrosis
  Fabry's disease
  Cystinosis
  Myeloma kidney
  Polycystic kidney
  Pyelonephritis
  Glomerulonephritis
  Congenital renal disease (aplasia/dysplasia; valves)

been reported by a number of investigators. The small caliber of vessels and active social behavior of children make their management on hemodialysis extremely difficult. Long-term immunosuppressive therapy is also thought to interfere with normal growth with resultant social problems. Long-term hemodialysis is seldom satisfactory, and a parent is almost always willing to donate a kidney. Several infants have had transplants, and at least one has survived for more than 1 year. The growth of children following transplantation has been the subject of several studies. Most children with allografts grow slightly more slowly than normal. The adolescent growth spurt is absent in children with transplants and adolescent growth is particularly depressed in girls.

This early cessation of growth causes the typical appearance of girls with transplants, who are short and more cushingoid than the boys. Attempts to correlate the amount of first-year posttransplant growth with the kidney donor, renal function, or prednisone dosage have been unsuccessful. No such correlations can be made, even though it is generally felt that prednisone interferes with growth.

Sexual maturation in boys appears to be normal, although the period of observation has been short. Similarly, some girls have failed to menstruate at the usual age despite relatively normal renal function and only moderate doses of prednisone. Most girls have resumed menstruating if previously mature, or they undergo a normal menarche upon reaching age thirteen or fourteen.

MULTIPLE TRANSPLANTS. A number of studies have shown that second and third transplants are less successful than the first, if the first was rejected soon after transplantation. The rejection of one transplant may sensitize the patient to a number of weaker histocompatibility antigens that cannot be easily detected by sensitive crossmatch techniques. In addition, such patients may have less compromised immune systems that permitted the rejection of the first transplant. By contrast, patients who have maintained a successful first transplant for several years will, after losing the first transplant, accept the second transplant more readily.

XENOGRAFTS

Xenografts between related species are rejected by the same immune mechanisms as are allografts. Xenografts between distant species are rejected by an additional mechanism—the reaction of the xenograft with preformed antibodies that then trigger the efficient complement and clotting cascades. In short, xenografts across distant species barriers are rejected like hyperacute rejections.

There is not much information about clinical xenografts, because, in general, they have not proved to be useful. Xenografts of calf skin have sometimes been used for burn dressings and appear to offer some advantage over other dressing material, although they are not as useful as allografts. Some xenograft calf heart valves have been placed in patients, although it seems likely that these will not be as successful as are allografts, and they might be expected to calcify and become incompetent over a period of years. One xenograft chimpanzee heart has been placed in a patient, but this functioned for only about an hour. Since allografted hearts are invariably rejected experimentally, it would be expected that cardiac xenotransplants would suffer the same fate even more quickly. Renal and heart xenografts using both chimpanzee and baboon donors have been done in a number of human beings, but this procedure has been abandoned. Surprisingly enough a few relatively long-term survivors were achieved with chimpanzee renal transplants that were considerably better tolerated than baboon transplants. Some testicular xenografts have been carried out in human beings in the past but have long since been abandoned. Bone and cartilage xenografts are still used from time to time but seem to offer no advantage over allografts. The use of organs from nonhuman species for extracorporeal perfusion, both kidneys and livers, has been tried but currently is of little value.

ORGAN PRESERVATION

The viable preservation of whole organs is one of the essential components of any transplantation program. Only cadaver donors can be used for some organs (heart

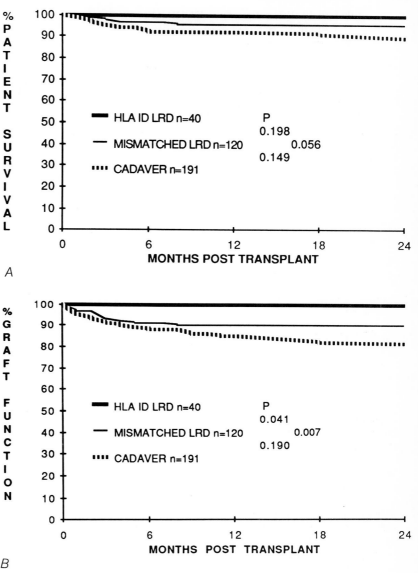

Fig. 10-44. *A* and *B*. Patient and graft survival rates in recipients according to donor source for all adult renal allografts transplanted from 1984 to 1986 at the University of Minnesota.

and liver), and even when the organ is expendable (as in one of a pair of kidneys), the use of cadaver donors avoids the risks inherent in surgical removal of the organ from living persons. If tissue typing and matching ever achieve their true potential, it may be necessary to store the organ until these matching procedures can be carried out. Even more time-consuming procedures, such as tolerance induction, may ultimately become available to pretreat the recipient and make him or her unresponsive to specific histocompatibility antigens. Table 10-19 lists some of those procedures that might be useful to carry out during organ preservation.

Methods of Viable Organ Preservation

The main problem associated with preservation of organs in a viable state seems to be hypoxia. When the organ is removed from its physiologic state, it is deprived of its normal oxygenation. The two major approaches to organ preservation have been what might be called metabolic inhibition and metabolic maintenance.

Metabolic inhibition seeks to prevent the normal catabolic processes from causing severe or irreversible damage to the tissues, during the period of preservation. It is currently best achieved by hypothermia, which protects the organ by slowing metabolic activity and decreasing oxygen need. Two techniques of cooling are currently available: (1) simple cooling of a kidney by immersing it

Table 10-19. PROCEDURES DURING
ORGAN STORAGE

A. Evaluation of the organ
  1. Typing and matching
    a. ABO typing
    b. Lymphocyte typing
    c. Organ cell typing
    d. Mixed lymphocyte culture with the recipient
  2. Diagnosis of disease in the donor or donor tissue
    a. Malignant tumors
    b. Infections
    c. Degenerative conditions
  3. Determination of functional state
  4. Restoration of normal function
B. Preparation of the recipient
  1. Induction of tolerance
  2. Immunosuppression
  3. Surgical procedures
C. Logistical procedures
  1. Stockpile various sizes and types
  2. Transport to a distant recipient
D. Modification of the immunogenicity of the organ

in, or flushing it with, a cold solution, which allows many hours of preservation and is almost always used for short periods of time, prior to transplantation of any organ; and (2) perfusion cooling, which allows longer periods of preservation.

Metabolic maintenance, the second approach to organ preservation, attempts to sustain a level of metabolic activity as close to physiologic normalcy as is feasible. Usually it implies perfusion of the organ in vitro with a carefully controlled fluid medium, although tissue oxygenation may be attempted. In practice metabolic maintenance is always best combined with perfusion cooling. The best system, at present, utilizes a pulsatile pump and pooled homologous plasma passed through a membrane oxygenator. Excellent transplantation results are obtained after perfusion as long as 72 h. These moderately long preservation periods provide adequate time for accurate matching of donors and recipients.

Not all organs can be perfused equally well by the same approach. Certain precautions are necessary. It is necessary *to maintain optimal organ function* up to and beyond the moment of clinical death. For kidneys, adequate hydration and maintenance of systemic blood pressure are recommended. Manipulation of the organ also contributes to vasospasm, and so surgical dissection should be as rapid and efficient as possible. The *period of time* between the cessation of blood flow through the organ and the establishment of the organ in its new environment (warm ischemia time) is critical in preservation studies. *Temperature* is also important. Successful perfusion systems have incorporated hypothermia to reduce the need for oxygen and metabolic nutrients. *Oxygenation* is also critical. Oxygen dissolves in aqueous solution more readily at lower temperatures; a membrane oxygenator is incorporated into the system.

The *flow rate* necessary at 37°C can be substantially reduced when metabolic activity is lessened by hypothermia; flow rates of one-fifth to one-third of normal have been satisfactory. The *viscosity of the perfusion fluid* may have some influence on perfusion pressure and flow rate. The perfusion pressure is significant. If the flow rate is adequate to provide the nutrients and waste removal, then the absolute level of pressure is not critical, but excessive perfusion pressure invariably causes transudation of the perfusate, tissue edema, and, ultimately, obstruction to the flow. Another factor is *pulsation.* Perfusion results in less damage when the flow is pulsatile, particularly at normothermic temperatures. The necessity for pulsatile flow during hypothermic perfusion is less well documented. It is probably not necessary to maintain any *venous pressure gradient.* The *perfusate composition* has apparent significance. Whole plasma probably is the most physiologic perfusate and contains most of the nutrient ingredients, including fatty acids, that might be required for the metabolic activity of organs. Many other formulations have been successful, including dextran, albumin, other plasma expanders, tissue culture media, and balanced salt solutions. *Osmolarity* is important. Crystalloids are poor perfusates and lead to edema. The perfusate must be maintained at "normal" pH range of 7.35 to 7.45. CO_2 buffering may be necessary with the addition of 2.5 to 5 percent of this gas to the oxygenator. Extremes of alkalosis and acidosis can be prevented with the addition of HCl or $NaHCO_3$ as necessary. A number of *additives* to the perfusate have been tried. These include membrane stabilizers, vasodilators, and anticoagulants. *Hyperbaric oxygenation* has also been used to prolong the viability and storage time of organs in conjunction with hypothermia or a combination of hypothermia and perfusion. Hyperbaric oxygenations will probably play no significant role in organ preservation, or at least its effects may not prove to be additive to those of hypothermia and perfusion.

There is evidence that an adequate flow rate during perfusion is a good prognostic sign of the viability and transplantability of the organ. The most significant indication of inadequate flow rate is the swelling caused by fluid retention. This edema is usually the result of anoxia with subsequent lysosomal and cellular damage. Poor perfusion itself can produce anoxia, so that a vicious cycle of edema-anoxia-edema can be started. Other possible causes of interstitial edema are perfusate osmolarity and excessive perfusion pressure. Even hypothermia alone may cause cellular swelling. Another important factor in the obstruction of flow is simple blockage of the microvasculature. The many causes of this blockage have been described in detail and include bubbles in the perfusion system, fibrin, red cell agglutination, the adherence of platelets and leukocytes to endothelial cells, cell breakdown due to mechanically imperfect pumps, crystal formation, and even agglutination of bacteria. Some of this blockage can be prevented with adequate filtration, but even blood-derived perfusion media like whole plasma have been shown to contain aggregates that appear during hypothermic perfusion. This aggregated material has been identified as lipoprotein. Fortunately, these substances can be removed from plasma quite easily by freezing, which causes flocculation of the lipoprotein, and by subsequent filtration and/or ultracentrifugation to remove the aggregates.

When plasma or plasma products are used as perfusates, immunologic damage is possible. This may be due to antibodies directed against organ antigens or to the precipitation of circulating antigen-antibody complexes within the organ. Although complement cannot be activated at hypothermic temperatures, bound antibody will activate complement within the recipient's body soon after transplantation. Although this has led to few recognized complications after renal transplantation, elimination of immunoglobulins from perfusates would be preferable.

One of the major problems in organ preservation research is the lack of methods to assay the functional state of organs in vitro and the consequent inability to measure the effectiveness of innovations in organ preservation techniques. Ultimately, of course, each preservation method must be tested by reimplantation of the organ. This is an all-or-none test that requires a large number of transplants in order to get statistically valid data. What is needed is an in vitro assay technique that can predict the transplantability of an organ and provide quantitative assessment of viability as the organ is subjected to the various preservation protocols. For practical purposes, such an assay should be utilized both before preservation (to determine whether postmortem changes have rendered the organ unfit for preservation) and immediately before transplantation (to determine whether the preservation efforts have been effective). As mentioned, the currently most popular technique involves the measurement of perfusate flow to the preserved kidney. Studies of enzymes or metabolites (like lactate) released from the graft appear promising.

Various pharmacologic agents have also been used as metabolic inhibitors. These include such drugs as magnesium sulfate, chlorpromazine, chloroquine, hydrocortisone, and diuretics such as mersalyl. Unfortunately, experiments utilizing such agents in addition to hypothermia show little additive effect. Most recently, however, allopurinol has been shown to protect against some of the anoxic damage to organs.

Storage of Nonviable Tissues by Freeze-Drying

Tissue grafts have been used in human reconstructive surgery for several decades. A majority of these grafts are from connective tissue and do not require that the graft be viable to function adequately. A major constituent of most of these tissues is collagen, which seems to maintain its integrity (or at least its strength) even after long-term storage by freezing or freeze-drying. Many thousands of patients each year receive bone, fascia, dura, tendon, heart valve, or skin grafts in treatment of traumatic or surgical defects. The architecture of these grafts is used as a framework for reconstruction as the host slowly replaces the tissue.

These tissues are probably best preserved by freeze-drying, which consists of rapid freezing of the tissue and the application of vacuum for removal of the water from the frozen state to the vapor state without permitting it to become liquid. Such a process usually results in maintenance of morphologic structure and therefore maintains the strength and structural integrity of the tissue. The rapidity of the initial freeze is important, as slow freezing can result in the formation of large ice crystals that can disrupt the tissue. This is apparently not a severe problem in tissues that consist largely of collagen. Other tissues, such as vascular grafts that contain elastic fibers, can show a disruption of these fibers due to crystal formation. In this instance, the most rapid freeze possible would be indicated to minimize crystal size. The graft is then dehydrated to a residual moisture of 5 percent. At this level it has been noted that tissues can subsequently be stored under vacuum at room temperature for years without further degradation or activation of metabolic processes. On reconstitution, it has been found preferable to inject water or saline solutions into a vacuum bottle containing tissue, so that the fluid can enter the tissue before it is exposed to air. Prior exposure to air apparently allows air molecules to enter the tissue and delays or prevents subsequent penetration of the water molecules necessary to rehydrate the tissue.

The usefulness of freeze-dried allografts is at least partly due to reduced antigenicity remaining in such grafts. The results of using freeze-dried allogeneic bone and autografting bone are not remarkably different. The dura has also been preserved by freeze-drying and functions extremely well when used to cover large cranial defects. Flexor tendon grafts of the hand have also been freeze-dried and used successfully, particularly when removed with their tendon sheaths intact. Many other freeze-dried tissues have been used with greater or lesser success. Cornea for nonpenetrating lamellar transplants, fascia, cartilage, heart valve, and nerve have all been tried.

Similarly, freeze-dried grafts have served as temporary biologic dressings to cover large burn wounds. In these instances the nonviable, freeze-dried graft "takes" and is even revascularized. It remains in place for several weeks or months, before it is finally sloughed. These grafts can be applied repeatedly without sensitization or acceleration of sloughing. Skin grafts have proved to be the best biologic dressing to prevent infection and to promote maximum granulation tissue formation in open skin wounds.

The usefulness of these techniques for the preservation of transplantable tissue has recently led to the organization of the American Association of Tissue Banks. The purpose of this organization is to encourage research into and to standardize successful methods for the harvest, storage, and distribution of tissues and organs to needy patients.

Bibliography

General

Abouna GM (ed): *Current Status of Clinical Organ Transplantation: With Some Recent Developments in Renal Surgery.* The Hague, Martinus Nijhoff, 1984.

Davis FD, Lucier JS, et al: Organization of an organ donation network. *Surg Clin North Am* 66:641, 1986.

Evans RS: Cost-effective analysis of transplantation. *Surg Clin North Am* 66:603, 1986.

Morris PJ (ed): *Kidney Transplantation: Principles and Practice.* New York, Grune and Stratton, 1984.

Morris PJ, Tilney NC (eds): *Progress in Transplantation.* Edinburgh, UK, Churchill Livingstone, 1985.

Najarian JS, Simmons RL (eds): *Transplantation.* Philadelphia, Lea & Febiger, 1972.

Park WE, Barber R, et al: Ethical issues in transplantation. *Surg Clin North Am* 66:663, 1986.

Penn I: Cancers following cyclosporine therapy. *Transplantation* 43:32, 1986.

Rapaport FT, Dausset J (eds): *Human Transplantation.* New York, Grune and Stratton, 1968.

Report of the Task Force on Organ Transplantation Issues and Recommendations: US Department of Health and Human Services, 1986.

Roberts AJ, Parnven GA (eds): Organ transplantation. *Surg Clin North Am* 55:1, 1986.

Simmons RL, Finch NL, et al (eds): *Manual of Vascular Access, Organ Donation and Transplantation.* New York, Springer-Verlag, 1984.

Simmons RG, Klein SK, et al: *Gift of Life: The Social and Psychological Impact of Organ Transplantation.* New York, Wiley, 1977.

Terasak PI (ed): *Clinical Kidney Transplants 1985.* Los Angeles, UCLA Tissue Typing Laboratory, 1985.

Tilney NL, Lazarus JM: *Surgical Care of the Patient with Renal Failure.* Philadelphia, Saunders, 1982.

Yunis EJ, Gatti RA (eds): *Tissue Typing and Organ Transplantation.* New York, Academic, 1973.

Transplantation Immunology

Calne RY (ed): *Transplantation Immunology: Clinical and Experimental.* Oxford, Oxford Medical, 1984.

deVries RRP, Van Rood JJ: Immunology of HLA class I and class II molecules. *Prog Allergy* 36:1, 1985.

Goldstein G: An overview of Orthoclone OKT3. *Transplant Proc* XVII:927, 1986.

Hayry P: Intragraft events in allograft destruction. *Transplantation* 38:1, 1984.

Hayry P, von Willebrand E: Transplant aspiration cytology. *Transplantation* 38:7, 1984.

Kahan BD: *Cyclosporine, Diagnosis and Management of Associated Renal Injury.* Orlando, FL, Grune and Stratton, 1985.

Kirkmon RL, Berrett LV, et al: Administration of anti-interleukin 2 receptor monoclonal antibody prolongs cardiac allograft survival in mice. *J Exp Med* 162:358, 1985.

Mason DW, Morris PJ: Effector mechanisms in allograft rejection. *Annu Rev Immunol* 4:119, 1986.

Murrach P, Kappler J: The T cell and its receptor. *Sci Am* 254:36, 1986.

Shevach EM: The effects of cyclosporine on the immune system. *Annu Rev Immunol* 3:397, 1985.

Strom TB: Clinical transplantation, in Stites DP, Stoles JD, et al (eds): *Basic and Clinical Immunology.* Los Altos, CA, Lange Medical, 1982.

Strom TB: Immunosuppressive agents in renal transplantation. *Kidney Int* 26:353, 1984.

Van Buren CT: Cyclosporine: Progress, problems and perspectives. *Surg Clin North Am* 66:435, 1986.

Liver Transplantation

Ascher NL, Simmons RL, et al: Host hepatectomy and liver transplantation, in Simmons RL, Finch ME, et al (eds): *Manual of Vascular Access, Organ Donation, and Transplantation.* New York, Springer-Verlag, 1984, p 255.

Cosmini AB, Cho SI, et al: A randomized clinical trial comparing OKT3 and steroids for treatment of hepatic allograft rejection. *Transplantation* 43:91, 1987.

Demetriou AA, Chowdrury NR, et al: New method of hepatocyte transplantation and extracorporeal liver support. *Ann Surg* 204:259, 1986.

Fath JJ, Ascher NL, et al: Metabolism during hepatic transplantations. Indicators of allograft function. *Surgery* 96:64, 1984.

Gordon RD, Shaw BW, et al: Indications for liver transplantation in the cyclosporine ERA. *Surg Clin North Am* 66:541, 1986.

Hood JM, Koep LJ, et al: Liver transplantation for advanced liver disease with alpha-1-antitrypsin deficiency. *N Engl J Med* 302:272, 1980.

Kam I, Lynch S, et al: Low flow venous bypasses in small dogs and pediatric patients undergoing replacement of the liver. *Surg Gynecol Obstet* 163:33, 1986.

Kretchtle SJ, Kolbeck PC, et al: Hepatic transplantation into sensitized recipients: Demonstration of hyperacute rejection. *Transplantation* 43:8, 1987.

Krom RAF, Kingma LM, et al: Choledococholedochostomy, a relatively safe procedure in orthotopic liver transplantation. *Surgery* 97:552, 1985.

Lerut J, Gordon RD, et al: Biliary tract complication following human orthotopic liver transplantation. *Transplantation* 43:47, 1987.

Perkins JD, Wiesner RH, et al: Immunohistologic labelling as an indication of liver allograft rejection. *Transplantation* 43:100, 1987.

So SKS, Platt JL, et al: Increased expression of class I MHC antigens on hepatocytes in rejecting human liver allografts. *Transplantation* 43:79, 1987.

Wall WJ, Grant DR, et al: Liver transplantation without veno veno bypass. *Transplantation* 43:56, 1987.

Pancreas Transplantation

Corry RJ, Nghiem DD, et al: Surgical treatment of diabetic nephropathy with simultaneous pancreatic duodenal and renal transplantation. *Surg Gynecol Obstet* 162:547, 1986.

Hullett DA, Faleny JL, et al: Human fetal pancreas—A potential source for transplantation. *Transplantation* 43:18, 1987.

Nghiem DD, Gonwa TA, et al: Metabolic effects of urinary diversion of exocrine secretion in pancreatic transplantation. *Transplantation* 43:70, 1987.

Prieto M, Sutherland DER, et al: Experimental and clinical experiences with urine amylase monitoring for early diagnosis of rejection in pancreas transplantation. *Transplantation* 43:73, 1987.

Sutherland DER: Pancreas and islet transplantation II. Clinical trials. *Diabetologia* 20:435, 1981.

Sutherland DER, Ascher NL, et al: Pancreas transplantation, in

Simmons RL, Finch ME, et al (eds): *Manual of Vascular Access, Organ Donation, and Transplantation.* New York, Springer-Verlag, 1984, p 237.

Sutherland DER, Kendall D, et al: Pancreas transplantation. *Surg Clin North Am* 66:557, 1986.

Bone Marrow Transplantation

Advisory Committee of the Bone Marrow Transplant Registry: Bone marrow transplantation from donors with aplastic anemia: A report from the ACS/NTH bone marrow transplant registry. *JAMA* 236:1131, 1976.

Beatty PG, et al: Marrow transplantation from related donors other than HLA identical siblings. *N Engl J Med* 313:765, 1985.

Bolman RM, Molina JE, et al: Heart transplantation, in Simmons RL, Finch ME, et al (eds): *Manual of Vascular Access, Organ Donation and Transplantation.* New York, Springer-Verlag, 1984, p 209.

Frazier OH, Cooley DA: Cardiac transplantation. *Surg Clin North Am* 66:477, 1986.

Gentry LO, Zelerff BJ: Diagnosis and treatment of infection in cardiac transplant patients. *Surg Clin North Am* 66:454, 1986.

Griffith BP, Trento AF, et al: Cardiac transplantation: Emerges from an experiment to a science. *Ann Surg* 204:308, 1986.

Modry DL, Oyer PE, et al: Cyclosporine in heart and heart/lung transplantation. *Can J Surg* 28:274, 1985.

Thomas ED: Bone marrow transplantation in hematologic malignancies. *Hospital Practice* 22:77, 1987.

Thompson CB, Thomas ED: Bone marrow transplantation. *Surg Clin North Am* 66:589, 1986.

Heart Transplantation

Andreone PA, Olivari MT, et al: Reduction of infectious complications following heart transplantation with triple-drug therapy. *J Heart Transplant* 5:13, 1986.

Bailey LL, Nehlsen-Cannarella SL, et al: Baboon-to-human cardiac xenotransplantation in a neonate. *JAMA* 254:3321, 1985.

Barnard CN: A human cardiac transplant. *S Afr Med J* 41:1271, 1967.

Baumgartner WA: Infections in cardiac transplantation. *J Heart Transplant* 3:75, 1983.

Bieber CP, Reitz BA, et al: Malignant lymphoma in Cyclosporin A treated allograft recipients. *Lancet* 1:43, 1980.

Billingham ME: Diagnosis of cardiac rejection by endomyocardial biopsy. *J Heart Transplant* 1:125, 1982.

Carrel A, Guthrie CC: The transplantation of veins and organs. Am Med 10:1101, 1905.

Cooper DKC, Novitzky D, et al: Are there indications for heterotopic heart transplantation in 1986? *Thorac Cardiovasc Surg* 34:300, 1986.

Dummer ST, White LT, et al: Morbidity of cytomegalovirus infection in recipients of heart or heart-lung transplants who received cyclosporine. *J Infect Dis* 152:1182, 1985.

Evans RW, Manninen DL, et al: Donor availability as the primary determinant of the future of heart transplantation. *JAMA* 255:1892, 1986.

Fuster V, Gersh BJ, et al: The natural history of idiopathic dilated cardiomyopathy. *Am J Cardiol* 47:525, 1981.

Hunt SA: Complications of heart transplantation. *J Heart Transplant* 3:70, 1983.

Lower RR, Shumway NE: Studies on orthotopic transplantation of the canine heart. *Surg Forum* 11:18, 1960.

Mammana RB, Peterson EA, et al: Pulmonary infections in cardiac transplant patients: Modes of diagnosis, complications, and effectiveness of therapy. *Ann Thorac Surg* 36:700, 1983.

Meister ND, McAleer MJ, et al: Returning to work after heart transplantation. *J Heart Transplant* 5:154, 1986.

Michler RE, Smith CR, et al: Reversal of cardiac transplant rejection without massive immunosuppression. *Circulation* 74(suppl III):68, 1986.

Pennock JL, Oyer PE, et al: Cardiac transplantation in perspective for the future. *J Thorac Cardiovasc Surg* 83:168, 1982.

Sadeghi AM, Robbins RC, et al: Cardiac xenotransplantation in primates. *J Thorac Cardiovasc Surg* 93:809, 1987.

Solis E, Kaye MP: The Registry of the International Society for Heart Transplantation: Third Official Report, June 1986. *J Heart Transplant* 5:2, 1986.

Heart-Lung

Burke CM, Baldwin JC, et al: Twenty-eight cases of human heart-lung transplantation. *Lancet* 1:517, 1986.

Burke CM, Theodore J, et al: Post-transplant obliterative bronchiolitis and other late lung sequelae in human heart-lung transplantation. *Chest* 86:824, 1984.

Griffith BP, Hardesty RL, et al: Asynchronous rejection of heart and lungs following cardiopulmonary transplantation. *Ann Thorac Surg* 40:488, 1985.

Hardesty RL, Griffith BP: Autoperfusion of the heart and lungs for preservation during distant procurement. *J Thorac Cardiovasc Surg* 93:11, 1987.

Hardesty RL, Griffith BP: Procurement for combined heart-lung transplantation: Bilateral thoracotomy with sternal transection, cardiopulmonary bypass, and profound hypothermia. *J Thorac Cardiovasc Surg* 89:795, 1985.

Haverich A, Scott WC, et al: Twenty years of lung preservation—A review. *J Heart Transplant* 4:234, 1985.

Jamieson SW, Stinson EB, et al: Operative technique for heart-lung transplantation. *J Thorac Cardiovasc Surg.* 87:930, 1984.

Painvin GA, Reece IJ, et al: Cardiopulmonary allotransplantation, a collective review: Experimental progress and current clinical status, *Tex Heart Inst J* 10:371, 1983.

Reitz BA, Burton NA, et al: Heart and lung transplantation: Autotransplantation and allotransplantation in primates with extended survival. *J Thorac Cardiovasc Surg* 80:360, 1980.

Reitz BA, Wallwork JL, et al: Heart-lung transplantation: Successful therapy for patients with pulmonary vascular disease. *N Engl J Med* 306:557, 1982.

Solis E, Kaye MP: The Registry of the International Society for Heart Transplantation: Third official report, June 1986. *J Heart Transplant,* 5:2, 1986.

Starkey TD, Sakakibara N, et al: Successful six-hour cardiopulmonary preservation with simple hypothermic crystalloid flush. *J Heart Transplant* 5:291, 1986.

Theodore J, Jamieson SW, et al: Physiologic aspects of human heart-lung transplantation: Pulmonary function status of the post-transplanted lung. *Chest* 86:349, 1984.

Single-Lung Transplantation

Dark JH, Patterson GA, et al: Experimental en bloc double lung transplantation. *Ann Thorac Surg* 42:394, 1986.

Dubois P, Choiniere L, et al: Bronchial omentopexy in canine lung allotransplantation. *Ann Thorac Surg* 38:211, 1984.

Goldberg M, Lima O, et al: A comparison between cyclosporine A and methylprednisolone plus azathioprine on bronchial healing following canine lung autotransplantation. *J Thorac Cardiovasc Surg* 85:821, 1983.

Jamieson SW, Ogunnaike HO: Cardiopulmonary transplantation. *Surg Clin North Am* 66:491, 1986.

Montefusco CM, Veith FM: Lung transplantation. *Surg Clin North Am* 66:503, 1986.

Nelems JM, Rebuck AS, et al: Human lung transplantation. *Chest* 78:569, 1980.

Toronto Lung Transplant Group: Unilateral lung transplantation for pulmonary fibrosis. *N Engl J Med* 314:1140, 1986.

Veith FJ: Lung transplantation in perspective. *N Engl J Med* 314:1186, 1986.

Veith FJ, Kamkolz SL, et al: Lung transplantation. *Transplantation* 35:271, 1983.

Veith FJ, Norin AJ, et al: Cyclosporine A in experimental lung transplantation. *Transplantation* 32:474, 1981.

Kidney Transplantation

Burlingham WJ, Grailer A, et al: Improved renal allograft survival following donor specific transfusions. II. *In vitro* correlates of early DST type rejection episodes. *Transplantation* 43:41, 1987.

Calne RY, Wood AJ: Cyclosporine in cadaveric renal transplantation: 3 year followup of a European multicenter trial. *Lancet* 2:549, 1985.

Canadian Multicentre Transplant Study Group: A randomized trial of cyclosporine in cadaveric renal transplantation. *N Engl J Med* 314:1219, 1986.

Casteneda-Zuniga WR (ed): *Radiographic Diagnosis of Renal Transplant Complications*. Minneapolis, University of Minnesota, 1986.

Chandler ST, Buckels J, et al: Indium labelled platelet uptake in rejecting renal transplants. *Surg Gynecol Obstet* 157:242, 1983.

Cho SI, Zalneraetes BP, et al: The influence of acute tubular necrosis on kidney transplant survival. *Transplant Proc* XVII:16, 1985.

Fryd DS, Sutherland DER, et al: Results of a prospective randomized study on the effect of splenectomy versus no splenectomy in renal transplant patients. *Transplant Proc* XIII:48, 1981.

Keown PA, Stiller CB: Kidney transplantation. *Surg Clin North Am* 66:517, 1986.

Malkowicz SB, Perloff LJ: Urologic consideration in renal transplantation. *Surg Gynecol Obstet* 160:579, 1985.

Mauer SM, Barbosa J, et al: Development of diabetic vascular lesions in normal kidneys transplanted into patients with diabetes mellitus. *N Engl J Med* 295:916, 1976.

Mendez–Picon G, Posner MS, et al: The effect of delayed function on long term survival of renal allografts. *Surg Gynecol Obstet* 161:351, 1986.

Monoco AP: Clinical kidney transplantation. *Transplant Proc* XVII:5, 1985.

Najarian JS, Fryd DS, et al: A single institution, randomized, prospective trial of cyclosporine, versus azathioprine-antilymphocyte globulin for immunosuppression in renal allograft recipients. *Ann Surg* 201:142, 1985.

Najarian JS, So SKS, et al: The outcome of 304 primary renal transplants in children (1968–1985). *Ann Surg* 204:246, 1986.

Najarian JS, Sutherland DER: The impact of transplantation on the understanding and treatment of diabetes and the pancreas. *Transplant Proc.* XII:634, 1980.

Novick AC (ed): Renal transplantation. *Urol Clin North Am* 10:203, 1983.

Opelz G: Correlation of HLA matching with kidney graft survival in patients or without cyclosporine treatment. *Transplantation* 40:240, 1985.

Opelz G: Current relevance of the transfusion effect in renal transplantation. *Transplant Proc* XVII:1015, 1985.

Ortho Multicenter Study Group: A randomized clinical trial of OKT3 monoclonal antibody for acute rejection of cadaveric renal transplants. *N Engl J Med* 313:37, 1985.

Report of the medical consultants on the diagnosis of death: Guidelines for determination of death. *JAMA* 246:2184, 1981.

Simmons RG, Anderson CR: Related donors and recipients: Five to nine years post-transplant. *Transplant Proc* XIV:9, 1982.

Simmons RL, Najarian JS: Kidney transplantation, in Simmons RL, Finch ME, et al (eds): *Manual of Vascular Access, Organ Donation, and Transplantation*. New York, Springer-Verlag, 1984, p 292.

Simmons RL, Sutherland DER: Transplant nephrectomy, in Simmons RL, Finch ME, et al (eds): *Manual of Vascular Access, Organ Donation, and Transplantation*. New York, Springer-Verlag, 1984, p 329.

So SKS, Simmons RL, et al: Improved results of multiple transplantation in children. *Surgery* 98:729, 1985.

Sommer BG, Henry M, et al: Sequential antilymphoblast globulin and cyclosporine for renal transplantation. *Transplantation* 43:85, 1987.

Starzl TE, Hakala TR: Variable convalescence and therapy after cadaveric renal transplantation under cyclosporin A and steroids. *Surg Gynecol Obstet* 154:819, 1982.

Stiller CR, Keown PA: Immunologic monitoring: Current perspectives and clinical implications. *Transplant Proc* XIII:1699, 1981.

Sutherland DER: International human pancreas and islet transplant registry. *Transplant Proc* XII:229, 1980.

Sutherland DER, Fryd DS, et al: The high-risk recipient in renal transplantation. *Transplant Proc* XIV:19, 1982.

Wing AJ, Broyer M, et al: Renal transplantation in Europe—Some comparisons between national programs. *Transplant Proc* XIV:5, 1982.

Transplantation of Other Organs

Baird RN, Abbott WM: Vein grafts: An historical perspective. *Am J Surg* 134:293, 1977.

Cohen Z, Wassef R, et al: Transplantation of the small intestine. *Surg Clin North Am* 66:583, 1986.

Friedlander GE, Mankin HJ, et al (eds): *Osteochondral Allografts*. Boston, Little, Brown, 1983.

Pritchford TJ, Kirkman RL: Small bowel transplantation. *World J Surg* 9:860, 1985.

Quilici PJ, Vieta JO, et al: The use of dura mater allografts in the surgical repair of the abdominal wall. *Surg Gynecol Obstet* 161:47, 1985.

Vrist MR: Practical application of basic research on bone graft physiology. Instructional course lectures. *Am Acad Orthoped Surg* 25:1, 1976.

Chapter 11

Anesthesia

Ronald D. Miller

INTRODUCTION

Anesthesia care involves care for the entire perioperative period, including preoperative evaluation, selection of appropriate monitoring for the perioperative period, administration of anesthesia, and postoperative care as it relates to anesthesia and surgery. Anesthesiologists also serve as consultants in the areas of chronic pain, critical care medicine, and respiratory therapy. In this chapter, the discussion will be limited to those aspects of anesthesia related to the perioperative period.

ANESTHETIC RISK

Anesthetic risk, per se, is difficult to determine because perioperative complications are usually a result of multiple causes related to concurrent disease, the complexity of surgery, and perhaps anesthesia itself. Examples of complications solely related to anesthesia are vomiting and aspiration of gastric contents and hypoxemia due to the inability to maintain a patent airway and/or adequate ventilation. Increasing emphasis has been placed on rare anesthetic mishaps, such as anesthetic overdose, undetected intubation of the esophagus instead of the trachea, and accidental disconnection of the ventilator from the endotracheal tube. It is extremely difficult to determine the true incidence and, therefore, risks of pure anesthetic complications that occur at such a low frequency. Taking all studies into account and despite the above stated limitations, death rates of 1 in 10,000 due entirely to anesthesia and about 2 in 10,000 in major part due to anesthesia appear to be reasonable estimates of overall anesthetic risks. These figures obviously do not take into account the multiple causes of morbidity, such as postoperative neurological complication, broken teeth, and many others. Despite the problems listed above, with proper care, anesthetic risk is extremely low.

The patient's physical status is usually classified according to the criteria in Table 11-1. This system does not specifically identify anesthetic risk but is often utilized for epidemiologic and descriptive purposes.

Table 11-1. PHYSICAL STATUS CLASSIFICATION OF THE AMERICAN SOCIETY OF ANESTHESIOLOGISTS

Class	Physical status
1	Patient has no organic, physiologic, biochemical, or psychiatric disturbances
2	Patient has mild to moderate systemic disturbance that may or may not be related to the disorder requiring surgery (e.g., essential hypertension, diabetes mellitus)
3	Patient has severe systemic disturbance that may or may not be related to the disorder requiring surgery (e.g., heart disease that limits activity, poorly controlled essential hypertension)
4	Patient has severe systemic disturbance that is life-threatening with or without surgery (e.g., congestive heart failure, persistent angina pectoris)
5	Patient is moribund and has little chance for survival, but surgery is to be performed as a last resort (resuscitation effort) (e.g., uncontrolled hemorrhage, as from a ruptured abdominal aneurysm)
E	Patient requires emergency operation

PREOPERATIVE EVALUATION

History and Physical

The history and physical examination is not meant to duplicate the surgeon's evaluation, but rather it is to specifically examine those areas relevant to anesthesia. Preoperative evaluation by an anesthesiologist is considered to be the standard of care in anesthesia. The history should include a review of the patient's previous hospitalizations, surgeries, and anesthesia, in an effort to identify clues that may influence anesthesia care, such as allergic reactions, delayed awakening, and jaundice. Concurrent diseases can have a tremendous influence on perioperative care, especially certain endocrine diseases (i.e., diabetes), cardiovascular disease (i.e., hypertension and myocardial infarction), respiratory disease (i.e., obstructive airway disease), coagulopathies (i.e., hemophilia), and abnormalities of vital excretory organs (i.e., kidney and/or liver disease).

Concurrent drug therapy must be reviewed because many drugs influence the response to anesthetic drugs. For example, echothiophate may prolong the response to succinylcholine. Various antihypertensive and other vasoactive drugs can alter the circulatory response to anesthetics (e.g., beta-adrenergic blocking drugs). Many drugs can either increase or decrease anesthetic requirement, including acute cocaine intoxication, tricyclic antidepressants, and antihypertensive drugs. Other drugs may prolong the neuromuscular blocking properties of nondepolarizing muscle relaxants, such as antibiotics and local anesthetics. Still other drugs may influence the metabolism of anesthetic drugs, increasing the possibility of a toxic reaction.

The physical examination should focus on those aspects that are important to the particular anesthetic being planned. If regional anesthesia is being planned, examination of the landmarks (and their accessibility) should be ascertained. For example, an epidural anesthetic may not be appropriate in an extremely obese patient in whom the vertebra cannot be palpated. In a more general sense, a physical examination should most assuredly include the cardiovascular system, lungs, and upper airway. Arterial blood pressure should often be determined in both the supine and sitting positions to ascertain whether postural hypotension is present, which serves to assess the presence of autonomic dysfunction and/or an inadequate intravascular volume. If abnormalities are found, additional tests (e.g., pulmonary function tests) may be indicated. Laboratory tests should not be ordered unless a specific diagnostic and therapeutic end point is defined. For example, in a patient with obstructive airway disease, pulmonary function tests may be indicated to ascertain whether any additional preoperative respiratory care is indicated (e.g., the response to bronchodilators) and to provide a baseline with which postoperative pulmonary care can be compared. Lastly, a limited neurological examination should be performed depending on the position and the type of anesthesia to be chosen. Certain intraoperative positions are well known to be associated with postoperative neuropathies.

Laboratory Tests

Traditionally, hospital rules and regulations dictated that certain minimal laboratory tests be obtained. Recognizing the expense of routine testing and with sophisticated cost-benefit analyses, many of these regulations are now realized to be inappropriate. In general, the history and physical examination are the most important guides as to whether certain laboratory tests are needed. In a patient who has a completely normal history and physical examination, our practice (at the University of California, San Francisco Medical Center) is not to automatically order any laboratory tests in adult men who are under the age of 40 years and have no history of problems with anesthesia or no abnormal findings upon physical examination. Women of this age and health status usually only require a hemoglobin determination.

Informed Consent

In general, an "informed consent" is difficult to define for both anesthesia and surgery. Theoretically, the patient should know of all possible risks associated with anesthesia. Yet, in many patients this presents an undue concern, especially if the risk is particularly tragic and extremely rare. It is not practical and it may even be harmful to cause undue worry. Also, the extent to which the complications are described depend on the necessity for surgery and anesthesia (e.g., minor cosmetic surgery versus an exploratory laparotomy for a ruptured appendix). Despite the above-stated limitations, patients should know what to expect from the administration of anesthesia and possible adverse effects and risks. Those areas that should receive particular attention include the timing and administration of preoperative medication, anticipated time of transport to the operating room, sequence of events prior to induction of anesthesia, anticipated duration of surgery, a description of where awakening from anesthesia will occur and whether catheters will be present, expected time of return to the hospital room, the likelihood of postoperative nausea and vomiting, and the measures that will be taken to deal with postoperative pain. A signed consent form should be obtained from the patient, and all the risks discussed with the patient should be noted in the patient's medical records.

Recently, there has been increasing concern whether a separate informed consent should be obtained for blood transfusions. While it is this author's belief that such a separate consent is unwarranted, clearly complications of blood transfusions should be discussed with the patient, especially recognizing the relatively high risk of hepatitis (e.g., 3 to 15 percent) and the rare problem associated with the acquired immunodeficiency syndrome (AIDS).

IMMEDIATE PREOPERATIVE CARE AND PREPARATION

Preoperative Medication

Preoperative medication is usually given to provide sedation and possibly induced amnesia. This combination generally will result in also alleviating anxiety. Because of the concern of vomiting and aspiration of gastric contents, another goal of preoperative medication is to decrease secretion of saliva and gastric juices and to elevate gastric pH. For inpatients, medication is usually given 1 to 2 h prior to the induction of anesthesia. The value and the selection of preoperative medication is largely subjective. Most commonly, sedation is provided with the oral administration of diazepam, although other drugs such as barbiturates and narcotics are frequently given intramuscularly. Gastric secretion can be reduced by H_2 receptor antagonist, such as cimetidine. Drying agents such as atropine or scopalomine are rarely indicated and in fact make the patient uncomfortable by providing excessive drying of the mouth. These drugs historically were necessary when anesthetics markedly increased salivary secretions (e.g., diethyl ether). Modern anesthetics, however, do not increase salivary secretions to an unusual degree.

A thoughtful and concerned conversation with the patient preoperatively can attenuate the need for preoperative medications regarding anesthesia and surgery. For patients who arrive the morning of surgery, premedications, if needed, can be given immediately prior to being taken into the operating room. For example, it is common to give midazolam, 1.0 to 4.0 mg/70 kg intravenously to provide a calming effect and a high incidence of amnesia. Often, concomitant narcotics are given if regional anesthesia is about to be performed.

Preparation for Administration of Anesthesia

GENERAL CONSIDERATIONS

When the patient arrives in the operative theater, he or she should be properly identified and the nurses' notes from the preceding evening should be reviewed to ensure that any unexpected changes in the patient's condition have not occurred. Also, the administration of preoperative medication should be verified. Lastly, all personnel in the operating room should be specifically instructed as to what requirements will be needed during induction of anesthesia (e.g., cricoid pressure during a rapid sequence induction of anesthesia).

ANESTHETIC MACHINE

The anesthetic machine and all associated equipment (e.g., suctioning device) must be checked immediately prior to inducing anesthesia. Rare anesthetic mishaps have been related to an unexpected malfunctioning of the anesthesia machine. This should not happen if the machine has been properly checked prior to induction of anesthesia.

MONITORING

Increasingly, standards are being set for monitoring that should apply to nearly all administrations of anesthesia. Several hospitals in the Harvard Medical School have established the minimum requirements listed in Table 11-2. An anesthesiologist or nurse anesthetist should be present in the operating-room theater at all times during the administration of general anesthesia, regional anesthesia, and monitored intravenous anesthetics. Occasionally a brief exit is tolerated when a known hazard, such as radiation, is being applied. Under most circumstances, heart rate and blood pressure should be monitored at a minimum rate of every 5 min. It is highly desirable to have the electrocardiogram continuously displayed from the induction of anesthesia until the patient is prepared for leaving the operating-room theater. Even though heart rate and arterial blood pressure are recommended to be measured every 5 min, measures should be taken to ensure that cardiorespiratory function is continuously moni-

Table 11-2. BASIC MONITORING REQUIREMENTS*

Anesthesiologist's or nurse anesthetist's presence in the operating room
Blood pressure and heart rate
Electrocardiogram
Continuous monitoring for cardiorespiratory function
Breathing system disconnection monitoring
Oxygen monitor
Temperature

* Adapted from Eichhorn JH, Cooper JB, et al: *JAMA* 256:1017, 1986.

tored. This may include palpation or observation of the reservoir breathing bag, auscultation of breath and heart sounds, or more sophisticated monitoring such as a tracing of an intraarterial blood-pressure line. When ventilation is controlled by an automatic mechanical ventilator, a device should be present to warn the anesthesiologist when the ventilator becomes accidentally disconnected from the endotracheal tube. An oxygen analyzer should be functioning during the administration of general anesthesia to ensure that hypoxic mixtures are not being administered. Lastly, although not a requirement in every patient, a means to measure body temperature should be available, especially to detect intraoperative hypothermia or the rare case of malignant hyperthermia.

POSITION

The patient must be positioned properly on the operating table in order to avoid physical and physiologic complications. Nerve damage can be caused by placing the patient in a position that stretches or applies pressure to the nerve. The most common peripheral nerve injuries are related to the brachial plexus and especially the ulnar nerve. Also, the patient's position can cause cardiovascular changes, such as hypotension when the patient is rapidly shifted from the supine to the sitting or prone position. Lastly, complications can occur from improper application of the anesthetic mask strap, or endotracheal tube connector. Necrosis of the bridge of the nose has occurred when the mask is applied with excessive pressure. Removal of the mask every 5 min and massaging the nose should minimize this complication. Also, patients have had loss of hair when their head has been in one position for several hours. This complication can be minimized by changing the patient's head position every 1 or 2 h.

INTRAOPERATIVE ANESTHESIA

General Anesthesia

GENERAL CONSIDERATIONS

Although the various inhaled and intravenous anesthetics have marked differences in pharmacologic activity, especially circulatory changes, the selection of anesthesia has never been demonstrated to be an important factor regarding overall outcome. The lack of influence of choice of anesthesia on outcome may be related to the greater importance of the anesthesiologist's skill rather than the specific agent chosen. Conversely, perhaps small differences in outcome are related to the choice of anesthesia but have not been demonstrated because of the lack of availability of large epidemiologic outcome-related studies.

Until the early 1960s, the potency of anesthetic drugs had not been precisely determined because of a lack of a suitable technique. Since then, the minimum alveolar anesthetic concentration (MAC) has been developed and utilized as a measure of anesthetic potency for the inhaled anesthetics. MAC is defined as that alveolar concentra-

tion at which 50 percent of the subjects move in response to a noxious stimulus. MAC has been determined in anesthetized patients by finding that concentration at which half of the patients do not move in response to a skin incision. This concept and measurement has allowed comparison of the pharmacologic and physiologic effects of various anesthetic drugs at equipotent concentrations. Also, MAC has allowed a more precise determination of those physiologic factors that may influence anesthetic requirements, including increasing age, debility, and the concomitant administration of other drugs. The determination of MAC was greatly facilitated by being able to measure the end-tidal anesthetic concentration, which is a direct reflection of the alveolar concentration and, therefore, the brain concentration at steady state. Studies are being conducted to provide comparable measurements of anesthetic potency for the intravenously administered anesthetics.

INDUCTION OF ANESTHESIA

Anesthesia can be induced by giving drugs intravenously, by inhalation, or by a combination of both. Two major factors govern the method by which anesthesia is induced. One is the necessity to protect the airway if a patient has recently eaten or has a condition known to facilitate vomiting and aspiration of gastric contents (e.g., pregnancy or ascites). The other factor is the physiologic status of the patient. If a patient is very fragile (e.g., a reduced intravascular volume, or elderly), anesthesia probably should be given very slowly so that the known cardiovascular depressant effects of most anesthetics do not become excessive.

Other than an awake endotracheal intubation, the airway is most rapidly protected by using a "rapid sequence" method of inducing anesthesia. This method of inducing anesthesia has the disadvantage of needing to administer large doses of anesthetic drugs with known adverse cardiovascular effects. Anesthesia is most commonly induced by the administration of an ultra-short-acting barbiturate (e.g., thiopental) followed by a depolarizing muscle relaxant (e.g., succinylcholine). This allows anesthesia to be induced rapidly and the trachea intubated within 30 to 90 s. If cricoid pressure is concomitantly administered, theoretically the airway should be completely protected from aspiration of gastric contents. Cricoid pressure needs to be precisely applied in order to occlude the esophagus and prevent gastric contents from entering the pharynx, and therefore the trachea. Oxygen is usually given via mask before inducing anesthesia to allow maximum time for intubation while the patient is apneic.

Anesthesia can be induced by inhalation of a potent volatile anesthetic (e.g., halothane, enflurane, or isoflurane) with or without nitrous oxide. Anesthesia can be induced within 3 to 5 min. This technique has the advantage of allowing careful titration of the anesthetic and the immediate withdrawal of the anesthetic if adverse effects, such as hypotension, occur. This technique has the disadvantage that induction of anesthesia is longer than by the intravenous route and requires a skilled anesthetist to administer the anesthetic while avoiding coughing and the excitement stage (i.e., stage II of anesthesia). After anesthesia has been induced, the trachea can be intubated with or without administration of a neuromuscular blocking drug. Attempting endotracheal intubation in a spontaneously breathing, unparalyzed, anesthetized patient is difficult. Although conditions for intubation may not be as good with this method, the patient will still be breathing if some difficulties with intubation prolong the time before complete airway control is achieved. If severe difficulties with airway control are anticipated, an awake endotracheal intubation should be considered, possibly with the aid of a fiberoptic bronchoscope.

Anesthesia is usually induced by intravenously administered anesthetics with or without the concurrent administration of an inhaled anesthetic. Thiopental undoubtedly is the most commonly administered intravenous anesthetic, although various narcotics (e.g., fentanyl, morphine, sufentanil) and benzodiazepines (e.g., diazepam and midazolam) have become increasingly popular. The intravenously administered anesthetic has the advantage of minimizing the discomfort of the anesthetic mask and inducing anesthesia very rapidly.

AIRWAY MANAGEMENT (ENDOTRACHEAL INTUBATION)

Although general anesthesia can be given without intubating the trachea, this is very uncommon. While the complications of endotracheal intubation are avoided, this approach has many disadvantages. The airway is unprotected in case the patient vomits. Also, the anesthesiologist must hold the mask with one hand during the entire procedure, which hinders the performance of many other tasks, including monitoring and blood or drug administration.

Endotracheal intubation is usually performed during general anesthesia to ensure a patent airway, to prevent aspiration of gastric contents, and to facilitate tracheal or bronchial suctioning and positive-pressure ventilation. Also, if the patient is in a position other than the supine or Trendelenburg position, it is very difficult to provide adequate ventilation via a mask, and endotracheal intubation is usually indicated.

There are several complications of endotracheal intubation. On an immediate basis, complications from direct laryngoscopy and insertion of the endotracheal tube often involves injuries to the teeth. If a tooth is dislodged, it must be removed. If the tooth cannot be located, radiographs of the chest and abdomen should be obtained to ascertain that the tooth has not passed into the airway via the glottic opening. Because endotracheal intubation is very stimulating, hypertension and tachycardia can occur. However, this is so transient that it is of rare clinical significance. It can be minimized by assuring that the depth of anesthesia is adequate and/or by administration of 100 mg/70 kg of lidocaine intravenously.

Intraoperatively, the endotracheal tube can be obstructed or accidentally removed. If it has been incorrectly inserted (e.g., into the esophagus) hypoxemia will result. If this is not detected soon enough, permanent adverse complications can occur (i.e., hypoxic brain damage). Auscultation of the lungs and stomach, and palpation of the endotracheal tube cuff in the trachea will assure proper placement of the endotracheal tube. Also, if too much pressure is applied to the balloon cuff of the endotracheal tube, the tracheal mucosa may be ischemic. This complication has been decreasing because of the use of ''low-pressure cuffs,'' which adapt to the irregularities of the tracheal wall and produce a seal at pressures of 15 to 30 mmHg (previous endotracheal tube cuffs required 80 to 250 mmHg of pressure to occlude the trachea). Still, ciliary denudation can occur over the tracheal rings with only 2 h of intubation and tracheal pressure less than 25 mmHg.

Upon completion of anesthesia, extubation of the trachea can be complicated by laryngospasm, aspiration of gastric contents, pharyngitis, laryngitis, and laryngo- or subglottic edema. The incidence of these complications can be reduced by using the low-pressure endotracheal tube cuff and performing prompt extubation when clinically possible.

MAINTENANCE OF ANESTHESIA

Intraoperatively, anesthesia must provide analgesia, unconsciousness, skeletal muscle relaxation, and control of the sympathetic nervous system responses to noxious stimulation. The inhaled and intravenous anesthetics can be given alone or together to achieve these ends. Monitoring depth of anesthesia is relatively straightforward in an unparalyzed patient. Movement, depth and rate of respiration, and many other physiologic responses to anesthesia can be monitored. However, when a patient is paralyzed by neuromuscular blocking drugs, such as pancuronium, many of the signs of anesthesia are absent. It is essential that the anesthesiologist continue to attempt to assess the depth of anesthesia to avoid having a patient be awake, but paralyzed, during the surgical procedure.

A major challenge for anesthesia, especially during intraabdominal cases, is to provide adequate relaxation by the administration of proper anesthetic and neuromuscular blocking drug doses. Monitoring with a peripheral nerve stimulator will guide the anesthesiologist as to whether an adequate neuromuscular blockade is present and to avoid excessive doses of neuromuscular blocking drugs. If excessive doses of neuromuscular blocking drugs are given, the patient may have prolonged postoperative paralysis. If anesthesia is sufficient, elimination of 90 percent of the response to peripheral nerve stimulation will usually ensure adequate relaxation. The effectiveness of the neuromuscular blocking drug and anesthesia is facilitated when the surgical team takes other measures to maximize exposure, such as correct positioning.

Regional Anesthesia

GENERAL CONSIDERATIONS

Regional anesthesia has several advantages. The concept of anesthetizing only that part of the body upon which surgery is being performed (e.g., brachial plexus for arm or hand surgery), rather than subjecting the entire body to the problems of general anesthesia is an attractive concept, although it is not clear that regional anesthesia will improve mortality and morbidity. Furthermore, regional anesthesia has the advantage that skeletal muscle relaxation is usually excellent if an appropriate dose of local anesthetic is administered. A major disadvantage of regional anesthesia is the occasional failure to produce adequate anesthesia, necessitating that additional anesthesia be given, usually by the inhalation or intravenous route. As far as operating-room efficiency is concerned, proper plans and logistics must be made, or regional anesthesia has the possibility of increasing time between cases.

Despite the limitations described above, there are some suggestions that regional anesthesia indeed does have advantages in certain situations. Blood loss from total hip arthroplasty and prostatectomy is clearly reduced by spinal or epidural anesthesia. Thromboembolic complications following total hip arthroplasty may be reduced by the use of a local anesthetic. Also, regional anesthesia may reduce postoperative impairment of pulmonary function. More recently, regional anesthesia has been shown to prevent postoperative impairment of some immune functions, although the relationship to postoperative infection has not been established. Lastly, the time of convalescence may be less with regional anesthesia. These proposed advantages require an epidemiologic study involving hundreds or perhaps thousands of patients to ascertain whether these and other advantages of regional anesthesia are in fact true. As indicated with general anesthesia, regional anesthesia is facilitated by an anesthesiologist skilled with these procedures.

SPINAL AND EPIDURAL ANESTHESIA

Spinal anesthesia is usually produced by inserting the local anesthetic into the lumbar intrathecal space. The local anesthetic then blocks nerve conduction in the spinal nerve routes, dorsal route ganglia, and probably the periphery of the spinal cord. Epidural anesthesia is accomplished by injecting the local anesthetic into the extradural space, usually in the lumbar area. Another form of epidural anesthesia is "caudal" anesthesia, in which the local anesthetic is deposited into the epidural space when the needle is introduced into the sacral hiatus. The epidural space is that compartment between the dura mater and the bony ligamentous walls of the spinal canal. It is a potential space filled with fat and the internal vertebral plexus of veins. Either spinal or epidural anesthesia has the advantage of providing anesthesia selectively in regard to the surgical site. In addition, the patient may be awake or sedated. As indicated above, profound muscle relaxation can be achieved without the use of neuromuscular blocking drugs, such as pancuronium or *d*-tubocurarine. The gastrointestinal tract is usually contracted, which facilitates exposure within the abdominal cavity for the surgeon. Despite these advantages, bias often exists against the use of spinal or epidural anesthesia. Often these biases are based on the patient's fear of being awake and the surgeon's concern that the block may be

inadequate, resulting in a delay in starting the operation while the anesthesiologist induces general anesthesia.

The circulatory responses to epidural and spinal anesthesia are a result of peripheral sympathetic nervous system blockade. Because the level of sympathetic blockade is about two dermatomes higher than that of a sensory blockade, a sensory level of T3 will result in a total sympathetic blockade. This will result in decreases in arterial blood pressure and central venous pressure. The decrease in blood pressure is primarily due to a decrease in cardiac output, secondary to pooling of blood in denervated veins. Treatment of hypotension during spinal anesthesia is to increase venous return, which facilitates cardiac output. This objective is best achieved by a modest Trendelenburg position, administration of crystalloids intravenously, or a small dose of a vasopressor, such as ephedrine, 10 to 25 mg/70 kg intravenously.

The most common complication of a spinal anesthetic is a postoperative headache. The mildest forms of postspinal headache can be treated conservatively by enforcing bed rest for 24 to 48 h. In severe cases, a "blood patch" epidural should be administered, in which 5 to 10 mL of the patient's own blood is introduced into the epidural space. This results in over 95 percent success of obliterating the postspinal headache. Urinary retention is also a complication; neurologic sequelae are extremely rare.

In most respects, epidural anesthesia is similar to spinal anesthesia, except that the circulatory responses are more gradual in onset. The major site of action of the local anesthetic placed in the epidural space is probably at the nerve roots and dorsal root ganglion beyond the point of the meningeal covering.

PERIPHERAL NERVE BLOCKS

The most common peripheral nerve blocks performed are those related to the upper extremity. The brachial plexus can be blocked by three approaches, namely, the axillary, supraclavicular, or interscalene. Also, the radial, ulnar, and median nerves can be blocked at the elbow or wrist. The upper and lower extremity can be blocked by the "Bier block." This block is performed by placing a tourniquet proximal to the site of an intravenous injection of an appropriate volume of local anesthetic. The local anesthetic effect can be terminated by releasing the tourniquet. Obviously a major hazard of this technique is the premature release of the tourniquet, allowing an excessive dose of local anesthetic to enter the circulation and, therefore, the brain, causing convulsions. However, if the tourniquet is properly applied, this complication is indeed rare.

Other nerve blocks performed less frequently include intercostal nerve blocks for postoperative pain relief and sciatic-femoral nerve block for surgery of the lower extremities. Unfortunately, peripheral nerve blocks are not a major component of anesthesia given intraoperatively because of the discomfort they cause when inexperienced individuals are administering them and the time they require.

Special Techniques

Several techniques that can be used in anesthesia may result in decreased blood loss and/or decreased metabolism. Recognizing the concern regarding the infectivity of blood transfusions (e.g., posttransfusion hepatitis and AIDS), the overall indications for blood transfusions intraoperatively have been reexamined, which is the subject of other chapters in this text. There are techniques that anesthesiologists can utilize to decrease the amount of blood lost, and therefore the amount of blood required during surgery.

METHODS TO DECREASE BLOOD TRANSFUSIONS

DELIBERATE HYPOTENSION. Deliberate (or controlled) hypotension is an anesthetic technique in which arterial blood pressure is decreased electively to decrease blood loss during surgery and to provide a dry surgical field for the surgeon. In certain operative procedures (e.g., plastic surgery) deliberate hypotension is said to facilitate the surgical procedure from a technical point of view. Numerous techniques and drugs have been used to lower arterial blood pressure, including ganglionic blockers and deep levels of general anesthesia. The most common operative procedures in which deliberate hypotension is used are neurosurgery, total hip arthroplasty, plastic surgery, and operations for head and neck cancer.

It is not known precisely what the absolute contraindications to this technique should be. For example, the brain can tolerate a mean arterial blood pressure of 55 mmHg, but the lower limits and the influence of specific diseases have not been defined. In general, patients who have had strokes, transient ischemic attacks, myocardial infarctions within the previous 3 years, renal disease, previous renal transplant, and untreated hypertension should not be considered for deliberate hypotension.

AUTOTRANSFUSION. Autotransfusion therapy is performed by using one of three approaches: preoperative removal and storage; immediate preoperative phlebotomy and hemodilution; and intraoperative blood salvage and retransfusion. The latter technique is of prime importance in terms of anesthesia involvement. The concept of transfusing a patient's own blood and retrieving it during surgery to maintain circulatory stability is attractive. However, this approach has been fraught with complications, including hemolysis, coagulation disorders, microembolism (fat, denatured protein, microaggregates such as platelets and leukocytes), air embolism, and sepsis and metastasis if used in patients with infection or malignancy.

The technology has improved so that the incidence of the first four complications listed above has been reduced or nearly eliminated with use of the appropriate blood-salvage apparatus. Obviously, the transmission of bacteria or cancer cells is still a problem.

HEMODILUTION. Hemodilution and autologous transfusions are now being used for open heart surgery. Basically, this is an extension of the preoperative form of autologous transfusion by infusion of a hemodiluent in one vein and simultaneous phlebotomy from another vein to produce a state of normovolemic anemia. Specifically, one or two units of blood from an arterial cannula can be withdrawn into plastic bags containing citrate phosphate dextrose solution. After phlebotomy, blood pressure and heart rate are maintained with crystalloid administration and, when needed, homologous blood. The autologous blood is then transfused at the end of perfusion after the administration of protamine. Many clinicians have reported successful use of this technique. Obviously, the value of hemodilution and autologous transfusion lies in the fact that significantly less homologous blood will be needed.

HYPOTHERMIA

When the body is cooled, the metabolism decreases at about 8 percent/°C to one-half normal at 28°C. Hypothermia is used clinically to reduce metabolic rate, rendering the brain and other metabolically active organs less susceptible to periods of ischemia or hypoxia. Hypothermia is used mainly for cardiac and neurosurgery.

Special Anesthetic Problems

ASPIRATION PNEUMONITIS

A major hazard of anesthesia is vomiting and aspiration of gastric contents during anesthesia. When the airway is unprotected, especially during induction and emergence from anesthesia, this complication is most likely to occur. Although undigested food may be aspirated, producing airway obstruction and respiratory distress, the more common problem is aspiration of gastric secretions, which have a pH below 2.5. Aspiration of such acid material can produce sudden bronchospasm, tachypnea, diffuse rales, cyanosis, and hypotension. Cardiac arrest may occur in severe cases.

The most important measure in preventing aspiration of gastric contents is to minimize the time that the airway is unprotected. Generally, any patient who has eaten within 8 h of surgery should be considered to have a full stomach and, therefore, to be at risk of vomiting during induction. In a patient who has pain or is pregnant, gastric emptying may be delayed, and the interval between eating and elective surgery probably should be lengthened to at least 12 h. Various antacids have been utilized to neutralize the gastric pH. Specifically, drinking sodium citrate will raise the gastric pH in most patients, but it must be given 45 to 75 min before induction of anesthesia. If time does not permit such a wait, either endotracheal intubation with the patient being awake or a rapid sequence induction of anesthesia should be performed.

MALIGNANT HYPERTHERMIA

Malignant hyperthermia can occur soon after the induction of anesthesia in patients with this inherited disease. The onset of malignant hyperthermia can be acute and rapid, particularly during induction of anesthesia with an inhaled anesthetic, or the use of succinylcholine. The course of malignant hyperthermia can be extraordinarily rapid, including a striking increase in metabolism, resulting in an intense production of heat, carbon dioxide, and lactate, and associated respiratory and metabolic acidosis. If untreated, the fatality rate is extremely high. Treatment should include all conceivable cooling measures and the administration of dantrolene up to 10 mg/kg intravenously.

Patients who require anesthesia and are known to be susceptible to malignant hyperthermia should be pretreated with dantrolene for 1 to 3 days, and given anesthetics known not to trigger the syndrome, which include narcotics, barbiturates, nitrous oxide, and ester local anesthetics.

HEPATOTOXICITY

Over 20 years ago, halothane administration was proposed to be unrelated to massive postoperative hepatic necrosis and to be safe for use in hepatobiliary surgery. Massive hepatic necrosis has been associated with other anesthetics and may be related to other conditions (i.e., blood transfusions, hypovolemic shock). Still, in the rare patient, halothane appears to cause a form of hepatitis. The most recent theory is that the cellular susceptibility to damage from halothane occurs after exposure to electrophilic drug metabolites. The predisposing factor is familial and constitutional, but presently there is no method of preoperatively identifying those rare patients who may be susceptible to developing massive hepatic necrosis from halothane.

RECURRENT MYOCARDIAL INFARCTION

If a patient has had a myocardial infarction preoperatively, he or she may have an increased risk of postoperative myocardial infarction. This increased risk is related to the time since the previous infarction. The risk of postoperative myocardial infarction decreases to about 5 percent (50 times the normal risk) 6 months after the first infarction. Therefore, elective surgery, especially thoracic and upper abdominal procedures, should be delayed for 6 months. The incidence of myocardial infarction is increased in patients having intrathoracic or intraabdominal operations lasting more than 3 h. There is no correlation between risk and the site of previous infarction, the site of surgery if less than 3 h in duration, or choice of anesthetic drugs or techniques. Close hemodynamic monitoring using intraarterial and/or pulmonary artery catheters and prompt treatment of hypotension or hypertension decrease the risk of periperative infarction in high-risk patients.

POSTANESTHETIC ROOM (RECOVERY ROOM)

General Considerations

The postanesthetic or recovery room is that area designated for the monitoring and care of patients who are re-

covering from the immediate physiologic derangements produced by anesthesia and surgery. This room should be staffed with specially trained nurses skilled in the prompt recognition of postoperative complications. Such complications include upper-airway obstruction, arterial hypoxemia, alveolar hypoventilation, hypotension, hypertension, cardiac dysrhythmias and agitation (emergence delirium). Location of the recovery room in close proximity to the operating rooms assures rapid access to physician consultation and assistance. Specifically, a qualified physician, usually an anesthesiologist, should be readily available and responsible to ensure the patient's safe recovery from anesthesia. Equipment and drugs must be available to provide routine care (supplemental oxygen, suction, monitoring of vital signs, electrocardiogram and advanced organ support, ventilators, transducers to monitor intravascular pressures, devices for continuous infusion of drugs). An electrical defibrillator and appropriate drugs to assist in the optimal provision of cardiopulmonary resuscitation must also be available. The recovery room should have good access to radiographic and arterial blood gas services. The size of the recovery room is determined by the number and type of operative procedures, with approximately 1.5 recovery room beds necessary for every operating room.

Pain Relief

Pain is a predictable response as the effects of anesthetic drugs wane in the early postoperative period. Postoperative pain is influenced by patient age and personal interaction of physicians and nurses with the patient. In general, greater personal contact between health care professionals and the patient will reduce the amount of pharmacologic pain relief required. Treatment of postoperative pain is usually with incremental doses of intravenous narcotics, usually morphine in a dose of 15 to 30 μg/kg. In the future, continuous intravenous infusion of a low dose of narcotic may be used to provide more consistent and optimal analgesia with minimal respiratory depression. Continuous thoracic or lumbar epidural blockade with a long-acting local anesthetic such as bupivacaine is also an effective method of providing postoperative analgesia.

The epidural administration of a narcotic, usually morphine, has proved to be an innovative method of producing postoperative analgesia. In this situation, patients can have complete relief of pain with no autonomic sensory or motor blockade. This technique has been limited because of the rare occurrence of postoperative respiratory depression several hours after the administration of the narcotic epidurally. Once this rare complication is eliminated, it is this author's opinion that this technique will become a dominant form of postoperative pain relief. Patient-controlled analgesia is frequently used, in which a dilute form of narcotic is infused by control of the patient using various devices that will not allow an excessive dose of narcotic to be administered.

MONITORED ANESTHESIA CARE (STANDBY ANESTHESIA)

Monitored anesthesia care, often termed standby anesthesia, refers to the intravenous administration of sedative hypnotics (e.g., diazepam or midazolam) and/or narcotics (e.g., fentanyl) while the surgeon uses local infiltration of local anesthetic. Often, these types of cases do not require an anesthesiologist. However, in the elderly or fragile patient (especially those with an unprotected airway), these cases can be as challenging or complex as those cases in which the patient undergoes general anesthesia. In such cases, anesthesiologists will monitor the patients and titrate the appropriate drugs to provide sedation. This is particularly challenging to administer the appropriate amount of sedative drugs in a patient whose airway is unprotected.

ANESTHESIA AND AMBULATORY SURGERY

Increasingly, surgery is being performed on a "come-and-go" basis. Approximately 20 to 40 percent of a hospital's inpatient surgery could be performed in an outpatient setting. Compared with inpatient surgery, the advantages of performing the same operation on an outpatient basis include a decrease in medical costs, increased availability of beds for patients who require hospitalization, protection from hospital-acquired infections, and avoidance of the disruption of the family unit attendant upon hospitalization. Patients who report to the hospital on the day of surgery must be given detailed instructions well in advance of surgery. Local or general anesthesia usually is used in ambulatory surgical procedures, although epidural anesthesia can be used. Spinal anesthesia is inadvisable because of the possibility of postanesthetic headache. Recovery from anesthesia is accompanied by a return of vital signs to a normal level of consciousness and the ability to walk without assistance. Nausea, vomiting, and vertigo should be absent, and the patient should not have excessive pain. The patient should be able to drink fluids.

The ambulatory surgical patient should be reminded that mental clarity and dexterity may remain impaired for a period of 24 to 48 h, despite an overall feeling of well-being. Driving motor vehicles or operating complex equipment should not be attempted during this period. Finally, the patient should be given the physician's telephone number and instructed to report any new symptoms or other concerns.

Bibliography

Anesthetic Risks

Davies JM, Strunin L: Anesthesia in 1984: How safe is it? *Can Med Assoc* J 131:437,1984.

Hamilton WK: Unexpected deaths during anesthesia: Wherein lies the cause? *Anesthesiology* 7:25, 1979.

Keats AS: What do we know about anesthetic mortality? *Anesthesiology* 50:387, 1979.

Keenan RL, Boyan CP: Cardiac arrest due to anesthesia: A study of incidences and causes. *JAMA* 253:2373, 1985.

Tinker JH, Roberts SL: Anesthetic risk, in Miller RD (ed): *Anesthesia,* 2d ed. New York, Churchill Livingstone, 1986, chap 10.

Preoperative Evaluation

Egbert LD, Battit GE, et al: The value of the preoperative visit by an anesthetist. *JAMA* 185:553, 1963.

Kaplan EB, et al: The usefulness of preoperative laboratory screening. *JAMA* 253:3576, 1985.

Immediate Preoperative Care and Preparation

Britt BA, Joy N, et al: Positioning trauma, in Orkin FK, Cooperman LH (eds): *Complications in Anesthesiology.* Philadelphia, Lippincott, 1983, chap 51.

Eichhorn JH, Cooper JB, et al: Standards for patient monitoring during anesthesia at Harvard Medical School. *JAMA,* 256:1017, 1986.

Roizen MF: Routine preoperative evaluation, in Miller RD (ed): *Anesthesia,* 2d ed. New York, Churchill Livingstone, 1986, chap 8.

Stone DR, Downs JB, et al: Adult body temperature and heated humidification of anesthetic gases during general anesthesia. *Anesth Analg* 60:736, 1981.

Intraoperative Anesthesia

Cutler BS: Avoidance of hemologous transfusion in aortic operations: The roles of autotransfusion, hemodilution, and surgical technique. *Surgery* 95:717, 1984.

El-Hassan KM: Venous pressure and arm volume changes during simulated Bier's block. *Anaesthesia* 39:229, 1984.

Fahmy NR: Nitroprusside versus nitroprusside-triemethophan mixture for induced hypotension: A comparison of hemodynamic effects and cyanide release. *Anesthesiology* 61:A40, 1984.

Farrell G, Prendergast D, et al: Halothane hepatitis: Detection of a constitutional susceptibility factor. *N Engl J Med* 313:1310, 1985.

Flacke JW, Bloor BC, et al: Comparison of morphine, meperidine, fentanyl, and sufentanil in balanced anesthesia: A double blind study. *Anesth Analg* 64:897, 1985.

Ghoneim MM, et al: Comparison of four opioid analgesics as supplements to nitrous oxide anesthesia. *Anesth Analg* 63:405, 1984.

Goldman L: Cardiac risk and complications of noncardiac surgery. *Ann Surg* 198:780, 1983.

Gronert GA: Malignant hyperthermia, in Miller RD (ed): *Anesthesia,* 2d ed. New York, Churchill Livingstone, 1986, chap 56.

Kehlet H: Does regional anesthesia reduce postoperative morbidity? *Intensive Care Med* 10:165, 1984.

Little PE, et al: Site of action of intravenous regional anesthesia. *Anesthesiology* 61:507, 1984.

Manchikanti L, Marrero TC, et al: Preanesthetic cimetidine and metoclopramide for acid aspiration phrophylaxis in elective surgery. *Anesthesiology* 61:48, 1984.

McAuley CE, Watson CG: Effective inguinal herniorrhaphy after myocardial infarction. *Surg Gynecol Obstet* 159:36, 1984.

Nilsson A, et al: Midazolam as induction agent prior to inhalational anesthesia: A comparison with thiopentone. *Acta Anaesthesiol Scand* 28:249, 1984.

Rao TKL, Jacobs KH, et al: Reinfarction following anesthesia in patients with myocardial infarction. *Anesthesiology* 59:499, 1983.

Rogers SN, Benumof JL: New and easy technique for fiberoptic endoscopy-aided tracheal intubation. *Anesthesiology* 59:569, 1983.

Schmidt JF, Schierup L, et al: The effect of sodium citrate on the pH and the amount of gastric contents before general anesthesia. *Acta Anaesthesiol Scand* 28:263, 1984.

Weymuller EA Jr, Bishop MJ, et al: Quantification of intralaryngeal pressure exerted by endotracheal tubes. *Ann Otol Rhinol Laryngol* 92:444, 1983.

Postanesthetic Room (Recovery Room)

Catley DM, Thornton C, et al: Pronounced, episodic oxygen desaturation in the postoperative period: Its association with ventilatory pattern and analgesic regimen. *Anesthesiology* 63:20, 1985.

Cucchieri RJ, Morran CG, et al: Postoperative pain and pulmonary complication: Comparison of three analgesic regimens. *Br J Surg* 72:495, 1984.

Glenski JA, Warner MA, et al: Postoperative use of epidurally administered morphine in children and adolescents. *Mayo Clin Proc* 59:530, 1984.

Rodriguez JL, Weissman C, et al: Morphine and postoperative rewarming in critically ill patients. *Circulation* 68:1238, 1983.

Slotman GJ, Jed EH, et al: Adverse effects of hypothermia in postoperative patients. *Am J Surg* 149:495, 1985.

Wallace LM: Surgical patients' expectations of pain and discomfort: Does accuracy of expectations minimize post-surgical pain and distress? *Pain* 22:363, 1985.

Anesthesia and Ambulatory Surgery

Carter JA, Dye AM, et al: Recovery from day-case anaesthesia: The effects of different inhalational anaesthetic agents. *Anaesthesia* 40:545, 1985.

Natof HE: Complications associated with ambulatory surgery. *JAMA* 244:1116, 1980.

Ryan JA Jr, Adye BA, et al: Outpatient inguinal herniorrhaphy with both regional and local anesthesia. *Ann J Surg* 148:313, 1984.

Chapter 12

Complications

Seymour I. Schwartz

GENERAL CONSIDERATIONS

Surgical care must encompass an appreciation and anticipation of postoperative complications that may result from the disease process per se, errors of omission, or errors of commission in technique. In regarding the patient postoperatively, any deviation from the anticipated norm for clinical evaluation and/or diagnostic findings should alert one to focus on complications of the disease and also to retrace the operative procedure. It is unusual, although certainly possible, that clinical and laboratory abnormalities may be caused by the chance occurrence of an unrelated disease during the postoperative period. Acute cholecystitis and appendicitis are two examples of diseases that may become manifest during the postoperative course of the patient.

CHRONOLOGIC CONSIDERATIONS. Fever that presents shortly after surgical treatment in a patient who was previously afebrile is generally related to atelectasis or aspiration. Fever may also appear early in the postoperative course secondary to urinary tract infection, particularly if the patient has been catheterized. Fever of wound infection and leakage of an intestinal anastomosis or closure more frequently become evident on the fourth to seventh postoperative day. Hypotension in the early postoperative phase may be due to continued hemorrhage or the effects of depressive drugs that have been administered during the recovery period. Hypotension later in the postoperative course in a patient with sepsis should alert one to the possibility of septic shock.

WOUND COMPLICATIONS

Wound Dehiscence

Wound disruption, or dehiscence, generally refers to a separation of an abdominal wound involving the anterior fascial sheath and deeper layers. The inaccuracy of computing the frequency of wound disruption is notorious; the incidence in the literature ranges from 0.5 to 3 percent, averaging 2.6 percent when all abdominal operations are considered collectively. The incidence is definitely related to age and is reported to be 1.3 percent for patients under forty-five years in contrast to 5.4 percent for those over forty-five years. There is a higher incidence in elderly, debilitated patients with poor nutrition and in the presence of significant ascites or jaundice. Carcinoma is also associated with an increased incidence. Over 5 percent of laparotomies in patients in whom cancer was found are reported to have wound disruption in contrast to a 2 percent incidence when laparotomy demonstrates a benign condition. Other general factors that have been implicated include hypoproteinemia and atelectasis with its associated coughing, which, along with retching and hiccuping, increases the intraabdominal pressure and puts a strain on the incision. Obesity is definitely associated with an increased incidence. A lack of correlation between anemia and wound disruption has been reported.

Local factors involved in wound disruption include hemorrhage, infection, excessive suture material, and poor technique. Several series have suggested that the incidence of wound dehiscence is increased with vertical incisions. Recently this has been refuted in a prospective randomized series. When an intestinal stoma or a drain is brought out through any incision, the incidence of wound dehiscence increases.

A multicentric randomized prospective trial compared continuous and interrupted sutures of polyglycolic acid with close midline abdominal incisions. The overall dehiscence rate was 1.6 percent in patients with continuous versus 2 percent in the patients with interrupted sutures. The dehiscence rate in the interrupted group was significantly higher than in the continuous group when the wounds were contaminated. No significant difference has been noted between polyglycolic acid and polygalactin sutures.

CLINICAL MANIFESTATIONS. Most disruptions are concealed in the deeper layers of the wound and do not manifest until the fifth postoperative day, although the separation may, in fact, occur in the operating room or recovery room. The presenting sign that precedes the diagnosis of dehiscence in about 85 percent of cases is serosanguineous drainage from the wound, and if this occurs more than 24 h postoperatively, it is virtually pathognomonic. Frequently, wound dehiscence becomes manifest when the skin sutures are removed and evisceration of intraperitoneal contents, either intestine or omentum, occurs. In some instances, wound disruptions remain concealed beneath an intact cutaneous closure and go unrecognized initially, only to become manifest later in the form of a postoperative ventral hernia.

TREATMENT. The management depends on the patient's condition. If the patient can tolerate the procedure, a secondary operative closure is indicated. The author prefers through-and-through horizontal mattress sutures placed superficial to the peritoneum or buried figure-of-eight monofilament stainless steel sutures to approximate the muscle and fascial layers. In some instances, it is preferable to treat the patient conservatively with an occlusive wound dressing and binder and to accept the complication of a postoperative hernia. If evisceration occurs, sterile moist towels should be applied to cover the extruded intestine or omentum, and the patient should be taken directly to the operating room. After general irrigation, the abdomen is closed with one of the two previously mentioned techniques.

The mortality associated with wound disruption depends on the patient's age and original pathologic condition. Although one recent series reported that 34 percent of patients died after operative closure of an abdominal wound evisceration, most authorities report that the mortality has been reduced to 0.5 to 0.3 percent in recent years. The main morbidity is prolonged hospitalization. The incidence of postoperative hernia is hard to define but has been reported to be at least 32 percent.

Wound Infection

Postoperative wound infection results when bacteria within the wound multiply, exciting a local reaction and, frequently, a systemic response. Most wounds become infected in the operating room while they are open, but the presence of bacteria in the wound at the end of the surgical procedure does not usually result in a wound infection. The bacterium most frequently implicated is *Staphylococcus aureus.* Enteric organisms are the causative agents when bowel operation has been performed, and hemolytic streptococci account for about 3 percent of infections. Other common pathogens include enterococci, *Pseudomonas, Proteus,* and *Klebsiella.*

The reported incidence of wound infection has a wide range. The Public Health Laboratory Service of England and Wales reported an overall wound infection rate of 9.7 percent. In a combined study conducted by the Division of Medical Sciences, National Academy of Science-National Research Council, and reported in 1964, the overall incidence of infection in five participating hospitals varied from 3 to 11.1 percent. Clean atraumatic and uninfected operative wounds in which neither the bronchi, nor the gastrointestinal tract, nor the genitourinary tract was entered and which were elective, primarily closed, and undrained had an overall incidence of definite infection of 3.3 percent, while similar wounds that were either not elective, or not primarily closed, or drained mechanically through the incision or via a stab wound had a 7.4 percent incidence of wound infection. Operative wounds in which the bronchus, gastrointestinal tract, or oropharyngeal cavity were entered but without unusual contamination had an overall incidence of infection of 10.8 percent. Open, fresh traumatic wounds, operations with a major break in sterile technique, and incisions encountering acute nonpurulent inflammation were associated with an incidence of wound infections of 16.3 percent. Old traumatic wounds and those involving abscesses of perforated viscera had the highest rate of infection (28.6 percent).

A variety of factors other than the nature of the wound also influence the incidence of infection. Age is a definite factor; the rate of wound infection rises steadily from 4.7 percent in the fifteen- to twenty-four-year-old group to 10.7 percent in the sixty-five to seventy-four-year-old group. There is virtually no difference in sex and race. The presence of diabetes is associated with an increase in infection rate, but when this is adjusted for age, there is no statistical significance to this figure. Steroid therapy affects the wound infection rate adversely; an incidence of 16 percent for patients receiving steroids has been contrasted with 7 percent for those not on such drugs. Patients who are extremely obese also have a more than doubled rate of wound infection when compared with control groups. In the combined study, patients with severe malnutrition also displayed a markedly increased rate of wound infection, but this was distorted by other factors, which, if corrected, cast doubt on the widely held belief that malnourished patients are intrinsically more susceptible. Patients who harbor infections remote from the operative incision have an increased infection rate. The duration of operation exerts a profound influence on wound infection, the incidence rising steadily from 3.6 percent for procedures lasting less than 30 min to 18 percent for those lasting over 6 h. The urgency of operation only indirectly influences the wound infection rate.

The use of a drain was associated with an 11 percent infection rate, whereas undrained wounds had a rate of 5 percent, but it could not be concluded that the drains themselves were responsible for the infection. Patients hospitalized for fewer than 2 days preoperatively had an infection rate of 6 percent, whereas those hospitalized for periods greater than 3 weeks preoperatively had a rate of 14 percent, and this relationship could not be explained on the basis of other associated factors. The prophylactic use of antibiotics was paradoxically associated with a much higher wound infection rate in the combined series, and similar findings were reported for orthopaedic cases. In contrast, Ketcham et al., in a double-blind study, reported a reduction of wound infection in patients with extensive cancer who were placed on prophylactic antibiotics. In addition preoperative and early postoperative use of cephalosporin or metronidazole reduced the incidence of wound infection in patients in whom segments of stomach or intestine were opened.

The two factors of importance in the genesis of infection are breaks in surgical technique and the host-parasite relationship. Two potential sources of contamination are patients themselves, particularly the gastrointestinal tract, and the environment of the operating room including the operating team. Carriers of *Staph. aureus* in the hospital population have become an increasing source. It has been demonstrated that patients who are nasal carriers of *Staph. aureus* have a higher incidence of wound infection than noncarriers.

CLINICAL MANIFESTATIONS. In a typical situation about 3 to 4 days following operation, there is some increase in pulse rate, and about the fourth postoperative day, a low-grade, intermittent fever is noted. Usually there is edema and redness of the wound, but the most important early sign is undue pain. In some types, marked thrombosis of surrounding blood vessels is an important feature. Wound dehiscence is usually not caused by infection per se unless the infection is neglected. The diagnosis is usually made on the fifth to seventh day, but this interval may be extended if the patient has been on antibiotics. At that time, the wound is commonly seen as a suppurative process, essentially an abscess. Systemic features of septicemia may be present.

TREATMENT. The most important prophylactic measure is excellent technique. In human volunteers, Elek and Conen have shown that the presence of suture material enhances the infective power of *Staph. aureus* 1000 to 10,000 times. Therefore, fine sutures and accurate hemostasis should reduce the incidence. It is generally felt that prophylactic antibiotics do not contribute to a reduction in the incidence of wound infection. In patients undergoing intestinal resections, wound irrigation with a cephalosporin has reduced the incidence of infection. Irrigation of subcutaneous tissue with povidone-iodine significantly reduced the incidence of wound infection following a variety of surgical procedures in one series. Other studies, however, have shown no greater protection than that achieved with saline irrigation and less than that with local cephaloridine.

Once diagnosed, the treatment consists of surgical drainage. The skin sutures should be removed and the wound irrigated with saline solution and lightly packed. As a general principle, antimicrobial drugs are not required unless the offending organism is *Streptococcus pyogenes* or hemolytic streptococci, which should be treated with penicillin for a period of at least 1 week. Also, patients with wound infections around the central area of the face should receive antimicrobial therapy to prevent intracranial extension. Finally, if the wound sepsis is associated with bacteremia or spreading cellulitis, antimicrobial therapy is also indicated. The antibiotic used is determined by culture and sensitivity studies of the infected wound.

See Chap. 5 for a discussion of specific infections, i.e., staphylococcal infections, streptococcal infections, anaerobic clostridial cellulitis, clostridial myonecrosis, streptococcal myositis, and tetanus.

Wound Hemorrhage, Hematoma, and Seroma (Accumulation of Serum)

Wound hemorrhage is generally related to an error in technique in which hemostasis is not accomplished. There is a higher incidence in patients with polycythemia vera, myeloproliferative disorders, or coagulation defects and in patients receiving anticoagulant therapy (see Chap. 3). Postoperative hemorrhage usually becomes manifest with a sensation of pressure or pain within the wound shortly after the patient awakes from anesthesia. There may be leakage of sanguineous or serosanguineous material at that time. To control bleeding from the wound edges, pressure may be applied initially, but if the bleeding continues, additional sutures or reexploration of the wound may be required.

The placement of drains in areas of anticipated wound bleeding is usually not indicated. If the bleeding is trivial, the drain is unnecessary; if the bleeding is severe, it will not evacuate the material. Drains or catheters connected to closed suction are appropriately used to evacuate serous fluid from underneath skin flaps, such as that associated with mastectomy or neck or groin dissection, in order to prevent the vicious cycle in which an expanding serous collection produces significant bleeding as it separates the wound. If a large skin flap has been raised, fluid will develop, and in order to facilitate apposition between the subcutaneous tissue and deep fascia, drainage should be effected. This obviates formation of a seroma.

Once a seroma develops, it should be aspirated initially; if multiple aspirations are required, a polyethylene catheter may be inserted and attached to negative suction. Prompt treatment is indicated, since the presence of contained serous fluid increases the incidence of subcutaneous infection. The same situation pertains to a subcutaneous hematoma, and drainage is required, since the blood affords an excellent culture medium and also prevents apposition between the two surfaces.

POSTOPERATIVE PAROTITIS

Postoperative parotitis is a serious complication and is associated with a high mortality related to it and to the primary disease with which it is associated. Recent reviews indicate a real recrudescence related to the increasing age of the surgical population. The right and left glands are involved equally, and in 10 to 15 percent of cases, the disease presents bilaterally. Seventy-five percent of patients are seventy years or older, and the overwhelming majority have associated diseases. Patients having major abdominal surgical treatment, fractured hip, debilitating diseases, and severe injury are among the most commonly afflicted.

The factors implicated in the etiology include poor oral hygiene, dehydration, and the use of anticholinergic drugs. In one large series, one-third of the patients with acute suppurative parotitis had carcinoma, and one-half had preexisting major infection elsewhere in the body. In only one-third of the cases in this series the acute suppurative process developed in the postoperative period.

The pathogenesis is thought to be a transductal inoculation of the parotid, and the majority of infections are due to staphylococci. The combination of poor oral hygiene and lack of oral intake to stimulate parotid secretions predisposes to bacterial invasion of Stensen's duct. The inflammatory lesions of early parotitis are confined to an accumulation of cells within the larger ducts. The parenchyma of the smaller ducts are initially spared, but once penetration of the parenchyma occurs, multiple abscesses form and later coalesce. If the process continues, the purulent material penetrates the capsule and invades the surrounding tissue along one of three routes: downward into the deep fascial planes of the neck, backward into the external auditory canal, or outward into the skin of the face.

CLINICAL MANIFESTATIONS. The interval between operation and the onset of parotitis varies from a few hours to many weeks. The patient initially presents with pain in the parotid region. The pain is usually unilateral but may become bilateral in a short period of time. Initially, inspection shows the gland to be slightly swollen, and palpation demonstrates exquisite tenderness. Because of the septate anatomy of the gland, fluctuance is rarely demonstrable. The course of postoperative parotitis is rapid and fulminating with severe cellulitis developing on the affected side of the face and neck. The temperature and leukocyte count may be extremely high. Obstruction of the airway may necessitate tracheostomy, and the abscess may rupture into adjacent structures of the ear, mastoid, pharynx, or anterior and posterior triangles of the neck. Parotitis is to be differentiated from benign postoperative swelling of the parotids, which occurs more frequently in Blacks and may be related to straining, atropine, and neuromuscular depolarizing drugs.

TREATMENT. Prophylactic therapy consists of adequate hydration and good oral hygiene that can be aided by allowing the patient to take ice chips and stimulating salivary flow. Prophylactic antibiotics are of no apparent value.

Once the diagnosis is entertained, pus should be expressed from Stensen's duct and culture and sensitivity tests performed. A broad-spectrum antibiotic that acts against the staphylococci should be started while awaiting results. In one series of 66 glands cultured, 64 contained staphylococci. In some cases, these were combined with streptococci, gram-negative bacilli, and pneumococci. If there is considerable pain and the disease is less than 48 h old, irradiation of the gland in small doses is indicated. Irradiation may provide symptomatic relief by reducing the secretions of the obstructed gland, but this type of therapy does not affect the course of the disease as much as antibiotics or surgical drainage.

Frequent observation of the patient is essential. If the disease persists or progresses, drainage should be considered as early as the third day. If there is moderate improvement, drainage may be delayed for a day or two, but in no circumstance should it be delayed beyond the fifth day. An incision is made anterior to the ear, extending down to the angle of the mandible, and flaps are reflected, exposing the gland. A hemostat is inserted through the capsule and opened in the direction of the course of the branches of the facial nerve. Multiple drainage sites are thus established, and the wound is packed lightly open. Deferring drainage until fluctuation is apparent is unwise. Stimulation of the salivary flow by massage of the gland or other means is contraindicated, once the inflammatory process is established.

PROGNOSIS. In a recent series, the mortality rate approximated 20 percent, but this was frequently related to the patient's basic disease. Thirty-six percent of the patients who died demonstrated active parotitis. In 80 percent of patients treated with incision and drainage, the parotitis was palliated or cured.

POSTOPERATIVE RESPIRATORY COMPLICATIONS

Respiratory Failure

Respiratory failure is the major cause of death after surgical or accidental trauma, accounting for 25 percent of postoperative deaths. It is a significant contributory factor in another 25 percent of postoperative patients. It can be defined as a situation in which the partial pressure of oxygen in arterial blood (Pa_{O_2}) is below 50 torr while the patient is breathing room air, or when the Pa_{CO_2} is above 50 torr in the absence of metabolic alkalosis.

PATHOPHYSIOLOGY. Physiologic causes of acute respiratory insufficiency following surgery include (1) hypoventilation, (2) diffusion defects, (3) abnormalities in the ventilation-perfusion ratio, (4) shunting that is either anatomic or related to atelectasis, (5) reduction in cardiac output with concomitant persistent shunt, and (6) alteration in the hemoglobin level and/or dissociation curve. Respiratory failure occurs when the functional residual capacity (FRC), i.e., the amount of air present in the lung at the end of a normal expiration, is reduced to a level that is associated with alveolar collapse and consequent intrapulmonary shunting that leads to hypoxemia.

A variety of measurements of ventilation and oxygenation have been applied to assess the pathophysiologic events. Ventilatory mechanics are evaluated by measuring the ventilatory rate, the vital capacity (VC), total volume (VT), and dead space (VD). VD/VT, which is also influenced by cardiac output, is used to assess CO_2 elimination. Compliance is a measurement of the distensibility of the lung.

The partial pressure of CO_2 in arterial blood (Pa_{CO_2}) can be considered as a reciprocal function of ventilation and is normally 40 torr. The adequacy of intrapulmonary blood-gas exchange is determined by measuring the Pa_{CO_2} and the Pa_{O_2} in relation to the inspired $F_{I_{O_2}}$. One method of estimating the efficacy of oxygen exchange in the lung is to measure the alveolar-arterial oxygen tension difference $[(A-a)D_{O_2}]$. Factors that influence the $(A-a)D_{O_2}$ include the degree of mismatching of ventilation to perfusion, shunts around the lung, the difference between the arterial and mixed venous oxygen content, the mixed venous oxygen content itself, which may reflect oxygen consumption, the cardiac output, the inspired oxygen concentration ($F_{I_{O_2}}$), the position of the oxygen hemoglobin dissociation curve, and the position of the Pa_{O_2} on the curve. A nomogram can be used to define the calculated amount of blood shunted around the lung as a fraction of the total cardiac output ($\dot{Q}_S/\dot{Q}_T$) based on the measurement of Pa_{O_2} and pulmonary alveolar oxygen tension (PA_{O_2}), as shown in Fig. 12-1. As can be seen, small changes in the $\dot{Q}_S/\dot{Q}_T$ are more readily detected when the patient is breathing 100% oxygen for 20 to 30 min. This may result in absorption atelectasis that will increase

$\dot{Q}_S/\dot{Q}_T$. Therefore, "shunt fraction" is usually measured at the inspired O_2 concentration ($F_{I_{O_2}}$) required to maintain an adequate arterial P_{O_2} (60 to 70 torr or greater). The ratio of arterial P_{O_2} to alveolar P_{O_2} tends to be independent of inspired $F_{I_{O_2}}$. Determinations are affected by alterations in the cardiac output and pH.

PATHOGENESIS. Hypoventilation may be related to thoracic trauma, muscle weakness, and deleterious changes in the respiratory mechanics, which have been shown to exist for several days following thoracotomy and laparotomy. The defects also may be related to the aspiration of gastric content, which is now appreciated to occur more commonly; an incidence of 10 percent has been reported for intubated patients undergoing elective operations, and a higher percentage for patients undergoing emergency operations. There is no evidence that tracheostomy completely protects against such aspiration. Oxygen itself has intrinsic toxicity, and when $F_{I_{O_2}}$ is over 50% for more than 2 to 3 days, destruction of respiratory epithelium may occur. Therefore, it is preferable to maintain patients with respiratory insufficiency at the lowest $F_{I_{O_2}}$ that still maintains a Pa_{O_2} of 70 torr rather than expose the airway to 100% oxygen for a long period of time. Fluid overload with pulmonary edema decreases compliance and impairs gas exchange. Other intrapulmonary lesions that may contribute to interference with oxygenation include microemboli, fat emboli, and pulmonary in-

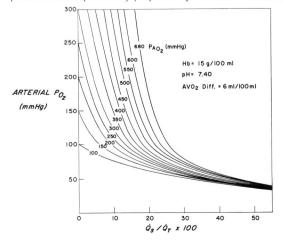

Fig. 12-1. Analog-computed relationship between percent right-to-left shunt ($\dot{Q}_S/\dot{Q}_T \times 100$), arterial P_{O_2}, and inspired oxygen or alveolar oxygen tension (PA_{O_2}). The alveolar-arterial oxygen tension gradient can be obtained by drawing a horizontal line from the ordinate (arterial P_{O_2}) to the appropriate PA_{O_2} line. For example, when $\dot{Q}_S/\dot{Q}_T \times 100 = 20$, and $PA_{O_2} = 680$ mmHg, then the arterial P_{O_2} is approximately 175 mmHg and the $(A-a)D_{O_2} = 680 - 175 = 505$ mmHg. Note that below a right-to-left shunt value of 30, small changes in $\dot{Q}_S/\dot{Q}_T \times 100$ can produce drastic alterations in arterial P_{O_2} particularly when the subject is breathing high concentrations of oxygen. The curves were drawn assuming a hemoglobin concentration of 15 g/100 mL, an arterial pH of 7.40, an $A - V_{O_2}$ difference of 6 mL/100 mL, and a standard oxyhemoglobin dissociation curve. (From: *Pontoppidan H et al: Adv Surg 4:163, 1970. Copyright 1970 by Year Book Medical Publishers, Chicago. Used by permission. Graphs kindly prepared by Dr. M. A. Duvelleroy.*)

fection. Abnormalities of the ventilation-perfusion ratio ($\dot{V}/\dot{Q}$) result when areas well perfused with blood are underventilated. Maintaining the patient in a supine position accentuates this maldistribution, and the resultant consequence of atelectasis is a significant contributor to increased $\dot{V}/\dot{Q}$. Other factors that alter the ventilation-perfusion ratio are obesity and upper abdominal operation with consequent collapse of the basal alveoli. Both atelectasis and reduced cardiac output result in intrapulmonary shunting. A shift in the oxygen-hemoglobin dissociation curve to the left decreases oxygen delivery to the tissues. This may be caused by respiratory alkalosis, by deficiency in 2,3-diphosphoglycerate, which results from transfusion of banked blood more than 3 days old, and by carbon monoxide poisoning, which is commonly present in patients with smoke inhalation associated with burns.

The term "shock lung" is inappropriate. Hemorrhagic shock unassociated with sepsis rarely causes acute pulmonary insufficiency. There is no distinct pathologic lung lesion in patients dying of hemorrhagic shock. $Na^+ - K^+$ transport and adenosine nucleotides in the lung are unchanged in hemorrhagic shock, indicating that cellular energy utilization or production in the lung is unchanged. Sepsis is the most common factor implicated in the development of adult respiratory distress syndrome (ARDS). Almost 20 percent of hospitalized patients with septicemia develop ARDS. The pulmonary insufficiency usually cannot be reversed unless sepsis is controlled. Severe pancreatitis and the fat embolism syndrome also are etiologic factors. ARDS in these patients is an ominous manifestation.

CLINICAL MANIFESTATIONS. Among the situations that should alert the observer to the development of the syndrome of postoperative pulmonary insufficiency are (1) congestive failure, (2) dyspnea, (3) cyanosis, (4) evidence of obstructive lung disease, (5) pulmonary edema, and (6) unexplained deterioration of arterial O_2 tension.

Tachypnea and hypoxemia are the earliest manifestations of respiratory insufficiency. Early in the evolution of the syndrome, the patient manifests hyperventilation associated with a reduction in Pa_{CO_2} below 35 torr that may minimize a significant reduction in Pa_{O_2}. Ultimately there is a reduction in Pa_{O_2} that becomes more significant when the patient does not respond to increases in $F_{I_{O_2}}$. Radiographic changes tend to occur late in the course of the condition and may represent the effects of therapy. These lesions are characteristically scattered, ill-defined, bilateral densities. A correlation exists between the extension of the densities and deterioration of pulmonary function. The diagnosis of ARDS is usually assigned when conservative measures such as oxygen by mask, pulmonary toilet, and/or bronchodilators fail to maintain the Pa_{O_2} above 60 torr.

TREATMENT. Control of postoperative pain can effect a significant reduction in the incidence of pulmonary complications following thoracic or upper abdominal operations. Epidural bupivacaine has been particularly effective. Continuous positive airway pressure (CPAP), administered with a mask, offers an advantage because it requires no effort from the patient, and it is not painful. But attention to respiratory therapy, regardless of the modality employed, may be the most important factor.

The treatment of acute respiratory insufficiency is based primarily on ventilatory support. Specific indications for ventilatory support are listed in Table 12-1. This is accomplished through either an endotracheal tube or a tracheostomy, since ventilation via a face mask or mouthpiece is rarely effective for more than short periods and puts the patient at risk for acute aspiration. Endotracheal intubation, preferably through the nose, is considered the technique of choice when control of airway is urgently required. Although endotracheal tubes are not tolerated as well as tracheostomy tubes and prolonged intubation is associated with laryngeal swelling, 6 days in adults and up to 3 weeks in children are regarded as reasonable periods

Table 12-1. INDICATIONS FOR RESPIRATORY SUPPORT

		Acceptable range	Chest physical therapy, oxygen, close monitoring	Intubation tracheostomy, ventilation
Mechanics	Respiratory rate	12–20	20–30	> 30
	Vital capacity, mL/kg	70–30	30–15	< 15
	Inspiratory force, cmH$_2$O	100–50	50–25	< 25
Oxygenation	$(A-a)D_{O_2}$, torr*	100–200	200–350	> 350
Ventilation	VD/VT	0.3–0.4	0.4–0.6	> 0.6
	Pa_{CO_2}, torr	35–45	45–50	> 50†
Functional residual capacity (% normal predicted value)		80–100	50–80	< 50
Pulmonary venous admixture (shunt) (Q_{SP}/Q_T) %		<5	15–20	> 20

* After 15 min of 100% O_2.
† Except in chronic hypercapnia.

of prolonged endotracheal intubation. In general, intubation via a nasotracheal route is tolerated better than via the orotracheal route, but insertion may be more difficult. Attempts at swallowing may make an oral tracheal tube advance into the right main stem bronchus, resulting in atelectasis of the left lung. The major advantage of endotracheal intubation is that the mortality is low, the complications are minimal, and the hazards associated with tracheostomy are avoided.

Tracheostomy is now generally reserved for the patient who requires prolonged ventilatory support and may be associated with the complications of stenosis generally related to cuff pressure. The introduction of low-pressure cuffs has reduced the incidence of this complication.

If patients have criteria that indicate the need for ventilatory support (Table 12-1), intubation is carried out and an $F_{I_{O_2}}$ greater than 0.5 may be temporarily required, but this should be rapidly reduced. PEEP is increased in 2 cmH$_2$O increments until a $Pa_{O_2}/F_{I_{O_2}}$ ratio of 250:1 is achieved or, preferably, until the intrapulmonary shunt fraction should be determined to be less than 25 percent. Civetta and associates advise the use of a pulmonary arterial catheter if there is compromise of cardiac function or if a PEEP of 15 cmH$_2$O does not achieve the desired $Pa_{O_2}/F_{I_{O_2}}$ ratio. Intermittent mandatory ventilation (IMV) is increased by two breaths per minute to maintain a pH of 7.35 to 7.45, and a Pa_{CO_2} of 45 torr or less. The ventilatory is set to deliver a volume of 12 to 15 mL/kg body weight. PEEP results in increased functional residual capacity, reduced normal negative intrathoracic pressure with, at times, conversion to positive values, increased venous pressure, and decreased venous return to the heart. PEEP ventilation is particularly effective in causing a rise in Pa_{O_2}, a fall in physiologic shunt, and a decrease in shunting across the lung. PEEP ventilation is preferred for patients with profound hypoxemia, significant physiologic shunting, atelectasis, and high cardiac output. It is particularly appropriate for patients with massive chest wall injuries. PEEP is usually contraindicated for conditions characterized by normal oxygenation, hyperexpansion of the lung, such as pulmonary emphysema, and low cardiac output. PEEP should be increased in increments of 2 to 3 cm of water until the intrapulmonary shunt is reduced to 15 percent. The Pa_{O_2} on 30 percent O$_2$ should reach about 100 torr.

Prolonged artificial ventilation has been characterized by the formation of edema and deterioration of blood-gas interchange, which is generally manageable by water restriction and the administration of diuretic agents. When there is objective evidence that lung function is adequate to permit transfer from artificial to spontaneous ventilation, a gradual weaning process is required. Difficulty in weaning can be attributed to abnormalities in blood-gas exchange, pulmonary mechanics, reduction in cardiac output, and general muscle weakness. A more gradual weaning, employing intermittent mandatory ventilation, may expedite the process. Weaning should be accomplished only with careful monitoring of blood-gas exchange; the pulmonary mechanics are indicated in Table 12-1.

In the weaning process the first priority is to reduce the $F_{I_{O_2}}$ to less than 0.5 to avoid maintaining the collapse of the alveoli. Next, the number of IMV breaths should be decreased to a level that permits a normal pH and a Pa_{CO_2} of 35 to 45 torr at a respiratory rate of less than 30 per min. This is continued until only two mechanical breaths per minute are required. PEEP is lowered in increments of 2 to 3 cmH$_2$O/min monitoring the Pa_{O_2}. When adequate oxygenation is maintained with a PEEP of 5 cmH$_2$O and the IMV is 0 and the CPAP is 5 cmH$_2$O, and the criteria in the early ARDS columns of Table 12-1 are met, the patient generally no longer requires ventilatory support.

Ancillary treatment consists of cardiovascular interventions directed at the preload, contractility, and afterload. Intravascular and extracellular fluid deficits should be corrected. Care is taken to avoid fluid overload of the patient and to maintain the colloidal osmotic pressure of serum. The administration of concentrated albumin solutions to reduce pulmonary edema is ill-advised because the albumin will merely pass into the extravascular spaces. If fluid therapy is necessary to restore ventricular filling pressure, balanced electrolyte solutions are preferable. The administration of diuretics may have a negative net effect on cardiovascular function.

Enhancement of cardiac contractility may be required. Dopamine and/or dobutamine are employed to increase contractility without causing a marked increase in oxygen requirements. Decreasing the afterload by reducing the impedance to cardiac outflow has an additive effect. Drugs such as sodium nitroprusside that decrease arteriolar resistance or venous capacitance may be required.

Atelectasis

Atelectasis comprises 90 percent of all postoperative pulmonary complications, but a lack of definition and difficulty in diagnosis has resulted in a wide range of reported incidences varying between 1 and 80 percent depending on the type of operation. It occurs more commonly after upper abdominal operations. The term "atelectasis" is derived from the Greek meaning "incomplete expansion" but is generally applied to the situation in which there are airless alveoli. Although collapse of alveoli may occur within definite anatomic units such as segments, lobes, or an entire lung, the most commonly encountered variety is platelike and subsegmental.

ETIOLOGY. The two major factors that have been implicated as causes of atelectasis are bronchial obstruction with distal gas absorption and hypoventilation or ineffectual respiration. The loss of chemical elements that stabilize the lung at low volumes by reducing alveolar surface tension, i.e., *surfactants,* has been implicated.

Obstruction of the tracheobronchial airway occurs secondary to changes in bronchial secretion, defect in the expulsion mechanism, and reduction in bronchial caliber. Subsequent to tracheobronchial obstruction by secretion, vomitus, blood, or tumor material, there is a period during which a change occurs in the composition of gases within the alveolus, following which the gas composition in the obstructed alveoli remains constant until absorption is complete. The rate of absorption is a function of the pressure difference between the gas in the alveoli and the gas in the blood, the absorption coefficient of the gas, and the rate and quantity of blood flow. Obstruction of a large conductive airway certainly leads to atelectasis of the distal lung segment. However, there are many observations that cast doubt on bronchial obstruction as the sole or major causative factor in postoperative atelectasis.

Currently, many feel that atelectasis usually consists of small and diffuse lesions that are nonobstructive in origin and are due to inspiratory insufficiency. Atelectasis has been thought to occur without airway obstruction as a result of a constant volume ventilation with volumes approximating normal tidal volume, and the process is reversible by hyperinflation.

A major cause of alveolar collapse is related to the surface forces acting at the gas-liquid interface within the alveolar units. Normally, there is a film, surfactant, which has the property of reducing surface tension when the alveolar volume is decreased. Increased surface tension of this film encourages collapse or decrease in the size of the alveolus and makes it more difficult to inflate. Regional changes in the pulmonary circulation may alter the characteristics of surfactant. Deep breathing mobilizes surfactant from within the alveolar cell to augment or replace the aging surfactant on the alveolar surface, maintaining stability and preventing atelectasis.

Many factors predispose to the development of postoperative atelectasis. There is an increasing incidence in patients who smoke and those who suffer from bronchitis, asthma, emphysema, or other chronic lung diseases. Anesthesia and postoperative narcotics depress the cough reflex, while chest pain, immobilization, and splinting with bandages reduce the effective nature of the cough. The incidence of atelectasis is related to the duration and depth of anesthesia, and although higher incidences have been reported with general anesthesia than with regional anesthesia, when the same postoperative care was applied to the two groups, the difference disappeared. Nasogastric tubes have been implicated because of the increased secretions and predisposition toward aspiration. Bronchospasm is a predisposing factor, but severe bronchospasm is rarely encountered during clinical anesthesia. Congestion of the bronchial walls due to edema represents another source of decrease in the bronchial lumen.

CLINICAL MANIFESTATIONS. Atelectasis usually becomes manifest in the first 24 h after an operation and rarely appears after 48 h. There is usually a sudden onset of fever and tachycardia. Frequently, the pulmonary manifestations are so minor that they are not recognized. Early findings include rales located posteriorly in the bases, diminished breath sounds, and bronchial breathing. With massive involvement, there may be a shift of the trachea, mediastinum, and heart to the involved side, but this is not present with the more common subsegmental lesions. Pronounced dyspnea and/or cyanosis are relatively uncommon. Radiographs may demonstrate areas of consolidation, but in early cases bronchial breathing is detected more frequently than radiographic changes. Determination of blood gases indicating intrapulmonary shunting of blood provides the diagnosis. Characteristically with atelectasis and significant shunting, the arterial Pa_{O_2} is decreased while the arterial Pa_{CO_2} may be normal or decreased. The ventilation is normal or increased.

If atelectasis persists, the clinical manifestations are those generally associated with pneumonia. The temperature increases to a greater extent, and there is increasing tachycardia, dyspnea, and cyanosis. It is felt that the great majority of postoperative pneumonias begin as atelectasis, since atelectatic areas are poorly drained and represent good sites for infection. In some instances, however, pneumonia may result from the aspiration of infected material. Another consequence of atelectasis is the development of lung abscess, which also may be initiated by the aspiration of foreign material, such as teeth or blood during tonsillectomy and purulent material from putrid abscesses in the mouth. Aspiration of gastric contents also represents a possible cause of lung abscess.

TREATMENT. Prophylaxis begins preoperatively by having the patient cease smoking, if possible, for at least 2 weeks prior to operation and instructing the patient in deep abdominal breathing and productive coughing. Postoperative prophylaxis includes the minimal use of depressant drugs, the prevention of pain that may limit respiration, frequent changes of body position, deep breathing and coughing exercises, and early ambulation. Sustained maximal inspiration, which can be accomplished with the aid of a variety of devices, is an important factor in the prevention and treatment of atelectasis.

Three groups of medications have been applied to the prophylaxis and therapy of atelectasis. These are (1) expectorants to provide more liquid and less viscous secretions, (2) detergents and mucolytic solutions to alter the surface tension of secretions and render their elimination more likely, and (3) bronchodilators used primarily by inhalation to provide increased size of the tracheobronchial tree and elimination of bronchospasm. The mucolytic agents, such as Mucomist or Alevaire, are indicated because inhaled air with a relative humidity lower than 70 percent inhibits ciliary activity and tends to desiccate secretions.

Once atelectasis becomes clinically manifest, coughing, clearing of secretions, and increase in depth of respiration may be stimulated by endotracheal suction with a soft rubber catheter or the instillation of 1 to 2 mL of saline solution directly into the trachea via an intracatheter polyethylene tube. If these measures are not successful, bronchoscopy may be required, and if multiple bronchoscopic aspirations are necessary, tracheostomy should be performed to facilitate subsequent aspiration.

Pulmonary Edema

Pulmonary edema may occur during or immediately after an operation. The increased use of massive blood transfusions, plasma expanders, and other fluids during operative procedures has resulted in an increased incidence of this complication. Circulatory overload represents the most common cause of pulmonary edema. Other factors that have been implicated include left ventricular failure, shift of blood from the peripheral to pulmonary vascular bed, negative pressure on the airway that increases the gradient between the transmural capillary pressure and the alveolar pressure favoring transudation, and injury to the alveolar membrane by noxious substances.

Although circulatory overload is most frequently due to infusion of fluid during operative procedure, it may also result from the absorption of solutions during irrigation of hollow viscera, such as the bladder, and is frequently associated with subclinical heart failure in those patients in whom pulmonary edema becomes manifest.

Incomplete cardiac emptying may be attributed to any anesthetic, narcotic, or hypnotic agent, since all are capable of decreasing myocardial contractility. Incomplete cardiac emptying may also be due to gross irregularities in rhythm. Left ventricular failure results in elevated left atrial and pulmonary artery blood pressures. Peripheral vascular beds may vasoconstrict, causing blood to shift centrally and result in pulmonary edema. A reflex mechanism of neurogenic origin that causes redistribution of blood from the periphery to the pulmonary bed has been reported to occur during manipulation of the brain and following head trauma.

Pulmonary edema caused by injury to the alveolar membrane is associated with the inhalation of noxious gases or vapors and the aspiration of gastric contents or chemicals, particularly kerosene, that are pulmonary irritants. Endotoxins released during gram-negative sepsis cause pulmonary edema by increasing pulmonary permeability. White blood cells sequestered in the lung with pulmonary emboli and hypoperfusion release vasoactive substances that effect these changes.

CLINICAL MANIFESTATIONS. The early disturbances of pulmonary edema are accumulation of fluid in the sheath around small pulmonary arteries and thickening of the capillary and alveolar membranes. In the early stage, the principal effect is widening of the $(A-a)O_2$ gradient. A reduction in lung compliance precedes evidence of carbon dioxide retention in the blood. Bronchospasm usually occurs and contributes further to reducing the compliance. As frank edema develops, a frothy pink-stained fluid appears in the alveoli, bronchi, and trachea, and at this time the problem is one of airway obstruction. Clinically, bronchospasm and marked reduction in lung compliance in a patient being ventilated should provide premonitory evidence and anticipate the development of dyspnea and cough. A few scattered rales may appear early, but as the process intensifies, bubbling rales and rhonchi are heard all over the chest. The systemic blood pressure is usually raised initially but may be normal or reduced, and characteristically there is a marked tachycardia. Shock may appear with signs of peripheral circulatory failure, and death may occur from asphyxia.

TREATMENT. Therapy is directed at (1) providing oxygen, (2) allowing oxygen access to the alveoli by removing obstructive fluid, and (3) correcting the circulatory

overload if present. Arterial oxygen saturation can be restored by increasing the concentration of oxygen in inspired air.

Measures to reduce the pulmonary capillary pressure include venous occlusion tourniquets, placing the patient in a head-up or sitting position to reduce the flow of venous blood to the heart, and phlebotomy. Since systemic vasoconstriction has been shown to be a precipitating cause, therapy may be indicated to reverse this mechanism. Spinal anesthesia has been applied successfully in the treatment of pulmonary edema, as have the ganglionic blocking agent Arfonad and afterload reduction with sodium nitroprusside.

Drug therapy includes furosemide or ethacrynic acid for rapid diuresis and digitalis glycosides for situations where myocardial failure and lower output coexist (particularly in mitral stenosis) or where there is arrhythmia such as flutter or fibrillation. Morphine has been shown to be of value, though its mode of action remains unclear. If applied early, CPAP can reverse the process; in the intubated patient PEEP is most effective.

CARDIAC COMPLICATIONS

This section considers cardiac arrhythmias and myocardial ischemia and infarction related to surgery. A discussion of cardiac arrest and the postcardiotomy syndrome is presented in Chap. 19.

Arrhythmias

Although cardiac arrhythmias are frequently associated with operative repair of congenital and acquired lesions of the heart (see Chaps. 18 and 19), they represent a potential complication of any surgical procedure. As the age of the surgical population increases, one should encounter an increasing incidence of these disturbances.

INCIDENCE. The incidence varies and is somewhat determined by whether sinus tachycardia is included in the series. In a recent review, Reinikainen and Pontinen report that the incidence of cardiac arrhythmias occurring during extrathoracic operative procedures ranged between 30 and 100 percent. During thoracotomies carried out under general anesthesia, incidences as high as 77 percent have been recorded. Heart diseases increased the incidence; in one series, in 51 percent of cardiac patients as contrasted with 20 percent of other patients, arrhythmia developed during anesthesia. Kuner and associates, monitoring continuous electrocardiographic signals on magnetic tape for prolonged periods of time, found the incidence of cardiac arrhythmia during anesthesia to be 61 percent. The arrhythmias that they noted most frequently were wandering pacemaker, atrioventricular (AV) dissociation, and nodal rhythm and premature ventricular systoles. Relating intraoperative arrhythmias to type of anesthesia, Reinikainen and Pontinen recorded arrhythmias in 24 percent of patients in whom operations were carried out under local anesthesia. The majority of these were of vagal origin and caused by the occulocardiac reflex. There were also ventricular systoles related to anxiety or fear. Under epidural anesthesia, the incidence was 23.5 percent, and this was frequently related to blood pressure reduction. With general anesthesia arrhythmias occurred during intubation in 29 percent and during maintenance of anesthesia in 13 percent of patients.

A study of over 3000 noncardiac cases revealed 2.4 percent had abnormal postoperative electrocardiograms. The majority of patients were asymptomatic, and most of the abnormalities were conduction disturbances. Buckley and Jackson studied 100 patients immediately after surgical treatment and noted sinus tachycardia in 32 percent, sinus bradycardia in 2 percent, sinus arrhythmia in 3 percent, occasional ventricular contractions in 7 percent, and trigeminy in 1 percent. Arrhythmias occur much more frequently following thoracic surgical procedures, with paroxysmal fibrillation and atrial flutter or fibrillation representing the most common types. The time of onset is variable, 30 percent occurring on the first postoperative day and 60 percent within 72 h of operation, though the onset has been noted as late as the eighteenth day. Wheat and Burford reported that 20 to 30 percent of patients recovering from thoracic operations exhibited cardiac arrhythmias. The site and extent of the procedure represented important factors. Arrhythmia occurred in 11 to 32 percent of cases following pneumonectomy and in only 5 percent following lobectomy or lesser resection procedures. When the thoracic lesions involved the vagus nerve, an increasing frequency was noted.

ETIOLOGY. Important predisposing factors include the patient's age and the presence of preexisting heart disease, arteriosclerosis, or hypertension. The highest incidence of arrhythmias occurs in patients over sixty, and it has been shown that the diseased heart is definitely more excitable. Other determining factors include the type of anesthetic, the duration of surgical procedures, the need for intubation, and hyperventilation. Halothane is usually associated with bradycardia and AV dissociation, and when vasopressors are used in combination with halothane, there is an increased incidence of paroxysmal arrhythmia. Atropine also has been noted to cause AV dissociation during anesthesia in patients undergoing breast and perineal surgery. There is a high incidence of sinus bradycardia during Pentothal induction. Serum electrolyte abnormalities during the postoperative course are contributory factors, particularly acidosis and hypokalemia. Hypercalcemia following parathyroid manipulation or with inappropriate intravenous calcium therapy may precipitate rapid ectopic atrial arrhythmia. Thoracic surgery is associated with an increased incidence of arrhythmias. During the postoperative period, myocardial infarction and pulmonary complications are frequently associated with ventricular arrhythmias.

Postoperative cardiac arrhythmias frequently have their genesis in the preoperative period. Atrial arrhythmias are usually due to vagal stimulation. Other provoking factors are hypotension, hypoxia, and hypercapnia, all of which may cause inhibition of the sinus node and activation of a local pacemaker or reentrant atrial mecha-

nisms. The most important reason for ventricular arrhythmia is increased excitability of the myocardium and specialized conduction pathways. This may be attributed to sympathomimetic drugs, such as epinephrine, and increase in blood pressure. It is generally held that some anesthetic agents like halothane and cyclopropane produce sensitization of the myocardium, making it more responsive to the catecholamines, thus potentiating the development of arrhythmia. Muscle of the diseased heart is also more excitable, and hypercapnia provokes ectopic rhythm by decreasing pacemaker activity. Electrolyte disturbances, particularly alterations in potassium concentration, can cause ventricular arrhythmia. The vasovagal cardiac reflex has been implicated in arrhythmias that develop during intubation, surgical manipulation of the lung, and operations on the gallbladder and stomach. Positive-pressure breathing mechanisms may induce a high resistance in the pulmonary circulation, reduce venous return, and stimulate ventricular arrhythmia. Specific diseases that have been implicated as causes of arrhythmia during operative procedures are thyrotoxicosis and pheochromocytoma with its high catecholamine concentration in the plasma.

TREATMENT. In view of the high incidence of arrhythmia in elderly patients undergoing thoracic surgical procedures, some have suggested prophylactic digitalization, and others have employed quinidine and procainamide therapy preoperatively. Lidocaine prophylaxis is reserved for patients with symptomatic ventricular arrhythmia. Digitalization is particularly applicable in patients with frequent atrial premature systoles, while withholding of digitalis is indicated in the presence of sustained or intermittent paroxysmal nodal rhythms. Many have advised discontinuing all myocardial depressant agents, including quinidine and procainamide preoperatively, and withholding all cardiac drugs in the operating room, unless an arrhythmia compromises cardiac output. A bipolar electrode may be inserted preoperatively into the apex of the right ventricle for emergency electronic pacing in patients with advanced second-degree heart block or third-degree AV block. The present consensus is that patients with fascicular blocks such as left anterior hemiblock and right bundle branch block are best managed without prophylactic pacing as long as they have 1:1 AV conduction.

Once an arrhythmia develops, if it is tolerated well by the patient, it may be simply observed, since a high percentage convert spontaneously. In general, therapy is directed at maintaining adequate cardiac output and coronary blood flow. Vasopressors may be administered to maintain the blood pressure while the definitive treatment is organized. If congestive failure threatens, digitalis is the treatment of choice. Digitalis is also the drug of choice in the presence of all supraventricular arrhythmias. For rapid digitalization of adult patients 1 mg of digoxin may be administered intravenously as a loading dose. However, paroxysmal and atrial tachycardia with block and nonparoxysmal nodal tachycardia may all be caused by inappropriate administration of digitalis. Although quinidine may convert atrial fibrillation to sinus rhythm, it does not represent the prime treatment in any real emergency. The safety and effectiveness of cardioversion has preempted the use of quinidine.

It is also unwise to administer calcium and depressant agents indiscriminately. If the arrhythmia is related to overdigitalization, potassium should be administered as 40 meq of potassium chloride in 50 mL of solution, limiting the dose to 20 meq/h. Lidocaine, 1 mg/kg intravenously administered rapidly or as a continuous drip of 1 to 2 mg/min, is preferred for ventricular arrhythmias. It has the advantage over procainamide that it is not associated with hypotension. Diphenylhydantoin (Dilantin) is effective as treatment for digitalis-induced supraventricular tachycardia and ventricular irritability. However, it may reduce myocardial contractility, increase AV block, and cause cardiac arrest. Propranolol, a beta-adrenergic blocker, is used for digitalis intoxication and for slowing ventricular rate in atrial flutter or fibrillation. The calcium channel blocker verapamil, in an intravenous dose of 5 to 10 mg, is especially useful for urgent conversion of reentrant supraventricular tachycardias unresponsive to the usual vagal maneuvers.

Sinus Tachycardia. By definition this disturbance in normal rhythm is not an arrhythmia. Sinus tachycardia is caused by increased sympathetic tone or decreased vagal tone frequently secondary to hypoxia, hypovolemia due to blood loss, and pain. Hypercapnia, dehydration, hyperthyroidism, and congestive heart failure are frequently associated with sinus tachycardia. A variety of drugs, including meperidine, atropine, theophylline, and epinephrine, all increase the heart rate, as does digitalis intoxication. Treatment is directed at the cause.

Paroxysmal Supraventricular Tachycardia. This is usually characterized by the sudden onset of a regular heart rate ranging between 140 and 220 beats per minute. An incidence of 0.2 percent during the postoperative period has been reported. The disturbance may be caused by digitalis or quinidine toxicity, myocardial infarction, congestive heart failure, thyrotoxicosis, and hypoxemia. The arrhythmia is more likely to occur in patients with a history of previous attacks.

The disturbance usually responds to carotid sinus stimulation; immediate therapy is required only with extremely rapid ventricular rates. Depressive drugs may increase vagal tone via the carotid, and aortic sinus reflex stimulation associated with elevated blood pressure and phenylephrine hydrochloride is effective in about 80 percent of cases. Treatment includes the use of intravenous verapamil, cardioversion, or rapid digitalization. Propranolol also has been effective in this situation.

Atrial Flutter. While the atrial rate resulting from ectopic stimuli ranges between 200 and 400 per minute, the ventricular rate is dependent upon the degree of heart block that characteristically occurs. The ventricular rate decreases with carotid sinus pressure only to increase again when the pressure is released, in contrast to the permanent conversion of an atrial nodal paroxysmal tachycardia to sinus rhythm. Atrial flutter occurs more frequently in elderly patients with cardiovascular disease and in patients undergoing intrathoracic surgical treatment. Vagal nerve stimulation, hypotension, and hypoxemia have all been considered as etiologic factors. Continued atrial flutter frequently causes congestive heart failure, particularly when the ventricular rate is rapid.

Digitalis is usually effective in converting the flutter to atrial fibrillation with a slower ventricular response. In the immediate perioperative period it may be difficult to control the heart rate with digitalis preparations. Quinidine also has been used therapeutically, but only after digitalization. Atrial flutter is readily cardioverted at relatively low energy settings, making cardioversion the treatment of choice.

Paroxysmal Ventricular Tachycardia. This is a rare disorder that has serious implications, since it is associated with a damaged myocardium. The pulse rate is usually between 140 and 180. There is no effect with carotid sinus pressure, and there may be some irregularities of rhythm. Ventricular tachycardia may represent one of the first findings in a patient with myocardial infarction. This disorder of rhythm has also been precipitated by hypercapnia and may progress rapidly to ventricular fibrillation.

Cardioversion or lidocaine given intravenously are the treatments of choice. If the disorder is related to digitalis intoxication, diphenylhydantoin and correction of hypokalemia may be therapeutic.

Sinus Bradycardia. This refers to irregular rhythm with a rate less than 60 per minute. The low rate is normal in young athletic patients. The bradycardia may also be induced by drugs such as neostigmine, quinidine, procainamide, digitalis, methoxamine, and levarterenol. Arrhythmia usually does not require treatment unless there is evidence of reduced cardiac output, in which case atropine may be indicated.

AV Nodal Rhythm. This arrhythmia is usually a temporary disturbance caused by vagal inhibition of the sinus node and may be manifest only by a slow pulse, 40 to 50 per minute. Pronounced jugular venous cannon waves may be noted. The rhythm may be caused by carotid sinus pressure, endotracheal intubation, digitalis, and the vasopressor drugs. It usually corrects itself spontaneously, and no treatment is necessary.

AV Block. Incomplete block is an uncommon arrhythmia that is due to organic or surgically induced disturbance of the conduction pathway. Vagal stimulation, carotid sinus pressure, and vasovagal reflexes have also been implicated, as have digitalis, quinidine, and morphine. The pulse is slow and regular, and the neck veins may demonstrate atrial pulsation. If the cause is reflex in origin, atropine is indicated, whereas if the condition is drug-induced, the drug should be withdrawn.

Complete AV block results in a ventricular rhythm of between 30 and 60 beats per minute and occasionally follows trauma to the conduction system during heart operation or intraoperative and postoperative septal infarction. Surgically induced blocks are best treated by a pacemaker.

Sinus Arrhythmia. This is more frequently noted in younger patients and children, and irregularity is characteristically associated with phases of respiration. It is occasionally seen in patients with digitalis toxicity. No treatment is required, though atropine will correct the abnormality, since it is related to vagal tone.

Sinoatrial Block. Either single beats drop out with regular sequence, or there are runs of two or three dropped beats. If the block is prolonged, nodal or ventricular escape occurs. The block is caused by increased vagal tone and depression of the sinus node impulse. It occurs during tracheobronchial suctioning, with carotid sinus pressure, and in hyperkalemia, and is associated with neostigmine administration. It may reverse itself spontaneously or with atropine administration.

Atrial Fibrillation. Atrial fibrillation with its characteristic irregular pulse most frequently appears postoperatively in arteriosclerotic patients subjected to thoracic surgical treatment. In early cases, the ventricular rate is usually rapid, but when digitalis has been given, a slow ventricular rate may be noted. In the absence of failure, no treatment is indicated, since spontaneous correction may occur. In the case of a paroxysmal atrial fibrillation, which may precipitate congestive heart failure, digitalis therapy is indicated. Quinidine or electric cardioversion may be used when there is no associated failure.

Premature Contractions. These represent the most common irregularities of the pulse, and they may originate from any portion of the conduction system. The premature beat characteristically occurs earlier than expected and is followed by a pause due to failure of the ventricle to respond to the next normal impulse. The abnormality occurs in 2 to 8 percent of postoperative patients. The occurrence has been associated with changes in posture, drug therapy with ephedrine and epinephrine, digitalis toxicity, and myocardial infarction. Usually premature contractions have no clinical significance and require no therapy, though if they occur with disturbing frequency, quinidine or lidocaine is recommended unless there is congestive failure, in which case digitalis is the drug of choice, provided it does not represent a possible cause.

Myocardial Infarction

The majority of patients who died suddenly during the operative and immediate postoperative period demonstrated coronary artery thrombosis or myocardial infarction at autopsy. The reported incidence for postoperative myocardial infarction is about 0.15 percent of all surgical patients; the incidence is ten times greater for patients over seventy years old. Eleven unsuspected acute myocardial infarctions were detected by routine postoperative electrocardiograms taken on 1000 patients in the recovery room.

Tarhan et al. recently assessed the significance of operative procedures under general anesthesia performed in patients who had previous myocardial infarction; 6.6 percent had another infarct in the first week after operation, and 54 percent of these died. Myocardial infarction after a major operation is more lethal than myocardial infarction alone. Reinfarction occurred most frequently after operations on the thorax or upper abdomen. In over one-third of patients operated on within 3 months of infarction, reinfarction occurred. This rate decreased to 16 percent in

patients at 3 to 6 months postinfarction and to 4 to 5 percent when infarction occurred more than 6 months prior to surgery. The cardiac risk of a noncardiac operation is definitely increased within 6 months following a myocardial infarction but may be lower than previously reported. Patients with congestive failure, significant valvular disease, and arrhythmias such as frequent premature ventricular contractions are also at increased risk, as are patients over seventy years. Stable angina and moderate hypertension are not significant risk factors. Goldman has developed a multifactorial assessment of risks in patients undergoing an operation (Table 12-2). High-risk patients have scores greater than 5. The risk of death from cardiac causes is increased in patients with scores exceeding 25.

CLINICAL MANIFESTATIONS. The majority of cases occur on the operative day or during the first 3 postoperative days, and although infarction has been associated with all anesthetics, the incidence is higher after general anesthesia for abdominal or pelvic surgical treatment. The most important precipitating factor is shock, either during the operation or in the early postoperative phase. The more prolonged the shock, the greater the risk of coronary thrombosis and myocardial ischemia. The electrocardiogram may show ST depression and T-wave flattening with the loss of as little as 500 mL of blood in patients with previous coronary occlusion.

The diagnosis may be difficult, because chest pain is often absent or obscured by narcotics. Chest pain occurred as a primary clinical manifestation in only 27 percent of patients, which is less than the 97 percent generally reported in patients in whom a coronary occlusion is

Table 12-2. COMPUTATION OF MULTIFACTORIAL INDEX SCORE TO ESTIMATE CARDIAC RISK IN NONCARDIAC SURGERY

	Points
S3 gallop or jugular venous distention on preoperative physical examination	11
Transmural or subendocardial myocardial infarction in the previous 6 months	10
Premature ventricular beats, more than 5/min documented at any time	7
Rhythm other than sinus or presence of premature atrial contractions on last preoperative electrocardiogram	7
Age over 70 years	5
Emergency operation	4
Intrathoracic, intraperitoneal, or aortic site of surgery	3
Evidence for important valvular aortic stenosis*	3
Poor general medical condition†	3

* Findings of a cardiologist's examination, noninvasive testing, or cardiac catheterization.

† As evidenced by electrolyte abnormalities (potassium, <3.0 meq/L: HCO_3, <20 meq/L), renal insufficiency (blood urea nitrogen, >50 mg/dL; creatinine, >3.0 mg/dL), abnormal blood gases (P_{O_2}, <60 mmHg; P_{CO_2}, >50 mmHg), abnormal liver status (elevated aspartate transaminase or signs at physical examination of chronic liver disease), or any condition that has caused the patient to be chronically bedridden.

SOURCE: Goldman L: *Ann Surg* 198:780, 1983, with permission.

not related to surgery. It is appropriate to consider routinely monitoring patients with previous infarction in an intensive care unit. The sudden appearance of shock, dyspnea, cyanosis, tachycardia, arrhythmia, or congestive failure should alert one to the diagnosis. The triad of dyspnea, cyanosis, and arterial hypotension requires a differential diagnosis between cardiac and respiratory problems. The electrocardiogram may provide the diagnosis with a characteristic infarction pattern. However, this is not an unequivocal finding, since, in older patients, ST segment and T-wave changes may be associated with myocardial ischemia, and the same changes may be observed with postoperative shock. A study of arterial gases may provide a differential diagnosis in reference to respiratory problems. Left ventricular failure with pulmonary edema is not generally accompanied by carbon dioxide retention, and, in contrast to airway obstruction and alveolar hypoventilation, there is usually a reduction in arterial carbon dioxide tension (Pa_{CO_2}) and respiratory alkalosis when cardiac failure accompanies myocardial infarction. The CPK-MB isoenzyme is the most precise method for detection of myocardial necrosis following operation. If myocardial infarction is suspected, serial studies, including ECG, SGOT, and CPK-MB, should be done daily. Isotope scanning of the myocardium using technetium pyrophosphate may detect a recent acute infarction.

TREATMENT (See Chap. 4). Preoperative preparation of patients with signs of cardiac insufficiency should include digitalization for patients with enlarged hearts or histories of previous cardiac failure. Routine digitalization is not indicated. Anemia, if present, requires treatment, and attention should be directed toward the regulation of fluid and electrolyte balance and hypovolemia. Patients on propranolol should continue to receive the drug until the morning of the operation. Operation is contraindicated for a period of at least 6 weeks and preferably 6 months following myocardial ischemia or infarction, except in an emergency. During the operation, a broad spectrum of factors that precipitate myocardial infarction should be avoided. These include anoxia, hypotension, hemorrhage, dehydration, electrolyte disturbance, and arrhythmias. The regulation of blood pressure during anesthesia is probably the most important measure in the prevention of myocardial ischemia and infarction. When the blood pressure falls significantly, in the absence of blood loss, the prompt correction of anoxia by adequate ventilation with oxygen and the administration of vasopressors is indicated. Digitalization may be required when shock is combined with heart failure. The administration of blood or fluid is indicated to maintain blood volume.

Treatment of myocardial infarction itself consists of relief of pain and anxiety using morphine and sedation. Relief of anoxia is accomplished with 33 to 50% oxygen delivered via a BLB mask or nasal catheter. Suctioning of the tracheobronchial tree may be required to clear obstructing secretions. Critically ill patients are best managed in an intensive care unit setting with invasive monitoring using arterial lines and a Swan-Ganz catheter. Shock is treated by vasopressor agents. Promptness in

instituting vasopressor therapy will increase the chances of its being effective. Rapid digitalization is applicable in treatment of shock when the myocardial insufficiency may be responsible for the severe hypotension. Digitalization is also indicated for the treatment of heart failure, which is a frequent manifestation of postoperative myocardial infarction. In addition to digitalization, parenteral diuretic therapy may be used in the treatment of cardiac failure. Some writers have advocated the use of anticoagulant therapy after the danger of excessive bleeding from an operative site ceases.

DIABETES MELLITUS

Diabetes mellitus occurs in 2 to 3 percent of the general population with a higher rate among older people. In two series, the disease was discovered in the perioperative period in 16 and 23 percent of patients. The most commonly associated operative procedures were related to vascular disease, but in a high percentage of patients diabetes was discovered prior to an emergency procedure. Diabetic patients represent a special challenge during total surgical care, because the impairment of the homeostatic mechanism for glucose may result in ketoacidosis if untreated or hypoglycemia if overtreated and also because of the associated incidence of generalized vascular disease.

PATHOPHYSIOLOGY. The basic defect is a lack of metabolically effective circulating insulin. The elevated blood sugar level is a result of deficient utilization on the part of peripheral tissues and an increased output of glucose by the liver. In diabetes, the breakdown of fatty acids is increased, and since the metabolism of the ketone bodies is limited, they accumulate in the bloodstream and are eliminated via the kidneys. Glycosuria itself produces an osmotic diuresis that is enhanced by the presence of ketone bodies and the associated loss of sodium and potassium. Evaluation of decompensated diabetes, therefore, includes not only measuring the blood glucose but also measuring acetone, electrolytes, and carbon dioxide–combining power of the serum.

The anesthetic agent may affect carbohydrate metabolism, in which case the hyperglycemia is related to an increased breakdown of liver glycogen and a concomitant catabolism of muscle glycogen with the formation of lactic acid. Also, the anesthetic agents affecting glucose catabolism cause an exaggerated hyperglycemic epinephrine response and an increased resistance to exogenously administered insulin.

The stress of surgical treatment aggravates hyperglycemia because of the increased secretion of epinephrine, growth hormone, and glucocorticoids. Increased epinephrine secretion results in an increased breakdown of liver glycogen to glucose, which is released into the general circulation. The glucocorticoids also increase hepatic glucose output via mobilized protein and exert an anti-insulin effect by stimulating a circulating insulin antagonist. The effects of both epinephrine and glucocorticoids are offset to some extent by an increased secretion of endogenous insulin in the normal person but may require the administration of larger doses of insulin in diabetic patients. Treatment is directed at preventing ketoacidosis, hyperosmolar nonketotic coma, decreased cardiac output with associated poor peripheral perfusion, electrolyte imbalance, impaired polymorphonuclear leukocyte phagocytosis, and decreased wound healing, all of which have been related to uncontrolled diabetes.

MANAGEMENT. In the diabetic patient, essential laboratory studies include hemoglobin determination, white cell count, urinalysis for sugar and acetone, fasting and timed postprandial blood glucose determination, blood urea nitrogen, and, in older patients, serum cholesterol determination and electrocardiography. Diabetic patients should have a preference for an early place on the operative schedule to minimize the effects of fasting and ketosis. Preoperative medication should be kept to a minimum, since diabetic patients, particularly elderly ones, are sensitive to narcotics and sedatives and there is a danger of hypercapnia and hypoxia. The choice of anesthesia should be determined by the operative procedure and the preference of the anesthesiologist. It should not be influenced by the presence of diabetes. Spinal anesthesia has little tendency to evoke hyperglycemia apart from the stress of the operation; among the inhalation anesthetics, nitrous oxide, trichloroethylene, and halothane have the least effect on carbohydrate metabolism. The degree of control during the perioperative period should be assessed by serial determination of the blood sugar and urinalysis for glycosuria and acetonuria. In general, it is safer to permit mild glycosuria and minimal elevation of the blood sugar level in the perioperative periods, particularly in the elderly and cardiac patients. In the patient with postoperative hypotension, blood glucose determination should be obtained to rule out hypoglycemia as an etiologic factor.

Mild diabetics frequently do not require insulin, and dietary control is sufficient. The cornerstone of all diabetic management is the dietary or parenteral intake. The preoperative diabetic intake should contain 140 to 200 g of carbohydrates, 60 to 100 g of protein, and adequate vitamins and minerals and should furnish 1200 to 2100 kcal daily. If parenteral fluids are required, there is a theoretical advantage to the use of fructose or sorbitol, which can be utilized in amounts up to 50 g daily in the diabetic patient. The goal of the dietary or parenteral fluid regimen is to keep the patient free of acetonuria and without excessive hyperglycemia. The patients in whom diabetes is well controlled with oral agents should continue the use of these drugs until the day prior to operation, particularly if the medication is tolbutamide or phenformin. With longer-acting agents, such as chlorpropamide, the drug should be discontinued 72 h preoperatively if the administration of insulin is contemplated. Galloway and Shuman stated that patients who take tolbutamide preoperatively usually require insulin during and immediately after major surgical treatment whereas patients receiving chlorpropamide usually do not require insulin during the immediate paraoperative period.

Insulin Therapy. A variety of programs for the administration of insulin have been proposed. One of the popular methods of treatment employs a regimen in which the daily carbohydrate requirement is divided into four equal doses and given parenterally as 5 to 10% dextrose in water every 6 h. This initiation of the parenteral glucose infusion is accompanied by the subcutaneous injection of unmodified regular insulin in doses equal to approximately one-fourth the dose of insulin that the patient required prior to operation. Urine is checked regularly, and supplementary doses of crystalline insulin are given as indicated. Based on the extent of glycosuria, 4 to 10 units of additional insulin is provided for each unit of positivity. Larger doses may be indicated when acetonuria, severe stress, infection, or marked hyperglycemia is present. The advantage of this method is that glucose and insulin are given at regular intervals, permitting adjustment in the dose during the day. It is preferable to monitor blood glucose levels. The major disadvantage is that inadvertent interruption of glucose infusion may result in hypoglycemia. With this regimen as with others, slight glycosuria is preferable provided there is no acetonuria.

The second basic regimen is directed at patients who are under control with single-injection therapy employing long-acting insulin and in whom a complicated postoperative course is not anticipated. On the day of operation, the patient receives 50 g of glucose in 1000 mL of solution, and at the time the intravenous solution is started, one-half the daily dose of insulin that previously was required is administered. Following operation and return to the recovery room or ward, the remainder of the usual daily dose of insulin is given subcutaneously. Thus, the amount of insulin given on the day of operation approximates that given the day before. On the day following operation, the usual dose of insulin is given in the morning prior to breakfast or at the time of starting an intravenous infusion. Modifications of this approach employ small doses of regular insulin subcutaneously during the postoperative period based on the extent of glycosuria or preferably the serum glucose level. In patients who have been treated with single daily injections and who are not under control prior to operation, conversion to a regimen of soluble insulin is indicated.

There is general agreement that severe hyperglycemia in patients undergoing major operations is more effectively managed with intravenous regular insulin. The problem of insulin absorption by the container has been overcome by the use of plastic containers, high concentrations of insulin, and flushing the system. A specific infusion protocol is outlined in Table 12-3.

A simplified protocol has been proposed by Woodruff et al. The patients receive their evening dose of insulin the preoperative day but no subcutaneous insulin on the morning of surgery. The patient is scheduled as the first case. Insulin and glucose are controlled with two separate infusion pumps; one infuses 5% dextrose in Ringer's lactate at 2 mL/(kg · h), while the other dispenses insulin from a plastic bag containing 250 mL sodium chloride to which 50 units of U-100 regular insulin was added. The rate of insulin infusion is based on the serum glucose level. Twenty units per hour is infused for glucose levels

Table 12-3. INSULIN INFUSION PROTOCOL IN MAJOR SURGERY IN DIABETIC PATIENTS

1. Day before surgery
   a. Obtain 5:00 P.M. plasma glucose STAT.
   b. Start intravenous infusion of 5% dextrose in water at the rate of 50 mL/h and maintain this rate until the patient is taking solid foods without difficulty postoperatively.
   c. "Piggy-back" to dextrose infusion an infusion of regular insulin using IVAC or other infusion pump. Preparation of insulin solution: 50 units in 250 mL 0.9% N saline; flush 60 mL of infusion mixture through system and discard before attaching.
   d. Set infusion rate with this equation:

$$\text{Insulin (units/hour)} = \frac{\text{plasma glucose (mg/dL)}}{100}$$

   (Divide by 150 rather than 100 if the patient is thin or is not taking corticosteroids.)
   e. Repeat glucose determination every 3 h as needed with appropriate insulin adjustments to obtain a plasma glucose level between 100 and 200 mg/dL.
2. Day of surgery
   a. Continue dextrose solution as above.
   b. Manage fluid and electrolyte requirements in peri- and postoperative periods with non-glucose-containing solutions *only*.
   c. Obtain plasma glucose STAT every 2 h during surgery and every 6 h for the rest of that 24-h period; adjust insulin accordingly.
3. Days after surgery
   a. Continue dextrose and other fluid replacement as on the day of surgery.
   b. Obtain daily fasting and afternoon plasma glucose values to assess insulin treatment and adjust as necessary.
   c. Hypoglycemia contingencies (plasma glucose less than 50 mg/dL):
      (1) Obtain STAT plasma glucose; decrease insulin rate accordingly; treat orally.
      (2) Give 15 mL intravenous bolus of 50% dextrose in water if oral therapy is insufficient.
      (3) Repeat steps 1 or 2 at 15-min intervals if symptoms persist or recur.
      (4) Determine cause of hypoglycemia and treat promptly.
   d. Discontinue infusion when patient is tolerating solid food.
      (1) Reinstitute appropriate twice-a-day insulin dosage.
      (2) Do not stop infusion completely without switching to insulin injections.

SOURCE: From Meyer EJ, Lorenzi M, et al: *Am J Surg* 137:323, 1979, with permission.

greater than 200 mg/dL, no insulin for levels below 80 mg/dL. The surgical procedure is not begun until the level is below 200 mg/dL. Insulin therapy during emergent surgery or surgery complicated by infection will require greater amounts of insulin to maintain serum glucose levels below 200 mg/dL. In extreme cases, bolus injection of 0.1 to 0.4 unit/kg may be required as an additive.

Management of Ketoacidosis. The preparation for surgical treatment of a patient with ketoacidosis is critical, and one should keep in mind that ketoacidosis itself may masquerade as a surgical emergency. The patient with frank diabetic coma is no candidate for surgical treatment regardless of the indication. Crystalline insulin should be used in all cases to establish control. Page et al. reported effective management of diabetic coma with continuous low-dose insulin infusion using an average of 7.2 units/h. Plasma glucose, ketone bodies, and free fatty acids decreased 58 percent in 4 h. There is an associated deficiency of dehydration and electrolyte abnormality that must be corrected, and the ordinary patient with advanced coma will require an average of 2 to 4 or more liters of fluid to overcome the dehydration. The serum potassium should be determined at 6- to 8-h intervals and potassium added to the fluid in quantities of 40 meq/L administered at a rate of no greater than 25 meq/h. Usually the need for potassium does not exceed 80 meq. There is generally no need to add glucose to intravenous fluid unless the blood glucose level falls below normal. Gastric atony is a frequent accompaniment of diabetic ketoacidosis, and suction is frequently required to minimize pulmonary aspiration. It is usually possible to correct ketoacidosis in sufficient time so that the patient's surgical status is not compromised.

Nonketotic Hyperglycemic Hyperosmolar Coma. Hyperosmolar dehydration and coma is a relatively uncommon syndrome that usually occurs in elderly diabetic or nondiabetic obese patients and patients receiving total parenteral nutrition. The blood sugar level is frequently above 1000 mg/dL, and ketone bodies are absent from the plasma and urine. Treatment consists of large amounts of hypotonic solutions plus intravenous insulin. Marked lowering of the blood sugar level may result with small doses of insulin, and it is recommended that a test dose of 10 units be given to determine responsiveness.

FAT EMBOLISM SYNDROME

Fat embolism is one of the important causes of increased morbidity and mortality in patients with fractures and extensive trauma. A distinction must be made between fat as a pathologically demonstrable phenomenon and fat embolism as a clinical entity. The presence of pulmonary fat embolism is a relatively common accompaniment of trauma, while the clinical entity is an infrequent occurrence. The pathologic entity of fat emboli in the pulmonary capillaries following trauma was described initially by Zenker in 1862. In World War I, 112 cases in which fat embolism was implicated as the cause of death had been reported. Mallory et al. reported that 65 percent of 60 patients who died of battle wounds in World War II had pulmonary fat embolism, and a similar finding was noted in 39 percent of 79 patients dying from war wounds in the Korean conflict. In 1962, Sevitt described 100 cases of fat embolism, 82 percent of which were related to long bone fractures.

The occurrence of the pathologic entity of fat embolization is correlated with the degree of injury and survival time. In a study of 300 accident victims, 80 percent of those dying immediately had embolization of varying degrees. In those living up to 6 h after accident, fat embolism was found in 96 percent of autopsies, and 12 h after a fatal accident from mechanical trauma, there was not a single case without fat embolism. Massive fat embolism occurred in 26 percent of the cases with one fracture and 44 percent of those with multiple fractures. Chan and associates reported that 8.75 percent of patients with fractures of the femur, tibia, and pelvis, or multiple fractures presented with overt clinical manifestations of the fat embolism syndrome.

In addition to fat embolization associated with extensive trauma, the clinical syndrome has been reported in blast concussion, with liver trauma, in burns, in severe infection (particularly that due to clostridia, which mediate alpha-toxins that disintegrate fat), in closed-chest cardiac massage, with the use of extracorporeal circulation, and following renal transplantation and high-altitude flights.

PATHOGENESIS AND PATHOPHYSIOLOGY. In the fat embolism syndrome there is an interaction between platelet aggregation, a coagulopathy, and circulating fats that result in diffuse organ changes, particularly in the lungs and central nervous system. There is disagreement as to whether the embolized fat originates from bone marrow and soft tissue or from circulating blood lipids. The most popular theory, which implicates mechanical causes, proposes that with trauma there is a liberation of liquid fat and intravasation of fat into the vascular channels. Bone, with its high fat content, vascularity, and rigidity, provides an ideal setting. Most of the cases of fat embolism occur after fracture of major long bones with high fat content, and occasionally hemopoietic marrow fragments have been found within the lung as an accompaniment of fat embolization.

It is also proposed that the normal emulsion of fat within the plasma is altered to allow coalescence of the chylomicrons into larger fat droplets with subsequent embolization. This is supported by the fact that emboli may be found in nontraumatic conditions and that the chemical makeup of the embolic fat more closely resembles circulating lipids than marrow or depot fat. Several contributing factors are important in the pathogenesis. These include shock, disseminated intravascular coagulation, sepsis, local pressure, and release of kinins.

Circulating fat macroglobules larger than 20 μm in diameter are the offending elements. The lung usually acts as a very effective filter, as evidenced by the observation that 95 percent of patients dying of injury had pulmonary involvement while only 23 percent demonstrated systemic fat embolism. Thus, in approximately three-fourths of the patients with fat embolism the lesion is confined to the lung. The first stage is hypoperfusion due to the mechanical effects of the macroglobules and adherent platelets, red cells, and fibrin plus the chemical effects of released serotonin and kinins. Local lipolysis leads to the second stage, chemical pneumonitis. Damage to the alveolar wall interferes with lung surfactant activity. Pathophysiologically, early hyperpnea leads to a transitory respiratory alkalosis, but combined respiratory and metabolic acidosis evolves rapidly. The cardiac effects are related primarily to the increased pulmonary vascular resistance and, to a lesser degree, to diffuse fat embolism

within the myocardium itself. If the fat emboli pass through the pulmonary filter to reach the circulation, they may lodge in the cerebral vessels, accounting for central nervous system manifestations, and in the skin, producing the characteristic petechial changes. Although the kidneys are involved quite regularly when there is systemic fat embolism, they are usually not severely damaged.

CLINICAL MANIFESTATIONS. Although pathologic pulmonary fat embolization is a common occurrence, the clinical manifestations are rare. Symptoms characteristically occur within 12 to 48 h but have been noted as late as 10 days following injury. The main manifestations relate to pulmonary pathology. Before symptoms become apparent, blood-gas determinations may define significant hypoxemia. Tachypnea and tachycardia are characterisic. Pulmonary infection may ensue and lead to augmented respiratory symptoms plus manifestations of sepsis. Rarely, massive pulmonary embolization of fat will result in the sudden onset of right heart failure.

Cerebral fat embolism usually does not occur without evidence of pulmonary involvement. Symptoms that suggest cerebral involvement include changes in personality, drowsiness leading to coma, muscle weakness, spasticity, or rigidity, diplopia or blindness, and, rarely, extreme pyrexia. The cerebral manifestations must be differentiated from delirium tremens, cerebral contusion, and epidural hematoma. The lucid interval with cerebral contusion is usually absent, whereas it characteristically lasts 6 to 10 h with epidural hematoma and 24 h with fat embolism. Coma may be present immediately with cerebral contusion and evolves rapidly with fat embolism and slowly with an epidural hematoma. Decerebrate rigidity occurs early in fat embolism and is a terminal event with epidural hematoma. Tachypnea and tachycardia are characteristic of fat embolism, whereas the pulse and respiratory rate are slow with epidural hematoma.

The classic physical finding of fat embolism is the appearance of petechial hemorrhages in the capillary plexus of the dermis. They occur in a distinctive pattern over the shoulders, chest, axilla, and, rarely, the abdominal wall and extremities. They may also be noted in the subconjunctival region and on the palate. Petechiae occur as early as the second or third day and as late as the ninth day after injury and are present in 20 percent of patients found at autopsy to have fat embolism. A counterpart to the petechial hemorrhages is evident on funduscopic examination as emboli within the retinal vessels, and there may be streaks of hemorrhage throughout the retina and macular edema. Renal involvement usually does not produce severe damage, and both gross hematuria and impaired function are rare occurrences. Recently, an association with acute peptic ulceration has been noted.

DIAGNOSTIC STUDIES. A sudden and precipitous drop in the hematocrit is frequently noted and has been related to trapping of red cells and occasionally an associated DIC within the pulmonary parenchyma. It may occur as early as the second or third day following injury, just prior to the onset of dyspnea, disorientation, and the appearance of petechial hemorrhages. Thrombocytopenia

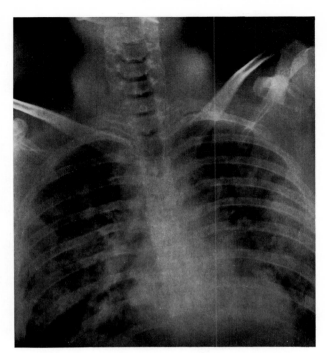

Fig. 12-2. Pulmonary fat emboli. Note bilateral extensive ill-defined nodular densities situated primarily in peripheral lung fields. Patient was in an automobile accident and fractured his femur and two metatarsals. Twenty-four hours after admission fever developed, and 3 days later hemoptysis and mental confusion. Changes were seen radiographically on the fourth day after trauma. There were lipid bodies in the urine, and the serum lipase level was elevated. The patient was treated with antibiotics, heparin, and dextran, and the symptoms subsided 7 days after therapy.

occurs less frequently. Radiographic pulmonary changes are noted in about 36 percent of the cases. The characteristic pattern is that of unevenly distributed areas of radiodensity, congestive hilar shadows, and increased bronchovascular markings with dilation of the right side of the heart (Fig. 12-2). Serial measurements of Pa_{O_2} offer a better index of the degree of pulmonary involvement. In one series, 64 percent of patients with clinical manifestations had a significant reduction in Pa_{O_2}. The electrocardiogram may reveal changes that reflect myocardial ischemia and right ventricular strain. These are usually noted 24 to 48 h after injury. The important findings are the sudden appearance of a prominent S wave in lead I and prominent Q waves in lead III. Inversion of the T wave indicates severe overloading of the right ventricle. Depression of the RS-T segments suggests subendothelial ischemia. There may be a right bundle branch block. Arrhythmias are frequent. The electroencephalogram may indicate a diffuse slow wave pattern.

Detection of Fat. A cryostat test has been applied to determine the presence of fat globules in blood. In one series the test was positive in 52 percent of symptomatic patients. Lipuria occurs in the first few days following injury and is usually associated with a serious degree of fat embolism. Free fat in the urine has been demonstrated in over 57 percent of cases in one series. Examination of

the urine is simple but must be precise. The collecting apparatus must be free of fat, and the bladder must be emptied completely, since the fat floats and the majority of globules remain in the bladder residue. The patient should be catheterized using a nonoily lubricant and the fluid collected in a volumetric flask. The meniscus may be skimmed, or, after centrifugation, the supranatant is smeared and stained with Sudan III. Deep-orange-colored droplets represent fat globules. Another method of demonstrating fat in the urine is the Scuderi "sizzle" test, which involves placing a wire loop containing the supranatant fluid over a flame and listening for a pop or sizzle produced by burning fat. The fat can be detected in concentrations as small as 1:1000. The demonstration of fat in the sputum has little diagnostic value, since it is a common phenomenon following trauma. Biopsy of petechiae may establish the diagnosis, and frozen section is mandatory to determine the presence of fat. Needle biopsy of the kidney also has been applied to demonstrate fat globules.

Serum Lipase. A serum lipase level elevation occurs in about 14 to 50 percent of the cases, the rise usually beginning on the third day and reaching a maximum on the seventh or eighth day after injury. An elevation greater than 1 mL is significant, and this determination is considered by Peltier to be the best laboratory test between the third and seventh day. The serum lipase level can be suppressed by the administration of ethyl alcohol and augmented by heparinization. Once elevated, the level is thought to reflect the prognosis, and elevations greater than 2 mL are associated with a higher incidence of favorable outcome. In a patient with extensive trauma, an elevated serum lipase level in the first 48 h is more suggestive of pancreatitis.

TREATMENT. Prophylaxis against potentiating fat embolization includes careful handling of the patient and early splinting of fractures. Vigorous applications of resuscitative measures are indicated to correct oligemic shock, since it has been demonstrated that fewer emboli may be lethal in the hypotensive than in the normotensive patient. High doses of corticosteroids (1.0 to 1.5 g hydrocortisone) administered during the first 2 days following injury may inhibit the pneumonitis or expedite its resolution. Pulmonary manifestations are treated with oxygen therapy, rapid digitalization, and intensive endotracheal suction to minimize the accumulation of secretions. IPPB or PEEP are frequently indicated. Pa_{O_2} should be monitored and maintained between 80 and 100 mmHg. Endotracheal intubation is preferred over tracheostomy, since the latter has been associated with a high mortality rate in these patients. Cerebral manifestations are treated with sedation and anticonvulsive therapy.

Trasylol, which inhibits the effects of kinins, has been beneficial in several instances. Heparin in doses that do not have an anticoagulant effect will clear lipemic plasma and stimulate lipase activity. A dose of 5000 units may be administered intravenously every 6 h. In the presence of acute systemic toxicity or a rapidly rising lipase level, the drug should be discontinued, since the release of fatty acids is undesirable. Low-molecular-weight dextran

(40,000) has been administered intravenously to counteract intravascular thrombosis. One thousand milliliters is administered per 24 h for 2 days. Ethyl alcohol, which may decrease the rate of hydrolysis of neutral fat and slow the release of toxic free fatty acids, has been used. Presently, this applicability of alcohol is debatable.

PROGNOSIS. Old age, preexisting lung disease, and reduced cardiac reserve have adverse effects. The early appearance of marked hypoxemia and the requirement of persistently high $F_{I_{O_2}}$ are bad prognostic signs, as is hypocalcemia resulting from ion binding by FFA, while a persistently high serum lipase level is a favorable sign. At the Birmingham Accident Hospital, a fatality rate of 12 percent has been reported for 25 cases diagnosed according to strict criteria (all had petechial rash). While the "pure" cerebral form of the fat embolism syndrome generally has a better prognosis, the presence of coma is a poor sign. Acute respiratory disease usually is self-limiting.

PSYCHIATRIC COMPLICATIONS

Severe psychiatric disturbances may occur any time during an illness, but their appearance in the postoperative period is particularly significant. The first account of postoperative psychiatric disturbance presented by a surgeon was that of Dupuytren who, in 1834, wrote that "the brain itself may be overcome by pain, terror, or even joy and reason leaves the patient at the instant when it is most necessary to his welfare that he should remain calm and undisturbed." In 1910, Da Costa indicated that the anticipated frequency for such complications is as high as 1 in 250 laparotomies, while Lewis, more recently, suggested an incidence of 1 in 1500. Scott described 11 cases in 2000 surgical procedures. The validity of any of these figures, however, is open to question, since "postoperative psychosis" per se does not appear in the standard nomenclature and is frequently not coded on the patient's record. Diagnostic criteria for psychosis have become more specific over the years. Also, surgeons may not be sensitive to the behavioral patterns that are psychodiagnostic.

The study of Titchener et al., who evaluated 200 patients admitted to the surgical service of the Cincinnati General Hospital utilizing interview and the Minnesota Multiphasic Personality Inventory to substantiate a psychiatric diagnosis, indicated that 86 percent of the sample had either distressing psychologic symptoms, disabling patterns of behavior, or both. The patients considered were in a municipal hospital and represented a lower socioeconomic group, but the figures of 21 percent having neuroses, 11 percent psychophysiologic reactions, 14 percent psychoses, 34 percent character behavior disorders, and 3 percent chronic brain syndrome are most impressive.

GENERAL CONSIDERATIONS. "Postoperative psychosis" cannot be considered as a distinct clinical entity. No single factor has been shown to be responsible, and the physical illness and operative procedure may merely bring to light a latent psychotic tendency. Both illness, particularly when prolonged, and surgical procedures represent threats to the integrity of the organism on somatic and psychologic grounds. In nearly every person informed of the need for a surgical procedure, some degree of anxiety arises. There may be fear of loss of life, of loss of body part or function, such as castration as with pelvic and hernia operations. The anxiety signal is assimilated and integrated by the patient in preparation for the surgical stress. Surgical intervention to cure, modify, or prevent illness is the beginning of a complicated and multifaceted process. The psychodynamic processes at work during the preoperative, postoperative, and convalescent periods may be classified as involving (1) psychophysiologic factors, (2) somatopsychic factors, or (3) psychosocial factors. Psychophysiologic factors represent processes originating from psychologic stress that act along neurogenic or humoral pathways to modify the healing process. A poorly functioning gastroenterostomy or marginal ulcer in a patient with emotional stress represents an example of this type. The somatopsychic factors have to do with the psychologic adaptation involved when the surgical procedure imposes a somatic defect, such as an ileostomy or colostomy. The psychosocial factors refer to patients' concern with the effects of their physical illness or surgical procedure on their ultimate position in society. All these may interplay and contribute to anxiety, neurotic symptoms, severe depression, and frank psychosis.

CLINICAL MANIFESTATIONS. The time of occurrence of psychiatric derangement during illness is variable, and the duration of latent interval between surgical treatment and the psychologic disturbance may be days to weeks. Winkelstein and associates reported that, in the recovery room, patients who had been subjected to surgical procedures under general anesthesia exhibited a lack of concern about the operation and an absence of affective response, despite the fact that they were sufficiently oriented to be interviewed. After 24 h the patients responded with these concerns and emotions that were so conspicuously absent in the immediate postoperative period. Both psychologic and pharmacologic factors are implicated in this response, since patients under spinal anesthesia exhibit immediate and overt emotional reaction.

The manifestations are extremely variable. Fear may be accompanied by depression or elation and overactivity. The clinical picture may be that of acute delirium with confusion and disorientation or merely a vague alteration in perception and mood. The manic type of reaction may incorporate psychomotor excitement, delirium, delusions, visual or auditory hallucinations, agitated depression, and feelings of persecution. The psychotic reactions that were observed in 44 of 200 patients in the Cincinnati series are indistinguishable from the range of psychoses observed under other circumstances. The acute brain syndrome, or delirium, was manifest in 20 patients.

Delirium may begin with an inappropriate remark or a dramatic agitated outburst and is frequently the first sign of continued mental deterioration leading to a chronic brain syndrome, particularly in an elderly patient. Therefore, delirium must be regarded as a potentially dangerous situation. It occurs most commonly in elderly patients who have lost closeness and support of family or friends and in patients who are immobilized for long periods of time.

Depressive reactions represented the second most important psychosis in surgical patients and occurred in 4.5 percent of patients in the Cincinnati series. The patient is characteristically uncooperative in an active way, or recovery may be impeded by listlessness, anorexia, and disinterest. The depressive reaction may be accompanied by physiologic changes; Moore et al. demonstrated the effects of emotion on the pituitary-adrenal axis during the immediate and subsequent postoperative period. Suicide is a major risk in patients with depressive reaction.

Another category includes the paranoid psychotic disorder. Although it is not rare for schizophrenic reaction to have its onset in the surgical patient, no acute breaks of the schizophrenic type were noted among the 200 patients studied by Titchener et al. Generally, there is no contraindication to surgical treatment of patients with schizophrenia. Manic excitement is a particularly difficult problem in the management of surgical patients and requires the close cooperation of psychiatrist, surgeon, and anesthesiologist.

MANAGEMENT. The first step in the management of psychiatric disturbances occurring in the course of the surgical illness or following surgical procedures is that of anticipation. Although Knox has indicated that the incidence of postoperative psychosis was not related to the duration of preoperative hospital stay, the duration of illness, particularly when prolonged, does determine the patient's psychologic reaction to surgical experience. At the other end of the spectrum, sudden emergency operation often results in reactions marked by acute anxiety, nightmares, insomnia, irritability, and protective withdrawal from all stimuli. Age is an important factor, the highest incidence occurring in children under the age of two and in the elderly patients. In the latter group, this is particularly true of patients who have lost their proximity to and support of family and friends, and who have not developed a close relation with the hospital personnel. Knox has presented evidence of constitutional predisposition, and although 17 percent of his patients had had previous surgical treatment uncomplicated by psychiatric disturbances, 11 percent did have a previous psychiatric illness. Twenty-two percent of patients had a family history of mental illness of serious proportion. There is an increasing incidence of delirium in response to anesthesia and surgical treatment in patients who are alcoholic, while patients suffering from extensive trauma may have organic psychosis. Acidosis, acetonuria, hyperglycemia, hypercalcemia, hypomagnesemia, and hepatic insufficiency may all cause postoperative mental aberrations, and cerebral hypoxia frequently results in behavioral changes. Medications, such as barbiturates, anticholinergics, and cortisone, also have been implicated.

There is an obvious need for integrating psychologic treatment with the management of surgical patients. As Titchener and Levine emphasize, it is not necessary, possible, or advisable for these needs to be turned over to psychiatrists, and it is frequently preferable that the measures be carried out by the surgeon in charge. Verbal communication between the surgeon and patient is the best means of overcoming emotional or mental difficulty. The anesthesiologist is regarded as an impersonal distant figure who carries out a task without emotional impact on the patient. The surgeon should become aware of the patient's feelings, attitudes, and needs for specific information, i.e., diagnostic procedures, operating approach, and postoperative possibilities. Information on expected feelings and sensations may have a direct effect on the adequacy of adjustment. Also, changes to increase the patients' positive adaptation to their illness should be constantly considered. The striking incidence of significant postoperative disturbance suggests the need for "mental check" to be incorporated into the usual postoperative surgical rounds. Efforts should be directed at removing toxic causes of the acute brain syndrome, removing undue stimuli without isolating the patient, and providing psychologic or pharmacologic tranquilization.

The physician's psychologic approach should include repeated explanation and inquiries about the patient's concerns. In some instances, specific counseling and directive treatment, which may require direct intervention in the patient's personal or family affairs and the assistance of the social service department, is indicated. The best prophylactic therapy, however, can be classified as supportive, in that surgeons allow themselves to be the object of dependency on the part of the patient. This relationship is fostered by interest on the part of the surgeon and trust on the part of the patient.

The provocative patient who emits anger or attempts to irritate others as a mechanism for covering fear or relieving guilt needs understanding of the emotional reason for the provocation and an attitude of firmness rather than anger from the physician. The attempt on the part of patients to sign out against advice is a mechanism of expressing anger or fear and should be handled by the surgeon in such a way that patients are allowed to change their minds without becoming embarrassed. In these and other situations, patients may hide their real feeling behind an intellectual screen. For understanding, patients should be encouraged to bring forth both the emotional and intellectual aspects of their personalities.

Consultation with a psychiatrist is indicated in the case of any acute and severe emotional disturbance, and the referral should be candidly discussed between the surgeon and the patient. Patients must come to the conclusion that they require expert help for their problems. Referral is also indicated for long-standing disturbances discovered during hospitalization and is frequently appropriate in patients with psychosomatic illness. Browning and Houseworth, in a study of patients with peptic ulcer, demonstrated that the removal of symptoms without altering the psychosomatic disorders led to the formation of a new spectrum of symptoms. The surgeon should be prepared to differentiate organic from functional disorders, psychosis, and depressive states since psychiatric consultation may not be available or may be refused by the patient. Specific drugs may be prescribed. Most postoperative traumatic neuroses, manifest by anxiety and reliving the operative experience, can be managed with minor tranquilizers, e.g., diazepam, lorazepam, or hypnotics such as flurazepam. Psychoses such as schizophrenia, mania, and depression may respond to a phenothiazine derivative. Benzodiazepine derivatives are preferable for nonpsychotic anxiety. Tricyclic antidepressants have an effect that can be delayed 1 to 3 weeks and are associated with acute cholinergic side effects and changes in cardiac conduction. These drugs are rarely used in the postoperative period.

Special Surgical Situations

The very young and old patients are particularly vulnerable to the development of psychiatric complications following surgical treatment. Psychotic disturbances have been found in 2 to 3 percent of patients following cataract extraction. The combination of surgical procedure and the awareness of the implications of the illness is critical in the patient with cancer. Because of the high incidence of emotional disorders following surgical procedures, special consideration is indicated for mastectomy and gynecologic procedures, cardiac surgical treatment, dialysis and transplantation, and prolonged periods in an intensive care unit. The management of drug addicts is assuming greater importance.

PEDIATRIC SURGERY

In children, severe anxiety states may be precipitated by the shock of operation. Levy reported that of a group of 124 children who had operations, 20 percent showed residual emotional disturbances. This occurred most frequently in the one- to two-year-old group; after the age of three there was a sharp decrease with age. The age distribution was attributed to a greater dependence on home and mother, and Levy went so far as to suggest postponement of elective surgical treatment until the child could comprehend something about the situation. Postoperative reactions consisted of negativism, disobedience, tantrums, defiance, destructive behavior, and dependency, as manifested by clinging to the mother or attendant. The responses have been related to a feeling of betrayal and the consequent desire for revenge and rebellion. When a child is suffering from fears engendered by an operation, a second operation usually intensifies the earlier fears.

Prophylactic therapy is important. The maturity of the child's emotional adaptation is more a factor in the response than the operation per se. Parental absence is frequently associated with emotional difficulty. Prugh and associates compared two groups, one treated without organized consideration for emotional needs and another in which these needs were considered and ample opportunity for play was provided. Moderate or severe anxiety reactions, immediately after leaving the hospital, were observed in 92 percent of the control group and in 68 percent of the experimental group, with a peak incidence in children under three. Three months after discharge, the incidence of persisting anxiety had fallen to 58 percent for the control group and 44 percent for the experimental group. The youngest children reacted more severely with

apprehension, feeding disturbances, and depression. The pattern for the four- to six-year-old group was a tendency toward obsessive worries, phobias, and accentuated aches and pains. The six- to ten-year-olds manifested conversion symptoms, compulsive behavior, and restlessness.

SURGERY IN THE AGED

Elderly patients are more prone to become emotionally disturbed when confronted with new situations, especially if they have inadequate comprehension and a generalized feeling of insecurity. The operative procedure also presents an obvious physical threat to the integrity of the nervous system. Titchener and associates reported a 25 percent incidence of significant and, at times, irreversible change in cerebral function in the patients in their group over the age of sixty-five. Some degree of depression was observed in 90 percent of the older patients, and this was of a disabling nature in about 50 percent. Indifference of the family, friends, and society contributed to the evolution of a paranoid cycle.

Attempts should be directed at limiting the physical insult to the brain, and postoperative mental evaluation is indicated on a routine basis in order to detect the early changes of the organic brain syndrome and delirium. Efforts should be made to familiarize the patients with the hospital and personnel, and visitors should be encouraged to maintain a human contact and prevent withdrawal. Collaboration with a social worker is frequently indicated for long-term rehabilitation.

GYNECOLOGIC AND BREAST SURGERY

Removal of the breast and a variety of gynecologic procedures are highly represented in most series of postoperative psychosis. Maguire and associates found that 1 year after mastectomy the women reported a 20 percent incidence of depressed feelings, a 10 percent incidence of anxiety, and 38 percent incidence of sexual difficulties. Contact with other mastectomy patients expedites psychologic rehabilitation. Routine counseling lowered the postoperative psychiatric morbidity from 38 to 12 percent. Hysterectomy is associated with emotional disturbance more frequently than other gynecologic operations, and the more the procedure antedates the menopause, the more the likelihood of associated psychologic disturbance. The loss of menstrual function is perceived by the woman as a blow to normal feminine esteem. Hollender reported that of 203 women admitted to psychiatric hospital, 9 had pelvic surgical treatment as a precipitating event, and this was in contrast to a total of 5 women admitted following operations of all other kinds. Lindemann noted that the relative frequency of restlessness, insomnia, agitation, and preoccupation with depressive thoughts was greater after pelvic operations than after cholecystectomy.

CANCER SURGERY

Cancer patients are exposed to two major threats, disease and extensive surgical treatment. They are concerned with death or injury during operation and disruption of their pattern of living as a result of the effects of cancer or the surgical procedure. Patients with emotional problems involving self-destruction are particularly vulnerable to preoperative anxiety concerning death and mutilation. This may be manifest by anorexia, insomnia, tachycardia, fear, and panic. Acute depression with suicidal tendencies has been reported in anticipation of surgical procedures. Postoperatively, depression is related to an anticipated interference with valued activities. Sutherland and associates have demonstrated that colostomy imposed on almost all patients a new order of living, and the subjects were powerfully motivated to avoid social rejection. A rigid life arose from the fearful expectation of rejection because of the colostomy combined with the fear of death from cancer. There is a tendency toward seclusion, withdrawal, and nonparticipation. Spells of depression are frequent, and Sutherland and his associates are of the opinion that loss of an important bodily part or function is more depressing than the fear or expectation of death. The management of patients with carcinoma must be based on an appreciation that they frequently suffer a sense of isolation, guilt, and abandonment.

CARDIAC SURGERY

Serious psychiatric disturbances have been observed to occur with considerable frequency following mitral valvulotomy and open heart surgery. Fox and associates and Bliss et al. reported, respectively, a 19 and 16 percent incidence of serious emotional disturbance following mitral valve surgery. Bolton and Bailey, however, in an evaluation of 1500 consecutive patients, noted an incidence of psychosis of 3 percent with no relation to age, sex, severity of heart disease, duration of failure, or complications of surgical treatment. Egerton and Kay noted delirium in 25 of 60 adults following open heart surgery.

Manifestations generally occur after an initial lucid interval 3 to 5 days after operation and clear shortly after the patient is transferred from an intensive care unit to a standard hospital ward. Postoperative incapacitation and increased time on the heart-lung machine apparently are factors increasing the likelihood of delirium, while age and sex do not alter the incidence. Zaks has suggested that cardiac operation may produce organic brain damage, thus sensitizing patients and increasing the incidence of postoperative psychologic symptomatology. A prediction equation was successful in differentiating reactors from nonreactors. Using the ego strength variable of the Minnesota Multiphasic Personality Inventory, there is a significant inverse correlation between the reaction and the incidence of acute psychotic episodes following cardiac operation. The incidence of psychoses is greater in males, older patients, and those expressing minimal preoperative anxiety. A preoperative psychiatric interview reduces the incidence of postoperative psychosis by 50 percent.

Following operations on the heart, the patients with emotional disturbances manifest perceptual distortion, visual and auditory hallucinations, disorientation, and paranoia. Twenty-eight percent of adult patients subjected to open heart surgery, as reported by Egerton and Kay, had delirious states ranging in duration from several nights to several weeks, averaging 5 days. The delirious patients had no psychologic sequelae, and no relation could be established between the incidence of delirium and the duration of cardiac bypass, but open heart procedures were more likely to produce delirium than other intrathoracic operations. The writers felt that the precipitating factors for delirium included dehydration, hyponatremia, and the performance of a tracheostomy, while the predisposing factors included a familial history of psychosis, previous brain damage, overwhelming personal problems, and the presence of a rheumatic valvular lesion. Other psychiatric disturbances noted in patients following open heart surgery were disabling anxiety state, conversion hysteria, tension headaches, and, in a surprising 5 percent of the operative cases, exacerbation of peptic ulcer. The almost total absence of delirium and other emotional disorders in children is of particular interest and may be related to the fact that the concept of death as a permanent biologic process usually does not develop until the age of nine.

DIALYSIS AND TRANSPLANTATION

A variety of emotional disturbances have been observed in patients undergoing hemodialysis. The suicide rate is 300 times greater than for a comparable healthy population. Uremia, debilitating disease, and the repeated technical procedures that are performed all constitute etiologic factors. Wright et al. followed 11 patients on chronic dialysis and noted a number of stresses affecting them, such as unpredictability of well-being, tensions arising in the marital situation from guilt and anger, effects of separation on the families, and financial anxiety. Following each episode of dialysis, the main patient response was one of relief. Cramond and associates noted that their patients at first denied their illness and later realized that they had lost their health and independence and their futures were uncertain. This has been referred to as a "mourning reaction." From time to time the patients wished to be dead. They felt that life dependent on chronic dialysis was not worth living. Some patients passed from the mourning reaction to a state of active depression.

All patients undergoing dialysis become extremely dependent on the staff and emotionally attached to them. The patients often react emotionally to a sense of loss when any replacement of staff occurs. During the course of the dialysis program, regression occurs relatively frequently and the patient becomes withdrawn and pretends to sleep. Insomnia and frightening dreams also occur, and the frequency with which emotional disturbances have been noted suggests that psychiatric assistance plays an important role in a dialysis program.

Two distinct groups of patients, the donors and recipients, must be considered in a renal homotransplantation program. Psychologic screening of the potential donors is indicated, and selection should be from individuals who are stable and who have mature judgment. Individuals with psychopathologic motives such as sacrifice or exhibitionism should be excluded, particularly when they are unrelated donors. It is to be emphasized that those who refuse to cooperate risk being rejected by the family and are frequently made to feel guilty. Therefore, when potential donors are rejected on psychiatric grounds, the rejection should be ascribed to a minor physical variation. In four of five cases, Cramond noted an ambivalent relationship between donors and recipients. Donors experienced emotional and physical investment in the patient and, at times, sought to overprotect the patient. They felt that their sacrificial gift was in jeopardy if the patient behaved in a manner of which they did not approve.

The recipient has been shown to be aware of an obligation to the donor and resents the dependency relationship. At times feelings of shame and guilt must be considered. Kemph, in a follow-up of recipients of renal homotransplants, has noted periods of severe depression and concern with bodily damage and sexual damage. After the operation the donors also experience depression. Many expressed the feeling that they were not attentively supported by the hospital personnel.

Some recipients regard the operation as symbolic of rebirth and may undergo a religious conviction. In some recipients, a graft from a donor of an opposite sex is considered a threat to sexual identity. All recipients demonstrate anxiety in reference to injury of the grafted kidney. Although severe depressions and emotional reactions are uncommon, psychologic adjustment takes longer than a year to accomplish. When given a choice, patients who have rejected their kidney transplants have almost uniformly chosen a second transplant over return to dialysis.

INTENSIVE CARE DELIRIUM

Delirium manifested by a wide variety of behavior patterns, ranging from apathy to restlessness and combativeness, is a common occurrence in intensive care units. Drugs are a common cause, but both environmental and metabolic factors also have been implicated. The former can be corrected by transferring the patient to a regular hospital ward or room as soon as possible. Katz et al. indicated a physiologic abnormality, such as hypoxemia or electrolyte or acid-base abnormality, as the cause in the great majority of patients. Preoperative discussion and support lowered the incidence of postcardiotomy delirium from 37 to 14 percent in one series.

DRUG ABUSE

Beebe and Keats have shown that not all narcotic addicts require detoxification associated with an operation. Methadone is the drug of choice for treating withdrawal. Haloxone may be preferable in an emergency situation. For patients on methadone maintenance, this drug can be stopped temporarily and frequent doses of conventional narcotics substituted during the early postoperative period. Withdrawal from barbiturates prior to elective operation may take 2 to 3 weeks. There is no physiologic addiction requiring maintenance of amphetamines or hallucinogens.

COMPLICATIONS OF GASTROINTESTINAL SURGERY

The complications considered in this section are divided into (1) vascular complications, including hemorrhage and gangrene; (2) mechanical problems of gastroenterostomy and enteroenterostomy, including stomal obstruction, the afferent, or blind, loop syndrome, extrinsic obstruction and internal hernia, and inadvertent gastroileostomy; (3) leakage of an anastomosis, including the duodenal stump blowout; (4) external fistulas and stomal problems; and (5) damage to adjacent organs, including postoperative pancreatitis and jaundice.

Vascular Complications

HEMORRHAGE

Gastrointestinal hemorrhage that occurs subsequent to a gastrointestinal anastomosis may become manifest postoperatively by hematemesis, melena, hematochezia, or, most frequently, the passage of bright blood via a nasogastric tube positioned in the stomach. Bleeding from the suture line is most commonly associated with gastric surgery, occurring in approximately 1 to 5 percent of patients following gastric resection, with a higher incidence in those patients in whom operation is performed for a duodenal ulcer. Bleeding from the suture line is apt to occur either immediately after the operation or on the first postoperative day, but a second minor peak in incidence has been noted between the seventh and tenth postoperative days. Bleeding arising from the suture line on the first postoperative day is usually minimal or moderate and requires no specific therapy, but if it is continuous, the stomach should be aspirated and irrigated with ice-cold saline solution. Hemorrhage that does not stop following conservative measures constitutes an indication for endoscopy. Endoscopically directed coagulation or laser therapy may effect control of a bleeding site. If bleeding continues, reoperation is indicated, at which time the suture line should be inspected. It may be preferable to enter the stomach above the line of anastomosis and ligate vessels from within. Bleeding later in the course of convalescence is usually due to sloughing from the suture line and generally responds to iced saline lavage. Significant hemorrhage from the suture line of small intestinal and large intestinal anastomoses is extremely rare. Upper gastrointestinal bleeding following a surgical procedure in a patient who is debilitated or in whom sepsis develops frequently indicates a stress ulcer (see Chap. 26).

GANGRENE

Gangrene is a rare complication of resection of a segment of gastrointestinal tract, since the intestine is supplied with a rich network of arteries. Necrosis of the gastric remnant has been reported following a high subtotal gastrectomy, particularly if the procedure incorporates ligation of the left gastric artery and concomitant splenectomy. Devascularization of the areas to be anastomosed should not occur following small intestinal surgical procedures if attention is directed toward the vascular supply. A precautionary measure is to slant the lines of incision so that more intestine is resected on the antimesenteric aspect. Small intestinal gangrene is more frequently due to mechanical strangulation, obstruction secondary to postoperative adhesions, volvulus, internal hernias, or vascular thrombosis. Gangrene of the segment of intestine may be apparent in the case of a colostomy in which an inadequate vascular supply has been provided. In each instance, the recognition of gangrene requires resection of the gangrenous segment of intestine or stomach and reestablishment of intestinal continuity or a colostomy in bowel that is viable.

Mechanical Problems

STOMAL OBSTRUCTION

Although obstruction of the stoma may follow any intestinal anastomosis as a result of technical factors, postgastrectomy stomal obstruction represents the most common type and is frequently related to local edema. Factors that have been implicated in the etiology of edema include electrolyte depletion, hypochloremia, incomplete hemostasis, hypoproteinemia, leakage from the anastomosis, inadequate proximal decompression, and incorporation of too much tissue within the sutures. Other causes include rotation of the jejunum on its long axis, obstruction by the transverse mesocolon, particularly in an obese patient, obstruction by a fatty omentum, effect of vagotomy, and, rarely, jejunogastric intussusception, which has been reported as a complication in slightly over 100 cases of Billroth II procedures.

Postgastrectomy stomal obstruction is a most troublesome complication, and the reported incidence has ranged between 1 and 3 percent. In a review of 648 partial gastrectomies, an incidence of 4.6 percent for patients requiring further operative therapy, 4.1 percent for Billroth II operations, and 3.5 percent for Billroth I types was recorded. In most instances in their series, the efferent loop was obstructed by the transverse mesocolon.

Symptoms usually occur on the third to fourth postoperative day, at which time there is abdominal fullness and increased return from the nasogastric suction. If the patient has been on oral intake, nausea followed by vomiting of large quantities of bile-colored gastric fluid occurs. Instillation of barium or Gastrografin via the nasogastric tube may reveal stomal obstruction or a patent stoma with distal loop obstruction. The symptoms usually persist for only short intervals and cause little disability, but occasionally they are prolonged and then have severe metabolic effects.

Prophylaxis is directed at avoiding the factors that have been implicated. Therapy of established stomal obstruction consists of adequate decompression and replacement of fluids and nutrients, while waiting for the obstruction to become relieved spontaneously. The course may be prolonged, extending over a period of several weeks.

Metaclopramide or bethanechol may be administered for several days in an attempt to improve gastric atony. If there is not relief after extended conservative management or if the patient's condition is deteriorating, operative intervention is indicated. Rarely, a simple release of adhesions may be therapeutic, but more often the anastomotic site requires revision, a procedure that is frequently difficult in view of the extensive reaction around the stoma. It is generally preferable to transect the proximal and distal loops of intestine at their entrance to and exit from the indurated mass. These are then anastomosed to one another, and the short segment of intestine and a cuff of stomach are removed with the gastroenterostomy. Continuity is reestablished with a long antecolic gastrojejunostomy.

AFFERENT (BLIND) LOOP SYNDROME

The afferent loop syndrome represents a complication of subtotal gastrectomy with Billroth II gastroenterostomy. The afferent loop consists of duodenum and a segment of jejunum of variable length. Acute or chronic obstruction can occur at any point proximal to the gastrojejunostomy. Blomstedt and Dahlgren reported an incidence of 18 percent with mild to moderate symptoms (type I and type II). The symptom complex of partial obstruction of the afferent loop was reported by Magnuson et al. to occur following gastrectomy in 4.2 percent of patients with gastric ulcer in contrast to 0.9 percent of patients with duodenal ulcer.

PATHOGENESIS. Normally after partial gastrectomy, biliary and pancreatic secretions enter the afferent loop, pass through the gastrojejunostomy to mix with gastric juice, and then pass through into the efferent loop. During a 24-h period, approximately 1 to 1.5 L of secretion enters the afferent loop. The afferent loop syndrome is caused by partial and, rarely, total obstruction of flow from the afferent loop. The pressure within the duodenum and segment of jejunum rises, and the loop becomes dilated by bile and pancreatic juice. After the ingestion of food, particularly a fatty meal, the duodenal contents increase rapidly, thus explaining the postcibal nature of the syndrome. With incomplete obstruction, pressure within the intestine eventually becomes sufficient to overcome resistance, and the contents are emptied into the stomach, causing variable amounts to be vomited. With total obstruction, the loop no longer has any communication with the stomach, and vomitus is free of bile.

CLINICAL MANIFESTATIONS. The symptoms of partial obstruction of the afferent loop occur most commonly in the early postoperative period. Two-thirds of the cases occur during the first week, but in some instances the syndrome becomes apparent months to years following gastrectomy. The symptoms vary in intensity and are characterized by postcibal vomiting. Mild symptoms consist of eructation of a mouthful of green biliary fluid within an hour and a half after a meal. Vomiting is generally preceded by the sensation of fullness and, at times, pain in the epigastrium. In some instances, the symptoms of chronic obstruction persist for several months, and the amount of biliary vomiting and antecedent epigastric pain are appreciable. With persistence of partial obstruction, the stools become bulky and gray and contain much fat. Radiographic examination may show passage of contrast material into the efferent loop, while the afferent loop, as a rule, fails to fill. Chronic partial obstruction is associated with anemia. Urinary excretion of B_{12} is reduced or absent and is unaffected by the administration of intrinsic factor, in contrast to pernicious anemia. However, following a course of 3 to 5 days of tetracycline, B_{12} urinary excretion returns to normal.

In the rare situation of the acute complete obstruction of the afferent loop, the patient becomes acutely ill with severe epigastric pain, and bile is characteristically absent from the vomitus. A mass may be felt in the upper abdomen. The patient's condition may deteriorate rapidly, and shock may occur as a result of compromise of the circulation of the duodenal wall and/or perforation with generalized peritonitis. Radiographs are of little diagnostic assistance. There may be delayed emptying of contrast material from the gastric remnant, and no barium enters the afferent loop. The amylase level may be markedly elevated.

TREATMENT. Incomplete obstruction generally subsides on a conservative regimen. Capper and Welbourn collected 44 cases requiring surgical intervention and reported that 36 of them had a good outcome. Surgical decompression of the afferent loop may be accomplished by anastomosis between the afferent and efferent loops, by employing a Roux en Y anastomosis or converting a gastrojejunostomy to a gastroduodenostomy. In the case of acute total obstruction, early operation with decompression of the afferent loop is mandatory.

INTESTINAL OBSTRUCTION

Intestinal obstruction in the immediate postoperative period is most frequently due to ileus or fibrinous adhesions. Following laparotomy the stomach usually recovers motor activity in hours, the small intestine within a day, and the colon in 30 days. In the face of peritonitis or mesenteric or retroperitoneal hematoma, ileus is usually prolonged. It may be impossible to distinguish postoperative ileus and mechanical obstruction. Following the progression of radiopaque material instilled via a nasogastric tube may distinguish the two disorders. Internal herniation represents a complication of subtotal gastrectomy, generally following a Billroth II antecolic anastomosis. Internal herniation of the small intestine may also take place through improperly closed mesenteric rents or when the mesentery of the ileum or colon is not tacked to the peritoneum in the course of an ileostomy or colostomy. Closed-loop obstruction generally results and may rapidly progress to compromise the vascular supply with ultimate perforation. Operative reduction and repair of an internal hernia are required. Adhesions and/or volvulus may occur in the postoperative hospitalization and require surgical intervention for relief of obstruction. The incidence is particularly high following resection for congenital atresia in infancy, especially when the proximal dilated bowel is not resected. Postoperative intussuscep-

tion, generally involving the small intestine, is also to be considered in the pediatric age group.

INADVERTENT GASTROILEOSTOMY

The error of anastomosing the stomach to the ileum rather than the jejunum is fortunately uncommon. The situation results in a malabsorption syndrome that begins as soon as the patient is allowed to eat solid food. Diarrhea, weight loss, and inanition in the absence of abdominal pain are characteristic. The stool contains a high percentage of undigested food and a large quantity of unabsorbed fat. Fecal vomiting and hemorrhage occasionally occur, and an ulcer may develop at the site of the ileum, in which case abdominal pain may be present. The diagnosis can be established radiographically by demonstrating a rapid transit and short distal intestine. The error should be avoided by using the ligament of Treitz as a landmark in establishing a gastroenterostomy; in the absence of a ligament of Treitz an anomaly of rotation should be suspected, and the loop of intestine for anastomosis should be selected by tracing the duodenum distad or the small bowel proximally from the cecum. The preoperative management of patients with gastroileostomy requires a vigorous preparation with TPN, or a preliminary feeding jejunostomy is of value. A block resection of the gastroileostomy is advocated for patients who have had subtotal gastric resection, while, in the absence of gastric resection, the ileostomy may be taken down directly. A gastrojejunostomy and reconstitution of intestinal continuity are then performed.

Anastomotic Leak

Suture line leakage represents a potential complication of any intestinal anastomosis. The three prime etiologic factors are (1) poor surgical technique, (2) distal obstruction, and (3) inadequate proximal decompression. Leak from an enteroenterostomy becomes manifest as localized or generalized peritonitis. Small leaks with localized response may be treated by proximal decompression and administration of appropriate antibiotics, while large leaks and diffuse peritonitis frequently require surgical intervention. Fistulization may develop as a tract becomes established between the point of leakage and the skin. A leak from the line of anastomosis is a relatively rare complication following gastroenterostomy. Such leakage occurs more frequently when there has been impairment of the blood supply of the residual gastric pouch and a concomitant splenectomy has been performed. A common point at which leaks develop has been referred to as the "angle du mort," where the residual gastric pouch of a Hofmeister closure meets the line of anastomosis of the small intestine.

Duodenal stump leakage (blowout) is a more frequent and critical complication of gastric resection. A review of gastrectomies performed at the Mayo Clinic in 1956 revealed that 4.5 percent of patients subjected to the procedure for gastric ulcer had some evidence of leak, while 5.6 percent of patients in whom the same procedure was carried out for duodenal ulcer revealed similar evidence. In that study, drains had been inserted into the stump region, and in many patients increased drainage represented the evidence of a leak. Edmunds et al. reported a 1.1 percent incidence of dehiscence of the stump, the mortality due to this cause was 0.6 percent.

Duodenal stump leakage occurs most commonly after operation for a duodenal ulcer and frequently when gastrectomy is performed as an emergency procedure to stop hemorrhage. In a great majority of cases, the leak arises as a result of technical error and failure of the suture line. A scarred and edematous duodenum predisposes to the complication as does obstruction of the afferent loop and local pancreatitis. Complications of duodenal leakage include peritonitis, subhepatic abscess, pancreatitis, sepsis, and establishment of an external fistula with fluid and electrolyte abnormalities.

Specific measures can be taken to avoid this complication. In the face of marked inflammatory disease in the duodenal region, vagotomy and gastroenterostomy definitely represent safer procedures. When resection has been undertaken and duodenal closure is difficult, catheter duodenostomy may be used as an adjunct. Rodkey and Welch reported that in 51 cases with difficult duodenal stump closures in whom planned duodenostomy was carried out, there was only one death, and only five patients had drainage from the fistula that lasted more than 48 h after the catheter was removed. As a compromise between primary closure and planned duodenostomy, some surgeons have advised drainage of the right upper quadrant placed in the region of the duodenal stump in the hope that if perforation occurs, the contents will discharge along the tract. However, this does not provide the safety factor of planned duodenostomy, since the drain tract may wall off from the stump before the perforation becomes established.

Duodenal blowout is a major catastrophe that is most likely to occur between the second and seventh postoperative day, and becomes manifest by sudden pain, elevation in temperature and pulse rate, and general deterioration of the patient's condition. Adequate drainage must be instituted at once and is best accomplished by an incision below the right costal margin and insertion of a large sump catheter that is passed down to the duodenal stump area, with constant suction applied. Attention must be directed toward fluid and electrolyte therapy, and TPN should be instituted. Fistula closure can be anticipated within 2 to 3 weeks. Another area in which leaks are a major concern is low colon anastomoses; incidences of 5 to 51 percent have been reported. Pedicled omentum may be applied to seal the anastomosis. The mortality rate in patients with major colon leaks is extremely high, and this has led to a resurgence of enthusiasm for protective transverse colostomy if the anastomosis appears compromised.

External Fistulas and Stomal Complications

FISTULAS

External fistulas may arise from the stomach and duodenum, the small intestine, or the colon. In one series of 157 patients, there was equal distribution of fistulas from the three major segments of the intraabdominal alimentary tract. Surgical procedures have been implicated as etiologic factors in 67 to 80 percent of cases.

Gastric and Duodenal Fistulas

The incidence of gastrojejunal or duodenal stump fistulas following subtotal gastrectomy has been reported to be 1 to 2 percent, approximately one-quarter of which originated from the gastrojejunostomy. Suture line failure accounted for 82 percent of all gastroduodenal fistulas. The causes of fistulas arising from the gastrojejunostomy may be related to the suture line containing tumor, ischemia of the gastric stump due to high ligation of the gastric artery and vasa brevia, stomal obstruction, and pancreatitis or tension on the suture line. The causes of duodenal stump fistula have been referred to in the previous section on stump leakage. The complications of an established gastric or duodenal fistula include electrolyte abnormalities and malnutrition, sepsis, intraperitoneal abscesses and wound infection, jaundice, and pancreatitis.

Treatment. Intensive fluid, electrolyte, and nutritional therapy is frequently required. This may be facilitated by TPN or enteral feeding with elemental diet delivered distally via a jejunostomy or a nasogastric tube advanced beyond the area of the fistula. Large amounts of drainage can usually be collected with a well-fixed appliance; continuous suction is rarely employed. Skin care is an essential factor; autodigestion can be prevented with a variety of barrier powders or sheets. The majority of fistulas that close spontaneously do so within 6 weeks.

An established gastric fistula may require resection and correction of distal obstruction if the latter is present. Fistulas arising at the site of a gastrojejunostomy generally require resection and establishment of a new gastroenterostomy. Duodenal fistulas are generally not amenable to direct closure. Tarazi and associates recently reported an experience with 47 patients, 18 with gastric and 29 with duodenal fistulas, and they reviewed other series. The mortality of gastric fistulas was 22 percent compared with reported percentages of 15 to 50 percent. The mortality of lateral duodenal fistulas was 25 percent compared with other reports of 0 to 67 percent. The mortality of duodenal stump fistulas ranged from 12 to 50 percent. The incidence of spontaneous closure ranged from 25 to 54 percent of gastric fistulas and from 37 to 100 percent for duodenal fistulas. When operation was performed for duodenal fistula, the authors noted a success rate of less than 50 percent; others have reported excellent results with a jejunal or ileal serosal patch or a Roux en Y anastomosis to the defect.

Small Bowel Fistulas

Seventy-two percent of the 46 fistulas in this group reported by Edmunds et al. represented surgical complications secondary to dehiscence of anastomoses or inadvertent injury during dissection or closure of an abdominal incision. Although jejunal and proximal ileal fistulas are frequently characterized by profuse drainage, the fluid loss is generally less than that associated with duodenal fistulas, and therefore fluid and electrolyte abnormalities occur less frequently. Malnutrition must be aggressively combated in these patients, and sepsis is a major complication. A large number of intraperitoneal abscesses develop. Skin digestion is a frequent occurrence, and many of these patients eventually develop a ventral hernia due to wound complications.

Many factors influence the outcome of treatment of enterocutaneous fistulas. Jejunal fistulas have a poorer prognosis than ileal fistulas; high-output fistulas are also associated with a greater mortality rate. Intraabdominal sepsis, anemia, and malnutrition all have adverse effects. Series reported since 1970 indicate medical regimens effect cures in an average of 62 percent of cases and are associated with an average mortality rate of 13 percent.

Treatment. Supportive management of small bowel fistulas is similar to that outlined for gastroduodenal fistulas. This includes maintenance of fluid and electrolyte balance and nutrition. An elemental diet may be applicable particularly for low output fistulas. TPN may be applicable. In the case of a proximal jejunal fistula, a distal feeding jejunostomy is frequently indicated to permit adequate fluid and nutritional intake. Oral feeding of low-residue diets is feasible with ileal fistulas. Control of fluid loss and diarrhea may be accomplished with the use of Lomotil, Kaopectate, and opiates plus nonabsorbable antibiotics when indicated. Protection of the skin in the region of the fistula is indicated.

Operative procedures include direct attack on a fistula with resection both of the fistula and the segment of intestine from which it arises or an indirect attack through a clean abdominal incision with a bypass operation or complete exclusion of the fistula by means of end-to-end anastomosis of the proximal and distal intestine. The excluded loop is then decompressed completely through a large fistula by exteriorizing the ends of the intestine to prevent later blowout. Definitive operations should be performed only in sepsis-free patients in wound nutritional status.

Colonic Fistulas (See Chaps. 27 and 28)

These are generally caused by anastomotic leaks or inadvertent trauma to the segment of intestine. Anastomosis in the region of tumor or inflammation and distal partial obstruction are predisposing factors. Fluid and electrolyte abnormalities are uncommon, while the incidence of infection is extremely high. This includes peritonitis, intraperitoneal abscesses, and wound infections. Significant skin digestion and irritation are rare.

Treatment. The patients can generally be managed on a low-residue or elemental diet, using enteric or parenteral antibiotics when indicated. Spontaneous healing of fistulas in these regions is the rule rather than the exception, but defunctionalizing colostomies for descending colon fistulas or ileal transverse colostomies for ascending colon and distal ileal fistulas may be indicated. Medical management is generally indicated for about 6 weeks to permit any active inflammation to subside. Definitive surgical treatment is indicated for fistulas that fail to progress satisfactorily after 6 weeks. If the fistula is accompanied by generalized peritonitis, early emergency resection is

indicated and frequently should be accompanied by a proximal defunctionalizing procedure. Definitive operations include a turn-in procedure or resection that may be coupled with a temporary protective colostomy or bypass. Seventy-five percent of patients with no operation experienced spontaneous cure; 74 percent of chronic fecal fistulas treated by turn-in or resection were cured.

EXTERNAL STOMAL COMPLICATIONS (See Chap. 28)

Ileostomy

Ileostomy performed for ulcerative colitis may be associated with complications related to technical factors, presence of disease, and the nature of the intestinal contents that are discharged. The location of ileostomy is critical to permit application of an effective collecting device, while the method of fixation of the ileal mesentery is important to prevent internal herniation. Formation of the ileostomy itself is important in reducing the incidence of complications. The technique of operative maturation by everting the mucosa reduces the incidence of serositis and peritonitis. The liquid nature of the ileostomy discharge requires that measures be taken to avoid excoriation of the skin, which is usually due to delayed application of the bag and a poor fit. When excoriation appears, it is generally wise to discontinue the use of cement and apply a soothing powder. The patient may be placed in a prone position on a frame so that the ileal contents are allowed to drain into a container and contact with the skin is avoided. The complication of prolapse, which requires revision, should be seen infrequently if the mesentery has been fixed. Fistulas that develop at or below the skin level are an indication for early revision of the ileostomy.

Cecostomy and Colostomy

Cecostomies generally demand more attention than colostomies, and frequent irrigation is indicated. Subsequent to removal of the cecostomy catheter, spontaneous closure is to be anticipated, but in unusual circumstances, surgical closure is required. Complications following colostomy include ischemia, gangrene, bleeding, wound abscesses, stenosis, or retraction of the stoma. In the case of a terminal colostomy, fixation and maturation during the operative procedure should prevent retraction. If either retraction or gangrene becomes evident, immediate operation is indicated to revise the colostomy using viable bowel of sufficient length. A paracolostomy hernia may require direct fascial repair.

Bibliography

General Considerations

Artz CP, Hardy JD: *Complications in Surgery and Their Management.* Philadelphia, Saunders, 1967.

Wound Complications

Alexander HC, Prudden J: The causes of abdominal wound disruption. *Surg Gynecol Obstet* 122:1223, 1966.

Banerjee SR, Daoud I, et al: Abdominal wound evisceration. *Curr Surg* 40:432, 1983.

Elek SD, Conen PE: The virulence of *Staphylococcus pyogenes* for man: A study of the problems of wound infections. *Br J Exp Pathol* 38:573, 1957.

Fagniez J–L, Hay JM, et al: Abdominal midline incision closure. *Arch Surg* 120:1351, 1985.

Gammelgaard N, Jensen J: Wound complications after closure of abdominal incisions with Dexon or Vicryl. *Acta Chir Scand* 149:505, 1983.

Goligher JC, Irvin TT, et al: A controlled clinical trial of three methods of closure of laparotomy wounds. *Br J Surg* 62:823, 1975.

Greenburg AG, Saik RP, Peskin GW: Wound dehiscence. *Arch Surg* 114:143, 1979.

Halasz NA: Dehiscence of laparotomy wounds. *Am J Surg* 116:210, 1968.

Pemberton LB, Manax WG: Complications after vertical and transverse incisions for cholecystectomy. *Surg Gynecol Obstet* 132:892, 1971.

Pollock AV, Froome K, Evans M: The bacteriology of primary wound sepsis in potentially contaminated abdominal operations: The effect of irrigation, povidone-iodine and cephaloridine on the sepsis rate assessed in a clinical trial. *Br J Surg* 65:76, 1978.

Sindelar WF, Mason GR: Irrigation of subcutaneous tissue with povidone-iodine solution for prevention of surgical wound infections. *Surg Gynecol Obstet* 148:227, 1979.

Wolff WI: Disruption of abdominal wounds. *Ann Surg* 131:534, 1950.

Postoperative Parotitis

Hemenway WG, English GM: Surgical treatment of acute bacterial parotitis. *Postgrad Med* 50:114, 1971.

Krippaehne WW, Hunt TK, Dunphy JE: Acute suppurative parotitis: A study of 161 cases. *Ann Surg* 156:251, 1962.

Lary BG: Postoperative suppurative parotitis. *Arch Surg* 89:653, 1964.

Petersdorf RG, Forsyth BB, Bernake D: Staphylococcal parotitis. *N Engl J Med* 259:1250, 1958.

Postoperative Respiratory Complications

Adriani J, Zepernick R, et al: Iatrogenic pulmonary edema in surgical patients. *Surgery* 61:183, 1967.

Ashbaugh DG, Petty TL: Positive end-expiratory pressure: Physiology, indications, and contraindications. *J Thorac Cardiovasc Surg* 65:165, 1973.

Civetta JM, Augenstein JS: Acute respiratory failure following surgery and trauma, in Greenfield LJ (ed): *Complications in Surgery and Trauma*. Philadelphia, Lippincott, 1984, chap 21, pp 243–259.

Clements JA: Surface phenomena in relation to pulmonary function (sixth Bowditch lecture). *Physiologist* 5:11, 1962.

Cuschieri J, Morran G, et al: Postoperative pain and pulmonary complications: Comparison of three analgesic regimens. *Br J Surg* 72:495, 1985.

Davis HA, Pollak EW: Adult respiratory distress syndrome in postoperative patients: Study of pulmonary pathology in "shock lung" with prophylactic and therapeutic implications. *Am Surg* 41:391, 1975.

Joffe N: Roentgenologic findings in post-shock and postoperative pulmonary insufficiency. *Radiology* 94:369, 1970.

Laver MB, Bendixen HH: Atelectasis in the surgical patient: Recent conceptual advances. *Prog Surg* 5:1, 1966.

Neely WA, Robinson TW, et al: Post-operative respiratory insufficiency. *Ann Surg* 171:679, 1970.

Norwood SH, Civetta JM: Ventilatory support in patients with ARDS. *Surg Clin North Am* 65:895, 1985.

Peters RM, Hilberman M, et al: Objective indications for respiratory therapy in post-trauma and postoperative patients. *Am J Surg* 124:262, 1972.

Pontoppidan H, Geffin B, Lowenstein E: Acute respiratory failure in the adult: Trends in treatment of acute respiratory failure. *N Engl J Med* 287:690, 1972.

Pontoppidan H, Geffin B, Lowenstein E: Acute respiratory failure in the adult: Assessment of respiratory function. *N Engl J Med* 287:743, 1972.

Pontoppidan H, Geffin B, Lowenstein E: Acute respiratory failure in the adult: Effect of mechanical ventilation and airway pressures on circulation and blood gas exchange. *N Engl J Med* 287:799, 1972.

Pontoppidan H, Laver MB, Geffin B: Acute respiratory failure in the surgical patient. *Adv Surg* 4:163, 1970.

Rinaldo JE, Rogers RM: Adult respiratory distress syndrome. Changing concepts of lung injury and repair. *N Engl J Med* 306:900, 1982.

Sayeed MM, Chaudry IH, Baue AE: Na$^+$–K$^+$ transport and adenosine nucleotides in the lung in hemorrhagic shock. *Surgery* 77:395, 1975.

Shoemaker WC: Controversies in the pathophysiology and fluid management of postoperative adult respiratory distress syndrome. *Surg Clin North Am* 64:931, 1985.

Staub NC: Pulmonary edema due to increased microvascular permeability. *Annu Rev Med* 32:291, 1981.

Stock MC, Downs JB, et al: Prevention of postoperative complications with CPAP, incentive spirometry, and conservative therapy. *Chest* 87:151, 1985.

Cardiac Complications

Buckley JJ, Jackson JA: Postoperative cardiac arrhythmias. *Anesthesiology* 22:723, 1961.

Dreifus LS, Rabbino MD, et al: Arrhythmias in the postoperative period. *Am J Cardiol* 12:431, 1963.

Goldman L: Cardiac risks and complications of noncardiac surgery. *Ann Surg* 198:780, 1983.

Mauney FM Jr, Ebert PA, Sabiston DC Jr.: Postoperative myocardial infarction: A study of predisposing factors, diagnosis, and mortality in a high risk group of surgical patients. *Ann Surg* 172:497, 1970.

Merideth J: Cardiac arrhythmias in the postoperative patient. *Surg Clin North Am* 49:1083, 1969.

Reinikainen M, Pontinen P: On cardiac arrhythmias during anaesthesia and surgery. *Acta Med Scand Suppl* 457, 1966.

Singh BN, Ellrodt G, Peter CT: Verapamil: A review of its pharmacological properties and therapeutic use. *Drugs* 15:169, 1978.

Tarhan S, Moffitt EA, et al: Myocardial infarction after general anesthesia. *JAMA* 220:1451, 1972.

Wroblewski F, LaDue JS: Myocardial infarction as a postoperative complication of major surgery. *JAMA* 150:1212, 1952.

Diabetes Mellitus

Galloway JA, Shuman CR: Diabetes and surgery: A study of 667 cases. *Am J Med* 34:177, 1963.

Gastineau CF, Molnar GD: The care of the diabetic patient during emergency surgery. *Surg Clin North Am* 49:1171, 1969.

Kidson W, Casey J, et al: Treatment of severe diabetes mellitus by infusion. *Br Med J* 2:691, 1974.

Marble A, Steinke J: Physiology and pharmacology in diabetes mellitus: Guiding the diabetic patient through the surgical period. *Anesthesiology* 24:442, 1963.

Meyer EJ, Lorenzi M, et al: Diabetic management by insulin infusion during major surgery. *Am J Surg* 137:323, 1979.

Page M McB, Alberti KGMM, et al: Treatment of diabetic coma with continuous low dose infusion. *Br Med J* 2:687, 1974.

Woodruff RE, Lewis SB, et al: Avoidance of surgical hyperglycemia in diabetic patients. *JAMA* 244:166, 1980.

Fat Embolism Syndrome

Ashbaugh DG, Petty TL: The use of corticosteroids in the treatment of respiratory failure associated with massive fat embolism. *Surg Gynecol Obstet* 123:495, 1966.

Benoit PR, Hampson LG, Burgess JH: Value of arterial hypoxemia in the diagnosis of pulmonary fat embolism. *Ann Surg* 175:128, 1972.

Chan KM, Tham KT, et al: Post-traumatic fat embolism—its clinical and subclinical present status. *J Trauma* 24:45, 1984.

Evarts CM: The fat embolism syndrome: A review. *Surg Clin North Am* 50:493, 1970.

Palmovic V, McCarroll JR: Fat embolism in trauma. *Arch Pathol* 80:630, 1965.

Pazell JA, Peltier LF: Experience with sixty-three patients with fat embolism. *Surg Gynecol Obstet* 135:77, 1972.

Sevitt S: *Fat Embolism*. London, Butterworth Scientific Publications, 1962.

Shier MR, Wilson RF: Fat embolism syndrome: Traumatic coagulopathy with respiratory distress. *Surg Annu* 12:139, 1980.

Weisz GM: Fat embolism. *Curr Probl Surg* November 1974.

Psychiatric Complications

Altschule MD: Postoperative psychosis. *Surg Clin North Am* 49:677, 1969.

Beebe HG, Keats NM: Surgical patients and drug abuse syndrome. *Am Surg* 39:88, 1973.

Bolton HE, Bailey CP: Surgical aspects in psychosomatic aspects of cardiovascular surgery. in Cantor AJ, Foxe AN (eds): *Psychosomatic Aspects of Surgery*. New York, Grune & Stratton, 1955, chap 3.

Donovan JC: Some psychosomatic aspects of obstetrics and gynecology. *Am J Obstet Gynecol* 75:72, 1958.

Egerton N, Kay JH: Psychological disturbances associated with open heart surgery. *Br J Psychiat* 110:433, 1964.

Fox HM, Rizzo ND, Gifford S: Psychological observations of patients undergoing mitral surgery: Study of stress. *Psychosom Med* 16:186, 1954.

Hackett TP, Weisman AD: Psychiatric management of operative syndromes. I. The therapeutic consultation and the effect of noninterpretive intervention. *Psychosom Med* 22:267, 1960.

Hackett TP, Weisman AD: Psychiatric management of operative syndromes. II. Psychodynamic factors in formulation and management. *Psychosom Med* 22:356, 1960.

Howell JG: *Modern Perspectives and Psychiatric Aspects of Surgery*. New York, Brunner-Mazel, 1976.

Johnson JE, Leventhal H: Contribution of emotional and instrumental response processes in adaptation to surgery. *J Pers Soc Psychol* 20:55, 1971.

Katz NM, Agle DP, et al: Delirium in surgical patients under intensive care: Utility of mental status examination. *Arch Surg* 104:310, 1972.

Kemph JP: Renal failure, artificial kidney and kidney transplant. *Am J Psychiat* 122:1270, 1966.

Knox SJ: Severe psychiatric disturbances in the postoperative period: A five-year survey of Belfast hospitals. *J Ment Sci* 107:1078, 1961.

Kornfeld DS, Zimberg S, Malm JR: Psychiatric complications of open-heart surgery. *N Engl J Med* 273:287, 1965.

Layne OL Jr, Yudofsky SC: Postoperative psychosis in cardiotomy patients: The role of organic and psychiatric factors. *N Engl J Med* 284:518, 1971.

Maguire P, Tait A, et al: The effect of counselling on the psychiatric morbidity associated with mastectomy. *Br Med J* 281:1454, 1980.

Meyer BC: Some psychiatric aspects of surgical practice. *Psychosom Med* 20:203, 1958.

Prugh D, Staub E, et al: A study of the emotional reactions of children and families to hospitalization and illness. *Am J Orthopsychiatry* 22:70, 1953.

Spiro HR: Psychiatric reactions associated with surgery. in Condon RE, DeCosse JJ (eds): *Surgical Care*. Philadelphia, Lea & Febiger, 1980.

Titchener JL, Levine M: *Surgery as a Human Experience: The Psychodynamics of Surgical Practice*. Fair Lawn, NJ, Oxford University Press, 1960.

Titchener JL, Zwerling I, et al: Psychosis in surgical patients. *Surg Gynecol Obstet* 102:59, 1956.

Weiss SM: Psychological adjustment following open-heart surgery. *J Nerv Ment Dis* 143:363, 1966.

Winkelstein C, Blacher RS, Meyer BC: Psychiatric observations on surgical patients in recovery room: Pilot study. *NY J Med* 65:865, 1965.

Wright RG, Sand P, Livingston G: Psychological stress during haemodialysis for chronic renal failure. *Ann Intern Med* 64:611, 1966.

Zaks MS: Disturbances in physiologic functions and neuropsychiatric complications in heart surgery, in Luisada AA (ed): *Cardiology: An Encyclopedia of the Cardiovascular System*. New York, McGraw-Hill, vol 3, 1959.

Complications of Gastrointestinal Surgery

Blomstedt B, Dahlgren S: The afferent loop syndrome. *Acta Chir Scand* 120:347, 1961.

Brooke BN: Management of an ileostomy including its complications. *Lancet* 2:202, 1952.

Capper WM, Welbourn RB: Early postcibal symptoms following gastrectomy. *Br J Surg* 43:24, 1955.

Devlin HB, Elcoat C: Alimentary tract fistula: Stomatherapy techniques of management. *World J Surg* 7:489, 1983.

Dietel M: Elemental diet and enterocutaneous fistula. *World J Surg* 7:451, 1983.

Edmunds LH Jr, Williams GM, Welch CE: External fistulas arising from the gastro-intestinal tract. *Ann Surg* 152:445, 1960.

Fazio VM: Alimentary tract fistulas—an introduction. *World J Surg* 7:445, 1983.

Fischer JE: The pathophysiology of enterocutaneous fistulas. *World J Surg* 7:446, 1983.

Gleysteen JJ, Sillin LF, Condon RE: Delayed gastric emptying, in Condon RE, DeCosse JJ (eds): *Surgical Care*. Philadelphia, Lea & Febiger, 1980, chap 2.

Herrington JL Jr, Sawyers JL: Complications following gastric operations, in Schwartz SI and Ellis H (eds): *Maingot's Ab-*

dominal Operations. Norwalk, Appleton Century Crofts, 1985, pp 897–942.

Hill GL: Operative strategy in the treatment of enterocutaneous fistulas. *World J Surg* 7:495, 1983.

Johnson CL, McIlrath DC: Management of patients with enterocutaneous fistulas. *Surg Clin North Am* 49:967, 1969.

Malangoni MA, Madura JA, Jesseph JE: Management of lateral duodenal fistulas: A study of fourteen cases. *Surgery* 90:645, 1981.

Magnuson FK, Judd ES, Dearing WH: Comparison of postgastrectomy complications in gastric and duodenal ulcer patients. *Am Surg* 32:375, 1966.

Morgenstern L, Yamakawa T, et al: Anastomotic leakage after low colonic anastomosis. Clinical and experimental aspects. *Am J Surg* 123:104, 1972.

Pettersson S, Wallensten S: Leakage at suture lines after partial gastrectomy for peptic ulcer. *Acta Chir Scand* 135:229, 1969.

Rodkey GV, Welch CE: Duodenal decompression in gastrectomy. *N Engl J Med* 262:498, 1960.

State D: Immediate complications of gastric surgery. *Surg Clin North Am 44:371, 1964*.

Tarazi R, Coutsoftides T, et al: Gastric and duodenal cutaneous fistulas. *World J Surg* 7:463, 1983.

Woods JH, Kowalske M, DeCosse JJ: The new stoma: Ileostomy and colostomy, in Condon RE, DeCosse JJ (eds): *Surgical Care*. Philadelphia, Lea & Febiger, 1980, chap 6.

Chapter 13

Physiologic Monitoring of the Surgical Patient

Louis R. M. Del Guercio and John A. Savino

INTRODUCTION

Among the 14 definitions of the word "monitor" that appear in one dictionary, three appear applicable to medicine: "Something that serves to remind or give warning"; "A device or arrangement for observing or recording the operation of a machine or system, especially an automatic control system"; and "To observe, record, or detect an operation or condition with instruments that have no effect on the operation or condition."

The last definition offers the key to a basic problem of all patient monitoring, i.e., that the measuring system tends to change the measurements. The application of electrodes, cannulas, mouthpieces, and other paraphernalia definitely has psychologic and physiologic effects on the patient. From this it follows that the ideal monitoring system should be noninvasive and unobtrusive.

The most sophisticated and advanced electronic system can never substitute for close surveillance by an experienced and qualified health professional. Monitors in surgery are worthwhile only if they provide information about the patient that cannot be detected by the five senses of a physician or nurse. In addition, the transducers, signal processors, or readout devices should not so encumber the patient as to interfere with essential nursing care.

There is a tendency to think of monitoring in terms of complicated electronic devices and computers; in fact, the serial recordings of temperature, pulse, respiratory rate, and blood pressure are forms of clinical monitoring in common use for decades. This approach to monitoring was observed by Harvey Cushing on a visit to Italy, and overcoming considerable resistance, he introduced routine blood-pressure recording to the United States in 1903. These simple techniques served the surgeon fairly well until the advent of cardiopulmonary bypass and open-heart surgery. At that point, it was recognized that optimum clinical care in the period following what could be considered at best a controlled physiologic insult required a better assessment of the cardiovascular and respiratory status of the patient. Decisions regarding therapy had to be made rapidly on the basis of reasonably accurate measurements of physiologic variables.

This led in the early 1960s to the clinical use of central venous pressure and cardiac output determinations. The invention of the densitometer for the continuous recording of indicator dilution and of electrodes for the rapid determination of the partial pressures of oxygen and carbon dioxide in whole blood provided the technical impetus for the modern era of clinical monitoring.

Subsequently, many specialized diagnostic and treatment centers established within the hospital have included physiologic monitoring as an adjunct to patient care. Coronary care units, respiratory care centers, burn centers, neurosurgical intensive care units, pediatric and neonatal intensive care units, renal dialysis centers, and surgical intensive care units all utilize some forms of patient monitoring. Only in the coronary care unit, however, can it be statistically documented that lives are saved by monitoring. In this case, the electrocardiograph is an almost ideal monitor because it is safe, noninvasive, and specific for the physiologic aberration of cardiac arrhythmias that kills most myocardial infarction victims.

This chapter summarizes the usefulness and indications of various monitoring modes, from routine screening techniques to advanced cardiorespiratory monitoring of high-risk surgical patients preoperatively, intraoperatively, and postoperatively.

A review of the fundamental and basic monitoring techniques utilized in most intensive care units as well as an elaboration of physiologic principles regarding oxygen delivery to the tissues will be provided. Subsequently, invasive and noninvasive techniques will be discussed. Special emphasis will be placed on the use of invasive hemodynamic monitoring techniques to preoperatively evaluate high-risk surgical patients.

BASIC MONITORING

The ultimate improvement in patient outcome or decision-making ability results from increased information. The broad spectrum from noninvasive to highly invasive monitoring is shown in Table 13-1. Measurements that are appropriate for the surgical patient with multiple organ abnormalities and that directly or indirectly provide information about organ function in most ICU settings are listed in Table 13-2. Not all of these measurements are necessary in every surgical patient being monitored. Selection of tests should be made based on the likelihood that the information generated will be valuable for clinical decision making. Selected variables, their units, formulas, and normal values are presented in Table 13-3.

Table 13-1. MONITORING PROCEDURES

Noninvasive procedures
  Physical examination
  Electrical sensing with surface electrodes, e.g., ECG and EEG
  Impedance phlebography
  Arterial tonometry
  Gas sampling using skin surface probes
  Radiologic examination
  Bedside mass spectrometry
  Expired gas analysis
Invasive procedures
  Intravenous injection and blood sampling from capillaries and peripheral veins
  Cutaneous needle electrodes for ECG and EEG
  Rectal probe for temperature
  Bladder catheter for renal function
  Tissue oxygen probe
  Intraarterial and venous gas tension and pH analysis
Highly invasive procedures
  Arterial and central venous catheter
  Intracardiac probes
  Transcardiac probes for pulmonary artery catheter for pressures and flows
  Subarachnoid probes for pressure
  Intracranial probes for CSF pressures and flows

Table 13-2. PHYSIOLOGIC VARIABLES (IN ORDER OF INCREASED SPECIFICITY)

1. Arterial blood pressure
2. Heart rate, respiratory rate
3. Temperature
4. Hematocrit and hemoglobin concentration
5. Urine output rate
6. Central venous pressure (CVP)
7. Electrocardiogram (ECG), chest x-ray
8. Serum electrolytes: Na^+, K^+, Cl^-, HCO_3^-, BUN, creatinine
9. Arterial blood gases—pH
10. Tidal volume (V_T), respiratory rate (f), minute volume (MV)
11. FeNa, RFI, creatinine clearance
12. Plasma and urine osmolalities, osmolar and free water clearances
13. Electroencephalogram (EEG)
14. Intracranial pressure (ICP)
15. Pulmonary arterial and capillary wedge pressures (PAP and PCWP)
16. Cardiac output and hemodynamic variables
17. O_2 transport variables: O_2 delivery, O_2 consumption (V_{O_2}), and O_2 extraction rate
18. End-tidal CO_2 (PET_{CO_2}), V_{CO_2}, V_D/V_T, $P(A-a)D_{O_2}$
19. Mass spectrometry
20. Transcutaneous O_2 and CO_2

VITAL SIGNS. Arterial pressures, heart rate, temperature, and respiratory rate, the so-called vital signs, are the simplest, most easily measured, and most commonly monitored variables. They are a useful screening technique and, as such, are a part of the admission note, physical exam, and daily nursing routine. Vital signs are recorded more frequently during critical periods to provide a running graphic record for frequent evaluations of the patient's condition. Arterial pressures and the other vital signs are monitored in routine hospital and ICU admissions; in preoperative, intraoperative, and postoperative patients, in patients with suspected acute circulatory problems, and patients with myocardial infarction, sepsis, or blood loss; in cases of major trauma, head injury, or blunt injury to chest or abdomen; in shock syndromes; and in other life-threatening conditions or emergencies.

Frequent observation of a patient's mental status can provide important clues to the presence of hypoxemia, hypercapnia, and acidosis. Restlessness and confusion can be early warning signs of sepsis and low output status. Careful attention to the skin can yield valuable clues to the presence of anemia (pallor), severe hypoxemia (cyanosis), and decreased perfusion (decreased temperature or diaphoresis or both). These plus the fundamentals of physical examination can yield a tremendous amount of information rather inexpensively and without risk in an era of sophisticated ICU care.

ARTERIAL PRESSURE. Arterial pressure, the most frequently monitored circulatory variable, reflects the overall circulatory status but lacks diagnostic specificity. Pressures fall after hypovolemia from blood or fluid loss, during cardiac failure, and in the terminal stage of most

Table 13-3. SELECTED VARIABLES: THEIR UNITS, FORMULAS, AND NORMAL VALUES

Abbreviation	Variable name	Formula	Normal values	Unity
MAP	Mean arterial pressure	MAP = diastolic + 1/3 pulse pressure	89–95	mmHg
CVP	Central venous pressure	Direct measurement	0–10	cmH_2O
Hb	Hemoglobin concentration	Direct measurement	12–15	g/dL
MPAP	Mean pulmonary arterial pressure	Direct measurement	10–18	mmHg
PCWP	Pulmonary capillary wedge pressure	Direct measurement	2–12	mmHg
CI	Cardiac index	Cardiac output/ body surface area	2.5–3.5	L/min/m²
LVSW	Left ventrical stroke work	$LVSW = \dfrac{SI \times MAP \times 13.6}{HR}$	44–68	$g \cdot m/m^2$
TPR	Total peripheral resistance	TPR = 80 (MAP − CVP)/CI	1200–1800	$dynes \cdot s/cm^5 \cdot m^2$
PVR	Pulmonary vascular resistance	PVR = 80 (MPAP − WP)/CI	150–250	$dynes \cdot s/cm^5 \cdot m^2$
HR	Heart rate	Direct measurement	65–80	beats/min
Temp	Temperature	Direct measurement	98–98.6; 37	°F; °C
O_2	O_2 availability	O_2 avail = $CI \times Ca_{O_2} \times 10$	500–700	mL/min/m²
V_{O_2}	O_2 consumption	$V_{O_2} = CI \times (Ca_{O_2} - Cv_{O_2}) \times 10$	180–200	mL/min/m²
O_2 ext	O_2 extraction	$O_2\ ext = \dfrac{Ca_{O_2} - Cv_{O_2}}{Ca_{O_2}}$	20–30	
V_D/V_T	Dead space/tidal	$V_D/V_T = \dfrac{PA_{CO_2} - PE_{CO_2}}{PA_{CO_2}}$ or $\dfrac{Pa_{CO_2} - PE_{CO_2}}{Pa_{CO_2}}$	1.30	
P_{osm}	Plasma osmolality	Direct measurement	279–295	mO/kg
PA_{O_2}	Alveolar oxygen tension	$PA_{O_2} = (P_B - 47)\, F_{iO_2} - \dfrac{PA_{CO_2}}{R}$	5–20	mmHg
Q_s/Q_t	Physiologic shunt	$Q_s/Q_t = \dfrac{C_{CO_2} - Ca_{O_2}}{C_{CO_2} - Cv_{O_2}}$	3–5	Percent

diseases. Decreased blood pressure indicates circulatory decompensation or failure of a specific therapy; increased pressure may indicate improved circulatory function or sympathetic neurohormonal response, unless the elevation of pressure is produced by vasopressor therapy.

Arterial pressures do not directly measure reductions of blood flow and volume, but rather the failure of circulatory compensations. Since blood pressure, flow, and volume interactions are extremely complex, only the grossest aspects of the circulatory status are reflected by serial blood-pressure measurements. In short, arterial-pressure measurements are very useful for screening and for rapid assessment of trends in emergency conditions, especially trauma and gastrointestinal bleeding, but in and of themselves are of dubious physiologic import.

Normal arterial blood pressure taken by sphygmomanometer cuff is approximately 120/80 mmHg for healthy young adults; this increases gradually with age. As a rough estimate, the upper limit of normal for systolic pressures over 160 and diastolic pressures over 90 mmHg are considered hypertensive. Young adults, especially teenage females, may normally have pressures as low as 90/60 mmHg. It is important to know the patient's base-

line preillness pressure to properly treat those individuals whose normal pressures are not within the standard range.

The pulse pressure, which is the difference between systolic and diastolic pressures, often is more informative than the latter two pressures. Decreased pulse pressure often precedes a decrease in diastolic pressure in patients developing hypovolemic shock and is one of the first clinical signs of blood volume loss; increased pulse pressure is an early sign of volume restoration.

Mean arterial pressure (MAP) is the diastolic pressure plus one-third of the pulse pressure; alternatively, it may be expressed as one-third the sum of the systolic pressure plus twice the diastolic pressure. MAP is also measured directly in various recording systems as a dampened electrical mean of the systolic and diastolic pressures.

Intraarterial pressure, obtained by a system of intraarterial catheters, pressure transducers, and a continuous recording system that has been zeroed and calibrated, is more accurate than cuff pressure. In normal conditions, pressures obtained from intraarterial catheters are about 2 to 8 mmHg higher than cuff pressures. In critically ill patients, intraarterial pressures may be 10 to 30 mmHg higher than cuff pressure. Furthermore, cuff pressures are often inaccurate when there is severe vasoconstriction with low stroke volume. Arterial pressures of 50 to 60 mmHg have been noted by intraarterial catheter and transducers when the cuff pressures were unobtainable.

Therefore, the indications for this type of continuous pressure recording are shock, critical illness, intraoperative and postoperative monitoring in extensive operations, marked peripheral vasoconstriction, and high-risk conditions. In these cases, accurate, continuous arterial-pressure display is needed for trend analysis and for assessment of therapy. Moreover, the presence of an arterial catheter allows frequent arterial blood-gas measurements.

Because specific unilateral arteriosclerotic or traumatic vascular lesions may produce 10 to 20 mmHg differences between the left and right sides, early in the patient's hospital course pressures should be taken in both arms. Similarly, in trauma to the aorta or femoral artery, there may be differences in the cuff pressures of each leg or each arm; usually the femoral arterial pressures are 5 to 10 mmHg higher than brachial pressures.

Arterial pressures decrease during shock and trauma states; however, these decreases are nonspecific and only poorly and belatedly reflect deficits in blood volume or cardiac function; this is because compensatory neurovascular reactions sustain pressures in the face of falling blood flow. Usually, arterial pressure decreases after the compensations are exhausted, which may be long after the precipitating event. Severely reduced cardiac output has been documented for periods of 40 min to 2 h before a significant reduction in arterial pressures was observed.

Intraarterial catheters may be placed in the femoral, radial, brachial, or axillary arteries. The femoral artery was frequently used in the past, but it makes nursing care difficult and limits and patient's ability to move about, sit up, or ambulate. Further, its placement near the groin risks infection. The radial artery is probably the most commonly used site for continuous arterial pressure monitoring. The brachial artery is most frequently used for cardiac catheterization; however, clotting at the catheter site is likely to jeopardize the limb's circulation during long-term monitoring.

Complications of arterial puncture or arterial catheterization are infrequent but may include hematoma and bleeding at the catheter site; puncture and penetration of the posterior arterial wall; dissection of the intima of the posterior wall by the needle or Seldinger wire; arteriovenous fistula and pseudoaneurysm; arterial spasm; arterial thrombosis; arterial occlusion, ischemia, or gangrene; arteritis; foreign body from sheared-off end of catheter; and cardiac arrest.

The rate of catheter-associated sepsis (demonstrated by positive cultures of blood and the catheter tip that yield the same organism, with no other of infection) is about 4 percent. Sepsis is more likely with surgical cutdowns if the catheter is left in place for more than 4 days or if evidence of local inflamation is present. The pressure transducer or flushing solution can also become infected if left in place more than 48 h.

To minimize the risks with arterial lines, one must perform Allen's test to ensure the patency of the ulnar circulation. Other procedures that will minimize the risk of thrombosis and infection include percutaneous insertion rather than surgical cut-down, changing the entire infusion apparatus every 48 h, using a No. 20 rather than a No. 18 catheter, and removing the catheter within 4 days if at all possible. Continual observation for skin mottling or decrease in temperature of the patient's hand mandates immediate catheter removal.

HEART RATE. The indications for measuring heart rate (pulse) are the same as those for arterial pressure. Arterial pressures and heart rate are routinely taken together and graphically recorded daily or twice daily on the vital signs sheet of the patient's chart.

Heart rate is usually counted by manual palpation of the radial artery just above the wrist, for at least 30 s. When there are premature ventricular contractions (PVCs), skipped beats, or other irregularities, the heart rate is counted by auscultation of the apex; the difference between apical and radial rates is the number of dropped beats. Heart rates may also be measured automatically from either the ECG wave or the arterial-pulse wave.

Heart rate is a very nonspecific cardiorespiratory variable. Its increase suggests blood flow and blood volume deficits; the faster the heart rate, the greater the hypovolemia or cardiac impairment. However, heart rate also increases with infection, anxiety, stress, nonspecific fever, exercise, pain, and discomfort. Tachycardia is a heart rate over 100 beats/min. With irregularities of heart rate, apical as well as radial rates should be compared.

A slow heart rate, or bradycardia, may occur with inferior myocardial infarction when occlusion of the right coronary artery produces ischemia and block of the sinatrial node, and with certain types of arteriosclerotic heart disease. Bradycardia during low cardiac output is an ominous sign suggesting inadequate coronary blood flow. Dysrhythmias associated with cardiac problems require ECG and other methods of specific diagnosis.

TEMPERATURE. Body temperature is taken routinely with the blood pressure, pulse, and respirations. Usually, it is taken rectally in ill patients or orally when significant elevations are not expected. On occasion, thermocouples may be used to take temperatures orally and at the skin of the big toe to obtain the toe-oral temperature gradient, and at the tympanic membrane or midesophagus to assess more accurately the central body core temperature. Pulmonary arterial temperatures, which also reflect core temperature, are routinely available with the pulmonary-artery thermodilution catheter. With a respiratory rate of 40/min, the oral temperature may underestimate the rectal temperature by 3°C.

Temperature elevations are most often associated with infection, tissue necrosis, late-stage carcinomatosis, Hodgkin's disease, leukemias, hyperthyroidism, and other hypermetabolic states. Low-grade fever is also present after accidental or surgical trauma, particularly with hematomas, foreign bodies, fistulae, urinary extravasation, or stasis of urinary or bronchial secretions. Hypothermia may occur in a small percentage of patients with septic shock, reduced metabolism associated with hypothyroidism, malnutrition, and cold exposure. Like arterial pressure and heart rate, temperature is a very useful but nonspecific screening test of little direct physiologic meaning.

RESPIRATORY RATE. One of the earliest responses to a decrease in Pa_{O_2} or a rise in Pa_{CO_2} is an increase in respiratory rate. The normal range is 10 to 16/min, and a rate over 20/min should be viewed as abnormal, particularly if an upward trend continues. Rates over 30/min indicate severe respiratory distress and may produce severe hypocarbia. A sudden increase in respiratory rate may be the first detectable sign of sepsis or a pulmonary embolization.

Observation of the patient's respiratory pattern can yield valuable information. Rapid, shallow respirations are common with interstitial edema, whereas large tidal volumes are typical of pulmonary vascular disease, metabolic acidosis, and sepsis. Rates of less than 12 suggest central-nervous-system depression. Irregular respiratory patterns (Cheyne-Stokes and Biot's respirations) may indicate central-nervous-system or cardiovascular disease.

BODY WEIGHT. An accurate record of daily weight is often the most important indicator of fluid balance. Patients receiving only intravenous fluids usually lose 0.3 to 0.5 kg (0.6 to 1 lb) per day. Weight loss greater than this amount is excessive. Unless a patient is receiving substantial intravenous or enteral alimentation, stable weight or a weight gain indicates retention of water.

HEMATOCRIT. The hematocrit, which is a measure of the percentage of red cells in a sample of venous blood, has been widely used to assess blood loss after trauma and surgery. In general, hematocrit values are decreased by hemorrhage and increased by dehydration.

The hematocrit is measured in routine admissions; emergency conditions, including trauma and hemorrhage or suspected hemorrhage; dehydration, fever, or other suggested water loss; suspected overtransfusion; suspected overhydration; hemolysis or destruction of red cells from fresh-water drowning, envenomation, or consumption coagulopathies, including disseminated intravascular coagulopathies, postoperative states, especially when intraperitoneal bleeding is suspected; and acute illnesses, circulatory shock, and sepsis.

A decreased percentage of red blood cells is an indirect effect of blood loss produced by compensatory transcapillary refilling of the plasma volume from the extracellular water. It takes time for this compensation to occur. If a patient rapidly exsanguinates in a few minutes, the first and last drops of blood will have nearly the same hematocrit. However, a 500-mL blood loss in human volunteers will be replaced by interstitial water over an 18-h period. Replacement occurs at about 1 mL/min for the first few hours and then at successively decreasing rates. For these reasons, serial hematocrits at 4-h intervals are useful in the early period of traumatic shock when covert blood loss is suspected.

Decreases in serial hematocrits of postoperative and posttraumatic patients can signal intraabdominal hemorrhage, but this test is nonspecific and has severe limitations. Since the hematocrit represents a static measurement of red cell concentration in a sample of venous blood, it is affected by a gain or loss of plasma water as well as a gain or loss of red cells. However, it cannot distinguish among the effects of fluids administered intravenously, fluids leaking from the plasma to the interstitial space, red cells being transfused, and other red cells forming aggregates and microthrombi and dropping out of the circulation. Therefore, after the patient has been given large volumes of crystalloids and colloids, as well as multiple transfusions, changes in hematocrit may be misleading and are extremely difficult to interpret. Although the hematocrit may be a reasonably good screening test for gross changes in early stages of hemorrhage, it is not generally a reliable estimation of the blood volume status.

URINE OUTPUT RATE. The rate of urine output is easily measured at minimal expense. The patient is catheterized, preferably with a Foley catheter, and the urine is collected in a closed sterile system; output is usually recorded hourly. The catheter must be irrigated with aseptic precautions at regular intervals, since the most common cause of low urine output, or anuria, in the hospitalized patient is an occluded catheter. (Normal output = $\frac{1}{2}$ mL/kg/min.)

The hourly rate of urine output obtained using an indwelling urethral catheter is a reasonable measure of the perfusion of one vital organ, provided the patient has an adequate blood volume and no preexisting renal disease. In resuscitation from acute injury, decreased urine flow may reflect low blood volume, poor perfusion of the kidney, or the onset of acute renal failure. Other measures of renal function, such as osmolar and free water clearance, are presented below.

Urine output provides a good estimate of the adequacy of renal perfusion, and urine specific gravity reflects renal concentrating ability. Serum creatinine and blood urea nitrogen (BUN) levels are traditionally used to monitor renal function; however, other less frequently used tests may also be useful, since the BUN and creatinine values are not abnormal until 70 percent of renal function is lost. An early sign of relative hypovolemia may be a falling urine sodium concentration and/or a rising urine osmolality. Urine sodium less than 10 to 20 meq/L or urine osmolality greater than 450 mO/L suggests hypovolemia. A urine sodium greater than 40 meq/L suggests acute tubular necrosis and a urine osmolality less than 300 mO/L suggests antetubular necrosis (ATN).

Renal function also can be monitored by measurement of plasma (P_{osm}) and urine (U_{osm}) osmolality as well as calculation of osmolar and free water clearance. The U_{osm}/P_{osm} ratio is calculated, and if it is greater than 1.7, good concentrating ability is present. The osmolar clearance (C_{osm}) is calculated according to the following equation:

$$C_{osm} = \frac{U_{osm}}{P_{osm}} \times \text{Urine output (1 h)} \qquad N\text{: } 100\text{--}125 \text{ mL/h}$$

The osmolar clearance reflects the rate of removal of solutes from plasma. Normal osmolar clearance is 120 mL/h and is decreased in renal failure. Free water clearance is calculated by subtracting the C_{osm} from the 1-h urine output. The free water clearance (C_{H_2O}) usually is negative (-125 to -100 mL/h), and the values close to zero or above precede acute renal failure.

The creatinine clearance (C_{cr}) reflects the glomerular function, since this substance is neither excreted nor absorbed by the tubules. Clearance results are normalized and expressed as milliliter per minute per 1.73 m^2.

$$C_{cr}: \frac{U_{cr} \times U \text{ vol (1 h)} \times 1.73}{P_{cr} \times 60 \times \text{body surface area}}$$
$$N: 100\text{--}125 \text{ mL/min/1.73 m}^2$$

$$C_{Na}: \frac{U_{Na} \times U \text{ vol (1 h)} \times 1.73}{P_{Na} \times 60 \times \text{body surface area}}$$
$$N: 3\text{--}4 \text{ mL/min/1.73 m}^2$$

Excretion data include the fractional excretion of sodium (F_eNa) and renal failure index (RF_i), which allow differentiation between reversible prerenal azotemia and antetubular necrosis.

$$F_eNa(\%): \frac{U_{Na} \times P_{cr} \times 100}{P_{Na} \times U_{cr}} \quad \begin{array}{l} < 1 = \text{prerenal} \\ >1 \text{ or } >3 = \text{ATN} \end{array}$$

$$RF_i(\%): \frac{U_{Na} \times P_{cr}}{U_{cr}} \quad \begin{array}{l} < 1 = \text{prerenal} \\ >3 = \text{ATN} \end{array}$$

Urinary indices have long been utilized for diagnosis of prerenal failure, or ATN. In prerenal azotemia, tubular function remains intact, and reabsorption of sodium and water is characteristic of this period. Hence urinary sodium <20 meq/L, $U_{osm} > 450$ mO, U/P creatinine >40. In acute tubular necrosis the concentration ability is impaired owing to tubular damage, resulting in $U_{Na} >40$ meq/L, $U_{osm} < 300$ mO, U/P creatinine < 20. F_eNa and RF_i are found to be below 1 percent in prerenal azotemia and above 3 percent in ATN.

Normal osmolality of body fluids is 275 to 295 mO/L H_2O. Plasma osmolality is calculated by the following formula:

$$P_{osm} \text{ (mO/L)} = 2 \times \text{sodium (meq/L)}$$
$$+ \frac{\text{glucose (mg/dL)}}{18} + \frac{\text{BUN (mg/dL)}}{2.8}$$

An osmolality above 320 mO/L generally is tolerated poorly, and levels greater than 350 mO/L may be fatal. The calculated serum osmolality is normally 5 to 8 mO less than the measured osmolality. This difference is called the osmolar discriminant and is due to the presence of anions, e.g., lactate or phosphate. An increased osmolar discriminant is usually associated with increased lactate production and a poorer prognosis.

The advantages of utilizing a renal profile, especially if computerized, is that the clinician is provided with all the parameters that need to be evaluated to differentiate acute tubular necrosis from an oliguric prerenal state. By utilizing a multiple-parameter approach, an earlier diagnosis of acute tubular necrosis can be made. The comput-

erized method provides the clinician with all the parameters that usually require tedious calculations rapidly and expeditiously. Vo et al. have previously described the automated renal profile.

ARTERIAL BLOOD-GAS ANALYSIS AND PULMONARY MONITORING

Arterial blood-gas tensions are determined by the composition of alveolar gas and the efficiency of gas transfer between the alveoli and pulmonary capillary blood. Alveolar gas tension depends on the mixture of inspired gas, ventilation and blood flow (V/Q), and the composition of mixed venous blood gases. Because mixed venous P_{O_2} usually varies with cardiac output, significant arterial hypoxemia can result from shunting of venous blood with a low P_{O_2} through the pulmonary circulation. Failure to recognize this nonpulmonary cause of arterial hypoxemia may cause a clinician to falsely ascribe a falling Pa_{O_2} to deteriorating pulmonary function.

Pulmonary abnormalities that may result in hypoxemia, alone or in combination, include diffusion block, ventilation-perfusion inequality, intrapulmonary shunting, and hypoventilation. Diffusion abnormalities lead to hypoxemia if pulmonary end-capillary blood fails to equilibrate fully with alveolar gas. Such conditions are probably a very uncommon cause of hypoxemia except in patients with chronic lung disease during exercise or exposure to a decreased F_{iO_2} at high altitude.

Although bulk oxygen is carried in combination with hemoglobin, delivery to tissue depends on its partial pressure in the blood, which also reflects the amount of oxygen available to be delivered from hemoglobin. A fall in Pa_{O_2} without a change in Pa_{CO_2} suggests that blood oxygenation is deteriorating despite constant alveolar ventilation. In the acutely ill patient, this finding usually is due to ventilation-perfusion imbalance or intrapulmonary shunting. An important feature of shunting is that hypoxemia cannot be abolished by the administration of 100 percent oxygen because the chemoreceptors sense any elevation in Pa_{CO_2} and reflexly induce an increase of ventilation.

When patients hypoventilate while breathing ambient air, hypoxemia results from an increase in alveolar P_{CO_2}. Calculation of the alveolar oxygen tension and determination of the alveolar-arterial ($A-a$) oxygen tension difference $P(A-a)D_{O_2}$ allows separation of hypoventilation from other causes of hypoxemia. With hypoventilation, the $A-a$ oxygen gradient is normal; with other causes of hypoxemia, it is increased. The alveolar oxygen tension can be estimated from the following abbreviated formula, which is adequate for clinical purposes:

$$PA_{O_2} = P_{iO_2} - \frac{Pa_{CO_2}}{R}$$

P_{iO_2} is equal to the barometric pressure (P_B) minus the water vapor pressure (47 mmHg at 37°C) multiplied by the F_{iO_2}. The respiratory quotient (R) is approximately 0.8 in the steady-state resting condition. It is assumed to be

0.8 in respiratory failure, although this assumption is not always valid.

The correction for R varies depending on the inspired oxygen concentration (F_{iO_2}), as can be seen from the nonsimplified alveolar air equation:

$$PA_{O_2} = F_{iO_2} (P_B - 47) - PA_{CO_2} \left(F_{iO_2} + \frac{1 - F_{iO_2}}{R} \right)$$

Although this equation appears formidable, if Pa_{CO_2} is used rather than PA_{CO_2}, and 100 percent oxygen is inhaled, solution of the equation is simply the difference between inspired P_{O_2}. For clinical purposes, it is important to appreciate the small but definite error if PA_{O_2} is calculated using the abbreviated formula at different inspired oxygen concentrations.

The $P(A-a)D_{O_2}$ in normal human beings breathing room air varies between 10 and 15 mmHg. Half of this venoarterial admixture is caused by true shunting of desaturated blood into the left atrium, and the other half by ventilation-perfusion imbalance. When the patient with normal cardiorespiratory function breathes pure oxygen for 15 or 20 min, the alveolar-arterial gradient is between 25 and 65 mmHg. Barometric pressure, less carbon dioxide tension, less water vapor pressure, less the normal gradient yields a value of around 630 mmHg for arterial oxygen tension while breathing pure oxygen. In this condition the gradient represents both anatomic shunting and perfusion of total nonventilated alveoli. Patients are ready to begin to be reversed from the ventilator when their gradient of alveolar to arterial oxygen is less than 350 mmHg while they are receiving 100 percent oxygen (indicating that they could be maintained on 50 percent oxygen).

The arterial oxygen tension divided by the alveolar oxygen tension is called the a/A ratio. This ratio is relatively stable with a varying F_{iO_2}, unlike the classic alveolar-arterial gradient. Thus it is a useful index of changes in lung function when a patient's inspired oxygen concentration is changed. The normal a/A ratio is 0.75. The ratio can also be used to predict the new Pa_{O_2} that results from a change in inspired oxygen concentration.

Another nonpulmonary factor that can significantly affect gas exchange is the level of CO_2 production (V_{CO_2}). The amount of CO_2 produced by the body is a function of the metabolic rate and the substrate(s) used as fuel. CO_2 production varies from 70 to 100 percent of the O_2 consumption as the fuel is switched from fat to carbohydrate. When caloric input exceeds metabolic needs, excess calories are converted to fat, which further increases CO_2 production.

Measurements of CO_2 production by indirect calorimetry may be helpful in patients receiving hyperalimentation. Although nutritional support is vital in the critically ill patient, it may sometimes raise CO_2 production above base-line levels. Thus, patients may require higher levels of ventilation to eliminate CO_2. If the ventilation cannot be increased, arterial partial pressure of CO_2 will rise. Decreasing CO_2 production in the patient who is difficult to wean may make weaning easier by reducing the requirements for ventilation. Although one obviously does not want to eliminate essential nutrients, the administration of fat instead of some of the glucose will help to lower the CO_2 production.

Agarwal et al. have developed a computerized automated metabolic profile that provides the physician with a comprehensive review and graphic display of a patient's nutritional status, energy expenditure, substrate utilization, and nutritional requirements. Utilizing indirect calorimetry, the nutritional management of patients requiring ventilatory support can be optimized according to their needs with facility. Savino et al. have demonstrated with indirect calorimetric techniques that the work of breathing can be quantitated more accurately.

Monitoring P_{50} (P_{O_2} at 50 percent oxyhemoglobin saturation) may also be helpful in assessing oxygen delivery. A right-shifted curve (e.g., higher P_{50}) assists in delivery of oxygen to tissues. The significance of shifts of the oxyhemoglobin curve on overall tissue oxygenation remains a topic of active investigation. Rightward shifts are commonly seen in conditions associated with decreased oxygen delivery, e.g., anemia and chronic hypoxemia. Beneficial effects of decreased oxygen affinity are difficult to demonstrate experimentally. Increased mortality and decreased oxygen consumption and cardiac output have been associated with a low P_{50} in experimental studies. These findings are of clinical significance to patients receiving large transfusions of stored blood or others who develop respiratory alkalemia or metabolic alkalosis, resultant leftward shift of the oxyhemoglobin dissociation curve and decreased P_{50}. As these patients are more likely to have limited cardiac reserve because of acute illness, they are least able to compensate by an increase in cardiac output or a shift in blood flow to tissues utilizing high extraction ratios to meet required oxygen demands. Organs such as the heart and brain are particularly vulnerable.

Marked changes in Pa_{O_2} in critically ill patients that may be missed by intermittent sampling occur during the administration of drugs, suctioning, and changes in body position. The frequency with which arterial blood gases should be measured depends on the clinical situation. In patients with severe chronic obstructive pulmonary disease and impending respiratory failure, arterial blood gases may need to be measured every 30 to 60 min. Continuous monitoring of Pa_{O_2} by electrodes in the femoral, radial, and brachial arteries as well as the P_{O_2} in mixed venous blood in the pulmonary artery has been reported. Obviously these techniques have the same problems as other invasive techniques, and further experience is needed before it can be concluded that such monitoring is indicated in the management of critically ill patients.

Because of the intermittent nature of blood-gas measurement and the lag in reporting results, considerable effort has been directed to developing noninvasive continuous monitoring of blood- and tissue-gas values. On occasion, ear oximetry allows continuous monitoring of oxygen saturation, the values obtained reflecting changes in arterial oxygen saturation. Artificially low readings are recorded in patients with jaundice and when oxygen saturation is lower than 65 percent. Artificially high values are obtained when levels of carboxyhemoglobin are higher than 3 percent. When they are accurately calibrated, ear oximeters can markedly decrease the number of needed blood-gas measurements and reflect changes in the patient's hemodynamic status. Unfortunately, ear oximetry is less valuable in unstable patients with rapidly changing hemodynamic parameters. Transcutaneous oxygen measurements are less accurate because the values vary with skin thickness, blood volume, and flow. With a normal cardiac output, transcutaneous oxygen tracks partial pressure of arterial oxygen, whereas with diminished cardiac output, it tracks oxygen delivery.

The measurement of the peak expired CO_2 is directly related to the Pa_{CO_2}, which in turn is primarily related to the CO_2 production, alveolar ventilation, and pulmonary capillary blood flow. End-tidal CO_2 analysis allows the clinician to change Pa_{CO_2} during mechanical ventilation. Currently two methods of CO_2 analysis are commonly used, infrared spectroscopy and mass spectrometry. With infrared spectroscopy absorption of infrared energy by a given gas such as CO_2 produces an infrared spectrum consisting of a number of energy bands, whereby the identity and concentration of CO_2 are discerned by the end-tidal gas monitor. Mass spectrometers, unlike infrared monitors, typically monitor multiple different expired gas tensions simultaneously, including CO_2.

End-tidal CO_2 monitoring is extremely useful as a diagnostic tool in several situations unique to anesthesia. The most important role of end-tidal CO_2 monitoring is in the verification of intratracheal placement of breathing tubes, particularly in infants, obese patients, and patients with craniofacial or anatomical airway abnormalities. Once the tube has been inserted, if CO_2 is present in expired gases in the appropriate concentration of 4 to 6 volumes percent (28 to 42 mmHg), then intratracheal-tube placement and pulmonary ventilation are assured.

Blockage of the pulmonary circulation by air emboli results in an increase in dead space, thus reducing alveolar and end-tidal CO_2 concentration. This form of monitoring is recommended in neurosurgical cases requiring the sitting position.

End-tidal CO_2 monitoring can be an extremely valuable diagnostic tool for detecting malignant hyperthermia. In a number of documented cases the initial presenting sign of this pharmacogenic disease was an unexplained increase in the end-tidal CO_2 concentration in the face of unchanged ventilation.

Decreases in cardiac output are associated with corresponding decreases in the end-tidal CO_2. Thus capnography can serve as an additional monitor of cardiovascular function and signal the need for an appropriate therapeutic intervention. Certainly this form of monitoring is invaluable in detecting anesthesia-machine malfunction during surgery but it can also be utilized in the ICU environment as a ventilator disconnect alarm as well as a system to determine ventilator malfunction.

Unfortunately, with obstructive airway disease and resultant abnormalities in the distribution of ventilation, and with rapid shallow respirations, it is difficult to deter-

mine the end-tidal partial pressure of carbon dioxide accurately. As technology improves, this method may become a valuable noninvasive method of monitoring ventilation.

Two of the most practical instruments for measuring ventilatory parameters are the Wright and Drager respirometers. Low tidal volumes associated with tachypnea increase dead-space ventilation. The product of rate and tidal volume is minute volume, a useful measure of total ventilation. High minute ventilation suggests severe hypocarbia or decreased dead space and respiratory work that may lead to exhaustion. A tidal volume greater than 5 mL/kg and a vital capacity greater than 10 mL/kg may be useful guidelines for predicting successful weaning from mechanical ventilation. Vital-capacity levels below 15 mL/kg are often associated with an inadequate cough, and below 10 mL/kg hypercarbia develops. Measurement of minute volume and maximum inspiratory pressure is also employed. Sahn and Lakshminarayan showed that a resting minute volume of less than 10 L and the ability to double the resting minute volume on command predicts success in weaning patients on ventilators. Inspiratory force is normally less than −80 cm of water. Values below −20 cm of water are usually adequate to maintain normal minute ventilation.

In the spontaneously breathing patient it is important to monitor trends in blood gases and mechanics in order to predict and treat acute respiratory decompensation. In general there are four reasons to intubate a patient:

1. For oxygenation when a patient is unable to maintain a Pa_{O_2} of 70 mmHg with 100 percent O_2 administered through a face mask, nasal prongs, with a reservoir bag;
2. For ventilation when respiratory acidosis develops;
3. For protection of the airway from aspiration;
4. For management of excessive secretions. Patient selection is extremely important, but frequently in order to diminish stress one may opt for sedation and early controlled ventilation.

The ventilator in a patient who is intubated is a readily available source of monitoring of the patient's ventilatory mechanics and oxygenation. Physiologic dead space is the portion of the tidal volume that does not participate in gas exchange. In the healthy adult the physiologic dead space is approximately 150 mL at rest (about 20 to 30 percent of each tidal volume). This value represents the anatomic dead space from the mouth, pharynx, larynx, trachea, bronchi, broncholes, as well as a contribution from the alveoli that are overventilated with respect to perfusion. Positive pressure alone can increase dead space.

With respiratory failure the physiologic dead space is increased because of continued ventilation of the alveoli whose perfusion is either absent or decreased. The ratio of dead space to tidal volume (V_D/V_T) can be calculated by measuring the arterial and mixed expired CO_2 tension ($P\overline{E}_{CO_2}$) by the Bohr equation:

$$\frac{V_D}{V_T} = \frac{PA_{CO_2} - P\overline{E}_{CO_2}}{PA_{CO_2}}$$

The Enghoff modification of the Bohr equation is often used clinically:

$$\frac{V_D}{V_T} = \frac{Pa_{CO_2} - P\bar{E}_{CO_2}}{Pa_{CO_2}}$$

If the end-tidal P_{CO_2} is substituted for the Pa_{CO_2}, anatomic dead space can be calculated, requiring only expired air (eliminating arterial blood sampling). A correction for dead space due to the expansion of the tubing in mechanically ventilated patients should be made. Ratios of dead space to tidal volume reflect the amount of wasted ventilation; rising values are usually associated with respiratory failure and progressive involvement of the pulmonary vascular bed. Values above 0.6 are usually not compatible with adequate spontaneous ventilation.

Volume change per unit of pressure change is compliance, a useful measure of the elastic properties of the body. The compliance of the normal lung is approximately 200 mL/cmH$_2$O. Particularly important in monitoring pulmonary mechanics is peak inspiratory pressure, which should be monitored at least hourly. Increases in the peak inspiratory pressure and correspondingly in the dynamic compliance [tidal volume/(plateau pressure − PEEP)] may indicate the presence of an obstructed or misplaced endotracheal tube, mucous plugging, bronchospasm, and pneumothorax. Measurements of static compliance [tidal volume/(plateau pressure − PEEP)] can be obtained by adding a respiratory pause. Changes in static compliance can reflect atelectasis or an increase in the amount of lung water. Monitoring static compliance is useful in evaluating the course in patients with the adult respiratory distress syndrome and during PEEP trials in order to determine the appropriate levels of PEEP. Compliance measurements are a good indication of the patient's work of breathing.

Normal compliance of the lung and chest wall in the mechanically ventilated patient is about 70 mL/cmH$_2$O. When the static compliance of the lung and chest wall is less than 25 mL/cmH$_2$O, as in severe respiratory failure, difficulties in weaning are common because of the high work of breathing.

If one ventilates the lungs at various tidal volumes and records the peak and plateau pressure for each volume, dynamic and static curves can be quickly graphed; the former correlates with airway resistance and the latter is a measure of lung stiffness.

Two errors in these measurements are possible with unrelaxed respiratory muscles. If the patient is resisting mechanical ventilation, the total pressure developed by the ventilator will be greater than that required to inflate the lungs of the relaxed patient. Also, if the patient is actively inspiring, the pressure developed by the ventilator will be less than the total pressure required.

Elucidation of the mechanical function of the lung requires the continuous recording of pressure and flow during the respiratory cycle. Flow usually is measured by a pneumotachograph, which senses the differential pressure across a resistance in most cases. Inspiratory and expiratory pneumotachographs are a part of some single-patient monitoring systems, as in the Siemens-Elema ventilator. With in-line pneumotachographs, expired volume measurements that include volume expended by compression in the expansion of the ventilator circuit are less of a problem. Incorporation of pneumotachographs into the ventilator system introduces an entirely new set of problems, however, ranging from incorrect information because of mucous plugging of the pneumotachograph to problems of calibration changes caused by varying gas concentration. Because of problems with constant measurements using the Fleish pneumotachograph, other flow-measuring devices have been developed, including the variable-orifice flowmeter, ultrasonic flowmeter, and turbulent flowmeter. These flowmeters are presently undergoing clinical trials, and their accuracy and durability are still to be determined.

The pneumotachograph must be frequently calibrated to avoid error, usually with a 1- to 3-L syringe in line with a standard spirometer. Because pneumotachographs are sensitive to temperature, humidity, and flow, they should be calibrated under clinical conditions for reliable results. Flow rates should be linear over a range of 0 to 3 L/s, and appropriate pneumotachographs should be used in those patients. In automated systems, airway pressure is measured by reliable strain gauges that provide a linear electrical output spanning a range of 0 to 200 cmH$_2$O.

A Fleish pneumotachograph with pressure- and gas-sampling lines leading to a mass spectrometer and computer allows simultaneous measurement of inspired and expired gases and mechanics.

To measure lung compliance rather than lung and chest wall compliance, transpulmonary pressure must be determined. Respiratory pressure fluctuations reflected by an esophageal balloon or from the proximal port of a thermodilution Swan-Ganz catheter or a central venous catheter can be used for this purpose. Esophageal balloons are now available that attach to standard nasogastric tubes. If an esophageal balloon is used, a differential pressure transducer is needed to measure intrapleural pressure relative to mouth pressure. Lung plus chest wall compliance measured from airway pressure of the ventilated patient is affected by muscle contractions. The direct measurement of lung compliance thus adds both specificity and resolution.

Cardiovascular Physiology in Acute Illness

The overall assessment of oxygen transport, or the delivery of oxygen from the atmosphere to the mitochondria of the body cell mass, can be used as a model to evaluate the abilities of particular monitoring systems to detect critical events and trends. This process involves many organ systems and complicated feedback loops for regulation and compensation. It is imperative for the survival of the individual that the oxygen transport system continue in operation without interruption.

Many factors are capable of influencing an individual

patient's metabolic response to acute illness. The period immediately after acute injury is characterized by a systemic O_2 consumption (V_{O_2}) that may be less than normal. This period of initial resuscitation is quickly followed by a time when the metabolic rate, hence V_{O_2}, is increased and when the host's response is now primarily devoted to ensuring appropriate tissue repair. An increase in systemic V_{O_2} is, therefore, a characteristic response to injury and the early stages of sepsis. Wilmore has determined that the elevation in systemic V_{O_2} in such cases is related to a rise in body temperature, increased mechanical work (for example, heart and lungs), and increased synthetic work (for instance, protein). The range of changes noted in systemic V_{O_2} from base line depends upon the primary illness itself, as well as on associated complications. For example, patients with severe burns usually have the greatest increase in V_{O_2}, but, when these patients have the complication of acute respiratory failure, the systemic V_{O_2} will rise to even greater levels because of the additive metabolic load imposed on the patient secondary to an increase in mechanical work of the respiratory musculature.

Actively metabolizing cells require nutrients (for example, glucose) as well as O_2. Ranges in the internal milieu of the gluconeogenetic hormones usually favor maintenance of adequate glucose calories in the early hypermetabolic stages of trauma and sepsis. Hence, the concentration of essential nutrients may not be as potentially rate-limiting in the critically ill patient as is the supply of cellular oxygen. In summary, critically ill patients demonstrate a range of systemic V_{O_2} that depends upon the metabolic stress of the underlying illness. Traumatized patients and those with sepsis demonstrate a need for a greater oxygen delivery (D_{O_2}) than do cardiac patients because of the increased metabolic rate characteristic of the former groups compared with the latter.

To ensure survival, microcirculatory D_{O_2} must, therefore, balance systemic V_{O_2}. Anything less is reflected in the definition of heart failure, which is an inability of the ventricles to deliver adequate quantities of blood (e.g., oxygen) to the metabolizing tissues at rest or during normal activity. Failure to balance the metabolic demands of peripheral tissues will result in a shift from aerobic to the inefficient anaerobic use of O_2. If uncorrected, lactic acidosis will ensue as a result of cellular hypoxia, and a sequence of events will then develop that eventuates in cellular metabolic failure, characterized by an inability of the cell to use available O_2 and finally by death of the organism. Heart failure is functionally not defined in terms of the level of a cardiac output (CO) or of a pulmonary capillary wedge pressure (PCWP), but rather in terms of the heart's ability to support the metabolic needs of the body adequately, regardless of the demands imposed by the systemic V_{O_2}.

In the presence of an increased O_2 demand (V_{O_2}) by the periphery, there are local and systemic adaptive responses that will assist in increasing cellular O_2 availability. Locally, improved cellular O_2 transport may occur as a consequence of:

1. Peripheral vasodilation, with a consequent increase in the surface area of the microcirculatory bed across which oxygen may diffuse to the cell;
2. A rightward shift of the oxyhemoglobin dissociation curve, which will facilitate the peripheral unloading of oxygen from hemoglobin, both of which will result in increased oxygen extraction down the concentration gradient provided between oxygen tension within the cell and the microcirculation.

The natural affinity of hemoglobin for oxygen is decreased by heat, hydrogen ions, carbon dioxide (Bohr effect), and red cell diphosphoglycerate (DPG). These agents act at a stereochemical level to help form a hemoglobin molecule that is more stable in its unsaturated state. The heat of working tissues, hypoxic acidosis, and carbon dioxide from cellular metabolism all tend to shift the oxyhemoglobin dissociation curve to the right where more oxygen is released at a higher tissue oxygen tension. The relative position of the oxyhemoglobin dissociation curve is identified by the P_{50} value, the partial pressure of oxygen at which the hemoglobin is half saturated at 37° and pH 7.4.

When adaptation by the local factors to maintain cellular O_2 supply is exhausted, and compensatory acute changes in the systemic control of O_2 transport are likewise stressed, selective vasoconstriction in some organs will follow in order to divert O_2 to critical areas, such as the heart and brain, but at the expense of reduced O_2 supply to teleologically noncritical organs, such as skin and skeletal muscle. Other factors may also operate at a local level to enhance cellular O_2 availability (for example, changes in the rheologic properties of blood), although their role is not as well defined in the critically ill as the aforementioned.

Systemically, delivery of O_2 to the periphery is a direct function of the cardiac output and the arterial oxygen content (Ca_{O_2}) which represents the oxygen bound to hemoglobin (1.34 mL/g). O_2 delivery (D_{O_2}) = [flow (cardiac output)] × [(Hb)(Sa_{O_2}) + 0.0031(Pa_{O_2})]. The importance of three major organ systems in ensuring O_2 availability within the peripheral microvasculature is emphasized in this equation: the cardiovascular system to subserve tissue perfusion, the respiratory system to oxygenate venous blood, and the hematopoietic system to provide adequate hemoglobin to carry O_2. In patients with a normal hemoglobin and with a Pa_{O_2} greater than 70 mmHg, there is little remaining compensation acutely available to augment D_{O_2} by changes in Ca_{O_2}. Chronically, however, polycythemia and an increase in 2.3-diphosphoglycerate (2.3-DPG) would assist in improving CO (for instance, in chronic airflow limitation). Therefore, in acute disease states characterized by a heightened systemic V_{O_2}, in which an increase in CO is a requirement to ensure metabolic survival of the organism, an increase in the systemic flow, i.e., increased cardiac output, is likely to be the most important and immediate mechanism available to the organism to ensure an appropriate increase in systemic O_2 delivery. As a result, "the appropriate" hemodynamic response to any critical illness typified by a heightened systemic V_{O_2} may be defined as a high cardiac output, nonhypotensive state. Initial studies of patients with systemic sepsis complicated by adult respiratory distress syndrome (ARDS) identified a positive correlation between the ability of the myocardium to sustain a high cardiac output state and ultimate survival; regarding systemic sepsis, Weil and colleagues noted that the mortality rate was greater in patients with underlying cardiac disease than in those without preexisting ischemic heart disease.

The correlation between survival and a high cardiac output, or "hyperdynamic," response may be analyzed further in those disease states characterized by an increased systemic V_{O_2}. The appropriate cardiovascular response is the one that assists in improving D_{O_2} to the cell and hence prevents the development of an anaerobic state. In this regard, the need to match D_{O_2} with systemic V_{O_2} in patients with sepsis or trauma is no different from the systemic response to strenuous exercise. Strenuous exercise is not reflective of the sustained demand on D_{O_2} that diseases may be. In some acute disease states there seems to be a defect in the maximal use of the peripheral mechanisms potentially available to improve cellular D_{O_2}. Specifically, O_2 extraction may not be as sufficient within the periphery in patients with ARDS as in patients with acute cardiac illnesses. Therefore, to maintain the balance between cellular D_{O_2} and systemic V_{O_2}, and hence to prevent the development of anaerobiosis, more dependence is apparently placed on the systemic adaptive mechanisms for increasing cellular O_2 delivery. The correlation between survival and the level of the CO in the critically ill thereby reflects a positive correlation between survival and the ability of the host to increase systemic D_{O_2}, accomplished primarily by an elevation in the CO. In a description of the hemodynamic sequelae of critical illness, emphasis must, therefore, be placed on understanding those factors that may influence the biventricular response to the particular disease, since an appropriate response is the one that ensures that CO, hence D_{O_2}, will vary according to the total metabolic demands imposed on the patient by the underlying illness.

SERUM LACTATE LEVELS. Arterial blood lactate levels have been found to be of great assistance to the clinician in circumstances of impaired tissue perfusion by providing an index of the severity of shock. Serum lactate has also been found to be a prognostic indicator in the early stages of a clinical course, as well as a monitor of the success of various therapeutic maneuvers.

Blood lactate levels are normally 0.7 to 1.8 mmol/L. During impaired perfusion, tissue hypoxia stimulates anaerobic metabolism with subsequent overproduction of lactate from pyruvate, although reduced splanchnic renal flow may impair lactate clearance by the liver and kidneys. Studies of lactate levels have been performed in both hypovolemic and septic shock. In hemorrhagic shock lactate is an indicator of the degree of anaerobic metabolism consequent upon oxygen deficiency. The situation in septic shock is much more complex, with impaired tissue perfusion existing as only one factor together with biochemical alterations at the cellular level

that may influence lactate production, and hepatic effects that may determine lactate clearance.

In septic shock, a hyperdynamic circulation with elevated cardiac output frequently exists. Oxygen consumption in this situation may be normal, elevated, or reduced in the presence of raised serum lactate levels. This suggests that the tissues are unable to extract the optimum amount of oxygen from the blood in the face of increased demands related to fever, tissue inflammation, and increased circulating catecholamines. Anaerobic metabolism thus ensues despite increased oxygen delivery. This failure to utilize oxygen in sepsis has been attributed to an inhibiting effect of endotoxin, lysosomal enzymes, and acidosis on mitochondrial function together with the presence of arteriovenous shunts.

Although anatomical shunts have not been demonstrated, it is known that maldistribution of tissue perfusion may occur, with blood traversing preferred route capillaries rather than nutrient vessels.

Rashkin recently attempted to define the critical level of oxygen delivery in critically ill patients and found that survival was good, together with lactate concentration in or near the normal range of oxygen delivery greater than 8 mL/kg/min. Below this level survival was poor and blood lactate markedly increased. He suggested that an oxygen delivery of greater than 8 mL/kg/min is probably sufficient to sustain organ function. However, measurement of oxygen delivery necessitates invasive procedures and blood lactate is a more convenient indicator of tissue oxygenation and metabolism.

Recent studies have suggested that serial lactate measurements could be used as a useful adjunct to the clinical evaluation of the critically ill patient and that consideration should be given to a change in therapy should a fall in lactate not be demonstrated during the early stage of treatment.

Waxman and colleagues demonstrated that despite attempts to maintain cardiac output during the intraoperative period at or above preoperative levels, the magnitude of this increase appeared to correlate with the degree of intraoperative reduction in oxygen consumption. These data suggested that a metabolic debt usually accumulates intraoperatively from inadequate tissue oxygenation. The hyperdynamic and hypermetabolic postoperative period may then represent a compensatory state necessary to repair intraoperative cellular and organ damage resulting from inadequate cellular oxygenation.

In a subsequent study sequential arterial blood lactate concentrations were determined pre-, intra-, and postoperatively in 12 high-risk surgical patients. These levels were correlated with simultaneous measurements of arterial blood pressure, cardiac index, and oxygen consumption. There was a marked increase in lactate values intraoperatively. This increase did not correspond to decreases in either mean arterial pressure or cardiac index but did appear to correlate with decreased intraoperative oxygen consumption. Postoperatively lactate levels remained elevated, and this elevation appeared to correlate with an estimation of intraoperative oxygen deficit.

Postoperatively cardiac index and oxygen consumption were increased.

While decreased oxygen consumption during operation has been previously recognized, it has usually been attributed to decreased demands caused by anesthetic agents and intraoperative hypothermia. Elevated lactate values, however, suggest that the oxygen consumption may be reduced beyond the reduction in metabolic demands, such that inadequate tissue oxygenation may be occurring. This inadequate tissue oxygenation is occurring despite therapy to maintain systemic blood flow. This implies impaired cellular utilization of oxygen, caused by either microcirculatory flow maldistribution, impairment of oxyhemoglobin dissociation, or a direct impairment of mitochondrial functions. An alternative explanation is that lactate clearance decreased intraoperatively and that this represents the pathophysiology of the increased levels rather than increased lactate production.

The persistently elevated levels of lactate into the postoperative period suggests that the metabolic deficit may persist into that period. Presumably, this supports the concept of the hyperdynamic postoperative state based on increased circulatory and metabolic demands because of a persistent metabolic deficit from the operation. Athletes, similarly, have increased cardiac output and oxygen consumption after exercise. A quantitative relationship between intraoperative oxygen deficit and postoperative lactate concentration was demonstrated. Potentially, lactate levels postoperatively may indicate the degree of the metabolic insult that the patient has suffered intraoperatively. Patients with more intraoperative oxygen deficit and higher postoperative lactate levels may require higher and more prolonged increases in cardiac index and oxygen consumption to recover.

The Waxman data also imply that the commonly monitored intraoperative clinical signs such as arterial pressure, heart rate, ECG, and CVP appear to be inadequate in detecting deficiencies of tissue oxygenation. Monitoring methods and systems that more directly address tissue oxygenation are needed. Lactate determinations may be very useful both in assessing the degree of accumulated oxygen deficit and in titrating therapy to support the necessary physiologic compensations.

Cowan and colleagues supported the idea that serial lactate measurements were better at predicting outcome than single measurements, when they demonstrated a fall in blood lactate during the first 3 h of resuscitation from shock in association with an improvement in the clinical condition. Statistical analysis of results, however, suggested that serial measurements of simple hemodynamic variables such as urine output, core-peripheral temperature gradient, or mean arterial pressure may be more valuable in predicting outcome than serial blood lactate.

CARDIOVASCULAR MONITORING

In considering the physiology of body blood flow, two important points must be made: the cardiac output alone is not an indicator of myocardial contractility, and arterial blood pressure alone is not an indicator of blood flow. Myocardial contractility refers to the state of health of the heart muscle and the rate at which the muscle fibers can shorten circumferentially around the bolus of blood within the ventricles. As will be seen later, myocardial contractility is intimately involved with myocardial oxygen transport (Fig. 13-1).

Cardiac output, the actual amount of blood ejected by the heart, is related to three other factors besides contractility: preload, afterload, and pulse rate. The preload is the degree of muscle fiber stretch imposed by filling of the ventricles during diastole. According to Starling's law of the heart, this varies directly with cardiac output (Fig. 13-2). The afterload is the impedance to cardiac ejection during systole imposed by vascular resistance, blood pressure, and blood viscosity (Fig. 13-3). The stroke output of the heart varies inversely with the afterload. The cardiac output varies directly with the pulse rate up to a level of 160, at which point there is insufficient time for complete ventricular filling. Any monitoring system designed to assess the state of the myocardium must include these factors. The Sarnoff ventricular function curve is a plot of stroke work (the product of stroke volume and mean aortic blood pressure) against ventricular end-diastolic pressure or end-diastolic volume. It provides a good evaluation of myocardial contractility because it includes consideration of afterload and preload. The bedside determination of fundamental hemodynamic variables such as cardiac output and PCWP is essential for the proper management of severely ill surgical patients.

Catheterization of the central venous system or right side of the heart for manometry, injection of indicator, or mixed venous sampling is used as an integral part of many

Fig. 13-1. Determinants of stroke volume, cardiac output, and arterial pressure.

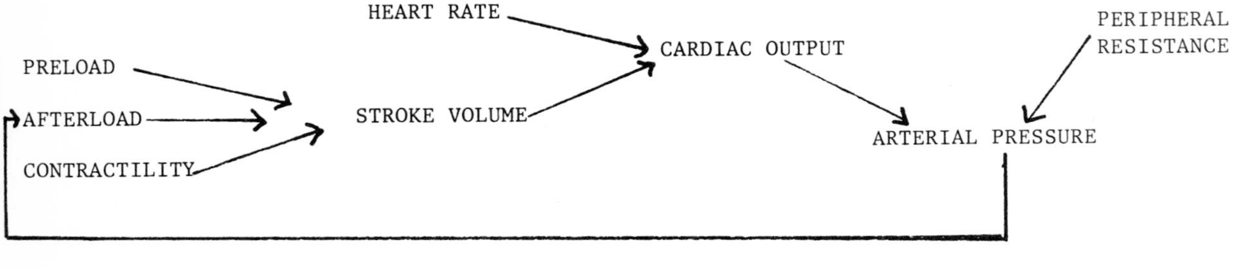

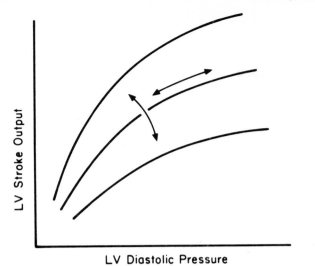

Fig. 13-2. Relationship between stroke output and diastolic pressure (Starling's law).

surgical monitoring systems. There are several routes of access to the central venous system. In order of increasing risk these are the median basilic vein in the the antecubital fossa, the external jugular vein, the internal jugular vein, and the subclavian vein. The femoral vein is seldom used because of contamination and thrombophlebitis. The median basilic vein directs the catheter directly into the subclavian vein and superior vena cava if the arm is extended laterally during the procedures, whereas the cephalic vein is difficult to negotiate at the shoulder. The external jugular vein is best approached with the neck extended, turned to the opposite side and lower than

Fig. 13-3. Relationship between afterload and contractility.

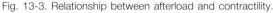

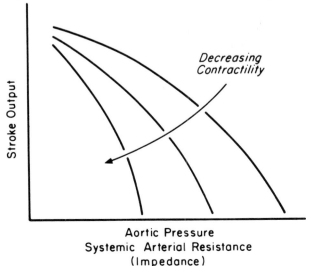

Aortic Pressure
Systemic Arterial Resistance
(Impedance)

heart level (to fill the vein and prevent air embolism). The vein can also be steadied and distended by proximal pressure at the neck. As with the antecubital approach, venisection is best done before the vein is damaged with multiple puncture attempts. If there is difficulty passing the jugular-subclavian junction, the catheter may pass if the shoulder is depressed. The internal jugular vein can be cannulated percutaneously above the clavicle. The puncture is made immediately lateral to the pulsation of the common carotid artery through the lateral head of the sternocleidomastoid muscle. The distance to the proper position in the superior vena cava requires a catheter 20 cm long.

Puncture and catheter introduction into the subclavian vein involves a slightly greater risk of pneumothorax, but its ease of access makes it popular in emergency situations. As with the other sites, local anesthesia should be used as well as complete sterile precautions. Skin puncture is done just inferior to the clavicle at the junction of the middle and inner thirds, with the needle aimed at a point behind the manubrium. The catheter should not be threaded through or over the needle until venous blood is easily aspirated. When threaded through the needle, the catheter should never be withdrawn separately because of the danger of shearing it off with the sharp edge of the needle. Some commercial sets have protective sleeves that can be extended beyond the needle point to prevent cutting the catheter. A chest radiograph should always be obtained following central venous catheterization to check for pneumothorax and ascertain the position of the catheter tip. If a nonradiopaque catheter is used, it can be filled with contrast medium during the exposure. A number of commercial intravenous catheter sets are available that are ingeniously designed to facilitate advancement of the catheter without contamination or kinking (Fig. 13-4).

The proper interpretation of central venous pressure or pulmonary artery wedge pressure for monitoring surgical patients requires an understanding of all factors that may cause elevated readings. Artifacts such as inaccurate zero level, blockage, or kinking should be excluded by observation of 1- to 2-cm pressure fluctuations with the respiratory cycle and careful sighting of the zero level at the midaxillary line. The zero level should correspond to the point of projection of the posterior leaflet of the tricuspid valve on the right chest wall. Noncardiac factors that increase central venous pressure are hypervolemia, vasoconstrictor drugs (metaraminol and mephentermine constrict the veins as well as arterioles), positive-pressure ventilation, pneumothorax, hydrothorax, flail chest, and mediastinal compression. If none of these factors exists, normal readings vary between 0 and 9 cm of water for central venous pressure and 5 to 12 mmHg PCWP. Elevated values suggest the inability of either ventricle to handle its venous return. Filling pressure alone is not a measure of ventricular function or myocardial contractility, because afterload and ventricular work are unknown quantities. A high central venous pressure does serve as a warning that volume infusion should be continued with extreme caution. However, in situations such as pericardial tamponade or pulmonary embolism, a high central

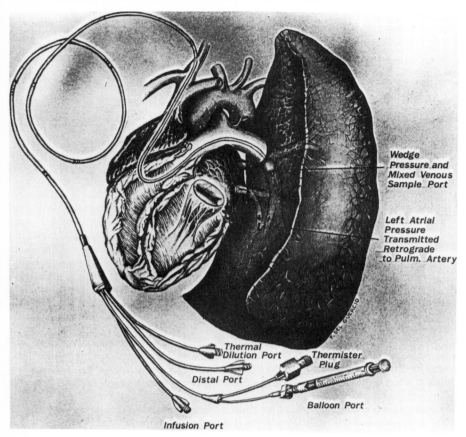

Fig. 13-4. Balloon catheter for invasive studies.

venous pressure is essential to maintain an adequate cardiac output until definitive therapy is used to relieve the obstruction. The most logical use of central venous pressure or PCWP as a guide to fluid replacement in seriously ill patients is the observation of the response to challenge with 100 mL increments of volume infusion. Infusion is stopped when a sharp rise in pressure occurs.

Equating wedge pressure with left atrial pressure assumes an open circuit from the catheter tip to the left atrium. This is not the case if the vessel is filled with blood clots or if the catheter is located in zones I and II in the pulmonary vascular bed, where alveolar pressure is greater than arterial pressure (zone I) or venous pressure (zones I and II) (Fig. 13-5).

In zone III, where both arterial and venous pressures exceed alveolar pressure, there is continuous flow, and conditions are met for accurate measurement of pulmonary-capillary wedge pressure. Fortunately, most of the lung enters zone III when the patient is supine, and most pulmonary-artery catheters will float into zone III since most of the blood is flowing into this zone. When vascular pressures are very low (hypovolemic shock) or when PEEP increases alveolar pressure, zone III may be converted to zone II. It has been shown that if the tip of the catheter is at or below the left atrium, the conditions in zone III exist even if PEEP values are as high as 30 cm

H_2O. If one finds that the wedge pressure has increased almost as much as the PEEP has, this increase suggests that the catheter has slipped into zone II or I. A cross-table, lateral chest film should confirm the location of the catheter tip relative to the left atrium. If the tip is above the atrium, the catheter should be repositioned.

Left atrial pressure does not equal left ventricular end-diastolic pressure in the presence of mitral-valve disease or markedly reduced ventricular compliance, in which atrial contraction can cause an appreciable increase in left ventricular end-diastolic pressure. In such a setting the pulmonary-capillary wedge pressure will still be an accurate monitor for cardiogenic pulmonary edema but will be less helpful in assessing left ventricular function. One must also realize that the left ventricular end-diastolic pressure may not be an accurate reflection of left ventricular end-diastolic volume. Very stiff noncompliant ventricles may allow a high end-diastolic pressure to accompany a normal end-diastolic volume. PEEP may increase end-diastolic pressure without increasing end-diastolic volume. Thus, although pulmonary-capillary wedge pressure usually reflects left ventricular end-diastolic pressure, it may not reflect actual preload.

There are additional problems due to PEEP-induced changes in vascular and pleural pressures. During spontaneous breathing the measured pulmonary-capillary wedge

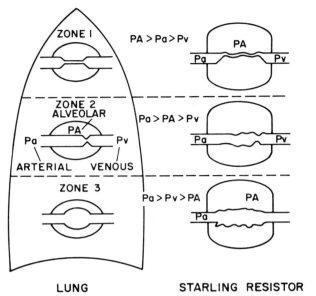

LUNG   **STARLING RESISTOR**

Fig. 13-5. The pulmonary capillary bed has flow characteristics of a Starling resistor, which consists of a length of flaccid collapsible tubing passing through a rigid chamber. In the Starling resistor, when chamber pressure (*PA*) exceeds the downstream pressure (*pv*), flow is independent of downstream pressure. However, when downstream pressure exceeds the chamber pressure, flow is determined by the upstream-downstream difference. The alveolar pressure is the same throughout the lung. The pulmonary artery pressure (*Pa*) increases down the lung. Zone 1 exists when alveolar pressure exceeds pulmonary arterial pressure and no blood flow occurs. This might occur when the pulmonary arterial pressure is decreased, as in hypovolemia, or when alveolar pressure is increased, as with the application of positive end-expiratory pressure. Zone 1 functions as alveolar dead space. In zone 2, pulmonary arterial pressure increases and exceeds alveolar pressure. In zone 2, blood flow is determined by the difference between arterial and alveolar pressures. In zone 3, blood flow is determined by the arteriovenous pressure difference. (From: *Bone RC: The treatment of severe hypoxemia due to the adult respiratory distress syndrome. Arch Intern Med 140:85, 1980, with permission.*)

pressure approximates the transmural pulmonary-capillary wedge pressure (measured value minus value for pleural pressure) because pleural pressure is small. This may not be true during breathing under PEEP, which may increase pleural pressures. Furthermore, some of the PEEP may be directly transmitted to the vessel itself. The application of PEEP can lead to artificially high intravascular-pressure readings if transmural pressures are falling. The amount of pressure transmitted to the pleural space and intrathoracic vessels depends on the compliance of the lungs and chest wall. When the lungs are very compliant and the chest wall is very stiff (e.g., as in emphysema), more pressure will be transmitted, making interpretation of pressure measurements quite difficult.

How does one cope with the above uncertainties? In general, if the level of PEEP is below 10 cmH$_2$O, there is no difference between pulmonary-capillary wedge pressures measured during ventilation and without ventilation. One study found that PEEP up to 30 cmH$_2$O did not markedly affect pressures in patients with very poor lung

compliance. Other studies, however, suggest that even in patients with stiff lungs, measured vascular pressures may increase with increasing PEEP and transmural pressures may actually decline.

There are two potential solutions to this problem, short of inserting pleural catheters in all patients. One is to disconnect the patient from the ventilator and measure all the pressures. This is not a practical approach. Although ventilation with 100 percent oxygen through one hand is probably safe, it may not always be. Moreover, the patient needs the ventilator. The second solution is to place the pulmonary-artery line in zone III of the lung and to keep the level of PEEP below 10 cmH$_2$O. If the PEEP level is higher, the measured vascular pressures may rise 1 to 2 mmHg for every 5 cm of PEEP applied to 10 cmH$_2$O. Although a pulmonary-capillary wedge pressure of 18 mmHg in a patient breathing spontaneously would be associated with interstitial pulmonary edema, it may be an acceptable value in a patient receiving PEEP at 20 cmH$_2$O. One must take readings consistently at end expiration, be sure that all the equipment is properly calibrated, and be careful not to overinterpret pressure readings in patients receiving PEEP.

Bedside monitoring of left ventricular dynamics by right-sided catheterization was facilitated by the development of the balloon-tipped Swan-Ganz catheter. With the balloon inflated, the catheter sails through the right side of the heart into a wedge position in the pulmonary artery in less than 1 min. In the absence of pulmonary vascular disease, pulmonary capillary wedge pressure is a reliable guide to left atrial and, in turn, left ventricular end-diastolic pressure. Without the wedge position, the pulmonary artery end-diastolic pressure is an acceptable indicator of mean left atrial pressure. Central venous pressure alone has been found to be an unreliable index of left ventricular function, since filling pressure in the left side of the heart may rise sharply and pulmonary edema may occur without significant increase in right atrial pressures.

The right ventricle is bound by a convex septal wall and a concave free wall, which enclose a crescent-shaped slit between them. In the right ventricular cavity a relatively narrow space is therefore confined between two broad surfaces, so that the surface area of the chamber is great in relation to the volume. Therefore, the configuration of the right ventricle is ideally suited to the ejection of large volumes of blood with minimal amounts of myocardial shortening. This architectural design is not conducive to the development of high intraventricular pressures. Anatomically, the pericardium surrounding the right and left ventricles may have a substantial effect on ventricular function, as this rather still membrane is not capable of acute rapid expansion.

Considerable "interdependence" exists between right and left ventricular function. In a noncompliant nondistensible pericardium, an acute increase in right ventricular end-diastolic volume may result in a shift of the interventricular septum toward the left ventricular cavity with a consequent reduction in the left ventricular end-diastolic volume. In this instance, assessment of left ventricular preload may not be accurately measured as the pulmonary artery wedge pressure due to the decrease in left ventricular compliance.

The development of pulmonary artery hypertension is a common denomination in severe cases of acute respiratory failure during critical illness. The pulmonary vascular bed provides the impedance to ejection (afterload) faced by the right ventricle. The physiologic consequences of increased impedance on right ventricular function have been well described. Initially an increase in systolic force of right ventricular contraction is noted with increased right ventricular systolic pressures. Subsequently, an increase in the right ventricular diastolic pressure may be followed by right ventricular failure.

Recently, some of the pathophysiologic consequences of pulmonary hypertension and right ventricular function have been defined. Initially, increased force of right ventricular ejection is allowed by an increase in right ventricular end-diastolic volume. The use of the Starling relationship in this circumstance results in a maintenance of right ventricular ejection. As the compliance characteristics of the right ventricle are altered, the increased end-diastolic volume results in increased intracavitary pressures. During diastole, such increased pressures exceed left ventricular end-diastolic pressures, and the septum will therefore be shifted toward the left ventricular cavity. Septal shift may then affect left ventricular function by reducing the volume (preload) of the left ventricle. Therefore, an adaptive response on the right side of the heart to pulmonary hypertension may result in left ventricular dysfunction.

The critically ill patient, most especially during sepsis, may show evidence of pulmonary hypertension associated with higher right ventricular end-diastolic volume, intracavitary pressure, septal shift, and reduced left ventricular function. The right and left ventricular dysfunction may be accentuated by the application of positive-pressure ventilation, particularly with use of positive end-expiratory pressure.

CENTRAL VENOUS OXIMETRY. The mixed venous oxygen level reflects the extent to which the body must call upon the blood oxygen stores in states of cardiovascular stress. The value of right heart oxygen saturation monitoring during surgery has been demonstrated (Fig. 13-3). Changes in cardiac output secondary to hemorrhage and other problems are reflected by early changes in right atrial oxygen saturation, usually before changes in arterial blood pressure, venous pressure, or heart rate. Changes in arterial oxygen content secondary to pulmonary shunting or decreased oxygen-carrying capacity also promptly affect mixed venous oxygen saturation. It was originally thought that pulmonary arterial samples would be necessary for this type of monitoring, but experience has shown that, in the stressed patient, right atrial or right ventricular samples correlate well with those from the pulmonary artery. Saturations below 50 percent from these sites are a bad prognostic sign and indicate either severe arterial hypoxemia or very significantly decreased cardiac output.

In a recent study by Nelson, continuously measured mixed venous oxygen saturation (Sv_{O_2}) was a reliable predictor of Sv_{O_2} measured intermittently by in vitro methods. In critically ill surgical patients, Sv_{O_2} does not correlate highly with the individual determinants of oxygen transport but rather correlates with the oxygen utilization coefficient (V_{O_2}/D_{O_2}) and therefore reflects the overall balance between oxygen consumption and delivery.

To understand this concept clearly, the components of the Fick equation must be analyzed and rearranged. The Fick equation relates cardiac output, tissue oxygen consumption, and the arterial-venous oxygen content difference.

$$V_{O_2} = C(a - v)_{O_2} \times CO \times 10$$

Other cardiopulmonary parameters that are calculated include:

$$Ca_{O_2} = (Sa_{O_2} \times Hb \times 1.34) + (Pa_{O_2} \times 0.0031)$$
$$Cv_{O_2} = (Sv_{O_2} \times Hb \times 1.34) + (Pv_{O_2} \times 0.0031)$$
$$C(a - v)_{O_2} = Ca_{O_2} - Cv_{O_2}$$
$$D_{O_2} = CO \times 10 \times Ca_{O_2}$$
$$OUC = V_{O_2}/D_{O_2}$$

where Ca_{O_2} = arterial oxygen content (mL/dL), Sa_{O_2} = arterial oxygen saturation (fraction), Hb = hemoglobin concentration (g/dL), Pa_{O_2} = arterial oxygen tension (mmHg), Cv_{O_2} = venous oxygen content (mL/dL), Sv_{O_2} = mixed venous oxygen saturation (fraction), Pv_{O_2} = mixed venous oxygen tension (mmHg), $C(a - v)O_2$ = arterial-venous oxygen content difference (mL/dL), D_{O_2} = oxygen delivery (mL/min), CO = cardiac output (L/min), V_{O_2} = oxygen consumption (mL/min), OUC = oxygen utilization coefficient (fraction).

When the terms of the Fick equation are rearranged, it may be seen that the determinants of Sv_{O_2} are the components of oxygen delivery and oxygen consumption:

$$\frac{V_{O_2}}{CO \times 10} = C(a - v)_{O_2}$$

$$\frac{V_{O_2}}{CO \times 10} = Ca_{O_2} - Cv_{O_2}$$

$$\frac{V_{O_2}}{CO \times 10} - Ca_{O_2} = -Cv_{O_2}$$

$$Cv_{O_2} = Ca_{O_2} - \left[\frac{V_{O_2}}{CO \times 10} \right]$$

$$\frac{Cv_{O_2}}{Ca_{O_2}} = 1 - \left[\frac{V_{O_2}}{CO \times 10 \times Ca_{O_2}} \right]$$

If $Sa_{O_2} = 1.0$, then

$$Sv_{O_2} = \frac{Cv_{O_2}}{Ca_{O_2}}$$

$$Sv_{O_2} = 1 - [V_{O_2}/(CO \times 10 \times Ca_{O_2})]$$

$$Sv_{O_2} = 1 - \frac{V_{O_2}}{D_{O_2}}$$

From the foregoing formulas only three mechanisms can account for a decrease in the venous oxygen content (Cv_{O_2}): a decrease in the arterial oxygen content (Ca_{O_2}), oxygen consumption (V_{O_2}), and total cardiac output (CO). Similarly, provided there is no change in the other components in the equation, an increase in the oxygen consumption (V_{O_2}) or a decrease in the cardiac output (CO), hemoglobin concentration (Hb), or arterial oxygen saturation (Sv_{O_2}) will produce a decrease in the Sv_{O_2}.

A major development in pulmonary-artery catheters has been the addition of a channel including two fiberoptic bundles for light transmission, allowing continuous measurements of oxygen saturation of the mixed venous blood by an oximeter. The insertion of fiberoptic catheters is not afflicted with additional difficulties, despite the fact that the optic fibers are relatively fragile and can easily be fractured. A major problem lies in the high cost of the catheter and the oximeter. Continuous Sv_{O_2} display, however, can limit the number of venous blood gas and cardiac output determinations. As an online parameter, it is undoubtedly an invaluable indicator of acute cardiorespiratory disturbance in severely ill patients.

While continuously measured Sv_{O_2} may correlate with hemodynamic changes (cardiac output) in some groups of patients, the nonsteady nature of critical illness has taught us not to expect that arterial oxygen saturation, hemoglobin concentration, or oxygen consumption will remain stable, and therefore changes in Sv_{O_2} will not necessarily reflect changes in cardiac output in these patients. Nelson indicated that, although there is some statistical correlation between Sv_{O_2} and both cardiac output and oxygen delivery, the correlation coefficients are so small that the use of Sv_{O_2} as a predictor of cardiac output is unreliable. Similarly, correlations could not be established between Sv_{O_2} and arterial oxygenation, oxygen consumption, or arterial-venous content difference as independent variables. The high degree of inverse correlation between Sv_{O_2} and oxygen utilization ratio makes this relationship clinically useful.

The goal of many interventions in critically ill patients is to ensure that oxygen delivery to the tissue meets or exceeds the oxygen demand of that tissue. Our clinical ability to monitor this relationship is severely lacking. While we can measure total body oxygen uptake by the patient with reasonable reliability, oxygen uptake is equal to oxygen consumption only in the steady state. To make matters worse, oxygen consumed by the patient is not necessarily equal to the oxygen demand by the tissues of the patient. Normally, oxygen consumption increases when oxygen demand increases. Oxygen consumption may increase through an increase in the extraction of oxygen from arterial blood as it traverses the capillary bed [(i.e., an increase in $C(a - v)_{O_2}$] or through an increase in blood flow (i.e., cardiac output). Both of these factors may increase by approximately threefold in normal subjects, allowing a ninefold increase in oxygen consumption to meet the oxygen demand of the tissue. Critically ill patients may not be capable of increasing cardiac output spontaneously and therefore may have a markedly diminished "safety factor" in regard to increasing oxygen

consumption. When oxygen demand exceeds oxygen consumption, anaerobic metabolism ensues and lactic acidosis results, as previously described.

In the normal resting state, the entire body consumes only 25 percent of the oxygen transported to it by the cardiac output. Normal mixed venous blood is found to be 75 percent saturated with a partial pressure of 40 mmHg. An additional complicating factor is the fact that oxygen consumed by the various tissues differs, and it is not possible at this time to measure clinically oxygen demand or consumption of individual organs. For example, at rest myocardial oxygen extraction is near maximal while renal oxygen extraction is very low. At times of stress when myocardial oxygen demand increases, oxygen consumption can increase only by increases in myocardial blood flow. During this same period of stress, renal blood flow may actually decrease dramatically and renal oxygen consumption may be maintained by increased oxygen extraction in the renal capillary bed. Mixed venous blood represents a "flow-weighted average" of the blood returning from all perfused tissues. That is to say, the magnitude of the effect of oxygen extraction by any organ on Sv_{O_2} is proportional to the blood flow to that organ so that low-consumption, high-flow organs (kidneys) have a greater effect on Sv_{O_2} than do high-consumption, low-flow organs (myocardium).

Since our goals are not necessarily to provide the highest oxygen delivery but rather to bring into balance the relationship between oxygen consumption and oxygen delivery, it seems apparent that continuously measured Sv_{O_2} is at this time the best indicator clinically available to assure that this goal has been attained.

A low or rapidly decreasing Sv_{O_2} indicates an imbalance between oxygen consumption and oxygen delivery that requires further investigation of the determinants of these parameters. A low or falling Sv_{O_2} does not tell us which therapy is appropriate in a given situation but rather tells us that more information is needed to assess the problem. The falling Sv_{O_2} may indicate a decrease in hemoglobin concentration, arterial oxygen content, or cardiac output, or an increase in tissue oxygen consumption. When a low or decreasing Sv_{O_2} is encountered, the clinician may obtain an arterial blood-gas analysis, hemoglobin value, and hemodynamic assessment of the patient to select the most appropriate intervention that may restore the balance between oxygen consumption and delivery. This function has been described by Watson as the "early warning system" of cardiorespiratory imbalance.

CARDIAC-OUTPUT DETERMINATIONS

Invasive Techniques

In spite of various questions regarding accuracy in high- or low-flow states, the description of indicator-dilution curves from central circulation remains the basic method for monitoring cardiac output. The technique involves the injection of an indicator into the right side of the heart and continuous determination of its concentration as it mixes with the cardiac output somewhere downstream. Any indicator can be used, as long as it does not affect hemodynamics or disappear from the blood before the concentration is measured. It can best be understood as a variation of the Fick principle, where the known amount of indicator is equivalent to a fixed amount of oxygen consumption, and the mean concentration of indicator after mixing is equivalent to the arteriovenous oxygen difference. It follows, then, that the faster the volume of blood flow, the lower the arteriovenous oxygen difference and mean concentration of indicator. All methods for the calculation of cardiac output from both continuous and single-bolus injection of indicator use this principle in analyzing the time-concentration curves to obtain the mean concentration of indicator. The number of milligrams of indicator injected divided by the mean concentration of indicator gives the volume of flow during the time of the indicator-dilution curve. Thermal dilution curves are similar in principle, with use of cold saline solution as the indicator. They are popular because of their simplicity and the availability of bedside computers, but the required flow-directed balloon-tipped thermistor catheters are expensive. Since cardiac output is usually expressed as flow per minute, the volume of flow during description of the curve is multiplied by 60 and divided by the number of seconds of duration of the curve.

Intracardiac and arterial blood-pressure data, cardiac output data, and electrocardiograph tracings combined with arterial and mixed venous blood-gas data permit calculation of a number of derived cardiorespiratory variables of physiologic significance. A microprocessor-controlled printer located right in the intensive care unit gives all professional personnel immediate access to a comprehensive display of cardiovascular performance, pulmonary function, and oxygen transport. A programmed instruction feature makes it easy to use.

Several hand-held calculators with program cards specifically made up for shock-cart calculating are available. The primary data obtained from the recorder and blood-gas machines are entered on the keyboard, and the derived values are immediately computed. Civetta's and Shoemaker's groups have made available magnetic card programs for the rapid automatic calculation of up to 27 derived cardiorespiratory variables, using Hewlett-Packard and Texas Instrument calculators, respectively.

Data become information only in the brain of the beholder. The average physician is "turned off" by a column of numbers representing cardiac index, stroke index, right and left ventricular stroke work, pulmonary and systemic vascular resistance, ventricular function indices, intracardiac and systemic pressures, arteriovenous oxygen difference, venoarterial admixture, oxygen consumption, P_{50}, serum lactate, and arterial base excess or deficit. In an attempt to make dull data attractive, Cohn and Del Guercio devised a system for displaying these derived variables on an easily scanned, logically organized, barchart format. Arterial and mixed venous blood-gas and saturation values along with cardiac output, temperature, height, weight, and inspired oxygen concentration are entered on the keyboard of a minicomputer, and within seconds the derived variables are drawn on a preprinted sheet by an X-Y alphanumeric recorder. This system, called the automated physiologic profile, is a compromise between the hand-held calculator approach and the very expensive built-in digital computer monitors. The profile serves as a useful permanent record of cardiorespiratory status before and after therapeutic interventions.

The example shown in Fig. 13-6 demonstrates a number of points regarding monitoring of the critically ill patient. This was a study, with Swan-Ganz thermistor catheter and radial artery cannula, of a young man who suffered a 30 percent burn and smoke inhalation. The physiologic assessment was done 24 h after injury and showed a "normal" cardiac index and blood pressure with an increase in oxygen consumption resulting from a widened arteriovenous oxygen content difference. Why, then, was there evidence of anaerobic metabolism and hypoxic acidosis with twice normal serum lactate levels and a base deficit of 6 meq/L? Because the patient's oxygen needs were even greater, and had the state of increasing oxygen debt continued, the patient surely would have died. The ventricular function curve in the lower right quadrant shows why the patient could not increase his cardiac output enough to supply his increased oxygen needs. The plot, representing the Starling-Frank relationship, is significantly below the zone of normal ventricular function. The cause for this cardiac failure could have been circulating myocardial depressant factors, known to be associated with burns, early sepsis, or poisoning of myocardial mitochondrial cytochromes by the high level of carbon monoxide (S_{CO}), which probably had been much higher on admission. The high right atrial and pulmonary artery wedge pressures indicate that both ventricles had more than adequate preload. Since total peripheral vascular resistance was normal, that determinant of cardiac output (afterload) also was not the limiting factor. It was obvious from this physiologic profile (but not from the ECG, PCWP, or systemic BP) that the patient would not survive unless inotropic therapy could stimulate the myocardium to at least normal contractility. This was accomplished with digitalis, dopamine, and GIK (glucose, insulin, potassium).

At the same time, the profile also illustrated the need for a volume-cycled respiratory with PEEP to reduce the severe pulmonary shunting (venoarterial admixture) caused by the smoke inhalation. The most appropriate setting of end-expiratory pressure (optimum PEEP) was determined by performing automated physiologic profiles sequentially at increased levels of PEEP. Beyond a certain level, reduced cardiac output, resulting from restricted preload, produced a net decrease in oxygen transport, even though arterial oxygen content continued to improve. Had it not been for the information provided by the monitoring of these derived cardiorespiratory variables, it is unlikely that lifesaving therapeutic decisions could have been made in time.

The effect of the 15% carboxyhemoglobin concentration on the position of the oxyhemoglobin dissociation curve is also shown. The P_{50} STD value of 30.2 excludes the effect of carbon monoxide, and the P_{50} STDX value of

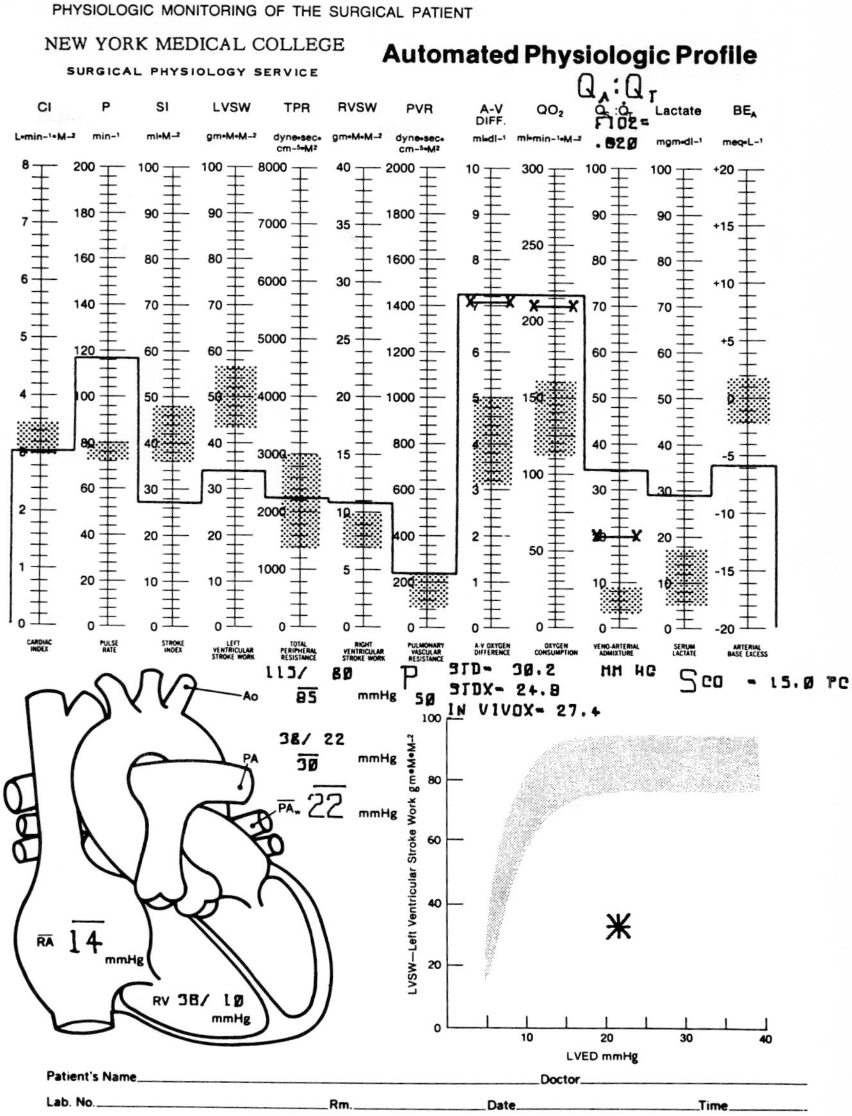

Fig. 13-6. Automated physiologic profile.

24.9 indicates the shift to the left caused by carboxyhemoglobin. The lines with the X's on the bar charts for "A-V Diff," Q_{O_2}, and Q_a/Q_t indicate those values at the patient's actual P_{50} compared with what they would have been had the P_{50} been normal (26 to 27 mmHg). This type of calculation is of value clinically, since it is possible to manipulate the P_{50} by pharmacologic means in order to improve oxygen transport. Harken's recent review of this aspect of monitoring emphasizes the importance of dissociation-curve shifts in clinical syndromes.

The automated physiologic profile is in use in many institutions, including a number of community hospitals, where it has been proved cost-effective, particularly when used for preoperative assessment and physiologic fine tuning in the high-risk patient, which will be discussed later (Fig. 13-7).

There are other monitoring systems that involve the use of catheter-tip sensors. One measures pressure and electromagnetic flow velocity. When threaded retrograde into the left ventricle, this sensor permits the on-line recording of the left ventricular pressures, left ventricular pressure acceleration (dp/dt), intracardiac heart sounds, ascending aortic blood velocity, and ascending aortic blood acceleration. If the cross-sectional area of the aorta is known, total flow can be calculated. All these serve as very useful indices of left ventricular function, particularly following myocardial infarction. The problem of calibration of the electromagnetic flowmeter probe without a zero-flow calibration point is a serious one, as it is for all clinical studies involving electromagnetic flowmeters.

A disposable, very thin polarographic oxygen-sensing electrode can be used for mixed venous oxygen tension

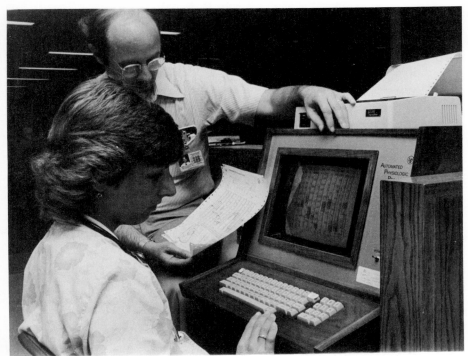

Fig. 13-7. Hardware for automated physiologic profile.

monitoring. The miniature sensor is fabricated by dip-coating or painting the various insulators, diffusion membranes, and buffers directly onto the central wire electrode. Other similar devices are available complete with compact solid-state battery-powered recorders for use at the bedside.

The insertion of a long catheter from the radial artery up to the region of the aortic arch permits a detailed analysis of the aortic pulse contour. Warner has perfected this technique for clinical monitoring. Stroke volume is computed from the pulse contour on a beat-by-beat basis. This, combined with pressure variables, provides an almost instantaneous cardiovascular assessment. Unfortunately, McDonald et al. have pointed out, the method depends upon a stable vascular impedance, which is seldom the case in critically ill patients. For this reason, the technique is not in general use.

Preoperative Hemodynamic Assessment

There is evidence that preoperative hemodynamic assessment of patients is applicable to specific situations. Using pulmonary-artery catheters, Corlon and associates have revealed seriously impaired hemodynamic function in many patients. Patients with abnormal cardiac function had a postoperative mortality rate approximately 100 times higher than the average for all patients in that institution. Patients readmitted to the ICU postoperatively who received extensive hemodynamic monitoring and management had substantially better results than those not readmitted.

Del Guercio and associates have used right-sided heart balloon flotation catheters for arterial sampling to determine the physiologic variables representing left and right ventricular function, oxygen transport, and metabolic parameters of ventricular function curves in a group of elderly patients. Invasive preoperative assessments of these elderly patients disclosed a high percentage of serious physiologic abnormalities requiring a delay of operation in some and cancellation in others. The frequent observation of subtle underlying defects in cardiac reserve in patients who otherwise appeared healthy to the clinician precipitated the opening of a preoperative assessment unit at the Westchester County Medical Center. Preoperative assessment of patients who underwent gastric partition procedures for morbid obesity demonstrated that although there was no clinical evidence of congestive heart failure and there was no evidence of abnormality in the arteriovenous oxygen content differences, the left ventricular function was reduced to 57 percent of normal.

Circulatory response to trauma of a major operation, performed with general anesthesia, consists of two phases—the operative phase and the postoperative phase. The first phase is characterized by depressed cardiac output and cardiac index, and the second by an elevation of the cardiac output and index, particularly in the immediate postoperative period. The first phase response is more marked in obese patients and the increase characteristic of the second phase is less than that noted for nonobese patients. The abnormal response of the second phase is an important contributing factor to the increased operative mortality in the morbidly obese patients. Vascular disorders in which there is frequent coexistence of heart disease, hypertension, diabetes, stroke, as well as the usual high-risk factors of advanced age also benefit from preoperative evaluation. The study by Barber et al. indicates that only one-third of patients undergoing preoperative evaluation for a vascular operation had normal left ventricular function and required no therapeutic intervention before the operative procedure. About one-quarter of patients with impaired left ventricular function responded to preload augmentation, 40 percent required inotropic support, 13 percent needed afterload reduction, and about 10 percent required a combination of a change in preload inotropic support and afterload reduction. It is also appropriate to perform a preoperative physiologic profile on patients with acute limb ischemia because low cardiac output with or without excessive SVR is present in about 10 percent. The ischemia resulting from the low flow portends a dire prognosis, and a discernible improvement in the circulatory status in the limbs coincided with the correction of low-flow states by appropriate hemodynamic maneuvers. Preoperative physiologic assessment of patients with hip fractures and optimizing the hemodynamic status reduce mortality and morbidity. This circumstance also pertains to elderly patients undergoing urologic procedures.

Studies have concluded that right heart catheterization is indicated for severely ill hemodynamically unstable patients who do not respond to therapy deemed appropriate after clinical evaluation. The clinical states that benefit most and have more clearly defined indications for the use of invasive pulmonary catheter monitoring are listed in Table 13-4.

Table 13-4. INDICATIONS FOR PULMONARY-ARTERY CATHETERS

1. Myocardial infarctions complicated by
   a. Hypotension unresponsive to volume challenge
   b. Marked hemodynamic instability requiring intravenous inotropic or vasoactive drugs or mechanical assist devices
   c. Hypotension and congestive heart failure
   d. ?Cardiac tamponade (equalization of end-diastolic pressures)
   e. ?Acute mitral regurgitation (giant V waves)
   f. ?Ruptured interventricular septum (step-up in oxygen saturation)
2. Unstable angina requiring intravenous nitroglycerin (most patients)
3. Congestive heart failure unresponsive to conventional therapy, to guide preload and afterload therapy
4. Pulmonary hypertension, for diagnosis and monitoring during acute drug therapy
5. Distinguishing cardiogenic from noncardiogenic pulmonary edema
6. Optimizing PEEP and volume therapy in the adult respiratory-distress syndrome
7. Resolving doubts about volume or cardiovascular status if a diuretic or fluid challenge would be unsafe or would yield equivocal results
8. Preoperative assessment of high-risk patients

Noninvasive Techniques

As more sophisticated noninvasive techniques develop in the next decade, the use of invasive techniques will diminish. At the present time preoperative Swan-Ganz catheter insertion can be performed safely and efficiently, and also provides the surgeon and anesthesiologist an on-line continuous monitoring mode of hemodynamic parameters intraoperatively and postoperatively.

Assessment of right ventricular function is made difficult by the complex geometry and shape of the right ventricle. The thermodilution techniques used to measure cardiac output with the pulmonary-artery catheter can now also determine right ventricular ejection fraction quite easily if a fast-response thermistor is used. An essential advantage of this measurement is the ability to repeatedly evaluate right ventricular function during the course of disease, and also to assess the effects of therapeutic interventions. These catheters are about 20 percent more expensive than standard ones, and the cardiac-output computers needed for calculation of the right ventricular ejection fraction cost twice as much as standard cardiac-output computers.

All the methods of estimating cardiac output described thus far are invasive to varying degrees and therefore present some risk and considerable expense because they require skilled personnel for their application. A number of promising noninvasive adaptations of the indicator-dilution principle are in clinical use. Included in this category are gamma densitometry (quantitative angiography), videodensitometry, isotope-dilution analysis, fluorescence excitation analysis, and magnetic fluid tracer dilution.

Information regarding flow rates, vascular volumes, distribution of pulmonary transit times, intracardiac and pulmonary shunting, and right or left ventricular ejection efficiency is theoretically contained in the shapes of indicator-dilution curves. With the conventional indocyanine green dye technique, sampling rates are too slow, and the injection and sampling sites are too far apart for complete interpretation of the physiologic events that create the shape of the curve. Catheter lag between the sampling point and the densitometer cuvette also produces distortion of the curves and loss of potential information. Gamma densitometry, in which the indicator is a small bolus of radiopaque contrast medium and the blood vessels or cardiac chambers serve as the densitometer cuvettes, avoids these problems. Gamma rays or x-rays, projected through the cardiac silhouette, produce high-dynamic-response indicator time-concentration curves through the detection of changes in gamma photon density related, according to Beer's law, to the concentration of radiopaque indicator in the blood. In clinical practice, solid-state radiation detectors are placed behind the patient as in a portable x-ray unit. Five milliliters of Hypaque is then injected into the central venous catheter, and six simultaneous contrast dilution curves are recorded from the heart and great vessels. Analysis of these curves permits calculation of pulmonary circulation time, pulmonary blood volume, right and left ventricular ejection fraction, and other useful variables. More sophisticated interpretation requires electronic data processing for transfer-function analysis.

Videodensitometry and digital subtraction angiography are similar in principle to gamma densitometry, except that an actual angiocardiogram is performed and recorded. The advantages are that, at leisure, an infinite number of curves can be obtained from any point in the cardiac silhouette as the tape is played over and over. Disadvantages include great expense, lack of portability, and low signal-to-noise ratio requiring signal processing to obtain recognizable curves.

Isotope dilution analysis has made a great leap forward with the development of the Anger scintillation camera and other rapid-response isotope scanning devices. The ability to image and quantify the distribution of a radioactive tracer second by second through the heart and lungs adds a new dimension of considerable value to surgical cardiovascular monitoring. High-photon-yield isotopes are injected intravenously and the gamma camera images are recorded on magnetic tape. Later, specific areas can be analyzed to produce indicator-dilution curves that can be related to changes in size and position of the cardiac chambers. Jones et al. have produced good indicator-dilution curves for the right and left sides of the heart using an autofluoroscope. Spatial resolution and dynamic response, however, can never be as good as that obtained with the linear interrogating beams of radiation used in gamma densitometry.

With the advent of the radionuclide gated blood-pool scans, one could determine the left ventricular ejection fraction very accurately in critically ill patients in the intensive care unit. The scan relies upon technetium 99 pyrophosphate to label circulating erythrocytes, and the tracer quantity of radionuclide produces an image that is gated to an electrocardiogram to provide a very accurate measure of left ventricular ejection fraction and continuous motion of the heart chambers. The latter method allows one to evaluate ventricular wall motion by performing simultaneously a radionuclide scan and thermodilution cardiac index. One can calculate the end-diastolic volume index using the following formula:

$$\text{LV end-diastolic volume} = \frac{\text{stroke volume index}}{\text{LV ejection fraction}}$$

where LV is left ventricular, stroke volume index is determined from the thermodilution cardiac output, and the left ventricular ejection fraction is determined from the radionuclide scan. Because the tracer remains in the bloodstream for 6 or more hours with a single radionuclide injection, one can determine the left ventricular ejection fraction for this 6 h. Thus, if a base-line scan and output are performed, one can calculate the ventricular volumes serially for 6 h in response to a volume infusion, pressors, or vasodilator administration.

It is also possible to tag flowing blood in vivo by reversing the magnetic alignments of hydrogen nuclei in the water of the plasma by applying a powerful external magnetic field. These effects are detected farther downstream by means of magnetic resonance imaging. Magnetic resonance imaging devices are currently available. The technique, as described by Singer, is totally noninvasive.

It is obvious that noninvasive techniques for describing indicator-dilution curves will play a prominent role in surgical monitoring for years to come. Surgeons will be provided information regarding cardiac and circulatory function in their patients that will permit management of critical states on a firm physiologic basis.

The determination of systolic time intervals provides an external assessment of left ventricular function based entirely on intrinsic electrical and mechanical events. The methodology is gaining in popularity because it is physiologically sound and has been largely validated by extensive comparative clinical studies including catheterization of the left side of the heart.

Simultaneous recordings of the electrocardiogram, phonocardiogram, and external carotid pulse tracing are analyzed for the following time variables: total left ventricular systolic time (QRS complex to second heart sound), left ventricular ejection time (duration of carotid pulse upstroke), and preejection period (the difference between total left ventricular systolic and left ventricular ejection times). Although the calculations are straightforward, placement of the carotid pulse sensor and phonocardiogram microphone on the neck and chest is critical. With technical care in the performance of the recordings, remarkably good correlation with direct measures of the dynamics of the left side of the heart can be shown. Weissler et al. have found that the ratio of the preejection period to left ventricular ejection time (PEP/LVET) is relatively constant around 0.35 in patients with normal hearts. With failure of the left side of the heart, the PEP becomes longer and the LVET shorter, increasing the ratio. Serial studies reveal good correlation between the PEP/LVET ratio and left ventricular ejection fraction, end-diastolic volume, and end-diastolic pressure. This noninvasive approach, which requires inexpensive equipment, is useful for the continuous bedside monitoring of left ventricular function.

Alterations of left ventricular conduction, however, as in left bundle branch block, prolong the PEP selectively with no apparent change in LVET. Changes in peripheral impedance or vascular runoff, as occur in septic shock, may alter the relation between the PEP/LVET ratio and cardiac performance.

The application of ultrasound to clinical monitoring is undergoing a period of rapid growth according to Feigenbaum. Both industrial and academic sectors have developed methods for cardiovascular assessment based on interrogating beams of high-frequency sound waves (less than 1 mm wavelength). Ultrasonic energy can penetrate all tissues except bone and air-filled structures and provide good spatial resolution for diagnostic studies. Thus far, at the levels of energy needed for clinical work, there has been no suggestion of injury to living tissue, not even the fetus. The lack of hazard and the reasonable cost of the equipment required have led to more clinical studies than with any other technique aside from electrocardiography.

There are two basic methods of operation of ultrasound for diagnostic purposes—the pulse-echo mode (sonar) and the backscatter frequency-shift mode (Doppler effect). In the former, the distance between the emitter and any sound-reflecting interface deep within the body is measured in terms of the transit time of bursts of ultrasound to and from the tissue. An A scan device is held stationary against the body and a recording of the depth of structures in the path of the beam is made on the basis of the known speed of sound in tissue. The B scan is produced if the ultrasonic emitter is traversed across the body while echo-ranging, in order to produce a picture of the tissue cross section.

Not only is ultrasound less harmful than ionizing radiation, but it is capable of revealing internal surfaces that are invisible to x-rays. These include the internal structures of the heart and blood vessels. In addition, devices using the Doppler principle can detect rapid motions within the body. This makes them useful for studies of peripheral blood flow and cardiac valve function.

In echocardiography for ultrasonic determination of cardiac chamber size and stroke volume, a transducer is applied to the chest over the cardiac area. Sound in the 1- to 5-MHz frequency is delivered through the chest in on-off bursts about 1500 times per second. Echoes are detected during the off periods and recorded in terms of time lag (distance). The distances between the intraventricular septum and the posterior endocardial wall of the left ventricle are recorded at end diastole and end systole. The calculations of end-diastole and end-systolic volumes are made on the assumption that the shape of the chamber is a prolate ellipse. The results from a number of investigators are remarkable. The left ventricular volumes measured by echocardiography and by biplane angiocardiography were very similar over a wide range of values (correlation coefficient .97). The problem with this technique for surgical monitoring is that operators must be highly skilled and experienced in aiming the transducer and recognizing on the scan the exact structures they wish to measure. The device cannot be simply strapped on and left alone for 24 h to record left ventricular function. Some method will have to be devised for the ultrasonic beam to "lock on" to the left ventricular wall reflections.

The Doppler flowmeter has achieved considerable sophistication as a clinical tool in the past few years. Readout varies from a simple audible signal related to pulse velocity to signals combining vessel cross section and velocity to provide actual flow measurements. These techniques cannot yet be applied to aortic flow determination, but the entire field of ultrasonics offers many possibilities for the evolution of the perfect cardiovascular monitor.

The concept of measuring pulse volume on the basis of the electrical properties of blood goes back 40 years, but practical instruments for measuring electric impedance related to movement of electrolyte of the electromagnetic field have only recently been developed. In the instrument developed by Kubicek et al., two electrodes are placed around the neck and two around the abdomen just below the chest. The volume of blood between the electrodes decreases as the stroke volume flows up the carotids and down the aorta. This produces a decrease in electric impedance in the thorax. Since this cyclic change in impedance, compared with total chest impedance, is equivalent to less than one part in a thousand, considerable electronic sophistication is required for its detection. Alternating current is sent through the outer electrodes, and the change in voltage between the inner electrodes measured during cardiac systole indicates the impedance change due to left ventricular ejection. The problem is that venous inflow occurs more or less continuously, so that a net stroke volume during maximum ejection is measured. Great hopes were held for thoracic impedance plethysmography as a relatively inexpensive noninvasive means of monitoring cardiac output and ventricular function. Unfortunately, electrode motion artifacts and lack of correlation with other methods for the estimation of cardiac output in nonsteady states have dampened enthusiasm for this class of instruments.

There is no more consistently accurate method of measuring cardiac output than a properly calibrated electromagnetic flowmeter placed firmly around the ascending aorta. This approach is accepted as the standard against which other cardiac output monitoring equipment is evaluated for accuracy. Electromagnetic flowmeters can be used only for assessing vascular operations.

The nuclear probe (nuclear stethoscope, bios) has been developed as a modification of the equilibrium blood-pool scan (MUGA). This device consists of a collimated single-crystal nuclear probe or camera and a dedicated computer (Fig. 13-7).

The nuclear probe study has several advantages over other nuclear techniques—true portability, decreased cost, superior detector sensitivity and temporal resolution, and a reduced radionuclide dose requirement. There is, however, no imaging to guide the user to areas of interest. Instead, characteristics of the ventricular volume (or time activity) curve along with the length of an indicator bar are used to identify the left ventricle and background positions.

The nuclear probe or stethoscope provides a nonimaging assessment of left ventricular performance with a simple means of quantifying various systolic and diastolic parameters. Its portability and ease of handling add to the attractiveness of serial determinations over long- or short-term intervals. Accepted clinical applications have included arrhythmia analysis, assessment of myocardial infarction, shock, heart failure, and postoperative states, as well as drug-response patterns (e.g., doxorubicin toxicity).

MONITORING OF TISSUE METABOLISM

Under certain conditions, such as hypoxemia or septic shock, a high cardiac output is no guarantee of adequate delivery of oxygen to the cells. Couch and colleagues have succeeded in developing a practical and simple solution to the problem of an early warning system for tissue hypoxia. With an electrometer and right-angle pH electrode, skeletal muscle surface pH is continuously monitored. A 2-cm incision through skin, subcutaneous tissue, and fascia is required for placement of the electrode in gentle contact with the surface of the biceps muscle in adults and the quadriceps in children. Clinical monitoring by this technique has been continued for as long as 8 days.

The rationale for this approach is that with tissue deprivation of oxygen, oxidative phosphorylation ceases, and pyruvate is converted to lactic acid rather than carbon dioxide and water. Diffusion of the hydrogen ions and lactate across the cell membranes into the extracellular fluid is passive and rapid. Extracellular fluid acidosis related to anaerobic glycolysis precedes arterial pH depression because of a number of factors: in low-flow states there is a delay of acid metabolite washout into the peripheral circulation; arterial pH will change only after the hemoglobin-, bicarbonate-, and phosphate-buffering capacity of the blood is exceeded; and metabolism of lactate by the heart and liver tends to reduce the peripheral lactate levels until late in shock.

Skeletal muscle itself offers several advantages for surveillance of overall oxygen transport. Since it can tolerate hypoxia, its blood supply tends to get shut off early in critical states, and it tends to shift readily into anaerobic glycolysis and lactate production because of its high glycogen content. The surface of the muscle rather than the interior is monitored to avoid artifacts due to hematoma formation. Studies in human beings have shown that muscle surface pH is a sensitive indicator of muscle metabolism and as such is valuable as a practical monitoring instrument to alert against hypoxia of more vital tissues. The normal resting biceps pH is 7.38, slightly below arterial pH. When the normal oxygen gradient to the muscle cells is restored after the circulatory crisis is over, pH promptly returns to the normal resting level.

Couch's group has also done redox potential measurements of muscle as an indicator of balance between oxygen delivery and tissue needs. Redox potential of tissue reflects the overall balance of electron transfer, which shifts toward the negative or reduced state with prolonged hypoxia. Although the trends were found to be similar to the surface pH changes, absolute redox potential values were not as reliable indicators as pH changes. Muscle surface pH monitoring provides a good early warning of disaster during and after surgery. The small incision certainly can be justified in high-risk patients or those undergoing formidable operations.

Woldring et al. developed a mass spectrometer as previously described, which accurately records partial pressures of oxygen, carbon dioxide, or other gases, sampled through plastic or rubber membranes mounted on a catheter tip. Using a mass spectrometer, Owens et al. measured intracerebral gas tensions continuously across a heparinized silastic membrane on a perforated cannula. The measurements represent the gas tensions in the extracellular fluid surrounding local tissue injury rather than intact cells. Other problems are related to changes in membrane permeability due to fibrin deposits and protein denaturation.

Bioengineers are looking for noninvasive methods of scanning cellular bioenergetics. Huckabee had defined hypoxia as the "condition which exists when the supply of oxygen to the exterior of living cells is reduced to a rate insufficient for their current metabolic needs, with the result that various cellular oxidation-reduction systems must shift toward more reduced state." Detection of this state by a safe external sensor is the ultimate goal.

A number of attempts in this direction are in progress. One involves the stimulation of intracellular oxygen molecules with modulated soft x-rays. The stimulated emission of oxygen is in the microwave area of the 0.5-cm band and can be detected externally with a suitable waveguide and amplifier system. This approach would offer some degree of spatial discrimination of tissue hypoxia in specific organs. Another experimental method is a cross between Chance's fluorescence-emission technique and thermography. Energy transfers within living cells emit specific wavelengths of electromagnetic radiation according to quantum bioenergetic laws. Energy dissipation associated with inefficient anaerobic metabolism or uncoupling of oxidative phosphorylation should be detectable by suitable instrumentation. Such a system has been developed to detect and identify narrow-band and line spectra associated with abnormal tissue states. These signals in a physiologic situation are superimposed on the broad-band (black-body) radiation of the skin or organ surface along with the far-infrared spectral pattern of cellular water and carbon dioxide. The desired signals are somewhat analogous to the Fraunhofer lines of the solar spectrum due to absorption in the sun's mantle. The approach differs from conventional infrared thermography in that the strategy is to analyze the spectral pattern rather than to determine the energy level within a specified wavelength. A Fourier interferometer, which is about the size of a bread box, is used to scan the patient at the bedside. The recorded interferogram is then transmitted by a time-shared system over telephone lines to a computer for Fourier transform and a signature analysis. Emission power spectral density tracings have been obtained from human limbs as well as other tissues and superficial carcinomas. Cross-correlation techniques have been used to establish significant differences. Alterations in infrared emission spectra reflect changes in tissue metabolism from analysis of the frequencies of radiation corresponding to molecular vibrations and rotations. Although highly experimental, this is a good example of monitoring at the business end of the oxygen transport chain.

Biosensors are an emerging technology that combines advances in biology and electronics to produce devices capable of measuring minute quantities of substances within the body. The term refers to a broad base of devices that will enable the detection, in vivo and in vitro, of a variety of physiologic parameters that were previously either impossible to acquire or could be obtained only with difficulty. Additionally, these devices are likely to provide data in real time, so that biological activity can be continuously monitored—and on a remote basis if so desired. They will also be used for closed-loop drug-administration systems that deliver medication automatically in direct response to body requirements.

Biosensors generally rely on a selective mechanism such as an enzyme or antibody to selectively detect a substance or react with it to determine and quantify its presence. When the chemical or biologic detector is attached to a transducer, the chemical reaction is converted into electronic signals and passed along to a monitor. The electronic signal is proportional to the concentration of a substance within the body.

Biosensors offer the potential not only for detecting and quantifying the presence of various substances within the body but also for regulating the action of implantable devices that could deliver drugs or electrical charges selectively to various sites. Theoretically, in addition to the pacemaker-control function, coronary vasodilators could be delivered through a closed-loop system measuring myocardial oxygen consumption in angina. A barosensor implanted within the vascular system could measure blood pressure, causing release of antihypertensive medication from a reservoir implanted within the body in cases of severe hypertension, thus affording optimal control compared with present methods. Arrhythmias theoretically could be better controlled by pharmacologic means if medication could be immediately released from an internal reservoir at the instant one developed. Individuals known or thought to be at risk of acute sudden death are also likely to benefit from this type of technology.

Bibliography

Basic Monitoring

Baek SM, Brown RS, Shoemaker WC: Early prediction of acute renal failure and recovery. *Ann Surg* 177:253, 1973.

Band JD, Maki DG: Infections caused by arterial catheters used for hemodynamic monitoring. *Am J Med* 67:735, 1979.

Bedford RF: Wrist circumference predicts the risk of radial-arterial occlusion after cannulation. *Anesthesiology* 48:377, 1978.

Bedford RF, Wollman H: Complications of percutaneous radial-artery cannulation: An objective prospective study in man. *Anesthesiology* 38:228, 1973.

Brown RS, Babcock R, et al: Renal function in critically ill postoperative patients: Sequential assessment of creatinine, osmolar and free water clearances. *Crit Care Med* 8: 68, 1980.

Davis FM, Stewart JM: Radial artery cannulation: A prospective study in patients undergoing cardiothoracic surgery. *Br J Anaesth* 5241, 1980.

Dunea G, Freedman P: Renal clearance studies. *JAMA* 205:170, 1968.

Espinel CH: The FeNa test. *JAMA* 236:579, 1976.

Gardner RM, Schwartz R, et al: Percutaneous indwelling radial-artery catheters for monitoring cardiovascular function: Prospective study of the risk of thrombosis and infection. *N Engl J Med* 290:1277, 1974.

Hermreck AS: The pathophysiology of acute renal failure. *Am J Surg* 144:605, 1982.

Hilberman M, Meyers BD, et al: Acute renal failure following cardiac surgery. *J Thorac Cardiovasc Surg* 77:880, 1979.

Lucas CE: The renal response to acute injury and sepsis. *Surg Clin North Am* 56:953, 1976.

Maki DG, Hassemer C: Endemic rate of fluid contamination and related septicemia in arterial pressure monitoring. *Am J Med* 70:733, 1981.

Miller TR, Anderson RJ, et al: Urinary diagnostic indices in acute renal failure. *Ann Intern Med* 89:47, 1978.

Shoemaker WC: Monitoring of critically ill patient, in Shoemaker WC (ed): *Textbook of Critical Care*. Philadelphia, Saunders, 1984, pp 905–120.

Stott RB, Cameron JS, et al: Why the persistently high mortality in acute renal failure? *Lancet* 2:75, 1972.

Vo NM, Savino JA, et al: The automated renal profile. *J Clin Engr* 8:4, Oct–Dec 1983.

ABG and Pulmonary Monitoring

Agarwal NR, Savino JA, et al: The automated metabolic profile. *Crit Care Med* 11:546, 1983.

Askanazi J, Norderstrom J, et al: Nutrition for patients with respiratory failure: Glucose vs. fat. *Anethesiology* 54:373, 1981.

Askanazi J, Rosenbaum SJ, et al: Respiratory changes induced by the large glucose loads of parenteral nutrition. *JAMA* 243:1444, 1980.

Bland R, Shoemaker WC, Czor LSC: Evaluation of the biological importance of various hemodynamic and oxygen transport variables. *Crit Care Med* 7:424, 1979.

Bone RC: Diagnosis of causes for acute respiratory distress by pressure-volume curves. *Chest* 70:740, 1976.

Bone RC: Monitoring respiratory function in the patient with adult respiratory distress syndrome, in Decker BC (ed): *Adult Respiratory Distress Syndrome. Seminars in Respiratory Medicine*. Vol 2, 1981, p 140.

Bone RC: Treatment of respiratory failure due to advanced obstructive lung disease. *Arch Intern Med* 140:1018, 1980.

Danek SI, Lynch JP, et al: The dependence of oxygen uptake on oxygen delivery in the adult respiratory distress syndrome. *Am Rev Respir Dis* 22:387, 1980.

Downs JB, Douglas ME: Assessment of cardiac filling pressure occurring in continuous positive pressure ventilation. *Crit Care Med* 8:285, 1980.

Fox MG, Brady JS, Weintraub LR: Leukocyte larceny: A case of spurious hypoxemia. *Am J Med* 676:742, 1979.

Gilbert F, Keightley JF: The arterial/alveolar oxygen tension ratio: an index of gas exchange applicable to varying inspired concentrations. *Am Rev Respir Dis* 109:142, 1974.

Luterman A, Horowitz JH, et al: Withdrawal from positive end-expiratory pressure. *Surgery* 83:328, 1978.

Newell JC, Shah DM, et al: Pulmonary pressure-volume relationships in traumatized man. *J Surg Res* 26:114, 1979.

Peabody JL, Willis MM, et al: Clinical limitations and advantages of transcutaneous oxygen electrodes. *Acta Anesth Scand* (suppl) 68:76, 1978.

Popovich J, Bone RC, et al: Mass spectrometry. *Respir Ther* 10:50, 1980.

Sahn Sa, Lakshminarayan S: Bedside criteria for discontinuation of mechanical ventilation. *Chest* 63:1002, 1973.

Savino JA, Dawson J, et al: The metabolic cost of breathing in critical surgical patients. *J Trauma* 25:1126, 1985.

Savino JA, Vo N, et al: Monitoring respiratory complications in critically ill patients. *Infect Surg* 2(8):585, August 1983.

Savino JA, Vo NM, et al: Automated respiratory profile. *J Clin Engr* 9(1): Jan–Mch 1984.

Savino JA, Vo NM, et al: Systemic organ assessment using computerized profiles. *Med Instrum* 17(6):433, 1984.

Shimada Y, Yoshiga I, et al: Evaluation of the progress and prognosis of adult respiratory distress syndrome: Simple physiologic measurement. *Chest* 76:180, 1979.

Suwa K, Hedley-White J, Bendixen HH: Circulation and physiological dead space changes on controlled ventilation of dogs. *J Appl Physiol* 231:1855, 1966.

Sweet SJ, Glenney JP, et al: Effect of acute renal failure and respiratory failure in the surgical intensive care unit. *Am J Surg* 141:492, 1981.

Tremper KK, Waxman K, et al: Transcutaneous oxygen monitoring during arrest and CPR. *Crit Care Med* 8:377, 1980.

Tremper KK, Waxman K, Shoemaker WC: Effects of hypoxia and shock on transcutaneous PO_2 values in dogs. *Crit Care Med* 7:526, 1979.

Turney SZ, McAslan TC, Cowley RA: The continuous measurement of pulmonary gas exchange and mechanics. *Ann Thorac Surg* 13:229, 1973.

Versmold HT, Linderkamp O, et al: Limits of the $tCPO_2$ monitoring in sick neonates: Relation to blood pressure, blood volume, peripheral blood flow and acid base status. *Acta Anaesth Scand* (suppl) 68:88, 1978.

Wagner PD: Diffusion and chemical reaction in pulmonary gas exchange. *Physiol Rev* 57:257, 1977.

Wagner PD, West JB: Effects of diffusion impairment on O_2 and CO_2 time courses in pulmonary capillaries. *J Appl Physiol* 33:62, 1972.

Wagner PD, Saltzmann HA, West JB: Measurement of continuous distributions of ventilation-perfusion ratios: Theory. *J Appl Physiol* 36:588, 1974.

West JB, Wagner PD: Pulmonary gas exchange, in West JB (ed): *Bioengineering Aspects of the Lung*. New York, Marcel Dekker, 1977.

Wilson RS: Monitoring the lung: Mechanics and volume. *Anesthesiology* 45:135, 1976.

Zwillich CW, Pierson DJ, et al: Complications of assisted ventilation. *Am J Med* 57:161, 1974.

Cardiovascular Response to Acute Illness

Abraham E, Bland RD, et al: Sequential cardiorespiratory patterns associated with outcome in septic shock. *Chest* 85:65, 1983.

Aubier M, Viires N, et al: Respiratory muscle contribution to lactic acidoses in low cardiac output. *Am Rev Respir Dis* 126:648, 1982.

Braunwald E: Heart failure, in Wintrobe MM, Thorn G, Adams R et al (eds): *Harrison's Principles of Internal Medicine*, 7th ed. New York, McGraw-Hill, 1974, pp 1117–25.

Bursztein S, Taiterman U, et al: Reduced oxygen consumption in catabolic states with mechanical ventilation. *Crit Care Med* 6:162, 1978.

Cain SP: Peripheral oxygen uptake and delivery in health disease. *Clin Chest Med* 4:139, 1983.

Clowes GH, Del Guercio LRM, Braiunsky J: The cardiac output in response to surgical trauma. *Arch Surg* 81:212, 1960.

Connors AF Jr, McCafree DR, Gray BA: Evaluation of right-heart catheterization in the critically ill patient without acute myocardial infarction. *N Engl J Med* 308:263, 1983.

Cryan L, Ledingham IM: Significance of blood lactate in intensive care. *Intensive Crit Care Dig* 5:15, 1986.

Danek SJ, Lyncy JP, et al: The dependence of oxygen uptake on oxygen delivery in the adult respiratory distress syndrome. *Am Rev Respir Dis* 122:387, 1980.

Dawkins KD, Jamieson SW, et al: Long-term results, hemodynamics and complications after combined heart and lung transplantation. *Circulation* 71:919, 1985.

Enger EA: Cellular metabolic response to regional hypotension and complete ischemia in surgery. *Acta Chir Scand* (suppl) 178:481, 1977.

Finch CA, Lenfant C: Oxygen transport in man. *N Engl J Med* 268:407, 1972.

Forrester JS, Diamond G, et al: Filling pressures in the right and left sides of the heart in acute myocardial infarction: A reappraisal of central-venous pressure monitoring. *N Engl J Med* 285:190, 1971.

Greene NM: Lactate, pyruvate and excess lactate in anesthetized man. *Anesthesiology* 22:404, 1961.

Laver MB, Strauss HW, Pohost GM: Right and left ventricular geometry: Adjustments during acute respiratory failure. *Crit Care Med* 7:509, 1979.

Lowenstein E, Teplick R: To (PA) catheterize or not to (PA) catheterize—that is the question (editorial). *Anesthesiology* 53:361, 1980.

MacLean LD, Mulligan WG, et al: Patterns of septic shock in man—a detailed study of 56 patients. *Ann Surg* 166:543, 1967.

Rhodes GR, Newell JC, et al: Increased oxygen consumption accompanying increased oxygen delivery with hypertonic mannitol in adult respiratory distress syndrome. *Surgery* 84:490, 1978.

Robin ED: Of men and mitochondria: Coping with hypoxic dysoxia. *Am Rev Respir Dis* 122:517, 1980.

Schwager O, Howland WS, et al: The effect of ether and halothane on blood levels of glucose, pyruvate, lactate and metabolites of the tricarboxylic acid cycle in normotensive patients during operation. *Anesthesiology* 28:814, 1967.

Shoemaker WC: Cardiorespiratory patterns in complicated and uncomplicated septic shock: Physiologic alterations and their therapeutic implications. *Ann Surg* 174:119, 1971.

Shoemaker WC, Appel P, et al: Pathogenesis of respiratory failure (ARDS) after hemorrhage and trauma: 1. Cardiorespiratory patterns preceding the development of ARDS. *Crit Care Med* 8:504, 1980.

Shoemaker WC, Priten KJ, et al: Hemodynamic patterns after acute anesthetized and unanesthetized trauma. *Arch Surg* 95:492, 1967.

Shoemaker WC, Montgomery Ed, et al: Physiologic patterns in surviving and nonsurviving shock patients. *Surg Gynecol Obstet* 152:633, 1981.

Sibbald WJ: Myocardial function in the critically ill: Factors influencing left and right ventricular performance in patients with sepsis and trauma. *Surg Clin North Am* 65:867, 1985.

Silverman WA: *Retrolental fibroplasia: A Modern Parable*. New York, Grune & Stratton, 1980.

Waxman K, Nolan LS, Shoemaker WC: Sequential perioperative lactate determination. Physiological and clinical implications. *Crit Care Med* 10:96, 1982.

Waxman K, Lazrove S, Shoemaker WC: Physiologic responses to operation in high risk surgical patients. *Surg Gynecol Obstet* 152:633, 1981.

Weil MH, Nishijima H: Cardiac output in bacterial shock. *Am J Med* 64:920, 1978.

Wilmore DW, Aulick LH: Systemic response to injury and the healing wound. *J Parenter Enterol Nutr* 4:147, 1980.

Wilson RF, Thal A, et al: Hemodynamic measurements in septic shock. *Arch Surg* 91:121, 1963.

Cardiovascular Monitoring

Alderman EL, Glantz SA: Acute hemodynamic interventions shift the diastolic pressure-volume curve in man. *Circulation* 54:662, 1976.

Archer G, Cobb LA: Long term pulmonary artery pressure monitoring of mixed venous oxygen saturation in critically ill patients. *Anest Analg* 61:513, 1982.

Baele PL, McMichan JC, et al: Continuous monitoring of mixed venous oxygen saturation in critically ill patients. *Anest Analg* 61:513, 1982.

Birdman H, Haq A, et al: Continuous monitoring of mixed venous oxygen saturation in hemodynamically unstable patients. *Chest* 86:753, 1984.

Civetta JM: Continuous mixed venous saturation: Neither too little nor too much. *Soc Crit Care Med* (panel). May 1985, Chicago.

Civetta JM: Critical illness: The nonsteady state. *Surg Forum* 23:153, 1972.

DeCampo T, Civetta JM: The effect of short-term discontinuation of high-level PEEP in patients with acute respiratory failure. *Crit Care Med* 7:47, 1979.

Elliott CG, Zimmerman GA, Clemmer TP: Complications of pulmonary artery catheterization in the care of critically ill patients: a prospective study. *Chest* 76:647, 1979.

Feliciano DV, Mattox KL, et al: Major complications of percutaneous subclavian vein catheters. *Am J Surg* 138:869, 1979.

Forrester JS, Diamond G, et al: Filling pressures in the right and left sides of the heart in acute myocardial infarction: A reappraisal of central-venous pressure monitoring. *N Engl J Med* 285:190, 1971.

Gore JM, Sloan K: Use of continuous monitoring of mixed venous saturation in the coronary care unit. *Chest* 86:757, 1984.

Hynes JB, Carson SD, et al: Positive end-expiratory pressure shifts left ventricular diastolic pressure-area curves. *J Appl Physiol* 48:670, 1980.

Jamieson WRE, Turnbull KW, et al: Continuous monitoring of mixed venous oxygen saturation in cardiac surgery. *Can J Surg* 25:538, 1982.

Jernigan WR, Gardner WC, et al: Use of the internal jugular vein for placement of central venous catheter. *Surg Gynecol Obstet* 130:520, 1970.

Kazarian KK, Del Guercio LRM: The use of mixed venous blood gas determinations in traumatic shock. *Ann Emerg Med* 9:179, 1980.

Nelson LD: Continuous venous oximetry in surgical patients. *Ann Surg* 203:329, 1986.

Pinilla JC, Ross DF, et al: Study of the incidence of intravascular catheter infection and associated septicemia in critically ill patients. *Crit Care Med* 11:21, 1983.

Puri VK, Carlson RW, et al: Complications of vascular catheterization in the critically ill: A prospective study. *Crit Care Med* 8:495, 1980.

Qvist J, Pontoppidan H, et al: Hemodynamic responses to mechanical ventilation with PEEP: The effect of hypervolemia. *Anesthesiology* 42:54, 1975.

Roy R, Powers SR Jr, et al: Pulmonary wedge catheterization during positive end-expiratory pressure ventilation in the dog. *Anesthesiology* 46:385, 1977.

Shasby DM, Daube IM, et al: Swan Ganz catheter location and left atrial pressure determine the accuracy of the wedge pressure when positive-end-expiratory pressure is used. *Chest* 80:666, 1981.

Swan HJC, Ganz W, et al: Catheterization of the heart in man with use of a flow-directed balloon-tipped catheter. *N Engl J Med* 283:447, 1970.

Todd TRJ, Baile EM, Hogg JC: Pulmonary arterial wedge pressure in hemorrhagic shock. *Am Rev Respir Dis* 118:613, 1978.

Tooker J, Huseby J, Butler J: The effect of Swan-Ganz catheter height on the wedge pressure-left atrial pressure relationship in edema during positive-pressure ventilation. *Am Rev Respir Dis* 117:721, 1978.

Waller JL, Bauman DI, Craver JM: Clinical evaluation of a new fiberoptic catheter oximeter during cardiac surgery. *Anesth Analg* 61:676, 1982.

Watson CB: The PA catheter as an early warning system. *Anesth Rev* 10:34, 1983.

West JB, Dollery CT, Naimark A: Distribution of blood flow in isolated lung: Relation to vascular and alveolar pressures. *J Appl Physiol* 19:713, 1964.

Zapol WM, Snider MT: Pulmonary hypertension in severe acute respiratory failure. *N Engl J Med* 296:476, 1977.

Cardiac-Output Determinations—Invasive Monitoring

Askanazi J, Koenigsberg DI, et al: Echocardiographic estimates of pulmonary artery wedge pressure. *N Engl J Med* 305:1566, 1981.

Civetta JM: Cardiopulmonary calculations: A rapid, simple and inexpensive technique. *Intensive Care Med* 3:209, 1977.

Cohn JD, Engler PE, Del Guercio LRM: The automated physiologic profile. *Crit Care Med* 3:51, 1975.

Del Guercio LRM: Contrast dilution analysis. *Trans NY Acad Sci* 33:387, 1971.

Del Guercio LRM, Cohn JD: Monitoring methods and significance. *Surg Clin North Am* 56:977, 1976.

Ganz W, Swan HJC: Measurement of blood flow by thermal dilution. *Am J Cardiol* 29:241, 1972.

Shabot MM, Shoemaker WC, State D: Rapid bedside computation of cardiorespiratory variables with a programmable calculator. *Crit Care Med* 5:105, 1977.

Shoemaker WC, Chang P, et al: Cardiorespiratory monitoring in postoperative patients: II Quantitative therapeutic indices as guides to therapy. *Crit Care Med* 7:243, 1979.

Siegel JH, Fabian M, et al: Clinical and experimental use of thoracic impedance plethysmography in quantifying myocardial contractility. *Surgery* 67:907, 1970.

Siegel JH, Greenspan M, et al: A bedside computer and physiologic nomograms: Guides to the management of the patient in shock. *Arch Surg* 97:480, 1968.

Weissler AM, Harris WS, Schoenfield CD: Bedside techniques for the evaluation of ventricular function in man. *Am J Cardiol* 23:577, 1969.

Cardiac-Output Determinations—Noninvasive Monitoring

Berger HJ, Davis RA, et al: Beat-to-beat left ventricular performance assessed from the equilibrium cardiac blood pool using a computerized nuclear probe. *Circulation* 63:133, 1981.

Bourguignon MH, Wagner HN Jr: Noninvasive measurement of ventricular pressure throughout systole. *Am J Cardiol* 44:466, 1979.

Hansen RM, Viquerat CE, et al: Poor correlations between pulmonary arterial wedge pressure and left ventricular end-diastolic volume after coronary artery bypass graft surgery. *Anesthesiology* 64:764, 1986.

Kay HR, Afshari M, et al: Measurement of ejection fraction by thermal dilution techniques. *J Surg Res* 34:337, 1983.

Marushak GF, Schauble JF: Limitation of thermodilution ejection fraction degradations of frequency response by catheter mounting of fast-response thermistors. *Crit Care Med* 13:679, 1985.

Natanson C, Fink MP, et al: Gramnegative bacteremia produces both severe systolic and diastolic cardiac dysfunction in a canine model that simulates human septic shock. *J Clin Invest* 78:259, 1986.

Parrillo JE, Burch C, et al: A circulating myocardial depressant substance in humans with shock. *J Clin Invest* 76:1539, 1986.

Strashun A, Horowitz S, et al: Noninvasive detection of left ventricular dysfunction with a portable electrocardiographic gated scintillation probe device. *Am J Cardiol* 47:610, 1981.

Vincent JL, Thirion M, et al: Measurement of right ventricular ejection fraction with a modified pulmonary artery catheter. *Intensive Care Med* 12:33, 1986.

Wagner N: Monitoring ventricular function at rest and during exercise with a nonimaging detector. *Am J Cardiol* 43:975, 1979.

Wagner HN Jr: Use of the nuclear stethoscope to monitor ventricular function. *Practical Cardiol* 7:113, 1981.

Preoperative Assessment

Agarwal N, Shibutani K, et al: Hemodynamic and respiratory changes in surgery of the morbidly obese. *Surgery* 92:226, 1982.

Alexander JK, Peterson KL: Cardiovascular effects of weight reduction. *Circulation* 45:310, 1972.

Babu SC, Sharma PV, et al: Monitor-guided responses. *Arch Surg* 115:1384, 1980.

Babu SC, Shah PM, Clauss RH: Unappreciated causes of ischemia in the leg. *Am J Surg* 144:225, 1982.

Barrera F, Reidenberg MM, Winters WL: Pulmonary function in obese patients. *Am J Med Sci* 254:785, 1967.

Catenacci AJ, Anderson JD, Boersma D: Anesthetic hazards of obesity. *JAMA* 175:657, 1961.

Clowes GHA Jr, Del Guercio LRM, Barowinsky J: The cardiac outpatient in response to surgical trauma. *Arch Surg* 81:212, 1960.

DeAngelis J, Chang P, et al: Hemodynamic changes during prostectomy in cardiac patients. *Crit Care Med* 10:38, 1982.

Del Guercio LRM, Savino JA, Morgan JC: Physiologic assessment of surgical diagnosis-related groups. *Ann Surg* 212:519, 1985.

Del Guercio LRM, Cohn JD: Monitoring operative risk in the elderly. *JAMA* 243:1350, 1980.

Douglas FG, Chong PY: Influence of obesity in peripheral airway patency. *J Appl Physiol* 33:559, 1972.

Dremick EJ, Bole GS, et al: Assessing mortality and causes of death in morbidly obese men. *JAMA* 243:443, 1980.

Graham JP Jr, Covel JW, et al: Control of myocardial oxygen consumption: Relative influence of contractile state and tension development. *J Clin Invest* 47:374, 1968.

Grindlinger GA, Vegos AM, et al: Volume loading and vasodilators in abdominal aortic aneurysmectomy. *Am J Surg* 139:480, 1980.

Jabbour I, Savino JA, et al: Pneumatic antishock garments detrimental in elderly with diminished myocardial reserve. *Curr Surg* November–December 43:498, 1986.

Kaufman BJ, Ferguson MH, Cherniak RM: Hypoventilation in obesity. *J Clin Invest* 38:500, 1959.

Prem KA, Menshala MN, McKelvey JL: Operative treatment of endometrium in obese women. *Am J Obstet Gynecol* 93:16, 1965.

Rochester DF, Enson NY: Current concepts in the pathogenesis of the obesity-hypoventilation syndrome: Mechanical and circulatory factors. *Am J Med* 57:402, 1974.

Savino JA, Del Guercio LRM: Preoperative assessment of high risk surgical patients, *Surg Clin North Am* 65:763, 1985.

Savino JA, Agarwal N, et al: Invasive preoperative hemodynamic monitoring superior to clinical risk factors in predicting ICU stay. *Crit Care Med* (abstract), April 1986.

Savino JA, Jabbour I, et al: Overinflation of pneumatic antishock garments (PASG) detrimental in elderly. *Am J Surg.* (In press.)

Schultz RJ, Whitfield GF, et al: Role of physiologic monitoring in patients with hip fractures. *J Trauma* 25:309, 1985.

Vaughn RW, Engelhardt RC, et al: Postoperative hypoxemia in obese patients. *Ann Surg* 180:877, 1974.

Vaughn RW, Wise L: Intraoperative arterial oxygenation in obese patients. *Ann Surg* 184:35, 1976.

Monitoring of Tissue Metabolism

Cohn JD, Del Guercio LRM, et al: Infrared emission spectroscopy from human limbs. *Proc 25th Conf Engineering Med Biol* 1972, p 55.

Cohn JD, Del Guercio LRM, et al: Infrared spectral analysis of metabolic function. *Fed Proc* 31:350, 1972.

Del Guercio LRM, Cohn JD, et al: Noninvasive assessment of cellular function and organ perfusion, in *Advances in Automated Analysis: Diagnostic Medicine, Biomedical Profiling,* vol 2. Tarrytown, NY, Mediad, 1973.

Kreisberg RA: Lactate homeostasis and lactic acidosis. *Ann Intern Med* 92:227, 1980.

Laks H, Dmochowski JR, Couch NP: The relationship between muscle surface pH and oxygen transport. *Ann Surg* 183:193, 1976.

Owens G, Belmusto L, Woldring S: Experimental intracerebral PO_2 and PCO_2 monitoring by mass spectroscopy. *J Neurosurg* 30:110, 1969.

Shoemaker WC, Vidyasagar D (eds): Symposium issue, transcutaneous 02 and CO2. Monitoring of the adult and neonate. *Crit Care Med* 9:689, 1981.

Woldring S, Owens G, Woolford DC: Blood gases: Continuous in vivo recording of partial pressures by mass spectroscopy. *Science* 153:885, 1966.

Chapter 14

Skin and Subcutaneous Tissue

R. Christie Wray, Jr.

PHYSIOLOGY

The skin, which is the largest organ in the body, represents more than a structure covering vital organs and separating them from the environment. It is a complex organ that possesses unique physical properties and physiologic functions.

Physical Properties

Both *tension* and *elasticity* are physical properties that are related to structural macromolecules, collagen, and elastin within the skin. Tension is the characteristic that accounts for the fact that the skin resists stretching by weak forces; the maximal deforming force that is resisted by the skin, expressed in dynes per centimeter, is a measurement of tension. Tension varies in different areas and is most marked where the skin contains dense elastic fibers, particularly in regions where the skin is thin. The direction of the tension also varies anatomically and forms the basis of the line system described by Langer in 1861. The tension of skin is greater in young than in elderly patients. Elasticity refers to the skin's ability to resume its original shape after an external force has been applied to cause deformation. This also varies with age, being less in the elderly and also in patients with edema.

Quantification of the physical properties of the skin has been made by determining the *tensile strength,* or the resistance of skin to tearing under tension. The average tensile strength of the adult skin, without fat, is approximately 1.8 kg/m². This is significantly reduced in infants up to three months of age, and the lowest values are found in multiple forms of the Ehlers-Danlos syndrome, which is characterized by a reduction of elastic fibers and collagen defects. In patients with Cushing's syndrome or those taking high doses of cortisone for prolonged periods of time, the tensile strength of skin is significantly less than normal, and there is also a low modulus of elasticity.

The electrical behavior of skin has been the subject of much investigation. The skin generates polarization currents that provide great resistance to external electric forces. The intensity of imposed current passing through the skin is therefore very low. The skin also offers a resistance to alternating currents by its property of impedance.

Functions of Skin

Important physiologic functions of skin include (1) percutaneous absorption, (2) an important role in the circulatory system, (3) serving as an organ of senses, (4) secretion of sweat, (5) providing an avenue for the insensible loss of water, and (6) contributing to thermal regulation.

PERCUTANEOUS ABSORPTION. This refers to the penetration of substances through the skin, permitting them to enter the bloodstream. The stratum corneum is the major barrier to diffusion. It has been shown that radioactive water, applied either as a vapor or as a solution, appears in both the circulation and the urine. If the skin is warmed after exposure, the concentration in the urine increases rapidly. Electrolytes applied to the skin in aqueous solution either do not penetrate or may enter in small amounts via the appendages. The skin is impermeable to sodium and calcium when these are applied to the skin in the form of a chloride solution. However, there is some evidence that the iodide ion may enter the skin either because it increases the negative electric charge of skin or because it penetrates via appendages. When radioactive electrolytes are rubbed onto the skin, they are absorbed, and the absorption is increased if the skin is abraded or has been shaved.

Lipid-soluble substances are fairly rapidly and completely absorbed through the skin, and absorption appears to be faster if the substances are also soluble in water to some degree. In the latter instance, the penetration is so rapid that the rate of absorption is comparable with gastrointestinal absorption and even absorption of the material injected subcutaneously. The percutaneous absorption of phenol has been recognized for many years, and fatal poisoning may be associated with the application of carbolic acid to large areas of skin. Salicylic acid also penetrates with great ease from alcoholic and aqueous solutions as well as from ointments. Estrogenic hormones, testosterone, progesterone, and deoxycorticosterone all penetrate the intact skin rapidly. Hydrocortisone may be therapeutically effective by percutaneous application, while cortisone acetate applied locally is poorly absorbed. Water-soluble hormones, which are large-molecule proteins, generally are not absorbed. Lipid-soluble vitamins are absorbed with ease, while water-soluble vitamins do not penetrate the skin. Heavy metals may be absorbed to some extent.

Substances in the gaseous form, with the exception of carbon monoxide, penetrate the skin easily. Oxygen, nitrogen, and carbon dioxide are examples of gases that perfuse readily. Carbon tetrachloride is also readily absorbed through the skin. The absorption of pharmaceutic agents through the skin has been employed by using dimethyl sulfoxide as a vehicle.

CIRCULATION AND VASCULAR REACTIONS. The cutaneous vascular system is extremely complex and contributes significantly to the general circulation and vascular reactions. Direct visualization of flow in minute vessels can be carried out by observing the capillary circulation of the base of the nail. The color of the skin, which is related to melanin and carotene pigments, is also dependent upon the quantity of blood in the subpapillary plexus of vessels, particularly in the Caucasian. The skin temperature depends chiefly on the rate of flow through the whole skin. The range of pressure in human skin capillaries is between 12 and 45 mmHg, and the average capillary pressure is equivalent to the colloid osmotic pressure of plasma proteins. Arteriovenous anastomoses of digital skin play an important role in temperature regulation and are implicated in the formation of the glomus tumor.

Local vascular responses may result from direct action on the vessel wall or its contractile elements. Local vasoconstriction follows gentle stroking. If the mechanical stimulus is of greater intensity than that which causes constriction, a red local reaction may develop secondary to dilatation of small vessels. Circumscribed superficial edema of the skin in areas responsive to stimuli is referred to as a "wheal" and is due to leakage of plasma from dilated blood vessels into the extracellular space. There are two distinct steps in the formation of the wheal: (1) local dilatation and (2) increased capillary permeability. Stimulation of the sympathetic fibers supplying the skin causes vasoconstriction of the cutaneous vessels, while interruption of these fibers results in dilatation of the small arteries and arterioles. The cutaneous circulatory system also responds to chemical agents. Acetylcholine causes vasodilatation, while norepinephrine and epinephrine are important vasoconstricting drugs. Vasopressin is also an active vasoconstrictor. Nicotinic acid and nitrites cause flushing and warmth, increased temperature, and increased blood flow. Smoking paradoxically results in decreased blood flow to the skin. This decrease becomes most significant in patients undergoing an operation involving large skin flaps or digital replantation. In both groups of patients gangrene is more common in chronic heavy smokers. For an elective operation, if the patient stops smoking for as little as 1 week the likelihood of skin flap gangrene will decrease. Ergot alkaloids act as vasodilators by their sympatholytic action, but the drugs also directly constrict the muscles of the peripheral arterioles, and the net effect is a decrease in blood flow.

SENSORY FUNCTION. The skin's sensory functions pertain to the modalities of pain (including itching), touch, and temperature. Skin consists of a mosaic of multiple sensitive spots, the relative density of which varies with the region of body. Cold sensitivity is probably mediated by Krause's end bulbs, whereas Ruffini's endings are probably receptors for warmth. Meissner's corpuscles and Merkel's discs are implicated in the tactile sensation, and the Pacinian corpuscles are involved in the sensation of pressure. Pain is mediated by free nonmyelinated endings, which are in a plexiform arrangement. Following injury to the skin, there is a widespread area of hyperalgesia that radiates from the point of injury. A striking condition of increased pain and sensitivity accompanied by cutaneous vasodilatation may occur after nerve injury.

Originally described after injury of major nerves and called causalgia, it is now known to occur after injury to small unnamed branches following simple laceration or skin incision and is usually called reflex sympathetic dystrophy. In modern series, the most common cause of reflex sympathetic dystrophy is a prior operation (correction of carpal tunnel syndrome in the upper limb). Cure of the condition may be difficult; the cornerstone of success is early recognition and the institution of physical and occupational therapy. Intensive active use of the limb appears to be particularly beneficial. For more advanced cases, regional sympathetic nerve blockade (stellate ganglion for the upper limb) and intraarterial or intravenous reserpine may be used. If the condition is relieved by a stellate ganglion block but recurs despite repeated blocks, sympathectomy is frequently curative.

SWEAT SECRETION. The skin contains two types of sweat glands, eccrine glands, which are small sweat glands, and apocrine, or large, sweat glands. The eccrine glands are distributed all over the body and are the true secretory glands that produce clear, aqueous sweat responsible for heat regulation. The apocrine glands in the human being are almost rudimentary structures. If the environmental temperature rises above 31 or 32°C (90°F), there is a sudden outbreak of visible sweating over the entire body. The insensible sweat secretion constitutes one part of the total insensible water loss.

The distribution of sweat glands is such that the highest number per square inch are located in the palms and soles and are also more dense on the dorsum of the hand, forehead, and trunk. There are fewer glands in the lower extremity than in the upper extremity. In most instances, sweating is almost exclusively the result of nervous impulses, but the glands are able to respond directly to application of heat if it is sufficiently intense. The nonnervous sweat response is strictly limited to the local area of stimulation. The nervous response is almost entirely mediated over sympathetic nerves and results from the pharmacologic action of parasympathetic substances. The nerve fibers to the sweat glands liberate acetylcholine at their endings upon stimulation. Atropine and other anticholinergics block the receptor sites so that they are unable to respond and thus interfere with secretion. Hyperhidrosis (increased sweating) may result from an abnormal increase in nerve impulses as in central nervous system lesions or emotional states. Increased tonicity of the sweat fibers may intensify the sweat response to normal nervous and nonnervous stimuli.

Primary hyperhidrosis usually presents as excessive sweating noted early in life. Mild cases can be managed with anticholinergic drugs and antiperspirant creams. Sympathectomy at T_2 to T_4 or T_5 abolishes eccrine sweating in the involved areas of the upper extremity. A modified Hurley-Shelley operation is used for axillary hyperhidrosis. The hair-bearing axillary skin is excised, and the ganglia at T_2 and T_3 are removed for accompanying hand sweating.

Eccrine sweat is a clear aqueous solution containing 99 percent water and 1 percent solids, half of which are inorganic salts and half organic compounds. Under normal circumstances it is hypotonic, but at high rates of sweating it depends on material within the bloodstream; it is not a simple ultrafiltrate of plasma but represents an active secretion. The concentration of sodium and chloride is lower than that in plasma, while the concentration of potassium is somewhat higher. The concentration of chloride depends on many factors and is usually in the range of 15 to 60 meq/L. The sodium concentration is almost always entirely equivalent to that of chloride and varies in a parallel fashion. Chloride and sodium concentrations rise with prolongation of sweating and with the rate of sweating and temperature of the skin. The salt concentration of sweat also depends on the intake, and an adequate supply of drinking water depresses the concentration. The loss of potassium through the skin ranges between 2.7 and 3.1 meq/L.

Nitrogen compounds are also lost transdermally, and the concentration of urea in sweat is twice as high as that in the blood. Creatinine is present in sweat in only a minute amount, and amino acids have also been noted. Ammonia is a primary constituent of sweat, and it can be concentrated by the sweat glands with nearly the same efficiency as the renal excreting unit. Large amounts of lactic acid and lactate have been demonstrated in sweat, particularly during heavy muscular exercise and in association with thermogenic sweat. The concentrations are ten to twenty times higher than that in the blood, and it is felt that the lactic acid originates from breakdown of glycogen within the sweat glands.

Sweat provides the skin with an "acid mantle." The average pH of freshly secreted sweat is 5.7 to 6.4. As the sweating progresses, the acidity decreases, but considerable amounts of acid are still lost with profuse thermal sweating. There is increasing acidity with evaporation of water from the sweat. The acidity modulates the growth of many bacteria that reside in the inner keratin layers, glands, and hair follicles.

In contrast to the eccrine glands, which develop as separate downgrowths from separate anlagen in fetal epidermis, the apocrine glands are formed from follicular epithelium, as are sebaceous glands. Like sebaceous glands and hair follicles, the apocrine glands have major development during puberty. They are greater in number in females and respond to autonomic nervous stimulation rather than thermal stimulation. They function by producing a somewhat viscous milklike droplet.

INSENSIBLE WATER LOSS. Sweat secretion provides but one of two separate mechanisms contributing to insensible loss of water through continuous evaporation that occurs at all environmental temperatures. The other mechanism is that of loss through the epidermis which, unlike sweat secretion, is not affected by atropinization. Water loss through the epidermis is contrasted with sweat because it does not contain salts or other solutes. The total insensible water loss through skin and lungs is constant under basal conditions and amounts to about 200 g/m² every 24 h, 60 percent of which is cutaneous loss. Total cutaneous water loss in the adult at rest without visible sweating is about 500 to 700 mL daily. The insensible loss from both the skin and the lungs shows a linear relationship to the basal metabolic rate. Water intake has no effect on cutaneous loss in the adult but does increase it in children. In hypothyroidism, the water loss is conspicuously low, whereas in thyrotoxicosis, total insensible perspiration is greatly increased. The stratum corneum acts as the rate-determining layer.

THERMOREGULATION. The skin plays an important role in the regulation of body temperature. Heat is lost through the skin under the processes of radiation, convection, conduction, and evaporation. Sweating is a useful process only when the sweat can evaporate. It is therefore very efficient as a regulatory mechanism in a dry, hot environment, but with increased humidity the efficiency decreases markedly. Humidity begins to be of importance between 30 and 31°C (86 to 88°F) air temperature, at which point the difference between 50 and 100 percent relative humidity decides whether the person will be comfortable or hyperthermic. If heat production is raised or atmospheric temperature is raised, there is a shift of blood flow from the interior to the skin. The converse is also true, and this process is carried out reflexly.

Cold stimuli of a moderate degree result in the production of pallor. After the stimulus has ceased, there is reactive arterial vasodilatation. Cold stimuli of long duration are associated with livid discoloration as a result of paresis in the venous limbs of the capillaries. With extreme stimuli, there may be a reddish discoloration due to dilatation of the arterioles. The condition, however, is not associated with increased blood flow, and skin temperature does not rise. Further cooling causes the skin to become frostbitten. The reduction in temperature is also accompanied by interference with the utilization of oxyhemoglobin. Immersion foot, or "trench foot," occurs when the skin is exposed for long periods of time to cold water. There is vasoconstriction and capillary damage, and if the skin's temperature is returned to normal rapidly, reactive hyperemia and blistering result. Thrombosis may complicate the situation. Exposure to the cold (frostbite or immersion foot) should be treated by immersion of the involved portion of the limb in water at a temperature of 40°C. The role of sympathectomy early in the course of frostbite has been debated.

Heat exhaustion refers to a syndrome characterized by excessive loss of salt and water when people are exposed to high temperatures. A sweat retention syndrome has been recognized among troops in hot, humid climates. The common name "heat stroke" may be applied either to heat exhaustion or to the sweat retention syndrome. In the latter situation, the high humidity prevents the effective cooling of the body by evaporation of sweat. The patients develop exhaustion, headache, palpitation, dizziness, and confusion. Moderate hyperthermia may progress to extreme hyperthermia and death if environmental conditions are unchanged and insufficient salt and water intake persists. Treatment is immediate cooling by evaporation (pouring water on the victim and fanning) or by the application of ice. Simultaneously, intravascular volume replacement with fluids is indicated.

PRESSURE SORES

Pressure on an area of skin for 2 or more hours, particularly in patients with impaired nutritional status, may result in sufficient ischemia to cause a decubitus ulcer. The ulceration usually occurs over bony prominences. Preventive measures include a nutritive diet, correction of anemia, and relief of pressure over the area. Routinely turning the patient and using special mattresses is effective. Surgical therapy is indicated in most patients who are generally suitable for rehabilitation. This requires sharp debridement to excise the ulcer and underlying fascia and necrotic material. The bony prominence frequently requires modification; the aim is to remove the most prominent portion of the bone, thereby increasing the surface area and decreasing the pressure. Enough bone is removed to maximize the surface area of the remaining bone. Following hemostasis, the bony prominence is usually covered with a flap. Recently myocutaneous flaps have gained popularity. The muscular portion may be more effective in treating infected bone. The popularity of myocutaneous flaps compared with skin flaps is due to the lower necrosis rate of the former.

HIDRADENITIS SUPPURATIVA

This is a chronic acneform infection of the cutaneous apocrine glands, subcutaneous tissue, and fascia. It is generally confined to areas in which these glands are found, namely, the axilla, areola of the nipple, groin, perineum, and circumanal and periumbilical regions. The disease was first described by Velpeau in 1839, and clinical manifestations vary with the duration of the lesion. At first, there is a slight subcutaneous induration, and as the lesion enlarges, the process advances to the skin, which becomes inflamed and adherent. Suppuration eventually develops, and cellulitis surrounds the abscess. At this stage, pain is often severe. Incision and drainage at this point result in a few drops of thick, viscous, purulent material. The process may subside after 2 or 3 days, only to recur. In the chronic stage, the patient presents with multiple painful cutaneous nodules that coalesce and are surrounded by fibrous reaction. The pathologic picture is a combination of that seen in acute pyogenic infection and chronic inflammation of the skin, but involvement of the apocrine glands establishes the diagnosis. Culture of the pus yields a variety of saprophytic and pathogenic bacteria with a preponderance of staphylococci and streptococci.

Cures can be achieved early in the course of the disease by improved hygiene and incision and drainage. Mild cases respond to high dosages of tetracyclines. Once the chronic inflammation and pattern of recurrent, acute inflammation is established, curative treatment can be obtained only by operation. Complete excision of the involved area is necessary. In the axilla, advancement flaps combined with adduction of the arm obtain better results than skin grafting. Localized areas in the perineum can also be treated by excision and advancement flap or primary closure. More extensive areas require split-thickness skin grafting.

CYSTS

Epidermal Inclusion Cyst

When the epithelium of the skin is trapped subdermally as a result of trauma or for other reasons, it may continue to grow and desquamate. This creates a cyst lined by epidermal cells and filled with keratin and desquamated cells (Fig. 14-1). The cysts may occur anywhere in the body, but the vast majority of patients who desire removal have cysts on the head and neck. Occasionally cysts on the hand limit the ability to make a fist. If the cyst becomes infected, incision and drainage is indicated. Incision and drainage is temporarily beneficial, but cyst elements usually persist and repeat infection is likely. Both for the noninfected cyst and for those previously infected, cure is effected by complete removal of the cyst.

Sebaceous Cyst

Sebaceous glands are most numerous on the face and in the midline of the trunk, and they are generally associated with hair follicles and a keratinizing epithelium. They produce sebum, an oily material, which serves as a natural dressing for the hair and skin. If the exit of sebum is blocked, the material accumulates and a cyst is formed. True sebaceous cysts are very rare. In 15 years of practice I have removed over 1000 epidermal (or keratinous) cysts, but not a single sebaceous cyst. Sebaceous cysts are often incorrectly diagnosed; the presence of glandular epithelium lining is necessary for the diagnosis.

Dermoid Cyst

This is usually a congenital lesion that does not manifest until early childhood. The primary clinical differentiation between dermoid and epidermal cysts is age of presentation. Dermoid cyst present in the first few years of life and epidermal inclusion cysts appear in early to late adulthood. Cutaneous openings connecting to the cyst are somewhat more common in epidermal than in dermoid cysts. Dermoid cysts generally occur in the midline of the body, the lateral eyebrow (Fig. 14-2A and B), on the scalp over the occiput, on the nose, and in the abdominal and sacral regions. They are considered to be occlusion cysts, taking their origin from an embryonic process. Although it has been suggested that malignant degeneration may occur, no authentic case has been reported. Surgical excision is the treatment of choice. Communication of the dermoid with the central nervous system is extremely rare in any location but more common with those located in the nasal region. For this reason a CT scan should be obtained preoperatively before excision of a nasal dermoid.

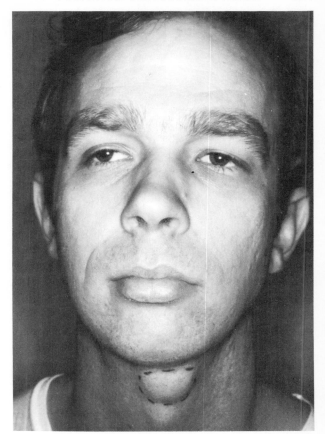

A

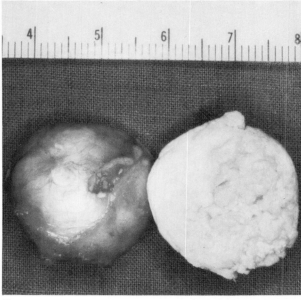

B

Fig. 14-1. *A.* Epidermal inclusion cyst. Subepidermal swelling in anterior neck is marked. *B.* Cut cross section of lesion on left and external surface of lesion on right.

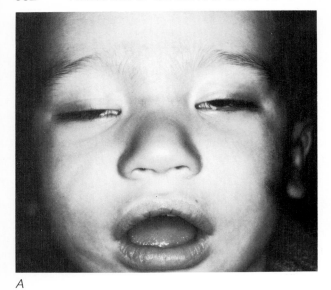

A

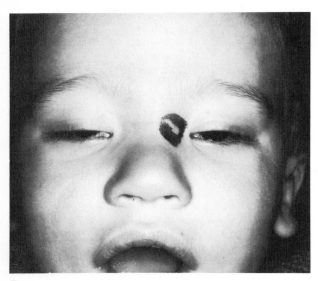

B

Fig. 14-2. *A.* Dermoid cyst. Note slight asymmetry of medial canthal region. *B.* Site of subepidermal mass marked.

Pilonidal Cyst and Sinus

These are common malformations that occur over the sacrococcygeal region. Their origin is associated with the neurenteric canal, and it is thought that their development is related to blockage of a congenital coccygeal sinus that is a vestige of this canal. This is substantiated by evidence that some of the pilonidal cysts and sinuses result from penetration of local skin by growing hairs (Fig. 14-3*A* and *B*). The ingrowth of such hairs sets the stage for cyst formation and repeated infection. The lesions may often be present from birth but are usually not manifest until the late adolescent or early adult years. The disease has been referred to as "jeep-driver's disease," and it is

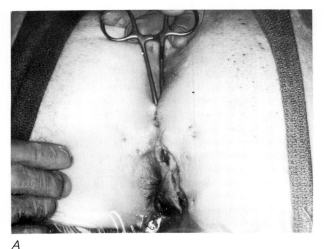

A

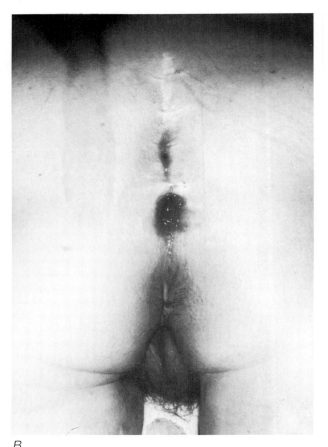

B

Fig. 14-3. *A.* Typical interconnecting pilonidal disease with a clamp showing site of interconnection. *B.* Pilonidal disease recurrent despite six operations.

thought that the bumpy driving merely aggravates a congenital condition. Histologically, both the cysts and sinuses are lined with the stratified squamous epithelium.

The clinical manifestations vary from a barely perceptible dimple at the superior end of the buttock crease to an obvious sinus tract or cyst at this site. The sinus may chronically drain or become infected. The cyst also gradually increases in size and is susceptible to secondary infection. There have been rare reports of escape of cerebrospinal fluid from the pilonidal sinuses and equally rare instances of meningitis resulting.

TREATMENT. If the cyst is acutely infected, tender, and erythematous, incision and drainage are indicated. Secondary removal of the cyst or sinus is then planned after the infection has subsided. Elective surgical removal must be complete, and methylene blue may be injected as a guide to determine the extent of arborization of the sinus tract. Following excision of the sinus, closure may be accomplished either primarily or by granulation and epithelialization from the wound margins. If there is obvious infection, it is preferable to leave the wound open, unroofing all the tracts and allowing it to heal by secondary intention. In some instances, a very thin split-thickness graft (0.008 to 0.01 in.) may be used to achieve early closure. The thin skin graft permits the desirable contracture of the wound that accompanies the open technique. Primary closure of skin and subcutaneous tissue is usually successful for previously untreated patients. For treatment of recurrent lesions three additional approaches are useful. Simple gluteus muscle advancement and closure in the midline, gluteous myocutaneous flaps, or a z-plasty procedure to move the scar out of the midline are procedures of choice.

Ganglia

Ganglia are areas of mucoid degeneration of retinacular structures. They are tense, subcutaneous cystic masses occurring most commonly over the dorsum of the wrist and over tendon sheaths of the hands and feet (Fig. 14-4). They grow very slowly and are usually associated with only minimal discomfort. The lesions consist of a wall of collagenous tissue that may or may not have synovial cells. The cysts contain thin clear collagenous fluid similar to joint fluid. They have been related to trauma, either accidental or occupational.

Aspiration of the ganglion or deliberate rupture by the physician are temporarily effective but usually associated with about a 75 percent recurrence rate. The recurrence rate after iatrogenic rupture is very low for palmar ganglia or ganglia arising from the digital flexor sheath. For the latter lesions, destruction of the ganglion with a needle is usually curative. Surgical excision after exsanguination and application of a tourniquet to permit precise dissection is curative for the other ganglia. The ganglia that are closely adherent to a tendon sheath are relatively easy to remove, but those that communicate with the synovium of a joint require excision of a portion of the joint capsule to protect against recurrence.

BENIGN TUMORS

Warts

The common wart, or verruca vulgaris, is caused by a variety of viruses and is both contagious and autoinoculable (Fig. 14-5A and B). Lesions may occur on any part of the body but are most common on the hand and the soles of the feet. They appear as circumscribed intraepidermal tumors that may be elevated or flat. Verruca plantaris (plantar wart) is the most troublesome variety and is located on the soles of the feet in the region of the metatarsal heads or over the os calcis. These warts may become quite tender and painful.

Verruca vulgaris may be treated by a variety of simple methods including freezing with liquid nitrogen, and caustic agents, e.g., 40% salicylic acid plaster. In general, however, electrodesiccation under local anesthesia is the most efficacious treatment. All treatments have been fol-

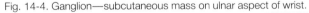

Fig. 14-4. Ganglion—subcutaneous mass on ulnar aspect of wrist.

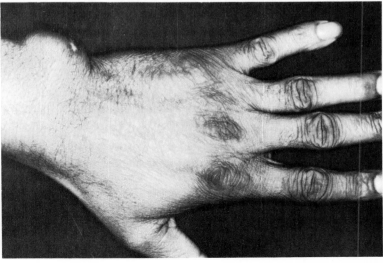

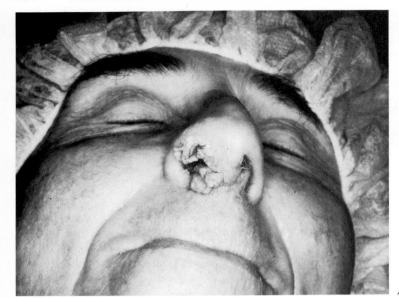

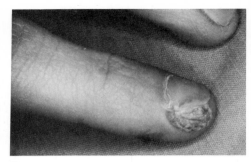

A

Fig. 14-5. *A.* Verruca vulgaris. Rough-surfaced lesion on inferior aspect of alar rim and columella. *B.* Recurrent verruca vulgaris on radial aspect of index finger after 10 previous attempts at removal.

lowed by a finite rate of recurrence due to the infectious nature of the lesion. The symptoms of plantar warts may be relieved by using pads or metatarsal bars to remove direct weight bearing from the wart area. Chemotherapy and surgical paring have also been used, and injection of local anesthesia into the base of the wart has achieved some success. Hyfercation has been very effective. It is difficult to evaluate therapy of these lesions, since the clinical course is extremely variable and spontaneous disappearance, formation of daughter warts, and recurrence challenge conclusions.

Keratosis

This represents hypertrophy of the epidermis and is considered a precancerous lesion. Clinical classification includes senile keratosis, arsenical keratosis, and seborrheic keratosis.

Senile keratoses develop most commonly in individuals with fair complexion and characteristically present as multiple lesions in the sixth, seventh, and eighth decades. Lesions proved benign by biopsy may be treated with liquid nitrogen, trichloracetic acid, topical 5-fluorouracil, or electricodesiccation. Lesions suspected of being malignant should be treated by surgical excision.

Seborrheic keratoses (Fig. 14-6) develop in middle-aged or older people as multiple lesions occurring chiefly on the trunk. They appear as thickened areas and are usually brown but may be gray or black. They are often great in number and may be confluent. The darker lesions have been mistaken for melanotic tumors. Histologically, they may be differentiated from senile keratoses and remain benign. Treatment is usually conservative, employing shaving and electrocoagulation.

Fig. 14-6. Seborrheic keratoses: pigmented, greasy lesions that, when solitary, may be mistaken for melanotic tumors.

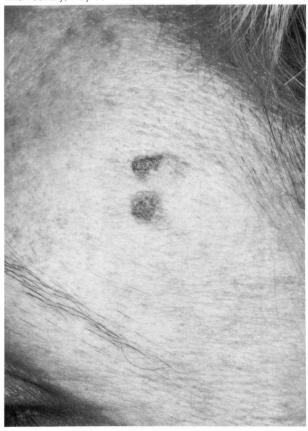

Keloid

The term is derived from the Greek word meaning "crab's claw" and refers to a dense accumulation of fibrous tissue that extends above the surface of the skin and also circumferentially beyond areas that were originally traumatized or incised and sutured. Keloids are usually erythematous in their early stages and hyperpigmented in the later stages (Fig. 14-7). Current research indicates the defect is a failure of collagen breakdown and not an increase in collagen production. Keloids are most common in blacks and progressively less common in Orientals, dark-skinned Caucasians, and light-skinned Caucasians. Keloids may occur anywhere in the body but are frequent in the skin over the shoulder and sternum particularly in young females. Because of their visibility, keloids on the head and neck are frequently presented for treatment. Keloids distal to the knee are rare and those of the palm and soles extremely rare. Recurrence following simple excision is common.

The first line of treatment of keloids or hypertrophic scars is steroid injection. Steroid injection is effective in relieving the burning and itching sensation and may produce actual shrinkage of the lesion. The most definitive treatment is excision combined with steroid injection at the time of operation and postoperatively. Formerly, intralesional excision (leaving a margin of keloid unexcised) was recommended. No data support intralesional excision, however. Admonitions against subcuticular sutures are voiced, but no study has clearly demonstrated them

Fig. 14-7. Keloid of ear originally following small laceration on helical rim. Three previous attempts at removal.

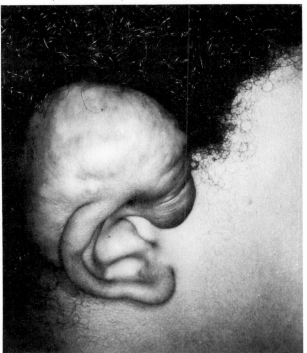

detrimental. If primary closure is not possible, split-thickness skin grafting may be needed. The use of postoperative radiation therapy is controversial. No controlled study has demonstrated benefits from postoperative radiation therapy. Knowledge of the long-term ill effects of radiation has mandated against its use in recent years.

Vascular Tumors

Classically the terminology of vascular tumors has been quite confusing. Different authors have used the same name for different lesions. Recently Mulligan has developed a more rational classification based on the endothelial features of cutaneous vascular tumors. This has allowed division into two major categories based on the rate of endothelial turnover. Hemangiomas are vascular tumors with increased endothelial turnover during their proliferative phase; they may have a normal endothelial turnover during their stable or involutional phase. Vascular malformations are tumors with a normal endothelial cell turnover rate throughout their lifetime.

CAPILLARY (PORT WINE) MALFORMATION

The lesion is made up of closely packed, dilated abnormal capillaries in the subpapillary, dermal, or subdermal region of the skin. Clinically, there is no elevation or contour change but rather a reddish or purplish patch of staining (Fig. 14-8). Growth parallels that of the involved area. If the lesion is small, it may be treated by excision and closure with excellent results. Larger lesions, however, are most difficult to treat, since the entire dermis is involved and excision results in a contour defect and scar. Argone laser treatment is currently accepted as the most useful for larger lesions. Results have ranged from marked to minimal improvement. The degree of improvement seems to increase when there are more vessels located just beneath the skin and the lesion is more nearly purple than pink. Owing to the development of hypertrophic scarring, laser treatment is generally recommended only in patients older than 14 years.

HEMANGIOMA (STRAWBERRY MARK) (Fig. 14-9)

This appears in infancy and undergoes a remarkable change with the growth of the child. The lesion generally enlarges, sometimes quite dramatically, during the first several months to 1 year, subsequent to which spontaneous regression usually occurs. Clinically, immature hemangiomas are raised and irregular, with some bright-red areas. They are compressible and may show superficial areas of opacity suggesting the beginning of regression. Regression takes the form of increasing opacity and whitening of the surface with progressive thickening and flattening. The hemangioma may become ulcerated if it is in an area subjected to trauma, but hemorrhage from these lesions is not common and is generally readily controlled by pressure. Such episodes of ulceration, minor hemorrhage, or superficial infection may actually hasten spontaneous resolution. Treatment in large part consists of

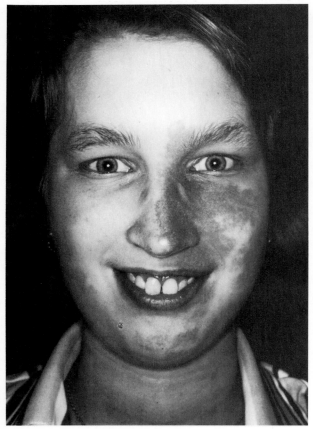

Fig. 14-8. Capillary (port wine) malformation. Note discoloration in forehead, nose, cheek, and upper lid area. Limited almost precisely to the midline.

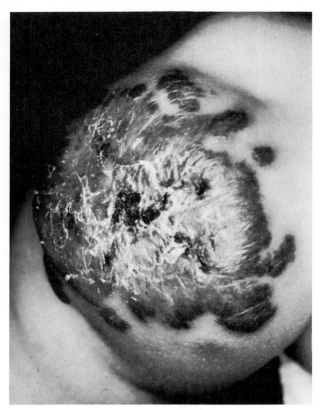

Fig. 14-9. Immature hemangioma (strawberry mark). Note opacification in the center. Lesion is undergoing spontaneous resolution.

reassuring the parents that spontaneous resolution will occur by about age seven in over 90 percent of the lesions. Rapidly growing tumors in childhood that involve the eyes, mouth, or ears may require treatment. These hemangiomas may stop expanding or regress on a high-dose oral prednisone regimen (2 to 3 mg/kg).

ARTERIOVENOUS MALFORMATION

These lesions have been called cavernous hemangiomas by many authors. The lesions are full-sized in proportion to the child at birth and do not undergo changes with rapid growth or spontaneous regression. They consist of mature vessels and may include multiple arteriovenous communications.

Arteriovenous malformations frequently involve deep tissues, such as muscles and even the central nervous system. They may also be combined with lymphatic malformation elements. Treatment of cavernous hemangiomas that invade deep to the subcutaneous tissue is extremely difficult. Wide local excision is the treatment of choice, but involvement of vital structures, particularly in the head and neck, frequently prevents complete excision. An encouraging new therapy involves preoperative embolization of feeding vessels using selective radiography followed by wide local excision. Despite this combination of techniques, incomplete excision is frequent. Incomplete excision almost inevitably leads to a recurrence equaling or exceeding the size of the original.

GLOMUS TUMOR

The glomus tumor is a benign, rare, and exquisitely painful small neoplasm of the skin and subcutaneous tissue occurring usually on the extremities and particularly in the nail beds of the hands and feet (Fig. 14-10). The tumor is derived from the glomic end organ apparatus consisting of arteriovenous anastomoses that function normally to regulate the blood flow in the extremity. The organ contributes to the regulation of local and general body temperature through the dissipation or conservation of heat.

The tumors vary in structure but resemble the normal glomus unit and have often been referred to as *angiomyoneuroma*. The layers of circular muscle of the vessels may be separated from the endothelium by collagenous membrane, or the endothelium may be bordered directly by the so-called glomus epithelioid cells. In some tumors, the blood vessels are so enlarged that they resemble true angiomas. The glomus cells are supplied by nonmyelinated nerve fibers, which accounts for the pain-

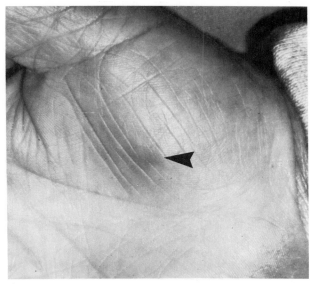

A

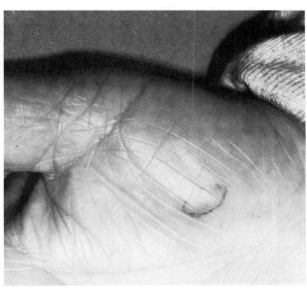

B

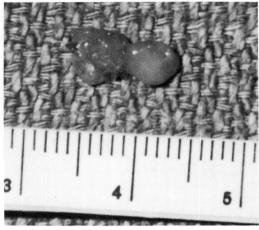

C

Fig. 14-10. *A.* Area glomous tumor—area of discoloration in proximal aspect of thenar eminence. *B.* Area of discoloration outlined. *C.* Cross section and external surface of tumor—scale in centimeters.

ful nature of the lesion. Although the tumor per se is benign, a malignant counterpart exists and is referred to as a *hemangiopericytoma.*

Glomus tumors are usually single, but a familial multicentric form, which is usually painless, occurs. The color varies from deep red to purple or blue, and there is variation in color with changes in temperature. The patients usually present in the fifth decade, but the tumor has been reported at all ages. The pain associated with the lesion is the most prominent symptom and may occur either spontaneously, with pressure, or in association with trauma. The pain, which is described as stabbing, lancinating, and radiating from the tumor, may be intermittent in character or may occur only when the lesion is touched. The glomus tumor is radioresistant. Encapsulated tumors may be shelled out, but when an obvious capsule is not seen, wide excision is indicated.

LYMPHATIC MALFORMATIONS

Lymphatic malformations are congenital in origin. The most common type is deep and cavernous, consisting of lymph-filled spaces with thin-walled septums and some areas of fibrosis. A superficial variant presents as circumscribed lesions that appear as small blisters and slightly elevated skin patches. When deep lesions are present in the neck, mediastinum, and axilla, they are referred to as *cystic hygroma* (see Chap. 39) (Fig. 14-11). The treatment is surgical excision which, although frequently incomplete, is rarely associated with recurrence. As with arteriovenous malformations, if the lymphatic malformation invades deep to the subcutaneous tissue, complete excision is virtually impossible. Truly massive lymphangiomas may be impossible to cure.

Dermatofibroma

This is actually a subepidermal nodular fibrosis that occurs chiefly on the extremities and may be related to trauma. Most patients, however, are unable to remember any specific episode of trauma. The tumor presents as a small nonpainful nodule, and the overlying epidermis may be pigmented in such a manner that the lesion is often mistaken for malignant melanoma (Fig. 14-12). The treatment is surgical excision.

Fat Tumors

LIPOMA

This is an extremely common subcutaneous lesion composed of fat and at times difficult to distinguish from the normal subcutaneous adipose tissue. Usually, how-

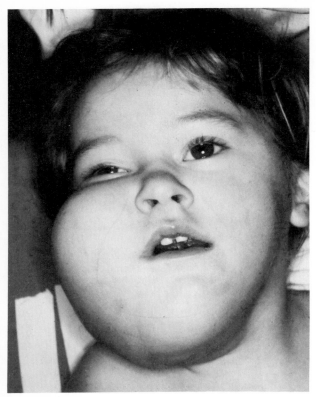

Fig. 14-11. Lymphangioma, diffuse enlargement of inferior one half of right cheek and upper neck.

ever, there is a thin, fibrous capsule, and the lesion can be enucleated from surrounding normal fat. Benign lipomas occur more frequently over the back, between the shoulders, and on the back of the neck, and liposarcomatous transformation is extremely uncommon. Treatment is surgical excision.

Fig. 14-12. Dermatofibroma—darkly pigmented intradermal mass.

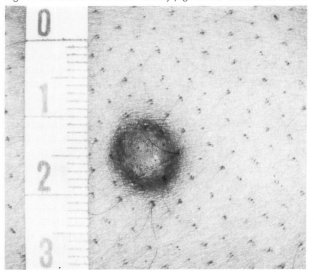

WEBER-CHRISTIAN DISEASE

This is an uncommon inflammatory lesion of the subcutaneous fat characterized by painful reddened areas involving the panniculus. The diagnosis is made by biopsy and is based on the presence of inflammatory cells in the adipose tissue. Many lesions so classified represented facticial dermatitis or skin manifestations of fat necrosis associated with pancreatitis.

Neural Tumors

Neurilemmoma and neurofibroma are the two benign tumors of neural origin. Neurilemmomas arise from the sheath cell of Schwann. Neurofibromas contain the element of peripheral nerves, neurons, Schwann cells, fibroblasts, and perineural cells. Neurilemmomas frequently arise from relatively small nerves and do not produce much pain. Treatment is surgical excision. Neurofibromas may be multiple and may be associated with von Recklinghausen's disease, including café au lait spots and scoliosis. Patients with neurofibromatosis are prone to develop meningiomas, gliomas, and pheochromocytomas; eventual sarcomatous degeneration occurs in approximately 10 percent.

MALIGNANT TUMORS

Carcinoma of the skin occurs predominantly in exposed areas, most frequently in weather-beaten skin. Factors indicted as causes of skin cancer are ultraviolet light, ionizing radiation, chemicals such as tars and pitch, and immunologic and genetic defects. It is generally a low-grade malignant tumor that may metastasize late, in which case the metastasis is usually to regional lymph nodes, so that curability is high compared with that of other tumors.

Basal Cell Carcinoma

This is a localized malignancy that grows slowly, at times taking 1 or more years to double in area. Basal cell carcinoma is more common than the squamous cell tumor, accounting for at least three-fourths of all cases in most clinical series. Lesions may be found over most areas of the body and are waxy, grayish yellow, pink, or translucent, often with telangiectasia below the surface (Fig. 14-13A and B). About 75 percent of basal cell carcinomas are located on the head and neck, 10 percent on the trunk, and 15 percent on the limbs. In some instances, the tumors are darkly pigmented and difficult to distinguish from melanoma (Fig. 14-13B). Basal cell carcinoma may extend deeper subcutaneously than is initially apparent, and extensive ulceration into the deep tissue without marked induration or infiltration has been referred to as rodent ulcer. If the tumor is not treated, it may erode into the deep structures including the skull, orbit, or brain. Less commonly, basal cell carcinoma may appear fungoid and grow large externally.

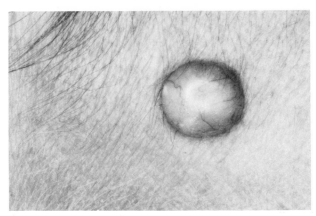

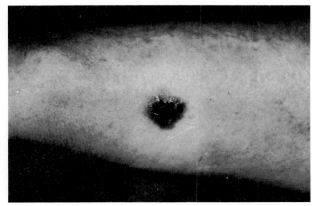

A

B

Fig. 14-13. *A.* Basal cell carcinoma of cheek—even more typical is a depressed center. *B.* Pigmented basal cell carcinoma. Note characteristics of melanotic tumor.

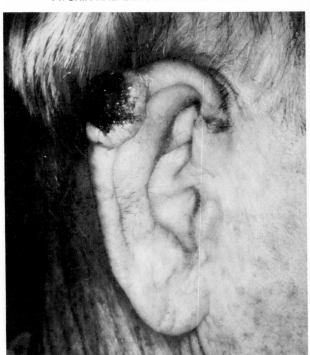

Fig. 14-14. Typical squamous cell carcinoma of ear with raised rolled edges and evidence of recent hemorrhage.

Squamous Cell Carcinoma

Squamous cell carcinoma presents in a fashion quite similar to basal cell carcinoma. Either may present as a nodule with a translucent surface and telangiectasia. Ulceration may occur in both lesions. Squamous cell carcinoma tends to grow more rapidly, and if an accurate history can be obtained, this may allow differentiation on a clinical basis. Biopsy is necessary for accurate differentiation. Squamous cell carcinoma is both relatively and absolutely less common on the head and neck than is basal cell carcinoma. About 65 percent of squamous cell carcinoma occurs on the head and neck, 30 percent on the limbs, and 5 percent on the trunk (Fig. 14-14).

The primary lesion of the squamous cell carcinoma is occasionally surrounded by satellite nodules, and central ulceration may occur. The degree of induration around the lesion is significant. The center gradually deepens into a crater with an irregular base that is covered by crust. Small pearls may be expressed from the ulcer, and rolled margins surrounding the ulcer contribute to the lesion's resembling a small volcanic crater. Growth may be superficial, or the lesion may burrow into deeper tissue with minimal effect on the cutaneous surface. Squamous cell carcinoma is more malignant than the basal cell variety and will metastasize to regional glands more rapidly.

Squamous cell carcinoma is particularly common in the lip at the vermillion border and in the folds of the paranasal area or in the axilla. Lesions occur more frequently in blond individuals with thin, dry skin that is subjected to frequent irritation by rubbing or shaving. Squamous cell carcinoma is also particularly likely to originate in actinic keratosis, atrophonic epidermis, xeroderma pigmentosa, or cutaneous horns, and it develops at the site of postradiation dermatitis and ulcerations in old burn scars (Marjolin's ulcer). The incidence is also higher in people exposed to arsenicals, nitrates, and hydrocarbons.

At times the appearance of *keratoacanthoma* mimics that of both squamous and basal cell carcinoma. Keratoacanthoma presents as a papule with a central keratinous plug and raised rolled edges (Fig. 14-15). Keratoacanthomas are probably derived from hair follicles and are most commonly located on the head and neck. Keratoacanthomas straddle the boundary between benignity and malignancy. The base of a classic-appearing keratoacanthoma may show changes of squamous cell carcinoma. Lacking such changes, local recurrence is possible but not distant metastasis. Although spontaneous resolution will occur in a small percentage of keratoacanthomas, owing to the possibility of malignant changes, surgical excision is the treatment of choice.

Bowen's disease is slowly growing squamous cell carcinoma in situ for which excision is recommended (Fig. 14-16). Adenoacanthoma, which frequently develops on

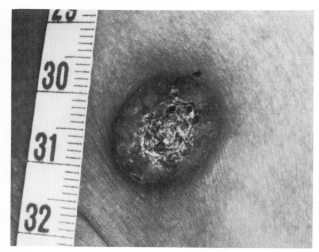

Fig. 14-15. Keratoacanthoma—typical lesion of trunk with keratinous plug surrounded by viable tissue.

the face or ear, is characterized grossly by a verrucous appearance and microscopically by desquamated cells. Local excision only is indicated, since it rarely metastasizes.

Sweat Gland Carcinoma

This rare tumor usually occurs in the sixth and seventh decades of life, but it has been reported in adolescents. Characteristically, a soft tissue mass has been present for

Fig. 14-16. Bowen's disease—erythematous plaque on ventral aspect of penile shaft.

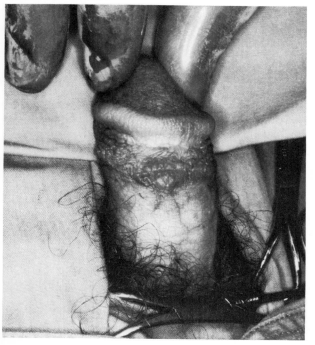

many years. Therapy consists of wide local excision with consideration of lymphadenectomy, since regional lymph nodes are involved in about half the cases. Following treatment, the reported 5-year survival is 38 percent for all patients and 24 percent for those with lymph node involvement.

TREATMENT. Electrodesiccation and Curettage. Electrodesiccation and curettage are applicable for superficial nonrecurrent basal cell carcinomas. Such treatment is not appropriate for squamous and other skin carcinomas. Electrodesiccation and curettage are performed under local anesthesia and consist of treating the surface of the lesion with electrocautery followed by scraping. Traditionally, this sequence is repeated three times at the same sitting. Healing is by secondary intention, and a hypopigmented scar results.

Cryosurgery. After a biopsy to provide diagnosis, cryosurgery, to cure the tumor, is applicable to those lesions treatable by curettage; for palliation it is also applicable to lesions that recur after radiation therapy or curettage. Anesthesia is usually not necessary because the liquid nitrogen freezes the nerve endings. The area treated should extend 2 to 3 mm beyond the margins of the lesion.

Chemosurgery. Mohs originally described a technique of serial excision using zinc chloride paste. His original technique has largely been abandoned and replaced by a fresh-frozen technique. In this technique the lesion is excised under local anesthesia and frozen sections are taken of the entire surface of resection. This is unlike conventional frozen section where only portions of the margin of resection are sampled. For recurrent carcinoma, four to five resections combined with examination of the margin of resection are usually necessary to obtain complete excision. The procedure is repeated until the margins show only healthy tissue. The advantage of this method is the possibility of eradicating small extensions of the central lesion with certainty. The granulation tissue below the lesion heals rapidly and becomes epithelialized. Mohs has achieved 93 percent cures for carcinoma of the skin in all locations on the surface of the body and 87.5 percent cures for carcinoma of the lip. Similar cure rates have been reported following radiation therapy or surgical excision of basal cell and squamous cell carcinoma. The results in *recurrent* basal cell or squamous cell carcinomas reported by Mohs are the best ever reported.

Radiation Therapy. Both basal and squamous cell carcinomas of the skin can be cured by this modality. The site of the lesion may constitute an indication for radiation therapy in that it may provide a better cosmetic result with less effort. It is less appropriate than surgical excision for cancers arising in burn scars or in previously irradiated regions and for tumors invading underlying cartilage or bone.

Surgical Therapy. The advantage of this approach is that the lesion can be completely removed and the extent of the tumor can be assessed. Surgical treatment for carcinoma of the skin should include complete excision of all malignant tissue and a sufficient margin of normal tissue. The acceptable margin of normal tissue to be removed at the margin of the cancer is controversial. Classic recommendations have been 0.5 cm about basal cell carcinomas, and 1 cm about squamous cell carcinomas. More recent evidence indicates that a margin of 3 mm around primary basal cell carcinomas and a margin of 0.5 cm about primary squamous cell carcinomas is sufficient. These margins must extend both laterally and in depth beyond the lesion. For recurrent lesions, the margins of 0.5 cm for basal cell carcinoma and 1 cm for squamous cell carcinoma are indicated. In recurrent lesions, frozen section or permanent section determination of tumor-free margins should precede definitive reconstruction. Primary closure is the treatment of choice. If the dimensions of the lesion physically prevent primary closure or if primary closure distorts normal features (particularly on the head and neck) additional reconstructive technique is useful. Local flaps are the first choice; additional reconstructive technique, at times full-thickness skin grafts, distant flaps, or free flaps may be necessary. Regional lymph-node dissection is performed only for clinical evidence of node involvement.

Treatment of patients with positive margins at the time of resection of basal cell carcinoma is controversial. Only about one-third of patients with positive margins after resection of basal cell carcinoma will ever develop recurrent tumor. If the patient is reliable in returning for follow-up, simple observation may be all that is indicated. If the patient is unreliable, resection of recurrent basal cell carcinoma or any squamous cell carcinoma demands treatment. Repeat surgical excision is usually the best treatment, but at times radiation therapy is indicated.

PROGNOSIS. This is difficult to evaluate, but recurrence rates are very low. A cure rate of about 99 percent for primary basal cell carcinoma should follow either surgical excision, radiation therapy, or electrodesiccation and curettage. About 80 percent of squamous cell carcinomas are cured by surgical excision and a somewhat lower percentage by radiation therapy. About 90 percent of recurrent basal cell carcinoma and 70 percent of recurrent squamous cell carcinoma can be cured by a repeat surgical excision. Mohs has reported about a 95 percent cure rate for recurrent basal cell carcinoma and a 75 percent cure rate for recurrent squamous cell carcinoma.

Other Tumors

Since the dermis has a mesodermal origin, it is logical that sarcomas should develop, and the skin represents the site of origin of 6 percent of all cases of sarcoma. Primary sarcomas vary in degree of malignancy and in histologic characteristics. Excision is associated with an overall incidence of recurrence of 61 percent.

FIBROSARCOMA

This occurs most commonly in women in the buttocks, thigh, and inguinal regions and it occurs particularly frequently in scars. The tumors are usually of relatively low-grade malignancy and are radioresistant. Wide surgical excision is the treatment of choice, but it is followed by a high incidence of recurrence. In one series, 56 percent survived 10 years without recurrence. Distant spread occurs in 25 percent.

HEMANGIOPERICYTOMA

This is a malignant tumor of angioplastic origin and is considered a malignant variant of the glomus tumor. The lesions are extremely malignant, and the prognosis is poor, with only 27 percent surviving 5 years without evidence of disease. Surgical excision has proved unsatisfactory for larger tumors, and x-ray therapy is considered the treatment of choice.

KAPOSI'S SARCOMA

The etiology and pathogenesis of this lesion have not been resolved. It occurs more commonly in men. In Western countries there is a predilection for Jews, Italians, and Prussians. The tumor is prevalent in equatorial Africa. A markedly increased incidence has been noted in homosexuals. Acquired immunodeficiency syndrome (AIDS) is not infrequently associated with Kaposi's sarcoma. Currently the majority of patients with Kaposi's sarcoma also have AIDS. The tumor usually starts in the hands or feet as multiple plaques that are reddish-to-purple and may be flat, ulcerated, or polypoid. The lymph nodes may be involved, and obstruction of the lymph nodes may result in lymphedema.

X-ray may retard the growth of the lesion, but wide surgical excision is also useful. A more extensive operation, such as amputation, is probably not warranted because the skin lesion is merely the manifestation of a systemic disease. Total body radiation followed by bone marrow transplantation is an occasionally successful experimental approach. Patients with florid lesions respond well to actinomycin D (dactinomycin). The prognosis is poor, although some cases have survived for prolonged periods of time. In the terminal stages, the tumor extends to the mucous membranes and portions of the gastrointestinal tract.

OTHER SARCOMAS

A wide variety of other tumors having origin in different cells has been described. Dermatofibrosarcoma protuberans represents one tumor with relatively low-grade malignancy that generally occurs on the trunk. The tumors are radioresistant but respond to surgical excision, and 70 percent have been reported to be free of the disease for at least 5 years. Widespread dissemination is rare, but local recurrence may occur repeatedly.

Lymphangiosarcoma is almost always associated with chronic lymphedema. A review included 186 cases; 162 cases occurred postmastectomy an average of 10 years after operation, with a range of 1 to 26 years. All patients had had radical mastectomy, and the overwhelming majority had received postoperative irradiation. Only 9 percent of the patients survived 5 or more years, and only 2 of 24 patients with nonpostmastectomy lymphangiosarcoma were alive at 5-year follow-up. Amputation gave significantly better results than radiation therapy.

MELANOMA AND OTHER PIGMENTED LESIONS

General Considerations

Since melanoma is a relatively uncommon disease, occurring in 0.0018 percent of the general population, while the average Caucasian adult has 15 to 20 nevi, it is obvious that removal of all moles is not advisable. On the other hand, about 25 percent of patients who have malignant melanoma recall having had a "mole" at the site of origin of the malignant lesion. Therefore, in dealing with pigmented lesions, the surgeon must be aware of characteristics that should arouse suspicion of malignancy or premalignancy.

Benign Pigmented Lesions

These include the intradermal nevus, or common mole, the junctional nevus, compound nevus, juvenile melanoma, and freckles. The *intradermal nevus* is characterized by nests of melanoblasts that are confined to the dermis. The lesions are smooth or papillary and rarely occur on the soles or palms. The presence of hair is strong presumptive evidence of the diagnosis. In the case of the *junctional nevus,* the proliferation of melanoblasts originates in the basal layer of the epidermis and extends down into the dermis. The lesions are smooth, flat, or slightly raised. They occur on the genitalia, soles, palms, nail beds, and mucous membranes. The *compound nevus* is formed from junctional and intradermal elements. It is smooth, elevated, occasionally papillary, and hairless. *Juvenile melanomas* are nevi that occur prior to puberty, and although the microscopic picture is similar to that of melanoma, the lesions are clinically benign. They may be purplish red, brown, or black; they are generally smooth and hairless with irregular edges. The majority occur on the face and enlarge slowly. *Freckles* occur most commonly in blond and red-headed people on exposed portions of their bodies and represent pigment in the basal layer and upper dermis. They are not of clinical significance.

DIFFERENTIAL DIAGNOSIS. Although the classic mole has a characteristic appearance, the differential between benign pigmented skin lesions, and melanoma may be quite difficult. Other lesions that cause particular confusion are (1) seborrheic and senile keratoses (Fig. 14-6) and (2) pigmented basal cell tumors (Fig. 14-13*B*). Small intradermal hematomas may have an appearance similar to melanomas, and subungual hematomas have been mistaken for melanomas. High-speed dental drills may force silver fillings into the buccal mucosa, and the appearance mimics that of melanoma.

TREATMENT. If the pigmented lesion is considered a junctional nevus, excision is advisable. Various characteristics of any pigmented lesions are indications for excision. These include change in color or pigment distribution; development of erythema; change in size or consistency; change in the surface characteristic, i.e., scaling, oozing, bleeding, crustings or erosion; subjective symptoms such as pain, numbness, burning, itching, diffusion of pigment into normal skin; satellite nodules; and regional lymphadenopathy.

The *Hutchinson freckle* (lentigo maligna) is worthy of special note. This is a circumscribed precancerous melanosis of the face, generally occurring in elderly people. There are two stages of disease: In the macular stage, the lesion is smooth and light brown with irregular borders and uneven color. About one-third of the lesions then evolve into a tumor stage characterized by induration and all the histologic features of melanoma, but the behavior is similar to the most superficial melanomas. The prognosis is excellent when the lesion is excised from the face, but it is guarded when the lesion is found in other body areas, in which case it should be treated as a melanoma. Excision of any suspicious lesion should be complete and should include a margin of normal skin.

Melanoma

By definition the term *melanoma* refers to a malignant lesion originating in the melanoblast of the skin. The tumor may develop in any area of the skin, mucous membrane, or pigmented region of the eye. There is almost an equal distribution between the head and neck, lower extremities, and trunk, each accounting for approximately 25 percent of cases. About 11 percent occur in the upper extremities, and the remainder involve the genitalia or represent cases in which the primary lesion is never determined. The typical skin lesion (Fig. 14-17) is darkly pigmented, smooth, firm, and nonhairy. Subungual melanomas in whites are more frequent than pigmented nevi in this region, but may be difficult to distinguish from subungual hematoma and chronic paronychial infection (Fig. 14-18). The presence of black stripes subungually is very unusual in whites, but is common in blacks. All melanomas originate from the melanoblast at the dermal-epidermal junction, but the cell does not contain melanin at all times, and therefore, some lesions may be amela-

Fig. 14-17. Typical malignant melanoma. Note central darkly pigmented elevation and surrounding halo of superficial satellite extensions. Sudden change in appearance and growth brought the patient to the doctor.

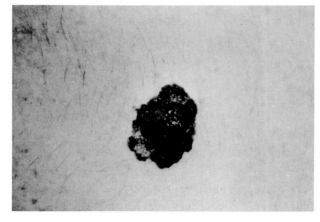

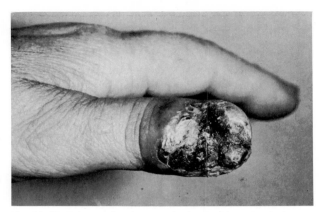

Fig. 14-18. Subungual melanoma. Lesion had been treated as an infection for nearly 1 year. Note pigmentation and replacement of nail. X-rays showed destruction of the distal phalanx. Axillary metastases were evident by this time.

notic. The cells are characterized by a dopa-positive reaction.

Microstaging has been determined by direct measurement, or according to Clark's levels of invasion (Fig. 14-19). Level I (in situ) applies when all tumor cells are above the basement membrane. Level II has tumor extension into the papillary but not the reticular dermis. Level III refers to tumor cells in the ill-defined interface between the papillary and reticular dermis. Level IV is characterized by tumor cells in the reticular dermis. Level V has invasion into the subcutaneous fat. Breslow introduced staging that uses an occulomicrometer. The

Fig. 14-19. Clark's levels of invasion. Papillary and reticular dermis of normal skin of the right upper arm; hematoxylin and eosin stain. The tissue just below the epidermis is pale and delicate, without obvious collagen bundles. Deep to this, collagen is organized into bundles, and the upper part of this zone forms an almost straight line with the papillary dermis (small arrows). Piling up of cells at this interface constitutes level III invasion. The arrows and their respective roman numerals indicate invasion levels. Level V (not shown) is into fat.

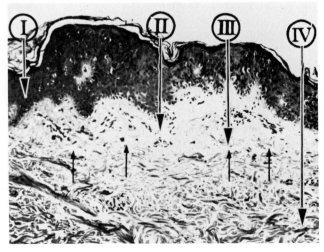

maximal thickness of the lesion is measured in slides from the top of the granular cell layer to the deepest point of invasion. If the lesion is ulcerated, the ulcer base over the deepest point of invasion is used rather than the top of the granular cell layer. The specific measurements should be recorded, but for staging purposes the lesions are categorized as (1) 0.75 mm or less, (2) 0.76 to 1.50 mm, (3) 1.51 to 3.0 mm, and (4) greater than 3.0 mm. Although both Clark's and Breslow's methods of tumor evaluation are generally reported, Breslow's technique has gained wider acceptance. Less interobserver variation of classification follows the use of Breslow's technique because of less subjective criteria. Breslow's classification is usually used for critical decisions about therapy.

Clinically, staging relates to the presence or absence of nodal and distal involvement. Stage I refers to a lesion with isolated skin involvement. Stage II refers to lesions with involvement of regional lymph nodes. Stage III includes lesions with distal metastases.

NATURAL HISTORY. There is a rising incidence of cutaneous melanoma and a consequent increase in mortality related to the lesion. Increased exposure to solar radiation in light-skinned races has been suggested as an explanation. The low incidence of melanoma in darkly pigmented races, and the tendency for the lesions in these individuals to develop in relatively nonpigmented areas, suggests that melanin may have a protective effect. Ultraviolet light is regarded as a stimulus that enhances the mitotic potential of melanocytes. In patients with xeroderma pigmentosum, a rare genetic recessive disorder associated with hypersensitivity to ultraviolet light, there is a marked increase in the incidence of epidermoid and basal cell carcinomas; melanoma develops in approximately 3 percent of patients.

The majority of melanomas are associated with a preexisting nevus or pigmented lesion. Over two-thirds of melanomas arise in a congenital mole or in a long-standing mole; only one-third appear de novo. Melanomas generally arise in those nevi that exhibit junctional activity. The junctional nevus, either alone or as part of a compound nevus, has been implicated more frequently than the pure intradermal nevus. The blue nevus is rarely the source of melanoma, and the development of malignancy in the small congenital hairy nevus is even more unusual. The incidence of malignant melanoma in giant pigmented nevi has been reported to vary between 0 and 44 percent. Although the exact incidence cannot be defined, the best available figure is about 8 percent. Nevi of the palms, soles, nail beds, genitalia, and mucous membranes retain functional elements that are more prone to be the source of melanoma than moles at other sites. In blacks the palms and soles are the most common sites of melanoma. Malignant melanoma rarely occurs in prepubertal children.

The histologic type of lesion affects the natural history. Four histologic types may be considered: (1) superficial spreading melanoma, (2) nodular melanoma, (3) lentigo maligna melanoma (melanoma arising in Hutchinson's freckle), and (4) acral-lentiginous melanoma. The latter

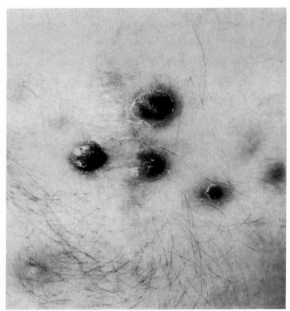

Fig. 14-20. Recurrent satellite nodules. These followed inadequate excision of a malignant melanoma that was thought to be a simple nevus. Note the characteristic deep-black color and emergence of lesions from the subcutaneous tissues to and through the skin.

may occur in the palms, soles, and subungual areas and has a histology similar to the lentigo maligna melanoma. Superficial spreading melanoma is characterized by intradermal spreading that may be present from 1 to 5 years before vertical dermal invasion occurs. It accounts for 60 to 70 percent of all cutaneous melanomas, and has an equal distribution in both sexes. Nodular melanoma, by contrast, has little radial growth, and the size of the lesion is smaller than that of the superficial spreading melanoma. It occurs most commonly on the back, the head, and the neck, and has a predilection for men; it accounts for about 12 percent of all melanomas. Lentigo maligna melanoma constitutes about 10 percent of all cutaneous melanomas, occurs in older age groups, and has the most indolent course. This lesion is twice as common in women. The histologic description of melanoma in the four categories given above has largely been supplanted by Breslow's measurement of tumor thickness. There is some cross correlation, however, and a nodular melanoma and superficial spreading melanoma of equal thickness do have different prognoses. The prognosis of nodular melanoma is significantly worse.

SURGICAL TREATMENT. Surgical excision represents the primary therapeutic modality in the treatment of skin lesions and metastases to regional lymph nodes. Surgical biopsy provides the definitive diagnosis, and permits evaluation of the depth of involvement. Excisional biopsy, with a margin of 2 to 5 mm, is indicated for most pigmented lesions. Incisional biopsy may be required for lesions that are extremely large, and there is no evidence to suggest that this increases the incidence of dissemination.

When all tumor cells are above the basement membrane level and the lesion can be categorized as Clark's Level I excisional biopsy with a very small margin of normal skin is all that is required. The ideal limits of excision of normal tissue about the melanoma have not been defined. Recent evidence indicates that for tumors less than 0.75 mm in thickness, a margin of 2 cm is certainly adequate; data currently being gathered may eventually demonstrate that a 0.5-cm margin is adequate. For lesions 0.76 to 1.5 mm in thickness, a 2-cm margin is probably adequate. For thicker lesions, a 4-cm margin is adequate. The need to remove the underlying fascia has not been resolved. To meet the requirements for wide excision, amputation of a digit is indicated when the lesion is located in the distal part of the finger or toe. When the lesion is located in the proximal half of the digit, disarticulation is performed at the level of the corresponding tarsometatarsal or carpometacarpal joint. The rate of local recurrence for clinical Stage I (Fig. 14-20) malignant melanomas of the limb is approximately 2 percent.

One of the points of contention about the treatment of melanoma relates to the removal of regional lymph nodes. There is no controversy regarding the need to dissect obviously involved nodal areas when other signs of dissemination are not present. There is a question whether lymph-node dissection should be performed in continuity with resection of primary melanoma, particularly in the distal part of the extremities. Some authors have reported an increased incidence of in-transit metastasis after discontinuous lymph-node dissection; other authors have not been able to confirm these findings.

The major problem regarding the surgical treatment of lymph nodes focuses on the uninvolved regional lymph nodes; the problem is whether the surgeon should perform an immediate elective node dissection as soon as the diagnosis of malignant melanoma is made or wait for clinical evidence of node involvement. The chance of having lymph node containing tumor correlates well with tumor thickness. Tumors less than 0.76 mm thick or between 0.77 and 1.5 mm have about a 15 percent association with positive lymph nodes. Lesions between 1.6 and 3.7 mm in thickness have about a 35 percent association with positive lymph nodes. About half the patients with tumors thicker than 3.7 mm have positive lymph nodes. A prospective randomized study by the World Health Organization showed no survival improvement for patients who had undergone elective node dissection. A number of other studies have failed to show any improved survival for prophylactic lymph-node dissection when the melanoma is located on the trunk or limbs. One study has demonstrated a slightly improved survival if prophylactic lymph-node dissection is done for head and neck melanomas. Prophylactic lymph-node dissection does give valuable prognostic information regardless of the location of the melanoma. Veronesi and Cascinelli have suggested that elective regional lymph node dissection be confined to those patients for whom follow-up is a problem. It should also be used when the melanoma originates in the skin covering a lymph node basin, since the postoperative changes following excision of the primary melanoma may

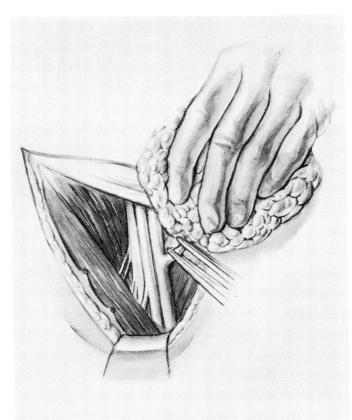

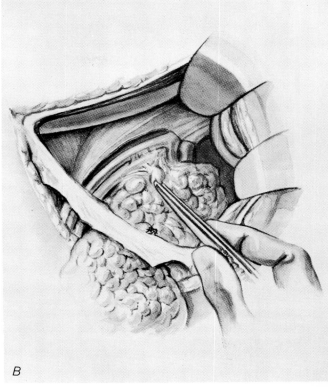

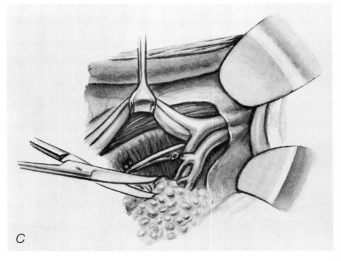

Fig. 14-21. Groin dissection. *A.* Dissection of upper thigh and sheath of femoral triangle. *B.* Dissection of inguinal region including excision of endopelvic fascia. Note exposure of iliac vessels. *C.* Dissection of obturator fossa containing medial chain of obturatory lymph nodes. Note that external iliac vein is elevated and obturator nerve is isolated from the fascia.

complicate the clinical evaluation of lymph nodes. They also feel that if the primary melanoma is classified Level V, prophylactic resection of regional lymph nodes seems to increase the chance of cure.

Groin Dissection (Fig. 14-21). Groin dissection is performed preferably through a vertical incision centered over the inguinal lymph nodes. All lymph node bearing tissue in the area of the saphenous vein is removed as well as the subcutaneous tissue extending superiorly on the lower abdominal wall. The saphenous vein is transected. All the fatty tissue about the femoral artery and vein is removed.

Iliac node dissection for melanoma was formerly popular, but recent evidence indicates there is little therapeutic benefit to adding complete iliac node dissection to the groin dissection. Morbidity (lower limb lymphedema) is considerably increased by adding the iliac node dissection. Sampling of the most inferior iliac node is performed by separating the attachment of the transversalis fascia to the inguinal ligament, division of the inferior epigastric

artery and vein, and reflection of the peritoneum. If the most inferior iliac node contains tumor on frozen section, iliac node dissection may be beneficial. The transversalis fascia is reattached to minimize hernia formation. The origin of the sartorius muscle is transected and reflected mediad to cover the femoral artery and vein. The wound is closed over suction catheters.

ADJUNCTIVE TREATMENT. Adjunctive therapy includes regional perfusion with hyperthermic chemotherapeutic

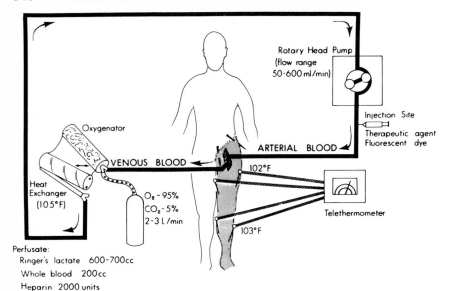

Fig. 14-22. Diagram illustrating flow scheme for extremity perfusion.

agents as well as local and systemic immunotherapy and systemic chemotherapy.

Regional Chemotherapy and Hyperthermia. Isolated regional perfusion with the temperature of the perfusate elevated so that the monitored limb temperature is approximately 40°C has been applied to the management of melanoma (Fig. 14-22). The chemotherapeutic agent most commonly used is melphalan. Excisional surgery and adjunctive perfusion in 286 patients with Stage I disease resulted in cumulative survival rates of 87 percent at 5 years and 75 percent at 10 and 15 years. Hyperthermic chemotherapy is probably beneficial only in those patients whose tumor is thicker than 3.7 mm. With recurrent or metastatic regional disease, treated by perfusion alone, or in combination with surgical excision, the survival rates were 36, 34, and 31 percent, at 5, 10, and 15 years, respectively. In patients with nodal and soft tissue involvement, the survival rates were 22.5 percent at 10 and 15 years. For patients in whom isolation perfusion therapy is not suitable, continuous intraarterial infusion of chemotherapeutic agents has achieved objective responses in over half the patients treated.

Immunotherapy and Chemotherapy. Immunotherapy with a variety of agents has temporarily controlled accessible cutaneous melanoma metastases. Approximately 20 percent of patients with metastases limited to the skin were brought into remission with local intralesional BCG immunotherapy. Immunotherapy, used either alone or in combination with chemotherapeutic agents, has shown little or no activity in the treatment of metastatic malignant melanoma. The results of chemotherapy in the treatment of advanced and disseminating melanoma have been disappointing.

PROGNOSIS. The 10-year survival rate for patients with Stage I cutaneous melanoma ranges between 80 and 95 percent, depending on the Clark-Breslow microstaging of the lesion. The 5-year cure rate for lesions smaller than 0.76 mm in thickness is about 95 percent. For lesions between 0.76 and 1.5 mm it is 85 percent, and for lesions between 1.6 and 3.0 mm it is 60 percent; for those thicker than 3.0 mm the rate is 45 percent. The survival rate in the Stage II melanoma depends on the extent of lymph node involvement. In a series reported by Das Gupta and associates, the 5-year survival in Stage II melanoma patients with Level III primary lesions was 100 percent if the lymph node metastases were clinically undetectable, and 50 percent in patients with macroscopic disease. In the World Health Organization study, survival was similar for patients who had positive nodes whether a node dissection had been done electively for presumed microscopic disease in clinical Stage I patients or therapeutically for macroscopic disease in clinical Stage II patients. The 5-year survivals were approximately 35 percent in each group.

Bibliography

General

Fitzpatrick TB, Eisen AZ, Wolff K, Freedberg IM, Austen H (eds): *Dermatology in General Medicine.* 2d ed, New York, McGraw-Hill, 1979.

Physiology

Ellis H, Morgan MN: Surgical treatment of severe hyperhidrosis. *Proc Roy Soc Med* 64:768, 1971.

Hartfall WG, Jochimsen PR: Hyperhidrosis of upper extremity and its treatment. *Surg Gynecol Obstet* 135:586, 1972.

Rothman S: *Physiology and Biochemistry of the Skin.* Chicago, The University of Chicago Press, 1954.

Pressure Sores

Herceg SJ, Harding RL: Surgical treatment of pressure sores. *Pa Med* 74:45, 1971.

Hidradenitis Suppurativa

Conway H, Stark RB, et al: The surgical treatment of chronic hidradenitis suppurativa. *Surg Gynecol Obstet* 95:455, 1952.

Knaysi GA Jr, Cosman B, Crikelair GF: Hidradenitis suppurativa. *JAMA* 203:19, 1968.

Cysts and Benign Tumors

Brasfield RD, Das Gupta TK: Von Recklinghausen's disease: A clinicopathological study. *Ann Surg,* 175:86, 1972.

Brown SH Jr, Neerhout RC, Fonkalsrud EW: Prednisone therapy in management of large hemangiomas in infants and children. *Surgery* 71:168, 1972.

Conway H: *Tumors of the Skin.* Springfield, IL, Charles C Thomas, 1956.

Dwight RW, Maloy JK: Pilonidal sinus: Experience with 449 cases. *N Engl J Med* 249:926, 1953.

Hvid-Hansen O: Treatment of ganglions. *Acta Chir Scand* 136:471, 1970.

Mandel SR, Thomas CC Jr: Management of pilonidal sinus by excision and primary closure. *Surg Gynecol Obstet* 134:448, 1972.

Mulliken JB: Cutaneous vascular lesions of children, in Serafin D (ed): *Pediatric Plastic Surgery.* St Louis, CV Mosby, 1984.

Strahan J, Bailie HWC: Glomus tumor: A review of 15 clinical cases. *Br J Surg* 59:91, 1972.

Malignant Tumors

Andrade R, Gumport SL, et al (eds): *Cancer of the Skin.* Philadelphia, Saunders, 1976, pp 755–781.

Castro El B, Hajdu SI, Fortner JG: Surgical therapy of fibrosarcoma of extremities: A reappraisal, *Arch Surg* 107:284, 1973.

El-Domeiri AA, Brasfield RD, et al: Sweat gland carcinoma. *Ann Surg* 173:270, 1971.

Epstein E: Sarcoma involving the skin. *Arch Dermatol,* 60:1130, 1949.

Futrell JW, Krueger GR, et al: Carcinoma of sweat glands in adolescents. *Am J Surg* 123:594, 1972.

MacDonald EJ: Epidermiology of skin cancer, 1975, in *Neoplasms of the Skin and Malignant Melanoma.* Chicago, Year Book Medical Publishers, 1976, pp 27–42.

McLean DI, Haynes HA, et al: Cryotherapy of basal-cell carcinoma by a simple method of standardized freeze-thaw cycles. *J Dermatol Surg Oncol* 4:175, 1978.

Mohs F: *Chemosurgery.* Springfield, IL, Charles C Thomas, 1978.

Sharp GS, Binkley FC: The treatment of carcinoma of the skin. *Am J Roentgenol Radium Ther Nucl Med* 67:606, 1952.

Vogel CL, Templeton CJ, et al: Treatment of Kaposi's sarcoma with actinomycin-D and cyclophosphamide: Results of a randomized clinical trial. *Int J Cancer* 8:136, 1971.

Woodward AH, Ivins JC, Soule EH: Lymphangiosarcoma arising in chronic lymphedematous extremities. *Cancer* 30:562, 1972.

Melanoma and Other Pigmented Lesions

Benjamin RS: Chemotherapy of malignant melanoma. *World J Surg* 3:321, 1979.

Bluming AZ, Vogel CL, et al: Immunologic effects of BCG in malignant melanoma: Two modes of administration compared. *Ann Intern Med* 76:405, 1972.

Breslow A: Thickness, cross sectioned area and depth of invasion in the prognosis of cutaneous melanoma. *Ann Surg* 172:902, 1970.

Briele HA, Das Gupta TL: Natural history of cutaneous malignant melanoma. *World J Surg* 3:255, 1979.

Clark WJ Jr, From L, et al: The histogenesis and biologic behavior of primary human malignant melanomas of the skin. *Cancer Res* 29:497, 1969.

Das Gupta TK: Results of treatment of 269 patients with primary cutaneous melanoma. *Ann Surg* 186:201, 1977.

Davis NC: Cutaneous melanoma: The Queensland experience. *Curr Probl Surg* XII: 5, 1976.

Goodnight JE, Morton DL: The role of immunotherapy in the management of patients with malignant melanoma. *World J Surg* 3:309, 1979.

Greeley PW, Middleton AG, Curtin JW: Incidence of malignancy in giant pigmented nevi. *Plastic Reconstr Surg* 36:26, 1965.

Harris MN, Gumport SL, Maiwandi H: Axillary lymph node dissection for melanoma. *Surg Gynecol Obstet* 135:936, 1972.

Knutson CO, Hori JM, Spratt JS Jr: Melanoma. *Curr Probl Surg* December 1971.

Krementz ET, Carter RD, et al: The use of regional chemotherapy in the management of malignant melanoma. *World J Surg* 3:289, 1979.

MacDonald EJ: Epidemiology of melanoma. *Ann NY Acad Sci* 100:4, 1963.

Milton GW, McCarthy WH, et al: Prophylactic lymph node dissection in clinical stage I cutaneous malignant melanoma: Results of surgical treatment in 1319 patients. *Br J Surg* 69:108, 1982.

Morton DL, Eilber FR, et al: BCG immunotherapy of malignant melanoma: Summary of 7-year experience. *Ann Surg* 180:635, 1974.

Raven RW: The clinicopathological aspects of malignant melanoma. *Ann NY Acad Sci* 100:142, 1963.

Spratt JS Jr, Shieber W, Dillard BM: *Anatomy and Surgical Technique of Groin Dissection.* St Louis, CV Mosby, 1965.

Stehlin JS, Giovanella BC, et al: Eleven year's experience with hyperthermic perfusion for melanoma of the extremities. *World J Surg* 3:305, 1979.

Veronesi U, Cascinelli N: Surgical treatment of malignant melanoma of the skin. *World J Surg* 3:279, 1979.

Wanebo HJ, Woodruff J, Fortner JG: Malignant melanoma of the extremities: A clinicopathologic study using levels of invasion (microstage). *Cancer* 35:666, 1975.

White LP: The role of natural resistance in the prognosis of human melanoma. *Ann NY Acad Sci* 100:115, 1963.

WHO Collaborating Centers for Evaluation of Methods of Diagnosis and Treatment of Melanoma (Bufalino R, Cascinelli N, Morabito A, Preda F): Register: Analysis of 4739 cases, 1977.

Chapter 15

Breast

Benjamin F. Rush, Jr.

The breast is a human being's insignia of membership in the class Mammalia. It is somewhat humbling to reflect that this badge of status had its origin as a modified sweat gland. In the male the breast is, with few exceptions, a dormant structure. In the female, from puberty to death, the breast is subjected to a constant dynamic role of physical changes related to the menstrual cycle, pregnancy, lactation, and the menopause. Associated with this active role are numerous malfunctions and dysfunctions that make diseases of the breast common clinical problems.

EMBRYOLOGY

The human breast makes its first appearance in the sixth week of embryonic development as an ectodermal thickening extending from the axilla to the groin, a distinct linear elevation called the *mammary ridge,* or *milk line.* Lens-shaped thickenings appear along the milk line, presaging the sites of developing breasts. In human beings the caudal two-thirds of the line disappears rapidly,

and the pectoral thickening progresses with the ultimate formation of a breast primordium. Human beings share this pectoral location of the breasts with other primates and with the elephant and sea cow, in contrast to the multiple breasts of the dog and pig and the inguinal location in the cow, goat, and whale.

In the fifth month of embryonic development the human primordial breast develops 15 to 20 solid cords that fan out beneath the skin in the underlying connective tissue. These primary milk ducts branch, and the ends develop club-shaped dilatations. During the seventh or eighth month the ducts hollow to develop lumina. During this same period the point in the skin corresponding to the nipple develops a small depression. At birth the breast is represented by a slight pit pierced by 15 to 20 openings into the primary milk ducts. The areola is a slight thickening in the skin that contains a few glands (of Montgomery). Shortly after birth the nipples become everted, and the areola is distinguished by a slight increase in pigmentation.

A few days after birth, bilateral or unilateral enlargement of the breast occurs in 70 percent of infants. In half the infants the swelling is accompanied by the secretion of a cloudy fluid similar to colostrum, the "witch's milk" of folklore. Histologically, these changes are associated with hypertrophy of the duct system, the appearance of acini, and an increased vascularity of the stroma. These alternatives are considered an indirect effect of the high level of maternal estrogens in the infant's circulating blood. Following birth the falling estrogen level stimulates the hypophysis to produce prolactin, resulting in the mammary changes. These changes occur equally in male and female infants and regress spontaneously by the second or third week of life. Attempts to strip the breasts of their milk, as advocated by some superstitions, provoke the breasts to remain in the secretory state. Hyperplasia of the infant breast persisting over many months with persistent secretions has resulted from such manipulations.

CLINICAL CORRELATIONS. A number of developmental errors of the breast are of clinical importance. Most often observed is the persistence of one or more of the additional nipples in the milk line. These are commonly mis-

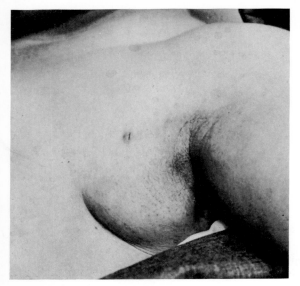

Fig. 15-1. Supernumerary breast.

taken for moles. A rare anomaly is the occurrence of ex-tramammary breast tissue, usually seen in the axilla or over the upper abdomen (Fig. 15-1), often not appearing until the tissue is stimulated by pregnancy and lactation. Excision of these supernumerary structures is the treatment of choice. Absence of one or both nipples or of one or both breasts occurs, though rarely. While these conditions are serious cosmetic and functional defects, a more important functional deficiency is the often associated absence of the underlying pectoralis muscles and chest wall.

Occasionally the nipple fails to evert following birth and remains retracted or inverted throughout life. This is a serious functional problem when the patient attempts to nurse a child.

In some infants the collecting ducts fail to open onto the apex of the nipple, opening onto the areola instead. In a few instances collecting ducts are observed to empty onto the skin of the breast, failing entirely to traverse the nipple. These nippleless collecting ducts recapitulate the normal anatomy of the nippleless breast of the duckbill platypus.

ANATOMY AND DEVELOPMENT

Except for the neonatal period of hypertrophy and a period of slight hypertrophy occurring at puberty, the male breast undergoes little change throughout life. The female breast shows little change through infancy and childhood, but in the prepubertal period and throughout the remainder of life the breasts undergo numerous gross and microscopic changes (Fig. 15-2).

ADOLESCENCE. During the prepubertal period (from eleven to fifteen years) growth of the breast begins with the development of the prepubertal ''bud.'' The areola becomes elevated and forms with the nipple a small coni-

cal protuberance. Histologically, the rudimentary primary ducts begin a rapid process of elongation and terminal branching, pushing down through the subcutaneous tissue toward the pectoral fascia and carrying with them sheaths of periductal connective tissue. A firm plaque of fibrous breast tissue forms as the lobes of the breasts develop, crowding out the subcutaneous fat. Radiographs of the breast at this period show a featureless, fibrous mass without trabeculae. Lobules do not form, however, until ovulation begins. Following ovulation at age fourteen to fifteen the breasts mature into their normal nulliparous form.

THE YOUNG ADULT. Anatomic Limits. The breast is suspended from the anterior chest wall, extending from the second to the sixth rib. The medial boundary is at the lateral border of the sternum, and the lateral border stretches to the anterior axillary line (Fig. 15-3).

Areola and Nipple. The areola in the young female is convex and lens-shaped, surmounted at its center by the nipple. The areola gains a slight amount of pigmentation during adolescence, and although its surface is hairless, a few hairs may appear at the skin of the periphery. Both

Fig. 15-2. Gross and microscopic appearance of breast at different stages of development. Central pictures show three-dimensional projection of microscopic structure. *A.* Adolescence. *B.* Pregnancy. *C.* Lactation. *D.* Postmenopausal period.

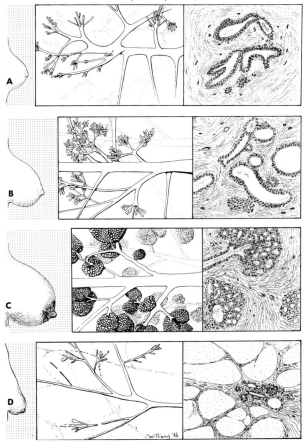

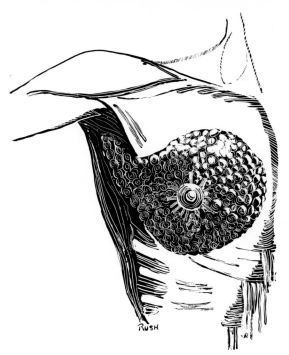

Fig. 15-3. Normal distribution of mammary tissue of adult female breast. Note long tail of Spence extending into axilla.

the subareolar area and the nipple contain much smooth muscle. The fibers of the areola are arranged in concentric rings as well as radially and are inserted into the base of the dermis. They function to contract the areola and to compress the base of the nipple. The bulk of the nipple is made up of smooth muscle fibers arranged both circularly and longitudinally. The nipple is made erect, smaller, and firmer by contraction of these fibers, and this involuntary action serves to aid in emptying the intrapapillary ducts. This response is evoked by sucking or by tactile stimuli. Sir Astley Cooper, a pioneer in describing the anatomy and diseases of the breast, first pointed out that the nipple lies to the lateral side of the center line of the breast and that its axis points upward and outward. The teleologic assumption is that this arrangement is for the convenience of the suckling child.

Glandular Tissue. The functional portion of the breast is a modified cutaneous gland, an appendage of the skin. It is enclosed between the superficial and deep layers of the superficial fascia. The glandular portion of the breast spreads out widely as a layer over the chest wall beneath the integument. It is roughly circular in outline except at the upper outer quadrant, where the axillary tail of Spence extends toward the axilla (Fig. 15-3). The tip of the axillary tail intrudes through an opening in the deep fascia of the axilla, Langer's foramen, to lie well up within the axilla. Neoplasms or deformities in this tail are sometimes mistaken for enlarged axillary nodes.

Portions of the fibrous tissue of the breast parenchyma extend from the surface of the glandular breast anteriorly to intermingle with the superficial layer of the superficial

fascia. Similar processes arise from the deep surface of the gland to cross the retromammary space and fuse with the pectoral fascia. The anterior ligaments were described by Cooper, who noted, "The breast is slung upon the fore part of the chest, for [the ligaments] form a movable but very firm connection with the skin so that the breast has sufficient motion."

Blood Supply and Venous Drainage. Three major arteries generously supply the breast with blood. The perforating branches of the internal mammary artery pass through the first, second, third, and fourth intercostal spaces just lateral to the sternum to penetrate and pass through the origin of the pectoralis major muscle and enter the medial edge of the breast, supplying more than 50 percent of the blood to this organ. The lateral thoracic artery arises from the axillary artery and courses down along the lateral border of the pectoralis minor muscle. Its external mammary branches provide the second largest source of blood to the breast. The third artery of importance is the pectoral branch of the acromiothoracic artery, also a branch of the axillary artery. The pectoral artery is given off by the acromiothoracic at the medial edge of the pectoralis minor muscle. In its course between the pectoralis major and minor muscles, the pectoralis artery gives off branches to the posterior surface of the breast. The superior branch of the axillary artery, the lateral perforating branches of the intercostal arteries, and branches of the subscapular artery also contribute minor amounts to the blood supply.

The mammary glands have a rich, anastomosing network of superficial subcutaneous veins. These veins become markedly dilated during pregnancy and may sometimes become quite prominent over an area of underlying neoplasm. The majority of the superficial veins drain to the internal mammary vein. In some individuals these veins drain into the superficial veins of the lower neck.

The deep veins of the mammary gland drain along routes roughly corresponding to the arterial blood supply. Thus one major route is through the anterior intercostal perforating veins to the internal mammary veins. Another is by way of multiple branches to the axillary vein. A third route is by way of posterior branches anastomosing with the intercostal veins. This last route has special significance, since the intercostal veins communicate with the vertebral veins. This anastomosis with the vertebral veins is offered by Batson as the explanation for the often capricious metastasis of mammary cancer to the vertebral bodies or even the sacrum or pelvis without the presence of metastatic deposits in the lung. He holds that the wide variation in pressure within the thoracic cavity induced by straining or coughing may change the flow patterns within the valveless anastomosing veins so that blood from the breast draining through the lateral perforators to the intercostal vessels is forced down along the vertebral plexus.

The Lymphatics. A generous lymphatic plexus drains the skin and glandular tissues of the breast (Fig. 15-4). The lymphatic vessels empty into two main depots represented by the axillary and the internal mammary lymph nodes. There are an average of 53 lymph nodes in the

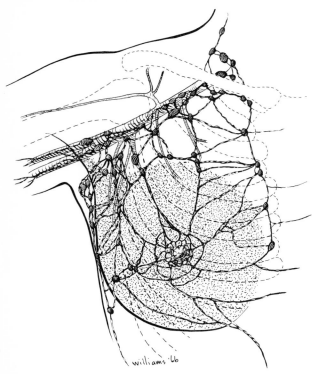

williams '66

Fig. 15-4. Lymphatic drainage of breast. Nipple drains both laterally and medially. Medial side of breast drains to small internal mammary lymph nodes.

axillary fossa, arranged along the course of the arteries and veins. Lymph from the lower outer quadrant of the breast drains to the lateral and inferior axillary nodes, while lymph from the areola, the upper outer quadrant of the breast, and the axillary tail drains to the medial superior axillary nodes. Within the axilla, lymph passes from the lateral inferior to the medial superior nodes at the apex of the axilla. Lymph then courses through lymphatic channels under the clavicle to the supraclavicular lymph nodes and by major lymphatic trunks to the junction of the subclavian and jugular veins. On the right, lymph enters the blood directly through these lymphatic trunks as they join the veins. On the left these trunks may first join with the thoracic duct, which shortly communicates with the venous system.

The internal mammary lymph nodes are much fewer in number than the axillary nodes, averaging but three or four nodes on each side lying along the internal mammary vessels, usually in the first, second, and third interspaces. Despite the scarcity and tiny size of these lymph nodes, most of the lymph from the upper and lower inner quadrants of the breast drains by this channel. Lymph from the nipple and areola may drain to both the internal mammary and the axillary nodes. The internal mammary lymphatic trunks eventually empty into the great veins of the neck, usually by way of the thoracic duct or of the right lymphatic duct.

Histology of the Resting Mammary Gland. Each lobe of the mammary gland is an independent compound alveolar gland. The mammary gland is a conglomeration of a variable number of such independent glands, each with its own excretory duct that has its separate opening on the surface of the nipple. The excretory ducts measure from 0.4 to 0.7 mm in diameter at the nipple surface and run perpendicularly through the nipple to turn and radiate out toward the periphery of the breast. Beneath the areola they dilate into a short fusiform area called the *milk sinus.* Beyond the milk sinus the excretory ducts begin to subdivide into smaller and smaller branches forming the lobules of the lobe. Within the lobules the ducts subdivide further, forming terminal, elongated tubes, the alveolar ducts, which are covered by round evaginations, the alveolae. Lobules are peripheral and scanty in the nulliparous breast (Fig. 15-2A).

There is mild controversy as to whether alveolae are present in the resting mammary gland. Some claim that the resting gland is entirely a tubular structure and becomes tuboalveolar only during pregnancy. The majority opinion is that a few alveolae are scattered through the lobules in the resting state.

The walls of the alveolae and the alveolar ducts consist of a prominent basement membrane surrounding a layer of myoepithelial cells, which in turn lie beneath a layer of low columnar glandular cells. The myoepithelial layer is thin and difficult to identify in the acini and the alveolar ducts but becomes more prominent in the more major lobular ducts. These cells take a spiral course about the larger ducts and probably play a role in propelling milk from the acini to the nipple during lactation.

The collecting ducts are lined with a double layer of cuboidal to columnar epithelium until the milk sinus is reached. Here the lining changes to squamous epithelium. This continues through the milk sinus to the surface of the nipple.

Each lobule is surrounded by a coating of dense, firm, interlobular connective tissue, which is an intimate part of the breast parenchyma. The lobules are separated by a looser coating of less dense fibrous tissue, the interlobular connective tissue. This layer represents the supporting stroma of the breast. These layers are easily recognized histologically, but grossly the various lobules are intimately and firmly bound together and cannot be dissected apart.

Cyclic Changes of the Breast. Beginning about the eighth day of the menstrual cycle the female breast gradually increases in size, the volume often increasing by 50 percent by the immediate premenstrual period. At this point the breast is tense and may be somewhat tender. Part of the increase in size is due to interlobular edema and increasing congestion of the vasculature. Ingleby and Gershon-Cohen state that there is also a proliferation of the parenchyma, with the appearance of new lobules. These lobules then regress and fibrose during menstruation. Congestion and edema subside, and the breast again reaches its smallest size on about the eighth day after the onset of menstruation.

PREGNANCY AND LACTATION. Implantation of the ovum initiates a profound change in the gross and histologic structures of the breast. Grossly there is a pronounced enlargement of the breast, progressing throughout pregnancy. The normal size may be increased as much as two or three times. The nipple and areola become more prominent and more deeply pigmented. The openings of Montgomery's glands on the areola become prominent and are called *Montgomery's tubercles.* Pigmentation may spread beyond the areola onto the skin, forming a "secondary areola." The veins are engorged, and striae are frequently visible in the skin.

Histologically, the epithelium of the lobular ducts and alveolar ducts proliferates, and new ducts covered with multiple alveolar outpouchings are generated. The total number of lobules increases greatly. By the end of the sixth month the glandular cells of the acini produce small amounts of secretion, colostrum, which increases toward the end of pregnancy (Fig. 15-2C).

Two or three days after delivery, globules appear in the supranuclear cytoplasm of the acinar cells. These push toward the cell lumen, increasing in size. The cell becomes tall and more columnar. Finally the globule is extruded into the lumen, and the cell shrinks to a cuboidal form, to begin the process again. The acini become distended with milk, which is propelled to the nipple during nursing. This process continues as long as suckling continues. When lactation ends, the extralobular tissue involutes, leaving small areas of fibrosis, and the breast gradually returns to the resting state. It never returns to the nulliparous form, however, but has the contour of maturity. The areola recedes into the breast tissue, with only the nipple projecting. Some of the darker pigmentation of the nipple and areola and residual skin striae persist.

MENOPAUSAL CHANGES. Following menopause the mammary gland gradually involutes (Fig. 15-2D). This change is slow and progressive, with gradual disappearance of lobules. Senile involution does not lead to complete extinction of mammary tissue; some lobules always remain, but they are scattered and small. In many areas only the larger lobular and collecting ducts may be found. The parenchyma and stromal fibrous tissue gradually blend together into a homogeneous mass, and the original lobular structure is almost completely lost. As the glandular tissues recede, there is a gradual invasion of fat, which aids in maintaining the breast outline, although in very thin women the breasts may become quite flabby as glandular tissue is lost.

CLINICAL CORRELATION. Both breasts of the adolescent girl usually develop at the same pace. Occasionally development is out of phase, and one breast will develop much more rapidly than the other, leading to distressing asymmetry (Fig. 15-5). The difference in size is usually repaired with time but occasionally persists. Patients complaining of asymmetric breasts during the adolescent period are advised to wait until maturation is complete. If asymmetry persists, a plastic surgical procedure may be required to adjust the difference.

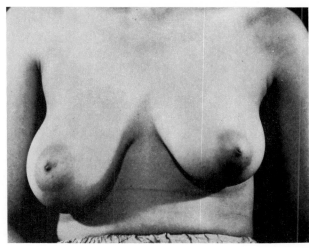

Fig. 15-5. Asymmetric breasts.

A slight swelling of the breasts is often seen in adolescent boys. This is called *gynecomastia* and is a physiologic response to the change in the hormonal milieu in the pubertal male (Fig. 15-6). This slight hypertrophy normally subsides spontaneously but occasionally persists, either unilaterally or bilaterally. Persisting gynecomastia in young manhood requires an evaluation to exclude the possibility of abnormal endocrine secretion. If no abnormalities are found, the small button of hypertrophied breast tissue may be removed surgically to repair an embarrassing cosmetic defect in a young man.

Occasionally the growth of the female breast at puberty fails to cease and the breasts become huge—so-called virginal hypertrophy (Fig. 15-7). Breasts weighing 40 to 50 lb and descending to the level of the genitalia are described.

Fig. 15-6. Gynecomastia.

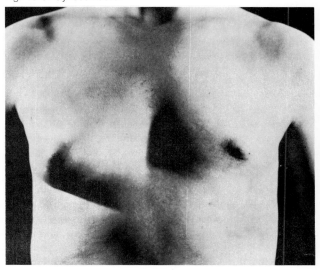

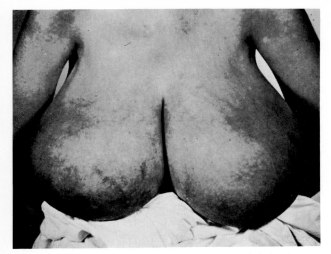

Fig. 15-7. Virginal hypertrophy. This growth occurred during 1 year in fifteen-year-old white girl and required plastic surgery for repair. *(Courtesy of Paul Weeks, M.D.)*

Spontaneous regression does not occur, and the only solution is plastic surgical repair. This rare defect is seen in pregnant females as well and requires the same treatment.

EXAMINATION

INSPECTION. Physical examination of the breasts should begin with the patient erect, usually sitting on the edge of the examining table. The breasts are observed for symmetry, dimpling of the skin, edema, deformity of outline, retraction of the nipple, or inflammation. Underlying masses will produce deformity or skin retraction, which is much more easily detected when the patient is erect and the breasts dependent. Haagensen suggests that the patient be allowed to lean forward to increase the breast dependency and further accentuate areas of deformity or dimpling.

PALPATION. Examination of the axillary and supraclavicular area is always part of a complete breast examination and is best done when the patient is erect. The axilla is examined with the humerus slightly abducted and the pectoralis muscle relaxed (Fig. 15-8*B*). The contents of the axilla are pressed gently against the rib cage, and the axilla is progressively palpated from apex to base. The apex of the axilla does not lie under the humeral head but anteriorly under the clavicle, where the axillary vein and artery pass under the clavicle to become the subclavian vessels. Palpation of lymph nodes at this level is of great importance in predicting the prognosis in a patient with cancer.

The supraclavicular area is palpated with the tips of the fingers, making sure that the fingers are pressed down well behind the clavicle to roll the supraclavicular structures against the scalene muscles. In a thin neck the transverse fibers of the posterior belly of the omohyoid are sometimes mistaken for an enlarged lymph node. This

can be differentiated by observing that a medial and lateral margin to the supposed node cannot be felt, although an upper and lower border are easily detected. Following palpation of the axilla and supraclavicular area, the breasts are also palpated, although masses in the breasts are best felt when the patient is supine.

After inspection and palpation with the patient erect, the entire mammary gland is palpated carefully with the tips of the fingers with the patient in the supine position, with the arm first over the head and then at the side (Fig. 15-8). This should be done systematically and in the same way in each examination so that the examiner follows a definite pattern. One may begin at the upper inner quadrant, gradually inspecting the breast tissue from above downward until the medial portion of the breast has been examined. The areolar area is then palpated. If the patient has complained of secretions or blood from the nipple, the areola should be stroked toward the nipple to see if this symptom can be reproduced. The lateral portion of the breast is palpated starting at the upper outer quadrant and completing the examination at the lower outer quadrant. The tail of the breast should also be examined as it extends into the axilla.

By self-examination a woman can usually detect a smaller mass in her own breasts than can a physician if she knows the proper methods to use. Since cancer of the breast is one of the major neoplasms in females, instruction in self-examination is a valuable addition to the physician's examination of the breast. A patient is instructed to emulate the physician's pattern of inspection and examination. She carries this out upon herself in both the erect and supine postions. Women thirty-five years of age

Fig. 15-8. Examination of breast. *A.* Observation with arms at side. *B.* Palpation of axilla. *C.* With arms raised. *D.* Palpation with patient supine.

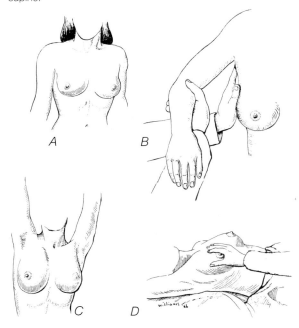

and older should conduct such an examination at home once monthly. Numerous studies show that breast cancers detected by women who practice breast self-examination are significantly smaller with fewer positive lymph nodes than cancers found in women who do not use this technique. Huguley and Brown point out that this method is safe and without cost. It has the potential for helping more women to find their breast cancer early than any other method now available and is feasible for widespread use.

MAMMOGRAPHY. Mammography is an x-ray examination of the breast. It requires special techniques and film, and a radiologist skilled in interpretation.

This technique is not a substitute for biopsy, which still provides definitive confirmation, but is a helpful adjunct in diagnosis. Mammography is especially useful in (1) follow-up examinations of the contralateral breast following radical mastectomy; (2) examination of an indeterminate mass that cannot be considered a dominant nodule, especially when there are multiple cysts or several vague masses and the indication for biopsy is uncertain; and (3) the large, fatty breast, when the patient has complaints but no nodules are palpated. Tumors cannot be easily felt in such breasts, but the mammogram is most accurate in the fatty breast.

A skilled radiologist can detect cancer of the breast

with a false-positive rate of 11 percent and a false-negative rate of 6 percent. A fine stippling of calcium on the radiogram in the area of the lesion is very suggestive of cancer. There is also a characteristic infiltration of the surrounding tissues; a typical skin thickening may be seen, and the density of the lesion itself is often helpful in interpretation (Fig. 15-9). Some radiologists believe that certain patterns in the breast parenchyma revealed by mammography are associated with a higher risk of cancer. The "Wolf classification" that describes these patterns is still under study but seems to be losing favor in recent reports.

Radiography of the breast can detect some cancers that cannot be found in any other way. It has been estimated that the lead time for treatment of lesions discovered at this small size is 1 or 2 years compared with cancers discovered by conventional palpation of the breast. Axillary nodal involvement is very rare in these early lesions, and preliminary results of follow-up indicate that 5-year survival rates for such tumors may exceed 90 percent. These data led to considerable activity in developing pilot mass screening programs for cancer of the breast that include mammography and careful physical examination.

In 1973 the American Cancer Society and the National Cancer Institute inaugurated a massive pilot program of breast screening, the Breast Cancer Detection Demonstration Program (BCDDP). Two hundred eighty thousand self-selected women were screened annually by mammography and breast examination. In 1975 considerable opposition developed to the use of mammography in women under fifty based on the fear that the cumulative

Fig. 15-9. Mammography of breast. *A.* Normal postmenopausal patient with atrophy of lobular tissue and ducts and predominance of fatty supporting tissue. *B.* Multiloculated cyst in menopausal patient. *C.* Scirrhous carcinoma in menopausal patient, demonstrating sunburst pattern; characteristic calcifications not present in this case.

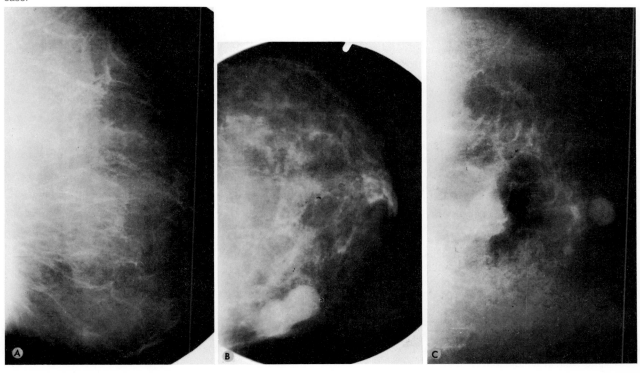

dose of radiation would incite breast cancer in some women. Rapid development of new radiological techniques reduced the absorbed dose of radiation to as little as 0.1 rad at midbreast, and cumulative dose became so small that today the radiation risk is considered negligible.

With the end of the pilot screening program in 1978, a vigorous follow-up program was inaugurated; it was concluded in 1985. Initial reports from this project indicate that screening of breast cancers in women under fifty years of age allows earlier diagnosis and treatment of breast cancer. Disease-free 5-year survival in this group was as high as 93.5 percent.

The American Cancer Society currently recommends that all women begin breast self-examination after the age of twenty, that they obtain a "base-line" mammographic examination some time between thirty-five and forty, that they consult their doctor about the need for regular mammographic screening between forty and fifty, and that they have annual mammographic screening thereafter. This fairly cautious recommendation may be extended even further for examinations in the forty- to fifty-year age group in the light of new findings that radiation exposure involves a risk of cancer induction in women under thirty but that the risk is virtually zero in the cancer age group. Prospective randomized studies of routine mammographic screening have shown 40 percent reduction of Stage II and greater cancers in the screened group and a 30 percent increase in survival in those patients found to have cancer.

Xeroradiography of the breast is basically a radiographic technique that is carried out in exactly the same way as mammography, except that the image is recorded on a xerographic plate instead of the conventional x-ray transparency. The image is positive rather than negative and appears easier to read to the untrained eye. Unfortunately, a badly exposed xeroradiograph, too poor for proper interpretation, is harder to recognize than a poor radiomammograph and may fool the unwary physician.

THERMOGRAPHY. The skin over malignant tumors of the breast is usually warmer than the surrounding areas. Using special heat scanners it is possible to delineate these "hot spots" on film. This method may help to differentiate malignant and benign tumors. Infection may be associated with a false positive, and, conversely, not all cancers are "hot" and so false negatives may occur. The BCDDP abandoned the use of thermography after 3 years because the incidence of false positives and negatives was too high. Research continues to improve the technique, but it is still investigational and not considered a reliable screening method.

ULTRASONOGRAPHY. Ultrasound used in diagnosis of breast lesions is highly effective in differentiating a cystic from a solid mass. It is unsatisfactory for detecting early breast cancers owing to the inability to visualize microcalcification. It is also unlikely to discriminate lesions smaller than 5 mm. While ultrasonography is an excellent method for diagnosing a cyst, needle aspiration as described on page 562 is usually just as effective and a much simpler and less expensive office procedure.

OTHER METHODS. The explosion in technology that has occurred in the past few years has introduced computed tomography (CT), magnetic resonance imaging (MRI), and digital subtraction angiography to the differentiation of breast lesions. In a recent report all of 20 carcinomas of the breast showed an enhanced image when examined with MRI whereas dysplastic or scar tissue enhanced slightly or not at all. This technique has the advantage of avoiding any exposure to radiation. Further experience will be required to determine the incidence of false negative and positive rates for these procedures.

DISEASES OF THE BREAST

Neoplasms

From the standpoint of morbidity and mortality, cancer is by far the most important clinical problem that concerns the breast today. Most benign neoplasms of the breast would have little clinical importance if it were not for the difficulty in differentiating them from cancer. To emphasize this relationship, benign neoplasms are discussed in the section on differential diagnosis of cancer.

In recent years four major controversies have surfaced concerning breast cancer: (1) the relation of treatment to the natural history of the disease; (2) the role of mammography in diagnosis, and especially in screening programs; (3) the appropriate operation for treatment; and (4) the use of postoperative chemotherapy as an adjuvant to primary therapy.

INCIDENCE

Cancer of the breast is the commonest form of cancer in females. The American Cancer Society estimates that 130,000 women in the United States will develop breast cancer in 1987. According to the excellent cancer registry systems in Connecticut and upper New York State, the age-adjusted incidence of new cases has been increasing steadily since the middle 1940s. In the 1970s the chance of developing breast cancer among United States women was estimated at 1 in 13; in 1980 it was 1 in 11, and now it is 1 in 10.

Worldwide figures show that 541,000 cases were diagnosed in 1975 and that the number may approach one million by the year 2000. The Dutch have the highest national mortality of cancer of the breast, with 24.19 patients per 100,000 population. The United States ranks ninth, with 21.38 cases per 100,000 population. The Japanese rank lowest among all nations with reliable statistics, with an incidence of 3.76 per 100,000 population. The factors leading to this wide range of incidence are unknown, although studies seeking an answer are in progress.

ETIOLOGY

Sex is certainly an important contributing factor in this disease, since it is very rare in males. Maleness is not a complete protection, however; there is 1 carcinoma of the breast in men for every 100 carcinomas of the breast in women.

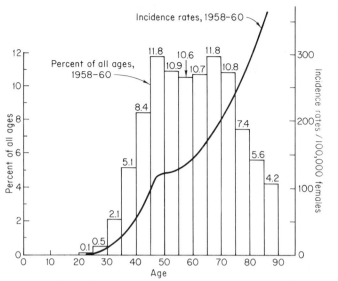

Fig. 15-10. Newly diagnosed breast cancer among women, 1958–1960: percentage distribution and incidence rates by age. Note plateau in incidence between ages forty-five and fifty-five.

The age of the patient is also important (Fig. 15-10). Breast cancer is almost unknown in the prepubertal female and is very rare under the age of twenty. From the age of twenty onward there is a gradually increasing incidence, which reaches a plateau between the ages of forty-five and fifty-five at about 125 new cases each year for every 100,000 females of the age range. After fifty-five the incidence begins to rise again quite sharply, so that the annual risk of developing breast cancer for women eighty to eighty-five is twice as high as for women sixty to sixty-five (312 versus 153 new cases per 100,000 women per year). Some suggest that the plateau of incidence during the menopausal age period reflects the effects of a changing hormonal pattern in women at this time.

Genetic factors play a role in the development of this cancer, though the genetic effect does not seem to be strong and more than one allelic gene must be involved. When the mother has had a breast cancer, the chance of cancer of the breast developing in the daughter is two to three times greater than would be expected in the general population, but no specific pattern of inheritance is evident. Some hypothesize that there is a genotype that has a predisposition to the formation of cancer but that must interact with some nongenetic agent before cancer develops.

Patients in whom breast cancer develops and who have positive family histories for the disease are generally younger and have a higher frequency of bilaterality than breast cancer patients with negative family histories. Blood type O, benign breast disease, and ovarian cysts and tumors also tend to be more common in patients with early diagnosis of breast cancer. Blood type A, diabetes, hypertension, and uterine disorders are more common in those who are older at the time of diagnosis.

Interlinked with factors of age, sex, national origin, and

inheritance in the development of breast cancer is the important role played by hormonal environment. Some breast cancers are highly susceptible to changes in the patient's hormonal pattern and will regress for a time when hormones of various types are given. Mammary cancer can be induced in the mouse and rat by repeated injections of estrogens and in the rat by a combination of estrogen and progesterone. There is a vast literature concerning both experimental and clinical induction and extinction of tumors with hormonal agents. The exact role of hormones in human cancer still remains elusive. It is not known whether hormonal maladjustment is responsible for human breast cancer or what predisposing causes may be required to produce a susceptibility to hormonal change.

Breast cancer may well be multifactorial. Other interesting correlations with breast cancer include the incidence of coronary artery disease, which has a positive correlation with breast cancer death rates in 24 parts of the world. Hems has concluded that "early" breast cancer (age group forty to forty-four) appears to be genetically influenced, while "late" breast cancer (age group sixty-five to sixty-nine) is more closely associated with environmental factors, such as diet. Among younger women, higher risk is associated with late first pregnancy, while among women over fifty years of age the risk appears to increase with weight and the relation of weight to height. Zippin and Petrakis have reported an association between wet cerumen, or earwax, and breast cancer rates in diverse population groups, and breast cancer mortality is closely associated with wet cerumen. Such an association is plausible since the mammary and ceruminous glands are histologically of the apocrine type and have many similarities in their secretions. Cerumen exists in two phenotypic forms, wet and dry, which are controlled by a pair of genes in which the allele for the wet type is dominant over that of the dry type. The dry is homozygous recessive and is highly prevalent in the mongoloid population of Asia and in American Indians. The wet type predominates in Western Europeans, Caucasian Americans, and Negro Americans. These findings support the hypothesis that genetic variations in the apocrine system may influence susceptibility to breast cancer.

Diet in terms of the consumption of animal fat is strongly correlated with breast cancer incidence. Rose and associates plotted correlation of animal fat consumption in 32 countries with incidence of breast cancer and found a highly significant direct relationship (R = 0.74).

It has long been known that breast cancer in mice is related to a viral factor transmitted in the milk. Considerable excitement has attended the discovery of particles in human milk with the same morphologic characteristics as those found to be associated with breast cancer in mice. Antigens to these viral particles have been identified in human plasma. These particles have been found in the milk from the breasts of 60 percent of American women with family histories of breast cancer compared with 5 percent of women without positive family histories. The milk of 39 percent of Parsi women in India also was found to contain these particles. The group of Parsi women is of particular interest because of their endogamous history over the centuries, resulting in an inbred population. Breast cancer accounts for approximately half of the cancers among Parsi women in contrast with Connecticut women, for example, in whom breast cancer represents one-fourth of all cancers.

NATURAL HISTORY

A typical carcinoma of the breast is a scirrhous adenocarcinoma beginning in the ducts and invading the parenchyma (80 percent). Beginning in the upper outer quadrant (40 to 50 percent), it grows slowly, doubling its volume every 2 to 9 months in 70 percent of patients. Starting from a single cell, it takes 30 doubling times for a tumor to attain a size of 1 cm—the smallest tumor of the breast normally found on physical diagnosis. Thus even the fastest-growing tumor of the more common type may require 5 years before it becomes clinically palpable. The use of doubling times to calculate the preclinical course of tumors of the breast is subject to many errors, the most obvious being that growth rates are not always constant, varying with areas of necrosis within the tumor and hormonal changes in the patient. Laboratory and clinical observations indicate, however, that growth rates are more consistent than is usually appreciated, especially during the first 30 doublings. The concept of the origin of these tumors in a single cell with increase in size by doubling is a useful model and suggests the long occult period that probably is present in many tumors before they are diagnosed and treated. Cancers of the breast are often multicentric (15 to 40 percent), but each tumor is assumed to have started from its own individual cell.

A characteristic of malignant cells is the lack of adhesion to adjacent tissue. As the small mass of tumor increases in size, increasing numbers of tumor cells shed into the intercellular spaces to be taken up by the lymphatics. At about the twentieth doubling, the still tiny tumor mass acquires its own blood supply as a network of new capillaries forms. Tumor cells can now be shed directly into the bloodstream. Fisher notes that the cells entering the lymphatic network can cross over into the bloodstream by lymphaticovenous communications. Successful implantation of shed cells is another matter, however, and depends on the number of cells shed, special characteristics of the shed cells, and the resistance of the host. Empiric clinical data indicate that successful implantation of metastatic cells from breast cancer rarely occurs until the primary lesion is larger than 0.5 cm in diameter, or about the twenty-seventh doubling.

Fisher has also introduced the important concept that the appearance of gross tumor in the axillary nodes is an index of the failure of host resistance and that such nodal involvement indicates a probability of disseminated malignant disease. The chance of dissemination is roughly correlated with the number of nodes involved.

As the tumor increases in size and invades the surrounding glandular tissue, the accompanying fibrosis tends to shorten Cooper's ligaments, producing the characteristic dimpling in the skin (Fig. 15-11). Cords of tumor

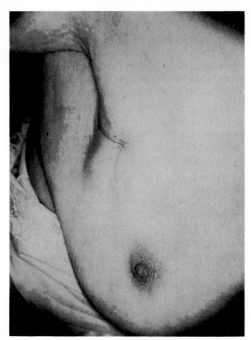

Fig. 15-11. Dimpling of skin over primary carcinoma of breast in upper outer quadrant. Slowly growing lesion in seventy-year-old patient; dimpling had been present for 2 years.

cells grow out along lymphatics, ultimately invading the skin itself. This invasion is preceded by localized edema of the skin as many lymphatic avenues are blocked and drainage of fluid from the skin is impeded. Eventually tumor cells replace the skin, which breaks down to form an ulcer. The tumor increases in size, and new areas of skin invasion may occur, indicated by small satellite nodules adjacent to the ulcer crater. Blood vessels are invaded, and additional tumor cells seed into the circulation, passing into axillary or intercostal veins to be scattered through the pulmonary circuit into the lungs or by way of the vertebral veins up and down the vertebral column.

As the breast tumor extends toward the skin, tumor cells simultaneously pass along the lymphatic vessels from the upper outer quadrant to the axillary nodes, where they implant and grow. As the axillary nodes enlarge, they are at first shotty and fairly soft, then firm and hard as they are increasingly replaced by tumor. Eventually the nodes adhere to one another in a large conglomerate mass, and as the tumor breaks out of the lymphatic capsule the mass of nodes becomes fixed to the medial wall of the axilla. As the axillary nodes become choked with tumor, cells are passed along the chain to the supraclavicular nodes, which also enlarge. Other cancer cells pass by way of the right lymphatic trunk or the thoracic duct into the bloodstream, heart, and lungs. Systemic spread is the rule, and 95 percent of patients who die of uncontrolled breast cancer have distant metastases. Lung (65 percent), liver (56 percent), and bones (56 percent) are the commonest sites for these deposits.

Patients today are rarely allowed to proceed through all stages of carcinoma without some therapeutic intervention. Data are available, however, from the latter half of the 1800s and the first few years of this century indicating the normal course of events in untreated tumors. The excellent report in 1962 by Bloom and associates summarizes much of the data. They cite the experience of the Middlesex Hospital in London, where in 1791 a cancer charity was founded to which patients were admitted to "remain an unlimited time, until either relieved by art or released by death." From the well-preserved records of this charity it was possible to collect a series of 250 advanced cases of untreated breast cancer seen between 1805 and 1933 (Fig. 15-12). All the patients reported died in the hospital, and in every case an autopsy was performed. In the last 86 cases, histologic sections were available. The mean survival in this series and for over 1000 untreated cases collected from the literature was 38.7 months, with a range from 30.2 to 39.8 months. It must be noted that in all reports of untreated patients survival is calculated from the onset of the first symptom. Fifty percent of the patients died in 2.7 years (median survival); 18 percent survived 5 years, 3.6 percent 10 years, and 0.8 percent 15 years. The longest survivor in the group died in the nineteenth year after onset of symptoms. Histologic grading indicated that for 23 patients with grade 1 tumors the mean survival was 47 months. Autopsies indicated that 95 percent of the women died of their carcinoma, only 5 percent of intercurrent disease. Nearly three-fourths of the patients had ulceration of the breast at death, and in 21 percent this was very extensive, sometimes destroying the entire breast and excavating the chest wall. Bloom concluded that treatment of patients with breast cancer appeared to increase the length and improve the quality of survival.

DIAGNOSIS AND STAGING

The normal breast is a nodular structure by virtue of its lobular architecture, and this lobularity may be accentuated during the later portion of the menstrual cycle, pregnancy, or lactation. To the inexperienced examiner the normal nodularity may feel faintly suspicious throughout, although no obvious lesion can be felt. Palpation of the typical carcinoma of the breast normally leaves little doubt in the examiner's mind: the lesion is hard, almost cartilaginous; the edges are distinct, serrated, and irregular. This is true for the 75 to 80 percent of breast tumors associated with productive fibrosis. It is the remaining 20 to 25 percent of tumors, those associated with little fibrosis and those with a medullary or a colloid element or other less typical lesions, which form the spectrum of neoplasms most difficult to distinguish from benign lesions.

Physicians would prefer to have only the clues provided by the local mass to make the physical diagnosis of carcinoma, for it is only when the mass is localized to the breast that one can assume an "early" lesion and expect the best possible chance of long survival. Too often the later signs of breast cancer are present to confirm the di-

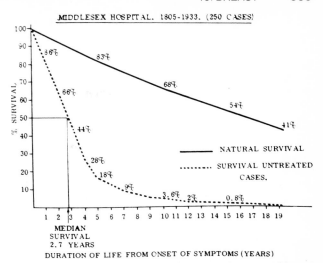

Fig. 15-12. Survival of patients with untreated cancer of breast compared with natural survival. (From: *Bloom HJG, Richardson WW, Harries EJ: Br Med J 5299:213, 1962, with permission.*)

agnosis. As indicated previously, these are skin dimpling or nipple retraction, satellite skin lesions, edema or ulceration, and ipsilateral enlarged axillary or supraclavicular nodes. Signs of even wider spread may be present such as a history of back or leg pain, an enlarged and nodular liver, or perhaps a complaint of dyspnea associated with physical findings of fluid in the chest.

The physical examination of a patient with breast cancer should include an attempt on the part of the examiner to classify and record the stage of the patient's disease specifically. Only consistent classification can make possible clear conclusions concerning prognosis and type of treatment. The problem of comparing the results of treatment from institution to institution and among different operators has been impaired for years by a lack of adequate classification or by varying standards of classification. At present the only acceptable method of classification is a standard system devised by the American Joint Committee on Cancer Staging and End Results Reporting, based on a system proposed by the International Union against Cancer in 1958. This system of classification is called the TNM Classification, the T standing for "tumor," the N for "nodes," and the M for "metastasis." The system is very precise but also complex. If a patient's cancer is staged, it is best to use a staging form as shown in Table 15-1.

DIFFERENTIAL DIAGNOSIS (BENIGN LESIONS)

CHRONIC CYSTIC MASTITIS. Chronic cystic mastitis was first described in the medical literature in the last two decades of the nineteenth century, by Reclus (1883), Brisaud (1884), Schimmelbusch (1890), and König (1893). For a time the disease was known as either Reclus' or Schimmelbusch's disease, but use of these eponyms dwindled following the introduction of the term *chronic cystic mastitis* by König. He chose this term to describe a

Table 15-1. STAGING OF BREAST CARCINOMA

Definitions for all time periods

Primary tumor (T)
☐ TX   Tumor cannot be assessed.
☐ T0   No evidence of primary tumor.
☐ TIS Paget's disease of the nipple with no demonstrable tumor.
NOTE: Paget's disease with a demonstrable tumor is classified according to the size of the tumor.
T1* Tumor 2 cm or less in greatest dimension.
☐ T1a No fixation to underlying pectoral fascia or muscle.
☐ T1b Fixation to underlying pectoral fascia and/or muscle.
   (Check below in addition to T1a or T1b)
      ☐ I tumor ≤ 0.5 cm.
      ☐ II tumor > 0.5 ≤ 1.0 cm.
      ☐ III tumor > 1.0 ≤ 2.0 cm.
T2* Tumor more than 2 cm but not more than 5 cm in its greatest dimension.
☐ T2a No fixation to underlying pectoral fascia or muscle.
☐ T2b Fixation to underlying pectoral fascia and/or muscle.
T3* Tumor more than 5 cm in its greatest dimension.
☐ T3a No fixation to underlying pectoral fascia or muscle.
☐ T3b Fixation to underlying pectoral fascia and/or muscle.
T4 Tumor of any size with direct extension to chest wall or skin.
NOTE: Chest wall includes ribs, intercostal muscles, and serratus anterior muscle, but not pectoral muscle.
☐ T4a Fixation to chest wall.
☐ T4b Edema (including peau d'orange), ulceration of the skin of the breast, or satellite skin nodules confined to the same breast.
☐ T4c Both of the above.

Lymph nodes (N)
        Definitions for clinical-diagnostic stage
☐ NX Regional lymph nodes cannot be assessed clinically.
☐ N0 Homolateral axillary lymph nodes not considered to contain growth.
☐ N1 Movable homolateral axillary nodes considered to contain growth.
☐ N2 Homolateral axillary nodes considered to contain growth and fixed to one another or to other structures.
☐ N3 Homolateral supraclavicular or infraclavicular nodes considered to contain growth, or edema of the arm.†

Lymph nodes (N)
        Definitions for surgical evaluative and postsurgical treatment-pathologic
☐ NX Regional lymph nodes cannot be assessed (not removed for study or previously removed).
☐ N0 No evidence of homolateral axillary lymph node metastasis.
☐ N1 Metastasis to movable homolateral axillary nodes not fixed to one another or to other structure.
 ☐ N1a Micrometastasis ≤ 0.2 cm in lymph node(s).
 ☐ N1b Gross metastasis in lymph node(s).
   ☐ I   Metastasis more than 0.2 cm, but less than 2.0 cm in one to three lymph nodes.
   ☐ II Metastasis more than 0.2 cm, but less than 2.0 cm in four or more lymph nodes.

☐ III Extension of metastasis beyond the lymph node capsule (less than 2.0 cm in dimension).
☐ IV   Metastasis in lymph node 2.0 cm or more in dimension.
☐ N2 Metastasis to homolateral axillary lymph nodes that are fixed to one another or to other structures.
☐ N3 Metastasis to homolateral supraclavicular or infraclavicular lymph node(s).

Distant metastases (M)—All time periods
☐ MX Not assessed.
☐ M0 No (known) distant metastasis.
☐ M1 Distant metastasis present.
        Specify: _____

Tumor size: _____ × _____ × _____ cm.
Predominate lesion
  Measured on: ☐ Patient   ☐ Mammogram
               ☐ Pathological specimen
Location   ☐ OUQ   ☐ Nipple/areola
(Multiple when ☐ OLQ   ☐ IUQ   ☐ ILQ
 necessary)

Lymph nodes: Total No. _____   No. with met. _____

Performance status _____ (see reverse side.)

Examination by _____ M.D.

Date _____

STAGE:
☐ Clinical-   ☐ Postsurgical
  diagnostic   treatment-
                                                 pathologic

☐ Stage TIS—In situ				Stage TIS	☐
☐ Stage X—Cannot stage (unstageable)				Stage X	☐
☐ Stage I	☐ T1ai	N0	M0 ☐	Stage I	☐
	☐ T1aii	N0	M0 ☐		
	☐ T1aiii	N0	M0 ☐		
	☐ T1bi	N0	M0 ☐		
	☐ T1bii	N0	M0 ☐		
	☐ T1biii	N0	M0 ☐		
☐ Stage II	☐ T0	N1a or 1b	M0 ☐	Stage II	☐
	☐ T1a or T1b	N1a or 1b	M0 ☐		
	☐ T2a or T2b	N0	M0 ☐		
	☐ T2a or T2b	N1a or 1b	M0 ☐		
☐ Stage IIIa	☐ T0	N2	M0 ☐	Stage IIIa	☐
	☐ T1a or T1b	N2	M0 ☐		
	☐ T2a or T2b	N2	M0 ☐		
	☐ T3a or T3b	N0	M0 ☐		
	☐ T3a or T3b	N1	M0 ☐		
	☐ T3a or T3b	N2	M0 ☐		
☐ Stage IIIb	☐ Any T	N3	M0 ☐	Stage IIIb	☐
	☐ Any T4	Any N	M0 ☐		
☐ Stage IV	☐ Any T	Any N	M1 ☐	Stage IV	☐

* Dimpling of the skin, nipple retraction, or any other skin changes except those in T4b may occur in T1, T2, or T3 without affecting the classification.
NOTE: Cases of inflammatory carcinoma should be reported separately.
 † Edema of the arm may be caused by lymphatic obstruction and lymph nodes may not then be palpable.
SOURCE: American Joint Committee on Cancer—1982.

group of pathologic lesions found in the breast because he thought they were due to a "vicious cycle of secretion and irritation." While the disease is indeed chronic, it may not be cystic and is certainly not inflammatory, so this old name is at least two-thirds in error. Nonetheless, attempts to introduce more accurate or at least other nomenclatures have failed. Fibrocystic disease, fibroadenosis, mastopathy, nodular hyperplasia, cyclomastopathy, adenofibromatosis, mazoplasia, cystiphorous epithelial hyperplasia, adenocystic disease, and mammary dysplasia have all been offered, but chronic cystic mastitis is still the most widely used designation.

The term chronic cystic mastitis describes a family of lesions found in the breast. Pathologists disagree as to which lesions are legitimate family relations, so the morphology of the disease, like the terminology, appears rather fuzzy to the casual observer. Foote and Stewart have named 10 lesions often described as members of this group: cysts, papillomatosis, blunt duct adenosis, sclerosing adenosis, apocrine metaplasia, stasis and distention of ducts, periductal mastitis, fat necrosis, hyperplasia of duct epithelium, and fibroadenoma. These writers accept, however, only the first five of this group as being related lesions and forming part of chronic cystic mastitis; the others are held to represent different disease entities. They refer to the first five as the cystic and proliferative group, assuming that the proliferative lesions are responsible for the subsequent formation of cysts. A majority of pathologists accept this list, though some have argued for the inclusion of fibroadenoma. In addition, epithelial hyperplasia is usually accepted as part of the complex, with papillomas representing an advanced manifestation of hyperplasia.

The lesions of chronic cystic mastitis begin to appear in the breasts of a few women in their late twenties. The incidence is greater in the thirties and forties. Originally it was thought that the incidence of these lesions decreased after the menopause, but careful autopsy studies indicate that the lesions are common in the older age groups and may continue to increase in frequency with age. Frantz et al. found a 71 percent incidence of cystic and proliferative lesions in women over seventy years of age. Sandison noted epithelial hyperplasia of the ducts in 7 percent of women in their twenties and in 33 percent of women in their eighties. Rush and Kramer in 1963 reviewed step sections from the breasts of 20 women over seventy years of age. Approximately 100 sections were reviewed per patient, and with this close scrutiny two or more lesions of cystic mastitis were found in all the patients. Moderately severe epithelial hyperplasia was found in 14 of the 20 (Fig. 15-13). A case may be made for considering the lesions of cystic mastitis somewhat as one considers arteriosclerosis: a pathologic process that varies in degree and in time of onset but that is found to some degree in all adult females as they age.

Most of the lesions making up the complex of chronic cystic mastitis are proliferative, and almost from the first recognition of this disease there has been a suspicion that these lesions may represent a premalignant condition. Follow-up studies of patients shown by biopsy to have

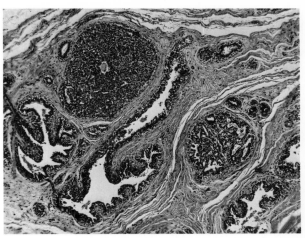

Fig. 15-13. Benign marked intraductal hyperplasia in eighty-eight-year-old female. (Hematoxylin and eosin; ×32.) (From: *Rush BF Jr, Kramer WM: Surg Gynecol Obstet 117:425, 1963, with permission.*)

chronic cystic mastitis uniformly indicate that cancer subsequently occurs three to five times more often in these patients than in the general population.

If one assumes that all women eventually develop some degree of chronic cystic mastitis, how can one conclude that the finding of chronic cystic mastitis on biopsy is associated with an increase in the incidence of cancer of the female breast compared with patients in the general population? Recent studies clearly show that only a small subgroup of lesions, those with severe hyperplasia or atypism, are associated with an increased risk of cancer. All other lesions of the complex have no associated increase in risk. The term fibrocystic *condition* has been proposed to avoid any stigma of premalignancy. This has practical importance, since some insurance companies attempted to raise their rates when the diagnosis of fibrocystic disease was made.

The lesions of chronic cystic mastitis that are most likely to present a problem in differential diagnosis and to require biopsy are cysts, fibroadenoma, ductal papilloma, and sclerosing adenosis.

Treatment. The most important aspect of this condition is the differentiation of the diffuse nodularity of the breast from carcinoma. However, many women suffer associated symptoms of tenderness and swelling of the nodules that occur most commonly during menstruation. Some claim that abstaining from coffee and other xanthine-containing substances will ameliorate the syndrome. Benefits are also claimed for high doses of vitamin E. Neither of these treatments is established as clearly effective. Danazol, a synthetic androgen analog that suppresses follicle-stimulating hormone and luteinizing hormone, is highly effective although expensive. From 100 to 400 mg, given in two divided doses daily, will usually abolish pain and tenderness within a month. Nodularity will diminish and disappear in 2 to 6 months. About half of the patients will show evidence of recurrence of symptoms within a year following the end of therapy. Treatment may be re-

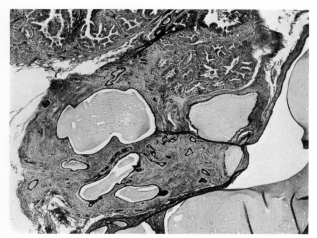

Fig. 15-14. Cystic disease with apocrine metaplasia in seventy-three-year-old female. (Hematoxylin and eosin; ×32.) (From: *Rush BF Jr, Kramer WM: Surg Gynecol Obstet 117:425, 1963, with permission.*)

peated. The antiestrogen tamoxifen is also said to be effective but is not yet FDA-approved for the treatment of this condition.

CYSTS. The cystic component of chronic cystic mastitis is most prominent in patients in their thirties and forties. The cysts may vary in size from microcysts of 1 to 2 mm to large masses several centimeters in diameter (Fig. 15-14). They are felt in the breast substance as firm, round, fairly distinct masses, often with a rubbery feeling indicative of their cystic nature. Lesions in the anterior and dependent portions of the breast may be transilluminated. They are sometimes tender and, like many of the other lesions of this complex, may increase in size toward the end of the menstrual period.

If a lesion in a patient's breast is clearly suggestive of a cyst, aspiration is a good method for confirming the diagnosis. This technique should not be used unless the rules for its employment are clearly understood. The fluid obtained should be the characteristic clear, brown-green fluid of a cyst. When the cyst is aspirated dry, no underlying mass should be palpable. If a residual mass remains after aspiration or if the fluid is bloody, biopsy must be done. The patient should be followed at intervals for a month or two after aspiration; if the cyst reappears, biopsy is also indicated. Approximately half the cysts treated by aspiration will disappear, and fluid will not reaccumulate.

FIBROADENOMAS. These lesions are most common in the twenties and early thirties. They present as lobular but not serrated masses with a firm, rubbery consistency. Their edges are sharply defined. Most commonly solitary, they may occasionally be multiple. They are differentiated from cancer by the smooth rather than irregular lobulations and by the age group in which they occur. Although a skilled examiner can probably detect a fibroadenoma with an accuracy of 80 to 85 percent, biopsy is mandatory.

DUCTAL PAPILLOMA. The hallmark of the ductal papilloma is abnormal secretion from the nipple, which is often blood-stained. In 30 percent a small nodule, 3 or 4 mm in diameter, will be palpated in the major ducts underlying the areola. In the absence of a palpable nodule the papilloma's general position can often be detected by stroking the areola toward the nipple with the tips of the fingers, carefully working around the areola in a clockwise direction until an area is discovered which on pressure results in secretion from the nipple. A bloody nipple discharge may also be indicative of an intraductal carcinoma or even a deeper-lying infiltrating ductal carcinoma. The incidence of malignancy in the presence of this physical finding is 20 to 30 percent. Diagnosis is confirmed and treatment accomplished by excision of that portion of the collecting duct system shown on physical examination to be responsible for the secretion. Urban and Baker propose that the entire collecting duct system should be excised en bloc, since these lesions are often multiple and a partial excision of the duct system will often result in the retention of other lesions which will lead to further bloody secretions later.

SCLEROSING ADENOSIS. These lesions can sometimes result in an area of fibrosis within the mammary tissue that is firm and irregular and impossible to differentiate clinically from an ordinary scirrhous carcinoma. Biopsy is required to make the differential diagnosis.

OTHER BENIGN LESIONS. Fat necrosis, thrombophlebitis of the breast, and granular cell myoblastoma are three benign lesions of the breast that can be confused on physical examination with malignant growths. All three are uncommon. Fat necrosis is the most common of the group and is probably due to trauma, although only half the patients who have this lesion recall a trauma of the breast. The breasts are in an exposed position, however, and may be hurt at the time of a larger accident when the injury to the breast is overshadowed by more serious injuries. The lesions are always superficial and often near the areola. In 40 to 50 percent of patients with this lesion, accompanying ecchymoses are lingering stigmata of previous trauma. In one-third of the patients there is a history of pain or tenderness. Retraction of the skin over the lesion is seen in 50 to 60 percent. Retraction is due to the fibrosis and scarring in the fatty lobules that involve Cooper's ligaments. As the scarring progresses and matures, skin retraction, which may first be seen within 2 weeks of the original injury, becomes more prominent. The mass of subcutaneous scar tissue that forms is distinct, irregular, and often very firm. It is easy to understand how such a mass associated with skin retraction may be mistaken for carcinoma, and in every instance a biopsy specimen of the lesion must be examined histologically. In decades past, many unnecessary radical mastectomies were done in patients with fat necrosis. Today, the practice of routinely examining frozen sections of biopsy material and most often waiting for final histologic sections prevents this tragedy.

Granular cell myoblastomas occur most commonly in the tongue but may also occur in the breast. The clinical importance of this rare tumor is that it can produce all the clinical signs of early cancer of the breast. The lesion is hard and relatively fixed to the breast tissue surrounding it. It sometimes causes dimpling of the overlying skin. Moreover, on gross examination of the specimen at operation the lesion looks and cuts like a scirrhous carcinoma of the breast. Only frozen or permanent sections can confirm that one is dealing with a benign rather than a malignant lesion.

Thrombophlebitis of a superficial vein of the breast, called *Mondor's disease,* may rarely be mistaken for a tumor because of the dimpling of the skin it produces. The tubular shape of the thrombosed vein and the accompanying tenderness usually indicate the diagnosis, but biopsy is often required for confirmation.

BREAST BIOPSY

Breast biopsy is a procedure with little risk and can be done under local anesthesia. It was the general custom to do the biopsy under general anesthesia and proceed to a definitive cancer operation if the frozen section of the lesion indicated malignancy. However, there is an increasing trend to do the biopsy under local anesthesia, often in an outpatient setting, and to continue with the larger operation, if indicated, a few days later. This delay in definitive operation has no effect on the recurrence or survival rates. A curvilinear incision in the direction of the skin lines is made over the suspicious mass. If the lesion is small, total excision is preferred, but if a large lesion is encountered, a small incisional biopsy of the main mass is done.

The nonpalpable lesion discovered by mammography presents a special problem for the surgeon. Such lesions must be marked before biopsy so that the operator can be sure that the proper tissue is removed. Marking is done by injection of a dye or insertion of a wire guide under x-ray control.

Needle biopsy of breast masses is done in many institutions and is very satisfactory if the pathologist is familiar with this type of material. Negative needle biopsies have no significance, however, since an adequate sample may not be obtained.

These biopsies were mainly done with a trocarlike needle such as a Vim-Silverman or "True-cut" that yielded a core of tissue that could be fixed and mounted. Currently, biopsy with a thin or "skinny" needle, usually 20 to 22 gauge, is gaining popularity. The thin needle is thrust several times through the tumor while suction is exerted on the attached syringe. The material obtained is spread on a slide and fixed. This is a cytologic rather than a histologic technique. Cancer cells are much less adherent to adjacent tissue than normal cells, and the thin needle seems to dislodge them preferentially so that the smaller specimens obtained yield equivalent and perhaps superior results to a trocar. In addition, patients find the thin needle a less painful and more tolerable method.

HISTOPATHOLOGY

Malignant neoplasms of the breast, with few exceptions, are adenocarcinomas. The histologic features of these lesions vary considerably, and a number of classifications are available. The following was proposed by Foote and Stewart:

HISTOLOGIC CLASSIFICATION OF CANCER OF THE BREAST

A. Paget's disease of the nipple
B. Carcinomas of mammary ducts
  1. Noninfiltrating
  2. Infiltrating
    a. Papillary carcinoma
    b. Comedocarcinoma
    c. Carcinoma with productive fibrosis
    d. Medullary carcinoma with lymphoid infiltrate
    e. Colloid carcinoma
    f. Tubular carcinoma
C. Carcinomas of mammary lobules
  1. Noninfiltrating
  2. Infiltrating
D. Relatively rare carcinomas
E. Sarcoma of the breast

PAGET'S DISEASE OF THE NIPPLE. This constitutes 1 percent of all breast carcinomas but has attracted an inordinate amount of attention and speculation, since for many years there was confusion as to whether this lesion arose primarily in the skin or in the mammary ducts. It is now generally accepted that this is a primary carcinoma of the mammary ducts of the nipple that has subsequently invaded the skin. The lesion presents as a scaling, eczematoid, and quite innocent-appearing lesion of the nipple (Fig. 15-15). In most instances it has a slow natural history, and the skin lesion may be the only evidence of neoplasm for many years. Ultimately an underlying mass will develop if the lesion is untreated. Any eczematoid lesion

Fig. 15-15. Typical scaling eczematoid lesion of Paget's disease; frequently misdiagnosed and treated by salves and ointments, with long delay in proper diagnosis.

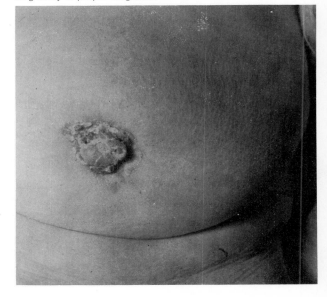

of the nipple in a postmenopausal female that persists for more than a few weeks should be biopsied to exclude the possibility of Paget's disease. Adequate histologic studies of surgical specimens almost always reveal underlying carcinomas of the mammary ducts. Invasion of the skin by these cells produces the interesting Paget's cell, a large cell with clear cytoplasm and commonly with binucleation. This is associated with evidence of chronic inflammation and a surface crust. Robbins and Berg's study of 89 cases indicated that one-third of the patients showed noninfiltrating carcinoma, and in this group the survival rate was 100 percent at 5 years. The remaining patients had infiltrating carcinoma. The overall survival rate for the group was 64 percent, indicating a better prognosis for this lesion than for the average carcinoma of the breast.

NONINFILTRATING CARCINOMAS OF THE MAMMARY DUCTS. These constitute 1 percent of carcinomas of the breast. It is unfortunate that more cancers are not seen at the noninfiltrating stage, since these lesions are carcinomas in situ and operation should result in 100 percent 5-year survival. That this is not the case, 5-year survival being about 90 percent, reflects the fact that the breast is a large organ and that lesions that appear to be noninfiltrating may in fact be infiltrating at some area that the pathologist has not examined. Foote and Stewart report that they have traced progression of intraductal carcinoma from benign papillary hyperplasia through atypism to noninfiltrating intraductal carcinoma and ultimately to infiltrating carcinoma throughout a breast specimen. They state that while this may be one route for the development of cancer of the breast, cancer may arise from normal intraductal cells directly. The differentiation of a noninfiltrating intraductal carcinoma from a benign hyperplasia may be difficult; areas of atypism can blend gradually from one state into the other. Histologically, the duct epithelium is usually seen to be thrown up into papillae that show a loss of cohesiveness and disorientation of cells, with pleomorphism and occasionally mitotic figures but without evidence of invasion of the basement membrane. A more dramatic form is the noninfiltrating comedocarcinoma, in which hyperplasia is more extreme, choking the entire duct for long distances with masses of cells. These lesions commonly develop central necrosis of the cells. A gross section of such a lesion will extrude small cores of tissue from the ducts very much as the core is extruded from a comedo when it is squeezed, thus giving rise to the term comedocarcinoma.

INFILTRATING PAPILLARY CARCINOMA. Presumably a later stage or a more aggressive form of the noninfiltrating papillary lesion, these carcinomas still tend to evolve slowly and have a better 5-year survival rate than the average carcinoma of the breast. They produce a mass rather soft to palpation compared with the typical hard, fibrous lesion usually associated with breast cancer. They may reach large size before metastasizing to the axilla. Dimpling and skin edema are less commonly seen, another index of the late infiltration of the lymphatics and of the failure to stimulate a fibrous response. Noninfiltrating papillary carcinomas are often seen in association with the infiltrating form.

Infiltrating comedocarcinomas comprise approxi-

mately 5 percent of all breast cancers. They are often found in association with other forms of adenocarcinoma that result in productive fibrosis, and the presence of comedocarcinoma together with other elements of carcinoma of the breast does not significantly alter the prognosis from the average.

INFILTRATING DUCT CARCINOMA WITH PRODUCTIVE FIBROSIS. This is the commonest form of breast cancer, constituting 78 percent of the specimens seen. There is a tremendous variation in the amount of fibrosis. The lesion has been termed *scirrhous carcinoma, fibrocarcinoma,* and *sclerosing carcinoma.* The desmoplastic response to the invading cancer cells accounts for the remarkable hardness of the average breast cancer. Grossly the lesions have uneven serrated edges. They cut with great resistance and often with a rather gritty feeling as the knife edge passes through them. Histologically the lesions may vary from scattered, well-differentiated adenomatous clusters and a massive amount of fibrostroma to dense cellular aggregates with only minor amounts of fibroplasia (Fig. 15-16). Electron microscopic examination of these tumors indicates that they originate in the myoepithelial cells of the mammary duct.

MEDULLARY CARCINOMAS. Five percent of carcinomas of the breast assume this pattern, and the diagnosis indicates a favorable prognosis for the patient. Even in the presence of metastatic disease the prognosis remains favorable; the 5-year overall survival rate for the lesion is 85 to 90 percent. These lesions are soft, bulky, and often large. Necrotic areas of varying size are usually present. Occasionally one finds a lesion that is almost totally infarcted. On physical examination these tumors are freely movable, and smaller tumors are likely to be diagnosed clinically as cysts or fibroadenomas. Histologically the tumors are made up of large rounded or polygonal cells with an abundant cytoplasm arranged in broad or narrow plexiform masses anastomosing with one another. Electron microscopic and histochemical evidence suggests that these cells originate in the ductal epithelium. There is

Fig. 15-16. Intraductal carcinoma with stromal invasion in eighty-three-year-old female. Field shows almost entire extent of this very early lesion. (Hematoxylin and eosin; ×32.)

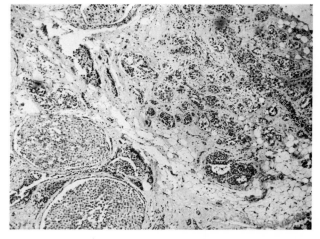

an abundant lymphoid infiltrate. Plasma cells are often seen and are sometimes very prominent. Axillary metastases occur less frequently than in the ordinary carcinoma of the breast but are not uncommon, occurring in about 40 percent. Metastasis frequently involves only a single node.

COLLOID CARCINOMA. This is an infrequent mammary cancer constituting about 1 percent of all breast cancers. The lesions contain a much greater amount of mucin than the usual adenocarcinoma and may be frankly gelatinous on cut section. Clinically these lesions are soft and ill defined and, like the medullary lesions, may be quite bulky before detection. Histologically the predominant picture is of large mucinous lakes in which epithelial aggregates float. Patients with these lesions have a better-than-average survival rate.

TUBULAR CARCINOMA. Also known as "well-differentiated" or "orderly" carcinoma, this lesion has only recently received attention. It may mimic sclerosing or blunt duct adenosis and is made up of tubular structures, typically lined by a single layer of well-differentiated epithelium. It occurs in pure form in only 1.2 percent of cases but may be combined frequently with other histological forms. If a breast carcinoma contains 90 percent or more of the tubular lesion, long-term survival approaches 100 percent.

CARCINOMA OF THE MAMMARY LOBULES. This lesion arises in the mammary lobules from the cells of the acini and the terminal ducts. Most of the acini of a lobule are involved. Lobules may be of normal size or enlarged, with an unsystematic hyperplasia of the lining cells until the lumen is plugged. At the in situ stage of development these are the only changes, and simple mastectomy at this point should produce cure. The lesion subsequently becomes infiltrative and ultimately may give rise to regular scirrhous carcinoma.

Multicentricity and bilaterality are important features of lobular carcinoma. Eighty-eight percent of breast specimens removed for in situ lobular carcinoma show other in situ lesions scattered throughout the specimen. Examination of the contralateral breast has demonstrated in situ lesions in from 35 to 59 percent of specimens.

SARCOMA OF THE BREAST. Sarcomas of the breast are very rare. The commonest sarcoma seen is cystosarcoma phylloides, but only one in ten of these is truly malignant, the great majority being a benign variant of fibroadenoma. Great confusion is created because both the benign and malignant form are called "cystosarcoma." When Müller first described and named the lesion in 1838 he was aware of its predominantly benign nature. At that time "sarcoma" meant simply a fleshy tumor and did not carry the meaning of malignancy that it does today. Modern synonyms for the benign lesion are *giant intracanalicular or pericanalicular fibroadenoma* and *intracanalicular myxoma*. The malignant variant has been called *adenocarcinoma*.

Cystosarcoma phylloides occurs at an older average age (forty), is larger, and has a more cellular stroma than fibroadenoma. When first seen clinically these tumors average 5 to 10 cm, have a firm and rubbery consistency, and may have a bosselated surface. In cut section the

tumors have a discrete capsule. Small lesions present leaflike intracanalicular protrusions, and larger lesions have cystic spaces into which project densely packed polypoid masses.

The malignant variant metastasizes most commonly to the lungs, bones, and subcutaneous tissues. Axillary metastasis is so uncommon that simple mastectomy is an adequate procedure for both the benign and the malignant forms.

PRIMARY TREATMENT

The first historical reference to cancer of the breast appears in the Edwin Smith Surgical Papyrus (3000 to 2500 B.C.). The patient described is a man, but the description suggests most of the clinical features of breast cancer. The author concludes that "there is no treatment." References to cancer of the breast are scattered and brief over the following 2500 years. Even in that large body of writings concerning Greek and Roman medicine, the Corpus Hippocraticum, direct reference to the treatment of breast cancer is absent, although it is clear that the condition was recognized.

Celsus, a Roman of the first century, spoke of operation and advised limiting it to early lesions: "None of these can be removed but the cacoethes [early lesion], the rest are irritated by every method of cure. The more violent the operations are, the more angry they grow." Galen, in the second century, inscribed one of the classic clinical observations:

We have often seen in the breast a tumor exactly resembling the animal the crab. Just as the crab has legs on both sides of his body, so in this disease the veins extending out from the unnatural growth take the shape of a crab's legs. We have often cured this disease in its early stages, but after it has reached a large size no one has cured it without operation. In all operations we attempt to excise a pathological tumor in a circle in the region where it borders on the healthy tissue.

Although Galen spoke of operations for tumors, his system of medicine ascribed the disease to an excess of black bile, and logically excision of a local outbreak could not cure the systemic imbalance. The Galenic theories dominated medicine until the Renaissance. Most established physicians looked down on attempts at operative treatment as misdirected and futile. Only when it was again established that a cancer could arise in a part as a local disorder quite separate from a systemic imbalance could excision of the tumor be recognized as rational therapy. Morgagni's definitive study of gross pathology, appropriately entitled *The Seats and Causes of Disease*, supplied this new rationale. Radical mastectomy until recently was the standard treatment for operable cancer of the breast in the United States. This operation involves the removal of the entire breast with a generous portion of overlying skin, all the underlying pectoralis major and minor muscles, and the entire lymphatic and fibrofatty contents of the axilla.

This procedure evolved slowly from simple amputation of the breast. LeDran in the eighteenth century repudiated Galen's humoral theory and stated that cancer of the breast was a local disease that spread by way of the lymphatics to the regional nodes. He removed enlarged axillary nodes in his operations on patients with breast cancer. In the nineteenth century, Moore of Middlesex Hospital, England, emphasized wide removal of the breast and felt that when there was neoplasm in the axilla, the axillary contents should be removed in one block together with the breast. In a presentation before the British Medical Association in 1877, Banks supported Moore's concepts and advocated that axillary nodes should always be removed in one block with the breast tissue whether there were palpable nodes present or not, since occult involvement of the axillary nodes was so often present.

As Lewison notes, it remained for Halsted, the new professor of surgery at a young school called The Johns Hopkins Medical School, to "culminate the operation and germinate the present modern method." Halsted proposed a standard procedure, removing all the structures in one block. His first operation was performed about 1882, and he reported 13 cases in 1890. The procedure was almost exactly as it is today except that the pectoralis minor muscle was not removed. In 1894 he reported more than 50 cases over the preceding 12 years. In the same year Herbert Willy Meyer of New York reported six patients operated upon by a technique he had evolved independently. This procedure, almost a duplicate of the Halsted mastectomy, added the removal of the pectoralis minor muscle. Halsted subsequently accepted this addition, and the modern radical mastectomy is often attributed to both these men. This procedure and the wide-block excision that it incorporated was soon adopted widely and for the following 60 years was the only operation used by the well-trained surgeon for treatment of breast cancer.

Halsted's operation proved so successful because it provided highly reliable locoregional control of breast cancer in an era when almost all patients presenting for treatment had neglected, far-advanced cancer (Stage III or IV) by modern standards. Every one of Halsted's first 50 patients had involved axillary nodes, and he considered a 6-cm mass to be "small." By the middle of this century the situation changed markedly. The average size of lesions when first seen was much smaller, and these were patients with axillary nodal metastasis. As we shall explore in the section on selection of the operation, this greatly expanded the possible procedures available and markedly diminished the role of radical mastectomy.

SELECTION OF PATIENTS. When radical mastectomy was the only treatment available, surgeons attempted to exclude from the operation those patients who would almost certainly develop distant metastasis at a later date. The generally accepted "criteria of inoperability" include fixation of the local breast lesion to the chest wall, fixation of the involved lymph nodes in the axilla, and inflammatory carcinoma of the breast. Haagensen compiled the following detailed list of criteria:

1. Extensive edema of the skin over the breast (Fig. 15-17)
2. Satellite nodules in the skin over the breast
3. Carcinoma of the inflammatory type (Fig. 15-18)
4. Parasternal tumor nodules
5. Proved supraclavicular metastases

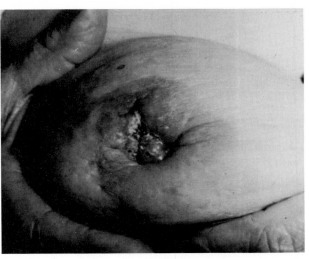

Fig. 15-17. Large cancer of breast with retraction of nipple, skin edema, and several satellite skin nodules.

6. Edema of the arm
7. Distant metastases
8. Any two or more of the following grave signs of locally advanced carcinoma:
   a. Ulceration of the skin
   b. Edema of the skin of limited extent (less than one-third of breast skin involved)
   c. Solid fixation of tumor to the chest wall
   d. Axillary lymph nodes measuring 2.5 cm or more in transverse diameter
   e. Fixation of the axillary nodes to the skin or deep structures of the axilla

At one time these criteria excluded more than 25 percent of patients from surgical treatment. In the average

Fig. 15-18. Inflammatory carcinoma of breast. Bright pink to red suffuses area of skin involvement, reflecting inflammatory response to extensive scattering of tumor cells in subcutaneous tissues. Large skin lesion above nipple is congenital pigmented nevus unrelated to the cancer.

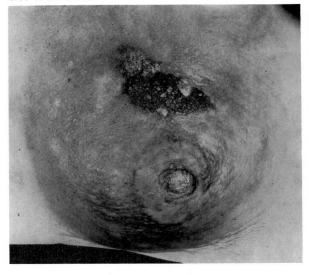

community hospital today less than 15 percent of patients would be found with such advanced tumors. In addition, the successful use of adjuvant chemotherapy has greatly changed our attitude toward patients with a high likelihood of disseminated disease, and if no clinical metastasis is found on initial clinical work-up, most patients will have an operation designed to eradicate the locoregional disease.

Every effort should be made to identify patients with distant metastasis. Search for metastatic lesions preoperatively should include a chest film and liver chemistries. If liver chemistries are altered, a liver scintiscan should be done. If the patient has symptoms of bone pain, a bone scintiscan is indicated. A large number of serum markers for breast carcinomas, both primary and metastatic, are currently under investigation but have yet to emerge into clinical practice.

SELECTION OF THE OPERATION. For the past 20 years a controversy has been raging about the appropriate operation for patients with operable breast cancer. The debate was initially between radical mastectomy and total ("simple") mastectomy plus radiation therapy; then between radical mastectomy and total mastectomy alone; and finally between radical mastectomy alone and partial mastectomy or "lumpectomy" with or without radiation therapy. While these have been the major themes, some minor variations of radical mastectomy also were proposed, either a little less than the radical mastectomy, sparing the pectoralis major (Patey's operation) or both pectoral muscles (Madden's operation), or a little more than the radical mastectomy, taking the internal mammary lymph nodes and adjacent chest wall (Urban's operation). Even more minimal operations include local excision of the breast mass with complete or partial resection of axillary nodes and finally incisional or needle biopsy of the primary lesion with subsequent radiation therapy to the breast and axilla.

The arguments for the various procedures have been remarkably bitter at times, with charges of bias, the citing of incomplete data, and irrationality being hurled not only in the scientific but in the lay press as well. Carter notes that "some women's groups have viewed the discussions about various treatment options in terms of feminist issues. The radical and modified radical mastectomy have been portrayed as procedures devised by male surgeons insensitive to the mutilating effects on women." He compares this with the debate about radical prostatectomy versus radiation for local control of primary prostate cancer "which is not tinged with anything like the emotionalism that similar options evoke for primary breast cancer."

American surgeons have remained reasonably levelheaded during this period, most influenced by maturing data from large, prospective, randomized trials. At first they adhered to the traditional radical mastectomy. After all, the advantages of doing lesser operations were functional and cosmetic, while the penalty of being wrong was the life of a patient. A survey of New Jersey surgeons in 1971 showed that 75 percent would do a radical breast dissection and 15 percent a modified radical operation for

a 2-cm lesion in the upper outer quadrant of a fifty-year-old woman. In 1977, surgeons in the same state indicated that approximately 40 percent would do a radical mastectomy, 40 percent a modified radical mastectomy, 15 percent a total mastectomy, and 5 percent some other procedure. By 1982, 90 percent of these surgeons had adopted modified radical mastectomy (Fig. 15-19) for Stage I breast cancers but very few were doing lesser procedures.

Operations for Early Breast Cancer. Stages I and II breast cancers make up 80 to 85 percent of cases now seen in most hospitals in this country. The general consensus until recently was that modified radical mastectomy was the procedure of choice for these lesions, and Maddox reported that a randomized trial showed no significant difference in survival when this procedure was compared with the classic radical mastectomy.

In 1980 Veronesi reported the results of a large, randomized, prospective trial in Italy in which breast tumors 2 cm or less with palpable axillary nodes were randomized to treatment either with radical mastectomy or with "quadrantectomy" (the quadrant of breast in the area of the tumor was removed) plus total axillary node dissection and radiotherapy. Local recurrence rates and survival were the same in both groups. In 1985 Fisher reported the results of the National Surgical Adjuvant Breast Project (NSABP) study that compared three arms of therapy for lesions 4 cm or smaller in diameter with or without palpable axillary lymph nodes. The treatment modalities were modified radical mastectomy, removal of the tumor with a rim of normal tissue, plus removal of lower axillary nodes, plus postoperative radiotherapy; the third group was like the second except that radiation was omitted. Survival and local recurrence were statistically the same in both the first and second arm. In the third arm, patients with local excision and removal of the lower axillary nodes, but without radiation therapy, had a very high local recurrence rate of 24 percent in lymph node negative patients and 36 percent in node positive patients (Fig. 15-20). This finding seems to support the multicentric nature of breast cancer and to indicate that the entire breast on the involved side should be treated. The choice of such treatment may have to be left to bias of the surgeon and the wishes of the patient. The conclusions of the NSABP study are based on 5-year actuarial results and will be firmer if they hold up over time. Past experience from other series suggests that the results will continue to be valid (Fig. 15-21).

The great advantage of sparing the breast by using local excision is the encouragement it gives patients to approach diagnosis and treatment early enough to be eligible for such treatment.

In addition to excision of the local breast mass, the axillary lymph nodes should be removed. The value of removing axillary contents has been defended in the past on the claim of improved survival. The results of controlled cooperative clinical trials indicate that treatment of the axilla does not change survival in patients with clinical Stage I tumors. On the other hand, the added information gained by knowing whether or not axillary nodes are his-

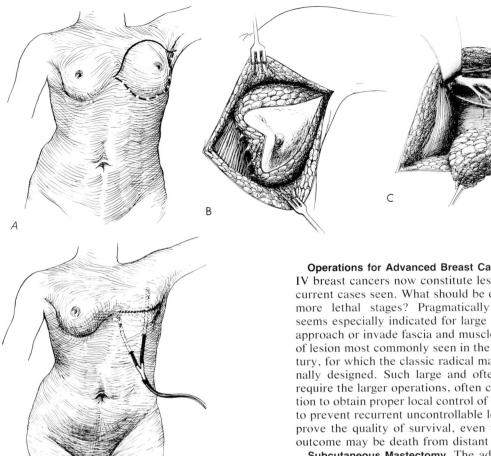

Fig. 15-19. Technique of total mastectomy and axillary dissection (modified radical mastectomy). *A.* Transverse elliptical incision facilitates subsequent reconstruction. *B.* Development of skin flaps. *C.* Clearing of the axillary vein and axilla en bloc with breast. This provides optimal sampling of lymph nodes. The pectoralis major and minor muscles are retracted medially. *D.* Suction drainage obviates accumulation of fluid beneath flaps and allows a small dressing.

tologically involved by malignancy is of enormous value to surgeons and patients, both in rendering an accurate prognosis and in influencing the trend of future therapy. The addition of axillary dissection to breast resection adds very little in risk or morbidity, and the dividend in "staging" the extent of the disease is well worth the price whether survival is improved or not. While "sampling" the lower axilla has been suggested as adequate, several studies indicate that accurate staging is correlated with the completeness of the axillary dissection. In patients treated by local excision and radiation, complete removal of the axillary nodes obviates the need for axillary, supraclavicular radiation, greatly simplifying the radiotherapeutic approach.

Operations for Advanced Breast Cancer. Stages III and IV breast cancers now constitute less than 20 percent of current cases seen. What should be done for these much more lethal stages? Pragmatically, muscle resection seems especially indicated for large or deep tumors that approach or invade fascia and muscle. This was the type of lesion most commonly seen in the late nineteenth century, for which the classic radical mastectomy was originally designed. Such large and often ulcerated tumors require the larger operations, often combined with radiation to obtain proper local control of tumor. The object is to prevent recurrent uncontrollable local disease and improve the quality of survival, even though the eventual outcome may be death from distant metastasis.

Subcutaneous Mastectomy. The advent of mammography has led to an increasing diagnosis of in situ (TIS) and very small microinvasive cancers (T1a). This has coincided with the introduction of subcutaneous mastectomy, a technique in which most of the mammary tissue is removed but the skin of the breast is preserved. Contour is restored by inserting a silastic prosthesis into the subcutaneous pocket left by the excision of breast tissue or now, more commonly, under the pectoralis major muscle. It is impossible to remove all breast tissue by this method, and 1 or 2 percent remains in the subcutaneous layer near the skin even if the nipple is sacrificed. Development of cancer in this residual mammary tissue has been reported, and in view of the multifocal nature of breast cancer, it is expected that some of the foci may be left behind. The risk benefit ratio of this approach remains to be established, and while it is a very attractive alternative for women with in situ cancer of the breast, the accepted procedure for such lesions in the United States is still total mastectomy or possibly radiation therapy.

The Problem of Bilateral Mastectomy. Foote and Stewart have observed that "the most frequent precancerous lesion of the breast is a cancer of the opposite breast." Berg and Robbins noted that the incidence of occurrence of cancer in the contralateral breast following radical mastectomy was approximately 1 percent per year, so that

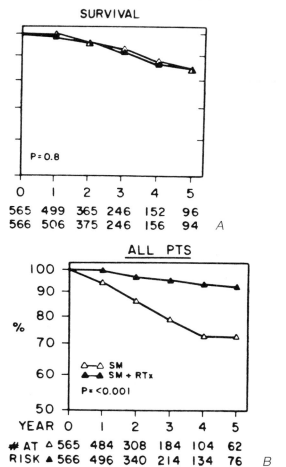

SURVIVAL

P = 0.8

	0	1	2	3	4	5
	565	499	365	246	152	96
	566	506	375	246	156	94

A

ALL PTS

△—△ SM
▲—▲ SM + RTx

P = <0.001

YEAR	0	1	2	3	4	5
# AT △	565	484	308	184	104	62
RISK ▲	566	496	340	214	134	76

B

Fig. 15-20. *A.* Survival in patients with segmental mastectomy compared with segmental resection plus radiation. The curves are virtually identical. *B.* Disease-free survival in patients with segmental mastectomy alone, compared with patients with segmental mastectomy plus radiation. (From: *Fisher B et al: N Engl J Med 312:655, 1985, with permission.*)

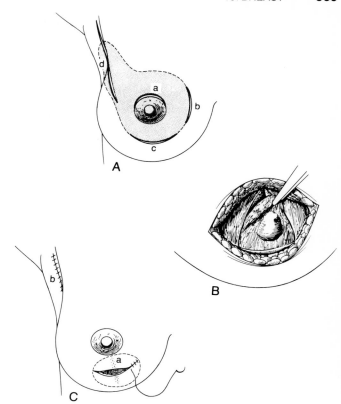

A

B

C

Fig. 15-21. Technique of segmental mastectomy. *A.* Because of the circumferential skin lines of the breast a circumferential incision gives the best cosmetic results. If the tumor is relatively small and close to the nipple, a periareolar incision, as shown in Aa, is chosen; otherwise circumferential incisions directly over the main body of the tumor as shown in Ab and c should be used. Tumors in the upper outer quadrant, especially close to the axillae, can best be approached through an incision that lies along the tail of the breast and extends into the axillae, parallel to the fibers of the pectoralis major muscle. This incision gives the best access to the outer quadrant, tail of the breast, and axillary contents simultaneously. *B.* This illustrates the approach to a breast tumor through a circumferential incision. Dissection is carried down through the fat until the breast tissue is revealed. Skin and fat are undermined in a radial direction, both away and toward the nipple. A wedge-shaped excision of the full thickness of breast tissue containing the tumor with a 1- to 2-cm margin of normal tissue is removed. *C.* Closure of the incision. The excision of breast tissue has left a wedge-shaped defect in the disclike breast. Rotating the two cut edges of the breast toward each other will result in a nice anatomical closure along a radial line. (a) The skin and fat must have been undermined sufficiently so that the breast tissue will slide together without distorting the skin. The skin is then closed in a circumferential direction using subcuticular sutures. Note that the axillary dissection is not done in continuity except for lesions of the upper outer quadrant. An incision slightly posterior and parallel with the upper lateral border of the pectoralis major muscle (b) provides the best cosmetic approach since it is totally hidden from view and also provides the best exposure to all levels of the axillae.

the cumulative risk of cancer in the remaining breast among patients surviving radical mastectomy for 20 years was as high as 20 percent. As long ago as 1951, Pack published a plea for routine simple mastectomy of the remaining breast at the time of mastectomy for cancer. Presumably because of the psychologic blow to a woman who is asked to lose both her breasts, this approach has rarely been advocated by surgeons, and the usual routine after mastectomy has been to follow the contralateral breast with special care in the ensuing years. The recognition of the high risk of contralateral cancer in patients with in situ lobular carcinoma has caused a change in attitude toward this particular form of the disease. Currently recommended treatment for patients with either in situ or invasive lobular cancer of the breast is total mastectomy of the contralateral breast. Treatment of the other breast with radiation therapy instead may be effective since the

NSABP study seems to establish the effectiveness of radiation therapy for microscopic disease. This inference has not been established by any clinical trials. Should this recommendation be refused, the patient is requested at least to permit a biopsy of the remaining breast. If this biopsy reveals in situ lobular cancer, a total mastectomy is carried out. If invasive lobular cancer is found, modified radical mastectomy is done. If the biopsy is negative, a very careful follow-up is recommended, with mammography and careful breast examination at least twice yearly.

A minority of physicians recommend a "watch" policy for in situ lobular carcinoma. They reason that only one-third of these lesions ultimately become invasive, and that even the invasive lesions of this tumor have a better prognosis than the usual invasive ductal lesion. Close follow-up would thus preserve a substantial number of women from what might be an unnecessary mastectomy. This view of therapy has not proved popular among patients and surgeons. Most women are uneasy about harboring a malignant breast lesion even if it is preinvasive, and most surgeons share this feeling. Moreover, the transition from preinvasive to invasive may go undetected for long periods, since it is not necessarily accompanied by any clinical signs.

OPERATIVE MORTALITY. This is very low for all the various types of mastectomy. Kennedy and Miller reported no deaths following 212 simple mastectomies; Handley and Thackray reported no deaths following 143 modified radical mastectomies; Butcher reported 0.7 percent mortality in 425 radical mastectomies; and Haagensen and his associates had no deaths in 556 radical mastectomies. In all these series any death of a patient up to 3 months after operation was considered an operative death. Even among patients with extended mastectomy, mortality is low. Sugarbaker reported 1 postoperative death in 250 patients with this procedure.

ADJUVANT THERAPY FOLLOWING OPERATIONS FOR BREAST CANCER. The most rewarding event in breast cancer therapy in recent years is the demonstration that adjuvant chemotherapy in high-risk patients contributes substantially to relapse-free long-term survival. This has served as a model for trials of adjuvant therapy in other cancers as well. Fisher deserves the chief credit for first recognizing that early trials of a very brief course of triethylene ethiophosphonamide (Thiotepa) given during and immediately after operation produced a decrease in recurrence rate in long-term follow-up of a small subset of younger patients. As principal investigator of the National Surgical Adjuvant Breast Project (NSABP), he conducted extensive adjuvant studies of a single drug L-PAM (L-phenylalanine mustard), which confirmed his early observation. Bonadonna and his group at the Milan Tumor Institute then found that a three-drug combination of methotrexate, cytoxan, and 5-fluorouracil (CMF) was also effective, and Fisher confirmed in comparative trials that a two-drug combination of L-PAM and 5-FU was superior to L-PAM alone for adjuvant therapy. When several drugs are used in adequate dosages, it also appears that patients in all age groups benefit, rather than only the younger patients who responded to the older one-drug protocols (Fig. 15-22). Bonadonna and others have reported that 6 months of postoperative adjuvant therapy with CMF is as effective as 12 months. The impressive benefit of adjuvant therapy is demonstrated by a report from the South Western Oncology Group (SWOG) in which multidrug adjuvant therapy consisting of CMF plus vincristine and prednisone produced a 5-year relapse-free survival rate of 88 percent in women with one to three positive axillary nodes compared with the 50 percent relapse-free survival rate that occurs in this group without adjuvant treatment. Currently the most frequently used adjuvant therapy following operations for breast cancer is CMF. While this was originally recommended only for women with three or more positive axillary nodes, the present trend has been to use it in any patient with one or more grossly positive axillary nodes. Adjuvant chemotherapy of patients with low-risk Stage I lesions is not recommended, since the mortality due to cancer in this group is less than 10 percent at 5 and 10 years, and long-term hazards of chemotherapeutic drugs, especially the alkylating agents, have not been fully determined. There is some evidence that these are carcinogenic and may themselves induce some cancers. However, considerable effort is being expended to identify subsets of patients at high risk for recurrence. Even when the lesion is Stage I, such patients would be likely candidates for adjuvant therapy.

If a postmenopausal patient has an estrogen-receptor positive tumor, the adjuvant treatment of choice is the antiestrogen, tamoxifen, which will confer a survival advantage at least as good as and probably better than chemotherapy in such patients. Current recommendations of a consensus panel at the NIH for adjuvant therapy for women not on a clinical trial are: for premenopausal node positive women, chemotherapy; for premenopausal node negative women, no adjuvant therapy; for node positive, ER positive, postmenopausal women, tamoxifen; for postmenopausal node negative or node positive, ER negative women, no therapy.

For many decades radiotherapy was the conventional adjuvant therapy used in all patients following radical mastectomy when axillary nodes were found to contain tumor. Multiple randomized clinical trials carried out in the 1950s and 1960s revealed that such radiotherapy had no effect on relapse-free survival or on mortality. Local recurrence rates were favorably affected, with reductions of as much as 50 percent. Most recently the trend has been to advise radiotherapy following operation only in patients at high risk for local recurrence. Even this practice is now debated because a randomized trial indicates that multiple-drug chemotherapy given postoperatively is a substantially superior adjuvant treatment compared with the same drugs given after radiotherapy.

PROGNOSIS

The arguments for and against different forms of therapy in breast cancer are mainly statistical and are chiefly based on survival figures. Before an observer can appreciate this debate, a clear understanding of the data is required. The accurate comparison of results in different series demands that there be a common denominator.

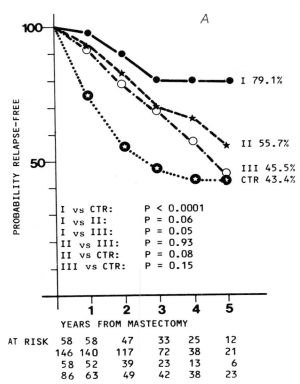

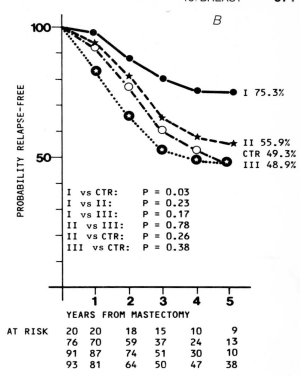

Fig. 15-22. *A.* Relationship of relapse-free survival to dose level in 348 premenopausal patients. The dose levels are indicated by I (>85 percent of the optimal calculated dose), II (65 to 84 percent), and III (<65 percent); CTR denotes controls. The percentages beside the dose levels show the proportion of patients who did not have relapses during the 5 years. *B.* Relationship of relapse-free survival to dose levels in 280 postmenopausal patients; abbreviations are the same as in *A.* Significantly superior and comparable survival occurred in both premenopausal and postmenopausal patients when adequate dosages of CMF were used. (From: *Bonadonna G et al: Cancer Treat Rep 65:61, 1981, with permission.*)

There is great variation in the base line of many published series, and astute investigation is often necessary to determine whether two sets of figures are truly comparable.

An older method of standard reporting required that all patients seen at an institution be reported in the final results, whether they were treated or not. This was called the "absolute," or "crude," survival figure. It had the advantage of indicating the effect of patient selection on the surgical, or "definitive," survival figures. Its disadvantage was that the total experience at different institutions varied greatly. Private hospitals and clinics have a much greater number of early and operable cases compared with cancer hospitals and charity institutions.

Favorable attention has been given to methods of clinical evaluation of the stage of the tumor. By this method the results in patients at an equal stage of disease can be compared among institutions. An advantage of this approach is that since the evaluation is based on pretreatment clinical findings, it is possible to compare the results in patients treated by radiation, radical mastectomy, simple mastectomy, or extended radical mastectomy even though microscopic evaluation of lymph node involvement is available with some forms of treatment and not with others. Disadvantages are that judgment of the extent of involvement is subjective and classification depends greatly on the skill and consistency of the examiner. The system of staging recommended by the American Joint Committee on Cancer Staging and End Results Reporting is most widely accepted (Table 15-1). Other systems include the Columbia classification, the Manchester classification, and the Steinthal classification; these are now obsolete.

New diagnostic methods, especially mammography, have provided a new group of lesions not previously considered by any of the staging methods. Termed by some "minimal breast cancer," these are in situ and microinvasive lesions so small that they are not detectable by conventional palpation of the breast. Current data indicate that 5-year survivals in this group exceed 90 percent.

The best way to evaluate methods of treatment is by cooperative programs among many institutions in which all factors are governed by the same rules and in which random selection of patients for the different methods of therapy is used. Even these trials are not an easy solution to the problem. Such trials tend to be biased toward false-negative results. Only in the largest of the cooperative trials is the chance of error in a negative result reduced to under 10 percent.

NO TREATMENT. In 1951 Park and Lees in a statistical analysis of 5-year survival figures for breast carcinoma tried to show that the course of the disease was not affected by operation. They regarded the improvement in 5-year survival seen following operation as an artifact introduced by operating upon patients earlier in the natural course of the disease. There are now available a number of studies of large groups of patients with untreated breast cancer. Survival computed from the onset of symptoms averages 19 percent at 5 years, 2.5 percent at 10 years. If one computes survival from onset of diagnosis, a figure more comparable with the situation in surgical series, the 5- and 10-year survivals average 8.6 percent and 1.2 percent, respectively. Bloom et al. found that untreated patients with histologically low-grade (grade 1 of 3) neoplasms had survivals of 22 percent, 9 percent, and 0 at 5, 10, and 15 years, respectively. They compared these with survivals of 82, 56, and 37 percent at the same time intervals for lesions of comparable histologic grade in their own treated series (Fig. 15-12).

OPERATIVE THERAPY. If survival data following operative therapy from the introduction of the radical mastectomy to the present are examined, one may wonder why there has been argument and confusion (Fig. 15-23). Dean Lewis and William Reinhoff reported in 1942 that the overall 5-year survival of 393 patients treated at the Johns Hopkins Hospital between 1889 and 1931 was 18 percent, little better than Bloom et al.'s untreated patients. In 1973 the American Joint Committee on Cancer Staging reported in a collected series of 2424 patients treated from 1950 to 1957 an overall survival of 61 percent. Haid and Zuckerman examined the results in 560 patients between

1973 and 1977 and found the 5-year survival was 81 percent. In the first two series the standard operation was radical mastectomy; in the last group most patients underwent modified radical mastectomy. Early diagnosis appears a major factor influencing the change in mortality. The Joint Committee patients had Stage I lesions in 17 percent, while the Haid and Zuckerman patients were classified Stage I in 51 percent. Only 19 percent of their patients were Stage III or IV. Even in this last group there was an improvement in survival, probably because 78 of 288 Stages II and III patients received multidrug therapy following operation. The end result is that the National Cancer Institute and a number of state tumor registries have reported small but steady increases in 5-year survivals in patients with both regional and localized disease since about 1950. Epidemiologic reports from Connecticut and Saskatchewan, Canada, establish a significant increase in the incidence of breast cancer in the last several decades accompanied by a decrease in mortality, thus implying an increase in survival (Fig. 15-24). This trend has continued to the present.

Survival for 5 years following radical mastectomy does not provide the same assurance against recurrence that it does for some other cancers. The risk of death continues higher than for the general population for at least 25 years after the operation, although this risk gradually diminishes with time. According to Berg and Robbins, change in risk over the postoperative period follows a log-normal curve. From this model it can be predicted that after operation the risk of recurrence and death will continue to decrease but will always be present, being about 1 percent in the decade from 30 to 40 years after operation and 0.5 percent from 40 to 50 years after operation.

Our attitudes concerning survival and prognosis continue to be conditioned by our beliefs concerning the natural history of the disease. Mueller has reported data indicating that survival following treatment of breast cancer follows an exponential curve, that is, that the annual risk of recurrence and death remains constant and if patients lived long enough all would eventually die of their tumor. If true, this would imply that all tumors have disseminated and metastasized before clinical detection and treatment. In this circumstance treatment is effective only by altering the slope of the curve and delaying the ultimate death due to the cancer, long enough, it may be hoped, so that the patient dies of other "more natural" causes. This hypothesis is in conflict with the data of Berg and Robbins cited above and those of Blackwood and Rush, who indicated that the hazard function or risk of annual recurrence decreases significantly over time, following a well-known survival curve called the Weibull distribution. Duncan and Kerr have examined a large series of patients treated in the 1940s with a follow-up of 20 or more years. Their data indicate that the "curability" of Stages I and II patients in their era was 30.5 percent (Fig. 15-25). If only lesions of 1 cm were considered without positive nodes clinically, 20-year survival was 90 percent.

Koscielny and his coauthors suggest that there is a critical volume or threshold for each tumor at which the first

Fig. 15-23. This graph illustrates the startling increase in 5-year survival in patients with "operable" (i.e., Stages I, II, and III) breast cancer in the past century regardless of the mode of therapy. The Hopkins series, the Haagensen series, and the American Joint Committee on Cancer series were treated by radical mastectomy; McWhirter's patients were treated with total mastectomy and radiation therapy; and those in the Haid series were treated with modified radical mastectomy, and in some patients adjuvant chemotherapy was used.

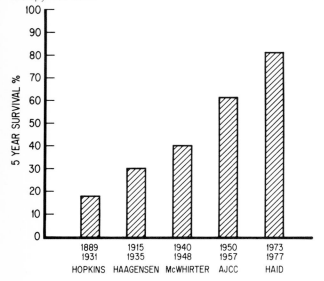

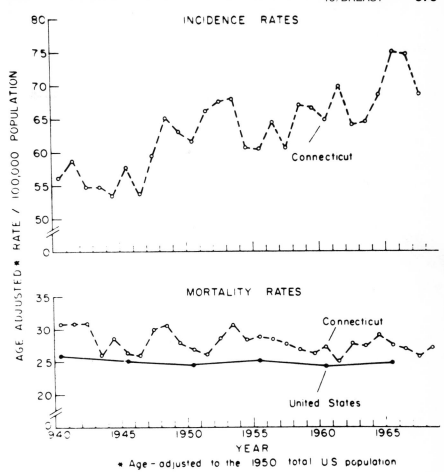

Fig. 15-24. Contrary to past reports data from large population groups now indicate an increasing incidence and a decreasing mortality rate for breast cancer. (From: *Cutler SJ, Christine B, Barcley THC: Cancer 28:1376, 1971, with permission.*)

Fig. 15-25. ''Curability'' of breast cancer as determined in a group of patients treated 20 or more years. Survival rate in Stages I and II patients parallels the normal population at 20 years, and projection to the base line indicates that 30.5 percent of such patients are curable. (From: *Brinkley D, Haybittle JL: World J Surg 1:287, 1977, with permission.*)

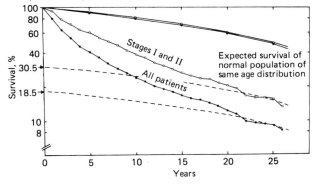

remote metastasis is initiated. The smaller and more well differentiated a tumor is the less likely it is that distant spread will have occurred and the more likely that locoregional methods will cure the lesion.

Radical mastectomy is no longer the routine treatment for all patients with cancer of the breast, and most agree that there is a group of smaller cancers that can be treated by lesser procedures. It is still, however, the reference procedure, the operation with which we have the most experience over the greatest period of time. Comparisons between institutional series have little or no statistical validity at this level of discrimination, and one must turn to the rapidly accumulating data from controlled cooperative clinical trials.

Prognosis for Early Breast Cancer. The current outlook for patients with Stage I breast cancer treated by radical or modified radical mastectomy is remarkably good. Haid and Zuckerman found a 5-year survival of 95 percent in patients with Stage I lesions and 80 percent in patients with Stage II lesions; modified radical mastectomy was the treatment in both groups. The availability of effective adjuvant chemotherapy has provoked an intense search for subsets of patients with early breast cancer who have a poorer prognosis than expected and who would be candidates for adjuvant therapy. Nealon et al. used four histologic criteria to define such high-risk patients: poor cytologic differentiation, lymphatic permeation, blood vessel invasion, and poor circumscription (invasion of tumor into surrounding soft tissues). Using these criteria in a retrospective analysis of patients with negative axillary nodes and tumors 2 cm or less in diameter, they found that all 83 patients classed as low risk survived 10 years and only one had recurrence of disease. Of those with one or more risk criteria, 50 percent had recurrence of tumor within 10 years.

Other criteria of high risk and a poor prognosis not included in the TMN clinical system are rapid growth rate either by history or by evidence of a high thymidine labeling index (indicating an increased number of dividing cells); youth of the patients (the younger the patient the higher the risk); and estrogen receptor negativity.

There are only a few randomized trials that compare the results of different forms of purely *surgical* treatment. Of these the most convincing were those of the NSABP-05 trial in which total mastectomy was compared with radical mastectomy in clinical Stage I patients. Results were identical in both groups up to 10 years after operation. Forrest et al. reported the same outcome in a similar study that differed only in that patients were staged by a partial excision of axillary nodes. Helman's study from South Africa was negated because the project was stopped after 3 years. This was the only study in which clinically positive axillary nodes were *not* treated by either operation or radiation. Subsequent growth of nodes in Stage II patients caused the investigators to abandon the protocol.

Until recently the operation of choice for early cancer of the breast in this country was modified radical mastectomy. A randomized trial comparing this procedure with radical mastectomy has shown that radical and modified radical operations produce the same results.

The psychologic effects of operation would be reduced and early treatment encouraged if sacrifice of the breast were not required. This can be achieved by confining operation to partial mastectomy alone or by combining local excision or simple biopsy of breast cancer with radiation therapy.

A randomized trial of the NSABP compared two surgical arms, lumpectomy and axillary dissection, and total mastectomy with axillary dissection with a combination of lumpectomy and axillary dissection plus irradiation. Omission of treatment of the whole breast by either operation or radiation resulted in a high rate of local recurrence at 5 years, 24 percent for Stage I lesions and 38 percent for Stage II. When radiation of the breast was added to lumpectomy and axillary resection, the local recurrence was 6 percent. In addition, survival rates were slightly but significantly better in the lumpectomy and irradiation treatment arm compared with the other two. This report, together with Veronese's data from Italy, seem to support the use of lumpectomy, axillary resection, and irradiation for breast cancer tumors equal to or smaller than 4 cm in size.

Prognosis in Advanced Breast Cancer. Advanced breast cancers now constitute less than 20 percent of cases and are the lesions that fall into the Joint Committee Stages III and IV. In the recent past prognosis for these patients was bleak, averaging 15 to 20 percent survival at 5 years, little different from the survival of untreated patients. Most of these patients satisfy Haagensen's criteria of inoperability and would previously have been referred for radiation with or without a preceding total mastectomy. The use of adjuvant chemotherapy has cast a new and more hopeful light on this group. Excluding patients with overt distant metastasis (Stage IV), the prognosis for 5-year survival may be doubled in this group. Some of these patients may benefit from radical mastectomy, especially those with large local cancers but few or no axillary nodes. The possibility of controlling disseminated micrometastasis makes a strenuous effort to eliminate gross locoregional disease a rational component of therapy.

The new experiences with control of inflammatory carcinoma of the breast in premenopausal women, the most lethal of all breast cancers, may be an example of the advantages of combining numerous forms of local and systemic therapy. In a sequential series of patients at the MD Anderson Hospital, all 10 patients with inflammatory breast cancer treated by radiotherapy alone suffered relapse by 19 months (median relapse-free survival 9 months). All nine patients treated by chemotherapy and radiation relapsed by 25 months (median relapse-free survival 17 months). Seven patients were treated with chemotherapy followed by extended total mastectomy followed by immunotherapy, maintenance chemotherapy and radiation therapy. After an average follow-up of 21 months, only two patients had relapsed. A more recent report indicates a 5-year survival rate of 74 percent.

Advice to Patients. Carter has observed that controversies about the treatment of primary breast cancer have become so visible to the public that state governments are now entering the picture. In California a new law requires that breast cancer patients be informed by their physicians of the "alternative and effective methods of treatment with an explanation of their risks, advantages and disadvantages." The failure of a physician to so inform a patient would be grounds for a charge of unprofessional conduct. Massachusetts has passed a similar law, and other states are considering like measures.

Medical, surgical, and radiation oncologists are likely to deliver the message concerning breast treatment somewhat differently. In addition there are at least 90 different options for the therapy of Stage I cancer alone. In any case, my advice to patients is to accept those therapies tested by randomized clinical trials as proved effective and regard those therapies not so tested as still experimental. By these standards, total mastectomy or modified radical mastectomy are proved treatments for clinical Stage I cancer, equal in effectiveness to radical mastectomy. Partial mastectomy or lumpectomy is proved effective for tumors 4 cm or less when combined with axillary node dissection and postoperative radiation. Every pa-

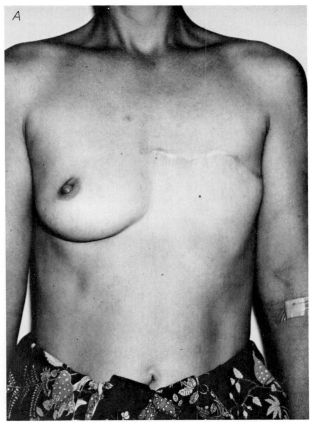

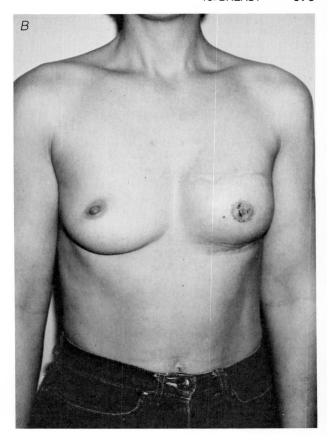

Fig. 15-26. *A.* Postoperative result following modified radical mastectomy with transverse incision. *B.* Reconstruction of the breast with subpectoral silastic implant and of the nipple using skin from the inner thigh. *(Provided by Carl G. Quillen, M.D.)*

tient with clinical Stages I and II breast cancer should have a total removal of axillary lymph nodes, not because it is a proved treatment, but because it is a proved method for effectively staging breast cancer and bringing into the treatment regimen suitably selected adjuvant therapy.

REHABILITATION. Most women require instruction in exercising the arm on the side of operation following radical mastectomy. Proper physical therapy in the immediate postoperative period should ensure complete return to normal function. Following operations that spare the pectoral muscles, full function of the arm usually returns promptly with little or no special help. Psychologic support is also important in restoring the patient's self-image and her confidence that she is still desirable to a present or future companion, or, if the breast has been preserved, that her chances of long survival are good. The Reach to Recovery program of the American Cancer Society has been most successful in providing advisors to the recent mastectomy patient from the ranks of women who have previously had the same operation.

Many women are interested in the possibility of subsequent reconstruction of the excised breast. If the previous operation was radical mastectomy, reconstruction is complex, but good restoration can be accomplished using a myocutaneous latissimus dorsi graft. In patients who have had modified radical or total mastectomy, especially if the operation was performed through a transverse incision, reconstruction with a silastic implant placed under the pectoralis major muscle is a relatively simple and feasible technique (Fig. 15-26). The result is never a perfect match for the remaining breast, and decisions about which patients will find these reconstructions worthwhile must be individualized.

TREATMENT OF RECURRENT CANCER

Prior to the 1950s recurrent cancer of the breast was treated either with radiation or operation or not at all. Radiation remains an extremely useful agent for painful osseous metastases and small subcutaneous lesions. Operation also may be useful for small local lesions. The basic problem in the patient with recurrent cancer is most often wide dissemination, and systemic agents, hormone therapy, and chemotherapy are the treatments of choice.

Selection of hormonal therapy or chemotherapy as the initial treatment of recurrent disease depends on whether the patient's tumor is hormonally sensitive. For decades the only index of hormonal sensitivity was the patient's

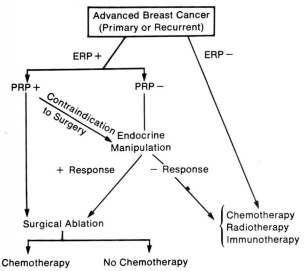

Fig. 15-27. Schema for the treatment of patients with recurrent breast cancer when determinations to estrogen receptors and progesterone receptors are available. Patients who are estrogen receptor–positive (ERP) and progesterone receptor–positive (PRP) have an 80 percent response rate to surgical ablation. (From: *Degenshein GA et al: Breast 3:29, 1977, with permission.*)

response to a trial of hormonal treatment. We now know that the response of breast cancers to hormones is dependent on the presence of hormone receptors in the substance of cancer cells. Hormonal receptors for estrogens, prolactin, progesterone, and corticosteroids have been identified. Dependable clinical tests for estrogen receptors (ER) are now widely available, and all primary cancers should be submitted for testing when first removed; 50 percent of these tumors will prove to be ER-positive. Progesterone receptors (PR) also appear to have a predictive value. Eighty percent of patients with breast cancers that have both ER and PR will respond to hormonal manipulation. Breast cancers that are ER-positive but PR-negative respond in 27 percent, those that are ER-negative and PR-positive (rare) respond in 45 percent, and those that are ER-negative and PR-negative respond in less than 10 percent. A schema for treatment of patients tested for both ER and PR is shown in Fig. 15-27. The presence of hormone receptors is a marker indicating a more differentiated tumor. Such tumors respond to all forms of therapy better than receptor-negative breast cancers.

TREATMENT OF ESTROGEN RECEPTOR–POSITIVE RECURRENT TUMORS. The choices of hormone manipulation are (1) ablation, the removal of estrogen-generating tissue by operation; (2) additive (paradoxically treatment with high doses of estrogens or progesterone is also effective); and (3) antiestrogens. All these techniques produce the same approximate result, regression in about 60 percent of ER-positive patients. Many still consider oophorectomy the therapy of choice for the menstruating pa-

tients; risk is minimal, and there is no concern about compliance over the long term. Favorable response averages 1 year in duration and predicts probable responses to further endocrine maneuvers.

For postmenopausal patients, either naturally or surgically induced, the choice is between additive and antiestrogen therapy. Of these, tamoxifen, an antiestrogen that acts by blocking estrogen receptor sites, is the current favorite. Side effects are minimal, consisting of hot flashes and a mild cytopenia in 10 to 15 percent of patients that does not become clinically important. Diethylstilbesterol, the previous drug of choice, is cheaper but produces nausea in 50 percent of patients, vomiting in 25 percent, and edema in 50 percent. Aminoglutethimide blocks the conversions of cholesterol to pregnenolone and thus inhibits the production of adrenal steroids. It also inhibits the aromatization of androsteredione to estrone in peripheral tissues. When compared with tamoxifen in randomized trials, response rates and durations of survival are similar. Toxicity, consisting of lethargy and a morbilliform rash in about 8 percent, is greater than for tamoxifen. However, patients failing tamoxifen may respond to aminoglutethimide, and it is probably useful as a secondary hormonal treatment. If aminoglutethimide is used, the patients must also receive replacement hydrocortisone or dexamethasone. The effect of aminoglutethimide is often referred to as "medical adrenalectomy," and it seems to eliminate the need for operative adrenalectomy.

TREATMENT OF ESTROGEN RECEPTOR–NEGATIVE RECURRENT TUMORS. Patients who have tumors that are estrogen receptor–negative rarely respond to estrogen ablative therapy (10 percent or less). Such patients, together with the 40 percent who fail to respond to a therapeutic trial of estrogen ablation or antiestrogens, are candidates for cancer chemotherapy. Multiple-drug regimens spaced at much longer intervals than the older single-drug programs are the current mode and have produced a doubling and even tripling of the improvement in the old results with single drugs. Arrest of tumor growth, partial remission, and even complete remissions can be expected in 65 percent of patients so treated. Because of the rapid improvement in the results of chemotherapy, there is now some controversy as to whether hormonal therapy should precede or follow chemotherapy. Wilson and Moore, among several clinicians, have combined total operative estrogen ablation with almost simultaneous cancer chemotherapy in patients with recurrent breast cancer. They suggest that the two forms of therapy work synergistically, with a better response for combination than for sequential use of these techniques when compared with historical controls. No controlled clinical trials are available to confirm this observation, and hormonal therapy remains the first treatment of recurrence at the present. Both therapies are palliative and not curative measures, and most patients will eventually receive most or all of the agents currently available. The aim of therapy is to improve the quality of life and the length of survival, but not as yet to provide cure.

Infection

ACUTE INFECTION

Bacterial infections almost always occur in the lactating breast in the first month or two following delivery. The portal of entry is an abrasion or fissure in the nipple. The best treatment is prevention, with the nursing mother carefully cleaning and drying her nipples after nursing. In general, cleanliness is important. Infections are also seasonal, being more common in the hot summer months.

The milk-containing ducts and acini of the lactating breast are a perfect culture medium, and infection, having gained access, often progresses rapidly through inflammation to suppuration. This is accompanied by extreme pain in the breast, and a good diagnostic sign of abscess is the patient's rapid withdrawal when the physician attempts to palpate the involved breast. The breast is red and the area of abscess indurated and firm. The tendency is to underestimate the size of the abscess on physical examination.

An abscess may be aborted by the use of systemic antibiotics given in the presuppurative period. Treatment of abscess, once it forms, is by surgical drainage. Antibiotics will suppress the process for a time, but it will flare up again when they are discontinued. A curvilinear transverse incision is made in the dependent portion of the breast and the gloved finger or a clamp is used to break up the many septa that separate the cavity into loculations. A rubber drain is left in the wound. Culture of the pus usually demonstrates *Staphylococcus aureus*. Pain is relieved promptly by drainage, and the surrounding inflammation subsides rapidly.

CHRONIC INFECTION

Chronic infection of the breast is now rare. Tuberculosis is the major cause, and as the incidence of this disease has decreased, so have breast lesions caused by it. The index of suspicion for this lesion should still be high in patients with AIDS or those from third world countries. The genesis of breast tuberculosis is either pleural or, more commonly, the breaking down of a mediastinal node to involve one of the costal cartilages. Infection simmers in the cartilage for long periods, giving rise to lesions in the breast, which eventually form one or several fistulas to the skin. Antituberculosis drugs are now the primary treatment for this disease, but care of the breast lesion usually requires excision of the affected costal cartilage.

Bibliography

General

Haagensen CD: *Diseases of the Breast,* 2d ed. Philadelphia, Saunders, 1971.

McKenna R, Murphy G: *Fundamentals of Surgical Oncology.* New York, Macmillan, 1986.

Nealon T: *Problems in General Surgery: Controversies in Cancer of the Breast and Colon.* Philadelphia, Lippincott, 1985.

Anatomy and Development

Batson OV: The function of the vertebral veins and their role in the spread of metastasis. *Ann Surg* 112:138, 1940.

Cooper Sir AP: *The Anatomy and Diseases of the Breast.* Philadelphia, Lea and Blanchard, 1845.

Ingleby H, Gershon-Cohen J: *Cooperative Anatomy: Pathology and Roentgenology of the Breast.* Philadelphia, University of Pennsylvania Press, 1960.

Taylor GT: Anatomy of the breast with particular reference to lymphatic drainage, in Parson WH: *Cancer of the Breast.* Springfield, IL, Charles C Thomas, 1959.

Examination

Clark RL, Copeland MM, et al: Reproducibility of the technic of mammography (Egan) for cancer of the breast. *Am J Surg* 109:127, 1965.

Fagerberg G, Baldetorp L., et al: Effects of repeated mammographic screening on breast cancer stage distribution. Results from a randomized study of 92,934 women in a Swedish county. *Acta Radiol (Oncol)* 24:465, 1985.

Gershon-Cohen J, Berger SM: Detection of breast cancer by periodic x-ray examinations: A five-year survey. *JAMA,* 176:1114, 1961.

Gershon-Cohen J, Berger SM, Klickstein HS: Roentgenography of breast cancer moderating concept of "biologic predeterminism." *Cancer* 16:961, 1963.

Gershon-Cohen J, Ingleby H: Roentgenography of unsuspected carcinoma of breast. *JAMA* 166:869, 1958.

Heywang S, Hahn D, et al: MR imaging of the breast using godolinium DTPA. *J Comput Assist Tomogr* 10:199, 1986.

Horwitz R, Lamas A, Peck D: Mammographic parenchymal patterns and risk of breast cancer in postmenopausal women. *Am J Med* 77:621, 1984.

Ingleby H, Moore L, Gershon-Cohen J: A roentgenographic study of the growth rate of six "early" cancers of the breast. *Cancer* 11:726, 1958.

Snyder RE: Mammography and lobular carcinoma in situ. *Surg Gynecol Obstet* 122:255, 1966.

Treves N, Holleb AI: Cancer of the male breast: a report of 146 cases. *Cancer* 8:1239, 1955.

Watt C, Ackerman L, et al: Differentiation between benign and malignant diseases of the breast using digital subtraction angiography of the breast. *Cancer* 56:1287, 1985.

Neoplasms

Abramson DJ: Delayed mastectomy after outpatient breast biopsy. *Am J Surg* 132:596, 1976.

Adair F, Berg J, et al: Long-term follow-up of breast cancer patients: The 30-year report. *Cancer* 33:1145, 1974.

Baclesse F: Five-year results in 431 breast cancers treated solely by roentgen rays. *Ann Surg* 161:103, 1965.

Baker LH: Breast cancer detection demonstration project: Five-year summary report. *CA* 32:194, 1982.

Barrows G, Anderson T, et al: Fine needle aspiration of breast cancer: Relationship of clinical factors to cytology results in 689 malignancies. *Cancer* 58:1493, 1986.

Berg JW, Robbins GF: Factors influencing short and long-term survival of breast cancer patients. *Surg Gynecol Obstet* 122:1311, 1966.

Blackwood JM, Seelig RF, et al: Survival distribution in breast cancer. *Surgery* 82:443, 1977.

Bloom HJG, Richardson WW, Harries EJ.: Natural history of untreated breast cancer (1805–1933): Comparison of untreated and treated cases according to histological grade of malignancy. *Br Med J* 5299:213, 1962.

Bloom JR, Cook M, et al: Psychological response to mastectomy: A prospective comparison study. *Cancer* 59:189, 1987.

Bluming AZ: Treatment of primary breast cancer without mastectomy. *Am J Med* 72:820, 1982.

Bonadonna G, Rossi A, et al: Adjuvant combination chemotherapy for operable breast cancer. Trials in progress at the Istituto Nazionale Tumori of Milan. *Cancer Treat Rep* 65:61, 1981.

Branfield JR, Fingerhut AG, Warner NE: Lobular carcinoma of the breast—1969: A therapeutic proposal. *Arch Surg* 99:129, 1969.

Brinkley D, Haybittle JL: The curability of breast cancer. *World J Surg* 1:287, 1977.

Butcher HR Jr: Effectiveness of radical mastectomy for mammary cancer: An analysis of mortalities by the method of probits. *Ann Surg* 154:383, 1961.

Butcher HR Jr: Radical mastectomy for mammary carcinoma. *Ann Surg* 157:165, 1963.

Caceres E, Lingan M, Delgado P: Evaluation of dissection of the axilla in modified radical mastectomy. *Surg Gynecol Obstet* 143:395, 1976.

Cancer Research Campaign Trial: Management of early cancer of the breast. *Br Med J* 1:1035, 1976.

Cant EL, Smith AF, et al: "Superstaging" in breast cancer: A correlation of lymph node histology and investigations designed to detect occult metastatic disease. *World J Surg* 1:303, 1977.

Carpenter JT, Maddox WA, et al: Favorable factors in the adjuvant therapy of breast cancer. *Cancer* 50:18, 1982.

Carter SK: The California breast cancer law and government-mandated patient education. *CA* 32:173, 1982.

Chang JC, Wergowske G: Correlation of estrogen receptors and response to chemotherapy of cyclophosphamide, methotrexate, and 5-fluorouracil (CMF) in advanced breast cancer. *Cancer* 48:2503, 1981.

Chu AM, Kiel K: Comparison of adjuvant postoperative radiotherapy and multiple-drug chemotherapy (CFM-VP) in operable breast cancer patients with more than four positive axillary lymph nodes. *Cancer* 50:212, 1982.

Cooper MR, Rhyne AL: A randomized comparative trial of chemotherapy and irradiation therapy for stage II breast cancer. *Cancer* 47:2833, 1981.

Cronin TD, Upton J, McDonough JM: Reconstruction of the breast after mastectomy. *Plast Reconstr Surg* 59:1, 1977.

Cukier DS, Lopez FA, Maravilla RB Jr: One-view follow-up mammogram: Efficacy in screening for breast cancer. *JAMA* 237:661, 1977.

Cuzick J, Stewart H, et al: Overview of randomized trials comparing radical mastectomy without radiotherapy against simple mastectomy with radiotherapy in breast cancer. *Cancer Treat Rep* 71:7, 1987.

Danforth DN Jr, Findlay PA, et al: Complete axillary lymph node dissection for stage I-II carcinoma of the breast. *J Clin Oncol* 4:655, 1986.

Degenshein GA, Bloom N, et al: Estrogen and progesterone receptor site studies as guides to the management of advanced breast cancer. *Breast* 3:29, 1977.

DeGroote R, Rush BF Jr, et al: Interval breast cancer: A more aggressive subset of breast neoplasias. *Surgery* 94:543, 1983.

Duncan W, Forrest APM, et al: New Edinburgh primary breast cancer trials: Report by co-ordinating committee. *Br J Cancer* 32:628, 1975.

Duncan W, Kerr GR: The curability of breast cancer. *Br Med J* 2:781, 1976.

Fisher B: Laboratory and clinical research in breast cancer—a personal adventure: The David A. Karnofsky Memorial Lecture. *Cancer Res* 40:3863, 1980.

Fisher B, Bauer M, et al: Five year results of a randomized clinical trial comparing total mastectomy and segmental mastectomy with or without radiation in the treatment of breast cancer. *N Engl J Med* 312:655, 1985.

Fisher B, Fisher ER, Redmond C, Participating NSABP Investigators: Ten-year results from the National Surgical Adjuvant Breast and Bowel Project (NSABP) clinical trial evaluating the use of L-phenylalanine mustard (L-Pam) in the management of primary breast cancer. *J Clin Oncol*, 4:929, 1986.

Fisher B, Ravdin RG, et al: Surgical adjuvant chemotherapy in cancer of the breast: Results of a decade of cooperative investigation. *Ann Surg* 168:337, 1968.

Fisher B, Slack NH, et al: Ten year follow-up results of patients with carcinoma of the breast in a co-operative clinical trial evaluating surgical adjuvant chemotherapy. *Surg Gynecol Obstet* 140:528, 1975.

Fisher B, Wolmark N, et al: Findings from NSABP Protocol No. B-04: Comparison of radical mastectomy with alternative treatments. II. The clinical and biologic significance of medial-central breast cancers. *Cancer* 48:1863, 1981.

Fisher B, Wolmark N, et al: Lumpectomy and axillary dissection for breast cancer: Surgical, pathological, and radiation considerations. *World J Surg* 9:692, 1985.

Fisher ER, Gregorio RM, et al: The pathology of invasive breast cancer. A syllabus derived from findings of the National Surgical Adjuvant Breast Project (Protocol No. 4). *Cancer* 36:1, 1975.

Foote FW, Stewart FW: Comparative studies of cancerous versus noncancerous breasts: I. Basic morphology characteristics. *Ann Surg* 121:6, 1945.

Foote FW, Stewart FW: Comparative studies of cancerous versus noncancerous breasts: II. Mammary carcinogenesis: Influence of certain hormones on human breast structure. *Ann Surg* 121:197, 1945.

Forrest APM, Roberts MM, et al: Simple mastectomy and pectoral node biopsy. *Br J Surg* 63:569, 1976.

Gardner B: Cancer revisited. *JAMA* 232:742, 1975. (Editorial.)

Gibson EW: Reconstruction of the breast after mastectomy for cancer. *Clin Plast Surg* 3:371, 1976.

Haagensen CD: The choice of treatment for operable carcinoma of the breast. *Surgery* 76:685, 1974.

Haid M, Zuckerman L: Breast carcinoma: Expected results with prevailing therapy. *J Surg Oncol* 19:52, 1982.

Handly RC, Thackray AC: Conservative radical mastectomy (Patey's operation). *Ann Surg* 157:162, 1963.

Hayes DF, Zurawski VR, Kufe DW: Comparison of circulating CA15-3 and carcinoembryonic antigen levels in patients with breast cancer. *J Clin Oncol* 4:1542, 1986.

Hayward JL: The Guy's trial of treatments of "early" breast cancer. *World J Surg* 1:314, 1977.

Hems G: Epidemiological characteristics of breast cancer in middle and late age. *Br J Cancer* 24:226, 1970.

Henderson IC, Gelman R, et al: Prolonged disease-free survival in advanced breast cancer treated with "super-CMF" Adriamycin: An alternating regimen employing high-dose methotrexate with citrovorum factor rescue. *Cancer Treat Res* 65:67, 1981.

Holland JF, Glidewell O, Cooper RG: Adverse effect of radiotherapy on adjuvant chemotherapy for carcinoma of the breast. *Surg Gynecol Obstet* 150:817, 1980.

Horsley JS III, Newsome HH, et al: Medical adrenalectomy in patients with advanced breast cancer. *Cancer* 49:1145, 1982.

Hortobagyi GN, Aman UB: Progress in inflammatory breast cancer: Cause for cautious optimism. *J Clin Oncol* 4:1727, 1986.

Huguley CM, Brown RL: The value of breast self-examination. *Cancer* 47:989, 1981.

James F, James VHT, et al: A comparison of in vivo and in vitro uptake of estradiol by human breast tumors and the relationship of steroid excretion. *Cancer Res* 31:1268, 1971.

Kaae S, Johansen H: Breast cancer: A comparison of simple mastectomy with postoperative roentgen irradiation by the McWhirter method with those of extended radical mastectomy. *Acta Radiol (Stockh)* 155(suppl):185, 1959.

Kaae S, Johansen H: Simple mastectomy plus postoperative irradiation by the method of McWhirter for mammary carcinoma. *Ann Surg* 157:175, 1963.

Kay S, Poulos NG: Evaluation of the criteria of operability of carcinoma of the breast. *Surg Gynecol Obstet* 113:562, 1961.

Kennedy BJ, Meilke PW Jr, Fortuny IE: Therapeutic castration versus prophylactic castration in breast cancer. *Surg Gynecol Obstet* 118:524, 1964.

Kennedy CS, Miller E: Simple mastectomy for mammary carcinoma. *Ann Surg* 157:161, 1963.

Koscielny S, Tubiana M, et al: Breast cancer: Relationship between the size of the primary tumour and the probability of metastatic dissemination. *Breast Cancer* 84:12, 2.

Kraft RO, Block GE: Mammary carcinoma in the aged patient. *Ann Surg* 156:981, 1962.

Kramer WM, Rush BF Jr: Mammary duct proliferation in the elderly: A histopathologic study. *Cancer* 31:130, 1973.

Kusama S, Spratt JS Jr, et al: The gross rates of growth of human mammary carcinoma. *Cancer* 30:594, 1972.

Lacour J, Bucalossi P, et al: Radical mastectomy versus radical mastectomy plus internal mammary dissection: Five-year results of an international cooperative study. *Cancer* 37:206, 1976.

Lavigne JD, Minet P: Conservative surgery for stage I and II breast cancers. Results at 5 years. *Lyon Chir* 77:145, 1981.

Legha SS, Carter SK: Antiestrogens in the treatment of breast cancer. *Cancer Treat Rev* 3:205, 1976.

Letton AH, Mason EM: Five-year-plus survival of breast screenees. *Cancer* 48:404, 1981.

Levitt SH, McHugh RB: Radiotherapy in the postoperative treatment of operable cancer of the breast: Part I. Critique of the clinical and biometric aspects of the trials. *Cancer* 39:924, 1977.

Levitt SH, McHugh RB, Song CW: Radiotherapy in the postoperative treatment of operable cancer of the breast: Part II. A re-examination of Stjernsward's application of the Mantel-Haenszel statistical method: Evaluation of the effect of the radiation on immune response and suggestions for postoperative radiotherapy. *Cancer* 39:933, 1976.

Lewison EF: *Breast Cancer and Its Diagnosis and Treatment.* Baltimore, Williams & Wilkins, 1955.

Lewison EF: The results of treatment of breast cancer at the Johns Hopkins Hospital 1941–1945, with a discussion. *Surg Gynecol Obstet* 107:313, 1958.

MacDonald I: The natural history of mammary carcinoma. *Am J Surg* 111:435, 1966.

McWhirter R: Treatment of cancer of the breast by simple mastectomy and roentgenotherapy. *Arch Surg* 59:830, 1949.

Madden JL: Modified radical mastectomy. *Surg Gynecol Obstet* 121:1221, 1965.

Maddox WA, Carpenter JT, et al.: A randomized prospective trial of radical (Halsted) mastectomy versus modified radical mastectomy in 311 breast cancer patients. *Ann Surg* 198:207, 1983.

Missakian MM, Witten DM, Harrison EG Jr: Mammography after mastectomy: Usefulness in search for recurrent carcinoma of the breast. *JAMA* 191:1045, 1965.

Moore DH, Sarkar NH, et al: Some aspects of the search for a human mammary tumor virus. *Cancer* 28:1415, 1971.

Moore FD, Van Devanter SB, et al: Adrenalectomy with chemotherapy in the treatment of advanced breast cancer: Objective and subjective response rates; duration and quality of life. *Surgery* 76:376, 1974.

Moore SW, Lewis RJ: Carcinoma of the breast in women 30 years of age and under. *Surg Gynecol Obstet* 119:1253, 1964.

Mouridsen HT, Palshof T, et al: Evaluation of single-drug versus multiple-drug chemotherapy in the treatment of advanced breast cancer. *Cancer Treat Rep* 61:47, 1977.

Mueller CB, Jeffries W: Cancer of the breast: Its outcome as measured by the rate of dying and causes of pain. *Ann Surg* 182:334, 1975.

Murray JG, MacIntyre J, et al: Cancer research campaign study of the management of "early" breast cancer. *World J Surg* 1:317, 1977.

Nealon TF Jr, Nkongho A, et al: Treatment of early cancer of the breast ($T_1N_0M_0$ and $T_2N_0M_0$) on the basis of histologic characteristics. *Surgery* 89:279, 1981.

Nevin JE, Baggerly JT, Laird TK: Radiotherapy as an adjuvant in the treatment of carcinoma of the breast. *Cancer* 49:1194, 1982.

Nissen-Myer R, Kjellgren K, Mansson B: Preliminary report from the Scandinavian adjuvant chemotherapy study group. *Cancer Chemother Rep* 55:561, 1971.

Oberman HA: Sarcomas of the breast. *Cancer* 18:1233, 1965.

Owen HW, Dockerty MB, Gray HK: Occult carcinoma of the breast. *Surg Gynecol Obstet* 98:302, 1954.

Pack GT: Argument for bilateral mastectomy. *Surgery* 29:929, 1951. (Editorial).

Park WW, Lees JC: Absolute curability of cancer of the breast. *Surg Gynecol Obstet* 93:129, 1951.

Pater JL, Mores D, Loeb M: Survival after recurrence of breast cancer. *Can Med Assoc J* 124:1591, 1981.

Pennisi VR, Capozzi A, Perez FM: Subcutaneous mastectomy data. *Plast Reconstr Surg* 59:53, 1977.

Pichon MF, Milgrom E: Characterization and assay of progesterone receptor in human mammary carcinoma. *Cancer Res* 37:464, 1977.

Priestman T, Baum M, et al: Comparative trial of endocrine versus cytotoxic treatment in advanced breast cancer. *Br Med J* 1:1248, 1977.

Ribeiro GG, Swindell R: The prognosis of breast carcinoma in women aged less than 40 years. *Clin Radiol* 32:231, 1981.

Robbins GF, Berg JW: Curability of patients with invasive breast carcinoma based on a 30-year study. *World J Surg* 1:284, 1977.

Robbins GF, Brothers JH III, et al: Is aspiration biopsy of breast cancer dangerous to the patient? *Cancer* 7:774, 1954.

Rosato FE, Fink PJ, et al: Immediate postmastectomy reconstruction. *J Surg Oncol* 8:277, 1976.

Rosen PP, Fracchia AA, et al: "Residual" mammary carcinoma following simulated partial mastectomy. *Cancer* 35:739, 1975.

Rosen PP, Saigo PE, et al: Axillary micro- and macrometastases in breast cancer. *Ann Surg* 194:585, 1981.

Rosen PP, Snyder RE, et al: Detection of occult carcinoma in the apparently benign breast biopsy through specimen radiography. *Cancer* 26:944, 1970.

Rosner D: Ultrasonography in diagnosis and management of palpable breast masses. *NY State J Med* 81:1066, 1981.

Ross MB, Buzdar AU, Blumenschein GR: Treatment of advanced breast cancer with megestrol acetate after therapy with tamoxifen. *Cancer* 49:413, 1982.

Rush BF Jr: Axillary dissection in breast cancer: A staging procedure. *Surgery* 77:478, 1975.

Rush BF Jr, Kramer WM: Proliferative histological changes and occult carcinoma in the breast of the aging female. *Surg Gynecol Obstet* 117:425, 1963.

Sacks H, Chalmers TC, Smith H Jr: Randomized versus historical controls for clinical trials. *Am J Med* 72:233, 1982.

Sandison AT: An autopsy study of the adult human breast, with special reference to proliferative epithelial changes of importance in the pathology of the breast. *Natl Cancer Inst Monogr* 8, June 1962.

Schottenfeld D, Nash AG, et al: Ten-year results of the treatment of primary operable breast carcinoma: A summary of 304 patients evaluated by the TNM system. *Cancer* 38:1001, 1976.

Shimkin MB: Cancer of the breast: Some old facts and new perspectives. *JAMA* 183:358, 1963.

Shimkin MB, Koppel M, et al: Simple and radical mastectomy for breast cancer: A re-analysis of Smith and Meyer's report from Rockford, Illinois. *J Natl Cancer Inst* 27:1197, 1961.

Shingleton WW, Sedransk N, Johnson RO: Systemic chemotherapy for mammary carcinoma. *Ann Surg* 173:913, 1971.

Silvestrini R, Daidone MG, Gasparini G: Cell kinetics as a prognostic marker in node-negative breast cancer. *Cancer* 56:1982, 1985.

Strax P: New techniques in mass screening for breast cancer. *Cancer* 28:1563, 1971.

Sugarbaker ED: Extended radical mastectomy: Its superiority in the treatment of breast cancer. *JAMA* 187:95, 1964.

Surgical Adjuvant Chemotherapy Breast Group: Breast adjuvant chemotherapy: Effectiveness of thio-tepa (triethylenethiophosphoramide) as adjuvant to radical mastectomy for breast cancer. *Ann Surg* 154:629, 1961.

Tabár L, Dean PB: Mammographic parenchymal patterns. *JAMA* 247:185, 1982.

Tellem M, Prive L, Meranze DR: Four-quadrant study of breast removed for carcinoma. *Cancer* 15:10, 1962.

Teramoto YA, Mariani R, et al: The immunohistochemical reactivity of a human monoclonal antibody with tissue sections of human mammary tumors. *Cancer* 50:241, 1982.

Urban JA: Bilaterality of cancer of the breast: Biopsy of the opposite breast. *Cancer* 20:1867, 1971.

Urban JA, Baker HW: Radical mastectomy in continuity with en bloc resection of the internal mammary lymph-node chain: A new procedure for primary operable cancer of the breast. *Cancer* 5:992, 1952.

Vana J, Bedwani R, et al: Trends in diagnosis and management of breast cancer in the U.S.: From the surveys of the American College of Surgeons. *Cancer* 48:1043, 1981.

Veronesi U, Cascinelli N, et al: A reappraisal of oophorectomy in carcinoma of the breast. *Ann Surg* 205:18, 1987.

Veronesi R, Saccozzi R, et al: Comparing radical mastectomy with quadrantectomy, axillary dissection, and radiotherapy in patients with small cancers of the breasts. *N Engl J Med* 305:6, 1981.

Veronesi U, Rossi A, Bonadonna G: Adjuvant combination chemotherapy with CMF in primary mammary carcinoma. *World J Surg* 1:337, 1977.

Wanebo HJ, Huvos AG, Urban JA: Treatment of minimal breast cancer. *Cancer* 33:349, 1974.

Ward RM, Evans HL: Cystosarcoma phyllodes: A clinicopathologic study of 26 cases. *Cancer* 58:2282, 1986.

Watts GT: Restorative prosthetic mammaplasty in mastectomy for carcinoma and benign lesions. *Clin Plast Surg* 3:177, 1976.

Williams IG, Curwen MP: Total mastectomy with axillary dissection and irradiation for mammary carcinoma. *Ann Surg* 157:174, 1963.

Willis KJ, London DR, et al: Recurrent breast cancer treated with the antiestrogen tamoxifen: Correlation between hormonal changes and clinical course. *Br Med J* 1:425, 1977.

Wiseman C, Jessup JM, et al: Inflammatory breast cancer treated with surgery, chemotherapy and allogeneic tumor cell/BCG immunotherapy. *Cancer* 49:1266, 1982.

Wynder EL, Rose DP, Cohen L: Diet and breast cancer in causation and therapy. *Cancer* 58:1804, 1986.

Zafrani B, Fourquet A, et al: Conservative management of intraductal breast carcinoma with tumorectomy and radiation therapy. *Cancer* 57:1299, 1986.

Zippin C, Petrakis NL: Identification of high risk groups in breast cancer. *Cancer* 28:1381, 1971.

Benign Lesions

Banerjee SN, Ananthakrishnan N, et al: Tuberculous mastitis: A continuing problem. *World J Surg* 11:105, 1987.

Davis HH, Simons M, Davis JB: Cystic disease of the breast: Relationship to carcinoma. *Cancer* 17:957, 1964.

Frantz VK, Pickren JW, et al: Incidence of chronic cystic disease in so-called "normal breasts": A study based on 225 postmortem examinations. *Cancer* 4:762, 1951.

Grow JL, Lewison EF: Superficial thrombophlebitis of the breast. *Surg Gynecol Obstet* 116:180, 1963.

Urban JA: Excision of major ducts of the breast. *Cancer* 16:516, 1963.

Chapter 16

Tumors of the Head and Neck

Benjamin F. Rush, Jr.

HISTORICAL BACKGROUND

The head and neck are such public regions of the anatomy that one would expect ancient medical manuscripts to give considerable attention to tumors affecting these parts. Strangely, the ancient writers rarely mention such lesions. The Smith Papyrus (2300 B.C.) mentions wounds of the head frequently, but not a single tumor of the area is discussed. The Ebers Papyrus (1500 B.C.) contains references to "eating ulcer" of the gums and "illness of the tongue," but the descriptions are too brief to be adequately interpreted. Celsus (A.D. 178) is often credited with devising an operation for cancer of the lower lip. Martin notes that Celsus recognized and described cancer of the skin or the face, but his operation on the lower lip was for repair of a "mutilation," probably a war wound.

A perusal of *The Surgery of Theodoric* (A.D. 1267) in the translation of Campbell and Colton gives an interesting perspective of the personal experiences of a master surgeon of the era who had a profound knowledge of the writings of preceding centuries. Theodoric describes numerous lesions about the head and neck, mostly of minor significance, i.e., wens, "white pustules or spots which appear by the nose and over the cheeks," "lumps or swellings occurring on the head called horns," "nodes or wens which are formed on the eyelids," lipoma, pustules on the face, freckles, brown patches, wrinkles, and black and blue spots on the face. There is a lengthy section on "the scrofula." He had a much clearer concept of cancer than most of his contemporaries, but in his entire writing he does not mention the treatment of a single lesion of the lip or intraoral area.

This frequent failure to single out cancerous lesions in this area reflects the inability of our medical ancestors to differentiate grossly between chronic infections and cancer. Certainly some miraculous cures were achieved by ointments and spells applied to hard, round ulcers which, in fact, were chronic infections. An early, operable lesion was certain to be treated at length with salves and potions, and when it was evident beyond doubt that the treatment had failed, it was too late to do anything else.

Galen had established firmly the concept that cancer was a systemic disease, an oversupply of black bile. It made more sense by this concept to treat the systemic cause of the affliction by "proper balancing of the constitution" with bleeding or purging or hot and cold baths than it did to attack directly a symptom of the internal problem that happened to occur on the face or in the mouth. The beginnings of rational operations for cancer awaited the discovery of cancer's primary origin in the various organs and the ability to differentiate cancer grossly and microscopically from other confusingly similar diseases.

In addition to the problems of diagnosis, extensive cancer operations were impossible without anesthesia. Even minor operations about the head and neck were few when the patient had to be conscious to witness them. The gruesome habit of excising the tongue for torture and punishment is as old as man, but the first such excision for cancer is attributed to Marchette in 1664. Avicenna (980–1037) described excision of tumors of the lip, the wound being left open to heal by secondary intention, but the classic V excision for cancer of the lip was not described until the first part of the nineteenth century. Tracheotomy to relieve laryngeal obstruction was described by Galen and through the ages was occasionally used to prolong somewhat the lives of those with carcinoma of the larynx, but laryngectomy was not accomplished until the late nineteenth century.

With the advent of anesthesia and microscopic pathology in the mid-1800s, operative attack upon cancer in all areas moved swiftly forward. This was especially true of tumors of the head and neck, since they involved easily seen structures and were so readily diagnosed and the suffering of the untreated patients was so apparent. Surgeons of the German school introduced an array of new techniques for operations upon the tongue, gingiva, mandible, maxilla, and larynx. Partial laryngectomy was introduced by Gurdon Buck in 1853, and total laryngectomy for cancer was first accomplished by Billroth in 1873.

In general, the results of these new procedures were more horrifying than gratifying. Operations in a septic field and without antibiotics produced a postoperative complication rate close to 100 percent with cellulitis, sepsis, abscess, pneumonia, and death the common results. Mortality rates exceeded 50 percent. Moreover, the results of many of the early and unsophisticated operations were not much better than if the cancer had not been treated. Billroth's famous first laryngectomy left the patient with an open pharyngostome and esophagostome, so that he constantly drooled saliva over his neck and had to feed himself with a rubber tube during the entire 8 months that he survived operation.

Operative excision was usually confined to the primary lesion, and in many of the patients fortunate enough to survive the initial operation metastatic disease subsequently developed in cervical nodes. Kocher and Butlin recognized this problem early and recommended excision of the lymphatic contents of the anterior triangle of the neck together with the removal of the primary lesion in the mouth.

At the turn on the century Crile devised radical neck dissection, removing all lymphatic tissue in both the anterior and posterior triangles of the neck together with the jugular vein and the sternocleidomastoid muscle. The basic elements of his classic procedure remain valid to the present.

Patients were willing to risk the high morbidity and mortality of operations in this region because the relentless progress of untreated disease offered a slow death by asphyxia, malnutrition, and eventual hemorrhage. Even the slimmest chance of avoiding this terrible triad seemed worthwhile.

As Crile was developing his operation for treating the cervical lymph nodes, radiation therapy for cancer was introduced. This, it was quickly apparent, offered a preferable alternative to operation, especially for primary lesions of the skin and oral cavity. Until the end of the 1930s most radical operations for cancers of the head and neck were abandoned, and the primary therapy was radiation. Techniques of radiation therapy became more refined and more successful. External radiation replaced radium as the treatment of choice, and fractionated therapy replaced the use of single applications of radium or a single dose of external therapy. With each refinement the percentage of patients who were cured increased. It was soon found that metastatic deposits in the neck did not respond as well to radiation as to operation, and radical neck dissection remained in use. Occasionally, patients who failed to respond to radiation or who had recurrent cancers were submitted to one or another of the old radical procedures. But when these operations were performed in a heavily irradiated fibrotic field, wound breakdown and complications often resembled the results of surgical treatment of the prior century.

In the 1940s, the introduction of endotracheal anesthesia, liberal use of blood transfusions, and antibiotics markedly changed the ability of surgeons to operate in and about the oral cavity. Postoperative morbidity and mortality dropped to a reasonable level. Radiation therapy, so long dominant in the treatment of oral lesions, seemed at a plateau with much dissatisfaction concerning the morbidity of overtreatment. These factors led to a reevaluation of operation. Grant Ward of The Johns Hopkins Hospital and Hayes Martin of the Memorial Center for Cancer led in devising combined operations whereby the primary lesions and the cervical contents were removed in a single block.

Application of this principle improved substantially the prognosis of patients with head and neck carcinomas, especially large lesions involving the oral cavity, hypopharynx, and larynx. In some institutions the pendulum swung from almost exclusive use of radiotherapy to almost exclusive use of operation. Increasing application of these combined operations during the 1950s made possible an evaluation of their mortality, morbidity, and effectiveness. By the end of the decade the place for surgical control of head and neck lesions was much more clearly defined and accepted.

Because of the late development of operative therapy after the long period of dormancy during the radiation era, this field of surgery is still something of a frontier with rapid developments of new techniques and the evolution of new ideas and approaches.

In the meantime, radiation therapy also acquired new techniques. Supervoltage radiation, originally with cobalt 60 and later with linear accelerators, delivered higher doses of therapy with a decreased morbidity, especially sparing the patient's skin and leaving a field more suitable for operation when this was required. Radiotherapists and surgeons who previously tended to disparage the results of each other's methods and to advance their own techniques as the primary treatment for tumors suddenly found that there was considerable common ground for the two methods and that there were patients who frequently could benefit from both operation and radiation as a planned course of integrated treatment.

Detection of most lesions of the head and neck is relatively easy, since the majority are readily available to the eye and the examining finger. Even so, it is tragic to find how often malignant lesions of this area are overlooked, not only lesions more difficult to diagnose, as in the maxillary sinuses and hypopharynx, but lesions readily visualized, such as tumors or the floor of the mouth, tongue, and tonsil.

DIAGNOSIS

Physical Examination

SKIN. The skin (see Chap. 14) of the face and neck should be closely scrutinized, keeping in mind that basal and squamous carcinomas of the skin are the most common of all cancers and that the most common site for such lesions is the area of the head and neck. Seborrheic keratosis, senile keratosis, and patches of atrophic skin often appear side by side with skin neoplasms. Differential diagnosis may be difficult, and biopsy is often required. Pigmented lesions must be examined closely to determine the presence of bleeding ulceration or satellitosis indicating melanoma. All lumps should be palpated to observe their firmness, whether they have a cystic or solid quality, and whether they are fixed to the underlying tissues.

ORAL CAVITY. The oral cavity is often neglected in the course of a complete physical examination. It is said that the internist looks at the top of the tongue depressor, the otolaryngologist looks at the tonsils, and the general surgeon may not look at all. There is no excuse for this neglect, since the oral cavity is a rich source of pathologic processes, not only of local lesions, but often of lesions reflecting pathologic conditions elsewhere in the body.

Proper examination requires the use of a tongue depressor, finger cot or glove, and good lighting. If the examiner is skilled with the use of a head mirror, this will provide ideal illumination. However, there are numerous electric headlights that work equally well and that can be used at different points in the office or at the bedside without requiring an elaborate setup.

With the patient's mouth open, the light is directed into the oral cavity. If the patient has dentures of any sort, they should be removed. The examiner begins by looking at the anterior floor of the mouth and the openings of Wharton's ducts. Then the floor of the mouth is observed, progressing posteriorly along the gingivolingual gutter to the tonsillar pillars on either side. The undersurface of the anterior and lateral tongue can also be observed. This is a good place to detect early jaundice.

The lower gingiva and teeth are examined next. The condition of the teeth and the presence or absence of sepsis are considered. The gingivobuccal gutters are often the hiding place of small malignant lesions and should be inspected thoroughly.

The buccal mucosa can be examined next. Patches of hyperkeratosis are often seen here. The examiner looks for the nipple indicating the opening of Stensen's duct. Pressure on the parotid should express saliva from the orifice. The position and mobility of the tongue are observed. A deviated tongue may indicate injury to the hy-

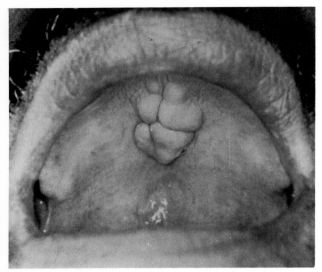

Fig. 16-1. Torus, a congenital lesion formed along the median raphe where the palatine processes of the maxilla join. These protuberances are normally smooth; the lobulation seen here is unusual.

poglossal nerve or a previous stroke. Numerous longitudinal fissures reflect previous syphilis, a condition now rarely seen. Malignant lesions are normally found on the edges or at the tip of the tongue.

Occasionally, a patch of dirty fibers will occupy the surface of the tongue. This condition, called "hairy tongue," often occurs in a dry mouth with impaired salivary secretion. Vitamin deficiencies are reflected by an atrophy of the taste buds with a flat, smooth, erythematous mucosa.

The tonsils and soft palate are considered next. The presence or absence of the tonsils or tonsillar tags should be noted. If the patient gags, the posterior tonsillar pillars rotate toward the midline, better exposing the tonsillar fossa itself. The anterior tonsillar pillar is a common site for patches of hyperkeratosis, or sometimes for very early carcinomas. Inappropriate hypertrophy of one tonsil may reflect a lymphoma. Paralysis of one side of the soft palate is often seen in patients who have had a cerebrovascular accident. Large tumors in the nasopharynx may push the soft palate forward and down.

The examiner can complete the observation with inspection of the hard palate. A smooth or occasionally lobular elevation running down the midline of the palate is usually a torus, a harmless, congenital deformity (Fig. 16-1). Tori of the mandible also occur, projecting into the mouth bilaterally at the level of the canine tooth. They have no particular importance except to the frightened patient who may notice them for the first time in adulthood and mistake them for new growths. Occasionally, patients with atrophied lower alveoli following total loss of the lower teeth will have a spur that projects backward from the midline into the floor of the mouth. This represents a prominence of the symphysis made detectable by the absorption of the surrounding bone.

Palpation is equal in importance to inspection. Many early lesions of the oral cavity cannot be detected except by the sense of touch. This is especially true of lesions buried within the substance of the tongue or in the salivary glands. The gloved finger is passed over the tongue, the floor of the mouth, and the gingivobuccal gutters. Any mass encountered can be made more prominent by bimanual or bidigital palpation, pressing the mass inward from the cheek or submental area toward the oral cavity. If the patient can tolerate it, palpation of the lateral pharyngeal wall may reveal masses in the deep lobe of the parotid. If the index of suspicion is high concerning lesions in the nasopharynx or base of tongue, these areas should be palpated as well.

NECK. Inspection and palpation of the cervical area are done methodically, keeping in mind a distinct list of structures to be felt. These should include the larynx, thyroid, trachea, sternocleidomastoid muscle, lymph node–bearing areas, and salivary glands. The submental area is examined for the presence of enlarged lymph nodes and the size and consistency of the submaxillary glands. In the older patient they may hang low in the anterior cervical triangle as the enveloping fascia becomes lax with age. In this location they often are mistaken initially for enlarged lymph nodes. The presence of any enlarged or firm lymph nodes incorporated within the substance of the submaxillary gland should be noted. Bimanual palpation through the floor of the mouth helps greatly.

The angle of the jaw is a common site for enlarged lymph nodes or not infrequently of a tumor in the tail of the parotid gland. The anterior border of the sternocleidomastoid may overlap a cystic mass representing a branchial cleft cyst. Cystic or fluctuant masses in the posterior cervical triangle may represent a lipoma or a cystic lymphangioma.

The most important consideration in the adult is the presence of enlarged lymph nodes. A number of structures in the neck deceive the novice and at first appear to be enlarged lymph nodes when in fact they are normal structures. The carotid bulb is commonly so mistaken, especially in older patients in whom arteriosclerosis has diminished or obliterated the pulse at the bulb. The tip of the hyoid bone adjacent to the carotid bulb sometimes fools the unwary, unless they are clever enough to palpate for this structure bilaterally. The posterior belly of the omohyoid muscle as it crosses the posterior triangle in the thin patient can mimic a fusiform node until the examiner realizes that the ends of the apparent node cannot be felt. Also in thin patients the tips of the transverse process of the second cervical vertebra are felt posterior to the ascending ramus of the mandible and may seem like a lymph node until it is realized that the structures are bony in consistency and bilateral.

Masses in the thyroid are best felt if the examiner stands behind the patient and palpates the lobes of the gland between thumb and forefinger. A midline mass just above the isthmus of the thyroid may represent an enlarged lymph node, a pyramidal lobe of thyroid, or a thyroglossal duct cyst.

PARANASAL SINUSES. The paranasal sinuses are relatively inaccessible to physical examination. Neoplastic

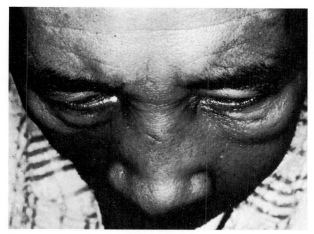

Fig. 16-2. Early swelling of the maxilla, seen best from above, as shown here. The patient had a space-occupying lesion within the sinus that was not as well appreciated in the frontal view.

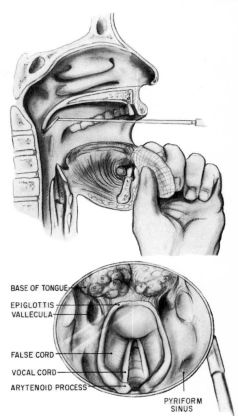

Fig. 16-3. Laryngeal mirror examination of the larynx. Cross section of the oral cavity illustrates the relation of the mirror to the larynx. Insert: View seen by the examiner. Note the epiglottis hiding the anterior portion of the cords.

lesions often hide within these recesses and are not manifest until quite late. Bulging, particularly asymmetric bulging of one maxillary sinus, can best be appreciated by observing the cheeks from above either by having the patient lean toward the examiner or by standing above the patient and looking down (Fig. 16-2). Palpation of the maxillary, ethmoid, or temporal areas may elicit tenderness or a sense of fullness. Transillumination of the sinuses by a bright light placed within the oral cavity of a patient in a dark room may reveal opacification of one or more of the sinuses. This is a relatively crude method of examination compared with x-ray examination.

INDIRECT LARYNGOSCOPY. There is a common misconception that indirect laryngoscopy is an examination to be performed only by specialists. Hoarseness and throat pain are such common symptoms and cancer of the pharynx and larynx so frequent that indirect laryngoscopy should be part of the armamentarium of any physician and part of the routine general physical examination.

The patient is seated in a chair slightly higher than the chair or stool of the examiner. The examiner sits opposite him with his right thigh and knee parallel and immediately adjacent to the right thigh and knee of the patient. The patient should extend his neck, thrusting his chin straight forward, as though he had just finished sneezing. The patient's tongue is wrapped in a gauze sponge, and the examiner, if he is right-handed, grasps the tip of the tongue between the thumb and second finger of the left hand, using the first finger to elevate the patient's upper lip. The tongue is drawn forward, and the patient is instructed to breathe rapidly in short, quick breaths, to "pant like a dog." As long as the patient continues to breathe in this fashion, gagging is inhibited. The examiner inserts a medium to large laryngeal mirror, previously flamed to keep it from fogging, into the oropharynx and shines the headlight on the mirror, reflecting a spot of light down into the hypopharynx (Fig. 16-3).

If one is a novice with the head mirror, an electric head lamp should be used. With the mirror in the oropharynx

and directed downward, the posterior third of the tongue, the lateral pharyngeal wall, the posterior pharyngeal wall, the epiglottis, the valleculae, and the pyriform sinuses can all be examined thoroughly. The epiglottis will usually hide most of the glottic opening, and only the posterior portions of the arytenoids may be seen at first. The patient is told to breathe deeply several times. This often throws the uvula forward until more of the glottic opening and a little of the subglottic space is seen. The patient is asked to attempt to enunciate an "ee" sound. This throws the epiglottis even farther forward and usually brings the entire glottis, including the anterior commissure, into view.

The false cords, aryepiglottic folds, and posterior epiglottis can now be examined. The movement of the cords is considered, to determine whether both are moving adequately and whether they meet in the midline. Paralysis of one cord may indicate a malignant lesion in the mediastinum or cervical area or may be related to previous operation or cerebrovascular accident. If nodules in the pharynx or posterior tongue are noted, they should subsequently be palpated. As the examiner acquires skill in this procedure, most of these examinations can be accomplished without local anesthesia. Topical anesthesia

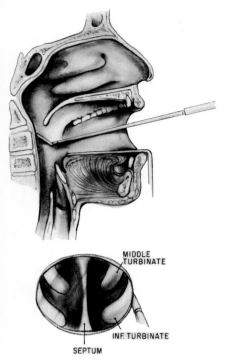

MIDDLE
TURBINATE

INF TURBINATE

SEPTUM

Fig. 16-4. Mirror view of the nasopharynx. Soft palate is drawn forward, and the mirror in the oropharynx is directed upward. Insert: View seen in the mirror.

with lidocaine 1% should be used by the beginner. Although expensive and somewhat fragile, the flexible fiberoptic nasopharyngoscope is a very handy office instrument and may give novice examiners a better view of the larynx than indirect laryngoscopy.

In one or two patients out of every twenty, examination is incomplete or impossible because of a hypersensitive gag reflex or an acquired or congenital malformation of the epiglottis that makes visualization of the glottis impossible. In such instances, direct laryngoscopy must be used. While direct laryngoscopy is the more sophisticated and complex procedure, indirect laryngoscopy actually gives a better overall picture of the larynx and pharynx. The chief reason for resorting to direct laryngoscopy other than the above is the necessity of biopsy of lesions deep in the larynx. Direct laryngoscopy is sometimes performed using a *suspension laryngoscope,* which, once the cords are visualized, can be fixed in place so that operators do not have to use their hands to hold the laryngoscope. This technique can be combined with the use of an optical device that greatly magnifies the cords so that small irregularities and tiny lesions may be examined. Occasionally in patients with unexplained hoarseness this approach will reveal early localized benign and malignant changes.

NASOPHARYNGOSCOPY. The mirror used for indirect laryngoscopy may be turned over and directed upward. The examiner, standing at the patient's shoulder and depressing the tongue with a tongue blade, may shine the headlight on the mirror and gain a fairly spacious view of

the nasopharynx. In most instances the space between the soft palate and posterior pharyngeal wall is too small for the nasopharynx to be adequately visualized in this fashion. If physical findings or the history so indicate, complete examination of the nasopharynx is done by inserting a soft rubber #10 French catheter through either nasal passage, drawing its tip out through the mouth and retracting the soft palate forward, revealing the entire nasopharynx for indirect examination by the mirror (Fig. 16-4). The torus tubarius, the openings of the eustachian tubes, the posterior surface of the soft palate, the posterior aspect of the nasal septum arching back toward the sphenoid sinus, and the posterior tips of the turbinates are seen. The normal lymphatic tissue of the adenoids may lend a granular appearance to some of the posterior and superior mucosal surfaces.

The direct nasopharyngoscope is an instrument that can be used in the office. It is a small instrument like a miniature cystoscope and has a Foroblique or right-angled lens. The diameter of the tube is 5 to 8 mm, and the visual field is quite small and easily obscured by mucus or blood. Use of this instrument is a valuable adjunct to indirect inspection of the nasopharynx and is particularly helpful in searching for small neoplasms.

Introduction of the fiberoptic laryngoscope has made it possible to examine both the nasopharynx and larynx with the same instrument. This thin, flexible instrument is inserted through the nostril and is easily tolerated by the patient. In many offices it is supplanting indirect laryngoscopy.

Diagnostic Studies

RADIOGRAPHY. Most of the bones of the face and neck are adjacent to air-filled cavities or are air-containing, creating an excellent situation for diagnostic radiographs. Lesions of the paranasal sinuses, nasal cavity, orbit, mandible, and larynx are readily revealed.

Arteriography. Injection of contrast medium into the vessels is a useful maneuver for evaluating tumors within the cranium or evaluation of tumors in this region. The rare carotid body tumor can be nicely outlined by the use of radiopaque medium injected into the appropriate common carotid artery, and its appearance when examined in this fashion is pathognomonic. At times, arteriography is useful to outline the extent of a hemangioma of the face or oral cavity (Fig. 16-5).

Laminography. This technique is of great usefulness in examinations of the head and neck, especially for minute examination of the bony walls of the paranasal sinuses. Usually, the clouding of a paranasal sinus by tumor and by infection cannot be differentiated by x-ray unless obvious evidence of bone erosion is seen. Early detection of such erosions is best seen in laminograms. Tumors of the larynx are easily seen from above by indirect laryngoscopy, but their inferior extent is hidden from view unless the lesion is very small. Laminograms and lateral soft tissue views of the larynx play a useful role in revealing the extent of subglottic extension and often the degree of involvement of the pyriform sinuses, which may not other-

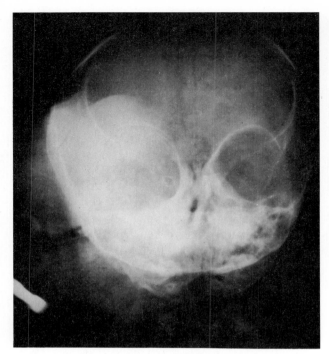

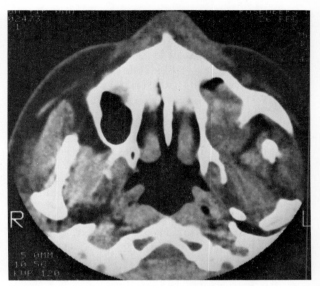

Fig. 16-6. Computer tomography of a squamous cell carcinoma in the left maxillary sinus. Posterior extent of this lesion with perforation of the maxillary wall and proximity to surrounding structures is clearly shown by this technique.

Fig. 16-5. Arteriographic demonstration of hemangioma of the oral cavity. On physical examination, only the cheek appeared involved. In the x-ray view, involvement of the lateral pharyngeal wall and oral cavity is noted. (From: *Rush BF Jr: Ann Surg 164:921, 1966, with permission.*)

wise be detectable. Details of retropharyngeal and esophageal tumor spread can be seen on the lateral soft tissue view. Laryngograms are performed by the application of barium to the back of the tongue, cords, epiglottis, and all of the intrinsic larynx. A very clear examination of laryngeal structures can be obtained that offers excellent correlation with other diagnostic methods available.

Computer Tomography. This intriguing technique has found applications throughout the body and is especially useful in the head and neck. The true extent of large tumors of this area is best defined by the multisectional studies offered by computer tomography. This is especially true of tumors in the nasopharynx, paranasal sinuses, and the larynx. In these areas the new technique is superior to and is supplanting laminography (Fig. 16-6); when it is used with vascular contrast, enlarged cervical lymph nodes can be detected before they are palpable.

Magnetic Resonance Imaging. Images in the head and neck area provided by this method demonstrate the most detail in soft tissues of any technique available. There is superior differentiation of abnormal from normal tissue. In addition, vascular structures are revealed without having to inject contrast material. Since MRI does not require the use of radiation, it may eventually take the place of arteriography, laminography, and even computer tomography except for very special applications.

BIOPSY. The vast majority of head and neck lesions can be easily biopsied in the office or clinic. The tools required are simple, and the procedure is short and uncom-

plicated. Lesions of the lip, skin, gingiva, floor of the mouth, tongue, and buccal mucosa can quickly be biopsied with a 4-mm dermatologist's skin punch. The area to be biopsied is cleansed with an antiseptic agent infiltrated with a small amount of local anesthesia, and the skin punch is pressed into the lesion to a depth of 4 to 6 mm, cutting a small disc of the tumor, and is withdrawn. The core of tissue that is still connected at its base is grasped with forceps, pulled up until the base is flush with the surface tissues, and cut off with a small pair of scissors. A silver nitrate stick thrust into the depth of the remaining cavity and mild pressure for a minute or two control bleeding in almost all instances. Lesions of the soft palate, tonsillar pillar, or posterior tongue that cannot be reached with a skin punch can often be biopsied easily and quickly with a cervical biopsy forcep; the techniques of anesthesia and hemostasis are essentially the same as described above.

If skill is obtained with indirect laryngoscopy, lesions of the lateral pharyngeal wall, pyriform sinus, epiglottis, and aryepiglottic folds can often be quickly biopsied in the office. While similar biopsies of the true and false cords sometimes can be achieved with skillful manipulation of the indirect mirror, such procedures are best carried out under direct laryngoscopy. Manipulation of biopsy forceps immediately above the cords is much more difficult for the patient to tolerate and may stimulate laryngeal spasm and bleeding at a site where aspiration of blood into the trachea is likely.

Biopsy of the primary lesion is always preferable, but sometimes although cervical nodes are enlarged, no primary tumor can be found. If so, needle biopsy of cervical nodes is indicated and is a rewarding procedure when the node contains metastatic squamous carcinoma. This neoplasm is easily diagnosed even with the smallest fragments of tissue. Nodes involved by lymphoma, on the other hand, are virtually impossible to diagnose by needle biopsy. Positive results of needle biopsy are useful and timesaving; the negative result of a needle biopsy has no significance and must be followed by open biopsy.

Needle biopsy has been rediscovered several times in the 50 years since it was first described. In the last decade there has been considerable excitement over "skinny needly biopsy," biopsy with needles of 20 to 24 gauge. This is a cytologic method, and the fine needles remove cells and tissue fluid rather than any bits of organized tissue. Because tumor cells are less adherent than normal cells, the small needle will often harvest many more abnormal than normal cells, an advantage over the core biopsies taken with larger needles.

There has been much controversy concerning the tendency to spread tumor cells with the use of needle biopsies, and certainly it seems likely that tumor cells are spread into the needle tract by this manipulation. However, this is of greater theoretical than practical importance. Long experience with this technique at a number of major centers has not produced any gross difference in survival rates on long-term follow-up either in the head and neck or elsewhere. Open biopsy of a lymph node seems just as likely to scatter tumor cells, and even more widely.

VITAL DYES. Many cancers of the oral mucosa in their early stages are soft and superficial. They may have an erythematous appearance rather than a white color as usually thought and can easily escape detection even in a careful examination. If suspicion is aroused by a vaguely erythematous patch, the application of toluidine blue will aid in making the diagnosis. This technique will distinguish areas of dysplasia and carcinoma in situ as well as frank carcinoma of the mucosa. The method has its chief use in mapping out the full extent of dysplastic areas or areas of intraepithelial carcinoma.

CYTOLOGY. As used in the oral cavity, exfoliative cytology is a superficial biopsy, since it does not reflect collection of fluid from the entire oral cavity but involves scraping a specific lesion with a spatula and spreading this scraping on a slide. Such cytologic examinations, therefore, require a specific area of suspicion compared with sampling of an entire anatomic area such as in the cervix or bronchial tree. If a specific lesion is present, it is best evaluated by an actual biopsy. The chief virture of oral cytology is that physicians who cannot bring themselves to use office biopsy techniques or who feel they are beyond their competence can still have the opportunity to obtain a histologic specimen from the lesion in question. Unlike biopsy, cytology has no significance when it is negative. Thus, cytology will establish the presence of a lesion but cannot be relied on to rule that a questionable lesion is not malignant.

Tumor Markers. Substances produced by tumor or antigens to these substances sometimes appear in the serum. Few of these appear at an early enough stage in the growth of tumors to be much use in diagnosis, but if they are elevated when the tumor is found, increase or decrease in the marker usually is correlated with increase or decrease in tumor mass. Some head and neck tumors secrete a parahormone-like substance that is associated with an elevated calcium in about 10 percent of Stages III and IV tumors. This finding usually reflects a grim prognosis. Reduction of tumor mass by operation, chemotherapy, or radiation will return the calcium level to normal. Carcinoembryonic antigen (CEA) is sometimes elevated in head and neck tumors and can be used to follow therapy. Squamous cell carcinoma–associated antigen (SCCA) is elevated in 60 to 70 percent of Stages III and IV cancers of the head and neck. Its usefulness as a monitor for therapeutic response is currently under investigation.

CANCER STAGING. An important facet of diagnosis is staging the clinical extent of the tumor. The efforts of the American Joint Commission for Cancer Staging have introduced the now widely accepted TNM system of staging in which T stands for tumor, N for regional lymph nodes, and M for metastasis. In 1987 this system was brought into agreement with the system of the Union Internationale Contre Cancrum (UICC), so there is now a single worldwide staging system. Proper description of each aspect of a malignant lesion permits more precise comparison between series of patients and better evaluation for prognosis. The committee has a book available in which all the major areas for staging in the head and neck are covered. The system has great value but is complex enough that patients should never be staged from memory but only with the staging reference available. Staging may be either clinical, based entirely on the physical examination, or pathologic, based on gross and microscopic examination of the specimen. Recent studies show that thickness of an oral lesion is more important than the area covered when predicting subsequent involvement of cervical nodes and survival.

LIP

Squamous cell carcinomas of the lip are one of the common malignant tumors of the oral cavity, constituting 15 percent of all such lesions and 2.2 percent of all cancers. Basal cell carcinoma is much less frequent; only about 3 are seen for every 100 squamous cell carcinomas of the lip. Benign lesions that are occasionally seen in the lips include mucous cysts, tumors of the minor salivary glands, hemangiomas, lymphangiomas, venous lakes, fibromas, fissures, and hyperkeratosis.

ETIOLOGY. Like tumors of the skin, there is an important relationship between tumors of the lip and exposure to sunlight. About one-third of patients have a history of working outdoors, and the incidence of malignant squamous cancers of the lip increases progressively the farther south the latitude of the patient population being considered. Thus, in the United States the highest incidence is in Florida and Texas. Actinic rays are stronger at higher altitudes and in dryer air, and in areas having these features the incidence of lip (and skin) cancer is increased. Fishermen, sailors, and farmers are among the occupational groups with an increased incidence.

Complexion also plays a role. Susceptible types are fair-skinned, light, blond or ginger-haired, and blue-eyed, with the kind of complexion that freckles and burns rather than tans on exposure to the sun. Resistant people have the opposite characteristics: they are brunet and dark-skinned; blacks are rarely affected.

While there is a relation between lip cancer and tobacco, the exact cause for this is less apparent than in patients with lesions of the intraoral area, larynx, or lungs. The average cigarette smoker receives almost no carcinogen from tobacco directly to the lips, since the smoke is drawn into the oral cavity and tracheobronchial tree without passing over the mucosa of the lips themselves. Some feel that the inmates of nursing homes and institutions are more prone to have carcinoma of the lip from cigarette smoking. Smokers in this population usually treasure their cigarettes, smoking them down to the smallest possible butt. Macerated, moist tobacco and heat are directly applied to the lips.

Reports in the literature implicating pipe smoking as a cause of lip cancer have been appearing since 1795, and the Advisory Committee to the Surgeon General on Smoking and Health has accepted the causal relationship as established. Pipestems of wood and clay that soak up tobacco tars directly and apply a ''tar poultice'' to the lips have been viewed with special suspicion. In any case, such stems are little used now, and indeed the incidence of cancer of the lip in the United States has been gradually decreasing over the past 30 years. One may speculate whether this reflects the decrease in pipe smoking, outdoor work, use of wood and clay pipestems, or a combination of these and other factors.

Cancer of the lip in women is very rare, occurring in only 1 woman for every 20 to 30 men.

Benign Tumors

The mucosa of the inner surface of the upper and lower lips is subject to the same benign lesions as those throughout the mucosa of the oral cavity. These are discussed in greater detail in the following section, Oral Cavity, and include such lesions as mucous cysts, hemangiomas, tumors of the minor salivary glands, hyperkeratosis, and inflammatory hyperplasia. Specific benign lesions that involve the exposed borders of the lips include venous lakes, pigmented spots, hemangiomas, and very rarely neuromas. Venous lakes are a telangiectasis, usually of the lower lip, occurring in older individuals as a small bluish spot. They appear to have no pathologic significance. The other three lesions all have interesting systemic correlations. Multiple pigmented spots of the lips may be associated with Peutz-Jeghers syndrome and denote the presence of multiple small intestinal polyps, which sometimes lead to bleeding and intussusception but are rarely malignant. Scattered small hemangiomas of the lip may be associated with similar lesions elsewhere in the oral cavity and gastrointestinal tract, those of Rendu-Osler-Weber disease. Neuromas of the lips, particularly at the commissures, suggest a neuroendocrine dysplasia, a fascinating syndrome associated with pheochromocytomas, medullary carcinoma of the thyroid, hyperparathyroidism, and hypertrophy of the gastrointestinal myenteric plexus.

Hyperkeratosis

This is a premalignant condition of the lips, usually associated with long exposure to sunlight. It typically occurs in fair-skinned individuals in their sixties or seventies who have long histories of outdoor employment. The normal distinct line marking the mucocutaneous border becomes indistinct and gradually retreats, indicating a metaplasia of the outer portion of the mucosa to a keratosquamous epithelium. The mucosa of the lip becomes paler, thinner, and more fragile. There may be perpendicular cracks and fissures. On this base, a white film indicative of early hyperkeratosis appears. This may grow gradually thicker and more exophytic as the condition progresses (Fig. 16-7) or may remain stationary for many years. Gradually, a small area of scabbing and ulceration occurs. This breakdown within the hyperkeratotic tissue represents a failure of the less resistant areas of hyperkeratosis to tolerate normal wear and tear. When such areas of ulceration appear, they continue to break down and heal and often give rise to carcinoma in situ and eventually invasive carcinoma. Persistent hyperkeratosis is a distinct premalignant lesion, and 35 to 40 percent of all carcinomas of the lip are preceded by this condition. Cancers arising on such a base can be prevented by excising the entire exposed mucosa of the lip, elevating the protected mucosa of the inner lip, and advancing it over the bed of the excised mucosa to form a new lining for the

Fig. 16-7. Hyperkeratosis of lower lip. This degree of hyperkeratosis merits serious concern. The entire lower lip is involved and should be treated by excision (lip stripping) and advancement of the mucosa of the inner lip to cover the defect.

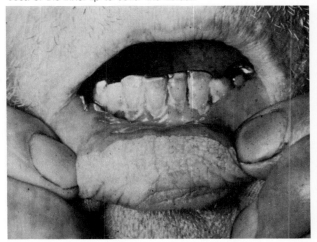

lip. This procedure is called a *lip stripping and resurfacing*.

Carcinoma of the Lip

Most cancers of the lip are squamous carcinomas. When basal cell carcinomas appear, they usually involve the skin of the lip beyond the vermilion border and probably should be considered with the cancers of the skin of the face. Ninety-three percent of the squamous cancers occur on the lower lip. These are usually low-grade, well-differentiated lesions, 80 percent being grade 1 or grade 2. The lesions most frequently start on the outer edge of the mucosa at the vermilion border and seem to favor the middle two-thirds of the lip somewhat more frequently than the commissures (Fig. 16-8).

The natural history of these lesions is of slow but relentless growth. Some grow to great size, destroying the entire lip without ever metastasizing, but the incidence of metastasis gradually increases with the increasing size of the tumors (Fig. 16-9). About 5 to 10 percent of all patients with lip cancer have cervical lymph node metastasis, and in half of these patients only one lymph node is involved. The normal spread of cancer from the lower lip is by way of lymphatics to the submental node on the side of the lesion. Metastases do not involve the opposite submental node unless the primary lesion crosses the midline. Lesions of the upper lip drain to lymph nodes in the anterior portion of the submaxillary gland.

An ulcer of the lip that fails to heal is soon detected by patients or their friends, and in most urban populations such lesions quickly come to the attention of physicians. In rural populations it is surprising how long patients will carry these ulcerations before seeking medical aid.

Treatment for carcinoma of the lip has remained a topic of controversy between radiotherapists and surgeons for many decades. Recent controlled series comparing treatment by both modalities in randomly selected patients

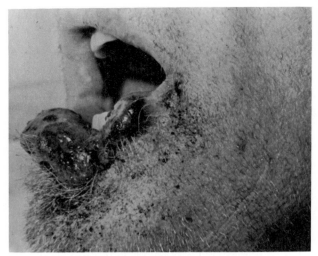

Fig. 16-9. Neglected carcinoma of the lip. A metastatic node is present along the line of the mandible. The chance of cure for this type of lesion is 50 percent or less.

indicate that there is no statistical difference between the two methods in terms of cure rate. The choice for therapy must be made on other grounds. Small lesions of the lip can usually be excised under local anesthesia with little or no hospitalization time. Good radiation therapy producing maximal regression with minimal residual scarring requires 2 to 4 weeks of outpatient therapy. Medium-sized lesions require the use of flaps from the upper lip or elsewhere for closure, and for these lesions radiotherapy often requires the same or less time and less morbidity. For very large lesions that have destroyed most of the lip and are associated with metastasis to the neck, subsequent repair of the lip will be required under any circumstance as well as probable radical neck dissection for removal of cervical nodes; for these major lesions an integration of radiation and surgical therapy may be used to improve cure rates, which are relatively low for either radiation or operation alone. A final consideration is that most carcinomas of the lip are related to solar radiation. Since radiotherapy increases the sensitivity of tissues to such exposure, it is best to avoid radiotherapy in patients who expect to return to outdoor occupations.

Prognosis for lip cancers of 1 cm or less is excellent, ranging from an 87 to 95 percent 5-year survival rate without recurrence. Neglected lesions, especially with associated cervical metastasis, do much more poorly, with a 5-year survival of 50 percent.

ORAL CAVITY

The oral cavity includes the buccal mucosa, upper and lower gingivae, anterior two-thirds of the tongue (that portion anterior to the circumvallate papillae), floor of the mouth, and hard palate.

INCIDENCE. Eight percent of all malignant tumors occur in this area, 95 percent of such tumors being squamous

Fig. 16-8. Squamous carcinoma of lip. Any patient with a chronic ulcer of this sort should seek medical advice. The chance of cure at this early stage approaches 100 percent.

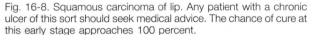

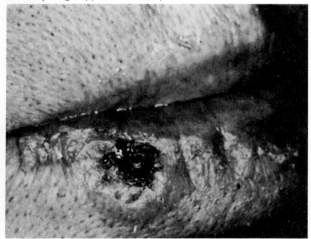

carcinomas. The risk of carcinomas developing here in a male is approximately 1 percent in a lifetime. The risk in females is far less: oral cancer develops in about 1 woman for every 10 males. Benign tumors of the oral cavity are common in both sexes.

ETIOLOGY. Some benign lesions have a specific cause, which will be discussed with the descriptions of the lesions below. Contributing causes to squamous carcinoma are smoking, a heavy intake of alcohol, poor oral hygiene, and syphilis. While cancer often occurs without the presence of any of these factors, they are associated with a majority of the lesions seen.

The *Report on Smoking and Health* by the Advisory Committee to the Surgeon General notes a suggestive relationship between smoking and oral carcinoma. This is especially true in pipe and cigar smokers, where oral cancer has the highest mortality ratio, 3.3,* of all causes of death compared with the nonsmoking population. There are a number of exotic cancers of the oral cavity that serve to indicate the relationship of tobacco to cancer. In Andhra Pradesh, a state in India, the habit of smoking a cigar (i.e., *chutta*) with the burning end inside the mouth is widespread. Carcinoma of the palate, called *chutta cancer,* is common. Presumably, repeated thermal trauma and/or tobacco smoke provide the carcinogenic agents.

In Uttar Pradesh and Bihar, a mixture of tobacco and slaked lime is habitually sucked by men of the districts. The quid is kept in the lower gingivolabial fornix for many hours during the day; a high incidence of carcinoma is found at this site. This has come to be called *khaini cancer,* from the name of the tobacco-lime mixture.

Betel-nut chewing is a common habit among the Indians, Javanese, and Malayans. The chew is made of a mixture of ground betel nut, slaked lime, and spices, such as ginger or pepper. These are wrapped in a betel leaf and chewed. The Indians add tobacco to their betel preparations and have a high incidence of oral cancer, whereas the incidence is low among the Javanese and Malayans, who consume their betel nut without benefit of the tobacco additive. Among betel nut–tobacco chewers, oral cancer comprises 36 percent of all cancers.

Alcoholism has a highly suggestive role in oral cancer. As many as 42 percent of all patients so afflicted have a history of alcoholism. As a corollary, cirrhosis of the liver is a common finding in patients with oral cancer, 20 percent having cirrhosis as compared with 9 percent in a control population. It has been proposed that alcohol acts as an adjuvant to the use of tobacco in producing oral cancer. This is a difficult point to prove, since finding a control population of patients who drink heavily but do not smoke is virtually impossible.

The roles of poor oral hygiene and oral sepsis, mentioned for decades as etiologic agents for oral cancers, are also difficult to evaluate. These conditions are seen most

---

* That is, 3.3 times as many pipe and cigar smokers died of oral cancer as did nonsmokers in the same age group. The mortality ratio for cancer of the lung in pipe smokers was 1:1, no different from that of the nonsmokers.

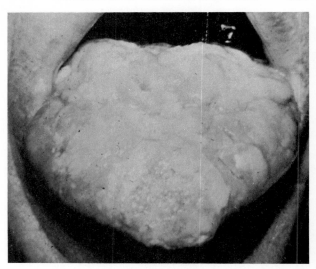

Fig. 16-10. Syphilis of the tongue. The dense, white patches are sometimes mistaken for "geographic tongue." Cancers of the dorsal surface often follow this condition.

commonly in patients at the lower end of the social scale and in the ward population rather than in private practice. Oral hygiene is poor in this group, but it cannot be said whether poor hygiene or social level or other correlated factors are responsible.

Syphilis has a direct relation to cancer of one specific site in the oral cavity, the tongue. When syphilitic glossitis, a lesion of late syphilis, heals, it often leaves the tongue fibrotic and scarred with longitudinal fissures and thick hyperkeratotic plaques. It is on this base that lingual cancer develops (Fig. 16-10). In the days of Bloodgood (1921), 21 percent of American men with lingual cancer had syphilis. Willis still calls this condition "the most clearly established causative factor in European males."

Benign Lesions

Common benign tumors of the oral cavity are inflammatory hyperplasias and cysts. Less commonly seen are giant cell granulomas, salivary tumors, granular cell myoblastomas, dermoids, and hemangiomas.

INFLAMMATORY HYPERPLASIA

The oral mucosa is subject to a number of irritating conditions producing tumorlike projections that are not true neoplasms. Patients develop the nervous habit of sucking a portion of mucosa from the cheek, tongue, or lip between the teeth or through an interdental or edentulous space. The traumatized mucosa becomes edematous and prominent, and the irritation may be compounded by the patient who bites as well as sucks on the offending mucosal fold. Initially, the overlying mucosa is swollen, and eventually this undergoes metaplasia to squamous epithelium. The tissue underlying the elevated mucosa changes from edematous connective tissue to a denser and more fibrotic collection of collagen. At this stage the

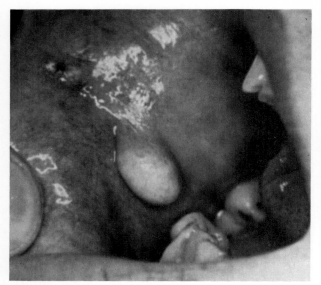

Fig. 16-11. Irritation fibroma. The lesion seen here was caused by persistent sucking and irritation of mucosa through the edentulous space, which can be seen adjacent to this polyp. *(Courtesy of Sheldon Rovin, D.D.S.)*

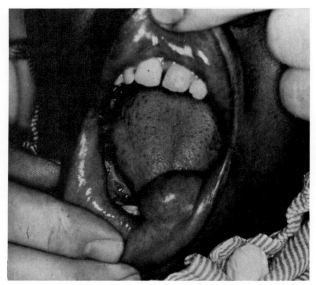

Fig. 16-12. Mucous cyst of the lip, the most common location for this lesion. This mucocele has resulted from rupture of a minor salivary gland duct with spillage of mucus into the surrounding tissue.

lesion may be termed a *fibroepithelial polyp* (Fig. 16-11). Similar lesions are often seen in the gingivobuccal gutter and on the palate in patients with ill-fitting dentures. Those lesions that occur along the vestibular mucosa next to the gingiva in this relation are sometimes called *epulis fissurata*. Another appropriate term, more descriptive of the later stages of these lesions when the fibrosis and scarring has advanced, is *irritation fibroma*. In the early inflammatory phase of these lesions, the overlying mucosa is friable and bleeds easily.

The chief responsibility of the examiner who has recognized the lesion is to reassure the patient that it is not malignant. Although these lesions are usually not ulcerated and are easily recognized, diagnosis should be confirmed by biopsy. Treatment is by correction of the causative factor, either by the design of new dentures or by discouraging the patient from manipulating and traumatizing the area involved. Excision may be necessary, but if the basic problem is not abolished, recurrence is prompt.

CYSTS

Mucous cysts are a common oral lesion occurring on the posterior surface of the lip, floor of the mouth, tongue, and buccal mucosa. These cysts arise from the salivary gland–bearing areas of the oral mucosa and were thought to be due to obstruction of the excretory duct of minor salivary glands. It has been found, however, that these cysts have no epithelial lining and that they result from a rupture of the excretory duct. Saliva spills from the defect in the duct and begins to collect in the tissues. At first it forms a diffuse lesion, but soon a circumscribed cyst with a wall of granulation tissue develops. These mucoceles measure from 1 or 2 mm to 1 or 2 cm in diameter and appear as elevated, translucent, bluish lesions of the mucosa (Fig. 16-12). They frequently rupture, discharging sticky mucoid material, and then recur as the laceration in the overlying mucosa heals. Treatment consists of wide surgical unroofing of the lesion.

A somewhat larger and more dramatic mucocele may result from obstruction and rupture of the major excretory ducts in the floor of the mouth, ducts of the lingual or submaxillary glands. Except for size, these lesions resemble in every way the lesions that result from obstruction of the minor salivary glands but have received the special name of *ranula*.

Dermoids may develop in the floor of the mouth and the base of the tongue along the midline. If neglected, these lesions grow slowly as they accumulate the sloughed-off cells, secretion, and hair of the epidermal lining. They present as both a swelling in the submental triangle and an elevation of the floor of the mouth (Fig. 16-13). They will eventually elevate the floor of the mouth and tongue until it touches the palate and interferes with speech. Treatment consists of operative excision of the cyst, which may be done either intraorally or extraorally. The lesion has a definite, thick capsule and can be shelled out with ease from its relatively avascular midline location.

PERIPHERAL GIANT CELL REPARATIVE GRANULOMA

These benign tumors occur on the gingivae, affecting the maxillary or mandibular gingiva with equal frequency. Grossly, they appear as a slow-growing, reddish, smooth sessile tumor that bleeds easily. They often occur at an area of an interdental papilla (Fig. 16-14) but may also arise in edentulous patients. Histologically, the lesion is covered by stratified squamous epithelium. Endothelial

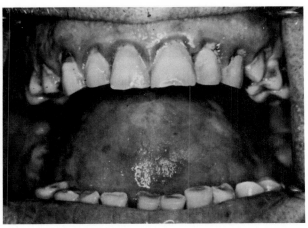

Fig. 16-13. Dermoid of the mouth. This huge dermoid has elevated the floor of the mouth until the tongue is forced against the hard palate and in this illustration is out of sight behind the cyst.

and fibroplastic proliferations, multinucleated giant cells, and extracellular and intracellular hemosiderin are diagnostic microscopic criteria. Multinucleated giant cells are distributed unevenly throughout an area of rich fibroblastic proliferation. Some lesions show spicules of bone tissue. In general, the lesion closely resembles the giant cell tumor of bone seen in hyperparathyroidism. The descriptive term *peripheral* indicates that the lesion is of soft tissue, while the so-called central giant cell reparative granuloma is an intraosseous form found in the mandible or maxilla.

When these lesions arise in the mandible or maxilla, they may be confused with the giant cell tumors of long bones. The distinction between the two lesions must be made, since the oral lesions have no propensity for malignant transformation, as have the lesions seen elsewhere.

Fig. 16-14. Peripheral giant cell tumor. These often arise in interdental spaces, as seen in photograph.

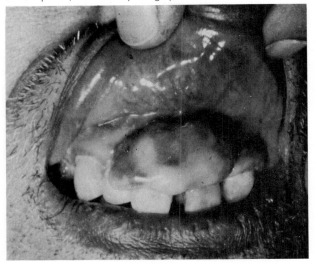

Treatment of the soft tissue lesions is by complete excision. Inadequate removal may result in recurrence.

PERIPHERAL FIBROMA

These are also lesions of the gingiva and are in many respects similar grossly to the giant cell granuloma. They are usually firmer and under the microscope are made up of dense connective tissue. They may also contain bone spicules and may be calcified. One can speculate as to the relation of these lesions to the giant cell granuloma. They may represent a later stage of this lesion or may be a late stage of inflammatory hyperplasia. Excision is usually curative.

GRANULOMA PYOGENICUM

This is an elevated pedunculated or sessile lesion that may occur on the lips, tongue, buccal mucosa, or gingiva. It bleeds readily on being traumatized. Histologically it is made up of edematous, fibrous connective tissue with a prominent endothelial component arranged in lobules of varying sizes separated by bands of collagen. Numerous blood vessels are scattered throughout the tumor. No cause is known for the lesions of the lips, buccal mucosa, and tongue, but lesions of the gingiva are often associated with pregnancy. Thirty to forty percent of pregnant women show some degree of gingival enlargement. Of these, about 1 percent will have an isolated "tumor." These lesions in the pregnant female have been called "granuloma gravidarum." They appear about the third month of pregnancy and increase in size throughout the growth of the child in utero. They usually diminish in size and disappear following delivery, although with a subsequent pregnancy they may appear again in the same location. Lesions unassociated with pregnancy may be treated by excision. It is usually advisable to wait until the end of pregnancy to treat granuloma gravidarum.

SALIVARY TUMORS

Pleomorphic adenomas (mixed tumors) occasionally arise from any of the 400 to 700 minor salivary glands. Occurring most commonly on the lips, tongue, and palate, they can be found anywhere in the oral cavity where minor salivary glands are found. They are usually slow-growing, round masses of a rather rubbery consistency (Fig. 16-15). They have the potential of becoming malignant and if simply enucleated without adequate excision have a marked propensity for local recurrence. Treatment, therefore, is by wide local excision.

HEMANGIOMA

Capillary hemangiomas, not unlike the strawberry hemangioma of the skin, are sometimes seen in the mucous membranes of the oral cavity in infants. Like the lesions of the skin these lesions regress spontaneously, and unless they are so large that they interfere with function, they should be left to regress at their own pace. In most instances they will undergo involution by the end of the fifth year. Unlike the skin lesions they do not disap-

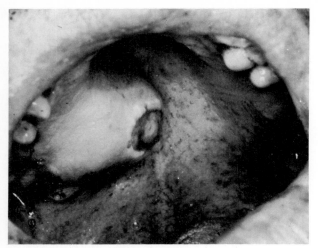

Fig. 16-15. Mixed tumor of palate. This is a benign lesion. Adequate removal to ensure prevention of recurrences includes resection of the underlying hard palate and gingiva.

pear completely and may still be seen as a small, dark lesion underneath the mucosa (Fig. 16-16). It is likely that the transparent nature of the mucosa reveals the sclerosed remnant in a manner that is not seen if the lesion is under the more opaque skin. The sclerosed hemangioma will remain visible throughout life but has no significance and does not require treatment. Rarely, large regional vascular malformations will involve the entire side of the mouth, including the tongue, gingiva, and buccal mucosa. Such lesions do not regress spontaneously. Their treatment is difficult, often requiring multiple plastic procedures to excise the hemangiomatous tissue and to return the contours of the mouth and oral cavity to normal.

GRANULAR CELL MYOBLASTOMA

This is a rare and interesting lesion that occurs most commonly within the muscle of the tongue, presenting as a small, firm spheroid mass detected best by manual palpation. These lesions have no malignant potential but may gradually increase in size with functional impairment. Treatment is by simple excision.

Hyperkeratosis and Erythroplasia

The gross finding of white patches on the oral mucosa elicits the diagnosis of leukoplakia from the clinician. "Leukoplakia" roughly translated means "white patches," so physicians need not feel too proud of their accomplishment; they have only managed to translate English into Latin. To some "leukoplakia" means a specific premalignant lesion. This meaning is not inherent in the original use of this term. Most pathologists adhere to a more rigid description of such lesions and describe the underlying microscopic changes: hyperplasia, keratosis, and dyskeratosis. White patches in the oral cavity may be associated with any or all of these basic changes (Fig. 16-17). Inflammation in this area often stimulates marked hyperplasia of cells, sometimes to the point where they resemble epidermoid tumors and are spoken of as *pseudoepitheliomatous hyperplasia*. Keratosis is a common response of the buccal mucosa and may appear in the presence of lichen planus, chronic dyscoid lupus, and Darier's disease, as well as be a possible accompaniment of malignant change.

Dyskeratosis, the loss of normal stratification or orientation of cells together with irregularity in the size and shape of cells and abnormal staining characteristics, is a much more predictable lesion and much more likely to announce malignant disease. A reddened area in the mucosa or erythroplasia is the earliest indication of dysplasia

Fig. 16-16. Fibrosing hemangioma. Lesions in the mucosal area remain visible under the buccal mucosa, whereas similar lesions may not be discernible under the skin.

Fig. 16-17. Hyperkeratosis of mucosa. The white mucosa in the gingivobuccal gutter of the patient is due to an ill-fitting denture causing hyperkeratosis, a normal response of the oral mucosa to irritation. *(Courtesy of Sheldon Rovin, D.D.S.)*

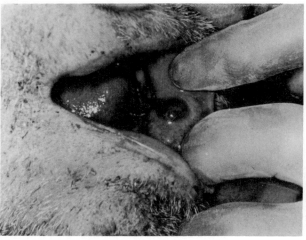

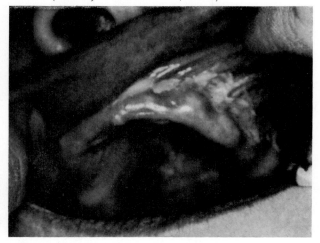

and is the earliest indicator of a malignant or premalignant lesion in the oral cavity. An overproduction of keratin, hyperkeratosis, is a much less common companion (4 percent) of dyskeratosis than it is on the lips, where hyperkeratosis often accompanies dyskeratosis, probably because the squamous cells of the vermilion border normally produce more keratin than the cells of the oral mucosa. Erythroplasia of the oral cavity occurs most commonly in the floor of the mouth, the lingual border, and the anterior tonsillar pillars and may signal not only dysplasia but frank carcinoma in situ and even microinvasive carcinoma. Since erythroplasia is such a definite sign of premalignant or malignant change, all such lesions should be excised promptly. Multiple lesions are common and patients are subject to the appearance of other lesions in the oral cavity and for that matter in the entire aerodigestive tract. Sometimes the dysplastic process will cover a major area such as the entire soft palate or floor of the mouth. Excision, in this case, is futile and radiation of the oral cavity is required after appropriate biopsy.

Malignant Tumors

PATHOLOGY. Low-grade epidermoid carcinomas make up the overwhelming majority of all carcinomas of the oral cavity, varying from highly differentiated tumors, difficult to tell histologically from inflammatory hyperplasia, to less well-organized but still obvious epidermoid tumors usually with associated squamous pearls. Highly undifferentiated and anaplastic lesions are rare. The few adenocarcinomas found are derived from minor salivary glands. The occasional adenoid cystic carcinomas and mucoepidermoid carcinomas seen also arise from salivary tissues.

In the southern United States a very low-grade cancer, verrucous carcinoma, is occasionally seen. This is an exophytic, shaggy white lesion usually found in the gingivobuccal gutter of patients who are tobacco chewers or "snuff dippers." Unless treated by radiation, the lesion never metastasizes, although it frequently invades surrounding tissues, including the mandible.

In general, lesions of the oral cavity are better differentiated and less malignant than lesions occurring in the oropharynx.

TONGUE

Carcinoma of the tongue commonly begins at the tip or along the free borders. It often starts in an area of hyperkeratosis and gradually develops as an ulcerated lesion with a moderately exophytic undermined border. The area of ulceration is related to the rest of the tumor as the tip of an iceberg is to its main mass, and palpation of the tongue may indicate that invasion has occurred deeply throughout underlying muscle (Fig. 16-18). Carcinomas beginning in an area of syphilitic glossitis are exceptions to the normal pattern and occur on the dorsal glossal surface.

Cancer of the tip of the tongue (Fig. 16-19) metastasizes to submental nodes, often bilaterally, while lesions along

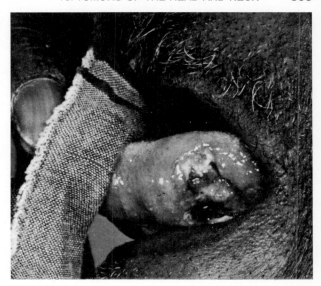

Fig. 16-18. Squamous carcinoma of the lateral border of the middle third of the tongue. The lesion is deeply invasive and much larger than the area of ulceration would indicate. The curled raised border is characteristic.

the borders of the tongue metastasize to ipsilateral submandibular nodes and occasionally to nodes at the angle of the mandible.

These lesions are quick to metastasize, and 40 percent of patients have nodes in the neck when first seen. In another 40 percent nodes develop at some point during therapy or during follow-up. For this reason therapy is designed to attack not only the primary lesion but also the nodes of the ipsilateral neck, as well. Combined operation including wide resection of the oral lesion together with radical neck dissection has been our treatment of choice in the past. More recently we have added either pre- or

Fig. 16-19. Squamous carcinoma of the tip of the tongue. An exophytic, fairly superficial lesion that histologically shows a well-differentiated structure. The prognosis for such a lesion is excellent.

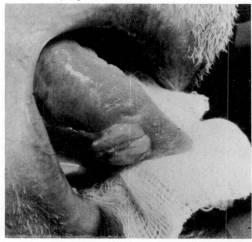

postoperative radiation therapy. The horizontal ramus of the mandible must be resected together with the tumor if the oral cancer has come in contact with the periosteum of the mandible at any point. Such contact seeds the periosteal lymphatics with tumor cells and makes resection of bone mandatory. The determinate 5-year survival for cancer of the tongue is 32 to 40 percent. If no palpable lymph nodes are present, the 5-year survival rate is 53 percent.

FLOOR OF THE MOUTH

The floor of the mouth is that portion of the oral cavity between the tongue and the inner surface of the mandible. This crescentic area of the mucosa lies over the sublingual and submaxillary salivary glands and contains their excretory ducts. It is divided into two halves by the frenulum, a fold of mucosa lying in the midline and extending to the tongue.

Squamous carcinomas developing in this area tend to develop a "run-around" extending anteriorly and posteriorly around the rim of the mandible, and if they are neglected long enough, the entire floor of the mouth becomes involved. This pattern of growth results in common bilateral involvement at the anterior floor of the mouth (Fig. 16-20) with frequent bilateral cervical metastases. These lesions tend to be less well differentiated than lesions of the tongue or gingiva and rapidly invade the surrounding structures, especially the periosteum of the adjacent mandible and the tissues of the submaxillary space. Metastases occur first to the submaxillary lymph nodes and are frequent. Taylor and Nathanson observed that 60 percent of these patients had palpable cervical metastases on admission, and in 90 percent cervical lymph node involvement had developed within a year of diagnosis.

The primary symptoms of these neoplasms are often neglected for some time, since they are quite minimal. Eventually the patient complains of pain, swelling of the tongue, and difficulty in eating and speaking. Early lesions are usually discovered by patients themselves while inspecting the mouth or have been noticed by an alert dentist or physician. Rarely, very early lesions may be seen involving only the superficial mucosa.

Large lesions of the floor of the mouth require wide excision in continuity with resection of a portion of the mandible and radical neck dissection. The neck dissection is done whether lymph nodes are palpable or not, in view of the high incidence of positive cervical nodes. Operative therapy may be integrated with pre- or postoperative radiation in the larger lesions. The much less common superficial and in situ lesions can be treated by local excision only. The 5-year survival rates for cancers in this site are comparable with those for cancer of the tongue. James reports an average determinate survival of 37 percent, and the Tumor Registry of the Memorial Center for Cancer reports a 5-year survival rate of 39 percent.

GINGIVAE

Cancer of the gums is better differentiated and slower in its pattern of growth than lesions of the tongue and floor of the mouth. Patients first note a mass (Fig. 16-21) of slight tenderness of the gum, sometimes with loosening of teeth in the area of the tumor. This often leads them to consult their dentist, who, if not alert to the problem, may extract the teeth under the mistaken impression that the patient has an underlying abscess or cyst. As the lesion progresses, it ulcerates, bleeds, and interferes with mastication. As a neoplasm invades the underlying bone, it can involve the mandibular nerve with the appearance of numbness in the mental and submental areas. Extraction of a tooth often accelerates the invasion of the mandible.

Treatment of cancer of the lower gingiva requires resecton of the involved mandible and overlying gum together with a radical neck dissection. Metastases from cancers at this site are usually to the submaxillary lymph nodes and are present in about half the patients at their first visit. Epidermoid cancers of the upper gingiva are less common and better differentiated than cancers of the

Fig. 16-20. Squamous carcinoma of the floor of the mouth. This lesion is in a typical location in the midline with spread in both directions around the curve of the mandible. It has invaded deeply into underlying structures.

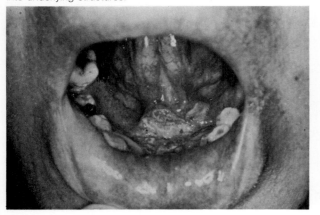

Fig. 16-21. Carcinoma of the gingiva. The adjacent teeth are loose and easily removed. The underlying mandible is already invaded.

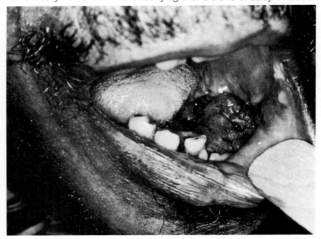

lower gingiva. Metastases to cervical nodes are much less common. Therefore, treatment is restricted to local excision. Radical neck dissection is deferred until there is evidence of palpable cervical node involvement.

The definitive 5-year survival rate following treatment for carcinoma of the gingiva averages 45 percent.

HARD PALATE

The hard palate is the U-shaped area enclosed by the upper gingiva and bounded posteriorly by the attachments of the soft palate. It consists of the palatine processes of the maxillary bones in its anterior two-thirds and of the horizontal portions of the palatine bones in its posterior third.

The most common malignant lesions of the hard palate are tumors of the minor salivary glands. Adenoid cystic carcinomas (Fig. 16-22) and adenocarcinomas occur in almost equal number; malignant mixed tumors are somewhat less frequent. Epidermoid carcinomas primary in the hard palate are rare, although carcinomas primary in the maxillary sinus will occasionally invade the hard palate and perforate into the oral cavity.

The primary symptom is a mass usually noted first by the patient. There is no tenderness or other associated symptom until fairly late in the course of the tumor. As in most salivary malignant tumors, growth is very slow and metastases occur quite late, so that involved cervical lymph nodes are not found initially. Salivary neoplasms respond poorly to radiation therapy, and primary treatment is excision. The chief fault in treatment is underestimation of the extent and potential of these lesions. They are usually fixed to the underlying periosteum, and adequate excision must include resection of the hard palate together with the tumor mass. An attempt to enucleate

the tumor from the underlying bone almost ensures a local recurrence. Excision with a wide margin including the bony palate leaves a substantial palatal defect requiring repair by either surgical reconstruction or the use of an upper plate constructed by a prosthodontist with an obturator that will plug the defect.

Despite the phlegmatic nature of these tumors, complete excision and complete eradication of the lesions are often elusive. The lesions tend to be of a higher grade than malignant lesions of the major salivary glands. Five-year survival rates between 30 and 40 percent are reported, but the incidence of new disease between the fifth and fifteenth year is frequent.

BUCCAL MUCOSA

The lateral walls of the oral cavity are formed by the cheeks, which consist of the buccinator muscle covered on its inner surface by a layer of mucosa extending from the upper to the lower gingivobuccal gutters and from the lateral commissure of the lips anteriorly to the ascending ramus of the mandible posteriorly. Lymphatics from this area pass through the buccinator muscle and follow the facial vein to end in the submaxillary and upper cervical lymph nodes.

The natural evolution of epidermoid carcinoma of the buccal mucosa varies according to the grade of the tumor. About half of the lesions are rather undifferentiated and associated with ulceration, rapid invasion of the cheek, and sometimes even perforation of the skin and formation of an orocutaneous salivary fistula (Fig. 16-23). The majority of such lesions are accompanied by enlarged submaxillary lymph nodes when first seen.

A less aggressive form of buccal cancer is also encountered, especially in patients who are tobacco chewers and "snuff dippers." This is the so-called verrucous carcinoma, which tends to occur in the gingivobuccal gutter and progresses very slowly, sometimes over a period of

Fig. 16-22. Adenoid cystic carcinoma of the hard palate. Although this lesion is much smaller than the mixed tumor in Fig. 16-15, it is malignant. Treatment is by wide excision, including the underlying bone.

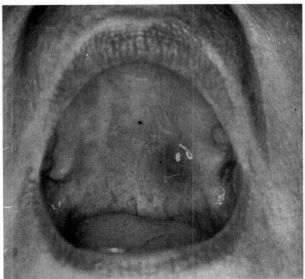

Fig. 16-23. Carcinoma of buccal mucosa. A well-differentiated and slowly growing lesion that was neglected and mismanaged for many years. (From: *Rush BF Jr: Curr Probl Surg May 1966*, with permission.)

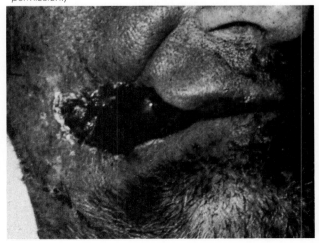

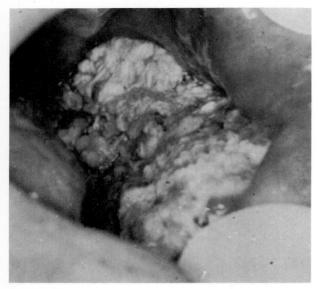

Fig. 16-24. Verrucous carcinoma. The shaggy white plaque along the gingivobuccal gutter is typical. The patient is seventy-five years old and has chewed tobacco for over 50 years.

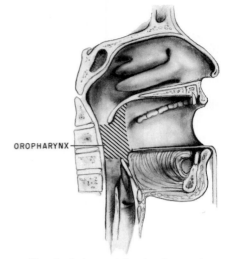

Fig. 16-25. Oropharynx. The shaded area delineates the oropharynx. The nasopharynx is located above, and the hypopharynx and larynx are located below.

years. The tumor is locally invasive, but metastases have never been reported except in patients who have received previous irradiation. Verrucous lesions are easily recognized by their exophytic form and shaggy white appearance (Fig. 16-24). They may cover a wide area, sometimes the entire buccal surface, and have a propensity for bony invasion, often involving a large portion of the mandible or occasionally the maxilla.

Treatment of buccal carcinoma is dictated by the type of lesion encountered. External radiation therapy alone does not eradicate the less well-differentiated lesions, although it has been combined with interstitial therapy with some success. The highly differentiated verrucous carcinomas are fairly radiosensitive but have a marked tendency to recur following an early gratifying regression. In addition, the distressing propensity of these lesions for developing a higher grade of malignancy with metastases after being exposed to radiation is a unique characteristic that has discouraged many from using radiation in treatment. Therefore, the initial therapy for verrucous lesions is wide excision. Since cervical metastases are not ordinarily found, an accompanying radical neck dissection is not done.

For the high-grade lesions, block dissection of the cheek with radical neck resection is the operative treatment of choice. Additional benefit may be derived from combining this with preoperative radiotherapy; this type of combined treatment is still undergoing evaluation. James reported 5-year survival rates in 181 patients with carcinoma of the buccal mucosa of all types as 54.4 percent. The prognosis for the well-differentiated lesions, such as the verrucous carcinoma, should be much better than this.

OROPHARYNX

The oropharynx is the region of the mouth posterior to the anterior tonsillar pillars and the circumvallate papillae of the tongue (Fig. 16-25). It contains the soft palate, tonsil and tonsillar fossa, posterior third of the tongue, anterior surface of the epiglottis, and surrounding pharyngeal walls. The most common site for malignant tumors in this area is the tonsil.

TONSIL

The most common benign lesion of the tonsil is, as every layman knows, inflammatory swelling. This can lead to confusion in diagnosing nonulcerated tumors of these organs. Common malignant lesions are high-grade epidermoid carcinomas (78 percent) and lymphosarcomas (16 percent). A large group of miscellaneous tumors are found, including hemangiomas, neurofibromas, and salivary gland tumors. High-grade epidermoid carcinomas in this area are often described as lymphoepitheliomas and transitional cell carcinomas. It is our feeling that these are simply microscopic variants of highly undifferentiated epidermoid carcinomas.

The frequent first symptom of carcinoma of the tonsil is a slight feeling of tenderness in the area, a typical sore throat. This is easily ignored by the patient for long periods until its persistence finally forces a consultation with the physician. Even then the evidence of a growing tumor may be overlooked and the patient treated for some time with mouthwashes and antibiotics. The lesion will appear grossly as a swelling of the tonsil with a central ulcer. Palpation reveals firmness and induration spreading well beyond the area of ulceration. Trismus and pain in the ear are common complaints. The metastatic spread from this area is to the tonsillar node at the angle of the mandible,

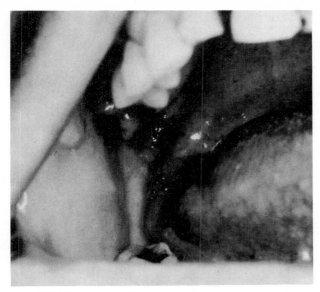

Fig. 16-26. Carcinoma of the anterior tonsillar pillar. These tiny lesions are invasive areas of carcinoma. Despite their size, the patient already had metastatic disease in the ipsilateral neck.

so often enlarged in children who have tonsillitis. The tonsil is a common site for very tiny "occult" carcinomas, which lead to large cervical masses and must be inspected minutely when one is searching for a primary site for cervical metastases (Fig. 16-26). Lymphosarcomas of the tonsil usually present with a more bulky primary lesion and are not as inclined to ulceration. The primary lesions may be bilateral with involvement of both tonsils.

Treatment of tonsillar carcinoma by either radiation or operation has never been very satisfactory. Lymphosarcomas are quite radiosensitive and, if localized, should be treated primarily by radiation. Carcinoma, on the other hand, yields poorly to either form of therapy. Integrated therapy with pre- or postoperative radiation to the tonsil with resection in continuity with a radical neck dissection seems to produce the best results. The definitive 5-year survival following treatment of cancer of the tonsil is 25 percent.

POSTERIOR THIRD OF THE TONGUE

Tumors in the posterior third of the tongue differ markedly in their natural history from those in the anterior two-thirds. Whereas the anterior lesions tend to be well differentiated, remain confined to the primary site, or involve only high cervical nodes for long periods, lesions in the posterior third are of much higher grade, often being classified as *lymphoepitheliomas,* or *transitional cell tumors.* They spread rapidly to the cervical nodes and often beyond to distant sites. A frequent initial symptom of carcinoma of the posterior third of the tongue is a large cervical lymph node accompanied by the complaint of pain on swallowing. Unfortunately, this is a fairly silent area, and lesions may attain considerable size before

causing pain or dysfunction. Wide ulceration causes a malodorous breath and dysphasia. Weight loss is prominent. Treatment has been highly unsatisfactory in the past. Radiation therapy infrequently controls the primary lesion. Operation often results in total loss of the tongue, an overwhelming psychologic and functional deficit. Since these lesions are often across the midline, bilateral neck dissection must be combined with resection of the tongue. Initial experience with combined radiation and operation indicated that occasionally the lesions can be reduced in size sufficiently by preoperative radiation to permit a more conservative resection of the posterior tongue, leaving a functional anterior tongue behind.

SOFT PALATE

Malignant tumors of the soft palate are almost always epidermoid carcinomas. These tend to be well differentiated, slow-growing, and late to metastasize. They are generally superficial lesions spreading over the anterior surface of the soft palate and down the tonsillar pillars. Often it is difficult to determine whether the lesions arose in the tonsil or in the soft palate. Spread may be extensive, covering much of the soft palate, the tonsillar fossa, and the tongue. Pain and dysphagia are the usual first symptoms. Diagnosis by inspection and palpation is a simple matter, and biopsy is easily accomplished.

Response to radiation therapy is only fair. Resection is more likely to produce a cure but often leads to a difficult functional defect, since the patient is unable to close the nasopharynx and will tend to regurgitate food through the nose on swallowing. This is a situation where the clever prosthodontist can help greatly by installing an adequate extension on an upper plate that extends backward into the pharynx to seal the palatal defect. An even more convenient method of closing the palatal defect is to raise a flap from the posterior pharynx and swing it forward to close the defect at the time of the original operation. Prognosis is difficult to determine, since these tumors are usually classed in the literature with tumors of the tonsil or of the hard palate.

EPIGLOTTIS

Malignant tumors of the anterior surface of the epiglottis are usually exophytic and well differentiated and have a slow, natural evolution. Dysphagia and aspiration are early symptoms. Treatment by radiation therapy is quite successful. Hemilaryngectomy of the upper larynx above the cords has also produced good results. Patients who have had resection of the epiglottis must relearn swallowing, and this requires a reasonable level of intelligence. Senile patients or those with poor learning ability should be treated by either radiation or total laryngectomy.

LARYNX

When describing the site of tumors of the larynx, the terminology can be confusing and frustrating. According to current usage, the larynx is made up of those structures lying both above and below the true vocal cords. Thus, the mucosa of the larynx extends along the posterior surface of the epiglottis including its tip, along the aryepiglottic folds, and over the arytenoid cartilages posteriorly. It covers the inner surface of the aryepiglottic folds, the false vocal cords, and the ventricles. All of the larynx thus far described constitutes the supraglottic larynx, i.e., that which is above the true vocal cords. The glottic portion of the larynx is that portion made up of the true cords themselves. The mucosa lining the area underneath the true cords down to the lower border of the cricoid cartilage covers the infraglottic portion of the larynx.

In the past the area just described was called the "endolarynx," or the "intrinsic larynx," although the latter term gradually came to mean the true cords alone. Tumors taking their origin on the outside of the larynx for many years were designated as arising from the "extrinsic larynx." However, this term came to be used for supraglottic lesions as well, so this usage has now been abandoned. Lesions involving any portion of the exterior of the larynx are now spoken of as "hypopharyngeal" or, by some, "laryngopharyngeal."

INCIDENCE AND ETIOLOGY. Cancer of the larynx accounts for 1.62 percent of all cancers in men and only 0.14 percent of all cancers in woman; thus the ratio of incidence favors the male sex over 11:1. The report of the Advisory Committee to the Surgeon General on Smoking and Health reviewed 10 retrospective studies and 7 prospective studies on the relationship of smoking to carcinoma of the larynx. There was a statistically positive relationship in every study. In the prospective studies the mortality ratios for smokers averaged 5.4 times greater for cigarette smokers than for nonsmokers and 2.8 times greater for cigar and pipe smokers than for nonsmokers. Laryngeal cancer mortality has increased somewhat over the past three decades, but the increase has been much less than that for lung cancer. It appears that the induction of carcinoma of the larynx cannot occur solely as a result of tobacco tars but that a further agent, or cocarcinogen, is needed. One such agent may be alcohol, since a high percentage (30 to 40 percent) of patients with carcinoma of the larynx are alcoholics and come from population groups where the risk of alcoholism is great, such as bartenders and entertainers. Cirrhosis of the liver is a common complaint among patients with carcinoma of the larynx; this may be a secondary relationship due to the frequency of alcoholism in this group.

CLASSIFICATION. As it has for other cancers, the American Joint Committee on Cancer Staging and End Results Reporting has developed a TNM system for carcinomas of the larynx. Because of differences in prognosis at different sites the committee has divided the larynx into its three major areas: the supraglottic (posterior surface of the epiglottis, aryepiglottic folds, arytenoids, false cords, ventricles); the glottic (right and left vocal cords and anterior glottic commissure); and the subglottic (subglottic region exclusive of the undersurface of the true cords and down to the lower margin of the cricoid cartilage). About 56 percent of squamous epidermoid cancers of the larynx

occur in the glottic region, 42 percent occur in the supraglottic region, and the remaining 2 percent are subglottic. The combination of topographic spread (T), nodal involvement (N), and distant metastasis (M) in a description of three separate anatomic sites results in a complex system, yet it is the most precise method whereby lesions can be classified and comparisons between institutions adequately made as to the results of treatment.

PATHOLOGY. Polyps, papillomas, granulomas, cysts, and areas of hyperkeratosis make up the common benign lesions of the cords. Rarely hemangiomas and chondromas of the laryngeal cartilages are seen. Ninety-nine percent of the malignant lesions of the larynx are epidermoid carcinomas, and most of these are of the ordinary cornifying (squamous cell) type. These lesions arise from the squamous epithelium of the cords themselves or from areas of metaplasia in the mucosa of the endolarynx. On the cord, carcinoma may be preceded by hyperkeratosis and stages of transition from hyperkeratosis to dyskeratosis, carcinoma in situ, and microinvasive carcinoma. Glottic cancers are usually very well differentiated, slow-growing, and late to metastasize. Supraglottic and infraglottic cancers are less well differentiated and more likely to have spread to lymph nodes when first seen.

DIAGNOSIS. Space-occupying lesions of the larynx produce initial symptoms through interference with phonation and respiration. Hoarseness, the usual first symptom, may be slight and intermittent but gradually becomes constant. What begins as a slight huskiness gradually progresses, until sounds are produced with difficulty. Respiratory obstruction is a later sign, although small lesions on the true cords will produce a greater degree of obstruction than somewhat larger lesions in the supraglottic or infraglottic area. Obstruction progresses in severity until the patient may respire with visible effort, using accessory muscles to force air through the cords, sometimes with audible stridor. At this point the patient's life is in jeopardy. At any moment the slightest additional swelling or edema can cut off breathing completely. The use of sedatives in patients at this phase of obstruction is fraught with danger. Under sedation the patient's tired muscles may fail, with a rapid shallowing of respiration, progressive anoxia, and cardiac arrest. The finding of a tumor on the cord associated with stridor, retraction, or the use of accessory muscles to breathe indicates immediate tracheostomy. It is far better to elect a tracheostomy done in the operating room than to be forced into an emergency tracheostomy in the ward or in the emergency room under much less favorable circumstances.

Late signs of malignant lesions of the larynx are a malodorous breath, pain on swallowing, weight loss, and hemoptysis.

Any patient who has persistent hoarseness for more than 3 or 4 weeks should have a careful inspection of the vocal cords by indirect laryngoscopy. If this reveals no pathologic condition but hoarseness persists, direct laryngoscopy should be used to examine the cords even more closely.

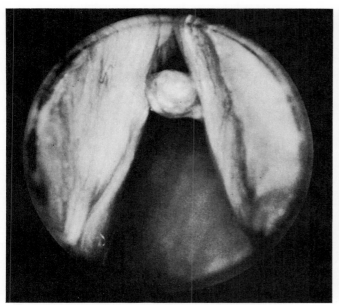

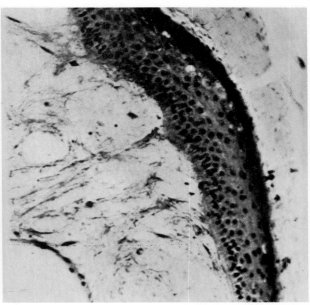

Fig. 16-27. Pedunculated polyp of the right vocal cord arising at the junction of the anterior and middle thirds. (From: *Holinger PH et al: Ann Otol Rhinol Laryngol 56:583, 1947, with permission.*)

Benign Tumors

POLYPS

According to Holinger, 43 percent of all benign lesions of the larynx are simple polyps. These arise on the phonating edge of the cord at the junction between the anterior one-third and the posterior two-thirds (Fig. 16-27). Their cause is obscure. Treatment is by removal with a cupped forceps at direct laryngoscopy.

VOCAL NODULES

The second most common benign tumor of the larynx, these are usually bilateral and, like polyps, occur at the junction of the anterior one-third with the posterior two-thirds of the cords. They are often called "singer's nodules" but certainly are not confined to singers and can occur in any occupational group. Treatment is by removal with the biopsy forceps.

RETENTION CYSTS

About half of these occur on the vocal cords, the remainder being found in the aryepiglottic folds, arytenoids, or epiglottis. They appear to occur as a result of the obstruction of small mucous glands. These lesions can reach considerable size and offer marked embarrassment to respiration.

HYPERKERATOSIS

Hyperkeratosis can affect the vocal cords as it does any of the mucosal areas of the lips, oral cavity, or pharynx.

These lesions are evidence of a premalignant change and should be stripped off the cord with the use of the biopsy forceps. Patients who have developed hyperkeratosis should be followed at twice yearly intervals to guard against recurrence or the appearance of a frank carcinoma.

PAPILLOMAS

These multiple lesions are found most often on the true cords but may appear on any portion of the larynx or pharynx and even on the soft palate. While they are most commonly reported in children prior to adolescence, some adults are also affected. Like warts, these tumors appear to be caused by viruses. Frequently the growths cover the mucosa of the cords in great profusion, causing severe respiratory embarrassment and requiring tracheostomy. They can persist for many years; during this period the patient often must continue to wear a tracheostomy tube while papillomas are cleared from the airway by frequent excisions through the laryngoscope. Repeated excision is the only effective treatment to date. The large number of other forms of therapy attempted indicates the generally unsatisfactory state of therapy. Eventually, after a period of months or years of repeated excisions, the lesions gradually disappear.

Malignant Lesions

Carcinoma of the true cords (Fig. 16-28) is a lesion that should be easily detected. It gives warning of its presence at an early stage through hoarseness and grows slowly enough so that early therapy should be rewarded by a 90 percent or better 5-year survival rate. In many urban areas over half of the lesions of the true cords are stage 1

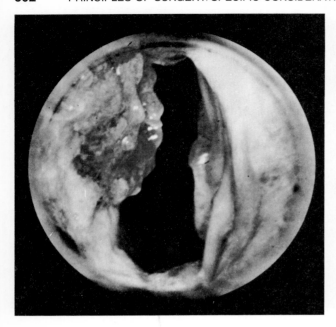

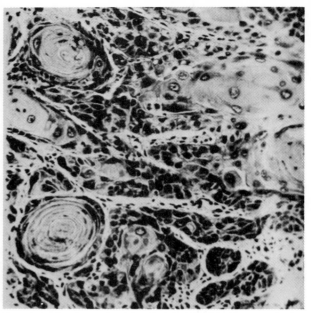

Fig. 16-28. Carcinoma involving the left side of the larynx and anterior commissure. (From: *Holinger PH et al: Ann Otol Rhinol Laryngol 56:583, 1947, with permission.*)

lesions confined entirely to the cord. In contrast, some rural areas report that in only 5 percent of patients reaching the physician the lesions are still in Stage I. As the tumor grows, it extends off the cord, either up into the supraglottic area or less commonly inferiorly into the infraglottic region. Invasion occurs slowly but relentlessly, eventually with perforation of the thyroid cartilage and direct invasion of the soft tissues of the thyroid gland and of the neck.

If cancer remains confined to the true cords, a high percentage of 5-year survivals can be obtained following treatment by radiotherapy alone. Holinger noted that in a series of 102 patients with cordal lesions treated with cobalt irradiation, only 9 patients had residual or recurrent cancer that required subsequent laryngectomy. None of the patients in this series died of carcinoma. Loss of the larynx is such a major functional and psychologic disability that if excellent results can be obtained by irradiation, this should be the treatment of choice.

Cancers that have invaded areas beyond the cord have a much different outlook. Involvement of cervical nodes becomes an important problem, and the ability to eradicate the disease by radiation alone is greatly decreased. For Stages II, III, and IV cancers, partial or total laryngectomy is mandatory. In addition, a radical or modified radical neck dissection on the side of the lesion is often performed, even though palpable nodes are not present. Using this approach, Norris has reported a 70 to 75 percent 5-year survival rate for Stages II and III lesions of glottic and supraglottic origin. Some feel that if no nodes are palpable prophylatic radiation to the neck will suffice. The very large Stage IV lesions do very poorly with surgery alone, with a 5-year survival rate of only 21 percent. Combined radiation therapy and operation in treatment of advanced cancers of the larynx improves the long-term

survival rate. Our recent experience with adding chemotherapy to the integrated treatment of Stage IV lesions indicates a further improvement in survival to as high as 50 percent.

The major problem for the patient after laryngectomy is to regain a useful voice. About half of all such patients will learn to use effective esophageal speech, meaning they can communicate understandably with strangers and casual acquaintances. An additional 25 percent can make themselves understood to members of their family but find that their esophageal speech is too distorted to be useful in the general community. The remaining 25 percent of patients will be unable to conquer the technical problems of learning this method of conversation.

Esophageal speech is by far the most useful technique for speaking after laryngectomy, since it requires no additional paraphernalia and can be refined to the point where it very closely resembles the tone and expression of ordinary speech. It is produced by swallowing air and regurgitating it, creating a vibration in the pharynx—probably at the level of the cricothyroid muscle. The oral cavity modulates this tone just as it would a tone from the larynx.

For the 50 percent of patients who are partly or completely unable to learn esophageal speech, electric vibrating devices can be used to provide a tone in the oral cavity that is modulated by the patient's oral structures, giving a fairly reasonable method of communication.

The realization that any fistula between the trachea and pharynx that permits passage of air from the lungs to the mouth will produce easily understood and controlled speech has led to the development of the Singer-Blom prosthesis. This is a silicone valve that is placed in a passage connecting trachea and pharynx and allows air to

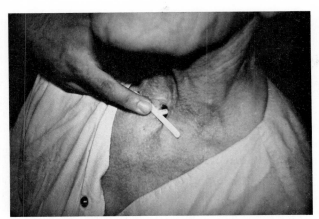

Fig. 16-29. A Singer-Blom prosthesis placed in the fistula between the trachea and pharynx in a laryngectomized patient. The patient will speak by occluding the trachea with a finger, redirecting air from the lungs through the prosthesis into the pharynx. Vibrations induced by pharyngeal structures produce sound that is modulated by the oral cavity to produce excellent speech in most instances.

pass into the pharynx and mouth but prevents saliva from passing into the trachea. With this device successful speech has been reported in from 60 to 90 percent of patients (Fig. 16-29). The principle employed by the Blum-Singer prosthesis has been recognized for many years and operative attempts to create a valved fistula between trachea and pharynx have appeared sporadically for many decades and with increasing frequency in the last 10 years. The major problem has been in establishing a competent valve that prevents aspiration of saliva. Figure 16-30 shows an example of one such operation developed in our clinic that has had some success but requires further development.

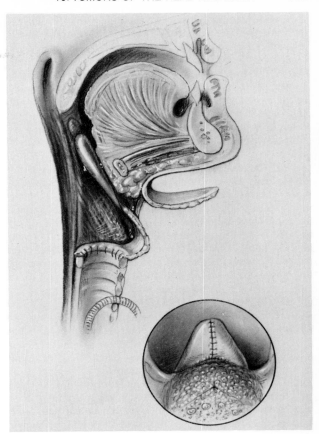

Fig. 16-30. A valved tracheopharyngeal fistula that is formed by a flap turned in from the neck following laryngectomy. Part of the flap forms a "neoepiglottis" (inset) that serves as the valve to close the newly formed glottis when the patient swallows and prevents aspiration. To speak, the patient occludes the tracheostomy, directing air into the pharynx and opening the valve.

HYPOPHARYNX

The hypopharynx is that area of the throat which surrounds the larynx. It is made up of the piriform sinuses on either side, the exterior portions of the aryepiglottic fold, and the lateral and posterior pharyngeal walls. It includes the mucosa overlying the posterior portions of the cricoid cartilage.

INCIDENCE. Cancer of the hypopharynx is three to four times as common as cancer of the larynx and constitutes 4.05 percent of all cancers in males. It is three times more common in men than in women. These tumors appear to be related to smoking. The correlation is stronger with pipe and cigar smoking than with cigarette smoking. Another etiologic factor is the Plummer-Vinson syndrome, found most commonly in Scandinavian women. This deficiency syndrome, now gradually disappearing, is clearly related to carcinoma of the hypopharynx and posterior tongue. At the Radiumhemmet in Stockholm carcinomas of the hypopharynx are seen more frequently in women than in men, and most of these cases are associated with a Plummer-Vinson syndrome.

PATHOLOGY. The great majority of these tumors are epidermoid carcinomas and compared with the oral cavity and endolarynx tend to be of a higher grade with a preponderance of grades 3 and 4 lesions. Better-differentiated forms are seen, however, most commonly on the exterior portions of the aryepiglottic folds and in the postcricoid area. Spread of the tumor occurs promptly and usually by way of the lymphatic channels that drain the hypopharynx, exiting between the lateral portion of the hyoid bone and the upper edge of the thyroid cartilage to travel with the superior thyroid artery to the midjugular chain of lymph nodes. Unlike most head and neck cancers, distant metastases are more common with involvement of mediastinal nodes, lung, liver, and other distant viscera.

DIAGNOSIS. Since these lesions arise outside the endolarynx away from major paths of respiration and speech, hoarseness or dyspnea are uncommon findings until late in the growth of the tumor. Interference with swallowing, on the other hand, is the most common early symptom and is associated with choking and aspiration.

Aspiration pneumonia may be the illness that first brings the patient to the physician. The lesions seem to have a long silent period and can grow to considerable size in the depths of the piriform sinus or on the pharyngeal walls before the first definite symptoms appear. Not uncommonly, the first sign is the appearance of a midjugular cervical node. The better-differentiated lesions invade and ulcerate widely, so that a malodorous breath is a common associated finding. Diagnosis is confirmed by indirect laryngoscopy and biopsy through a laryngoscope.

TREATMENT. Until recent years this was a highly lethal tumor with few cures either by operation or by irradiation. The introduction of wide radical excision with removal of the larynx and hypopharynx and en bloc radical neck dissection increased the cure rate perceptibly. This may be another area where judicious combination of irradiation and operation can improve the cure rate even more. Five-year survival rates with the older form of therapy were no more than 10 to 15 percent. With more aggressive operative approaches, cure rates in the vicinity of 30 percent have been reported.

Rehabilitation following these massive resections has been a very difficult problem requiring restoration of the digestive tract between the oral pharynx and cervical esophagus. Many techniques have been tried including myocutaneous skin flaps, free transfer of segments of small bowel with arterial microanastomosis in the neck, and transfer of a loop of the colon. The current favorite is the "gastric pull-up" whereby the stomach is freed in the abdomen and the fundus is pulled up through the anterior or posterior mediastinum and attached at the base of the tongue. The blood supply is excellent, anastomosis is very reliable, and fistula formation is rare. This procedure is done immediately following resection of the hypopharynx and larynx so that when the patient awakes all continuity has been restored.

NASOPHARYNX

The nasopharynx is at the top of the pharynx, just underneath the base of the skull. The body of the sphenoid bone forms a roof for this cavity, while its floor is formed by the soft palate. There is no anterior wall as such except for the posterior openings of the nasal passage together with the posterior aspects of the nasal septum and the turbinates. The roof of the cavity slopes into the posterior wall made up of the basiocciput and the atlas and the overlying covering of muscle and mucosa. Each lateral wall contains the opening of a eustachian tube guarded by a small prominence, the torus tubarius. The only structure lying within the nasopharynx is the lymphoid tissue of the adenoids scattered on the posterior and superior walls.

INCIDENCE. These tumors are uncommon but not rare, constituting about ½ percent of all cancers. They are somewhat more common in males than in females (2.4:1). There is an interesting relation to race. This is a frequent tumor in the Near East, among the Filipinos, Malays, and Dayaks, and especially among the Chinese. This cancer accounts for 30.4 percent of all cancers in males in Taiwan. The incidence among the Chinese born in the Far East is more than thirty times greater than in this country, while the incidence among American-born Chinese is about six times as common as the incidence among the other racial groups here. This shift in pattern would suggest that both genetic and environmental causative factors are operating.

Benign Lesions

These include hypertrophied lymphatic tissue, juvenile nasopharyngeal hemangiofibroma, Rathke's pouch cyst, dermoids, and mixed tumors. Of these, hypertrophied adenoids occur commonly, and hemangiofibroma and Rathke's pouch cyst have a special predilection for this site.

Any enlarging, space-occupying lesion of the nasopharynx calls attention to itself by respiratory obstruction and nasal stuffiness. Obstruction to the eustachian tubes provokes earaches and often chronic ear infection. As the lesion encroaches on the soft palate, deglutition is disturbed with pain on swallowing or regurgitation of food and fluids into the nasopharynx and out of the nose.

HYPERTROPHIED ADENOIDS

The adenoids represent a portion of the large circle of lymphatic tissue surrounding the oral respiratory passageway at the level of the posterior tongue and tonsils. Chronic upper respiratory tract infections in infants and children often cause marked and persistent hypertrophy of some of this rim of tissue. In past decades resection of the adenoids and tonsils was one of the most common of operations in children. With the advent of the antibiotics the need for these procedures has diminished markedly. Nonetheless, in an occasional child a persistent hypertrophy of the adenoids will develop that disturbs the breathing pattern, causing mouth breathing, or more importantly will obstruct the eustachian tubes, leading to chronic ear infections with a threat to the child's hearing. These symptoms are adequate indication for operative excision.

JUVENILE NASOPHARYNGEAL HEMANGIOFIBROMA

Made up of a hard stroma of fibrous tissue, richly interlaced with capillaries and cavernous sinuses, this rare and interesting tumor appears to originate on the roof of the nasopharynx perhaps from the periosteum of the sphenoid bone (Fig. 16-31). It increases in size slowly but relentlessly and eventually begins to erode the anterior structures, obstruct the nasal passages, and enter the maxillary sinus on one or both sides. The first symptom may be nasal obstruction but is usually epistaxis, which can be very profuse and even life-threatening.

This lesion is found exclusively in males, usually in the preadolescent or adolescent age groups. In some instances as the boy matures, the lesion appears to regress spontaneously. Just as often it persists, and heman-

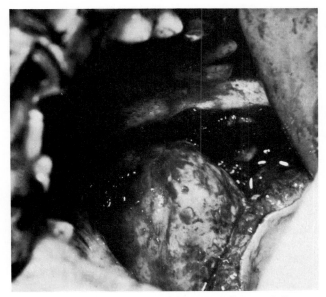

Fig. 16-31. Juvenile nasopharyngeal hemangiofibroma. A fibrous, highly vascular lesion on the posterior wall of the nasopharynx. This was first noted because of epistaxis. Exposure was obtained by an incision between the hard and soft palate with retraction of the soft palate downward.

giofibromas of the nasopharynx have been described in males in their twenties and thirties, either persisting from childhood or appearing for the first time.

The progressive destruction of surrounding bone by pressure and the continuing threat of major hemorrhage require prompt treatment, preferably before the lesions grow too large. Radiation therapy is ineffective, and operative excision appears the only mode of treatment. There is a tendency toward local recurrence following excision, and these patients must be followed carefully for some years after operation.

Malignant Lesions

These are epidermoid carcinoma, lymphosarcoma, adenoid cystic carcinoma, cervical chordoma, sarcoma, and myeloma. The only lesions occurring with any frequency are epidermoid carcinoma and lymphosarcoma.

EPIDERMOID CARCINOMA

These develop from areas of metaplasia in the respiratory epithelium of the nasopharynx and are moderately to highly undifferentiated. There is a liberal amount of lymphoid tissue in the nasopharynx, and frequently malignant epithelial cells are seen mixed with a prominent lymphoid stroma. This mixture of epidermoid and lymphoid cells gave rise to the term ''lymphoepithelioma'' introduced by Regaud and Schmincke. Many pathologists feel there is no place for this special term, since these tumors are probably highly anaplastic epidermoid carcinomas and the lymphoid element may not constitute an actual malignant part of the growth. Some feel that a large

percentage of lymphoid intermixing indicates a more radiosensitive and more radiocurable tumor.

In addition to the obstructive symptoms described for benign tumors, the invasive qualities of malignant lesions produce a number of characteristic signs and symptoms. These lesions invade the roof of the nasopharynx entering the cavernous sinus with paralysis of the IIId, IVth, Vth, and VIth cranial nerves. The VIth nerve is usually paralyzed first; this is frequently accompanied by pain in the distribution of the supraorbital and infraorbital branches of the Vth nerve. The tumor reaches these nerves by spreading along the eustachian tube into the space between the pharynx and the maxilla, then extending upward through the suture line between the petrous portion of the temporal bone and the lateral wing of the sphenoid. Thus, the symptom complex is called the *petrosphenoidal syndrome*. Metastatic nodes in the retropharyngeal space tend to spread into the area along the base of the skull medial to the parotid gland, where they compress the IXth, Xth, XIth, and XIIth cranial nerves. This causes difficulties with deglutition from hemiparesis of the superior constrictor muscle, a perversion of the sense of taste in the posterior third of the tongue, and hypesthesia of the mucous membranes of the soft palate, pharynx, and larynx. Paralysis of the trapezius muscle, the sternocleidomastoid, the soft palate, and one side of the tongue may also occur. These signs may be associated with Horner's syndrome from compression of the cervical sympathetic chain. Invasion of the orbit and displacement of the globe will cause double vision and proptosis.

Unfortunately, the nasopharynx is a silent area, and tumors here can reach considerable size before any symptoms are evident. The early signs of nasal obstruction or brief episodes of epistaxis are easily ignored. In two-thirds of the patients, by the time diagnosis is made, invasion of the sphenoid bone and base of the skull or nerve paralysis is present. Not infrequently, the primary growth will remain small, even microscopic, and is announced by its cervical metastases. These occur in a characteristic location, high in the neck behind the lower portion of the ear with additional involved nodes scattered along the path of the spinal accessory nerve as it courses down the trapezius muscle (Fig. 16-32). Cervical metastases are found in 50 percent of patients when first seen and are the presenting symptom in one-third.

There is no acceptable way of obtaining an adequate margin of resection when operating upon lesions of the nasopharynx, and the only operative procedure used is biopsy. Treatment of the primary lesion and usually of the metastases is by radiation therapy. Considering the advanced state of most of these lesions when first seen, the 5-year survival rate as a result of therapy is remarkably good, with an overall absolute survival of 28 percent. For the occasional patient who does not have evidence of cervical node metastasis at the beginning of treatment the 5-year survival rate is 55 percent.

LYMPHOSARCOMA

Lymphosarcomas of the nasopharynx tend to occur at the extremes of age in childhood and in the seventh and

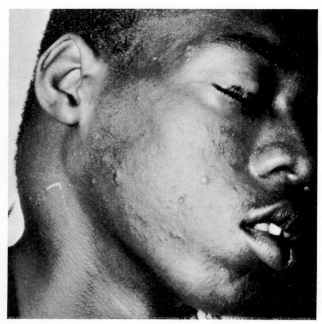

Fig. 16-32. Metastatic lymph nodes in the neck from lymphosarcoma of the nasopharynx. Note the characteristic location behind and inferior to the ear.

eighth decades. These are nearly always non-Hodgkin's lymphomas. The majority of these lesions announce their presence by the occurrence of cervical node metastases, which are usually bulky with a rubbery consistency; the nodes mat together but are less inclined to be invasive and fixed than nodes involved by carcinoma. While lymphosarcoma may mimic all the symptoms produced by epidermoid carcinomas, they invade bone infrequently, and paralysis of nerves is much less common. If there is no evidence of spread beyond the area of the head and neck, the radiotherapist usually administers a high level of therapy in the vicinity of 6000 rad of high-energy (cobalt or linear accelerator) radiation to both the nasopharynx and the cervical lymphatic tissues bilaterally. If the lesions have spread beyond the head and neck or if systemic symptoms are present, chemotherapy is the treatment of choice. Five-year survival in these highly radiosensitive tumors is slightly better than for epidermoid carcinoma, averaging 35 to 40 percent.

NASAL CAVITY AND PARANASAL SINUSES

The position of the eight nasal sinuses surrounding the nasal cavity is often poorly appreciated. The maxillary sinuses lateral to the nasal cavities and beneath the orbits are the largest and most important of the sinus structures. The ethmoid air cells occupying the space between the orbit and the upper nasal cavity are much smaller and are less commonly involved by tumors. The frontal sinuses bilaterally above the orbits are the second largest set of sinuses. The paired sphenoid sinuses divided by a thin septum just below the pituitary and over the roof of the nasopharynx are the most remote of the sinuses. The frontal and sphenoid sinuses are rare primary sites for tumors.

INCIDENCE. Tumors of the nasal cavity and paranasal sinuses represent about 1 percent of all cancer seen. Malignant lesions are found here three times as commonly in men as in women. With the exception of the esthesioneuroblastoma no specific cause is known for lesions arising here.

Benign Tumors

Polyps of the nasal cavity and maxillary sinus are the most common growths seen. These are usually associated with chronic inflammation or, occasionally, allergy. Sometimes the underlying infection may be due to a tumor, so that the discovery of polyps should not be considered an adequate diagnosis until the possibility of an underlying tumor has been ruled out. While polyps can be eradicated by simple excision, they will usually re-form unless the basic pathologic condition leading to their growth has been determined and corrected. This may be allergy, septal deviation, or other factors that obstruct adequate drainage and promote infection.

Malignant Tumors

Of 293 patients with neoplasms of the nasal cavity and paranasal sinus examined at the Mayo Clinic approximately 50 percent had epidermoid carcinomas, 10 percent had lymphomas, and 20 percent had tumors that probably arose from minor salivary tissue. The remaining 20 percent had various soft tissue sarcomas such as fibrosarcoma, chondrosarcoma, neurofibrosarcoma, and osteogenic sarcoma. Among 648 patients seen in Sweden with epidermoid carcinomas arising from the paranasal sinuses, the average age ranged from fifty to seventy years, and the vast majority of the lesions arose in the maxillary sinus (Fig. 16-33). None of these tumors occurred in the sphenoid sinus and only one in the frontal sinus.

Tumors, whether benign or malignant, are announced by pain, nasal obstruction, and persistent nasal secretion. Fifty percent of the patients present with one or more of these three symptoms. Unfortunately, these are also the presenting symptoms of sinusitis; patients may be treated with antibiotics and other measures for long periods before the more serious nature of the disease is realized. Repeated epistaxis is more likely to suggest the presence of tumor but occurs in only 10 percent as a presenting symptom. Swelling or ulceration of the hard palate or gingiva, swelling of the cheek, or ocular symptoms are evidences of a much more advanced stage of tumor growth yet constitute the presenting symptom in 25 to 30 percent of patients (Fig. 16-34). Bone destruction seen on radiographic examination is almost certain evidence of a tumor and unfortunately is also a late sign. Absence of bone destruction does not rule out a malignant tumor. All tissue removed when polyps of the nose or maxillary sinus are treated or when the maxillary sinus is drained should

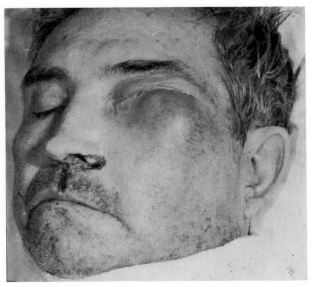

Fig. 16-33. Squamous carcinoma of the maxilla. The lesion had its origin in the upper portion of the maxillary sinus and invaded the floor of the orbit.

Fig. 16-34. Squamous carcinoma of the ethmoid sinuses. This lesion began in the left ethmoid and invaded the nasal cavity and right ethmoid sinus.

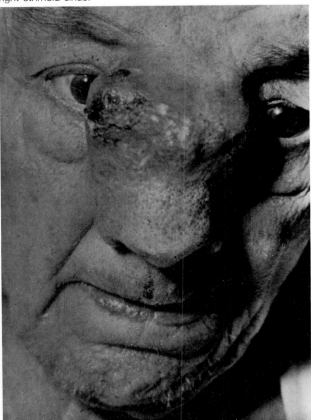

be submitted for histologic examination. Not infrequently this is the first evidence of the presence of an underlying carcinoma and may be the only opportunity for diagnosis of such lesions at an early state.

TREATMENT. Electrosurgical therapy, radiation therapy, and operative excision have all been used to treat these tumors. Lymphomas are ordinarily treated by radiation alone or, depending on type, with appropriate chemotheraphy. Epidermoid carcinomas of this site are refractory to either irradiation or operation. Integration of irradiation preoperatively with operative excision has been used for many years and has gained wide acceptance. This approach yields a 5-year survival rate of 30 to 35 percent for lesions of the maxillary sinuses. Cervical lymph nodes are involved late, and radical neck dissections are not done unless palpable nodes are present.

MANDIBLE

Tumors of the mandible arise from two main sources, from the tooth-forming (odontogenic) tissue and from bone.

Odontogenic Tumors

These neoplasms arise from ectodermal odontogenic tissue, mesodermal odontogenic tissue, or a mixture of both. They are invariably benign. The lesions most commonly seen are ectodermal odontogenic cysts: the follicular and radicular cysts. A rare and intriguing tumor is the ameloblastoma. Other odontogenic tumors are too rare to merit consideration here.

FOLLICULAR CYST

Some cysts are derived from the dental lamina and outer enamel epithelium of developing teeth. Remnants of this tissue sequestered during development may undergo proliferation and cystic change. Microscopically, they have fibrous walls usually lined by squamous epithelium. Occasionally remnants of odontogenic epithelium are present from which ameloblastomas may develop. Often the cyst envelops an unerupted tooth. A pathognomonic x-ray finding is the appearance of a smooth symmetric cyst in the mandible containing an unerupted tooth in its cavity. Clinically the tumor is found as a mass causing enlargement of the ramus of the mandible or the rim of the gingiva. Treatment is by intraoral excision, removing the top of the cyst and excising its entire lining membrane.

RADICULAR CYST

Infection of the dental pulp is the most common cause of this frequent cyst. A dental granuloma forms when epithelial remnants of the sheath about the tooth root are entrapped. Nests of epithelial tissue proliferate to line a central lumen usually at the apex of the infected tooth (Fig. 16-35). Cysts may vary in size from 1 to several centimeters. Microscopically, there is a dense, fibrous connective tissue lining covered internally by squamous epi-

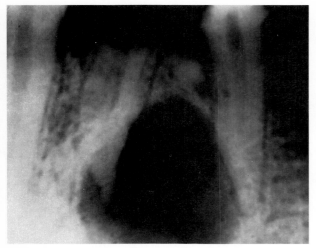

Fig. 16-35. Radiograph of a radicular cyst. Note the root of the tooth from which the cyst took origin. *(Courtesy of Sheldon Rovin, D.D.S.)*

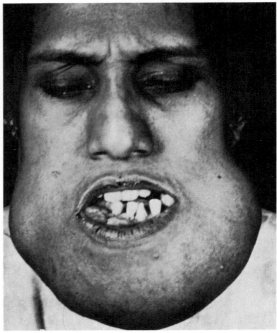

Fig. 16-36. Ameloblastoma. These lesions can grow to fantastic size, as shown here. Aside from the mass and functional disability, they are painless and never become malignant. *(Courtesy of Sheldon Rovin, D.D.S.)*

thelium. Frequently, a generalized inflammatory reaction in the cyst wall is seen. Treatment is by extraction of the tooth involved and excision of the cyst with its lining.

AMELOBLASTOMA

Although very uncommon, this is the most frequent solid tumor of the mandible. It usually appears in the body of the mandible at its junction with the ramus. Growth is slow, and the lesion is relatively asymptomatic, although it may expand the bone about it and eventually attain enormous size, encroaching on soft tissues of the face and neck (Fig. 16-36). Microscopically, the tumor presents interlacing strands and nests of odontogenic epithelium enmeshed in a connective tissue stroma with numerous areas of cystic degeneration. Treatment is by segmental resection of the portion of the mandible affected by the tumor including a centimeter or two of normal bone on either side. Unless the wide excision is accomplished, recurrence is common. The adjacent soft tissues need not be resected, and a good bed is usually left for reconstruction of the mandible.

Osteogenic Tumors

The mandible is affected by the same group of benign and malignant tumors that affect other bones in the body. Benign lesions include exostosis (torus mandibularis), fibrous dysplasia, Paget's disease, and giant cell tumor. Primary malignant lesions are multiple myeloma, Ewing's sarcoma, osteogenic sarcoma, chondrosarcoma (Fig. 16-37), and periosteal fibrosarcoma.

Giant cell tumors of the mandible are often referred to as *central* reparative giant cell tumors and are equivalent to the peripheral giant cell tumors of the gingiva. Although this lesion grows slowly and expands the surrounding bone, it never appears to have the malignant potential of giant cell tumors seen elsewhere in the skeleton and may have a different histogenesis. Microscopically, no distinction can be made between mandibular giant cell tumors and giant cell lesions of other bones. Treatment is usually by unroofing the tumor and curetting its tissue from the bony cavity.

Fig. 16-37. Chondrosarcoma of the mandible. This is a slowly developing lesion and was present in this patient for 9 years before medical aid was sought. The pressure of the upper gingiva has caused the groove that is seen in the dorsal surface of the tumor. Even at this late date, the tumor had not metastasized, and the patient was still alive and well 5 years after resection. (From: *Rush BF Jr, Trinkle K: South Med J 60:714, 1967, with permission.*)

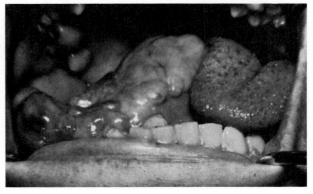

SALIVARY GLANDS

Salivary tissue is found in the parotid gland, the submaxillary gland, the lingual gland, and the numerous salivary glands. The parotid gland is a unilobular structure that is bent in a U shape about the posterior portion of the mandible in such a way that the larger external portion of the gland is often called the *superficial lobe* and the smaller internal portion lying on the internal surface of the ascending ramus is called the *deep lobe*. The VIIth nerve exiting from the skull by way of the stylohyoid foramen crosses the space between the mastoid and the ascending ramus of the mandible and plunges into the parotid gland at the point where it turns the corner around the posterior edge of the ascending ramus. The VIIth nerve usually bifurcates within the substance of the parotid. Each bifurcation further subdivides, and the branches eventually lie between the parotid gland and the underlying masseter muscle. The relationship of the VIIth nerve to the parotid gland is of clinical importance, since tumors of the parotid lie most commonly in the external portion of the gland; on excising such tumors great care must be taken not to cut the branches or the main trunk of this nerve.

The submaxillary gland is an ovoid structure lying in the submaxillary fossa beneath the horizontal ramus of the mandible. It is bounded by the anterior and posterior portions of the digastric muscle, thus occupying most of the digastric triangle in the neck. The important relationships of this gland are to the ramus mandibularis, the lowest branch of the VIIth nerve that courses over the upper portion of the gland. Injury to this nerve blocks innervation of the inferior quarter of the orbicularis oris on the side of the nerve and deprives patients of the ability to pucker their lips normally. The lingual nerve, deep to the upper inferior surface of the submaxillary gland, provides the gland with some small branches. In addition, the lingual nerve parallels the course of Wharton's duct, which conducts saliva from the submaxillary gland to the mouth. When the gland is removed, injury to the lingual nerve can occur either when Wharton's duct is clamped or when the gland is pulled down into the neck dragging the lingual nerve along by its nerve attachments.

The lingual gland is the smallest of the three major salivary glands. It lies beneath the mucosa of the anterior floor of the mouth.

The minor salivary glands are small deposits of salivary tissue that are scattered throughout the mucosa of the oral cavity, maxilla, and nasopharynx. The term *ectopic salivary tissue* is sometimes used but carries an incorrect connotation, since this salivary tissue is a normal finding in all individuals and is not the result of an error in development.

INCIDENCE. About $\frac{1}{3}$ percent of all malignant tumors occurs in the salivary tissues. These tumors are equally common in men and women. About 60 percent of these lesions occur in the parotid glands, which is not surprising, since this is the largest single collection of salivary tissues. The second largest concentration of tumors is found in the submaxillary gland and the third largest in the minor salivary glands. Tumors of the lingual glands are rare. No specific cause is known for any of the benign or malignant tumors of the salivary glands other than the occasional congenital or obstructive cyst. Women with malignant tumors of the salivary glands are known to have a higher incidence of cancer of the breast.

Benign Lesions. A variety of lesions may arise in salivary tissue.

Mixed Tumors. The most common lesion of the salivary glands is the mixed tumor (pleomorphic adenoma). Fifty percent of all tumors of the salivary glands and over 80 percent of all benign tumors are mixed tumors. These probably originate from adult glandular epithelium and, as their name implies, have an extremely diverse structural pattern. In 90 percent of the tumors one finds areas where the tumor grows in a network of strands made up of spindle and stellate cells not always connecting and sometimes lying entirely detached. In about a third of all cases this loose myxoid pattern predominates but is by no means the sole structural component. Half the tumors have pseudocartilaginous structures. Twenty percent show tissue closely resembling hyaline cartilage. Well-formed tubular structures are common and present a wide variety of patterns. The lining epithelium may be single-layered, conspicuously double-layered, stratified, or pseudostratified. Some areas of metaplasia into squamous epithelium may be seen, and well-differentiated squamous epithelium can be found in about a fourth of the cases.

Papillary Cystadenoma Lymphomatosum (Warthin's Tumor). These curious lesions occur only in parotid salivary tissue and almost exclusively (95 percent) in males. About 10 percent of them are bilateral. Characteristically they are made up of a papillary epithelial component intermingled with well-developed lymphoid tissue commonly containing germinal centers. Their histogenesis is uncertain, but many feel they represent parotid duct tissue sequestered in lymph nodes within the parotid gland. They represent the second most common benign tumor of salivary tissue but are a poor second to mixed tumors, which are at least eight times more common.

Mikulicz's Disease. This disease is characterized by a dense infiltration of lymphocytes occasionally arranged in follicles throughout the salivary tissues. This is accompanied by atrophy and disappearance of acinar tissue. Scattered throughout the lymphoid tissue are foci of epithelial and myloepithelial cells in close relationship to distal structures. The more popular modern term for this lesion is *benign lymphoepithelial lesion,* and many feel it represents a phase of the larger disease complex *Sjögren's syndrome.* The diffuse lymphocytic infiltrate, much as one sees in lymphomatous thyroiditis, suggests the possibility of an autoimmune disease. While several of or all the major salivary glands may be involved, a single parotid gland is the most frequent site (80 percent). The highest incidence of the disease is in patients between thirty-one and forty years of age.

Asymptomatic Enlargement of Salivary Tissue. This affection is usually observed in both parotid glands but may involve all the major salivary glands. The characteristic microscopic findings are an increase in size of the glandular acini due to swelling of the individual acinar cells. There is an increase of the secretory granules, a fatty infiltration, and a moderate fibrosis. These changes seem associated with nutritional deficiencies and have been found in patients suffering from cirrhosis of the liver, kwashiorkor, and diabetes mellitus. It also has been found in whole populations suffering from malnutrition in India, in Greece during the occupation of World War II, and in the inmates of German concentration camps. Katsilambros believes that this is a fundamental response to a deficiency of vitamin A and has duplicated his findings in vitamin A-deficient rats.

Other Lesions. Cysts of the parotid glands are seen quite rarely and in some instances may represent cysts of the first branchial cleft. Hemangiomas in children have a predilection for the area of the parotid gland and sometimes persist into adulthood. Neurofibromas and lipomas of the parotid gland have been described.

Malignant Lesions. About 75 percent of all malignant salivary tumors arise from the parotid gland, and 25 percent of all parotid tumors are malignant. Ten percent of malignant salivary lesions arise in the submaxillary gland and an additional 12 percent in the minor salivary glands. The incidence of malignant lesions in the submaxillary and minor salivary glands compared with benign lesions is somewhat higher than in the parotid gland, averaging one-third to one-half of all lesions seen. Roughly one-third of the malignant lesions of salivary tissue arise from the acinar epithelium and are adenocarcinomas. Another third arise from the ductal epithelium as various forms of epidermoid carcinomas. The remaining third appear either as highly anaplastic and unclassified lesions or as malignant mixed tumors.

Epidermoid Carcinoma. The most frequent of these are the mucoepidermoid carcinomas originally identified as a special group by Stewart et al. in 1945. These interesting tumors are made up, as the name indicates, of epidermoid cells and mucus-containing cells. The name falls short of being completely descriptive, since there is a third cell called an "intermediate" cell, smaller than either of the other two, that closely resembles certain cells of the salivary gland duct. They are commonly seen in stratifications lining dilated ductlike structures. Stewart et al. suggest that this intermediate cell is capable of differentiation into mucinous cells or into epidermoid and even squamous cells.

Mucoepidermoid carcinomas are usually divided on the basis of the microscopic appearance into low-grade and high-grade tumors. Low-grade tumors contain a large portion of mucus-secreting cells, often with the presence of microcysts and large amounts of mucoid material that may leak diffusely through the tissues, generating variable degrees of inflammatory reaction. In the highly malignant tumors epidermoid and intermediate cells dominate the picture. Pseudoglandular formation is fairly frequent, and the growth pattern is commonly sheetlike or in coarse plugs.

Squamous cell carcinomas like mucoepidermoid carcinomas must certainly originate in the ductal epithelium,

and the ability of salivary duct epithelium to undergo squamous metaplasia is well known. Stewart et al. suggest that most squamous cell carcinomas represent diffuse squamous cell overgrowth of tumors that were fundamentally mucoepidermoid. Microscopically, these lesions share the usual features of squamous cell carcinomas seen in the skin, oral cavity, and elsewhere. In this location, however, they are usually more malignant, and local and regional metastases are common.

Adenocarcinoma. Adenoid Cystic Carcinoma (Cylindroma). The chief histologic feature of these lesions is the arrangement of rather small, darkly staining cells with relatively low cytoplasm in anastomosing cords between which are acellular areas that may contain mucous, hyaline, or mucohyaline material. The cystic components of an adenoid cystic carcinoma usually stain positively with mucicarmine, indicating the presence of mucin. While the lesions are of sluggish evolution, metastases to cervical lymph nodes develop in 30 percent of the cases.

Acinar Cell Adenocarcinoma. These histologically distinct tumors are of low-grade clinical malignancy and fairly rare. They appear to arise from the acinar cells of salivary tissue and to be limited to the parotid gland. In the usual microscopic arrangement rounded or polygonal cells with a dark eccentric nucleus and a finely granular basophilic cytoplasm are packed closely together, sometimes in crude, acinar groups. While low-grade, these lesions are capable of metastasis both regionally and to distant locations.

Miscellaneous Adenocarcinomas. Adenocarcinomas may have a trabecular pattern and may be anaplastic or resemble adenocarcinomas of the gastrointestinal tract. These are usually highly malignant with a high degree of local invasiveness and regional and distant metastases.

Malignant Mixed Tumors. It is usually assumed that malignant mixed tumors arise from a neoplastic transformation of a previously benign mixed tumor. Patients who demonstrate these lesions are generally older than those with benign mixed tumors and have had a mass in the parotid for a longer period. Moreover, the malignant lesions are usually larger than the benign. In general, the microscopic picture is of a definite mixed tumor that contains within it malignant elements that may be adenocarcinomas, squamous cell carcinomas, or a malignant spindle cell alteration. The malignant component of a mixed tumor may so greatly overgrow the area of origin that it is extremely difficult to identify the previous benign mixed tumor.

NATURAL HISTORY. With the exception of the mixed tumor the common benign lesions of salivary tissue have no malignant potential. While the mixed tumor may have a very long history without malignant transformation and may grow for 20 to 30 years at a slow pace (Fig. 16-38), a rapidly growing and even anaplastic component can suddenly develop that markedly changes its course. On rare occasions mixed tumors have been found that have metastasized to local nodes without apparent histologic change and in their new location have pursued a slow course of growth. The most common pattern, however, is the development of a squamous cell carcinoma, adeno-

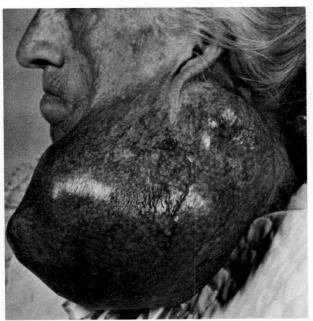

Fig. 16-38. Giant mixed tumor of the parotid. This lesion had been present for 29 years. It was still benign and was excised without evidence of recurrence in a 5-year follow-up. (From: *Rush BF Jr, Trinkle K: South Med J 60:714, 1967, with permission.*)

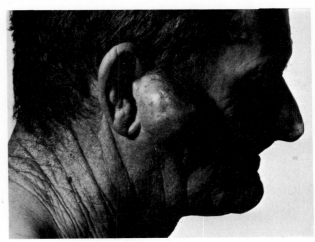

Fig. 16-39. Multilobulated mixed tumor of the parotid. The lesion presents in the upper pole of the superficial portion of the gland.

carcinoma, or other tumor that rapidly overgrows the original mixed tumor. Some very slowly evolving "chronic" carcinomas are known to develop from salivary tissue. Notable among these are the adenoid cystic carcinomas, which may develop their metastases 10, 15, and even 20 years after treatment of the primary tumor.

Many such tumors have been reported in which metastatic nodules in the lungs have been observed growing very slowly, at times appearing almost stationary for 10 and 15 years. The mucoepidermoid carcinoma, while not as slow-growing as the adenoid cystic carcinoma, is rather slowly progressive; however, this trait is offset by its great degree of local invasiveness, especially by perineural invasion. The chances for local recurrence are great even after wide local excision. Squamous cell carcinomas and adenocarcinomas of the salivary glands are almost always highly malignant, quick to invade and metastasize, and fatal in a high percentage of the patients affected.

DIFFERENTIAL DIAGNOSIS. Most tumors of the salivary glands appear as painless, slowly growing nodules (Fig. 16-39). Lesions of the parotid are bound by the heavy cervical fascia that splits on either side of the gland and invests it with a strong capsule. This dense covering obscures the actual size of the underlying tumor, and the surgeon may be surprised by the size and extent of a lesion at operation. Paralysis of the VIIth nerve is indicative of a malignant tumor and usually of a highly malignant lesion such as squamous carcinoma or adenocarcinoma. Mucoepidermoid carcinomas of the low-grade type or adenoid cystic carcinomas frequently spare the nerve

until quite late in their course. Fixation of the gland to underlying structures and palpable nodes in the neck are also more commonly seen with the tumors of higher grade. Since there is nothing that can distinguish the benign mass in the salivary gland from an early malignant tumor, excision of the mass and histologic examination are indicated in every case.

TREATMENT. Benign mixed tumors, the most common solid tumors of salivary gland origin, are so easily disseminated that incisional biopsy is never indicated. In earlier decades the technique of choice for removal was enucleation. Follow-up of patients so treated indicated that local recurrence was late and slow to develop and occurred in as many as 50 percent. Attempt at excision of these lesions with a cuff of surrounding normal tissue was accompanied by a high rate of injury to one or more branches of the VIIth nerve.

Through these painful experiences the present method of therapy was developed. After isolation of the VIIth nerve, the superficial portion of the parotid gland is dissected from the underlying tissues and removed with the tumor contained within it, assuring against injury of branches of the facial nerve and against dissemination and local recurrency of the tumor.

Frozen section of the lesion should be done at operation. If a low-grade malignant lesion such as an acinar cell adenocarcinoma, a low-grade mucoepidermoid carcinoma, or an adenoid cystic carcinoma is identified, the remainder of the gland and probably the VIIth nerve should be removed. If a high-grade lesion such as an anaplastic adenocarcinoma or squamous carcinoma is identified, a radical neck dissection should accompany the procedure. Aside from the problem of dealing with the VIIth nerve, the same general rules apply for lesions in the submaxillary gland.

Most of the tumors of salivary glands have a reputation for being poorly radiosensitive; however, the more malignant the lesion, the less likely this is to be true. Many high-grade mucoepidermoid carcinomas, squamous carcinomas, and even an occasional adenocarcinoma will demonstrate considerable sensitivity to x-ray therapy.

PROGNOSIS. Benign mixed tumors will recur in 40 to 50 percent of patients if improperly excised. If excision is by superficial lobectomy, the recurrence rate should be 5 percent or less. Five-year survival rates tend to be misleading, particularly in the chronic, slow-growing tumors. Adenoid cystic carcinoma has an 86 percent 5-year survival rate but a 57 percent 10-year survival. Malignant mixed tumors may have a 5-year survival of 87 to 90 percent and a 10-year survival of 60 to 70 percent.

AIDS-RELATED TUMORS

The epidemic of acquired immunodeficiency syndrome (AIDS) arose through the introduction of human T-cell lymphotrophic virus III (HTLV-III) into the homosexual and drug cultures of this country little more than half a decade ago. It now appears to be spreading through heterosexual contact as well and the case load is believed to be doubling each 6 months. Although patients may have suffered for some time with systemic symptoms of the AIDS-related complex, they may come for initial treatment because of the appearance of tumors, often first noted in the head and neck. The purple-black lesions of Kaposi's sarcoma often appear in the oral cavity where the half palate is the most common site. This tumor may also present on the tonsillar pillars, buccal mucosa, and tongue.

Cervical lymphadenopathy may reflect the persistent generalized adenopathy of the complex or may announce the appearance of a lymphoma. These are usually either B-cell immunoblastic lymphoma or small cell, noncleaved lymphoma (either Burkitt's or Burkitt's-like). Biopsy of the lesions establishes the diagnosis. Treatment with radiation and/or chemotherapy is palliative since the tumors and the syndrome are uniformly fatal.

Patients with AIDS or AIDS-related complex who have malignancies normally unassociated with AIDS may find the course of their tumors greatly altered. In a recent report a patient with AIDS-related complex and a basal cell carcinoma of the chin exhibited diffuse skeletal metastasis.

TUMORS OF THE NECK

Palpable or visible cervical swellings are a common complaint. Two to three percent of all admissions to hospital surgical services are for this condition. About half of these lesions occur in the thyroid gland; the remainder are due to a wide range of malignant, congenital, or inflammatory swellings.

Inflammation

Inflammatory swelling in the adult neck is now a rare hospital problem. Skandalakis and coworkers, in reviewing 1616 nonthyroid masses of the neck, found that only

3.2 percent were inflammatory, whereas 84 percent were neoplastic and 12 percent congenital or miscellaneous. The inflammatory lesions requiring hospitalization of adults are largely acute, often resulting from drainage from infection elsewhere. A common source is an infected tooth draining to the nodes in the submandibular area and causing an abscess. Only two patients in Skandalakis' entire series had tuberculous adenitis (scrofula). This was once the most common cause of neck masses, but with the tuberculin testing of cows and the pasteurization of milk, bovine tuberculosis has virtually disappeared in this country.

Malignant Tumors

The vast majority of cervical masses in adults are due to neoplasms. About 80 percent of these are metastatic from some other site, while the remainder occur from primary lesions in the neck. Primary cervical neoplasms either occur in the major salivary glands (40 percent) or are lymphomas primary in the cervical lymph nodes (60 percent). At one time it was proposed the squamous carcinomas arose primarily in the neck from the lining of branchial cleft cysts. This diagnosis was often made only to discover at a later date that the lesion was actually a metastasis from the oral cavity, nasopharynx, or laryngeal area. While there is some evidence that branchiogenic cysts become malignant, the reported, provable cases number only a handful.

A knowledge of the statistics quickly indicates that a clinician's first suspicion concerning any nonthyroid, cervical mass in adults is of a malignant tumor. He may also suspect that it is metastatic and from a site at some point above the clavicle, since 85 percent of all metastatic cervical lesions come from a supraclavicular site.

When a firm to hard cervical node that suggests malignancy is found, the first responsibility of clinicians is a thorough exploration of possible sites of origin. Cervical tumors appearing below and behind the ear and along the cervical chain are more likely to come from the nasopharynx or lateral pharyngeal walls. Swollen lymph nodes at the angle of the mandible or in the area of the submaxillary gland are most commonly from lesions in the tonsillar area, buccal mucosa, floor of the mouth, and gingiva. Swelling of the lymph nodes in the submental area should provoke a thorough examination of the tip of the tongue, lower lip, and anterior gingivobuccal gutter. Lymph nodes involved by neoplasms that appear in the middle third of the neck should cast suspicion first on the hypopharynx, piriform sinus, larynx, or thyroid.

Only when enlarged lymph nodes appear in the supraclavicular area does metastasis from below the clavicle become a major possibility. These may stem from carcinoma of the upper lobes of the lung or mediastinum or, in women, from carcinoma of the breast. The left supraclavicular nodes are frequently involved by malignant tumors metastatic from the abdomen (Virchow's node). Advanced adenocarcinoma of the stomach, pancreas, biliary tree, and even large bowel metastasize to this site.

If a thorough search of all sites reveals no possible

source of a primary lesion, biopsy of the cervical node is usually carried out. If this confirms the clinical impression of malignancy, further attempts to find the primary lesion are indicated. This can include surgical exploration of the maxillary sinuses. If all avenues have been searched thoroughly and no primary lesion has been found, the problem of local treatment still remains. The best course is to treat the lesion to achieve cure. If operation is chosen, it should be a radical neck dissection; if radiation therapy is used, it should be a full course of therapy. Since lymph nodes involved by metastatic disease respond poorly to radiation, the treatment of choice is normally operation. In the presence of advanced lesions a combination of radiation and operation may be used.

If a group of these patients treated without a known primary lesion is followed for 5 years, 80 percent of the patients will ultimately manifest the primary lesion. In some instances this may subsequently be resected for cure. A few patients may die over this period without ever demonstrating the source for the metastatic lesion, and even at postmortem examination it may not be found. Even more interesting, about 20 percent of the patients survive 5 or more years with apparent ''cure'' of their metastatic lesion even though the presumed primary lesion has not been found or treated. In those patients who received radiation therapy, either together with operation or alone, it may be that the port included the primary lesion as well. In those patients who are treated by operation alone, the fate of the primary lesion remains a mystery. A few of these patients may represent true branchiogenic carcinoma, or possibly the primary lesion regresses spontaneously.

Other Lesions

A host of other tumors, found infrequently in the area of the neck, present problems in differential diagnosis. Dermoids occur in the midline, most commonly in the submental area and sometimes along the line of the clavicle. Sebaceous cysts are common, especially in men, and probably are related to the trauma of shaving.

Carotid body tumors (chemodectomas) are rare tumors of the paraganglionic tissue found at the carotid bifurcation. Another lesion with a slow evolution, it gradually increases in size over many years, enveloping the bifurcation and slowly compressing the adjacent nerves including the hypoglossal, vagus, and sympathetic chain. For many periods, the only symptom is the mass in the neck. Eventually nerve paralysis, dysphagia, and pain appear. Malignant transformation is rare, but early removal is indicated to avoid the late symptoms. Small lesions can be removed easily (Fig. 16-40), but advanced large tumors require resection of the carotid artery with the risk of subsequent hemiparesis.

TUMORS OF THE NECK IN CHILDREN

The order of frequency of masses in the neck in children differs markedly from that found in adults. Inflam-

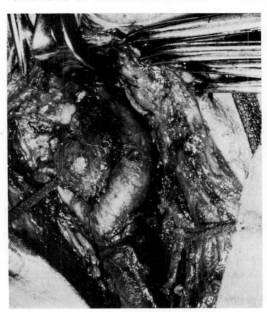

Fig. 16-40. Carotid body tumor of moderate size. The lesion lies between the internal and external branches of the carotid arteries; the adventitial layer binding it to the carotid bulb has been removed. (From: *Rush BF Jr: Ann Surg 157:633, 1963, with permission.*)

matory lesions are by far the most common, often coming from related infections of the tonsils. The most common malignant lesion is the lymphoma, and the second most common is carcinoma of the thyroid. Congenital lesions, of course, are much more common in children than in adults.

CHEMOTHERAPY AND IMMUNOTHERAPY

In the past decade it has been discovered that certain types of neoplasms commonly found in the head and neck area can be cured by chemotherapy. Burkitt's lymphoma, a rare neoplasm in the United States but common in some parts of Africa, was the first such cancer. It became apparent that a predictable and consistent percentage of patients with this disease could be cured by the use of *systemic* chemotherapy alone. Recently we have also learned that squamous cancer of facial skin and of the lips, while in the in situ microinvasive and superficial stages, can be cured by the topical application of 5-fluorouracil used as a cream or paste. These lesions are multiple and often tedious to eradicate by operation or radiation. A third head and neck lesion in which chemotherapy has become important is embryonal rhabdomyosarcoma, an uncommon lesion found in infants and children. Cure of this lesion occasionally has been obtained by combining radiation, chemotherapy, and operation.

Epidermoid cancers of the head and neck respond transiently to a number of single agents. Methotrexate has been the most extensively used. Response rates range from 15 to 57 percent. Bleomycin has also been found to have significant activity, comparable with methotrexate, with reported responses ranging from 15 to 50 percent. Other, less effective, single agents are cyclophosphamide (36 percent), vinblastine (29 percent), hydroxyurea (39 percent), 5-fluorouracil (15 percent), and procarbazine (10 percent). Reports of many of these latter drugs are based on small series and represent, at best, rough estimates. The most recent drug to excite interest in treatment of these tumors is *cis*-dichlorodiamine platinum (II) (DDP or cisplatin), which appears to match or exceed methotrexate and bleomycin in activity, especially when used in high doses with mannitol-induced diuresis to avoid renal injury.

Arterial infusion for the treatment of cancer in the head and neck area has received much attention. This involves the introduction of chemotherapy, usually methotrexate or 5-fluorouracil, into the external carotid artery via a catheter. The agents are administered either continuously or intermittently over 1 to several weeks. At present, this technique is known to produce a substantial to complete regression of the lesions in a large percentage of patients— as high as 50 percent in some series. Unfortunately, the response is usually transient, and the cancers return to continued growth within 2 to 3 months after treatment is discontinued. Long-term regression is uncommonly seen, and the period of regression obtained is rarely worth the morbidity and complications of the treatment itself. Nonetheless, these observations continue to tantalize clinical investigators seeking a clue that will lead to longer or even permanent remissions.

The recent introduction of an implantable, subcutaneous, long-term infusion pump may reduce morbidity, increase convenience, and make this technique more practicable.

The growing body of knowledge concerning the interrelationships between cancer and the body's immune system has touched the field of head and neck cancer through the work of Chretian and others. Squamous carcinoma of the tongue has been found in young men with acquired immune deficiency syndrome. At least half the patients with epidermoid cancer of the oral cavity, hypopharynx, and larynx show some degree of immune incompetence. Moreover, this incompetence is correlated with treatment failure following either radiation or operation. Immune competence can be restored in a number of these patients by improving nutrition, by the use of immunostimulant agents such as BCG or c-Parvum, and by "reconstitution" agents such as levamisole, thymosin, and transfer factor. Trials to determine the effectiveness of manipulations of the immune system in the immune-incompetent patient have so far shown either no or only marginal benefit.

The rapid expansion in our knowledge of the immune system has introduced a new generation of immunogenic agents that are much more specific in their effects. These include interferon, leukocyte-activated natural killer cells, and monoclonal antibodies to specific tumor antigens. The role of these new modalities and how they should be combined with other therapeutic agents remains to be developed.

Combined forms of treatment for head and neck cancers, which include chemotherapy and immunotherapy as well as radiation and operation, have enjoyed marked clinical and investigative interest in the past several years. The more our knowledge of the natural history of tumor growth develops, the more rational and logical it appears to combine available treatment methods.

Multinodal systemic chemotherapy will double or triple the partial and complete regression rates when the drugs are given as the first part of a therapeutic regimen to patients with previously untreated tumors (Table 16-1). Our current experience suggests that far-advanced (Stage IV) head and neck tumors have double the 2-year disease-free survival if chemotherapy precedes preoperative radiation and operation as compared with preoperative radiation and operation alone (66 vs. 35 percent). This is especially impressive when one realizes that Stage IV tumors ordinarily have a 5-year survival rate of 0 to 15 percent depending upon site (Fig. 16-41).

The practice of using chemotherapy as the first step in the course of multimodal treatment has been called "neoadjuvant" therapy. Several uncontrolled studies have claimed improved survival for late tumors with this technique. On the other hand, several prospective randomized studies report significant early tumor regression but no overall benefit in terms of survival. Since this approach appears to rescue some patients who are otherwise untreatable for cure, it is still under intensive study.

OPERATIONS OF THE HEAD AND NECK

The most commonly performed major operation for cancer of the head and neck is radical neck dissection.

Table 16-1. MULTIDRUG CHEMOTHERAPY FOR UNTREATED HEAD AND NECK CANCER

Drugs	Cycles	No. of pts.	50% Responses	Complete responses	Total responses	Author
DDP, VB, Bleo	3	106	44	22	66	Perry
DDP, MTX	4	82	62	4	66	Tejada
DDP, 5FU	2	26	69	19	88	Kish
DDP, Adra, Bleo, CTX	2	18	33	67	100	Feldman
VCR, Bleo, MTX, 5FU, HYD	2	200	61.5	6.5	67	Price

Abbreviations: DDP = cisplatin; MTX = methotrexate; VCR = vincristine; CTX = cytophosphamide; 5FU = 5-fluorouracil; Bleo = bleomycin; HYD = hydrocortisone; VB = vinblastine; Adra = Adriamycin.

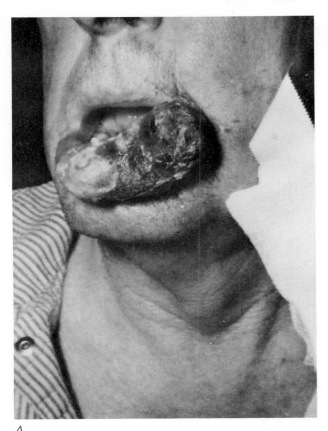

A

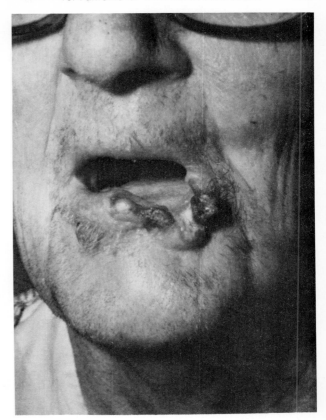

B

Fig. 16-41. Effect of chemotherapy upon squamous carcinoma of the lip. *A.* Lesion prior to treatment. *B.* Lesion following 2d cycle (approximately 4 weeks of treatment) of cisplatin, methotrexate, and bleomycin, 95+ percent regression. Patient had complete regression in another 4 weeks and continued treatment with radiotherapy, operative excision, and reconstruction.

This procedure was originally designed by Crile to eradicate the cervical lymphatic network, thereby eliminating sites of metastasis from cancer of the oral cavity, pharynx, paranasal sinuses, or other areas of the head and neck. In the early days of head and neck surgery radical neck dissections were usually performed after the primary lesion had been controlled through the use of radiation therapy. Today, we are more inclined to combine radical neck dissection with a simultaneous resection of the primary lesion. This is sometimes preceded by a course of radiation therapy to the primary area as part of a planned program of tumor treatment. Combined operations have been called by a number of terms including *composite resections* and *commando operations*. Other common operations in this area are superficial resection of the parotid gland, V excision of carcinoma of the lip, and resection of the maxillary antrum.

Radical Neck Dissection

Incisions for radical neck dissection are numerous and include a T-shaped incision originally used by Crile, a Y incision described by Ward, and a double Y incision described by Martin (Fig. 16-42). We prefer a hockey-stick shaped incision with the ascending limb along the posterior border of the sternocleidomastoid muscle and the horizontal portion crossing the neck about 2 or 3 cm above the clavicle (Fig. 16-43). This last approach has the advantage of being outside areas of radiation when the neck has had previous exposure to radiation therapy and of being a simple linear incision avoiding small triangular-shaped flaps, which have a tendency to slough. The skin flap is reflected mediad, including the underlying platysma muscle, and dissection of neck structures begins in the posterior triangle, dissecting the fibroareolar tissue of this space away from the trapezius muscle and the underlying brachial plexus and scalene fibers. The portion of the dissection is carried mediad until the phrenic nerve lying on the anterior scalene muscle is identified.

The lower end of the sternocleidomastoid muscle is transected and the jugular vein identified and ligated. The accompanying vagus nerve next to the jugular vein in the carotid sheath is identified and spared. Dissection is then carried up the neck, gradually dissecting the lymph node chain free from underlying fascia and beneath the carotid artery. Just above the level of the carotid bulb the hypoglossal nerve is identified. In the upper portion of the neck the sternocleidomastoid muscle is again transected at the level of the mastoid together with the tip of the

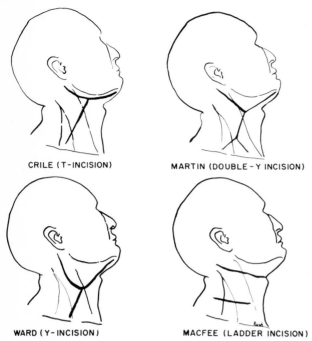

CRILE (T-INCISION)   MARTIN (DOUBLE-Y INCISION)

WARD (Y-INCISION)   MACFEE (LADDER INCISION)

Fig. 16-42. Common operative incisions for radical neck dissections. (From: *Rush BF Jr: Curr Probl Surg May 1966, with permission.*)

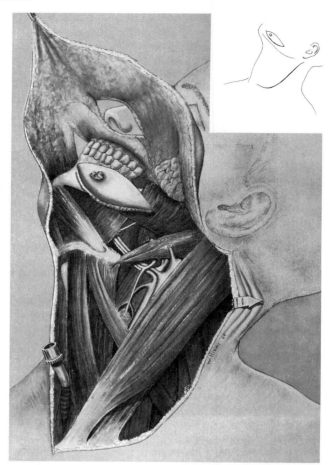

Fig. 16-43. Radical neck dissection through a hockey-stick incision (shown in insert) combined with an exposure of the mandible. The tumor has grown through the mandible and presented on the cheek so that a portion of the skin of the cheek has been left on the specimen. Structures of the neck are shown exposed and intact prior to the start of radical neck dissection. (From: *Rush BF Jr: Surg Gynecol Obstet 121:353, 1965, with permission.*)

parotid gland. The submaxillary gland is dissected free from the digastric fossa and included with the specimen. The lingual nerve and artery in the depths of the submaxillary fossa are visualized and left intact. Care is taken to identify the ramus mandibularis, the tiny fiber of the VIIth nerve that innervates the lower lip, and to reflect this above the submaxillary gland so that its continuity is maintained. The spinal accessory nerve is usually sacrificed, being cut in the lower neck where it enters the trapezius muscle and in the upper neck where it enters the sternocleidomastoid muscle. The operation is completed with the transection of the jugular vein at the point where it leaves the base of the skull (Fig. 16-44). If a radical neck dissection alone is performed, the operation is ended at this point by closing the skin flaps. Multiperforated catheters are left underneath the flaps and are connected to suction. This helps to draw the flap firmly to the structures of the neck and eliminates the problem of fluid collecting under the flap.

MODIFIED RADICAL NECK DISSECTION

This operation is still ill-defined. To some it means preserving the spinal accessory nerve but otherwise doing a complete radical neck. At the other extreme some surgeons spare all the ''functional'' structures in the neck including the sternocleidomastoid muscle, the spinal accessory nerve, and the jugular vein, removing mainly the lymphoareolar tissue of the anterior and posterior triangle and the submaxillary gland. Our preference is to spare the sternocleidomastoid muscle and the XIth nerve but to

remove the jugular vein. There is little morbidity incurred by removing the vein, and the lymphatic tissues of the neck are closely associated with the vein. The indication for limiting radical neck dissection to a modified operation is a negative neck without clinically positive nodes in the presence of a primary lesion with a high risk of occult nodal metastasis.

COMBINED OPERATION

If a radical neck dissection is to be combined with the removal of structures within the oral cavity or tonsillar area, the contents of the neck dissection are left attached to the horizontal ramus of the mandible. The mandible is frequently divided. If the lesion is in the floor of the mouth or tongue, the horizontal ramus of the mandible may be resected. If the lesion is in the tonsillar fossa, the ascending ramus of the mandible is removed. If the lesion

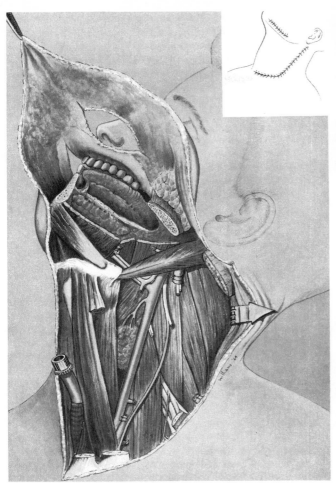

Fig. 16-44. Radical neck dissection completed, combined with excision of the horizontal ramus of the mandible. The jugular vein and sternocleidomastoid muscle have been removed. The phrenic nerve and the common carotid artery are seen coursing across the operative field. The closure of the neck incision is seen in the insert. (From: *Rush BF Jr: Surg Gynecol Obstet 121:353, 1965, with permission.*)

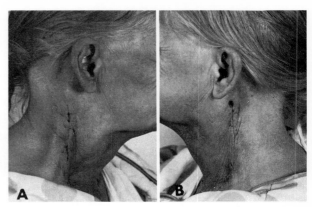

Fig. 16-45. Mandibular resection, 8 days after bilateral neck dissection and partial mandibulectomy on the left, with resection of a portion of the floor of the mouth and the anterior half of the tongue for carcinoma of the tongue. The portion of the jaw was replaced with a Steinmann pin. At 3 years postoperatively there still was no recurrence. Note that it is difficult to determine on which side the mandible was resected. (From: *Rush BF Jr: Curr Probl Surg May 1966, with permission.*)

BILATERAL RADICAL NECK DISSECTION

Lesions that are in the midline of the oral cavity often spread bilaterally, and it is necessary to remove lymph nodes on both sides of the neck. Simultaneous bilateral neck dissections are feasible with an acceptable mortality; however, the postoperative course is likely to be prolonged, since there is a period of marked facial edema following this extensive resection that can persist for several weeks. Some operators will spare the jugular vein on one side when a bilateral neck dissection is done in order to decrease the amount of postoperative edema. Others stage the dissection, allowing a delay of several weeks before operating on the second side.

Parotidectomy

Most lesions in the superficial lobe of the parotid gland are removed by superficial parotidectomy. This operation is designed to give maximal safety in operating about the branches of the VIIth nerve (Fig. 16-46). The VIIth nerve pierces the parotid gland at its posterior margin and lies underneath the gland on the muscles of the face. A Y-shaped incision is made with the lower limb lying behind the angle of the mandible and the arms of the Y on either side of the lobe of the ear. Dissection is carried down to identify the main trunk of the VIIth nerve, which lies in the space between the mandible and the mastoid bone approximately one fingerbreadth below the external auditory meatus. Once the main trunk is identified, dissection is carried along the external surface of the nerve and its branches, gradually separating away the overlying portion of the parotid gland. Stensen's duct is identified at the most medial portion of the midpoint of the parotid gland and is ligated. This technique sometimes causes temporary weakness in the fibers of the VIIth nerve but prevents transecting any of the major trunks of the nerve.

in the oral cavity is quite large, total removal of the hemimandible on the side of the lesion may be necessary. Resection of the mandible is done to remove bone involved by tumor and sometimes to obtain a closure of the oral cavity that would not be feasible without removing a portion of the bony framework. Mandibular resection can be done with the acceptable cosmetic and functional result, especially when the anterior portion of the mandible is preserved (Fig. 16-45). The more anteriorly the mandible is resected, the more likely there is to be facial deformity. If the primary site of the tumor is in the larynx or thyroid, then these structures may also be removed with the radical neck dissection. The mortality for radical neck dissection alone is less than 1 percent. If neck dissection is combined with en bloc excision of a primary lesion, then mortality rates range from 2 to 5 percent.

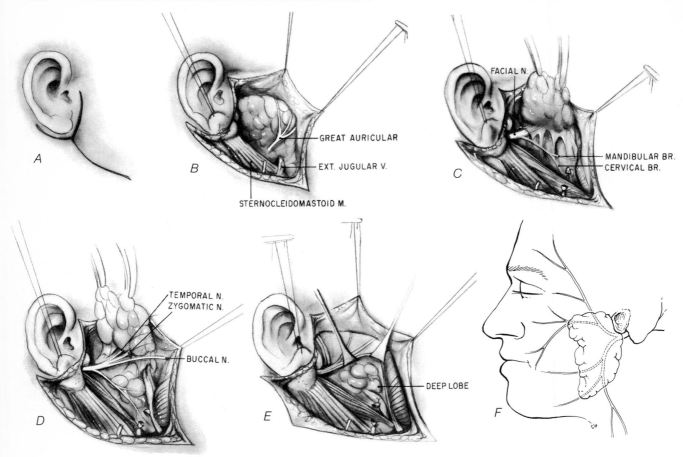

Fig. 16-46. Superficial parotidectomy. *A.* Incision. *B.* Skin flaps established and fascia incised; greater auricular nerve transected and external jugular vein identified. *C.* External jugular vein transected; superficial lobe is being reflected anteriorly, and facial nerve with its mandibular and cervical branches are shown. *D.* Dissection continued anteriorly, demonstrating temporal, zygomatic, and buccal branches. *E.* Superficial lobe removed; if excision of the deep lobe is indicated, the facial nerve can be retracted craniad and the remaining parotid removed. *F.* Relationship of facial nerve and parotid gland. The nerve branches lie between the deep and superficial lobes of the parotid. *(Courtesy of Robert Chase, M.D.)*

Recovery of function in all branches is ensured by the knowledge that they are intact and usually occurs within a week or two following completion of the operation.

V Excision of the Lip

Most cancers of the lower lip are removed with the use of V excision. Between one-fourth and one-third of the lower lip can be easily resected by simple excision without resulting in residual deformity or interference with function. While we refer to this excision as a V, a much better cosmetic result is obtained if the outline of the incision resembles that of a shield. A true V excision results in some flattening of the lower lip with a loss of normal eversion. If a shield-shaped incision is used, the lip will evert normally.

If the tumor involves more area than can be excised with a V excision, a flap is migrated from the upper lip. This involves outlining a V-shaped flap in the upper lip that is left attached at its lower medial corner and is then rotated into the defect in the lower lip. Using this type of closure excision of up to two-thirds of the lower lip can be accomplished without difficulty.

Maxillectomy

Cancer of the hard palate or the lower maxilla requires subtotal excision of the maxillary sinus. Cancer in the upper maxilla involving the orbital plate requires total excision of the maxillary sinus together with an exenteration of the orbital contents. While these excisions are basically mutilating, they can be accomplished with little visible external deformity. The Weber-Fergusson incision is used. This begins at the midpoint of the upper lip, extends to the columella of the nose, and is carried around the edge of the nose and up to the corner of the eye. A horizontal portion continues laterally from the inner canthus to a point just beyond the outer canthus and about 2 or 3 mm below the palpebral fissure. The skin and muscles of the cheek are undermined laterally, so that the entire cheek is turned outward, opening a door to the maxillary sinus. The bony attachments of the maxillary sinus are divided, including the midline of the hard palate, the zygoma, the pterygoid plates; if the orbital plate is to be removed, the bony walls of the medial and lateral orbit are also transected. When this is accomplished, the entire maxillary sinus can be lifted like a small box from its normal position. The inner surface of the Weber-Fergusson flap is covered with a split-thickness skin graft, and the incision is closed. Because it falls in the normal skin lines and about the normal structures of the face, this incision is often difficult to detect after it has healed as long as the structures have been replaced precisely and in good apposition. This operation leaves a large defect in the hard palate on the side of the procedure. This is occasionally closed by subsequent operations, but more commonly a dental prosthesis with a large obturator that fits into the defect is constructed by the prosthodontist. This restores normal speech and relatively normal mastication for the patient.

Total Laryngectomy

Total laryngectomy is traditionally accomplished through a midline longitudinal incision. We have found definite advantages in accomplishing this procedure through a transverse incision in the lower neck very much like the typical thyroidectomy incision. The incision is made 4 cm above the clavicles and approximately 4 cm beyond the edge of the sternocleidomastoid muscles on either side; it is carried down through the platysma muscle, and the upper flap is then developed. The upper limit of dissection is approximately 1 cm above the hyoid, and at this point the entire group of strap muscles and the midportion of the hyoid are exposed. In cancer operations for glottic tumors of any size, all the anterior strap muscles are removed. Occasionally at the election of the operator in the presence of somewhat smaller lesions, the strap muscles on the side contralateral to the lesion may be preserved, or, rarely, the larynx is skeletonized with the preservation of strap muscles on both sides. In the ordinary instance, however, the sternothyroid and sternohyoid muscles are transected at the level of the cricoid, the digastric and mylohyoid muscles are separated from the hyoid above, and the body of the hyoid bone is cut at the junction of the attachments to the lateral wings on either side. The larynx is rocked laterally exposing the pharyngeal constrictors, which are cut at the lateral edge of the thyroid cartilages bilaterally. One can now enter the pharynx laterally, usually on the side opposite the tumor, so that proper visualization of the area can be obtained, and an adequate margin of excision of pharyngeal mucosa will be developed around the tumor. Once the pharynx is entered, it is possible for the surgeon to operate both outside and inside the pharynx. The remaining muscles of the tongue are severed from the hyoid, and the larynx is pulled forward. The vascular pedicles containing the laryngeal arteries and the superior laryngeal nerves

are ligated bilaterally. An incision is made in the pharyngeal mucosa just posterior to the arytenoids, entirely circumscribing the point at which the larynx projects into the pharynx. As all pharyngeal mucosa is now separated from the larynx, the larynx is pulled forward, and a plane of dissection is developed between the larynx and the anterior esophageal wall. This dissection is carried inferiorly until the only remaining structure holding the larynx in place is the trachea. This is then divided obliquely around the site of the tracheostomy (if one has been done previous to the operation), or if an endotracheal tube has been used in anesthesia, this is now removed, and a tube is placed in the severed trachea so that anesthesia can be continued. After the larynx has been removed, the defect in the pharynx is closed transversely with an inverting Connell stitch. This is reinforced by interrupted sutures of 4-0 silk which are used to imbricate the constrictor muscles up and around the pharyngeal closure. This closure may further be reinforced by stitches that catch the platysma muscle and draw it down snugly along with the overlying skin. A generous circular portion of skin is removed in the lower midline; this measures about 3 to 4 cm in diameter with three-quarters of the circle lying above the transverse skin incision and one-quarter of the circle lying below. The beveled end of the trachea is then drawn up to the skin by interrupted sutures of nylon. Every attempt is made to obtain a delicate mucosa to skin closure, since the smaller the size of the scar at the junction between mucosa and skin, the less likely there is to be subsequent stenosis of the tracheal opening. The generous amount of skin excised tends to evert the trachea in a slighty "trumpet-like" manner, and this too ensures against subsequent stenosis. This type of trachea skin closure can be maintained without the use of an indwelling tracheostomy tube except for the first 24 h or so postoperatively. The remainder of the wound is closed with interrupted sutures to the platysma muscle and skin. Two suction catheters are left in place on either side of the neck and are usually removed in 24 to 36 h. The patient is maintained on postoperative feeding through a nasal tube made up of a #18 whistle-tip red rubber catheter inserted at the time of operation through the nose and into the esophagus before the pharyngeal defect is closed. This tube is sutured to the nasal columella. The patient is maintained on nasal tube feedings for about 10 days. A liquid diet is usually begun on the fifth or sixth day, and the patient may take solid food on the ninth or tenth day. The nasal tube is removed as soon as it is apparent that patients can well maintain their own nutrition.

Partial Laryngectomy and the Neolarynx

In the past all lesions extending beyond the true cords have been treated by the total laryngectomy. The functional importance of the voice and the great benefit of preserving it for the patient has led to an evaluation of cancer operations that do not remove the entire larynx. Ogura and Biller have led this effort and have proposed a number of new operations that involve removal of most or all of the larynx above the cords (supraglottic laryngectomy) or excision of most of one side of the larynx (hemilaryngectomy) for lesions that are confined enough in their growth to be suitable for this technique. This approach requires careful selection of patients who are young and flexible enough to overcome some of the swallowing and aspiration difficulties that often arise postoperatively. Since the resected margin around the tumor may be very limited, careful diagnostic techniques must be used to identify the outer margins. This technique is almost always combined with preoperative radiation therapy to ensure a lesser threat from residual cells at the periphery of the tumor that may be left by the surgeon. Using these techniques in patients with tumors advanced enough to cause fixation of the cord, Ogura and Biller have reported a 77 percent 3-year survival.

An alternative method for preserving the voice, especially in patients with lesions not amenable to partial laryngectomy, is creation of a pseudolarynx. The most popular method for this procedure is that of Staffieri, in which the open stump of the trachea is covered by a flap of pharyngeal mucosa and a very small mucosa-lined fistula is created connecting the trachea to the pharynx. The patient speaks by occluding a lateral tracheostoma with a finger and diverting air from the lungs into the pharynx and mouth. Aspiration is avoided by the very small size of the fistula but may be a problem in a substantial number of these patients. Attempts at developing a valve of tissue to cover the fistula are in progress, as previously mentioned (Fig. 16-30).

POSTOPERATIVE CARE FOLLOWING HEAD AND NECK OPERATIONS

Tracheostomy is performed at the time of operation in any patient in whom a portion of the mandible is removed or when there is extensive removal of oral structures. Postoperative edema plus the tendency for the larynx to shift position following sacrifice of many of its suspensory muscles predispose to aspiration and obstruction. Catastrophic anoxia may supervene rapidly, with little apparent warning. The tracheostomy tube must be aspirated frequently. This requires the presence of well-trained nursing personnel. If a patient appears to be accumulating unusual amounts of tracheal secretions, it is probable that saliva is being aspirated through an incompetent larynx. This can be controlled by diligent suctioning. In extreme instances, a cuffed tracheostomy may be required temporarily.

The patient with a tracheostomy has lost the usual humidifying effects of the nasal and pharyngeal passageways. The best way to provide humidity for the patient's trachea is to tie an umbilical tape about the neck above the tracheostomy and to hang a moistened 4 by 4 sponge over this tape very much in the manner that a towel is hung over a rail. The sponge must frequently be moistened, and after the first day or two patients can be taught to moisten their own sponges and arrange them for themselves.

There is no need to leave the tracheostomy in place for prolonged periods. As soon as the patient is found to be maintaining a dry, unobstructed airway and the skin flaps are sealed, the tracheostomy tube is covered with a piece of adhesive tape. This is done about 5 days postoperatively. If the patient tolerates the covering of the tracheostomy tube for 24 h, it can be removed. This tube should always be removed in the morning, so that the patient can be observed during the daylight hours following removal.

Patients who have undergone combined resections have had extensive superficial operation, but the body cavities have been undisturbed, and the normal function of the gastrointestinal tract resumes almost immediately. A nasoesophageal tube consisting of a #16 French urethral catheter is left in place at the end of the operative procedure. The tip of the standard urethral catheter reaches to the lower third of the esophagus but does not traverse the esophagocardiac junction. Such tubes can be left in place for long periods without the risk of acid regurgitation and peptic esophagitis. The patient receives fluids intravenously on the day of operation, but on the first postoperative day nasal feedings of half-strength milk are given. On the second postoperative day a nasal formula consisting of a blenderized regular diet diluted with milk is begun. This is continued until the fifth or sixth postoperative day or until patients show evidence that they can tolerate an adequate diet by mouth.

Except for the different flora encountered, there is little difference in the principles of operating on the mouth and other areas in the gastrointestinal tract. This is a contaminated area, and numerous tissue planes are open to this contamination. All patients should be placed on appropriate antibiotics postoperatively. Ketcham et al. demonstrated in a controlled study the advantages of prophylactic antibiotics in these patients.

The mental stress in patients undergoing an oral operation of any magnitude is considerable. They awaken unable to speak because of the tracheostomy. They are unable to control their saliva and find that they are constantly aspirating small amounts of mucus. Their necks and shoulders are completely numb and boardlike because of the section of all cervical sensory nerves on the side of the lesion, and while they have little or no sharp pain, they have a pounding and persistent headache due to the ligation of the jugular vein and concomitant rise of spinal fluid pressure. In a day or two they look into the mirror and may not recognize the swollen, edematous, and possibly deformed face that stares back. It would be abnormal if they were not depressed under these circumstances. Support for the patient depends on good preoperative preparation. The patient must understand clearly what to expect in the postoperative period. Patients do not panic if they understand their problems and realize that most of their deficiencies are reversible as edema subsides and the tracheostomy tube is removed.

REHABILITATION

As Shedd has pointed out, progress in medicine often brings new problems. In head and neck oncology the suc-

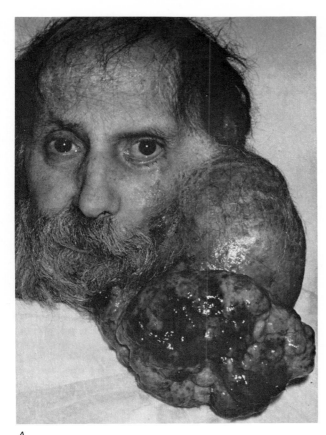

A

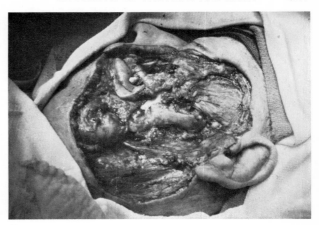

B

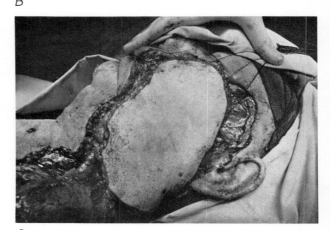

C

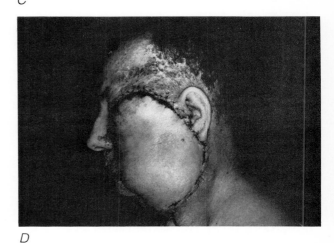

D

Fig. 16-47. Pectoralis myocutaneous flap in repair of a facial defect: *A.* Large neglected malignant mixed tumor of parotid with necrosis and ulceration of lower pole. *B.* Operative field after removal of tumor. Ascending ramus of mandible with anterior half removed is in center of field. Tongue is visible at 11 o'clock following removal of entire left cheek and buccal mucosa. Anterior wall of maxillary sinus has been removed. *C.* Pectoralis myocutaneous flap brought up to fill defect. *D.* Seven days after operation, myocutaneous flap in place, slight bulge in lower neck indicates site of muscle pedicle providing blood supply to the flap.

cessful control of major cancers may leave a considerable number of patients whose posttreatment life involves a significant degree of disability. Major impairment in appearance, swallowing, taste, and speech all reduce the quality of life and the effectiveness of treatment. While the field of rehabilitation of these patients is too broad to detail here, the major thrust of recent years has been to accomplish as much of the rehabilitation as possible on the operating table at the primary procedure.

The development of free flaps and myocutaneous flaps is a major advance in the reconstruction of head and neck defects. For the first time an adequate source of soft tissue and even bone is immediately available for rapid one-stage reconstruction of operative defects. Myocutaneous flaps are constructed by freeing up one end of a muscle and leaving the blood supply to the other end intact. All or any part of the overlying skin can be brought up with the muscle pedicle to fill the operative defect. The skin obtains its blood supply from the underlying muscle. While there are many muscles that can be used in head and neck reconstructions including the trapezius, sterno-cleidomastoid, and latissimus dorsi, the favorite has become the pectoralis major, which can reach any part of the face and can be fashioned to fill large and small defects (Fig. 16-47*A, B, C,* and *D*).

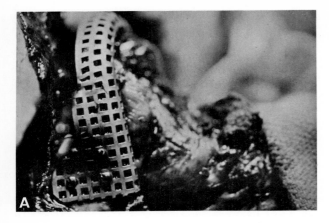

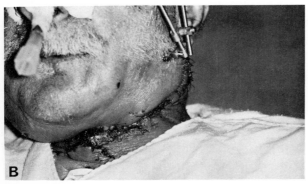

Fig. 16-48. *A.* Resection of the entire anterior mandible is one of the most devastating procedures for patients both cosmetically and functionally. Attempts at immediate reconstruction include use of a tantalum tray as shown here filled with cancellous bone chips. *B.* The tray is incorporated in a flap of cervical skin from the anterior neck, which also is used to line the residual tongue and floor of the mouth. The remaining mandible is immobilized with external pins. Immediate appearance and function are very acceptable.

Free flaps or grafts are areas of tissue removed with an associated artery and vein. The vessels must be large enough to permit microvascular reanastomosis to vessels of the head or neck. These operations are long and arduous, requiring great skill and patience in isolating and anastomosing the vascular structures so that myocutaneous flaps have preference in most cases. Free grafts of small bowel for one-stage replacement of the cervical esophagus and pharynx after major resections have gained some advocates, although many prefer to bring up the stomach through the anterior mediastinum and use the fundus of the stomach in restoring these structures. In any case the use of skin tubes for this purpose has been totally superseded.

Transplantation of generous amounts of fresh tissue with a new blood supply into operated areas of the head and neck has made possible major reconstructions even after high-dose radiation has preceded the operation. Total replacement of the mandible by transplanted bone or metal prosthesis has a much higher success rate in this setting (Fig. 16-48).

The maximum results of rehabilitation are usually ob-tained by a team effort incorporating the skills of the head and neck surgeon, plastic surgeon, oral surgeon, speech therapist, and psychotherapist.

Bibliography

General

Advisory Committee to the Surgeon General on Smoking and Health: Report on smoking and health. *Public Health Serv Publ* 1103, 1964.

Arons MS, Smith RR: Distant metastases and local recurrence in head and neck cancer. *Ann Surg* 154:235, 1961.

Baker H: Oral cancer: A six part series. *CA,* pt. I: January–February, 1972; pt. II: March–April, 1972; pt. III: May–June, 1972; pt. IV: July–August, 1972; pt. V: September–October, 1972; pt. VI: January–February, 1973.

Baker HW: The staging of head and neck cancer. *Adv Oncol* 3:1, 1987.

Brody WR, et al: Intravenous arteriography using digital subtraction techniques. *JAMA* 248:671, 1982.

Dorman EB, Yang FH, et al: The incidence of hypercalcemia in squamous cell carcinoma of the head and neck. *Head Neck Surg* 7:95, 1984.

Glazer HS, Niemeyer JH, et al: Neck neoplasms: MR imaging. Part I. Initial evaluation. ICRDB, Series CT11 86:12, 1986.

Gowen GF, deSuto-Nagy G: The incidence and sites of distant metastases in head and neck carcinoma. *Surg Gynecol Obstet* 116:603, 1963.

Kaplan MH, Susin Y, et al: Neoplastic complications of HTLV-III infection. *Am J Med* 82:3, 1987.

LoVerme PJ, Rush BF Jr, et al: Combined therapy in advanced squamous cell carcinoma of the head and neck. *Am Surg* 48:197, 1982.

Mashberg A: Tolonium (toluidine blue) rinse—a screening method for recognition of squamous carcinoma. Continuing study of oral cancer IV. *JAMA* 245:2408, 1981.

Mashberg A, Barsa P: Screening for oral and oropharyngeal squamous carcinomas. *CA* 34:5, 1984.

Montgomery WW: *Surgery of the Upper Respiratory System.* Philadelphia, Lea & Febiger, 1979, vol I.

Moore C: Smoking and cancer of the mouth, pharynx and larynx. *JAMA* 191:107, 1965.

Rubin P: Current concepts in cancer: Cancer of the head and neck. *JAMA* 221:68, 1972. (First of a continuing series of articles.)

Rush BF Jr, Chambers RG, Ravitch MM: Cancer of the head and neck in children. *Surgery* 53:270, 1963.

Rush BF Jr, Horie N, Klein NW: Intra-arterial infusion of the head and neck: Anatomical and distributional problems. *Am J Surg* 110:510, 1965.

Rush BF Jr, Trinkle K: The management of low-grade, neglected neoplasms. *South Med J* 60:714, 1967.

Schottenfield D: Cancer of the buccal cavity and pharynx: A review of end results of primary treatment in 2877 cases 1949–1964. *Clin Bull Memorial Hosp.* 2:51, 1972.

Schuller DE, Fritsch MH: An assessment of the value of triple endoscopy in the evaluation of head and neck cancer patients. *J Surg Oncol* 32:156, 1986.

Serafini I: Larengectomia totale con mantenimento della respirazoine per via naturale (resoconto sul primo case recentemente operato con technica personale). *Min Otorinolarin* 20:73, 1970.

Shedd DP: Rehabilitation problems in head and neck patients. *J Surg Oncology* 8:11, 1976.

Sitz KV, Keppen M, Johnson DF: Metastatic basal cell carcinoma in acquired immunodeficiency syndrome–related complex. *JAMA* 257:3, 1987.

Vega MF: Larynx reconstruction surgery. A study of three-year findings: A modified surgical technique. *Laryngoscope* 85:866, 1975.

Willis RA: *Pathology of Tumors*. London, Butterworth, 1960.

Historical Background

Absolon KB, Rogers W, Aust JB: Some historical developments of the surgical therapy of tongue cancer from the seventeenth to the nineteenth century. *Am J Surg* 104:686, 1962.

Campbell E, Colton J: *The Surgery of Theodoric*. New York, Appleton-Century-Crofts, 1955.

Fletcher GH, Jesse RH Jr: The contribution of supervoltage roentgenotherapy to the integration of radiation and surgery in head and neck squamous cell carcinomas. *Cancer* 15:566, 1962.

Lip

Ashley FL, McConnell DV, et al: Carcinoma of the lip: A comparison of five year results after irradiation and surgical therapy. *Am J Surg* 110:549, 1965.

Blackerby JN, Hamilton JE: Carcinoma of the lip. *Surgery* 51:591, 1962.

Stephens FO, Harker GJS, Hambly CK: Treatment of advanced cancer of the lower lip—the use of intraarterial or intravenous chemotherapy as basal treatment. *Cancer* 48:1309, 1981.

Oral Cavity

Evans JF, Shah JP: Epidermoid carcinoma of the palate. *Am J Surg* 142:451, 1981.

Fayos JV, Lampe I: Treatment of squamous cell carcinoma of the oral cavity. *Am J Surg* 124:493, 1972.

Helfrich GB, Nickels ME, et al: Management of cancer of the floor of the mouth. *Am J Surg* 124:559, 1972.

Kraus FT, Perez-Mesa C: Verrucous carcinoma: Clinical and pathologic study of 105 cases involving oral cavity, larynx, and genitalia. *Cancer* 19:26, 1966.

Marchetta FC, Sako K, Murph JB: The periosteum of the mandible and intraoral carcinoma. *Am J Surg* 122:711, 1971.

Martin HE: The history of lingual cancer. *Am J Surg* 48:703, 1940.

O'Brien PH, Catlin D: Cancer of the cheek (mucosa). *Cancer* 18:1392, 1965.

Rush BF Jr: Combined procedures in the treatment of oral carcinoma. *Curr Prob Surg* May 1966.

Rush BF Jr, Humphrey L: Primary repair of full thickness excision of the cheek. *Am J Surg* 114:592, 1967.

Sandler HC: Oral cytology. *CA* 16:97, 1966.

Schottenfeld D: Snuff dipper's cancer. *N Engl J Med* 304:778, 1981.

Silver CE, Glackin BK, et al: Surgical treatment of oral cavity carcinoma. *Head Neck Surg* 9:13, 1986.

Southwick HW, Slaughter DP, Trevino ET: Elective neck dissection for intraoral cancer. *Arch Surg* 80:905, 1960.

Spiro RH, Spiro JD, Strong EW: Surgical approach to squamous carcinoma confined to the tongue and the floor of the mouth. *Head Neck Surg* 9:27, 1986.

Stecker RH, Devine KD, Harrison EG Jr: Verrucose "snuff dip-
per's" carcinoma of the oral cavity: A case of self-induced carcinogenesis. *JAMA* 189:144, 1964.

Yarington CT Jr: A rational approach to carcinoma of the tongue. *Am Surg* 9:381, 1981.

Yonemoto RH, Ching PT, et al: The composite operation in cancer of the head and neck (commando procedure). *Arch Surg* 104:809, 1972.

Oropharynx

Baker RR, Weiner S: The clinical management of tonsillar carcinoma. *Surg Gynecol Obstet* 121:1035, 1965.

Barkley HT, Fletcher GH, et al: Management of cervical lymph node metastasis in squamous cell carcinoma of the tonsillar fossa, base of tongue, supraglottic larynx and hypopharynx. *Am J Surg* 124:464, 1972.

Dasmahapatra KS, Mohit-Tabatabai MA, et al: Cancer of the tonsil: Improved survival with combination therapy. *Cancer* 57:3, 1986.

McIlrath DC, ReMine WH, et al: Tumors of the parapharyngeal region. *Surg Gynecol Obstet* 116:88, 1963.

McNeill R: Surgical management of carcinoma of the posterior pharyngeal wall. *Head Neck Surg* 3:389, 1981.

Perez CA, Ackerman LV, Mill WB: Malignant tumors of the tonsil: Analysis of failures and factors affecting prognosis. *Am J Roentgenol Radium Ther Nucl Med* 114:43, 1972.

Rush BF Jr, Reynolds G, Greenlaw R: Integrated irradiation and operation in treatment of cancer of the larynx and hypopharynx: A preliminary report. *Am J Roentgenol Radium Ther Nucl Med* 102:129, 1968.

Larynx

Baker RR, Cherry J: Carcinoma of the larynx: Results of therapy in 209 cases. *Arch Surg* 90:449, 1965.

Biller HF, Lawson W: Partial laryngectomy for vocal cord cancer with marked limitation or fixation of the vocal cord. *Laryngoscope* 96:61, 1986.

Donegan WL: An early history of total laryngectomy. *Surgery* 57:902, 1965.

Flynn MB, Jesse RH, Lindberg RD: Surgery and irradiation in the treatment of squamous cell cancer of the supraglottic larynx. *Am J Surg* 124:477, 1972.

Goldman JL, Cheren RV, et al: Combined irradiation and surgery for cancer of the larynx and laryngopharynx, in Conley J (ed): *Cancer of the Head and Neck*. Washington, Butterworth, 1967.

Holinger PH: Cancer of the larynx: Classification and partial laryngectomy, in Conley J (ed): *Cancer of the Head and Neck*. Washington, Butterworth, 1967.

Johns ME, Cantrell RW: Voice restoration of the total laryngectomy patient: The Singer-Blom technique. *Otolaryngol Head Neck Surg* 89:82, 1981.

Krause LG: Clinical review of carcinoma of the larynx: Experience of a large cancer hospital. *Am J Surg* 111:206, 1966.

Lundgren JA, Van Nostrand P, et al: Verrucous carcinoma (Ackerman's tumor) of the larynx: Diagnostic and therapeutic considerations. *Head Neck Surg* 9:19, 1986.

Ogura JW, Biller HF: Preoperative irradiation for laryngeal and laryngopharyngeal cancer. *Laryngoscope* 80:802, 1970.

Ono J, Shigejo S: Endoscopic microsurgery of the larynx. *Ann Otol Rhinol Laryngol* 80:479, 1971.

Powell RW, Redd BL, Wilkins SA Jr: An evaluation of treatment of cancer of the larynx. *Am J Surg* 110:635, 1965.

Rush BF Jr: New voices for old: Attempts to create a new larynx. *Surg Rounds* 4:16, 1981.

Rush BF Jr, Swaminathan AP, et al: Construction of a neolarynx after radiation and laryngectomy. *Am J Surg* 138:619, 1979.

Shahrokh DK, Devine KD, Harrison EG Jr: Statistical evaluation of 115 cases of carcinoma of the epiglottis (1943 to 1952). *Am J Surg* 102:781, 1961.

Shedd DP: Role of surgical measures in voice restoration after laryngectomy, in *Symposium on Malignancies of The Head and Neck*. St Louis, Mosby, 1975.

Spalt L, Greenlaw R, Rush BF Jr: Integrated therapy for carcinoma of the larynx, in Rush BF Jr, Greenlaw RH (eds): *Integrated Radiation and Operation in Cancer Therapy: A Symposium*. Springfield, IL, Charles C Thomas, 1968.

Vuyk H, Tiwara R, Snow GB: Staffier's procedure revisited. *Head Neck Surg* 8:21, 1985.

Nasopharynx

Jesse RH: Preoperative versus postoperative radiation in the treatment of squamous carcinoma of the paranasal sinuses. *Am J Surg* 110:552, 1965.

Moench HC, Phillips TL: Carcinoma of the nasopharynx: Review of 146 patients with emphasis on radiation dose and time factors. *Am J Surg* 124:515, 1971.

Thomas JE, Waltz AG: Neurological manifestations of nasopharyngeal malignant tumors. *JAMA* 192:103, 1965.

Nasal Cavity and Paranasal Sinuses

Kurohara SS, Ellis F, et al: Role of radiation therapy and of surgery in the management of localized epidermoid carcinoma of the maxillary sinus. *Am J Roentgenol Radium Ther Nucl Med* 114:35, 1972.

Moseley HS, et al: Advanced squamous cell carcinoma of the maxillary sinus. Results of combined regional infusion chemotherapy, radiation therapy and surgery. *Am J Surg* 141:522, 1981.

Rush BF Jr, Knightly JJ, Jewell W: Transoral and transverse incision for excision of the maxillary sinus. *J Surg Oncol* 3:53, 1971.

Tabah EJ: Cancer of the paranasal sinuses: A study of the results of various methods of treatment in fifty-four patients. *Am J Surg* 104:741, 1962.

Mandible

Bernier JL: *Tumors of the Odontogenic Apparatus and Jaws*. Washington, Armed Forces Institute of Pathology, 1960.

Cramer LM, Culf NK, et al: Reconstruction management of the mandible in the treatment of head and neck, in *Symposium on Malignancies of The Head and Neck*. St Louis, Mosby, 1975.

Khanna S, Khanna NN, et al: Primary tumors and tumor-like conditions of the mandible. *J Surg Oncol* 16:365, 1981.

Salivary Glands

Beahrs OH, Woolner LB, et al: Surgical management of parotid lesions. *Arch Surg* 80:890, 1960.

Bhaskar SN, Bernier JL: Mikulicz's disease. *Oral Surg* 13:1387, 1960.

Connell HC, Evans JC: Mucoepidermoid carcinoma of the salivary glands. *Am J Surg* 124:519, 1972.

Foote FW, Frazell EL: *Tumors of the Major Salivary Glands*. Washington, Armed Forces Institute of Pathology, 1954.

Gates GA: Current concepts in otolaryngology. Malignant neoplasms of the minor salivary glands. *N Engl J Med* 306:718, 1982.

Grage TB, Lober PH: Benign lymphoepithelial lesion of the salivary glands. *Am J Surg* 108:495, 1964.

Grage TB, Lober PH, Shahon DB: Benign tumors of the major salivary glands. *Surgery* 50:625, 1961.

Katsilambros L: Asymptomatic enlargement of the parotid glands. *JAMA* 178:513, 1961.

Reynolds CT, McAuley RL, Rogers WP Jr: Experience with tumors of minor salivary glands. *Am J Surg* 111:168, 1966.

Rosenfeld L, Sessions DG, et al: Malignant tumors of salivary gland origin: 37-year review of 184 cases. *Ann Surg* 163:726, 1966.

Stewart FW, Foote FW, Becker WF: Mucoepidermoid tumors of salivary glands. *Ann Surg* 122:820, 1945.

Stuteville OH, Corley RD: Surgical management of tumors of intraoral minor salivary glands: Report of eighty cases. *Cancer* 20:1578, 1967.

Suen JY, Johns ME: Chemotherapy for salivary gland cancer. *Laryngoscope* 92:235, 1982.

Winsten J, Ward GE: The parotid gland: An anatomic study. *Surgery* 40:585, 1956.

Tumors of the Neck

Albers GD: Branchial anomalies. *JAMA* 183:399, 1963.

Hoffman E: Branchial cysts within the parotid gland. *Ann Surg* 152:290, 1960.

Jesse RH, Neff LE: Metastatic carcinoma in cervical nodes with an unknown primary lesion. *Am J Surg* 112:547, 1966.

MacComb WS: Diagnosis and treatment of metastatic cervical cancerous nodes from an unknown primary site. *Am J Surg* 124:441, 1972.

Marchetta FC, Murphy WT, Kovaric JJ: Carcinoma of the neck. *Am J Surg* 106:974, 1963.

Mohit-Tabatabai MA, Dasmahapatra KS, et al: Management of squamous cell carcinoma of unknown origin in cervical lymph nodes. *Am Surg* 52, 1986.

Mooney CS, Jewell W, et al: Simultaneous bilateral radical neck dissection following high level radiation therapy. *J Surg Oncol* 1:335, 1969.

Razack MS, Sako K: Carotid artery hemorrhage and ligation in head and neck cancer. *J Surg Oncol* 19:189, 1982.

Roseman JM, James AG: Metastatic cancers to the neck from undermined primary sites long-term follow-up. *J Surg Oncol* 19:247, 1982.

Rush BF Jr: Current concepts in the treatment of carotid body tumors. *Surgery* 52:679, 1962.

Rush BF Jr: Familial bilateral carotid body tumors. *Ann Surg* 157:633, 1963.

Skandalakis JE, Gray SW, et al: Tumors of the neck. *Surgery* 48:375, 1960.

Suarez Nieto D, Estevan Solano JM, et al: Invasion of the carotid artery in tumors of the head and neck. *Clin Otolaryngol* 6:29, 1981.

Chemotherapy and Immunotherapy

Adams GL, Berlinger NT, et al: Immunologic assessment of regional lymph node histology in relation to survival in head and neck carcinoma. *Cancer* 37:697, 1976.

Alexander JC Jr, Chretien PB, et al: Viral-specific humoral immunity to herpes simplex-induced antigens in patients with squamous carcinoma of the head and neck. *Am J Surg* 132:541, 1976.

Blackshear PJ, et al: An implantable pump for long-term intravascular drug infusion. *Med Instrum* 15:226, 1981.

Connors JM, Andiman WA, et al: Treatment of nasopharyngeal carcinoma with human leukocyte interferon. *J Clin Oncol* 3:6, 1985.

Couture J, Deschenes L: Intra-arterial infusion: An adjuvant to the treatment of oral carcinoma. *Cancer* 29:1632, 1972.

Cvitkovic E, Gerold FP, et al: cis-Dichlorodiamineplatinum (II) in the treatment of epidermoid carcinoma of the head and neck. *Cancer Treat Rep* 61:359, 1977.

Dasmahapatra KS, Citrin P, et al: A prospective evaluation of 5-fluorouracil plus cisplatin in advanced squamous-cell cancer of the head and neck. *J Clin Oncol* 3:11, 1985.

Decker DA, et al: Adjuvant chemotherapy with high-dose bolus cis-diamminodichloroplatinum II (CDD) and 120-hour-infusion 5-fluorouracil (5-FU) in stage III and IV squamous cell carcinoma of the head and neck. *Proc Am Soc Clin Oncol* 1:195, 1982.

Ervin TJ, Clark JR, et al: An analysis of induction and adjuvant chemotherapy in the multidisciplinary treatment of squamous-cell carcinoma of the head and neck. *J Clin Oncol* 5:1, 1987.

Feldman J, et al: Up front bleo-cap chemotherapy produces a 100% rate (33%) complete response in previously untreated advanced head and neck cancer. *Proc Am Soc Clin Oncol* 1:193, 1982.

Freckman HA: Results in 169 patients with cancer of the head and neck treated by intra-arterial infusion therapy. *Am J Surg* 124:501, 1972.

Frei Emil II: The national cancer chemotherapy program. *Science* 217:600, 1982.

Holden C: New disease baffles medical community. *Science* 217:618, 1982.

Horn Y, et al: Long-term remission of an advanced head and neck tumor following intra-arterial infusion with *cis*-dichlorodiammineplatinum. *J Surg Oncol* 18:189, 1981.

Kish J, et al: Clinical trial of cisplatin and 5-FU infusion as initial treatment for advanced squamous cell carcinoma of the head and neck. *Cancer Treat Rep* 66:471, 1982.

Milazzo J, Mohit-Tabatabai MA, et al: Preoperative intra-arterial infusion chemotherapy for advanced squamous cell carcinoma of the mouth and oropharynx. *Cancer* 56:1014, 1985.

Perry DJ, Davis RK, Weiss RB: Combined modality treatment with combination chemotherapy for advanced squamous cell carcinoma of the head and neck. *Proc Am Soc Clin Oncol* 1:193, 1982.

Price LA, Hill BT: Safe and effective combination chemotherapy without *cis*-platinum for squamous cell carcinomas of the head and neck. *Cancer Treat Rep* 65 (suppl. 1):149, 1981.

Richman SP, et al: Chemotherapy versus chemoimmunotherapy of head and neck cancer: Report of a randomized study. *Cancer Treat Rep* 60:535, 1976.

Tannock IF, Browman G: Lack of evidence for a role of chemotherapy in the routine management of locally advanced head and neck cancer. *J Clin Oncol* 4:7, 1986.

Tejada F, Chandler JR: Combined therapy for stage III & IV head and neck cancer (H&N). *Proc Am Soc Clin Oncol* 1:199, 1982.

Williams AC: Topical 5 FU: A new approach to skin cancer. *Ann Surg* 173:864, 1971.

Woods JE: The influence of immunologic responsiveness on head and neck cancer. *Plast Reconstr Surg* 56:77, 1975.

Operations of the Head and Neck

Achauer BM, Salibian AH, Furnas DS: Free flaps to the head and neck. *Head Neck Surg* 4:315, 1982.

Frazell EL, Moore OS: Bilateral radical neck dissection performed in stages: Experience with 467 patients. *Am J Surg* 102:809, 1961.

Pradhan SA: Gastric pull-up for cancers of the hypopharynx and cervical esophagus: Our experience. *J Surg Oncol* 26:149, 1984.

Smith PG, Sharkey DE, et al: The infratemporal fossa approach to neoplastic and arterial lesions of the lateral skull base. *Surg Rounds* 9:63, 1986.

Wilson JS, Yiacoumettis AM, O'Neill T: Some observations on 112 pectoralis major myocutaneous flaps. *Am J Surg* 147:273, 1984.

Chapter 17

Chest Wall, Pleura, Lung, and Mediastinum

Thomas C. King and Craig R. Smith

INTRODUCTION

Life depends on a delicate sequence of events that moves air to blood and blood to tissues. The cardiorespiratory system functions to assure those events occur dependably; the margin of error is extremely small. The analysis and management of surgical concerns involving the chest and its contents, whether relating to tumors, trauma, or infection, all focus on the mechanical transport of oxygen to the vital organs and the necessary exchange of gases. Air with adequate oxygen content must pass through the upper airway, the trachea, and the bronchi to reach the alveoli properly warmed and humidified for movement across alveolar membranes. Those membranes must be in condition to allow efficient diffusion of oxygen and carbon dioxide. Blood with sufficient oxygen-carrying capacity must be circulating through the alveolar capillaries in adequate volumes and at the proper speed to allow pickup of oxygen and discharge of carbon dioxide; it must also be at the proper pH and temperature and must have the proper biochemical characteristics for optimum exchange. The vascular system must have the appropriate integrity, pressure gradients, volume, and flow dynamics to traverse the pumps and conduits from alveolar capillaries to vital organ capillaries and back. At the vital organ interface, the characteristics for release from the blood to the tissues of oxygen, and recapture of carbon dioxide must be present. Irreparable damage to vital organs may occur in minutes if any part of the system fails.

Near normal physiologic cardiopulmonary function must continue during surgical procedures involving the chest. Preexisting impairment of pulmonary function, operative removal of tissue from the chest wall or lungs, and postoperative pain are routine hazards to the patient's ability to continue adequate respiratory exchange following operation. The development of thoracic surgery has followed the development of anesthesiology: techniques for tracheal intubation and positive-pressure ventilation. Prior to this recent development, surgeons' efforts were largely limited to the management of trauma, and the history of the field is closely linked to the history of weaponry. Management of chest wounds received in battle was recorded in very ancient writings, including the *Iliad* (ca. 950 B.C.). Galen described a patient who recovered after partial excision of the sternum and pericardium for recurrent abscess due to an injury. Writing about chest wounds in the thirteenth century, Theodoric noted that "the stitches should be placed . . . so that the natural heat cannot escape in any way nor the air outside be able to enter."

The introduction of firearms in the fourteenth century complicated the management of chest wounds because of uncertainty about the intrathoracic damage, and the proper care of the open pneumothorax. Many felt the wound should be kept open for drainage of blood. Consistent with many of his other revolutionary insights, Napoleon's surgeon, Baron Larrey, confirmed the sporadic observations of other surgeons about the lifesaving value of closing an open wound of the thorax. His de-

scription of the cardiopulmonary effects of an open chest wound can hardly be improved upon:

A soldier was brought to the hospital of the Fortress of Ibrahyn Bey, immediately after a wound penetrated the thorax, between the fifth and sixth true ribs. It was about 8 cm in extent. A large quantity of frothy and vermilion blood escaped from it with a hissing noise at each inspiration. His extremities were cold, pulse scarcely perceptible, countenance discolored, and respiration short and laborious; in short, he was every moment threatened with a fatal suffocation. After having examined the wound, the divided edges of the part, I immediately approximated the two lips of the wound, and retained them by means of adhesive plaster and a suitable bandage around the body. In adopting this plan, I intended only to hide from the sight of the patient and his comrades, the distressing spectacle of a hemorrhage, which would soon prove fatal; and I, therefore, thought that the effusion of blood into the cavity of the thorax, could not increase the danger. But the wound was scarcely closed, when he breathed more freely, and felt easier. The heat of the body soon returned, and the pulse rose. In a few hours he became quite calm, and to my great surprise grew better. He was cured in a very few days, and without difficulty.

The history of elective thoracic surgery is the history of airway management. By the late nineteenth century, open thoracic procedures on large animals were successfully performed along with experimentation on mechanical maintenance of ventilation. In 1904, Sauerbruch developed a negative-pressure chamber in which the operating team and the patient could be housed during operation. Under these conditions, the lung would not collapse when the chest was open. Though animal experiments gave some success, operations on patients were not rewarding. Positive-pressure systems with endotracheal intubation were also actively evolving during this fertile period of development. Orotracheal intubation with metal tubes for the treatment of croup and for the prevention of aspiration during oral surgical procedures provided the early experience that led to endotracheal anesthesia for thoracic surgery. An artificial respiration device consisting of a hand bellows and a tracheostomy tube were introduced by Fell in 1893, and modified by O'Dwyer in 1896. The latter substituted an orotracheal tube and a foot bellows with a greater volume capacity. Rudolph Matas in New Orleans advocated the use of the Fell–O'Dwyer apparatus to allow a more general availability of thoracic surgical techniques, and he introduced his own modification of the equipment in 1900. These early techniques to ventilate during thoracotomy were associated with hazards of their own. Consequently, individual surgeons were devising and reporting makeshift techniques to control the open pneumothorax associated with chest wall resections through the first third of this century. These included various packing techniques, preoperative pneumothorax for "conditioning," and suturing the lung to the parietal pleura. Improvements in laryngotracheal intubation techniques, in design and materials of tracheal tubes, and in anesthesia gradually displaced these local improvi-

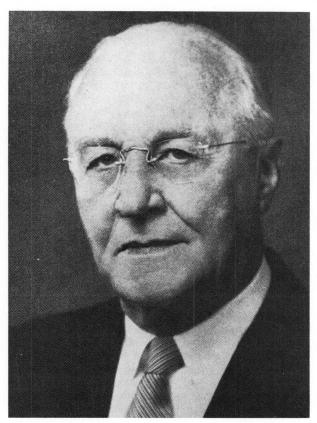

Fig. 17-1. Evarts Ambrose Graham (1883–1957). A dominant figure in the development of the field of thoracic surgery. He performed the first successful pneumonectomy (for bronchogenic carcinoma) on April 5, 1933.

dominate clinical practice as the long-predicted increase in cancers among smoking women has finally succeeded in making lung cancer the most common cancer killer of women as well as men. There is increasing evidence implicating side-stream smoke in health problems of nonsmokers, particularly children. New developments in imaging techniques, particularly involving computer-assisted tomography and nuclear-magnetic resonance are making important improvements in the accuracy of diagnosis and staging of intrathoracic diseases. Our evolving skills in fiberoptic endoscopy have opened new diagnostic and therapeutic opportunities in airway, esophageal, and pleural disorders. These techniques are resulting in early detection and surgical resection of some tumors in a preclinical stage and yielding "cure" rates previously considered to be unobtainable. Some unanticipatedly encouraging results are appearing following multimodal therapy with chemotherapy and radiation therapy as pre- or postoperative adjuvant therapy for patients with lung cancer. The diagnostic and/or therapeutic role of immunohistochemical techniques, including monoclonal antibodies, remains uncertain, though recent research in the field presents some exciting theoretic potential for important future contributions. Several centers are now reporting success with heart-lung transplantation applied to the management of young patients with a variety of end-stage cardiopulmonary diseases.

ANATOMY OF THE THORAX AND PLEURA

Anatomic correlation with clinical diagnosis in chest disease is improved because many of the bony parts of the thoracic cage are palpable and cardiac and breath sounds are transmitted through the chest wall. There are a number of anatomic factors, however, that can be quite misleading and lead to errors of analysis and judgment. The "squaring off" effect of the shoulder girdle gives the chest the physical appearance of a rectangle, tempting the examiner to forget that the skeletal chest wall is conical in shape, tapering quite sharply in the upper chest. The diaphragm rises as high as the level of the nipple; the upper part of the abdomen is overlapped by six of the ten anterior ribs and the lower four posterior ribs. The lung apices rise well above the level of the clavicles anteriorly and the scapular posteriorly. These easily overlooked anatomical facts can lead to serious errors, especially in patients with blunt trauma (Fig. 17-2). The lower ribs and costal margin overlap the liver, spleen, stomach, the upper pole of both kidneys, and the distal part of the pancreas.

The framework of the thoracic cage consists of the sternum, twelve thoracic vertebrae, ten pairs of ribs that end anteriorly in segments of cartilage, and two pairs of floating ribs (Fig. 17-3). The thoracic inlet is characterized by having a rigid structural ring formed by the sternal manubrium, the short, semicircular first ribs, and the vertebral column. As a result of its articulation with the manubrium and the attachment of the costoclavicular ligament, the clavicle participates in providing protection for the underlying vascular and neural structures that traverse the tho-

sations. A pivotal figure in most of this evolution of the field of thoracic surgery was Evarts Graham (Fig. 17-1). While a captain in the Army in 1918, he served as chairman of the Empyema Commission and made fundamental observations and recommendations about the cause and care of intrapleural infections, a major cause of death following the disastrous worldwide influenza epidemic at that time. In 1933, he performed the first successful pneumonectomy. The patient was a long-term survivor of lung cancer. Shortly following that dramatic success, the majority of thoracic surgical techniques in use today for noncardiac disease were developed, refined, and widely implemented. He was also among the first to clearly recognize the central role tobacco addiction played in the etiology of most pulmonary diseases and tumors. It is ironic that he died of the consequence of his tobacco addiction (lung cancer) even though he had quit smoking as soon as he recognized the correlation between smoking habits and lung cancer.

Though somewhat overshadowed by the dramatic developments in cardiac surgery, significant recent diagnostic, technical, and therapeutic progress has been occurring in other areas of thoracic surgery. The terrible public health consequences of tobacco addiction continue to

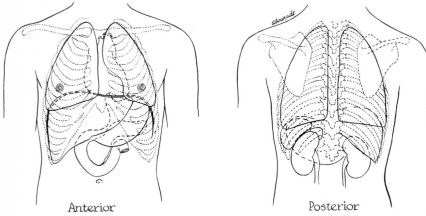

Anterior   Posterior

Fig. 17-2. The relationship of the thoracic cage to the upper abdominal viscera must be remembered to avoid overlooking concomitant abdominal injuries in patients with thoracic trauma.

racic inlet. The same rigidity that provides protection from trauma, however, leaves little room for pathologic swelling, enlarging masses, or postural adjustments with age.

The cartilages of the first six ribs have separate articulations with the sternum; the cartilages of the seventh through the tenth ribs fuse to form the costal margin before attaching to the lower margin of the sternum. As there is significant flexibility of the chest wall in children, serious trauma can be transmitted to the intrathoracic structures with little injury to the bony framework. Even though this flexibility decreases progressively with age, surprising damage can occasionally occur in the chest of adults without evidence of skeletal injury.

The pectoralis major and minor muscles constitute the principal muscular covering of the anterior thorax, and the lower margin of the pectoralis major forms the anterior axillary fold. Auscultation of the chest in the axilla often allows the best determination of breath sounds,

Fig. 17-3. The radiolucent costal cartilages and the poor projection of the sternum on anteroposterior chest x-rays make it difficult to demonstrate major injuries or abnormalities of the anterior part of the chest wall.

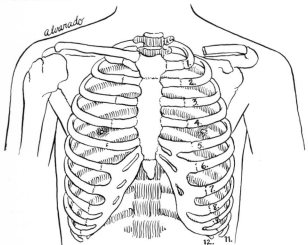

because the thoracic cage is covered only by the origins of the serratus anterior muscle in that location. The long thoracic nerve passes vertically on the axillary surface of that muscle—a point to be remembered when doing a thoracentesis or tube thoracostomy. A convergence of the latissimus dorsi and teres major muscles forms the posterior axillary fold on each side. The triangle of auscultation can often be palpated near the inferior medial border of the scapula, but the latissimus, trapezius, rhomboid, and other shoulder girdle muscles form a strong muscular coat for the posterior thorax. A disadvantage of the heavy muscle coat is the difficulty in accurately identifying specific ribs by palpation of the posterior chest wall.

The sternal angle is almost always palpable, and this allows quick identification of the second rib because of its articulation with the sternum at this location. A plane that is parallel to the floor and passes through the sternal angle of an upright patient will also pass through the fourth or fifth thoracic vertebra. The tracheal bifurcation lies in this same plane, while the apex of the aortic arch is located slightly higher. There is a gradual increase in the length of ribs from the first to the seventh and a progressive lateral displacement of the rib–costal cartilage junctions. Because of the radiolucency of the cartilages, standard anteroposterior chest x-rays may fail to document injury to the thoracic cage even though a severe blunt injury to the chest has disarticulated and fractured multiple costal cartilages.

The pleura is a serous membrane of flat mesothelial cells overlying a thin layer of connective tissue in which a vascular and lymphatic network is distributed. That part covering the lungs is referred to as the visceral pleura, and it is continuous over the pulmonary hilus and the mediastinum with the parietal pleura, which covers the inside of the chest wall and the diaphragm. While it is convenient to consider the pleura as a closed sac around the pleural cavity, that model encourages a static model that misrepresents a highly dynamic structure. The pleural surfaces behave more like a flowing syncytium across which fluids actively move (from visceral pleura to parietal pleura), actively phagocytosing cells and debris and sealing air leaks and capillary leaks. It is this physiologically active membrane that contributes to the general resistance of the pleural space to infection and the lung's remarkable ability to tolerate the trauma of surgery or injury with such a low frequency of persisting air-leak problems. With normal lung expansion the pleural cavity is completely filled and only a potential space exists. As shown in Fig. 17-4, the line of pleural reflection extends slightly beyond the lung border in each direction. This is expected because of the dynamic process of respiration and the need for the pleural sac to accommodate maximum lung expansion with deep inspiration. Conversely, with acute decreases in lung volume, such as that with lobar atelectasis, there is a limit to the pleural accommodation and fluid may be drawn into the pleural cavity to replace partially the lost lung volume.

There is no communication between the pleural cavities, but the anteromedial borders of the two pleural sacs come nearly into apposition behind the sternum. The interior border of each pleural cavity is located at the ninth rib in the midaxillary line, and the borders continue posteriorly in the eleventh intercostal space. Occasionally the pleural sac extends as low as the twelfth rib. Posteriorly, the margins of the two pleural sacs lie on the anterolateral surfaces of the vertebrae, separated by the esophagus. A retroesophageal recess is occasionally formed when the pleural margins are in near apposition, and pulmonary lesions arising in the recess are easily mistaken for mediastinal tumors or cysts. At the inferior margin of the lung hilus on each side, a double layer of mediastinal pleura is formed, the inferior pulmonary ligament.

The structures that occupy the intercostal spaces have considerable significance in relation to thoracic function,

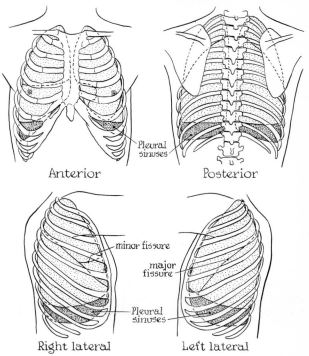

Fig. 17-4. The relation of the pulmonary lobes and pleural sinuses to the chest wall.

disease, and diagnostic procedures. The parietal pleura, for example, is well supplied with nerve endings for pain, while the visceral pleura is insensitive. Only when pulmonary disease extends to involve the parietal pleura or chest wall is pain produced. Figure 17-5 shows the structures in an intercostal space and emphasizes the layering effect of the muscles and fascia. Three layers of intercostal muscles are present in a major part of the thoracic wall, but some anatomists consider the innermost and the

Fig. 17-5. An illustration of the structures within an intercostal space. (Modified from: *Blevins CE: Anatomy of the thorax and pleura, in Shields TW (ed): General Thoracic Surgery, 2d ed. Philadelphia, Lea & Febiger, 1983, with permission.*)

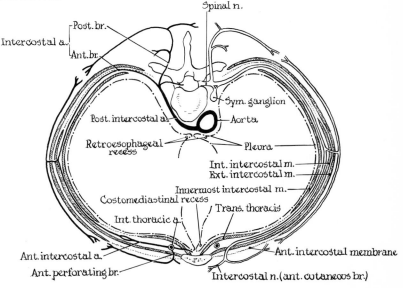

internal intercostals to be a single muscle entity. With quiet respiration the ribs are elevated by synchronous contraction of the intercostal muscles. Because the ribs of each side move as a unit in respiration, a localized painful lesion may eliminate effective function of the entire side. During quiet respiration, however, movements of the diaphragm provide approximately 75 percent of pulmonary ventilation, and temporary loss of unilateral intercostal muscle function is not a threat to breathing. With labored breathing, the muscles of the upper extremity and those cervical muscles that attach to the chest wall assist in elevation and expansion of the thorax.

The endothoracic fascia is a layer of light areolar tissue subjacent to the parietal pleura. At the apex of each hemithorax it is thickened into a more substantial layer referred to as Sibson's fascia.

The vein, artery, and nerve of each interspace are located deep to the external and internal intercostal muscles and lie just behind the lower margin of the rib. For most interspaces a smaller collateral artery runs along the top border of the rib below. There is significant overlap of neural supply by adjacent nerves, and complete anesthesia in an interspace will generally not occur unless the intercostal nerve of the adjacent space above and below and the space in question are anesthetized. To minimize the risk of lacerating the intercostal artery, a thoracentesis needle or a clamp used to perforate the pleura for insertion of a catheter should be passed across the top of the lower rib of the selected interspace.

The lymphatic drainage of the chest wall extends in both anterior and posterior directions. Lymph draining from the anterior region of the first four or five intercostal spaces passes to lymph nodes along the internal thoracic arteries. These nodes may be connected by cross anastomoses before draining into a single or double trunk that joins the thoracic duct, a right lymphatic duct, or a bronchomediastinal trunk. Lymphatics that drain the posterior and lateral regions of the intercostal spaces are tributary to lymph nodes that lie near the vertebral ends of each interspace. In the lower part of the thorax these nodes join the drainage from the posterior mediastinum to contribute to the cisterna chyli. The posterior lymph nodes of the upper thorax drain into the thoracic duct or a right lymphatic duct.

A musculofibrous floor is provided for the thorax by the diaphragm. The peripheral muscular portions of the diaphragm arise from the lower six ribs and costal cartilages, from the lumbar vertebrae (right and left crus), and from the lumbocostal arches. Additional fibers arise from the xiphoid cartilages, and all the muscular elements converge into the central tendon. The central part of the tendon underlies the pericardium, while the right and left divisions extend posteriorly. Some of the lower intercostal nerves are thought to contribute to the sensory innervation of the diaphragm, but motor innervation is supplied by the phrenic nerve on each side.

Of the three major openings in the diaphragm the aortic hiatus is most posterior. The aorta, azygos vein, and thoracic duct pass through this opening. The esophageal hiatus transmits the esophagus and vagus nerves, and only

the inferior vena cava goes through the foramen of that name.

Contemporary imaging techniques (including computer-analyzed tomographic and nuclear-magnetic resonance scanning) have increased the clinician's ability to identify anatomic relationships and their clinical significance. They have dramatically altered the preoperative assessment of both pulmonary and mediastinal lesions.

Figure 17-6 shows the cross-sectional anatomy at four different levels in the thorax associated with identifiable topographical landmarks. These studies provide considerable anatomic clarification of intrathoracic problems.

THORACIC INCISIONS

A basic knowledge of the incisions used to perform thoracic operations is helpful in understanding the postoperative course of patients and the management of complications. Because of the rigidity of the thoracic cage, most incisions for major procedures are relatively large and disrupt the integrity of muscles and bone, or cartilage, though contemporary anesthetic intubation techniques allowing single-lung anesthesia are making less destructive incisions feasible in selected cases. The extensive division of tissues and the distortion or stretching associated with the use of strong mechanical retractors often result in severe postoperative pain.

There are two principal incisions: (1) lateral thoracotomy, performed as either an anterolateral, midlateral (modified transaxillary), or posterolateral incision, and (2) median sternotomy, performed as a vertical, sternal splitting incision. Other incisions are infrequently used, either because experience has shown them to be inferior, or because they are used in unusual circumstances. The thoracoabdominal incision combines an upper abdominal incision with an incision in a lower intercostal space (sixth, seventh, or eighth) that may be carried as far posteriorly as the posterior axillary line. The costal margin and diaphragm are divided to provide an extensive exposure of the upper part of the abdomen and the retroperitoneal and posterior thoracic structures. Prolonged pain associated with incomplete healing of the costal margin, as well as complicated wound management involving two body cavities if infection occurs, has reduced the enthusiasm for this incision. Though elective use of this disabling incision is becoming less common, it is still useful for certain operations involving retroperitoneal structures (kidney, thoracoabdominal aorta), and it may be appropriate for hepatic or thoracoabdominal trauma under emergency conditions.

A bilateral transverse thoracotomy incision with transection of the sternum is rarely used at present but was employed for routine operative approach to the heart and mediastinum before confidence was gained in the median sternotomy incision. The incision generally extends from one anterior axillary line to the other, in either the third or the fourth intercostal space. For reduced exposure needs the incision may be started on the side where the principal dissection will be done and extended only a short distance

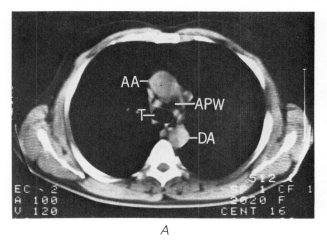

A

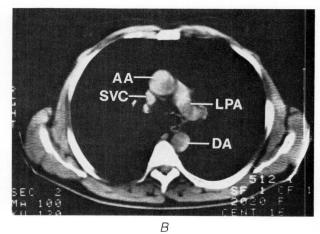

B

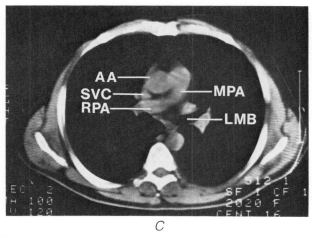

C

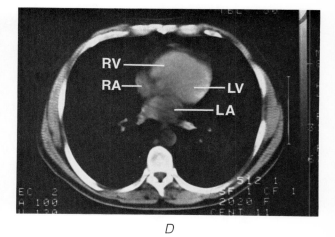

D

Fig. 17-6. Transverse sectional anatomy at four levels as shown by a CT scan of the thorax in a normal person. *A.* A transverse section at the level of the tracheal bifurcation outlines the aortico-pulmonary window, a frequent site of mediastinal lymph-node metastases in patients with bronchogenic carcinoma arising in the left lung. *B.* A section 1 cm inferior to *A* shows the origin of the left pulmonary artery and an air bubble in the esophagus as it lies immediately posterior to the origin of the left main-stem bronchus. *C.* The origin and course of the right pulmonary artery are shown at this level, and the left-upper-lobe bronchus is seen at its origin from the left main bronchus. *D.* At a lower level in the thorax the more complex mediastinal anatomy gives way to the cardiac chambers and pulmonary veins. AA = ascending aorta, DA = descending aorta, APW = aortico-pulmonary window, T = trachea, SVC = superior vena cava, LPA = left pulmonary artery, MPA = main pulmonary artery, RPA = right pulmonary artery, LMB = left main bronchus, RA = right atrium, RV = right ventricle, LA = left ventricle.

into the opposite hemithorax after transection of the sternum. The disadvantages of this incision include the longer time required to make the incision and to close the chest, compared with the median sternotomy incision. Both pleural cavities are usually entered with the transverse incision, but this may be avoided with the median sternotomy approach. In unusual circumstances, where the instruments necessary to perform median sternotomy are not available and there is urgent need to have access to

both sides of the mediastinum, this incision may still be quite useful. It also provides some cosmetic advantage in young women where bilateral submammary incisions leave much less disfiguring scars than the median sternotomy. The sternotomy can be carried out through a submammary incision with large skin flaps, though an anesthetic nipple is a relatively frequent complication of this approach.

The anterolateral and posterolateral thoracotomy incisions are used most frequently for general thoracic operations. Each one requires division of one or more major shoulder-girdle muscles, and this results in voluntary restriction of shoulder motion in the early postoperative period. Because they function as accessory muscles of respiration, it is possible that the selection and placement of the incision to minimize muscle injury could be important in an occasional patient with need for maximal muscle preservation. All patients must be encouraged to begin active shoulder and arm motion after operation, but elderly patients are especially likely to develop a restricted range of shoulder motion if not supervised carefully. The distal parts of the transected muscles lose their nerve supply and atrophy to a significant degree postop-

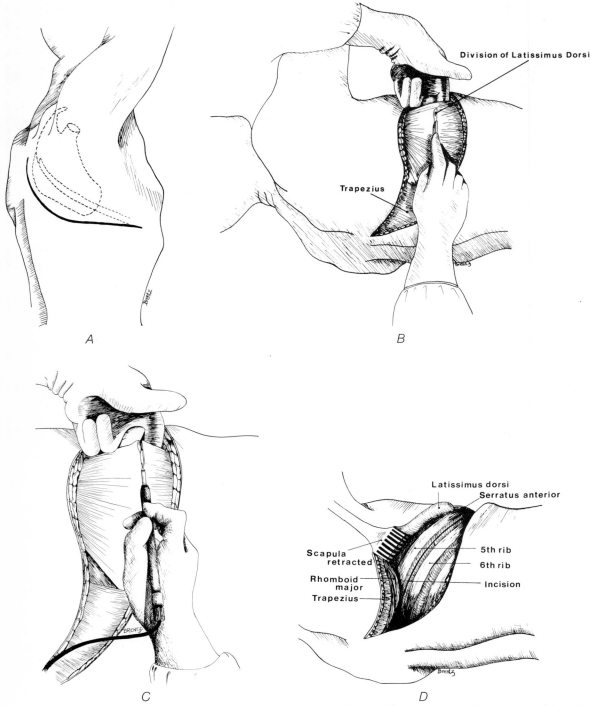

Fig. 17-7. The posterolateral thoracotomy incision. *A.* The skin incision begins near the anterior axillary line and curves posteriorly around the vertebral border of the scapula. *B.* The skin and muscle incisions are located in approximately the same position, whether the pleural cavity is entered in the fourth, fifth, or sixth intercostal space. *C.* Division of the shoulder-girdle muscles with the electrocautery may reduce blood loss and operating time. *D.* The pleural cavity is entered by dividing the intercostal muscles along the lower margin of the interspace.

eratively. Commonly, patients note a zone of reduced sensation in the skin on the caudal side of the incision for months after operation.

The posterolateral thoracotomy is used for the majority of pulmonary resections (except lung biopsy), for esophageal operations, and for the approach to the posterior mediastinum and the vertebral column (Fig. 17-7). When the intent is to enter the pleural cavity in the fifth intercostal space, the most common selection, the skin incision is begun at the anterior axillary line just below the nipple level in the male, and at the corresponding position in the female. The incision extends posteriorly below the tip of the scapula and ascends midway between the vertebral border of the scapula and the spinous processes of the vertebrae. To expose the thoracic cage it is necessary to divide part of the serratus anterior, latissimus dorsi, trapezius, and rhomboid major muscles. The pleural cavity may be entered by dividing the intercostal muscles in the chosen interspace, or by resecting the posterior two-thirds of the corresponding rib. The division of the rib posteriorly before the mechanical rib spreader is put in place may avoid accidental fracture of one or more ribs or a costochondral separation by the instrument. The injury to the rib or cartilage may increase postoperative incisional pain and prolong the restricted motion of the chest cage.

Two advantages of the anterolateral thoracotomy may be important in trauma victims and in patients with an unstable cardiovascular system. The incision can allow rapid entry into the chest, and the patient may be placed in the semisupine position on the operating table. This is tolerated better than the lateral decubitus position, and it gives the anesthesiologist the maximum control over the patient's cardiorespiratory system. The incision may be used for mediastinal operations, for some cardiac procedures, and for wedge resections of the upper and middle lobes of the lung. It is preferable to make a submammary skin incision starting at the sternal border overlying the fourth intercostal space and extending to the midaxillary line. The pectoralis major muscle and part of the pectoralis minor are divided at the level of the fourth or fifth intercostal space, and the incision is extended into the serratus anterior. By extending the chosen intercostal muscle incision posteriorly along the top of the subjacent rib it is possible to obtain a wider opening in the chest than the length of the skin incision would suggest. Still further exposure may be obtained by transecting the sternum.

As most advances in thoracic surgery have followed improvements in techniques of managing the airway, the recent widespread introduction of the double-lumen endotracheal tube has made it possible to utilize a less destructive midlateral thoracotomy incision. This incision is a modification of the transaxillary approach through the bed of the third rib that has been used extensively in some clinics for upper-lobe biopsies, for resection of small apical pulmonary blebs and pleural abrasion in patients with recurrent pneumothorax, for upper thoracic sympathectomy, and for biopsy of upper mediastinal lymph nodes or masses. By moving down the lateral chest wall several ribs, and with the advantage that single-lung anesthesia allows, good exposure can be obtained for most pulmonary resections and hilar dissections. The incision has the advantage that it requires cutting no major muscles, can be rapidly made and closed, and results in significantly less postoperative discomfort. An important requirement for adequate exposure in the incision is proper positioning of the patient. The patient is placed in a straight lateral

position with the arm at right angles (in order to facilitate mobility of the scapula). The skin incision parallels the course of the fifth rib extending from a few centimeters anterior to the middle of the lateral border of the scapula forward toward the submammary fold. The latissimus dorsi is elevated along its entire anterior border, as is the pectoralis major along its axillary border. The serratus is separated from its insertion into the fifth rib, which is removed after the periosteum is stripped. Two Tuffier retractors are placed at right angles to one another, one retracting the two muscle groups anteriorly and posteriorly and one retracting the ribs caudad and cephalad. The upper lung is allowed to collapse as dissection proceeds. Depending on the exposure desired, the skin incision parallels the course of the third, fourth, or fifth rib extending from the middle of the anterior border of the scapula at the posterior axillary fold to the anterior axillary fold (Fig. 17-8).

A hazard that is common to all the lateral thoracotomy incisions is the potential for injury to the brachial plexus and the axillary neurovascular structures from excessive displacement of the shoulder in positioning the patient on the operating table after anesthesia has been induced. By preventing posterior displacement of the shoulder this complication can be minimized.

The median sternotomy incision provides optimum exposure for anterior mediastinal lesions, and it is the principal incision used for cardiac operations. Either pleural cavity may be entered, or incision into the pleural cavity may be avoided if it is unnecessary. Disadvantages of the incision include an increased risk of infection if it is necessary to do a tracheostomy within a few days after operation, and the protracted course that occurs with infection because of involvement of the sternal fragments. An occasional patient who develops an acute wound infection also develops a severe mediastinitis associated with dehiscence of the sternal wound. The mortality rate for this complication is high but has decreased with the evolution of effective treatment.

The skin incision extends from just below the suprasternal notch to a point several centimeters below the xiphoid process (Fig. 17-9). Either an oscillating saw or a Lebsche knife and mallet may be used to split the sternum. A mechanical retractor is used to spread the incision, but the retractor blades may fracture the sternal halves with excessive pressure. Less commonly, there may be injury to the $C_8–T_1$ component of the brachial plexus, thought to be due to excessive spreading of the sternal halves and high placement of the retractor blades. In some instances a posterior fracture of the first rib can be demonstrated with special rib radiographs. After operation, patients who have had a sternotomy have less pain and less interference with pulmonary function than those who have had a lateral thoracotomy.

The pleural cavity is usually drained with one or two chest tubes connected to an underwater seal system at the conclusion of the intrathoracic portion of the operation. Each chest tube should be brought through a separate stab wound in the chest wall at least two interspaces away from the incision. If the pleural cavity is not entered in operations through a median sternotomy, it is advisable

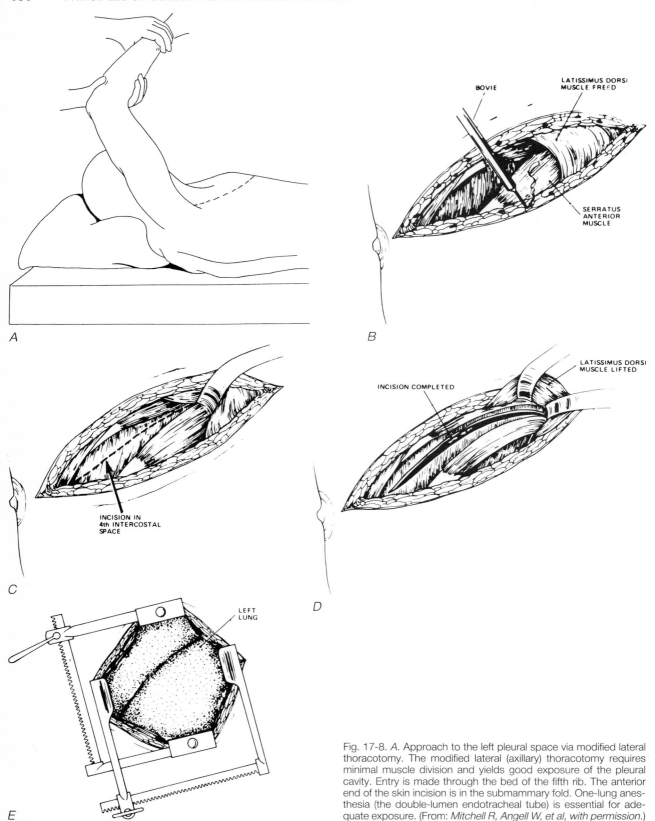

A

B

LATISSIMUS DORSI MUSCLE FREED

BOVIE

SERRATUS ANTERIOR MUSCLE

C

INCISION IN 4th INTERCOSTAL SPACE

D

INCISION COMPLETED

LATISSIMUS DORSI MUSCLE LIFTED

E

LEFT LUNG

Fig. 17-8. *A.* Approach to the left pleural space via modified lateral thoracotomy. The modified lateral (axillary) thoracotomy requires minimal muscle division and yields good exposure of the pleural cavity. Entry is made through the bed of the fifth rib. The anterior end of the skin incision is in the submammary fold. One-lung anesthesia (the double-lumen endotracheal tube) is essential for adequate exposure. (From: *Mitchell R, Angell W, et al, with permission.*)

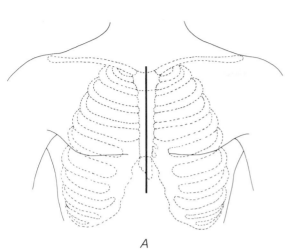

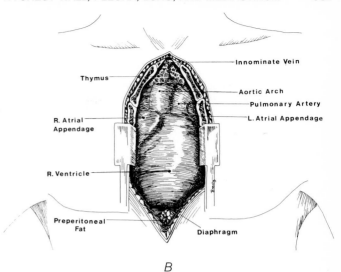

A

B

Fig. 17-9. *A*. A median sternotomy incision is outlined. *B*. Exposure of a pleural space would be made optimum by placement of mechanical retractor, rotating the patient slightly, and the use of single-lung anesthesia.

to drain the retrosternal space for 24 h with an intercostal tube that is brought out through a stab wound in the epigastrium.

PATIENT EVALUATION

As diagnostic procedures are being completed in the patient with a thoracic lesion, it is important to assess the ability of the patient to undergo operative treatment. The surgical lesion should be evaluated sufficiently to plan the soundest and most effective operative procedure. Since all operations on the chest result in some short-term respiratory disability, and many require removal or permanent alterations in function of intrathoracic organs, the surgeon must make a careful assessment of the patient's ability to withstand the contemplated procedure. This assessment includes most components of the patient's overall state of health.

The surgeon must make a preliminary decision based on an evaluation of the patient's health, the operation that would be required, the patient's age, and the complications or disability that may occur postoperatively; the potential benefit from operation must be weighed against the involved risk.

The history and physical examination, with the consequence of thoracotomy in mind, constitute the foundation of each patient's evaluation. If the patient is found to be in good health, is young, and has normal values for the hospital admission blood tests and urinalysis, little further evaluation may be necessary. Most candidates for operation, however, have a pulmonary or esophageal neoplasm, or are cigarette smokers with symptoms of chronic bronchitis, and are at least middle-aged. If the patient is a satisfactory candidate for operation, a procedure will be

required that will interfere with cardiopulmonary function, at least temporarily. During an operation, one lung will be either retracted or displaced and will contribute little, if any, to respiratory gas exchange. Further, it may be necessary to retract intermittently against the pericardium interfering with venous return to the atria or precipitating brief arrhythmias. Therefore, the functional status of the contralateral lung and the presence of preexisting cardiac disease are major determinants of the safety of the operation.

MALNUTRITION. Malnutrition increases the morbidity and mortality rate of any major surgical procedure, and an assessment of the preoperative nutritional state is important. While most emphasis has been placed on preexisting protein deficits, both fat and carbohydrate can spare protein and therefore have an effect on nitrogen balance. In clinical practice it may be difficult to separate the effects of total calorie deficit from a deficiency of protein alone. Even so, much of the data relating nutritional deficiency to postoperative complications are based on experimental or clinical effects of hypoproteinemia. There is a reduced blood volume and reduced tolerance for intraoperative bleeding in hypoproteinemic patients. Impaired antibody production, decreased lymphocyte proliferative response, and depression of the delayed skin reactivity to antigens are associated with weight loss and hypoalbuminemia and reduced host resistance to infection.

Particularly important in thoracic surgical patients are the adverse effects of protein depletion on pulmonary functions and ventilatory capacity. As skeletal muscle is catabolized during starvation, the muscle groups in the thorax, abdomen, shoulder, and diaphragm that are involved in respiration and coughing share in the unselective loss of strength that is seen in all muscles. Coupled with the increased tendency for interstitial edema associated with hypoproteinemia, the effects of protein depletion can significantly increase the risk of a major thoracic operation.

The assessment of nutritional status begins with the history and physical examination, keeping in mind that evidence of malnutrition may be quite subtle. This is especially true in the elderly and in individuals who have followed self-prescribed diets for cosmetic or social reasons. A history of weight loss, anorexia, or altered gastrointestinal function should signal the need for a more complete evaluation. The physical examination may show signs of weight loss, or suggest vitamin and mineral deficiencies. An occasional patient, however, may appear well nourished even though an underlying pathologic process has produced a serious negative nitrogen balance and early malnutrition.

Search for other evidence of deficiency should also be made. In addition to the routine hemoglobin, hematocrit, and base-line coagulation studies, particular attention should be paid to the measurement of serum proteins, electrolytes, and liver enzymes. A total lymphocyte count below 1500 cells/mm^3 should be followed up by skin testing to determine if the patient is anergic. Postoperative and posttraumatic anergic patients are at increased risk for sepsis and mortality. Any evidence of significant malnutrition, anergy, or hypoproteinemia should result in a concerted effort to correct the deficit before subjecting the patient to operation.

CARDIAC EVALUATION. The need for preoperative cardiac evaluation is based on the expected postoperative demand for increased cardiac output, the frequency of coincidental cardiac disease, and the likelihood of cardiopulmonary complications after thoracic operations. Because cardiac symptoms are sometimes masked by the symptoms of the primary thoracic disease for which the patient is being considered, the screening evaluation must be precise. A preoperative electrocardiogram must be obtained. If the history, examination, or electrocardiogram reveals any abnormality, a consultation with a cardiologist is usually in order. The development of nuclear medicine techniques for myocardial imaging and for gated radionuclide angiocardiograms has provided noninvasive methods for evaluation of suspected myocardial ischemia and for determination of ventricular functions such as cardiac output, stroke volume, and ejection fraction. Echocardiography can also be used for estimates of ventricular function, but it is not considered as reliable. For patients with evidence of significant coronary artery occlusive disease it may be appropriate to proceed to coronary arteriography if the circumstances suggest that coronary revascularization may be necessary.

In a study of 1001 patients over forty years of age subjected to noncardiac operations Goldman and associates developed a multifactorial index to estimate the risk of cardiac complications. The investigators identified nine independent correlates of life-threatening and fatal cardiac complications, shown in Table 17-1. A cardiac risk index was then computed, with each significant factor assigned a point value as illustrated in Table 17-2. By computing each patient's point total it was possible to define four risk categories. The incidence of life-threatening complications varied from 0.7 percent in Class I to 22 percent in Class IV, while cardiac deaths varied from 0.2

Table 17-1. PREOPERATIVE FACTORS RELATED TO THE DEVELOPMENT OF POSTOPERATIVE LIFE-THREATENING OR FATAL CARDIAC COMPLICATIONS

S_3 gallop or jugular-vein distention on preoperative examination
Myocardial infarction in preceding 6 months
Rhythm other than sinus, or premature atrial contractions on preoperative electrocardiogram
> 5 premature ventricular contractions/min documented at any time before operation
Intraperitoneal, intrathoracic, or aortic operation
Age >70 years
Important valvular aortic stenosis
Emergency operation
Poor general medical condition*

* Partial pressure of oxygen <60 torr, partial pressure of carbon dioxide >50 torr, potassium <3.0 or bicarbonate <20 meq/L, blood urea nitrogen >50 or creatinine >3.0 mg/dL, elevated transaminase, signs of chronic liver disease or patient bedridden from noncardia causes.
SOURCE: Reproduced from Goldman L, Caldera DL, et al: Multifactorial index of cardiac risk in noncardiac surgical procedures. *N Engl J Med* 297:845, 1977, with permission.

to 56 percent, respectively, in the same classes. On the basis of these results the investigators recommend that only truly lifesaving operations be performed on patients with risk index scores of 26 points or more.

It should be noted from Table 17-2 that 28 of the 53 points are potentially controllable, and therefore the risk of cardiac complications may be reduced by appropriate corrections. While elective operations should ordinarily

Table 17-2. COMPUTATION OF THE CARDIAC RISK INDEX

Criteria	Points
History	
Age over 70 years	5
Myorcardial infarction in previous 6 months	10
Examination	
S_3 gallop or jugular venous distention	11
Significant valvular aortic stenosis	3
Electrocardiogram	
Premature atrial contractions or rhythm other than sinus	7
More than 5 premature ventricular contractions per minute	7
General status	
P_{O_2} < 60 or P_{CO_2} > 50 torr	3
Potassium < 3.0 or HCO_3 < 20 meq/L	
BUN > 50 or Cr > 3.0 mg/dL	
Chronic liver disease	
Operation	
Intraperitoneal, intrathoracic, or aortic	3
Emergency operation	4
Total possible	53 points

SOURCE: Reproduced from Goldman L, Caldera DL, et al: Multifactorial index of cardiac risk in noncardiac surgical procedures. *N Engl J Med* 297:845, 1977, with permission.

be delayed for 6 months after a myocardial infarction, use of the cardiac index allows patients with a recent infarction to be separated into high-risk and low-risk groups.

OTHER ORGAN SYSTEMS. The preoperative evaluation should include screening tests for renal and hepatic function even in the absence of historical data that would suggest disease of those organs. Under ordinary circumstances a hospital admission biochemical profile that includes measurements of blood urea nitrogen, creatinine, serum proteins, transaminases, lactic dehydrogenase, alkaline phosphatase, and bilirubin is adequate for initial investigation. The discovery of any abnormality mandates a more detailed evaluation.

PULMONARY FUNCTION. The major consideration in evaluating the potential thoracotomy patient is whether or not the pulmonary function is adequate to tolerate the operation and the handicaps of the postoperative period. When the planned operation will result in a loss of functioning pulmonary tissue (lobectomy, pneumonectomy), there is a significant hazard of postoperative respiratory insufficiency if the patient's preoperative pulmonary function is already compromised. With rare exceptions, it is desirable to obtain objective measurements of pulmonary function. This allows the most accurate interpretation of data and provides a permanent record for comparison measurements.

No single test is available that provides an overall evaluation of lung function that would be adequate for surgical patients. Measurements of value include lung volumes, mechanics of breathing, regional lung function ("split function"), diffusion capacity, and arterial blood gases. Carefully performed spirometry forms the basis of the pulmonary-function data most used by thoracic surgeons, and the advances in technology with automated data processing allow most hospitals to have excellent pulmonary-function capability. Also, the development of electronic spirometers for office use makes it possible to perform screening tests during outpatient evaluation. If a patient has reduced pulmonary function, it is possible to begin a plan of management and determine progress before hospitalization.

Spirometry. Figure 17-10 illustrates the subdivisions of lung volume in relation to a spirographic tracing. Functional residual capacity (FRC) and residual volume (RV) may be measured either by gas-dilution techniques or by body plethysmography. Body plethysmography has the additional advantage of permitting measurements of airway resistance and compliance.

Vital capacity (VC), the amount of air that can be forcefully expelled from a maximally inflated lung position, can be a useful determination if its limitations are accepted. The predicted value decreases with age, and its measurement requires understanding as well as full cooperation from the patient. While VC is found to be normal or near-normal in patients with moderately severe obstructive airway disease, it is reduced in individuals with restrictive pulmonary disease and those with neuromuscular disease.

The mechanics of breathing permit dynamic measurements of a patient's ability to move volumes of air during

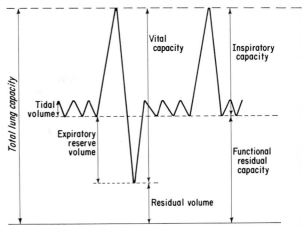

Fig. 17-10. The lung volumes and their subdivisions related to a spirograph tracing. Functional residual capacity and residual volume must be measured by other techniques.

units of time. Individual laboratories vary in the panel of function tests that are performed, sometimes on the basis of an interest in a specific part of the expiratory flow curve of the spirogram. The forced expiratory volume in 1 s (FEV_1) is the commonest flow measurement, and it seems unlikely that measurements of an earlier portion of the curve, i.e., $FEV_{0.5}$, offer any advantage over FEV_1. The FEV_3 may be useful for detecting abnormalities in airflow that are not detected by the FEV_1. For example, small-airway disease is not generally detected at high lung volume flow, which is that part specifically measured by the FEV_1. In practice the FEV_1 is usually reported as a percentage of the VC (FEV_1/VC) as well as an actual volume. It is important to note its value both ways. If the VC is significantly reduced, the ratio FEV_1/VC may be satisfactory while the actual volume exhaled is markedly abnormal. The FEV_1 is reduced in obstructive airway disease, but the degree of reduction may vary from day to day or week to week in the same individual. The FEV_1 may be the most useful test to monitor in patients with marginal pulmonary function who are being prepared for operation by aggressive respiratory therapy programs.

The forced expiratory flow 25 to 75 percent (FEV_{25-75}) is derived from the midportion of the spirogram curve and is considered to be relatively effort-independent. It is also designated as the maximum midexpiratory flow rate (MMFR), and it is recorded in liters per second. For surgical patients any flow rates below 1 L/s suggest caution in considering thoracotomy without an effort to improve pulmonary function.

A test that is effort-dependent is the maximal voluntary ventilation (MVV), performed by having the patient inhale as deeply and rapidly as possible for 10, 12, or 15 s. Although FEV_1 and MVV are expressed in volumes, they are really flow rates since they are measurements per unit of time. The MVV measures the status of the respiratory muscles, the compliance of the lung-thorax system, and airway resistance. Because of relatively large variations in normal values, only large reductions in MVV are truly

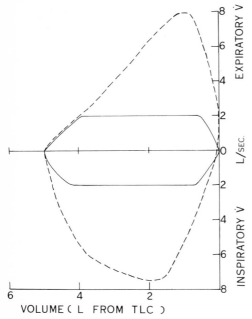

Fig. 17-11. A fixed obstruction in the trachea markedly alters the maximum expiratory flow-volume curve (MEFV). The normal MEFV is shown by the interrupted line. (Reproduced from: *Hyatt RE: Evaluation of major airway lesions using the flow-volume loop. Ann Otol Rhinol Laryngol 84:635, 1975, with permission.*)

significant. Moderate or severe obstructive airway disease invariably decreases the MVV, but patients with pure restrictive lung disease may have normal values for this test. The MVV usually correlates well with the FEV_1, and the expected relationship is $FEV_1 \times 34$ for males, $FEV_1 \times 40$ for females. If the actual measured value fails to correlate with the calculated value, it suggests a poor effort or a fatigued patient. In most laboratories the patient is given an aerosol of a sympathomimetic amine bronchodilator and the spirometry is repeated. An improvement, sometimes significant, in flow rates and in VC may occur. A failure of severely decreased function values to improve does not mean that the patient has irreversible pulmonary disease. Aggressive therapy with the patient's cooperation can often improve pulmonary function, a benefit both to the patient's comfort and to the operative procedure.

The significance of early small-airway disease that is not demonstrated by standard spirometry has not been defined for thoracic surgical patients. Nevertheless, there is interest in two tests that provide data useful in the understanding of pulmonary function. The maximal expiratory flow-volumes curve (MEFV) is inscribed from a plot of airflow against the volume of vital capacity. This relationship of the data may provide information not given by a spirogram. Major airway lesions may distort the MEFV curve; Fig. 17-11 shows the abnormality seen with fixed obstruction of the trachea. The closing volume (CV) depends on the fact that gravity results in a greater negative pressure at the apex of the lung than at the base in an upright person. That lung volume at which lung units in

the dependent regions of the lung cease to ventilate, presumably because of airway closure, is referred to as the CV. The measurement can be made by monitoring the concentration of nitrogen in the exhaled gas during a vital-capacity maneuver after inspiration of a bolus of 100% oxygen. ^{133}Xe or another gas may be used as the marker. An abrupt increase in the marker concentration in the terminal portion of the vital-capacity curve is the CV, and the value is expressed as a percentage of the vital capacity. Normally, VC is above the RV and below the end-tidal point. The CV increases with age, and it is increased in smokers, in peripheral obstructive airway disease, and in congestive heart failure.

The pulmonary-function values obtained with spirometry in the individual patient must be compared with those obtained from other individuals of the same sex, age, and height who are known to be free of pulmonary disease. Data obtained from the spirometric studies in hundreds of normal males and females form the basis for prediction nomograms that facilitate that comparison. Figure 17-12 shows a prediction nomogram developed from studies of 422 normal adult males in a Veterans Administration–Army Cooperative Study of Pulmonary Function. To demonstrate the considerable information about the individual patient's pulmonary function that may be accumulated, Table 17-3 lists the values for a healthy young male breathing air at sea level. In addition to the studies shown, patients with marginal pulmonary function may require measurements of diffusing capacity, regional lung function with radionuclides, and exercise testing.

Blood-Gas Determination. A measurement of the arterial blood gases and pH should be routine in the preoperative evaluation of a candidate for thoracic surgery. It would be an unusual situation in which the decision to advise operation depended solely on a single measurement of arterial oxygen or carbon dioxide tension. Even so, an occasional patient is discovered to have hypoxemia or CO_2 retention that was not suspected on the basis of clinical examination or spirometry. A measurement of the Pa_{CO_2} provides an immediate indication of the patient's alveolar ventilation; any value above 46 torr means that there is hypoventilation. There are multiple causes for this, and the specific reason should be sought in each patient. The ability of the lungs to excrete CO_2 is remarkable, and any persistent elevation of Pa_{CO_2} in a patient who might other-

Fig. 17-12. A prediction nomogram for pulmonary function in men. FRC, functional residual capacity; TLC, total lung capacity; RV, residual volume; $FEV_{0.5}$, 0.5-s forced expiratory volume; MVV_F, maximal voluntary ventilation (free); FEV_1, 1-s forced expiratory volume; FVC, forced vital capacity. The predicted values for FRC and TLC can be read directly from the left-hand scale, based on the patient's height. The scale at the bottom is for convenience in converting centimeters to inches. RV/TLC (%) may be used directly from the age scale. For the other predicted values, lay a straightedge between patient height and age. Predicted normal values can be read directly from the joints where the straightedge crosses the RV, $FEV_{0.5}$, MW_F, FEV_1, and FVC scales. (Reproduced from: *Boren HC, Kory RC, Syner JC: The Veterans Administration–Army Cooperative Study of Pulmonary Function: II. The lung volume and its subdivisions in normal men. Am J Med 41:96, 1986, with permission.*)

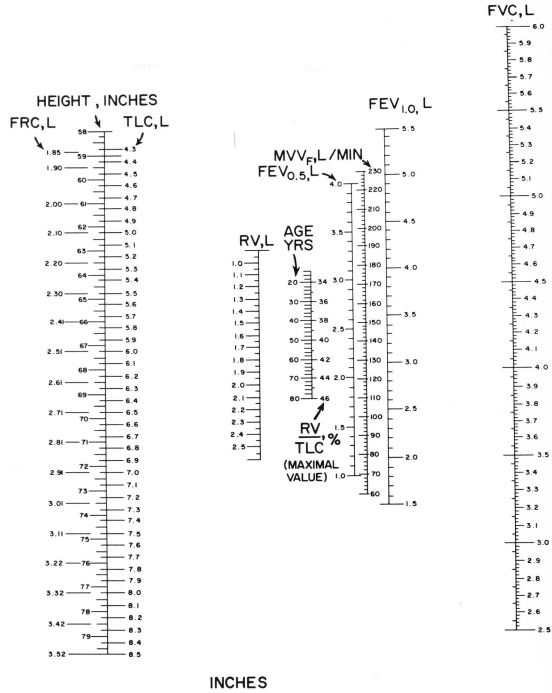

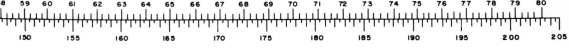

Table 17-3. TYPICAL VALUES IN PULMONARY
FUNCTION TESTS*

Lung volumes:	
Inspiratory capacity, mL	3600
Expiratory reserve volume, mL	1200
Vital capacity, mL	4800
Residual volume (RV), mL	1200
Functional residual capacity, mL	2400
Thoracic gas volume, mL	2400
Total lung capacity (TLC), mL	6000
RV/TLC ×100, %	20
Ventilation:	
Tidal volume, mL	500
Respiratory dead space, mL	150
Respirations/min	12
Minute volume, mL/min	6000
Alveolar ventilation, mL	4200
Mechanics of breathing:	
Maximal voluntary ventilation, L/min	125–170
Forced expiratory volume, % in 1 s	83
Forced expiratory volume, % in 3 s	97
Maximal expiratory flow rate (for 1 L), L/min	400
Maximal inspiration flow rate (for 1 L), L/min	300
Compliance of lungs and thoracic cage, L/cmH$_2$O	0.1
Compliance of lungs, L/cmH$_2$O	0.2
Airway resistance, cmH$_2$O/L/s	1.6
Alveolar ventilation/pulmonary capillary blood flow:	
Alveolar ventilation, L/min/blood flow, L/min	0.8
Physiologic shunt/cardiac output ×100, %	<7
Physiologic dead space/tidal volume ×100, %	<30
Arterial blood:	
Oxygen tension, torr	100
Carbon dioxide tension, torr	40
Oxygen tension (100% inhaled oxygen), torr	640
Alveolar-arterial P_{O_2} difference (100% inhaled oxygen), torr	33
Oxygen saturation (% saturation of hemoglobin)	97.1
pH	7.4

* The values shown are those of a resting young male, 1.7 m^2 body surface area, breathing room air at sea level, except where specified otherwise.
SOURCE: Modified from Comroe JH Jr: *The Lung,* 2d ed. Year Book Medical Publishers, Chicago, 1962, with permission.

wise be considered a candidate for a major thoracotomy suggests serious abnormalities in distribution of ventilation and perfusion. Most operations will temporarily increase the ventilation-perfusion abnormality. A mild elevation of the Pa_{CO_2} in a patient with chronic lung disease may be treated aggressively to improve pulmonary function and allow the patient to be considered for operation. If pulmonary resection is contemplated in such an individual, the risk of postoperative respiratory failure is high

and the decision to operate may depend on whether functioning pulmonary tissue would be removed.

The measurement of arterial Pa_{O_2} is valuable in the preoperative assessment of pulmonary function, but the number reported must be viewed with a consideration of the possibilities for error in its measurement. At sea level the normal Pa_{O_2} is above 85 torr. It is remarkable, however, how seldom one sees a patient with even minimal pulmonary disease who has an arterial oxygen tension in the normal range. The majority of patients considered by a thoracic surgeon have a Pa_{O_2} of 80 torr or below, and values in the range of 70 to 80 torr do not suggest unusual risk in the absence of other signals of caution. If the Pa_{O_2} is below 70 torr, an attempt should be made to determine the cause and to improve the patient's respiratory exchange. The possibilities include right-to-left shunting as a result of the thoracic disease for which the patient is being considered, uneven distribution of ventilation and perfusion, or diffusion barrier. More sophisticated pulmonary function tests may be indicated, including determination of alveolar-arterial oxygen difference, calculation of right-to-left shunt fraction, and split pulmonary function.

Other Specialized Tests. A specialized test of lung function that has been especially helpful for patients with compromised pulmonary reserve determined by spirometry is radionuclide perfusion scanning for regional lung function. This technique has replaced bronchospirometry for measuring the separate contributions of the right and left lungs to overall pulmonary function, and the method is often referred to as a "split-function" study. The data can be obtained by comparing the counts over each lung during 99 mTc perfusion scanning, or more detailed information may be utilized if both ventilation and perfusion scanning are performed.

The practical value of the split-function studies is that postoperative VC and FEV$_1$ can be predicted for the patient who may require pneumonectomy for adequate resection of a bronchial neoplasm (predicted postoperative FEV$_1$ = preoperative FEV$_1$ × percent perfusion in noninvolved lung). Even though a patient may require only a lobectomy for resection of a pulmonary neoplasm, the effects of a major thoracotomy can be likened to a "functional pneumonectomy" in the early postoperative period and can be expected to reduce pulmonary function by approximately 50 percent. This is particularly true if there is significant preoperative reduction in pulmonary function.

In an important prospective study Boysen and associates demonstrated the validity of the split-function concept in a group of patients with impaired ventilatory function (preoperative FEV$_1$ <2.0 L). If the predicted postoperative FEV$_1$ exceeded 800 mL, they considered the patients to be acceptable candidates for pulmonary resection up to and including a pneumonectomy. The perioperative mortality in their series was 15 percent, a figure considered acceptable for major pulmonary resections in extremely high-risk patients. Other investigators have corroborated their data and have shown the measured values for FEV$_1$ after a pneumonectomy correlated closely with the predicted values. Figure 17-13 illustrates the use of a split-function study to decide that a patient with severely decreased pulmonary function is a reasonable risk for pneumonectomy.

In recent years there has been increasing interest in exercise testing for patients who are candidates for pulmonary resection but have impaired pulmonary function. It is particularly indicated for those patients who have reasonable exercise capability despite severe obstructive airway disease. It may be performed as a simple graded exercise test using a treadmill, or it may be done as progressive incremental exercise on a bicycle ergometer with simultaneous respiratory gas analysis. With the treadmill test, the speed is increased every 2 min until 3 mi/h is reached. The elevation is raised in increments to 10°, and patients who complete the test are good risks to tolerate pneumonectomy even with significant impairment on spirometry. By combining respiratory gas analysis with ergometer testing, more sophisticated data can be obtained for correlation of oxygen consumption with work capacity.

Unilateral balloon occlusion of the pulmonary artery with right-heart catheterization is only rarely indicated in the preoperative evaluation of patients who require a major pulmonary resection. Normally, pulmonary vascular resistance decreases with exercise and with pneumonectomy the remaining lung accepts the entire pulmonary blood flow without development of pulmonary hypertension. In a very occasional patient, occlusion of one pulmonary artery results in pulmonary hypertension to levels above 30 torr, and this has been correlated with excessive mortality after pneumonectomy. This test is only done in circumstances where there is conflicting information from the other tests of pulmonary function.

Years of experience and numerous studies have shown that there is no data-analysis technique that will absolutely separate the operable patient from the inoperable. Instead, the goal of preoperative evaluation is to separate patients into low- and high-risk groups. Of the standard function tests, surgeons have come to place the greatest reliance on the expiratory flow rates and MVV as the critical determinants of operability for the patient with reduced function from respiratory disease, advanced age, or chronic illness. Mittman reported a 9 percent cardiopulmonary mortality rate in patients with a maximum breathing capacity (MBC—now called the maximal voluntary ventilation) greater than 50 percent of the predicted value. Those patients whose MBC was less than 50 percent had a 45 percent cardiopulmonary mortality rate after thoracotomy. Miller reported similar results for patients who underwent pneumonectomy, with a slightly lower mortality for those who had a lobectomy.

Other studies have failed to support a precise correlation between a given level of reduced pulmonary function and an expected mortality risk. The continuing improvements in facilities and technology for postoperative care have influenced surgeons to become more aggressive in advising thoracotomy for patients with compromised pulmonary function. In a recent report, Peters and associates presented their results with pulmonary resection in a

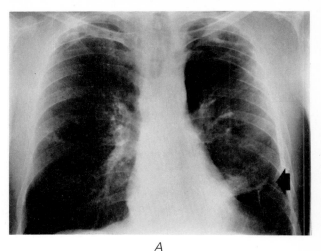

A

Patient - 58 y.o. white male

Spirometry	Measured	Predicted	% Predicted
FEV_1	1.72 liters	3.14 liters	55
FVC	2.47	4.37	57
Peak Flow	2.90 liters/s	8.63 liters/s	34
MVV	66.0 liters/min	130.0 liters/min	49

B

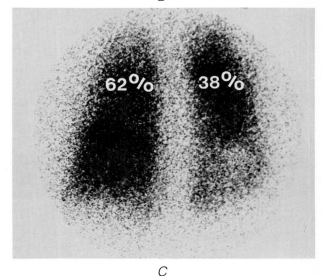

C

Fig. 17-13. An example of the use of radioisotope lung scanning for the prediction of postpneumonectomy pulmonary function. *A*. The P-A chest x-ray of a fifty-eight-year-old man with a recurrent bronchiolo-alveolar cell carcinoma in the left lower lobe. *B*. The results of preoperative spirometry show marked reduction in measured values for expiratory flow rates, vital capacity, and maximum voluntary ventilation. *C*. A lung perfusion scan with macroaggregated radioalbumin shows that approximately 62 percent of pulmonary blood flow is directed to the right lung. Therefore, the predicted values for postoperative vital capacity and FEV_1 after left pneumonectomy would be 1.5 and 1.0 L, respectively. These values were marginal but acceptable, and the patient underwent successful pneumonectomy. The actual measured FEV_1 2 weeks after operation was 1.02 L.

group of 22 patients with impaired pulmonary function (FEV_{25-75} less than 1 L/s and FEV_1 less than 70 percent) and recorded only two postoperative deaths. Neither was caused by pulmonary insufficiency. The authors speculated that the low mortality rate was due to the fact that vital capacity was preserved in these patients despite major obstructive disease of the airways. An earlier report by Bryant also suggested a critical relationship between vital capacity and operative results in patients with compromised pulmonary function.

The interest in providing a satisfactory evaluation of the patient before thoracic operation must not obscure the ultimate purpose of the evaluation—to provide the patient with whatever physical and mental preparation is needed. Many patients are smokers, and every effort should be made to persuade them to stop smoking before operation, preferably for 2 weeks or more. All authors agree that the character and amount of bronchial secretions have major impact on postoperative morbidity. Aggressive attention to reducing the amount and tenacity of the secretions must be made before the operation. The etiology of pulmonary infection should be identified and treated intensively, using respiratory therapy, physical therapy, or appropriate techniques. Thoracic operations often are associated with prolonged stays in intensive care units, with multiple chest tubes, with invasive catheters of several types, and with considerable pain. All patients deserve a full explanation of what to expect from the operation, presented in a way that assures them of excellence in their medical care and concern for their well-being.

POSTTHORACOTOMY CONSIDERATIONS (See Also Chapter 12)

PULMONARY FUNCTION CHANGES. Significant pathophysiologic changes in pulmonary function follow major thoracic and abdominal operations. Upper abdominal procedures and thoracic operations produce similar changes in pulmonary function and have similar complications. The magnitude of the changes is affected by preexisting bronchopulmonary disease, length of the operation, postoperative analgesics, and immobilization in bed. Patients without pulmonary disease develop similar changes and are subject to similar complications. The pulmonary changes seen relate to: (1) lung volumes, (2) ventilatory patterns, (3) respiratory gas exchange, and (4) defense mechanisms.

Lung Volume. Total lung capacity and each of its subdivisions are significantly reduced after abdominal or thoracic operations. Vital capacity is reduced by 25 to 50 percent or more, with the maximum reduction occurring during the first 4 days after operation. Similarly, functional residual capacity and expiratory reserve volume are decreased, with a gradual return toward normal beginning in the second week after operation. If a pulmonary resection has been performed, the magnitude of change is even greater and is proportional to the amount of functioning lung that was removed. The reduction in

lung volumes is often accompanied by an increase in the closing volume to potentiate the development of atelectasis.

Ventilatory Pattern. The sedative effect of the anesthetic agent and the postoperative analgesics, combined with the severe pain of the thoracotomy incision, produces sharp reductions in tidal volume after operation. The expected response is an increase in respiratory rate sufficient to maintain minute ventilation. Unfortunately, the parenteral narcotics ordinarily used to manage postoperative pain all depress the respiratory center, inhibiting the rate increase and leading to carbon dioxide retention and hypoxemia.

An equally important effect of the changes in ventilatory pattern is the sharp reduction or elimination of the normal periodic hyperinflations (sighs). Normal adults sigh at the rate of nine or ten times per hour under quiet conditions. With loss of periodic hyperinflations, there is closure of lung units and a reduction in compliance.

Gas Exchange. Decreases in Pa_{O_2} and mild elevations of Pa_{CO_2} are frequent as patients recover from anesthesia. However, Pa_{CO_2} generally returns to normal or below normal in the early postoperative period, while Pa_{O_2} remains depressed during the first week. The factors responsible for reduction in the Pa_{O_2} include abnormal ventilation-perfusion relationships and intrapulmonary shunting associated with closure of terminal lung units.

Pulmonary Defense Mechanisms. The lung is normally protected against inhaled particulate matter and microbes by several mechanisms. The cough reflex defends the upper airways against inhaled or aspirated material in the tracheobronchial tree. Clearance of inhaled particles and microbes from the lower airways is dependent on the mucociliary system, and the alveoli are defended by mucociliary transport, lymphatic drainage, and the alveolar macrophages. Since coughing is inhibited by several mechanisms in the postoperative period, there is significant impairment of that defense mechanism. Ciliary function is decreased, and multiple factors, including arterial hypoxemia, depress the activity of alveolar macrophages. Finally, the composition and physical properties of mucus are altered in a way that reduces the effectiveness of the mucociliary transport system.

COMPLICATIONS. Pulmonary complications of thoracic operations have their origins in these changes and usually begin in the operating room or soon thereafter. The principal pulmonary complications consist of obstructive atelectasis and respiratory infections, and it is possible to consider each of these problems in terms of the complex of factors that contribute to their development.

Atelectasis means closure of lung units, and it exists as microatelectasis, a diffuse sublobular form not visible on chest x-rays, and macroatelectasis, the collapse of a segment, lobe, or entire lung. The three mechanisms that are considered responsible for atelectasis are accentuations of the postoperative pathophysiologic changes described earlier: (1) retained bronchopulmonary secretions, (2) decreased sighing, and (3) decreased expiratory reserve volume.

Retention of secretions is a major cause of atelectasis in

patients with chronic bronchitis. It is more subtle in patients with normal lungs though they also develop either microatelectasis or macroatelectasis. Decreased sighing and reduced tidal volume contribute to the reduced compliance in the postoperative period. Unless reversed by voluntary efforts at deep breathing, induced coughing, or attentive respiratory care techniques, these changes will contribute to the development of both forms of atelectasis. Similarly, the postoperative reductions in lung volumes are related to airway closure that is associated with the changes in ventilatory pattern. The critical relationship may be between the reduced expiratory reserve volume (ERV) and CV. Normally, CV is above residual volume but below the end-tidal point. In the postoperative state with the expected reduction in ERV, the CV may exceed the ERV and be located above the end-tidal point. Under these circumstances, the peripheral airways are subjected to compression and closure during tidal breathing. For some patients the risk of atelectasis is greater because of preexisting abnormalities in ERV and CV. For example, elderly patients and smokers have an increased CV and patients with obstructive airway disease have an increased CV and a decreased ERV. These circumstances potentiate the opportunity for airway closure and significant atelectasis.

Postoperative bronchopulmonary infectious complications consist of tracheobronchitis and pneumonitis. While these complications occur in normal persons, their incidence is higher in patients with preexisting chronic airway disease. Decreased cough, atelectasis, reduced mucociliary clearance of inhaled particles and bacteria, pain, and analgesic drugs all contribute to these infectious complications. Interference with the mucociliary clearance mechanism leads to rapid bacterial proliferation distal to obstruction in an area of atelectasis. Of equal importance has been the demonstration that the respiratory tract becomes colonized with gram-negative bacilli, particularly in the presence of tracheal intubation, coma, hypotension, hypoxia, acidosis, and azotemia. Many of these conditions exist in the postoperative period of patients subjected to major thoracic procedures.

PAIN CONTROL. In the first few postoperative days effective management of incisional pain is of central importance in the maintenance of adequate ventilation. The pain that accompanies the thoracotomy is severe and disabling. Unless well managed, it will cause hypoventilation, retention of secretions, atelectasis, hypoxia, hypoxemia, shallow and ineffective respiratory effort, and pneumonia. It is a constant challenge to find the delicate balance between giving patients enough pain medication so that they are able to cough, without giving them so much that they lose their drive to do so.

In most centers, pain is managed by parenteral narcotics administered intramuscularly or intravenously, on a fixed schedule (by-the-clock) or on-demand (p.r.n.). Particularly when given p.r.n., these techniques are associated with the likelihood of swings in levels from obtundation with respiratory depression and suppression of cough to frightened and agitated patients who hurt too much to move. If parenteral narcotics are to be the primary means

for postthoracotomy pain control, they should probably be given by I.V. drip in a dose carefully regulated by observation to provide adequate continuous pain relief without allowing undue somnolence. Success with this approach requires careful preoperative education of the patient and close nursing care. Nausea and vomiting are frequent side effects.

Some surgeons have reported success with intraoperative intercostal blocks. Either short-acting (lidocaine) or long-acting (bupivacaine) agents can be given but great care must be taken to avoid inadvertent intravascular or subdural injection. Severe vasomotor hypotension has occasionally been reported following this technique, and the patient should be monitored closely whenever it is used. More recently, several investigators have advocated intercostal nerve cryoanalgesia and have reported excellent incisional pain relief by this nerve-freezing approach. Maiwand et al. have reviewed their experience in 600 consecutive cases; the technique is now routine in their unit. Just before the chest is closed, each appropriate nerve receives one 30-s exposure to the probe. While pulmonary function and gas exchange were not uniformly improved over that expected from more conventional management, patients were more comfortable and active, and analgesic medication usage was reduced.

In the mid-1970s opiate receptors were identified in the spinal cord and their specific mediators, endorphins and enkephalin, were characterized. Since that time, active investigation on both sides of the Atlantic has resulted in many highly encouraging reports advocating the use of continuous epidural infusion of preservative-free morphine in doses near 0.1 mg/h. The narcotics can be administered through either a thoracic or a lumbar epidural catheter. While early reports suggested that the obviously more comfortable patients had improved postoperative ventilation characteristics, in a recent controlled, comparative study, Larsen and his group failed to confirm that expectation. Analog pain scores were ordinarily greatly improved, but the profound postoperative decrease in the forced vital capacity and other pulmonary function parameters and the drop in arterial oxygen tension occurred equally in all groups.

Advances in anesthesia techniques, particularly improvements in the design of the various double-lumen endotracheal tubes used with or without high-frequency jet ventilation, have offered the surgeon new options for reducing postthoracotomy pain. The need for wide exposure for delicate hilar dissection was clear when the dissection was carried out around a retracted but filled, moving lung. The ability to work in the chest with a fully deflated lung is encouraging surgeons to seek less traumatic means for entry into the chest. Urschel has reported a large series of lobar resections in both chest cavities through a median sternotomy. The extensive experience with this incision in the open-heart surgery population has demonstrated that it is much less painful and much better tolerated physiologically. Others have worked to improve the straight lateral, or modified axillary incision to allow major resections without the necessity of dividing the muscles to the shoulder girdle. In that lateral incision no major muscles need be cut, as the latissimus is elevated and retracted posteriorly, and the serratus is split at its insertion into the rib overlying the periosteal bed (usually the fifth) through which the chest is to be entered. This incision is rapidly opened, rapidly closed, and leaves a chest wall with more functional integrity. Successful use of either of these incisions requires one-lung anesthesia.

THORACIC INJURIES

General Considerations

The leading cause of death, hospitalization, and short- and long-term disability for all ages from the end of the first year through the forty-fifth year of life is trauma. Twenty-five percent of all trauma deaths are due to chest injuries alone, and respiratory problems contribute significantly in 75 percent of traumatic deaths. It is not surprising that this should be so, for the respiratory system is basically a simple mechanical system of bellows, pumps, and hydraulics that requires smooth coordination of all its elements and that works on a very small margin of safety. Physical disruption of the integrity of the system, as may be expected in trauma, must be corrected rapidly or irreversible damage resulting from hypoxia in vital structures will occur. With complete loss of oxygen and with normal tissue oxygen demands (e.g., normal ambient temperature), such damage occurs after only 4 min. Lesser disruptions of delivery extend the tolerance time, but it should be apparent that accurate diagnosis of the failing or disrupted elements of the system and their prompt correction is delayed at progressive peril to the patient.

PROGRESSING TRAUMA. Trauma is a dynamic event. Injury does not stop at the moment of impact or penetration. Continued muscular effort by the patient, or movement of disrupted parts during resuscitation or transport, can quickly convert a stabilized cardiorespiratory system into an unstable one with the development of new life-threatening factors. There is always some progressive evolution of the acute injury that can create tension or fluid in spaces unable to accommodate them without dire consequences. In assessing and managing the patient with chest injury, it is especially important to recognize this propensity for continuing alterations in physiology and function.

The general considerations regarding the management of the injured patient are discussed in Chapter 6. The pre-injury cardiopulmonary functional status must be carefully considered. The rib fracture or modest pneumothorax that is well tolerated without hospitalization in a healthy young man may lead to pneumonia, empyema, or death in an older patient with chronic airway disease. The patient with preexisting cardiac disease is particularly vulnerable to the development of pulmonary edema and hypoxia that may occur with the rapid administration of intravenous fluids during resuscitation.

A rapid but perceptive overall evaluation of the patient must be carried out whether the injury is thought to be serious or not. Chest trauma is usually associated with other injuries, and the overlap of the upper part of the abdomen by the thoracic cage provides a border zone difficult to assess and often the site of combination injuries. Particularly challenging are those patients who cannot describe symptoms, because of associated head injuries or profound shock. The importance of attending to the whole patient and the other progressive or subtle injuries must be emphasized, but this section will focus on those problems that result from injuries to the chest and most of its contents.

TYPES OF INJURIES. Injuries to the chest are often classified according to the type of insult that caused the damage. Depending on the setting (military or civilian, urban or rural), the predominant injury will differ. High-velocity penetrating wounds produce most of the military injuries; low-velocity gunshot wounds are replacing knife wounds as the most common in urban civilian populations; blunt injuries from motor vehicular accidents make up the majority of nonurban injuries. Penetrating wounds are becoming more frequent in suburban and rural areas as violent personal crimes increase, and blunt injuries are increasing in frequency in urban areas as the incidence of falls and jumps from buildings increases.

The mortality rate of major blunt injuries has been reduced steadily during the past quarter century, but complications and death associated with pulmonary contusion, posttraumatic pulmonary insufficiency, and trauma to the heart and great vessels are still impressive. It is especially characteristic of blunt injuries that the maximal extent of cardiopulmonary functional loss and often the complete diagnosis require several days for development.

Among the penetrating wounds that are especially treacherous are those in the lower thoracic region. The diaphragm rises to the level of the nipples in normal expiration and management of penetration in this region is dominated by concern that subdiaphragmatic viscera may have been penetrated. Some surgeons believe that a stab wound of the left lower part of the chest mandates early abdominal exploration on the basis that the knife may have injured the spleen, stomach, or colon. As the negative pressure in the chest aspirates fluid into the chest through the diaphragm wound, the abdominal findings in these cases may be missing or late in coming and peritoneal lavage is notoriously misleading. The consequence of error is costly. Because the liver is usually the abdominal structure injured by right-sided stab wounds that penetrate the diaphragm, it may be reasonable to delay exploration until the patient is more stabilized. Early abdominal exploration is indicated if there is evidence of continuing blood loss. The late consequence of holes in the diaphragm probably justifies operative repair as soon as safe in all but a few highly selected patients.

Whatever the cause, the principles of management should remain focused on the mechanical systems involved: the pump (the heart, see Chapter 19), the hydraulics (the vessels, see Chapter 20), and the bellows (the suction-blow system that draws atmospheric air into the alveoli and expels it). We will discuss the problems associated with traumatic failure of the bellows and the deliv-

Aligning the airway for intubation

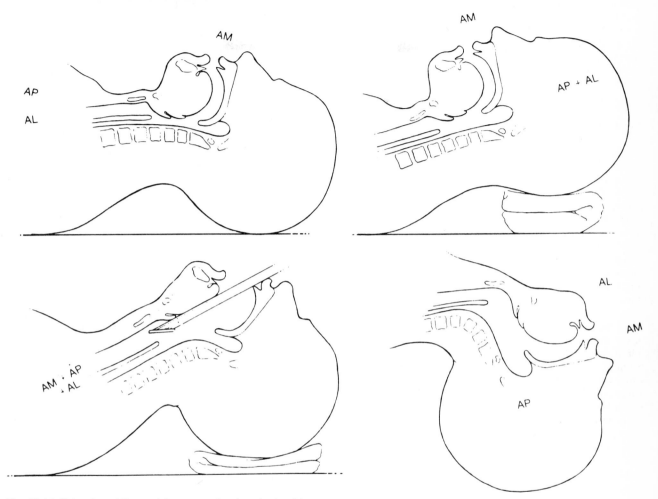

Fig. 17-14. Extension of the neck is commonly misunderstood to be the proper position for airway access. As shown, the neck should be *flexed* with the chin elevated in order to straighten the airway for visualization of cords of optimum clearing of supralaryngeal obstructions.

ery and removal of certain gases to and from the blood, but obviously the pump must be working and the vessels must have the integrity and suitable contents to transport the gases to and from the tissues.

Conditions Requiring Urgent Correction

AIRWAY OBSTRUCTION. Most patients with major disruption of the airway leading to obstruction will not survive initial accident; the leading cause of death at the accident site is airway obstruction. At any stage of the early resuscitation and transportation of the patient, correctable airway obstruction may occur. The oropharynx should be cleared of mechanical debris and the chin and neck positioned to facilitate opening the posterior pharynx. Until the stability of the cervical vertebrae has been

ascertained, the neck should only be positioned by an anterior chin-thrust motion while applying continuous cephalad traction to the head (Fig. 17-14). If the upper airway remains at risk after clearing and positioning, access to the endotrachea for control is indicated. If cervical spine injury is suspected and midface soft tissue damage is not extensive, nasotracheal intubation is preferred, even though the small caliber of the nasotracheal tube prevents subsequent flexible bronchoscopic examination. If it can be safely done, orotracheal intubation with a size 8 mm or larger endotracheal tube is indicated.

If the equipment or expertise is not available, or if the upper airway injury precludes safe access to the cords from above, cricothyroidotomy should be performed. If high-pressure oxygen is available, catheter jet ventilation may be used (percutaneous passage of cricothyroid membrane catheter, 12 gauge or larger) while the patient is being stabilized and arrangements for tracheal intubation are being completed.

TENSION PNEUMOTHORAX. When an injury to the lung parenchyma has occurred that allows air to enter the pleural space with each respiratory effort, and when the flap-valve effect of the injury prevents that air from reentering the bronchial tree for egress through the trachea during expiration, tension develops within the pleural space until equilibration with the negative pressures the patient is able to generate is reached; at that time effective ventilation ceases and venous blood can no longer enter the chest. The mechanics of a developing tension pneumothorax may not be obvious when the patient is first seen. Pain may be the primary complaint, with no evidence of respiratory distress. But if the lung wound is behaving as a check valve, some air will escape into the pleural cavity with each inspiration or with each cough. Gradually, intrapleural pressure will build up, the lung collapses, and tension pneumothorax may develop. A shift of the mediastinum and compression of the large veins result in a decreased cardiac output that may lead to sudden death.

The diagnosis should be instantly made by the observation of a patient with dilated neck veins making respiratory effort but not respiratory motions, and unable to move air. It is immediately confirmed by the hyperresonant percussion note over the injured hemithorax and absent or distant breath sounds. The immediate release of the tension by placement of a large-bore needle followed immediately by insertion of a thoracostomy tube is lifesaving.

OPEN PNEUMOTHORAX. The sucking chest wound is one in which a segment of the chest wall has been destroyed such that negative intrapleural pressure sucks air directly through the chest wall defect rather than through the trachea into the alveoli. Whenever the cross-sectional area of the defect exceeds that of the trachea, the undesirable preferential air movement takes place. It occurs most commonly after shotgun blasts, explosions with flying debris, or impalement injuries. It may or may not be associated with underlying parenchymal damage.

The diagnosis can be made by noting a patient with normal or collapsed neck veins who is making respiratory motions but not moving air. Confirmation is immediate on inspection of the patient's chest and observation of the wound. The patient is stabilized by any mechanical covering over the open wound. As soon as convenient, a watertight dressing should be placed and an intercostal catheter inserted into the pleural cavity. Early debridement and closure of the wound should then be scheduled.

MASSIVE FLAIL CHEST. Whenever severe blunt injury results in two-point fractures of four or more ribs, a large segment of the chest wall becomes flail. On inspiratory effort, the negative pressure in the chest pulls the unstable segment of the wall inward in a paradoxical motion. The patient may be unable to develop sufficient intratracheal negative pressure to maintain adequate ventilation, and atelectasis, hypoxia, and hypercapnia occur. A patient who is conscious may splint the segment sufficiently to make it inapparent to cursory examination, but the continuing extra effort in the attempt to move air soon leads to tiring and may result in sudden respiratory de-

compensation. The progressing failure is aggravated by the developing pulmonary contusion that accompanies blunt trauma sufficient to break that many ribs. In the unconscious patient, the lesion may be less dangerous, because it is more readily recognized and more apt to be treated early.

In the massive flail chest, the diagnosis may be difficult unless the chest wall is visualized during the respiratory effort. If unconscious, the patient is ordinarily making vigorous respiratory motions, but moving little air; the paradoxical segment should be obvious. The patient who is awake may exhibit a very rapid shallow breathing pattern at or above 40 breaths per minute. Other aspects of the management of lesser flail injuries are discussed below, but when massive flail is diagnosed, endotracheal intubation and positive-pressure controlled ventilation is mandatory.

MASSIVE HEMOTHORAX. When 1500 mL or more of blood is acutely removed from the pleural space as a thoracostomy tube is placed, Rene has shown that urgent thoracotomy will find a surgically correctable lesion in a high proportion of the cases. If a patient with penetrating injury or multiple rib fractures is found to have a complete hemithorax dull to percussion in association with hypotension, a chest tube should be inserted. If massive hemothorax is found, the patient should be taken directly to the operating room as blood volume resuscitation is taking place.

Conditions Requiring Urgent Thoracotomy

CONTINUED INTRAPLEURAL BLEEDING. If bleeding continues from a thoracostomy tube after initial placement at a rate exceeding 100 mL/h for 6 h or more, most surgeons would now agree that a surgically correctable lesion is present. Ordinarily it will be a bleeding intercostal vessel, since bleeding from the lower-pressure pulmonary system will almost always stop when the lung is reexpanded after the pleural space is evacuated. The rate and pattern of bleeding are more important than the amount in deciding to explore.

MASSIVE AIR LEAK. This is an increasingly commonly recognized injury resulting from steering wheel compression of the trachea against the vertebral bodies following high-speed head-on collisions. Complete disruption of the trachea or a major bronchus may occur. The injury is often fatal but may be surprisingly well tolerated for a brief period. All levels of the trachea and all major bronchi have been involved; however, greater than 80 percent of these injuries are within 2.5 cm of the carina. Patients with intrathoracic tracheal or central bronchial disruption may exhibit a variety of signs and symptoms depending on whether there is free communication between the site of injury and the pleural cavity. A particularly important diagnostic finding is complete unilateral atelectasis in the face of a large air leak, or the symmetrical downward displacement of the bilateral hila. Distal injuries often result in pneumothorax, which is manageable by tube thoracostomy alone since the air leak is small. Lazar and King have reported a case in which a complete tracheal disruption just above the carina with 6 cm of discontinuity was tolerated in a young athlete for 24 h before accurate diagnosis and repair. Extreme care must be taken in the evaluation of patients with massive air leaks, since overly aggressive diagnostic bronchoscopy or endotracheal intubation and positive-pressure ventilation before accurate location of the defect and careful operative preparation for approaching it have been made could result in rapid death. Occasionally, as in other tracheobronchial injuries discussed below, an injury may seal itself off and fail to be recognized until severe stenosis develops.

OTHER INDICATIONS. Several other important causes are listed here, but discussed elsewhere.

Acute or rapidly recurring pericardial tamponade
Acute heart failure secondary to valve or septal injury
Widened or widening mediastinum
Perforation of the intrathoracic esophagus

Dangerous but Less Compelling Injuries

DIAPHRAGM RUPTURE. Urgent repair of massive diaphragmatic rupture is sometimes necessary if high-volume herniation of abdominal contents into the chest prevents adequate ventilation. Ordinarily, however, the acute problems associated with diaphragm rupture are related to the associated injuries to abdominal viscera resulting from the force necessary to rupture the diaphragm. Penetrating trauma to the lower chest or upper abdomen and crush injuries, most often secondary to automobile accidents, are the usual causes of traumatic rupture of the diaphragm. The left hemidiaphragm is ruptured more frequently by blunt trauma than the right, the ratio being about 9:1. The right hemidiaphragm is said to be protected by two mechanisms: the liver on the right and the heart in the center have a buffering effect that diffuses the sudden increase in intraabdominal pressure; and cadaver studies have shown an inherent weakness in the posterior lateral aspect of the left diaphragm. When rupture of the right side does occur, the liver is usually the only abdominal structure that herniates into the chest early, though gradual aspiration of the stomach into the right chest through the diaphragmatic defect can occur over time. With rupture of the left hemidiaphragm, the stomach, spleen, left transverse colon, and omentum in any combination may enter the left pleural cavity. When the diagnosis is delayed for several days or longer, there is often a progressive displacement of the abdominal viscera into the chest or progressive gaseous distention of the herniated stomach. The latter may occur despite an indwelling nasogastric tube, and it may precipitate respiratory distress (Fig. 17-15).

Patients with diaphragmatic rupture due to blunt trauma usually have associated injuries that demand first attention and prevent a detailed initial evaluation. The first chest x-ray after rupture of either hemidiaphragm may show nothing more than a blurring of the diaphragm with or without evidence of a small hemothorax. In some patients the diagnosis is made very early because the nasogastric tube is seen to lie within the confines of the left pleural cavity. Injection of air through the nasogastric

tube during auscultation of the left side of the chest may add support to the diagnosis.

Penetrating diaphragmatic injuries rarely produce early symptoms except those related to other structures that may be injured. After several months or years, gastrointestinal obstruction may develop and lead to strangulation of herniated viscera. The hole in the diaphragm is small, and herniation occurs slowly. Early transabdominal operation is indicated when the diagnosis is confirmed, and associated intraabdominal injuries may be repaired at the same time. The wound in the hemidiaphragm may vary from a simple radial tear to an extensive and complex laceration. Repair can usually be accomplished by direct suture, but a prosthetic patch is occasionally required. If the diagnosis is delayed, a transthoracic approach may be preferred. It provides better exposure to (1) reduce the hernia, (2) free adhesions between the abdominal viscera and intrathoracic structures, and (3) repair the defect in the diaphragm.

PNEUMOTHORAX. Pneumothorax is usually the result of injury to the lung or the tracheobronchial tree. Esophageal perforation may be followed by a pneumomediastinum that ruptures into the pleural cavity. Whether the pneumothorax is associated with blunt injury and fractured ribs or is due to a penetrating wound, there is a variable amount of bleeding into the pleural cavity. The decision to use the term hemopneumothorax depends on the amount of blood in the pleural cavity and the likely consequences. If sufficient blood is present to require a concerted effort to assure its removal, or if its loss from the circulating volume requires transfusion replacement, it seems proper to use the double term.

Pneumothorax varies from that which is so slight that it may be missed on the initial x-ray examination to a massive, continuing air leak that displaces the mediastinum, depresses the diaphragm, and compresses the opposite lung, the tension pneumothorax discussed previously (Fig. 17-16). A pneumothorax due to a parenchymal lung injury tends to be self-limited because the developing lung collapse combines with blood clotting in the wound for a sealing effect. For some patients extensive adhesions already present between the visceral and parietal pleura may localize the pleural air and prevent a collapse of the lung (Fig. 17-17).

With any chest injury it is wisest to presume that a pneumothorax is present until proved otherwise. Because of pain and limited chest motion on the injured side, physical examination may be inadequate for diagnosis of a minimal pneumothorax. Since attention may be diverted to the management of other injuries, and because of the risks of tension developing should a general anesthetic with positive-pressure ventilation be given, prophylactic thoracostomy catheters should usually be placed whenever there is significant chest injury. The catheter is usually best placed in the lateral axillary line, just above the fifth rib, after finger exploration has induced a temporary pneumothorax or otherwise assured the pleural space to be free at the site of insertion.

Treatment of the more usual pneumothorax depends on symptoms of respiratory insufficiency, the extent of the

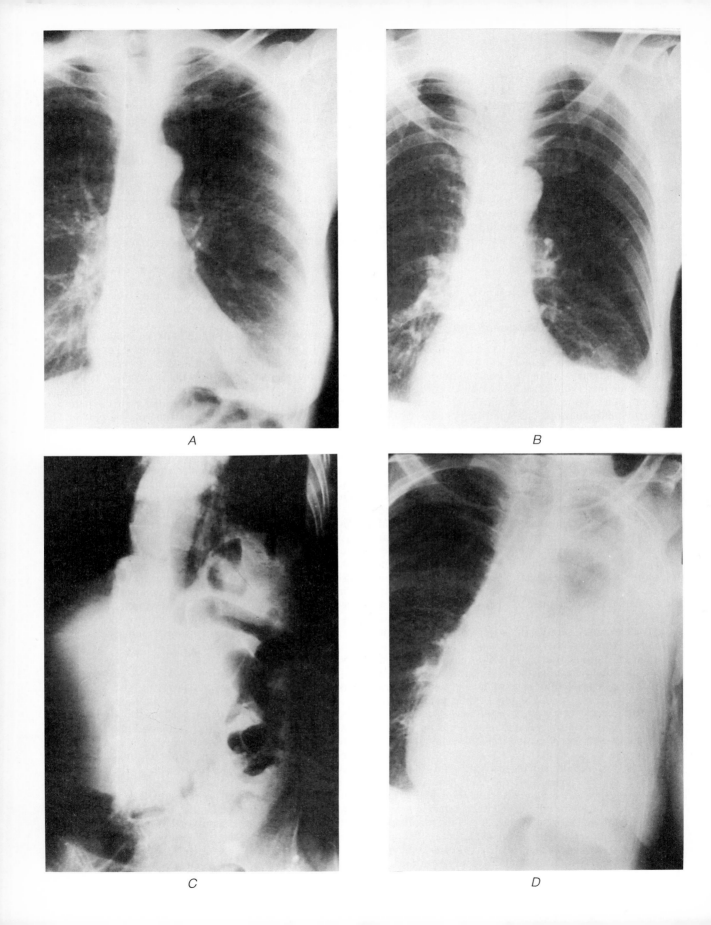

A

B

C

D

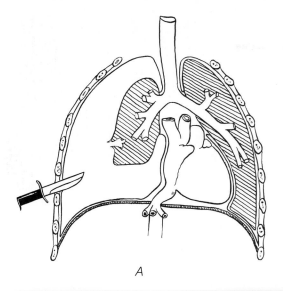

A

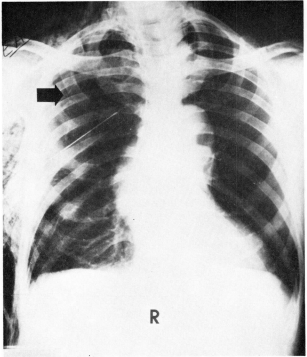

C

B

Fig. 17-16. *A.* In a tension pneumothorax there is compression of the contralateral lung and a displacement of the mediastinum that may sharply reduce venous return to the atria. *B.* If the diagnosis is strongly suspected, needle aspiration of the pleural space should be done without waiting for the chest x-ray. In this patient, the tension pneumothorax developed slowly and became symptomatic shortly after this film was taken. The lower arrow points to the displacement of the right heart border, and the lung is completely collapsed *(upper arrow). C.* Following needle aspiration a large intercostal tube was put in place, but a major air leak continued for several days and eventually required insertion of an additional chest catheter. The arrow points to the visceral pleura, showing incomplete expansion of the lung.

◀ Fig. 17-15. *A–D.* Traumatic rupture of the diaphragm can present rapidly progressive and life-threatening complications early or late after injury. The patient whose films are pictured here developed increasing herniation of abdominal contents into the left chest over a 3-day period before findings led to urgent thoracotomy for removal of infarcted small intestine. *(Courtesy of Dr. John H.M. Austin.)*

pneumothorax, and the presence of significant hemothorax. There is a tendency to think of pneumothorax in terms of a two-dimensional concept that is conveyed by the anteroposterior chest x-ray. Instead, the hemithorax must be considered a modified cone, and when the lung surface is separated from the chest wall by 3 cm or more, the patient may have a 50 percent lung collapse (by volume) rather than the 25 or 30 percent collapse that the chest x-ray suggests. With a pneumothorax that is less

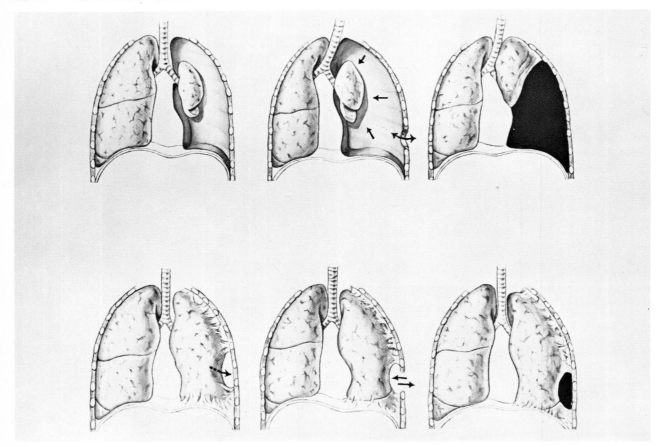

Fig. 17-17. A free pleural space will allow the development of a complete pneumothorax or a massive hemothorax. These potentially fatal complications cannot occur in patients with an obliterated pleural space. (Reproduced from: *Naciero EA: Chest Injuries. New York, Grune & Stratton, 1971, with permission.*)

than this amount, due to a nonpenetrating injury (theoretically, no contamination of the pleural space), and not accompanied by significant blood or fluid in the pleural cavity, treatment may not be required. A decision not to remove the pleural air implies that the patient has had a simple injury and that conditions for observation are ideal. Approximately 1.25 percent of the air will be absorbed each day, with full expansion expected in 3 to 6 weeks.

Aspiration of the air with a needle and insertion of an intercostal catheter only if lung collapse recurs is a reasonable method of treatment advocated by some physicians even when the pneumothorax amounts to as much as 50 percent. In all cases with greater than 50 percent collapse, in those with hemopneumothorax, and in patients whose pneumothorax is the result of penetrating trauma, an intercostal catheter should be inserted and attached to a water seal with 10 to 25 cmH$_2$O negative pressure. In the majority of patients, lung reexpansion and cessation of the air leak will occur within a few hours or a few days. If not, a major bronchial injury may be present, and a thoracotomy may be required after appropriate diagnostic procedures.

The use of prophylactic systemic antibiotics in patients with chest trauma is a subject of current debate, but their use in cases of nonpenetrating trauma seems unjustified. The simple insertion of an intercostal catheter does not justify prescribing antibiotics.

Interstitial Emphysema. Disruption of the respiratory tract at any level will result in the passage of air into the surrounding tissues. Mediastinal emphysema occurs when air enters the areolar tissue planes from a tracheobronchial wound or from a perforation of the esophagus. Occasionally, blunt injuries to the chest may disrupt the integrity of a group of bronchioles or alveolar units without disrupting the visceral pleura. As air escapes into the pulmonary interstitium, it dissects centrally along the bronchi and pulmonary vessels to reach the mediastinum. When the mediastinal pleura remains intact, progressive loss of air into the tissue carries the dissection into the neck, where the air escapes the deep tissue planes and spreads in the subcutaneous tissue. The development of subcutaneous emphysema may cause marked distortion of the patient's appearance, but there is no reason to "treat" the condition, except to take whatever steps are appropriate to stop the air leak. The source of the leak must be found, since some potential causes (esophageal perforation or major bronchial injury) require early intervention.

RIB FRACTURES AND LESSER FLAIL INJURIES. The most common injury of the chest is a fracture of one or more ribs, including fracture at the costochondral junction ("separation"). Children seem less liable to rib fractures, but chest x-rays are made less frequently in those young age groups with minor trauma. Fractures occur most commonly in the middle and lower ribs with blunt trama, but the distribution with penetrating wounds varies with the distribution of the penetrating objects.

First Rib Fractures. First rib fractures have historically been associated with high probability of associated upper rib fractures and major vessel injuries. Recent reports by many authors, however, have demonstrated isolated first rib fractures without other significant injuries in the thoracic outlet in a wide variety of patients. Because of the relative high frequency in association with cranial and maxillofacial injuries, and in the "surfer's" rib (an injury occurring in surfers performing the so-called lay-back maneuver), it seems probable that isolated first rib injuries are secondary to avulsion of the first rib by its muscular attachments rather than direct trauma to the relatively protected first rib. There is inconclusive evidence that a direct relationship exists between first and second rib fractures and trauma to major vessels at the apex of the hemithorax (Fig. 17-18). Lazroni et al. recommend arteriography in stable patients with first rib fracture who have (1) absent or decreased upper extremity pulses, (2) hemorrhage, especially large extrapleural hematoma or hemothorax, and (3) brachial plexus injury. Additional criteria for angiography include displacement of fragments and multiple thoracic injuries.

Multiple Fractures. The problem of massive flail chest has been briefly discussed previously. Lesser degrees of flail occur whenever there are multiple fractures of the chest wall skeletal structure. Flail chest is appropriately diagnosed whenever there is paradoxical respiratory movement in a segment of the chest wall. This generally requires at least two segmental fractures in each of three adjacent ribs or costal cartilages or other multiple combinations of rib or sternal fractures with costochondral or chondrosternal separations. Posterior flail segments, in the absence of disrupted intrathoracic structures, are easier to manage because of the strong muscular and scapular support, and because of patients' natural tendency to lie with their backs against the mattress.

Chest wall stabilization and reduction of respiratory dead space are major goals of treatment. Improvements in respiratory therapy, including bedside measurements of pulmonary mechanics and the widespread availability of arterial blood-gas determinations, have allowed greater individualization in the treatment of patients with flail-chest injuries. For many years endotracheal intubation or early tracheostomy has been recommended for the management of patients with flail chest, because it allows easy access for tracheobronchial suctioning, it reduces dead space, and it facilitates internal stabilization of the chest wall through mechanical ventilation. Intubation is often delayed now until evidence of a need for ventilatory

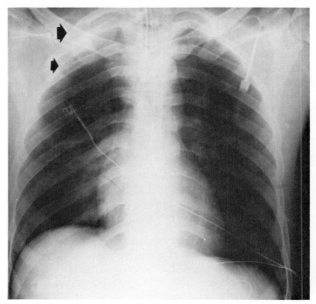

A

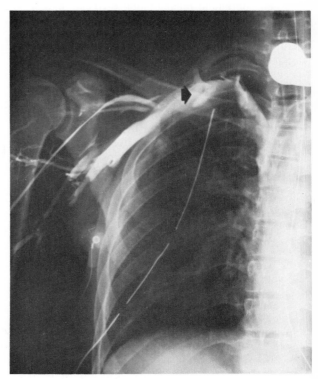

B

Fig. 17-18. *A.* The first chest x-ray of a twenty-five-year-old man who was injured in a motorcycle accident shows a fracture of the right first rib (upper arrow) and a small extrapleural hematoma at the right apex (lower arrow). *B.* A subclavian arteriogram and venogram were done 3 days after admission because of the sudden development of a massive hemothorax (2000 mL blood) on the right side. Bleeding stopped spontaneously, and the venogram shows a tear in the subclavian vein at the rib fracture site.

support develops: a respiratory rate of 40 breaths per minute, a falling Pa_{CO_2} is evidence of excessive work of breathing to maintain adequate oxygenation, or a Pa_{O_2} below 60 torr on inspired oxygen fractions of over 0.5. Other techniques for stabilizing the flail segment, such as the use of external compression dressings or the application of traction by encircling the fractured ribs with towel clips or wire, are historical oddities. For some patients with a small flail area and minimal pulmonary injury, close observation alone may allow satisfactory recovery without the use of assisted ventilation. In these patients treatment should be directed at the respiratory dysfunction rather than at stabilizing the area of paradoxical motion. A rare patient presents with localized chest wall fractures amenable to direct operative stabilization. When feasible, this approach can considerably shorten convalescence.

Several long-term follow-up studies have recently been published analyzing the late consequences of flail-chest injuries. Significant disability was reported in from 50 to 64 percent of the patients with pain as the common residual complaint. In one study, 40 percent of examined patients had found it necessary to change their life style as a result of the chest injury. Much better attention to the early and continuing rehabilitation of these injured patients is undoubtedly indicated by these findings.

Other Rib Fractures. An inward displacement of the fracture fragments at the time of injury may lacerate the lung parenchyma and produce a pneumothorax with bleeding into the pleural cavity. With a single rib fracture the incidence of pneumothorax is not high, but there is an increasing likelihood of this complication as the number of fractured ribs increases. The occurrence of pneumothorax may be delayed for some hours or even days after the injury has occurred. As noted previously, hemothorax of a significant degree occurring with rib fractures is usually due to laceration of an intercostal artery rather than to bleeding from the lung. Again, bleeding may be delayed in onset or it may recur after an interval of several days, and it may be life-threatening. Especially in the patient who has multiple rib fractures with segmental fractures of one or more ribs, a delayed pneumothorax or hemothorax may coincide with some shift of the rib fragments demonstrated in serial chest x-rays.

In elderly or chronically ill patients rib fractures may occur with severe coughing or hard straining. The occurrence of a spontaneous fracture should alert the physician to the possibility of a bone abnormality such as metastatic neoplasm or hyperparathyroidism. Pneumothorax and hemothorax are infrequent with rib fractures that do not result from external trauma.

The diagnosis of a rib fracture may be implied from the pleuritic type of pain and marked tenderness over the fracture area. A sharply localized contusion of the chest wall structures may mimic the findings, including shallow respirations with chest wall splinting. Green-stick fractures are those not associated with separation of the fragments, and they may not be demonstrated by the initial chest x-ray examination. Several weeks may elapse before a suspected fracture is confirmed. When the patient

has two or more adjacent fractured ribs, especially if the ribs are broken in more than one place (segmental fractures), the diagnosis is made with greater certainty by examination alone. Cartilage fractures and separation from either the rib or sternum are not demonstrated by chest x-rays. In a recent review of emergency room practice, Thompson and his coworkers emphasized how infrequently management is influenced by rib radiographs and urged higher reliance on physical findings and avoidance of efforts to obtain confirmatory radiographs, unless findings might alter treatment.

The principal goal of treatment for patients without serious injury is relief of pain. If this is accomplished, patients may resume their normal activities except those that require a vigorous work effort. Adhesive strapping of the chest or chest binders to splint the fracture area should be avoided in all but the very young. In the majority of other patients, an adequate oral analgesic or an intercostal nerve block plus oral analgesics provides reasonable pain relief with minimal risk of side effects (Fig. 17-19). Binders or strapping are particular hazards in the elderly and in patients with chronic lung disease. The nerve block may need to be repeated once daily for several days, but a single injection may suffice for individuals whose injury does not require hospitalization. A patient whose rib fractures are accompanied by minimal pneumothorax (less than 1.5 cm separation between the lung and the inner chest wall by x-ray) may be treated as an outpatient under ideal conditions of observation and follow-up.

Sternal Fractures. Any major blunt trauma to the anterior chest wall may cause a fracture of the sternum. Such fractures may occur alone or in combination with multiple rib fractures. The fractures are usually transverse and most often occur in the body of the sternum at or near the junction with the manubrium (Fig. 17-20). The injury is extremely painful and can usually be pinpointed by the conscious patient. The diagnosis should be made on physical examination and confirmed by lateral x-rays of the sternum or tomography. It is essential to rule out significant injury to underlying structures, especially the heart. In the absence of other major injury, the treatment of the fracture is aimed toward relief of pain and observation for signs of respiratory embarrassment. In patients with compromised pulmonary function or obvious instability of the fragments, more vigorous treatment is required, e.g., positive-pressure ventilation and/or operative reduction and stabilization of the fragments. When the pain of a sternal fracture persists for a long period of time, a nonunion should be suspected. Most often, this is the result of persistent displacement of the proximal fragment. In this instance open reduction is usually required.

HEMOTHORAX. Intrathoracic bleeding occurs with any form of chest injury that disrupts the tissues. Hemothorax usually develops at the time of injury, but the bleeding may be delayed for several days. Occasionally an extrapleural hematoma will break into the pleural cavity and give the impression of delayed hemorrhage.

Bleeding from the lung as a result of a rib fractures, stab wounds, or small-missile wounds will generally stop

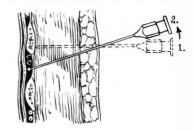

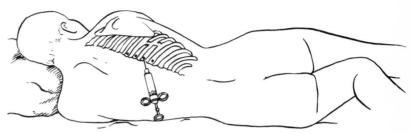

Fig. 17-19. Intercostal nerve blocks may be very effective in relieving the pain of rib fractures. The nerves above and below the fractured ribs must be blocked, in addition to those corresponding to the ribs fractured.

Fig. 17-20. A lateral chest x-ray demonstrates the type of sternal fracture that occurs when the driver of a car is thrown against the steering wheel.

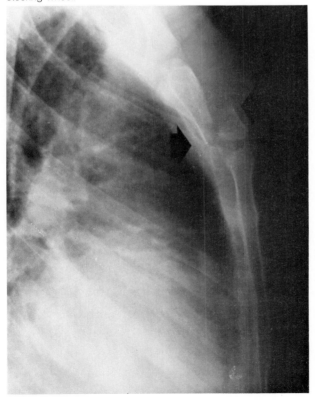

before a sufficient volume has been lost to mandate an emergency thoracotomy. From accumulated military and civilian experience it can be estimated that slightly more than 10 percent of patients with traumatic hemothorax will require thoracotomy for control of bleeding or determination of the extent of injury.

Movement of the diaphragm and thoracic structures causes partial defibrination of blood that is shed into the pleural cavity, and clotting is usually incomplete. Sufficient coagulation does occur to interfere with efficient drainage of the pleural blood through intercostal catheters, and the latter often become plugged with blood clot. Pleural enzymes begin to produce clot lysis within a few hours after bleeding stops, and the process of hemolysis with protein breakdown increases the osmotic pressure. Unless the pleural space is drained adequately, the transudation of fluid into the space can produce a significant compression of the lung and a shift of the mediastinum toward the opposite hemithorax.

The main diagnostic concerns in the management of the patient with traumatic hemothorax are how much bleeding has occurred, is it continuing, and, if stopped and clotted, when should clot be removed. Consideration of the type and extent of injury, general signs of blood loss, physical signs of fluid in the pleural cavity, and chest x-ray findings are guides to the assessment of the extent of hemothorax. Four to five hundred milliliters of blood may be hidden by the diaphragm on the upright chest x-ray, and 1 L or more may be overlooked on a supine film. A large hemothorax may even be missed on the upright chest x-ray unless the observer is aware of the phenomenon of subpulmonary trapping of the blood (Fig. 17-21). Lateral decubitus x-ray can confirm the diagnosis of hemothorax and guide placement of an appropriate drainage catheter.

A small hemothorax that produces little more than blunting of the costophrenic angle on the chest x-ray does

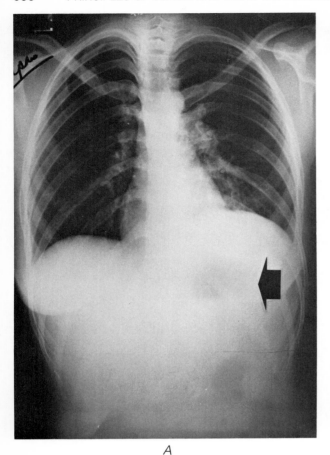

A

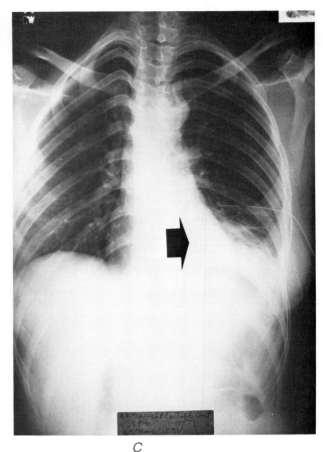

C

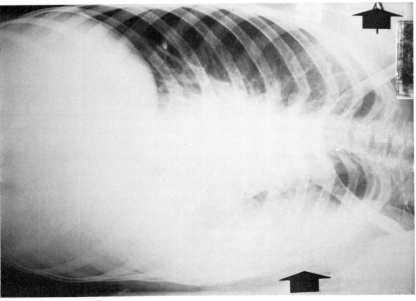

B

Fig. 17-21. Traumatic hemothorax due to a stab wound of the left chest in a thirty-two-year-old woman. *A.* The first chest x-ray suggests an elevation of the left diaphragm, and the emergency-room physician did not suspect a hemothorax. The surgical consultant was suspicious of subpulmonary trapping of a hemothorax because of the distance between the top of the apparent diaphragm and the gastric air bubble *(arrow)*. *B.* A lateral decubitis x-ray shows a large collection of blood in the left hemithorax. *C.* Insertion of an intercostal tube resulted in drainage of 600 mL of blood. However, the chest x-ray suggests the presence of residual blood and clots in the pleural cavity *(arrow)*.

not require initial treatment; follow-up x-rays at appropriate intervals will assist with the decision to drain the pleural cavity if there is a progressive accumulation. When the hemothorax exceeds an amount that fills the costophrenic sulcus, or when there is associated pneumothorax, one or more large catheters should be placed in the pleural cavity through the seventh, eighth, or ninth intercostal space in the posterior-axillary line. Underwater drainage alone may be sufficient, but low suction applied to the catheters is often helpful when combined with active efforts at stripping the tubes of blood clot. If the initial drainage of blood is followed by continued bleeding in the absence of a clotting defect, a decision to operate must be made, with a broad consideration of the possible sources of the bleeding.

With a major hemothorax the success of tube drainage is often frustrated by extensive clot that obstructs the tubes. An attitude should be adopted that a nonfunctioning chest tube represents a liability to the patient because of discomfort and the risk of carrying infection from the skin wound into the pleural clot. Especially with penetrating trauma, a hemothorax that fails to drain adequately through intercostal catheters may develop into empyema. An additional hazard is the organization of residual clot to form a fibrothorax. Coselli and his colleagues in Houston have recently reviewed their experience with clotted hemothorax and have found early thoracotomy substantially reduces hospitalization time and empyema rates.

TRACHEOBRONCHIAL INJURY. The management of massive tracheobronchial injuries is discussed above. For small penetrating injuries of the intrathoracic trachea and major bronchi, tracheostomy and effective pleural decompression may provide satisfactory definitive treatment. Those injuries which are associated with an actual defect in the tracheobronchial wall, including partial disruption, require operative exploration and repair. Tracheostomy may be necessary to prevent high intratracheal pressures and to allow tracheal care postoperatively, but positive-pressure assisted ventilation should be avoided.

Penetrating injuries of lobar or segmental bronchi may produce a similar clinical picture to proximal tracheobronchial injuries. Bilateral pneumothorax is rare, and the principal immediate problem is to begin management of the major air leak and confirm the presence of a major bronchial injury. The bronchial air leak often stops soon after an intercostal catheter is put in place. The definitive diagnosis may be delayed if the bronchus becomes obstructed by blood clot or mucus and the air leak ceases. Under these conditions the pulmonary lobe or segment becomes atelectatic and resists conservative methods to produce reexpansion. If infection does not occur, the injured bronchus may heal with significant distortion and obstruction, or the atelectasis may persist and lead subsequently to a correct diagnosis. Operative repair of the disrupted bronchus can be achieved even years after injury. If infection occurs at the site of the bronchial injury, the patient may develop pneumonia, distal bronchiectasis, and empyema. Resection of the bronchus and the involved pulmonary lobe is then required.

PULMONARY INJURY. The lungs have a remarkable ability to tolerate penetrating injuries and blunt trauma without long-term residual effects. Civilian gunshot wounds of the chest penetrate a lung more frequently than any other structure, but the majority of patients with no other significant injury can be treated without a thoracotomy. Any penetrating object produces an air leak with a variable degree of pneumothorax. The disruption of tissue along the missile track causes bleeding, which usually ceases as the damaged parenchyma becomes swollen and filled with blood clot. With small-caliber and low-velocity bullet wounds that pass through the lung periphery, the amount of tissue damage produced may be sufficiently small that late follow-up chest x-rays fail to demonstrate the area of injury. With high-velocity bullets, the tissue destruction extends more widely, and even a peripheral bullet pathway may result in irreversible damage to a lobar or lung hilus.

The immediate management of the patient with a penetrating injury is the insertion of at least one intercostal catheter for evacuation of the associated hemopneumothorax. Serial arterial blood gases and frequent evaluation of the patient's ventilatory ability allow an overall estimate of the effect of the injury on respiratory exchange. Civilian penetrating wounds rarely require ventilatory assistance. Only rarely is there a need for thoracotomy to control bleeding or to perform pulmonary resection for an irreversibly injured lung.

PULMONARY CONTUSION. Pulmonary contusion is the consequence of blunt trauma to the lung. The frequent causes of contusion include rapid deceleration of the chest against an automobile steering wheel, falls from a height, and blast injuries. Particularly in young persons, severe pulmonary contusion can occur by transmission of force through the chest wall with minimal fractures of the ribs or sternum. In middle-aged or elderly persons significant pulmonary contusion is usually accompanied by multiple fractures of the thoracic cage.

The contused lung is characterized by capillary disruption that results in intraalveolar and interstitial hemorrhage, edema, protein and fluid obstruction of small airways, and leukocyte infiltration. Serial chest x-rays begun right after injury show a fluffy infiltrate that progresses in extent and in density over a period of 24 to 48 h. Although the maximum lung injury is directly related to that region of the chest wall that receives the trauma, a "countrecoup" effect may be responsible for a wider distribution of the pulmonary damage. Unless the contusion involves only a small region of one lung, it may result in serious loss of respiratory function. The associated injury to the chest wall is aggravated by the loss of pulmonary compliance, increasing the work of breathing. Small areas of atelectasis become confluent, and progressive hypoxia further diminishes the patient's ability to compensate for the loss of function.

Pulmonary contusion is often part of a major chest injury that includes one or more fractures of the thoracic cage, pneumothorax, and hemothorax. If not present initially, a pneumothorax may subsequently develop from actual disruption of the contused pulmonary parenchyma.

Although it is infrequent in patients who survive to reach the hospital, a major pulmonary laceration may represent the maximum extent of pulmonary contusion. In some instances the tissue disruption is the result of extensive penetration by rib fragments, but in others the causative factor is probably a severe shearing force. The clinical and x-ray findings suggest a serious chest injury but do not differentiate the patient with a major lung laceration from those with pulmonary contusion and associated hemopneumothorax. Continued or uncontrolled hemorrhage and massive air leak generally mandate an early thoracotomy. A major pulmonary resection is often necessary, and the mortality rate is high.

Treatment of pulmonary contusion must include an accurate clinical assessment of the patient's respiratory exchange and careful monitoring by serial measurements of the arterial blood gases. Steroids probably have no role in the management of pulmonary contusion.

A high percentage of patients require temporary assisted ventilation, and it may be evident at the time of admission that endotracheal or nasotracheal intubation should be performed. Without question, aggressive respiratory therapy, including ventilatory support, should be initiated before cardiopulmonary decompensation requires treatment measures that add additional risks. Criteria for instituting assisted ventilation are shown in Table 17-4. For most patients the need for assisted ventilation does not extend beyond 48 to 72 h unless there is major injury to the chest wall or to other body regions.

POSTTRAUMATIC PULMONARY INSUFFICIENCY. The development of acute respiratory failure can be expected in a high percentage of patients who suffer major thoracic trauma. Preexisting pulmonary status will influence the severity of respiratory insufficiency, and the extent of actual pulmonary damage will determine whether the patient survives. An initial evaluation of respiratory exchange and ventilatory ability, confirmed by measurement of pulmonary mechanics and arterial blood gases, should be followed by serial reevaluations.

Especially in patients who have suffered multiple trauma, a respiratory-distress syndrome may develop that is out of proportion to the extent of thoracic injury. A series of terms has evolved over the years to designate several forms of respiratory insufficiency that follow trauma and may be associated with a constellation of causative factors. Such terms as "wet lung," "shock lung," "congestive atelectasis," and "adult respiratory-distress syndrome" reflect some principal features that seemed to be characteristic of the cases that came to the attention of those who coined the terms. There is certainly some overlap in the causation of the several forms of respiratory failure that follow major trauma, and it is important to determine the specific causes in individual patients. Blaisdell and Lewis have presented a thorough discussion of posttraumatic pulmonary insufficiency, choosing the term respiratory-distress syndrome of shock and trauma for those cases not due to a specific cause. They suggest that eight different explanations for respiratory failure other than the respiratory-distress syndrome occur with reasonable frequency in patients who suffer major injury. These include aspiration, simple atelectasis, lung contusion, fat embolism, pneumonia, pneumothorax, pulmonary edema, and pulmonary embolism.

On the basis of their experience with a large number of cases, Blaisdell and Lewis have concluded that the respiratory-distress syndrome (RDS) is one and the same as the fat-embolism syndrome. Originally thought to result from fat embolism from fracture of long bones, the syndrome consists of pulmonary, neurologic, and systemic manifestations. The pulmonary manifestations appear first, generally within 24 to 36 h after injury, and consist of dyspnea, tachycardia, fever, and cyanosis. Documentation that much of the fat that appears in the blood following injury represents a mobilization of free fatty acids from body neutral fat as a result of shock and increased levels of catecholamines has helped in understanding the mechanism of this condition. Because some degree of intravascular coagulation can be demonstrated in all cases, this is almost certainly a factor in development of the syndrome.

For patients who suffer major chest injury it may be impossible to define what part of their respiratory failure is a result of direct trauma and how much is a consequence of the RDS. Treatment must be based on correction of the direct results of injury and on the anticipation or early recognition of respiratory insufficiency. The radiologic changes of RDS, consisting of diffuse lung infiltrates that progress to become confluent, may be super-

Table 17-4. CRITERIA FOR ASSISTED VENTILATION

Function	Normal values	Ventilate
Pulmonary mechanics:		
Respiratory rate	12–20	>35
Vital capacity, mL/kg	65–75	<15
Maximum inspiratory force, cmH$_2$O (negative values)	75–100	<25–35
Gas exchange		
Pa_{O_2}, torr	76–100 (room air)	<65–70 (added oxygen)
Alveolar-arterial oxygen difference, torr (100% oxygen)	30–70	>350
Pa_{CO_2}, torr	35–45	>50
Dead space/tidal volume ratio	0.25–0.40	>0.6

imposed on the effects of pulmonary contusion and atelectasis. Changes observed on serial chest x-rays lag behind the changes in pulmonary function, and a patient may be in critical respiratory failure before the films suggest a progressive pulmonary lesion.

Management of the RDS requires maintenance of good cardiovascular function and prompt institution of ventilatory support. An adequate volume replacement for external fluid and blood losses is complicated by the internal fluid losses due to increased capillary permeability in the lung, in all areas of direct tissue trauma, and to a varying degree throughout the body. Monitoring central venous pressures is the minimum for guidance of fluid and diuretic therapy in these patients, but placement of a Swan–Ganz catheter to allow left atrial and pulmonary artery pressures is superior. The need for inotropic myocardial support can be detected earlier by this access to left-sided heart pressures.

Ventilatory support techniques have advanced to allow a wider selection of ventilators and methods of assisted respiration. Attention to detail can offer the patient a maximum chance of survival with a minimum risk of complications. An unanswered question is the place of steroid therapy. The experience with these agents has been variable, and their employment is generally delayed until the patient appears to be nearing an irreversible state of progressive respiratory failure. This is probably too late for a reasonable drug effect. Sladen has described an approach that probably justifies a clinical trial. He used pharmacologic doses of methylprednisolone (30 mg/kg) intravenously every 6 h for 48 h in combination with ventilatory support and reported a significant reduction in mortality rate when compared with historical controls.

CHEST WALL

Congenital Deformities

PECTUS EXCAVATUM

The most common congenital deformity of the chest wall is pectus excavatum, in which the body of the sternum is displaced posteriorly to produce a funnel-shaped depression (Fig. 17-22). The etiology is not certain, but most authors ascribe to the notion that overgrowth of the lower costal cartilages and ribs is responsible. The defect varies widely in expression. The depression is most often centered at the xiphisternal junction but may extend to the manubrium in rare cases. In lateral extent the presentation varies from a narrow central cleft to a broad dish-shaped defect extending from nipple to nipple. The depth of the depression is equally variable, with the sternum reaching or even overlapping the spine in extreme forms. Asymmetry is common, and always involves greater depression of the right costal cartilages with rotation of the sternum to the right. Several authors have attempted to classify the severity of defects based on radiographic findings. One method uses the sternovertebral distance measured on a lateral chest x-ray to classify the defects

as slight (>7 cm), moderate (5 to 7 cm), and severe (<5 cm), and others use a ratio of sternovertebral distance to transthoracic diameter. Computed tomography (CT) scanning may allow better quantitative volumetric analysis but has not been widely applied.

Pectus excavatum is present at birth and progresses at a variable and unpredictable rate through childhood. Infants and young children often have a protuberant abdomen that accentuates the deformity. Later in childhood a characteristic posture has been described, with rounded and forward-sloping shoulders, forward angulation of the head and neck, and dorsal kyphosis of the spine. Breast development in young women is frequently asymmetric, with a smaller breast on the right.

Although most cases appear in isolation, a familial tendency has been noted, and the defect is frequently seen in more than one sibling. The anomaly is about three times more frequent in males. Pectus excavatum is frequently seen in Marfan's syndrome and is one of a variety of chest wall deformities seen with increased frequency in patients with congenital heart disease.

That pectus excavatum produces a cosmetic deformity is not a matter of debate. Thirty to seventy percent of patients are reported to be symptomatic, with a broad range of presentations including exercise intolerance, atypical chest pain, dyspnea, bronchospasm, poor feeding, and arrhythmias. In all reported series, symptoms are almost always relieved by operative correction. Systolic ejection murmurs are frequently reported, and are thought to reflect compression of the right ventricular outflow tract. Electrocardiographic abnormalities are frequent and usually resolve after repair, but are thought to reflect changes in axis due to rotation and displacement rather than any fundamental electrophysiologic disturbance.

Whether or not a physiologic defect is responsible for the characteristic symptomatology is still quite controversial. Although most studies of cardiorespiratory function in pectus excavatum have placed patients in the normal or low-normal range, there have been notable exceptions. Weg found a decrease in forced expiratory flow and maximum voluntary ventilation in 25 young men with pectus excavatum. Blickman et al. recently demonstrated abnormal xenon ventilation scintigraphy in 12 of 17 patients before repair, which resolved in 7 of the 12 postoperatively. Perfusion and ventilation-perfusion ratios were abnormal preoperatively in 10 of 17 patients and normalized postoperatively in 6 of the 10. Not surprisingly, the defects were in the lower left lung. The authors did not address the clinical significance of the findings. Cahill et al. recently reported a small improvement in total lung capacity, a significant improvement in maximal voluntary ventilation, and an improvement in exercise performance after repair of pectus excavatum in 14 patients, supporting their belief that a dynamic restrictive pulmonary defect exists in symptomatic pectus excavatum that is reversible with repair.

Indices specific for cardiac performance have also been studied. A diastolic dip-and-plateau configuration in the right ventricular pressure tracing has been occasionally

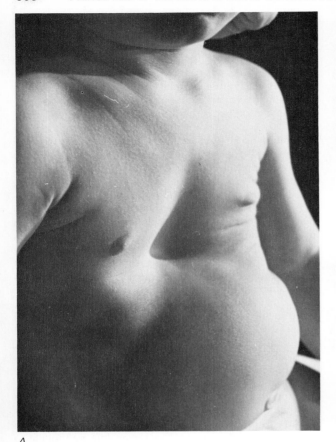

A

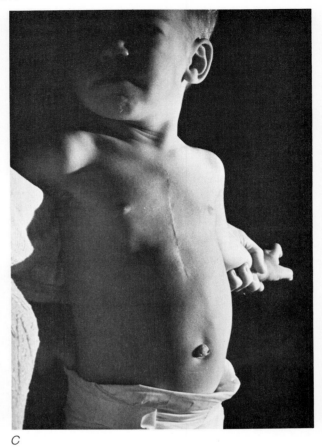

C

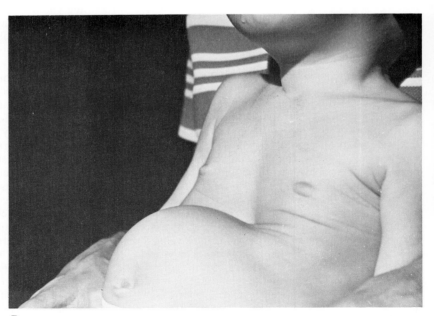

B

reported, suggesting a constrictive effect on the right ventricle. Beiser et al. reported normal exercise cardiac index in six supine patients with pectus excavatum that decreased significantly during upright exercise, although the cardiac index during upright exercise was within the reported normal limits in four patients. Of only three patients studied postoperatively, only two had an abnormal exercise cardiac index preoperatively, one of whom continued to be abnormal. In spite of the somewhat confusing findings in a small number of patients, this report has been frequently cited as evidence of abnormal cardiac exercise performance in pectus excavatum.

The largest group of patients (13) with pectus excavatum in whom cardiac performance has been studied was reported in 1985 by Peterson et al. First-pass radionuclide studies during upright rest and bicycle exercise were performed before and at least 6 months after pectus repair. Eighty-five percent of the patients were symptomatic, and all demonstrated striking subjective improvement after repair, correlating with a marked decrease in symptoms during a regulated exercise protocol. Objectively, however, left ventricular ejection fraction and cardiac index were normal before and after repair. Left ventricular end-diastolic volume index and stroke volume index increased at rest after operation, and resting right ventricular end-diastolic volume increased markedly, associated with a decrease in right ventricular ejection fraction. Although the data showed no impairment in exercise cardiac function before or after pectus repair, the increase in ventricular volumes suggested that some degree of cardiac compression was relieved by repair.

Two conclusions are possible. One is that no significant functional disturbance is associated with pectus excavatum. Another is that the methods available to study functional performance are too insensitive to detect the abnormalities that account for the pervasive symptomatology. Underlying the entire controversy is the fact that the anatomic spectrum is very broad and the number of patients available for study comparatively small. Objective study may be further confounded by psychological factors associated with an obvious cosmetic defect.

OPERATIVE TREATMENT. Most authors recommend operative correction during the preschool years (before five years of age) but not before 18 months. Operation at that age is thought to prevent the secondary postural and psychological consequences of the defect. Correction in adolescence or early adulthood is just as frequently performed, and with equal justification based on the desire to wait until evolution of the defect with growth is complete.

Fig. 17-22. A two-year-old child with moderate pectus excavatum. *A.* The posterior displacement of the sternum appears to start at the level of the third chondrosternal junction. *B.* The potbelly that accompanies pectus excavatum in the young child is accentuated in the sitting position. *C.* The postoperative photograph shows an excellent cosmetic result. Either a vertical incision (shown) or a bilateral submammary transverse incision can be used for the repair. *(Photographs courtesy of Dr. Harold A. Albert.)*

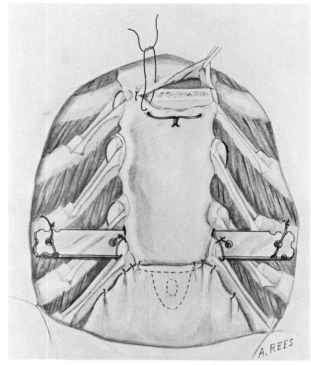

Fig. 17-23. Operative correction of pectus excavatum. The distorted medial portions of the costal cartilages have been resected and a steel bar has been placed behind the lower end of the sternum to decrease the possibility of late posterior sagging of the bone. From 9 to 12 months after operation the steel bar is removed through a small incision at the lateral ends. (From: *Holcomb GW Jr: Surgical correction of pectus excavatum. J Pediatr Surg 12:295, 1977, with permission.*)

The technique most widely used is that described by Ravitch. All the deformed costal cartilages are excised, the xiphisternal joint is disarticulated, and intercostal muscle bundles are separated from the sternum, and transverse posterior osteotomy of the sternum is performed above the point of depression. The osteotomy is combined with a forward fracture of the sternum and insertion of a bone wedge in the osteotomy site to provide an overcorrection of the deformity. Early results are 80 to 90 percent satisfactory.

The few long-term (20-year) results available suggest a disappointing tendency for the defect to slowly recur, and a number of modifications have been developed to counteract this tendency. Holcomb has described such a modification using a metal strut that is removed several months after the repair (Fig. 17-23). Wesselhoeft and Deluca have described a simplified procedure in which the deformed costal cartilages are resected subperichondrially through individual incisions in the pectoral muscles, without mobilizing the sternum from the intercostal muscles. A malleable metal strut is passed transsternally and placed beneath the pectoral muscles laterally. The strut is removed in 4 to 6 months, frequently under local anesthesia. Seventy of seventy-five children followed more than 5 years had an excellent cosmetic result.

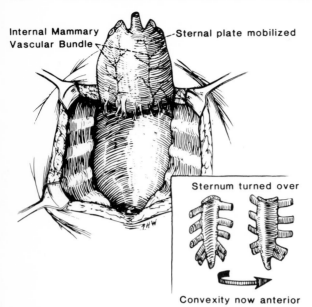

Internal Mammary Vascular Bundle — Sternal plate mobilized

Sternum turned over

Convexity now anterior

Fig. 17-24. Sternal eversion technique for repair of pectus excavatum. *A.* The sternum is divided transversely just above the beginning of the deformity. The costal cartilages are divided vertically, just lateral to the beginning of the cartilaginous deformity. *B.* The sternal plastron is elevated and rotated so that the convexity is now anterior. The authors prefer to preserve one mammary pedicle. (From: *Hawkins JA, Ehrenhaft JL, et al: 1984, with permission.*)

Kirschner wires, autologous rib struts, Marlex mesh, and other devices have also been described, without reported results that would convincingly favor the use of any particular method.

Sternal eversion is a method that has been widely used in Japan by Wada, who reported satisfactory results in 97 percent of 199 patients over a 15-year experience. A smaller series from Iowa with similar results was reported by Hawkins et al. in 1984. The technique involves transverse division of the sternum, division of the costal cartilages, 180° axial rotation of the sternum (sternal eversion), and suture reattachment. In essence, the concave deformity is made convex. The sternal plastron can be rotated on a mammary artery vascular pedicle or as a free graft (Fig. 17-24).

Surgeons who prefer to focus on the cosmetic defect have used silicone implants to remodel the external appearance of the chest wall, with cosmetically satisfying results. Such a method is not applicable until growth has ceased, and would seem inappropriate in patients whose symptoms or findings suggest a physiologic impairment.

PECTUS CARINATUM

The protrusion deformities of the sternum are much less common than pectus excavatum, accounting for less than 10 percent of patients presenting for repair. Two principal types have been distinguished by Ravitch, although there is considerable variation from patient to patient. The most common type has been called the

"chicken breast" type by Ravitch and is characterized by a deep depression of the costal cartilages along each side of the sternum, accentuating mild protrusion of the sternum by creating an illusion of greater anterior projection relative to the ribs. The deformity is usually developed maximally below the nipple level, involving the fourth through the seventh or eighth costal cartilages. As with pectus excavatum, asymmetry is common, most often producing mild rotation of the sternum to the right.

The second type Ravitch has called the "pouter pigeon" variety, characterized by a double angle in the sternum. The manubrium and upper costal cartilages project forward, while the body of the sternum first angulates posteriorly for a variable distance, then sharply reverses to project anteriorly. A depression is created in the lower part of the sternum that resembles pectus excavatum.

Although symptoms reminiscent of pectus excavatum have been associated with the protrusion defects, it appears that most are asymptomatic, and the condition has seldom been studied physiologically. Operative correction is done through a curved submammary incision that allows broad exposure of the deformed cartilages and costochondral junctions (Fig. 17-25). Subperichondral and subperiosteal resection of all deformed cartilages and ribs is performed throughout the length of their deformity. The excessive length of each perichondral bed is obliterated with reefing sutures, and the sternal contour is adjusted with a transverse osteotomy if necessary. Correction of the "pouter-pigeon" variety requires less lateral dissection but does require osteotomy at each of the two sternal angulations.

STERNAL FISSURES

The sternum is formed when two lateral plates of mesoderm fuse in the midline during the tenth week of embryonic development. The clavicular heads also contribute primordia to the manubrium. Failure of fusion can be complete, or it can be confined to the superior end or the inferior end of the sternum.

SUPERIOR STERNAL CLEFT. In this type of defect the cleft is broad and U- or V-shaped, usually extending down to about the fourth costal cartilage (Fig. 17-26). The prominent pulsations of the heart, which is covered only by thoracic fascia and skin, create the illusion of cardiac displacement into the neck. In fact, the heart usually lies in approximately normal position, and the two separate halves of the sternum can be located at the periphery of the defect and reapproximated. Osteotomies in each half, or distal transection of each half is usually necessary to

Fig. 17-25. A fourteen-year-old boy with pectus carinatum. *A.* The preoperative lateral chest x-ray shows remarkable anterior projection of the sternum. *B.* A line drawing demonstrates the forward projection of the sternum that is accentuated by the prominence of the knoblike costal cartilages. *C.* The postoperative photograph of the patient demonstrates a very satisfactory result. *D.* The postoperative lateral chest x-ray contrasts sharply with the preoperative film.

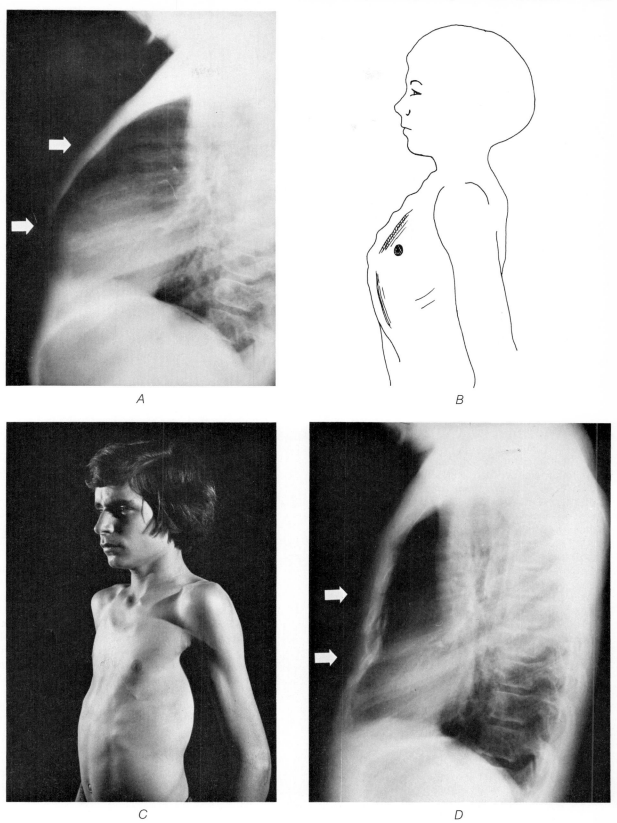

A

B

C

D

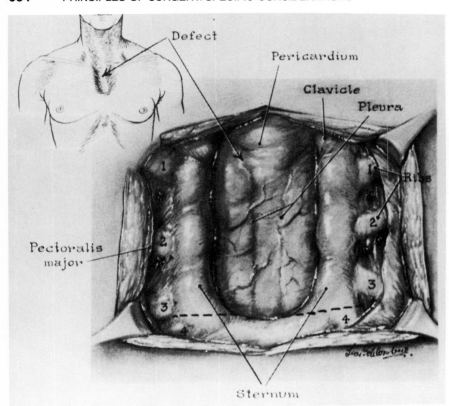

Fig. 17-26. A superior sternal cleft, presenting clinically with striking pulsation at the base of the neck, where the pericardium bulges out through the defect. It is frequently possible to pull the two sternal halves together by transecting the inferior end of the defect (dotted lines), combined with oblique chondrotomies of the costal cartilages. In the case illustrated, an eleven-year-old girl, reduction was not possible, and the defect was successfully repaired with a steel wire mesh covering. (From: *Ravitch MM, with permission.*)

bring them together. In some cases, especially those repaired after infancy, there will not be room for the heart, and coverage with prosthetic material is required.

DISTAL STERNAL CLEFT. A defect in the distal sternal is almost invariably part of a syndrome called Cantrell's pentalogy, which consists of the following five components: (1) a cleft distal sternum, (2) a ventral abdominal wall defect that may be a true omphalocele, (3) an anterior crescentic deficiency of the diaphragm, (4) communication between the parietal and peritoneal cavities through the diaphragm, and (5) congenital heart disease, usually with a ventricular septal defect and a left ventricular diverticulum.

Operative correction requires a staged approach taking into account the priorities of each defect. The omphalocele is usually repaired first. As with other forms of sternal cleft, early reconstruction offers the best chance for primary closure.

COMPLETE STERNAL CLEFT. In this rarest form of sternal cleft, failure of midline fusion is complete, leaving the mediastinal contents bulging through a thin covering of skin and fascia. In the few cases described, an associated failure of midline abdominal fusion has been frequent, and communication between the peritoneum and pericardium common. Repair in infancy is highly desirable and can be quite satisfactory.

MISCELLANEOUS ANOMALIES OF RIB AND COSTAL CARTILAGE

The simplest anomalies consist of deformed, deficient, or enlarged cartilage or rib presenting as an isolated finding in an asymptomatic patient. More complex anomalies include absence or wide divergence of one or more lower ribs and are commonly associated with hemivertebrae, fused bony paravertebral bars, and progressive scoliosis. The chest wall defect can manifest obvious paradoxic respiratory motion and even true lung herniation, but the spinal anomalies are usually more functionally significant and demand more therapeutic attention.

Poland's syndrome consists of absence or hypoplasia of the pectoralis major and minor muscles, breast hypoplasia, and partial absence of the upper costal cartilages (Fig. 17-27). Brachysyndactyly, ectrodactyly, and ectromelia are frequently described associations. It is invariably unilateral. Depending on the extent of cartilage deficiency there may be an impressive lung hernia, paradoxical respiratory motion, or simple flattening of the

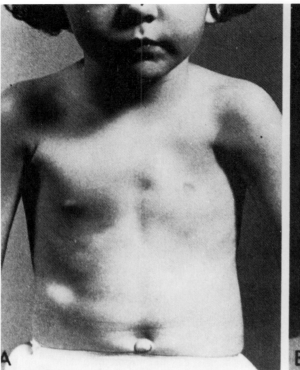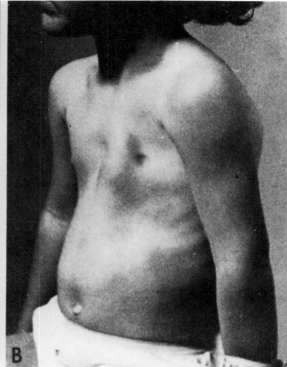

Fig. 17-27. Poland's syndrome in a child. The sternocostal portion of the pectoralis major, the pectoralis minor, and cartilages 2 to 4 are absent on the left side. The nipple, breast, and subcutaneous tissue are hypoplastic. (From: *Ravitch MM, with permission.*)

anterolateral chest wall. When the anomaly is on the left side, the underlying heart and lung are significantly vulnerable, since they are covered only by skin, fascia, and pleura. As the child grows, the concavity tends to become more severe on either side.

Operative reconstruction is recommended for cosmetic reasons, to eliminate paradoxical motion, and to protect intrathoracic structures. Staged procedures involving split rib grafts from the contralateral side combined with Teflon felt or Marlex mesh have been advocated in the past. A logical outgrowth of the increasing popularity of pedicled myocutaneous flaps has been their application in the reconstruction of this anomaly. Urschel et al. described successful single-stage reconstruction in two patients using a lattisimus dorsi flap and simultaneous augmentation mammoplasty.

Thoracic Outlet Syndrome

The thoracic outlet is a tight anatomic space with rigid delimiters and much crowding of the important neurovascular components that must traverse the space. These structural components are subject to a variety of congenital, traumatic, and degenerative abnormalities that may impinge on the vessels and nerve trunks that have low tolerance for compression without symptoms. Osteopo-

rotic or arthritic degenerative changes in cervicothoracic vertebra, callus-rich healing of first rib or clavicular fractures, developmental or fibrotic variations in the course or insertion of the scalene family of muscles, the skeletal anomalies that occur in the first thoracic rib, and the relatively frequent finding of one or more cervical ribs all may contribute to symptomatic neurovascular compression syndromes. Over the past few decades, the several more specific anatomic structures believed to be causing the compression have been labeled "syndromes" embracing the symptoms, but currently the cervical rib, scalenus anticus, hyperabduction, costoclavicular, pectoralis minor, and first rib syndromes have all been subsumed under the more general concept of the thoracic outlet syndrome.

Cervical Ribs

Perhaps because they are anatomically easy to demonstrate, the cervical rib anomalies have received a disproportionate attention in symptomatic patients. Cervical ribs occur in about 1 percent of the population, but only a small minority of those (less than 10 percent) have symptoms attributable to the extra ribs. Bilateral in 80 percent of cases, the anomaly is characterized by significant anatomic variation, including variation between the two sides in the same person (Fig. 17-28) and the symptoms may be unilateral, correlating poorly with the extent of anatomic abnormality. In most large series of patients with thoracic outlet syndrome, less than 15 percent are found to have a cervical rib. In the simplest form, Type I, the rib is a short bar of bone that extends only a few millimeters beyond the transverse process of C_7 vertebra and is completely enveloped in cervical and scalene muscles. A Type III cervical rib extends to and joins the superior surface of the first rib at or near the scalene tubercle by a synchondrosis. Cervical ribs of intermediate length between Types I and III are designated as Type II, and they often

have a fascial condensation that extends as a ligament from the anterior tip to the superior surface of the first rib. The rare Type IV cervical rib is a complete rib articulating by a costal cartilage with the sternum. The lowest trunk of the brachial plexus (C_8 and T_1 nerve roots), the subclavian artery, and occasionally the subclavian vein may course over the superior surface of the cervical rib, or over the ligament from the tip of the rib to the first thoracic rib. In symptomatic individuals it is most often the pressure on the lowest trunk of the plexus, particularly those fibers giving rise to the ulnar nerve, that causes progressive discomfort.

SYMPTOMS. Symptoms of neurovascular compression at the thoracic outlet may occur whether or not a cervical rib is present. The compression usually results from the small space between the first thoracic rib and the clavicle. When a cervical rib is present, it may aggravate the symptoms by further reducing the space. Other potential sites of compression are the scalene triangle and the pectoralis minor space. Symptoms are much more frequent in women, with a high proportion appearing in the osteoporosis years. Patient complaints will vary depending on whether the structures compromised are primarily vascular or neural. While poststenotic dilation of the subclavian artery with peripheral embolization or other evidences of vascular insufficiency do occur, in over 90 percent of cases, the symptoms are neurogenic in nature. Symptoms are variable but generally include aching in the base of the neck, shoulder, or arm with paresthesias down the medial side of the arm, forearm, and hand. Intermittent weak-

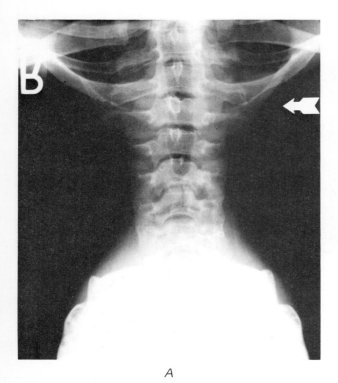

A

Fig. 17-28. A thirty-two-year-old woman with severe symptoms of thoracic-outlet compression syndrome in the left upper extremity. *A.* The cervical spine x-ray shows a Type III cervical rib on the left side *(arrow)* and a Type II cervical rib on the right. *B.* A selective left subclavian arteriogram shows compression of the artery at the point where it passes between the clavicle and the first rib. However, the patient's symptoms were predominately neurologic.

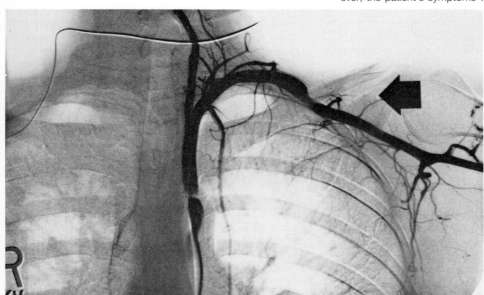

B

ness in grip may cause the patient to drop things or to develop hand and forearm fatigue quickly when doing manual work. Symptoms of arterial compression include numbness of the hand, pallor, fatigue, vague diffuse discomfort, coolness, occasionally a sensitivity to cold, and aggravation by postural elevation of the extremity. When venous compression occurs, the patient notices intermittent swelling and bluish discoloration of the extremity.

DIAGNOSTIC FINDINGS. Attention should be given to those factors in the history that might predispose to anatomic changes in the shoulder girdle. Trauma, particularly clavicular fractures, activities in occupation or exercise that might increase compression in the outlet (overhead hand-arm work or the ''milk-pail'' carrying position), and progressing sagging-shoulder posture are among the suggestive historical findings.

The majority of patients demonstrate little objective evidence of nerve compression on physical examination. If compression of the brachial plexus has been progressive, the patient may demonstrate atrophy and weakness of the intrinsic muscles of the hand, and eventually weakness of the forearm. If a cervical rib is discovered by x-ray examination in the absence of other explanations for their symptoms, the extra rib is too frequently assigned the causative role. Whether or not the extra ribs are present, it is often difficult to distinguish symptoms representing brachial plexus compression from those caused by cervical nerve root pressure or cervical disc disease. Moore, in his review of the experience at a large metropolitan hospital, has recently emphasized how frequently trauma to the neck or shoulder may precede the development of thoracic outlet symptoms and may be an unrecognized factor in those cases resistant to treatment. Capistrant, in reporting 35 cases of thoracic outlet syndrome complicating whiplash or cervical strain injury, described both an acute group and a group of patients with chronic symptoms. After etiologies such as trauma and cervical rib or other osseous abnormalities have been considered, there remain a large number of patients for whom there is no obvious explanation of the onset of symptoms. It is for these patients particularly that the physician must be cautious and conservative in approaching the diagnostic evaluation and treatment.

A lack of conclusive evidence by physical examination that neurovascular compression at the thoracic outlet is responsible for a patient's symptoms is not unusual. In slender patients a large cervical rib may be palpable, but the most consistent physical finding, whether or not an extra rib is present, is distinct tenderness over the brachial plexus in the supraclavicular space. Table 17-5, taken from Roos' extensive experience, lists the features of physical examination that are helpful in establishing the diagnosis of brachial plexus compression. Roos feels that an elevated arm exercise test is especially helpful in the clinical diagnosis if it reproduces the patient's symptoms. The test is performed by having patients hold their arms at right angles to the thorax with the forearms flexed at 90° and the elbows braced posteriorly. Patients are then asked to open and close their fists at moderate speed for 3 min.

Table 17-5. TESTS TO ESTABLISH THE DIAGNOSIS OF NEUROLOGIC THORACIC-OUTLET SYNDROME

1. Percussion pain
   Supraclavicular over brachial plexus
   Infraclavicular
   Ipsilateral side of neck
2. Thumb pressure (30 s)
   Pain and tenderness over brachial plexus (supraclavicular)
   Gradual reproduction of usual symptoms down the arm
3. Weak muscles
   Grip
   Triceps (innervated by seventh cervical nerve)
   Interosseous hand muscles (innervated by eighth cervical and first thoracic nerve roots)
4. Hypesthesia to touch and pinprick
   Inner forearm (eighth cervical, first thoracic dermatomes)
   Ulnar side of hand and fingers
   Occasionally radial dermatome, dorsum first web
5. Elevated arm exercise test (3 min)
   Early fatigue and heaviness of involved arm
   Gradual onset of numbness and tingling in hand
   Increasing vocal complaints
   Crescendo of distress of entire upper extremity
   Sudden dropping of limb into lap (''completely shot'')

SOURCE: Modified from Roos DB: Congenital anomalies associated wtih thoracic outlet syndrome. Anatomy, symptoms, diagnosis and treatment. *Am J Surg* 132:771, 1976, with permission.

Because pulse changes are easily documented, and even though only 5 to 10 percent of symptomatic patients suffer from vascular compromise, most of the diagnostic tests in use focus on compression of the subclavian artery by the clavicle, first rib, scalenus anticus, or pectoralis minor tendon. In the *Adson maneuver,* the first rib is elevated by a deep breath, the scalene is contracted by turning the head to the examined side and stretched by extending the neck; loss of the pulse is a positive finding. By assuming the exaggerated military position (the *costoclavicular maneuver*), the clavicle is pulled down toward the first rib to directly compress the subclavian artery; again the pulse may be reduced or obliterated. In the *hyperabduction maneuver,* the vessel is compressed (by passively hyperabducting the arm) by the tendon of the pectoralis muscle. Unfortunately all these maneuvers may reduce or obliterate the pulse in a high proportion of asymptomatic people, and a significant group of patients with advancing neurogenic symptoms may retain a pulse during the examinations. A vascular bruit may be heard over the subclavian artery, particularly with the shoulders in hyperabduction.

Whether or not vascular lesions are found, careful documentation of neurologic abnormalities should be sought. With the often confusing complaints and the overlapping of symptoms, it may be difficult to identify those patients who may have cervical nerve root compression, carpal tunnel syndrome, or other neurovascular abnormalities, rather than the thoracic outlet syndrome. Apically situated peripheral lung cancers (the Pancoast tumor) may present with symptoms suggestive of the thoracic outlet syndrome. Patients may have median nerve compression at the wrist and brachial plexus compression at the thoracic outlet simultaneously.

Several objective tests have been recommended as confirmatory evidence supportive of a clinical diagnosis of thoracic outlet syndrome. While some groups have found the ulnar nerve conduction velocity to be a good predictor of success from surgical approach, others have reported excellent symptomatic relief in some patients with normal preoperative values. Jerrett has added somatosensory evoked potentials (SEPs) to the electrophysiologic evaluation and finds it to be a reliable, sensitive, quantitative, and noninvasive diagnostic tool. Plethysmography, angiography, computer-assisted tomography, and other imaging techniques are all useful in selected cases to confirm the presence of anatomical abnormalities, but astute evaluation of the symptoms remains most important in diagnosis because of the frequency of successfully treated symptoms in the absence of any detectable structural abnormality, the frequency of the anatomic abnormalities in the absence of symptoms, and the occasional persistence of symptoms after surgical correction of apparent physical compression.

TREATMENT. The treatment of thoracic outlet syndrome depends on the severity of symptoms, the apparent cause, and the presence of complications such as subclavian artery aneurysm. It now seems clear that, in the basence of clearly identified significant vascular problems, most patients should initially be treated nonoperatively with a reasonable expectation that a majority will achieve acceptable symptomatic relief. Treatment should be started with the use of shoulder girdle exercises and postural correction. This is based on the concept that an elevated and abducted shoulder girdle decreases compression of the neurovascular bundle at the costoclavicular space. If the patient presents with severe pain and muscle spasm, it may be appropriate to initiate treatment in the hospital with appropriate analgesics, moist heat, muscle relaxants, and a progressive program of physical therapy.

Many patients complain of waking from sleep with pain and paresthesias in the affected arm. McGough and his associates incorporate an attempt to manage sleeping posture in their regimen of nonoperative treatment. This involves a three-pillow positioning technique that attempts to maintain the shoulder girdles in an abducted and slightly elevated position during sleep. A majority of patients should respond to conservative treatment even though 6 weeks to 3 months may be required to achieve significant relief. The highest failure rate for nonoperative treatment has been in those patients with Type III cervical ribs or a trauma etiology.

Since Clagett's provocative presentation in 1962, the basic surgical treatment for thoracic outlet syndrome has consisted of resection of the first rib along with any cervical rib or abnormal congenital bands that may be present. Removal of the first rib results in the simultaneous division of the anterior and middle scalene muscles and the "dropping" of the floor, thereby opening the compression compartment. Strong advocates for each of several surgical approaches to the first rib have presented their preferences over the past two decades. The transaxillary approach has resulted in excellent results in experienced hands, but considerable skill is required to do an adequate resection of a cervical rib through this approach. Clagett's posterior parascapular incision allows good exposure of the brachial plexus and is especially helpful for reoperation. If a subclavian artery aneurysm must be treated, an anterior incision is required, often with partial resection of the clavicle. In most reports, approximately 80 percent of patients have excellent relief of symptoms following operation, while 5 to 10 percent continue to experience significant discomfort. Qvarfordt et al. have urged a combined supraclavicular scalenectomy (and cervical rib resection if indicated) and transaxillary first rib resection. In their 94 patients, the precise assessment of the anatomy was associated with a low failure rate and few postoperative complications.

First rib resection may not be the operation of first selection for all patients who require surgical treatment for thoracic outlet compression symptoms. In a group of patients with a history of neck trauma preceding the onset of symptoms, Sanders and his associates report success following anterior approach to anterior and middle scalenectomy without rib resection. Particularly where vascular reconstruction may be necessary, anterior approaches that allow adequate exposure of the subclavian vessel are essential. Scher, Veith, et al. analyzed the uncommon arterial complications associated with cervical ribs, recommending simple rib removal for stenosis with mild poststenotic dilation (Stage I). When intrinsic arterial damage is detected (Stage II), rib resection and arterial (or aneurysm) resection and reconstruction is indicated. Stage III lesions are those in which arterial thrombosis or peripheral embolization has developed. In these cases thrombectomy and embolectomy should be added to rib resection and arterial reconstruction. Blank and Connar have emphasized that cervical ribs are present in almost all patients who develop a vascular complication.

Chest Wall Tumors

In reviewing this topic in 1949, Brian Blades observed, "Available statistical data concerning the exact incidence of thoracic wall tumors are incomplete and probably unimportant. Moreover accurate histological classification of the tumors is often confusing." Now as then, many reports in the literature are limited case reports, the few larger series are reported from major tertiary referral hospitals, and the available statistical data relating to the frequency of the various types probably remain inaccurate. Depending on the referral characteristics of the reporting institution, the incidence of primary malignancy in recent reviews of chest wall tumors ranges from 13 percent (Cavanaugh) to over 50 percent (Sabanathan). Since most published cases are from the large referral centers, it seems likely that the true incidence of malignancy in the general population may be nearer the lower figure. Whatever the true frequency, malignancies are common enough and clinical or laboratory findings are sufficiently uncertain that speculating about the probabilities of any given chest wall mass being benign or malignant is usually an unimportant exercise. It should be considered malignant until proved otherwise by detailed analysis by an experienced surgical pathologist.

The reported experience from those centers confirms that malignancies in this location are easily and often mismanaged. Biopsies are untrustworthy, fears about chest wall reconstruction difficulties occasionally encourage inadequate local resection, and recurrence after inadequate initial resection is a common cause of failure. The risk of tumor implantation following needle or incisional biopsy has been widely cited. For these reasons, and because of the strong advocacy and excellent results reported from several centers, generous excisional biopsies have been widely recommended as the preferred first invasive diagnostic procedure. More recently several authors have emphasized that some of the assumptions that establish the rationale for that approach may no longer be applicable. For several tumors (e.g., Ewing's sarcoma, osteogenic sarcoma) chemotherapy plays an important, perhaps dominant, role. Contemporary diagnostic capabilities of surgical pathologists (e.g., electron microscopy, immunohistochemical techniques, special stains) have improved diagnostic accuracy. As pointed out by Benfield, the accumulating experience in most cancer centers in recent years has failed to support the hypothesis that implantation occurs following carefully done incisional biopsies. With advances in reconstruction techniques (e.g., myocutaneous flaps, improved synthetic materials), virtually any defect in the chest wall can be repaired and the complete removal of biopsy sites is less troublesome. Though the controversy is not fully resolved, a logical approach at present would seem to call for an aggressive effort to ascertain an accurate diagnosis before embarking on extensive ablative surgical therapy and to consider a multimodal approach, attending to advances taking place in oncology. Accurate diagnosis requires adequate tissue; needle biopsies should be avoided and frozen sections should be performed on removed tissue before leaving the operating room, not to establish a diagnosis but to be sure suitable tissue for eventual diagnosis has been submitted. Metastatic tumors, especially to the ribs, and direct invasion of the chest wall from primary lung and breast carcinomas easily outnumber the tumors arising from the chest wall. Therefore, while the biopsy is being processed, careful search for primary neoplasm elsewhere should be made. Thyroid, breast, and kidney are the most common to metastasize to the ribs.

The primary tumors that occur in the chest wall are those, both benign and malignant, that occur in the soft tissue and skeletal structures that are present there. Resection of cavernous hemangiomas, hemangiopericytomas, rhabdomyosarcomas, for example, have special significance when management of these tumors results in removing large segments of the bony thorax with the physiologic consequences that follow.

The clinical manifestation of a chest wall neoplasm is most often either pain, a palpable mass, or an abnormality detected on a chest x-ray. Surprisingly, with either benign or malignant lesions the discomfort is relatively mild, and patients often present with tumors that have been enlarging for months or years. Many patients will attribute the tumor origin to some episode of localized trauma, or they will state that they discovered the mass while rubbing their chest after a minor injury. A differential diagnosis will include the less frequent pulmonary infections that invade the chest wall, such as actinomycosis and nocardiosis, tuberculous chondritis, costochondral separation, and Tietze's syndrome (nonspecific chondritis). A suspicion of fluctuation in the mass and a corresponding pulmonary lesion may suggest that a diagnostic aspiration should be done in instances of probable infection. A true history of trauma and the ability to reproduce a clicking sensation with local pressure may reinforce the diagnosis of a suspected costochondral separation.

Work-up of the patient with a chest wall mass should focus on a search for other areas of neoplastic involvement by radioisotope studies and other imaging studies along with careful computer-assisted tomographic scans to accurately map the local extent of the tumor invasion and to plan resection and reconstruction of the chest wall defect. It must also include evaluation of pulmonary function and assessment of the patient's ability to tolerate the physiologic deficit that might result from the procedure. Since histological identification of the tumor type is essential in virtually all cases of chest wall mass, refining the clinical characteristics that might improve the diagnostic guess is less important than in some other circumstances.

BENIGN TUMORS

Among the more likely benign tumors are fibrous dysplasia, eosinophilic granuloma, osteochondroma, desmoid tumor, and chondroma.

Fibrous Dysplasia. The ribs are the most common site of solitary fibrous dysplasia (osteofibroma, bone cyst). Located most frequently in the posterior or lateral portion of a rib, it usually presents as a slowly enlarging nonpainful mass. Diagnostic radiographs show expansion and thinning of the bony cortex, with a central trabeculated appearance. Fibrous dysplasia in ribs as well as other bones forms part of Albright's syndrome, a condition that includes skin pigmentation and precocious puberty in girls.

Eosinophilic Granuloma. The lesions of eosinophilic granuloma are sometimes part of a disease that includes pulmonary lesions called histiocytosis X or eosinophilic granuloma of the lung. When it occurs in a rib, the granuloma is a solitary destructive process, often associated with pain and localized tenderness. Radiographs reveal a punched-out osteolytic lesion, which, when subjected to excision and microscopic examination, is found to consist of a chronic granuloma. Healing may occur spontaneously, or a pathologic fracture may develop through the area of osteolysis.

Osteochondroma. These slow-growing tumors generally arise from the cortex of a rib. As with other neoplasms, the occurrence of pain may signal accelerated growth, which produces concern over the possibility of malignant change. The radiographic appearance is often that of a distorted rib cortex with an overlying mass that has a thin rim of calcification.

Chondroma. They occur at the costochondral junction, primarily in children or young people, and may be difficult to differentiate from chondritis or the sequela of traumatic costochondral separation. Chest and rib x-rays show an expansion of bone with thinned but intact cortex. Probably because of the abundance of cartilage in the chest wall, chondromas and chondrosarcomas are the most common benign and malignant tumors of the skeletal components of the thorax. Chondrosarcoma is usually a well-differentiated tumor easily misdiagnosed as a benign chondroma resulting in inadequate local resection and consequent local recurrence.

Desmoid Tumors. Whether these tumors are a form of benign fibromatosis or a low-grade fibrosarcoma, they have a high propensity to recur locally and should be resected with the same wide margins recommended for primary malignant tumors.

MALIGNANT TUMORS

The optimum management of the malignant tumors of the chest wall may be influenced by accurate diagnosis. Those most likely to be found are fibrosarcoma, chondrosarcoma, Ewing's sarcoma, osteogenic sarcoma, and myeloma (plasmacytoma).

Fibrosarcoma. Fibrosarcomas may arise in the soft tissues of the chest wall or from the periosteum of the bony thoracic skeleton. Involvement of the skin and subcutaneous tissue occurs and metastases to the lungs are characteristic of the terminal stages. Wide surgical resection preceded and/or followed by chemotherapy is currently recommended treatment.

Chondrosarcoma. This relatively slowly growing malignancy occurs most commonly in the anterior part of the thorax in the third through fifth decades of life. The tumor may extend either internally or outwardly into the soft tissue of the chest wall. Because of a varied histologic picture that often fails to provide proof of malignancy, a simple biopsy of a chondrosarcoma may not be used to guide treatment unless it is interpreted as malignant. The performance of a wide excision of the tumor with a generous margin of surrounding tissue is the proper treatment for chondrosarcoma. It is the relatively frequent undertreatment of these tumors that provides the best argument for wide excisional biopsy as a preferred primary treatment for chest wall tumors.

Osteogenic Sarcoma. This tumor may exhibit extremely rapid growth, particularly in young people. The case depicted in Figs. 17-29 and 17-30 was believed to be a walnut-sized breast mass 4 months before the CT scan was taken. Resection required complete removal of ribs 4 through 11 along with the lateral portion of the diaphragm and a wedge of lung. The predominant component may be cartilaginous, bony, or fibrous, and the lesion may result in both bone destruction and bone production. There is often an early development of pulmonary metastases in osteogenic sarcoma, and in occasional instances it may be proper to resect the metastases at the same time that the

primary tumor is treated. Drawing from the experience with long bone osteogenic sarcoma in children, preoperative chemotherapy, occasionally combined with rapid-fraction irradiation, followed by wide surgical excision seems to be the most promising approach to this aggressive tumor. It is the relatively encouraging early results from this multimodal therapy that argues for accurate diagnosis by generous incisional biopsy before extensive surgery.

Ewing's Sarcoma. The appearance of a rapidly enlarging painful mass during the first two decades of life characterizes Ewing's tumor. Fever and malaise are common systemic symptoms. Radiographs may show a characteristic onion-skin appearance that is due to elevation of the periosteum as the tumor enlarges. Spread to other bones occurs early in a high percentage of patients, but the tumor is generally radiosensitive. If the diagnosis is made by biopsy, the choice of treatment may be irradiation alone or radical excision combined with the irradiation. Unfortunately, the prognosis is poor regardless of the treatment chosen.

Myeloma. Plasma cell myeloma is more frequently a generalized disease than a solitary tumor affecting a single rib. When a solitary plasmacytoma does occur in the thoracic cage, the serum proteins are generally normal and Bence–Jones proteins are not found in the urine. In general, myeloma is a disease of the elderly, and most who present with a solitary lesion will eventually develop systemic myeloma. Chest x-rays show the solitary lesion as a punched-out defect in the rib, with expansion and thinning of the cortex. The clinical course of patients with a solitary myeloma is markedly different from that of patients who first appear with multiple lesions. The latter are almost always dead within 2 years after the diagnosis is made, but those who have a solitary lesion initially may live for many years without evidence of other disease. A careful survey for other sites of disease should be made in patients who present with a solitary lesion, and if none is found, the involved rib should be resected.

Chest Wall Reconstruction

Because of the high rate of malignancy in chest wall neoplasms, there is need for an aggressive attitude toward management of any mass that likely represents a primary tumor. When malignancy is suspected, preliminary plans must be made for chest wall reconstruction that will allow resection of a generous margin of normal tissue around the neoplasm. The resection should include at least one normal adjacent rib above and below the tumor with all intervening intercostal muscles and pleura. In addition, it is often necessary to include an en bloc resection of overlying chest wall muscles such as the pectoralis minor or major, the serratus anterior, or the latissimus dorsi. When the periphery of the lung is involved with the neoplasm, it

Fig. 17-29. Preoperative CT and first postoperative chest x-ray of explosively enlarging chest wall tumor (osteogenic sarcoma) in the left chest of a forty-year-old woman. Only 4 months earlier a small nodule thought to be a breast tumor was felt.

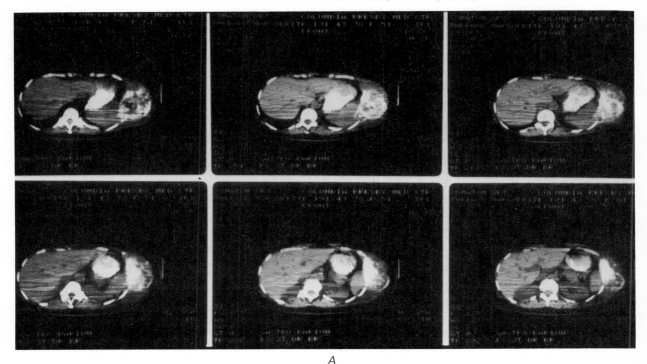

A

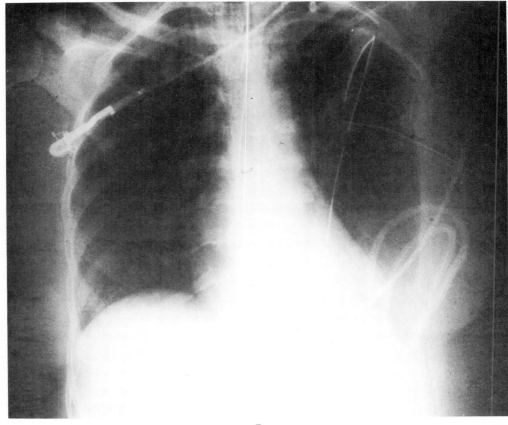

B

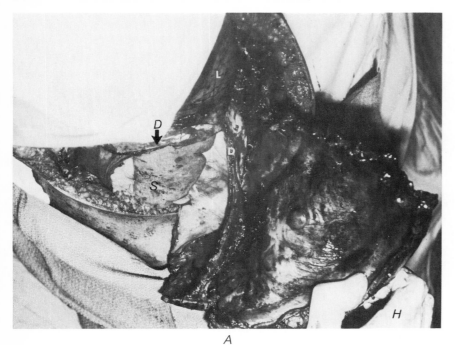

A

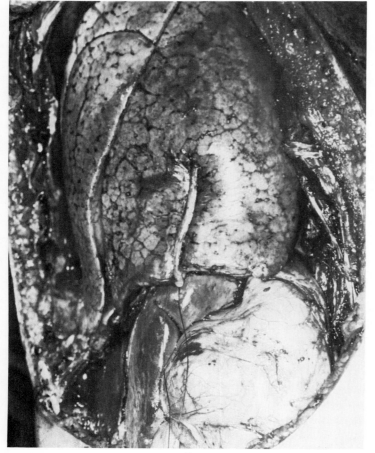

B

Fig. 17-30. Photographs taken in the operating room from the case noted in Fig. 17-29. *A.* The tumor is being resected with two grossly normal ribs above and below the lesion. This required removal of most or all of ribs 3 through 10. H indicates the surgeon's hand retracting the lesion; D marks the cut edge of the diaphragm on both specimen and patient side; S indicates the spleen; L is the lung. *B.* A wedge of lung was removed where pleural adhesions attached to the tumor. The large defect included the lateral third of the diaphragm. This operative view reveals the spleen and abdominal viscera and huge chest wall defect that existed after resection. *C.* The resected specimen. *D.* The prosthesis has been sewn in place. The line of reattachment of the diaphragm is seen in the lower third of the prosthesis. A myocutaneous flap from the left rectus muscle was used to close the skin defect.

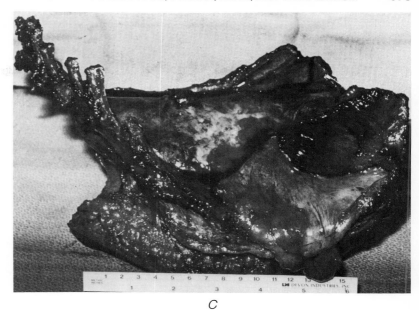

C

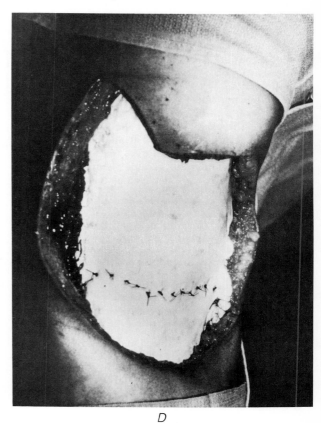

D

Fig. 17-30 *C,D.* Continued.

is appropriate to resect the adjacent part of the pulmonary lobe in continuity (Fig. 17-30*C*). Involvement of the sternum by a malignant tumor requires a total resection of the sternum with the adjacent cartilages. Techniques for postoperative respiratory support are sufficiently good

that resection should not be compromised because of a concern about the patient's ability to ventilate adequately in the early postoperative period.

Reconstruction of a large defect in the chest wall requires the use of some type of material to prevent lung herniation and to provide stability for the chest wall (Fig. 17-30*D*). Mild degrees of paradoxical motion are often well tolerated if the area of instability is relatively small. Pairolero and Arnold have recently reported an extensive experience at the Mayo Clinic of over 200 chest wall reconstructions following removal of significant portions of the bony thorax. They emphasize that both adequate resection and dependable reconstruction are essential ingredients to a successful operation and express the strong belief that a thoracic surgeon–plastic surgeon team is an important collaboration if these complicated problems are to be undertaken. While a wide variety of materials has been used to reestablish chest wall stability including rib autografts, steel struts, acrylic plates, and various synthetic meshes, their current preference is to use a 2-mm-thick polytetrafluoroethylene (Gore–Tex) soft tissue patch with rotation or myocutaneous flaps for coverage.

DISEASES OF THE PLEURA AND PLEURAL SPACE

The inner surface of each hemithorax has a mesothelial lining, the parietal pleura, which is invaginated at each pulmonary hilum to form the visceral pleura. The two surfaces are normally in apposition, lubricated by a thin layer of serous fluid secreted by the mesothelium, so that the steady motion of normal respiration is accomplished without friction. Therefore, the pleural ''space'' is normally only a potential space lying between the visceral pleura investing the lung and the parietal pleura of the chest wall. The elastic recoil of the lung and the rapid continuous absorption of fluid from the pleural space create a balance of opposing forces that favor apposition of the visceral pleura to the parietal pleura. The introduction of fluid or air breaks this dynamic coupling and converts the potential space to a real space. Normal respiratory mechanics are impaired in proportion to the size of the space created and the pressure within it. Many of the processes affecting the pleural space are essentially mechanical, such as spontaneous pneumothorax or congestive heart failure, and are not associated with any pathologic alteration in either pleural surface. However, virtually any chronic form of pleural space disturbance is associated with pathologic changes that produce thickening and adherence of the visceral and parietal surfaces. The end results vary from a few filmy adhesions of no consequence to a dense fibrous and calcific obliteration of the pleural space with a permanent restrictive defect in pulmonary function.

Pleural Effusion

A pleural effusion is an accumulation of fluid in the pleural space. It is not a disease entity but signals the effect of pleural or systemic disease on the normal daily passage of fluid through the pleural space. Normally, the balance of hydrostatic and colloid osmotic forces favors movement of fluid from systemic capillaries in the parietal pleura to pulmonary capillaries. It is estimated that

Table 17-6. CAUSES OF TRANSUDATIVE EFFUSION

Congestive heart failure
Nephrotic syndrome
Cirrhosis
Hypoproteinemia
Myxedema
Peritoneal dialysis

between 5 and 10 L of protein-free fluid traverses the pleural space in 24 h. Simultaneously, lymphatics drain smaller volumes of fluid containing protein, which would otherwise remain in the pleural space as a source of colloid osmotic pressure favoring retention of fluid. Alterations in systemic hydrostatic or colloid osmotic pressure that disturb the balance of forces across normal pleural surfaces produce an effusion consisting of a protein-poor ultrafiltrate of plasma classified as a transudate. Changes in capillary permeability caused by inflammation or infiltration of the pleura produce a protein-rich effusion classified as an exudate. Common causes of transudates and exudates are listed in Table 17-6 and Table 17-7. The distinction between transudate and exudate has diagnostic relevance, as noted in one series in which effusions were malignant in 42 percent of patients with an exudate and were caused by congestive heart failure in 83 percent of patients with a transudate.

Characteristics of fluid obtained by diagnostic thoracentesis that can help to make the distinction between transudative and exudative effusions are summarized in Table 17-8. Few findings are independently diagnostic, with the exception of positive cultures (empyema) and positive cytology (malignancy). Certain gross findings can be nearly diagnostic, such as the milky white fluid of chylothorax or the foul purulence of an empyema. Other findings can narrow the possibilities considerably. For example, grossly bloody fluid (red cell count >100,000 per mm^3) is almost always caused by trauma, pulmonary infarction, or malignancy. Markedly elevated amylase can be found in sympathetic effusions associated with pancreatitis, pancreatic pseudocyst, and esophageal perforation. Pleural fluid pH <7.20 (with an arterial pH >7.35) strongly suggests bacterial infection, and may appear before culture and Gram's stain are positive in some cases. Low pH has also been reported in some malignant effusions, and in effusions associated with connective tissue disease.

Table 17-7. CAUSES OF EXUDATIVE PLEURAL EFFUSION

Malignancy (primary and metastatic)
Infection
Infarction
Sympathetic (pancreatitis, subphrenic abscess, etc.)
Traumatic
Collagen vascular diseases (rheumatoid arthritis, lupus)

Table 17-8. SOME DISTINGUISHING CHARACTERISTICS OF TRANSUDATE AND EXUDATE

	Transudate	*Exudate*
Color	Clear, serous	Cloudy, tan
WBC count	<1000/mm³	>10,000/mm³
RBC count	<10,000/mm³	>10,000/mm³—blood tinged >100,000/mm³—grossly bloody
Glucose	Normal	Low in certain conditions
Protein	<3.0 g/dL	>3.0 g/dL
Protein ratio*	<0.5	>0.5‡
Specific gravity	<1.016	>1.016
LDH	Normal	>67% of upper limit of normal‡
LDH ratio†	<0.6	>0.6‡
pH	Same as arterial	<7.20 suggests empyema
Culture	Negative	May be positive (empyema)
Cytology	Negative	May be positive (malignant)

* Pleural fluid protein divided by serum protein.
† Pleural fluid LDH divided by serum LDH.
‡ From Light RW, MacGregor MI, et al.

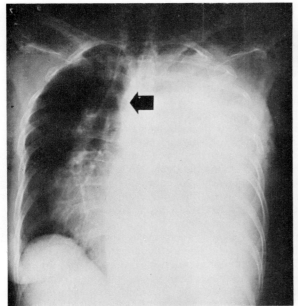

Fig. 17-31. A massive pleural effusion due to metastases from breast carcinoma. *A.* The arrow shows the tracheal displacement to the opposite side. *B.* The malignant effusion has been completely evacuated with a thoracostomy tube, and the mediastinum has shifted back to the midline. The left hemidiaphragm is elevated because of phrenic nerve invasion by pleural metastases.

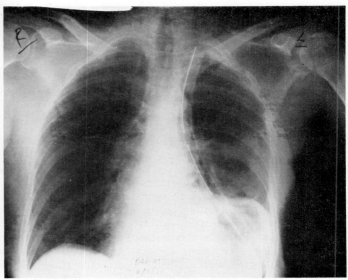

A

B

There can be considerable overlap in the findings ostensibly separating exudate from transudate, and any chronic effusion tends to develop "exudative" characteristics. Too much can be made of laboratory distinctions, and it is rare for pleural effusion to be the sole manifestation of disease such that diagnosis hinges exclusively on pleural fluid analysis. The etiology of most effusions is best recognized by simply looking carefully at the rest of the patient.

A concave meniscus in the costophrenic angle on an upright chest x-ray suggests the presence of at least 250 mL of pleural fluid. A lateral decubitus view can detect a smaller volume, and confirms that the fluid is free in the pleural space if it is shown to layer out along a dependent surface. In some cases an effusion is completely contained between the base of the lung and the diaphragm (a subpulmonic effusion), and can be difficult to distinguish from an elevated hemidiaphragm or a subdiaphragmatic process. When this occurs on the left side the position of the stomach bubble can provide a useful clue. On a supine film a small to moderate effusion will be completely inapparent, and a large effusion only produces a uniform hazy appearance of the affected hemithorax that can be difficult to detect unless the process is unilateral. A very large effusion can produce complete opacification of one hemithorax that does not change in appearance with changes in position (Fig. 17-31). Adhesions can compartmentalize an effusion into loculations that assume a wide variety of radiographic configurations, frequently requiring multiple views or CT scanning for definition. Presence of an air-fluid level has specific connotations, since the air can only come from the tracheobronchial tree, from the esophagus, or directly through the chest wall.

Thoracentesis is the mainstay of diagnosis. Needle biopsy of the pleura can provide diagnostic tissue but has a high frequency of false negative results because of sampling difficulties in diseases that do not involve the pleura uniformly. Thoracoscopy can increase the specificity of pleural biopsies in selected cases.

Pleural effusions can produce dyspnea but can also be surprisingly asymptomatic at rest. Therapeutic drainage is rarely indicated for transudative effusions since the fluid will rapidly reaccumulate until the underlying condition is improved. Most exudative effusions warrant a more aggressive approach. The treatment of hemothorax is considered elsewhere, and empyema, malignant effusion, and chylothorax are considered separately below. A variety of nonmalignant, uninfected exudative effusions are frequently treated as if they were transudative; examples include collagen vascular disease, pulmonary infarction, and sympathetic effusion secondary to abdominal pathology.

MALIGNANT PLEURAL EFFUSION

More than half of all patients with malignancy will have a pleural effusion at some time in their course. The effusion is frequently massive and symptomatic. The pathophysiology is thought to be interference with venous and lymphatic drainage by direct tumor invasion. Although pleural biopsy is most often normal, the fluid contains malignant cells in at least 80 percent of the patients. Lung carcinoma is the most common primary, with breast and gastrointestinal malignancies close behind. The fluid is exudative in character, and often bloody. Grossly bloody fluid (red cell count >100,000/mL) has a 90 percent probability of being malignant, once trauma and pulmonary infarction are excluded. The presence of a malignant effusion is a poor prognostic sign, with mean survival after diagnosis of 3 to 11 months in most series.

TREATMENT. Treatment is palliative. Repeated thoracentesis has a high failure rate. Chest wall radiation, thoracotomy with decortication and pleurectomy, and even pleuropneumonectomy have been described but carry unacceptable mortality and morbidity to be considered standard treatment. At present the standard therapy is tube thoracostomy and pleurodesis.

Pleurodesis creates an inflammatory fusion between visceral and parietal pleura that eliminates the potential pleural space. An essential first step is complete evacuation of the fluid and reexpansion of the lung (Fig. 17-31), accomplished by inserting a chest tube connected to a water seal drainage system (Fig. 17-32). If loculations or inaccurate tube placement prevent complete fluid removal and lung expansion, pleural symphysis will not occur uniformly and pleurodesis is much less likely to succeed; this is probably more important than the choice of the chemical agent used in the next step. Innumerable agents have been used to induce the inflammation, including talc, nitrogen mustard, Adriamycin, quinacrine, and tetracycline. Recently a preparation of heat-killed, freeze-dried *Corynebacterium parvum* has been tried, reportedly with great success. Tetracycline is the agent most commonly used in the United States. The agent selected is usually administered through the chest tube,

which is removed shortly thereafter. Although each agent has its staunch advocates, reported results suggest that the effusion will not recur in 60 to 90 percent of patients, regardless of which agent is used.

Use of an indwelling shunt connecting the pleural cavity to the peritoneum through a one-way valve has received attention recently. The system is analogous to a LaVeen or Denver shunt, except that the normal pressure gradient between the abdomen and chest is overcome with a subcutaneous squeeze bulb pump. The method has the theoretical disadvantage of continuously circulating malignant cells but does appear capable of producing satisfactory palliation in refractory cases.

EMPYEMA

Empyema is a suppurative infection confined to a natural anatomical space by normal epithelial boundaries; in the thoracic cavity this is the potential space existing between visceral and parietal pleura. Empyema was carefully studied 2400 years ago by Hippocrates, who first described open drainage with rib resection. In the early 1900s empyema complicated pneumonia in 5 to 10 percent of cases, and Sir William Osler required open drainage and rib resection in 1919 for a postpneumonic empyema.

In the postantibiotic era, empyema has become a less frequent complication of pneumonia, now occurring in about 1 percent of cases, and the bacteriologic spectrum has shifted from *Pneumococcus* and *Streptococcus* to *Staphylococcus, Streptococcus,* and gram-negative organisms. Although pneumonia is the most frequent association with empyema, it can also occur following trauma, pulmonary infarction, or pulmonary resection, and can be caused by spread from an intraabdominal source.

Infection of the pleural space initially produces a large, exudative effusion with a high concentration of leukocytes. In hours to days fibrinous adhesions succeed in limiting involvement to one or more loculated compartments. The ability of the lung to expand and obliterate potential space becomes very important in confining the infection, and prevents formation of a fibrous "peel" over the visceral pleura that can permanently restrain the lung in a partially collapsed configuration ("trapped lung"). The pleura actually has remarkable ability to resolve infection when assisted by an expanded lung. A persistent air leak (bronchopleural fistula) potentiates infection both by providing a route for constant inoculation of the pleural space, and by promoting lung collapse. The difficulty of obliterating space following pulmonary resection, particularly pneumonectomy, accounts in part for the seriousness of postresection empyema.

CLINICAL MANIFESTATIONS. Empyema should be suspected in a patient with a febrile illness and pleural effusion on chest x-ray. Thoracentesis with Gram's stain and culture of the fluid obtained confirms the diagnosis and guides selection of antibiotics. The gross appearance of the fluid is usually unambiguous, although some seropurulent parapneumonic effusions are sterile. In such cases pleural fluid of pH <7.20 is considered suggestive of empyema. Radiographic findings of loculated fluid or

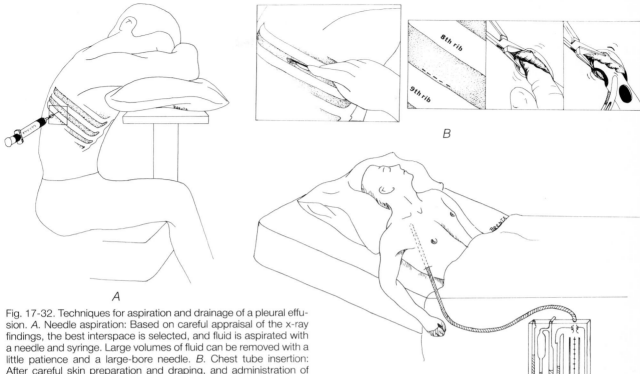

Fig. 17-32. Techniques for aspiration and drainage of a pleural effusion. *A.* Needle aspiration: Based on careful appraisal of the x-ray findings, the best interspace is selected, and fluid is aspirated with a needle and syringe. Large volumes of fluid can be removed with a little patience and a large-bore needle. *B.* Chest tube insertion: After careful skin preparation and draping, and administration of local anesthesia, a short skin incision is made over the correct interspace. The incision is deepened into the intercostal muscles, and the pleura is penetrated, usually with a clamp. When any doubt exists about the status of the pleural space at the site of puncture, the wound is enlarged bluntly to admit a finger, which can be swept around the immediately adjacent pleural space to assess the situation and break down any adhesions. The tube is inserted, with the tip directed toward the optimum position suggested by the chest x-rays. In general, a high anterior tube is best for air (pneumothorax) and a low posterior tube is best for fluid. A 28 to 32F tube is adequate for most situations. A 36F tube is preferred for hemothorax or for a viscous empyema. Many surgeons prefer a very small tube (16 to 20F) for drainage of simple pneumothorax. *C.* The tube is connected to a water seal drainage system. Suction is added if necessary to expand the lung, and will usually be required in a patient with a substantial air leak (bronchopleural fistula).

presence of an air-fluid level also suggest empyema in a clinical setting otherwise consistent with infection but can be difficult to distinguish from a lung abscess, an infected congenital cyst, or an infected bulla (pyocyst). A chest CT scan can be very helpful in avoiding inadvertent tube drainage of parenchyma.

TREATMENT. Successful treatment depends upon early recognition of the problem, selection of appropriate antibacterial therapy based on identification of the organism, and complete obliteration of the emypema space (Table 17-9). Thoracentesis alone has provided adequate treatment in only 9 to 12 percent of two large recent series, and success with this method depends on early treatment of relatively mild infections. Thoracentesis along had a 10 percent success rate even in the preantibiotic era.

A more aggressive form of drainage than thoracentesis is usually required. The first step is insertion of a chest tube connected to a closed drainage system. Suction is applied as necessary to obliterate the cavity and promote lung expansion, which is especially important in the presence of a bronchopleural fistula. Chest tube drainage of most early, moderate infections will result in rapid cessation of drainage and air leak, and obliteration of the cavity within several days. In such cases it is usually possible to simply remove the tube(s).

If early resolution does not occur, drainage of purulent material will continue, usually associated with radiographic evidence of a persistent cavity. It is a simple matter to convert closed-tube drainage to open-tube drainage by cutting the tubes off near the skin and allowing drainage to continue into dressings. With any form of open drainage, suction cannot be applied to the space, so that dependent position of the tube(s) becomes very important. Over a period of weeks to months, the cavity will shrink and eventually obliterate, slowly extruding the tubes, which are progressively shortened.

Conversion to open drainage cannot be done before pleural symphysis at the margins of the cavity has developed enough to prevent pneumothorax when the tube is disconnected from water seal, a process that requires at least 10 to 14 days. If this rule is violated and the lung is allowed to collapse, breaking down the immature symphysis, the empyema can spread rapidly to become a much more serious infection of the entire pleural space. A simple test is to disconnect the tubes and repeat a chest

Table 17-9. TREATMENT OPTIONS FOR EMPYEMA

1. Antibiotic alone
2. Thoracentesis
3. Closed-tube thoracostomy (drainage to water seal, +/− suction)
4. Closed-tube/catheter drainage with antibiotic irrigation
5. Closed-tube thoracostomy converted to open drainage (no water seal, tubes cut off at the skin and slowly extruded)
6. Formal open drainage with rib resection
7. Thoracotomy and decortication
8. Thoracotomy, decortication, pulmonary resection, thoracoplasty, intrathoracic rotation of pedicled muscle flaps

x-ray. If the space is ready for conversion to open drainage, the x-ray will be unchanged. Conversion to open drainage is also less attractive in the presence of an air leak, because the bronchopleural fistula is converted to a more chronic bronchopleurocutaneous fistula. In correctly selected patients, a combination of closed- and open-tube drainage is successful in at least 60 percent of cases.

Formal open drainage with rib resection (Fig. 17-33) was done more frequently in the preantibiotic era but is still useful today in the treatment of chronic, mature empyemas with a thick fibrous capsule (Fig. 17-34). Drainage is assured by marsupialization of the empyema cavity. The same cautions important in conversion of closed-tube to open-tube drainage still apply—the cavity must be mature, the drainage site should be dependent, and production of a bronchopleurocutaneous fistula is best avoided. The larger wound allows easier access to the cavity, and drainage can be augmented with irrigation.

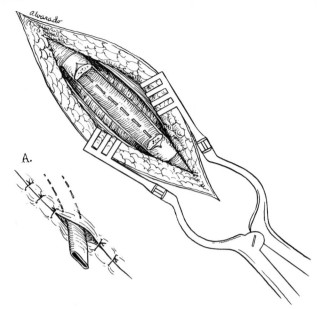

A.

Fig. 17-33. Open drainage through the bed of a resected rib. For an empyema dependent drainage is important and the site is selected accordingly. A tube can be left in place as shown to prevent closure of the skin opening, or the skin edges can be sewed to the parietal pleura to create an epithelialized tract (a modification of an Eloesser flap). Progress can be gauged by periodically measuring the volume of the cavity, which can be done simply by measuring the volume of saline required to overflow it.

A method that appears to be gaining in popularity combines closed-tube drainage with antibiotic irrigation. Results with this method were quite good in two series reported recently from England. Hutter et al. emphasized

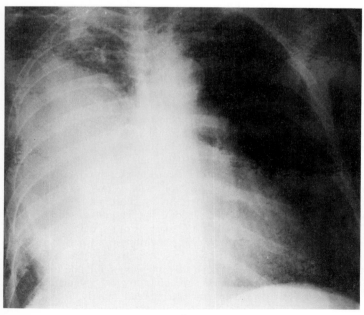

A

Fig. 17-34. *A.* This fifty-four-year-old homeless man presented to the emergency room with a massive consolidation of the right lung. *B.* On antibiotics the radiographic picture slowly evolved into a large cavity with an air-fluid level. *C.* Uncertainty about whether the cavity might be a large lung abscess or infected bulla was largely relieved by the CT scan, which shows a plate of consolidated lung compressed medially by a large empyema cavity. Note the degree of pleural thickening, which contributed to the difficulty encountered obtaining adequate drainage with thoracostomy tubes. Formal open drainage with rib resection was ultimately performed, with gradual resolution of the cavity over several months. At operation the fibrous wall of the cavity was 2 to 3 cm in thickness, precluding any thought of decortication.

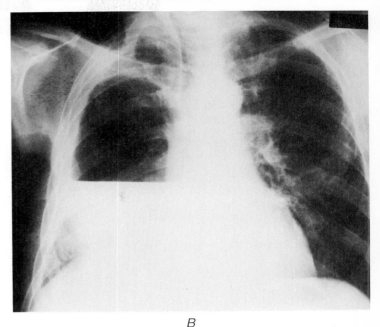

B

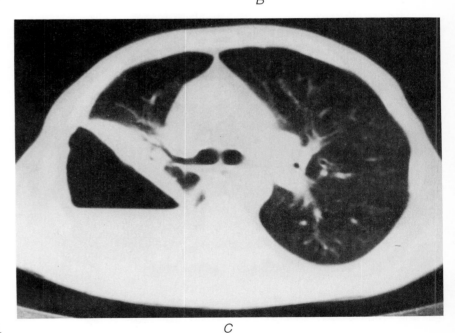

C

Fig. 17-34 *B,C.* Continued.

the role of thoracoscopy in this technique, which they feel is an important aid in achieving optimal tube position and lysis of intracavitary loculations.

If drainage fails to expand the lung, a permanent restrictive defect in ventilation on the affected side is likely to result as the inflammatory membrane heals and contracts over the surface of the lung. Failure of expansion is frequent with a bronchopleural fistula. Four to seven days of high-suction drainage is generally considered an adequate trial, after which thoracotomy and decortication should be performed (Fig. 17-35). The empyema space is completely evacuated under direct vision, and drainage tubes are accurately placed in the most dependent position. The inflammatory "peel" is tightly adherent to the visceral pleura and should be entirely removed, a tedious process that must be done carefully to prevent development of new air leaks from tears in the lung. When an intraparenchymal abscess coexists with a large air leak,

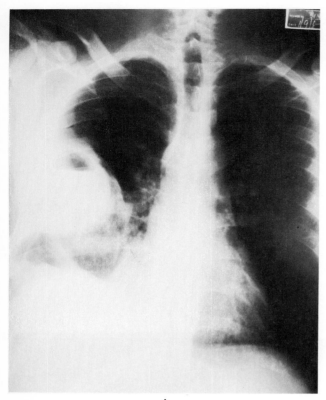

A

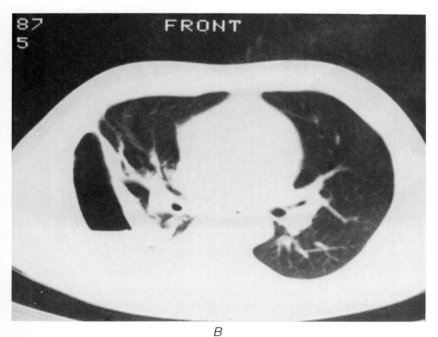

B

Fig. 17-35. *A.* This thirty-seven-year-old intravenous drug abuser presented with pneumonia that evolved into a cavitary process in the right lung, thought to be a lung abscess. *B.* The CT scan showed consolidated right lung compressed medially by a large, thick-walled empyema cavity with an air-fluid level. A decortication was performed through a right posterolateral thoracotomy with excellent results.

pulmonary resection is necessary. Thoracoplasty and intrathoracic rotation of muscle flaps can be added to help obliterate the remaining space.

Decortication has been successful in 80 to 100 percent of cases in reported series, and often shortens hospitalization. It has the disadvantage of requiring general anesthesia and a thoracotomy in patients who frequently have limited ventilatory reserve and are suffering the systemic consequences of chronic infection. Even so, with good anesthesia and aggressive postoperative care, thoracotomy is often better tolerated in the long run than a chronic, draining infection, even one that is slowly improving.

PLEURAL PLAQUES AND CALCIFICATION

Pleural plaques are idiopathic thickenings of parietal pleura, usually smooth and white, and frequently calcified. Most are small (1 to 5 mm) and irregular densities that are frequently bilateral and symmetric and do not occur at the apex or on the visceral pleura. They have no documented relationship to mesothelioma or other neoplasms. Localized inflammatory or traumatic events can heal with production of calcified plaquelike lesions, but they are usually larger and unilateral.

Chronic pleuritis can result in diffuse, remarkably uniform thickening and calcification of parietal pleura. The original pleuritis may result from an unresolved hemothorax, from tuberculous or nontuberculous empyema, and from viral or bacterial pleuritis or pleuropneumonitis. When the wall of a chronic but active empyema becomes calcified, resolution by drainage alone will never occur, and resection, decortication, pleurectomy, and thoracoplasty are likely to be required.

CHYLOTHORAX

Leakage of lymphatic fluid (chyle) from the thoracic duct produces a characteristic milky effusion called a chylothorax. The most common cause is surgical trauma to the thoracic duct, most frequently seen following procedures that involve dissection in the vicinity of the proximal descending thoracic aorta and left subclavian artery (Fig. 17-36), such as ligation of patent ductus or Blalock-Taussig shunt. However, the complication has also been described following a wide range of thoracic, cervical, and even abdominal procedures. Noniatrogenic trauma to the duct is a less common cause of chylothorax, thought to result from hyperextension of the spine producing stretch and rupture of the cysterna chyli over the vertebral bodies. Nontraumatic chylothorax is least common, is associated with malignancy or systemic pathology, and is frequently accompanied by chylous ascites. In nontraumatic cases the pathophysiology is more obscure but is thought to be related to obstruction or erosion of lymphatic channels.

Aspiration of milky-white, odorless fluid from the pleural space is virtually diagnostic. Pseudochyle, which has a similar appearance, is a rare source of confusion seen in certain malignancies, infections, and connective tissue diseases. In comparison with chyle, pseudochyle has a lower fat content and lymphocyte count, and its opalescent appearance is caused by the presence of lecithin-globulin complexes. If the patient is not eating, or if a coexisting problem could significantly dilute the chylous drainage, the gross appearance of the fluid may not be distinguishable from many other effusions. Table 17-10 summarizes characteristics of chyle that can be diagnostically helpful when gross appearance is ambiguous. The

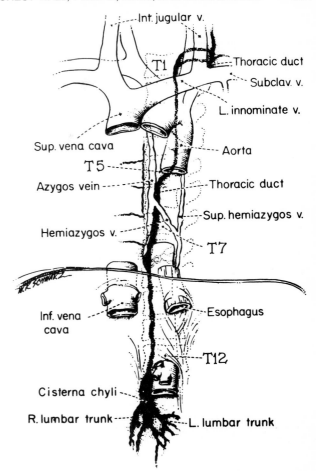

Fig. 17-36. The most common anatomy of the thoracic duct is shown. Anomalous patterns are frequently encountered. After passing through the diaphragm at the aortic hiatus, the duct lies between the aorta and the azygous vein on the anterior surface of the vertebral column, behind the esophagus. Ligation of the duct is most easily performed just above the diaphragm on the right. Although it can be ligated from the left side, the aorta must be mobilized for exposure. At about T_5 the duct crosses to the left side and ascends in the posterior mediastinum, where it is vulnerable to injury during any procedure involving dissection behind the distal transverse aorta. (From: *Bessone LN, Ferguson TB, et al, with permission.*)

lymphocyte count and triglyceride level are most useful. Lymphangiography will occasionally define the site of leak with precision, and is most useful in cases of nontraumatic chylothorax. It is rarely indicated in the traumatic variety.

Normal chyle flow ranges between 1.5 and 2.5 L/day but can vary much more widely depending on diet and on the fat content of the diet. During starvation or intravenous feeding flow falls to about 250 mL/day of clear fluid. Chylothorax is frequently massive (Fig. 17-37) and symptomatic, and significant volume losses can occur through thoracentesis or chest tube drainage. In one recent series, the average amount of fluid lost per day was 756 mL, ranging up to 1720 mL in one nine-year-old patient. Dehy-

Table 17-10. NORMAL COMPOSITION AND CHARACTERISTICS OF CHYLE

General:
  Opaque, milky, odorless
  Opacity clears with alkali/ether extraction
  Sterile
  pH 7.4–7.8
  Specific gravity 1.012–1.025
  Total protein 2.20–5.98 g/dL
  Glucose 48–200 mg/dL
Cell counts:
  Lymphocytes 400–6800/mm³ (average 70% of total WBC
    count)
  Erythrocytes 50–600/mm³
Fats:
  Fat globules stain with Sudan III
  Total fat 0.4–6.0 g/dL
  Triglycerides: Higher than serum value
                  Average 10-fold higher than upper limit of
                    normal
  Cholesterol: Same or lower than serum value
  Triglyceride/cholesterol ratio: >1
Electrolytes:
  Sodium   104–108 meq/L
  Potassium   3.8–5.0 meq/L
  Chlorine   85–130 meq/L
  Calcium   3.4–6.0 meq/L
Total protein 2.20–5.98 g/dL
Glucose 48–200 mg/dL

dration, nutritional losses, and a steady decline in circulating lymphocytes can produce significant disability and an increased susceptibility to infection.

TREATMENT. Until Lampson described successful treatment of chylothorax by ligation of the thoracic duct in 1948, mortality for the condition averaged 50 percent. Since that time, better understanding of fluid and electrolyte management, and the development of total parenteral nutrition have introduced additional options. Spontaneous resolution can occur, so a trial of nonoperative treatment is usually justified. Conservative treatment has two goals: one is to decrease chyle production; the other is to keep the lung expanded against the mediastinum. Maximal reduction in chyle production is achieved by eliminating oral intake, while the patient is supported by total parenteral nutrition. A defensible compromise is to replace all dietary fat with medium-chain triglycerides, which are not absorbed by lymphatics. Fluid can be removed intermittently by thoracentesis, but continuous evacuation with a chest tube is much more effective. It is generally accepted that a 2-week trial of drainage and diet manipulation is justified. Experience in renal transplantation has shown that thoracic duct drainage produces measurable immunosuppression after 2 weeks. An occasional patient will have such massive drainage that persistence for more than a few days is unacceptably debilitating. A commonly accepted criterion is that drainage exceeding 500 mL/day in an adult or more than 100 mL/day/year of age in a child is an indication for abandonment of conservative therapy.

If conservative treatment is unsuccessful, pleurodesis with any of the sclerosing agents used for treatment of malignant effusions can be attempted, although the success rate is quite low. Etiology has some bearing on choice of treatment. For the common iatrogenic variety of chylothorax, for example, that seen as a complication of patent ductus ligation, the preferred approach is to explore the left chest and identify and control the site of leakage. This is rarely as easy as it sounds, even when chyle production is increased by feeding the patient cream in the operating room. When the site of injury cannot be clearly identified, the thoracic duct is ligated at its entrance into the thorax, and a pleural abrasion is per-

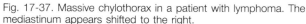

Fig. 17-37. Massive chylothorax in a patient with lymphoma. The mediastinum appears shifted to the right.

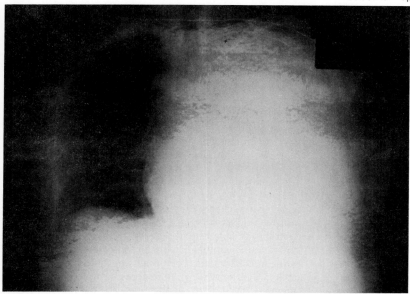

formed. Ligation of the duct is most easily done through a right thoracotomy, but it can be accomplished through a left thoracotomy when necessary. If the problem is bilateral, the right side is approached first, since ligation will usually resolve the problem on both sides. Direct operative approaches through thoracotomy are successful in approximately 80 percent of cases. Treatment failures are most common in nontraumatic chylothorax.

The use of a pleuroperitoneal shunt has been added recently to the list of effective treatment options for chylothorax. Fluid is pumped from the pleural cavity to the peritoneal cavity with a small subcutaneous squeeze bulb on a one-way valve. Early reported experience suggests that drainage will frequently cease over time, allowing eventual removal of the apparatus.

Tumors

MESOTHELIOMA

Mesothelioma is a neoplasm originating in the mesothelial lining of serosal cavities. Tumor presents in the pleura in 80 percent and in the peritoneum in 20 percent of cases. Although mesothelioma is a rare tumor (2.2 cases/million per year), an increased incidence has been anticipated since an association with asbestos exposure was recognized in the 1970s. In several large series, a history of asbestos exposure has been documented in 10 to 77 percent of patients. The disease has been most widely recognized in geographical areas having local industries associated with high risk of exposure, such as shipbuilding or manufacturing processes using asbestos. Exposure to asbestos particles carried on the clothing of workers at risk has been implicated as a cause of increased incidence of mesothelioma in family members. The epidemiology is complicated by the fact that asbestos is nearly ubiquitous in any urban environment, and the characteristic refractile particles can be identified in many people without disease. Some evidence has suggested that smoking is an important etiologic cofactor, and the latency period from exposure to clinical disease is very long.

Mesothelioma exists in a benign and malignant form. The benign form accounts for only 10 to 15 percent of the total, presents as an intrathoracic mass on chest x-ray, and is usually asymptomatic. Pleural effusion is rare. Pathologically the tumor arises from visceral or parietal pleura as an encapsulated mass that is pedunculated (Fig. 17-38). Resection is the treatment of choice, if only because thoracotomy has almost always been required for accurate diagnosis.

In contrast, malignant mesothelioma is a locally aggressive neoplasm usually appearing after age forty, with a male predominance of more than 2:1. The tumor usually appears to be multicentric, with multiple pleural-based nodules coalescing to form sheets of desmoplastic mass separated by loculated, cystic spaces. There are two cell types: fibrosarcomatous and epithelial. The fibrosarcomatous variety is less common and has a better prognosis.

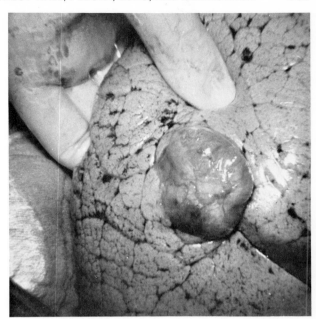

Fig. 17-38. A localized benign mesothelioma arising from the juncture of the right upper and lower lobes. The tumor was removed by wedge resection with a margin of normal lung.

Although hematogenous and lymphatic spread occur in at least one-third of cases, the predominant feature is aggressive tissue invasion. Involvement of lung, chest wall, diaphragm, and mediastinal structures is common. In one series of 69 patients only 3 of 14 patients autopsied had disease limited to the thorax, and 9 patients developed tumor in a needle biopsy tract. Local spread can produce a Horner's syndrome and spinal cord compression. Most patients die of the primary tumor rather than metastases. For unexplained reasons, thrombocytosis is frequently seen and may account for a high incidence of thromboembolic complications. In one series the platelet count was more than $400,000/mm^3$ in 90 percent of patients and greater than $1,000,000/mm^3$ in 14 percent.

CLINICAL MANIFESTATIONS. Chest pain, dyspnea, or both are present in virtually all patients with malignant mesothelioma. Pleural effusion is present at some time in 85 to 95 percent of cases, although as the disease progresses the pleural space tends to become obliterated with solid tumor. Radiographic findings other than effusion cover a wide spectrum including pleural thickening, lung nodules, chest wall masses, and mediastinal masses (Fig. 17-39). CT scan of the chest can add important anatomic detail regarding mediastinal involvement or contralateral pleural involvement, and one should always be obtained unless no treatment is planned (Fig. 17-40).

A tissue diagnosis is difficult to obtain without thoracotomy. In a series of 123 patients reported by Brenner et al. thoracentesis in 60 patients revealed malignant cells in only 22, and a definitive diagnosis of mesothelioma could only be made in 7. Needle biopsy and thoracoscopy have similar yield, and bronchoscopy almost never provides diagnostic tissue. Unless a representative specimen of

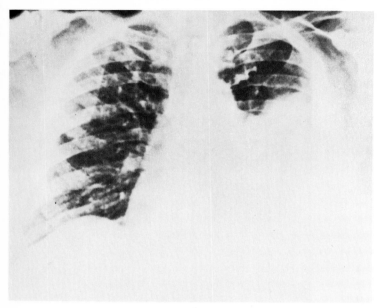

A

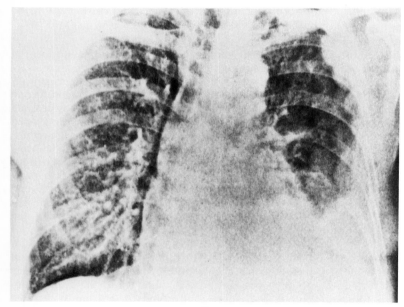

B

Fig. 17-39. Three common radiographic presentations of malignant mesothelioma. *A*. Large pleural effusion without a discrete mass. *B*. Multiple pleural-based masses without an effusion. While the appearance of the left lower lung field is consistent with effusion or mass, the two can be distinguished on the basis of lateral decubitus views and CT scan. *C*. Large pleural-based mass with pleural effusion and thickening. (From: *Martini N, McCormack PM, et al: Ann Thorac Surg 43:113, 1987, Fig 3A–C, p 116, with permission.*)

adequate size is obtained, the epithelial cell type in particular can be easily confused with adenocarcinoma.

TREATMENT. For benign mesothelioma, resection is the treatment of choice and is generally curative. For diffuse malignant mesothelioma treatment is controversial. Since thoracotomy is likely to be required for accurate diagnosis, careful preoperative clinical staging (Table 17-11) should be done to help estimate prognosis. Stages II to IV have a dismal prognosis regardless of treatment, with median survival measured in months. In such cases radiotherapy and chemotherapy are usually given, but proto-

cols with significant benefit have not been established. Even in Stage I disease, a 1986 retrospective analysis of 328 Canadian patients demonstrated median survival of only 17 months regardless of treatment.

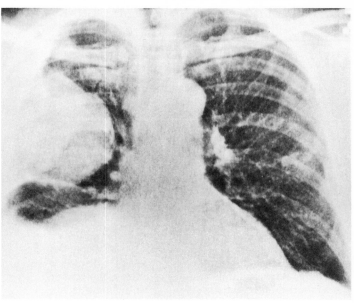

Fig. 17-39 *C.* Continued.   *C*

Radical surgery in Stage I disease is favored by some authors, who feel that meaningful palliation and an occasional long-term survival can be achieved with acceptable mortality and morbidity. At the most radical extreme, DaValle et al. recently reported their experience with 33 patients treated with extrapleural pneumonectomy, including resection of pericardium and diaphragm; 8 patients (24 percent) survived more than 24 months, and 5 survived more than 36 months. Operative mortality was 9 percent, and serious complications occurred in 24 percent. A less radical approach is favored at Memorial Sloan-Kettering Cancer Center in New York, where pleuropneumonectomy has been abandoned in favor of radical pleurectomy, preserving the lung but resecting diaphragm and pericardium when necessary. They emphasize the importance of combined treatment with systemic chemotherapy and radiation, administered as a combination of intraoperative implantation of radioactive material and postoperative external beam. In 94 patients there was no operative mortality, 40 percent survived more than 2 years, and median survival was 21 months.

Fig. 17-40. CT scan of a diffuse pleural mesothelioma encasing the lung and extending into the major fissure, but without evidence of mediastinal involvement. (From: *Martini N, McCormack PM, et al: Ann Thorac Surg 43:113, 1987, Fig 3A–C, p 116, with permission.*)

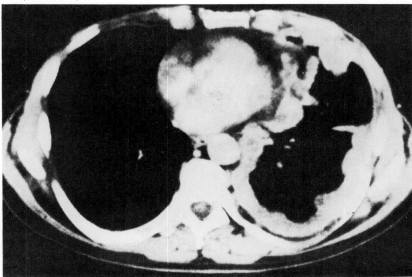

Table 17-11. CLINICAL STAGING OF MALIGNANT MESOTHELIOMA

Stage I:	Tumor confined to ipsilateral pleura or lung
Stage II:	Tumor involving chest wall, mediastinum, pericardium, or contralateral pleura
Stage III:	Tumor on both sides of the diaphragm, or in lymph nodes outside the thorax
Stage IV:	Hematogenous metastases outside the thorax

All authors agree that long-term survival in malignant mesothelioma remains a rare occurrence.

METASTATIC PLEURAL TUMORS

Over 90 percent of pleural tumors are metastatic. Lung and breast carcinoma are the most common primaries. In more than half of all cases, gross tumor is not visible but produces a malignant pleural effusion, which is discussed elsewhere. When multiple nodules or diffuse obliterative spread occur, differentiation from mesothelioma is impossible without biopsy.

Spontaneous Pneumothorax

Nontraumatic pneumothorax most commonly results from rupture of a pulmonary bleb or bulla. Negative intrathoracic pressure throughout the respiratory cycle favors movement of air into the pleural space, with egress prevented by the ball-valve effect of collapsing tissue during expiration. The pneumothorax will continue to progress until the leak seals with fibrin, at a rate directly related to the size of the bleb. Large leaks can produce life-threatening tension pneumothorax. Spontaneous resolution can occur once the leak stops, but the gas in the space is mostly nitrogen and is very slowly reabsorbed by the pleural surfaces.

Up to 80 percent of patients with spontaneous pneumothorax are young adults, usually male, without clinically significant pulmonary disease. A tall, asthenic habitus is common. In 85 percent of cases blebs or bullae of varying size are found in the lung apices (Fig. 17-41), and it is not known whether their origin is congenital or acquired. After the first episode the chance of ipsilateral recurrence is 50 percent, and the risk rises with each recurrence to 62 percent after a second episode and 80 percent after a third episode. The risk of a contralateral pneumothorax after the first episode is about 10 percent.

In patients over age forty, significant pulmonary disease is usually present, most frequently emphysema in a tobacco addict. Catamenial pneumothorax is a rare condition in which pneumothorax occurs predictably within a few days of menses, usually in women over thirty, and almost always on the right side. The mechanism is not known. The two most frequently cited possibilities are pleural endometriosis and small perforations of the diaphragm.

CLINICAL MANIFESTATIONS. Chest pain is the most common presenting symptom, followed by dyspnea. If the lung is more than about 25 percent collapsed, a decrease in breath sounds will be evident to auscultation, and the affected side will be hyperresonant to percussion. Young patients without underlying lung disease can be asymptomatic at rest with nearly complete collapse of one lung, and arterial blood gases will be nearly normal. A more dramatic presentation, including tachypnea, cyanosis, and hypoxia, is seen in patients with underlying lung disease and limited ventilatory reserve. An occasional patient with extensive lung disease and a pleural space obliterated with adhesions will present with massive subcutaneous emphysema and pneumomediastinum, because air escaping from the ruptured bleb follows the path of least resistance retrograde through the peribronchial soft tissue.

Fig. 17-41. An operative photograph showing a giant bulla arising from the upper lobe of an eighteen-year-old man with no symptoms of obstructive airway disease.

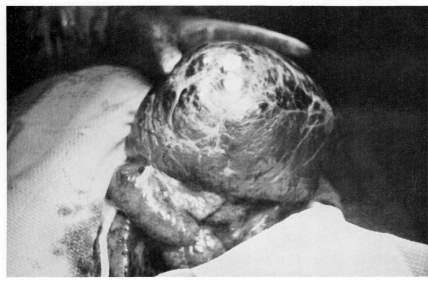

The characteristic radiographic finding is absence of lung markings and a faint visible line defining the edge of the lung. When the lung collapses almost completely, it is visible as an irregular density attached to the hilum (Fig. 17-42). Presence of a small amount of fluid with an air-fluid level is common. The fluid is usually serosanguinous and insignificant. On occasion bleeding from a torn pleural adhesion will produce a large and increasing hemothorax that can require urgent exploration. The lung fields must be closely examined for evidence of gross abnormalities, such as apical blebs or bullae. Although blebs and bullae are frequently obvious at thoracotomy, only about 15 percent are visible radiographically.

An asymptomatic or mildly symptomatic pneumothorax with less than 30 percent collapse that is shown not to increase in size over 6 to 8 h can safely be observed. Simple needle aspiration of the air space can nearly eliminate the space in a stable pneumothorax and will greatly reduce the amount of time required for spontaneous resolution. Needle aspiration of a tension pneumothorax can be a lifesaving temporizing manuever.

Thoracostomy tube drainage is the most common treatment. The tube is inserted either anteriorly (second interspace, midclavicular line) or laterally in a lower interspace (mid to anterior axillary line), with the tip directed toward the apex. The tube is connected to water seal, to which suction can be added to increase the gradient favoring removal of air from the pleural space. Water seal alone will suffice in many cases. As the lung reexpands, the patient will feel pain as the visceral and parietal surfaces reoppose. The pain gradually subsides but is usually much more acute and severe when suction is applied initially. Some authors favor attaching the tube to a one-way flutter valve (Heimlich valve) that permits outpatient treatment of a pneumothorax in a reliable patient with a small leak.

Serial check x-rays are followed to assess reexpansion, and the size of the air leak is monitored by observing the rate of bubbling in the water seal chamber. Air will cross the water seal only with cough or valsalva in a pneumothorax caused by a leak that has already sealed, and the bubbling will usually cease altogether within 24 h. At the opposite extreme, continuous bubbling occurring through both phases of respiration reflects a large active leak that may take days to seal, if it will seal at all. With large air leaks a single tube may be inadequate. If two tubes connected to suction still fail to expand the lung, thoracotomy is required. Even a large leak can seal if the lung can be fully expanded, which promotes adhesion formation between parietal pleura and the site of the leak in the visceral pleura.

Operation is indicated for a massive air leak with failure of lung reexpansion or for a smaller leak that has persisted for more than a week. Because of the frequency of recurrence after one episode, operation is recommended after any second episode and in any patient with a previous contralateral pneumothorax. Operation might be recommended after a first episode to anyone with large apical bullae visible on chest x-ray, to persons likely to be exposed to dangerous changes in atmospheric pressure (airline pilots, scuba divers), or to persons living in re-

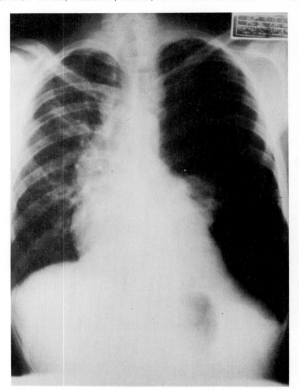

Fig. 17-42. Spontaneous pneumothorax in a young male. The lung is visible as a density collapsed against the mediastinum. The mediastinum is shifted to the right, the diaphragm is pushed down, and the intercostal spaces are wider on the left than on the right—findings that suggest an element of tension pneumothorax. In fact, the patient was hemodynamically stable and only mildly symptomatic.

mote areas. Complications such as empyema or hemothorax occasionally develop and mandate operation. In general, conservative treatment is continued as long as possible in older patients with underlying lung disease because of their limited ventilatory reserve.

At thoracotomy the site of the leak can almost always be identified (Fig. 17-43) and resected, oversewn, or closed with staples. Pleural abrasion should also be performed to promote formation of adhesions between visceral and parietal pleura, an especially important manuever if no leak site can be identified. Pleurectomy, accomplished by stripping all of the parietal pleura off the underlying ribs and intercostal muscles, is undeniably effective but has substantially greater morbidity and is reserved for extreme cases. Either method is 90 to 95 percent effective.

LUNG

Development and Anatomy

In the 4-mm (3-week) embryo, an outpouching from the primitive foregut appears caudad to the paired pharyngeal pouches and bifurcates into the right and left primitive

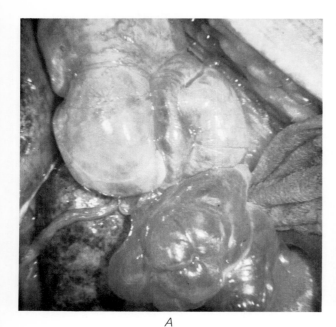

A

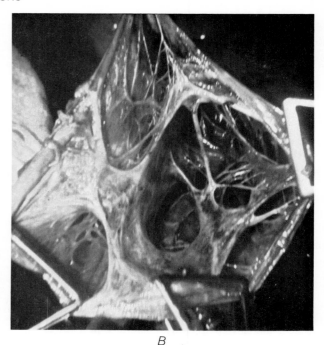

B

Fig. 17-43. This thirty-one-year-old salesman had three episodes of spontaneous pneumothorax over a 2-year period. *A.* At operation multiple bullae were found at the apex of the right upper lobe. *B.* The open bullae reveal a typical cavernous interior trabeculated by bands of fibrous tissue. The involved areas were removed with a wedge resection.

bronchial buds. Over the next two weeks, further branching occurs with 10 segmental tubes on the right and 8 on the left, providing an early indication of the lobar development that will continue in each lung. Progressive branching of epithelial tubes results in a rich arborization of bronchioles, and alveolar ducts and sacs. It is estimated that 300 million alveolar sacs eventually develop. As the structural maturation is taking place, histologic differentiation progresses from the cuboidal epithelium that lines the terminal buds during the first four fetal months to the flattened epithelium present at birth. Boyden and Tomsett have identified 23 to 27 branching generations in infants, adolescents, and adults, supporting the concept that the basic architecture of the lungs is completely developed at birth. As the lungs grow, they bulge into the lateral pleural cavities, leaving a dorsal mesentery to encase the developing mediastinal structures. The most caudal pair of aortic arches (the sixth) gives rise to the pulmonary arteries, with the remnant of the left sixth arch persisting as the ductus arteriosus. Vascular sprouts from the unilocular atrium fuse with the developing capillary vasculature in the lung mesenchyma to become the pulmonary veins.

Although the number of respiratory units may not increase after birth, it does seem apparent that the newborn's lung is structurally immature. In place of alveoli, the lungs are made up of primitive air sacs that differentiate into alveolar ducts and sacs. Alveoli develop by outpouching and compartmentalization, and maturation continues throughout the first eight years of life. The fully developed alveoli give a surface area of 70 to 80 m^2 at three-fourths maximal inflation of the adult lung.

SEGMENTAL ANATOMY. The segmental anatomy of the lungs and bronchial tree is illustrated in Fig. 17-44. Although there is continuity of the pulmonary parenchyma between adjacent segments of each lobe, the separation of the bronchial and vascular stalks allows subsegmental and segmental resections whenever the clinical situation requires or allows preserving lung tissue. This may be particularly important in patients with impaired pulmonary function or in those with disease processes that are apt to be or to become multifocal, requiring multiple resective procedures. Less-than-lobar resections are desirable when dealing with localized inflammatory diseases such as tuberculosis and bronchiectasis that characteristically involve segmental units of the upper and lower lobes, respectively, but often do so in a way that leaves one or more segments of the same lobe unaffected. Both these diseases, as well as metastatic pulmonary neoplasms, may involve more than one pulmonary lobe, either synchronously or metachronously. For many years, Jensik and others have raised questions regarding the necessity of extending the resection of primary lung neoplasms beyond the field necessary for adequate margins around the tumor. The advantages of a segmental concept of surgical treatment are important in all these circumstances.

LYMPHATIC DRAINAGE. Abundant lymphatic vessels are located beneath the visceral pleura of each lung, in the interlobular septums, in the submucosa of the bronchi, and in the perivascular and peribronchial connective tis-

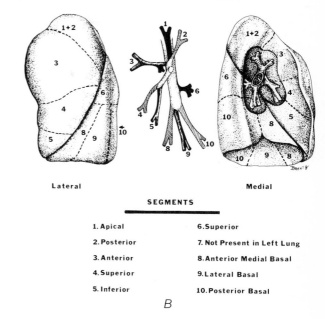

RIGHT LUNG AND BRONCHI

Lateral   Medial

SEGMENTS

1. Apical	6. Superior
2. Posterior	7. Medial Basal
3. Anterior	8. Anterior Basal
4. Lateral	9. Lateral Basal
5. Medial	10. Posterior Basal

A

LEFT LUNG AND BRONCHI

Lateral   Medial

SEGMENTS

1. Apical	6. Superior
2. Posterior	7. Not Present in Left Lung
3. Anterior	8. Anterior Medial Basal
4. Superior	9. Lateral Basal
5. Inferior	10. Posterior Basal

B

Fig. 17-44. *A* and *B*. The segmental anatomy of the lungs. An appreciation of these anatomic divisions often makes it possible to preserve pulmonary tissue by performing segmental resections for localized disease.

sue. The lymph nodes that drain the lungs are divided into two large groups, the pulmonary lymph nodes and the mediastinal nodes, referred to as N1 and N2 nodes, respectively, in the American Joint Committee Tumor-Nodal Involvement-Metastasis (TNM) system of staging of lung cancer (Fig. 17-45). In turn, the pulmonary lymph nodes consist of (1) intrapulmonary, or segmental, nodes that lie at points of division of segmental bronchi or in the bifurcations of the pulmonary artery, (2) lobar nodes that lie along the upper-, middle, and lower-lobe bronchi, (3) interlobar nodes, situated in the angles formed by the bifurcation of the main bronchi into lobar bronchi, and (4) hilar nodes located along the main bronchi.

The interlobar lymph nodes lie in the depths of the interlobar fissure on each side and have special surgical significance because they constitute a lymphatic sump for each lung, referred to as the lymphatic sump of Borrie (Fig. 17-46). This designation results from the fact that all the pulmonary lobes of the corresponding lung drain into that group of nodes. On the right side the nodes of the lymphatic sump lie around the bronchus intermedius, bounded above by the right-upper-lobe bronchus, and below by the middle lobe and superior-segmental bronchi. The lymphatic sump on the left side is confined to the interlobar fissure, with the lymph nodes disposed in the angle between the lingular and lower-lobe bronchi, and in apposition to the pulmonary artery branches.

The mediastinal lymph nodes consist of four principal groups: (1) anterior mediastinal, (2) posterior mediastinal, (3) tracheobronchial, and (4) paratracheal. The anterior mediastinal nodes are located in association with the

upper surface of the pericardium, the phrenic nerves, the ligamentum arteriosum, and the left innominate vein. Within the inferior pulmonary ligament on each side are found the paraesophageal lymph nodes that constitute a major part of the posterior mediastinal group. Additional paraesophageal nodes may be located more superiorly between the esophagus and trachea in the region of the arch of the azygos vein.

The tracheobronchial lymph nodes are made up of three subgroups that are located about the bifurcation of the trachea. Included are the subcarinal nodes, the lymph nodes lying in the obtuse angle between the trachea and each main-stem bronchus, and a few nodes that lie anterior to the lower end of the trachea. The paratracheal lymph nodes are located in proximity to the trachea in the superior mediastinum. Those on the right side form a chain with the tracheobronchial nodes inferiorly and with some of the deep cervical nodes above. A few of the latter are referred to as the scalene lymph nodes because they lie on the anterior scalene muscle. Lymphatic drainage of the right lung is ipsilateral except for an occasional incidence in which drainage to the superior mediastinum is bilateral. Drainage from the left lung to the superior mediastinum is as frequently ipsilateral as it is to the opposite side.

Diagnostic Evaluation

Two factors make diagnostic evaluation of disorders of the lung more logical than is often the case in other anatomic regions. There is direct communication between the oropharynx and the respiratory system, and the contrasting densities of the contents of the thorax provide exceptional opportunities for a variety of imaging tech-

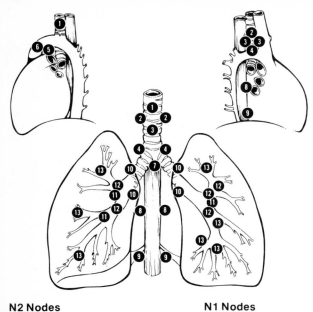

N2 Nodes

- Superior Mediastinal Nodes
  1. Highest Mediastinal
  2. Upper Paratracheal
  3. Pre- and Retrotracheal
  4. Lower Paratracheal
     (including Azygos Nodes)

- Aortic Nodes
  5. Subaortic (aortic window)
  6. Para-aortic (ascending aorta or phrenic)

- Inferior Mediastinal Nodes
  7. Subcarinal
  8. Paraesophageal (below carina)
  9. Pulmonary Ligament

N1 Nodes

10. Hilar
11. Interlobar
12. Lobar
13. Segmental

Fig. 17-45. The American Joint Committee classification of regional lymph nodes. (From: *Staging of Lung Cancer, American Joint Committee for Cancer Staging and End-Results Reporting, Task Force on Lung Cancer, Chicago, 1979, with permission.*)

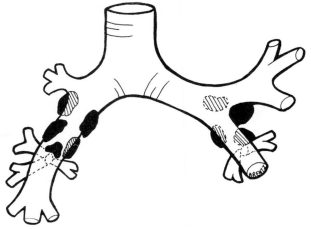

Fig. 17-46. The lymphatic sump of Borrie represents those lymph nodes on each side that receive lymphatic drainage from all lobes of the corresponding lung.

niques. The first factor allows collection of secretions, abnormal drainage or purulent material, and desquamated cells that may provide a definitive diagnosis. It also allows an orderly sequence of progressively more invasive diagnostic endoscopic procedures for visualization, culture, or biopsy. The "window" into the thoracic cavity provided by fluoroscopy, conventional radiography, computed tomography (CT), and magnetic resonance imaging (MRI) allows remarkably clear anatomical definition, opportunities for serial observations, and precise guidance of biopsy needles and forceps.

AIRWAY INVESTIGATION. In most acquired pulmonary diseases sputum collection and examination are indicated as an initial diagnostic procedure. The specific etiologic agent of infections is sought by examination of smears and by culture techniques. The flora of the upper part of the respiratory tract stops abruptly at the level of the larynx, and the tracheobronchial tree is normally sterile. Not frequently, either the patient's sputum is scant, or because it is mixed with saliva and an oral bacterial flora,

its diagnostic usefulness is reduced. To bypass these problems, percutaneous transtracheal aspiration may be performed through the cricothyroid membrane. A 16- or 14-gauge intracatheter needle is used for the procedure after preparation of the skin with soap or iodine solution and local infiltration anesthesia with lidocaine. Coughing may be induced by injecting 5 to 10 mL sterile saline solution without preservative into the trachea. Aspiration of the diluted secretions into a 10- or 20-mL syringe should be followed by immediate delivery of the material to the laboratory.

Bronchoscopy. Whenever malignancy is a diagnostic consideration, or when the preceding studies have failed to yield adequate information, direct visual examination of the tracheobronchial tree is indicated. Information can be gained from this procedure that is available from no other source: cell type of bronchial neoplasms by direct biopsy, mobility of surrounding structures, extent of endobronchial involvement in neoplasms and inflammatory disease, and on occasion, source of bleeding. In addition, the therapeutic aspects of bronchoscopy should not be overlooked. The removal of thick, inspissated secretions from the postoperative patient can be lifesaving. The benefit of foreign body extraction by endoscopic means is obvious.

While the vast majority of endotracheal endoscopic examinations are now made with the flexible bronchoscope, there are still some important uses for the rigid scope, particularly for the removal of certain foreign bodies and the performance of endobronchial resections. The rigid scope provides a large, controlled airway with superb suction capabilities, and room for limited use of snares, scissors, and forceps. In small children, the restricted caliber of the airway may require use of the rigid scope.

The introduction of the flexible bronchoscope in 1967 by Ikeda has greatly extended indications for this procedure. Optically enhanced visualization of tracheobronchial tree to the subsegmental level is now possible and with the addition of fluoroscopic guidance, brush biopsy of many peripheral lesions has become practical.

Both rigid and flexible bronchoscopy may be performed using either topical or general anesthesia, on conscious or unconscious patients, and with patients breathing either spontaneously or with ventilator support. With the rigid scope, a ventilating scope is used that has a side arm for attachment of the ventilator connectors. A size 8 or larger endotracheal tube will allow passage of the flexible scope through a special attachment. Topical anesthesia is the preferred method under most circumstances. The flexible scope can play a major therapeutic role in intubated patients in an intensive care setting where specific suctioning of the segmental bronchi can prevent obstructive atelectasis and provide specific culture information by gathering secretions from localized infected areas. The sputum coughed up immediately after bronchoscopy is especially valuable for cytologic examinations. Chest physical therapy, ultrasonic nebulizers, and bronchodilators are additional techiques to facilitate the collection of sputum.

IMAGING. The juxtaposition in the chest of tissues of widely differing densities makes radiography especially useful in the diagnosis of diseases involving the thorax and its contents. The standard posteroanterior (PA) chest film along with a companion lateral view, each taken at 6-m tube-to-film distance, remains the most frequently used study. When correlated with symptoms, physical findings, and previous radiographs, it provides most of the information needed for the diagnosis and management of a high proportion of disorders of the lung and its major support systems. With the addition of computed tomography (CT) and magnetic resonance imaging (MRI), the ability to accurately map and characterize abnormalities in the lung parenchyma, pleura, and hilar and mediastinal nodal areas is excellent and the wide application of these techniques has simplified significantly the work-up and preoperative staging of patients with intrathoracic neoplasm. Gamsu has recently reviewed the role of these techniques in the staging of lung cancer and has suggested some useful simplifying generalizations. CT has been found to be reasonably sensitive and specific for diagnosing hilar and mediastinal metastases: nodes over 1.5 cm in diameter are definitely abnormal. It is not possible to discriminate between neoplastic and inflammatory enlargement, however. MRI is better at differentiating nodal tissue from fat or vessels and can readily detect encasement or invasion of mediastinal or hilar vessels by tumor (see Fig. 17-96). As cardiac and pulmonary gating become more widely available and as experience grows with the MRI techniques, there is reasonable probability that the improved resolution of fat, vessel, and node will improve our ability to discriminate between malignant and benign masses. Most recently published comparative reviews of the relative merits of the two techniques in their present generations of development conclude that they are roughly equivalent in their ability to assess the extent of hilar and mediastinal tumor, with the exception of the resolution of hilar vessels by MRI. The increased time it takes to perform MRI sequences gives CT a decided ad-vantage in most clinical settings, particularly when, as is usually the case, it is desirable to evaluate the upper abdominal organs to which lung tumors commonly metastasize (liver and adrenal glands).

The indications for other more invasive radiographic procedures have been sharply reduced by these new techniques. Bronchography is still occasionally useful in the assessment of bronchiectatic dilations or in demonstrating occult esophageal fistulae. Pulmonary angiography has been disappointing as a general diagnostic technique, but it can be important in defining congenital abnormalities. Bronchial arteriography can be a useful technique in the diagnosis and treatment of chronic or massive hemoptysis. Intractable hemoptysis associated with chronic pulmonary inflammatory diseases such as bronchiectasis, cystic fibrosis, or tuberculosis may be due to an eroded bronchial artery. In carefully selected cases, selective bronchial arteriography may identify the site of bleeding and allow embolic occulsion of the bleeding vessel through the arteriographic catheter.

Nuclear medicine has played an increasingly important role in clinical diagnosis and in the evaluation of the patient with neoplastic disease. Lung ventilation and perfusion scanning has been important in the diagnosis of pulmonary embolism and for evaluation of split-pulmonary function. While some groups advocate a program of routine multiorgan scanning to evaluate potential lung cancer patients, most clinics have concluded that only in the presence of symptoms focusing on a specific organ should radionuclide scans be done.

BIOPSIES. There are many indications for biopsy of intrathoracic tissues for the diagnosis of nonneoplastic diseases. There are also several research protocols involving pretreatment of patients with certain stages of lung cancers. In each of those clinical situations, efforts to obtain diagnostic tissue and to sample certain lymph-node beds seem clearly indicated. It is logical to outline a sequence of biopsy efforts based on the invasiveness and risk of the studies. The usual approaches to obtaining that information are discussed below. Some controversy exists, however, concerning the appropriateness of preoperative invasive procedures if they will not alter the immediate operative plan. Metastatic disease in the mediastinum sharply worsens the prognosis for lung cancer patients. There is little consensus among thoracic surgeons, however, regarding the impact this observation should have on the initial clinical management of the individual patient. Several have reported 5-year survival of up to 28 percent in patients with positive mediastinal nodes, and have urged that the presence of nodes in that area does not indicate unresectability. These surgeons would emphasize that the most economical, expeditious, and accurate staging can be done at the time of thoracotomy for resection. They would suggest that, once the probability of extra thoracic metastases has been assessed and the appropriate search has been made, it is best to proceed directly with exploration for resection and staging. While this controversy has not been resolved, it seems likely that as multimodal therapy becomes a more usual approach to neoplastic disease, careful staging and preoperative planning will justify efforts to establish the extent of the disease at the onset of therapy.

Needle Biopsies. Advances on many fronts have made the use of needle biopsy techniques an increasingly productive diagnostic tool. Our surgical pathology colleagues have become extremely skillful in obtaining information from isolated cell clusters. Instrumental advances have created a variety of flexible and highly versatile needles: the Type I is a single-lumen fixed 22-gauge needle with a side channel to allow aspiration of the cytopathological specimen; the Type II double-lumen retractable needle has an outer protective sheath. Radiologists can assist us with accurate mapping of the mediastinal and parabronchial nodes, and with fluoroscopic guidance to high-yield areas. With careful techniques, tissue samples can be obtained that are sufficient to allow diagnosis of diffuse pulmonary diseases such as sarcoidosis, pulmonary alveolar proteinosis, and *Pneumocystis carinii* pneumonia. The morbidity rate of transbronchial lung biopsy has been low, with pneumothorax as the principal complication. Though the incidence of pneumothorax has varied from 5 to 20 percent, few patients require active treatment.

After substantial experience in Europe, the percutaneous transthoracic needle biopsy (TTNB) is gaining advocates on this side of the Atlantic. Stimulated primarily by the work of Dahlgren and Nordenstrom, several investigators in this country have reported diagnostic accuracy of 80 to 90 percent in accessible parenchymal lesions. Whether the patient has a diffuse lung disease or a tumor, needle biopsy can provide a rapid diagnosis that expedites overall evaluation and avoids the need for diagnostic thoracotomy in those individuals for whom operation is not indicated. For the patient who is a candidate for operative treatment, some would recommend proceeding with the thoracotomy without biopsy, since negative results cannot be relied upon. On the other hand, if the needle biopsy confirms a suspected primary malignancy, the established diagnosis allows surgeons to plan the operative procedure and fully inform patients of their plans; the psychological climate provided by certainty in diagnosis may be very important for some patients.

Figures 17-47 and 17-48 show the close correlation between cytologic material obtained with needle biopsy and the histology of the resected specimens. In reporting on a large experience with TTNB, Todd and associates noted particularly the ability of their cytologists to distinguish between primary and secondary malignancies and to indicate the exact tissue of origin in 46 percent of the metastatic lesions.

TTNB is performed under local anesthesia, usually with fluoroscopic control. Aspirated material must be immediately smeared or cultured, but pathology departments vary somewhat in their preference for the handling of tissue removed with cutting needles. The complications include hemoptysis, pneumothorax, and rarely hemothorax. Although an incidence of pneumothorax as high as 30 percent has been reported, only an occasional patient requires tube thoracostomy for treatment. The theoretic possibility of implanting the needle track

through the chest wall with malignant cells has not been confirmed by the extensive experience in a number of major cancer centers.

Both aspirating and cutting needles are available, but the Tru-cut disposable needle should only be used for shallow biopsies of pulmonary lesions that appear to be adherent to the chest wall. Contraindications to needle biopsy include (1) coagulopathies, (2) pulmonary hypertension, (3) severe bullous lung disease, (4) a patient receiving continuous positive-pressure breathing, and (5) a suspected vascular lesion.

Mediastinoscopy. Following its introduction by Carlens in 1959 and until the recent increasing dependence on CT scanning or oblique tomography of the mediastinum, mediastinoscopy gained increasing use as a technique for exploring the routes of mediastinal spread of pulmonary neoplasms. Considerable controversy exists among thoracic surgeons regarding the significance of positive mediastinal nodes. For those who would alter their management with confirmation of tumor involvement in the mediastinum, and when the imaging studies identify enlarged (>1.5 cm) nodes in the paratracheal (particularly on the right side) and the anterior subcarinal areas, these nodes can be satisfactorily explored and biopsied by passing a mediastinoscope or laryngoscope along the pretracheal plane for direct visualization and sampling of the suspicious nodes. The procedure is usually performed under general endotracheal anesthesia and utilizes a small transverse incision in the suprasternal notch. Digital exploration is carried inferiorly in the plane between the anterior surface of the trachea and the posterior surface of the innominate artery and the aorta. The paratracheal, tracheobronchial, and subcarinal lymph nodes are accessible to visualization and biopsy through the mediastinoscope, and tumor masses such as thymomas or thyroid lesions may be biopsied directly. The technique provides a positive diagnosis in almost all patients with lymphoma who have radiographic evidence of enlarged mediastinal lymph nodes, and the yield is similarly very high for patients with infectious granulomatous disease. Mediastinoscopy is considered the procedure of choice for diagnosis of sarcoidosis in most institutions, and it has largely replaced scalene lymph-node and fat-pad biopsy for both benign and malignant lesions (Fig. 17-49). Unfortunately, metastases to lymph nodes between the trachea and esophagus and to posterior mediastinal lymph nodes cannot be determined by mediastinoscopy. Similarly, suspected lesions on the left side are difficult to evaluate by this technique owing to the location of the aortic arch.

Parasternal Mediastinotomy. Additional methods for exploring the mediastinum have been developed, and the procedure referred to as anterior mediastinotomy has been used most frequently. Through either a transverse or vertical parasternal incision the second costal cartilage is removed on the side of the lesion. An effort is made to avoid opening the pleural cavity as the mediastinal pleura is freed from the undersurface of the sternum and dissected away from the mediastinum. By additional removal of the third costal cartilage a wider exploration can be performed, the object being to sample mediastinal

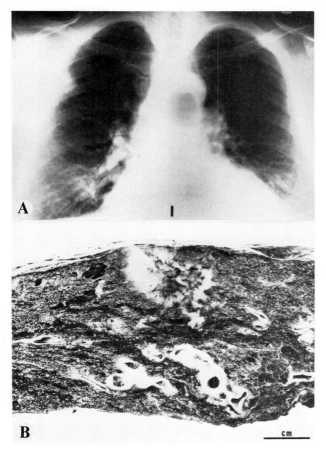

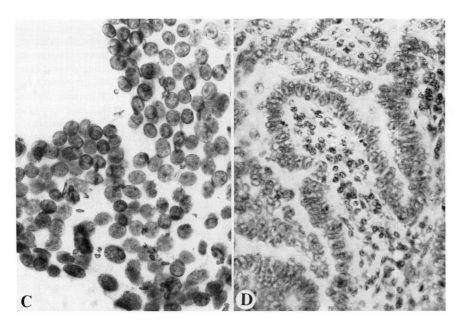

Fig. 17-47. A sixty-three-year-old male with an adenocarcinoma of the right upper lobe of the lung. *A.* The P-A chest x-ray shows a peripheral mass near the lateral chest wall in the right upper lobe. *B.* The right-upper-lobe specimen shows a 2-cm subpleural mass arising from within an anthracotic scar. *C.* Chiba fine-needle aspiration cytology from percutaneous needle biopsy: adenocarcinoma showing a papillary projection extending from a sheet of overlapping large cells with bland vesicular nuclei, prominent nuclear rim, and conspicuous nucleoli. (×471.) *D.* Tissue section histology: papillary adenocarcinoma, showing a papillary fibrovascular core lined by an irregular border of malignant epithelial cells. (×471.)

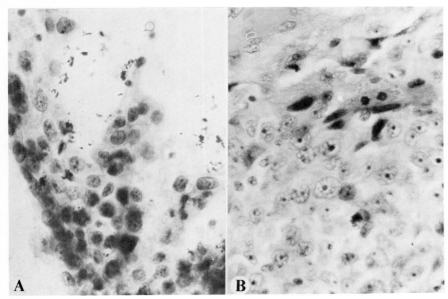

Fig. 17-48. Percutaneous needle biopsy and histology of the resected specimen from a fifty-five-year-old male with a right-lower-lobe mass. *A.* The Chiba fine-needle aspiration cytology shows a mosaic sheet of large pleomorphic cells with irregular, hyperchromatic granular nuclei and macronucleoli, interpreted as squamous carcinoma. (×471.) *B.* Resection specimen tissue histology: squamous carcinoma showing large pleomorphic cells with macronucleoli and a contrasting smaller population of cells with angular hyperchromatic nuclei and cytoplasmic keratinization. (×471.)

lymph nodes and determine the extent of mediastinal spread of a centrally located bronchial neoplasm. If it is pertinent to the confirmation of the diagnosis, the mediastinal pleura can be opened to allow direct lung or pleural biopsy. Several authors have recommended the combination of the parasternal approach to the mediastinum with the mediastinoscopic examination for improved exposure, control, and flexibility in evaluating suspicious mediastinal findings. The left mediastinotomy is particularly useful for the evaluation of nodes in the left aortic window, and in the right and left hila.

Fig. 17-49. This chest x-ray of a twenty-four-year-old woman shows bilateral hilar masses that could be lymphoma or sarcoidosis. Mediastinoscopy was performed to obtain tissue that confirmed the diagnosis of sarcoidosis.

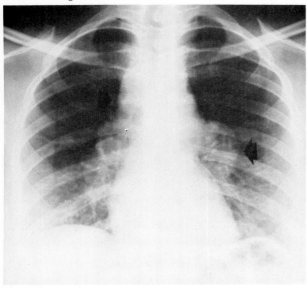

Thoracoscopy. In 1910, H.C. Jacobaeus adapted the cystoscope to investigate ''pleurisy,'' to biopsy pleural masses, and to lyse adhesions to facilitate the therapeutic induced pneumothorax then being used as collapse therapy for tuberculosis. With improved optics and growing experience with endoscopy in other areas over recent years, a sharply renewed interest in this procedure has occurred. It has been found useful in diagnosing chronic or recurrent pleural effusions that remain enigmas after pleurocenteses and needle pleural biopsies, in visualizing and obtaining tissue samples from pleural masses, in staging tumors, in removing foreign bodies, in assisting in therapeutic pleurodesis for malignant effusions or resistant pneumothorax, and in evacuation of posttraumatic clotted hemothorax when indicated. LoCicero has recently presented some encouraging experience in the laboratory utilizing low-energy carbon dioxide laser irradiation to ''seal'' experimentally induced air and blood leaks from the lung surface. When this work becomes clinically applicable, it could provide an important new tool for the management of some difficult persisting air-leak problems in the postresection, posttrauma, and resistant spontaneous pneumothorax patient.

The thoracoscope is usually passed after the patient has been intubated with a double-lumen tube and is under general anesthesia. The lung on the ipsilateral side is selectively deflated, and a rigid Stortz thoracoscope is inserted; a large (8 mm) bronchoscope or sigmoidoscope

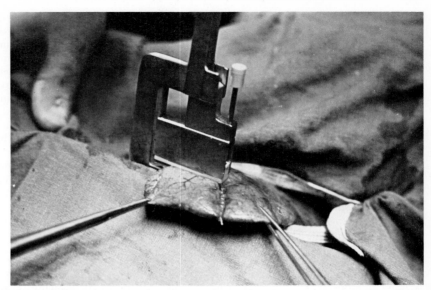

Fig. 17-50. Open lung biopsy is performed by delivering a margin of a pulmonary lobe through the small thoracic incision and applying the automatic stapler across the parenchyma, as shown here. The first line of staples has been applied, and the stapler is in place for the second line. A wedge of pulmonary parenchyma can then be amputated for appropriate studies.

may also be effectively used. The scope is usually best placed through a 2- to 3-cm incision in the midaxillary line through a sheathed trocar, after radiographic mapping and digital exploration has confirmed that the lung falls freely away from the intubation site. The scope can be removed and replaced through the trocar as needed; the flexible bronchoscope can be effectively used along with the rigid scope whenever it might add to the visualization. In extensive series reported by various authors, complications have been exceedingly rare, usually minor and non-life-threatening.

Open Lung Biopsy. The chief indications for open lung biopsy are failure of less invasive closed methods for diagnosis, including needle biopsy, or the presence of a small localized lesion that should be totally removed by the biopsy. An example of the latter circumstance is presented by the patient with a solitary pulmonary nodule and a previously controlled malignancy in another body region. Occasionally there is a need to remove a larger amount of tissue than can be obtained by needle biopsy in patients with either diffuse or localized disease.

Open lung biopsy is performed as a formal operation under general anesthesia, and the patient should be made to understand that it is not a minor procedure. The open lung biopsy may be carried out through a limited anterolateral or axillary thoracotomy, depending on the location of the tissue most desirable for sampling. One or more wedges of pulmonary tissue are removed with an automatic stapler or a careful suture technique to reduce the likelihood of postoperative air leak from the lung (Fig. 17-50). Since a leak does occur in a few patients, an intercostal tube is placed at the time of operation and removed the next day if possible. The morbidity of open lung biopsy is minimal, and patients can often be discharged from the hospital in 48 to 72 h if they require no further in-hospital procedures. The need for close follow-up must be emphasized to the patient when early discharge is allowed.

The indications for open biopsies in immunocompromised patients have been sharply reduced in recent years, partly because of the success of the transbronchial biopsy in diagnosing *Pneumocystis carinii,* and partly because of the various reports, such as that by McKenna and the group at M.D. Anderson Tumor Institute, noting that open biopsies infrequently lead to any change in therapy which beneficially affects the patient's clinical course.

Congenital Lung Lesions

DEVELOPMENTAL ANATOMY. The respiratory system begins to differentiate in the third week of gestation as an outpouching in the floor of the primitive foregut. As the outpouching lengthens it bifurcates into two distinct buds, which promptly elongate and begin to form the secondary buds that will become the lobar and segmental bronchi. Rapid dichotomous branching of the terminal bud proceeds such that the lobes of each lung are well defined by 12 weeks, and by 16 weeks development of the bronchial system is complete.

Alveolar development proceeds more slowly. The alveolar or terminal sac stage of development only begins in about the seventh month of gestation, when primitive air sacs surrounded by capillary loops can be identified. Most alveolar development occurs after birth. At birth, the lung contains approximately 20 million large, thick-walled terminal air sacs, which proliferate rapidly until 300 million alveoli have been formed, with most of the increase occurring during the first 4 years of life, and with no further proliferation after about 10 years of age.

The pulmonary arterial circulation begins in a rich capillary network surrounding the developing lung buds, which is joined by the primitive pulmonary arteries budding off the sides of the aortic sac at about 5 weeks of gestation. The left sixth aortic arch extends to join the developing pulmonary artery, and persists as the ductus arteriosus. Each pulmonary artery develops in close relationship to the bronchi, and follows the course of the branching airways, although it gives off many more branches than the airway it accompanies. Normally, the only persistent connections with the aorta are the ductus arteriosus and the bronchial arteries.

ANATOMIC VARIANTS. The most common variation of segmentation is the azygous lobe, which is present in about 0.5 percent of routine chest x-rays. In this anomaly the azygous vein lies in the substance of the right upper lobe, on a pleural mesentery that separates the azygous lobe from the remainder of the lung. It appears on chest x-ray as an "inverted comma" in the medial apex of the right upper lobe. On rare occasions an azygous lobe can be the site of an infection or neoplasm that does not involve the remainder of the right upper lobe.

Situs inversus is a rare entity in which the thoracic viscera alone (situs inversus thoracis) or the thoracic and abdominal viscera (situs inversus totalis) undergo complete mirror-image reversal in position during development. The anomaly may exist in isolation or may be associated with other conditions. One example of the latter is Kartagener's syndrome, a familial association of situs inversus with sinusitis and bronchiectasis. Abnormal ciliary function is thought to explain the syndrome.

Aberrant origin of a normal major bronchus is infrequent but can have major significance when pulmonary resection is required for another reason. The most common example is origin of the right upper lobe bronchus or the apical segmental bronchus from the lateral wall of the trachea just above the carina.

DEVELOPMENTAL ANOMALIES

Agenesis. Many tracheobronchial anomalies reflect an arrest in embryonic development. The most complete example is bilateral pulmonary agenesis, which is obviously incompatible with life and is often seen in anencephalic monsters. Unilateral pulmonary agenesis has a low survival rate when associated with other congenital anomalies, which are present in about 50 percent of cases. When seen as an isolated lesion it is compatible with relatively normal life. Seventy percent of cases occur on the left side. The single lung fills both hemithoraces, and the condition is often detected in otherwise normal individuals by findings suggesting mediastinal shift or asymmetric thoracic development. Pulmonary arteriography demonstrating single pulmonary artery confirms the diagnosis in such patients and may protect them against therapeutic misadventures. Lobar agenesis is rarely reported and is most often discovered during evaluation for other conditions.

Hypoplasia. Hypoplasia of the lung is most often seen in association with anomalies that compete with the lungs for space, such as diaphragmatic hernia. It has been postulated that the defect arises from arrested alveolar development occurring during the last 2 months of gestation. The scimitar syndrome is a condition difficult to classify, which has as one of its features hypoplasia of the right lung. The syndrome takes its name from the radiographic finding of a scimitar-like shadow running parallel to the right heart border that represents an anomalous pulmonary vein entering the inferior vena cava. The hypoplastic right lung also has an aberrant pulmonary arterial origin from the aorta.

Tracheoesophageal Fistulas. See Chap. 39.

Diverticula. These are usually asymptomatic, small, and in free communication with the airway, usually the distal trachea.

Cystic Adenomatoid Malformation. Cystic adenomatoid malformation is one cause of respiratory distress in the newborn period that can require emergent operation. Other congenital anomalies, prematurity, and stillbirth are common associations. Surviving neonates present with acute respiratory distress in the first few hours of life. The chest x-ray shows a multicystic "swiss cheese" configuration with overexpansion of the involved region and mediastinal shift toward the normal lung. The pattern on chest x-ray can be confused with dilated loops of intestine suggesting diaphragmatic hernia. Any lobe of either lung can be involved, although the process has a predilection for the lower lobes. About half the reported cases have escaped crisis in the newborn period to present later in infancy or during childhood with a more indolent course of chronic recurrent pulmonary infection, and can be difficult to distinguish clinically from sequestration, infected congenital cysts, and bronchiectasis.

Thoracotomy reveals a dense, meaty mass studded with cysts that may appear to be partially aerated but have no ventilatory function. Anomalous vessels are very rare. Histopathology reveals multiple components of respiratory tissue including a maze of irregular tubules resembling fetal bronchioles lined with disorganized respiratory epithelium that can resemble an adenoma. Lobectomy is the treatment of choice, although pneumonectomy has been necessary in some cases. The prognosis is excellent with a successful early operation.

Pulmonary Sequestration. A portion of lung may be isolated during development from the remainder of the lung and receive its blood supply from an aberrant branch of the aorta instead of the pulmonary artery. Intralobar sequestrations rest within a lobe and do not have their own visceral pleural envelope, but usually have a communication with the tracheobronchial tree producing a cystic appearance. They occur invariably in the posterobasal portion of the lower lobes, most frequently on the left side. The sequestered lung is supplied by an anomalous branch of the aorta that is usually tortuous and disproportionately large, arising from the thoracic aorta in 70 percent of cases and from the abdominal aorta or its branches in the remainder. The vessel reaches the sequestered lung by passing through the inferior pulmonary ligament. Venous drainage is through the pulmonary veins. The radiographic appearance is that of a dense

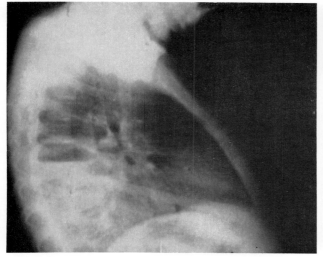

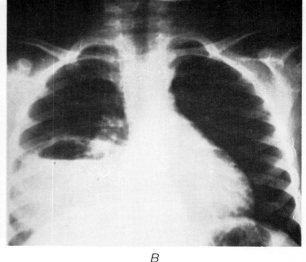

A   *B*

Fig. 17-51. An example of intrapulmonary sequestration. Consolidation and an air-fluid level are evident posteriorly in the right lower lobe. Lobectomy revealed an infected sequestration.

mass usually containing cysts with air-fluid levels, not distinguishable from cystic adenomatoid malformation or other congenital cystic abnormalities without an arteriogram (Fig. 17-51). Intralobar sequestration often remains asymptomatic until childhood or young adulthood, when it presents as pulmonary infection.

Extralobar sequestration is a much less common entity in which the sequestered lung is enclosed by a separate pleural envelope sitting in the inferoposterior mediastinum adjacent to lung and esophagus, usually on the left side (Fig. 17-52). Association with other congenital anomalies, especially diaphragmatic hernia, occurs in over 50 percent of patients. Although tracheobronchial communication is said not to occur, an esophageal communication is occasionally seen. Extralobar sequestration is more likely to be detected early in childhood, appearing as an unexplained dense triangular mass in the posterior lower lung field (Fig. 17-53). Venous drainage is to the azygous or portal venous system.

If either type of sequestration is suspected an arteriogram should be done to confirm the diagnosis and define the aberrant systemic blood supply (Fig. 17-53). A barium esophagram should be done to exclude the possibility of a communication with the esophagus. CT scanning can help to define lobar and mediastinal relationships. The treatment of choice is lobectomy for the intralobar types, and resection for the extralobar types.

An accessory lobe is distinguished from sequestration by the fact that it communicates with the trachea or a major bronchial branch, most commonly on the left side. The accessory lobe can be supplied by either the pulmonary or systemic circulation.

Congenital Cysts. These are a diverse group of abnormalities that can be single or multiple, and vary greatly in size. They are usually confined to a segment or lobe and almost invariably present with infection (Fig. 17-54). Eti-

ology is poorly understood and may be equally diverse. Unilateral absence of a pulmonary artery branch may produce hypoplastic development of the lung, leading to cystic transformation. The lesions may begin as intrapulmonary bronchogenic cysts, which are thought to represent remnants of developing bronchial buds pinched off in the lung periphery. A region of cystic lung can develop distal to congenital or acquired bronchial obstruction. The cysts are typically lined with respiratory epithelium and are filled with a viscid opaque fluid until they develop communication with the airway, after which they become partially air-filled and infected. The presence of respira-

Fig. 17-52. Artist's conception of an extralobar sequestration as seen at operation through a left posterolateral thoracotomy. Anterior is to the left. Note the anomalous systemic artery arising directly from the aorta, a feature common to both extralobar and intralobar sequestrations. (From: *Ferguson TB, in Gibbon's Surgery of the Chest, 4th ed, Fig 22-28, p 685, with permission.*)

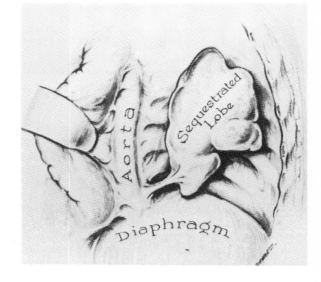

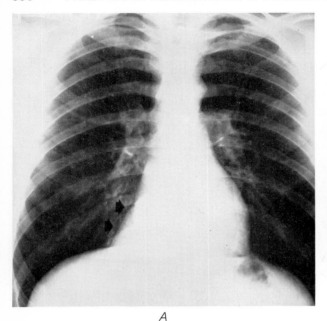

A

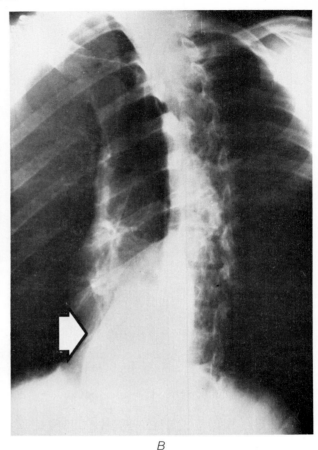

B

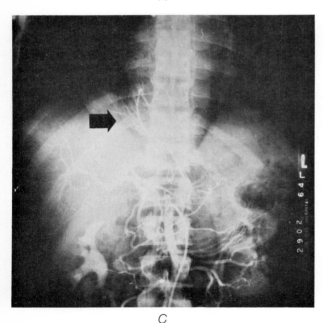

C

Fig. 17-53. An extrapulmonary sequestration discovered on a routine chest x-ray in a twenty-year-old male. *A.* The posteroanterior chest x-ray shows a triangular density adjacent to the right heart border and based on the diaphragm. *B.* An oblique view shows the density to be a large mass with sharp borders. *C.* An aortogram shows several arteries passing retrograde from the infradiaphragmatic aorta to supply the sequestration.

tory epithelium is thought to indicate true congenital origin, but once chronic infection destroys the epithelium it becomes impossible to separate a congenital cyst from a chronic pulmonary abscess or bronchiectasis, grossly or histopathologically. Resection is indicated for large or chronically infected cysts. Preoperative evaluation includes bronchoscopy and arteriography, to exclude sequestration.

Arteriovenous Malformation. Pulmonary arteriovenous malformation is a fistula between pulmonary arteries and pulmonary veins. One or more thin-walled saccular chan-

nels with an endothelial lining are present, without reaction in the surrounding lung tissue. The lesions are somewhat more frequent in the lower lobes. Multiple small (<1 cm) lesions associated with capillary abnormalities elsewhere, a feature of hereditary hemorrhagic telangiectasia (Osler–Weber–Rendu syndrome), account for half of all reported cases. In the other half the lesions are singular or few in number, and larger (1 to 5 cm) in size. Although the vascular pattern is variable, one afferent pulmonary arterial branch with two or more efferent venous branches is the most common arrangement (Fig. 17-55). The lesions are frequently very superficial and vulnerable to erosion, and can present with spontaneous hemothorax.

Diagnosis is easiest in the 20 percent of patients presenting with cyanosis, polycythemia, and clubbing. Cyanosis is said to develop when the shunt fraction exceeds 25 percent of the total blood flow and is usually not seen until adolescence or early adulthood. There is an interesting difference between the right-to-left shunt seen

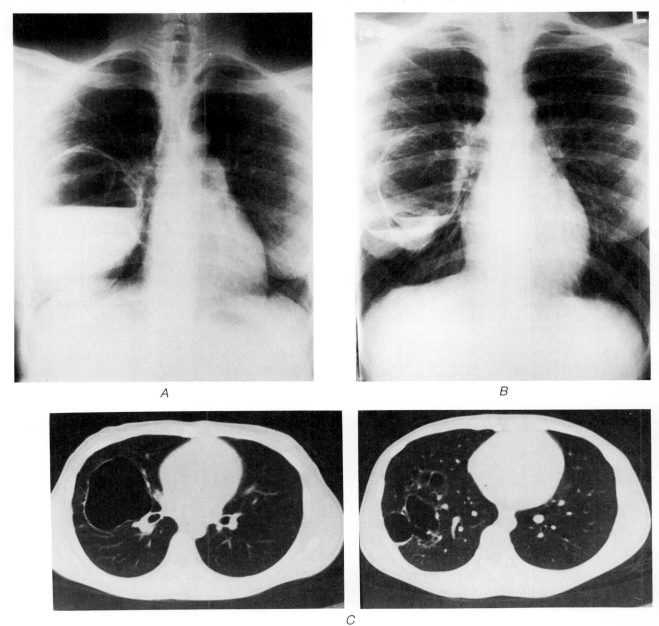

A

B

C

Fig. 17-54. *A.* This young woman had a long history of recurrent respiratory infections with foul, copious sputum production. *B.* The large cavity in the right lung would partially empty after each period of aggressive medical management, revealing a more complex array of cystic spaces with air-fluid levels. *C.* A similar appearance is evident on CT scan. After several years the patient was persuaded to undergo surgery. A preoperative arteriogram did not demonstrate anomalous vessels, suggesting sequestration. At operation, only the right upper lobe could be salvaged.

in congenital heart disease and that seen with a pulmonary arteriovenous malformation. In the latter condition, vascular resistance in both the pulmonary capillary bed and the fistula are negligible, so that the total volume returned to the left atrium is not increased, it is simply de-

saturated in proportion to the amount of flow going through the fistula. Therefore, in contrast to the patient with an intracardiac shunt, the patient with the fistula has normal cardiac output, pulse, blood pressure, venous pressure, electrocardiogram, and heart size. No murmur is audible over the heart, but in over half the cyanotic patients a continuous murmur can be heard peripherally over the fistula. Patients with either condition have arterial desaturation and polycythemia.

Diagnosis is more difficult in the asymptomatic, acyanotic patient. Small, single malformations can be indistinguishable from all other solitary pulmonary nod-

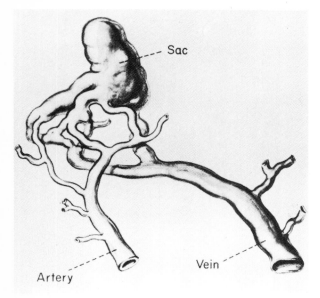

Fig. 17-55. Anatomy of a typical arteriovenous fistula in the lung. (From: *Ferguson TB, in Gibbon's Surgery of the Chest, 4th ed, Fig 22-42, p 694, with permission.*)

ules. Larger lesions may have a more characteristic lobulated appearance, and the afferent and efferent vessels can often be demonstrated on plane tomography or CT scan. Pulmonary angiography confirms the diagnosis (Fig. 17-56). Both lungs should be examined carefully for multiple lesions.

Significant complications occur in at least 25 percent of all patients, and in a higher percentage of patients with hereditary telangectasis and multiple fistulas. Complications can be local effects such as hemothorax, but conse-

quences of polycythemia, such as cerebral thrombosis, are more common. Resection is indicated in all patients with solitary nodules, and in selected patients with multiple nodules when adequate lung tissue can be preserved. Cyanotic patients with widespread multiple small fistulas are inoperable, although improvement with embolization has been reported in a few cases.

Lobar Emphysema. Lobar emphysema presents with massive distention of a lobe or segment that shifts the mediastinum and compresses the contralateral lung. It is the most common of the four structural lesions usually considered in the differential diagnosis of respiratory distress in the newborn. The other three are sequestration, cystic adenomatoid malformation, and bronchogenic cyst. Etiology has been a matter of continuing debate, and the clinical syndrome may represent the final common pathway of several distinct processes. Dysplasia of bronchial cartilage has been most frequently recognized, occurring in about 25 percent of cases. Acute bronchiolitis, extrinsic compression by lymph nodes or anomalous vessels, bronchial atresia, and several other possible causes of bronchial obstruction have been cited. No specific cause can be identified in more than 50 percent of cases. Associated malformations, mostly cardiovascular, are present in about 40 percent of patients, a fact that some authors interpret as support for a congenital etiology.

Respiratory distress typically appears from 4 days to 6 months postpartum. Half of all reported cases have occurred within the first 4 weeks of life. Physical findings of hyperresonance and decreased breath sounds mimic

Fig. 17-56. *A.* Three lesions *(arrows)* thought to be compatible with pulmonary arteriovenous aneurysms are visible on the chest x-ray in this eight-year-old boy. *B.* A pulmonary arteriogram confirms the diagnosis. The lesions were subsequently removed through staged bilateral thoracotomies.

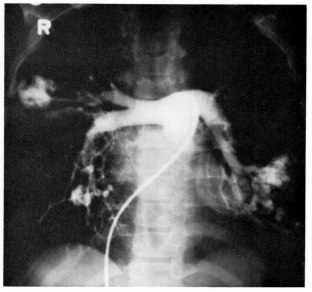

A

B

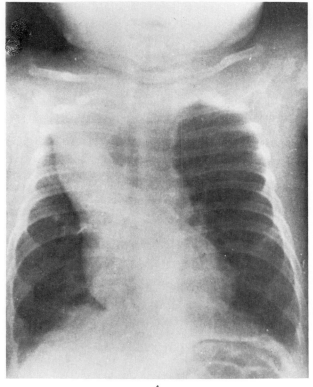

A

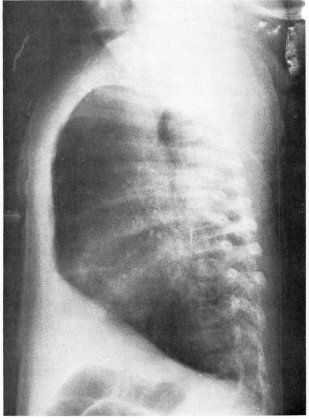

B

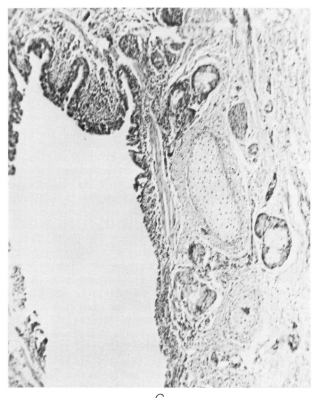

C

Fig. 17-57. Infantile lobar emphysema. *A.* The anteroposterior chest x-ray shows marked overinflation of the left upper lobe, with mediastinal shift to the right and compression of the right upper lobe. *B.* The lateral x-ray shows that most of the hyperinflation is anterior. *C.* Histologic examination of the resected left-upper-lobe bronchus shows incomplete cartilage development. (From: *Michelson E: Clinical spectrum of infantile lobar emphysema. Ann Thorac Surg, 24:182, 1977, with permission.*)

pneumothorax, which is a dangerous misapprehension if it leads to impulsive chest tube insertion. The chest x-ray can also mimic pneumothorax because the distended lung is very hyperlucent. Another common misinterpretation occurs when the compressed normal lung is thought to be atelectatic and the distended lung compensatory. An important radiographic clue is that the diaphragm is usually depressed on both sides with lobar emphysema but is normal or elevated on the side of primary atelectasis (Fig. 17-57).

In an infant with florid, progressive respiratory distress and a characteristic chest x-ray, emergency thoracotomy and lobectomy is indicated without further study. In such circumstances the mortality without operation approaches 50 percent. Involvement of an upper lobe or the right middle lobe is the most frequent finding. Lower lobe involvement is rare. Resection is ordinarily straightforward anatomically and completely curative. When the clinical presentation is less fulminant, the decision is more difficult. There is no question that varying degrees of lobar emphysema can be produced by aspiration of mucus or amniotic fluid, or by acute bronchiolitis. In such cases the emphysema almost always resolves in a few days with appropriate medical therapy.

Emphysematous Blebs and Bullae

Emphysema is characterized by enlarged air spaces produced by a complex process of elastic tissue destruction, alveolar wall breakdown, and coalescence of damaged alveoli, resulting in impaired alveolar ventilation and gas exchange. The disease represents one characteristic expression of advanced chronic obstructive pulmonary disease, overlapping considerably with the secretory, fibrotic bronchiolar obstructive pattern of chronic bronchitis, and with the reactive, atopic pattern of asthma. Pathogenetic differences promoting a predominant pattern of alveolar breakdown are difficult to isolate, and the response to a common mechanism of injury such as cigarette smoking is not predictable. An exception is the emphysematous pattern produced by the loss of normal restraints on tissue destruction seen in alpha$_1$-antitrypsin deficiency.

The surgeon has the luxury of ignoring the confusion of pathogenesis in this complex disorder to concentrate on the parts of the spectrum that have surgical significance. Emphysema is usually not truly diffuse, and involved areas may be quite localized into collections of small cysts (blebs) or very large ones (bullae). Blebs are usually subpleural, do not extend deeply into more central parenchyma, and consequently may have little effect on gas exchange or overall pulmonary function, even when multiple discrete collections of considerable size are present. Their chief significance relates to their potential for rupture with production of pneumothorax. The localized collection of blebs frequently encountered in the apices of otherwise normal lungs in healthy young individuals with spontaneous pneumothorax bear an uncertain pathogenic relationship to emphysema and may be in some way congenital. Although most blebs are apical, the blebs encountered in typical chronic pulmonary disease are more likely to be multiple and in other parts of the lung.

Bullae result from a much larger coalescence of destroyed alveolar septae and tend to develop deep within the lung parenchyma, compressing and distorting adjacent normal lung. They may assume the form of a single large cyst, or remnants of interstitium may remain to form a multiloculated space. Many bullae will remain stable or will increase in size slowly over many years, but they have the potential for rapid expansion, producing acute respiratory distress. An enormous single bulla may be very difficult to distinguish from a tension pneumothorax clinically or radiographically.

Diffuse emphysema is characterized by a uniform destructive process producing profound effects on pulmonary function and gas exchange. The full-blown clinical presentation includes extreme dyspnea, with a barrel chest and attenuation of intercostal and diaphragmatic musculature. Lungs with diffuse emphysema frequently contain areas of bleb or bullous disease as well.

SURGICAL CONSIDERATIONS. The surgeon confronts emphysema in two principal situations: in operations performed on patients with emphysema, and in operations performed for emphysema. In the former category, patients with emphysema undergoing procedures with general anesthesia have an increased operative risk due to their abnormal gas exchange and are at higher risk for barotrauma during mechanical ventilation. Postoperative pulmonary toilet can be a major challenge in a patient with greatly reduced expiratory forces whose ability to cough is further compromised by postoperative pain. Every surgeon has seen patients with marginally compensated emphysema become ventilator-dependent, with a tracheostomy and bilateral chest tubes, following routine abdominal surgery. Elective operation in such patients requires cautious assessment of risks and careful attention to preoperative pulmonary physiotherapy.

Thoracic operations designed to correct specific manifestations of emphysema carry similar risks but also offer the expectation of improvement. The history of operations for emphysema illustrates the danger of allowing surgical intuition to precede an understanding of pathophysiology. Some of the earliest procedures were designed to "make room" for the hyperinflated lung by further enlarging the barrel chest with sternotomy or chondrectomy. Upon observation that such procedures were ineffective at best, attempts were made to decrease lung volume by phrenic nerve destruction or thoracoplasty, with counterproductive results that would be considered predictable today.

Selection for operation is directed toward identifying patients in whom resection of localized bullous disease is likely to improve pulmonary function. Ventilation-perfusion scans and pulmonary angiography can help define areas of normal lung adjacent to large bullae that are compressed and nonventilated but normally perfused (Fig. 17-58). The most favorable patients are young (under age fifty-five years), with unilateral disease and marked asymmetry of function, recently progressive symptoms, well-defined bullae, and evidence of crowded vessels in adjacent parenchyma. Large bullae displacing more than half the hemithorax are more likely to produce symptomatic improvement after resection than smaller bullae.

In all patients every effort is made preoperatively to maximize pulmonary function and eliminate chronic bronchial infection. The disease is usually approached through a posterolateral thoracotomy, although some authors have favored median sternotomy for anterior and superior bullae, claiming that postoperative morbidity is reduced. The resection is carefully tailored to preserve all adjacent vascularized parenchyma. Mechanical stapling devices are extremely helpful. Planes of division through emphysematous lung are friable and prone to air leak. Elimination of any residual pleural space by careful placement of chest tubes and judicious use of pleural tents or thoracoplasty can be essential to success.

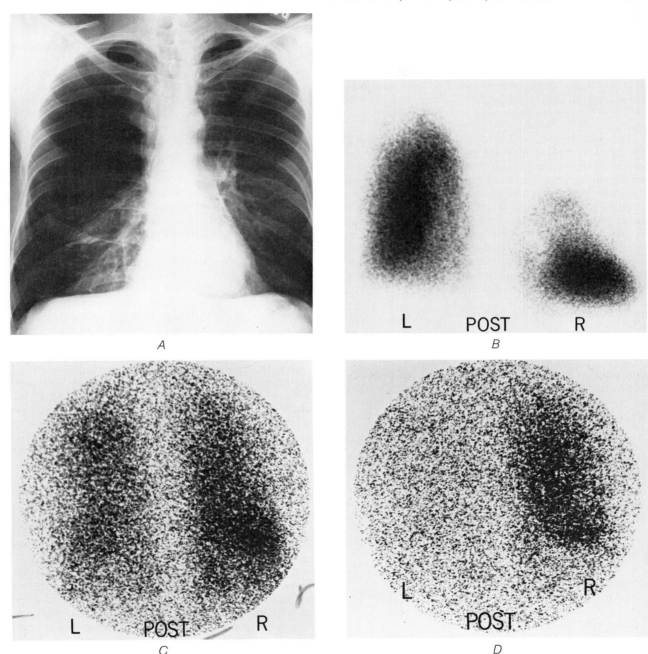

Fig. 17-58. A forty-nine-year-old man with obstructive airway disease (FEV_1 = 50% of predicted) and dyspnea with minimal exertion. *A.* The chest x-ray shows marked radiolucency in the upper half of the right hemithorax, due to giant bullae compressing the remaining normal parenchyma into the lower part of the hemithorax. *B.* A lung perfusion scan with ^{99m}Tc macroaggregated albumin shows loss of perfusion in the right upper and middle lobe regions. *C.* The ventilation scan with ^{33}Xe shows early delay in washout of the radioisotope from the right lung after equilibration. *D.* After 3 min of the washout phase of the ventilation scan, there is marked trapping of the radioisotope in the giant bullae of the right lung. The patient underwent successful resection of the bullae with considerable subjective improvement in symptoms.

Pulmonary Infections

As recently as the early 1960s, thousands of patients each year in the United States required pulmonary resection for lung abscess, bronchiectasis, and chronic granulomatous disease. Since that time effective antibiotics, aggressive methods for accurate early diagnosis, an increased standard of living, and public health programs are among the factors that have diminished the surgeon's role dramatically. Fifteen or twenty years ago it seemed reasonable to hope that suppurative pulmonary infections would remain a common surgical problem only in areas of the world with limited medical technology and limited access to antibiotics. Ironically such problems are becoming increasingly frequent at the high-technology frontiers—patients immunosuppressed following transplant or as part of cancer chemotherapy, and patients with AIDS all too commonly develop serious pulmonary infections.

The pathologic spectrum of pulmonary infections is very broad, ranging from the indolent bronchiolar and peribronchial suppuration of bronchiectasis, to the contained parenchymal necrosis of lung abscess, to the pleural space infection of empyema. The clinical expression of pulmonary infection is determined by the route of inoculation, the competence of host defenses, and the specific organism(s) involved, which can include aerobic and anaerobic bacteria, viruses, and fungi, often in synergistic combinations. This broad spectrum of pathology has an equally broad spectrum of treatment in which surgical management remains important.

LUNG ABSCESS

SPECTRUM OF DISEASE. Lung abscess may be defined as a focus of infection with parenchymal necrosis, usually with cavitation. Distinction between a lung abscess and a consolidated pneumonia is made as areas of cavitation appear on the chest x-ray, and as the peripheral margins of the infection develop sharper definition. Lung abscess and empyema can coexist as confluent or separate processes. Causes of lung abscess are outlined in Table 17-12.

Lung abscess is most commonly a complication of necrotizing pneumonia. Aspiration of gastric contents or sa-

Table 17-12. CAUSES OF LUNG ABSCESS

I. Primary necrotizing pneumonia
    A. Aerobic infection
        1. *Staphylococcus aureus*
        2. *Klebsiella, Pseudomonas,* other gram negatives
        3. *Mycobacteria (M. tuberculosis* and atypical *Myobacteria)*
    B. Anaerobic infection
        1. *Bacteroides (B. fragilis, B. melaninogenicus)*
        2. *Fusobacterium* species
        3. *Actinomyces*
    C. Parasitic infection
        1. *Entameba histolytica*
        2. *Echinococcus (E. granulosus, E. multilocularis)*
II. Aspiration pneumonia
III. Bronchial obstruction
    A. Neoplasm
    B. Foreign body
IV. Complication of systemic sepsis
    A. Septic pulmonary emboli
    B. Seeding of pulmonary infarct
V. Complication of pulmonary trauma
    A. Infection of hematoma or contusion
    B. Contaminated foreign body or penetrating injury
VI. Direct extension from extraparenchymal infection
    A. Pleural empyema
    B. Mediastinal, hepatic, subphrenic abscess

liva produces an infectious focus with enzymatic tissue degradation, mixed aerobic and anaerobic bacterial contamination, and frequently particulate matter that combine to promote abscess formation. Aspiration remains the most common single cause of lung abscess, and has a well-recognized association with altered states of consciousness (Fig. 17-59). Alcoholic stupor is most frequently cited, but drug overdosage, head trauma, cardiopulmonary resuscitation, and general anesthesia can also set the stage for aspiration leading to lung abscess. Because most episodes of aspiration occur with the person supine, the abscess is characteristically located in the lung segments that are dependent in the supine position— the posterior segments of the upper lobes, and the superior segments of both lower lobes. Bacteriologically the infection is usually mixed, with anaerobic mouth organisms such as *Bacterioides* species frequently predominating.

The tissue necrosis that is the hallmark of "necrotizing" pneumonia is a function of the specific organism involved, and is most prominent with *Klebsiella, Pseudomonas,* and other gram-negative organisms. Tissue necrosis is rare with Group B streptococcal pneumonia (*Pneumococcus*), whereas necrosis and abscess formation are frequent with *Staphylococcus aureus* and Group A streptococci. Staphylococcal lung abscess is most common in the first year of life and has characteristic pathology, most frequently with pyopneumothorax and pneumatoceles. The latter are large cystic spaces, typically not containing true pus, that are thought to result from air trapping distal to bronchiolar obstruction. Staphylococcal lung abscess in infancy is also characterized clinically by a remarkable tendency to resolve completely with antibiotics alone, even when temporary drainage of the pleural space has been required.

Establishment of a gram-negative pneumonia begins with major alteration in the bacteriologic composition of upper respiratory flora. The mechanisms that reduce gram negatives to transient visitors in normal individuals are seriously impaired in many hospitalized patients. For example, experiments in mice suggest that an *Escherichia coli* peritonitis interferes with recruitment of polymorphonuclear leukocytes in the lung, increasing susceptibility to gram-negative (*Pseudomonas*) but not to gram-positive infections. Over half the pneumonias seen in seriously ill hospitalized patients are gram-negative, and a significant proportion of such patients manifest a necrotizing infection leading to lung-abscess formation.

Systemic sepsis can produce multiple bilateral foci of parenchymal infection that are radiographically quite discrete, and are most frequently caused by *Staphylococcus* and other gram-positive organisms. One or more of the foci can become an abscess, although most resolve without a trace. Unlike staphylococcal pneumonia of tracheobronchial origin, hematogenous infection does not tend to form pneumatoceles and can be seen in septic patients of any age. Lung abscess developing in a pulmonary infarction following pulmonary embolus is most frequently a special case of hematogenous infection seeding an area of devitalized or injured tissue.

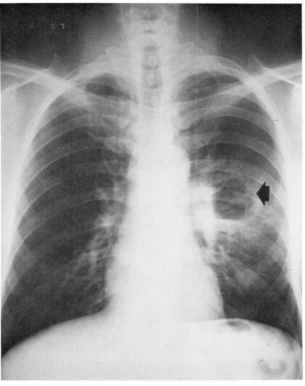

A

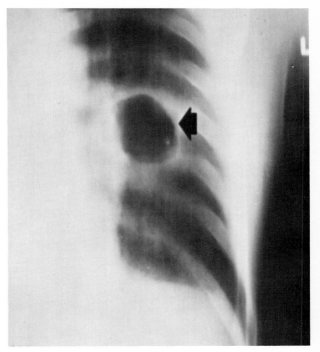

B

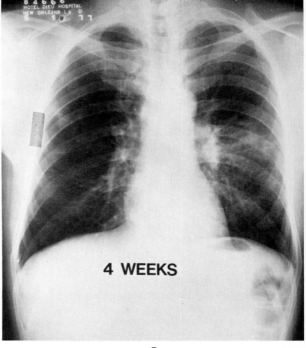

4 WEEKS

C

Fig. 17-59. Lung abscess due to vomiting and aspiration after an alcoholic binge. *A.* The chest x-ray shows an abscess cavity in the superior segment of the left upper lobe. *B.* A tomogram confirms the thin wall of the abscess, reducing the probability that the lesion could be a cavitated carcinoma. *C.* After 4 weeks of antibiotic therapy and postural drainage the abscess cavity appears to be healing.

A cavitary necrotizing infection can also form distal to an obstructive lung carcinoma or intrabronchial foreign body (Fig. 17-60), a reminder that bronchoscopy is an important diagnostic manuever. Not infrequently a carcinoma becomes visible as the distal infection responds to antibiotic treatment.

In certain parts of the world parasitic infection is a common cause of lung abscess. *Entameba histolytica* can produce lung abscess by hematogenous spread or by direct extension from the liver, in which case it is almost always associated with empyema. Metronidazole is usually effective treatment, and operative intervention is rarely required. Hydatid infection (*Echinococcus* species) is associated with lung abscess in some cases (Fig. 17-61). Intraabdominal pathology is much more prominent. Treatment with oral mebendazole has been moderately successful, but resection has frequently been required. Albendazole is currently in clinical trial and appears to offer the possibility of better results without operation.

CLINICAL MANIFESTATIONS. Regardless of etiology, the clinical presentation is relatively uniform. The patient appears chronically ill, is likely to be febrile, and will often describe recent onset of copious foul sputum pro-duction, reflecting decompression of the abscess into the airway. Whether the initial infection originated from the airway or the bloodstream, the necrotizing process tends to find its way into the tracheobronchial tree, a develop-

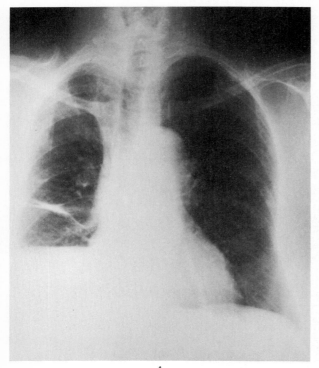

A

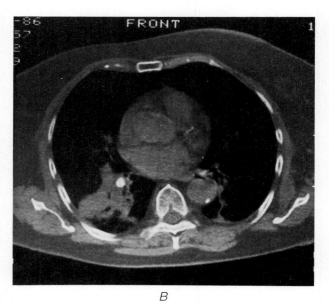

B

Fig. 17-60. *A.* This seventy-two-year-old woman presented with a clinical picture of slowly progressing pneumonia, and chest x-ray revealed right lower lobe consolidation with a pleural effusion. *B.* CT scan demonstrated a large area of consolidation and early abscess formation in the right lower lobe, and a small bone-density mass lying medially within. An obstructing chicken bone was identified by bronchoscopy but could not be removed. A successful right lower lobectomy was performed.

ment heralded radiographically by the appearance of cavitation on chest x-ray. Because of the necrotizing, erosive nature of the communication with the airways, hemoptysis can occur and can be massive. In contrast to pneumonia, dyspnea is not a prominent symptom. Auscultatory findings, if any, are more likely to be attributable to coexistence of a pleural effusion or empyema than to the presence of lung abscess. In the acute phase of abscess development, constitutional symptoms will overlap with those of acute pneumonia. As the process becomes more chronic symptoms frequently ameliorate as the abscess becomes walled off.

In a febrile patient with copious production of foul sputum, the differential diagnosis can be reduced to three entities: lung abscess, bronchiectasis, and cavitating carcinoma. Chronic copious sputum production is most characteristic of bronchiectasis; the other two entities tend to have acute or episodic sputum production. A dramatic febrile illness is most consistent with lung abscess, reflecting its origins in a necrotizing pneumonia, although bronchiectasis and carcinoma can have febrile episodes associated with exacerbations of the inflammatory process surrounding the primary pathology. A chest x-ray showing a well-delineated cavity is against bronchiectasis alone, but the chest x-ray is usually of little help in distinguishing carcinoma from lung abscess, for which bronchoscopy and biopsy are essential. Bronchiectasis is confirmed by bronchography.

TREATMENT. The options for treatment of lung abscess are outlined in Table 17-13. Primary treatment consists of

antibiotics and drainage. Antibiotics are administered intravenously in high doses and should be selected based on the sensitivities of the infecting organism. In the most fortunate cases, spontaneous drainage by expectoration is adequate. More commonly, drainage must be achieved by other means, the least invasive of which is bronchoscopic aspiration. Proponents of nonoperative treatment favor at least 8 weeks of antibiotics and ''internal'' (cough and bronchoscopy) drainage before proceeding to external drainage or resection. Such methods are successful in more than 75 percent of all patients with lung abscess (Fig. 17-59), although convalescence can be prolonged. In one representative nonoperative series the average duration of therapy was 4 months. Numerous surgical series have demonstrated that convalescence can be shortened dramatically in properly selected patients.

The guiding principle governing operative treatment of lung abscess is the establishment of drainage. When internal drainage has been ineffective, external drainage can be established in one of two ways. (1) Tube pneumonostomy is percutaneous insertion of a drainage tube into the abscess cavity, connecting the tube to a water-seal drainage system. The alternative is (2) pneumonotomy, an open drainage procedure that opens the abscess cavity

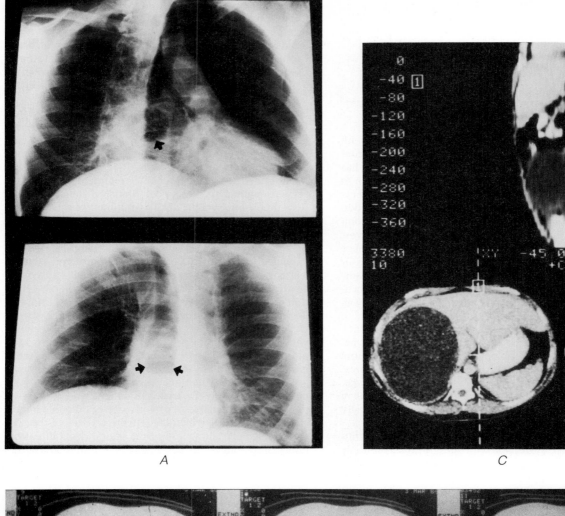

Fig. 17-61. *A.* This forty-eight-year-old Yugoslavian immigrant was completely asymptomatic until he presented with a transient episode of copious, foul productive cough. A mediastinal cavity is visible in the oblique views shown *(see arrows). B.* A CT scan of the chest shows the cavity lying just below the right main stem bronchus, and showed that the mediastinal cavity did not communicate with the abdomen. *C.* A CT scan of the abdomen shows further evidence of widespread infection with *Echinococcus granulosus.* The sagittal view shows a large pelvic mass, and the transverse section shows a huge mass in the right lobe of the liver, containing several daughter cysts.

directly to the outside through a generous incision and short rib resection.

Both methods bear obvious superficial resemblance to procedures performed for treatment of empyema. However, there are important differences that are crucial to success and safety. Most fundamentally, both procedures depend on pleural symphysis occurring between the parietal pleura and the visceral pleural surface closest to the

Table 17-13. OPTIONS FOR TREATMENT OF
LUNG ABSCESS

---

1. Antibiotics and internal drainage (cough, bronchoscopy)
2. External drainage
   a. Pneumonostomy
   b. Pneumonotomy
3. Pulmonary resection

---

abscess cavity. This commonly occurs in association with infection, and allows drainage to the outside without contamination of the free pleural space. After the body has succeeded in localizing a serious necrotizing infection to an abscess in the lung parenchyma, spilling the contents into the free pleural space can be catastrophic. In addition, the center of an abscess cavity in the lung can communicate directly with large-caliber bronchioles and vascular structures capable of producing major hemorrhage and/or a large bronchopleurocutaneous fistula (a large air leak), especially if the tube penetrates the soft inner surface of the abscess cavity. Therefore, it is critical to accurately localize the abscess in relationship to the chest wall and identify the site where pleural symphysis is likely to have occurred. Unlike drainage of empyema, dependency is not important. Abscess cavities close to the lung periphery are most likely to stimulate an aggressive pleural reaction, are least likely to be lined with major structures, and will be the ones most suitable for external drainage. Fortunately, most abscesses are more peripheral than central; this is particularly true of the common variety caused by aspiration.

Accurate localization of the abscess is obviously critical, and complete evaluation with chest x-rays in multiple views is the minimum required. Chest CT scan should be obtained if possible, it allows placement of skin markers over what appears to be the best drainage site. Ultrasound can be equally helpful and can be used during tube insertion. An essential preliminary step in any method of external drainage is location of the cavity with an aspirating needle inserted along the path proposed for drainage.

If the external drainage procedurre accidentally contaminates the free pleural space, separate drainage of the pleural space is established with a separate tube and drainage system. In performing a pneumonotomy, if inspection through the incision suggests that adequate symphysis has not occurred, the wound can be packed open down to the level of the external surface of the parietal pleura. After several days this usually results in an exuberant pleural reaction and symphysis allowing safe access to the abscess cavity

Choosing between pneumonotomy and pneumonostomy is a purely clinical judgment. Closed-tube drainage (pneumonostomy) is generally adequate and is enjoying a resurgence of popularity in the 1980s (Fig. 17-62), especially in children, based on the impressive results reported in several small series. Tube drainage is theoretically limited by the viscosity and particulate content of the pus. Even so, percutaneous drainage through small-caliber pigtail catheters inserted by invasive radiologists

has had some reported success as well, and seems likely to become a more common practice. On the other hand, the presence of a foreign body in the abscess cavity is thought to increase the risk of erosion and hemorrhage. Pneumonotomy unquestionably provides the swiftest and most reliable drainage, and for that reason might be favored for cavities containing large volumes of especially viscid pus mixed with a large amount of necrotic debris, but open drainage also leaves the patient with a large wound that must eventually heal. It is important to recognize that either method can be complicated by major hemorrhage or the development of a chronic bronchopleurocutaneous fistula.

The most definitive operative treatment for lung abscess is pulmonary resection. Standard indications for resection are chronicity with symptoms, serious hemorrhage, and suspicion of associated carcinoma. Lobectomy is ordinarily preferred to simplify dissection and preserve protective tissue planes. Resection has the advantage of removing the entire infection promptly, and is less hazardous than external drainage when the abscess is very large or centrally located. On the other hand, resection does not eliminate the risk of pleural space contamination. It can be technically difficult to remove a thin-walled abscess presenting close to the visceral pleura without spillage, and empyema following lobectomy is far more serious than primary empyema. Anesthetic technique and patient positioning are critical to prevent spillage of pus through the tracheobronchial tree across to the dependent lung. In the past, the patient was often positioned prone or supine. Currently use of a double-lumen endotracheal tube, which can effectively isolate the two sides, generally allows use of the lateral decubitus position. Safety can be further augmented by frequent intraoperative bronchosopy performed from the head of the table through the endotracheal tube, providing accurate irrigation and aspiration of the airways.

Life-threatening hemorrhage requires prompt resection once the bleeding site is unequivocally localized by bronchoscopy. Unfortunately, this complication most frequently arises in patients least able to tolerate thoracotomy, who are often bleeding because of coagulopathy secondary to sepsis and multiple organ failure. Acceptable temporizing measures designed primarily to protect the uninvolved lung include insertion of a double-lumen endotracheal tube, placement of a bronchial blocker on the affected side, and aggressive toilet of the unaffected side with rigid or flexible bronchoscopy. Bronchial artery embolization is worth consideration but is limited by the rich collateral circulation of the lung.

ACQUIRED IMMUNE DEFICIENCY SYNDROME (AIDS)

Cancer chemotherapy and organ transplantation are creating a steadily increasing population of immunologically compromised individuals who would not have been alive 20 years ago. Patients nursed through major trauma or complications of surgery exhibit a characteristic spectrum of immunologic compromise. As if the increasing numbers put at risk iatrogenically were not enough, pa-

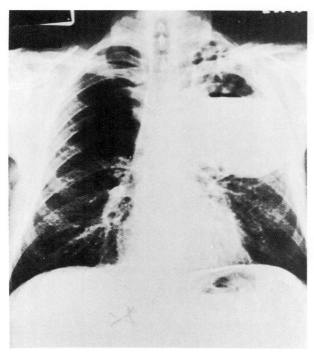

A

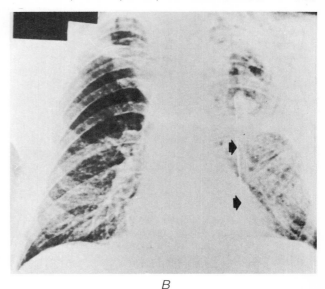

B

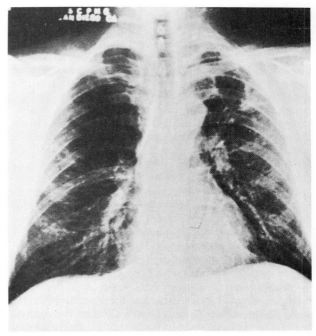

C

Fig. 17-62. *A.* Chest x-ray shows a large abscess cavity in the left upper lobe. The abscess appeared very anterior and adherent to the parietal pleura in lateral views (not shown), making it ideal for percutaneous drainage. *B.* At the bedside, a chest tube *(see arrows)* was inserted in the abscess cavity, and drained 900 mL of thick pus in the first 48 h. After 1 week the tube was amputated, leaving a short segment in the cavity as a straight drain. The patient was discharged on oral antibiotics, and the tube was removed 4 weeks later. *C.* A chest x-ray done 3 months after discharge showed mild residual scarring and a vague outline of the cavity in the left upper lobe. (From: Mengoli L: *J Thorac Cardiovasc Surg 90:189, 1985, Figs 8, 9, 10, with permission.*)

tients with the acquired immune deficiency syndrome (AIDS) are beginning to crowd wards in New York City, San Francisco, and elsewhere. All these kinds of susceptible patients share a predilection for pulmonary infections caused by some familiar agents, but even more so by organisms rarely seen in healthy individuals. Perhaps reflecting the fact the lung is the only organ capable of presenting pathogens to a delicate nonsquamous epithelium many times each minute, pulmonary infections are the most common infections seen in immunocompromised patients.

AIDS was defined in 1981 in a group of previously healthy homosexual men with *Pneumocystic carinii* pneumonia and mucosal candidiasis. The causative agent, a retrovirus named the "human T-lymphotrophic virus type III (HTLV-III)," was identified in 1983. By early 1986 over 17,000 cases had been reported with 9000 deaths, and it has been predicted that there will be at least 50,000 cases with 31,000 deaths by the end of 1987, and 270,000 cases with over 160,000 deaths by 1991. There are few examples of infectious disease with a higher case fa-

tality rate in previously healthy individuals. At present the average survival from the time of diagnosis is about 12 months, and the mortality for the disease appears to be virtually 100 percent. The syndrome appeared initially to be confined to highly specific groups (73 percent are homosexual males and 17 percent are intravenous drug abusers), but persons outside those groups are legitimately alarmed by the increasing evidence of the disease in the general population. Transmission by heterosexual contact and by blood transfusion has been especially disquieting. Adding to the anxiety is uncertainty concerning

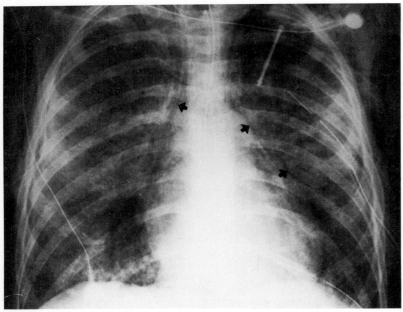

Fig. 17-63. This thirty-one-year-old male homosexual with AIDS developed *Pneumocystis* pneumonia. The typical bilateral hazy, diffuse infiltrates are clearly evident. In spite of having one chest tube on the right side and two on the left side, the patient has large amounts of subcutaneous and mediastinal air (see arrows), as well as a persistent pneumothorax at the left apex. The patient expired with *Pseudomonas* and *Staphylococcus aureus* superinfection and a total of six chest tubes in place.

the frequency of conversion from a positive HTLV-III titer to active disease, although current estimates are cause for concern—it appears that at least 30 percent of positive titers without disease will convert to active disease each year.

Opportunistic infection and Kaposi's sarcoma are the hallmarks of active disease, usually preceded by a febrile prodrome of weeks to months. *Pneumocystis carinii,* the most common pulmonary pathogen, is present in 50 to 60 percent of all patients. Cytomegalovirus (CMV) is being recognized with increasing frequency and may prove to be nearly universal. CMV nearly always coexists with other pathogens and probably has an important role as a potentiator of immune suppression by an unknown mechanism. Other organisms seen include all of the *Mycobacteria,* all fungi, protozoans such as *Toxoplasmosis,* and an assortment of bacteria rarely seen in normal hosts.

Pneumocystis. *Pneumocystis carinii* is a protozoan originally thought to be a trypanosome, and not recognized in human beings until 1938. Characteristic interstitial pneumonitis thought to be caused by *Pneumocystis* was recognized in epidemics among undernourished infants and among the very elderly. In the United States *Pneumocystis* emerged as an infection confined to iatrogenically immunosuppressed patients on chemotherapy, until its dominant role as a pulmonary pathogen in AIDS was recognized in 1981. The characteristic clinical presentation consists of diffuse interstitial infiltrates on chest x-ray, dyspnea, and an increased A-aO2 gradient. Trimethoprim-sulfasoxisole (TMP-SFX) is effective treatment in the majority of cases occurring in transplant recipients, in part because the degree of immunosuppression can be modulated, especially in kidney recipients. Pentamidine is also effective but is ordinarily reserved for resistant cases or patients allergic to TMP-

SFX. Medical treatment of *Pneumocystis* is considerably less successful in AIDS, with mortality reported up to 62 percent.

Treatment. For obvious reasons operation seldom provides definitive therapy for pulmonary infection in the immunocompromised patient. Operation is sometimes a necessary aid to diagnosis and can provide effective treatment for some of the manifestations of infection. It is now clear that transbronchial biopsy combined with alveolar lavage can establish a specific infectious diagnosis in 85 percent of cases. These methods are usually not able to diagnose pulmonary Kaposi's sarcoma. The predictably high frequency of *Pneumocystis* infection also makes it possible to treat most infections with a suggestive presentation empirically with TMP-SFX. Currently open lung biopsy is reserved for confusing mixed infections with inadequate response to empirical treatment, for the rare patient with a true contraindication to transbronchial biopsy and lavage, and for the patient in whom pulmonary Kaposi's syndrome is suspected.

Therapeutic procedures are most often palliative. Especially in patients with AIDS, the most common procedure is chest tube insertion for control of an air leak. Pneumothorax is common during infectious episodes, and the air leaks respond slowly to chest tube drainage. Frequently, several tubes are required (Fig. 17-63), and on occasion a thoracotomy for direct control of the leak and pleural abrasion will be justified (Fig. 17-64). One case of

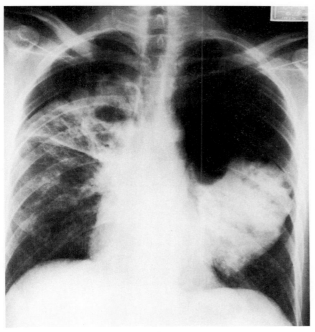

A

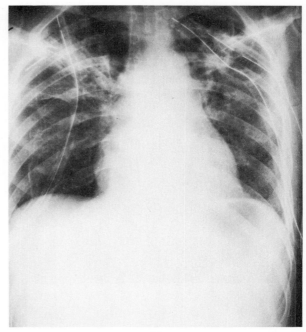

B

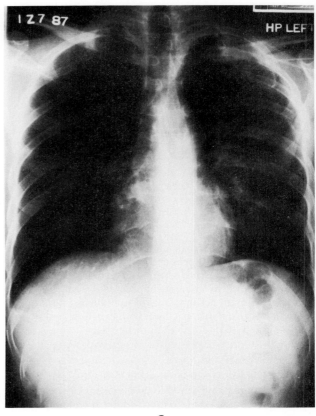

C

Fig. 17-64. *A.* This twenty-four-year-old male homosexual and intravenous drug abuser with AIDS developed *Pneumocystis* pneumonia and bilateral pneumothoraces. *B.* With two chest tubes on
each side, the right side eventually resolved. A large air leak persisted on the left. Because the infection was resolving remarkably
well on medical treatment, operation was elected. Through a left
thoracotomy a large collection of leaking apical blebs were stapled,
and pleural abrasion was performed. *C.* This chest x-ray obtained
after discharge from the hospital shows an unusually successful
early result in the treatment of AIDS.

lobectomy for AIDS-related bronchiectasis and one case
of esophagogastrectomy for adenocarcinoma have been
reported, but such procedures should remain rare until
expected survival improves.

Operation on patients with AIDS is frequently regarded
as hazardous for the medical personnel involved, and in
many institutions elaborate precautions are taken to reduce the risk of infection. Double gloving, gas sterilization of all instruments, and disposable drapes and anesthesia gas tubing are probably prudent precautions. The
risk of infection is thought to be very small, and much
smaller than the risk of acquiring hepatitis B. On the other
hand, the mortality of the disease is so high that fastidious
behavior is easily justified.

Operative therapy in immunocompromised patients
without AIDS can be applied with greater optimism. The
spectrum of infections includes *Pneumocystis* and the
other organisms seen in AIDS but also includes a greater
number of infections with more common pyogenic bacteria and *Aspergillus*. The role of open biopsy is controversial, with opinion dividing between those favoring initial
reliance on empiric therapy and those whose open biopsy
results alter therapy in up to 65 percent of cases. Empyemas and intraparenchymal infections should be ap-

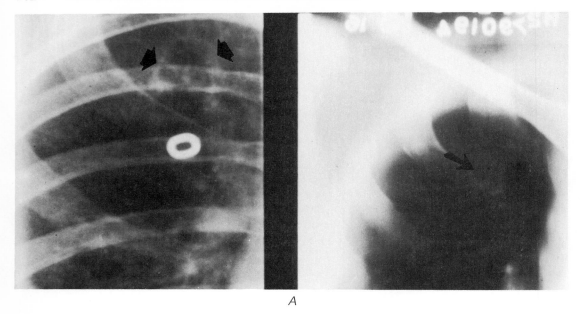

A

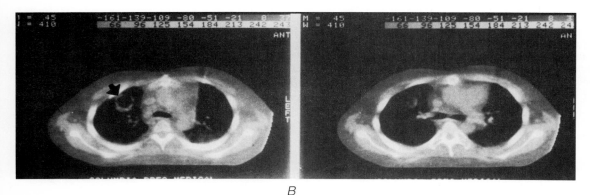

B

Fig. 17-65. *A.* Eight months following cardiac transplant this nineteen-year-old man developed a thin-walled cavity in the right upper lobe, seen (see arrows) in a magnified view of the right apex on the left, and in a tomogram on the right. *B.* CT scan of the lesion (see arrows). The cavity began to grow rapidly, and a right upper lobectomy was performed. The lesion proved to be an aspergilloma. *C.* A thoracoplasty was eventually required for control of a persistent air leak and pneumothorax. A late postoperative chest x-ray is shown. The infection never recurred and the patient was able to resume near-normal activity.

proached aggressively using indications for operation that are the same as those applied to normal hosts with similar infections. Although mortality and morbidity has generally been higher in immunosuppressed patients, it has been possible to perform major pulmonary resection, thoracoplasty, and decortication with excellent long-term results (Fig. 17-65).

BRONCHIECTASIS

Bronchiectasis is characterized by bronchial dilatation, a chronic course, and variable involvement of surrounding parenchyma. Second- to fourth-order segmental bronchi in the basal segments of the lower lobes, the right middle lobe, and the lingula are most frequently involved. Isolated upper-lobe involvement is very rare and is usually associated with tuberculosis or bronchial obstruc-

tion. Approximately one-third of bronchiectasis is unilobar, one-third is unilateral bilobar, and one-third is bilateral. Although the bronchial mucosa usually remains intact and lined with pseudostratified columnar epithelium, the bronchi are filled with mucus, pus, and an occasional broncholith. The changes vary in degree from mild tubular dilation to cystic or saccular changes with almost unrecognizable gross architecture (Fig. 17-66). Collateral

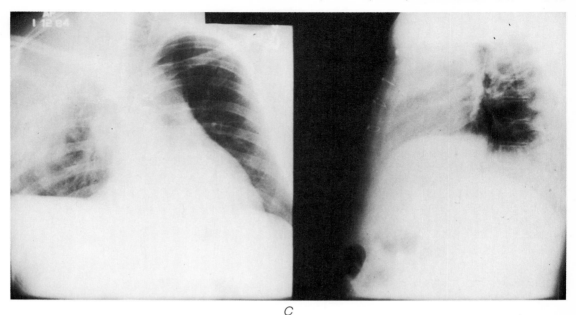

C

Fig. 17-65 *C.* Continued.

air circulation is only partially effective in maintaining expansion of alveoli distal to chronically obstructed segments, and a resected lobe will usually be shrunken and fibrotic. Hypertrophy of bronchial arteries occurs as part of the inflammatory process, producing a locally extensive precapillary left to right shunt into the pulmonary venous system, and laying the substrate for erosive hemorrhage and hemoptysis.

Fig. 17-66. The cut section of this right lower lobe shows one of several cystic bronchiectatic cavities with surrounding localized pneumonia.

In most cases the disease has to be considered idiopathic. It is occasionally associated with chronic bronchial obstruction by tumor, foreign body, or bronchostenosis. Immune deficiency states have been implicated in certain instances. Kartagener's syndrome (situs inversus, pansinusitis, bronchiectasis) is a rare congenital disorder possibly related to a defect in ciliary function. In many patients afflicted during childhood a history of recurrent bronchitis and bronchopneumonia, presumed to be viral, is present. Bronchiectasis frequently develops during the course of cystic fibrosis.

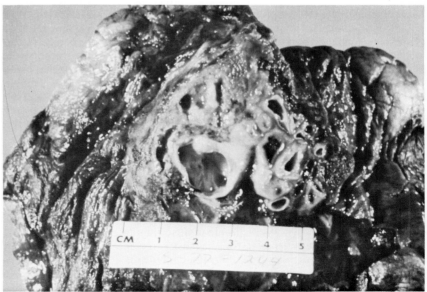

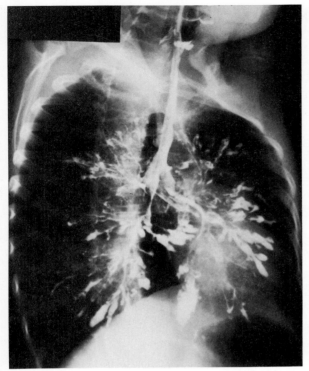

Fig. 17-67. Bronchogram obtained in an eight-year-old Alaskan native, demonstrating widespread saccular and cystic bronchiectasis. This otherwise normal child had a history of repeated respiratory infections, presumed to be viral, during infancy and early childhood. *(Courtesy of JP Wilson.)*

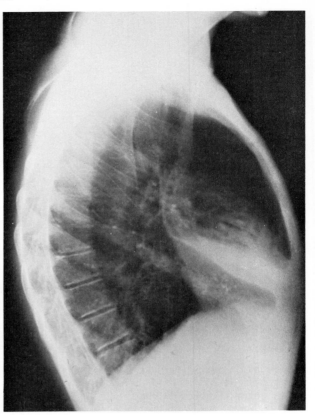

Fig. 17-68. This lateral chest x-ray shows a wedge-shaped density overlying the cardiac shadow and corresponding to a collapsed middle lobe. Resection of the fibrotic lobe showed marked bronchiectasis of the segmental bronchi (middle-lobe syndrome).

CLINICAL MANIFESTATIONS. The clinical picture is dominated by cough and production of mucopurulent sputum, varying in volume from scant to as much as 500 to 1000 mL/day. Fever is usually low-grade with acute exacerbations. The systemic effects of chronic infectious illness can dominate the picture to produce a broad spectrum of constitutional symptoms, weight loss, and retarded development. The disease can occur at any age and is seen equally in both sexes. In the United States an unusually high incidence has been identified in Alaskan Native children, many of whom have required aggressive surgical treatment (Fig. 17-67). Dyspnea is not common except in diffuse disease or in late disease with cor pulmonale. Hemoptysis occurs in about 50 percent of patients, usually late in the disease, and is only major in about 10 percent. Serious hemoptysis is more frequent in association with lung abscess than with bronchiectasis.

Physical findings are dominated by stigmata of chronic disease, and can include digital clubbing and pulmonary osteoarthropathy, even though cyanosis is rare. Auscultatory findings are primarily related to presence or absence of associated pneumonitis and to the effectiveness of pulmonary toilet. A history of chronic profuse sputum production will strongly suggest the diagnosis, and in children associations such as cystic fibrosis, immune deficiency, and alpha$_1$ antitrypsin deficiency should be

ruled out. Chest x-rays tend to be nonspecific but may show linear streaking and volume loss in the affected areas. Bronchiectasis is one possible explanation for the "middle-lobe syndrome," which is isolated middle-lobe atelectasis (Fig. 17-68). Bronchoscopy should be done to exclude the rare case of correctable bronchial obstruction or carcinoma, to obtain accurate cultures, and to aspirate the tracheobronchial tree. Careful bronchoscopic pulmonary toilet can achieve surprisingly durable symptomatic benefit. Complete bronchography remains the definitive test, and is essential to define the anatomy if resection is contemplated (Fig. 17-67). Even bilateral bronchography is usually well tolerated but can produce a febrile response due to chemical and bacterial pneumonitis. It should not be done within about 3 months of an acute episode of pneumonia to reduce this risk, and to avoid overinterpretation of changes that may be reversible.

TREATMENT. The majority of patients with bronchiectasis do not require operative treatment. Postural drainage and chest physical therapy (Fig. 17-69) minimize retention of purulent sputum, and antibiotic treatment of all episodes of pneumonitis should be pursued indefinitely. When debilitating effects of chronic infection become prominent, the anatomy should be carefully defined with

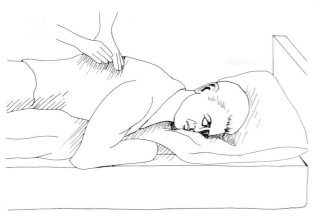

Fig. 17-69. Postural drainage combined with chest physical therapy is important in the medical management of bronchiectasis and in the preoperative care of patients who require pulmonary resection.

bronchography, and resection planned. When extensive saccular disease is confined to one lobe or segment in a sufficiently symptomatic patient, resection is a clear choice. In children, interference with growth should suggest resection. Frequent hemoptysis associated with localized disease deserves operation. Patients with diffuse bilateral disease, of which cystic fibrosis is usually a good example, should be approached cautiously by the surgeon.

All patients should receive a maximal preoperative effort to reduce sputum volume and infection. Care must be taken during anesthesia to prevent spillage of infected secretions into uninvolved segments. A double-lumen endotracheal tube can be used to protect the contralateral lung, and intraoperative flexible fiberoptic bronchoscopy can be used to aspirate uninvolved segments in the ipsilateral lung. As with operation for lung abscess, the risk of postoperative empyema is higher than for clean surgery, and considerable effort must be expended in postoperative pulmonary toilet to assure that residual infected secretions are not allowed to pool in the bronchial stump. The operative strategy is to remove as little normal lung as possible without entering the central focus of infection. This usually requires segmentectomy or lobectomy. Disease so localized as to be treatable with wedge resection probably should not come to operation. Pneumonectomy is almost never indicated for bronchiectasis.

As with many clinical situations in which choice of therapy is based largely on quality of life decisions, there are no prospective controlled series to compare relative benefits of medical versus surgical treatment. In one recent series of 40 patients, the 24 patients resected had an 80 percent chance of becoming nearly or totally asymptomatic. Viewing the group as a whole, the authors estimated that 70 percent of patients with symptomatic bronchiectasis will develop persistent or progressive symptoms on medical therapy. Similar conclusions have been reached in a number of series reported by surgeons, and it is probably fair to say that operation offers the greatest chance for achieving normal or near normal life, if the analysis is confined to the kinds of patients who tend to come to the attention of surgeons with an interest in bronchiectasis.

TUBERCULOSIS

Sanskrit written in 6000 B.C. refers to tuberculosis as the "King of Diseases." Tuberculosis, then called "phthisis," was well known to Hippocrates. A generation beginning to face an uncertain battle with the AIDS complex would do well to recall that pulmonary tuberculosis was epidemic in Europe during the eighteenth and nineteenth centuries and took an extraordinary toll on young adults in the prime of life. In the United States in the 1940s pulmonary resection for tuberculosis carried a mortality rate of about 25 percent, and effective chemotherapy did not exist until streptomycin was discovered in 1944. Tuberculosis remained epidemic in part of the United States (Alaska) as recently as the early 1960s. Yet in a little over 20 years the treatment of tuberculosis has largely been reduced to a straightforward recipe of medical therapy. In spite of such astounding progress, however, about 30,000 new cases are diagnosed each year, and a fraction of these will continue to present operative challenges that are characteristic of the disease.

PATHOPHYSIOLOGY AND CLINICAL MANIFESTATIONS. In broad outline a pulmonary infection with *Mycobacterium tuberculosis* behaves like a lung abscess, with notable differences based primarily on the peculiar growth characteristics of the organism and the nature of the host response. The disease usually becomes clinically apparent when a previously acquired and quiescent infection is reactivated, usually in the apical or posterior segments of an upper lobe or in the superior segment of a lower lobe. In an immunocompetent host the characteristic cycle of caseous necrosis and scar formation will eventually produce what amounts to a tuberculous lung abscess. Just as with pyogenic lung abscess, the smouldering central focus of infection tends to find communication with the tracheobronchial tree, providing a route for drainage and expectoration of purulent sputum loaded with tubercle bacilli, and allowing ingress of air to produce cavitation. The ultimate extent of infection is determined by the size of the inoculum, the immune competence of the host, and the success of antituberculous drugs. Rapid progression can produce a tuberculous empyema surrounding a destroyed lung. If growth of the bacillus is controlled, the cavity may collapse and obliterate or may remain open indefinitely. Such cavities ("open negative") are no longer sites of tuberculous infection but remain potential sites for secondary infection, the classic example of which is an *Aspergillus* "fungus ball" (mycetoma).

As with lung abscess and bronchiectasis, the intense inflammatory process in the periphery of a cavity tends to promote hypertrophy of bronchial arterial and pulmonary arterial branches. These may be eroded by the necrotizing process in the center of the cavity to produce hemoptysis, which can be life-threatening. The vessel responsi-

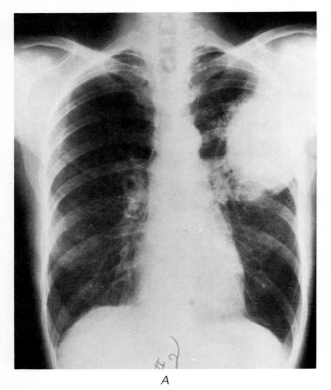

A

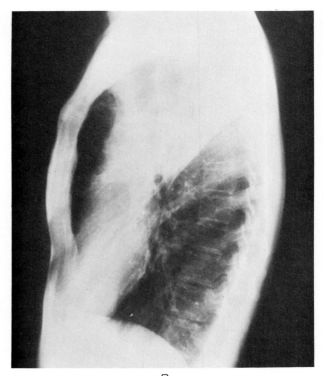

B

Fig. 17-70. Pulmonary tuberculosis, active. *A* and *B*. A large mass in the left upper lobe that was associated with marked atypia of cells obtained by bronchoscopy, and negative sputum smears for acid-fast bacilli. The resected lobe showed active tuberculosis without cavitation.

ble is most frequently a dilated pulmonary arterial branch, referred to as a Rasmussen aneurysm. The management of massive tracheobronchial hemorrhage has been discussed in connection with lung abscess. Because a tuberculous cavity is likely to be more chronic, when major hemoptysis occurs the vessel involved is likely to be larger than that seen in a pyogenic lung abscess, and emergency pulmonary resection is often necessary.

On occasion the most intense inflammatory process is confined to regional lymph nodes, which can enlarge enough to produce bronchial stenosis and distal atelectasis—one cause of the middle-lobe syndrome. If this occurs distal to an evolving cavity, rapid expansion can occur due to air trapping, to produce a "tension cavity." The responsible nodes are choked with caseating granulomata. Discrete bronchial stenosis can also be seen without evidence of extrinsic compression, in which case it is usually ascribed to an intense tuberculous bronchitis occurring in a segment draining an active parenchymal infection.

In a typical case of pulmonary tuberculosis the diagnosis is easily made on the basis of characteristic cavitary changes in an upper lobe on chest x-ray, occurring in a patient with a positive PPD whose sputum has grown *Mycobacterium tuberculosis*. A suggestive x-ray without positive cultures does not confirm the diagnosis, and a negative PPD does not rule out active tuberculosis. Definitive diagnosis rests on growth of the organism in culture (Fig. 17-70). A positive acid-fast stain provides a highly suggestive provisional diagnosis but cannot discriminate completely between *Nocardia* and *M. tuberculosis*.

Culture also allows identification of "atypical" *Mycobacteria*, which deserve special mention. Clinically and pathologically, infection with an atypical *Mycobacterium* can be indistinguishable from infection with *M. tuberculosis*. Resistance to multiple antituberculous drugs is common among the atypical *Mycobacteria*, and chances for a nonoperative cure depend on accurate assessment of appropriate medical therapy. Culture becomes important for identification of a specific species, and for characterization of its drug sensitivities. Even with successful medical treatment the use of three or four drugs for 2 to 4 years can be anticipated. Because of drug resistance, a higher proportion of atypical than of typical mycobacterial pulmonary infections will require operation. *Mycobacterium kansasii* and *M. intracellulare-avium* are the species most often associated with pulmonary disease (Table 17-14).

TREATMENT. Operative treatment of tuberculosis is ordinarily an elective procedure performed after a period of treatment with antituberculous drugs. Emergency operation is only required for life-threatening hemorrhage or massive air leak with tension pneumothorax. The procedure of choice is almost always lobectomy or segmentomy. The technical precautions necessary to minimize

Table 17-14. CLASSIFICATION OF ATYPICAL MYCOBACTERIA

Group	Example	Principal lesion
I. Photochromogens	*Mycobacterium kansasii*	Pulmonary disease
II. Scotochromogens	*Mycobacterium scrofulaceum*	Cervical lymphadenitis
III. Nonchromogenic	*Mycobacterium intracellulare* (Battey bacillus)	Pulmonary disease
IV. Rapid growers	*Mycobacterium marinum*	Swimming pool skin granuloma

the risk of tracheobronchial or pleural spread of infection are the same as those discussed with regard to resection for lung abscess. Noncontroversial indications for resection include (1) extensive pulmonary destruction with bronchopleural fistula and empyema, (2) persistently active disease with drug-resistant organisms, (3) inability to rule out coexisting bronchogenic carcinoma, (4) pulmonary hemorrhage, and (5) posttuberculous bronchostenosis with recurrent nontuberculous infection. There has always been some controversy regarding resection of an "open negative" cavity. In these patients with negative sputum, the goal of treatment is to ensure that the cavity itself is made truly negative. There is considerable evidence that well-managed long-term medical therapy can produce results at least as good as those following resection. Partial adherence to a drug regimen can encourage emergence of resistant strains, so that noncompliant patients are poor candidates for medical treatment of large residual cavities and should have a resection. This discussion applies equally to typical and atypical Mycobacterial infections.

An occasional patient will have persistent active infection but such limited ventilatory reserve that resection would not be tolerated. Under these circumstances thoracoplasty remains a valid alternative. Thoracoplasty is designed to collapse the affected lung, which can be remarkably effective. Collapse is achieved without entering the pleural space by performing an extrapleural resection of the first five ribs, followed in 10 to 14 days by resection of the sixth and seventh ribs. Although this procedure has its origins in the treatment of tuberculosis, the principle of chest wall collapse is occasionally used to obliterate pleural space following pulmonary resection as well.

FUNGAL INFECTIONS

By about 1900 all the major fungal pathogens had been isolated and named, but recognition of their role in disease underwent a very characteristic evolution. They were initially thought to be rare and fatal infections, but as diagnostic acumen increased, it became clear that mild asymptomatic infection was far more common. Now the pendulum is beginning to swing back somewhat, as fungal infections find their way into our enlarging reservoir of iatrogenically immunocompromised patients. Features common to all fungal infections include protean manifestations in compromised hosts, sensitivity to amphotericin B, and mimicry of carcinoma and tuberculosis. Amphotericin B is a very important drug that has rendered most

fungal infections medically treatable, but it is also a highly toxic drug that cannot be administered as casually as antituberculous drugs are given.

ACTINOMYCOSIS. For many years the actinomycetes were misclassified as fungi because they form branching hyphae and spores. Only in the past 20 years has it been recognized that the actinomycetes are bacteria. This taxonomic distinction has therapeutic relevance, because the pathogens in this group are sensitive to penicillin and sulfonamides but not to amphotericin B.

Actinomycosis is caused by *Actinomyces israelii,* an anaerobic filamentous bacillus that is not found in nature but is a normal commensal inhabitant of the oral cavity and tonsillar crypts. It is not known what causes this organism to become an invasive pathogen, but in about three-fourths of cases some kind of predisposing factor can be identified, such as immunosuppression or breakdown of local tissue barriers (i.e., tooth extraction). About 60 percent of cases are cervicofacial, and only 15 percent are thoracic. Thoracic infection is presumed to result from aspiration of infected secretions. Classically the disease is characterized by suppuration, abscess and sinus tract formation, and relentless invasion with complete disregard for tissue planes. Multiple sinus tracts are observed today in only one-third of cases, and the lesion is more commonly seen as a parenchymal process mimicking bronchogenic carcinoma. Nonetheless, when involvement of ribs or extension into mediastinal structures is seen, actinomycosis must be high on the list of possible causes (Fig. 17-71).

Expectorated sputum, material from a sinus tract, and biopsy material can demonstrate sulfur granules, which are yellow-brown clusters of microcolonies. This finding is highly suggestive, but since *Nocardia,* certain fungi, and *Staphylococcus aureus* are also capable of producing clumps of material resembling sulfur granules, diagnostic confirmation rests on identification of the bacillus within the granules, for which special stains are required. Cultures are positive in only about one-fourth of cases.

The organism is sensitive to penicillin, although large doses are required to penetrate the dense colonies, and medical treatment is most often quite successful. Therefore, the surgical strategy is to make an accurate diagnosis at an early stage of disease. Because the disease can have gross resemblance to fungal infections and to carcinoma, and because tissue stains are essential to the diagnosis, operation is frequently required to obtain adequate biopsy material. Successful diagnosis is followed by high-dose intravenous penicillin and a long subsequent course of oral administration. Resection should rarely be neces-

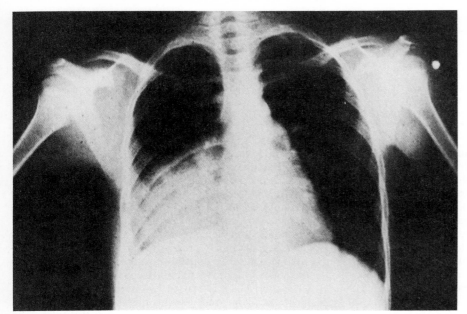

A

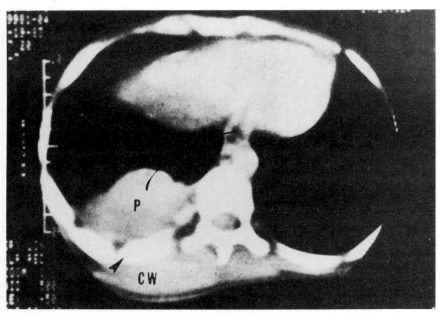

B

Fig. 17-71. A fourteen-year-old boy presented to his local hospital complaining of a ''lump'' on his back that had been growing for about 1 month. He recalled an episode of right lung pneumonia 10 months previously. *A.* Chest x-ray on admission showed a density in the right lower lung field and mild levoscoliosis. *B.* A CT scan of the lower thoracic region revealed a mass involving the pleura (P) and the chest wall (CW) with thickening of the eighth rib (arrow). CT sections of the first lumbar vertebra showed lucent bony lesions (not shown). *C.* Biopsy of the mass revealed the characteristic clumped colonies of *Actinomyces*. The patient was treated with 6 weeks of intravenous and 12 months of oral penicillin. The chest x-ray was normal in 3 months. (From: *Golden N, Cohen H, et al: Clin Pediatr 24:646, 1985, Figs 2, 3, 5, with permission.*)

sary except in unusually advanced presentations with an inadequate response to penicillin.

Nocardiosis. Nocardiosis is caused by *Nocardia asteroides,* an aerobic acid-fast filamentous bacillus widely distributed in nature as a saprophyte in soil and domestic animals. It is a rare pathogen except in an immunocompromised host and is most often thoracic, beginning as a pneumonic process difficult to distinguish grossly from tuberculosis, fungal infections, and carcinoma. It can also closely mimic actinomycosis, with chest wall involve-

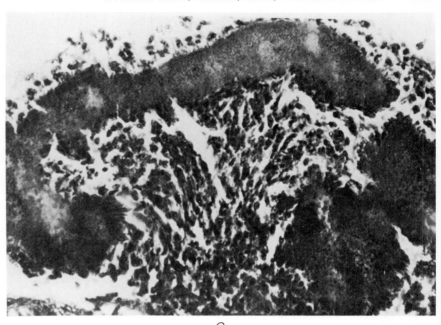

Fig. 17-71 *C*. Continued.   *C*

ment, sinus tract formation, and production of sulfur granules. The acute infection is often much more aggressive than actinomycosis, with extensive pulmonic necrosis and abscess formation, and metastatic dissemination to the central nervous system and elsewhere.

Nocardia is relatively easy to culture and to identify with standard stains, so that the diagnosis can frequently be made by brush or needle biopsy, and even from expectorated sputum. The organism is sensitive to sulfonamides, which usually provide successful therapy. Other drugs can be added in poorly responsive cases (trimethoprim-sulfamethoxasole, minocycline) with good results, and surgery remains purely adjunctive in the majority of cases. Pulmonary resection, drainage of empyema, and similar procedures can be performed safely when necessary.

Histoplasmosis. Histoplasmosis is the most common systemic fungal infection in the United States. *Histoplasma capsulatum* is a dimorphic fungus common in the great river valleys of the midwest, where it lives in mycelial form in soil, decaying organic material, and guano. It assumes yeast form in the cytoplasm of pulmonary alveoli after inhalation. It is extremely common in endemic areas as an asymptomatic infection; the severity of disease is determined by the size of the inoculum and the immune competence of the host. Release of a large inoculum can produce outbreaks of acute pneumonic illness in normal hosts, and usually occurs following an environmental disruption such as excavation or demolition. Such infections ordinarily resolve without specific treatment, but not before widespread lymphatic and hematogenous dissemination has occurred, apparent later as scattered calcific nodules in lungs, mediastinum, spleen, and liver. In symptomatic patients the disease can take many forms and is often distinguishable from tuberculosis only by culture. Skin testing reagents are available but are not as reliable as PPD. Serologic diagnosis is also available but is no more reliable and can be misleading if obtained following skin testing. As with tuberculosis, definitive diagnosis requires growth of the organism from pathologic specimens.

Amphotericin B is effective treatment in the majority of cases and is always the treatment of choice in a serious illness once the diagnosis is made. Most infections are asymptomatic or moderately symptomatic and self-limited, and chemotherapy is not recommended for skin test conversion as it is in tuberculosis. Operation is applied much as it is in tuberculosis. Cavitary disease is quite common, and in a recent large series from an endemic area (Tennessee) this was the most frequent indication for resection. Large, thick-walled cavities that have failed to improve after a course of amphotericin B are likely to progress and can be resected with low morbidity and mortality. Another frequent indication for operative intervention is inability to establish a definitive diagnosis, especially when the lesion presents as a solitary pulmonary nodule grossly consistent with carcinoma (Fig. 17-72). As in tuberculosis, hemoptysis can require operation, and bronchostenosis produced by extrinsic nodal compression can require resection. The lymphogenous phase of *Histoplasma* dissemination leads to remarkable nodal enlargement in some patients, producing symptoms related to compression of mediastinal structures, and a radiographic appearance resembling mediastinal malignancies. Mediastinal involvement can also produce a sclerosing mediastinitis with obstruction of the superior vena cava, pulmonary arteries or veins, esophagus, or tracheobronchial tree. The pathophysiology of

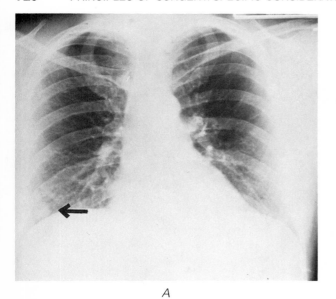

A

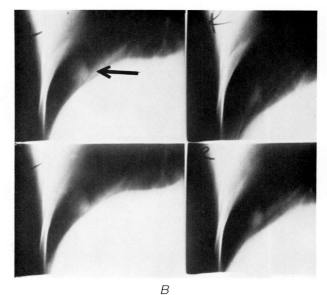

B

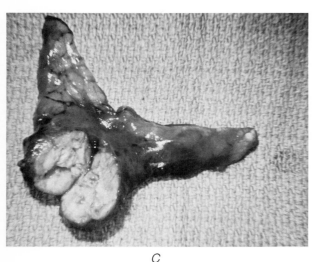

C

Fig. 17-72. Histoplasmosis. *A.* The chest x-ray shows a faint round lesion in the right lower lung field (arrow). *B.* Conventional tomography demonstrates the lesion clearly and shows that it has sharp borders. *C.* The lesion was removed by wedge resection; the cut surface shows a histoplasmoma.

this desmoplastic response to infection is not completely understood but appears to be an idiosyncratic reaction.

Coccidiomycosis. Coccidiomycosis is the second most common fungal infection encountered in the United States. *Coccidioides immitis* is a dimorphic fungus found in mycelial form as a saprophyte in the arid soil of the American Southwest. Arthrospores released by the hyphae are inhaled and initiate the parasitic phase by becoming spherules that release infective endospores. In the normal host most infections are asymptomatic, but some will manifest "valley fever," essentially a mild pneumonic form of the illness. The organism is not difficult to recover from sputum or pathologic specimens. The skin test and serologic titers are almost always positive in active disease but are more ambiguous in the more chronic and indolent forms of infection. Except for a propensity to form thin-walled cavities, the spectrum of

gross and microscopic pathology is similar to that seen in histoplasmosis, tuberculosis, and other fungal infections.

For patients with symptomatic illness requiring treatment, amphotericin B is the primary therapy. As with histoplasmosis, the lungs provide an effective barrier against serious systemic illness in most patients, and specific treatment is frequently not required. Aggressive necrotizing pulmonary infection and disseminated disease are usually seen in immunocompromised hosts, and require early and aggressive medical treatment.

Indications for operation are virtually identical to those applied to histoplasmosis. Resection of cavitary disease and resection for definitive diagnosis of a solitary pulmonary nodule are most frequently performed. Specific indications in cavitary disease include progressive enlargement, hemoptysis, rupture, and secondary infection.

Blastomycosis. Blastomycosis is caused by *Blastomy-*

ces dermatitidis, a round, single budding yeast endemic in the southeastern United States and other scattered areas. Although there is a common cutaneous form, the disease is always acquired through aspiration of spores into the lungs, where it can assume a variety of appearances— pneumonic infiltrates, cavitation, solitary granulomatous nodules, and disseminated disease. The cutaneous form is characterized by crusty, ulcerative lesions from the margins of which the organism can readily be cultured. Cutaneous and pulmonary infection can occur together, and the cutaneous form has a better prognosis. Diagnosis rests on identification of the organism, which can be done with a sputum Papanicolaou stain.

Although it can mimic tuberculosis and other fungal infections, in endemic areas it most frequently mimics bronchogenic carcinoma, and resection will frequently be required if a definitive diagnosis cannot be established (Fig. 17-73). Aggressive infection is treated with amphotericin B. Cutaneous infection and mild pulmonary infection also respond well to 2-hydroxystilbamadine. As with other fungal infections, treatment with amphotericin B can often be avoided in mild presentations of illness, especially in normal hosts during outbreaks in endemic areas.

Aspergillosis. *Aspergillus* is a filamentous fungus with septate hyphae that is ubiquitous in nature. Inhalation of spores from *A. fumigatus, A. niger,* and other species initiates infection in susceptible individuals. Aspergillosis presents in three forms: allergic bronchopulmonary, saprophytic, and invasive. The first is characterized by asthmatic symptoms resulting from host response to fungus in the airways and is of no surgical importance. The invasive form is usually seen in the immunocompromised host, can involve any organ system, and is almost always fatal. Surgical attention focuses on the saprophytic form, produced by colonization of a preexisting pulmonary cavity (an aspergilloma, mycetoma, or "fungus ball"). On chest x-ray the aspergilloma appears as a solid, rounded mass within a cavity, surrounded by a crescent of air between the fungus and the cavity wall (Fig. 17-74). *Aspergillus precipitins* are almost always detectable in patients with aspergilloma. Skin testing is available but is positive in only 30 to 75 percent of cases. The value of sputum cultures has been debated, but recent evidence suggests that two or more positive cultures carry excellent specificity and sensitivity.

For disseminated disease amphotericin B is the mainstay of therapy. Penetration of the drug into a cavity containing an aspergilloma is very poor, so that resection is considered the treatment of choice for a significant aspergilloma. Operative treatment most frequently requires lobectomy, segmentectomy, or pneumonectomy. Cavernostomy (open drainage through the chest wall) is occasionally performed in patients with poor ventilatory reserve and can be augmented by intracavitary instillation of antifungal agents. Operation is most often justified as prevention for hemoptysis, which occurs in 50 to 83 percent of cases and can be life-threatening in a fraction of that total. Even so, operation remains somewhat controversial because it is associated with considerable mortal-

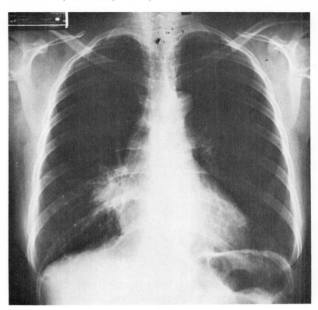

A

B

Fig. 17-73. North American blastomycosis. *A.* Chest x-ray shows a mass in the right lung field adjacent to the heart border. *B.* Conventional tomography defines the mass more clearly, but neoplasm cannot be excluded. A pulmonary resection revealed active blastomycosis in the right middle lobe.

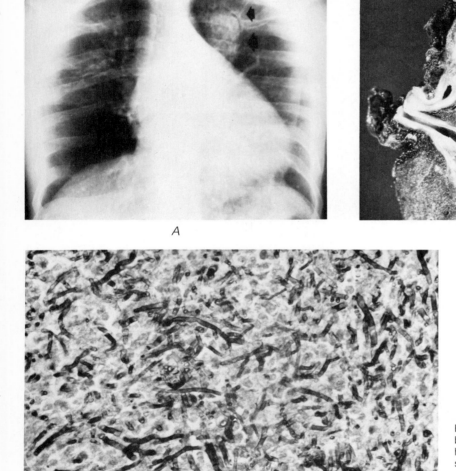

A

B

C

Fig. 17-74. A *Aspergillus fumigatus* "fungus ball." *A.* In a patient presenting with recurrent hemoptysis, a lordotic chest x-ray shows a solid mass within a cavity surrounded by a rim of air between the mass and the cavity wall *(arrows),* a finding highly suggestive of an aspergilloma. *B.* After resection of the left upper lobe, cut section reveals the fungus ball filling an old fibrotic cavity. *C.* The histopathology with special stains for fungus demonstrates mycelia infiltrating the tissue in the wall of the cavity.

ity and morbidity. This is related to the poor health of most susceptible hosts and the technical difficulty of resection through dense inflammatory tissue. In a recent series from the Mayo Clinic, for example, either underlying lung disease or immunologic risk factors were present in 92 percent of patients, and complications occurred in 78 percent of patients with complex aspergillomas. In this series and others, operative mortality has been 5 to 10 percent, and complications in "simple" aspergilloma resection have ranged from 25 to 34 percent. Nonetheless, in the Mayo Clinic series the late results were excellent in about 75 percent of cases. In conclusion it is probably prudent to observe small asymptomatic aspergillomas, but in most cases resection should be performed, accepting increased risk in favor of potential benefits (Fig. 17-65).

Cryptococcosis. Cryptococcosis is caused by *Cryptococcus neoformans,* a round, budding yeast found in soil and pigeon droppings. Infection occurs through inhalation of the organism and in most individuals produces a comparatively benign bronchopulmonary illness. The chief radiologic finding is a granulomatous complex with hilar node involvement, indistinguishable from the Ghon complex of tuberculosis. It is rarely of surgical significance except in the compromised host, when the entire spectrum of fungal pulmonary pathology seen in more inherently virulent infections can be seen on occasion (Fig. 17-75). The best-known disseminated manifestation is meningitis. Infection can be controlled in many cases with amphotericin B and 5-fluorocytosine, even with meningeal involvement.

Innumerable other fungi can be associated with pulmonary disease in human beings, but as the list diverges further and further from the recognized pathogens, it becomes increasingly confined to immunocompromised hosts. *Candida,* mucormycosis, sporotrichosis, monospirosis, *Torulopsis,* even *Penicillium*—all have been described. Surgical treatment is rarely indicated and seldom definitive.

Tumors

PRIMARY CARCINOMA

Tobacco addiction (cigarette smoking) is the predominant factor in the etiology of lung cancer. It must puzzle any logical person to observe the paradoxes in the way our society deals with its addiction problems. On the one hand are several substances that, though distressing in individual cases, pose a modest public health problem but are aggressively discouraged with heavy criminal sanctions against production, distribution, or use. On the other hand, we have long subsidized by tax dollars the production and distribution of an addicting drug that is by far this nation's most serious public health problem. How do we rationalize our bizarre tolerance of the "pushers" of this most costly and destructive of all addictive drugs? They spend $1.5 billion dollars each year (more than is spent to advertise any other product) to entice our children to become addicted in their teens to the drug that

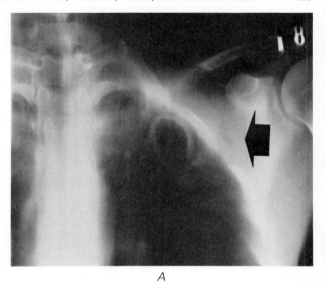

A

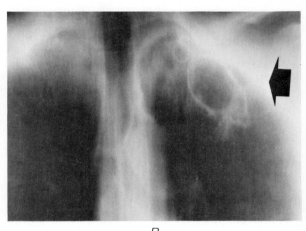

B

Fig. 17-75. *A.* Conventional tomography in a fifty-one-year-old man with hemoptysis showed cavitation within a pulmonary infiltrate in the left upper lobe. Bronchial washings returned a culture diagnosis of cryptococcosis. *B.* Despite two courses of amphotericin B and one course of ketoconazole, tomograms repeated 2 years later demonstrated progressive cavitation. A left upper lobectomy was performed for recurrent hemoptysis and failure of drug therapy.

now is responsible for killing more Americans annually than have been killed in all the wars of this century. Each year in the United States there are 350,000 excess and preventable deaths, and $65 billion in costs attributable to the use of tobacco. For smoker and nonsmoker alike, that represents $200 per person in extra taxes and health insurance premiums, $2.17 for each pack of cigarettes sold. The data from the Framingham study reveal that tobacco addicts are 9 to 10 times more likely to die before age seventy than are nonsmokers. There is no longer any reasonable doubt that those who live or work with tobacco addicts are forced to share a substantial health risk. Physicians must speak clearly on the importance of educating patients and public regarding the consequences of to-

CANCER DEATHS BY SITE AND SEX

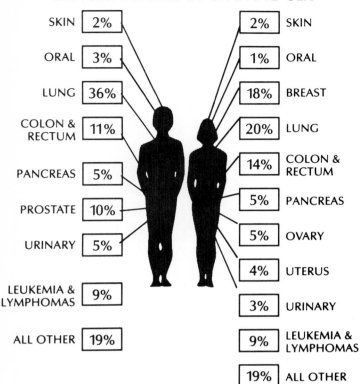

Fig. 17-76. Lung cancer has long been the leading cancer killer among men; by 1986 it had become the leading killer of women as well. (From: *American Cancer Society, with permission.*)

bacco addiction and on the importance of establishing a smoke-free environment in public and work places for the nonsmoking 70 percent of the population who must not be subjected to this unnecessary health hazard. Reports from Japan and Greece, along with Garfinkel and Auerbach's case control study of 134 cases of lung cancer in nonsmoking women, establish the association between those cancers and the smoking habits of spouses. Even with the best available air-moving and ventilating equipment, Environmental Protection Agency engineers demonstrated that it was not possible to reduce carcinogenic air contamination to an acceptable level for a nonsmoker sharing work space with a tobacco addict. Physical isolation of the addict while engaging in the habit is essential.

In a challenging recent editorial, William Pollin of the National Institute on Drug Abuse in reviewing U.S. statistics reminded us that tobacco addiction causes more excess deaths each year than all other drug and alcohol abuse deaths combined, seven times more than all automobile fatalities per year, more than a hundred times all deaths recorded through the end of 1986 caused by the acquired immunodeficiency syndrome, and more than all American military fatalities in this century put together.

From a trivial health problem at the beginning of this century, and a minor one by 1930 (a death rate of 5 per 100,000), lung cancer has now become the main cancer killer in both men and women (Figs. 17-76 and 17-77). With a death rate of 72 per 100,000 and over 130,000

deaths anticipated in 1986, nearly twice as many will die from lung cancer as will die from all accidents (63,000). A high proportion of those cancers will be in smokers or spouses and coworkers of smokers. Auerbach and his colleagues amplified the long-recognized statistical correlation of smoking and lung cancer by making a detailed analysis of histological changes in the bronchial mucosa of 117 autopsied males. They were able to accurately identify the premorbid smoking habits of the subjects by observing progressive mucosal changes from hyperplasia of the basal cells through stratification, squamous metaplasia, and finally carcinoma in situ. Several groups have closed the loop by producing invasive and metastatic bronchogenic cancers in animal models subjected to forced exposure to tobacco smoke over extended periods. The long exposure required for the development of malignancy provides important and reassuring information for the addict; those who stop smoking will sharply reduce their risk.

Along with tobacco, several other co-carcinogens have been incriminated. There is a potentiation of the cancer risk in tobacco addicts who work in environments contaminated by chromium, nickel, asbestos, mustard gas, arsenic, radioactive minerals, and polycyclic hydrocarbons. Some of the small proportion of lung cancers seen in reported nonsmokers occur in those subjected to these

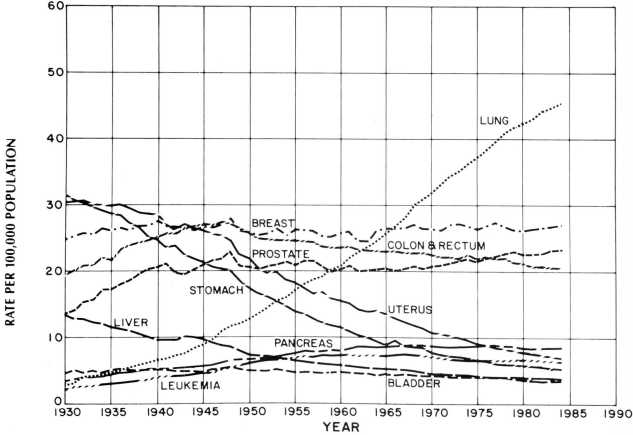

Fig. 17-77. Cancer death rates by site, United States, 1934–1984. Alarming rise in rate of death from lung cancer continues as all other causes of cancer deaths have stabilized or are falling. Rate for the population standardized for age on the 1970 U.S. population. Sources of data: National Center for Health Statistics and Bureau of the Census, United States. Rates for both sexes combined except breast and uterus female population only and prostate male population only. (From: *American Cancer Society, with permission*.)

workplace hazards, but most occur in wives or coworkers of heavily smoking addicts.

PATHOLOGICAL CLASSIFICATION. Several classification systems have been proposed for simplifying analysis and discussion of the various tumors that occur in the lung. Because of distinct differences in approach and management, the most rudimentary division is generally between non-small-cell lung cancer (NSCLC) and small-cell lung cancer (SCLC). Because they have a potential for cure by resection, the NSCLC group have more therapeutic interest to the surgeon. That group of tumors includes squamous cell (or epidermoid) carcinoma, adenocarcinoma, mixed adenosquamous, bronchoalveolar, and large-cell carcinoma.

The traditional histological classification of lung cancers has been based on morphological characteristics visualized by light microscopy. Benfield and Yellin have recently introduced a clinically useful, unifying nomenclature based on more sophisticated modern pathological

techniques, the electron microscope (EM), and immunohistochemistry (Fig. 17-78). These methods prove an interesting overlap among squamous cell carcinomas, adenocarcinomas, and small-cell undifferentiated carcinomas. These observations also clarify the recent reports that show a rising frequency of mixed adenosquamous carcinomas, previously representing under 4 percent of tumors but up to 46 percent in some current reviews. Accurate classification by a pathologist experienced in lung cancer and utilizing modern diagnostic tools is highly desirable.

Most primary bronchogenic carcinomas arise from basal or mucous cells in the surface epithelium of the bronchial tree. Tumors may also arise from the neurosecretory cells or the Clara cells of the distal bronchioles. Atypical epithelial proliferation may precede pulmonary neoplasms. The identification of these changes may provide the early diagnostic clues. Carcinoma in situ is probably a step in the chain of development from squamous metaplasia and dysplasia to invasive carcinoma. An atypical proliferation of Kultchitsky cells is associated with development of the carcinoid tumors.

Non-Small-Cell Lung Cancers (NSCLC). There is frequently a high degree of overlap in the histopathology of most of the various primary lung cancers. Particularly as they become less differentiated, many mixed elements

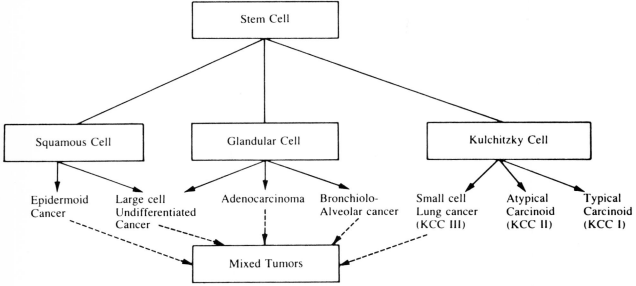

Fig. 17-78. Benfield and Yellin have presented a simplifying scheme for relating the patterns of histopathology seen in lung cancers. There is an increasing frequency of tumors with mixed elements in most current series. (From: *Benfield JR, Yellin A, with permission.*)

may appear that are suggestive of any of the NSCLCs. Except in the most typical situation, the classifications should not be overinterpreted. The therapeutic decisions are largely made on the basis of nodal metastases and other aspects of the clinical behavior of the tumor rather than the specific label assigned.

Squamous Cell Carcinomas. Though more common in upper lobes, bronchogenic carcinomas develop in all parts of the lung. In view of the long exposure to carcinogens in smoke that is required and the progressive mucosal abnormalities that occur, it is likely these cancers are very slow-growing and are present for several years before symptoms occur. It has been estimated that a tumor nodule must go through approximately 30 doublings to become 1 cm in diameter, a size that is large enough to be seen on the routine chest x-ray. This could mean pulmonary tumors may have been present for as long as 8 years before discovery. This slow growth is often a characteristic of squamous cell carcinoma, a tumor that seems to arise after a preliminary squamous metaplasia has replaced the normal respiratory pseudostratified epithelium. The degree of differentiation in squamous neoplasms varies widely. It is occasionally so highly anaplastic that its designation as a squamous tumor is speculative. Until recently, squamous cell carcinoma was the most prevalent type of lung cancer in the United States. Most recent reports documented a progressive increase in the incidence of adenocarcinoma. In many reports, it has now replaced squamous carcinoma as the leading pulmonary neoplasm. The reasons for this apparent change in pattern are unclear, though they may include modification of criteria for determining the histopathology of lung cancer.

Frequently slow-growing and late to metastasize, these tumors may present as central bulky masses obstructing bronchi or as expanding peripheral lesions with cavita-

tion. The centrally located tumors may invade the peribronchial and hilar lymph nodes by direct extension rather than by lymphatic permeation. Evidence of metastases may be absent even with tumors of very large size. When peripheral, the slow growth rate and late metastasis characteristic of these tumors may lead to extensive local chest wall invasion before metastases occur. The surgeons at several large cancer hospitals have recently reported 43 to 54 percent 5-year survival in $T_3N_0M_0$ lesions requiring extensive chest wall resection in continuity with the primary. The Pancoast syndrome represents a specific example of this circumstance wherein a tumor in the superior pulmonary sulcus may invade the brachial plexus, the upper two ribs or transverse processes, and the vascular structures at the thoracic apex.

Adenocarcinoma. These tumors generally arise in the subsegmental bronchi away from the pulmonary hilus. Growth is apt to be more rapid than in squamous tumors, and early metastasis by the vascular route is more common, particularly to the brain and adrenal. Since they are often anaplastic, the pathologist may have difficulty with clear-cut classification, and multiple sections from separate areas of the same neoplasm may suggest a different classification for each area, leading to the designation of adenosquamous carcinoma.

Bronchoalveolar Carcinoma. This variant of lung cancer has some interesting clinical and histopathological characteristics that may distinguish it from the other types. It also often has a more encouraging biologic behavior. It sometimes remains localized, developing as a well-differentiated peripheral tumor. Electron microscopy has been reported to show cellular features suggestive of alveolar origin in some instances, while other tumors have contained atypical Clara cells suggestive of an origin in bronchioles. Resection of the solitary or localized tumor has given a 5-year cure rate from 50 to 75 percent. This contrasts remarkably with the diffuse form of bronchioloalveolar cell carcinoma, in which there is rapid dissemination of the neoplasm in one or both lungs, with no possible consideration of operative treatment. The diffuse form of the neoplasm may be the result of aerogenic dissemination through the tracheobronchial tree from an initial single focus of tumor. In both forms of the disease, it may be possible to demonstrate the typical cells of the neoplasm distributed in alveoli of the surrounding lung parenchyma. Up to one-third of the patients with this relatively rare form of lung cancer may have no significant smoking history.

Scar Carcinoma. The term "scar carcinoma" has been used increasingly in recent years to refer to tumors that seem to arise at the site of previous pulmonary disease (Fig. 17-79). When a patient with previous pulmonary tuberculosis develops a neoplasm in the same area that was scarred by the tuberculosis process, there is generally a speculation about the cause-and-effect relationship. These lesions may be adenocarcinoma or bronchiolar cell carcinoma, and often are of mixed cellular appearance. There is a predominance of upper-lobe location.

Small-Cell Lung Cancer (SCLS). The small-cell anaplastic carcinoma, sometimes referred to as "oat cell carcinoma," is a highly malignant, rapidly growing neoplasm that is most often central in location because of origin from a proximal bronchus. In addition to early spread by hilar and mediastinal lymph-node involvement, this tumor aggressively invades local structures and is disseminated by early vascular invasion. Because of its rapid growth and spread, many consider the oat cell carcinoma to have no place among the bronchogenic tumors that are treated by surgical resection. It has become apparent that certain histologic subtypes of small-cell undifferentiated carcinoma have a better prognosis after curative resection (Fig. 17-80). A number of encouraging multimodal therapy investigative protocols are underway that provide some hope that short-term outlook might be better than has been believed. Surgical resection may still have an important role in the intermediate- (polygonal, fusiform) cell type of small-cell carcinoma, particularly when peripherally located without evidence of lymph-node spread. It is important for the pathologist to distinguish the variants of small-cell carcinoma, because the treatment may depend on the specific subtype.

STAGING. To share information and to standardize evaluation of protocols, the recommendations of the American Joint Committee on Cancer (AJCC) and the International Union Against Cancer (IUCC) have had their systems reconciled with Mountain's staging and the American Joint Committee Task Force on Lung Staging Revision. Recommended variations from the previous AJCC scheme include several modifications of the TNM descriptors. A T_4 category denoting local mediastinal, visceral, great vessel, or bony invasion, or the presence of

cytologically malignant pleural effusion has been added and N_3 has been redefined to include contralateral mediastinal, contralateral hilar, or scalene-supraclavicular nodal involvement. Stage III has been subclassified as a and b (b meaning T_4 or N_3 disease). Stage IV has been added to include all M_1 tumors.

Since this classification deviates from the more usually reported earlier AJCC classification, it is worth emphasizing several of the modifications from that version. Stage I no longer includes any patients with any nodal metastases. Stage III has been divided into one group with large locally invasive tumors but with nodes confined to the ipsilateral chest (IIIa) and a second group including contralateral nodal involvement or invasion of mediastinal viscera (IIIb). All tumors metastasizing beyond the thoracic and low cervical lymph nodes are now designated as Stage IV. Using the grading system, patients with NSCLC can be divided clinically into logical treatment groups, whatever the cell type. According to the NCI's current prognosis and treatment recommendations, Stages I and II tumors are usually surgically respectable. The prognosis in this group is 30 to 80 percent 5-year survival, with the range depending on a variety of tumor and host factors. If the patients in these groups have medical conditions that preclude an attempt at curative surgery, radiation therapy can be expected to result in a 20 percent survival at 5 years. A second group of patients with locally advanced cancers (T_3) or certain patterns of regional extension (N_2 or M_1 involving only the supraclavicular area) may respond favorably to extended local resection (the T_3 lesions) combined with radiation and/or chemotherapy, or curative radiation doses directed at the involved nodal areas. Though the overall 5-year survival for this group is 10 percent or less and the median survival is less than a year, as previously noted, several centers have achieved much better results in selected subsets of this group. In Stage IV patients (those with distant metastases at the time of diagnosis), radiation for palliation of symptoms from the primary tumor may be useful. Though progress is being made in the oncology field, at present chemotherapy has not produced much survival benefit. Patients with lung cancer who have extrathoracic disease rarely survive for any significant period. The median survival is less than 6 months.

CLINICAL MANIFESTATIONS. Bronchogenic carcinoma is seen predominantly in men of forty-five to sixty-five years of age, with a peak incidence at fifty-five to sixty years. It is not rare in men less than forty-five years old, and the diagnosis is being made with increasing frequency in women who are in their fifth decade. In a few cases, the disease is discovered incidentally in asymptomatic patients. Such discovery is by means of chest x-ray for the greatest number of patients, but sputum cytology occasionally leads to the eventual identification of an otherwise occult tumor.

Because intermittent or chronic cough is so common among tobacco addicts, it may be difficult to establish an onset of symptoms. Nevertheless, about three-fourths of patients with bronchogenic carcinoma must be said to

THE REVISED (1986) AJCC STAGING SYSTEM

Primary tumor (T)

TX	Tumor proved by the presence of malignant cells in bronchopulmonary secretions but not visualized roentgenographically or bronchoscopically, or any tumor that cannot be assessed as in a retreatment staging
T_0	No evidence of primary tumor
T_{is}	Carcinoma in situ
T_1	A tumor that is 3.0 cm or less in greatest dimension, surrounded by lung or visceral pleura, and without evidence of invasion proximal to a lobar bronchus at bronchoscopy
T_2	A tumor more than 3.0 cm in greatest dimension, or a tumor of any size that either invades the visceral pleura or has associated atelectasis or obstructive pneumonitis extending to the hilar region. At bronchoscopy, the proximal extent of demonstrable tumor must be within a lobar bronchus or at least 2.0 cm distal to the carina. Any associated atelectasis or obstructive pneumonitis must involve less than an entire lung.
T_3	A tumor of any size with direct extension into the chest wall (including superior sulcus tumors), diaphragm, or the mediastinal pleura or pericardium without involving the heart, great vessels, trachea, esophagus or vertebral body, or a tumor in the main bronchus within 2.0 cm of the carina without involving the carina
T_4	A tumor of any size with invasion of the mediastinum or involving heart, great vessels, trachea, esophagus, vertebral body, or carina, or presence of malignant pleural effusion

Nodal involvement (N)

NX	Minimum requirements to access the regional nodes cannot be met
N_0	No demonstrable metastasis to regional lymph nodes
N_1	Metastasis to lymph nodes in the peribronchial or the ipsilateral hilar region, or both, including direct extension
N_2	Metastasis to ipsilateral mediastinal lymph nodes and subcarinal lymph nodes
N_3	Metastasis to contralateral mediastinal lymph nodes, contralateral hilar lymph nodes, ipsilateral or contralateral scalene, or supraclavicular lymph nodes

Distant metastasis (M)

MX	Minimum requirements to assess the presence of distant metastasis cannot be met
M_0	No (known) distant metastasis
M_1	Distant metastasis present

Stage grouping

Occult stage	TX	N_0	M_0
Stage 0	T_{is}	N_0	M_0 (in situ)
Stage I	T_1	N_0	M_0
	T_2	N_0	M_0
Stage II	T_1	N_1	M_0
	T_2	N_1	M_0
Stage IIIa	T_3	N_0	M_0
	T_3	N_1	M_0
	T_{1-3}	N_2	M_0
Stage IIIb	Any T	N_3	M_0
	T_4	Any N	M_0
Stage IV	Any T	Any N	M_1

SUMMARY OF STAGING DEFINITIONS

Occult stage	Microscopically identified cancer cells in lung secretions on multiple occasions (or multiple daily collections); no discernible primary cancer in the lung
Stage 0	Carcinoma in situ
Stage I	Tumor surrounded by lung or visceral pleura arising more than 2 cm distal to the carina (T_{1-2}, N_0)
Stage II	Tumor not extending to adjacent organs, pleura, or chest wall, with hilar lymph-node involvement (T_{1-2}, N_1)
Stage IIIa	Tumor invading chest wall, pleura, or pericardium or within 2 cm but not involving carina; nodes in hilum or ipsilateral mediastinum (T_3, N_{0-1}; T_1, N_2)
Stage IIIb	Direct extension to adjacent organs (pleura, heart, chest wall, diaphragm, or mediastinum); or associated with contralateral mediastinal or supraclavicular lymph-node involvement (T_4 or N_3)
Stage IV	Any tumor with distant metastases (M_1)

have coughing as a principal symptom. Hemoptysis in the form of blood streaking of sputum occurs in about half of all patients, but massive hemoptysis or spitting of blood clots is unusual. Chest pain of dull, nonspecific type is described by some patients whose tumor is subsequently found to be free of chest wall involvement. When there is invasion of the parietal pleura or chest wall, the patient may have mild to severe pain that is either localized or radicular in form. Fever and purulent sputum may mark an increase of symptoms in the patient whose tumor is producing major bronchial obstruction, and wheezing or stridor may also be present.

Involvement of the left recurrent laryngeal nerve (rarely the right nerve), either by direct tumor invasion or by extension from a metastatic lymph node, may result in hoarseness that is often minimized by the patient. Direct tumor extension into the superior vena cava or its compression by the expanding neoplasm produces early symptoms of edema of the eyes and prominence or distension of the superficial veins over the upper part of the body. Dyspnea occurring as a symptom of bronchogenic carcinoma is usually associated with a large pleural effusion, paralysis of a hemidiaphragm due to phrenic nerve invasion, or major bronchial obstruction.

A loss of appetite accompanied by weight loss of more than a few pounds is an ominous sign in the patient with a bronchial neoplasm; such patients usually have either an unresectable tumor or systemic metastases. A deliberate search should be made for evidence of spread by isotope scanning and computed tomography. Because the metastatic spectrum of these tumors is so wide, almost any imaginable symptom can be produced. A rare patient may develop pulmonary hypertrophic osteoarthropathy with clubbing of the digits (Fig. 17-81). Evidence of metastases may be absent, and the process may be dramatically reversed when the tumor is resected.

A small percentage of patients with bronchogenic carcinoma present with extrapulmonary nonmetastatic manifestations that are considered due to elaboration of hor-

monelike substances by the neoplastic cells. The occurrence of these signs and symptoms does not imply systemic spread of the bronchogenic tumor, and resection of the lesion is generally associated with a regression of the symptoms. Ultrastructural studies have demonstrated the presence of neurosecretory-type granules in the cells of many anaplastic tumors, and the more striking clinical symptoms are associated with oat cell carcinomas. An example is a Cushing-like syndrome that differs from the classic Cushing's syndrome by an older age incidence, a greater frequency in males, and a more rapid clinical course. The ectopic adrenocorticotropic hormone that has been demonstrated in the oat cell tumors appears indistinguishable from the normal hormone. An inappropriate antidiuresis associated with the anaplastic small-cell carcinoma occasionally results in the symptoms of water intoxication with hyponatremia and increasing cerebral symptoms. The carinoid syndrome has been reported in a few patients with oat cell carcinoma, and either 5-hydroxytryptamine or 5-hydroxytryptophan may be secreted.

Hypercalcemia caused by a parathormone-like polypeptide has most often been associated with squamous bronchogenic carcinoma. Tender gynecomastia and ectopic gonadotropin secretion have been identified with large-cell anaplastic carcinoma. Satisfactory resection of the squamous neoplasm reverses the hypercalcemia, but it may return if the tumor recurs. A group of carcinomatous neuromyopathies is included in the nonmetastatic manifestations of lung cancer, and their incidence is thought to be as high as 15 percent. The symptoms may be subtle or somewhat overshadowed by the pulmonary complaints. The patient with bronchogenic carcinoma who mentions weakness along with his cough and chest pain is usually not questioned in detail about the characteristics of the weakness. This is the principal symptom, however, of a myasthenia-like syndrome that is probably due to a defect in neuromuscular conduction. Peripheral and central neuropathies also occur, and their differentiation from the symptoms of metastatic lesions can be im-

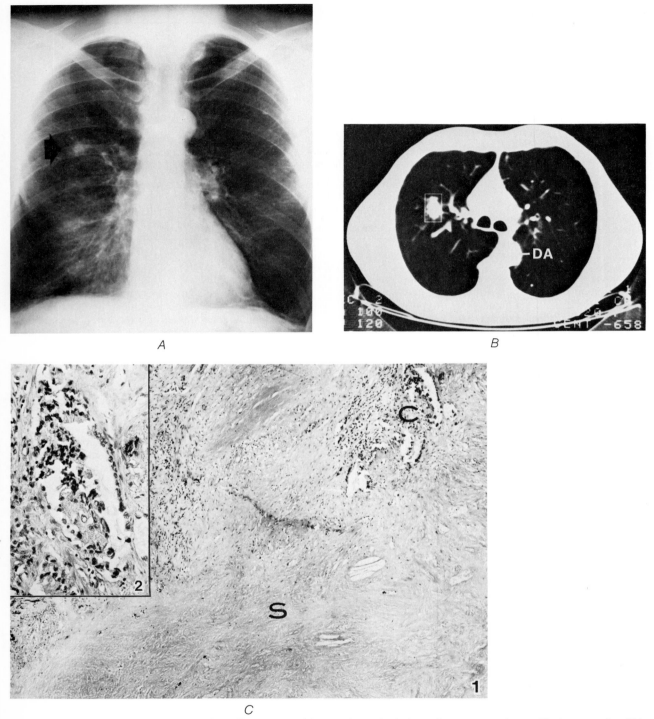

A

B

C

Fig. 17-79. A pulmonary scar carcinoma in a fifty-one-year-old man. *A.* The P-A chest x-ray shows an irregular density in the upper midlung field. *B.* A CT scan at the level of the main-stem bronchi shows a small dense mass in the parenchyma of the right upper lobe. *C.* The photomicrograph made from the resected upper lobe shows the lesion to be a scar carcinoma. The lower portion (S) is ancient hyalinized scar. In the upper right is a focus of adenocarcinoma (C) (×95). The insert is a higher magnification of the adenocarcinoma (×265).

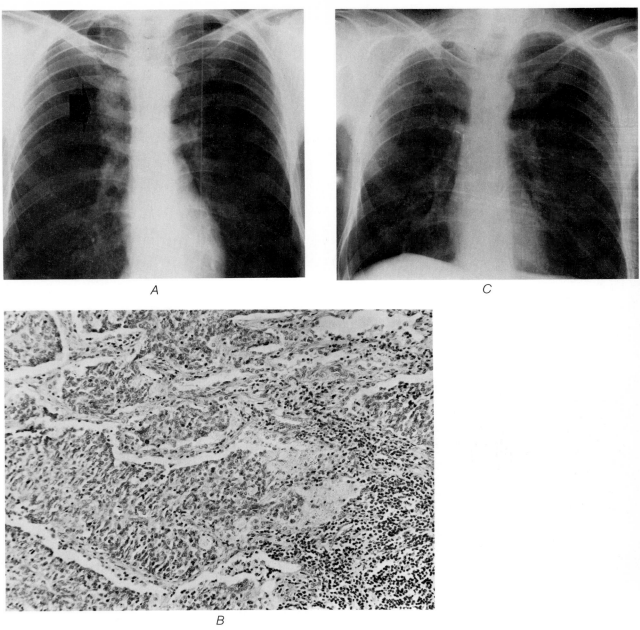

A

B

C

Fig. 17-80. Undifferentiated small-cell carcinoma, intermediate-cell type, in a fifty-five-year-old man. *A.* The preoperative chest x-ray shows a mass above the right hilus. Mediastinoscopy failed to show evidence of mediastinal lymph-node involvement, and the patient underwent right upper lobectomy. *B.* Histological examination of the resected lobe showed an undifferentiated small-cell carcinoma, intermediate-cell type, invading the lung parenchyma. Note the size of tumor cells in comparison with the mature lymphocytes in the lower right corner. (×188.) *C.* A follow-up chest x-ray 4 years after operation shows no evidence of tumor recurrence, and the patient is well.

portant. With the former, pulmonary resection may be possible and may result in disappearance of the symptoms.

DIAGNOSIS AND WORK-UP. Approximately 50 percent of patients with bronchogenic cancer are beyond consideration for operative treatment when the opportunity for definitive diagnosis is first presented. For this reason diagnostic evaluation must include an effort to determine whether localized or metastatic spread has occurred. The key to this effort is a meticulous history. If carefully sought, symptoms can almost always be found that will direct attention to involved organ systems. A thorough

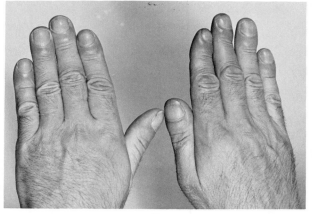

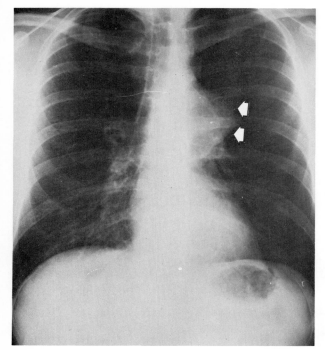

A

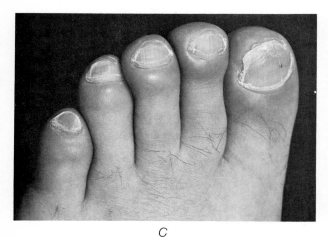

C

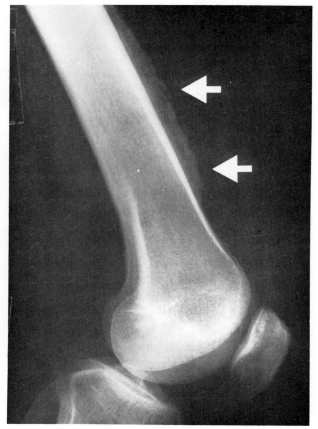

D

examination for suggestive lymph nodes must also be made. Though the yield is low in the absence of symptoms, any or all of the scanning techniques should be used to search for metastatic spread in the presence of suggestive symptoms, or if the patient's general condition suggests systemic spread. With any question of metastasis, an attempt at biopsy should be considered before treatment for the primary neoplasm is planned.

Whenever the differential diagnosis includes lung cancer, aggressive efforts to obtain cytologic or biopsy tissue diagnosis are indicated. Almost any type of pulmonary infiltrate, nodule, mass, or atelectasis should be considered cancer until it can be proved otherwise. This is particularly true if the patient is, has been, or lives with a

Fig. 17-81. Pulmonary hypertrophic osteoarthropathy associated with oat cell carcinoma. *A.* The chest x-ray in a thirty-nine-year-old man shows a left hilar mass that proved to be oat cell carcinoma on bronchial biopsy. *B.* Painful clubbing of the fingers and toes developed during an interval of approximately 3 months. *C.* A close-up of the patient's foot demonstrates clubbing of the toes. *D.* The arrow points to the new bone formation on the femur.

tobacco addict. As previously discussed, there is an orderly and progressively invasive series of investigative studies that can be undertaken to obtain diagnostic tissue. The degree to which a search should be made for extra thoracic disease is a matter of controversy among those who care for lung cancer patients. Radioactive scans of liver, brain, and bones are recommended by many, but evidence is lacking that such searches are fruitful in the absence of symptoms. In one recent analysis of a routine scanning program in patients without symptoms, 16 of 17 positive scans were false positive and 8 of 22 clinically evidence metastases were not detected. Recent reports in the radiology literature have indicated 5 to 20 percent occurrence of demonstrable adrenal metastases in lung cancer patients studied by CT. The demonstrated value of the CT in visualizing the mediastinum has greatly reduced the indication for staging mediastinoscopy, a procedure that had been gaining strong support until recently. Most surgeons now reserve exploration of the mediastinum for those patients with nodes identified on CT as being larger than 1 cm (Fig. 17-82).

Even before the general availability of computed tomography for careful preoperative evaluation of the mediastinum in lung cancer patients, there were differences of opinion about aggressive prethoracotomy staging by mediastinal exploration techniques. For some groups treating lung cancer, the attitude is that positive lymph nodes in the mediastinum preclude thoracotomy because of the very low 5-year survival with resection under these circumstances. Others, however, quoting reasonable survival figures, usually with postoperative adjuvant therapy, have concluded that ipsilateral mediastinal metastases are not a contraindication to pulmonary resection. Therefore, some of the latter surgeons do not feel that routine preoperative staging by mediastinal exploration is warranted.

Along with CT mapping, bronchoscopy is the fundamental diagnostic technique for patients with suspected carcinoma, and the development of the flexible fiberscope has increased the positive diagnosis yield to better than 70 percent in most centers. These results include bronchial brushing and cytologic studies of bronchial washings that may be obtained at the same time. The endoscopist must determine the proximal extent of a visualized neoplasm because the patient's operability may be governed by the closeness of the tumor to the tracheal carina. Murray and colleagues evaluated the relationship between positive bronchoscopy and lymph-node metastases in 42 consecutive patients with tumors of the right lower or middle lobe (Table 17-15). Bronchoscopy was considered positive when a visible endobronchial lesion was identified. When bronchoscopy was negative (21 patients), intraoperative evaluation and pathologic examination of the lymphatic sump of Borrie failed to demonstrate nodal metastases in 18 patients. Hilar nodes were positive in 2 patients, but no patient had mediastinal disease. Pneumonectomy was required in only 3 patients in the negative bronchoscopy group. Of the 20 patients with positive bronchoscopy 9 had metastases to the lymphatic sump and 2 had mediastinal metastases. There was a

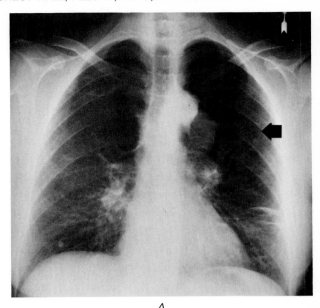

A

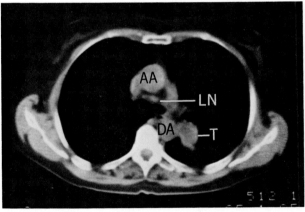

B

Fig. 17-82. The use of computed tomography for preoperative staging of bronchogenic carcinoma. *A.* The P-A chest x-ray in a sixty-two-year-old woman shows a mass between the aortic knob and the left hilus. On the lateral chest x-ray the mass was seen to be located in the posterior segment of the left upper lobe. *B.* A CT scan at the level of the tracheal carina shows the tumor in juxtaposition to the descending aorta. The lymph nodes just in front of the carina and posterior to the ascending aorta were interpreted to be at the upper limit of normal size. At operation all lymph nodes were negative for metastases, confirming the CT impression. AA = ascending aorta, LN = lymph nodes, T = tumor, DA = descending aorta.

marked superiority in survival in the negative bronchoscopy group.

A primary goal of the patient's work-up is to confirm the suspected diagnosis of carcinoma by means other than exploratory thoracotomy. Diagnostic procedures should be carried out as techniques for establishing the patient's suitability for operation are completed. Despite a proper application of all reasonable diagnostic proce-

Table 17-15. SIGNIFICANCE OF BRONCHOSCOPIC
FINDINGS IN THE EVALUATION OF EXTENT
OF DISEASE IN 41 PATIENTS WITH CARCINOMA
OF THE RIGHT LOWER OR MIDDLE LOBE

Evaluative evidence*	Bronchoscopy negative (21 pt)	Bronchoscopy positive (20 pt)
Mediastinal metastases	0	2
Lymphatic sump positive	0	9
Bronchial margin involved	0	3
Pneumonectomy required	3	10

* Includes clinical, surgical evaluative, and postsurgical treatment pathologic classification.
SOURCE: Murray GF, Mendes OC, Wilcox BR: Bronchial carcinoma and the lymphatic sump: Significance of bronchoscopic
findings. *Ann Thorac Surg* 34:634, 1982, with permission.

dures, 10 to 20 percent of patients usually undergo thoracotomy without a proved diagnosis before operation.

An infrequent but clinically frustrating dilemma occurs
when a patient is found to have recurring positive sputum
cytology without a visible lesion on the chest x-rays.
Other sources of the malignant cells, such as the nasopharynx or piriform sinuses, have to be eliminated, and
careful flexible bronchoscopic examination may need to
be performed at intervals of 4 to 8 weeks. Selective bronchial brushing or selective washing may localize the lesion, but exfoliated cells can become displaced into a
bronchus other than the one of origin. This suggests caution in planning a major resection on the basis of these
techniques alone. As new generations of CT scanners are
developed, it may become possible to localize a so-called
occult carcinoma by noninvasive techniques. The use of
photoelectric endoscopic markers has shown some promise in detecting early, occult cancers. Unfortunately, the
false positive rate is high since the agent used currently (a
hematoporphyrin derivative—HpD) is concentrated in
areas of atypical squamous metaplasia as well as in cancer tissue.

There is now less resistance to needle biopsy than there
used to be because of the decreasing fear of implanting
tumor cells in the needle tract. In some institutions, needle biopsy is among the first procedures performed in the
diagnostic work-up of the patient with a suspicious pulmonary lesion. Pneumothorax is the most frequent problem following needle biopsy, but less than half of the patients with this complication require treatment. In a series
of 5300 percutaneous biopsies performed in 2726 patients,
Sinner reported a definitive diagnosis in 90.7 percent,
with pneumothorax occurring in 27.2 percent. Two percent of the patients had hemoptysis, and one subcutaneous tumor implant occurred in the more than 1200 patients with malignant lesions.

A pleural effusion in the presence of a suspected or
confirmed pulmonary cancer is generally an indication of
extensive tumor that is producing pleural or mediastinal
invasion. An effusion can occur as a consequence of
bronchial obstruction with atelectasis or infection. The

fluid should be examined for the presence of blood and
malignant cells with a simultaneous pleural needle biopsy
if feasible. A demonstration of malignant cells in the effusion occurs in approximately half the patients with visceral or parietal pleural invasion by the neoplasm.

TREATMENT AND PROGNOSIS. An orderly approach to
consideration of treatment of lung cancer involves deciding what is best for the given tumor according to its stage
and cell type, and deciding what is best for the given patient according to the physical capabilities to withstand
what might be optimal tumor treatment. In general, results of standard treatment are discouraging except in the
most localized cancers. At this time, surgery is the only
therapeutic option with cure potential; though radiotherapy may provide occasional long disease-free survival, its
role is currently mostly adjunctive or palliative. It is likely
future treatment will combine surgery, radiotherapy,
chemotherapy, and immunotherapy.

The Tumor. The material in this section draws upon the
recommendations made by the National Cancer Institute
(NCI) and the National Library of Medicine (NLM) as
reported in their computer-based information resource,
PDQ. This excellent source of up-to-date information
reports *current research protocols* and consensus recommendations for therapy and outlook.

Non-Small-Cell Lung Cancer (NSCLC). *Occult NSCLC.*
Aggressive diagnostic efforts are required to define the
site and nature of the primary tumor since these tumors
are generally curable with surgery. Localized endoscopic
cytologic or photoactive marker methods may be useful.
Repeated chest imaging studies, at monthly intervals if
necessary, should be considered. Once properly staged,
appropriate therapy is as outlined below.
Stage I NSCLC. Five-year survival can be anticipated
in up to 80 percent of patients in this stage whose physical
condition permits surgical resection of the tumor. Medically inoperable patients with sufficient pulmonary reserve may be considered for radiation therapy with curative intent. Twenty percent 3-year survival results are
expected if 5500 to 6000 rad can be delivered with
megavoltage equipment (linear accelerator or cobalt) to
the tumor. Some now recommend prophylactic brain irradiation in patients with adenocarcinoma or large-cell carcinoma because of the high rates of cranial metastases in
those cell types. Attempts to improve survival by use of
adjuvant chemotherapy have failed, but new protocols
are under scrutiny. There has been no reported reproducible benefit from immunotherapy, though active investigation continues in that area as well.

Williams and associates have reported survival of 491
patients surgically treated for Stage I non-small-cell bronchogenic carcinoma, and projected a 5-year survival of 80
percent for those with small tumors without lymph-node
metastases ($T_1N_0M_0$). Figure 17-83, taken from their report, compares the survival according to TNM classification, and shows the effect of increasing size of tumor and
the effect of pulmonary lymph-node metastases. These
authors made several other comparisons by analysis of
this extensive experience. They found the survival of
women to be better than that of men in this series, and

LUNG CANCER SURVIVAL BY TN CLASSIFICATION

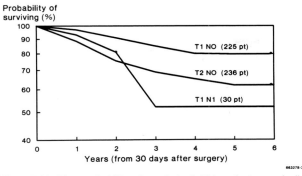

Fig. 17-83. The probability of survival of 491 patients surgically treated for Stage I bronchogenic carcinoma according to TN classification. (Reproduced from: *Williams DE, Pairolero PC, et al: Survival of patients surgically treated for Stage I lung cancer. J Thorac Cardiovasc Surg 82:70, 1981, with permission.*)

survival was better for patients less than seventy years of age than for those who were beyond seventy years. There were no overall significant differences in survival based on cell type, but those patients with bronchioloalveolar cell carcinoma had the highest 5-year survival at 81 percent. The 5-year survival for patients with squamous cell cancer was 70 percent, while the patients with adenocarcinoma and large-cell cancer had survival rates of 65 and 66 percent, respectively.

Stage II NSCLC. Surgery is also the treatment of choice for Stage II tumors, and 30 percent of resected patients should expect 5-year survival. As with Stage I patients, those who are medically unacceptable for surgery but who have sufficient pulmonary reserve to tolerate high-dose irradiation (5500 to 6000 rad) may anticipate up to 20 percent 3-year survival. Careful target volume definition and avoidance of critical normal structures is important for optimal results. In large-cell and adenocarcinoma prophylactic cranial irradiation is often considered.

Approximately 70 percent of surgically treated patients develop regional or distant metastatic disease. Therefore, most patients should be considered for adjuvant therapy, preferably through entry into an investigative clinical trial. As in several other controlled trials, Cox has shown a reduction in local recurrences following postoperative irradiation to N_1 patients, but failed to demonstrate a survival benefit in squamous cell tumors. Recent reports from the Lung Cancer Study Group, however, have shown increased disease-free survival and reduced deaths in controlled trials of adjuvant combination chemotherapy with cisplatin, doxorubicin, and cytoxan. Previous trials of other regimens had shown no significant benefit.

Stage IIIa NSCLC. The presence of lymph-node metastases has a profound effect on survival in bronchogenic carcinoma. Some groups have had such dismal results with resection in patients with mediastinal node metastases that they consider known metastases to be a contraindication to attempted surgical treatment. This is not the majority opinion, however, and other groups feel that

aggressive surgical and adjuvant therapy is warranted in the presence of positive mediastinal nodes. Recently, Martini and associates, in reporting on a group of 445 patients with clinically evident mediastinal lymph-node metastases, described 80 patients who had potentially curative resection of their primary tumor and all accessible lymph nodes. The majority of patients were also treated by postoperative external radiation therapy to the mediastinum. Included were 25 squamous cell carcinomas, 44 adenocarcinomas, 8 large-cell carcinomas, and 3 oat cell carcinomas. The survival rate was 49 percent at 3 years in those whose disease was completely removed. The authors concluded that there is a select group of patients with mediastinal node metastases who can benefit from surgical resection and radiation therapy.

Depending on clinical situation, some combination of radiation therapy and surgery is the mainstay in treating patients with locally or regionally advanced tumors. Surgery remains an important modality; the only chance for ''cure'' may be in those who have resectional surgery. Several groups have reported 5-year survival of approximately 50 percent in $T_3N_0M_0$ patients with chest wall invasion and wide resection. A special subset of these locally invasive tumors, the superior sulcus tumor (Pancoast tumor), have long been known to have a potential for satisfactory response to combined radiation and resection. In many reports of long-term survivors from large series, a few of the patients would appear to have had Stage III tumors. Though few patients achieve complete response to radiation, most have significant palliation and 5 to 10 percent will experience long-term survival benefit. Trials are in progress examining fractionation schedules, radiation sensitizers, radiolabeled antibodies, and combined modality approaches in efforts to improve regional control.

As with Stage II adenocarcinoma and large-cell undifferentiated carcinoma, the Lung Cancer Study Group has reported a regimen of chemotherapeutic agents (cisplatin, doxorubicin, and cytoxan) that increases survival and reduces deaths.

Mediastinal Involvement (N_2, M_0). Mountain and Martini have each presented persuasive series of patients with involved mediastinal lymph nodes who seem to have benefited from extended resection. Forty percent 5-year survival was achieved in patients with N_2 squamous cell cancers when the clinically negative mediastinal nodes were found by the pathologist to contain intranodal metastases. In Mountain's series, postoperative irradiation was not shown to improve the outcome over the results of resection alone. Other reports suggest postoperative radiation therapy may reduce local recurrences.

Stage IIIb NSCLC. In the special clinical setting of superior vena cava syndrome, prompt radiation therapy is indicated regardless of stage. Symptoms relating to specific local mechanical compression by growing tumor mass (tracheal, esophageal, bronchial, or superior vena caval obstruction, vocal cord paralysis, or hemoptysis) may respond to palliative radiation therapy. Appropriately timed radiation may maintain an acceptable lifestyle for a brief period in otherwise functional patients.

Stage IV (NSCLC). None of the currently reported therapeutic programs appear to offer any significant survival benefit for patients with distant metastases (M_1). The only justification for administering toxic chemotherapeutic agents to lung cancer patients with distant metastases at present is in those patients with good performance status who are able to be included in an investigational protocol. Only a small percentage of these patients can be expected to survive 5 years, though several selected subgroups may do reasonably well if aggressively treated, and an occasional long-term survivor is reported against all odds.

Small-Cell Lung Cancer (SCLC). The median survival following diagnosis of small-cell (oat cell) carcinoma is 2 to 4 months without treatment. It is almost always widely disseminated when diagnosed. Because of early metastases, localized treatment alone, such as surgical resection or radiation therapy or both, rarely produces long-term survival. Current treatment regimens, however, clearly prolong survival (four- to fivefold) compared with untreated patients. Five to ten percent of patients remain disease-free for up to 2 years form the start of therapy. Some of these patients may be cured of their small-cell cancer.

A few patients are found who have disease sufficiently localized to allow resection for cure by standard surgical criteria; these patients may have a reasonable prognosis. If the tumor has spread beyond the supraclavicular area, median survival of 6 to 12 months is all that can be achieved with currently available therapy; long-term disease-free survival is unusual. The prognosis for patients with small-cell lung cancer is unsatisfactory even though considerable improvements in diagnosis and therapy have been made over the past 10 to 15 years.

The role of surgical resection in small-cell undifferentiated carcinoma is presently undergoing reevaluation. In the 1970s, on the basis of several reports in which there were virtually no long-term survivors of pulmonary resection for this tumor, surgical intervention was largely abandoned. The poor results were due partly to the biologic behavior of small-cell carcinoma but also to poor selection of patients and failure to stage the patients preoperatively. Therefore, during the past decade the management of small-cell carcinoma has been provided by combination chemotherapy and radiation therapy. A few groups, however, have continued to operate on selected patients with small-cell carcinoma, often in combination with postoperative chemotherapy protocols. The reported 5-year survival rates of 25 to 48 percent have stimulated a general renewal of interest in surgical resection of carefully selected patients.

In their report on extended indications for resection in small-cell carcinoma, Meyer and his colleagues pointed out that the commonest single site of relapse in patients treated for clinically localized disease with chemotherapy and radiation therapy is within the chest. They suggest that complete surgical removal of the intrathoracic disease might offer the best chance to reduce this mode of relapse. On the basis of their remarkable results in patients with Stage I and Stage II disease treated by initial surgical resection and postoperative chemotherapy, they

have now begun a trial of resection in selected patients with Stage III disease who have no evidence of distant metastases. They state that in order for a known small-cell carcinoma to be classified as Stage I or II, the tumor must be peripheral, surrounded by clear lung, and undetectable by mediastinoscopy.

Shields and his colleagues have concluded that the patients with small-cell carcinoma who have the best prospect for long-term survival after primary resection are those with T_1 lesion without lymph-node metastases. They suggest that a central location of these small-sized tumors does not negate the possibility of a satisfactory result. Further, they recommend that patients selected for initial surgical resection should be classified as either $T_1N_0M_0$ or $T_2N_0M_0$. When the diagnosis of small-cell carcinoma is established preoperatively, either mediastinoscopy or mediastinotomy or both should be done, and bilateral iliac bone-marrow aspiration should be performed to rule out metastatic disease before resection is recommended.

The Patient. Careful preoperative assessment of the patient's overall medical condition and especially the patient's pulmonary reserve are critical issues in considering the benefits of surgery. Unfortunately, by the time the diagnosis is made the opportunity for curative surgery has passed in about half of all patients with bronchogenic carcinoma. These patients have centrally located neoplasms with evidence of mediastinal extension, symptoms of distant metastases, or compromised cardiopulmonary function that precludes a major pulmonary resection.

Factors such as the patient's age, impaired pulmonary function, and tumor extension outside the lung vary in their influence on the decision of individual surgeons to attempt pulmonary resection. Though there is increasing risk of morbidity and mortality for those who undergo major pulmonary resection after sixty years of age, it has been demonstrated that patients of seventy years and beyond tolerate lobectomy with an acceptable mortality rate (Table 17-16). Similarly, impaired pulmonary function does increase the risk of operation, but Peters and associates have demonstrated an acceptable mortality and complication rate by careful analysis of the pulmonary-function data to allow the selection of patients who can be brought through the surgical experience. Invasion of either the phrenic or recurrent laryngeal nerve is considered a contraindication to thoracotomy by most surgeons, but this is not totally accepted. In particular, phrenic nerve involvement is usually along its course over the pericardium, and some surgeons advocate an en bloc resection of the involved area along with the pulmonary resection.

SURGICAL CONSIDERATIONS. Several technical advances have made it possible to extend the indications for surgical resection to a higher-risk group of patients. Less physiologically damaging incisions (the median sternotomy and the straight lateral-modified transaxillary), better anesthetic tools (double-lumen tubes, jet ventilation), and the increasing use of parenchyma-saving resections (sleeve resections, wedge resections, and segmental resections) have made it possible to offer potentially cura-

Table 17-16. MORTALITY AND AGE-RISK FACTORS IN RESECTIONS FOR LUNG CANCER

LCSG mortality rates for pneumonectomy, lobectomy, and lesser resections

	No. of resections	Deaths	
		No.	Percent, %
Pneumonectomy	569	44	6.2
Lobectomy	1058	35	2.9
Lesser resection (segmentectomy or wedge excision)	143	2	1.4

$p < 0.001*$
$p = NS*$

* Chi square, NS = not significant.

Age-risk factors obtained from LCSG data

Age, years	Mortality rate, %
< 60	1.3
60–69	4.1
> 70	7.1

$p < 0.001*$
$p = 0.014*$

* Chi square.
SOURCE: From Ginsberg, Hill, et al, with permission.

tive operations to patients previously considered inoperable.

Within recent years, some chest surgeons have followed the trends established in some other areas of surgical oncology by reconsidering the question of extent of resection. Historically, the total pneumonectomy has been considered the optimal operation for lung cancer (Fig. 17-84), but the increased mortality and morbidity of that operation lead to the wide acceptance of the lobectomy as an acceptable compromise. As the evidence accumulated that the prognosis did not seem to be compromised by the lesser resection, the lobectomy became the operation of choice whenever it was possible to adequately remove the primary without pneumonectomy. As experience has grown with sleeve and segmental resections, largely stimulated by the work of Jensik, a similar evolution in thinking seems to be taking place. A dozen reports have appeared in the past several years indicating comparable survival figures in selected bad-risk patients undergoing lung-salvaging procedures because they could not safely undergo more extensive resections. As anticipated, the short-term survival was improved; less expected was the equivalent or improved long-term control of tumor. Particularly noteworthy has been the comparable incidence of local recurrence among these patients and those with more traditional resections.

ADJUVANT THERAPY. Multiple-agent therapy has shown considerable success in the control of small-cell carcinoma, particularly when combined with radiation therapy to the primary disease in the thorax and prophylactic radiation therapy to the brain. The current treatment protocols for small-cell carcinoma generally include cyclophosphamide, doxorubicin, and vincristine. VP-16 has become an important chemotherapeutic agent and is being evaluated in combination protocols with doxorubicin and vincristine.

Chemotherapy for non-small-cell bronchogenic carcinoma has appeared to be more effective for adenocarcinoma and large-cell carcinoma than for squamous tumors. Five-year survival rates of up to 20 percent have been reported in adenocarcinoma using combinations of radiation therapy and chemotherapy with cyclophosphamide, Adriamycin, methotrexate, and procarbazine. More recently, cisplatinum is being substituted for procarbazine in the four-drug regimens. Most studies have confirmed that if the patients with unresectable lung cancer have a good performance status, they are likely to benefit from carefully administered chemotherapy.

Immunodeficiency. Recent studies have emphasized the important but not clearly defined role of immunodeficiency in the prognosis of patients with many forms of cancer. An impaired reaction to delayed cutaneous hypersensitivity testing with 2,4-dinitrochlorobenzene has been demonstrated in many lung cancer patients, and those who are unable to become sensitized to this antigen often have unresectable neoplasms. Impaired lymphocyte transformation with in vitro stimulation by several antigens and mitogens has also demonstrated a marked decrease in immunocompetence in patients with pulmonary carcinoma. One of the mechanisms of immunodeficiency is thought to be the presence of circulating immunosuppressive factors in the serum of the lung cancer patient. Whether such factors might be produced by the neoplasm is only speculative. Some years ago the observation was made that patients who developed pleural empyema after pulmonary resection for bronchogenic carcinoma seemed to have a better survival. This was attributed to a nonspecific stimulation of the immune system. More recently, this purported increase in survival with postoperative empyema has been found not to be true.

Hyman and associates made some provocative inferences about the protective effect of blood transfusions on the host acceptance of renal transplants which led them to evaluate the effect of transfusions on survival of lung cancer. In their small series, intraoperative blood transfusion seemed to worsen prognosis, as predicted. If verified, this observation could have important implications for host defense relationship to early dissemination of tumor cells.

SOLITARY PULMONARY NODULES

Among those patients with lung cancer, the best survival can be expected from that group of patients where the cancer is first found as an asymptomatic solitary peripheral pulmonary nodule on the chest x-ray. Because of this relatively favorable outlook if the nodule is a cancer, and because of the variety of nonmalignant lesions that also present in this fashion, there is considerable interest in the differential diagnosis of these "coin lesions." For

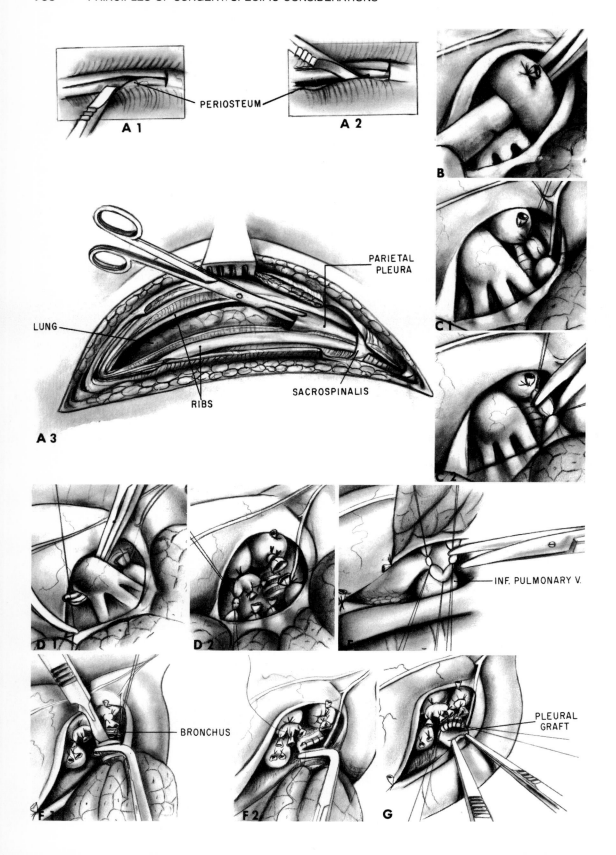

A 1

A 2

PERIOSTEUM

B

LUNG

PARIETAL
PLEURA

SACROSPINALIS

RIBS

A 3

C 1

C 2

D 1

D 2

INF. PULMONARY V.

F 1

BRONCHUS

F 2

G

PLEURAL
GRAFT

convenience in discussion the solitary pulmonary nodule (SPN) has been defined by general agreement to be an abnormal density up to 4 cm in diameter, rounded or ovoid in appearance (Figs. 17-85, 17-88), surrounded by a zone of lung tissue by x-ray, and free of cavitation or associated lung infiltrates. Eccentric flecks of calcium may be present, but lesions that are largely calcified or that have concentric calcium rings are not considered.

Whereas earlier reports suggested a malignancy rate of about 40 percent in the SPN, Francic and Zimmerman have recently reviewed the more current experience and found of 71 coin lesions seen in their clinic from 1982 to 1984, 48 were primary cancers and 6 were silent metastases—a 76 percent overall malignancy rate. In patients over fifty, 82 percent of all coin lesions were malignant. Only when the nodule is known to have been present for a long period with absence of growth and with a pattern of calcification characteristic of the several benign lesions that can occur should histologic diagnosis of these nodules be delayed.

Proof that the lesion is not of recent development requires inspection of old chest x-rays since faint, small lesions are frequently overlooked in screening films and a negative official report has often been found to be in error. Even when previous x-rays document radiologic stability of a solitary nodule for up to 2 years, malignancy must be suspected.

The differential diagnosis of an SPN includes many entities, among which are pulmonary hamartoma, granuloma, pulmonary arteriovenous fistula, pulmonary infarct, and several benign and malignant tumors. Since surgery is rarely indicated for the nonmalignant lesions under consideration, many clinics have recommended extensive diagnostic efforts to ascertain the correct diagnosis before thoracotomy. Unfortunately, there is a significant false negative rate in virtually all the studies short of excisional biopsy. With improving imaging techniques, the odds of a correct preoperative diagnosis are improving, but with the consequences of error so high and with the reasonably good results following surgical resection, many surgeons feel it is unwise to gamble on a determination of benignancy unless the lesion is in a young (under

35), nonsmoking patient with a known history of radiographic stability.

Where calcification is present, computed tomography is especially useful in improving the preoperative guess or in selecting the rare patient who can be safely observed. CT scans have the capacity to measure absorption coefficients and therefore indicate tissue density. Siegelman and associates used CT with thin sections to assess tissue density in 91 apparently noncalcified pulmonary nodules in 88 patients. They established a separation between benign and malignant lesions on the basis of high attenuation values in the benign SPN. The high values were presumably due to diffusely distributed calcium deposits within the lesions but not visible on standard radiographs. In the absence of calcium, however, benign SPN may have attenuation values in the same range as malignant lesions. Similarly, in a small proportion of cases, malignant lesions may have sufficient calcium to result in the high values characteristic of benign nodules.

For many years there has been a difference of opinion regarding the management of patients with solitary nodules with some groups advocating early thoracotomy with resection of the lesion for all patients above thirty-five years of age and others urging a more conservative approach with greater emphasis on diagnostic studies and observation. Though the resection policy did result in a 50 percent frequency of removal of benign lesions, excellent cure rates were expected if primary malignancies were found. With the sharply falling frequency of tuberculous granulomata and the continuing rise in lung cancer rates, current odds favor early resection unless there is strong evidence of a benign process. Sputum cytology, bronchoscopic washings and brushings, and percutaneous needle biopsies each provide clear-cut positive information if malignant cells are found but cannot exclude malignant disease.

If previous films are available for comparison, or if a course of observation is elected for other reasons, calculation of the time necessary for doubling of the tumor volume is a useful indicator of the nature of the lesion. Serial radiographs provide the data for calculation of growth rate, and it is generally possible to detect that a lesion is growing within a few weeks. The doubling time of malignant nodules is usually between 37 and 465 days. If the lesion is growing more slowly or more rapidly than this, the evidence is in favor of benignancy. Advocates of a conservative approach insist that present knowledge supports the concept that a pulmonary nodule can be watched safely for a period of time to determine whether it is growing.

A logical approach to the SPN at present would include early thoracotomy for lesions in known risk populations: age over fifty, smoking history, absence of certain knowledge of a similar lesion on chest film more than 2 years old. A careful review of systems for suggestion of symptoms that might justify a search for a primary elsewhere should be made, but extensive (and expensive) screening in asymptomatic patients is probably not warranted. If the patient is under thirty-five and a nonsmoker, and if the chance of malignancy is small, needle biopsy and

Fig. 17-84. Resection of lung. *A.* Opening into pleural cavity: (1) periosteum incised over the rib; (2) subperiosteal resection being performed; (3) pleura opened through bed of resected rib. *B.* Freeing of pulmonary artery from adjacent structures. *C.* Ligation and division of pulmonary artery: (1) artery doubly ligated with an adequate distance between the two ligatures; (2) artery transected between two ligatures. *D.* Peripheral dissection of pulmonary artery to increase safety factor: (1) branches of pulmonary artery and main pulmonary artery identified; (2) branches individually double-ligated and transected. *E.* Division of pulmonary vein. Double ligatures are on inferior pulmonary vein which is to be transected. *F.* Transection of bronchus. This is performed after ligation of pulmonary arteries and veins. Diagram indicates bronchial transection during a left pneumonectomy. (1) Clamp is applied to bronchus distad, and as the bronchus is transected, the proximal end is closed with interrupted sutures in order to avoid a widely open bronchus with its associated ventilatory disturbance; alternately, the bronchus may be closed with an automatic stapler. (2) Progression of bronchial transection. *G.* Pleural flap placed over sutured bronchial stump.

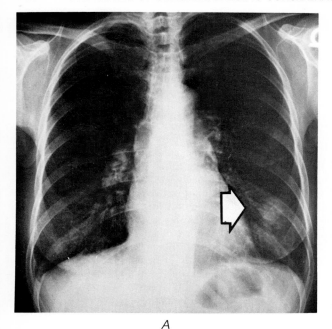

A

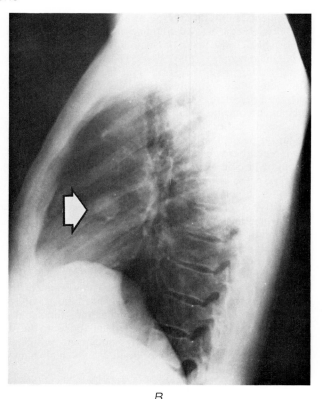

B

Fig. 17-85. A solitary pulmonary nodule. *A* and *B*. The posteroanterior and lateral chest x-rays show a round density in the lingula that had not been present on the patient's previous x-rays. *C*. The lesion is homogeneous, with smooth borders, on tomograms. A wedge resection showed the lesion to be a resolving pulmonary infarct.

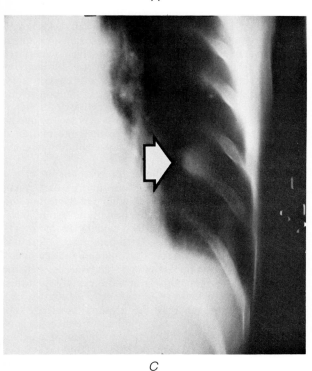

C

bronchial brush biopsy are appropriate, with watchful waiting and close observation for growth or change.

OTHER LUNG TUMORS

BRONCHOPULMONARY NEUROENDOCRINE TUMORS. Both Warren et al. and Benfield's group have recently presented analyses utilizing contemporary electron mi-croscopic and immunohistochemical techniques to demonstrate the continuum that exists from carcinoids to small-cell undifferentiated lung cancers (SCLC). It now seems clear that this group of tumors are all neuroendocrine neoplasms arising from Kulchitsky cells. At the benign end of the spectrum, the bronchopulmonary carcinoid histologically resembles the carcinoid tumors of the small intestine. Along with cylindroma and mucoepidermoid tumors, the bronchial carcinoid was formerly referred to as a bronchial adenoma. This designation was awkward because the term adenoma implied a fundamental quality of benignancy that was not in keeping with the high incidence of malignant behavior shown by cylindroma and mucoepidermoid tumors. Further, a small proportion of bronchial carcinoids will metastasize to regional lymph nodes, with the result that reference was occasionally made to "metastasizing bronchial adenomas."

Over 80 percent of carcinoids arise in proximal bronchi, but peripheral origin beyond cartilage-containing bronchi does occur. The tumors grow slowly and protrude into the bronchial lumen making signs and symptoms of bronchial obstruction the principal clinical presentation. Unusual vascularity may cause hemoptysis as

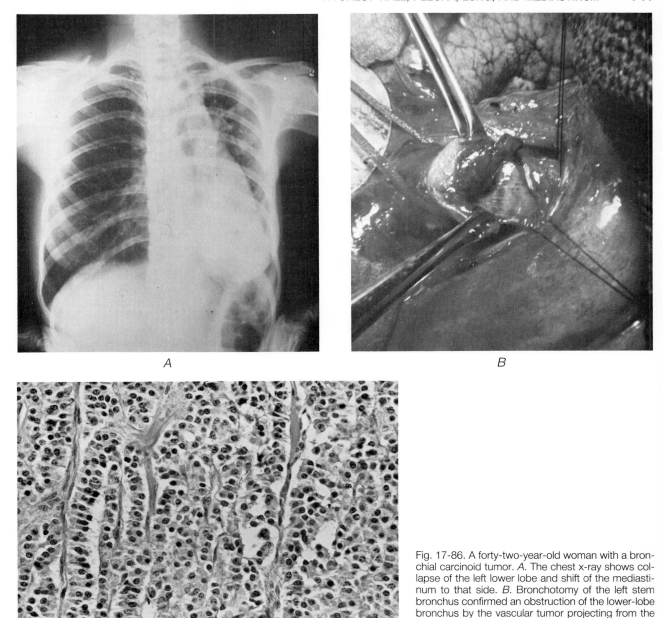

A

B

C

Fig. 17-86. A forty-two-year-old woman with a bronchial carcinoid tumor. *A*. The chest x-ray shows collapse of the left lower lobe and shift of the mediastinum to that side. *B*. Bronchotomy of the left stem bronchus confirmed an obstruction of the lower-lobe bronchus by the vascular tumor projecting from the bronchus between the Allis clamps. *C*. Histologic examination of the neoplasm showed it to be a benign carcinoid tumor. (×400.)

a presenting complaint (Fig. 17-86). The vascularity gives the tumor a deep pink or red color when visualized through a bronchoscope.

The extent of bronchial-wall involvement is variable, but there is usually invasion of the underlying cartilages. Rarely, direct extension through the bronchial wall can result in invasion of mediastinal structures. Regional lymph-node deposits are found in approximately 10 percent of patients, liver metastases more rarely. In keeping with the neuroendocrine origin of these tumors, a few patients with bronchial carcinoid have Cushing-like syndromes that seem attributable to the tumor.

Although the average age of patients with a carcinoid tumor is approximately forty years, the neoplasm does occur in children. Commonly, the clinical presentation is a result of bronchial obstruction with infestation and pulmonary atelectasis. Sputum cytology is negative, but more than 80 percent of the lesions can be visualized by bronchoscopy. The carcinoid syndrome is seen rarely and can occur without extrathoracic metastases. It is wise to

LEFT BRONCHIAL TREE

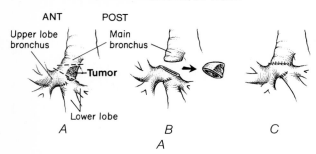

RIGHT BRONCHIAL TREE

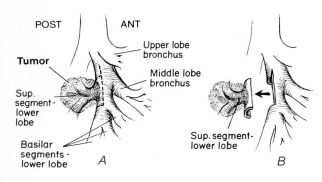

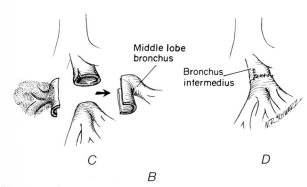

Fig. 17-87. Operative procedures to conserve pulmonary tissue in patients with bronchial carcinoid. *A.* Sleeve resection of tumor from left main bronchus. *B.* Superior segmentectomy and middle lobectomy with bronchial anastomosis. (From: *Jensik RJ, Faber LP, et al: Bronchoplastic and conservative resectional procedures for bronchial adenoma. J Thorac Cardiovasc Surg 68:556, 1974, with permission.*)

measure urinary 5-HIAA excretion and blood serotonin level, but these can be clearly elevated without corresponding symptoms.

The treatment for bronchial carcinoid tumor is surgical resection. Neither the primary neoplasm nor lymph-node metastases, when they occur, are sensitive to radiation therapy. Though lobectomy is an acceptable operation, most surgeons, in view of the low potential for malignancy of the carcinoid neoplasm, now recommend more conservative procedures such as sleeve resection or local bronchial excision with bronchoplasty whenever feasible (Fig. 17-87). The expected long-term survival rate is over 90 percent.

TUMORS OF BRONCHIAL GLAND ORIGIN. Cylindroma, or adenocystic carcinoma, and mucoepidermoid tumors are the commonest neoplasms arising from the bronchial glands. Their location is predominantly central, and they are said to take origin only from bronchi containing cartilage. Both neoplasms may show a spectrum of behavior from benign to malignant, with regional and distant metastases. The treatment is surgical resection, including en bloc removal of regional lymph nodes when possible. Though the long-term cure rate is considerably higher than that of primary carcinoma of the lung, it does not equal the results in bronchial carcinoid.

Other rare tumors of bronchial gland origin are occasionally reported; the majority seem to be forms of adenocarcinoma.

CARCINOSARCOMA. Making up less than 1 percent of lung cancers, the carcinosarcoma consists of both epithelial and mesenchymal types of tissue, and electron microscopy has confirmed that the sarcomatous elements are not simply transformed components of epithelial origin. The term blastoma has recently been used for some tumors that show histologic evidence of association with embryonal tissue.

Carcinosarcomas may be located in the lung periphery or in proximal bronchi, and they have been reported in a wide age range, including children. In a recent interview of the Mayo Clinic experience, Davis et al. found these tumors occurred typically in tobacco addicts in the sixth decade of life. Of their 17 patients, 15 were resected with curative intent; the median survival was 1 year and only two patients were alive to begin their second year following resection.

SARCOMA. A variety of mesodermal sarcomas and tumors of reticuloendothelial origin may occur in the lungs. As a group these tumors represent approximately 1 percent of all primary neoplasms removed at operation. The age range of presentation is considerably wider than that for bronchogenic carcinoma, and the tumors may arise anywhere in the lung or bronchial tree. Difficulty with true histologic identification of the neoplasms is not rare, and they may be mistaken for highly undifferentiated carcinomas or metastatic neoplasms.

In general, the symptoms may be the same as those expected with primary carcinomas, but there is no distinct association with cigarette smoking. When the tumors develop as intrabronchial polypoid neoplasms, the symptoms of bronchial obstruction lead to earlier diagnosis and, therefore, a relatively higher cure rate after resection. Leiomyosarcomas, for example, had a 5-year cure rate of approximately 40 percent in McNamara's report.

Lymphosarcoma and reticulum cell sarcoma may rarely develop in the lung without evidence of tumor elsewhere. Routine chest x-rays discover an asymptomatic pulmonary lesion in a number of patients; other lesions become symptomatic because of pressure of the growing tumor or lymph nodes on adjacent structures. There is no characteristic radiographic appearance, and the diagnosis is rarely suspected from sputum cytology or bronchoscopy. Percutaneous needle biopsy may give the diagnosis with either neoplasm.

A sufficient number of lymphosarcomas are localized to make the prognosis good after pulmonary resection. A 5-year survival exceeding 50 percent may be anticipated, but the results with reticulum cell sarcoma are not as good because the neoplasm is less often resectable.

Hodgkin's disease frequently involves the lung, and a rare patient is seen in whom a solitary pulmonary lesion is unassociated with other evidence of tumor. If resection has been performed, the patient should have complete staging of the disease so that decisions regarding additional therapy can be made.

Fibrosarcoma, rhabdomyosarcoma, neurofibrosarcoma, and other tumors of mesodermal origin may occur rarely in the lung but without specific clinical presentation. The treatment is surgical resection, and the prognosis depends on the stage at which the neoplasm was discovered.

BENIGN TUMORS. Primary or metastatic cancers make up 99 percent of all pulmonary tumors, and benign tumors are a relatively small fraction of the other 1 percent. Among that group of rare tumors, the hamartoma (chondroadenoma) is the commonest. Though occasionally seen in children, they usually appear in men in their fifth to sixth decades, produce no symptoms, and are found in the periphery of dependent portions of the lungs (Fig. 17-88). The characteristic marblelike feel of these cartilaginous tumors makes it is usually possible to simply enucleate them; wedge resection may be preferred if the physical findings leave the surgeon uncertain about the diagnosis. Epithelial elements are generally present, and there may be fat, muscular, or fibrous tissue interspersed.

Since benign tumors can theoretically occur wherever the cells from which they might arise are present, a wide variety of other exceedingly rare tumors are occasionally reported. They can be epithelial (tumorlet and papilloma), mesenchymal (fibroma, leiomyoma, lipoma, hemangioma, lymphangioma, neuroma, and rhabdomyoma), or lymphoid (plasmacytoma, lymphocytoma, plasma cell granuloma). Neurofibromas may occur, particularly in patients with neurofibromatosis. The significance of these tumors is almost exclusively related to the differential diagnosis from malignancies. When these neoplasms develop in a major bronchus, they may obstruct and present with the effects of chronic infection.

METASTATIC TUMORS

Metastases to the lungs are common during the clinical course of many uncontrolled primary neoplasms of extrathoracic origin. Metastases may become apparent some time after primary extrathoracic tumors have been controlled. Surgical resection of one or more pulmonary metastases can result in a significant 5-year survival rate for patients with several types of carcinomas or sarcomas.

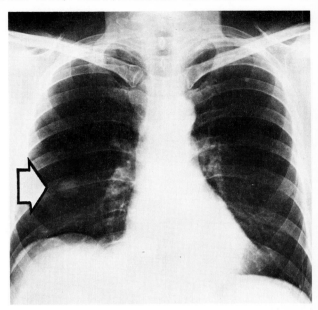

Fig. 17-88. This posteroanterior chest x-ray shows a smooth round density in the midlung field that proved to be a hamartoma when removed by wedge resection.

There has been an increasingly aggressive approach to the management of pulmonary metastases. Previously, recommendations for resection were made only when the metastases appeared a year or more after control of the primary tumor. Many have now reported 5-year survivors among patients who had pulmonary metastasis resected within several months after resection of the primary neoplasm. The cell type of the original tumor and its biologic behavior seem much more relevant in determining prognosis. Morton has shown that the measurement of the tumor doubling time (TDT) provides a clinically useful method for judging the biologic behavior of a neoplasm in the individual patient. From an experience with 60 patients who underwent resection for multiple pulmonary metastases, it was concluded that aggressive surgical resection is indicated when TDT is greater than 40 days. In that series, the estimated 5-year survival was approximately 60 percent for patients whose TDT exceeded 40 days.

Mountain has reviewed a 20-year experience during which 556 patients underwent 722 resections for pulmonary metastases noting an overall 35 percent 5-year survival. Table 17-17 summarizes their results with individual tumor types. In their patients, superior outcome followed use of planned adjuvant therapy. Others have confirmed the value of such adjuvant therapy, particularly in children with sarcomas.

The problem to be considered in a patient who presents with a solitary pulmonary nodule, either synchronous or metachronous with an extrathoracic cancer, is whether it is a metastasis, a primary pulmonary tumor, or a nonneoplastic lesion. In a report on 54 colon cancer patients who had a solitary lung shadow, 25 patients had colon cancer metastases and 29 had primary lung carci-

Table 17-17. SURVIVAL BY CELL TYPE
FOLLOWING RESECTION FOR METASTASES TO
THE LUNG

Cell type	No. of patients		Cumulative percent surviving 5 years
Carcinoma (N = 242)			
Squamous cell carcinoma	75		31.7
Adenocarcinoma	79		40.4
All other carcinoma	88		43.5
Embryoma		9	33.3
Transitional cell		14	41.3
Teratoma		9	63.5
Sarcoma (N = 141)			
Osteogenic sarcoma	56		50.7
Fibrosarcoma	16		37.5
All other sarcoma	69		26.9
Ewing's tumor		7	21.4
Rhabdomyosarcoma		6	16.7
Neurofibrosarcoma		5	60.0
Fibrohistiocytoma		8	37.5

SOURCE: From Mountain, McMurtrey, Hermes, with permission.

noma. Resection of the metastases resulted in a 35 percent 5-year survival. In the absence of strong evidence to support a conclusion that the pulmonary lesion is nonneoplastic, an aggressive surgical approach is warranted under these circumstances.

In the evaluation of patients to be considered for resection of pulmonary metastases, the exclusion of metastases to other sites should be as thorough as possible. Besides the standard radiographic and radioisotopic surveys for metastatic disease, other special procedures may be indicated, depending on the known biologic behavior of the primary neoplasm. Metastatic neoplasm results in positive sputum cytology or positive bronchial washings much less frequently than primary lung cancers. If preoperative confirmation of the diagnosis is imperative, percutaneous needle biopsy may offer the greatest chance for success.

It is always essential to assess the extent of the pulmonary lesions before operation. CT is currently the standard imaging approach to this assessment. Although the survival rate for individuals who had bilateral metastases were not found by Takita to be significantly different (statistically) from those with unilateral metastases, other factors are at play. Urschel and others have advocated a median sternotomy as the preferred approach to patients with bilateral lesions. The results achieved by Takita and his associates with a series of patients having simultaneous resection of bilateral metastases through this incision provide strong support for the single-stage operation.

The extent of pulmonary resection for metastatic lesions is determined by the location of the lesions, the patient's pulmonary function, and the number of metastases. In all cases, as much lung tissue as possible should be preserved. For the majority of patients with metastatic lesions, wedge resections or segmental resections are strongly preferred.

TRACHEA

ANATOMY. The trachea is a centrally located unpaired organ that shares with the heart singular importance in the physiologic matters of moment-to-moment survival. It follows an oblique course from a vulnerable superficial position in the neck deep into the cloistered recesses of the middle mediastinum. The adult trachea has an average length of 11 cm (range 10 to 13 cm) segmented by 18 to 22 cartilaginous rings, and has elliptical internal dimensions averaging 2.3 cm in lateral diameter and 1.8 in anteroposterior diameter. The cricoid cartilage of the larynx, which merges with the first tracheal ring, is the only complete cartilaginous ring. The membranous trachea is a flexible sheet of tissue forming the posterior wall of the trachea between the ends of the rings, and lies against the esophagus. The rigid rings of the anterior two-thirds of the trachea combined with the flexible posterior third impart great flexibility without collapse over a broad range of flexion, extension, and torsion, and maintains patency of the lumen through the extremes of coughing and forced respiration. The loss of cartilaginous support in tracheomalacia allows dynamic collapse and airway obstruction.

The important anterior relationships of the trachea are the thyroid isthmus, lying across the second to third rings, the innominate artery crossing obliquely several more rings distally, and the aortic arch crossing just above the carina. Laterally, the recurrent nerves lie close to the trachea in the tracheoesophageal groove, with the left recurrent following a longer course, joining the trachea just above the carina after passing around the ligamentum arteriosum. Since the blood supply enters laterally, dissection along the trachea is safest when confined to anterior and posterior planes. The major arterial inflow for the cervical trachea comes from the inferior thyroid artery. Lower portions of the trachea are supplied by branches of the bronchial arteries. Small branches from other mediastinal arteries can assume importance following tracheal division, as, for example, the coronary arterial branches that have been shown to provide blood supply to the tracheal anastomosis following heart-lung transplant.

Congenital Lesions

The most common congenital lesion involving the trachea is a tracheoesophageal fistula, the management of which is discussed in detail elsewhere. Congenital tracheal stenosis presents in several variants, all of which are uncommon. Simple weblike diaphragms can be seen, usually at the subcricoid level. Segments of functional stenosis due to tracheomalacia can be seen at sites of compression by a vascular ring or an anomalous pulmo-

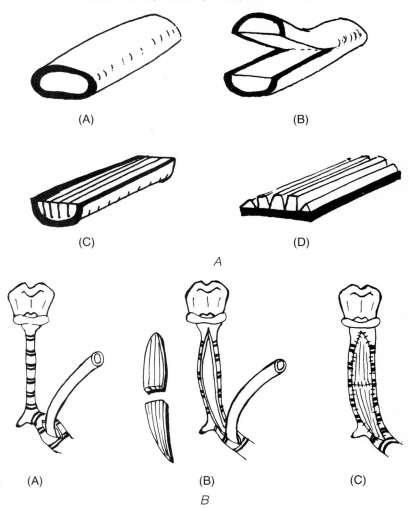

Fig. 17-89. One technique for reconstruction of congenital tracheal stenosis using autologous costal cartilage. *A.* The costal cartilage (A) is longitudinally split (B). Parallel longitudinal slits are made (C) to render the graft flexible (D). *B.* The stenotic trachea (A) is longitudinally opened (B), and the anterior wall reconstructed with the grafts (C). The long-term results with this method are not yet known. (From: *Kimura K, Mukohara N, et al: J Pediatr Surg 17:869, 1982, Figs 3 and 4, with permission.*)

nary artery (pulmonary artery sling). Another variant is characterized by absence of the membranous trachea with fusion of the cartilaginous rings posteriorly over a variable distance, presenting in three principal forms: (1) segmental stenosis; (2) funnel stenosis, in which the distal trachea tapers to a tight stenosis just above the carina; and (3) diffuse hypoplasia of the entire trachea.

DIAGNOSIS. Congenital stenosis should be suspected in any infant with noisy breathing, wheezing, and retractions occurring shortly after birth. The necessary diagnostic evaluation is exhaustive, reflecting the broad differential diagnosis and the association with other anomalies. Radiographic studies include chest films with magnification focused on the trachea, in inspiration and expiration, barium swallow, xeroradiography, CT scan of the neck and mediastinum, and angiography. Inspiratory and expiratory flow-volume curves, echocardiography, bronchoscopy, and bronchography are also frequently helpful. Great care is taken during bronchoscopy to prevent mucosal irritation and edema from converting partial to total obstruction.

TREATMENT. Therapy is individualized to suit the anatomy and the age of the child. Operative treatment is indicated if repeated dilatations or tracheostomy fail to allow growth, and every attempt is made to postpone reconstruction during infancy. When possible, the stenotic segment is resected and the trachea reconstructed with an end-to-end anastomosis. Diffuse involvement presents a greater technical challenge in which successful results have been rare, but recent reports by Nakayama et al. and Kimura et al. have shown that satisfactory reconstructions can be performed using splints constructed from rib or costal cartilage to patch the length of the stenotic segment (Figure 17-89). Perioperative airway management and the maintenance of lumenal patency during healing and remodeling pose major challenges. Relief of tracheal stenosis related to vascular anomalies requires more than simple correction of the vascular anomaly in

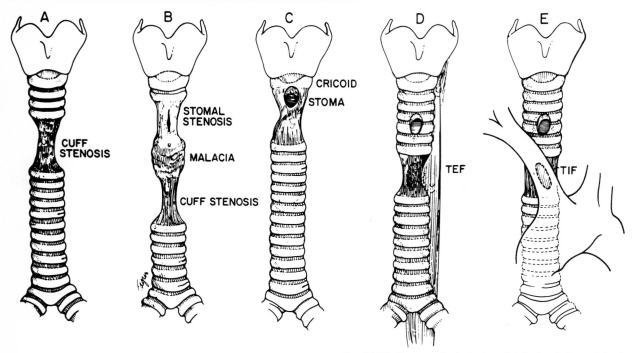

Fig. 17-90. Diagram of principal postintubation lesions. *A.* Lesion at cuff site in a patient who has been treated with an endotracheal tube alone. The lesion is high in the trachea and circumferential. *B.* Lesions that occur with tracheostomy tubes. At the stomal level, anterolateral stenosis is seen. At the cuff level, lower than with an endotracheal tube, circumferential cuff stenosis occurs. The segment between is often inflamed and malacic. *C.* Damage to the subglottic larynx. A high tracheostomy or one that erodes back by virtue of the patient's anatomy may damage the inferior cricoid and produce a low subglottic stenosis as well as an upper tracheal injury. *D.* Tracheoesophageal fistula (TEF). The level of fistulization is usually where the cuff has eroded posteriorly. Occasionally, angulation of the tip of the tube may produce erosion of the tip. There is also usually circumferential damage at this level by the cuff. *E.* Tracheoinnominate fistula (TIF). A high-pressure cuff frequently rests on the trachea directly behind the innominate artery. Erosion may occur, although rarely. The more common innominate artery injury is from a low tracheostomy where the inner portion of the curve of the tube rests in proximity to the artery and causes direct erosion. (From: *Grillo H: J Thorac Cardiovasc Surg 78:860, 1979, Fig 2, with permission.*)

about half of the cases. Simple congenital webs can occasionally be removed bronchoscopically.

Trauma

Blunt and penetrating trauma produce a spectrum of tracheal injury ranging from simple laceration or contusion to complete transection. Hemoptysis, stridor, wheezing, or the presence of subcutaneous air following trauma require that the possibility of tracheal injury be evaluated by bronchoscopy or exploration. Occasionally a primary reconstruction will be indicated, but the more conservative approach of inserting a tracheostomy tube at the site of injury is often more rational.

Currently the most common tracheal injury requiring treatment is that occurring as a complication of tracheal intubation for mechanical ventilation (Fig. 17-90). Modern endotracheal tubes and tracheostomy tubes with soft, low-pressure cuffs have reduced but not eliminated the problem. Ischemic necrosis at the site of the tube cuff or the tube tip can produce a segment of ischemic stricture, a segment of tracheomalacia with functional obstruction during expiration, or erosion and fistula formation with the esophagus or the innominate artery. At the site of a tracheal stoma, exuberant granulations can form a bulky obstruction, or cicatricial healing may form an anterolateral stricture.

Areas of stricture should be carefully defined with radiographic studies that include magnified air contrast examination of the trachea, xeroradiography, and CT scan of the cervical region and upper mediastinum. Particular attention is paid to definition of laryngeal function, which

can be done by fluoroscopy. Bronchoscopy is essential but is often deferred to the time of operation to avoid precipitation of tracheal obstruction in an uncontrolled setting.

TREATMENT. The operative approach for reconstruction of tracheal strictures is similar to that described below for the resection of tracheal neoplasms (Fig. 17-91). The endoscopic laser can be useful for removal of granulation tissue but has no place in the treatment of stricture. Tracheoesophageal and tracheoinnominate fistulas are repaired by separating the two structures, closing the defects, and interposing muscle. For tracheoinnominate fistulas it is usually not necessary to reconstruct the innominate artery; rather the involved segment is resected and the two ends ligated.

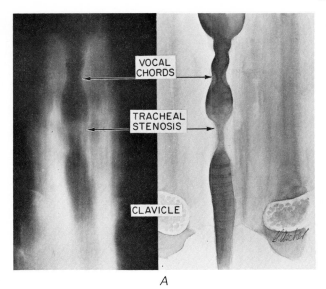

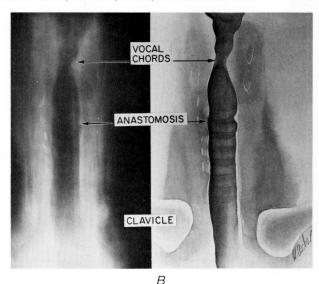

A   *B*

Fig. 17-91. Resection and the anastomosis of the trachea for tracheostomy stomal stenosis. *A.* A tomogram of the cervical trachea demonstrates the area of stenosis. *B.* A postoperative tomogram shows restoration of a normal tracheal lumen after resection and end-to-end anastomosis.

Neoplasms

Primary tracheal neoplasms are uncommon and are outnumbered by tumors that involve the trachea by direct extension from a bronchial, laryngeal, esophageal, or thyroid primary. More than 80 percent of primary tracheal neoplasms are malignant, with squamous cell carcinoma and adenoid cystic carcinoma accounting for the vast majority of histological types. Adenoid cystic carcinoma is radiosensitive and usually slow-growing, even when metastatic, so that resection combined with radiotherapy offers excellent long-term results. Squamous papillomas and fibromas are the most common benign tumors. A variety of rare benign and malignant neoplasms have been identified in the trachea, including carcinoid, chondroma, adenocarcinoma, mucoepidermoid carcinoma, and many others.

DIAGNOSIS. Symptomatic patients with tracheal tumors present with some combination of dyspnea, cough, wheezing, inspiratory stridor, hemoptysis, and recurrent respiratory infections. Chest x-rays can have the detrimental effect of delaying further evaluation because the lung fields are clear, but an alert physician will obtain magnification laminagrams of the trachea and a CT scan of the cervical region and upper mediastinum. Standard pulmonary function testing may be normal, but flow-volume loops can detect airway obstruction. Bronchoscopy is an essential part of the evaluation but is best approached cautiously after maximum information has been obtained from noninvasive methods, because of the potential for precipitation of acute airway obstruction. When approached carefully most tumors can be biopsied endoscopically and a tissue diagnosis confirmed before proceeding with further treatment.

TREATMENT. Resection, tracheostomy, and endoscopic ablation are the invasive options for treatment of tracheal neoplasms. Tracheostomy is pure palliation in patients with inoperable disease. Endoscopic ablation has been gaining favor in recent years because of advances in laser technology.

Laser Endoscopy. Developed in 1960, lasers produce coherent, low-divergence, high-intensity light capable of destroying tissue. As early as 1964, lasers were used experimentally to kill tumor cells. The CO_2 laser was the first of the five major types of laser to be used extensively for resection of neoplasms. The CO_2 laser is very effective for tissue cutting and vaporization, but use in the trachea requires a rigid bronchoscope because the beam cannot be passed through fiberoptic systems. The neodymium-yttrium aluminum garnet (Nd-YAG) laser is currently favored because it is almost as effective as the CO_2 laser and can be used through fiberoptic systems. In several large series recently reported, excellent results have been obtained in 58 to 69 percent of patients treated for unresectable obstructing tumors of the trachea, with quite low morbidity and mortality (Fig. 17-92). In spite of this surge in popularity, it remains unclear whether laser resection offers significant advantages over more traditional methods of palliative endoscopic resection using forceps and cautery, and it may be that laser will prove most useful as an adjunct to such methods. Use of laser ablation as the sole treatment for benign tracheal neoplasms is also controversial.

Another interesting application of laser technology as a preoperative means of increasing resectability has been reported recently by Kato et al. Hematoporphyrin derivatives, which are tumoricidal when stimulated by light and are reported to be preferentially retained by malignant tissues, were injected into 15 patients with lung cancer involving the proximal tracheobronchial tree. After 48 to 72 h photodynamic therapy was performed by directing an argon laser beam on the tumors. The authors assert

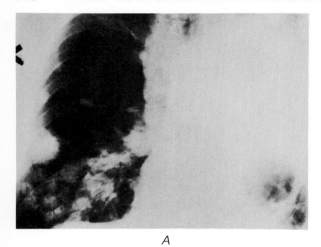

A

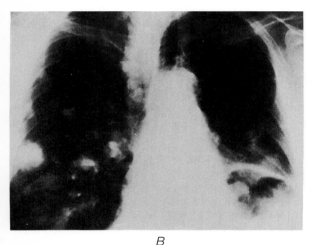

B

Fig. 17-92. *A.* Chest x-ray of a patient with metastatic renal cell carcinoma obstructing the left main-stem bronchus. Note the complete atelectatic opacification of the left lung, and the parenchymal metastases in the right lung. *B.* After Nd-YAG laser ablation of the bronchial lesion the left lung is reexpanded. (From: *Unger M, Atkinson GW: Nd:YAG applications in pulmonary and endotracheal lesions, in Joffe SN, Muckerheide MC, Goldman L (eds): Neodymium-YAG Laser in Medicine and Surgery, chap 9, p 78, Elsevier, 1984, with permission.*)

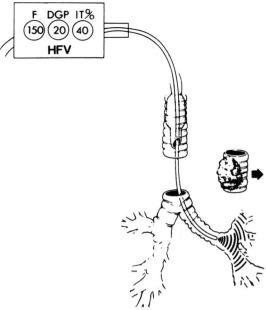

Fig. 17-93. Catheter for high-frequency positive-pressure ventilation ("jet" ventilation) shown passing through the endotracheal tube, across the tracheal lesion, and into the distal left main-stem bronchus. Ventilation is satisfactory with the trachea open, and the field is relatively unobstructed. In the illustration, the high-frequency ventilator (HFV) is set for a frequency of 150 breaths per minute. (From: *El-Baz N, Jensik R, et al: Ann Thorac Surg 34:564, Fig 4, with permission.*)

that four out of five originally inoperable cases became operable and that seven out of ten patients originally thought to require pneumonectomy were treated with lesser resections.

Operative Treatment. Operations on the trachea present both a surgical and an anesthetic challenge. Obstructing lesions make ventilation of the anesthetized patient difficult, and an endotracheal tube offers little advantage because its tip lies above the stenosis. Even when adequate ventilation can be maintained initially, operative manipulation can precipitate complete obstruction and an acute crisis of CO_2 retention, correctable only by the surgeon gaining rapid access to the airway distal to the obstruction. Furthermore, during reconstruction ventilation must be delivered to the lungs beyond the operative field without interfering with exposure. This has traditionally been accomplished by passing sterile endotracheal tubing off the field that can be placed in the distal airway through the open trachea or bronchus.

The ease of ventilation during tracheal reconstruction has been greatly facilitated by the development of high-frequency "jet" ventilation, which is delivered to the distal airway through a small catheter passed through the endotracheal tube (Fig. 17-93). A small tidal volume is delivered at high frequency (60 to 150 breaths/min), maintaining lung expansion, alveolar ventilation, and oxygenation in the normal range. The catheter is small enough to pass through most stenosis and interferes little with exposure.

The choice of incision for tracheal reconstruction depends on the level of involvement, and somewhat on the age of the patient. In a young patient hyperextension of the neck brings more than half the trachea above the suprasternal notch, accessible through a cervical incision. In older patients, it can be difficult to bring more than the first few tracheal rings above the notch. In general, lesions involving the upper half of the trachea are approached through a cervical collar incision, augmented as necessary with a midline upper sternal extension. Lesions involving the lower half can be approached through a

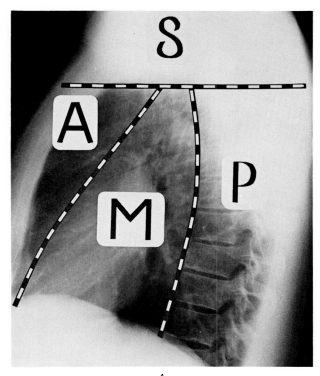

A

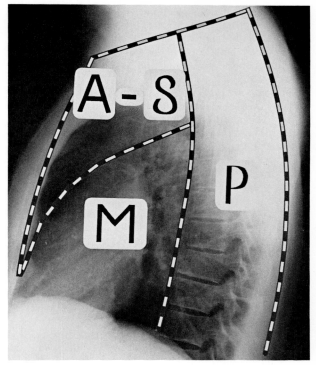

B

Fig. 17-94. The anatomic divisions of the mediastinum. *A*. The traditional classification divides the mediastinum into superior (S), anterior (A), middle (M), and posterior (P) compartments. *B*. A more clinically relevant classification divides the superior compartment between the anterior and posterior compartments. (From: *Burkell CC, Cross JM, et al: Mass lesions of the mediastinum, in Ravitch MM (ed): Current Problems in Surgery. Year Book Medical Publishers, Chicago, 1969, with permission.*)

right posterolateral thoracotomy (Grillo), entering the hemithorax at or above the fifth rib, or through a median sternotomy (Pearson). All cases are preceded by bronchoscopy in the operating room, at which time particularly tight stenoses (lumenal diameter <5 mm) should be dilated to temporarily facilitate anesthesia.

Surprising lengths of trachea can be resected and reconstructed with end-to-end anastomosis. Minimizing tension on the anastomosis is critical and is accomplished by holding the neck in hyperflexion for at least 7 days postoperatively, and by performing a laryngeal release procedure. Care is taken to avoid disturbance of the lateral blood supply, and only 1.5 cm of trachea should be circumferentially dissected on either side of the anastomosis. In most cases, 4.5 to 5 cm of trachea (at least eight rings) should be resectable. A wide variety of complex reconstructions involving the larynx, carina, and both main-stem bronchi have been described in detail by Grillo and others. The use of prosthetic materials for tracheal reconstruction remains anecdotal and experimental. Methods that appeared promising in series reported more than 10 years ago by Neville and by Moghissi have failed to achieve widespread application.

MEDIASTINUM

The mediastinum is the central cavity of the thorax, bounded on either side by the pleural cavities, bounded inferiorly by the diaphragm, and merging superiorly with the thoracic inlet. No compartment of the body carries more physiologic traffic. Many liters of blood pass through the mediastinum each minute, as liters of air, all ingested material and saliva, most autonomic nervous activity, and all of the body's lymphatic fluid pass through the same confined space. Much of the embryologic development of the circulatory, respiratory, and digestive systems takes place within the mediastinum. Congenital, traumatic, inflammatory, and neoplastic processes all find frequent expression in this complex compartment, and produce a broad spectrum of pathology in which anatomic relationships assume paramount importance.

The mediastinum is conveniently divisible along rough anatomic boundaries into subcompartments that contain characteristic lesions. The most traditional classification recognizing four spaces has largely given way to a system recognizing three spaces, which divides the highly overlapping contents of the superior compartment between the more surgically relevant anterior and posterior compartments (Fig. 17-94). In this system the anterior mediastinum lies anterior to the heart and extends cephalad into the anterior half of the thoracic inlet, where it meets the posterior mediastinum. The posterior mediastinum lies behind the heart, extending cephalad into the thoracic inlet where the anterior borders of the upper thoracic vertebrae form its boundary with the anterior mediastinum. The middle mediastinum is the wedge in between, with its base lying on the diaphragm and its apex at the top of the aortic arch.

The anterior mediastinum contains the thymus, along with a variable amount of adipose, areolar, and lymphatic tissue. The middle mediastinum contains the heart and pericardium, aorta, trachea and main-stem bronchi, and associated lymph nodes. The posterior mediastinum contains the descending aorta, the esophagus, autonomic nerve trunks, and the thoracic duct.

The great majority of mediastinal lesions appear as mass lesions radiographically, and most are neoplasms or cysts. A small number of mediastinal mass lesions are inflammatory or infectious. Vascular lesions, such as aneurysms, are considered elsewhere.

Tumors and Cysts

Mediastinal tumors and cysts in adults are distributed by type with similar frequencies in most large series. Neurogenic tumors are most common (about 20 percent), followed closely by thymomas, congenital cysts, and lymphomas. Most series in children from the 1960s and 1970s have reported a predominance of neurogenic tumors as well, followed by lymphoma and cysts, with thymomas rarely seen. In contrast, in a more recent large series of 188 children reported by the Mayo Clinic nearly half of the patients (87) had Hodgkin's or non-Hodgkin's lymphoma, with neurogenic tumors a distant second. Whether this truly reflects a shift in incidence remains to be confirmed. In adult series 25 to 35 percent of all primary tumors of the mediastinum are malignant, and in childhood series the figure is 25 to 45 percent. In either age group the most common malignant tumor is lymphoma, followed in adults in frequency by thymoma and mesenchymal tumors, and in children by neurogenic malignancies.

MANIFESTATIONS AND DIAGNOSIS. Mediastinal masses produce a wide variety of signs and symptoms, and half to one-third of patients are asymptomatic. The most common symptoms are nonspecific (chest pain, cough, dyspnea), and most can be ascribed to compression of adjacent structures, trachea and esophagus in particular. Superior vena caval obstruction, recurrent nerve palsy, and Horner's syndrome are less common examples, but their presence focuses diagnostic attention on the mediastinum. Certain mediastinal tumors are associated with symptomatic endocrine syndromes, such as hypertension (pheochromocytoma), hypercalcemia (parathyroid tumor), thyrotoxicosis (intrathoracic goiter), and gynecomastia (choriocarcinoma). In such cases symptoms have nothing to do with mediastinal location but are systemic consequences of the disease. Pel-Ebstein fevers associated with Hodgkin's disease are a similar example.

The presence of symptoms correlates with malignancy. Ninety-five percent of mediastinal masses that are discovered as incidental radiographic findings are benign, whereas symptomatic lesions are about half benign and half malignant. This correlation is less meaningful in children, whose airways are more vulnerable to compression. In a large series (188 children) from the Mayo Clinic, 78 percent of patients with benign mediastinal masses under age two had symptoms and signs of tracheal compression. Signs and symptoms of nerve compression, such as Horner's syndrome, vocal-cord paralysis, or hemiplegia usually reflect aggressive direct invasion and carry a poor prognosis.

Diagnostic evaluation begins with chest radiography in several views. Simply localizing the mass to one of the three subcompartments of the mediastinum narrows the possibilities (Fig. 17-95) and guides selection of further studies. In most patients the next step is computed tomography (CT), which can sort out the uniform radiographic densities of the mediastinum, identifying normal vascular and soft tissue structures with great cross-sectional clarity. CT of the mediastinum is most diagnostic of benign pathology, such as a cystic mass with an attenuation coefficient close to that of water. The CT appearance of solid malignancies is less definitive, but malignant characteristics such as extension, compression, or invasion are often readily demonstrated. The diagnostic power of CT can be further enhanced by intravascular or intraesophageal injection of contrast. In one series of children with mediastinal abnormalities, CT provided additional diagnostic information in 82 percent of patients, and in 65 percent the CT findings contributed to a change in clinical management.

Magnetic resonance imaging (MRI) is a noninvasive diagnostic modality thought to have great potential for imaging the mediastinum, especially for vascular lesions. Remarkable definition of vascular structures is obtainable in several views, entirely without the need for contrast injection (Fig. 17-96). Early experience has shown somewhat greater difficulty defining soft tissue masses, which tend to appear inhomogeneous or multifocal. The powerful magnetic field employed contraindicates the use of MRI in patients with pacemakers or cerebrovascular metal clips, and complicates examination of critically ill patients on monitors and elaborate life support systems. Fortunately, most metallic hardware likely to occur in the mediastinum (prosthetic valves, vascular clips, sternal wires) does not appear to pose a major hazard.

Plane tomography has been virtually replaced by CT and MRI but can still add useful information, especially in the vicinity of the pulmonary hila. A barium swallow can demonstrate invasion, compression, or displacement of the esophagus, resulting from intrinsic or extrinsic lesions. Arteriography is less frequently necessary with CT and MRI available, but contrast injection of the aorta or pulmonary artery provides information regarding blood supply and anatomic relationship to critical vascular structures that is sometimes not obtainable by any other method. For preoperative evaluation of major vascular disorders (aneurysms), which are discussed elsewhere, angiography is still the diagnostic standard. Venous angiography can provide specific information about the extent of involvement and nature of collateral channels in supe-

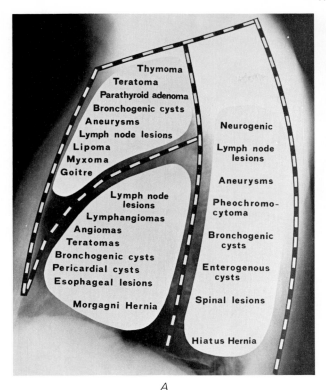

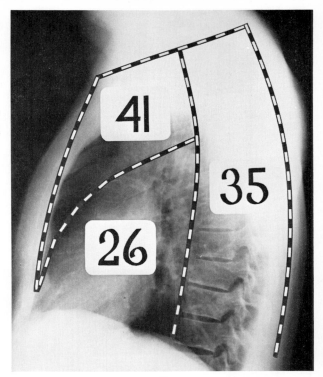

A

B

Fig. 17-95. *A.* Mediastinal lesions tend to occur within specific compartments, although some overlap is evident. *B.* The numbers shown indicate the distribution of lesions in 102 patients reported by Burkell and associates. (From: *Burkell CC, Cross JM, et al: Mass lesions of the mediastinum, in Ravitch MM (ed): Current Problems in Surgery. Year Book Medical Publishers, Chicago, 1969, with permission.*)

rior vena caval obstruction but is difficult to justify unless operation and reconstruction are anticipated. Myelography has been considered an essential part of the evaluation of posterior mediastinal tumors lying very close to the vertebral foramina, but this invasive procedure has also been replaced in many cases by CT of the spine.

Radioisotope scanning can provide very specific information when substernal goiter is suspected. Endoscopy of the esophagus or tracheobronchial tree can add observations on gross displacement or erosion by adjacent mass lesions and can occasionally provide biopsy material. Percutaneous needle biopsy, especially with direct fluoroscopic, ultrasonographic, or CT guidance, can be done safely in cases with favorable anatomy. Mediastinoscopy and mediastinotomy can also be employed for diagnosis.

Recitation of the expanding list of potentially applicable diagnostic procedures promotes the impression that operation is being avoided by assiduous diagnosis. On the contrary, there are still few mass lesions that do not come to operation. The operative mortality for resection of mediastinal lesions is quite low, amounting to 1.8 percent in one large series reported by Oldham and Sabiston. Operation provides definitive diagnosis and frequently

simultaneous definitive treatment, and remains an important part of most combined protocols for chemotherapy and radiation. In most cases the diagnostic armamentarium should be viewed as a means to a comprehensive preoperative evaluation.

NEUROGENIC TUMORS

Neurogenic tumors typically arise from sympathetic ganglia or intercostal nerves and are almost always found in the posterior mediastinum lying in the paravertebral gutter. Peak incidence is in adulthood. Since only 10 to 20 percent of adult neurogenic tumors are malignant, presentation as an incidental finding in an asymptomatic young adult is quite common. A higher proportion (20 to 40 percent) of childhood tumors are malignant. Chest wall pain due to nerve compression or bony erosion is the most common symptom. Hemiparesthesia, hemiparesis, and other signs of spinal cord compression can be seen in tumors with "dumbbell" extension through the intervertebral foramina. Hormonally active tumors are most often childhood malignancies, which can produce hypertension, flushing, diarrhea, diaphoresis, anorexia, and fever.

Neurilemmoma. Neurilemmomas (schwannomas) account for 40 to 60 percent of all neurogenic tumors. They arise from mature Schwann cells in intercostal nerves and have a hard, yellowish, well-encapsulated gross appearance consistent with the fact that most are benign. Some form dumbbell extensions through the intervertebral foramina (Fig. 17-97).

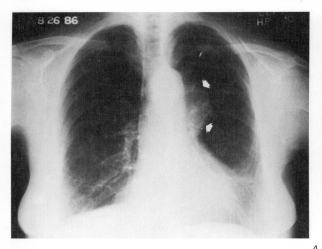

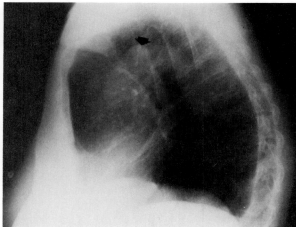

A

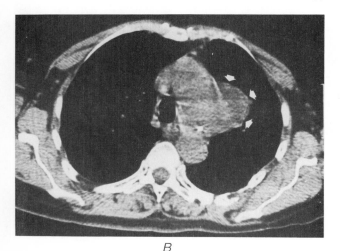

B

Fig. 17-96. *A.* This sixty-four-year-old woman was explored through a left thoracotomy for resection of the mass seen in the middle mediastinum on this chest x-ray *(arrows).* The gross findings were confusing to the surgeon, and the patient was closed and transferred to another institution. *B.* On CT scan the mass could be seen adjacent to the aorta *(see arrows). C.* An MRI scan demonstrated unequivocally that the mass was an aneurysm of the aortic arch, arising proximal to the left subclavian artery. 1 = ascending aorta, 2 = aneurysm, 3 = descending aorta, 4 = left subclavian artery, P = pulmonary artery, L = left atrium. The patient died suddenly while awaiting reoperation.

Neurofibroma. Neurofibromas contain elements of both nerve sheath and nerve cells, and account for about 10 percent of all neurogenic tumors. They are poorly encapsulated, but radiographically resemble neurilemmomas. Mediastinal neurofibromas can be one feature of generalized neurofibromatosis (von Recklinghausen's disease), in which case the risk of malignant degeneration to neurosarcoma is increased. Advanced age also increases the risk of malignancy. Malignancy is present in 25 to 30 percent of tumors of this type, and carries a poor prognosis because of rapid growth and aggressive local invasion.

Neuroblastoma. Neuroblastomas are the most poorly differentiated tumors arising from the sympathetic nervous system. Only about 10 percent occur as a primary lesion in the mediastinum. More than 75 percent occur in children under four years of age, and many are hormonally active, producing vanillylmandelic acid in sufficient quantity to present with a systemic symptom complex often consisting of hypertension, fever, vomiting, and diarrhea. Bone, liver, and lymph-node metastases, as well as direct spinal cord invasion with neurologic deficits, are not infrequent at the time of diagnosis. Tumors presenting in such advanced stages are usually unresectable, but the tumors are generally radiosensitive, and debulking followed by radiation therapy can produce long-term survival. Tumors presenting in the mediastinum and those presenting in the first year of life have a more favorable prognosis.

Ganglioneuroma, Ganglioneuroblastoma. Ganglioneuromas arise from mature nerve cells in sympathetic ganglia and are benign tumors that usually present in a younger age group than tumors of neural sheath origin. Radiographically, ganglioneuromas have a triangular configuration, with the base toward the mediastinum, and may be completely obscured by the vertebrae in the lateral projection. They tend to be poorly encapsulated and can be difficult to resect because of adherence to adjacent structures. Ganglioneuroblastomas consist of a mixture of mature and immature cells, and are rare tumors that share features of neuroblastoma. These are usually seen under three years of age, and are rare in adults.

Paraganglionic Tumors. Pheochromocytomas are chromaffin paraganglionic tumors that characteristically secrete catecholamines. Intrathoracic primaries are un-

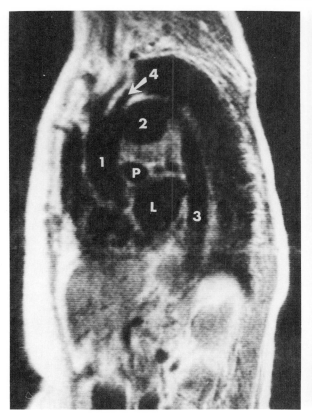
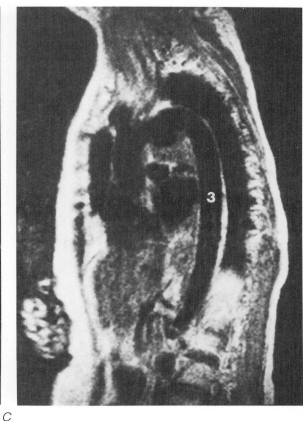

C

Fig. 17-96 *C.* Continued.

usual, occurring in about 1 percent of all pheochromo-cytomas. As with all extraadrenal locations, intraothoracic tumors are more frequently "silent" (nonsecreting) than their adrenal counterparts but are also more often malignant—about 30 percent of extraadrenal pheochromocytomas are malignant. Chemodectomas are nonchromaffin paraganglionic tumors that rarely secrete catecholamines, and arise from chemoreceptor tissue around the aortic arch, vagus, and aorticosympathetics. They are quite rare, and 15 to 30 percent are malignant.

TREATMENT. Operation is indicated in virtually all posterior mediastinal neurogenic tumors. The region is best approached through a standard posterolateral thoracotomy. Benign tumors should be completely excised. Preoperative evaluation of all posterior mediastinal tumors includes careful evaluation of the intervertebral foramina and vertebral bodies, which is most easily done initially with a CT scan, using magnified views as necessary. Myelography may still be required to confirm intraspinal extension (Fig. 17-97). When intraspinal extension exists, it is best to excise that portion first through a laminectomy, to avoid cord compression from intraspinal hemorrhage during the thoracic excision.

Malignant tumors are excised if possible. Radical operations for neuroblastoma are approached selectively, keeping clearly in mind the age of the patient, the radiosensitivity of the tumor, and the possibility of spontane-ous maturation. Resection of an active (secretory) pheochromocytoma requires attention to the perioperative medical management of paroxysmal hypertension.

THYMOMA

In adults thymoma is the most common anterior mediastinal mass, and ranks second in frequency among tumors and cysts of the mediastinum. Thymoma is rare in children and has equal sex distribution, with a peak age incidence between forty and sixty years. About one-third of patients are asymptomatic at the time of diagnosis. Symptomatic patients present either with mass effects on adjacent organs or with systemic effects referable to one of the paraneoplastic syndromes associated with thymoma. Of the former, common examples include cough, chest pain, dyspnea, and superior vena caval obstruction. Of the latter, myasthenia gravis is the most common, although hypogammaglobulinemia and red cell aplasia have been described. It is most often stated that the incidence of myasthenia gravis is 10 to 50 percent in patients with thymoma. Conversely, thymoma is seen in only 8 to 15 percent of patients with myasthenia gravis. Myasthenic patients with thymoma have a poorer prognosis than patients without thymoma, and are less likely to benefit from thymectomy.

Thymoma does not have a characteristic radiographic

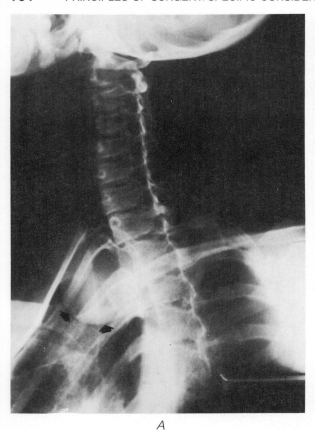

A

Fig. 17-97. This thirty-five-year-old woman complained of neck pain following a minor accident, and had x-rays taken of her cervical spine. *A*. The cervical spine was normal, but a smooth, hemispherical mass (see arrows) was noted incidentally in the apex of the right hemithorax. *B*. Standard views of the chest confirmed the presence of a mass lying high in the posterior mediastinum. *C*. The CT scan showed a homogeneous solid mass lying against the spine. Extension into the intervertebral foramen could not be excluded. *D*. A CT myelogram was obtained. The spinal cord (S) is the radiolucent circle in the center of the spinal canal, surrounded by the dense opacity of myelographic contrast medium. The mass (M) can be seen to enter the T2–3 neural foramen *(large arrow)*, but with no impingement on the spinal canal *(small arrow)*. The mass was resected uneventfully through a high right posterolateral thoracotomy. Pathologic examination proved it to be a neurilemmoma. *(Courtesy of Alfred Jaretzki III.)*

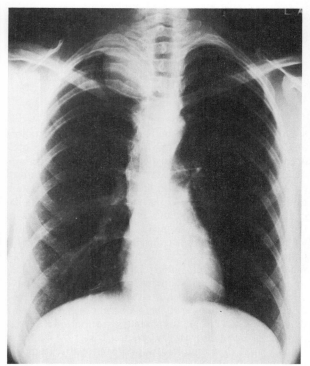

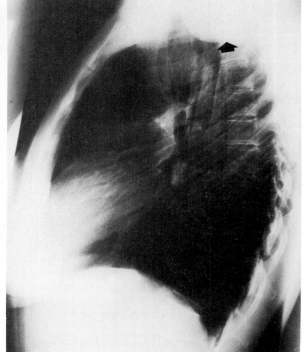

B

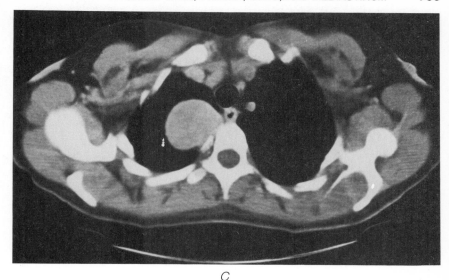

C

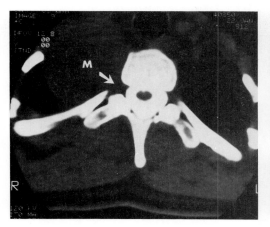

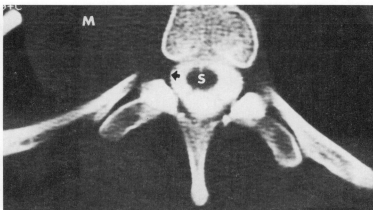

D

Fig. 17-97 *C,D.* Continued.

appearance, and diagnosis is usually made when the mass is excised (Fig. 17-98). The most prevalent histologic classification is based on the relative proportions of lymphocytic and epithelial elements, so that the tumor is described as lymphocytic, epithelial, or mixed. Histology, however, contributes nothing to the distinction between benign and malignant, which is based entirely on invasive gross characteristics. Distant metastases occur but are uncommon. CT scanning can add valuable preoperative radiographic evidence of invasive behavior. Biopsy is not usually recommended because of fear that violation of the capsule might promote invasive behavior, and because almost all such masses deserve an attempt at resection. When the findings suggest that complete resection might be difficult, it is perfectly rational to perform a biopsy followed by radiation or chemotherapy designed to shrink the tumor and simplify later resection.

In most cases resection through a median sternotomy provides the definitive diagnosis. Fifty to sixty-five per-

cent of thymomas are benign and subject to curative resection, which should encompass the entire thymus and all adjacent mediastinal adipose tissue. Truly complete resection is best accomplished with a generous extension into the neck to follow tongues of thymic tissue that commonly extent cephalad. All adjacent nonvital structures invaded by malignant thymoma should also be resected. Postoperative irradiation is of unproved benefit but is generally recommended for patients who have had incomplete resection of a malignant thymoma (Fig. 17-99).

LYMPHOMA

Mediastinal involvement is present in about 50 percent of patients with Hodgkin's and non-Hodgkin's lymphoma, and lymphoma is the most common mediastinal malignancy. Lymphoma is most frequently located in the anterior mediastinum (Fig. 17-100). Hilar nodes in the middle mediastinum are less commonly involved, and

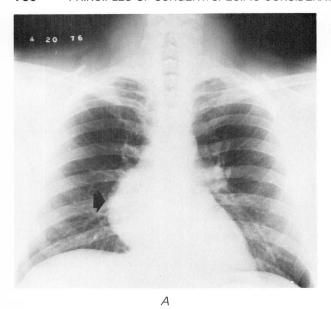

A

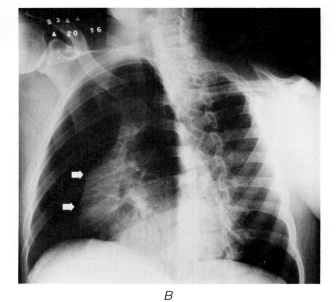

B

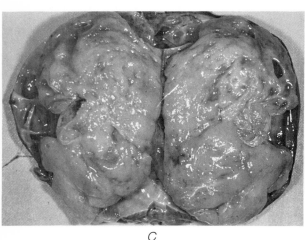

C

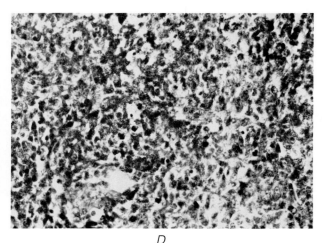

D

Fig. 17-98. A benign thymoma in a thirty-year-old man who presented with a persistent cough. *A.* Chest x-ray shows a large smooth mass contiguous with the right heart border. *B.* An oblique view suggests that the mass is closely related to the pericardium. *C.* The tumor was removed, along with remnants of the thymus, through a high right thoracotomy. This photograph of the bisected tumor shows that it was a well-encapsulated fleshy neoplasm. *D.* Histologic examination of the tumor shows a predominance of lymphocytic elements that justifies its classification as a lymphocytic type of thymoma.

posterior mediastinal location is rare. Radiation is the standard treatment for most lymphomas, and resection is indicated only for the 5 percent of patients with lymphoma whose disease is confined to the mediastinum, underscoring the importance of a thorough search for involved lymphatic tissue elsewhere.

TERATODERMOID TUMORS

Teratomas account for less than 10 percent of all mediastinal tumors, with almost all found in the anterior mediastinum. By definition teratomas consist of multiple tissue types not normally found at the site of the tumor. They are most often partially cystic and consist primarily of ectodermal elements that can include hair, teeth, and sebaceous glands. Teratomas are thought to arise from branchial cleft and pouch cells associated with the thymus. The mediastinum is second to the gonads as the

most frequent location of teratomas in adults. The sex ratio is roughly equal, and age distribution peaks in early adulthood.

In modern series about two-thirds of patients are asymptomatic at presentation, and the majority of symptoms are nonspecific mass effects such as chest pain, cough, and dyspnea. The classic pathognomonic presentation with cough productive of hair and sebum has become a rarity, as most tumors are detected before eroding

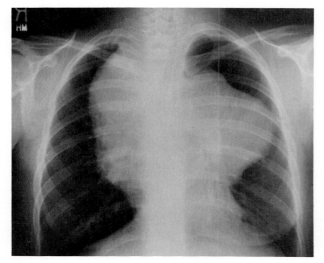

A

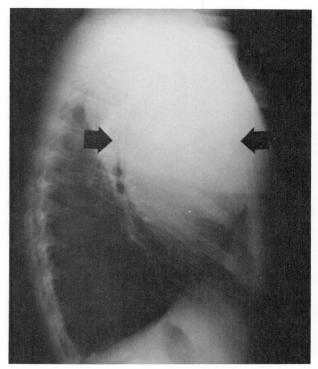

B

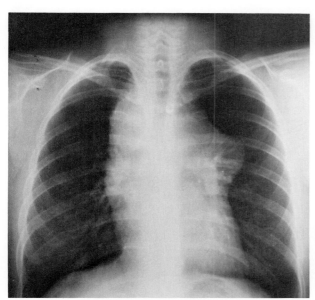

C

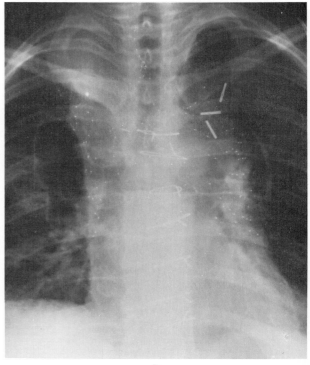

D

Fig. 17-99. A malignant thymoma in a twenty-nine-year-old woman who presented with superior vena caval obstruction and marked tracheal compression. *A*. The initial chest x-ray shows a huge mediastinal mass projecting into both hemithoraces. *B*. In lateral view the mass is seen to lie in the anterior mediastinum, compressing and posteriorly displacing the trachea. A mediastinal biopsy showed thymoma. *C*. After the patient received 2500 rad of external radiation therapy, a repeat chest x-ray shows a significant reduction in the size of the tumor. Symptoms were similarly improved. A subtotal resection was performed through a median sternotomy. The thymoma was found to invade the upper lobes of both lungs, the pericardium, and the areolar tissues of the mediastinum. Residual tumor was implanted with seeds of ^{125}I. *D*. A chest x-ray 1 month after operation shows further reduction in tumor size. The metallic markers of the isotope seeds can be seen throughout the tumor area. The patient has returned to work and is asymptomatic except for a chronic cough.

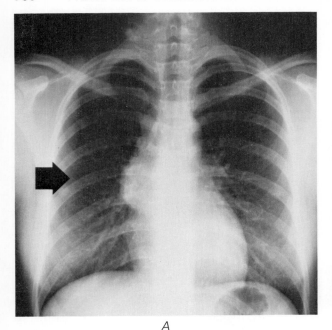

A

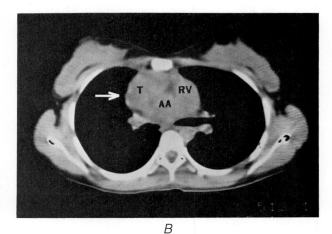

B

Fig. 17-100. Nodular Hodgkin's disease of the mediastinum in an eighteen-year-old woman. *A.* The chest x-ray shows a right mediastinal mass overlying the superior vena cava–right atrial junction. *B.* A CT scan section at the level of the right ventricular outflow tract (RV) shows the intimate relationship of the mass (T) to the ascending aorta (AA).

into the tracheobronchial tree. As with other neoplasms of the region, malignant teratocarcinomas are more likely to present with symptoms related to aggressive invasion of adjacent vital structures.

Typical radiographic appearance is that of a large, well-circumscribed anterior mediastinal mass. Twenty to forty percent of teratomas are calcified, most often appearing as a nonspecific opacity in the cyst wall, although occasionally due to the presence of teeth or bone. CT scanning

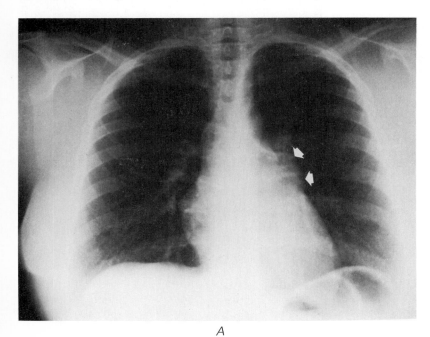

A

Fig. 17-101. *A.* Chest x-ray in an asymptomatic nineteen-year-old woman, demonstrating a mass along the left heart border in the vicinity of the left hilum *(see arrows).* The lateral (not shown) suggested that the mass was in the anterior mediastinum. *B.* A CT scan without contrast shows a mass with small islands of calcification lying in the anterior mediastinum against the left side of the heart. There is a faint lucency *(see arrows)* suggesting that pericardium separates the mass from the heart. *C.* A CT scan with intravascular contrast injection suggests that the mass (M) is adjacent to but separate from the pulmonary artery (P) and right ventricular outflow tract. Through a median sternotomy a benign teratoma was removed easily along with the left lobe of the thymus. *(Courtesy of Alfred Jaretzki III.)*

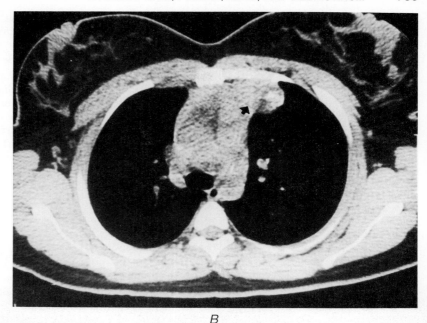

B

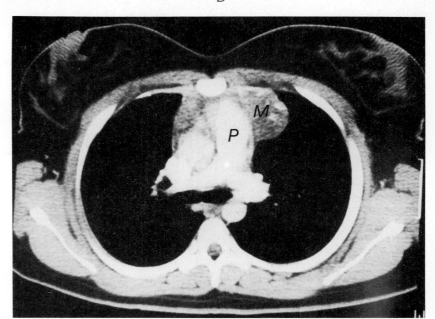

C

Fig. 17-101 *B,C.* Continued.

is very helpful in delineating involvement of adjacent structures, and in confirming fat density in the center of the cystic mass (Fig. 17-101). Elevated serum levels of alpha-fetoprotein and carcinoembryonic antigen suggest malignancy.

Surgical excision through a median sternotomy is the best method of diagnosis and treatment. Eighty percent are benign, and resection is curative. Even with benign forms resection is made more difficult by the tendency for the tumors to be densely adherent to surrounding struc-

tures, most commonly pericardium, lung, great vessels, and thymus, and incomplete resection is occasionally necessary. For benign tumors recurrence is rare even following partial excision. The prognosis for malignant tumors is poor because of local recurrence and distant metastasis.

GERM-CELL TUMORS

Primary extragonadal germ-cell tumors are rare. Although they can be seen in the pineal, sacrococcygeal, and paraaortic regions, they are most often found in the anterior mediastinum, where they comprise less than 1 percent of all mediastinal tumors. The histogenesis of germ-cell tumors outside the gonads is poorly understood, but a theory of origin from pluripotential primordial germ cells in the mediastinum is favored. Mediastinal teratoma should probably be viewed as the end point of benign differentiation in this germ-cell line but is usually considered separately because clinical behavior is quite different.

Five distinct cell types are recognized. Seminoma and embryonal cell carcinoma are most common, followed by choriocarcinoma, malignant teratoma, and endodermal sinus (yolk sac) carcinoma. These tumors are usually seen in young adults, with a male to female ratio of at least 4:1. Since the tumors are highly malignant, it is not surprising that 80 to 90 percent of patients are symptomatic when the diagnosis is made. The most frequent symptoms are nonspecific and result from tumor expansion encroaching on adjacent structures to produce cough, dyspnea, chest pain, or superior vena caval syndrome.

Standard posteroanterior and lateral chest roentgenograms will detect over 90 percent of such tumors. A CT scan can provide very helpful preoperative information regarding anatomic relationships and local invasion but does not substitute for exploration or biopsy. Serum tumor markers, while not specifically diagnostic, are important to obtain prior to treatment as a basis for monitoring relapse and response to treatment. All patients with choriocarcinoma have elevated serum human chorionic gonadotropin (HCG) levels, as will some patients with seminoma and embryonal cell carcinoma. Alpha fetoprotein levels can be elevated, most commonly in embryonal cell tumors, and carcinoembryonic antigen levels are occasionally elevated in all cell types.

The possibility of metastasis from a gonadal tumor must be excluded before a mediastinal germ-cell tumor is declared primary. Primary gonadal tumors rarely metastasize only to the mediastinum, and most often spread through retroperitoneal lymphatics. A gonadal primary can be excluded with reasonable accuracy if there is no evidence of retroperitoneal involvement by CT scan or lymphangiography, and if gonadal nodules are not detectable by palpation or ultrasound examination.

Most patients with mediastinal germ-cell tumors deserve exploration through a median sternotomy and an attempt at complete resection. In a recent large series from the Mayo Clinic, complete resection was achieved in 44 percent of 56 cases. The remainder frequently present with evidence of widespread local invasion or distant metastasis, and are subject to partial resection or to biopsy alone. It is important to separate seminoma from the other tissue types because of its radiosensitivity and generally better prognosis. Five-year survival is about 75 percent for seminoma treated with aggressive resection, followed by irradiation for local disease left behind, and chemotherapy for distant metastases. Prognosis remains poor in the other tissue types, although various protocols

of combination chemotherapy have provided increasingly successful palliation.

MESENCHYMAL TUMORS

Tumors of mesenchymal origin constitute about 7 percent of all mediastinal tumors and cysts, with most occurring in the anterior mediastinum. Lipomas are most common and are characteristically soft masses without fixation to surrounding structures that can reach enormous size without producing symptoms. Fibromas are more dense and less common but have similar clinical behavior. The malignant forms (liposarcoma and fibrosarcoma) are seen rarely.

Tumors of lymph-vascular and blood-vascular origin are also classified as mesenchymal neoplasms. Tumors of blood-vascular origin consist of hemangiomas (capillary, cavernous, and venous) and rare malignant hemangiopericytomas. The most common lymph-vascular tumor is a lymphangioma (cystic hygroma). Most vascular tumors present as smooth, often lobulated masses of uniform density on chest x-ray, and will appear as cystic masses on CT scan.

The complete list of mesenchymal mediastinal tumors also includes mesothelioma, hamartoma, myxoma, mesenchymoma, leiomyoma, and leiomyosarcoma, xanthogranuloma, and rhabdomyosarcoma.

ENDOCRINE TUMORS

Thyroid and parathyroid tumors appearing in the mediastinum are most properly considered within the context of their usual cervical manifestations. Less than 10 percent of parathyroid adenomas are located in the mediastinum, and most are approachable through a cervical incision. Because of their embryologic origin from the third branchial cleft they are usually in close association with the upper pole of the thymus gland. Parathyroid tumors rarely present as a mediastinal mass.

Similarly, mediastinal thyroid tissue is usually a direct substernal extension of the cervical gland. Aberrant mediastinal thyroid tissue with agenesis of the cervical gland is exceedingly rare but does provide the rationale for obtaining a radionuclide thyroid scan in any patient with an undiagnosed mass high in the anterior mediastinum.

MEDIASTINAL CYSTS

Congenital cysts constitute approximately 20 percent of all primary mediastinal mass lesions, and account for the vast majority of middle mediastinal primary lesions. On chest x-ray they appear as opaque densities that may be indistinguishable from neoplasms except on the basis of typical location. On CT scan a mass with near water density occurring in a characteristic location is virtually diagnostic, and provides a strong rationale for routine use of CT scanning in mediastinal lesions. In a recent review of experience with mediastinal cysts in 34 children, Snyder et al. found that the accuracy of their preoperative diagnosis increased from 50 percent before the use of CT scanning to 100 percent thereafter.

Pericardial Cysts. These cysts are the most common type occurring in the mediastinum. They are usually detected as an incidental finding in an asymptomatic patient, and very frequently appear at the right costophrenic angle as a smooth-walled cystic mass 3 to 6 cm in diameter. They contain a clear fluid and occasionally communicate with the pericardium. Histologically they are lined with a single layer of mesothelial cells. The location and appearance of pericardial cysts are so characteristic, especially on CT scan, that close observation is becoming a defensible option, although most are still resected for diagnosis.

Bronchogenic Cysts. Bronchogenic cysts are most frequently located just posterior to the carina or main-stem bronchi, although they can be found elsewhere in the mediastinum or more peripherally in the lung (Fig. 17-102). Communication with the tracheobronchial tree can occur to produce an air-fluid level, serving to distinguish them completely from pericardial cysts but allowing for confusion with lung or mediastinal abscess in certain cases. Chest x-ray and CT scan will usually demonstrate a cystic mass in the characteristic location, although bronchogenic cysts can contain a viscid fluid difficult to distinguish from a solid mass by CT scan alone. A contrast esophagram may show compression of the esophagus by an anterior mass. Histologically they are lined with ciliated respiratory epithelium, and contain varying amounts of cartilage, smooth muscle, and mucous glands. They are most frequently symptomatic in children, producing cough, dyspnea, and stridor in more than half. All bronchogenic cysts should be resected, and are usually approached through a posterolateral thoracotomy. Especially when they have formed a communication with the tracheobronchial tree, the chronic infection that frequently results can make resection through dense inflammatory adhesions very difficult.

Enteric Cysts. Enteric cysts are located in the posterior mediastinum adjacent to the esophagus. They are occasionally embedded in the muscularis of the esophagus but rarely communicate with the esophageal lumen. The cysts have a smooth wall with a muscular coat and a lining recognizable as intestinal mucosa, although it may be ciliated, and they contain a clear, colorless mucoid fluid. When lined with an aberrant gastric mucosa, peptic ulceration can lead to perforation of adjacent bronchus or esophagus, producing hemoptysis or hematemesis, and erosion into adjacent lung can produce a lung abscess. A rare association with vertebral anomalies has been described in which the enteric cyst is attached to the spinal cord of meninges, and a patent tract may exist that can be demonstrated by myelography.

Approximately 60 percent of enteric cysts are recognized under one year of age, when symptoms of tracheal and esophageal compression are prominent. Less than one-third of children with enteric cysts are asymptomatic. Complete evaluation of children with a suggestive presentation includes chest x-ray and esophagram followed by a CT scan with contrast in the esophagus. Resection is always indicated. The lesions are approached through a posterolateral thoracotomy with the choice of side determined by the level of involvement and the appearance of projection into either hemithorax.

Mediastinitis

ACUTE MEDIASTINITIS

Acute mediastinitis is a fulminant infectious process with high morbidity and mortality characterized by rapid spread through the areolar planes of the mediastinum. The mediastinal pleura confines the process to the mediastinum only temporarily, with a breach occurring into one or both pleural cavities early in the course of the infection in most cases, after which the negative pressure of the pleural space helps to rapidly spread the infection throughout. The rapid spread of infection is promoted by several factors. One is the separation of tissue planes produced by air forced into soft tissues adjacent to a perforated hollow viscus, most often the esophagus, further promoted by the digestive action of salivary and gastric enzymes. Another is the pressure gradient established from the atmosphere to the negative pressure of the pleural space once the pleura is penetrated, which tends to pull the infection through the mediastinum from its source and into the pleural space. A third factor is the presence of naturally continuous fascial planes connecting the deep cervical compartments with the mediastinum, along which oropharyngeal infection can spread.

The infection is initiated most frequently by esophageal perforation, resulting from instrumentation, trauma, foreign body, suture line leak, or spontaneous postemetic rupture (Boerhaave's syndrome). Tracheal rupture or perforation is a less common cause in which dissemination of air through the soft tissues is massive, and infection is likely to be a secondary development. Direct necrotizing spread of infection without violation of an intrathoracic viscus is seen most commonly with aggressive oropharyngeal infections involving the deep cervical space but has also been described in association with infections of ribs, sternum, and vertebrae.

Chest pain, dysphagia, respiratory distress, and cervical–upper thoracic subcutaneous crepitus are the chief hallmarks of the process during the earliest stages of infection, when it is most important to diagnose the problem and begin treatment. Evidence of fulminant systemic infection is certain to appear within 24 h, and florid sepsis with hemodynamic instability supervenes rapidly in untreated cases.

The chest x-ray may be normal very early in the process, although mediastinal and subcutaneous air becomes apparent in most cases. The mediastinal contour is usually wide, and pleural effusion with or without pneumothorax appears very frequently. A contrast esophagram, for which water-soluble contrast is usually recommended, is essential when esophageal perforation is known or suspected. Esophagoscopy is rarely indicated in acute perforation. Specific diagnostic and therapeutic

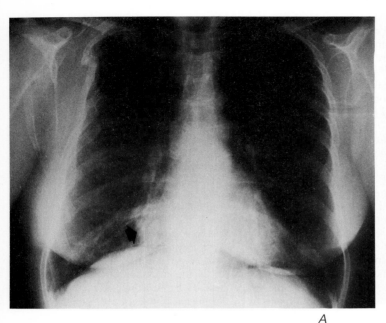

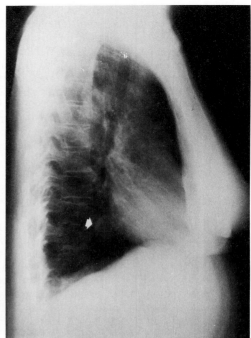

A

B

approaches to esophageal perforation are dealt with else-where.

Infections resulting from esophageal perforation and those descending from a perioral source are usually caused by a mixture of gram-positive and gram-negative aerobic and anaerobic organisms representing the spec-trum of oral flora. Initial antibiotic coverage should be broad enough to cover all possibilities until cultures are available.

Fig. 17-102. This forty-one-year-old woman had chest x-rays ob-tained during a mild respiratory illness. She was otherwise asymp-tomatic. *A.* A smoothly circumscribed mass is visible along the right heart border near the pericardiophrenic angle, and is seen in the middle mediastinum on the lateral view *(see arrows). B.* A magnified view from the CT scan shows a mass (M) of intermediate density lying just anterior to the spine, and just to the right of the aorta (A). The mass was resected through a right posterolateral thoracotomy, and was found to be a bronchogenic cyst, lined with respiratory epithelium. *(Courtesy of DM Carberry.)*

Treatment must be early and aggressive. Antibiotics and fluid resuscitation are begun immediately. Chest tubes are placed for pneumothorax or effusion. The primary problem, such as esophageal perforation, is treated according to accepted principles, either separately or in combination with drainage procedures. Direct drainage of the neck is occasionally required, entering the deep cervical space through an incision parallel to the sternocleidomastoid muscle and retracting the muscle laterally to expose the carotid sheath and pretracheal and retrovisceral spaces. Unilateral and often bilateral thoracotomy is frequently necessary for direct mediastinal drainage, debridement, and accurate placement of drainage tubes. In rare instances, especially in chronic contained posterior mediastinal infection, drainage is established by approaching the mediastinum extrapleurally through the bed of the posterior end of an overlying rib.

Mediastinitis is seen in 1 to 4 percent of patients following open heart surgery and has accounted for an increasingly large proportion of all cases of mediastinitis as open heart procedures have increased in frequency. It follows a more indolent course than the entities discussed above, is rarely associated with crepitus and mediastinal air on x-ray, and has the bacteriologic spectrum of other wound infections, with *Staphylococcus aureus* and *S. epidermidis* predominating. In recent years the use of muscle flaps rotated into the sternal defect has greatly improved the treatment of this complication, which is discussed more properly in detail as a specific complication of open heart surgery.

CHRONIC MEDIASTINITIS

Chronic inflammation and fibrosis in the mediastinum (sclerosing mediastinitis, fibrosing mediastinitis) are thought to result most often from granulomatous infection such as tuberculosis or histoplasmosis, although identification of an organism in individual patients is rare. It has been postulated that the process begins as an inflammatory reaction in the tissues surrounding involved lymph nodes. The process is likely to remain clinically silent unless it progresses to produce obstruction of the esophagus, airways, superior vena cava, or other mediastinal vascular structures. The chest x-ray may show mediastinal widening but is often normal. CT scanning combined with angiography may be necessary to define the process. Operative exploration is frequently required just to establish a diagnosis, and can also be undertaken to relieve obstruction.

Superior Vena Caval Obstruction

Superior vena caval obstruction is caused by bronchogenic carcinoma in 85 percent of cases. In the remainder the cause is another mediastinal tumor, fibrosing mediastinitis, thoracic aortic aneurysm, or caval thrombosis secondary to chronic indwelling catheters or instrumentation. At least 40 percent of bronchogenic carcinomas producing superior vena caval obstruction are small-cell tumors. Obstruction can be caused by compression or direct invasion. The clinical syndrome produced is easily recognizable, consisting of venous distention, facial edema, and plethora, often accompanied by headache and respiratory symptoms. In rare cases, associated airway compression or laryngeal edema can be life-threatening, but there is otherwise little evidence to support the commonly held notion that superior vena caval obstruction is inherently dangerous. Seizures, intracranial venous thrombosis, and other nonspecific cerebral consequences are unusual and highly associated with the presence of brain metastases. Survival in patients with obstruction due to carcinoma is usually measured in weeks to months, and it can be difficult to separate the dismal prognosis and aggressive behavior of the primary disease from the effects of superior vena caval obstruction alone. As with venous obstruction elsewhere in the body, compensatory venous collaterals develop promptly and largely ameliorate the condition, a fact that also complicates objective assessment of treatment modalities.

The vascular diagnosis can be confirmed by venography, but CT scanning with venous contrast is equally effective, and provides additional information regarding surrounding structures that can be diagnostically valuable. More invasive diagnostic procedures, such as mediastinoscopy, bronchoscopy, and lymph-node biopsy, have long been considered hazardous because of elevated venous pressure. A recent comprehensive review by Ahmann suggests that virtually all invasive procedures can be done with a low incidence of excessive bleeding. Respiratory complications related to venous engorgement and edema of the tracheobronchial mucosa can occur but are almost always manageable in the hands of a careful anesthesiologist. The very dominant clinical tradition favoring emergency radiation therapy for the clinical syndrome prior to obtaining a tissue diagnosis deserves reappraisal.

Especially since the vast majority of cases are caused by an incurable neoplasm, palliative radiation with or without combination chemotherapy is by far the most common treatment modality. The rare cases of benign etiology have occasionally been treated with venous bypass, but without large numbers of reportable patent conduits. Bypasses from the jugular vein to the atrium or distal superior vena cava have been accomplished with femoral vein and with a spiral graft constructed from excised saphenous vein (Fig. 17-103). Saphenojugular bypass has also been described, in which the saphenous vein is routed to the neck through a subcutaneous tunnel and left attached at the saphenous bulb for outflow. All invasive treatments have in common the difficulty of predicting which patients will be unable to establish sufficient venous collaterals over time without operation.

Bibliography

Introduction

Meade RH: *A History of Thoracic Surgery*. Springfield, IL, Charles C Thomas, 1961.
Ravitch MM: *A Century of Surgery 1880–1980*. Philadelphia, Lippincott, 1981.

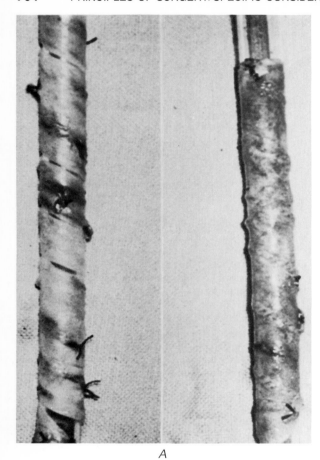

A

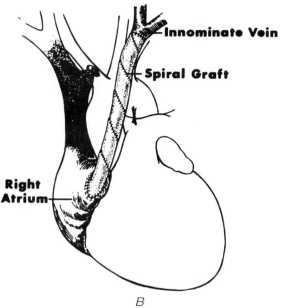

B

Fig. 17-103. Technique of spiral vein graft for bypass of superior vena caval obstruction. *A.* The spiral vein graft is constructed from a saphenous vein that has been opened from one end to the other and wrapped around a tubular stent (left). The opposing edges of vein are sewed together in a continuous spiral with fine monofilament suture (right). *B.* The spiral graft connects the innominate vein to the right atrial appendage. (From: *Doty DB, Baker WH: Bypass of the superior vena cava with spiral vein graft. Ann Thorac Surg 22:492, 1976, with permission.*)

Anatomy of the Thorax

Anderson JE: *Grant's Atlas of Anatomy,* 8th ed. Baltimore, Williams & Wilkins, 1983.

Blevins CE: Anatomy of the thorax and pleura, in Shields TW (ed): *General Thoracic Surgery,* 2d ed. Philadelphia, Lea & Febiger, 1983.

Thoracic Incisions

Asaph JW, Keppel JF: Midline sternotomy for the treatment of primary pulmonary neoplasms. *Am J Surg* 147:589, 1984.

El-Baz NM, Ivankovich AD: One-lung high-frequency ventilation, in Kittle RE (ed): *Current Controversies in Thoracic Surgery.* Philadelphia, Saunders, 1986.

Mitchell R, Angell W, et al: Simplified lateral chest incision for most thoracotomies other than sternotomy. *Ann Thorac Surg* 22:284, 1976.

Noirclerc M, Dor V, et al: Extensive lateral thoracotomy without muscle section. *Ann Chir Thorac Cardiovasc* 12:181, 1973.

Siegel T, Steiger Z: Axillary thoracotomy. *Surg Gynecol Obstet* 155:725, 1982.

Urschel HC Jr, Razzuk MA: Median sternotomy as a standard approach for pulmonary resection. *Ann Thorac Surg* 41:130, 1986.

Evaluation of the Thoracic Surgical Patient

Ali MK, Mountain CF, et al: Predicting loss of pulmonary function after pulmonary resection for bronchogenic carcinoma. *Chest* 77:337, 1980.

Bloomberg AE: Thoracoscopy in perspective. *Surg Gynecol Obstet* 147:433, 1978.

Boren HG, Kory RC, et al: The veterans administration—army cooperative study of pulmonary function: II. The lung volume and its subdivisions in normal men. *Med Clin North Am* 41:96, 1966.

Breyer RH, Karstaedt N, et al: Computed tomography for evaluation of mediastinal lymph nodes in lung cancer: Correlation with surgical staging. *Ann Thorac Surg* 38:215, 1984.

Doyle PT, Weir J, et al: Role of computed tomography in assessing "operability" of bronchial carcinoma. *Br Med J [Clin Res]* 292:231, 1986.

Gamsu G: Magnetic resonance imaging in lung cancer. *Chest* 89:242S, 1986.

Goldman L, Caldera DL, et al: Multifactorial index of cardiac risk in noncardiac surgical procedures. *Arch Surg* 101:140, 1970.

Mittman C: Assessment of operative risk in thoracic surgery. *Am Rev Respir Dis* 84:197, 1961.

Petty TL: *Pulmonary Diagnostic Techniques.* Philadelphia, Lea & Febiger, 1975.

Tisi GM: Preoperative evaluation of pulmonary function. *Am Rev Respir Dis* 119:293, 1979.

von Schulthess GK, McMurdo K, et al: Mediastinal masses: MR imaging. *Radiology* 158:289, 1986.

Postthoracotomy Considerations

Brynitz S, Schroder M: Intraoperative cryolysis of intercostal nerves in thoracic surgery. *Scand J Thorac Cardiovasc Surg* 20:85, 1986.

Conacher ID: Percutaneous cryotherapy for postthoracotomy neuraligia. *Pain* 25:227, 1986.

Cordell RA, Ellison RG: *Complications of Intrathoracic Surgery.* Boston, Little, Brown, 1979.

de la Rocha AG, Chambers K: Pain amelioration after thoracotomy: A prospective, randomized study. *Ann Thorac Surg* 37:239, 1984.

El-Baz NM, Faber LP, et al: Continuous epidural infusion of morphine for treatment of pain after thoracic surgery: A new technique. *Anesth Analg* 63:757, 1984.

Kirsh MM, Rotman H, et al: Complications of pulmonary resection. *Ann Thorac Surg* 20:215, 1975.

Larsen VH, Christensen P, et al: Postoperative pain relief and respiratory performance after thoracotomy: A controlled trial comparing the effect of epidural morphine and subcutaneous nicomorphine. *Dan Med Bull* 33:161, 1986.

Maiwand MO, Makey AR, et al: Cryoanalgesia after thoracotomy. Improvement of technique and review of 600 cases. *J Thorac Cardiovasc Surg* 92:291, 1986.

Mandal AK, Montano J, et al: Prophylactic antibiotics and no antibiotics compared in penetrating chest trauma. *J Trauma* 25:639, 1985.

Middaugh RE, Menk EJ, et al: Epidural block using large volumes of local anesthetic solution for intercostal nerve block. *Anesthesiology* 63:214, 1985.

Peters RM: Pulmonary resection and gas exchange. *J Thorac Cardiovasc Surg* 88:872, 1984.

Restelli L, Movilia P, et al: Management of pain after thoracotomy: A technique of multiple intercostal nerve blocks. *Anesthesiology* 61:353, 1984.

Thoracic Injuries

Albers JE, Rath RK, et al: Severity of intrathoracic injuries associated with first rib fractures. *Ann Thorac Surg* 33:614,1982.

Bailey P: Surfer's rib: Isolated first rib fracture secondary to indirect trauma. *Ann Emerg Med* 14:346, 1985.

Barone JE, Pizzi WF, et al: Indications for intubation in blunt chest trauma. *J Trauma* 26:334, 1986.

Beal SL, Oreskovich MR: Long-term disability associated with flail chest injury. *Am J Surg* 150:324, 1985.

Blaisdell FW, Lewis FR Jr: *Respiratory Distress Syndrome of Shock and Trauma.* Philadelphia, Saunders, 1977.

Chakravarty M: Utilization of angiography in trauma. *Radiol Clin North Am* 24:383, 1986.

Cole FH Jr, Miller MP, et al: Transdiaphragmatic intercostal hernia. *Ann Thorac Surg* 41:565, 1986.

Coselli JS, Mattox KL, et al: Reevaluation of early evacuation of clotted hemothorax. *Am J Surg* 148:786, 1984.

Hoekstra HJ, Kingma LM: Bilateral first rib fractures induced by integral crash helmets. *J Trauma* 25:566, 1985.

Johnson JA, Cogbill TH, et al: Determinants of outcome after pulmonary contusion. *J Trauma* 26:695, 1986.

Kelly JP, Webb WR, et al: Management of airway trauma. I: Tracheobronchial injuries. *Ann Thorac Surg* 40:551, 1985.

Landercasper J, Cogbill TH, et al: Long-term disability after flail chest injury. *J Trauma* 24:410, 1984.

Lazar HL, Thomashow B, King TC: Complete transection of the intrathoracic trachea due to blunt trauma. *Ann Thorac Surg* 37:505, 1984.

Neugebauer MK, Fasburg RG, et al: Routine antibiotic therapy following pleural space intubation. *J Thorac Cardiovasc Surg* 61:882, 1971.

Payne JH, Yellin AE: Traumatic diaphragmatic hernia. *Arch Surg* 117:18, 1982.

Poulton TJ, Haldeman LW, et al: Cardiopulmonary effects of severe thoracic subcutaneous emphysema. *J Trauma* 26:396, 1986.

Ross RM, Cordoba A: Delayed life-threatening hemothorax associated with rib fractures. *J Trauma,* 26:576, 1986.

Sladen A: Methylprednisolone. Pharmacologic doses in shock lung syndrome. *J Thorac Cardiovasc Surg* 71:800, 1976.

Symbas PN, Vlasis SE, et al: Blunt and penetrating diaphragmatic injuries with or without herniation of organs into the chest. *Ann Thorac Surg* 42:158, 1986.

Theriot BA, Gross BD, et al: Isolated fracture of the first rib associated with facial trauma. *J Oral Maxillofac Surg* 42:610, 1984.

Thompson BM, Finger W, et al: Rib radiographs for trauma: Useful or wasteful? *Ann Emerg Med* 15:261, 1986.

Chest Wall—Congenital Deformities

Beiser GC, Epstein SE, et al: Impairment of cardiac function with pectus excavatum with improvement after operative correction. *N Engl J Med* 287:267, 1972.

Blickman JG, Rosen PR, et al: Pectus excavatum in children: Pulmonary scintigraphy before and after corrective surgery. *Radiography* 156:781, 1985.

Cahill JL, Lees GM, et al: A summary of preoperative and postoperative cardiorespiratory performance in patients undergoing pectus excavatum and carinatum repair. *J Pediatr Surg* 19:430, 1984.

Hawkins, JA, Ehrenhaft, JL, et al: Repair of pectus excavatum by sternal eversion. *Ann Thorac Surg* 38:368, 1984.

Holcomb GW Jr: Surgical correction of pectus excavatum. *J Pediatr Surg* 12:295, 1977.

Marks MW, Argenta LC, et al: Silicone implant correction of pectus excavatum: Indications and refinement in technique. *Plast Reconstr Surg* 74:52, 1984.

Peterson RJ, Young WG, et al: Noninvasive assessment of exercise cardiac function before and after pectus excavatum repair. *J Thorac Cardiovasc Surg* 90:251, 1985.

Ravitch MM: Disorders of the sternum and the thoracic wall, in Sabiston DC, Spencer FC (eds): *Gibbon's Surgery of the Chest,* 4th ed. Philadelphia, Saunders, 1983.

Urschel HC Jr, Byrd HS, et al: Poland's syndrome: Improved surgical management. *Ann Thorac Surg* 37:204, 1984.

Wada J, Ikeda K, et al: Results of 271 funnel chest operations. *Ann Thorac Surg* 10:526, 1970.

Weg JG, Krumholz RA, et al: Pulmonary dysfunction in pectus excavatum. *Am Rev Respir Dis* 96:936, 1967.

Wesselhoeft CW Jr, Deluca FG: A simplified approach to the repair of pediatric pectus deformities. *Ann Thorac Surg* 34:640, 1982.

Chest Wall—Tumors and Thoracic-Outlet Syndrome

Blank RH, Connar RG: Arterial complications associated with thoracic outlet compression syndrome. *Ann Thorac Surg* 17:315, 1974.

Capistrant TD: Thoracic outlet syndrome in whiplash injury. *Ann Surg* 185:175, 1977.

Cavanaugh DG, Cabellon S Jr, Peake JB: A logical approach to chest wall neoplasms. *Ann Thorac Surg* 41:436, 1986.

Claggett OT: Presidential address: Research and prosearch. *J Thorac Cardiovasc Surg* 44:153, 1962.

King RM, Pairolero PC, et al: Primary chest wall tumors: Factors affecting survival. *Ann Thorac Surg* 41:597, 1986.

McGough EC, Pearce MB, Byrne JP: Management of thoracic outlet syndrome. *J Thorac Cardiovasc Surg* 77:169, 1979.

Moore M Jr: Thoracic outlet syndrome experience in a metropolitan hospital. *Clin Orthop* 207:29, 1986.

Pairolero PC, Arnold PG: Thoracic wall defects: Surgical management of 205 consecutive patients. *Mayo Clin Proc* 61:557, 1986.

Pairolero PC, Arnold PG: Chest wall tumors. Experience with 100 consecutive patients. *J Thorac Cardiovasc Surg* 90:367, 1985.

Qvarfordt PG, Ehrenfeld WK, et al: Supraclavicular radical scalenectomy and transaxillary first rib resection for the thoracic outlet syndrome. A combined approach. *Am J Surg* 148:111, 1984.

Roos DB: Congenital anomalies associated with thoracic outlet syndrome. Anatomy, symptoms, diagnosis and treatment. *Am J Surg* 132:771, 1976.

Sabanathan S, Salama FD, et al: Primary chest wall tumors. *Ann Thorac Surg* 39:4, 1985.

Sanders RJ, Monsour JW, et al: Scalenectomy versus first rib resection for treatment of the thoracic outlet syndrome. *Surgery,* 85:109, 1979.

Scher LA, Veith FJ, et al: Staging of arterial complications of cervical rib: Guidelines for surgical management. *Surgery* 95:644, 1984.

Diseases of the Pleura

Agostini E: Mechanics of the pleural space. *Physiol Rev* 52:57, 1972.

Azizkhan RG, Canfield J, et al: Pleuroperitoneal shunts in the management of neonatal chylothorax. *J Pediatr Surg* 18:842, 1983.

Bessone LN, Ferguson TB, et al: Chylothorax. *Ann Thorac Surg* 12:527, 1971.

Brenner J, Sordillo PP, et al: Malignant mesothelioma of the pleura. *Cancer* 49:2431, 1982.

Cattaneo SM, Sirak HD, et al: Recurrent spontaneous pneumothorax in the high-risk patient. *J Thorac Cardiovasc Surg* 66:467, 1973.

Chahinian AP, Pajak TF, et al: Diffuse malignant mesothelioma. *Ann Intern Med* 96:746, 1982.

DaValle MJ, Faber LP, et al: Extrapleural pneumonectomy for diffuse, malignant mesothelioma. *Ann Thorac Surg* 42:612, 1986.

de la Rocha AG: Empyema thoracis. *Surg Gynecol Obstet* 155:839, 1982.

DeMeester TR, Lafontaine E: The pleura, in Sabiston DC, Spencer FC (eds): *Gibbon's Surgery of the Chest,* 4th ed. Philadelphia, Saunders, 1983, chap 15.

Ferguson MK, Little AG, et al: Current concepts in the management of postoperative chylothorax. *Ann Thorac Surg* 40:542, 1985.

Fraedrich G, Hofmann D, et al: Instillation of fibrinolytic enzymes in the treatment of pleural empyema. *Thorac Cardiovasc Surg* 30:36, 1982.

Frimodt–Moller PC, Vejlsted H: Early surgical intervention in nonspecific pleural empyema. *Thorac Cardiovasc Surg* 33:41, 1985.

Ginsberg RJ: Diffuse malignant mesothelioma: A therapeutic dilemma. *Ann Thorac Surg* 42:608, 1986.

Hakim M, Milstein BB: Empyema thoracis and infected pneumonectomy space: Case for cyclical irrigation. *Ann Thorac Surg* 41:85, 1986.

Hutter JA, Harari D, et al: The management of empyema thoracis by thoracoscopy and irrigation. *Ann Thorac Surg* 39:517, 1985.

Lampson RS: Traumatic chylothorax. *J Thorac Surg* 17:778, 1948.

Light RW, MacGregor MI, et al: Pleural effusions: The diagnostic separation of transudates and exudates. *Ann Intern Med* 77:507, 1972.

Light RW, MacGregor MI, et al: Diagnostic significance of pleural fluid pH and P_{CO_2}. *Chest* 64:591, 1973.

Martini N, McCormack PM, et al: Pleural mesothelioma. *Ann Thorac Surg* 43:113, 1987.

McCormack PM, Nagasaki F, et al: Surgical treatment of pleural mesothelioma. *J Thorac Cardiovasc Surg* 84:834, 1982.

McLeod DT, Calverley PMA, et al: Further experience of corynebacterium parvum in malignant pleural effusion. *Thorax* 40:515, 1985.

Milsom JW, Kron IL, et al: Chylothorax: An assessment of current surgical management. *J Thorac Cardiovasc Surg* 89:221, 1985.

Reshad K, Inui K, et al: Treatment of malignant pleural effusion. *Chest* 88:393, 1985.

Robinson CLN: The management of chylothorax. *Ann Thorac Surg* 39:90, 1985.

Serementis MG: The management of spontaneous pneumothorax. *Chest* 57:65, 1970.

Strausser JL, Flye MW: Management of nontraumatic chylothorax. *Ann Thorac Surg* 31:520, 1981.

Wehr C, Adkins RB: Empyema thoracis: A ten-year experience. *South Med J* 79:171, 1986.

Lung—Anatomy and Diagnosis

Borrie J: Primary carcinoma of the bronchus: Prognosis following surgical resection. *Ann R Coll Surg Engl* 10:165, 1952.

Boyden EA, Tomsett DH: Congenital absence of the medial basal bronchus in a child: With preliminary observations on postnatal growth of the lungs. *J Thorac Cardiovasc Surg* 43:517, 1962.

Dahlgren S, Nordenstrom B: *Transthoracic Needle Biopsy.* Chicago, Year Book Medical Publishers, 1966.

Garfinkel L, Auerbach O, et al: Involuntary smoking and lung cancer. A case control study. *J Natl Cancer Inst* 75:463, 1985.

Garrison RJ, Castelli WP: Weight and thirty-year mortality of men in the Framingham study. *Ann Intern Med* 103:1006, 1985.

Graves WG, Martinez MJ, et al: The value of computed tomography in staging bronchogenic carcinoma: A changing role for mediastinoscopy. *Ann Thorac Surg* 40:57, 1985.

Hirayama T: Nonsmoking wives of heavy smokers have a high risk of lung cancer: A study from Japan. *Br Med J* 282:183, 1981.

LoCicero J 3d, Frederiksen JW, et al: Experimental air leaks in lung sealed by low-energy carbon dioxide laser irradiation. *Chest* 87:820, 1985.

Martin DH, Newhouse MT: Thoracoscopy: A clinical perspective, in Kittle RE (ed): *Current Controversies in Thoracic Surgery*. Philadelphia, Saunders, 1986.

Martini N, Heelan R, et al: Comparative merits of conventional, computed tomographic, and magnetic resonance imaging in assessing mediastinal involvement in surgically confirmed lung cancer. *J Thorac Cardiovasc Surg* 90:639, 1985.

McKenna RJ Jr, Mountain CF, et al: Open lung biopsy in immunocompromised patients. *Chest* 86:671, 1984.

Mutz N, Baum M, et al: Intraoperative application of high-frequency ventilation. *Crit Care Med* 12:800, 1984.

Oakes DD, Sherck JP, et al: Therapeutic thoracoscopy. *J Thorac Cardiovasc Surg* 87:269, 1984.

Pollin W, Ravenholt RT: Tobacco addiction and tobacco mortality. *JAMA* 252:2849, 1984.

Replace JL, Lowrey AH: An indoor air quality standard for ambient tobacco smoke based on carcinogenic risk. *NY State J Med* 85:381, 1985.

Ross JS, O'Donovan PB, et al: Magnetic resonance of the chest: Initial experience with imaging and in vivo T1 and T2 calculations. *Radiology* 152:95, 1984.

Shields TW: The dilemma of the mediastinal node, in Kittle RE (ed): *Current Controversies in Thoracic Surgery*. Philadelphia, Saunders, 1986.

Sinner WN: Complications of percutaneous transthoracic needle aspiration biopsy. *Acta Radiol (Diagn) (Stockh)* 17:813, 1976.

Todd TR, Weisbrod G, et al: Aspiration needle biopsy of thoracic lesions. *Ann Thorac Surg* 32:154, 1981.

Webb WR, Gamsu G, et al: Magnetic resonance imaging of the normal and abnormal pulmonary hila. *Radiology* 152:89, 1984.

Lung—Congenital Disorders, Emphysema

Brown SE, Wright PW, et al: Staged bilateral thoracotomies for multiple pulmonary arteriovenous malformations complicating hereditary hemorrhagic telangiectasis. *J Thorac Cardiovasc Surg* 83:285, 1982.

Dines DE, Arms RA, et al: Pulmonary arteriovenous fistulas. *Mayo Clin Proc* 49:460, 1974.

Ferguson TB: Congenital lesions of the lungs and emphysema, in Sabiston DC, Spencer FC (eds): *Gibbon's Surgery of the Chest*, 4th ed. Philadelphia, Saunders, 1983.

FitzGerald MX, Keelan PJ, et al: Long-term results of surgery for bullous emphysema. *J Thorac Cardiovasc Surg* 68:566, 1974.

Haller JA Jr, Golladay ES, et al: Surgical management of lung bud anomalies: Lobar emphysema, bronchogenic cyst, cystic adenomatoid malformation, and intralobar pulmonary sequestration. *Ann Thorac Surg* 28:33, 1979.

Iwa T, Watanabe Y, et al: Simultaneous bilateral operations for bullous emphysema by median sternotomy. *J Thorac Cardiovasc Surg* 81:732, 1981.

Michelson E: Clinical spectrum of infantile lobar emphysema. *Ann Thorac Surg* 24:182, 1977.

Tenholder MF, Jones PA, et al: Bullous emphysema: Progressive incremental exercise testing to evaluate candidates for bullectomy. *Chest* 77:802, 1980.

Wesley JR, Heidelberger KP, et al: Diagnosis and management of congenital cystic disease of the lung in children. *J Pediatr Surg* 21:202, 1986.

Lung—Pulmonary Infections

Alexander JC, Wolfe WG: Lung abscess and empyema of the thorax. *Surg Clin North Am* 60:835, 1980.

Amnest LS, Knatz JM, et al: Current results of treatment of bronchiectasis. *J Thorac Cardiovasc Surg* 83:546, 1982.

Battaglini JW, Murray GF, et al: Surgical management of symptomatic pulmonary aspergilloma. *Ann Thorac Surg* 39:512, 1985.

Confronting AIDS: *Directions for Public Health, Health Care, and Research*. Report of the Institute of Medicine, National Academy of Science, National Academic Press, Washington, 1986.

Cooper DKC, Lanza RP, et al: Infectious complication after heart transplantation. *Thorax* 38:822, 1983.

Cunningham RT, Einstein H: Coccidioidal pulmonary cavities with ruptures. *J Thorac Cardiovasc Surg* 84:172, 1982.

Daly RC, Pairolero PC, et al: Pulmonary aspergilloma. *J Thorac Cardiovasc Surg* 92:981, 1986.

Edson RS, Keys TF: Treatment of primary pulmonary blastomycosis. *Mayo Clin Proc* 56:683, 1981.

Elkadi A, Salas R, et al: Surgical treatment of atypical pulmonary tuberculosis. *J Thorac Cardiovasc Surg* 72:435, 1976.

Fuller J, Levinson MM, et al: Legionnaires' disease after heart transplantation. *Ann Thorac Surg* 39:308, 1985.

Golden N, Cohen H, et al: Thoracic actinomycosis in childhood. *Clin Pediatr* 24:646, 1985.

Glimp RA, Bayer AS: Pulmonary aspergilloma. *Arch Intern Med* 143:303, 1983.

Kosloske AM, Ball WS, et al: Drainage of pediatric lung abscess by cough, catheter, or complete resection. *J Pediatr Surg* 21:596, 1986.

Lacey SR, Kosloske AM: Pneumonostomy in the management of pediatric lung abscess. *J Pediatr Surg* 18:625, 1983.

Lemmer JH, Botham MJ, et al: Modern management of adult thoracic empyema. *J Thorac Cardiovasc Surg* 90:849, 1985.

leRoux BT, Mohlala ML, et al: Suppurative diseases of the lung and pleural space. Part I: Empyema. *Curr Probl Surg* 23:1, 1986.

Mammana RB, Eskild AP, et al: Pulmonary infections in cardiac transplant patients: Modes of diagnosis, complications, and effectiveness of therapy. *Ann Thorac Surg* 36:700, 1983.

McKenna RJ, Campbell A, et al: Diagnosis for interstitial lung disease in patients with acquired immunodeficiency syndrome (AIDS): A prospective comparison of bronchial washing, alveolar lavage, transbronchial lung biopsy, and open-lung biopsy. *Ann Thorac Surg* 41:318, 1986.

Mangoli L: Giant lung abscess treated by tube thoracostomy. *J Thorac Cardiovasc Surg* 90:186, 1985.

Miller JI: The thoracic surgical spectrum of acquired immune deficiency syndrome. *J Thorac Cardiovasc Surg* 92:977, 1986.

Newsom BD, Hardy JD: Pulmonary fungal infections. *J Thorac Cardiovasc Surg* 83:218, 1982.

Nonoyama A, Tanaka K, et al: Surgical treatment of pulmonary abscess in children under ten years of age. *Chest* 85:358, 1984.

Pass HI, Potter DA, et al: Thoracic manifestations of the acquired immune deficiency syndrome. *J Thorac Cardiovasc Surg* 88:654, 1984.

Pohlson EC, McNamara JJ, et al: Lung abscess: A changing pattern of the disease. *Am J Surg* 150:97, 1985.

Prager RL, Burney P, et al: Pulmonary, mediastinal, and cardiac presentations of histoplasmosis. *Ann Thorac Surg* 30:385, 1980.

Prober CG, Whyte H, et al: Open lung biopsy in immunocompromised children with pulmonary infiltrates. *Am J Dis Child* 138:60, 1984.

Rao RS, Curzon PGD, et al: Cavernoscopic evacuation of aspergilloma: An alternative method of palliation for haemoptysis in high risk patients. *Thorax* 39:394, 1984.

Rubinstein A, Morecki R, et al: Pulmonary disease in children with acquired immune deficiency syndrome and AIDS-related complex. *J Pediatr* 108:498, 1986.

Shamberger RC, Weinstein HJ, et al: The surgical management of fungal pulmonary infections in children with acute myelogenous leukemia. *J Pediatr Surg* 20:840, 1985.

Solomon NW, Osborne R, et al: Surgical manifestations and results of treatment of pulmonary coccidioidomycosis. *Ann Thorac Surg* 30:433, 1980.

Sterling RP, Bradley BB, et al: Comparison of biopsy-proven *Pneumocystis carinii* pneumonia in acquired immune deficiency syndrome patients and renal allograft recipients. *Ann Thorac Surg* 38:494, 1984.

Tokaro T, Sethi G, et al: Thoracic surgical infections, in Simmons RL, Howard RJ (eds): *Surgical Infectious Diseases.* New York, Appleton Century Crofts, 1982.

Tokara T: Lung infections and diffuse interstitial diseases of the lungs, in Sabiston DC, Spender FC (eds): *Gibbon's Surgery of the Chest.* 4th ed, Philadelphia, Saunders, 1983.

Treger TR, Visscher DW, et al: Diagnosis of pulmonary infection caused by Aspergillus: Usefulness of respiratory cultures. *J Infect Dis* 152:572, 1985.

Weber TR, Grosfeld JL, et al: Surgical implications of endemic histoplasmosis in children. *J Pediatr Surg* 18:486, 1983.

Weiland D, Ferguson RM, et al: Aspergillosis in 25 renal transplant patients. *Ann Surg* 198:622, 1983.

Weissberg D: Percutaneous drainage of lung abscess. *J Thorac Cardiovasc Surg* 87:308, 1984.

White JC, Nelson S, et al: Impairment of antibacterial defense mechanisms of the lung by extrapulmonary infection. *J Infect Dis* 153:202, 1986.

Wilson JF, Decker AM: The surgical management of childhood bronchiectasis: A review of 96 consecutive pulmonary resections in children with non-tuberculous bronchiectasis. *Ann Surg* 195:354, 1982.

Yellin A, Yellin EO, et al: Percutaneous tube drainage: The treatment of choice for refractory lung abscess. *Ann Thorac Surg* 39:266, 1985.

Young WG, Moor GF: The surgical treatment of pulmonary tuberculosis, in Sabiston DC, Spencer FC (eds): *Gibbon's Surgery of the Chest,* 4th ed. Philadelphia, Saunders, 1983.

Lung—Tumors

Aisner J, Whitacre M, et al: Combination chemotherapy for small cell carcinoma of the lung: Continuous versus alternating non-cross-resistant combinations. *Cancer Treat Rep* 66(2):221–230, 1982.

Auerbach O, Garfinkel L, et al: Scar cancer of the lung: Increase over a 21-year period. *Cancer* 43:636, 1979.

Belli L, Meroni A, et al: Bronchoplastic procedures and pulmonary artery reconstruction in the treatment of bronchogenic cancer. *J Thorac Cardiovasc Surg* 90:167, 1985.

Benfield JR, Yellin A: New horizons for lung cancer. *Surg Rounds* April 1985:26–52.

Breyer RH, Jensik RJ: Lung-sparing operations in elderly patients [letter]. *Ann Thorac Surg* 40:636, 1985.

Breyer RH, Zippe C, et al: Thoracotomy in patients over age seventy years. Ten-year experience. *J Thorac Cardiovasc Surg* 81:187, 1981.

Brock L: Long survival after operation for cancer of the lung. *Br J Surg* 62:1, 1975.

Cohen MH, Creaven PJ, et al: Intensive chemotherapy of small cell bronchogenic carcinoma. *Cancer Treat Rep* 61(3):349, 1977.

Cooper JD, Perelman M, et al: Precision cautery excision of pulmonary lesions. *Ann Thorac Surg* 41:51, 1986.

Cortese DA: Endobronchial management of lung cancer. *Chest* 89:234S, 1986.

Cox JD: Non-small cell lung cancer. Role of radiation therapy. *Chest* 89:284S, 1986.

Deslauriers J, Gaulin P, et al: Long-term clinical and functional results of sleeve lobectomy for primary lung cancer. *J Thorac Cardiovasc Surg* 92:871, 1986.

Eagan RT, Frytak S, et al: An evaluation of low-dose cisplatin as part of combined modality therapy of limited small cell lung cancer. *Cancer Clin Trials* 4(3):267, 1981.

Edell ES, Cortese DA: Bronchoscopic phototherapy with hematoporphyrin derivative for treatment of localized bronchogenic carcinoma: A 5-year experience. *Mayo Clin Proc* 62:8, 1987.

Errett LE, Wilson J, et al: Wedge resection as an alternative procedure for peripheral bronchogenic carcinoma in poor-risk patients. *J Thorac Cardiovasc Surg* 90:656, 1985.

Evans WK, Shepherd FA, et al: VP-16 and cisplatin as first-line therapy for small-cell lung cancer. *J Clin Oncol* 3(11):1471, 1985.

Faber LP, Jensik RJ, Kittle CF: Results of sleeve lobectomy for bronchogenic carcinoma in 101 patients. *Ann Thorac Surg* 37:279, 1984.

Feld R, Evans WK, et al: Combined modality induction therapy without maintenance chemotherapy for small cell carcinoma of the lung. *J Clin Oncol* 2(4):294, 1984.

Ferguson MK, Little AG, et al: The role of adjuvant therapy after resection of $T_1N_1M_0$ and $T_2N_1M_0$ non-small cell lung cancer. *J Thorac Cardiovasc Surg* 91:344, 1986.

Firmin RK, Azariades M, et al: Sleeve lobectomy (lobectomy and bronchoplasty) for bronchial carcinoma. *Ann Thorac Surg* 35:442, 1983.

Gail MH, Eagan RT, et al: Prognostic factors in patients with resected stage I non-small cell lung cancer: A report from the Lung Cancer Study Group. *Cancer* 54(9):1802, 1984.

Ginsberg RJ, Hill LD, et al: Modern thirty-day operative mortality for surgical resections in lung cancer. *J Thorac Cardiovasc Surg* 86:654, 1983.

Greco FA, Richardson RL, et al: Small cell lung cancer: Complete remission and improved survival. *Am J Med* 66(4):625, 1979.

Hansen HH, Dombernowsky P, et al: Chemotherapy of advanced small-cell anaplastic carcinoma: Superiority of a four-drug combination to a three-drug combination. *Ann Intern Med* 89(2):177, 1978.

Hardy JD, Ewing HP, et al: Lung carcinoma. Survey of 2286

cases with emphasis on small cell type. *Ann Surg* 193:539, 1981.

Hilaris BS, Gomez J, et al: Combined surgery, intraoperative brachytherapy, and postoperative external radiation in stage III non-small cell lung cancer. *Cancer* 55:1226, 1985.

Homes EC, Gail M: Surgical adjuvant therapy for stage II and stage III adenocarcinoma and large-cell undifferentiated carcinoma. *J Clin Oncol* 4(5):710, 1986.

Holmes EC, Hill LD, et al: A randomized comparsion of the effects of adjuvant therapy on resected stages II and III non-small cell carcinoma of the lung. The Lung Cancer Study Group. *Ann Surg* 202:335, 1985.

Hyman NH, Foster RS Jr, et al: Blood transfusions and survival after lung cancer resection. *Am J Surg* 149:502, 1985.

Ihde DC, Bunn PA, et al: Randomized trial of chemotherapy with or without adjuvant chest irradiation in limited stage small cell lung cancer, in Jones SE, Salmon SE (eds): *Adjuvant Therapy of Cancer IV*. New York, Grune & Stratton, 1984.

Immerman SC, Vanecko RM, et al: Site of recurrence in patients with stages I and II carcinoma of the lung resected for cure. *Ann Thorac Surg* 32:23, 1981.

Jensik RJ, Faber LP, et al: Segmental resection for bronchogenic carcinoma. *Ann Thorac Surg* 28:475, 1979.

Jensik RJ, Faber LP, et al: Survival following resection for second primary bronchogenic carcinoma. *J Thorac Cardiovasc Surg* 82:658, 1981.

Kirsh MM, Rotman H, et al: Carcinoma of the lung: Results of treatment over ten years. *Ann Thorac Surg* 21(5):371, 1976.

Kirsh MM, Tashian J, et al: Carcinoma of the lung in women. *Ann Thorac Surg* 34:34, 1982.

Kittle CF, Faber LP, et al: Pulmonary resection in patients after pneumonectomy. *Ann Thorac Surg* 40:294, 1985.

Komaki R, Cox JD, et al: Characteristics of long-term survivors after treatment for inoperable carcinoma of the lung. *Am J Clin Oncol* 8(5):362, 1985.

Komaki R, Roh J, et al: Superior sulcus tumors: Results of irradiation of 36 patients. *Cancer* 48(7):1563, 1981.

Kreyberg L, Liebow AA, Uehlinger EA: International histologic classification of tumours: No. 1. Histological typing of lung tumours. Geneva, World Health Organization, 2d ed, 1981.

Libshitz HI, McKenna RJ Jr, et al: Patterns of mediastinal metastases in bronchogenic carcinoma. *Chest* 90:229, 1986.

Maassen W, Greschuchna D, Martinez I: The role of surgery in the treatment of small cell carcinoma of the lung. *Recent Results Cancer Res* 97:107, 1985.

Martini N, Beattie EJ: Results of surgical treatment in Stage I lung cancer. *J Thorac Cardiovasc Surg* 74(4):499, 1977.

Martini N, Flehinger BJ, et al: Results of resection in nonoatcell carcinoma of the lung with mediastinal lymph node metastases. *Ann Surg* 198(3):386, 1983.

Martini N, Flehinger BJ, et al: Prospective study of 445 lung carcinomas with mediastinal lymph node metastases. *J Thorac Cardiovasc Surg* 80:390, 1980.

McCaughan BC, Martini N, et al: Chest wall invasion in carcinoma of the lung. Therapeutic and prognostic implications. *J Thorac Cardiovasc Surg* 89:836, 1985.

Meyer JA, Comis RL, et al: Phase II trial of extended indications for resection in small cell carcinoma of the lung. *J Thorac Cardiovasc Surg* 83:12, 1982.

Mountain CF, McMurtrey MJ, et al: Surgery for pulmonary metastasis: A 20-year experience. *Ann Thorac Surg* 38:323, 1984.

Mountain CF: The biological operability of stage III non-small cell lung cancer. *Ann Thorac Surg* 40:60, 1985.

Mountain CF: The new international staging system for lung cancer. *Chest* 89(4 suppl):225S, 1986.

Murray GF, Mendes OC, et al: Bronchial carcinoma and the lymphatic sump: Significance of bronchoscopic findings. *Ann Thorac Surg* 34:634, 1982.

Musset D, Grenier P, et al: Primary lung cancer staging: Prospective comparative study of MR imaging with CT. *Radiology* 160:607, 1986.

Osterlind K, Hansen HH, et al: Mortality and morbidity in long-term surviving patients treated with chemotherapy with or without irradiation for small-cell lung cancer. *J Clin Oncol* 4(7):1044, 1986.

Pairolero PC, Williams DE, et al: Postsurgical stage I bronchogenic carcinoma: Morbid implications of recurrent disease. *Ann Thorac Surg* 38:331, 1984.

Paladugu RR, Benfield JR, et al: Bronchopulmonary Kulchitzky cell carcinomas. A new classification scheme for typical and atypical carcinoids. *Cancer* 55:1303, 1985.

Paulson DL, Reisch JS: Long term survival after resection for bronchogenic carcinoma. *Ann Surg* 184:324, 1976.

Paulson DL: Carcinomas in the superior pulmonary sulcus. *J Thorac Cardiovasc Surg* 70(6):1095, 1975.

Pearson FG, De Larue NC, et al: Significance of positive superior mediastinal nodes identified at mediastinoscopy in patients with resectable cancer of the lung. *Thorac Cardiovasc Surg* 83:1, 1982.

Pearson FG: Lung cancer. The past twenty-five years. *Chest* 98(4 suppl):200S, 1986.

Perloff M, Killen JY, Wittes RE: Small cell bronchogenic carcinoma. *Curr Probl Cancer* 10:169, 1986.

Peters RM, Clausen JL, et al: Extending resectability for carcinoma of the lung in patients with impaired pulmonary function. *Ann Thorac Surg* 26:250, 1978.

Shields TW: The dilemma of the mediastinal node, in Kittle RE (ed): *Current Controversies in Thoracic Surgery*. Philadelphia, Saunders, 1986.

Shields TW, Higgins GA Jr, et al: Surgical resection in the management of small cell carcinoma of the lung. *J Thorac Cardiovasc Surg* 84:481, 1982.

Stair JM, Womble J, et al: Segmental pulmonary resection for cancer. *Am J Surg* 150:659, 1985.

Temeck BK, Flehinger BJ, et al: A retrospective analysis of 10-year survivors from carcinoma of the lung. *Cancer* 53:1405, 1984.

Warren WH, Gould VE, et al: Neuroendocrine neoplasms of the bronchopulmonary tract. A classification of the spectrum of carcinoid to small cell carcinoma and intervening variants. *J Thorac Cardiovasc Surg* 89:819, 1985.

Webb WR, Jensen BG, et al: Bronchogenic carcinoma: Staging with MR compared with staging with CT and surgery. *Radiology* 156:117, 1985.

Yellin A, Hill LR, Benfield JR: Bronchogenic carcinoma associated with upper aerodigestive cancers. *J Thorac Cardiovasc Surg* 91:674, 1986.

Zelen M: Keynote address on biostatistics and data retrieval. *Cancer Chemother Rep* 4(2):31, 1973.

Trachea

Ein SH, Friedberg J, et al: Tracheoplasty—a new operation for complete congenital tracheal stenosis. *J Pediatr Surg* 17:872, 1982.

El–Baz N, Jensik R, et al: One-lung high-frequency ventilation for tracheoplasty and bronchoplasty: A new technique. *Ann Thorac Surg* 34:564, 1982.

Grillo HC, Zannini P: Management of obstructive tracheal disease in children. *J Pediatr Surg* 19:414, 1984.

Grillo HC: Congenital lesions, neoplasms, and injuries of the trachea, in Sabiston DC, Spencer FC (eds): *Gibbon's Surgery of the Chest,* 4th ed. Philadelphia, Saunders, 1983, chap 11.

Grillo HC: Surgical treatment of postintubation tracheal injuries. *J Thorac Cardiovasc Surg* 78:860, 1979.

Kato H, Konaka C, et al: Preoperative laser photodynamic therapy in combination with operation in lung cancer. *J Thorac Cardiovasc Surg* 90:420, 1985.

Kimura K, Mukohara N, et al: Tracheoplasty for congenital stenosis of the entire trachea. *J Pediatr Surg* 17:869, 1982.

Kvale PA, Eichenhorn MS, et al: YAG laser photoresection of lesions obstructing the central airways. *Chest* 87:283, 1985.

Mehta AC, Golish JA, et al: Palliative treatment of malignant airway obstruction by Nd-YAG laser. *Cleve Clin Q* 52:513, 1985.

Moghissi K: Tracheal reconstruction with a prosthesis of marlex mesh and pericardium. *J Thorac Cardiovasc Surg* 69:499, 1975.

Nakayama DK, Harrison MR, et al: Reconstructive surgery for obstructing lesions of the intrathoracic trachea in infants and small children. *J Pediatr Surg* 17:854, 1982.

Neville WE: Prosthetic reconstruction of trachea: Technic and results in 54 patients. *Ann Chir Thorac Cardiovasc* 35:636, 1981.

Parr GVS, Unger M, et al: One hundred neodymium-YAG laser ablations of obstructing tracheal neoplasms. *Ann Thorac Surg* 38:374, 1984.

Pearson FG, Todd TRJ, et al: Experience with primary neoplasms of the trachea and carina. *J Thorac Cardiovasc Surg* 88:511, 1984.

Mediastinum

Allan A, Sethia B, et al: Investigation of superior vena caval obstruction. *Thorax* 39:878, 1984.

Aygun C, Slawson RG, et al: Primary mediastinal seminoma. *Urology* 23:109, 1984.

Baron RL, Levitt RG, et al: Computed tomography in the evaluation of mediastinal widening. *Radiology* 138:107, 1981.

Bechtold RE, Wolfman NT, et al: Superior vena caval obstruction: Detection using CT. *Radiology* 157:485, 1985.

Berry DF, Buccigrossi D: Pulmonary vascular occlusion fibrosing mediastinitis. *Chest* 89:296, 1986.

Cohen DJ, Ronnigen LD, et al: Management of patients with malignant thymoma. *J Thorac Cardiovasc Surg* 87:301, 1985.

Doty DB, Baker WH: Bypass of superior vena cava with spiral vein graft. *Ann Thorac Surg* 22:490, 1976.

Filler RM, Troggis DG, et al: Favorable outlook for children with mediastinal neuroblastoma. *J Pediatr Surg* 7:136, 1972.

Gladstone DJ, Pillai R, et al: Relief of superior vena caval syndrome with autologous femoral veni used as a bypass graft. *J Thorac Cardiovasc Surg* 89:750, 1985.

Ham RJ, Bulstrode C, et al: Saphenous jugular bypass for superior vena caval obstruction. *Br J Surg* 72:194, 1985.

King RM, Telander RL, et al: Primary mediastinal tumors in children. *J Pediatr Surg* 17:512, 1982.

Knapp RH, Hurt RD, et al: Malignant germ cell tumors of the mediastinum. *J Thorac Cardiovasc Surg* 89:82, 1985.

Lack EE, Weinstein HJ, et al: Mediastinal germ cell tumors in childhood. *J Thorac Cardiovasc Surg* 89:826, 1985.

Lewis BD, Hurt RD, et al: Benign teratomas of the mediastinum. *J Thorac Cardiovasc Surg* 86:727, 1983.

Livesay JJ, Mink JH, et al: The use of computed tomography to evaluate suspected mediastinal tumors. *Ann Thorac Surg* 27:305, 1979.

Monden Y, Nakahara K, et al: Myasthenia gravis with thymoma: Analysis of and postoperative prognosis for 65 patients with thymomatous myasthenia gravis. *Ann Thorac Surg* 38:46, 1984.

Parish JM, Marschke RF, et al: Etiologic considerations in superior vena cava syndrome. *Mayo Clin Proc* 56:407, 1981.

Sabiston DC, Oldham HN: The mediastinum, in Sabiston DC, Spender FC (eds): *Gibbon's Surgery of the Chest,* 4th ed. Philadelphia, Saunders, 1983.

Schaefer S, Peshock RM, et al: Nuclear magnetic resonance imaging in Marfan's syndrome. *J Am Coll Cardiol* 9:70, 1987.

Siegel MJ, Sagel SS, et al: The value of computed tomography in the diagnosis and management of pediatric mediastinal abnormalities. *Radiology* 142:149, 1982.

Snyder ME, Luck SR, et al: Diagnostic dilemmas of mediastinal cysts. *J Pediatr Surg* 20:810, 1985.

von Schulthess GK, McMurdo K, et al: Mediastinal masses: MR imaging. *Radiology* 158:289, 1986.

Wychulis AR, Payne WS, et al: Surgical treatment of mediastinal tumors. A 40-year experience. *J Thorac Cardiovasc Surg* 62:379, 1971.

Chapter 18

Congenital Heart Disease

Frank C. Spencer

INTRODUCTION

Because rheumatic fever is now rare, congenital heart disease is the most common form of heart disease seen in children. In several studies the frequency has been found to be 3 to 4 cases of congenital heart disease occurring in every 1000 live births. The frequency is about ten times greater in members of the same family than in the normal population. The risk of occurrence in younger siblings of a child with congenital heart disease is about 2 percent. In most patients the etiologic factor is unknown.

Rubella occurring in the first trimester of pregnancy is one of the few infectious diseases known to cause congenital heart disease. It produces the well-recognized syndrome of mental deficiency, deafness, cataracts, and congenital heart disease, usually a patent ductus arteriosus. Mongolism is another congenital abnormality associated with a high incidence of congenital heart disease. Usually congenital heart disease occurs as an isolated malformation resulting from defective embryonic development without known cause.

The surprisingly short period of time during which cardiac development occurs in uterine life should be emphasized, for virtually all fetal heart structures are formed between the third and eighth week of pregnancy, a time interval of only 5 weeks. Atrial or ventricular septal defects result from incomplete formation of the respective septa, while transposition and other anomalies of the aorta result from abnormalities in the spiral division of the primitive bulbus cordis. Although there are six branchial aortic arches, all atrophy with the exception of the fourth left arch, which becomes the aorta, and the sixth left arch, remaining as the ductus arteriosus. Vascular ring malformations arise from different remnants of these embryonic branchial arches.

The fetal circulation has several distinctive features that may influence association with congenital heart disease. In embryonic life the lungs are collapsed, with a high vascular resistance, and pulmonary blood flow is small. Most of the blood returning through the inferior vena cava to the right atrium goes through the foramen ovale into the left atrium and thence to the left ventricle. Also, most of the blood expelled from the right ventricle into the pulmonary artery is shunted through the ductus arteriosus into the descending thoracic aorta. At birth, with expansion of the lungs, there is a fall in pulmonary vascular resistance, although the vascular resistance does not decrease to that normally found in older individuals for the first 1 to 3 years of life. There is a corresponding persistence during this time of the fetal histologic structure of the pulmonary arteries, characterized principally by an abundance of smooth muscle in the media of the arterial wall. Persistence of the fetal histologic structure of the pulmonary arterioles is associated with pulmonary hypertension.

With expansion of the lungs, the ductus arteriosus normally closes in the first few days after birth. It remains patent in only a small percentage of individuals but is one of the most common forms of congenital heart disease. The foramen ovale is a slitlike channel that is automatically sealed when left atrial pressure becomes higher than right atrial pressure; it normally permits the flow of blood only from the right atrium to the left atrium, not in the reverse direction. Patency of the foramen ovale, usually an innocuous defect, remains throughout adult life in at least 10 to 20 percent of patients. With elevation of right atrial pressure above left atrial pressure from any cause, the foramen ovale may be stretched open and create a right-to-left shunt from the right atrium to the left atrium, resulting in cyanosis from shunting of unoxygenated blood. This characteristically occurs in patients with pulmonic valvular stenosis when right ventricular failure elevates right atrial pressure.

Although a large number of congenital heart defects have been recognized and classified, in a large pediatric cardiac clinic seven malformations will comprise the majority of abnormalities seen. Ventricular septal defect, with or without pulmonic stenosis, is by far the most common, representing 20 percent or more of all patients. The other six malformations, each occurring in 10 to 15 percent of patients, are atrial septal defect, pulmonic valvular stenosis, aortic valvular stenosis, patent ductus arteriosus, coarctation of the aorta, and transposition of the great vessels. The frequency of different defects varies somewhat with the age group evaluated; transposition of the great vessels is more common in the newborn but many do not survive beyond six months of age without an operation.

This gradual evaluation of symptoms is an important consideration in evaluating children with congenital heart disease, for parents are normally apprehensive about consenting to complex diagnostic studies or operative procedures on a child who seems, to the inexperienced eye, to have little disability. Postponing therapy until a child is disabled to a point that is clinically obvious may result in irreversible changes in ventricular muscle, for severe hypertrophy of the right or left ventricle often does not regress completely following surgical correction of the basic cause, such as pulmonic or aortic stenosis. Even more serious is an increase in pulmonary vascular resistance that is usually irreversible.

The three main physiologic disturbances resulting from congenital heart disease are (1) obstruction to emptying of the ventricles, (2) left-to-right shunts with increase in pulmonary blood flow and corresponding decrease in systemic blood flow, and (3) cyanosis. Each of these physiologic disturbances is considered in detail in subsequent sections. With almost all forms of congenital heart disease there is an increased susceptibility to bacterial endocarditis, because the anatomic malformation creates a localized turbulent flow of blood predisposing to local deposition of bacteria during a transient bacteremia.

OBSTRUCTIVE LESIONS. The most common disorders are pulmonic valvular stenosis, aortic valvular stenosis, and coarctation of the aorta. These impede emptying of the involved ventricular chamber, resulting in what has been termed "systolic" overloading and corresponding concentric hypertrophy of the ventricle. As the ventricular response is predominantly concentric hypertrophy, cardiac enlargement cannot be detected by clinical means, and often the chest radiograph is only slightly abnormal. The electrocardiogram and echocardiogram, however, can measure the degree of ventricular hypertrophy that has occurred. With progressive left ventricular hypertrophy angina pectoris may occur, with susceptibility to arrhythmias and even sudden death. Cardiac failure is a late and often preterminal manifestation.

LEFT-TO-RIGHT SHUNTS. As pressures in the left atrium and left ventricle are normally greater than those in the right atrium and right ventricle, a defect in either the atrial or ventricular septum results in a shunt of oxygenated blood from the left side of the heart to the right side. This causes pulmonary congestion from an increase in pulmonary blood flow and often a corresponding decrease in systemic blood flow. Cyanosis, of course, does not occur. With the increase in pulmonary blood flow there is a tendency to develop pulmonary hypertension, varying both with the type of defect and with the individual patient. The most common defects producing left-to-right shunts are atrial septal defects, with or without anomalous pulmonary veins, ventricular septal defects, and patent ductus arteriosus.

Pulmonary Congestion. A shunt becomes physiologically significant when the pulmonary blood flow is 1.5 to 2.0 times as great as the systemic blood flow. Large shunts may produce a pulmonary blood flow three to four times greater than systemic blood flow, with a pulmonary blood flow exceeding 10 to 15 L/min per square meter of body surface. The resulting pulmonary congestion produces a susceptibility to bacterial infection; recurrent bouts of pneumonia may occur in the first few years of life. Beyond early childhood, however, high pulmonary blood flows may produce surprisingly little disability for a period of time. With the increase in pulmonary blood flow there is a corresponding enlargement of the involved ventricle (right ventricle with atrial septal defect, left ventricle with patent ductus arteriosus, both ventricles with ventricular septal defect), resulting in so-called diastolic overloading of the ventricle, with cardiac dilatation rather than hypertrophy. The dilatation can be more easily recognized on clinical examination and on the chest radiograph than its counterpart, concentric hypertrophy. The changes in the electrocardiogram are often less prominent than those seen with concentric hypertrophy. But echocardiography can measure cardiac chamber size precisely. Cardiac failure tends to occur somewhat earlier in the course of the disease than with concentric hypertrophy, and the response to medical therapy is somewhat better than that for predominantly obstructive lesions.

Classification

Congenital heart disease may be classified by the type of anatomic abnormality present, which in turn produces a distinct physiologic disturbance. Four major groups exist: (1) obstructive lesions that restrict the flow of blood, with corresponding increased work loads on the obstructed ventricular chamber; (2) left-to-right shunts that occur through uncomplicated septal defects; (3) right-to-left shunts caused by the combination of a septal defect with obstruction to ventricular emptying; (4) complex malformations. These include abnormal origin or atresia of the aorta or pulmonary artery or hypoplasia or atresia of the right or left ventricle and the corresponding tricuspid and mitral valves.

Pathophysiology

Four degrees of severity of congenital heart disease can be recognized. The mildest form consists only of abnormal physical findings. In some instances, such as trivial pulmonic valvular stenosis, there may never be any sign of heart disease except the characteristic systolic murmur. In the second stage of severity, physiologic abnormalities, such as pressure gradients across stenotic pulmonic or aortic valves, increased blood flow through shunts occurring through atrial or ventricular septal defects, or elevation in pulmonary artery pressure, can be measured by cardiac catheterization. Eventually these physiologic abnormalities produce corresponding anatomic changes (the third stage in severity), manifested principally by cardiac enlargement with hypertrophy of the right or left ventricle, demonstrated by both the electrocardiogram and the radiogram. With the development of pulmonary hypertension, histologic changes occur in the media and intima of the pulmonary arterioles. Cardiac failure, the fourth stage, eventually results from the chronic increased work load on the heart, at times compounded by anoxia.

Increased Pulmonary Vascular Resistance. With the increase in pulmonary blood flow, pulmonary vascular resistance may increase. The mode of development remains incompletely determined. An excellent analysis of the functional pathology of the pulmonary vascular bed was published by Edwards in 1957. Pulmonary hypertension may result from at least three factors: (1) an increase in pulmonary blood flow, (2) histologic changes in the pulmonary vascular bed with corresponding anatomic restriction of distensibility of the pulmonary vessels, or (3) pulmonary venous obstruction. The most important consideration is the pulmonary vascular resistance, not the systolic pulmonary arterial pressure per se. Pulmonary hypertension resulting from an increase in pulmonary blood flow subsides as soon as the cardiac defect producing the increase in blood flow is corrected. Pulmonary hypertension due to increased pulmonary vascular resistance caused by thickening of the media and intima is often irreversible. When severe, surgical therapy is ineffective or contraindicated. Hence, in evaluating pulmonary hypertension, the significant physiologic measurement is the degree of change in the pulmonary vascular resistance, as calculated from the relation between flow and pressure, and not the absolute level of the pulmonary artery pressure per se.

Normally pulmonary arterioles are very distensible and can accommodate an increase in pulmonary blood flow up to three times normal values without any increase in pressure. Further distensibility is limited by the fibrous tissue in the adventitial sheath surrounding the arterioles. In infants and young children with pulmonary hypertension the prominent histologic change in the pulmonary arterioles is hypertrophy of the smooth muscle of the media of the arteriolar wall, which is similar to that normally found in embryonic life. Some consider these histologic changes a failure of involution of the normal fetal pattern. With more severe disease thickening of the intima occurs also. With associated fibrosis this has a serious prognosis, for such histologic changes are usually irreversible, remaining after the underlying cause has been corrected.

More significant than the increase in pulmonary blood flow, however, is the pressure under which blood is expelled into the pulmonary artery. Pulmonary hypertension is much more frequent with ventricular septal defects than with atrial septal defects that produce a similar increase in pulmonary blood flow. The incidence of hypertension with secundum atrial septal defects in children is about 5 percent, while the incidence is about 25 percent in men with ventricular septal defects.

There is also an individual variation in susceptibility to development of pulmonary hypertension. Some children with a large ventricular septal defect and a large increase in pulmonary blood flow will not develop any increase in pulmonary vascular resistance, while others with a smaller septal defect will develop significant pulmonary hypertension at an early age.

Defects such as truncus arteriosus or transposition may produce permanent injury in some infants before six months of age. Most lesions producing an increase in pulmonary vascular resistance, such as ventricular septal defect, patent ductus arteriosus, or atrioventricular canals should be surgically corrected in the first 6 to 12 months of life. The more serious defects, such as transposition or truncus arteriosus, may require operation in the first few weeks or months of life. With simple atrial secundum defect, however, operation at such an early age is virtually never necessary, illustrating the unknown etiologic factors in producing an increase in pulmonary vascular resistance.

Restriction in Systemic Blood Flow. With large left-to-right shunts there is often a decrease in systemic blood flow, frequently associated with a retardation in normal growth and development. This is more prominently seen in children with a patent ductus arteriosus or an atrial septal defect. The appearance of frail, underweight children with atrial septal defect has been termed the *gracile habitus.* Although mental retardation is slightly more common in children with congenital heart disease, beyond this association there is no evidence that congenital heart disease retards mental development. Unfortunately, correction of the cardiac defect does not result in any improvement in mental function. After operation there is often a substantial increase in growth and weight.

RIGHT-TO-LEFT SHUNTS. Right-to-left shunts of venous blood directly into the systemic circulation, producing arterial hypoxemia and cyanosis, result from the combination of an intracardiac septal defect with obstruction to normal flow of blood into the pulmonary artery. The classic example is the tetralogy of Fallot, a combination of ventricular septal defect and pulmonic stenosis. Other cyanotic disorders include the more complex malformations, such as transposition of the great vessels, tricuspid atresia, truncus arteriosus, and total anomalous drainage of the pulmonary veins. Right-to-left shunts produce a large number of physiologic disturbances because of the anoxia resulting from chronic hypoxemia. These are considered in detail in the following paragraphs. It should be emphasized that all these disturbances result from deficient oxygen transport to tissues of the body. With right-to-left shunts there is no increase in cardiac output; the pulmonary blood flow is usually less than normal. Hence cardiac failure is rare with an uncomplicated right-to-left shunt, in contrast to its inevitable eventual occurrence with left-to-right shunts.

Cyanosis. This is the most prominent feature of a right-to-left shunt. The degree of cyanosis depends upon both the degree of anoxia and the blood hemoglobin concentration, for the visible intensity of cyanosis is determined by the number of grams of reduced hemoglobin in the circulation. It has been estimated that about 5 g of reduced hemoglobin is required to produce visible cyanosis. Normally in the capillaries about 2.25 g of reduced hemoglobin is present, so with an average hemoglobin concentration of 15 g/dL of blood, a decrease in arterial oxygen from the normal range of nearly 95 to 75 percent is needed to produce visible cyanosis. In the presence of anemia, however, a more severe degree of anoxia is required to produce visible cyanosis, while with polycythemia and hemoglobin concentrations of 20 g/dL of blood or more, severe cyanosis occurs with lesser degrees of anoxia.

Cyanosis has been conveniently grouped into "central" and "peripheral" types. *Peripheral* cyanosis results simply from a decrease in cardiac output with sluggish regional flow of blood through the capillary circulation, as a result of which more oxygen is extracted and a greater amount of reduced hemoglobin is present. This type of cyanosis occurs with conditions producing a low cardiac output, such as mitral stenosis, and varies with the condition of the patient. It is usually more prominent in certain regions of the body, such as the tips of the fingers, the lips, or the lobes of the ears.

Central cyanosis results either from a defect in oxygenation of blood in the lungs or from an intracardiac shunt. Cyanosis resulting from ventilatory insufficiency can usually be recognized from its prompt improvement when the patient breathes 100% oxygen, increasing the efficiency of pulmonary ventilation. In the catheterization laboratory it can be recognized from the finding that oxygen saturation of blood in the left atrium is less than 95 percent. Pulmonary insufficiency from cardiac disease occurs only with severe pulmonary congestion from cardiac failure or far advanced pulmonary vascular disease.

An intracardiac shunt, permitting direct entry of venous blood into the systemic circulation, is the cause of central cyanosis in most patients. The intensity of the cyanosis is related to the volume of pulmonary blood flow, for ultimately cyanosis depends upon the relative proportions of unoxygenated and oxygenated blood in the arterial circulation. Even though a large intracardiac shunt is present, an increase in pulmonary blood flow to produce a larger amount of oxygenated blood can substantially reduce cyanosis and improve oxygen transport. This was dramatically demonstrated by Blalock with the systemic-pulmonary artery anastomosis for tetralogy of Fallot.

The two distinctive changes that inevitably appear with chronic cyanosis are clubbing of the digits and polycythemia. The triad of cyanosis, clubbing, and polycythemia is a familiar one in children with congenital heart disease. Clubbing of the digits, or hypertrophic osteoarthropathy, is an unusual change in the appearance and structure of the digits, consisting of a rounding of the tips of the fingers and toes, as well as a thickening of the ends, associated with deposition of fibrous tissue. In addition, there may be a pronounced convexity of the fingernails. Histologically, the fingers have increased numbers of capillaries, with a large number of tiny arteriovenous aneurysms. Clubbing is usually not prominent until a cyanotic child is one to two years of age, but in some instances of severe anoxia it may evolve within several weeks. It usually gradually subsides following correction of the intracardiac defect.

Polycythemia is a fortunate physiologic response of the bone marrow to chronic anoxia, as an increase in red cell and hemoglobin concentration increases the ability of the blood to transport oxygen. Hematocrits of 60 to 70 percent are frequent with chronic cyanosis: values exceeding 80 percent are noted in extreme cases. There is a parallel rise in viscosity of the blood, with restriction to the flow of blood as the hematocrit rises. Once the hematocrit exceeds 75 to 80 percent, the increased viscosity constitutes a significant hazard, for transitory dehydration in an infant with a hematocrit above 80 percent may precipitate cerebral venous thrombosis and permanent neurologic injury, apparently from formation of thrombi in the viscous blood.

Limitation of Exercise Tolerance. A decrease in exercise tolerance, with dyspnea on exertion, is characteristic of cyanotic heart disease, for the circulation is unable to increase oxygen transport with exercise. The severity of the disability, or its progression, can be conveniently measured in terms of the patient's ability to walk a measured distance. Associated with exertional dyspnea is squatting, a phenomenon first emphasized by Taussig. The cyanotic child quickly learns that dyspnea on walking can be lessened by assuming a squatting position. Physiologic studies indicate that squatting produces an increase in peripheral vascular resistance, with a corresponding increase in pulmonary blood flow. Squatting is most commonly seen in tetralogy of Fallot, less frequently in other cyanotic conditions.

Neurologic Damage. Periodic episodes of unconsciousness, termed *cyanotic spells,* are grave signs of cerebral anoxia. They often appear in the third to fourth month of life in severely cyanotic children, even in the first few weeks of life with extreme anoxia, but are rare after the fifth to sixth year of life. They characteristically occur at different times, not always associated with exertion, and evolve as episodes of crying, deepening cyanosis, and coma, lasting a few minutes to a few hours. Such episodes are extremely grave, for although recovery may ensue promptly, the spells are recurrent, and any spell may either terminate fatally or result in permanent neurologic injury. Emergency surgical treatment to improve the oxygen content of the arterial blood is strongly indicated.

Another cause of neurologic injury in cyanotic children is brain abscess, for which there is an increased susceptibility especially in children with tetralogy of Fallot. The increased susceptibility is partly related to direct access of bacteria in the venous circulation to the arterial circulation through the right-to-left shunt. This is probably not the entire explanation, however, for a similar increased frequency does not occur in other cyanotic conditions. A localized infarct with subsequent bacterial infection may explain the evolution in some patients.

Another rare cause of cerebral injury is paradoxic embolism through an intracardiac defect, in which a thrombus migrating in the venous circulation, which would normally produce a pulmonary embolus, traverses an intracardiac defect and lodges in the cerebral circulation. Hence permanent neurologic injury, most often seen as hemiplegia, is not uncommon in children with chronic severe cyanosis, constituting a strong indication for early surgical therapy when possible.

Other Changes. In older children with severe cyanosis there is a striking increase in bronchial circulation, apparently a compensatory response to the chronic decrease in pulmonary blood flow. The myriads of collateral vessels,

often constituting a mass of varicosities in the mediastinum, are principally of surgical significance because of the risk of bleeding during operation. They may be associated with epistaxis in some children, but hemoptysis is rare because the pulmonary blood flow is usually less than normal, even though the bronchial circulation is greatly increased.

Eventually, with chronic polycythemia in children older than ten to fifteen years of age, multiple defects in blood coagulation occur, with abnormalities in several components of the blood-clotting mechanism. Clinically this may result in mild gastrointestinal bleeding, but the major significance is the increased susceptibility to hemorrhage following surgical procedures.

Clinical Examination

HISTORY. In obtaining the history of a patient with congenital heart disease, the presence of abnormal factors during pregnancy, especially during the first trimester, should be noted. Rubella in the first trimester has been emphasized because of the high incidence of cardiac and other defects. In some disorders, notably hypertrophic muscular aortic stenosis, there is a definite familial history of the disorder. Also, with the majority of patients with congenital heart disease there is about a 2 percent associated occurrence of congenital heart disease in other members of the same family. In most patients, however, no etiologic factors can be found.

The age at which a cardiac murmur was detected for the first time should be carefully noted. Similarly the time of appearance of cyanosis is of significance, whether at birth or subsequently during infancy. Variations in the appearance of cyanosis, as well as its location, are also important. In some patients cyanosis may be recognized at birth, then disappear for months or years, and finally appear again.

A decrease in exercise tolerance, manifested by dyspnea on exertion, is a common symptom and a convenient indication of the severity of the disorder in patients with right-to-left shunts. Squatting can be readily identified by the parents. Symptoms of lesser degrees of restriction in physical capacity, such as undue fatigability or inability to participate in exercise, should be noted, although the ability of many children with large left-to-right shunts to participate vigorously in athletics is impressive. Feeding habits and the pattern of weight are also important features.

Previous neurologic episodes such as cyanotic spells, cerebral embolism, brain abscess, or other signs of cerebral injury should be noted.

An inquiry should be made about infections such as pneumonia, bacterial endocarditis, or rheumatic fever.

PHYSICAL EXAMINATION. Abnormalities in growth and development should be particularly assessed, because these are among the most common signs of cardiac disease. Cyanosis, with clubbing or polycythemia, may be obvious or may require close scrutiny for detection. On examination of the heart, any deformity of the left costal cartilages, indicating long-standing cardiac enlargement, should be noted. A palpable thrill is particularly important, for it almost uniformly indicates significant underlying cardiac disease. Cardiac size should be estimated, although this is difficult in small children and infants and is best determined by the x-ray and echocardiogram. Systolic murmurs are commonly found but often are of little diagnostic significance. Basal systolic murmurs occur with pulmonic stenosis, aortic stenosis, patent ductus in infants, and coarctation of the aorta. A murmur along the left sternal border is particularly prominent with ventricular septal defect. With systolic murmurs the type of murmur, location, and transmission are of particular importance. Diastolic murmurs are infrequent in infants but when present are especially significant. They may occur from aortic insufficiency with prolapse of an aortic cusp, with pulmonic insufficiency from long-standing pulmonary hypertension, or in association with a systolic murmur as the continuous murmur of a patent ductus arteriosus. The cardiac sounds, especially the second sound at the base, may be of importance in certain conditions. The pulmonic second sound is increased with pulmonary hypertension, decreased or absent with pulmonic stenosis or atresia. Variation in splitting of the second sound may be recognized by experienced observers and is of diagnostic importance, especially with atrial septal defect. Disturbances of rhythm are infrequent. The gallop rhythm with its ominous prognosis is seen in terminal forms of cardiac disease.

Examination of the lungs may detect rales from cardiac failure in large left-to-right shunts, but characteristically no abnormalities are found in the lungs with right-to-left shunts producing cyanosis. The hallmark of congestive failure in children is hepatic enlargement, occurring with surprising rapidity and regressing rapidly as failure improves. Hence estimation of the presence and extent of hepatic enlargement is of particular importance. Often hepatic enlargement precedes the detection of audible rales, in contrast to adult forms of cardiac disease. Similarly, edema is usually less prominent clinically than hepatic enlargement.

In the extremities, the presence and quality of the radial, femoral, and pedal pulses should be noted. Faint pulses are characteristic of aortic stenosis. With coarctation, radial pulses are prominent while femoral pulses are weak or absent. Easily palpable, bounding pulses are characteristic of defects producing an abnormal exit of blood from the aorta during diastole, such as patent ductus arteriosus, aortic insufficiency, or a ruptured aneurysm of the sinus of Valsalva. These are associated with an increase in pulse pressure, usually due to a decrease in diastolic pressure. Normally the systolic blood pressure in infants is in the range of 70 to 90 mmHg, rising to about 100 mmHg in the first 5 years of life and subsequently to the normal adult level of 120 mmHg in the next few years. Diastolic pressures are usually in the range of 55 to 60 mmHg.

Examination of the digits is particularly useful with cyanosis, because clubbing is inevitable with chronic severe cyanosis.

LABORATORY STUDIES. The basic noninvasive studies are the chest x-ray, electrocardiogram, and echocardiogram. On the chest x-ray, cardiac size, contour, and vascularity of the lung fields should be noted. Unusual abnormalities include pleural effusion and notching of the ribs, seen in coarctation of the aorta. Cardiac size is best expressed as the cardiothoracic ratio, with a ratio greater than 0.5 indicating cardiac enlargement. In oblique views, enlargement of specific cardiac chambers can be estimated, though this is more precisely done with echocardiography, measuring in centimeters the exact dimensions of the atria and ventricles. Enlargement of the left atrium occurs with mitral insufficiency, ventricular septal defect, patent ductus arteriosus, or any form of left ventricular failures. Left ventricular enlargement is characteristic of aortic disease, mitral insufficiency, coarctation of the aorta, patent ductus arteriosus, and ventricular septal defect. Right atrial enlargement is especially prominent in Ebstein's malformation and also occurs in tricuspid atresia, atrial septal defect, and pulmonic stenosis. Selective enlargement of the right ventricle is frequently seen with pulmonic stenosis, pulmonary hypertension from any cause, atrial septal defect, and ventricular septal defect.

Characteristic changes in contour are seen in certain malformations. The Sabot-shaped heart of tetralogy of Fallot results from hypertrophy of the right ventricle in association with a small pulmonary conus (Fig. 18-1). The egg-shaped heart of transposition of the great vessels (Fig. 18-2) is caused by enlargement of the right ventricle

Fig. 18-1. Chest radiograph of child with tetralogy of Fallot, showing typical cardiac silhouette (sabot-shaped heart). Features include heart of normal size with prominent apex from right ventricular hypertrophy. There is increased concavity at base of heart because pulmonic stenosis produces decrease in size or absence of shadow normally seen from pulmonary artery. Vascularity of lung fields may be normal or decreased. *(Courtesy of Dr. Raymond M. Abrams, Department of Radiology, New York University Medical Center.)*

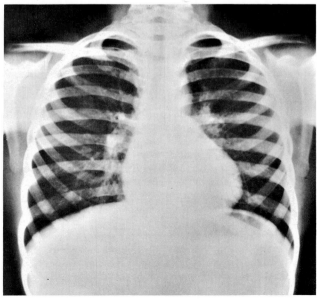

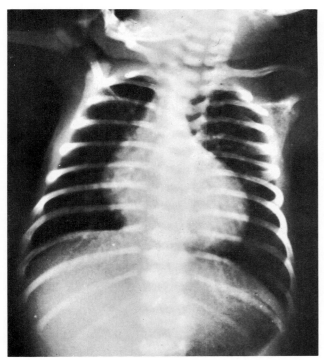

Fig. 18-2. Chest radiograph of child with transposition of great vessels, showing egg-shaped heart with large ventricular silhouette and small "waist," which results from abnormal location of aorta directly anterior to pulmonary artery. *(Courtesy of Dr. Raymond M. Abrams, Department of Radiology, New York University Medical Center.)*

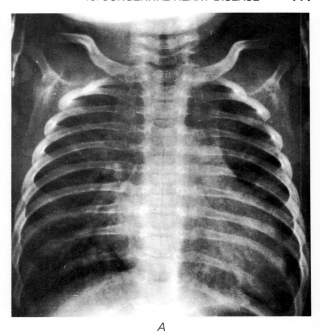

A

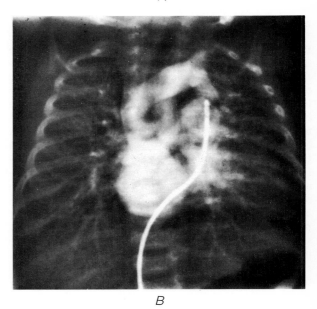

B

Fig. 18-3. *A.* Chest radiograph of child with total anomalous drainage of pulmonary veins through left superior vena cava. Shadow in left upper mediastinum is due to dilated left superior vena cava. *B.* Angiogram demonstrates left superior vena cava emptying into greatly dilated left innominate vein. This x-ray appearance is very suggestive of total anomalous drainage of pulmonary veins into left superior vena cava. *(Courtesy of Dr. Raymond M. Abrams, Department of Radiology, New York University Medical Center.)*

and right atrium, with a narrow shadow at the base from the anterior posterior relation between the aorta and pulmonary arteries. With total anomalous drainage of the pulmonary venous return, a figure of eight abnormality (Fig. 18-3), composed of a large left superior vena cava in the upper mediastinum separate from the cardiac shadow, is characteristic. The size of the pulmonary vessels and the pulmonary vascularity are also important. With left-to-right shunts producing a significant increase in pulmonary flow, the vessels are enlarged with engorgement of the lung fields. The appearance may be strikingly different from conditions with a normal or decreased pulmonary blood flow, as in tetralogy of Fallot.

The electrocardiogram is the best guide to the presence of ventricular hypertrophy. Selective hypertrophy of the left ventricle, as in aortic valvular stenosis, or selective hypertrophy of the right ventricle, as in pulmonic valvular stenosis, can be identified and correlated with the degree of stenosis.

The echocardiogram is often more precise, measuring the wall thickness of the involved chamber in millimeters. Very extensive developments have been made in the field of echocardiography over the past few years, as a result of which classic indications for cardiac catheterization are decreasing. With modern two-dimensional echocardiography, astonishingly clear images can be obtained of the different cardiac chambers. The noninvasive aspects

of echocardiography make it a particularly attractive diagnostic modality for prompt safe evaluation of many conditions, especially in seriously ill newborn infants. For many conditions catheterization with cineangiography is essential for complete evaluation because the measurements of intracardiac blood flow and pressures are far more precise than those that can be obtained by the two-dimensional echocardiogram with Doppler flow studies. With cardiac catheterization the intracardiac pressures can be determined, abnormal shunts of blood recognized, and the ratio between pulmonary and systemic blood flow determined. Mitral and aortic insufficiency are best evaluated by cineangiography.

In the normal heart the right atrial systolic pressure does not exceed 5 mmHg, while left atrial pressure is in the range of 5 to 12 mmHg. In the normal right ventricle systolic pressure ranges from 15 to 30 mmHg, while in the left ventricle pressures average 80 to 120 mmHg systolic and 5 to 12 mmHg diastolic. Continuous pressure recordings as a catheter is withdrawn from one cardiac chamber to another can readily detect the presence of stenosis; pulmonic stenosis can be measured as a catheter is withdrawn from the pulmonary artery to the right ventricle, and aortic stenosis as a catheter is withdrawn from the left ventricle into the aorta. Combined right- and left-heart catheterization is usually done with the introduction of a catheter through a systemic vein into the right side of the heart, combined with introduction of another catheter from a peripheral artery into the aorta and across the aortic valve into the left ventricle to obtain information from both the right and left sides of the heart simultaneously.

All variations from the normal pulmonary and systemic flow of 3 L/min per square meter of body surface may occur with intracardiac shunts. A rise in oxygen saturation of 1 volume percent between cardiac chambers is usually sufficient evidence to diagnose an intracardiac left-to-right shunt. Smaller shunts may be detected with a hydrogen electrode. A pulmonary blood flow one and one-half to two times greater than systemic blood flow is associated with mild physiologic disturbances and is on the borderline of indications for surgical correction. Defects producing greater pulmonary blood flows are usually recommended for operation. From the combination of pulmonary blood flow and pulmonary pressure, pulmonary vascular resistance can be calculated, which in the presence of pulmonary hypertension is one of the most significant physiologic measurements influencing prognosis.

The most precise physiologic evaluation of the degree of valvular stenosis is obtained by calculation of the functional cross-sectional area of the stenotic valve orifice. A normal mitral valve has a functional cross-sectional area of about 5 cm^2; mitral stenosis with an area of less than 1.5 cm^2 is functionally significant. In the aortic valve, normally with a cross-sectional area of 3 to 4 cm^2, a stenosis producing an opening of less than 0.8 cm^2 is functionally significant. Similarly, in the pulmonic valve, with a normal cross-sectional area of 2 to 4 cm^2, a stenosis producing an opening of less than 0.8 cm^2 is functionally significant.

Principles of Operative and Postoperative Care of Infants

Certain principles of management specifically pertain to infants undergoing cardiovascular surgery. For general

principles of operative monitoring, extracorporeal circulation, cardiac massage, and defibrillation, Chap. 19 on acquired heart disease should be consulted.

OPERATIVE MANAGEMENT. Four important aspects of operative care are temperature control, fluid administration, prevention of air emboli, and serial blood-gas monitoring. Temperature control is essential in infants, especially in air-conditioned operating rooms, because body temperature will quickly decrease to below 32°C when the infant is anesthetized and shivering mechanisms are abolished. Constant recording of the temperature with an electric esophageal or rectal probe is mandatory, and some method of warming the infant, preferably a water mattress, should routinely be employed.

Fluids must be administered with unusual precision; a 3-kg infant in cardiac failure should have no more than 20 to 40 mL of fluid in excess of measured losses during an operative procedure.

The danger of air embolism is frequently overlooked in cyanotic infants with right-to-left shunts, in whom air emboli can bypass the heart and lungs to enter the cerebral or the coronary circulation. With intravenous therapy, much care is required to prevent small air emboli, which can easily occur with the usual intravenous therapy during an operation. Only a few small bubbles, if lodged in a coronary artery, can precipitate ventricular fibrillation.

Serial measurement of the pH and the oxygen and carbon dioxide tensions of arterial and central venous blood, usually at 20- to 30-min intervals during an operation, is perhaps the most essential part of monitoring. Using a Swan-Ganz catheter, cardiac output and pulmonary wedge pressure can also be determined. Metabolic and respiratory acidosis are extremely frequent in seriously ill infants and may quickly become intensified with compression of the lung, ineffective cardiac contraction, or hypovolemia. A pH of central venous blood below 7.30 should be promptly corrected by appropriate ventilation, bicarbonate infusion, cessation of anesthesia, or other measures to increase cardiac output. In the author's experience, changes in pH almost always antedate cardiac arrest or ventricular fibrillation. With serial monitoring of blood-gas tensions during operation, desperately ill anoxic children may tolerate procedures that ordinarily would terminate in cardiac arrest or fibrillation.

POSTOPERATIVE CARE. Four important principles in a pediatric intensive care unit are constant observation, monitoring of the electrocardiogram, routine measurement of blood-gas tensions, and respiratory therapy.

Constant observation of the seriously ill infant by experienced staff on a 24-h basis is mandatory. This includes observation of adequacy of ventilation, blood-gas tensions, fluid therapy, and arrhythmias detected on the electrocardiogram. Ventricular fibrillation can appear virtually without warning but can be corrected, usually with electric cardioversion, if therapy can be started within 1 to 3 min. Hence, intensive care unit monitors with electrical alarms are essential.

Serial measurement of blood-gas tensions by analysis of blood samples withdrawn through arterial and central venous catheters is the best measurement of adequacy of ventilation and circulation. Arterial carbon dioxide tensions above 40 mmHg promptly develop with inefficient ventilation, and pH values below 7.30 quickly occur with either metabolic or respiratory acidosis. These changes far antedate any obvious clinical alteration in pulse or blood pressure and accordingly permit more effective therapy. Whether changes in pH and gas tensions are due to metabolic or respiratory causes can be determined by clinical evaluation and by gas analysis of peripheral arterial blood. Periodic measurement of cardiac output is a valuable guide in critically ill patients.

Proper ventilation may be a difficult postoperative problem in an infant following a thoracotomy or sternotomy. Secretions are difficult to remove, the tracheobronchial passages are so small that instrumental manipulation is difficult and can precipitate occlusive edema, and infants quickly develop cardiac arrest with transient anoxia or respiratory acidosis. Many advances in respiratory therapy of infants have been made in the past several years. These include mechanical respirators specifically designed for infants, the continuous positive-pressure breathing system developed by Gregory, and intermittent mandatory ventilation.

The following methods of management have been found useful, but the mode of application varies widely with individual patients. Adequate humidity, with the infant kept in a dense mist following operation, is essential. An endotracheal tube may be left in place for an indeterminate length of time following operation to assist ventilation and removal of secretions. Some have left endotracheal tubes in position for days or weeks, but the author prefers a much shorter period, usually less than 24 to 48 h. When an endotracheal tube is left in position, it may require changing every 6 to 12 h if inspissated secretions occlude the tip of the tube.

Translaryngeal aspiration of the trachea, accomplished with a laryngoscope to permit direct introduction of a soft catheter between the vocal cords into the trachea, is a valuable technique. It must be done by experienced personnel, otherwise trauma and edema of the vocal cords will quickly develop. The flexible bronchoscope is also being used with increasing frequency; it is far less traumatic than the rigid bronchoscope.

Tracheostomy should be avoided if possible but should be done if secretions cannot be adequately removed otherwise. With a precise technique avoiding excision of any tracheal cartilage, complications are far less frequent than in the past. An extensive experience with tracheostomy and mechanical ventilation for several weeks in the treatment of neonatal tetanus has clearly demonstrated the safety of a properly performed tracheostomy in infants.

OBSTRUCTIVE LESIONS

Pulmonic Stenosis

HISTORICAL DATA. In 1947–1948 Brock and Sellors independently performed the first successful valvulotomies for pulmonic valvular stenosis, using a valvulotome through a transventricular approach. A series of 19 patients was reported on by Blalock shortly thereafter. Open cardiotomy, using hypothermia and venous inflow occlusion, was first done in 1954 by Swan and Zeavin. Virtually all operations have been performed with extracorporeal circulation. In critically ill neonates, inflow occlusion and closed valvulotomy are still employed.

Recently, Srinivasan and Subramanian resurrected the concept of closed transventricular valvulotomy and reported survival in 14 of 16 patients less than three months of age. Ten additional infants over three months of age were operated upon using this technique. Late results were excellent in all but one.

INCIDENCE AND ETIOLOGY. Pulmonic stenosis is a common defect, constituting about 10 percent of all patients with congenital heart disease. It was once considered very rare. Taussig, a world-renowned authority, wrote in her classic monograph in 1947 that she had not had an opportunity to study a proven case herself. This astonishing statement indicates the degree to which knowledge of a disease is influenced by the diagnostic and therapeutic methods available. Usually there are no known etiologic factors. Rubella occurring during pregnancy has been implicated.

PATHOLOGIC ANATOMY. Pulmonic stenosis is a spectrum of disorders involving the pulmonary valve cusps, the valve annulus, the pulmonary artery, and the right ventricle. The most common variety results from fusion of the pulmonary valve cusps (Figs. 18-4 and 18-5). The severity varies widely, ranging from mild, clinically insignificant stenosis to "pinhole" stenosis requiring emergency care in neonatal life, to pulmonary atresia. Pulmonary atresia, fortunately, is uncommon, for it is a more severe malformation associated with varying degrees of

Fig. 18-4. Pulmonic valvular stenosis with fused valve cusps creating central stenotic opening. Annulus of pulmonic valve ring is normal. (From: *Cole WH, Zollinger RM: Textbook of Surgery, 8th ed. New York, Appleton-Century-Crofts, 1963, p 935, with permission.*)

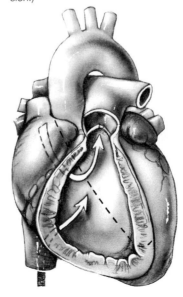

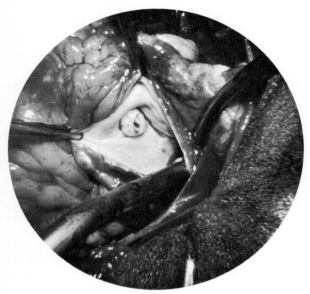

Fig. 18-5. Pulmonic valvular stenosis exposed at operation following incision of pulmonary artery. Dome-shaped structure produced by fusion of valve cusps, with small central opening, is clearly shown. Suction tip has been placed in distal pulmonary artery.

atresia of the right ventricle and malformation of the tricuspid valve. In the majority of patients with valvular stenosis, abnormalities in the right ventricle and tricuspid valve are not severe with the single exception of hypoplasia of the right ventricle in 10 to 15 percent of patients.

Hypoplasia of the annulus of the pulmonic valve, though uncommon, is most important to recognize because it mandates division of the annulus and insertion of a prosthetic patch to relieve the obstruction. A valuable nomogram, published by Kirklin, describes the normal relationships in children between cross-sectional areas of the pulmonic valve and body weight.

In pulmonary valvular dysplasia the obstruction is due to thickened shortened cusps, without any commissural fusion. Obstruction in the outflow tract of the right ventricle usually consists of diffuse muscular hypertrophy rather than a true hypoplasia. With severe chronic stenosis the hypertrophied right ventricular wall may be 1 to 2 cm thick, significantly decreasing right ventricular volume.

In 5 to 10 percent of patients an isolated infundibular stenosis is present (Figs. 18-6, 18-7). This type of stenosis is more commonly seen in association with ventricular septal defect, discussed in the section on tetralogy of Fallot.

Some degree of poststenotic dilatation of the pulmonary artery, especially the left, is seen in 60 to 70 percent of older patients. The foramen ovale is almost always patent, with the margins stretched apart because of the increased right atrial pressure.

PATHOPHYSIOLOGY. The obstruction to flow of blood produces elevation in right ventricular systolic pressure with a subsequent secondary hypertrophy of the right ventricle. The severity is most simply defined by deter-

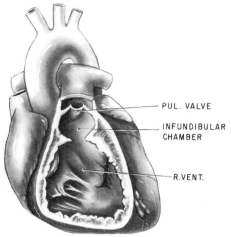

Fig. 18-6. Types of subvalvular or infundibular pulmonic stenosis. Infundibular stenosis may result in a discrete chamber between stenotic area and pulmonic valve. (From: *Cole WH, Zollinger RM: Textbook of Surgery, 8th ed. New York, Appleton-Century Crofts, 1963, p 936, with permission.*)

mining the systolic gradient between the right ventricle and the pulmonary artery. A gradient less than 50 mm is considered ''mild,'' while one greater than 80 mm is considered ''severe.'' With severe stenosis, high right ventricular systolic pressures may develop, reaching levels of 150 to 200 mmHg.

As the child grows, progressive hypertrophy of the right ventricle may increase the degree of obstruction present. If the stenotic pulmonary valve enlarges with

Fig. 18-7. Heart with infundibular stenosis. Site of infundibular stenosis is visible as area of constriction in outflow tract of right ventricle. Infundibular chamber, consisting of dilated right ventricular muscle, is located between infundibular stenosis proximally and pulmonary vein distad.

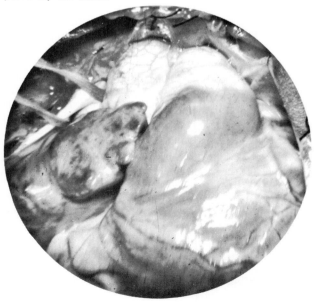

growth, the obstruction may remain stable or decrease; otherwise a small opening tolerated by a small child may produce serious obstruction subsequently. In some patients, severe elevation in right ventricular pressure is well tolerated for many years. In others, elevation of right atrial pressure produces a right-to-left shunt through the foramen ovale with resulting hypoxemia and cyanosis. Overt cardiac failure is uncommon after the first year of life. Right ventricular failure with hepatic enlargement and ascites is uncommon except in adults.

CLINICAL MANIFESTATIONS. Patients are often asymptomatic. Some dyspnea and easy fatigability are the most common symptoms. In a few patients, chest pain, apparently angina, is present.

On physical examination a harsh loud systolic murmur, heard best in the second left interspace, is characteristic. This is an ejection type murmur, the peak intensity varying with the severity of the stenosis. The pulmonic second sound is usually decreased or absent. Forceful contractions of the hypertrophied right ventricle may be palpable along the left sternal border.

The chest x-ray usally shows normal or decreased vascularity of the peripheral lung fields in association with prominence or overt poststenotic dilatation of the pulmonary artery. Enlargement of the right ventricle is usually prominent.

The electrocardiographic changes are those of right ventricular hypertrophy. The echocardiogram is virtually diagnostic, outlining both the location and severity of the obstruction. The severity of the obstruction, as well as associated abnormalities, are best defined by cardiac catheterization and angiography. Precise angiography is essential, noting the severity of hypertrophy in the right ventricular outflow tract, any focal obstruction, the pulmonic valve cusps, the diameter of the pulmonic annulus, and the size of the main pulmonary artery and its branches.

The diagnosis can be considered with reasonable certainty with the finding of a loud systolic murmur in the second intercostal space, combined with a weak pulmonic second sound. The noninvasive laboratory studies easily confirm the diagnosis. Until echocardiography and catheterization were performed, pulmonic stenosis with right-to-left shunting through a foramen ovale was confused with a tetralogy of Fallot.

TREATMENT. With mild pulmonic stenosis, no treatment is necessary. Often there are no cardiographic signs of hypertrophy of the right ventricle. With signs of significant right ventricular hypertrophy, cardiac catheterization should be done. Operation is usually performed if a systolic gradient greater than 50 mm is present between the right ventricle and the pulmonary artery.

In critically ill neonates, operation must be performed urgently within the first few days or weeks of life. Infusion of prostaglandin E_1 (PGE_1) in doses of 0.05 to 0.4 μg/kg per minute has become a valuable part of therapy, often significantly raising peripheral arterial saturation with immediate improvement in the infant's condition. In critically ill infants, the most popular approach is normothermic inflow occlusion for no more than 2 min, during which the stenotic valve can be quickly opened through a pulmonary arteriotomy. With the isolated exception of one report from the Boston Children's Hospital, however, mortality has remained distressingly high, 30 to 40 percent. Also there is little opportunity to correct a hypoplastic pulmonary annulus, dysplastic valve leaflets, or associated stenosis in the right ventricle. Balloon valvuloplasty is emerging as an alternate form of therapy in these critically ill infants. Though it has been employed in older patients, results with standard surgical techniques are so good that they are still generally applied. The different methods of therapy employed are well summarized by Coles and Trusler.

Operative Technique. Except for emergency operations performed in neonates (the first month of life), virtually all operations are performed with extracorporeal circulation through a median sternotomy. Careful study of the preoperative ventriculogram is most important to detect diffuse or focal stenosis in the right ventricle, hypoplasia of the pulmonic annulus, or focal stenosis in the main pulmonary artery or its branches. Cold potassium cardioplegia is routinely used. Valvulotomy is usually done through a longitudinal arteriotomy in the pulmonary artery dividing the fused commissures. Calibration of the annulus of the pulmonic valve with Hegar dilators is the best method for determining if significant hypoplasia is present, using the nomogram developed by Kirklin. Indications for performance of a ventriculotomy for diffuse obstruction are debatable, often based on the preoperative ventriculogram. If valvulotomy is employed as the standard procedure for all patients, 10 to 15 percent will require cooperation for infundibular stenosis.

The right ventricular incision may be longitudinal or transverse. If a longitudinal incision is made, a small prosthetic patch of dacron is used to close the ventriculotomy. At NYU considerable reliance has been placed on pressure gradients measured in the operating room to confirm relief of the obstruction. Others consider such pressure measurements of little value in deciding for or against resection of hypertrophied muscle. A foramen ovale, if present, is routinely sutured.

An alternate approach is the performance of valvulotomy with a valvulotome. The original Potts valvulotome is shown in Fig. 18-8. Subramanian reported good results with a valvulotome in a series of operations on critically ill infants.

Operative mortality is small, 1 percent or less after the first few months of life. Results are usually excellent. If signs of significant ventricular hypertrophy remain on the electrocardiogram after a few months, repeat catheterization should be done. Some degree of pulmonic insufficiency may be present, depending upon the abnormality in the fused valve cusps, but this is seldom of physiologic significance.

Congenital Aortic Stenosis

INCIDENCE AND ETIOLOGY. The condition is a common congenital abnormality, representing 8 to 10 percent of all patients with congenital heart disease. For unknown rea-

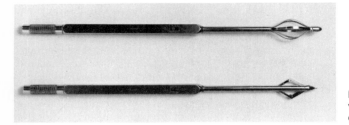

Fig. 18-8. Dilator and valvulotome developed by Potts for pulmonic valvulotomy. Calibrated swivel mechanism permits precise opening or closing of instruments.

sons, it is three to four times more frequent in males. Congenital aortic regurgitation, however, is uncommon. No causative factors are known. In the unusual variants of supravalvular or diffuse muscular stenosis associated factors suggest a genetic origin.

PATHOLOGIC ANATOMY. Over four types of congenital valvular stenosis have been described; the majority are either a bicuspid valve or a tricuspid valve with fusion of commissures. A bicuspid valve is a very common anomaly, occurring in nearly 2 percent of the normal population. A common variety of bicuspid valve is failure of separation of the right and left cusps, with the undeveloped commissure being represented by a median raphe that may or may not extend to the ventircular well. Thickening of the valve cusp is common and may, when severe, contribute to the stenosis. Calcification is frequent in adults but almost never seen before eighteen years of age. Mild poststenotic dilatation of the ascending aorta is common. In infants with severe valvular stenosis, more severe deformities are common, often a unicuspid valve. Other cardial malformations also commonly accompany this lesion, but subaortic stenosis is rare.

Subvalvular stenosis ranges from a narrow ring of fibrous tissue to a short fibromuscular tunnel in 15 to 20 percent of patients, with gradation between these two extremes. The discrete ringlike stenosis is present in about one-half of patients. The proximal aortic outflow tract is usually narrowed from muscular hypertrophy. Distally, the stenotic ring is adjacent to the base of the aortic cusp, often connected to the base of one cusp with a small raphe of fibrous tissue.

Two other anatomic relationships are of particular surgical importance. Beneath the noncoronary cusp the stenotic ring is attached to the ventricular septum, which can be perforated and the conduction bundle injured if appropriate landmarks are not observed. Beneath the left coronary cusp, the ring is attached to the base of the aortic leaflet of the mitral valve, which must be protected during excision.

Associated cardiac malformations are found in 15 to 20 percent of patients, more often with valvular stenosis. The most frequent ones are patent ductus, coarctation of the aorta, ventricular septal defect, and pulmonic stenosis.

PATHOPHYSIOLOGY. The physiologic abnormality is directly related to the severity of the obstruction. Mild stenosis of little physiologic significance can occur in the presence of typical physical findings. At the other extreme, severe obstruction can cause death from congestive heart failure in infants or sudden death in older children.

Cardiac catheterization easily quantifies the severity of the stenosis. This is usually expressed as peak systolic gradient between the left ventricle and aorta. A gradient less than 40 mmHg usually does not produce enough disability to require operation. The more precise measurement is to calculate the functional cross-sectional area of the aortic valve from the combination of pressure gradient and cardiac output. A cross-sectional area less than 0.5 cm/m^2 of body surface should be surgically corrected. Usually there is a systolic gradient of 50 to 75 mmHg with aortic stenosis of moderate severity, while severe stenosis produces gradients above 80 mmHg. Depending upon the degree of stenosis, there is a varying degree of hypertrophy of the left ventricle. Severe cardiac failure in infants is often fatal unless corrected.

Often between the ages of two and ten there are few signs of impaired ventricular function. As children grow, however, there may be a progressive decrease in cardiac reserve, with restriction of coronary and cerebral blood flow. Overt congestive failure, however, is rare. In some patients, as a consequence of fibrosis, there is an increase in the severity of the stenosis. Sudden death may occur, at times with a normal electrocardiogram. The risk of sudden death varies with different reports, and also with the signs of severity of obstruction. The mortality rate ranges from 4 to 9 percent.

In young adults with aortic stenosis calcification of the fused cusps develops with increasing frequency, approaching 100 percent in the third and fourth decades. Calcification superimposes rigidity of the leaflets onto the obstruction from the narrow orifice. Thus patients who have a history of an asymptomatic cardiac murmur during childhood may develop severe symptoms due to calcification. It is surprising how long some patients may function before calcification and rigidity precipitate cardiac failure. The author has frequently operated on patients over 70 years of age with calcific aortic stenosis and the classic commissural abnormalities of a congenital bicuspid valve.

Trivial aortic insufficiency is present in about 50 percent of patients with subaortic stenosis. This apparently arises from thickening of the aortic cusps. Fortunately, it is rarely of any consequence. Endocarditis is a rare complication, occurring in only 1 to 3 percent of patients.

CLINICAL MANIFESTATIONS. Symptoms. Many children with significant stenosis are asymptomatic, emphasizing the importance of catheterization to measure the severity of the abnormality. The most common symptoms are fatigue, dyspnea, angina, and syncope, found in 30 to 50 percent of patients. Usually these are found with a gradient above 50 mmHg.

Physical Examination. The four most frequent physical findings are a basal systolic murmur, a palpable thrill, a forceful left ventricular impulse, and a narrow pulse pressure. The systolic murmur is a harsh, ejection-type murmur heard best in the second right interspace, widely transmitted to the neck and arms. A palpable thrill is present in over 80 percent of patients. The left ventricular impulse is forceful and heaving. Pulse pressure is decreased in 30 to 40 percent of patients. An early diastolic murmur can be heard in 15 to 20 percent of patients; it is apparently of no physiologic significance.

LABORATORY FINDINGS. The electrocardiogram, indicating the severity of left ventricular hypertrophy, provides a moderately sensitive noninvasive guide to the severity of aortic stenosis, but has distinct limitations. The usual abnormalities are signs of left ventricular hypertrophy, and subsequent depression of the ST segment and inversion of T waves. With a gradient above 50 mmHg, a left ventricular strain pattern is common. Some patients may have severe obstruction with few electrocardiographic abnormalities.

The chest radiograph is frequently normal, because concentric hypertrophy of the left ventricle, rather than dilatation, is present. About one-half of patients will have a cardiothoracic ratio slightly greater than 50 percent. Mild dilatation of the ascending aorta is often noted. 2-D echocardiography is very useful. Doppler measurements define the gradient with reasonable accuracy.

Cardiac catheterization, measuring the systolic gradient between the left ventricle and aorta, readily establishes both the diagnosis and the severity. If the gradient is less than 50 mmHg, the functional cross-sectional area of the valve should be calculated. Valvular stenosis may be differentiated from subvalvular by angiography.

DIAGNOSIS. The diagnosis can be made with reasonable certainty with the findings of the characteristic systolic murmur, palpable thrill, left ventricular impulse, and narrow pulse pressure. Confirmatory evidence can be obtained from the chest radiograph and the electrocardiogram. Cardiac catheterization should be done to evaluate the severity of the obstruction. In infants the murmur may be loudest to the left of the sternum, requiring catheterization to establish the diagnosis. Critical aortic stenosis has been diagnosed by echocardiography in utero. A caesarean section was done and an aortic valvulotomy successfully performed 12 h later.

TREATMENT. In most children, operation is performed on an elective basis after catheterization has demonstrated the severity of the obstruction.

Operative Technique. The standard approach includes a median sternotomy incision, cardiopulmonary bypass with membrane oxygenator, and cardiac arrest produced by infusing cold blood with potassium to lower the myocardial temperature to below 15°C. The perfusate in the oxygenator is near 25°C. With this technique of myocardial preservation, periods of ischemia for as long as 60 to 90 min, fortunately rarely necessary, seem completely safe.

Once bypass has been established, and the heart cooled and arrested, a vent is inserted into the apex of the left ventricle to aspirate blood from the operative field. The ascending aorta is incised with a curved incision extending down into the noncoronary sinus. Calibrated Hegar dilators are useful for measuring the diameter of the stenotic orifice both before and after commissurotomy. Nomograms help estimate the length of commissural incision necessary to produce an adequate valve orifice. An opening larger than necessary should be made only if there is negligible risk of producing aortic insufficiency. In older children, the orifice should be enlarged so that a size 18 or 20 Hegar can be inserted. A smaller opening may be satisfactory in smaller children.

With valvular stenosis, the fused commissures are carefully incised with a small (#15) knife blade, carefully dividing the fused commissures exactly along the center of the fibrous raphe in order to leave a thick margin on each of the two cusps that are separated (Fig. 18-9). Inappropriate division of the fused commissures may result in an incision to one side of the area of fusion, increasing the likelihood of insufficiency. As far as possible, commissural incisions should be limited to where the commissures are well formed. When necessary, the incisions may be carried to the aortic wall. If not necessary, these may be terminated 1 to 3 mm from the wall.

With the classic bicuspid valve, the commissure be-

Fig. 18-9. *A.* Operative exposure of congenital aortic stenosis. Stenotic aortic valve has been exposed through longitudinal aortotomy. Fused commissures between three aortic cusps are clearly seen, with small central opening. *B* and *C.* Commissurotomy performed with knife, with center of fused commissures carefully incised and incision avoided in areas where commissures are not well developed. (From: *Spencer FC, Neill CA, Bahnson HT: The treatment of congenital aortic stenosis with valvulotomy during cardiopulmonary bypass. Surgery 44:116, 1958, with permission of CV Mosby, St Louis.*)

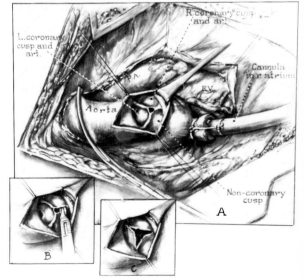

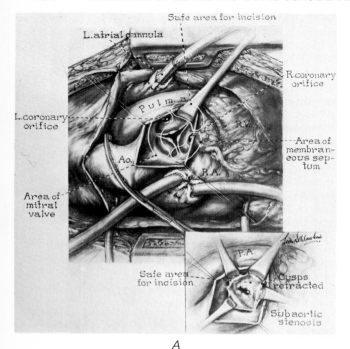

A

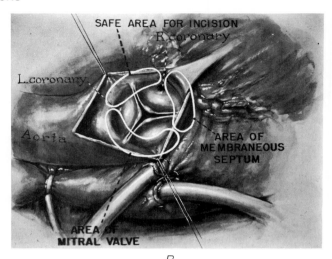

B

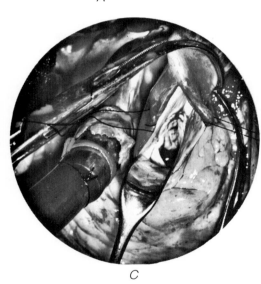

C

Fig. 18-10. *A.* Operative exposure of congenital subaortic stenosis. Valve cusps are normal. Insert shows membranelike subaortic stenosis exposed by retraction of valve cusps. (From: *Am Surg 26:210, 1960, with permission.*) *B.* Diagram of pertinent surgical anatomy with subaortic stenosis. Beneath noncoronary cusps and part of left coronary cusp is aortic leaflet of mitral valve. Beneath part of right coronary cusp is membranous septum. Only in area beneath commissure between right and left coronary cusps is limited zone where underlying ventricular muscle can be safely excised. Failure to observe these landmarks can result in injury to mitral valve or to membranous septum with conduction bundle. *C.* Subaortic stenosis exposed at operation. Aorta has been opened with longitudinal aortotomy and retractor inserted to retract normal aortic cusps. Diaphragmlike subaortic stenosis can be clearly seen with small pinpoint central opening. (From: *Spencer FC, Neill CA, Bahnson HT: The treatment of congenital aortic stenosis with valvulotomy during cardiopulmonary bypass. Surgery 44:117, 1958, with permission of CV Mosby, St Louis.*)

tween the right and left cusps is not well developed. Usually no incision at all is made in this area, leaving the valve as a bicuspid valve. Rarely, a short 2- to 4-mm incision may be cautiously made, but it has the hazard of producing insufficiency. *It is far better to leave some residual stenosis than to produce aortic insufficiency.* Long-term results have been disappointing if significant insufficiency was produced at operation, the patients often requiring aortic valve replacement within a few years because of cardiac failure.

In most patients the stenosis can be adequately relieved without producing significant insufficiency. The technique of commissurotomy has been emphasized in some

detail because most difficulties with aortic insufficiency following aortic valvulotomy have resulted from inept valvulotomies rather than from the pathologic anatomy.

With subvalvular stenosis, the valve cusps can be carefully retracted and the fibrotic ring excised. Excellent visualization is required to prevent injury to the base of the valve cusps. The ring may consist of thin, fibrous tissue, easily removed, or it may be a thick, fibrotic structure requiring excision with a knife and rongeur. Excellent exposure is required because the proximity of the mitral valve and the conduction bundle restricts excision of the ring out to the ventricular muscle to a narrow zone comprising less than 20 percent of the circumference of the ring. This "safe" area corresponds to the area beneath the commissures between the right and left coronary cusps (Fig. 18-10). An adequate rectangular block of hypertrophied muscle must be removed. Radical excision of the fibrotic ring beneath the left coronary cusp may perforate the aortic leaflet of the mitral valve, while radical excision beneath a noncoronary cusp may injure the ventricular septum, creating either a heart block or ventricular septal defect. A right-angled rongeur with a swivel permitting rotation of the instrument to an appropriate angle is particularly useful in small children (Fig. 18-11).

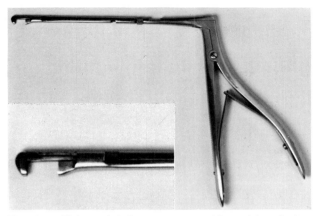

Fig. 18-11. Right-angled sharp rongeur used for excision of subaortic stenosis. Swivel mechanism permits rotation of instrument to obtain proper exposure.

With good exposure, an unhurried approach, and appropriate instruments, the area of stenosis can regularly be excised satisfactorily. Optical magnification and focal illumination with a headlight are excellent adjuncts in small children.

Subsequently the aortotomy is closed with a continuous Prolene suture, leaving a small opening for removal of air. Ventricular fibrillation is induced before removal of the clamp on the aorta, permitting the heart to fill with blood and displace air through the aortotomy and the left ventricular vent before the heart is allowed to beat. Following meticulous removal of air from the heart, defibrillation can be done. Following bypass, with a systemic pressure over 100 mmHg, the pressure gradient across the aortic valve should be measured by needle puncture, preferably obtaining a gradient well under 40 mmHg.

The risks of operation are small, about 1 percent, and the results good. Although several reports express pessimism with operations for aortic stenosis, considering them "palliative," our experience has been most favorable. In the past 15 years there have been no deaths following elective operation in patients with uncomplicated valvular or subvalvular stenosis. A satisfactory reduction in systolic gradient has been achieved in almost all patients; only a few had mild aortic insufficiency. Prosthetic replacement of the aortic valve has not been necessary in any patients in the primary operation, and to date has very rarely been necessary as a secondary complication in the 10 to 15 years years after the initial valvulotomy.

In 1986, Hsieh reported long-term results in 59 patients with a mean follow-up of 18 years. Forty-six patients were alive. Sudden death occurred in seven patients, at least four of whom were known to have significant residual disease. Actuarial analysis revealed the probability of reoperation to increase from 2 percent at 5 years to 44 percent at 22 years. Dobell had reported more discouraging results; one-third of the group required a repeat operation within 10 years.

Rarely emergency valvotomy is required in the first few days of life because of pinpoint life-threatening aortic stenosis. Usually, such operations have had a high mortality, 30 to 50 percent, but the report by Messina et al. is more encouraging. Eleven newborn infants underwent emergency valvotomy using a short period of cardiopulmonary bypass with only one operative death, and no late deaths.

In patients with severe hypoplasia of the left ventricular outflow tract, the best results follow the Konno procedure. Ebert and associates reported results for 14 patients with no operative deaths and one late death from bacterial endocarditis. This procedure seems to be preferable to the once popular insertion of an apical left ventricular-aortic conduit.

Subsequently the patient should be seen at periodic intervals indefinitely because of the abnormal valve. Long-term prognosis is uncertain, although some patients are now over 20 years since operation without subsequent problems. However, the reports cited in the earlier paragraphs indicate that in some centers 20 to 30 percent of patients have required a subsequent operative procedure within 10 years. In all likelihood, eventually fibrosis and calcification of the thickened aortic cusps will lead to stenosis or insufficiency.

SUPRAVALVULAR AORTIC STENOSIS

Supravalvular aortic stenosis is the rarest form of congenital aortic stenosis. Although the first successfully treated patient was reported by McGoon and Kirklin in 1956, 10 years later Rastelli et al., reporting a personal experience with 16 patients, could only find a total of 88 cases in the medical literature, 51 of which had been treated surgically.

There is considerable variation in the type of aortic obstruction in different patients. Peterson et al., reviewing 68 cases, found three types: hourglass, 45 cases; diffuse hypoplastic, 14 cases; membranous, 9 cases (Fig. 18-12). Associated abnormalities are frequent. In about one-third of the patients abnormalities of the aortic valve cusps are present, frequently consisting of adherence of part of one of the free margins of a cusp to the aortic wall, causing aortic regurgitation. Abnormal coronary arteries are found in over one-half of the patients. Often the right coronary artery is markedly dilated and tortuous. Focal stenotic lesions of branches of the aortic arch and peripheral branches of the pulmonary arteries have also been found.

The usual symptoms, as with other forms of aortic stenosis, are angina and syncope. Supravalvular aortic stenosis may be associated with an unusual "elfin" facies and mental retardation. Multiple peripheral pulmonary artery stenoses are also frequently noted. As physical examination provides no clues to the diagnosis except when the typical facies is present, aortography is required to establish the diagnosis. Sudden death is not uncommon in childhood, probably resulting both from the left ventricular outflow obstruction and from the coronary artery disease. It may be that most untreated patients, especially those with the characteristic facies, die before reaching adult life, because the syndrome is uncommon in adults.

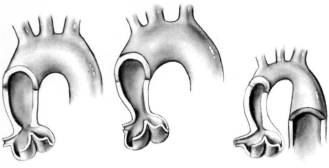

LOCALIZED   DIFFUSE

Fig. 18-12. Different types of supravalvular aortic stenosis, obstruction varying from localized constriction near aortic valve to diffuse hypoplasia of ascending aorta. (From: *Rastelli GC et al: J Thorac Cardiovasc Surg 51:878, 1966, with permission.*)

TREATMENT. With the hourglass type, widening the stenotic area by inserting a patch of Dacron or pericardium is satisfactory. Before the patch is inserted, the intimal ridge lying above the valve cusps should be excised as completely as possible (Figs. 18-13, 18-14). Sudden death has been described in some patients after operation, though the report by Rastelli et al. stated that a follow-up of 15 patients surviving operation found 13 with a good result. All 19 patients in the Kirklin/Barratt-Boyce series have had good short-term results.

Results have been less favorable with the diffuse hypoplastic type of obstruction. Enthusiasm has waned for a left ventricular-aortic conduit because of the high frequency of late complications. Extensive patch grafting of the ascending aorta and transverse aortic arch seems to be the most reasonable approach, though significant data are not available.

When a hypoplastic aortic annulus is present, the ingenious operation reported by Konno in 1975 seems the best approach. This involves extension of the aortotomy down

Fig. 18-13. Operation for localized supravalvular aortic stenosis. Stenotic area is widened by making longitudinal aortotomy and inserting Dacron patch. Partial excision of stenotic membrane is also shown. (From: *Rastelli GC et al: J Thorac Cardiovasc Surg 51:875, 1966, with permission.*)

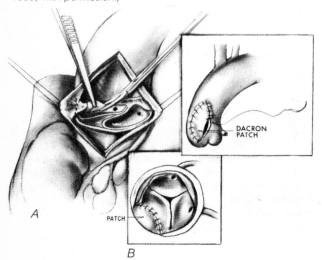

DACRON PATCH

PATCH

A

B

into the upper ventricular septum, with incision of the outflow tract of the right ventricle and the underlying ventricular septum. The complex aortotomy is then repaired with multiple patches after a prosthetic valve has been inserted (Fig. 18-15). Misbach et al. recently reported excellent results in 14 patients. A 23-mm prosthetic valve could be inserted in all patients. There were no operative deaths, one late death from endocarditis, and excellent results in the 13 survivors.

IDIOPATHIC HYPERTROPHIC SUBAORTIC STENOSIS

This disease is a hypertrophic myopathy of the left ventricular muscle, with secondary obstruction of the outflow tract developing from hypertrophy of the septum in about 20 percent of patients. The disease was first characterized in 1960. Diagnosis was greatly facilitated with the development of echocardiography which has recognized asymmetric septal hypertrophy and abnormal systolic anterior motion of the mitral leaflets as characteristic findings. Recognition of patients with few or no symptoms led to confirmation of the fact that the disease is almost always genetic.

Symptoms gradually increase with age, probably as the septal hypertrophy increases. The symptoms are similar to those associated with the more common forms of aortic stenosis and include syncope, angina, and dyspnea. A systolic murmur of medium intensity near the apex, but not prominent at the base of the heart, may be the first clue to the diagnosis. With progressive disease, atrial fibrillation systemic emboli, and sudden death are the most significant events. Sudden death is distressingly common, presumably from an arrhythmia. The chest radiograph and electrocardiogram are not diagnostic, but the 2-D echocardiogram precisely defines the abnormality and establishes the diagnosis. It can be further clarified with catheterization and angiography. On catheterization a gradient varying from 50 to 150 mmHg can be demonstrated in the proximal outflow of the left ventricle. The pressure gradient characteristically increases with the infusion of isoproterenol because of more forceful contraction of the left ventricle.

TREATMENT. Many patients are treated medically, reserving operation for those with symptomatic severe obstruction not improving with medical therapy. Beta

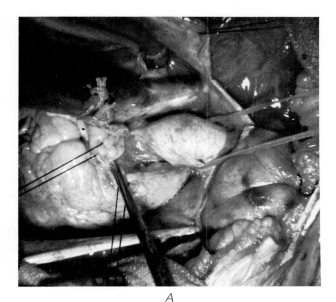

A

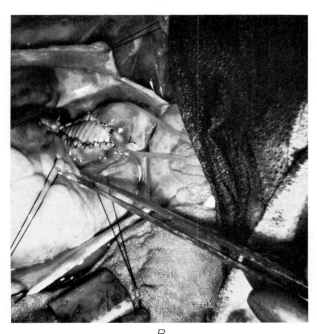

B

Fig. 18-14. *A.* Operative photography of the unusual lesion of supravalvular aortic stenosis. The waistlike narrowing of the ascending aorta just above the aortic valve can be clearly seen. *B.* Operative photograph of correction of supravalvular aortic stenosis by insertion of a Dacron patch to widen the area. The aortic valve gradient was reduced from 80 to near 30 mmHg.

blockade with drugs such as propanolol is usually employed.

Surgical myomectomy, as developed by Morrow, is clearly indicated with symptomatic patients and a gradient of 50 mm or greater. Although Morrow reported excellent results in a series exceeding 200 patients, and others have reported good results in smaller series, the

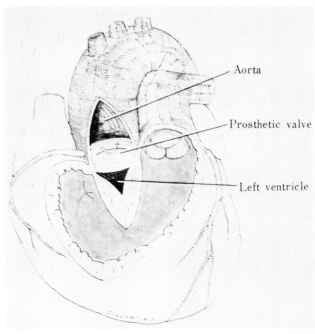

Fig. 18-15. Prosthetic valve is placed in subcoronary position. (From: *Konno S et al: J Thorac Surg 70:909, 1975, with permission.*)

operation is not widely used. Using a transaortic approach, a rectangular block of ventricular muscle is excised from the septum, extending down from the base of the aortic cusp into the ventricular cavity for several centimeters (Fig. 18-16). Late catheterization studies following the radical myomectomy clearly document permanent relief of the outflow tract obstruction.

Kirklin and Barratt-Boyes have reported a combined surgical experience including over 160 patients, with a low operative mortality and excellent long-term results. Symptoms are relieved. Sudden death continues to occur but much less frequently than in nonoperated patients.

Coarctation of the Aorta

HISTORICAL DATA. The characteristic features of coarctation were clearly outlined by Abbott in her classic analysis in 1928. In 1944 and 1945 Blalock and Park, Gross, and Crafoord and Nylin all independently contributed to the first surgical treatment of coarctation by excision and direct anastomosis. Subsequently Gross provided a strong stimulus to the study of vascular grafts by successfully using aortic homografts for patients with coarctation in whom direct anastomosis could not be done.

INCIDENCE AND ETIOLOGY. Coarctation is a common congenital malformation, occurring in 10 to 15 percent of patients with congenital heart disease. It is more common in males (3:1 ratio). Although the cause is unknown, the proximity of the coarctation to the ligamentum arteriosum supports the most plausible theory, that coarctation is an extension of the same fibrotic process that converts the patent ductus into a ligamentum arteriosum.

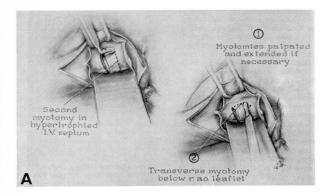

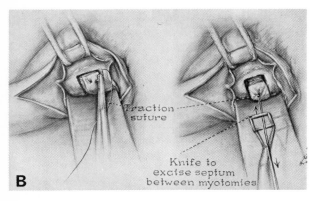

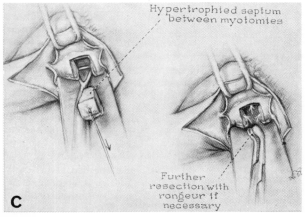

Fig. 18-16. *A.* Second myotomy is made about 1 cm to right (clockwise) of first. Incisions are then deepened if necessary by digital splitting of muscle fibers. Myotomies are usually 12 to 15 mm in depth at most prominent aspect of septum. Transverse incision is then made at base of valve leaflet connecting proximal portions of the myotomies. *B.* Bar of muscle isolated between incisions is held by traction suture as shown or by suitable clamp. Muscle is freed with rectangular knife (devised by Stinson) or with special angled rongeur. *C.* As traction is made on muscle bar, rectangular knife is pushed toward apex, freeing muscle bar from its anterior attachments to septum. Apical portion of resection is often more easily accomplished with rongeur, which may be introduced via aorta or via apical stab wound. In latter case, rongeur is positioned and directed by left index finger passed through valve ring. (From: *Morrow AG et al: Circulation 52:88, 1975, with permission.*)

PATHOLOGIC ANATOMY. In most patients the coarctation consists of a localized stenosis in the first 2 to 4 cm of thoracic aorta beyond the left subclavian artery. Usually there is a 1- to 3-mm lumen, though complete occlusion is present in 20 to 25 percent of patients. The ligamentum arteriosum is attached to the medial surface of the aorta near the site of coarctation. It clearly influences the coarctation, for when surgically divided, the two ends retract sharply, indicating the degree of tension previously exerted.

The stenotic area may have two or three component parts. The most frequent is a localized "shelf," consisting of an infolding of the aortic media into the lumen. This is most visible on the aortic wall opposite the ligamentum arteriosum. In the lumen, a thickened ridge of intima may be present and may increase the severity of the stenosis. In addition, a varying degree of "tubular hypoplasia" consisting of a narrowing of the aorta between the coarctation and the left subclavian artery, often the left common carotid artery, is common.

Distal to the coarctation, the aorta is usually dilated. In adults a true aneurysm forms in a small percentage of patients. Large, dilated intercostal arteries entering the distal aorta, providing collateral circulation around the site of obstruction, are a striking feature. In older patients these large arteries produce "notching" of the ribs. Ultimately they may become aneurysmal and rupture.

Unusual varieties of coarctation include a more proximal site of obstruction, involving the left subclavian artery, or even the left carotid and innominate artery. In some instances there is complete interruption of the aortic arch.

A rare severe anomaly, usually fatal in the first few months of life unless treated, is the so-called preductal coarctation. Usually other severe anomalies coexist. In this condition, a large patent ductus perfuses the distal aorta with blood from the pulmonary artery. The coarctation is located proximal to this. In the few patients who survive infancy without operation, cyanosis may be recognized as localized to the lower half of the body.

PATHOPHYSIOLOGY. In 5 to 10 percent of infants, left ventricular failure may be severe, even fatal, unless operation is performed. After the first year of life, congestive heart failure rarely occurs before the age of twenty.

The hypertension from the coarctation causes rapid degenerative changes in the proximal aorta. Children in their early teens often have obvious fibrosis rigidity in the aortic wall. Without treatment the average life expectancy is only 30 to 40 years. The four most common causes of death in unoperated patients are rupture of the aorta, cardiac failure, rupture of intracranial aneurysms, and bacterial endocarditis.

CLINICAL MANIFESTATIONS. Symptoms. Most children have minimal or no symptoms despite severe hypertension. The diagnosis is often made by a routine school physical examination uncovering hypertension. Headache, epistaxis, and leg fatigue are the most frequent symptoms. Claudication in the lower extremities is uncommon.

Physical Findings. The classic combination of hypertension in the upper extremities with absent or decreased pulses in the lower extremities in a child immediately suggests coarctation. If weak femoral pulsations are present, direct measurement of the blood pressure in the upper and lower extremities may be necessary to confirm the diagnosis. Prominent pulsations from collateral circulation may be visible in the neck and over the muscles of the shoulder girdle. A systolic murmur is usually audible over the left hemithorax.

LABORATORY STUDIES. In older patients the chest radiograph may automatically establish the diagnosis by demonstrating bilateral notching of the ribs posteriorly (Fig. 18-17). Notching is unusual before age six but is almost always present by age fourteen. The electrocardiogram characteristically shows signs of left ventricular hypertrophy, often left ventricular strain. In most patients the diagnosis can be made from the clinical findings in combination with the radiograph and electrocardiogram. 2-D echocardiography may be diagnostic. Cardiac catheterization and aortography should be done routinely to define the location and extent of the obstruction, as well as to detect additional anomalies.

Fig. 18-17. Chest radiograph in patient with coarctation of aorta, demonstrating classic notching of ribs from enlarged intercostal arteries. This x-ray appearance is virtually pathognomonic of coarctation of aorta, as it is rarely produced by any other condition. *(Courtesy of Dr. Raymond M. Abrams, Department of Radiology, New York University Medical Center.)*

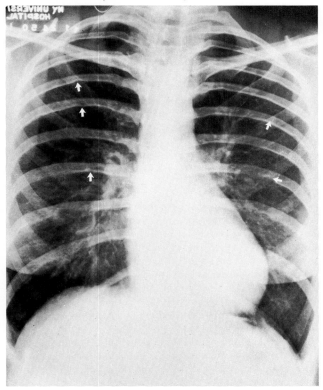

TREATMENT. The ideal age for operation is between three and four years. In infants with congestive failure, operation should be performed urgently, often within the first few weeks of life, because of the high fatality rate. With severe congestive failure, other cardiac anomalies are almost always present. These may require correction during the same hospitalization. When resection and end-to-end anastomosis is performed in infants, the coarctation may recur as the child ages. The subclavian flap technique is the procedure of choice in the first year of life (Fig. 18-18).

Operative Technique. A left posterolateral thoracotomy in the fourth intercostal space is used, dividing the fourth rib posteriorly in older patients (Fig. 18-19). The coarctation is usually readily seen, with the typical medial indentation at the site of insertion of the ligamentum arteriosum, with large, tortuous intercostal arteries entering the distal aorta (Fig. 18-20).

Initially the mediastinal pleura is incised, after which the vagus nerve is retracted medially, noting the course of the recurrent nerve encircling the ligamentum arteriosum. The aorta proximal to the left subclavian artery, the left subclavian, the ligamentum arteriosum, and the distal aorta are serially mobilized and encircled with tapes. Dissection should be kept in the adventitial plane next to the aorta. This minimizes bleeding and also avoids the occasional complication of inadvertent injury to the thoracic duct. Division of the ligamentum arteriosum facilitates dissection, as the aorta is more mobile once the tethering action of the ligamentum is removed.

Dissection of the distal aorta is hazardous in older patients when friable dilated intercostal arteries are present. Intercostal aneurysms, now rare, were found in 45 of 487 patients operated upon by Gross and associates. Usually the aorta can be mobilized sufficiently between the intercostal arteries, individually isolating these and separately occluding them during performance of the anastomosis. The intercostal arteries can also be divided, but this is seldom necessary.

Once the vessels have been adequately mobilized, the proximal aorta, the left subclavian, and the distal aorta are all occluded with vascular clamps, after which the coarctation is excised. The objective, of course, is to obtain an anastomotic lumen as large as the proximal aorta. In children, the widest anastomosis can be obtained by excising the aorta up to the level of the left subclavian. As much as 5 cm of aorta can be excised in a child (Fig. 18-21). In older children, as fibrosis decreases elasticity of the aorta, only 2.5 to 3 cm of aorta can be removed.

An end-to-end anastomosis is usually done with continuous sutures of polypropylene (Prolene) in the posterior row of the anastomosis. Interrupted mattress sutures should be used in small children in the anterior row to permit subsequent growth of the anastomosis.

Following completion of the anastomosis and removal of vascular clamps, the blood pressure should be measured proximal and distal to the anastomosis to confirm that no significant gradient remains. In addition, the circumference of the anastomosis should be measured and

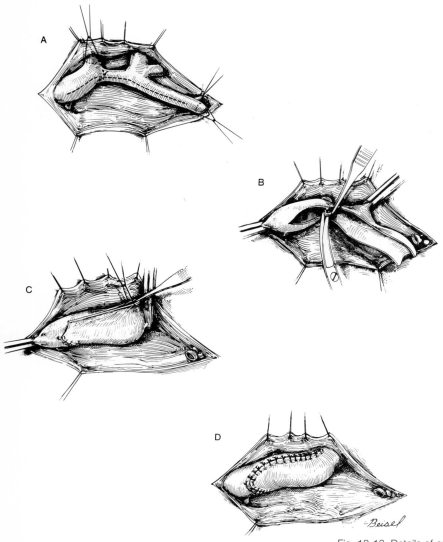

Fig. 18-18. Details of operation. (From: *Campbell DB, Waldhausen JA, et al: Should elective repair of coarctation of the aorta be done in infancy? J Thorac Cardiovasc Surg 88:929, 1984, Fig 2, with permission.*)

compared with that of the proximal aorta. When a gradient greater than 5 to 10 mmHg is present, especially with a circumference smaller than the proximal aorta, clamps should be reapplied after a short period of time, one or two sutures removed from the anterior suture line, and a short anterior arteriotomy made to permit insertion of an appropriate synthetic patch. The dimensions of the patch can be calculated to widen the lumen to the same size as the proximal aorta. This combination of anastomosis and selective patch grafting is a valuable technique, permitting complete correction of the obstruction without insertion of a vascular graft. Fewer than 10 percent of children have an obstruction so diffuse that primary insertion of a graft is necessary. Several reports have described the development of aortic aneurysm in patients 10 to 15 years after extensive patch grafting. We have not noted this development.

In adults, extensive degenerative changes in the aorta from calcification and fibrosis make insertion of a prosthetic graft necessary because direct anastomosis cannot be done. A simpler approach in such instances is to insert a bypass graft of Dacron around the obstruction, without attempting to excise the coarctation. This relieves the obstruction without risking the hazards of excision.

Postoperative Course. With present techniques, the risk of operation after one year of age is less than 1 percent. Antibiotics are given routinely during operation and postoperatively for 1 to 3 days. Patients usually recover rapidly and are discharged in 7 to 8 days.

The most feared operative complication is paraplegia. Current data indicate that paraplegia is due to ischemia of the spinal cord during cross-clamping in the majority of instances, and not due to ligation of interiostal arteries or other factors. In a survey of published reports by Brewer

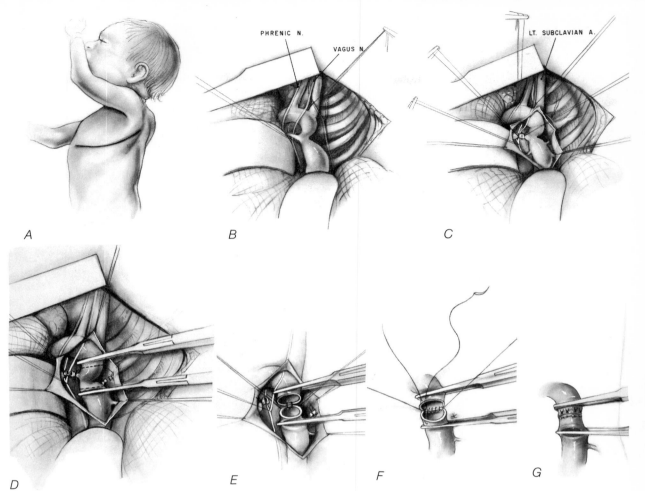

Fig. 18-19. Excision of coarctation of aorta. *A.* Chest is opened with posterolateral incision in fourth intercostal space. *B.* Once chest has been opened and lung retracted, site of coarctation is often visible where aorta is angulated inward toward mediastinum just distal to left subclavian artery. This is site where ligamentum arteriosum is inserted. *C.* After incision of mediastinal pleura overlying coarctation, vessels are isolated proximal and distal to coarctation and ligamentum arteriosum is mobilized and divided. Recurrent laryngeal nerve, often not seen during operative procedure, is displaced mediad with vagus nerve. *D.* After division of ligamentum arteriosum, vascular occlusion clamps are applied to aorta proximal and distal to site of coarctation. Often it is necessary to apply proximal clamp to aorta between left carotid and left subclavian arteries, separately occluding left subclavian artery, in order to excise widely the narrowed segment of aorta. *E.* End-to-end anastomosis is constructed with continuous or interrupted sutures of silk. *F.* After completion of posterior row of anastomosis, interrupted sutures are often used in anterior row in young children to permit growth of anastomosis. *G.* Final view of completed anastomosis.

et al., paraplegia was found to occur in approximately 0.5 percent of patients. The author has personally never had a postoperative neurologic complication following coarctation. For over a decade the pressure in the distal aorta has been continually monitored during excision of the coarctation by inserting a small catheter into the distal aorta before the aorta is clamped. Though it cannot be proved, it seems reasonable that neurologic injury probably should not occur if the distal aortic pressure remains above 60 mmHg. Distal aortic pressure following occlusions of the aorta and the left subclavian artery varies widely, from as low as 30 mmHg to levels greater than 60 mmHg.

Neurologic injury is virtually unknown if the aorta is occluded for less than 20 min. Hence, it seems wise to limit periods of aortic occlusion to less than 20 min if the distal pressure is less than 50 to 60 mmHg. Otherwise a temporary shunt should be used. When 103 patients were treated with those concepts, no neurologic problem occurred.

Often there is a ''paradoxical'' hypertension in the first 48 to 72 h after operation, occurring to a greater degree in older patients with a severe coarctation. Frequently this is associated with abdominal pain. This syndrome was first described by Sealy. It seemingly is related to an increase in arterial pressure in visceral arteries, previously functioning with a lower mean pressure. Rarely, serious problems such as intestinal necrosis can occur. Prompt treatment with appropriate hypertensive medications,

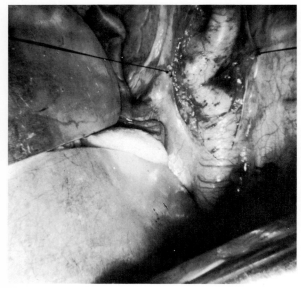

A

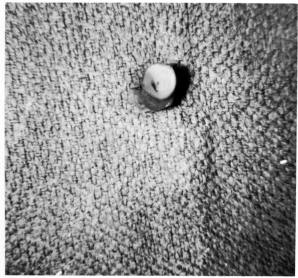

C

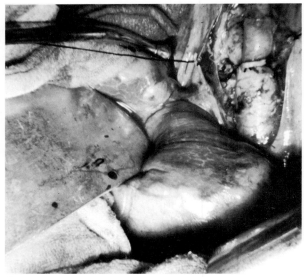

B

Fig. 18-20. *A.* Typical coarctation of aorta in child. Dilated subclavian artery is visible at top of field. At area of coarctation, aorta is angulated into mediastinum, where ligamentum arteriosum is inserted. *B.* Aortic anastomosis performed after excision of coarctation. Anastomosis is made at point of origin of left subclavian artery. *C.* Resected coarctation of aorta, showing narrow lumen that was present.

usually reserpine or nipride, virtually eliminates the problem.

Some residual hypertension is common in patients operated on after five years of age and seems to increase with age. Barratt-Boyes found that 90 percent of patients were normotensive 5 years after operation, but only 50 percent at 20 years and 25 percent at 25 years. A key question is whether residual hypertension will be significantly less in patients operated on at one to four years.

Vascular Rings

HISTORICAL DATA. The clinical significance of vascular rings was recognized by Abbott in her classical survey of congenital heart disease in 1932, but surgical therapy did not develop until 1945 when Gross successfully divided a double aortic arch. Gross subsequently developed most of the basic concepts of vascular rings, classifying and illustrating with clarity and precision the different anomalies found.

INCIDENCE AND ETIOLOGY. Vascular rings are uncommon but are quite significant because surgical therapy is effective with little morbidity or mortality. Embryologically, the vascular rings result from variation in the normal formation of the aorta and pulmonary artery from the six embryonic aortic arches. As six aortic arches exist in the embryo, it is somewhat surprising that such abnormalities are not more frequent. In normal embryonic life, the first two arches disappear, and the fifth never fully develops. The third, fourth, and sixth are significant in normal development. The right common carotid arises from the third arch, the innominate from the right fourth, while the left fourth contributes to the transverse aortic arch. The ductus originates from the sixth.

PATHOLOGIC ANATOMY. Five types of vascular anomalies of clinical significance have been recognized: (1) double aortic arch; (2) right aortic arch with left ligamentum arteriosum; (3) retroesophageal subclavian artery; (4) anomalous origin of innominate artery; and (5) anomalous origin of left common carotid artery. The last two conditions, anomalous origin of the innominate or the left common carotid, are very rare malformations in which the origin of the artery from the aortic arch is such that the trachea is compressed. The recommended method of surgical correction consists of mobilizing the anomalous

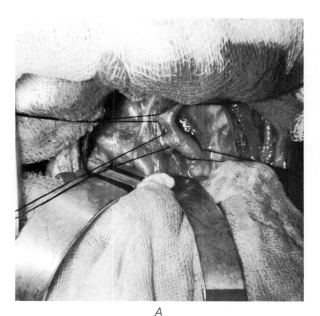

A

Fig. 18-21. *A.* Preductal coarctation exposed at emergency operation on thirteen-day-old infant. Large patent ductus equal in diameter to descending aorta is present. Proximal to patent ductus is coarctation of aorta with narrow proximal aortic segment and narrow subclavian artery. *B.* Appearance after excision of coarctation and suture of patent ductus arteriosus. Anastomosis was conducted proximally at point of origin of left subclavian artery from aorta.

vessel and suturing it into a more normal position. Actually, the mechanism of compression is less precise than in the other three conditions. Its clinical significance is not great.

A double aortic arch with one limb anterior to the trachea and the other limb posterior to the esophagus (Figs. 18-22 and 18-23) is the most severe of these malformations, producing symptoms in early infancy. Usually one limb is smaller than the other. Often the thoracic aorta descends on the right, rather than on the left. A right aortic arch with a retroesophageal ligamentum arteriosum or left subclavian artery is the other most frequent abnormality (Fig. 18-24). A retroesophageal subclavian artery, consisting of a right subclavian artery originating beyond the left subclavian artery and coursing posterior to the esophagus to the right upper extremity, is a common anomaly but usually does not cause symptoms (Fig. 18-25).

CLINICAL MANIFESTATIONS. Almost all symptoms from vascular rings result from compression of the trachea. Rarely is there difficulty in swallowing from compression of the esophagus.

Symptoms. Infants with a double aortic arch often develop difficulty breathing in the first few months of life and become critically ill. Stridor is the most frequent prominent symptom. Periodic episodes of serious respiratory distress, with ''crowing'' respirations, occur. During these attacks, the infant lies in hyperextension, gasping for breath. Feeding often precipitates such episodes, per-

A

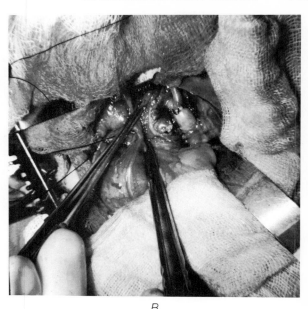

B

haps from flexion of the neck or aspiration. Infants quickly become underweight and malnourished.

Most patients requiring surgical treatment are seen in infancy. Those with mild symptoms developing after one year of age may spontaneously recover as they grow older. The most common symptoms are intermittent episodes of respiratory compression, at times with a respiratory infection; difficulty in swallowing, which, if present, is mild; and recurrent episodes of pneumonia, perhaps from aspiration. The mildest clinical picture is produced by the retroesophageal subclavian artery, which may cause mild, intermittent dysphagia. Some patients may be

Fig. 18-22. Double aortic arch with small anterior and large posterior limb. *A.* Anterior view of double aortic arch with small anterior limb *B.* Exposure after division of small anterior arch between left carotid and left subclavian artery, followed by displacement of carotid artery anteriorly toward sternum. (From: *Gross RE: The Surgery of Infancy and Childhood. Philadelphia, Saunders, 1953, p 917, with permission.*)

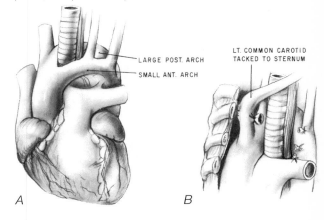

LARGE POST. ARCH
SMALL ANT. ARCH

LT. COMMON CAROTID TACKED TO STERNUM

A   *B*

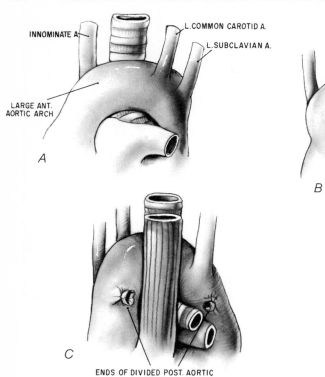

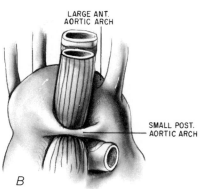

Fig. 18-23. *A.* Double aortic arch with large anterior arch. *B.* Small posterior arch, compressing esophagus. *C.* Appearance after division of small posterior arch. (From: *Gross RE: The Surgery of Infancy and Childhood. Philadelphia, Saunders, 1953, p 918, with permission.*)

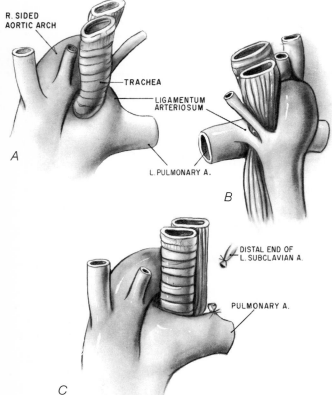

Fig. 18-24. *A.* Right aortic arch with left posterior ligamentum arteriosum. *B.* Posterior view of ligamentum arteriosum extending from right aortic arch to left pulmonary artery, compressing esophagus. Small left subclavian artery arising close to ligamentum arteriosum is also present. *C.* Appearance after division of ligamentum arteriosum and subclavian artery. (From: *Gross RE: The Surgery of Infancy and Childhood. Philadelphia, Saunders, 1953, p 923, with permission.*)

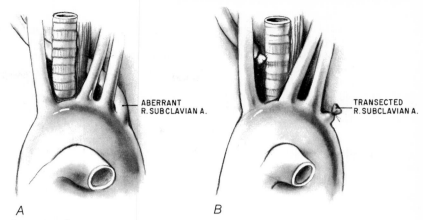

Fig. 18-25. *A.* Retroesophageal right subclavian artery, anomalous vessel arising from aortic arch distal to left subclavian artery. *B.* Appearance after division of anomalous vessel with retraction of distal stump to right of trachea. (From: *Gross RE: The Surgery of Infancy and Childhood. Philadelphia, Saunders, 1953, p 932, with permission.*)

symptomatic in infancy, and spontaneously recover with growth.

Physical Examination. No abnormalities are evident unless respiratory distress is present. If audible stridor is present, the diagnosis should be considered. During episodes of respiratory insufficiency, the infant lies with back arched and neck extended. Attempts to flex the neck may precipitate severe dyspnea and cyanosis.

LABORATORY STUDIES. Both the chest radiograph and electrocardiogram are normal unless aspiration pneumonia is present. Examination of the esophagus with a barium swallow usually establishes the diagnosis, demonstrating a typical area of compression from the retroesophageal artery, usually at the level of the third or fourth thoracic vertebra. This finding virtually confirms the diagnosis.

The precise nature of the obstruction can be defined with further studies. A tracheogram in the lateral view may provide further evidence of a vascular ring, demonstrating anterior compression of the trachea a short distance above the carina combined with posterior compression of the esophagus. Aortography can precisely delineate the abnormal arteries.

TREATMENT. Since a vascular ring has no physiologic significance, no treatment is needed in the absence of symptoms. If symptoms are mild, their origin may be uncertain, and a period of observation may be required to be sure that other difficulties are not responsible. If obvious respiratory compression is present, operation should be performed promptly, however, because death from airway obstruction can easily occur.

Operative Technique. The optimal incision varies with the type of anomaly. Usually an incision through the left four intercostal spaces is selected. An important principle is to dissect the aortic arch completely and identify the innominate artery, the left common carotid artery, and both subclavian arteries. Opening the pericardium facili-

tates identification of these vessels. The vagus nerve should be traced to the recurrent laryngeal nerve and the ligamentum arteriosum divided. Removal of part of the thymus gland will facilitate exposure. It should be emphasized that operative correction is more than simple division of an abnormal ring, because fibrosis surrounding the adventitia of the abnormal vessel may cause continued compression unless the vessels are widely mobilized and all possible compression is relieved.

With a double aortic arch, the smaller of the two arches should be divided. Usually, with a left descending aorta, the anterior arch is smaller and can be divided between the left common carotid and left subclavian artery, after which the mobilized anterior arch can be sutured to the posterior surface of the anterior chest wall to prevent compression of the trachea. If the posterior arch is smaller, it can be divided behind the esophagus. With a right descending thoracic aorta, almost always the posterior arch is the smaller of the two.

With a right aortic arch and a retroesophageal ligamentum arteriosum, division of the ligamentum arteriosum, combined with mobilization of the abnormal vessels, may be all that is necessary. In some patients the left subclavian artery may be in a retroesophageal location and should also be divided. A nubbin of aorta, constituting an aortic diverticulum, has been found in a retroesophageal location in some patients and may require amputation to relieve compression.

With a retroesophageal subclavian artery as an isolated anomaly, simple division of the artery is all that is necessary. Division of this artery through a cervical incision, followed by reimplantation into the right carotid artery, has been reported.

Postoperative Course. Postoperative care consists primarily of careful attention to respiration, with the infant kept in a highly humidified atmosphere and tracheal secretions aspirated. Tracheostomy is rarely necessary. If tracheal compression was present before operation, serious difficulties may develop afterward, probably from dissection around the trachea, creating postoperative edema. Unusually vigilant care for 24 to 72 h may be necessary. After recovery from operation, symptoms soon disappear. The risk of operation is primarily related to the age of the patient and the severity of compression of the trachea. Excellent results in a group of 70 patients have been reported by Gross, who had only 5 postoperative deaths, all of which occurred in a group of 26 infants with double aortic arches. Others have subsequently reported excellent results. By contrast, Bertrand et al. noted that 7 of 12 operated patients had residual symptoms.

LEFT-TO-RIGHT SHUNTS (ACYANOTIC GROUP)

Atrial Septal Defects

A variety of malformations involve the atrial septum or the pulmonary veins and result in a left-to-right shunt of blood from the systemic to the pulmonary circulation. These include atrial septal defects of the secundum type, anomalous drainage of the pulmonary veins, ostium primum defects, and atrioventricular canal malformations. These are individually discussed in the following sections. The physiologic abnormality is identical with secundum-type atrial defects and with partial anomalous pulmonary veins, consisting simply of a left-to-right shunt. Hence, these three anomalies are discussed together. Total anomalous drainage of pulmonary veins, a more complex anomaly, is discussed separately. With ostium primum defects and atrioventricular canals, mitral and tricuspid insufficiency are present in addition.

SECUNDUM DEFECTS

In 1953 Lewis successfully closed a defect under direct vision, using hypothermia and inflow occlusion. In the same year, Gibbon used the pump oxygenator successfully for the first time to suture an atrial septal defect. Gross in Boston developed the ingenious atrial well, which was used for several years. For the next 5 to 10 years patients were usually operated upon with hypothermia and circulatory arrest for 8 to 10 min, or the atrial well. As soon as extracorporeal circulation became safe, it was routinely adopted.

INCIDENCE AND ETIOLOGY. Atrial septal defects are among the most common cardiac malformations, representing 10 to 15 percent of all cases of congenital heart disease. They are more than twice as frequent in females. Embryologically, the secundum defects result from failure of the septum secundum to develop completely.

PATHOLOGIC ANATOMY. Atrial septal defects vary widely in size and location. A "high" defect near the orifice of the superior vena cava is commonly referred to as a sinus venosus type of defect because it is usually associated with anomalous entry of one or more superior pulmonary veins into the vena cava. The majority of secundum defects are located in the midportion of the atrial septum. "Low" defects are near the point of entry of the inferior vena cava, as a result of which right-to-left shunting occurs. Defects vary from as small as 1 cm in diameter to virtual absence of the atrial septum, but most are 2

to 3 cm. A foramen ovale should not be considered an atrial septal defect, for it is a normal opening in 15 to 25 percent of adult hearts. Because of its slitlike construction, a normal foramen ovale allows shunting of blood only from right to left. Unusual defects include different forms of "unroofing" of the coronary sinus. Multiple defects are very rare.

Anomalous pulmonary veins are found in 10 to 15 percent of patients. Anomalies of the right pulmonary veins are twice as common as those of the left. Anomalous right pulmonary veins may enter the superior vena cava inferior to the point of entry of the azygos vein, the right atrium, or the inferior vena cava. Left pulmonary veins may enter the innominate vein or the coronary sinus. Usually, anomalous drainage involves only the veins.

A very detailed report of the pathologic anatomy of anomalous pulmonary veins was published by Blake and Manion. A total of 27 different variations were found. Anomalous veins entering the superior vena cava are usually associated with a characteristic high atrial septal defect, termed a sinus venosus defect. Pulmonary veins entering the right atrium directly are usually found with a septal defect in a posterior location. It is most unusual for anomalous pulmonary veins to occur with an intact atrial septum, but when present, the physiologic abnormality of a large left-to-right shunt is identical. Pulmonary veins entering the inferior vena cava usually communicate through a single channel with the inferior vena cava near the diaphragm.

An unusual variant of anomalous pulmonary veins entering the inferior vena cava has been described as a "scimitar" syndrome, emphasizing a characteristic radiologic appearance resulting from the shadow of the anomalous vein which is parallel to the right border of the heart. The malformation is associated with hypoplasia of the right lung and anomalous origin of the pulmonary arteries from the aorta.

A rare variant of atrial septal defect is a secundum defect combined with mitral stenosis, the Lutembacher's syndrome. The mitral stenosis retards flow of blood from the left atrium to the left ventricle and produces an enormous left-to-right shunt through the septal defect, with massive dilatation of the pulmonary arteries. Some mitral valve prolapse occurs in 15 to 20 percent of patients, part of whom have significant mitral insufficiency that must be corrected at operation. Otherwise, simply closing the septal defect may precipitate fatal pulmonary edema.

PATHOPHYSIOLOGY. An atrial septal defect results in a left-to-right shunt of blood from the left atrium to the right atrium because of the pressure-volume characteristics of the left and right ventricles. The thick-walled left ventricle is less distensible than the right ventricle; with a closed atrial septum, left atrial pressure is normally 8 to 10 mmHg, while right atrial pressure is normally 4 to 5 mmHg. This difference in distensibility of the two ventricles results in a left-to-right shunt when an atrial septal defect is present. However, during infancy and the first few years of life the structure of the right ventricle more closely resembles the left ventricle, so the volume of the left-to-right shunt remains small until compliance of the right ventricle decreases 2 or more years after birth. Vascular resistance in the pulmonary bed also decreases.

The volume of the left-to-right shunt depends primarily on the pulmonary vascular resistance and the compliance of the two ventricles. The size of the defect exerts little influence. Most significant shunts have a pulmonary blood flow two to four times greater than systemic flow. Systemic blood flow is decreased and may result in retardation of normal growth and development, the so-called gracile habitus seen in some children with a large defect. The large pulmonary blood flow increases susceptibility to pneumonia and also causes dyspnea on exertion. For unknown reasons patients are susceptible to rheumatic fever, but bacterial endocarditis is rare.

With the increased pulmonary blood flow, pulmonary vascular resistance in children is usually less than normal. Pulmonary hypertension is found in less than 5 percent of children but occurs in 10 to 15 percent of adult patients, as pulmonary vascular resistance increases. Cardiac failure is unusual in children but becomes more frequent in early adult life. Arrhythmias become more common during the third decade. Without treatment it has been estimated that 75 percent of patients would die by age fifty, 90 percent by age sixty.

Some patients are initially seen in their fourth, fifth, or sixth decade with a previously undetected atrial septal defect. In these patients, arrhythmias are common, a result of long-standing hypertrophy of the right atrium. Even in patients over sixty to seventy years of age a good result may be obtained following operation if pulmonary vascular resistance is not greatly increased. Arrhythmias, however, often continue.

CLINICAL MANIFESTATIONS. Symptoms. Symptoms are uncommon in the first few years of life because the shunt is small until the right ventricular hypertrophy of infancy has subsided. Frequently children with large shunts are physically active and asymptomatic. In a report of 275 surgically treated patients, Sellers et al. found 113 asymptomatic. The most frequent symptoms are fatigue, palpitations, and exertional dyspnea. Slow growth and development may also occur. In adults, overt signs of congestive heart failure gradually appear, often with the first pregnancy.

Physical Examination. A soft systolic murmur is usually audible in the second or third left intercostal space. In the first few years of life this murmur may be faint or considered a functional murmur. The murmur arises at the pulmonary valve from the increased flow of blood. The second pulmonic sound is characteristically widely split, and "fixed." Slight to moderate cardiac enlargement is present with large defects. Patients are often thin, with long, narrow bones and limited muscular development—the gracile habitus.

LABORATORY FINDINGS. The chest radiograph shows mild to moderate cardiac enlargement, principally due to a large ventricle. The pulmonary right atrium and artery is prominent, with increased vascularity in the lung fields. The electrocardiogram is usually characteristic, with a right axis deviation with a right bundle branch block. 2-D echocardiography is usually diagnostic; cardiac catheterization is often not done in routine patients. If omitted, particular care must be taken at operation to explore the heart for additional anomalies, especially aberrant pulmonary veins.

DIAGNOSIS. Certain diagnoses in infancy may not be possible on clinical examination because the systolic murmur is not distinctive. In older children the diagnosis can be made with reasonable certainty from the combination of a soft systolic murmur with fixed splitting of the pulmonic second sound. These auscultatory findings, combined with the chest radiograph and electrocardiogram, virtually establish the diagnosis. A left axis deviation on the electrocardiogram immediately suggests that an ostium primum malformation is present.

TREATMENT. Indications. Since many children are asymptomatic, operation is frequently recommended on the basis of clinical findings and the demonstration on catheterization of a large shunt. Operation is usually performed if the pulmonary blood flow is more than 1.5 to 2.0 times greater than systemic flow. The only contraindication to operation is a severe increase in pulmonary vascular resistance, equaling or exceeding systemic vascular resistance (the Eisenmenger syndrome). This condition is very rare in children but is an ever-present danger after the third decade. Operation in patients with a pulmonary vascular resistance near systemic resistance is hazardous and may produce little improvement.

Operative Technique. All patients are operated on with extracorporeal circulation. A sternotomy or a right thoracotomy in the fourth intercostal space is used. Once bypass has been established, a finger is introduced into the right atrium through a stab wound to identify the pathologic anatomy, noting the atrial septal defect, the coronary sinus, the location of the pulmonary veins, the mitral and tricuspid valves, and the ventricular septum. Palpation beforehand minimizes the need for exploration of the heart once it has been opened and similarly lessens the hazards of air embolism.

The heart is then arrested with the cold blood–potassium technique, a perfusate temperature of 28°C, and a myocardial temperature of 15°C or less. The atrium is then opened widely (Fig. 18-26). Small defects can be closed with a simple continuous suture, usually polypropylene. Larger defects can be sutured, but patch closure with autogenous pericardium or Cacrom seems safer.

Aspiration of blood from the left atrium is avoided to protect from air embolism. As the suture line is completed, fibrillation is induced; the aorta is unclamped to expel blood from the left atrium into the right atrium and to protect from air embolism. The lungs are greatly ventilated. Gentle suction is also kept on a plastic needle vent in the ascending aorta for a short time after the heart starts to beat.

Subsequently, after bypass has been stopped, correction of the left-to-right shunt can be confirmed by aspirating blood from the superior vena cava and pulmonary artery and demonstrating similar oxygen concentration in the two samples. Left atrial pressure should be measured afterward and serially monitored if elevated.

Anomalous veins entering the right atrium can be cor-

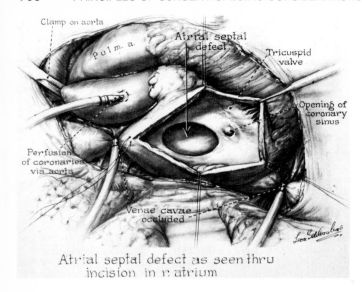

Fig. 18-26. Atrial septal defect of secundum type exposed at operation. Operation illustrated was performed under hypothermia before 1960 with perfusion of aorta with oxygenated blood. After 1961, all operations were performed with cardiopulmonary bypass. Large oval opening in atrial septum superior to coronary sinus is the type usually found with secundum-type defects.

rected by insertion of a prosthetic patch so the defect is closed and the pulmonary veins enter the left atrium. Pulmonary veins entering the superior vena cava with a sinus venosus defect require a more complex correction to avoid obstructing either drainage of the anomalous veins or the superior vena cava. This can be done satisfactorily with application of a pericardial patch. This is sutured superiorly around the point of entry of the anomalous veins and a baffle constructed that channels the blood from the pulmonary veins through the atrial septal defect into the left atrium (Fig. 18-27). Anomalous veins entering the inferior vena cava, the most unusual type, are usually treated with construction of an appropriate intraatrial pericardial baffle.

Postoperative Course. Postoperative convalescence is uncomplicated and recovery from any cardiac disability is prompt. The risk of operation with extracorporeal circulation is surprisingly small. Several groups have reported series of more than 100 patients operated upon with a mortality of 1 to 3 percent. In the author's experience with more than 100 secundum defects, mortality has been near zero for over 15 years.

TOTAL ANOMALOUS DRAINAGE OF PULMONARY VEINS

PATHOLOGIC ANATOMY. A classic pathologic study was reported by Brody in 1942, studying 100 cases of anomalous pulmonary venous drainage, 35 of which were total anomalous drainage. The anomalous veins are supracar-

Fig.18-27. *A.* Sinus venosus type of atrial septal defect located near junction of superior vena cava with right atrium. Defect is partly obscured by crescentic lower margin. Anomalous pulmonary veins from right upper lobe enter superior vena cava near its junction with right atrium. *B.* Prosthetic patch can be applied to encompass both atrial septal defect and ostia of anomalous pulmonary veins, avoiding undue constriction of point of entry of superior vena cava into right atrium. *C.* Final view of prosthetic patch that excludes anomalous veins and atrial septal defect from right atrium. (From: *Benson CD et al: Pediatric Surgery, vol 1. Chicago, Year Book Medical Publishers, 1962, p 439, with permission.*)

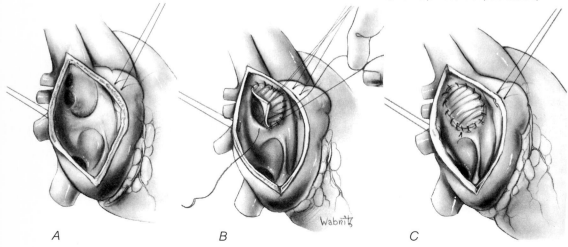

A   *B*   *C*

diac in about 45 percent of cases, cardiac in 25 percent, infradiaphragmatic in 25 percent, and mixed in about 5 percent. In almost all cases, the anomalous veins enter a common pulmonary venous sinus, which in turn enters the right side of the heart. With supracardiac drainage, the most common drainage is into a left vertical vein, which in turn enters the left innominate vein. Rarely, the common venous trunk may drain directly into the superior vena cava. With paracardiac drainage, anomalous veins may enter the right atrium directly or through the coronary sinus. With infracardiac drainage, the common venous trunk traverses the diaphragm and connects with the portal vein or adjacent structures. An atrial septal defect and a patent ductus arteriosus are almost always present.

PATHOPHYSIOLOGY. The disability is a severe one, producing death in 50 percent of untreated infants within 3 months, about 80 percent within the first year. Some degree of obstruction to pulmonary venous drainage is usually present, always so with infradiaphragmatic drainage. This venous obstruction in turn produces severe pulmonary hypertension.

In the fortunate 10 to 20 percent of infants without significant venous obstruction and with an adequate atrial septal defect, the patients may do surprisingly well for several years, the disability resembling that from a large atrial septal defect.

CLINICAL MANIFESTATIONS. Severe tachypnea is the dominant symptom in a seriously ill infant. The diagnosis is often initially unclear so total anomalous drainage must be considered in any severely tachypneic infant. Cardiac murmurs are not diagnostic. Cyanosis and signs of congestive failure vary in severity.

The chest radiograph may show definite abnormalities when there is significant dilatation of the common pulmonary vein in adjacent structures. With supracardiac drainage, a well-recognized double contour is visible on the x-ray, termed the "snowman" appearance (Fig. 18-3). This double contour is produced by dilatation of the left innominate vein and right superior vena cava.

2-D echocardiography can often establish the diagnosis and outline the abnormal channels, but cardiac catheterization and angiography should be done to delineate the abnormal anatomy. At catheterization a classical finding is that blood from the right atrium, pulmonary artery, and femoral artery have a similar oxygen content because of mixing of oxygenated and unoxygenated blood in the right atrium before entering the left atrium through the atrial septal defect.

TREATMENT. Successful total correction with bypass was reported byKirklin in 1956 and also by Cooley. Mortality remained quite high, however, for over a decade but decreased markedly after the introduction of the technique of profound hypothermia and circulatory arrest by Barratt-Boyes around 1969.

Operation must be performed urgently in critically ill infants. It is usually done with the technique of hypothermia and low flow or total circulatory arrest. Surgical correction includes construction of a large (2.5 to 3.0 cm) side-to-side anastomosis between the common venous

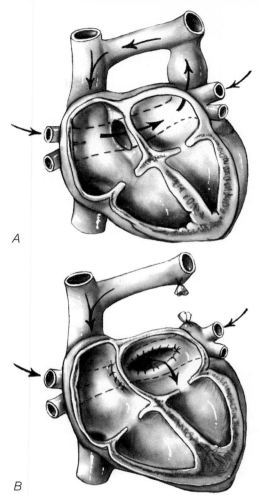

Fig.18-28. *A.* Abnormal physiology with anomalous drainage of pulmonary veins into left superior vena cava. All pulmonary venous blood flows through left innominate vein into large right superior vena cava and can enter systemic circulation only through atrial septal defect, usually foramen ovale. *B.* At operation, wide opening is made between posteriorly located common pulmonary venous trunk and left atrium, after which opening in atrial septum is closed and left superior vena cava divided. (From: *Benson CD et al: Pediatric Surgery, vol I. Chicago, Year Book Medical Publishers, 1962, p 446, with permission.*)

trunk and the left atrium (Fig. 18-28), followed by closure of the atrial septal defect and ligation of the left vertical vein. When anomalous veins enter the coronary sinus, surgical reconstruction is simpler, consisting of creation of a large opening between the coronary sinus and the left atrium. Operative mortality is between 15 and 20 percent in infants. The patients subsequently have almost normal cardiac function. During the first postoperative year, close observation is necessary because stricture of the anastomosis between the venous trunk and the left atrium occurs in 5 to 10 percent of patients.

In the 15 to 20 percent of patients with a large pulmonary blood flow who are operated on after one year of age, operative mortality is very low, approaching that of atrial septal defect.

PARTIAL ATRIOVENTRICULAR CANAL DEFECT (OSTIUM PRIMUM)

These defects are uncommon, occurring in 4 to 5 percent of patients with defects in the atrial septum. They are especially common in children with Down's syndrome, occurring with a frequency of 20 to 25 percent. Except for this unusual association, no etiologic factors are known.

At least three terms have been used interchangeably: ostium primum, partial atrioventricular canal, or partial endocardial cushion defect. "Ostium primum" is an older term, commonly used before the relation to complete atrioventricular canals was recognized. The proper generic name is either endocardial cushion defect (partial or complete) or atrioventricular canal (partial or complete).

PATHOLOGIC ANATOMY. The two significant defects are a defect (cleft) in the anterior leaflet of the mitral valve and a low, crescent-shaped defect in the atrial septum (Fig. 18-29). The sicklelike superior border of an ostium primum defect can be easily recognized on palpation at the time of operation. The cleft in the anterior leaflet of the mitral valve may be partial, extending for a short distance from the ventricular septum, or complete, separating the mitral valve leaflet into anterior and posterior halves.

Chordae tendineae are usually attached to the margins of the cleft constituting a "trileaflet valve," with little or no mitral insufficiency. In other patients, abnormal chordae tendineae are present.

An associated partial or complete cleft in the tricuspid valve is also frequent. As described by Perloff, failure of the endocardial cushions to fuse produces an abnormally low position of the atrioventricular valves with an abnormally high anterior position of the aortic valve, resulting in the characteristic "gooseneck" deformity seen on the left ventricular angiogram.

The defect in the atrioventricular septum results in inferior displacement of the conduction system, which, in turn, produces characteristic abnormalities on the electrocardiogram.

Primum defects are anatomically distinguished from the more severe atrioventricular canal malformation by the presence of distinct, separate mitral and tricuspid valve rings and an intact ventricular septum. Complete atrioventricular canals have an absence of the atrioventricular septum with free communication between the atrial and ventricular cavities.

PATHOPHYSIOLOGY. The physiologic abnormalities are a left-to-right shunt combined with mitral insufficiency. When mitral insufficiency is minimal, physiologic abnormality is identical to that of a large atrial septal defect of the secundum type. When mitral insufficiency is severe, left ventricular failure and pulmonary hypertension appear early in life and produce a <u>much more</u> severe impairment of cardiac function than is seen in secundum-type septal defects. Increase in pulmonary vascular resistance with pulmonary hypertension may develop but is more frequent with atrioventricular canals.

CLINICAL MANIFESTATIONS. Symptoms. A variety of clinical profiles occur, varying with the degree of mitral insufficiency. When mitral insufficiency is minimal, the clinical picture is similar to that of atrial septal defect of the secundum type. With significant mitral insufficiency, cardiac failure with pulmonary congestion and dyspnea may be fatal in the first year of life unless surgically corrected.

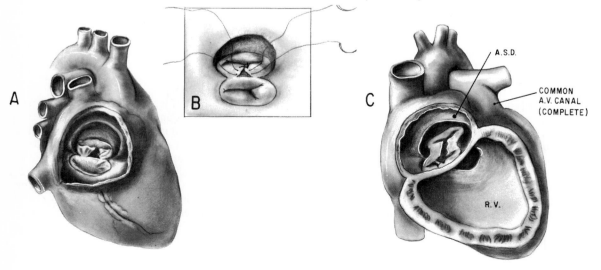

Fig.18-29. *A.* Ostium primum type of atrioventricular canal. There is a cleft in anterior mitral leaflet, but ventricular septum is intact. *B.* Method of repair of cleft valve with interrupted sutures to produce competent mitral valve. Classic crescent-shaped atrial septal defect superior to valve ring is shown. *C.* Appearance of complete atrioventricular canal, showing complete division of mitral and tricuspid valves in association with atrial septal defect and ventricular septal defect. (From: *McGoon DC et al: Am J Cardiol 6:598, 1960, with permission.*)

Physical Examination. Moderate cardiac enlargement is often present, with a thrill near the apex. A harsh apical systolic murmur from mitral insufficiency is usually obvious and should arouse suspicion of an ostium primum defect. An additional systolic murmur may be heard along the left sternal border. The intensity of the pulmonic second sound is often increased. With cardiac failure, signs of pulmonary congestion and hepatic enlargement are found. Growth is frequently retarded.

LABORATORY FINDINGS. The chest radiograph usually shows a moderate cardiac enlargement, involving both the right and the left ventricle. Increased pulmonary vascularity is common. The most useful diagnostic clues are found in the electrocardiogram and the vector cardiogram. The former shows abnormalities with a "left axis deviation," while the latter shows an abnormality in the frontal plane, a counterclockwise loop, that is almost pathognomonic. The 2-D echocardiogram shows classic abnormalities. Some clinicians feel that these findings are sufficient to confirm the diagnosis and do not routinely perform cardiac catheterization.

Cardiac catheterization, however, defines the characteristic left-to-right shunt at the atrial level with the associated increase in pulmonary blood flow and pulmonary hypertension. Mitral insufficiency is best evaluated with the left ventriculogram.

TREATMENT. In most patients operative correction of the defect should be performed between the ages of one and four years. With pulmonary hypertension and cardiac failure, operation may be necessary in infancy. Rarely, an adult is seen in the third or fourth decade with a history of little disability from a primum defect. These patients are those in whom mitral insufficiency has been minimal, with a clinical course similar to a secundum-type defect. In most patients the combination of a left-to-right shunt with mitral insufficiency results in progressive cardiac enlargement and failure in childhood.

Operative Technique. Operation is performed with extracorporeal circulation, using a median sternotomy incision. The three principal objectives are correction of the mitral insufficiency, closure of the septal defect, and avoidance of the production of heart block from injury to the conduction bundle along the posterior margin of the septal defect.

Cardiac arrest is produced by the cold blood–potassium technique. The right atrium is widely opened, and the septal defect, cleft in the mitral valve, associated cleft in the tricuspid valve, and ventricular septum are carefully examined. Initially the cleft in the mitral valve is closed with interrupted sutures placed from the ventricular septum out to the free margin of the mitral orifice (Fig. 18-29*B*), the points of insertion of the chordae tendineae being carefully noted. After repair of the cleft mitral valve, the septal defect is repaired with a patch of pericardium inserted with interrupted sutures. Along the posterior rim near the condition bundle the sutures are inserted superficially to the left of the rim of the defect along the annulus of the mitral valve. It is usually not necessary to repair any abnormalities in the tricuspid valve.

Postoperative Course. If adequate correction of the mitral insufficiency is accomplished and production of heart block avoided, postoperative recovery is usually uneventful and similar to that for closure of other septal defects. Heart block is rare, occurring in less than 5 percent of cases. Some mitral insufficiency remains in 15 to 20 percent of patients. When significant or progressive, this may require reoperation in later years. The functional results in the majority of patients, however, are satisfactory. At the Mayo Clinic, McGoon and associates in 1973 reported long-term results in 232 patients, the majority of whom had maintained an excellent result following operation. The operative mortality is less than 5 percent.

Goldfaden et al. reported long-term evaluation of 39 patients operated upon more than 5 years earlier. Eighteen percent had significant mitral regurgitation, severe in only two. Significant arrhythmias were present in 18 percent. The estimated actuarial survival at 13 years was 88 percent but the likelihood of being free of any type of late complication at 13 years was only about 52 percent.

In early experiences with surgical repair, an unusual syndrome of severe hemolytic anemia was recognized in a small percentage of patients following repair of an ostium primum defect. This striking clinical picture resulted from residual mitral insufficiency accidentally oriented so that the regurgitant jet of blood struck the prosthetic patch closing the septal defect and intermittently dislodged fibrin from the surface of the patch with each systolic jet. Although rare, such a syndrome should be recognized, for prompt reoperation and correction of the residual insufficiency is curative.

COMPLETE ATRIOVENTRICULAR CANAL

This severe malformation results from extensive failure of development of the endocardial cushions, resulting in a large atrioventricular defect involving both the atrial and ventricular septums with defects in the mitral and tricuspid valves (Fig. 18-29*C*). The great variation in valve deformities was well described by Rastelli in 1966 in an analysis of 30 postmortem specimens. Subsequently, the deformity present was often classified into one of three groups, a Rastelli type A, B, or C. The physiologic defect is a left-to-right shunt at both the atrial and ventricular levels, resulting in pulmonary hypertension and cardiac failure in infancy. The severity of the malformation depends upon the extent of the mitral insufficiency and the size of the ventricular septal defect. In infants with severe deformities the course is a severe one, with death in the first few months of life, unless operation is performed.

A complete atrioventricular canal, rather than a partial one, may be suspected from the malignant clinical course of severe cardiac failure in infancy. Diagnosis is established principally by the electrocardiogram and the echocardiogram. Cardiac catheterization should also be done for a complete evaluation.

TREATMENT. Operation is indicated in the first year of life, usually at six months of age when repair can be done electively. With refractory congestive failure, repair must be done earlier. The corrective procedure consists of insertion of a large prosthetic patch that initially is attached to the underlying ventricular septum, taking precautions to avoid injury to the conduction bundle. The abnormal mitral and tricuspid leaflets are then reconstructed and attached to the patch at an appropriate level, following which the atrial septal defect is closed.

For several years operative results were poor, with a mortality exceeding 75 percent in infants. Great advances were subsequently made with the techniques of surgical correction developed by Rastelli, McGoon, and Kirklin. Operative mortality is now between 5 and 15 percent, varying with the severity of the abnormality present.

Ventricular Septal Defect

HISTORICAL DATA. The description by Roger in 1879 of two patients with ventricular septal defect is a medical classic. It led to the designation *Roger's disease,* focusing emphasis upon the asymptomatic nature of the disease when the ventricular septal defect is small. Surgical closure became possible with the development of cardiopulmonary bypass in 1954–1955.

INCIDENCE AND ETIOLOGY. Ventricular septal defect is a common form of congenital heart disease, constituting 20 to 30 percent of congenital defects. There are no known etiologic factors.

PATHOLOGIC ANATOMY. Four major anatomic types of ventricular septal defect have been recognized, depending upon the location in the ventricular septum: perimembranous septal defect, outflow defect anterior to the crista supraventricularis, inflow defects near the tricuspid, and muscular defect in the muscular ventricular system. Defects in the membranous septum are by far the most frequent (80 percent of patients).

Perimembranous septal defects (Fig. 18-30, type B) are located in the membranous septum and often extend into adjacent structures. The bundle of His, of critical importance to the surgeon, is located at the posterior, superior rim of the defect, where it bifurcates into the right and left conduction bundles. The defect is located beneath the aortic cusps, which are often visible through the defect.

Outflow (infundibulum) septal defects (Fig. 18-30, type A) are anterior to the crista supraventricularis near the pulmonic valve. Surgical closure is simple because the defect is safely away from the conduction bundle. Inflow septal defects (Fig. 18-30, type C) are posterior to the papillary muscle of the conus, beneath the tricuspid valve.

Muscular ventricular septal defects (Fig. 18-30, type D) are located inferiorly in the ventricular septum and are often multiple. A common variety, the "Swiss cheese" type of septum, consists of many serpentine communications making surgical closure difficult, perhaps impossible. An approach through the left ventricle has been used as a last resort in some complex lesions but has the serious hazard of permanent left ventricular dysfunction.

Left ventricular–right atrial defects are the rarest of all, consisting of a communication between the left ventricle and the right atrium through the membranous septum superior to the annulus of the tricuspid valve. Although the defects are small, the resulting shunt is large because of the great difference in pressure between the left ventricle and right atrium. Closure can be easily done by direct suture.

The size of septal defects varies from as small as 3 to 4 mm to greater than 3 cm. Such defects are commonly classified as "restrictive" or "nonrestrictive," depending upon whether the defect is smaller than the orifice of the aortic valve. In nonrestrictive defects, right and left ventricular systolic pressures are equal, and flow is influenced by pulmonary vascular resistance. Small restrictive defects have a normal right ventricular systolic pressure with little or no hemodynamic disturbances. In larger "restrictive" defects right ventricular systolic pressure is increased but does not equal that in the left ventricle. The hemodynamic significance of nonrestrictive defects is determined by the pulmonary vascular resistance, normally 4 units per square meter body surface. A mild elevation in vascular resistance is near 6 units; a moderate elevation 6 to 10; a severe, 10 or more units.

With nonrestrictive defects and a right ventricular systolic pressure equaling that in the left ventricle, deadly histologic changes soon develop in the pulmonary arterioles, at times appearing in the first year of life. These were classically described by Heath and Edwards in 1958. The initial change is hypertrophy of the smooth muscle in the media, followed by proliferation in the intima, unfortunately, the intimal changes seem irreversible. The early evolution of these irreversible changes is the major reason for performance of operation in patients with nonrestrictive defects during the first year of life.

Associated anomalies are common. These include patent ductus arteriosus, coarctation, atrial septal defect, mild infundibular stenosis of the right ventricle, and aortic insufficiency from prolapse of an aortic valve cusp into the ventricular septal defect.

Fig.18-30. Common types of ventricular septal defect. Most common is type B, with defect lying just proximal to crista supraventricularis. Type A defects are located immediately proximal to pulmonic valve. Type C defects are located beneath septal leaflet of tricuspid valve. Type D defects are in muscular part of ventricular septum and are often multiple. (From: *Kirklin JW et al: J Thorac Surg 33:45, 1957, with permission.*)

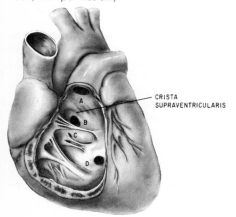

CRISTA
SUPRAVENTRICULARIS

PATHOPHYSIOLOGY. The two major consequences of a ventricular septal defect are cardiac failure and pulmonary hypertension. Normally systolic left ventricular pressure is about four times greater than systolic right ventricular pressure. Hence, a ventricular septal defect results in a left-to-right shunt of blood from the left ventricle into the pulmonary circulation, producing an increased pulmonary blood flow. The size of the left-to-right shunt varies with both the size of the defect and the pulmonary vascular resistance.

A small increase in pulmonary blood flow is well tolerated, but a pulmonary blood flow more than twice systemic flow may produce cardiac failure. With large nonrestrictive defects, pulmonary blood flow may be four to five times greater than systemic flow, producing severe pulmonary congestion and heart failure in infancy.

After the first year of life, overt cardiac failure is uncommon, but large defects produce chronic pulmonary congestion with recurrent episodes of pneumonia and limitation of growth and development.

The other major pathologic change is an increase in pulmonary vascular resistance, produced by the changes in the media and intima of the pulmonary arterioles described in the previous paragraphs. As pulmonary vascular resistance rises, the left-to-right shunt gradually reverses with an increasing degree of right-to-left shunting, producing arterial hypoxemia. Eventually this produces a "balanced" shunt, and then progresses to *reversal* of the shunt with severe cyanosis. This condition exists when pulmonary vascular resistance has increased to levels greater than systemic vascular resistance. The classic term "Eisenmenger's syndrome" refers to this pathologic condition. It is inoperable by present techniques except for heart-lung transplantation. It apparently can develop in 10 percent or more of untreated nonrestrictive septal defects.

Small restrictive septal defects, not increasing right ventricular systolic pressure, have no known physiologic handicap except a small increase in susceptibility to bacterial endocarditis, apparently resulting from the jet of blood through the defect striking the right ventricular wall. The endocarditis usually responds to antibiotic therapy.

The life expectancy of adult patients with a ventricular septal defect depends upon the pulmonary blood flow. The only known hazard with small defects is endocarditis. With large defects the critical question is the pulmonary vascular resistance. Patients with a significant increase in pulmonary vascular resistance may progress to the complete Eisenmenger's syndrome. The natural history of such patients has been well documented by Wood. Death usually occurs near forty years of age, often from massive hemoptysis. At present heart-lung transplantation has been used for a few such patients with encouraging short-term results. Patients with a large defect without increased pulmonary vascular resistance usually have a pulmonary blood flow over twice normal. They gradually develop cardiac enlargement and cardiac failure, much like patients with moderate aortic insufficiency.

CLINICAL MANIFESTATIONS. Patients with small defects are usually asymptomatic even though a loud murmur and thrill are present. With large defects, dyspnea on exertion with pulmonary congestion, often with frequent episodes of pneumonia, are common. Severe cardiac failure usually occurs only in infants or adults. Patients with a large increase in pulmonary vascular resistance are deceptively asymptomatic for several years until cyanosis and hemoptysis evolve as the shunt reverses and produces peripheral hypoxia.

A loud harsh pansystolic murmur is usually present along the left sternal border in the third and fourth intercostal spaces, often with a thrill. With pulmonary hypertension the pulmonic second sound is increased. Growth retardation may be significant with chronic congestive failure, accompanied by cardiac enlargement, rales, and hepatic enlargement. Basal diastolic murmurs are infrequent but can originate from two sources. A murmur of aortic insufficiency may develop from prolapse of an aortic cusp into the underlying septal defect. Alternately, a murmur from pulmonic insufficiency may appear with pulmonary hypertension.

The chest x-ray with small defects is normal, while in large defects, enlargement of both ventricles occurs, especially with a rise in pulmonary vascular resistance. Enlargement of the pulmonary arteries with pulmonary congestion is often prominent. The electrocardiogram shows signs of left ventricular hypertrophy and also right ventricular hypertrophy with pulmonary hypertension. The 2-D echocardiogram is of particular value, for the location and size of the septal defects may be determined with reasonable accuracy. The most precise information is obtained by cardiac catheterization, documenting the volume of the shunt and the pulmonary vascular resistance, and by selective angiography.

TREATMENT. Small defects should simply be observed because 60 to 70 percent will close in early life. The risk of endocarditis is small. Over half of such defects close before three years of age, about 90 percent by eight years. Closure most commonly occurs with membranous and muscular defects, rarely with inflow or outflow defects.

The treatment of large defects depends upon the presence of cardiac failure or increasing pulmonary vascular resistance. Severe cardiac failure in infancy may be fatal unless operation is performed in the first few weeks or months of life. Banding of the pulmonary artery was popularly used for such critically ill infants for some years but is now used with decreasing frequency because of the safety of operation in infants. Infants with significantly increased pulmonary vascular resistance should be operated upon promptly, no later than six to eight months of age. Barratt-Boyes has clearly documented irreversible changes in the pulmonary vascular bed of some infants who were operated upon even during the first year of life. With the safety of operation, and the ominous uncertain course of an increase in pulmonary vascular resistance, it is becoming increasingly clear that most infants with a large ventricular septal defect should be operated upon during the first year of life. This is a significantly earlier age than previously recommended, based upon both the safety of operation and the realization of the early devel-

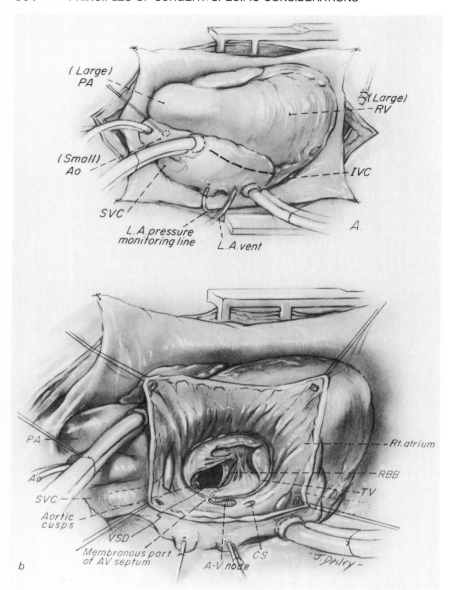

(Large)
PA

(Large)
RV

(Small)
Ao

SVC

IVC

L.A.pressure
monitoring line

L.A.vent

A.

PA

Rt. atrium

Ao

RBB

SVC

TV

Aortic
cusps

VSD

Membranous part
of AV septum

A-V node

CS

J. Desley

b

Fig.18-31. Repair of a perimembranous VSD from the right atrium. As, aorta; AL, anterior leaflet; AV node, atrioventricular node, CS, coronary sinus; IVC, inferior vena cava; PA, pulmonary artery; RBB, right bundle branch, SVC, superior vena cava; TV, tricuspid valve. [From: *Kirklin JW, Barratt-Boyes BG: Ventricular septal defect, in Kirklin JW, Barratt-Boyes BG (eds): Cardiac Surgery. New York, Wiley, 1986, chap 20, pp 629–630, with permission.*]

opment of pulmonary hypertension. When pulmonary vascular resistance is increased to near systemic levels (8 to 10 resistance units), the hazard of operation is increased and the benefit decreased. Criteria of inoperability vary significantly. In general, in about one-third of patients successfully operated upon with a major increase in pulmonary vascular resistance, the changes continue nonetheless, producing death within a few years. A significant percentage of the other patients remain with a permanent increase but without progression, while a small group have a decrease in resistance, either for regression of the existing changes or from the growth of new arterioles.

Technique of Operation. Operation is performed through a median sternotomy with extracorporeal circulation. If a

patent ductus is present, it must be closed at the beginning of operation. The defect may be closed through a right atrial approach or through a short transverse ventriculotomy (Figs. 18-31, 18-32). A prosthetic patch is routinely used. The critical part of the operation is to avoid heart block by identifying key anatomical guides at the posterior superior margin of the defect. A useful surgical guide was described by Barratt-Boyes. With a still dry field, the fibrous trigone located at the bottom of the

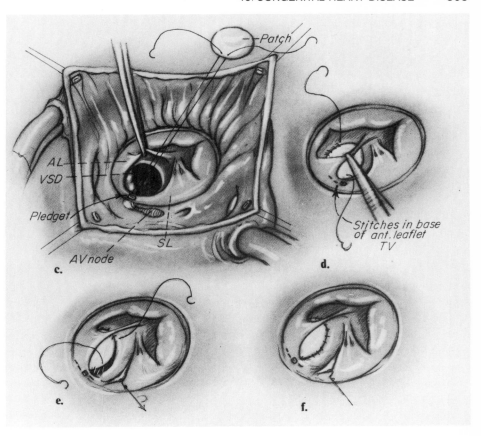

Fig. 18-31. Continued.

noncoronary sinus can be identified on inspection through the ventricular septal defect. The conduction bundle passes through this trigone and then along the area where the membranous septum joins the muscular septum posteriorly. Placing sutures to the right of an imaginary line projected between the fibrous trigone and the papillary muscle of the conus usually avoids injury to the conduction bundle. With present techniques, the risk of heart block is very small.

After closure of the defect, if a left ventricular vent has been inserted, saline can be injected forcefully through the vent into the left ventricle while the aorta is clamped, distending the ventricular septum. Residual shunts can be easily detected. This is especially valuable with multiple muscular defects. The editor has used this technique for over 10 years with excellent results.

Following bypass, residual shunts may also be detected by measurement of oxygen content of blood samples drawn simultaneously from the right atrium and pulmonary artery. Outflow defects (infundibular) can be readily repaired with a prosthetic patch because there is no danger of injury to the conduction bundle.

A small percentage of patients with ventricular septal defects develop severe aortic insufficiency from prolapse of an aortic valve cusp into the underlying defect. The lesion is a progressive one as the aortic cusp herniates to a greater degree, often virtually tamponading the underly-

ing septal defect. Surgical correction can often be done without insertion of a prosthetic aortic valve. A detailed report of the experience of the author and associates was published in 1973 (Fig. 18-33). Subsequent experience has remained quite satisfactory.

Defects in the muscular septum may be single or multiple. Extensive muscular defects have been described as a "swiss cheese septum." Successful closure of these defects requires careful preoperative study, combined with evaluation at operation of the presence of residual defects. Such defects often originate from only one opening in the left ventricle, providing a better surgical approach, but unfortunately left ventriculotomy may produce significant ventricular injury. Hence, different forms of approach through the right ventricle are preferred, utilizing a left ventriculotomy reluctantly after other methods have been found unsatisfactory.

Rizzoli and associates reported in 1980 that in the past 5 years only one death occurred among 94 patients with a single large ventricular septal defect, and only one death (7 percent mortality) in 14 patients with multiple ventricular septal defects. There was only one death in 35 infants less than one year of age. Neither the location of the ventricular septal defect nor the surgical approach (via the right atrium or right ventricle) were significant factors. Only one heart block developed among 261 patients. Richardson et al. also described excellent results follow-

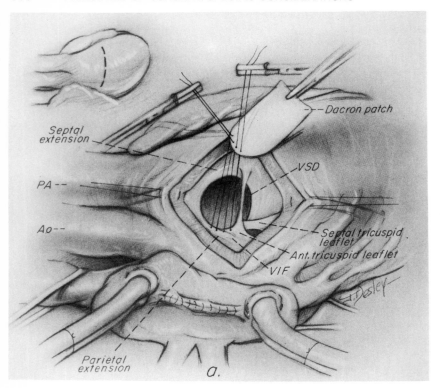

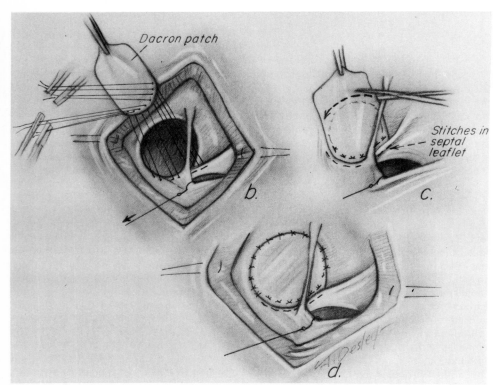

Fig. 18-32. Repair of a peri-membranous VSD from the right ventricle. Ao, aorta; PA, pulmonary artery; VIF, ventriculoinfundibular fold; VSD, ventricular septal defect. [From: *Kirklin JW, Barratt-Boyes BG: Ventricular septal defect, in Kirklin JW, Barratt-Boyes BG (eds): Cardiac Surgery. New York, Wiley, 1986, chap 20, pp 631–632, with permission.*]

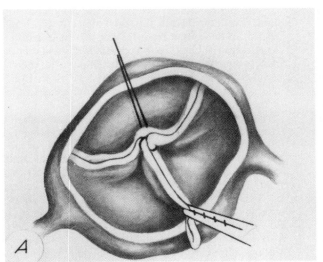

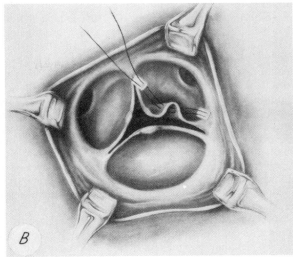

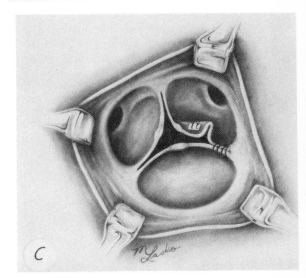

Fig. 18-33. The technique of cusp plication. *A.* The distance from corpus arantii to commissural margin is adjusted to equal that of the opposing cusp. The free edge of the elongated cusp is shortened to appose the normal cusp. *B.* The plicated cusp with its mobility preserved. Separate repair of the abnormal commissure is then carried out. (From: *Spencer FC, Doyle EF, et al: Long-term evaluation of aortic valvuloplasty for aortic insufficiency and ventricular septal defect. J Thorac Cardiovasc Surg 65:15, 1973, pp 16–17, with permission.*)

ing operation upon 32 infants between one and twenty-four months of age. In 1984, Yeager reported operative experiences with 128 patients less than one year of age with a hospital mortality of 7.8 percent.

Following recovery from operation, patients without a marked increase in pulmonary vascular resistance usually have a dramatic regression of all signs of cardiac disease. Heart size and vascularity of lung fields both return to normal. A right bundle branch block usually remains on the electrocardiogram. Life expectancy appears to be that of a normal person. If there is a persistent increase in pulmonary vascular resistance following recovery from operation, long-term prognosis is much less favorable. Regression of the increased pulmonary vascular resistance occurs in about one-third of patients; there is no significant change in about one-third, and a gradual increase in the remainder, probably representing an inherent disease in the pulmonary vasculature separate from that due to the previous left-to-right shunt.

Patent Ductus Arteriosus

HISTORICAL DATA. Gibson, in Edinburgh, in 1900 described the clinical features of a patent ductus arteriosus. In 1937 Strieder first attempted ligation of the ductus in a patient with bacterial endocarditis. This patient died on the fourth postoperative day, but the following year Gross successfully ligated the patent ductus of a seven-year-old girl.

INCIDENCE AND ETIOLOGY. Patent ductus arteriosus is one of the most common forms of congenital heart disease, occurring once in about every 2000 births and constituting about 10 percent of all cases of congenital heart disease. It is two to three times more frequent in females than in males.

The patent ductus arteriosus, which develops as an embryologic remnant of the sixth left aortic arch, is an important normal fetal pathway connecting the pulmonary artery at its bifurcation to the aorta just beyond the origin of the left subclavian artery. Through this channel in embryonic life blood bypasses the collapsed lungs, flowing directly from the pulmonary artery into the aorta. With the expansion of the lungs at birth, the ductus normally closes within a few days, becoming the fibrotic ligamentum arteriosum. The physiologic stimuli responsible for closure of the ductus have been studied in detail. Apparently changes in oxygen tension of the arterial blood exert a profound stimulus on the closure. The most important cause of closure, however, is probably related to the distinctive histologic structure of the wall of the ductus, which is different from that of either the pulmonary artery or the aorta. As the ductus closes, the wall of the ductus contracts, the internal elastic membrane fragments, and smooth muscle projects into the lumen as progressive fibrosis obliterates the patent channel.

If rubella occurs during the first trimester of pregnancy, a well-recognized syndrome of congenital defects can occur, including mental retardation, cataracts, and a patent ductus. For the majority of patients, however, the cause of persistent patency is unknown.

PATHOLOGIC ANATOMY. The diameter of a ductus ranges from as small as 2 to 3 mm to greater than 1 cm. Usually it is 5 to 7 mm. The length ranges from 5 to 10 mm (Fig. 18-34).

Associated anomalies occur in approximately 15 percent of cases; the most common are ventricular septal defect and coarctation of the aorta.

PATHOPHYSIOLOGY. Depending upon the diameter of the ductus, a varying amount of blood is shunted from the

Fig. 18-34. Patent ductus arteriosus is regularly found just distal to left subclavian artery between aorta and pulmonary artery. It is encircled by recurrent laryngeal nerve, a useful surgical landmark in isolating patent ductus in mediastinal tissues. (From: *Gross RE: The Surgery of Infancy and Childhood. Philadelphia, Saunders, 1953, p 807, with permission.*)

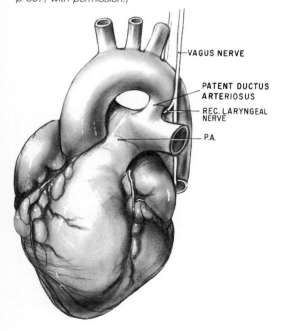

VAGUS NERVE

PATENT DUCTUS ARTERIOSUS

REC. LARYNGEAL NERVE

P.A.

aorta to the pulmonary artery, constituting a left-to-right shunt. In a large ductus, the shunt may constitute 50 to 70 percent of the output from the left ventricle, with resulting decrease of blood flow to other tissues and retardation of development. With such large shunts, the pulmonary blood flow may reach levels as high as 10 to 15 L/min. The symptomatology is directly proportional to the size of the shunt.

A large patent ductus in infants may result in serious or even lethal heart failure. Without surgical treatment, 25 to 30 percent of infants may die in the first year of life. Beyond one year of age, heart failure is rare until adult life.

In infancy the high pulmonary vascular resistance of fetal life subsides gradually in the first 1 to 2 years after birth. During this time only a systolic murmur may be audible. In some infants the increased pulmonary blood flow from the ductus causes the pulmonary vascular resistance to remain elevated and even increase, with resulting pulmonary hypertension. Usually the pulmonary vascular resistance will decrease to normal levels following surgical division of the ductus, but in older patients only a partial regression toward normal levels may occur. With a large patent ductus (diameter larger than the aorta) pulmonary vascular resistance may increase to exceed systemic vascular resistance, as early as five to six years of age. This produces a "reversed" ductus, with blood flowing from the pulmonary artery to the descending thoracic aorta to produce cyanosis in the lower half of the body (the Eisenmenger syndrome). With early diagnosis and treatment, this condition is now rarely seen.

An unusual feature of a patent ductus is susceptibility to development of bacterial endocarditis from *Streptococci viridoni*. This is most common after the first decade; it may occur rarely in children. It has been estimated that in untreated cases such an infection would ultimately develop in 20 to 25 percent of patients. The localization of the infection apparently is related to turbulent blood flow where blood forcefully ejected from the aorta through the ductus strikes the wall of the pulmonary artery. The vegetations of bacterial endocarditis usually begin in this location. Fortunately such infections can usually be promptly controlled with antibiotic therapy.

With the dual tendency to develop either heart failure or bacterial endocarditis, the estimated life expectancy of a seventeen-year-old patient with a patent ductus is approximately one-half that of a normal individual.

CLINICAL MANIFESTATIONS. Symptoms. In infants a large patent ductus may cause serious heart failure, and children over one year of age are usually asymptomatic. When symptoms are present, the most common are palpitations, fatigue, and dyspnea. Definite symptoms of congestive heart failure are usually seen only in adult patients. In the female these often appear during the first pregnancy. The author has successfully operated on one patient over sixty years of age after congestive failure.

Physical Examination. The hallmark of a patent ductus is the continuous murmur, one of the most distinctive signs in clinical medicine. Usually a patent ductus can be diagnosed with certainty simply on this basis. Because of the continuous quality of the murmur it is often described as a

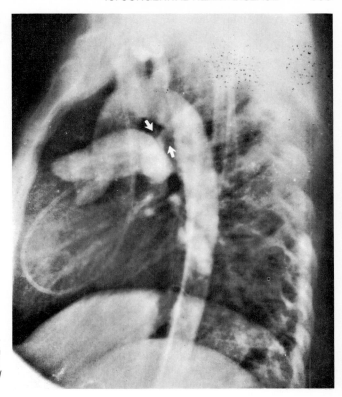

Fig. 18-35. Aortogram performed by injection of dye into aorta demonstrates patent ductus arteriosus, as indicated by arrows, with opacification of pulmonary artery. *(Courtesy of Dr. Raymond M. Abrams, Department of Radiology, New York University Medical Center.)*

''machinery'' murmur. It is a harsh, rasping sound, accentuated in systole and diminishing in diastole. It is best heard in the second left intercostal space but is normally widely transmitted over the chest and into the neck. In many patients the murmur is so loud that it is associated with a palpable thrill. Often in infants either no murmur or only a systolic murmur can be heard until the age of one or two years, after which a continuous murmur is audible. The absence of the diastolic component of the murmur during infancy is due to persistent elevation of the pulmonary vascular resistance, which limits flow of blood through the ductus during diastole.

A wide pulse pressure is usually found with a large ductus, produced by a decrease in diastolic pressure. In the extremely large ductus the diastolic pressure may approach very low levels and be associated with peripheral vascular findings similar to those of severe aortic insufficiency.

Cyanosis is never present with an uncomplicated patent ductus. The presence of cyanosis indicates either an associated cardiac anomaly, such as tetralogy of Fallot, or a marked increase in pulmonary vascular resistance from progressive sclerosis of the pulmonary arteriolar bed.

LABORATORY FINDINGS. With a small patent ductus the chest radiograph may be normal. With a larger ductus the pulmonary conus is prominent, the left ventricle is enlarged, and the pulmonary vascular markings are increased, all indicating a large left-to-right shunt. The electrocardiogram is often normal with a small ductus but will show left ventricular hypertrophy with a larger one. 2-D Doppler echocardiography may outline the size and shunt pattern with reasonable accuracy. Cardiac catheterization can readily localize the left-to-right shunt to the pulmonary artery and differentiate the condition from a ventricular septal defect or an atrial septal defect. Often with appropriate manipulation the cardiac catheter can be passed through the patent ductus, visually confirming the diagnosis. Aortography is the most definitive diagnostic measure, visually demonstrating the flow of dye from the aorta through the ductus into the pulmonary arteries (Fig. 18-35). It is of particular value with severe pulmonary hypertension, when only a systolic murmur may be audible.

DIAGNOSIS. In most patients the diagnosis can be made with confidence from the clinical findings combined with the chest radiograph, the electrocardiogram, and the echocardiogram. Cardiac catheterization with aortography should then be done both for confirmation and for detection of additional anomalies.

There are several rare conditions that may produce a continuous murmur simulating a patent ductus arteriosus, requiring cardiac catheterization and angiography for differentiation from a patent ductus. These include an aortic-pulmonary window, a ventricular septal defect with a prolapsed cusp causing aortic insufficiency, a ruptured aneurysm of the sinus of Valsalva, and a coronary arteriovenous fistula. Most of these conditions create a physiologic left-to-right shunt and hence a continuous murmur simulating a patent ductus.

TREATMENT. Infants with congestive failure should be operated on promptly. Otherwise, operation can be electively performed between one and two years of age. The operative risk approaches zero, and the results are excellent.

The only contraindication to operation, rarely seen, is cyanosis. Cyanosis may be due to an associated cardiac anomaly such as tetralogy of Fallot, in which case the patent ductus is an important ancillary source of blood flow to the lungs. Cyanosis can also develop with a reversed ductus when pulmonary vascular resistance has increased to exceed systemic vascular resistance, as a result of which blood flows from the pulmonary artery to the aorta and creates cyanosis in the lower half of the body. A reversed ductus cannot be safely closed, for the patent ductus partly decreases the pulmonary hypertension, shunting blood from the pulmonary artery to the aorta. Attempted surgical closure usually results in immediate death. Fortunately, with early operations for patent ductus, such advanced pulmonary vascular disease is almost unknown.

With bacterial endocarditis, intensive antibiotic therapy will effect cure in most patients; operation can then be more safely performed several weeks later. It is rarely necessary to operate in the presence of active infection.

Operative Technique. The operation is preferably done through a posterolateral thoracotomy in the fourth intercostal space, although a left anteriolateral thoracotomy in the third intercostal space has been satisfactorily used in previous years. The author's preferred operative technique is shown in detail in Fig. 18-36.

Patients in the third and fourth decade with pulmonary hypertension and sclerosis or calcification of the ductus constitute a difficult and dangerous technical problem because of friability of the ductus, especially at its junction with the pulmonary artery. Lacerations in this artery may quickly result in fatal hemorrhage. A temporary aortic shunt, either a left atrial–femoral artery bypass or a femoral-femoral bypass, can be employed to permit temporary occlusion of the aorta above and below the ductus, which can then be occluded with a single clamp placed near its junction with the aorta. The ductus can then be divided at its point of origin from the aorta. Alternately, the aorta can be incised and the orifice of the ductus obliterated with a patch applied from within the aorta. Barratt-Boyes has approached some patients through a sternotomy incision, using hypothermia and a brief period of ''low flow'' to permit opening the pulmonary artery and direct suture of the pulmonary orifice of the ductus.

Ligation of a patent ductus with multiple ligatures was developed and widely used by Blalock. It is now rarely used but is an effective technique in most patients. The original technique included four separate ligatures, with two purse-string sutures at the aortic and pulmonary artery ends of the ductus, followed by two transfixion ligatures.

The author treated a sixty-five-year-old patient with congestive failure and extensive calcification of both the aorta and a large patent ductus. Even simple application of vascular clamps to the calcified vessels seemed unusu-

ally hazardous. Accordingly, the ductus was effectively obliterated with multiple mattress sutures placed through Teflon felt surrounding the ductus. The patient has subsequently remained well.

As illustrated in Fig. 18-36, a valuable technical point for safe division of any patent ductus is the application of a vascular clamp tangentially onto the aorta a few millimeters from the ductus, rather than on the ductus itself. This method of application of the clamp avoids the problem of a short ductus.

Postoperative Course. With an uncomplicated ductus, the operative risk is near zero. As early as 1953 Gross reported experience with 611 patients, with a mortality rate of less than 0.5 percent in those with neither cardiac failure nor infection. Similar figures were described by Jones in a total series of 909 patients. At New York University there has been no mortality or serious complications following division of an uncomplicated patent ductus in the past 15 years.

Convalescence following operation is usually uneventful. A functional systolic murmur may remain audible in a few patients. The electrocardiogram usually returns to normal within a few months. From data now available from over 40 years' experience, it seems certain that cardiac function becomes normal once the ductus has been surgically obliterated.

PATENT DUCTUS IN THE PREMATURE INFANT

In recent years the frequency and significance of the patent ductus in premature infants has become widely recognized. Closure can be significantly hastened by the administration of indomethacin. Apparently, indomethacin acts by blocking the synthesis of prostaglandins, which normally influence contraction of the smooth muscle that obliterates the patent ductus. The frequency of patent ductus in premature infants varies inversely with the birth weight and gestational age, ranging from a frequency of 15 to 80 percent.

Diagnosis may be made from the widened pulse pressure detected through an umbilical arterial catheter. The echocardiogram may be helpful in confirming the diagnosis.

Most patients can be treated with medical therapy, combined with indomethacin when necessary. In the 1983 National Cooperative Study of 3559 patients, this therapy produced ductus closure in 79 percent of the group.

Fig.18-36. Division of patent ductus arteriosus. *A.* Chest is opened with left posterolateral incision in fourth intercostal space. *B.* Once lung has been retracted, mediastinal pleura is incised longitudinally parallel to vagus nerve. *C.* Initial dissection is along vagus nerve to expose widely the recurrent laryngeal nerve originating from vagus and passing beneath ductus. Wide exposure of recurrent laryngeal nerve is essential part of operative procedure. *D.* After dissection of recurrent laryngeal nerve, lappet of pericardium overlying ductus is freed by sharp dissection proximally to expose pulmonary artery. *E.* Subsequently ductus is encircled, and vascular occlusion clamps are applied. *F.* Ductus is gradually divided and sutured, employing two rows of sutures. *G.* Final view of divided ends of ductus with recurrent laryngeal nerve well exposed.

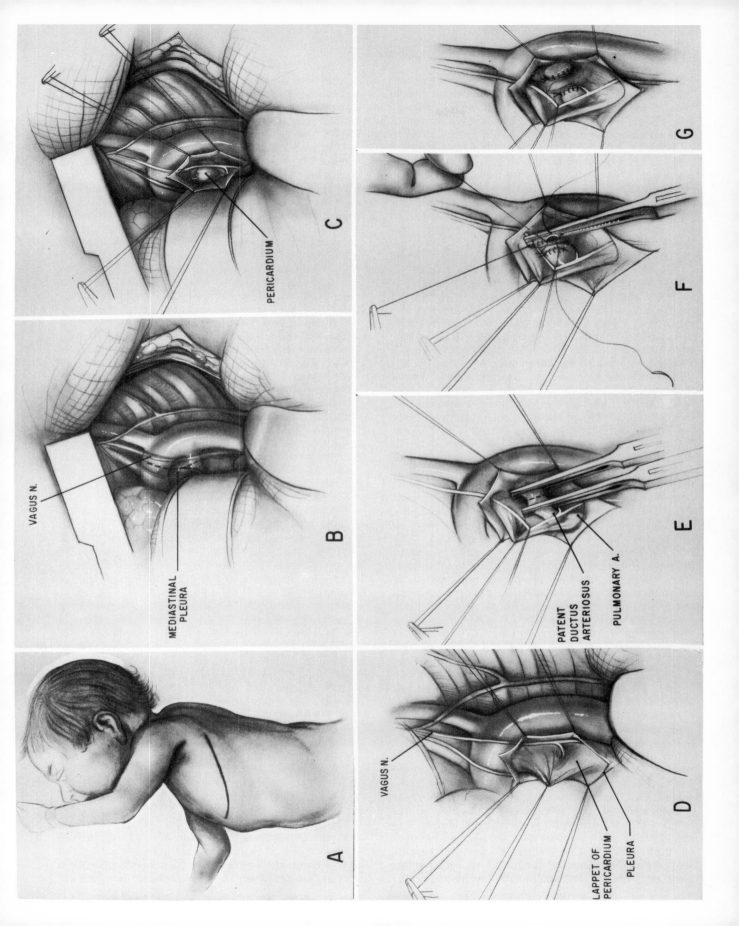

A

B

VAGUS N.

MEDIASTINAL
PLEURA

C

PERICARDIUM

D

VAGUS N.

LAPPET OF
PERICARDIUM

PLEURA

E

PATENT
DUCTUS
ARTERIOSUS

PULMONARY A.

F

G

Surgical occlusion is usually not the initial choice, because the ductus will eventually close in most patients. With severe respiratory insufficiency, however, an operation should be done. The ductus is exposed through a short lateral incision and occluded with a metallic clip; operating time is usually less than 30 min.

Operation is surprisingly safe. Mikhail reported experiences with 306 patients, average age eleven days, without any deaths.

RIGHT-TO-LEFT SHUNTS (CYANOTIC GROUP)

Tetralogy of Fallot

HISTORICAL DATA. Tetralogy of Fallot was described in 1673 by Steno, but became well known in 1888 when the combination of abnormalities regularly present was emphasized by Fallot, and subsequently known as the tetralogy. Effective therapy first became possible in 1944, when Blalock dramatically demonstrated that much benefit could be obtained by anastomosis of the subclavian artery and pulmonary artery to create an artificial ductus arteriosus. The operation was developed after the suggestion of Taussig, who had noted an increase in symptoms in infants when a patent ductus arteriosus spontaneously closed. Thereafter the procedure was termed the *Blalock-Taussig operation*. It constituted one of the milestones in cardiac surgery, far exceeding in importance the benefit for tetralogy patients. It demonstrated for the first time that complex cardiac procedures could be performed on cyanotic infants. This knowledge launched the modern era of cardiac and vascular surgery. Vascular prostheses, excision of aneurysms, hypothermia, and finally the heart and lung machine all evolved in the next 9 years. The Blalock-Taussig operation was done over 1500 times at the Johns Hopkins Hospital. Experience with these operations led to the development of many other aspects of cardiac surgery. With the development of extracorporeal circulation, correction became possible and was first performed by Lillehei in 1954.

INCIDENCE AND ETIOLOGY. Tetralogy of Fallot is one of the most common cyanotic malformations, constituting over 50 percent of all cases of cyanotic heart disease. Among cyanotic children who survive beyond the first 2 years of life, a tetralogy is present in 70 to 75 percent. There are no known etiologic factors.

PATHOLOGIC ANATOMY. The four features of tetralogy from which the name originates are obstruction of the outflow tract of the right ventricle, a ventricular septal defect, dextroposition of the aorta, and hypertrophy of the right ventricle. It is now known that these four abnormalities are not coincidental but result from a specific genetic abnormality—malalignment of the infundibular septum, the anatomic hallmark of tetralogy. In normal embryonic development the developing infundibular septum aligns inferiorly with the muscular septum. In tetralogy the infundibular septum deviates anteriorly and cephalad, creating the large ventricular septal defect at the point of nonunion. The anterocephalad rotation of the

septum both narrows the right ventricular outflow tract and enlarges the aortic root, hence the "overriding." The nonrestrictive ventricular septal defect results in systemic systolic pressure in the right ventricle with resulting concentric right ventricular hypertrophy.

The right ventricular obstruction may be produced by a wide variety of abnormalities. These include valvular stenosis or hypoplasia, diffuse hypoplasia of the right ventricular outflow tract, a localized infundibular stenosis, or pulmonary atresia. A discrete infundibular stenosis is present in about 15 percent, pulmonary atresia in about 20 percent. Pure valvular stenosis is unusual. In most patients a combination of infundibular and valvular stenosis is present (Fig. 18-37).

The ventricular septal defect is large, 2 to 3 cm in diameter, almost always located proximal to the crista supraventricularis in the membranous septum. The aortic cusps are readily visible through the defect, varying with the degree of dextroposition.

There is striking enlargement of the bronchial arteries, aortopulmonary collateral arteries, and other routes of collateral circulation to the lungs, creating extensive varicosities throughout the mediastinum and chest wall.

Anomalous coronary arteries are found in 5 to 10 percent of patients, especially in the outflow tract of the right ventricle, where they are of particular surgical significance. A right aortic arch, for unknown reasons, occurs in about 25 percent of patients. Atrial septal defect is found in 10 to 15 percent of patients. Such patients have been termed a pentology of Fallot, though the name has negligible physiologic significance. It is curious that although a patent ductus arteriosus may be essential to life, it gradually closes in most patients during the first few months of life, often with a disastrous increase in the severity of anoxia.

The pulmonary valve leaflets are often thickened, with fused commissures; in addition one or more leaflets may be tethered to the arterial wall with resulting limitation of motion.

PATHOPHYSIOLOGY. Physiologically, a tetralogy of Fallot is a combination of a large ventricular septal defect and an obstruction in the right ventricular outflow tract of sufficient severity to elevate right ventricular systolic pressure to equal left ventricular systolic pressure. Venous blood entering the right ventricle then is shunted directly into the aorta to produce cyanosis. In addition to cyanosis, the malformation decreases pulmonary blood flow and hence limits the capacity of the lungs to absorb oxygen. The inability to increase pulmonary blood flow constitutes the basis for the severe intolerance to exercise. The large ventricular septal defect has a separate influence, in that right ventricular pressure almost never exceeds left ventricular pressure, in contrast to isolated pulmonic valvular stenosis. *For this reason, cardiac enlargement and failure are rare.*

The severity of the anoxia varies with the degree of reduction in pulmonary blood flow. Arterial oxygen saturations of 70 to 85 percent are seen in older children, but in younger children, who may not survive infancy without operation, astonishingly low oxygen saturations are en-

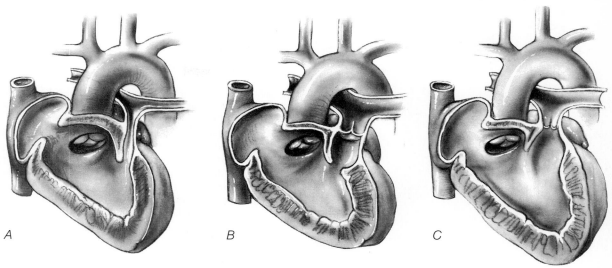

A   *B*   *C*

Fig.18-37. Different types of right ventricular obstruction in tetralogy of Fallot. *A.* Combined obstruction from hypoplasia of pulmonic annulus in association with diffuse stenosis of outflow tract of right ventricle. This type of diffuse stenosis is commonly found and often requires insertion of prosthetic patch to widen annulus. *B.* Localized stenosis of infundibulum of right ventricle, with "infundibular chamber" distal to this which is proximal to normal pulmonic valve. *C.* Pulmonic stenosis of valvular type in association with normal right ventricular outflow tract. (From: *Benson CD et al: Pediatric Surgery, vol I. Chicago, Year Book Medical Publishers, 1962, p 463, with permission.*)

countered. Saturations of 30 to 35 percent may be seen in patients who can walk only a short distance, and levels of 20 to 25 percent are found in some infants who are unable to walk. Saturations as low as 10 percent have been recorded, usually associated with loss of consciousness from cerebral anoxia. With exercise, there is often a precipitous fall in arterial oxygen saturation, decreasing from a resting level of 70 percent to 20 to 25 percent, clearly indicating the physiologic basis for exertional dyspnea.

Chronic anoxia produces compensatory polycythemia and eventual clubbing of the extremities. Polycythemia is seldom apparent until after two years of age, but later hematocrits from 60 to 75 percent are common. Wide variations in hematocrits are found, ranging from normal with mild tetralogies to levels as high as 85 to 90 percent in the most severe forms.

The degree of cyanosis increases significantly in the first few years of life, for visible cyanosis is proportional to the number of grams of unsaturated hemoglobin in the peripheral circulation as well as the actual oxygen concentration. Hence severe cyanosis is visible only after polycythemia has developed. The time of appearance has been used by Nadas for a convenient grouping of the clinical course of the disease. About one-third of patients are cyanotic at birth, another one-third become cyanotic in the first year of life, and one-third develop cyanosis in the next few years. Patients cyanotic at birth from severe anoxia often do not survive infancy unless operation is performed. Patients becoming cyanotic in the first year of

life have a milder course but are seriously disabled, while those who develop cyanosis in later years may have little incapacity and little polycythemia—a so-called pink tetralogy. These patients, of course, have only moderate reduction in pulmonary blood flow.

The main threat to life in the first year of life is cerebral infarction, from either thrombosis or anoxia. In severe cases, cyanotic "spells" are seen in which the infant becomes deeply cyanotic and comatose. Spontaneous recovery usually occurs, but death or hemiplegia may ensue. Such infants require emergency operation.

Brain abscess is another serious, often lethal, complication to which patients are peculiarly susceptible. The right-to-left shunt, bypassing the lungs and providing direct access for bacteria in the venous blood to enter the arterial circulation, is the most plausible explanation.

Cardiac failure is rare. Its presence always brings into question the accuracy of the diagnosis. Life expectancy without treatment is short. About 25 percent die in the first year, 40 percent by three years, and 70 percent by ten years. Formerly, only about 10 percent of patients reached twenty years of age.

CLINICAL MANIFESTATIONS. Symptoms. Almost all patients are symptomatic. Dyspnea and cyanosis, markedly aggravated by exertion, are the outstanding features. Two additional characteristics are cyanotic spells and squatting. Cyanotic spells are episodes of sudden increase in intensity of cyanosis, followed by unconsciousness, usually with spontaneous recovery within a few minutes or hours. Such episodes, representing acute cerebral anoxia, may be fatal or may result in hemiplegia. They are especially frequent between two and six months of age.

Squatting is an impressive characteristic, for children learn quickly to relieve dyspnea by assuming a squatting position. The physiologic benefit from squatting, apparently a redistribution of blood flow, is probably based on an increase in systemic vascular resistance. Walking for short distances, interrupted by squatting, is a well-recognized hallmark of the tetralogy. Hemoptysis is rare, oc-

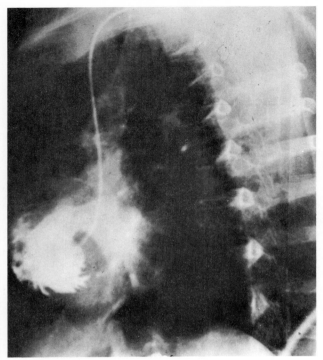

Fig.18-38. Cardiac angiogram in patient with tetralogy of Fallot, demonstrating large ventricular septal defect. Dye has been injected through catheter in right ventricle. Dye flows through large ventricular septal defect into left ventricle. Pulmonic stenosis that was present is not visible on this angiogram. *(Courtesy of Dr. Raymond M. Abrams, Department of Radiology, New York University Medical Center.)*

curring usually in older children with marked varicosities of the bronchial circulation.

Physical Examination. On physical examination the obvious features are cyanosis of varying severity and clubbing of the digits. The heart usually has a normal size, rate, and rhythm. A systolic murmur of grades II to III intensity is commonly present along the left sternal border at the third or fourth intercostal spaces, accompanied by a thrill in about one-half the patients. With severe pulmonic stenosis or pulmonary atresia, the murmur may be faint or absent because of absence of flow through the pulmonic orifice. The second pulmonic sound is weak or absent, while the aortic second sound is increased.

LABORATORY FINDINGS. The chest radiograph shows a heart of normal size with an unusual contour, termed the *coeur en sabot,* or sabot-shaped heart (Fig. 18-1). This unusual appearance results from the combination of a concave pulmonary artery segment, a horizontal ventricular septum produced by the concentric right ventricular hypertrophy, and a left ventricle that is smaller than normal. The lung fields show decreased vascularity.

The electrocardiogram is always abnormal, showing right ventricular hypertrophy of varying severity with right axis deviation. The echocardiogram is usually diagnostic. The most important data are obtained by cardiac catheterization and biplane angiography. Abnormalities

found at catheterization include the large left-to-right shunt with equal right and left ventricular systolic pressures. Pulmonary artery pressure is decreased, resulting in a large systolic pressure gradient between the right ventricle and pulmonary artery. Calculated pulmonary blood flow is decreased, varying with the severity of the disorder. The degree of decrease will parallel the severity of the arterial hypoxemia. Hematocrit is usually between 60 and 70 percent, ranging from 45 to 90 percent.

The biplane cineangiogram is the most important study, demonstrating all the key morphologic abnormalities when appropriate views are obtained. Essential information includes the type of abnormality in the right ventricular outflow tract, the pulmonary valve annulus, leaflets, main pulmonary artery and its branches. The typical ventricular septal defect is usually easily seen (Fig. 18-38); additional septal defects, if present, can also be identified. The coronary anatomy should be studied in detail for anomalous origin of the anterior descending from the right coronary.

DIAGNOSIS. The diagnosis can usually be made with reasonable certainty from clinical examination combined with radiograph, electrocardiogram, and echocardiogram. The important clinical features are cyanosis with severe exertional dyspnea and squatting. The important physical findings are a heart of normal size with a systolic murmur. Radiographic findings demonstrate a heart of normal size with decreased vascularity of the lung fields, while the electrocardiogram shows right ventricular hypertrophy.

TREATMENT. Indications for Operation. Infants with cyanotic spells require emergency operation to prevent death or hemiplegia. At present a shunt procedure seems preferable in the first 6 months of life, although a few surgeons use total correction. Although a wide variety of shunts have been used, the safest and most effective is either a subclavian pulmonary anastomosis (Fig. 18-39) or a subclavian-pulmonary Goretex interposition graft (Fig. 18-40). Operative risk with either type of shunt is very small, improvement is usually substantial, and removal of the shunt at the time of a subsequent corrective operation is not complicated.

Beyond six months of age, the increasing tendency is for a primary corrective operation rather than performance of a shunt. Excellent data have been reported from several centers supporting this approach.

Technique of Corrective Operation. A median sternotomy incision is preferred. Extracorporeal circulation with cold blood cardioplegia is used. If a previous shunt operation has been performed, the anastomosis is isolated before extracorporeal circulation is begun and subsequently occluded during bypass before the heart is opened. Once the pericardium has been opened, the outflow tract of the right ventricle is carefully examined for anomalous coronary arteries, choosing an approach that avoids dividing any such arteries.

Five potential zones of obstruction to flow of blood to the lungs should be considered for surgical correction, the location, the severity, and number varying with each patient. These include fusion of the pulmonary valve leaf-

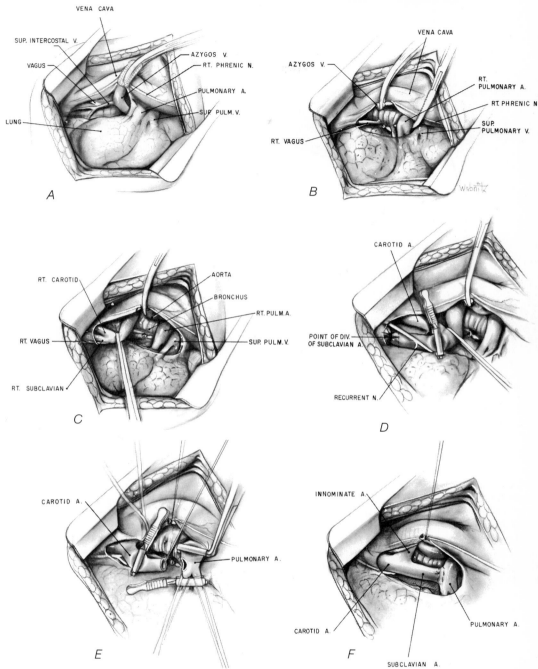

Fig.18-39. Blalock procedure. *A.* Dissection is begun by isolation and division of azygos vein, followed by incision of mediastinal pleura in front of pulmonary artery. *B.* Pulmonary artery is isolated in hilus, dissecting artery distally to beyond point of origin of upper lobe branch. Medially, artery is freed well into mediastinum in order to permit displacement of artery superiorly during construction of anastomosis. Traction on stump of divided azygos vein retracts superior vena cava to expose pulmonary artery in mediastinum. *C.* Subclavian artery is mobilized at apex of thorax, mobilizing carotid artery and subclavian artery down into mediastinum. Wide mobilization of carotid artery greatly facilitates subsequent performance of anastomosis. Vagus and recurrent nerves are protected during this dissection. *D.* After mobilization of carotid and subcla-vian arteries, tributaries of subclavian arteries are ligated, vertebral artery being ligated separately to avoid retrograde flow of blood from vertebral artery distad into arm, producing subclavian "steal" abnormality. *E.* After division of subclavian artery, longitudinal arteriotomy is made in pulmonary artery. Adventitia is carefully cleared from subclavian artery before performance of anastomosis. *F.* Appearance of completed anastomosis. Anterior row of anastomosis is usually made with interrupted sutures to permit growth of anastomosis. With wide mobilization of carotid artery superiorly and pulmonary artery inferiorly, satisfactory anastomosis can be accomplished with subclavian artery as short as 1 to 1.5 cm in length. Vein graft is rarely necessary.

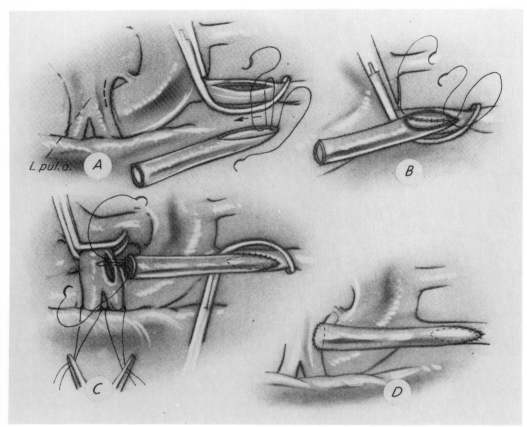

Fig. 18-40. Left Goretex interposition shunt. *A.* The Goretex graft has been trimmed for insertion. End-to-side anastomosis is made between the Goretex and the left subclavian artery. The first portion of the suture line is being made by sewing from within as shown. *B.* With the other end of the double-armed suture, the second portion of the suture is begun. *C.* The distal anastomosis is made in a similar fashion. The direction of suturing at both anastomoses minimizes the possibility of tearing the delicate subclavian or pulmonary artery. *D.* Completed anastomosis. [From: *Ventricular septal defect and pulmonary stenosis or atresia, in Kirklin JW, Barratt-Boyes BG (eds): Cardiac Surgery. New York, Wiley, chap 23, p 763, with permission.*]

lets; a hypoplastic pulmonic annulus; varying degrees of infundibular stenosis in the right ventricle, either fibrous or muscular; hypoplastic main pulmonary artery; or hypoplastic distal pulmonary arteries. The critical importance of these decisions emphasizes the crucial nature of preoperative selective angiocardiography.

The surgical approach may be through the right atrium or the right ventricle, varying with both the anatomy and the preference of the surgeon. The ventriculotomy may be transverse or a short (4 to 5 cm) high vertical one, stopping near the pulmonic annulus. A vertical ventriculotomy is routinely closed with an appropriate Dacron patch. Initially the large hypertrophied muscles of the crista supraventricularis are excised, providing better exposure of the ventricular septal defect (Fig. 18-41).

If the pulmonic valve ring is of adequate size, the fused commissures of the pulmonic valve may be divided through the ventriculotomy without opening the pulmonary artery. Otherwise a separate incision is made in the pulmonary artery to facilitate appropriate commissurotomies.

A crucial part of the operation is deciding whether the diameter of the pulmonic valve ring is adequate. Sizing of the diameter of the pulmonic ring with Hegar dilators is first done and then evaluated with the nomogram developed by Kirklin, describing normal relationships between

body weight and diameter of the pulmonic annulus. The measurements are particularly useful for smaller children. In larger children a pulmonic valve ring that will accommodate a size 16 Hegar dilator, representing a cross-sectional area slightly less than 2 cm^2, is satisfactory.

If the pulmonic annulus is hypoplastic, the ventriculotomy is extended accordingly across the annulus into the pulmonary artery and an appropriate patch applied.

Following correction of the infundibular obstruction, the ventricular septal defect is closed in a manner identical to that described previously for ventricular septal defect. Adequacy of closure is confirmed by retrograde injection of crystalloid solution through a left ventricular vent while the aorta is temporarily clamped. With the technique of closure of the septal defect as described, permanent heart block is very rare, now 1 percent.

If the diameter of the main pulmonary artery is less than 2 cm, it is also widened to an appropriate degree with a patch that may be extended when necessary beyond the bifurcation of the artery onto the left pulmonary artery.

Our preference for the prosthetic patch is a section of woven tubular Dacron graft. Pericardium is also a satisfactory material in most patients but has been associated with the subsequent formation of aneurysms in a small number of patients, usually with residual pulmonary hypertension.

Following bypass, intracardiac pressure is measured to confirm that right ventricular obstruction has been corrected. The right ventricular systolic pressure should be reduced to less than 60 to 70 percent of left ventricular systolic pressure. If right ventricular pressure is still elevated above this level, more adequate correction of the ventricular obstruction should be considered, though exact guidelines do not exist. Otherwise fatal depression of cardiac output from right ventricular failure may occur in the early postoperative course. In most patients following bypass a satisfactory result is obtained, with a systolic pressure near 100 mm, a right ventricular systolic pressure between 35 and 50 mm, and a pulmonary artery systolic pressure of 20 to 25 mm.

Postoperative Course. Following operation, particular attention is required in the first 24 h to intrathoracic bleeding, because older cyanotic patients have an increased hemorrhagic tendency from the long-standing polycythemia. Transfusion of fresh frozen plasma, often combined with platelet transfusions, is the best therapy. Close observation is necessary to detect intrathoracic accumulation of blood with cardiac tamponade.

Adequacy of cardiac output is monitored by direct measurement and indirectly by observing blood pressure, blood-gas concentrations in mixed venous blood, and urine output. Blood is transfused in sufficient amounts to keep left atrial pressure in the range of 10 to 15 mmHg if necessary, possibly at higher levels. If cardiac output is inadequate despite these measures, small amounts of inotropic drugs (dobutamine, dopamine, epinephrine, or isoproteronol) are infused. Assisted ventilation may be required for 12 to 24 h but seldom for longer.

The risk of operation varies with the age of the patient and the degree of cyanosis, reflecting the severity of the right ventricular obstruction. The risk is near 2 to 5 percent. Large clinical series showing low operative mortality have also been reported by Kirklin, Malm et al., Shumway et al., and McGoon et al.

Arciniegas et al. reported 209 patients in whom an outflow patch across the pulmonic annulus was employed in nearly 70 percent. Perioperative mortality was 5 percent and delayed mortality was 3 percent. Complete heart block occurred in only one patient. Late results were considered good in 87 percent of the patients.

Following recovery from operation, dramatic improvement is obvious. Cyanosis is, of course, absent, and exer-

Fig. 18-41. Right ventricular approach to ventricular septal defect. Ao, aorta; AV, atrioventricular; IVC, inferior vena cava; PA, pulmonary artery; PV, pulmoary valve; RBB, right bundle branch, SVC, superior vena cava; TSM, trabecula septomarginalis; TV, tricuspid valve; VSD, ventricular septal defect. [From: *Kirklin JW, Barratt-Boyes BG: Ventricular septal defect and pulmonary stenosis or atresia, in Kirklin JW, Barratt-Boyes BG (eds): Cardiac Surgery. New York, Wiley, chap 23, pp 732–734, with permission.*]

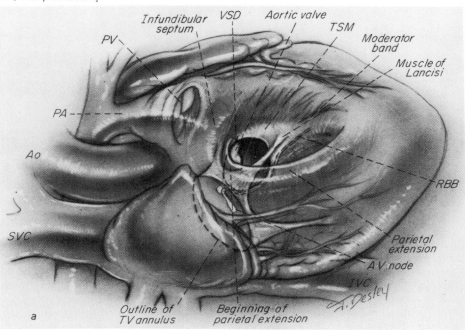

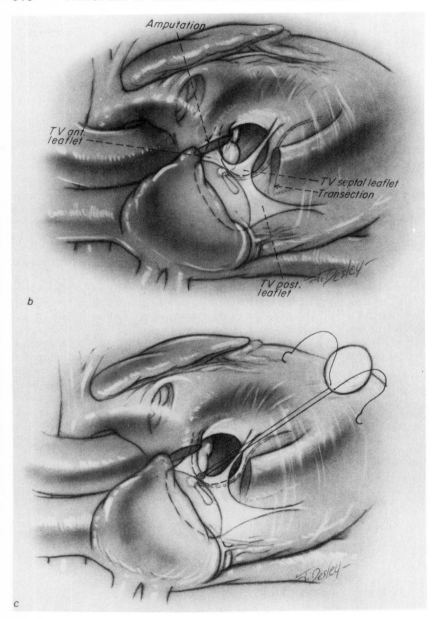

Fig. 18-41. Continued.

cise tolerance within a few months approaches that of a normal individual. If cardiac failure is significant following operation, convalescence may be slow for several weeks. Long-term studies show that most patients have excellent cardiac function.

The tolerance for pulmonic insufficiency after two to three decades is almost unknown, though Lillehei recently reported good long-term results in patients operated upon with a follow-up of more than 30 years. Ebert described repeat operations upon 24 patients who had been operated upon 1 to 21 years earlier. Several with severe pulmonary valve incompetence and right ventricular dysfunction were treated with insertion of a prosthetic valve.

COMPLEX MALFORMATIONS

Transposition of the Great Vessels

HISTORICAL DATA. The clinical syndrome of transposition of the great vessels was clearly described by Taussig in 1938. The first surgical procedure to achieve significant benefit, creation of an atrial septal defect, was reported in 1948 by Blalock and Hanlon. Because of the excellent results now obtained with balloon septostomy, developed by Rashkind in 1969, surgical creation of an atrial septal defect is now seldom performed. Another palliative surgical procedure, no longer used, was developed by Baffes around 1957. He transposed the inferior vena cava and

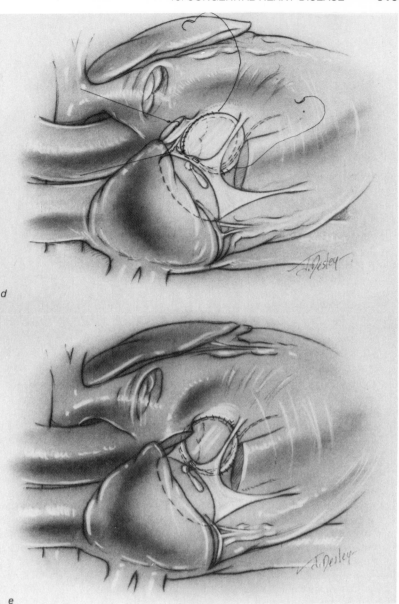

Fig. 18-41. Continued.

the right pulmonary veins. Senning, in 1957, first completely corrected transposition of the great vessels by repositioning the atrial septum, but mortality was prohibitively high. Further experience with a modification of the technique was reported by Senning in 1975. Mustard, in 1964, developed a method of reconstructing the atrial cavity that has produced the best clinical results to date. In the past few years a revised Senning procedure has been adopted by several groups as the procedure of choice.

INCIDENCE AND ETIOLOGY. Successful surgical correction of the transposed aorta and pulmonary artery, the "arterial switch" operation, was first successfully reported by Jatene in 1975. For the first few years, opera-

tive mortality remained excessive, but improved results in the last 3 to 4 years indicate that an arterial switch should be considered the primary operation in many patients. Quaegebeur reported in 1986 experiences with 66 patients with eight operative deaths and *no* late deaths among 33 patients followed for 1 to 8 years.

INCIDENCE AND ETIOLOGY. Transposition of the great vessels is a frequent disorder, representing 5 to 8 percent of all congenital cardiac malformations and accounting for about 25 percent of deaths in the first year of life. It is the most common cause of cardiac failure in the newborn. It results from abnormal division of the bulbar trunk in embryologic development, occurring between the fifth and seventh uterine week. Etiologic factors are unknown.

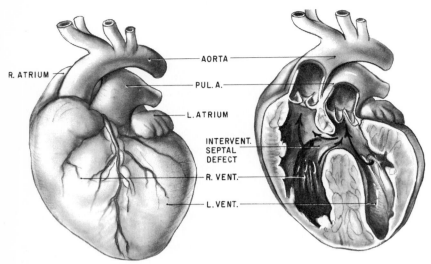

Fig.18-42. Transposition of great vessels, with aorta arising from right ventricle and pulmonary artery from left ventricle. Ventricular septal defect permits communication between pulmonic and systemic circulations; otherwise condition would be incompatible with life after birth. (From: *Taussig HB: Congenital Malformations of the Heart, 2d ed. Cambridge, Harvard University Press, 1960, p 149, with permission.*)

It is about four times more frequent in males than in females.

PATHOLOGIC ANATOMY. With transposition of the arteries, the aorta originates from the right ventricle and the pulmonary artery from the left ventricle (Fig. 18-42). As a result, venous blood returning through the venae cavae to the right atrium enters the right ventricle and is then ejected directly into the aorta. Oxygenated blood returning from the lungs through the pulmonary veins to the left atrium enters the left ventricle and is then expelled through the pulmonary artery to the lungs. This dual, parallel circulatory arrangement is obviously incompatible with life without communication between the pulmonary and systemic circulations. Three possible communications exist, a patent ductus arteriosus, an atrial septal defect or foramen ovale, or a ventricular septal defect. One or more of these, of course, must exist for the infant to survive even a few hours after birth. A patent ductus is present for a few weeks after birth in over one-half the patients. A foramen ovale is also frequent, and a ventricular septal defect occurs in 50 to 70 percent of patients.

Associated anomalies are common. One of the most frequent, pulmonic stenosis, occurs frequently enough to constitute a well-defined variant of the syndrome, because the prognosis is unusually favorable. A wide variety of other anomalies may occur, including coarctation of the aorta, pulmonary atresia, and dextrocardia.

PATHOPHYSIOLOGY. The two basic physiologic handicaps with transposition are severe anoxia from inability to transport oxygen from the lungs to the tissues of the body and progressive cardiac failure. The severe and rapidly progressive cardiac failure results partly from a high cardiac output and partly from the fact that the coronary arteries are filled with unoxygenated blood with resulting myocardial anoxia. The relative severity of the anoxia and the cardiac failure varies with the nature of the intracardiac communications and the adequacy of pulmonary blood flow. Nadas found cardiac failure at birth in 80 percent of live patients.

Transposition is a lethal condition. Patients with an intact ventricular septum, depending upon a foramen ovale to communicate between the two circulations, die most rapidly; 30 percent in 1 week, 50 percent in 1 month, 90 percent by 1 year. Those with a large ventricular septal defect develop pulmonary vascular changes at an astonishing rate, often within 6 to 8 weeks, with 80 percent dying within the first year.

Nadas conveniently grouped patients into three clinical categories related to prognosis. Those with an intact ventricular septum do poorly because of inadequate mixing of the pulmonary and systemic circulations. Similarly, those with a large ventricular septal defect do badly because of excessive pulmonary blood flow. Pulmonary vascular resistance rises very rapidly in this group. Patients with the most favorable prognosis have a ventricular septal defect combined with pulmonic stenosis. This combination permits mixing of the pulmonary and systemic circulations through the ventricular septal defect, while the pulmonic stenosis prevents excessive pulmonary blood flow with pulmonary congestion and secondary pulmonary hypertension.

CLINICAL MANIFESTATIONS. Symptoms. A high percentage of infants are cyanotic at birth. Over 90 percent are recognized the first day of life. Cardiac failure is similarly frequent. The combination of cardiac failure and cyanosis in a newborn suggests transposition. The most prominent symptoms are cyanosis and dyspnea.

Physical Findings. Cyanosis is usually obvious, often severe. Signs of congestive failure are almost always found, with cardiac enlargement, hepatomegaly, and pulmonary congestion. A systolic murmur is usually present but is variable and not diagnostic. It can result from any of the different intracardiac communications that may be present. Absence of a murmur, often indicating absence of an intracardiac communication, indicates a particularly unfavorable prognosis.

LABORATORY FINDINGS. The chest radiograph often shows three distinctive abnormalities. The contour of the heart has been described as "egg-shaped," resulting from the prominent right ventricle projecting into the left hemithorax and the dilated right atrium bulging into the right side. The base of the cardiac shadow, termed the "waist," may be unusually narrow because of the location of the aorta in front of the pulmonary artery, rather than the normal side-to-side relationship (Fig. 18-2). Pulmonary congestion is often marked.

The electrocardiogram consistently shows severe right ventricular hypertrophy. The presence of left ventricular hypertrophy depends on the pulmonary blood flow and the degree of pulmonary valvular stenosis. The echocardiogram is often diagnostic, outlining the transposed great arteries and the intracardiac communications.

Cardiac catheterization reveals several distinctive features. It may not be possible to enter all four cardiac chambers because of the malformations. The systolic pressure in the right ventricle is the same as in the aorta, while that in the left ventricle varies with the size of the ventricular septal defect and the presence of pulmonic stenosis. The oxygen saturation in the pulmonary artery is increased. A hallmark of the condition is the fact that oxygen saturation in the pulmonary artery is greater than that in the femoral artery. Varying degrees of arterial oxygen unsaturation are regularly found, ranging from as low as 12 percent to as high as 85 percent. Angiocardiography provides the best means for confirming the diagnosis, for it classically demonstrates the anterior origin of the aorta from the right ventricle, with the more faintly visualized pulmonary artery lying posteriorly.

DIAGNOSIS. The diagnosis of transposition can be immediately considered in a seriously ill, cyanotic infant with cardiac enlargement and congestive heart failure. In older children the retardation of physical development is striking. It must be differentiated from tetralogy of Fallot, tricuspid atresia, and total anomaly of venous return. Tetralogy of Fallot is readily identified in many patients by the normal cardiac size and the absence of cardiac failure. Tricuspid atresia is easily recognized by the characteristic left axis deviation on the electrocardiogram. Total anomalous drainage of the pulmonary veins may require cardiac catheterization to establish the diagnosis with certainty.

TREATMENT. Indications for Operation. In planning therapy transposition may be classified into four broad groups, as follows: (1) intact ventricular septum, patent foramen ovale; (2) ventricular septal defect; (3) ventricular septal defect and pulmonic stenosis; and (4) complex transposition, one of the previous three forms in association with other severe defects such as coarctation of the aorta.

The most critically ill infants are those with an intact ventricular septum, for the only communication between the pulmonary and systemic circulations is through the

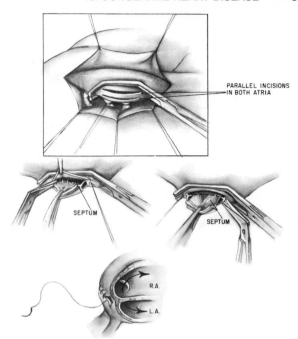

Fig. 18-43. Creation of atrial septal defect (Blalock-Hanlon technique). Right pulmonary veins are mobilized and occluded by traction on ligatures. Pulmonary artery and right main bronchus are also occluded to avoid congestion of lungs during occlusion of pulmonary veins. Tangential occlusion clamp is applied to right and left atria, enclosing atrial septum. Separate incisions are then made in right atrium and left atrium. Exposed atrial septum is then removed, temporarily releasing clamp in order to withdraw more septum from between its jaws and create larger defect. After excision of this septum, incision is sutured, creating large atrial septal defect. (From: *Cooley DA et al: Arch Surg 93:704, 1966, with permission.*)

foramen ovale. In these patients, balloon septostomy provides dramatic improvement. It should usually be done in the catheterization laboratory at the time the diagnosis is made.

Most infants improve dramatically after balloon septostomy, so elective operation can be done near three months of age. A few patients do not do well after balloon septostomy and may require a corrective operation at an earlier time. Creation of an atrial septal defect at operation with the original Blalock-Hanlon technique, illustrated in Fig. 18-43, is now seldom necessary.

Although elective repair was previously delayed until one or two years of age, the development of irreversible pulmonary vascular disease in some patients in the first year of life indicates that an earlier operation is preferable with present techniques. Operative risk is near 5 percent. Usually one of the two types of standard atrial switch operations is performed, either the Mustard procedure or the Senning. The latter seems to have a lower frequency of long-term complications, though excellent results have been reported with both techniques.

Infants with a large ventricular septal defect should be considered for definitive repair in the first few weeks of life because of the rapidity of development of pulmonary vascular disease. Either an atrial switch repair, combined with closure of the ventricular septal defect, or an arterial switch can be considered.

In patients with a ventricular septal defect and pulmonic stenosis, hypoxia may require use of a subclavian pulmonary shunt in the first few weeks of life. When older, the Rastelli procedure can be performed if the intracardiac anatomy is satisfactory.

Trusler et al. reported data from the institution in which the Mustard operation was developed. Only two deaths occurred in the last 100 operations. Modification in operative technique has decreased the frequency of pulmonary venous obstruction, caval obstruction, and arrhythmias; 89 percent of patients in the recent group maintained a sinus rhythm. At this time excellent long-term results have been reported with both the Mustard and the Senning methods of atrial correction. Increasingly good results have been reported with the arterial switch procedure.

If an arterial switch operation is performed, it must be done in the first 1 to 2 weeks of life in patients with an intact ventricular septum but may be delayed until about 3 months for those with a ventricular septal defect.

Tricuspid Atresia

HISTORICAL DATA. Systemic-pulmonary arterial shunts for tricuspid atresis were applied soon after their development in 1945–1947. There was significant short-term improvement, but long-term results were disappointing. A significant contribution was made by Glenn in 1958, with the development of the superior vena cava–right pulmonary artery anastomosis. The major advance, however, came in 1968 when Fontan successfully separated the right and left circulations in a patient for the first time, a physiologic concept that had seemed feasible in laboratory studies for over a decade but had never been successfully applied in human beings. In the last 15 years, the Fontan procedure has undergone several modifications but has been established clearly as the procedure of choice for this condition.

PATHOLOGIC ANATOMY. Tricuspid atresia is an important form of congenital heart disease, affecting 3 to 8 percent of children with cyanotic heart disease. The four basic abnormalities are atresia of the tricuspid valve, constituting complete obstruction to the flow of blood; an atrial septal defect; a varying degree of hypoplasia of the right ventricle; and a ventricular septal defect. The mitral valve and the left ventricle are usually normal. Blood enters the rudimentary right ventricle through a ventricular septal defect.

In about 70 percent of patients, the aorta and pulmonary artery are normally located, while in about 30 percent transposition is present. Hence, there are two major types of tricuspid atresia depending upon whether the great vessels are transposed or not. Each of these two major groups has been further subdivided into whether the pulmonary blood flow is normal or increased, decreased, or pulmonary atresia is present (Figs. 18-44, 18-45).

In the patients with normally related great vessels, the majority have a decreased pulmonary blood flow, while about 15 percent have a normal or increased pulmonary blood flow.

When the aorta and pulmonary artery are transposed, about 70 percent of patients have a normal or increased pulmonary blood flow.

Fig. 18-44. Three basic varieties of tricuspid atresia with normally related great arteries. Proximal to the mitral valve, anatomic arrangements are similar, with an interatrial communication providing the right atrium (RA) with its only outlet. Beyond the mitral valve, the anatomic patterns vary (LA-left atrium). *A.* When there is pulmonary atresia, i.e., no interventricular communication, all left ventricular blood enters the aorta (Ao). Pulmonary flow depends on a patent ductus arteriosus or systemic arterial collaterals. *B.* When there is pulmonic stenosis, the zone of obstruction typically consists of a slitlike ventricular septal defect that represents the only communication between the left ventricle (LV) and the small right ventricle (RV). The pulmonary trunk (PT) is normal or hypoplastic, and pulmonic valve stenosis may coexist. *C.* The absence of pulmonic stenosis signifies that there is a large ventricular septal defect with unobstructed flow into the pulmonary circulation. (From: *Perloff JK: The Clinical Recognition of Congenital Heart Disease. Philadelphia, Saunders, chap 25, p 555, with permission.*)

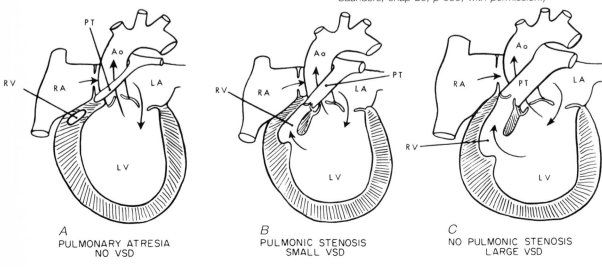

A
PULMONARY ATRESIA
NO VSD

B
PULMONIC STENOSIS
SMALL VSD

C
NO PULMONIC STENOSIS
LARGE VSD

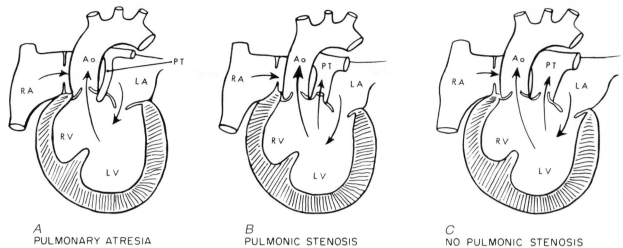

A
PULMONARY ATRESIA

B
PULMONIC STENOSIS

C
NO PULMONIC STENOSIS

Fig. 18-45. Three basic varieties of tricuspid atresia with complete transposition of the great arteries. Proximal to the mitral valve, the anatomic arrangements are similar, with an interatrial communication providing the right atrium (RA) with its only outlet. The ventricular septal defect is characteristically large so there is no obstruction to flow from left ventricle (LV) into the transposed aorta (Ao). Beyond this point the anatomic patterns vary. *A.* When there is pulmonary atresia (imperforate pulmonic valve and hypoplastic pulmonary trunk), all left ventricular blood enters the aorta. Pulmonary flow depends on a patent ductus arteriosus or systemic arterial collaterals. *B.* When pulmonic stenosis is present obstruction is either valvular or subvalvular. *C.* When there is no pulmonic stenosis, the pulmonary vascular resistance determines the amount of blood entering the lungs (RV = right ventricle; PT = pulmonary trunk; LA = left atrium). (From: *Perloff JK: The Clinical Recognition of Congenital Heart Disease. Philadelphia, Saunders, chap 25, p 555, with permission.*)

PATHOPHYSIOLOGY. The disability from hypoxia resulting from inadequate pulmonary blood flow is severe. This is most commonly due to restriction of flow of blood from the left ventricle through the ventricular septal defect and rudimentary right ventricle into the pulmonary artery. The ventricular septal defect usually decreases in size in the first year of life, further decreasing pulmonary blood flow, so over 90 percent of patients die before the first year unless operation is performed.

In the minority of patients with an increase in pulmonary blood flow, with either normal or transposed great arteries, congestive heart failure is present with gradual failure of the left ventricle. Only rarely is the pulmonary blood flow near normal.

CLINICAL MANIFESTATIONS. Disability is severe with cyanosis, usually obvious at birth. Over 50 percent of infants are correctly diagnosed during the first day of life. The clinical manifestations are usually those of severe cyanosis with anoxic spells often terminating in hemiplegia or death. In the few patients with an increased pulmonary blood flow, signs of pulmonary congestion and heart failure may predominate.

The physical examination is usually not diagnostic as the systolic murmur present varies widely, depending upon the size of the ventricular septal defect and the anatomical relationship of the great vessels. The chest roentgenogram shows decreased vascularity if pulmonary blood flow is decreased. Both the electrocardiogram and echocardiogram provide the diagnostic clues that establish the diagnosis. The electrocardiogram is strongly suggestive, showing a typical left axis deviation resulting from the underdevelopment of the right ventricle. The 2-D echocardiogram can often outline the atrial septal defect, the ventricular septal defect, and the relationships of the great arteries. Cardiac catheterization and angiography are required to precisely delineate these abnormalities.

TREATMENT. An emergency shunt is often necessary in the first few days or weeks of life to prevent death from anoxia. A Goretex interposition shunt, as described in the section on Tetralogy, is usually the simplest and most satisfactory.

In some patients, a small atrial septal defect (or foramen ovale) may restrict flow of blood from the right atrium to the left atrium. This can be determined at cardiac catheterization, measuring a gradient between the right and left atrium. If a gradient is present, a balloon septostomy can be performed at that time. Surgical enlargement of the atrial septal defect is almost never required at this time. After six to twelve months of age, a Fontan procedure can be performed, directing the venous blood into the pulmonary circulation.

This landmark procedure was first performed by Fontan in France in 1968 and has subsequently been widely used throughout the world with excellent results. Important modifications of the original Fontan concept were made by Kreutzer and by Bjork. At present, three varieties of connections between the right atrium and the pulmonary artery are performed. The simplest, when feasible, is establishment of a large direct communication between the right atrium and the main pulmonary artery, which is divided at its origin, mobilized, and anastomosed directly to a large circular opening in the right atrium. No valve is inserted (Fig. 18-46).

If the right ventricle is of significant size with a pulmonic valve, a conduit may be established from the right atrium to the right ventricle, either with or without a valve. In all procedures both the atrial and ventricular

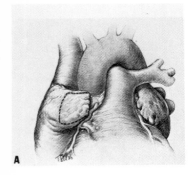
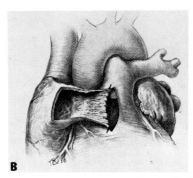
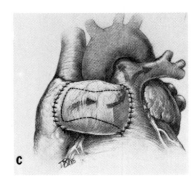

Fig. 18-46. Technique of anastomosing the right atrium to the right ventricle. *A.* An incision is made in the right atrial appendage to form a flap of the anterior wall. *B.* The cut edge of the flap is then sutured to the rightward edge of the longitudinal incision in the right ventricle to form the posterior wall of the tunnel. *C.* The procedure is completed by suturing a pericardial patch from the right atrial appendage to the right ventricle to form the anterior wall of the tunnel. Arrows indicate the flow of blood in the completed conduit. [From: *Stanton RE, Lurie PR, et al: The Fontan procedure for tricuspid atresia. Circulation 64(suppl 2):140, 1981, with permission.*]

septal defects are closed so the two circulations are separated. There are not adequate data at present to determine which of the techniques are preferable.

Operative risk in general is in the range of 5 to 15 percent with reasonably good results for at least 5 to 10 years after operation.

The operation physiologically depends upon using the venous pressure to perfuse the pulmonary vascular bed. This is usually satisfactory if the right atrial pressure remains below 15 mm. Higher levels result in severe problems such as chylothorax and protein-losing enteropathy. Hence, a contraindication to the Fontan procedure is an increase in pulmonary vascular resistance or hypoplasia of the pulmonary arteries.

In the minority of patients who were seen with refractory congestive failure from increased pulmonary blood flow in infancy, banding of the pulmonary artery can be done, followed later by a Fontan procedure and debanding after 1 to 2 years.

The Glenn procedure consists of anastomosis of the superior vena cava to the right pulmonary artery (Fig. 18-47). About 85 percent of patients survive 10 or more years, with generally satisfactory results. Symptoms tend to gradually recur, however, probably related to growth of the patient, development of collateral circulation, and the basic limitation that only part of systemic venous return has been directed into the pulmonary vascular bed.

RARE MALFORMATIONS

Cor Triatriatum

Cor triatriatum is a rare malformation. In 1960 a review by Niwayama found only 36 cases. Excellent embryologic and pathologic studies were reported by Van Praagh, and subsequently by Marin-Garcia.

PATHOLOGIC ANATOMY. The abnormality is best viewed as a variant of total anomalous pulmonary venous

Fig. 18-47. Anastomosis between superior vena cava and right pulmonary artery. *A.* Tangential clamp has been applied to superior vena cava to include origin of azygos vein. Right pulmonary artery has been divided, and end-to-end anastomosis will be constructed. *B.* Posterior row of anastomosis is constructed. *C.* Completed posterior row of anastomosis. *D.* Anterior row of anastomosis is constructed with interrupted sutures to permit growth of anastomosis. After removal of occluding clamps, superior vena cava is doubly ligated at point of juncture with right atrium. (From: *Glenn WWL: N Engl J Med 259:117, 1958, with permission.*)

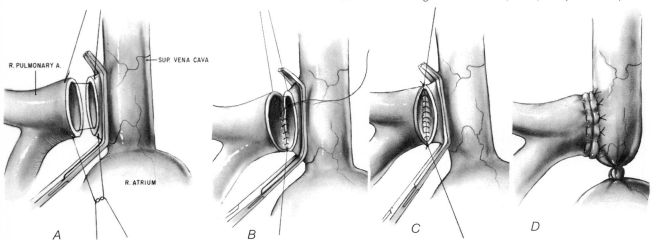

R. PULMONARY A.

SUP. VENA CAVA

R. ATRIUM

A   *B*   *C*   *D*

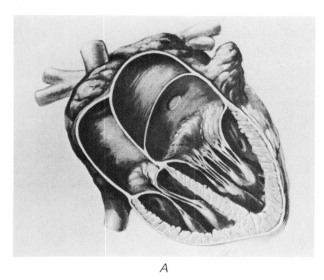

A

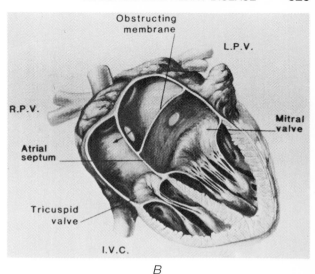

B

Fig. 18-48. *A.* Cor triatriatum with intact atrial septum (type A). *B.* Cor triatriatum with atrial septal defect between the proximal left atrial chamber and the right atrium (type A₁). (LPV = left pulmonary vein; RPV = right pulmonary vein; IVC = inferior vena cava.) (From: *Arciniegas E, Hakimi M, Green EW: Surgical treatment of cor tri-atriatum. Ann Thorac Surg 32:571, 1981, with permission.*)

drainage except that the unresorbed common venous sinus empties normally into the left atrium through a restricted aperture, rather than through abnormal channels to the right side of the heart. The common venous chamber is superior and posterior to the normal left atrium with a diaphragm separating this chamber from the true left atrium. The left atrial appendage enters the normal small left atrium. A small opening in a thick muscular diaphragm is the only communication between the two chambers.

This abnormality produces severe pulmonary hypertension, identical to mitral stenosis. Gradients as high as 20 mmHg have been recorded between the venous chamber and normal left atrium.

An atrial septal defect, usually a fossa ovalis, is present in about 70 percent of cases, generally entering the common venous chamber and resulting in a left-to-right shunt.

A classic malformation is shown in Fig. 18-48A. The most common variety, with an atrial septal defect between the common venous chamber and the right atrium, is shown in Fig. 18-48B.

CLINICAL MANIFESTATIONS. The disability is a severe one from pulmonary congestion, pulmonary hypertension, and heart failure. Without surgical treatment 70 to 75 percent of infants die in the first year of life. The clinical presentation is identical to that of mitral stenosis except that a typical diastolic murmur is often not present.

DIAGNOSTIC CONSIDERATIONS. The x-ray shows pulmonary congestion with right ventricular enlargement. Right ventricular hypertrophy is evident on the electrocardiogram, varying with the degree of pulmonary hypertension. 2-D echocardiography is diagnostic, outlining the abnormal chambers. Some investigators no longer consider cardiac catheterization necessary, although catheterization and angiography permits measurement of pulmonary artery pressure and more precise delineation of other associated anomalies. The classic physiologic abnormalities at catheterization are an elevated pulmonary artery pressure, an increased wedge pressure, and a *normal* pressure in the left atrium. The differential diagnosis includes the two other conditions that can commonly produce pulmonary venous hypertension, mitral stenosis, or stenosis of pulmonary veins.

TREATMENT. Operation should be performed promptly when the diagnosis is recognized in infancy because of the high mortality rate. With proper techniques of extracorporeal circulation, combined with hypothermia and circulatory arrest, operative results are usually excellent. The abnormal septum between the common venous sinus and the left atrium can be readily excised, eliminating the physiologic abnormality. An accompanying atrial septal defect can be closed at the same time. Usually an approach from the right side of the heart is preferable, though this varies with the precise abnormality present. Results in surviving patients are excellent.

Kirklin and Barratt-Boyes reported excellent results in a group of seven patients operated upon over a period of 30 years, emphasizing the rarity of the malformation. Oglietti reported experiences with 25 patients seen over a period of 21 years. The diagnosis was made preoperatively in 14, established at the time of operation for other abnormalities in 10. The anomalous membrane was excised in 18 patients with excellent results in all but one who required reoperation because of incomplete excision of the septum. Arciniegas reported on six patients ranging in age from one and one-half to ninety-three months. There was one postoperative death; the five surviving patients remained in excellent condition 4 years following operation.

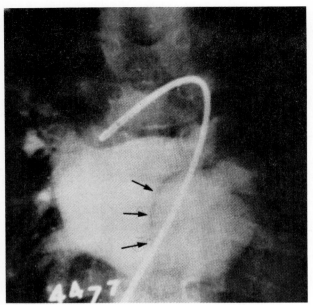

Fig. 18-49. Angiogram shows the subdividing left atrial membrane (arrows). The atrial septum was intact. Contrast material was injected into the pulmonary artery. (From: *Arciniegas E, Hakimi M, Green EW: Surgical treatment of cor triatriatum. Ann Thorac Surg 32:571, 1981, with permission.*)

Congenital Mitral Valve Disease

These abnormalities are rare, about 0.6 percent of all cases of congenital heart disease at autopsy, and about 0.3 percent of clinically diagnosed cases.

In 1967 a review by Tsuji found 131 reported cases, 41 of whom had been operated upon with 21 survivors. One of the most extensive experiences was described by Carpentier, reporting experiences with 47 children, in 14 of whom mitral stenosis was the dominant finding.

PATHOLOGY. Multiple abnormalities in the mitral valve apparatus are usually present. A distinct stenosing *supravalvular* ring has been described in a few patients. The mitral valve annulus is usually small. Usually there are multiple abnormalities in the leaflets with defective commissures. A few patients have a distinct isolated cleft causing insufficiency. The underlying chordae and papillary muscles are often malformed, producing either stenosis or insufficiency. One distinctive malformation, termed a "parachute" mitral valve, consists of a single papillary muscle with all chordae attached to this muscle.

Congenital mitral stenosis exists as an isolated lesion in about 25 percent of patients, in association with a ventricular septal defect in nearly 30 percent. Some form of left ventricular outflow tract obstruction is present in about 40 percent of cases. Van Praagh in 1978 reported an extensive pathologic study of 49 cases.

CLINICAL MANIFESTATIONS. Symptoms of pulmonary venous hypertension often appear in infancy and include dyspnea, orthopnea, and pulmonary edema. It has been estimated that about one-half of patients die within 6 months after symptoms appear. Those with less severe abnormalities are often seen between ages one and four; rarely symptoms may not become severe until ten to twelve years of age.

Chest x-ray and electrocardiographic abnormalities are similar to those of mitral stenosis. With 2-D echocardiography the diagnosis can usually be made with certainty and the precise abnormalities identified. Additional information can be obtained by subsequent cardiac catheterization and angiography (Fig. 18-49).

TREATMENT. Operation should clearly be postponed as long as possible because of the strong probability of the need for repeat operation as the child grows older. The feasibility of repair versus replacement depends upon the abnormality present. In the extensive experience reported by Carpentier, valve reconstruction was possible in 38 patients; valve replacement was necessary in 9; hospital mortality was 13 percent.

In patients in whom reconstruction was possible, some residual stenosis or insufficiency is usually present. Reasonable long-term results have been reported in the few patients surviving 10 years, with a 63 percent survival and about 80 percent remaining free of reoperation at 10 years.

Aortic-Pulmonary Window

This is a rare abnormality. At the Toronto Children's Hospital, only 23 of 15,000 patients with congenital heart disease who were seen over a period of 20 years had an aortopulmonary window. Synonyms referring to the same lesion include aortopulmonary fistula and aortic septal defect.

One case was treated by ligation by Gross in 1948, another by division and suture by Scott and Sabiston in 1951 (Fig. 18-50). Effective safe correction became possible only with the development of extracorporeal circulation.

PATHOLOGIC ANATOMY. Embryologically, the defect results from incomplete development of the spiral septum dividing the primitive truncus arteriosus into the aorta and pulmonary artery. Persistent truncus arteriosus is a more severe malformation of similar cause. The opening, or "window," between the aorta and pulmonary artery may vary in diameter from 5 to 30 mm. It is usually located proximally near the ostium of the coronary arteries. At least 30 percent of patients have a severe additional cardiac malformation.

PATHOPHYSIOLOGY. The large left-to-right shunt is similar to that of a large patent ductus arteriosus or ventricular septal defect. The course is a malignant one because an increase in pulmonary vascular resistance quickly occurs, similar to a large ventricular septal defect.

CLINICAL MANIFESTATIONS. The clinical findings may be identical to those of patent ductus arteriosus with a continuous murmur and wide pulse pressure. Often, however, only a systolic murmur is present because of the severe pulmonary hypertension. Differential diagnosis includes ventricular septal defect and truncus arteriosus.

LABORATORY FINDINGS. 2-D echocardiography can usually confirm the diagnosis. A CT scan is also usually

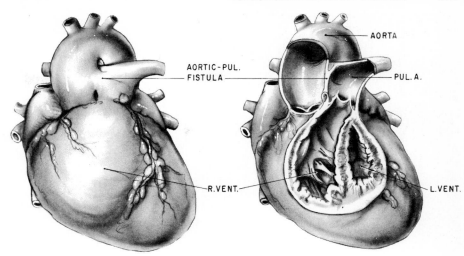

Fig. 18-50. Aortic-pulmonary fistula, showing large communication between aorta and pulmonary artery near base of heart. (From: *Scott HW, Sabiston DC: J Thorac Surg. 25:26 1953, with permission.*)

diagnostic. Cardiac catheterization and aortography should be done to define precisely the relationship to adjacent structures and also confirm that the aortic and pulmonic valve rings are intact. The degree of elevation of pulmonary vascular resistance can also be determined.

TREATMENT. Operation should be performed as soon as the diagnosis has been established because of the rapidity of development of irreversible pulmonary vascular disease. At operation a transaortic approach has usually been employed, closing large defects with a prosthetic patch. Care is taken to avoid injury to the coronary arteries or the pulmonary valve. In patients operated upon in infancy or before the development of severe pulmonary vascular disease, results have been excellent. Little information is available about those surviving with severe elevation in pulmonary vascular resistance.

Doty in 1983 reported 25 patients and reviewed 50 previous reported operative repairs. He concluded that a transaortic approach was preferable with patch closure of the defect. The risk of operation was proportional to the increase in pulmonary vascular resistance.

Ruptured Aneurysm of Sinus of Valsalva

This unusual abnormality produces a distinct syndrome that can be readily diagnosed and effectively treated. Before the development of extracorporeal circulation, it usually caused death from cardiac failure within 1 to 2 years after rupture. The natural history was well described by Sawyer in 1957, reviewing 47 reported patients. Successful operations with extracorporeal circulation were done by Lillehei and by Kirklin in 1956, and other successful care reports soon followed. By 1965 over 90 patients had been operated upon.

PATHOLOGIC ANATOMY. The basic abnormality is a thinning of the aortic media in the wall of the sinus of Valsalva. In embryonic development, the developing ventricular septum inferiorly meets the spiral septum superiorly which separates the aorta and the pulmonary arteries. Incomplete merger of these two structures results in a ventricular septal defect in the membranous septum. An aneurysm of the sinus of Valsalva results from a less severe malformation of a similar type, for the media of the aortic wall does not extend down to the annulus of the aortic valve ring. Hence, there is a spectrum of abnormalities, including ventricular septal defect, aortic valve abnormalities with aortic valve prolapse, and less frequently, pulmonic stenosis.

The right coronary sinus is involved in most patients with rupture into the right ventricle. The noncoronary sinus is involved in about 20 percent of patients, most commonly rupturing into the right atrium. Involvement of the left coronary sinus or rupture into the left atrium or left ventricle is very unusual, probably both because of the differences in anatomy and because of the high pressures in the left ventricle. The typical aneurysm is usually described as a "windsock" with a wide base at the aortic origin and a nipplelike apex projecting into a cardiac chamber where rupture eventually occurs.

CLINICAL MANIFESTATIONS. Until rupture occurs, there are no abnormalities unless an enlarging aneurysm distorts the aortic leaflets sufficiently to cause aortic insufficiency. The average age at rupture is 31 years. This is usually without known cause, although a few case reports describe the onset during physical exertion.

About one-third of patients develop acute symptoms at the time of rupture, with chest pain, soon followed by dyspnea and palpitation and the appearance of the characteristic murmur. In nearly one-half of patients, however, the onset is more gradual with progressive dyspnea, while a small percentage have very few symptoms when the cardiac abnormalities are detected. Death seldom occurs from right heart failure shortly following rupture, but over the ensuing weeks and months, cardiac failure relentlessly progresses with few patients tolerating the abnormality for more than 1 to 2 years.

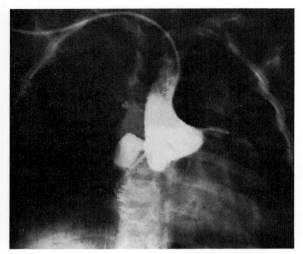

Fig. 18-51. Aortogram confirms diagnosis of ruptured aneurysm of sinus of Valsalva by demonstrating flow of dye from region of aortic sinuses to right atrium. *(Courtesy of Dr. Raymond M. Abrams, Department of Radiology, New York University Medical Center.)*

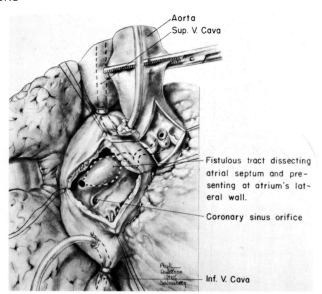

Fig. 18-52. Diagram of unusual type of ruptured aneurysm of sinus of Valsalva. Aneurysm arose from left coronary cusp and developed fistulous tract before rupture into right atrium. Operative closure was performed by opening aorta and closing opening directly. (From: *Ann Surg 152:965, 1960, with permission.*)

On physical examination the classical abnormality is a parasternal murmur, often with a thrill, loudest in the third or fourth interspace. This is often continuous, resembling a patent ductus, but is at a lower location. The usual hemodynamic abnormalities seen with a large patent ductus are present, including a wide pulse pressure, cardiac enlargement, and pulmonary congestion.

The diagnosis can readily be suspected from the history and the physical abnormalities. The chest x-ray shows cardiac enlargement and pulmonary congestion. Cardiac hypertrophy is evident on the electrocardiogram. With 2-D echocardiography the diagnosis can be promptly confirmed. Cardiac catheterization and angiography are usually performed to determine the site of origin, the cardiac chamber involved, and the presence of associated lesions, especially ventricular septal defect or aortic insufficiency (Fig. 18-51).

TREATMENT. Surgical correction, of course, should be performed promptly. The basic objective at operation is to close both the defect and any associated lesions (Fig. 18-52). An approach through both the aorta and the involved cardiac chamber is best, facilitating the correction of associated lesions such as a ventricular septal defect. The aneurysmal sac can be excised back to the aortic origin and closed, preferably with a prosthetic patch. Alternately, the aneurysm can be excised and sutured from within the ventricle, following which a prosthetic patch can be directly sutured over the aortic origin, avoiding any injury to the aortic cusps. The operative risk is small and reported results excellent.

Truncus Arteriosus

Truncus arteriosus is a rare malformation resulting from failure of division of the fetal arterial channel into the aorta and pulmonary arteries and the left and right ventricles. The embryonic origin of the malformation has been analyzed in detail by Rothko.

PATHOLOGIC ANATOMY. In this condition the entire circulation, including the coronary arteries, the pulmonary arteries, and the systemic arteries, arises from a common arterial trunk. There is always a ventricular septal defect. Only one semilunar valve is present, usually with three or four cusps.

In 80 to 85 percent of patients the pulmonary arteries arise from the truncus, either as a common stem or in close apposition. Infrequently, the origin of the two pulmonary arteries is separated a short distance, complicating the anatomic repair. In most patients the ductus arteriosus is absent; if present, it is usually large with corresponding decrease in size of the aortic isthmus (Fig. 18-53).

PATHOPHYSIOLOGY. The disability is a severe one with about 50 percent of patients dying in the first month of life, 90 percent within the first year, usually from congestive heart failure. The severe heart failure results from the large left-to-right shunt through the ventricular septal defect. Severe incompetence of the truncal valve, often from nodular myxomatous degeneration, may contribute significantly.

The blood entering the aorta is a mixture of blood from the systemic and pulmonary circulations, arterial oxygen unsaturation is always present, the degree varying with the volume of pulmonary blood flow. Usually, in infancy, the oxygen saturation is above 80 percent, so cyanosis is minimal. Severe pulmonary vascular disease develops rapidly, often before six months of age. As this progresses, arterial oxygen saturation decreases and cyanosis becomes more prominent.

The majority of infants are obviously seriously ill with congestive heart failure and an overactive heart with a wide pulse pressure. Murmurs are variable, not diagnos-

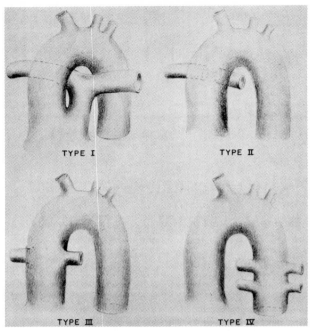

Fig. 18-53. Four anatomic types of truncus arteriosus. (From: *Poirier RA et al: J Thorac Cardiovasc Surg 69:169, 1975, with permission.*)

tic, unless a continuous murmur is audible. The chest x-ray shows cardiomegaly and pulmonary congestion. Both right and left ventricular hypertrophy are evident on the electrocardiogram. 2-D echocardiography is diagnostic, outlining the single vascular trunk originating from the base of the heart. Cardiac catheterization and angiography define the anatomy precisely, including the origin of the pulmonary arteries and the presence of insufficiency of the truncal valve. The pulmonary vascular resistance can be determined, indicating the gravity of the problem, and whether operation can be performed or not.

TREATMENT. Most modern treatment emerged from the excellent work of McGoon, who first successfully used a homograft conduit in 1967. In the procedure developed by McGoon the pulmonary arteries were detached from the truncus, the right ventricle opened, and the ventricular septal defect closed, after which the homograft conduit was inserted between the right ventricle and the distal pulmonary artery.

Most of the early operations were performed upon patients over two years of age, obviously a selective group as only about 10 percent of patients survive beyond the first year of life.

Current experiences at the Mayo Clinic were summarized by DiDonato in 1985, describing experiences with 167 patients over a 17-year period. There were 48 hospital deaths (29 percent mortality). Eighty-four percent of 119 surviving patients were alive at 5 years, 69 percent at 10 years.

In 1985, Sharma reported experiences with 23 patients, 16 of whom were less than one year of age. There were only three operative deaths, two of which occurred in

critically ill infants operated upon under one month of age.

As nearly 50 percent of infants die within 1 month, operation must clearly be performed in the neonatal period if heart failure is severe. Otherwise it may be delayed until three to six months of age, but further delay has the hazard of an irreversible rise in pulmonary vascular resistance.

In 1984, Ebert described experiences with 106 infants. One hundred were corrected by six months of age, with 11 operative deaths. Fifteen of the 86 long-term survivors have returned for change of the conduit because of body growth or pseudo-intimal proliferation in the conduit. There were no mortalities at the time of conduit change. A distinctive feature of the operative technique used by Ebert is minimizing the aortic cross-clamping, performing a significant part of the operation while the heart is beating.

The long-term course of surviving patients is unknown because to date there are few such patients. A progression in pulmonary vascular resistance has occurred in some patients. Another hazard in surviving patients is the development of insufficiency in the abnormal truncal valve.

Operative mortality has been low in the selective group of patients operated upon between five and ten years of age, in whom the pulmonary vascular resistance is less than 0.6 percent of systemic vascular resistance. However, this is a selective group because, as indicated earlier, there is both a high mortality in infancy and also rapid development of irreversible pulmonary vascular disease in many. These considerations were well reviewed in the reports by Poirier in 1975 and by Applebaum in 1976.

Banding of the pulmonary arteries in infancy to protect the pulmonary vascular bed has a surprisingly high mortality, nearly 50 percent from different reports according to Applebaum, and also a significant mortality at the time of attempted correction at a later date. Hence the increasing tendency is to perform corrective surgery with a valve conduit at an earlier age, probably between two and three years, or in the first years of life if symptoms are severe. This has been accomplished in several patients described by Ebert in 1976.

When a conduit is inserted in such small children, it will have to be replaced as the child grows older; Marcelletti and McGoon reported in 1976 that 22 aortic homograft conduits had been successfully replaced with a Dacron conduit, primarily because of deterioration of the aortic homograft.

Single Ventricle

A single ventricle is a severe malformation that fortunately is quite rare. Effective palliative surgery has become possible in a high percentage of cases. The long-term outlook has progressively improved with the effective development of cardiac transplantation.

PATHOLOGIC ANATOMY AND PATHOPHYSIOLOGY. A wide spectrum of abnormalities exists. The basic abnormality is a single functioning ventricle into which both atrioventricular valves empty. The variations include the type of functioning ventricular chamber (morphologically a "left" or a "right" ventricle), the type of hypoplastic ventricular chamber; different abnormalities in the atrioventricular valves; and the origin of the aorta and pulmonary artery from either the large ventricle or the hypoplastic one.

The two physiologic abnormalities are anoxemia from mixture of oxygenated and unoxygenated blood in the single ventricle before entering the aorta, and pulmonary congestion from the high pulmonary blood flow resulting from the origin of the pulmonary artery from the left ventricle. The degree of cyanosis present depends upon the pulmonary blood flow.

CLINICAL MANIFESTATIONS. About one-third of patients do not have significant pulmonic stenosis, so the resulting disability initially resembles that of a large ventricular septal defect with some cyanosis. At the other extreme, severe cyanosis is present from pulmonic stenosis, requiring an emergency shunt procedure in infancy.

In between these two extremes are patients with moderate pulmonic stenosis, often with a pulmonary blood flow about twice normal. Such patients may do reasonably well in the first few years of life.

In most patients the disability is severe, about 40 percent requiring operation in the first year of life, but only about 50 percent of patients alive at four years of age. Excellent morphologic and embryologic studies have been reported by both Van Praagh et al. and by Anderson et al.

CLINICAL MANIFESTATIONS AND DIAGNOSIS. The clinical picture varies with the pulmonary blood flow. Infants with an increased pulmonary blood flow are acyanotic but disabled from pulmonary congestion and cardiac failure. Such infants have been treated previously with pulmonary artery banding, which unfortunately results in subaortic stenosis in a high percentage of patients within the next 1 to 2 years. At the other extreme, with severely decreased pulmonary blood flow, cyanosis is severe so a shunt procedure is often required in infancy. The cardiac murmurs, x-ray, and electrocardiogram are usually diagnostic, but a precise diagnosis can be made by 2-D echocardiography, noting the absence of the normal ventricular septum. Catheterization with selective angiography can further delineate the precise abnormalities present.

TREATMENT. Urgent banding or shunting procedures have been used in infants, depending upon whether the pulmonary blood flow is increased or decreased. In older patients, surgically partitioning the ventricle or separating the two circulations with the Fontan procedure are the two procedures available. Which procedure is selected depends upon the abnormality present and the presence of increased pulmonary vascular resistance. Early experiences with partitioning of the ventricle were reported in four cases by Edie and Malm. In 1977, McGoon et al. reported experiences with 23 patients, obtaining satisfactory results in 61 percent. In 1984, Stefanelli et al. described experiences in 116 patients over a period of 15 years with a 10-year actuarial survival rate of 66 percent. Ventricular septation was performed in 36 patients with 15 deaths. The majority of patients developed complete heart block following septation, requiring a pacemaker.

A total of 73 patients underwent a Fontan-type procedure with a 22 percent mortality and a 10-year actuarial survival rate of 71 percent. Over 95 percent of surviving patients were reported as improving to a functional class I or II status.

A two-stage approach was described in five patients by Ebert, only partly closing the septal defect at the first operation. In this small group, all survived without any rhythm disturbances.

Ebstein's Anomaly

This unusual anomaly was described by Wilhelm Ebstein in 1866. The abnormality is uncommon, about 0.5 percent of all cases of congenital heart disease. There is a nearly 400 times increased frequency of Ebstein's malformation when the mother has taken lithium during the pregnancy.

PATHOLOGIC ANATOMY. The basic abnormality is a malformation of the septal and posterior leaflets of the tricuspid valve. The origin of the leaflets is displaced downward to a variable degree creating a third chamber on the right side of the heart. Both the leaflet tissue and its chordae are also abnormal. The anterior tricuspid leaflet is usually normal and may be unusually large and prominent, described as "sail-like" (Fig. 18-54). The segment of right ventricular wall between the true annulus of the tricuspid valve and the origin of the displaced leaflets becomes functionally part of the right atrium and has been termed the atrialized ventricle. There is a varying degree of hypoplasia of this segment in some patients resembling a true aneurysm that bulges paradoxically. In most patients, the atrialized segment has some muscle fibers with little paradoxical motion. The distal functioning right ventricle is small. Some investigators have felt that there is a true deficiency in the right ventricular fibers as well, contributing to the right ventricular dysfunction in this condition. A foramen ovale or ostium secundum defect are almost always present. The right atrium is usually dilated, often to a huge size in older patients.

The malformation varies widely in severity, ranging from relatively minor valvular abnormalities to virtual atresia of the valve leaflets.

PATHOPHYSIOLOGY. The main physiologic disturbance is inadequate cardiac output from the right ventricle, a result of both the tricuspid insufficiency and the dysfunction of the right ventricle. A variety of arrhythmias commonly occur in older patients; these are rarely fatal. Massive dilatation of the right atrium gradually develops in some patients. Cyanosis of moderate degree occurs in at least 50 percent of patients because of a right-to-left shunt through the foramen ovale. It gradually becomes more severe in older patients with progressive right ventricular failure.

CLINICAL MANIFESTATIONS. A significant percentage of infants present in the first month of life with tachypnea and cyanosis, probably a manifestation of the elevated pulmonary vascular resistance in the neonatal period. About one-half of patients who are severely symptomatic

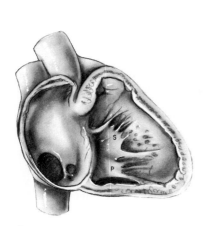
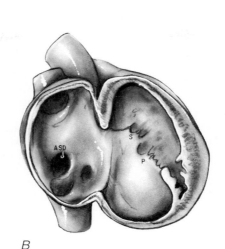
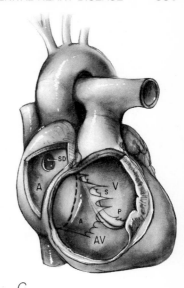

A   *B*   *C*

Fig. 18-54. *A.* Normal heart showing septal and posterior leaflets of tricuspid valve. *B.* Pathologic anatomy in Ebstein's malformation, with displacement of diminutive septal and posterior leaflets down into normal right ventricular cavity. Large anterior leaflet is not shown. *C.* Abnormal pathologic anatomy in Ebstein's malformation. There is large "sail-like" anterior leaflet with hypoplastic septal and posterior leaflets, which are often displaced downward into ventricle, creating third cardiac chamber interposed between right atrium and functioning right ventricle. (From: *Hardy KL et al: J Thorac Cardiovasc Surg 48:931, 1964, with permission.*)

in the first month of life subsequently die. After the first month, disability decreases, often with loss of cyanosis, so disability during childhood is often small. A mortality of about 15 percent has been estimated to occur between ages one and twenty. The course is a gradual one, so that the average age of diagnosis is in the midteens.

Many adults continue to function reasonably well, depending upon the presence of arrhythmias, cyanosis, and cardiac failure. A few patients have lived to beyond seventy years of age, but only about 5 percent of all patients live beyond fifty years.

DIAGNOSTIC CONSIDERATIONS. A variety of systolic and diastolic murmurs are present, though Nadas at one time stated that auscultatory findings were highly suggestive, emphasizing a slow cardiac rate with a triple or quadruple rhythm, a systolic murmur of tricuspid regurgitation, and often a low-pitched diastolic murmur.

The chest x-ray may show grotesque cardiac enlargement because of the huge right atrium and the atrialized right ventricle. Vascularity in the lung fields is usually decreased. Electrocardiographic abnormalities are considered typical with conduction disturbances, a prolonged PR interval, and partial right bundle branch block.

2-D echocardiography is virtually diagnostic, outlining the different abnormalities with surprising precision. Cardiac catheterization should be done carefully, for fatal arrhythmias have occurred. A right-to-left shunt at the atrial level with arterial hypoxemia is found in 25 to 50 percent of patients. The angiocardiogram is usually diagnostic.

TREATMENT. Only limited data are available because surgical treatment has only been used frequently in the past decade. Early corrective operations included prosthetic valve replacement by Barnard, and subsequently by Lillehei. Hardy reported a successful valvuloplasty in 1964, based upon concepts described by Hunter and Lillehei. Bahnson in 1965 reported successful reconstructive operations in two patients.

The best results have been reported by Danielson at the Mayo Clinic, who described in a 1985 report a total experience with 72 patients. Surgical intervention was recommended for all patients at a class III status, or in those with a cardiothoracic ratio enlarging beyond 0.65. In 81 percent of the group reconstruction of the tricuspid valve was possible, converting the valve to a monocusp valve with the functioning anterior leaflet. Prosthetic valve replacement was used in most of the other patients. There were five hospital and three late deaths. The 39 surviving operated patients were 87 percent class I or II at 5 years.

A different approach has been followed by Kirklin and Barratt-Boyes, employing valve replacement in 20 patients operated upon with an overall mortality of 20 percent. The editor feels the data of Danielson are quite convincing and would favor attempted valvuloplasty in the majority of patients operated upon.

At the time of operation the atrial septal defect is closed. Plication of the atrialized ventricle seems unnecessary in the vast majority of patients, employed only when the atrialized segment is clearly extremely thin and contracting paradoxically.

Amomalies of the Coronary Arteries

ANOMALOUS ORIGIN OF THE LEFT CORONARY ARTERY FROM PULMONARY ARTERY

This is a rare malformation, occurring about once in 300,000 live births and representing about 0.25 percent of patients with congenital heart disease. The clinical fea-

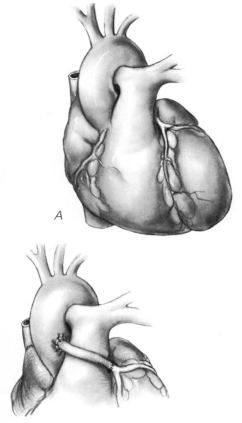

Fig. 18-55. *A.* Anomalous left coronary artery arising from pulmonary artery. *B.* Vein graft used to anastomose coronary artery to aorta. A graft of subclavian artery is preferable. (From: *Cooley DA et al: J Thorac Cardiovasc Surg 52:805, 1966, with permission.*)

tures were well described by Bland and associates in 1933, emphasizing the similarity of the syndrome to myocardial infarction in adults. A particularly significant contribution was made by Sabiston in 1959, conclusively demonstrating that the flow of blood in the anomalous left coronary artery was *retrograde* into the pulmonary artery. Ligation of the anomalous artery was subsequently performed. Reconstruction was first accomplished by Cooley by detaching the coronary artery and connecting it to the aorta with a saphenous vein graft (Fig. 18-55). Unfortunately, the vein graft in a few years became stenotic, so this is no longer considered a satisfactory operation.

PATHOLOGIC ANATOMY AND PHYSIOLOGY. The disability is a severe one, for myocardial infarction and left ventricular failure are commonly present within 3 months after birth. Only about 10 to 20 percent of untreated infants live more than 1 year, apparently because of abundant collateral circulation from the right coronary artery. Symptoms, if present, are usually mild for the first few weeks after birth, probably because of the elevated pulmonary vascular resistance in the neonatal period. Subsequently, symptoms progress with great rapidity. The classic symptom is poor feeding, as attempted feeding

produces severe distress. Signs of myocardial infarction or left ventricular failure are soon evident. Initially, only acute episodes occur with feeding, between which the infant may appear normal. During the acute episodes, there is apparently colicky pain, with tachypnea, cyanosis, pallor and sweating, probably angina pectoris, and progressive malnutrition. Subsequently, with chronic congestive failure, tachypnea becomes chronic. On physical examination there may be obvious cardiac enlargement with muffled heart sounds; no characteristic murmurs are found.

The chest x-ray may show extensive enlargement of the left ventricle with pulmonary congestion. Often the electrocardiogram is diagnostic with inverted T waves and prominent Q waves. 2-D echocardiography may confirm the diagnosis, demonstrating absence of the normal origin of the left coronary artery from the aorta, and at times actually demonstrating the anomalous origin from the pulmonary artery. Cardiac catheterization and angiography are diagnostic, demonstrating the abnormal origin of the left coronary artery and a small left-to-right shunt at the level of the pulmonary artery. When coronary angiograms are performed in older children, the right coronary is found dilated and tortous with dye filling the right coronary and subsequently opacifying the left coronary with retrograde flow into the pulmonary artery.

TREATMENT. Operation should be performed in symptomatic infants to prevent progressive myocardial infarction and death. Though reattachment of the coronary artery to the aorta is clearly the ideal operation, data do not clearly indicate better results with reconstruction as compared with simple ligation and interruption of retrograde flow. A mortality near 50 percent unfortunately is common. The ingenious tunnel operation of Takauchi is probably the preferred method of reconstruction, creating an intrapulmonary tunnel to connect the anomalous left coronary ostium to the aorta. If the abnormal anatomy is favorable, the left coronary may be detached from the pulmonary artery and anastomosed directly to the aorta as in the "arterial switch" operation for transposition. In older children a free graft of subclavian artery has been successfully used by several surgeons. A subclavian coronary artery bypass has been successfully performed in a few patients, though simpler techniques of reconstruction are probably preferable in the older patients in whom this type of bypass may be feasible.

In patients operated upon after one year of age, mortality is low and results excellent. The 18 long-term survivors reported by Kirklin were stated to be in excellent condition. Arciniegas reported experiences with 12 patients with only two deaths, but six seriously ill infants were not operated upon, all of whom died. If these six preoperative deaths are included, the total mortality is 40 percent among 20 patients, similar to that reported by other groups.

CORONARY ARTERIOVENOUS FISTULA

Familiarity with this unusual condition grew rapidly with the advent of cardiac angiography and open heart

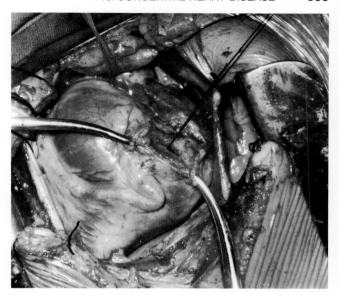

Fig. 18-56. Arteriovenous fistula of right coronary artery. Enlarged, tortuous right coronary artery is clearly visible over surface of right ventricle. Fistulous communication directly into right ventricle was found, as illustrated by ligatures, and ligated.

surgery. In 1960 Gasul found 52 cases in a collective review. At this time well over 300 surgical cases have been reported in the literature; and undoubtedly a much larger number have never been reported.

PATHOLOGIC ANATOMY AND PHYSIOLOGY. The right coronary is involved in about half of the cases, the left coronary in about a third, and both coronaries in only about 5 percent. The artery involved is usually a normal artery with a normal branching pattern. The fistula may be a "side-to-side" one with continuity of the vessel beyond the fistula, or "an end fistula" occurring where the vessel terminates. Over 90 percent of fistulas open into the right heart chambers or its connecting vessels, approximately 25 percent in the right atrium, 40 percent in the right ventricle, 15 to 20 percent in the pulmonary artery, and about 7 percent in the coronary sinus. Fistulas entering the left heart, left ventricle, or left atrium are uncommon. Usually a single fistulous opening is present, in the range of 2 to 5 mm. Rarely there are several openings or a localized angiomatous network. The involved coronary artery is dilated and elongated, at times growing to grotesque serpentine proportions. Actual rupture of an aneurysm, however, is rare (Fig. 18-56).

With fistulas entering the right heart, the resulting shunt is usually small. Only rarely is pulmonary blood flow increased to twice that of systemic flow. As with arteriovenous fistula elsewhere, the usual course is slow but progressive enlargement over decades so the volume of the shunt gradually increases with time.

Bacterial endocarditis may develop in a small percentage of cases, about 5 percent.

CLINICAL FEATURES. The majority of patients are asymptomatic, often evaluated because of the discovery of a continuous murmur. One report found that 80 percent of patients under twenty years of age were asymptomatic, decreasing to less than 50 percent in adults. Rarely, with huge fistulas, symptoms have appeared in the first year of life but are virtually unknown after that during childhood.

In adults the most common symptoms are dyspnea and fatigue from the left-to-right shunt. True angina occurs, probably a "coronary steal," in less than 10 percent. Eventually, congestive heart failure develops in 10 to 15 percent of patients, usually in older life as the shunt gradually enlarges in size.

The distinctive physical finding is a continuous murmur in a location that is unusual for a patent ductus arteriosus. The exact side of maximum intensity of the murmur varies with the cardiac chamber involved, whether it be right atrium, right ventricle, or pulmonary artery. The chest x-ray is either normal or shows slight enlargement with congestion of the lung fields from an increase in pulmonary blood flow. Changes in the electrocardiogram are usually minimal. Echocardiography may outline the dilated tortuous coronary artery. Cardiac catheterization and angiography readily establish the diagnosis and delineate the site of the fistula.

TREATMENT. As most patients are asymptomatic, small fistulas can probably be safely observed. Larger fistulas, however, should certainly be closed because the well-documented course is that of gradual enlargement with increasing disability, similar to that of a small atrial septal defect. The author has treated one patient over fifty years of age with congestive heart failure who subsequently remained in good condition over the next decade.

The present safety of cardiopulmonary bypass indicates that most procedures should either be performed with bypass or with bypass available if the location of the fistula precludes simple treatment without bypass. The fistula may be closed by opening the involved cardiac chamber and suturing the intracardiac communication, or with large fistulas by opening the coronary artery and suturing the opening directly. Preservation of distal coronary flow should be achievable in most patients as opposed to ligation. End fistulas, of course, can simply be treated by ligation.

Fistulas have been treated by placing multiple sutures

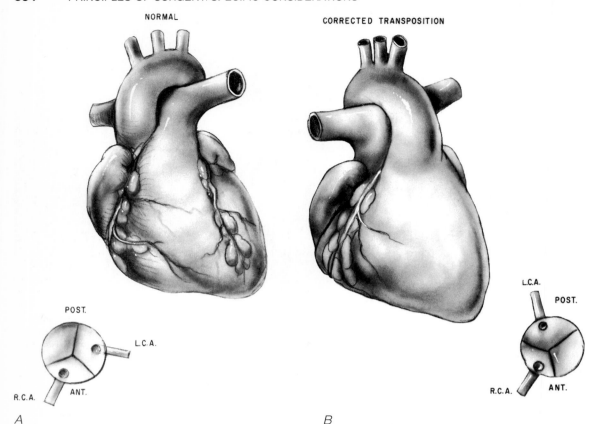

A   *B*

Fig. 18-57. *A.* Normal cardiac anatomy with pulmonary artery arising from right ventricle and aorta from left ventricle. Comparison with *B* shows that in corrected transposition, relative positions of aorta and pulmonary artery are reversed. *B.* In corrected transposition of great vessels, aorta arises anteriorly from ventricle that has anatomic characteristics of right ventricle. Pulmonary artery arises posteriorly and to right of aorta—reverse of normal anatomic arrangement. Insert depicts origin of coronary arteries in corrected transposition. (From: *Nadas AS: Pediatric Cardiology. Philadelphia, Saunders, 1964, p 714, with permission.*)

beneath the involved artery to obliterate the opening without precisely identifying it. Recurrences have been described, however, so this would seem to be a less desirable form of treatment.

In 1981, Lowe reported experiences with 28 patients. An additional 258 patients were reported by others. Operation was strongly recommended for there were no operative or late deaths and no recurrent fistulas over a period of 10 years. Urrutia reported experiences with 58 patients seen. There were no operative deaths in patients with isolated fistulas.

Corrected Transposition

The basic characteristics of this unusual malformation were described by Anderson in 1957 with additional contributions by Schiebler in 1961.

PATHOLOGIC ANATOMY AND PHYSIOLOGY. In this malformation the aorta and pulmonary artery are transposed to lie in a position exactly opposite of that normally occurring. The aorta arises from the anterior left border of the heart and the pulmonary artery from the right posterior area of the heart (Fig. 18-57). The ventricle from which the aorta arises is the morphologic right ventricle while that from which the pulmonary artery arises is the morphologic left ventricle. The atria and ventricle are also discordant; so blood from a morphologic right atrium reaches the pulmonary trunk by traversing a mitral valve

and a morphologic left ventricle, while blood from a morphologic left atrium reaches the aorta by traversing a tricuspid valve and a morphologic right ventricle. Hence, with the "double discordance" the basic circulation is normal. The anatomic relations of the coronary arteries are also altered with the right coronary artery arising anteriorly, the left coronary posteriorly, and the noncoronary sinus being located at the anterior left border of the heart.

The defect apparently arises from a malrotation of the embryonic heart tube, which bends to the left (L-ventricular loop). The significance of the malformation is primarily from the high incidence of associated abnormalities, for it has been estimated that only 1 to 2 percent of patients do not have an additional malformation. Four separate malformations commonly occur. The most frequent is a disturbance in conduction between the atrium and ventricle, originating from lack of normal continuity from the AV node to the ventricular septum. Normal AV conduction is present in less than one-half of patients.

A ventricular septal defect is present in the majority of patients, at least 80 percent. Some degree of pulmonic stenosis frequently occurs, which in some patients is of such severity that shunting must be performed in infancy. The fourth malformation, mitral insufficiency, gradually develops in older patients, perhaps a consequence of a tricuspid valve draining into the ventricle from which systemic pressure is generated.

A theoretical question arises from the altered physiology in this condition about whether a morphologic right ventricle can function for a normal lifespan. There are no significant data to indicate that this cannot occur, a particularly important long-term question for patients with transposition surgically corrected by the Senning or Mustard procedures. Most patients die before 50 years of age, usually from complications of the associated anomalies. Only one patient is known to have survived to age seventy-three.

CLINICAL MANIFESTATIONS. Conduction defects may cause problems in infancy as 5 to 10 percent of patients are born with a complete heart block, and subsequently heart block appears in about 2 percent of patients each year, with about 30 percent of patients eventually developing complete block.

Even though a large ventricular septal defect is present, some restriction to pulmonary flow commonly occurs so patients do not develop difficulty as rapidly as those with an uncomplicated large ventricular septal defect. Eventually severe pulmonary vascular disease develops unless significant pulmonic stenosis is present. In about one-third of patients the pulmonic stenosis is of such severity that a shunt must be surgically corrected in infancy or early childhood.

Physical examination is not diagnostic, though such patients have an unusually loud second sound to the left of the sternum, arising from the aortic valve. The chest x-ray characteristically has a narrow "waist" because of the abnormal location of the great arteries.

The electrocardiogram is almost always abnormal, often the first clue to the diagnosis. Characteristic abnormalities include the conduction disturbances and the unusual patterns of ventricular hypertrophy.

Echocardiography is usually diagnostic, but cardiac catheterization and angiography are routinely done to confirm the diagnosis and delineate the severity of associated abnormalities.

TREATMENT. Closure of the ventricular septal defect is technically difficult because a ventriculotomy through the anterior ventricle would injure the ventricle with systemic pressure. The preferred atrial approach is the transvalvular one through the atrium, incising the mitral valve leaflet for exposure if necessary. Heart block frequently occurs after operation, with a frequency of at least 10 to 20 percent. This is partly related to the abnormal location of the conduction bundle, located in the anterior rim of the ventricular septal defect. Pulmonic stenosis, when severe, is best corrected with an extracardiac conduit placed to the pulmonary trunk because the pathologic anatomy precludes an incision across the stenotic pulmonic valve.

The combined series reported in the Kirklin/Barratt-Boyes book total almost 100 patients with an operative mortality between 10 and 15 percent and a 10-year survival between 50 and 75 percent. Less favorable long-term results were reported by Metcalfe. Experiences with 19 patients treated over a decade included a high operative mortality, 37 percent, with only one patient asymptomatic 40 months following operation.

Theoretically, patients could get an excellent result if the ventricular septal defect is corrected before the development of severe pulmonary vascular disease, and conduction problems could be adequately treated with modern pacemakers.

Double Outlet Right Ventricle

This is a congenital malformation in which both great arteries are related to the morphologic right ventricle. It occurs in about 5 percent of all cases of congenital heart disease. Before open heart surgery became possible in 1954–1955, a few cases were reported, but modern knowledge of the condition emerged from surgical observations by Kirklin who, in 1957, first recognized the anatomic problem in the operating room and performed a surgical correction by creation of an intraventricular tunnel, similar to the treatment done today. The term double outlet right ventricle became established as the appropriate designation following a publication by Witham at that time. There are numerous subclassifications of this condition that are beyond the scope of this discussion.

Briefly, four types of relationships of the great arteries at the level of the semilunar valves have been described in this condition, varying with the relationship of the aorta to the pulmonary artery.

In addition, four separate anatomic locations of the ventricular septal defect have been described: subaortic, subpulmonic, beneath both great arteries ("doubly committed"), or beneath neither ("uncommitted"). Theoretically, the existence of two groups of four each creates 16 possible combinations of double outlet right ventricle. At one extreme the condition is that of classic transposition of the great vessels, while at another extreme the condition merges with tetralogy of Fallot. The classic case report by Taussig and Bing in 1949, leading to the eponym Taussig-Bing syndrome, described a double outlet right ventricle with a subpulmonic ventricular septal defect, occurring in about 8 percent of cases.

Clinically, three characteristic types of disability occur. With simply a large ventricular septal defect, the presentation is almost identical to that of a large ventricular septal defect. A high pulmonary vascular resistance develops in infancy with great rapidity. The second familiar clinical syndrome, pulmonic stenosis with a subaortic defect, is virtually identical to that of tetralogy of Fallot. A third variant is the Taussig-Bing, resembling classic transposition with severe disability in infancy from the combination of pulmonary congestion and hypoxemia.

Echocardiography can usually suggest the diagnosis, but precise biplane angiography is necessary for confirmation and delineation of exact details. With modern surgical techniques, most conditions can be corrected satis-

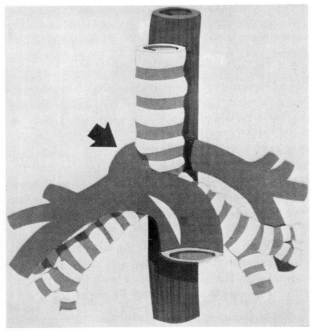

Fig. 18-58. Diagram of anomalous origin of left pulmonary artery from right pulmonary artery. Anatomic relationship of left pulmonary artery to trachea and esophagus is also shown. (From: *Grover FL et al: J Thorac Cardiovasc Surg 69:295, 1975, with permission.*)

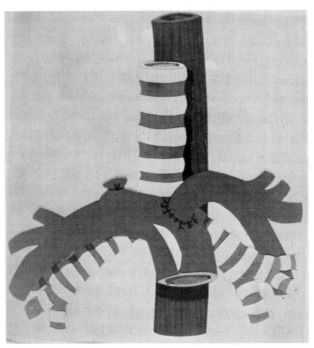

Fig. 18-59. Diagram of anatomy at completion of operation. Note that proximal stump of left pulmonary artery is to right of trachea after having been dissected free. Distal left pulmonary artery has been anastomosed to side of main pulmonary artery. (From: *Grover FL et al: J Thorac Cardiovasc Surg 69:295, 1975, with permission.*)

factorily with a precisely constructed intracardiac tunnel to channel blood from the left ventricle through the defect to the aorta. Excellent illustrations of the technique are present in the recent textbook by Kirklin and Barratt-Boyes.

In the Kirklin/Barratt-Boyes book, the combined experiences by the authors over a period of 15 years include 98 patients with an overall operative mortality of 30 percent. With the common simpler form, that with a subaortic VSD with or without pulmonic stenosis, operative mortality is now less than 10 percent.

Pulmonary Artery Sling

Vascular sling is a rare congenital malformation in which the left pulmonary artery arises from the right pulmonary artery and courses to the left between the trachea and esophagus to reach the left lung hilus, thus forming a sling around the trachea (Fig. 18-58). The term originated from a publication by Contro in 1958. Although the first patient was treated surgically by Potts in 1954, total reported surgical experience remains small. A review of Grover in 1975 described experiences with one patient and found a total of 63 patients reported by others. Twenty of 23 unoperated patients died.

The trachea is often narrowed at the site of compression and, in some patients, significant tracheal stenosis is present with complete cartilagenous rings. Other cardiac anomalies are present in nearly one-half of reported patients.

CLINICAL MANIFESTATIONS. Apparently, most infants

develop symptoms in the first few months of life, with wheezing, stridor, and choking. The diagnosis may be suspected from abnormalities visible on the chest x-ray, with a density separating the trachea from the esophagus on the lateral view. An esophageal barium swallow is usually diagnostic, showing anterior indentation of the esophagus just above the carina. A tracheogram and bronchoscopy should routinely be performed to evaluate the severity of associated tracheal malformations, one of the most important determinants of postoperative prognosis. A computerized tomogram will also confirm the diagnosis. Catheterization and angiography are routinely performed to confirm the diagnosis and detect additional anomalies.

The major decision before operation is evaluating the extent of inherent diseases in the trachea. Some infants with tracheal stenoses have ultimately died despite division of the sling and attempted correction of the tracheal malformation. Older patients are occasionally seen with minimal or no symptoms. Such patients often require no specific treatment.

TREATMENT. The operative procedure (Fig. 18-59) is a simple one, dividing the anomalous pulmonary artery at its origin, bringing it from behind the trachea and reanastomosing it to the main pulmonary artery. The ligamentum arteriosum is divided at this time. This has been done through a left lateral thoracotomy and also through a median sternotomy.

The prognosis following operation is determined principally by the inherent disease present in the trachea. Five patients were recorded by Kirklin/Barratt-Boyes, three of whom died after operation while the other two remain asymptomatic. Occlusion of the pulmonary artery has been subsequently found in some patients, probably a reflection of the technique of vascular anastomosis. Campbell, in 1983, reported two patients with good surgical results operating through a median sternotomy and also performing an "aortopexy" to minimize postoperative tracheal compression.

Bibliography

General

Abbott ME: *Atlas of Congenital Cardiac Disease.* New York, The American Heart Association, 1936.

Pulmonic Stenosis

Blalock A, Kiefer RF Jr: Valvulotomy for the relief of congenital valvular pulmonary stenosis with intact ventricular septum. Report of 19 operations by the Rock method. *Ann Surg* 32:496, 1950.

Brock RC: Pulmonary valvulotomy for the relief of congenital stenosis: Report of three cases. *Br Med J* 1:112, 1948.

Coles JG, Freedom RM, et al: Surgical management of critical pulmonary stenosis in the neonate. *Ann Thorac Surg* 38:458, 1984.

Griffith B, Hardesty R, et al: Pulmonary valvulotomy alone for pulmonary stenosis: Results in children with and without muscular infundibular hypertrophy. *J Thorac Cardiovasc Surg* 83:577, 1982.

Jonas RA, Castaneda AR, et al: Pulmonary valvulotomy under normothermic caval inflow occlusion. *Aust NZ J Surg* 55:39, 1985.

Sellors TH: Surgery of pulmonic stenosis. *Lancet* 1:988, 1948.

Srinivasan V, Konyer A, et al: Critical pulmonary stenosis in infants less than three months of age: A reappraisal of closed transventricular pulmonary valvotomy. *Ann Thorac Surg* 34:46, 1982.

Sullivan ID, Robinson PJ, et al: Percutaneous balloon valvuloplasty for pulmonary valve stenosis in infants and children. *Br Heart J* 54:435, 1985.

Congenital Aortic Stenosis

Brown J, Stevens L: Surgery for discrete subvalvular aortic stenosis: Actuarial survival, hemodynamic results, and acquired aortic regurgitation. *Ann Thorac Surg* 40:151, 1985.

Hsieh KS, Keane JF: Long-term follow-up of valvotomy before 1968 for congenital aortic stenosis. *Am J Cardiol* 58:338, 1986.

Hunta JC, Carpenter RJ Jr: Prenatal diagnosis and postnatal management of critical aortic stenosis. *Circulation* 75:573, 1987.

Konno S, Imai Y, et al: New method for prosthetic valve replacement in congenital aortic stenosis associated with hypoplasia of the aortic valve ring. *J Thorac Cardiovasc Surg* 70:909, 1975.

Messina LM, Turley K, et al: Successful aortic valvotomy for severe congenital valvular aortic stenosis in the newborn infant. *J Thorac Cardiovasc Surg* 88:92, 1984.

Misbach G, Turley K, et al: Left ventricular outflow enlargement using the Konno procedure. Paper presented at the American Association for Thoracic Surgery, Phoenix, Arizona, 1982.

Supravalvular Aortic Stenosis

Bernhard WF, Poirier V, LaFarge CG: Relief of congenital obstruction to left ventricular outflow with ventricular-aortic prosthesis. *J Thorac Cardiovasc Surg* 20:136, 1975.

Keane JF, Fellows KE, et al: The surgical management of discrete and diffuse supravalvular aortic stenosis. *Circulation* 54:112, 1976.

Peterson TA, Todd DC, Edwards JE: Supravalvular aortic stenosis. *J Thorac Cardiovasc Surg* 50:734, 1965.

Rastelli GC, McGoon DC, et al: Surgical treatment of supravalvular aortic stenosis: Report of 16 cases and review of literature. *J Thorac Cardiovasc Surg* 51:873, 1966.

Idiopathic Hypertrophic Subaortic Stenosis

Frye RL, Kincaid OW, et al: Results of surgical treatment of patients with diffuse subvalvular aortic stenosis. *Circulation* 32:52, 1965.

Kelly DT, Barratt-Boyes BG, Lowe JB: Results of surgery and hemodynamic observations in muscular subaortic stenosis. *J Thorac Cardiovasc Surg* 51:353, 1966.

Koch J, Maron H, et al: Results of operation for obstructive hypertrophic cardiomyopathy in the elderly. Septal myotomy and myectomy in 20 patients 65 years of age or older. *Am J Cardiol* 46:963, 1980.

Morrow A: Hypertrophic subaortic stenosis. Operative methods utilized to relieve left ventricular outflow obstruction. *J Thorac Cardiovasc Surg* 76:423, 1978.

Coarctation of the Aorta

Abbott ME: Coarctation of the aorta of the adult type: II. A statistical study and historical retrospect of 200 recorded cases, with autopsy, of stenosis or obliteration of the descending arch in subjects above the age of two years. *Am Heart J* 3:392, 1928.

Brewer LA III, Fosburg RG, et al: Spinal cord complications following surgery for coarctation of the aorta: A study of 66 cases. *J Thorac Cardiovasc Surg* 64:368, 1972.

Brom AG: Narrowing of the aortic isthmus and enlargement of the mind. *J Thorac Cardiovasc Surg* 50:166, 1965.

Campbell DB, Waldhausen JA, et al: Should elective repair of coarctation of the aorta be done in infancy? *J Thorac Cardiovasc Surg* 88:929, 1984.

Crafoord C, Nylin G: Congenital coarctation of the aorta and its surgical treatment. *J Thorac Surg* 14:347, 1945.

Fishman NH, Bronstein MH, et al: Surgical management of severe aortic coarctation and interrupted aortic arch in neonates. *J Thorac Cardiovasc Surg* 71:35, 1976.

Hehrlein FW et al: Instance and pathogenesis of late aneurysms after patch graft aortoplasty for coarctation. *J Thorac Cardiovasc Surg* 92:226, 1986.

Kirklin JW, Barratt-Boyes BG: *Cardiac Surgery.* Wiley, New York, 1986.

Krieger KH, Spencer FC: Is paraplegia after repair of coarctation of the aorta due principally to distal hypotension during aortic cross-clamping? *Surgery* 97:2, 1985.

Lerberg D, Hardesty R, et al: Coarctation of the aorta in infants and children: 25 years of experience. *Ann Thorac Surg* 33:159, 1982.

Perloff JK: *The Clinical Recognition of Congenital Heart Disease,* 3d ed. Philadelphia, Saunders, 1987.

Schuster SR, Gross RE: Surgery for coarctation of the aorta: A review of 500 cases. *J Thorac Cardiovasc Surg* 43:54, 1962.

Sealy WC, Harris JS, et al: Paradoxical hypertension following resection of coarctation of the aorta. *Surgery* 42:135, 1957.

Waldhausen J, Nahrwold D: Repair of coarctation of the aorta with a subclavian flap. *J Thorac Cardiovasc Surg* 51:532, 1966.

Yee ES, Soifer SJ, et al: Infant coarctation: A spectrum in clinical presentation and treatment. *Ann Thorac Surg* 42:488, November 1986.

Vascular Rings

Arciniegas E, Hakimi M, et al: Surgical management of congenital vascular rings. *J Thorac Cardiovasc Surg* 77:721, 1979.

Bertrand JM, Chartrand C, et al: Vascular ring: Clinical and physiological assessment of pulmonary function following surgical correction. *Pediatr Pul* 2:378, 1986.

Gross RE: Arterial malformations which cause compression of the trachea or esophagus. *Circulation* 11:124, 1955.

Idbeis B, Levinsky L, et al: Vascular rings: Management and a proposed nomenclature. *Ann Thorac Surg* 31:255, 1981.

Mahoney EB, Manning JA: Congenital abnormalities of the aortic arch. *Surgery* 55:1, 1964.

Roessler M, DeLeval M: Surgical management of vascular ring. *Ann Surg* 197:139, 1983.

Atrial Septal Defects: Secundum Defects

Freed MD, Nasas AS, et al: Is routine preoperative cardiac catheterization necessary before repair of secundum and sinus venosus atrial septal defects? *J Am Coll Cardiol* 4:333, 1984.

Paolillo V, Dawkins KD, Miller GA: Atrial septal defect in patients over the age of fifty. *Int J Cardiol* 9:139, 1985.

Sellers RD, Ferlic RM, et al: Secundum type atrial septal defects: Results with 275 patients. *Surgery* 59:155, 1966.

Sutton M, Tajik A, McGoon D: Atrial septal defect in patients 60 years or older: Operative results and long-term postoperative follow-up. *Circulation* 64:402, 1981.

Trusler G, Kazenelson G, et al: Late results following repair of partial anomalous pulmonary venous connection with sinus venosus atrial septal defect. *J Thorac Cardiovasc Surg* 79:776, 1980.

Anomalous Drainage of Pulmonary Veins

Bahnson HT, Spencer FC, Neill CA: Surgical treatment of 35 cases of drainage of pulmonary veins to the right side of the heart. *J Thorac Cardiovasc Surg* 36:777, 1958.

Blake HA, Hall RC, Manion WC: Anomalous pulmonary venous return. *Circulation* 32:406, 1965.

Brody H: Drainage of the pulmonary veins into the right side of the heart. *Arch Pathol* 33:221, 1942.

Turley K, Wilson J, Ebert P: Atrial repairs of infant complex congenital heart lesions. Emphasis on the first three months of life. *Arch Surg* 115:1335, 1980.

Ostium Primum Defect and Persistent Atrioventricular Canal

Berger T, Blackstone E, et al: Survival and probability of cure without and with operation in complete atrioventricular canal. *Ann Thorac Surg* 27:106, 1979.

Goldfaden D, Jones M, Morrow A: Long-term results of repair of incomplete persistent atrioventricular canal. *J Thorac Cardiovasc Surg* 82:669, 1981.

McGoon D, Puga F: Atrioventricular canal. *Cardiovasc Clin* 11:311, 1981.

McMullan MH, McGoon DC, et al: Surgical treatment of partial atrioventricular canal. *Arch Surg* 107:705, 1973.

Neill CA: Postoperative hemolytic anemia in endocardial cushion defects. *Circulation* 30:801, 1964.

Ventricular Septal Defect

Barratt-Boyes BG, Neutze JM, et al: Repair of ventricular septal defect in the first two years of life using profound hypothermia–circulatory arrest technics. *Ann Surg* 184:376, 1976.

Mattila S, Kostiainen S, et al: Repair of ventricular septal defect in adults. *Scan J Thorac Cardiovasc Surg* 19:29, 1985.

Otterstad JE, Erikssen J, et al: Long term results after operative treatment of isolated ventricular septal defect in adolescents and adults. *Acta Med Scan* 708(suppl):1, 1986.

Richardson J, Schieken R, et al: Repair of large ventricular septal defects in infants and small children. *Ann Surg* 195:318, 1982.

Rizzoli G, Blackstone E, et al: Incremental risk factors in hospital mortality rate after repair of ventricular septal defect. *J Thorac Cardiovasc Surg* 80:494, 1980.

Spencer FC, Doyle EF, et al: Longterm evaluation of aortic valvuloplasty for aortic insufficiency and ventricular septal defect. *J Thorac Cardiovasc Surg* 65:15, 1973.

Walker WJ, Garcia-Gonzalez E, et al: Interventricular septal defect: Analysis of 415 catheterized cases. *Circulation* 31:54, 1965.

Wood P: The Eisenmenger syndrome. *Br Med J* 2:701, 1958.

Yeager SB, Freed MD, et al: Primary surgical closure of ventricular septal defect in the first year of life: Results in 128 infants. *J Am Coll Cardiol* 3:1269, May 1984.

Patent Ductus Arteriosus

Blalock A: Operative closure of the patent ductus arteriosus. *Surg Gynecol Obstet* 82:113, 1946.

Gersony WM, Peckham GJ, et al: Effects of indomethacin in premature infants with patent ductus arteriosus: Results of a national collaborative study. *J Pediatr* 102:895, 1983.

Gold JP, Cohn LH: Operative management of the calcified patent ductus arteriosus. *Ann Thorac Surg* 41:567, 1986.

Gross RE, Hubbard JP: Surgical ligation of a patent ductus arteriosus: Report of first successful case. *JAMA* 112:729, 1939.

Jones JC: Twenty-five years experience with the surgery of patent ductus arteriosus. *J Thorac Cardiovasc Surg* 50:149, 1965.

Kitterman J: Patent ductus arteriosus: Current clinical status. *Arch Dis Child* 55:106, 1980.

Kron IL, Harman PK, et al: The adult ductus surgical results and longterm follow-up. *Am Surg* 49:546, 1983.

Mikhail M, Lee W, et al: Surgical and medical experience with 734 premature infants with patent ductus arteriosus. *J Thorac Cardiovasc Surg* 83:349, 1982.

Tetralogy of Fallot

Ebert PA: Second operation for pulmonary stenosis or insufficiency after repair of tetralogy of Fallot. *Am J Cardiol* 50:637, 1982.

Hammon JW, Henry CL, et al: Tetralogy of Fallot: Selected surgical management can minimize operative mortality. *Ann Thorac Surg* 40:280, 1985.

Kirklin JW, Blackstone E, et al: Risk factors for early and late failure after repair of tetralogy of Fallot and their neutralization. *J Thorac Cardiovasc Surg* 32:208, 1984.

Lillehei CW, Varco RL, et al: The first open heart repairs of ventricular septal defect, atrioventricular communis, and tetralogy of Fallot using extracorporeal circulation by cross-circulation: A 30 year follow-up. *Ann Thorac Surg* 41:421, 1986.

Roh MS, Hardesty R, et al: Blalock shunt: Procedure of choice in infants. *J Cardiovasc Surg* 25:1, 1984.

Transposition of the Great Vessels

Ashraf MM, Cotroneo J, et al: Fate of long-term survivors of Mustard procedure (inflow repair) for simple and complex transposition of the great arteries. *Ann Thorac Surg* 42:385, 1986.

Baffes TG, Riker WL, et al: Surgical correction of transposition of the aorta and the pulmonary artery. *J Thorac Cardiovasc Surg* 34:469, 1957.

Bender H, Graham T, et al: Comparative operative results of the Senning and Mustard procedures for transposition of the great arteries. *Circulation* 62(suppl 1):197, 1980.

Castaneda AR, Norwood WI, et al: Transposition of the great arteries and intact ventricular septum: Anatomical repair in the neonate. *Ann Thorac Surg* 38:438, 1984.

Hanlon CR, Blalock A: Complete transposition of aorta and pulmonary artery: Experimental observations on venous shunts as corrective procedures. *Ann Surg* 127:385, 1948.

Jatene AD, Fontes VF, et al: Successful anatomic correction of transposition of the great vessels: A preliminary report. *Arq Bras Cardiol* 28:461, 1975.

Jatene AD, Fontes VF, et al: Anatomic correction of transposition of the great arteries. *J Thorac Cardiovasc Surg* 83:20, 1982.

Mustard WT, Keith JD, et al: The surgical management of transposition of the great vessels. *J Thorac Cardiovasc Surg* 48:953, 1964.

Piccoli G, Wilkinson J, et al: Appraisal of the Mustard procedure for the physiological correction of ''simple'' transposition of the great arteries. *J Thorac Cardiovasc Surg* 82:436, 1981.

Quaegebeur JM, Rohmer J, et al: The arterial switch operation. An eight-year experience. *J Thorac Cardiovasc Surg* 92:361, 1986.

Senning A: Surgical correction of transposition of the great vessels. *Surgery* 59:334, 1966.

Stewart S, Alexson C, Manning J: Late results of the Mustard procedure in transposition of the great arteries. *Ann Thorac Surg* 42:419, 1986.

Trusler G, Williams W, et al: Current results with the Mustard operation in isolated transposition of the great arteries. *J Thorac Cardiovasc Surg* 80:381, 1980.

Turley K, Wilson J, Ebert P: Atrial repairs of infant complex congenital heart lesions. *Arch Surg* 115:1335, 1980.

Tricuspid Atresia

Bjork V, Olin C, et al: Right atrial-right ventricular anastomosis for correction of tricuspid atresia. *J Thorac Cardiovasc Surg* 77:452, 1979.

Fontan F, Baudet E: Surgical repair of tricuspid atresia. *Thorax* 26:240, 1971.

Fontan F, Deville C, et al: Repair of tricuspid atresia in 100 patients. *J Thorac Cardiovasc Surg* 85:647, 1983.

Girod DA, Fontan F, et al: Longterm results after the Fontan operation for tricuspid atresia. *Circulation* 75:605, 1987.

Glenn WW: Circulatory bypass with the right side of the heart shunt between superior vena cava and distal right pulmonary artery—Report of clinical application. *N Engl J Med* 259:117, 1958.

Kirklin JK, Blackstone EH, et al: The Fontan operation. *J Thorac Cardiovasc Surg* 92:1049, 1986.

Lee CN, Schaff HB, et al: Comparison of atrial pulmonary vs atrioventricular connections for modified Fontan–Kreutzer repair of tricuspid valve atresia. *J Thorac Cardiovasc Surg* 92:1038, 1986.

Trusler G, Williams G: Long-term results of shunt procedures for tricuspid atresia. *Ann Thorac Surg* 29:312, 1980.

Weinberg P: Anatomy of tricuspid atresia and its relevance to current forms of surgical therapy. *Ann Thorac Surg* 29:306, 1980.

Cor Triatriatum

Arciniegas E, Farooki A, et al: Surgical treatment of cor triatriatum. *Ann Thorac Surg* 32:571, 1981.

Marin-Garcia J, Tandon R, et al: Cor triatriatum: Study of 20 cases. *Am J Cardiol* 35:59, 1975.

Niwayama G: Cor triatriatum. *Am Heart J* 59:291, 1960.

Oglietti J, Cooley DA, et al: Cor triatriatum: Operative results in 25 patients. *Ann Thorac Surg* 35:415, 1983.

Ostman-Smith I, Silverman NH, et al: Cor triatriatum sinistrum: Diagnostic features on cross sectional echocardiography. *Br Heart J* 51:211, 1984.

Van Praagh R, Corsini I: Cor triatriatum: Pathologic anatomy and a consideration of morphogenesis based on 13 postmortem cases and a study of normal development of the pulmonary vein and atrial septum in 83 human embryos. *Am Heart J* 78:379, 1969.

Congenital Mitral Valve Disease

Grenadier E, Sahn DJ, et al: Two-dimensional echo Doppler study of congenital disorders of the mitral valve. *Am Heart J* 107:319, 1984.

Ruckman R, Van Praagh R: Anatomic types of congenital mitral stenosis: Report of 49 autopsy cases with consideration of diagnosis and surgical implications. *Am J Cardiol* 42:592, 1978.

Tsuji HK, Shapiro M, et al: Congenital mitral stenosis: Report of two cases and review of the literature. *J Thorac Cardiovasc Surg* 53:850, 1967.

Vitarelli A, Landolina G, et al: Echocardiographic assessment of congenital mitral stenosis. *Am Heart J* 107:319, 1984.

Aortic-Pulmonary Window

Doty D, Richardson J, et al: Aortopulmonary septal defect: Hemodynamics, angiography, and operation. *Ann Thorac Surg* 32:244, 1981.

Gross RE: Surgical closure of an aortic septal defect. *Circulation* 5:858, 1952.

Jolles PR, Shin MS, Jones WP: Aortopulmonary window lesions: Detection with chest radiography. *Radiology* 159:647, 1986.

Morrow AG, Greenfield LJ, Braunwald E: Congenital aortopulmonary septal defect: Clinical and hemodynamic findings, surgical technique, and results of operative correction. *Circulation* 25:463, 1962.

Scott HW, Sabiston DC: Surgical treatment for congenital aortico-pulmonary fistula. *J Thorac Cardiovasc Surg* 25:26, 1953.

Ruptured Aneurysm of Sinus of Valsalva

Heilman KJ III, Groves BM, et al: Rupture of the left sinus of valsalva aneurysm into the pulmonary artery. *J Am Coll Cardiol* 5:1005, 1985.

Lillehei CW, Stanley P, Varco RL: Surgical treatment of ruptured aneurysms of the sinus of valsalva. *Ann Surg* 146:459, 1957.

Sawyer JL, Adams JE, Scott HW: Surgical treatment for aneurysms of aortic sinuses with aorticoatrial fistula. *Surgery* 41:126, 1957.

Spencer FC, Blake HA, Bahnson HT: Surgical repair of ruptured aneurysm of sinus of valsalva in two patients. *Ann Surg* 162:963, 1960.

Truncus Arteriosus

Ceballos R, Soto B, et al: Truncus arteriosus. An anatomical-angiographic study. *Br Heart J* 49:589, 1983.

DiDonato RM, Fyfe DA, et al: Fifteen-year experience with surgical repair of truncus arteriosus. *J Thorac Cardiovasc Surg* 89:414, 1985.

Ebert PA, Turley K, et al: Surgical treatment of truncus arteriosus in the first 6 months of life. *Ann Surg* 200:451, 1984.

McGoon DC, Wallace RB, Danielson GK: The Rastelli operation: Its indications and results. *J Thorac Cardiovasc Surg* 65:65, 1973.

Rothko K, Moore G, Hutchins G: Truncus arteriosus malformation: A spectrum including fourth and sixth aortic arch interruptions. *Am Heart J* 99:17, 1980.

Sharma AK, Brawn WJ, Mee RB: Truncus arteriosus. Surgical approach. *J Thorac Cardiovasc Surg* 90:45, 1985.

Single Ventricle

Anderson RH, Becker AE, et al: Morphogenesis of univentricular hearts. *Br Heart J* 38:558, 1976.

Anderson RH, Macartney FJ, et al: Univentricular atrioventricular connection: The single ventricle trap unsprung. *Pediatr Cardiol* 4:273, 1983.

Ebert PA: Staged partitioning of single ventricle. *J Thorac Cardiovasc Surg* 88:908, 1984.

Edie RN, Malm JR: Surgical repair of single ventricle. *J Thorac Cardiovasc Surg* 66:350, 1973.

Freedom RM, Benson LN, et al: Subaortic stenosis, the univentricular heart, and banding of the pulmonary artery: An analysis of the courses of 43 patients with univentricular heart palliated by pulmonary artery banding. *Circulation* 73:758, 1986.

McGoon DC, Danielson GK, et al: Correction of the univentricular heart having two atrioventricular valves. *J Thorac Cardiovasc Surg* 74:218, 1977.

Stefanelli G, Kirklin JW, et al: Early and intermediate-term (10 year) results of surgery for univentricular atrioventricular connection ("single ventricle"). *Am J Cardiol* 54:811, 1984.

Van Praagh R, Ongley PA, Swan HJC: Anatomic types of single or common ventricle in man. Morphologic and geometric aspects of 60 necropsied cases. *Am J Cardiol* 13:367, 1964.

Van Praagh R, Van Praagh S, et al: Diagnosis of the anatomic types of single or common ventricle. *Am J Cardiol* 15:345, 1965.

Ebstein's Anomaly

Bahnson HT, Bauersfeld SR, Smith JW: Pathological anatomy and surgical correction of Ebstein's anomaly. *Circulation* 31(suppl 1):3, 1965.

Barbero-Marcial M, Verginelli G, et al: Surgical treatment of Ebstein's anomaly. Early and late results in twenty patients subjected to valve replacement. *J Thorac Cardiovasc Surg* 78:416, 1979.

Hardy, KL, May IA, et al: Ebstein's anomaly: A functional concept and successful definitive repair. *J Thorac Cardiovasc Surg* 48:927, 1964.

Mair DD, Seward JB, et al: Surgical repair of Ebstein's anomaly: Selection of patients and early and late operative results. *Circulation* 72:1170, 1985.

Radford DJ, Graff RF, Neilson GH: Diagnosis and natural history of Ebstein's anomaly. *Br Heart J* 54:517, 1985.

Anomalous Origin of the Left Coronary Artery

Bland EF, White PD, Garland J: Congenital anomalies of the coronary arteries: Report of an unusual case associated with cardiac hypertrophy. *Am Heart J* 787, 1933.

Donaldson RM, Raphael MJ, et al: Hemodynamically significant anomalies of the coronary arteries. Surgical aspects. *Thorac Cardiovasc Surg* 30:7, 1982.

Sabiston DC, Neill CA, Taussig HB: The direction of blood flow in anomalous left coronary artery arising from the pulmonary artery. *Circulation* 22:591, 1960.

Takauchi S, Imamura H, et al: New surgical methods for repair of anomalous left coronary artery from the pulmonary artery. *J Thorac Cardiovasc Surg* 78:7, 1979.

Vesterlund T, Thomsen PE, Hansen OK: Anomalous origin of the left coronary artery from the pulmonary artery in an adult. *Br Heart J* 54:110, 1985.

Coronary Arteriovenous Fistula

Gasul BM, Arcilla RA, et al: Congenital coronary arteriovenous fistula: Clinical, phonocardiographic, angiocardiographic, and hemodynamic studies in five patients. *Pediatrics* 25:531, 1960.

Lowe E, Oldham H, Sabiston D: Surgical management of congenital coronary artery fistulas. *Ann Surg* 194:373, 1981.

Lowe J, Oldham HN Jr, Sabiston DC Jr: Surgical management of congenital coronary artery fistulas. *Ann Surg* 194:373, 1981.

Urrutia SCO, Falaschi G, et al: Surgical management of 56 patients with congenital coronary artery fistulas. *Ann Thorac Surg* 35:300, 1983.

Corrected Transposition

Guit GL, Kroon HM, et al: Congenitally corrected transposition in the adult: Detection by radionuclide angiocardiography. *Radiology* 157:521, 1985.

de Leval M, Bastos P, et al: Surgical technique to reduce the risks of heart block following closure of ventricular septal defect in atrioventricular discordance. *J Thorac Cardiovasc Surg* 78:515, 1979.

Marcelletti C, Maloney J, et al: Corrected transposition and ventricular septal defect. Surgical experience. *Ann Surg* 191:751, 1980.

Metcalfe J, Somerville J: Surgical repair of lesions associated with corrected transposition. Late results. *Br Heart J* 50:476, 1983.

Schiebler GL, Edwards JE, et al: Congenital corrected transposition of the great vessels: A study of 33 cases. *Pediatrics* 27:851, 1961.

Vargas FJ, Kreutzer GO, et al: Repair of corrected transposition associated with ventricular septal defect and pulmonary stenosis. *Ann Thorac Surg* 40:509, 1985.

Waldo AL, Pacifico AD, et al: Electrophysiological delineation of the specialized A-V conduction system in patients with corrected transposition of the great vessels and ventricular septal defect. *Circulation* 52:435, 1975.

Double Outlet Right Ventricle

Anderson RH, Becker AE, et al: Surgical anatomy of double-outlet right ventricle—A reappraisal. *Am J Cardiol* 52:555, 1983.

Judson JP, Danielson GK, et al: Double-outlet right ventricle. *J Thorac Cardiovasc Surg* 85:32, 1983.

Kirklin JW, Pacifico AD, et al: Current risks and protocols for operations for double-outlet right ventricle. Derivation from an 18 year experience. *J Thorac Cardiovasc Surg* 92:913, 1986.

Luber JM, Castaneda AR, et al: Repair of double-outlet right ventricle: Early and late results. *Circulation* 68(2):II 144, 1983.

Pulmonary Artery Sling

Campbell DN, Lilly JR, et al: The surgery of pulmonary artery "sling." *J Pediatr Surg* 18:855, 1983.

Grover FL, Norton JB, et al: Pulmonary sling: Case report and collective review. *J Thorac Cardiovasc Surg* 69:295, 1975.

Gumbiner C, Mullins C, McNamara D: Pulmonary artery sling. *Am J Cardiol* 45:311, 1980.

King HA, Walker D: Pulmonary artery sling. *Thorax* 39:462, 1984.

Marmon LM, Bye MR, et al: Vascular rings and slings: Long-term follow-up of pulmonary function. *J Pediatr Surg* 19:683, 1984.

Chapter 19

Acquired Heart Disease

Frank C. Spencer

CLINICAL MANIFESTATIONS AND DIAGNOSTIC STUDIES

The standard methods for evaluating a patient with heart disease include the history and physical examination; the chest x-ray and electrocardiogram; and special diagnostic studies, especially echocardiography, cardiac catheterization and cineangiography, and special radionuclide studies. Fundamental general considerations are discussed in the following sections. More information is described in the specific section concerning different diseases in this chapter.

HISTORY. The frequent symptoms with cardiac disease include (1) symptoms of left heart failure: dyspnea, other symptoms of pulmonary congestion; (2) symptoms of right heart failure: edema from sodium retention, hepatomegaly and ascites; (3) angina; (4) arrhythmias; (5) syncope; and (6) fatigue. With the exception of angina, symptoms are usually a *late* sign of advanced cardiac disease. The initial change in most cardiac diseases is a rise in intracardiac pressure in the involved cardiac chamber, subsequently followed by cardiac enlargement, usually a combination of dilatation and hypertrophy. This is a manifestation of Starling's law of the heart; an increase in workload can be achieved by an increase in diastolic fiber length. These physiologic and anatomic changes are the early changes from heart disease. Symptoms develop subsequently as different compensatory mechanisms fail. This concept is an important one because abundant data indicate that operation should be considered for many diseases on the basis of physiologic abnormalities, such as reduction of cross-sectional area of an aortic or mitral valve below 1.0 cm^2, rather than the presence of symptoms. Delaying operation until symptoms are severe often results in irreversible ventricular injury, which in turn is a major cause of death in the first few years following operation.

Symptoms of Left Heart Failure. *Dyspnea.* The normal left ventricular end-diastolic pressure is less than 12 mmHg. Pressures in the range of 12 to 20 mmHg represent moderate disease, while pressures of 20 to 30 mmHg represent severe disease. The oncotic pressure of plasma is 30 to 35 mmHg. Hence, as left atrial pressure rises, pulmonary congestion develops as left atrial pressure approaches the colloidal osmotic pressure of plasma. The tolerance for pulmonary congestion depends upon several factors, including the capacity of the pulmonary lymphatics to resorb fluid. *Dyspnea* is one of the cardinal symptoms of left heart failure. It can be graded with the degree of exertion required to initiate dyspnea, as opposed to dyspnea at rest, which represents a severe form of heart disease. With mitral stenosis, dyspnea appears as an early sign because of restriction of flow from the left atrium into the left ventricle. With other forms of heart disease, however, dyspnea is a *late* sign as it develops only after the left ventricle has failed, with the end-diastolic pressure rising above 12 mm. Dyspnea with mitral insufficiency, aortic valvular disease, or coronary disease represents an advanced form of disease, in contrast to mitral stenosis.

A number of other respiratory symptoms represent different degrees of pulmonary congestion. These include orthopnea, paroxysmal nocturnal dyspnea, cough, hemoptysis, and pulmonary edema.

Symptoms of Right Heart Failure. Right atrial pressure is normally less than 5 mmHg. When right ventricular failure results in elevation of right atrial pressure above 5 mmHg, the earliest change is a retention of sodium, a complex homeostatic mechanism initiated by the liver, kidneys, and other organs, which increases blood volume and elevates venous pressure. Retention of more than 7 to 10 lb of fluid results in visible edema of the lower extremities. Hepatomegaly also develops. With chronic severe right heart failure fluid retention is severe, with marked deformities from accumulation of 20, 30, or more pounds of edema fluid, with ascites and massive hepatomegaly.

Angina. Angina is the hallmark of coronary artery disease, a symptom of myocardial anoxia with subsequent anaerobic metabolism. Classic angina is described as a precordial discomfort appearing with exercise, emotion, or eating, relieved by rest or nitroglycerin. This is discussed in more detail in the section on Coronary Artery Disease. It is present in the classic form in 70 to 75 percent of patients with coronary disease. When this history is elicited, the diagnosis of coronary disease can be made with a high degree of certainty. In perhaps 20 to 25 percent of patients, one of the numerous variations of angina occurs, so-called angina equivalents, with symptoms in the shoulders, arms, jaw, epigastrium, or other areas. Also, in a significant number of patients, the exact frequency of which is unknown, angina apparently does not develop, though "silent" ischemia is present.

Angina also is a typical symptom with aortic stenosis, resulting from the combination of decreased cardiac output and left ventricular hypertrophy. It is less common with other forms of heart disease.

With the exception of angina, other forms of pain from heart disease are uncommon; chest pain is usually due to musculoskeletal disorders in the chest wall, pericarditis, or pleural or esophageal disease.

Arrhythmias. Atrial fibrillation is usually one of the first cardiac abnormalities with mitral stenosis, resulting from left atrial hypertrophy evolving from the sustained elevation in left atrial pressure. With other forms of heart disease, arrhythmias are uncommon, occurring sporadically without any predictable consistency. They are more frequent with older patients, probably from intrinsic disease in the atrioventricular conducting mechanism, and in severe cardiac failure, probably a manifestation of generalized cardiac hypoxia.

Syncope. This is an important symptom with aortic stenosis, apparently from a transient decrease in cerebral blood flow. It is of particular importance because it indicates a severity of aortic stenosis that may unpredictably terminate with sudden death. It must be differentiated from syncope from other causes such as bradycardia or heart block.

Fatigue. This is a nonspecific symptom that may arise from many causes. In some patients it probably reflects a generalized decrease in cardiac output. Otherwise, its significance is vague.

PHYSICAL EXAMINATION. Only a few basic physical abnormalities are discussed in this short section, as abnormal physical findings are best discussed with the specific disease causing them. In some cardiac diseases, physical abnormalities are virtually diagnostic of both the disease and the severity of the problem, while in others, such as coronary disease or aortic stenosis, the paucity or absence of *any* physical abnormality can be seriously misleading.

Cardiac Cachexia. The muscular wasting that occurs from chronic congestive failure, reflected in a weight loss of 10 to 40 lb, is due to the long-standing changes of severe congestive failure in combination with a low cardiac output. In some patients, simply inability to eat may be an important cause, resulting in malnutrition from lack of calories and protein. Such patients are especially susceptible to infection following operation because of a generalized decrease in immunity.

Cardiac Size. When a valvular abnormality produces a significant change in intracardiac pressures, the initial physiologic adaptation is enlargement of the involved cardiac chamber, usually from a combination of dilatation and hypertrophy. A fundamental question in evaluation is, "Is there cardiac enlargement?" Accordingly, the finding of a forceful apical impulse in the anterior midaxillary line indicates advanced cardiac disease that usually requires prompt surgical treatment. Less obvious signs of cardiac enlargement may be seen on the chest x-ray, the electrocardiogram, or, most precisely, with the echocardiogram, which can define the exact size of the cardiac chamber and the thickness of the cardiac wall.

Cardiac Murmurs. Diastolic murmurs often establish the diagnosis. The apical diastolic rumble of mitral stenosis is virtually pathognomonic; the parasternal diastolic murmur of aortic insufficiency is also almost equally so.

Systolic murmurs are strongly supportive of the diagnosis of the underlying condition but not to the degree found with diastolic murmurs. These include the basal systolic murmur of aortic stenosis or pulmonic stenosis and the apical systolic murmur of mitral insufficiency.

DIAGNOSTIC STUDIES. Electrocardiography and Radiology. The electrocardiogram and the chest x-ray are the two standard diagnostic studies. The chest x-ray is one of the best guides for answering the basic question, "Is there cardiac enlargement?" Before the development of echocardiography, special oblique views and fluoroscopy provided supplemental information, but echocardiography is far more precise.

Analysis of the pulmonary circulation may show several abnormalities. Pulmonary venous congestion develops when left atrial pressure is chronically elevated above the upper normal limit of 12 mmHg, seen typically with severe mitral stenosis. The signs of pulmonary congestion include engorged pulmonary veins and congestion of pulmonary alveoli. Fluid accumulating in the interlobar planes forms transverse linear opacities perpendicular to the surface of the pleura, termed Kerley "lines." Their presence usually indicates a left atrial pressure exceeding 20 mmHg.

Marked enlargement of the pulmonary arteries may occur from an increase in pulmonary blood flow or an increase in pulmonary vascular resistance with pulmonary hypertension. Normally, the central pulmonary arteries are three to four times larger than the peripheral arteries. With an increase in pulmonary blood flow, as with an atrial septal defect, both central and peripheral arteries are symmetrically enlarged. With pulmonary hypertension, the central pulmonary arteries may become strikingly enlarged while the peripheral arteries are not.

Echocardiography, Cardiac Catheterization, and Cineangiography. Outstanding advances have been made with echocardiography over the past decade. The precise analysis of cardiac chambers, often combined with flow studies and gradient determinations with 2-D Doppler studies, have virtually made cardiac catheterization unnecessary in some conditions. Echocardiography is the most precise method for determining specific chamber enlargement, such as size of the left atrium or left ventricle. This is particularly important in serial evaluation of a patient over months or years, noting an asymptomatic progressive enlargement that could not be detected otherwise. Cardiac catheterization precisely establishes the presence and size of intracardiac shunts or stenoses, as well as the presence of serious physiologic changes of cardiac failure, such as an elevation in end-diastolic pressure or pulmonary hypertension. A sustained rise in left ventricular end-diastolic pressure above the normal upper limit of 12 mmHg is usually the hallmark of serious cardiac disease.

Cineangiography is the fundamental method for evaluation of coronary disease, also for aortic or mitral insufficiency. All three studies are usually performed in the evaluation of a patient with a serious cardiac problem.

PATHOPHYSIOLOGY: GENERAL PRINCIPLES

With valvular heart disease, "When should an operation be performed?" This basic question must be periodically evaluated during the medical therapy of any patient with cardiac valvular disease, because the disease process is usually a progressive one. As a result of several developments, surgical therapy is now being used at a much earlier stage of the disease than in previous years.

At present a decision for operation is best made from physiologic abnormalities found with diagnostic studies, such as cardiac catheterization, angiography, or radionuclide studies, rather than from the severity and disability from symptoms.

Several developments have combined to indicate that operation should be performed earlier. The safety of operative procedures has increased, with the risk of valve replacement now being in the range of 1 to 4 percent in good-risk patients. This is principally due to improvements in myocardial preservation with the widespread adoption of hyperkalemic cold cardiac arrest. The virtually indefinite durability of metallic prosthetic valves is now well established, though anticoagulation with coumadin is required.

Longevity following cardiac valve replacement is strongly influenced by the myocardial function at the time of operation. Patients with early disability (New York Heart Class II or early III) have a 5-year survival near 90 percent, but only 60 to 70 percent of patients with Class IV disability live 5 years. This striking difference is due to irreversible changes in myocardial function that existed before operation, indicating that operation should not be postponed until symptoms are disabling.

Aortic valve replacement should be seriously considered in asymptomatic patients if the orifice cross-sectional area has decreased to near 1.0 cm². An even more liberal indication should be used with mitral stenosis, considering therapy with an orifice cross-sectional area less than 1.5 cm² because a commissurotomy, rather than valve replacement, can usually be performed. The grave hazard always exists of cerebral embolism from thrombi developing in the left atrium, especially when atrial fibrillation has developed. The recent development of balloon valvuloplasty will undoubtedly further change the indications for early treatment.

With aortic and mitral insufficiency, selecting the proper time for operation is more difficult, as this depends upon the left ventricular function. The demonstration of a fall in left ventricular ejection fraction during exercise is probably the best currently available sign that operation should be done. Postponing operation until serious enlargement of the left ventricle develops or a permanent elevation in left ventricular end-diastolic pressure occurs is clearly a mistake because 5-year prognosis following successful operation is greatly decreased.

A patient with cardiac valvular disease is rarely inoperable. If the basic disease process is cardiac valvular disease, an operation, usually prosthetic valve replacement, can almost always be performed with current techniques of myocardial preservation with an operative risk no greater than 5 to 10 percent. Patients are still seen with far advanced Class IV failure and cardiac cachexia who simply have postponed operation for years with the concept that operation was "too dangerous." Some benefit will always result, because if a patient is alive with a malfunctioning valve, that patient will function better with a properly functioning prosthetic valve. The magnitude of benefit often cannot be predicted for some months, depending upon the unmeasurable irreversible loss of ventricular function. Realizing that the degree of improvement in left ventricular function cannot be predicted is an important consideration because the objectionable term "cardiac myopathy" implies that an irreversible disease is present. Except for the unusual type of intrinsic myocardial disease termed "myopathy," such a diagnosis implies a certainty that cannot be supported with objective data.

Pulmonary hypertension, seen especially with severe mitral stenosis, less commonly with chronic congestive failure from mitral or aortic insufficiency, almost always improves to a substantial degree following operation. With current techniques, the risk of an operation, even with a pulmonary artery systolic pressure above 100 mmHg is no more than 5 to 10 percent. This low mortality is a result of improvements in myocardial preservation, taking particular care to preserve the hypertrophied right ventricle. Unless massive pulmonary emboli have occurred, intractable right heart failure from pulmonary hypertension, the so-called cor pulmonale, is rare.

Survival following *prosthetic valve replacement* is primarily influenced by the left ventricular function beforehand. Either porcine or metallic prostheses have the permanent risk of endocarditis, a frequency near 1 percent per patient year. Porcine prostheses have a very low frequency of thromboembolism if arrhythmias or cardiac enlargement are not present, making anticoagulation unnecessary in a majority of patients, especially those with aortic prostheses. Their principal limitation is durability, currently excellent at 5 years but in the range of 80 to 85 percent near 10 years. As the rate of failure rises sharply per year after 7 or 8 years, the 15-year durability with porcine valves does not appear encouraging.

With metallic prostheses, the basic problems are thromboembolism and hemorrhage from anticoagulation therapy with coumadin. With proper anticoagulation, keeping the prothrombin time more than $1\frac{1}{2}$ times normal (above 20 s), thromboembolism is fortunately rare, a range near 1 to 2 percent per patient year. The role of antiplatelet therapy for prevention of thromboembolism is not clearly defined.

Anticoagulant hemorrhage remains a permanent hazard, occurring with a frequency of 1 to 4 percent in different series. The frequency of this problem is primarily related to patient compliance and supervision by the physician. With careful supervision based upon periodic prothrombin time measurements, significant hemorrhage from coumadin is uncommon. Conversely, anticoagulant hemorrhage can be a serious or lethal problem in a noncompliant patient with inadequate periodic evaluation. Hence, the basic decision in selecting a porcine versus a metallic prosthesis depends upon the patient's understanding and ability to take anticoagulant therapy safely and indefinitely.

EXTRACORPOREAL CIRCULATION

HISTORICAL DATA. The pioneering imagination and efforts of Gibbon were largely responsible for the development of extracorporeal circulation. In 1932, Gibbon initiated laboratory investigations that continued for over 20 years until the first successful open heart operation in human beings was performed by him in 1953. Subsequent developments were rapid, with brief use of cross circulation by Lillehei and associates in 1954, followed a short time later by the development of the bubble oxygenator by DeWall. The disc oxygenator was developed in Sweden by Bjork and Crafoord and introduced to the United States by Kay and Cross. For the past decade, diagnosable membrane and bubble oxygenation have been used almost routinely.

PUMPS. The majority of heart-lung machines utilize a simple roller pump, originally developed by DeBakey. The resulting flow is almost nonpulsatile, with a pulse pressure of about 15 mmHg. A variety of other pumps have been employed, with no clear demonstration of any advantages over the simple roller pump. A recurrent physiologic question has been the importance of a pulsatile flow in the normal circulation. Available experimental data indicate that over long periods of time a pulsatile flow may be of importance, but for periods up to 4 to 5 h, a nonpulsatile flow seems adequate. The gradual increase in vasomotor tone that occurs during extracorporeal circulation may be partly due to a physiologic response to nonpulsatile perfusion.

OXYGENATORS. Since 1970 the disposable membrane and bubble oxygenators have been the most widely used type (Fig. 19-1). Pump oxygenators in current usage usually require a priming volume in the range of 1500 to 2500 mL. Strenuous efforts are usually made to avoid the use of blood because of the risk of transmission of hepatitis or other infectious diseases; so the pump oxygenator system is usually filled with a crystalloid solution. At NYU a modified Ringer's lactate solution (Plasmalyte) is used that closely approximates the electrolyte composition of blood. A varying amount of serum albumin is added, keeping the oncotic pressure near 10 to 12 mmHg. The importance of albumin is uncertain, for some institutions seldom use albumin, accepting a much lower oncotic pressure during perfusion, as there are not clear data to indicate what degree of decrease in oncotic pressure is hazardous. If the hematocrit decreases below 20 to 25 percent, blood is added to the pump oxygenator.

TECHNIQUE OF PERFUSION. Sufficient heparin is given to elevate activated clotting time (ACT) well above 400 s, starting with a heparin dose of 4 mg/kg. Venous blood is aspirated by gravity drainage through large cannulae through the right atrium into the venae cavae. Oxygenated blood is returned to the arterial circulation, usually through a cannula in the ascending aorta. Perfusion is done at a flow rate of about 2.500 mL/m^2/min, providing a flow rate near 4 L/min for normal-sized adults. Oxygen flow rates through the oxygenator are adjusted to produce an arterial oxygen tension above 100 mmHg. Temperature is controlled with a heat exchanger in the circuit; it is usually lowered to 25 to 32°C. Intracardiac blood is aspirated with a suction apparatus, filtered, and returned to the oxygenator.

During perfusion a number of modalities are monitored. Arterial pressure and central venous pressure are monitored through intravascular catheters. At NYU a

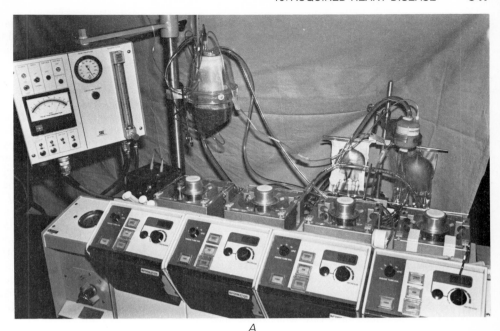

A

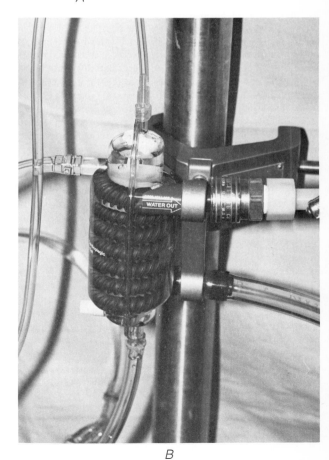

B

Fig. 19-1. *A.* Travenol membrane oxygenator showing the roller pumps used with the heart-lung machine. The membrane oxygenator is in the left upper portion of the photograph. The coronary suction device is in the center of the field. *B.* Buckberg-Shiley cardioplegia apparatus with heat exchanger. *(Photo courtesy of Joshua Heydemann.)*

Swan-Ganz catheter is almost always inserted in adults to monitor pulmonary artery pressures and cardiac output.

The blood pressure varies widely among different patients during perfusion. It usually decreases sharply with the onset of perfusion, apparently from vasodilatation, and then subsequently rises to above 60 mmHg. The importance of the actual level of mean arterial pressure, as long as flow rate is greater than 2 L/m^2/min, is uncertain. As cerebral autoregulation of blood flow becomes ineffective below a mean pressure of 50 to 60 mmHg, perfusion pressure is usually maintained above 50 mmHg, though with moderate hypothermia (25 to 30°C) an arterial pressure of 40 to 50 mmHg seemingly has no harmful physiologic effects. After 15 to 30 min of perfusion, perfusion pressure may gradually rise from progressive vasoconstriction.

Oxygen and carbon dioxide tensions are periodically measured in the venous blood returned to the oxygenator and the oxygenated blood returned to the patient. Preferably the arterial oxygen tension should be above 100 mmHg and the carbon dioxide tension 30 to 35 mmHg. Venous blood returning to the heart-lung machine with the described flow rate will usually have an oxygen saturation greater than 50 percent. With flow rates and oxygen saturations in this range, metabolic acidosis of significant degree does not occur.

Heparin is gradually metabolized by the body, and so additional heparin is given each hour of perfusion as necessary to keep the ACT above 400 s, usually 1 mg/kg of body weight. During perfusion the lungs are kept stationary in a partially inflated position.

Termination of Perfusion. As perfusion is slowed and stopped, blood is infused from the pump oxygenator to restore normal intracardiac pressures with maintenance of an adequate blood pressure and cardiac output. Left atrial pressure is routinely monitored through an indwelling catheter inserted as bypass is being stopped. Monitoring of left atrial pressure is usually the best guide to monitor infusion of fluids, noting what level of left atrial pressure is needed to maintain an adequate cardiac output.

At NYU an indwelling Swan-Ganz catheter in the pulmonary artery is routinely used to monitor pulmonary artery pressure and cardiac output for 24 to 48 h after operation. In many patients the pulmonary artery diastolic pressure, or wedge pressure, provides a reasonable guide to left atrial pressure.

Heparin is neutralized with protamine, giving sufficient protamine to return the activated clotting time as closely as possible to that existing before bypass. Usually this requires 3 to 4 mg of protamine, given in divided doses. If a coagulopathy is present, the activated clotting time may not return to prebypass levels, indicating the need for infusion of coagulation products, such as fresh frozen plasma, cryoprecipitate, or platelets.

Myocardial Preservation. The development of hyperkalemic hypothermic cardiac arrest for myocardial preservation was a major advance in cardiac surgery. This gradually evolved from laboratories throughout the world after 1975–1976. An unusually large number of substan-

tial contributions came from Buckberg and Maloney at UCLA and from Hirsch and Braimbridge in London. The improved myocardial protection, combined with the increased facility for performing complex cardiac procedures in a dry, quiet field, greatly augmented the safety and effectiveness of virtually all cardiac operations. The results from cardiac operations are now quite different from those obtained in the two decades between 1955 and 1975, when intermittent aortic occlusion was the most widely used technique. Many of the complications of that era were undoubtedly due to myocardial injury and infarction. The status of myocardial preservation in 1980 is well summarized in the Proceedings of the International Symposium on Myocardial Protection held in London that year.

Both crystalloid and blood cardioplegia are widely used, with the exact components of the cardioplegic mixture varying among different institutions. With periods of cardiac arrest for 60 to 90 min, there seems little measurable difference in the two techniques, but with the cold blood technique, regularly used at NYU, the heart can be safely arrested for a surprisingly long period of time, even more than 4 h.

The cardioplegia cold blood solution is that developed by Buckberg et al. with a blood temperature of 7 to 8°C, a potassium concentration near 30 meq/L, and a low calcium concentration.

After the aorta is clamped, blood is infused at a rate sufficient to produce an aortic root pressure initially of 80 to 100 mmHg (200 to 400 mL/min), infusing enough blood to lower myocardial temperature below 15°C, measured in different zones of the myocardium with a needle thermistor. With normal coronary arteries, this can be achieved with 1000 to 1500 mL of cold blood. When diffuse coronary disease produces maldistribution of blood flow, larger amounts may be required, as much as 2000 to 2500 mL. Subsequently, while the aorta is clamped, varying amounts of cold blood are reinfused every 20 to 30 min, usually in the range of 300 to 500 mL. Continuous topical hypothermia, constantly irrigating the pericardium with a 4°C electrolyte solution, is an important part of the procedure to keep the heart from being rewarmed as the temperature of the perfusate in the pump oxygenator is usually 25 to 30°C. With the combination of periodic infusion of cold blood and hypothermia, the myocardial temperature can easily be kept below 15°C.

TRAUMA FROM PERFUSION. Extracorporeal circulation inevitably produces some trauma to the blood, primarily from exposure of blood to gas in the oxygenator and from the use of suction to aspirate intracardiac blood. Minimizing the injury to blood during oxygenation, of course, is the basis for a membrane oxygenator rather than a bubble oxygenator. Trauma to blood from the blood pump itself is surprisingly small. At present, tolerance for long periods of perfusion, even 8 or 10 h, is surprisingly good. The minimal trauma from pump oxygenators is further demonstrated by the selective use of extracorporeal membrane oxygenators (ECMO) for infants with respiratory failure for periods of several days with surprisingly good results.

Studies of capillary microcirculation during perfusion often find a progressive sludging of blood elements, resulting in stasis and maldistribution of capillary blood flow. The clinical significance of these observations is uncertain. Microaggregates can be demonstrated in blood coming from the pump oxygenator, partly removed with filters in the pump circuit. At NYU a filter of 20 to 40 μm capacity is used.

Some derangement of normal clotting mechanisms invariably occurs, reflected by an increased bleeding tendency for 18 to 24 h, even though heparin activity has been neutralized. Such coagulation problems, however, are now far less severe than in previous years with the recognition of the vulnerability of platelets to injury from a wide variety of medications, combined with the availability of platelet transfusions, as well as specific transfusions of fresh frozen plasma or cryoprecipitate for specific coagulation disorders.

Except for the mild coagulation defect, other signs of injury following perfusion are mild. There may be a slight degree of renal insufficiency, manifested by a transient rise in blood urea nitrogen, returning to normal levels within 2 to 3 days. A number of organ systems may sporadically manifest injury with long periods of perfusion, but these are erratic and inconsistent. Respiratory insufficiency has become uncommon. Acute abdominal problems, such as pancreatitis, cholecystitis, or mesenteric infarction, occur in less than 1 percent of patients. With long perfusions, some changes occur in the central nervous system, almost all of which are transitory and of uncertain significance. Reports from England and from Scandinavia found a surprisingly high frequency of transient neurologic abnormalities following perfusion, though the origin and significance of these findings are currently unknown.

Risk of Perfusion. At present the inherent risk from extracorporeal circulation approaches zero, especially if blood transfusion is unnecessary. Large series of coronary bypass procedures have been reported, with an operative risk of less than 1 percent. Also, the risk of aortic valve replacement has decreased to less than 1 percent in several reports. This low risk represents an astonishing achievement, especially when less than four decades ago, 1950–1952, the entire concept of extracorporeal circulation was theoretical and conceived by many to be unachievable. Multiple organ injury was common in the first two decades of extracorporeal perfusion so that perfusion for longer than 1 to 3 h was regularly associated with signs of multiple organ injury. The gradual disappearance of these problems is a tribute to many contributions in the design and manufacture of the pump oxygenators currently used.

Postoperative Care and Complications

GENERAL PROCEDURES. Following a cardiac operation, patients are best kept in a specialized cardiac intensive care unit to permit appropriate monitoring of cardiac functions. With indwelling vascular catheters, the arterial pressure, central venous pressure, intracardiac pressures, and the electrocardiogram are usually displayed on an oscilloscope to permit continuous monitoring. Generally left atrial pressure and pulmonary artery pressures through an indwelling Swan-Ganz catheter are measured.

The key questions in the first 18 to 24 h following an open heart operation are (1) Is there intrathoracic bleeding? (2) Is the cardiac output adequate (near 2.5 L/m^2/min)? (3) Is there hypovolemia (manifested by low left atrial or central venous pressure)? (4) Is ventilation adequate? (5) Are any arrhythmias present?

Arterial and venous blood gas measurements (P_{O_2}, P_{CO_2}, and pH) are periodically measured, determining both the adequacy of ventilation and the adequacy of cardiac output. The oxygen tension (P_{O_2}) in mixed venous blood is particularly useful as a P_{O_2} near 30 mmHg indicates both adequate ventilation and adequate cardiac output while one near 25 mmHg or lower indicates that a serious circulatory ventilatory problem may be present.

POSTOPERATIVE COMPLICATIONS. Chest x-rays are periodically made to evaluate hemothorax and pulmonary function. The hematocrit and standard blood chemistries (sodium, potassium, carbon dioxide, chlorides, blood urea nitrogen) are serially measured.

Prophylactic antibiotics are regularly given during the operative procedure and for 24 to 48 h following operation, usually until indwelling intracardiac catheters have been removed. The prophylactic antibiotic used should be chosen on the basis of the most common organism causing infections in the hospital. Cefamandole has been one of the most popular antibiotics for the past few years.

With valvular prostheses, anticoagulant therapy with coumadin is usually begun 2 to 3 days after operation, keeping the prothrombin time slightly above 20 s, about $1\frac{1}{2}$ times normal.

Postoperative Bleeding. Blood coagulation mechanisms are abnormal for at least 18 to 24 h following bypass. With present pump oxygenators, blood loss is small, ranging from a total of 400 to 800 mL with different patients. A blood loss exceeding 1 L usually indicates active intrathoracic hemorrhage that requires return of the patient to the operating room. Unless known coagulation defects are present before operation, such as platelet abnormalities or deficient plasma coagulation factors secondary to liver disease, transfusion of platelets or fresh frozen plasma is seldom necessary.

Cardiac Tamponade. Cardiac tamponade is always a serious hazard in any patients following a cardiac operation. In the first 24 h, it may result from blood clots accumulating in the pericardium, or less commonly simply from myocardial edema with pericardial constriction. In subsequent weeks it may develop from a pericardial effusion; the possibility must be seriously considered with any circulatory problem occurring in a patient for several weeks following a cardiac operation. The classic findings of tamponade include elevated venous pressure, hypotension, and widening of the mediastinal shadow on the chest x-ray. Echocardiography is valuable for detection of pericardial effusions but not of much value for recognition of intrapericardial blood.

A particularly important point is that there is *no certain method* for excluding tamponade short of surgical reexploration. Grave tragedies have occurred from cardiac tamponade progressing to cardiac arrest because subtle findings are easily confused with a low cardiac output from cardiac failure. If a significant decrease in cardiac output is present that does not respond to appropriate treatment with infusion of fluids or inotropic agents, prompt surgical reexploration should be done to exclude cardiac tamponade.

Inadequate Cardiac Output. The adequacy of the cardiac output is the key question in any patient following a cardiac operation. Adequacy of cardiac output, of course, is reflected in the blood pressure and the urine output, but exact measurement of cardiac output is far more precise. This can be simply done with a thermodilution technique if a Swan-Ganz catheter has been inserted. This is the mainstay of treatment in any seriously ill patient. A normal cardiac output, of course, is a cardiac index near 3 L/m^2/min. An output between 2.0 and 2.5 L/m^2 represents moderate cardiac failure, while a decrease below 2 L/min is an ominous finding, often resulting in death from inadequate perfusion of peripheral organs unless cardiac output can be increased. The classic clinical findings of low cardiac output with inadequate oxygen transport are the familiar ones of hypotension, vasoconstriction, oliguria, and metabolic acidosis. Untreated cardiac output is ultimately fatal from either progressive renal failure or arrhythmias.

With treatment of a low cardiac output, the first consideration is to exclude cardiac tamponade or intrathoracic bleeding with hypovolemia. Once these two factors have been excluded, the three forms of therapy may be conveniently grouped as treatment of cardiac *preload, afterload,* and *inotropic agents* to improve cardiac contractility. Preload therapy consists of infusion of sufficient fluids to elevate left atrial pressure to an appropriate level; as defined with the Starling concept, cardiac output rises with a rise in left atrial pressure over a wide range.

Afterload reduction consists of reduction in peripheral vascular resistance with specific drugs to cause vasodilatation. If peripheral vascular resistance is elevated above the normal of 1000 to 1200 units, afterload reduction should be one of the initial forms of therapy. The most popular drugs for intravenous infusion are nipride or nitroglycerin.

A wide variety of inotropic agents have been used to augment myocardial contractility. Our preference is usually for dobutamine or dopamine in most instances, often augmented with small amounts of epinephrine.

If cardiac rhythm is not satisfactory, cardiac pacing should be used to maintain both an adequate rate and rhythm. If a sinus mechanism is not present, atrialventricular pacing is valuable.

An intraaortic balloon pump is a valuable form of assisted circulation that can be employed when simpler measures fail, as it augments cardiac output about 700 mL/m^2/min. The need for a balloon pump can easily be determined in the operating room by serial measurements of cardiac output following bypass, using an intraaortic balloon pump if cardiac index remains below 2.0 L/m^2. If this decision is properly made, insertion of an intraaortic balloon pump in the recovery room is seldom necessary. Usually an unexpected fall in cardiac output in the recovery room is due to some specific factor that can be corrected, either in the recovery room or by return of the patient to the operating room. The premature insertion of a balloon pump until all other possible causes of a low cardiac output have been eliminated is a serious error that may have fatal consequences if the basic cause is not recognized.

Cardiac Arrhythmias. An important component of postoperative care is constant, 24 h a day, monitoring of the cardiac rhythm on an oscilloscope for at least 2 to 3 days following operation. In an intensive care unit visual monitoring is satisfactory. Otherwise, some form of telemetry with an appropriate alarm mechanism is needed. Only by *constant* monitoring can serious arrhythmias be detected because such arrhythmias may develop unpredictably despite the presence of a normal cardiac output and without any other signs of circulatory failure. Delayed detection of a significant arrhythmia is a major cause of the rare but tragic unexpected death following cardiac operations. The prevalence of such arrhythmias is the reason that cardiac pacing wires are routinely left in the right ventricle and right atrium for several days following operation.

Ventricular extrasystoles are more serious because their appearance may herald the development of hazardous rhythms such as bigeminy, ventricular tachycardia, or fibrillation. Hypokalemia should always be considered because patients in cardiac failure preoperatively may have significant depletion of body stores of potassium from chronic diuretic therapy. The serum potassium should usually be kept well above 4.0 meq/L.

Intravenous lidocaine, 1 to 3 mg/m, is a valuable form of therapy for temporary control of arrhythmias, as the drug is quickly metabolized. Treatment of more complicated problems should be done in conjunction with a cardiologist. Methods of therapy include the use of digitalis, beta-blocking drugs such as propanolol, a calcium blocking drug such as verapamil, procaine-amide, or quinidine. Unfortunately, virtually all antiarrhythmic agents cause serious side effects in a small percentage of patients; so such patients require careful periodic monitoring. Electric cardioversion is a valuable technique for arrhythmias refractory to simpler forms of therapy.

Renal Failure. In the first 24 h after operation, baseline intravenous fluid therapy is usually in the range of 75 to 100 mL/h, providing a 24-h infusion of near 1500 mL/m^2 of body surface. Usually a limited oral intake of fluids is possible the day following operation; so intravenous therapy is needed for only a short period of time.

There is usually some degree of sodium retention for days or weeks following operation, especially in patients who have had chronic congestive failure beforehand. There is also a normal weight gain of five or more pounds following extracorporeal circulation because of the hemodilution used in the pump oxygenator. Moderate diuretic therapy is usually needed for a few days following operation, noting the change in daily body weight. If preoperative chronic cardiac failure was present, recording daily weight should be continued for weeks or months to permit appropriate adjustment of diuretic therapy.

Renal function is rarely a problem unless there is a persistently low cardiac output or serious preexisting renal disease, with a creatinine clearance less than 30 mL/min. Hourly urine output is carefully measured for 1 to 2 days, usually keeping an average output above 30 mL/h. A transitory elevation of blood urea nitrogen to 30 to 40 mg/dL commonly occurs but apparently is of no clinical significance.

Significant renal failure usually develops as a consequence of a persistent low cardiac output or in patients with minimal renal function before operation. This usually is manifested as a high-output renal failure, with a daily secretion of 1 to 2 L of dilute urine, associated with progressive elevation in blood urea nitrogen. The degree of renal insufficiency may be evaluated simply by performance of a urea clearance test, comparing the urea concentration in the blood and urine. Normally, urea concentration is fifteen to twenty times greater in the urine than in the blood; a urine urea concentration less than ten times that in the blood usually represents severe renal insufficiency.

If renal insufficiency evolves to produce a blood urea nitrogen above 50 to 60 mg/dL, peritoneal dialysis should be started promptly. This is a simple form of therapy that often controls the renal insufficiency until spontaneous recovery of renal function occurs. Permitting the blood urea nitrogen to rise to levels of 90 to 100 mg may precipitate serious cardiac arrhythmias and other metabolic disturbances such as gastrointestinal bleeding.

Oliguric renal failure of severe degree is a more ominous complication. If a short period of peritoneal dialysis is not satisfactory, hemodialysis is often necessary. Renal failure of such severity that hemodialysis is required is a very serious complication, as the mortality rate is at least 50 percent, often greater.

Respiratory Insufficiency. With current pump oxygenators, significant impairment of pulmonary function is uncommon except in patients with severe preexisting pulmonary disease or advanced cardiac failure. The simplest numerical expression of the pulmonary dysfunction is the alveolar-arterial oxygen gradient, representing impaired diffusion of oxygen from the alveoli into the pulmonary venous blood.

Ventilation through an indwelling endotracheal tube for 24 to 72 h is adequate for many patients. If longer periods of ventilation are necessary, a cricothyroidotomy or tracheostomy should be performed, although some patients may tolerate an indwelling endotracheal tube for several days. Removal of pulmonary secretions, however, a major cause of pulmonary infection, is done much better through a tracheostomy or cricothyroidotomy. Ventilatory support for more than a short time is seldom necessary except in chronically ill elderly patients in whom simple physical weakness may significantly impair the effectiveness of breathing and coughing. Such patients may require ventilatory support for days or even weeks.

Fever. A moderate temperature elevation to 100 to 101°F is common for 1 to 2 days following operation, probably reflecting both the operative trauma, impaired pulmonary function, and the products from the pump oxygenator. Fever persisting more than a few days is usually due to a pleural effusion or the so-called pericardiotomy syndrome. The pericardiotomy syndrome can develop in any patient in whom the pericardium has been opened; it is probably a reaction of a mesothelial lined surface to surgical trauma. The familiar clinical manifestations are fever, often in association with a pericardial friction rub, and pericardial or pleural effusions. The white blood cell count is usually near the normal range of 10,000/mm³.

Treatment with an anti-inflammatory agent, aspirin, or ibuprofen, is usually satisfactory. With more difficult problems, prednisone therapy may be given for a few days. Investigation should always be done for a bacterial source of infection. Common causes include atelectasis, urinary tract infection, or a wound infection. Blood cultures are usually routinely done to exclude the rare but serious development of endocarditis in patients with prosthetic valves. An infection of the sternotomy incision is a serious complication that requires prompt return to the operating room for treatment with either debridement and antibiotic drainage or debridement and closure with open muscle flaps in refractory cases. Such serious infections are rare, occurring in about 1 percent of all open heart operations.

Central Nervous System Complications. A stroke is perhaps the most serious complication following extracorporeal circulation, occurring with a frequency of 1 to 2 percent following open heart operations. The frequency is greater with older patients, almost surely because of the increasing frequency of atherosclerotic disease of the carotid and vertebral arteries in older patients. Possible causes of stroke that should be routinely investigated include carotid disease, emboli from the heart such as thrombi or calcium fragments from diseased valves, or air emboli from incomplete evacuation of air from the cardiac chambers. In the majority of patients, the cause simply remains unknown; so stroke remains a distressing serious cause of morbidity following any open heart operation. In recent years, at NYU, atherosclerotic disease in the aortic arch has been found by surgical exploration at operation in a significant number of older patients.

Prospective studies of cerebral function have been reported from England and Scandinavian countries in recent years that suggest a significant frequency of transient minor neurologic abnormalities with extracorporeal circulation presumably due to emboli of microaggregates. The significance of these observations is yet unknown.

Gastrointestinal Disturbances. The vast majority of patients recovery uneventfully. An acute abdominal problem has been reported to develop in about 1 percent of all patients following extracorporeal circulation. The specific disease varies widely and unpredictably, including acute cholecystitis, pancreatitis, perforated ulcer, gastrointestinal bleeding, or mesenteric infarction.

CARDIAC ARREST AND VENTRICULAR FIBRILLATION

Cardiac arrest and ventricular fibrillation are considered together because either catastrophe produces immediate cessation of the circulation. An injury causing generalized cardiac depression, such as anoxia, is more likely to lead to cardiac arrest, while agents increasing myocardial irritability, such as digitalis intoxication, are more likely to produce ventricular fibrillation. Diagnosis and treatment of the two conditions are, however, very similar.

HISTORICAL DATA. A successful cardiac resuscitation was performed in 1901 by Igelsrud in Norway, but for many years such experiences were very rare. The first successful case of electrical defibrillation was reported by Beck in 1947. In 1960 the most important advance in cardiac resuscitation occurred when Kouwenhoven, Jude, and Knickerbocker, at the Johns Hopkins Hospital, first introduced the concept of closed-chest massage. This launched the modern era of cardiopulmonary resuscitation, which quickly spread throughout the world. Over the past 10 to 15 years cardiopulmonary resuscitation (CPR) has been successfully taught in organized courses to large numbers of nonmedical personnel with widespread beneficial results. Cobb and associates reported that nearly 300 patients were successfully resuscitated each year. Subsequent studies found that nearly 80 percent had coronary disease but only 25 percent of these had a significant infarction; over 50 percent had no signs of infarction whatsoever, indicating the prevalence and importance of cardiac arrhythmias.

ETIOLOGY. Five frequent causes of cardiac arrest of fibrillation that should be routinely considered in the differential diagnosis are coronary occlusion, anoxia, electrolyte abnormalities, drugs, and arrhythmias.

Coronary Occlusion. Coronary disease is present in the majority of patients. An acute myocardial infarction is a common cause of fibrillation. When chronic coronary disease has produced significant ventricular scarring, cardiac arrhythmias may precipitate ventricular fibrillation in the absence of acute infarction.

Anoxia. Sustained anoxia may lead to ventricular fibrillation or cardiac arrest, both from the low arterial oxygen tension as well as the progressive metabolic acidosis that results. Inadequate ventilation from tracheobroncheal obstruction from aspiration of gastric contents or a foreign body is a frequent cause.

Electrolyte Abnormalities. Either a deficiency or an excess of potassium can cause cardiac arrest or fibrillation. A serum potassium below 4.0 meq or above 6.0 meq can be harmful, though the precise influence is determined by the coexisting concentration of calcium ions and the presence of acidosis or alkalosis.

Drugs. Several drugs may induce ventricular fibrillation or cardiac arrest, either from excessive amounts or from an abnormal sensitivity. Digitalis is one of the most frequent of this group because of its widespread usage. The sensitivity of the myocardium to digitalis varies with a number of factors, one of the most importance of which is the concentration of potassium. Quinidine is a familiar example of a drug that may cause a reaction from abnormal sensitivity, as an occasional patient develops ventricular fibrillation from a very small amount of quinidine.

Arrhythmias. A profound bradycardia, with a heart rate below 60 per minute, may result in ventricular fibrillation or cardiac arrest. This frequently occurs in patients with complete heart block. Ventricular arrhythmias from any cause may progress to bigeminy, ventricular tachycardia, and fibrillation. This well-known sequence is the reason for the fundamental importance of constant visual monitoring of the electrocardiogram on an oscilloscope in a cardiac postoperative unit.

DIAGNOSIS. The cerebral anoxia following circulatory arrest produces brain injury within 3 to 4 min, depending upon the temperature; so diagnosis must be made and treatment begun rapidly to avoid serious brain injury. Periods of anoxia for 6 to 8 min may produce extensive but reversible brain injury whereas longer periods regularly cause irreversible injury. When the diagnosis of cardiac arrest is considered, it should either be excluded within 30 to 60 s or treatment should be begun.

In most patients the diagnosis can be simply made. Loss of consciousness occurs within seconds, as well as absence of respiratory activity except for a few agonal gasps. The rapidity of loss of consciousness is awesome. Abruptly, without a sound or any other warning, the patient simply collapses. This is the reason alarm systems are essential in a busy intensive care unit, for otherwise cardiac arrest may not be recognized unless the patient is under direct visual observation. All peripheral pulses are absent, most easily confirmed by palpation of the femoral or carotid arteries. No cardiac sounds can be heard on auscultation of the chest.

Closed-chest massage should be started promptly, within 1 to 2 min. The electrocardiogram is of little value making a diagnosis of cardiac arrest, for some electrical activity may be visible on the electrocardiogram for a few minutes after effective cardiac contractions have ceased. The main value of the electrocardiogram is to demonstrate ventricular fibrillation, for cardiac arrest can be differentiated from ventricular fibrillation only by the electrocardiogram or by direct inspection of the myocardium.

The most common differential diagnosis from cardiac arrest is extreme bradycardia with hypotension, as in someone who has fainted or developed anaphylactic shock from a hypersensitivity syndrome. In such patients, though unconscious, there is slight respiratory activity and cardiac sounds are usually audible.

TREATMENT. Ventilation. The immediate first step in treatment is to provide adequate oxygenation (Fig. 19-2). Cardiac massage for more than a few seconds without ventilation of the lungs is futile. Ventilation is most quickly accomplished by mouth-to-mouth insufflation of the lungs. This can be begun immediately and continued until equipment for an oral airway or endotracheal intubation is obtained. With a laryngoscope, an endotracheal tube can easily be inserted readily by a physician or other trained personnel. In some patients, as in those with a short, thick neck, the anatomy is such that intubation is difficult, at times almost impossible by highly experienced staff. Unless intubation can be accomplished quickly and with certainty, oral insufflation should be continued until a cricothyroidotomy has been performed. A cricothyroidotomy is far simpler than a tracheostomy and equally satisfactory.

An infrequent but serious error occurs when the endo-

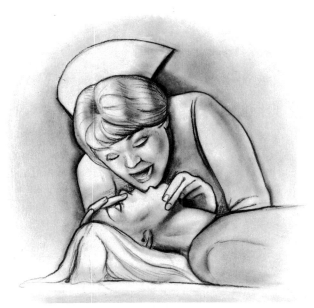

Fig. 19-2. Technique of mouth-to-mouth ventilation. The chin of the patient must be held forward with one hand to prevent obstruction of the nasopharynx by backward displacement of the tongue. The nostrils need to be occluded with the other hand. The head should be extended on the cervical spine to avoid obstruction in the nasopharynx.

tracheal tube is inadvertently placed in the esophagus. Determining whether the endotracheal tube has been placed in the trachea or not can be surprisingly difficult in some patients. If any uncertainty exists after brief auscultation of the lungs, a cricothyroidotomy should be done. A tightly fitting face mask can provide a method of temporary ventilation.

Fig. 19-3. A. Closed-chest massage. The heel of the hand should be used to compress intermittently the lower portion of the sternum toward the vertebral column. The effectiveness of the compression should be monitored by palpation of a peripheral pulse by another member of the team. Artificial ventilation must be performed at the same time. B. Cross section of chest showing the anatomic basis for closed-chest massage. The heart is seen suspended in the mid-thorax between the sternum anteriorly and the vertebral column posteriorly. The pericardium must be intact for closed-chest massage to be effective. C. Compression of the heart as the sternum is depressed downward toward the vertebral column.

Cardiac Massage. The effectiveness of closed-chest massage probably depends upon intermittent compression of the heart between the sternum and the vertebral column, with lateral motion of the heart limited by the pericardium. The patient must be on a firm surface, usually done by placing a board behind the back. The heel of the hand should be applied over the *lower third* of the sternum with the other hand above it to depress the sternum intermittently for 3 to 4 cm (Fig. 19-3). The sternal compression should be brisk, depress the sternum sharply and then releasing it to permit cardiac filling. Mechanical ventilation must be synchronized with massage.

Compression of the sternum near the xiphoid process may injure the liver; compression over the upper sternum or laterally over the chest wall may produce multiple fractures of the ribs. Massage should be at a rate of about 60/min; more than one person is required since the persons performing massage will fatigue quickly.

The amount of force applied should be judged by palpation of a peripheral pulse, usually the femoral. Caution is required to be certain that a regurgitant pulse in the femoral vein is not confused with a pulse in the femoral artery, for a strong retrograde pulse wave may be propagated down the vena cava during massage.

The influence of technique on effectiveness of massage can be easily judged when intraarterial pressure is visually displayed on an oscilloscope. Small adjustments in the technique of massage may change systolic blood pressure 40 to 60 mmHg.

Weisfeldt and associates proposed that the effectiveness of CPR depended upon the intrathoracic pressure rather than direct compression of the heart between the vertebral column and the sternum. Increasing intrathoracic pressure by inflating the lungs and compressing the abdominal wall with a binder substantially increased the effectiveness of cardiac massage, demonstrated by measuring both flow and pressure in the carotid artery.

If cerebral function is probably intact, massage should be continued as long as significant cardiac activity is present. Cardiac massage is seldom successful after about 15 min.

Retrospective analyses comparing patients who were and were not successfully resuscitated usually find certain basic differences. Patients successfully resuscitated

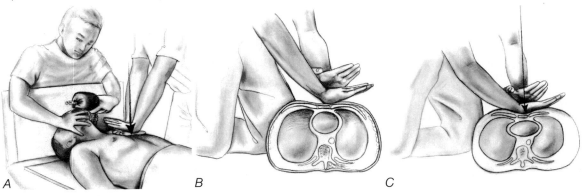

A   *B*   *C*

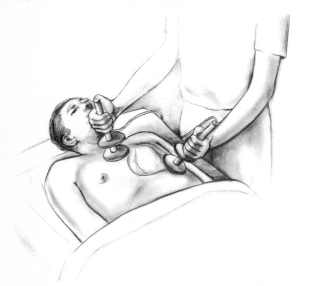

Fig. 19-4. Technique of closed-chest defibrillation. One electrode paddle is applied at the apex of the heart and the other at the base. The most common errors are inadequate electrical contact between the electrodes and the skin or inadequate amounts of current.

usually have an electrical failure, such as fibrillation or severe bradycardia, as opposed to a "power" failure from inherent myocardial injury, as with a massive infarction or terminal cardiac failure with anoxia and acidosis. In successfully resuscitated patients, resuscitation is started almost immediately.

Such observations characterize episodes of cardiac arrest from easily reversible causes, as opposed to those secondary to severe myocardial injury. A separate question is whether open-chest massage, mechanically more effectively, should be instituted earlier. This is commonly done in the postoperative recovery room if closed-chest massage does not produce an adequate blood pressure, because the surgical incision can be quickly reopened and tamponade or intrathoracic hemorrhage recognized. Geehr reported studies of the role of open heart massage instituted after initial closed-chest massage failed. His work and others indicate that open cardiac massage is far more effective if instituted promptly. Available data, however, do not support attempting open-chest massage after closed-chest massage has been ineffective more than 15 min. Rarely open-chest massage may be effectively continued for hours until the basic condition causing refractory fibrillation or arrest is corrected.

If a sternotomy incision has not been made previously, open cardiac massage is best performed through an anterolateral thoracotomy made in the left fourth or fifth interspace. The anterolateral fifth interspace may be opened in less than 1 to 2 min with an unsterile technique because there are no large muscles between the skin and the ribs.

Drugs and Fluids. Epinephrine, sodium bicarbonate, and calcium are the most useful agents. They are usually ineffective, however, if severe myocardial anoxia is pres-

ent. Anoxia can be corrected only by the combination of effective cardiac massage and ventilation. Excessive use of drugs before this has been accomplished is probably a futile diversion.

Epinephrine, 1 to 2 mL of 1:10,000 dilution, may be given intravenously or alternately by direct intracardiac injection. Calcium, 3 to 4 mL of a 10% solution, is another powerful stimulant of myocardial contraction. Calcium administration in cardiac arrest may be valuable in some circumstances, harmful in others. Calcium should not be used indiscriminately. Acidosis is usually present and may require intensive therapy to restore a normal pH. Large amounts of sodium bicarbonate, as much as 200 to 300 meq, may be required. Resuscitation is usually ineffective with a significant acidosis (venous blood pH near 7.20) before this has been corrected.

One or more liters of fluid should be rapidly infused, for vasodilatation is usually present. An intravenous infusion of a vasoconstrictor, norepinephrine or aramine, is often helpful as well.

Arterial and venous blood gas tension should be serially measured at 5- to 10-min intervals as soon as possible because acidosis invariably recurs with the low cardiac outputs produced by closed-chest massage.

Defibrillation. Ventricular fibrillation can be differentiated from cardiac arrest only by the electrocardiogram or by direct inspection of the myocardium. If closed-chest massage is not promptly effective and an electrocardiogram is not available, empiric defibrillation may be tried briefly because most resuscitations are effective when defibrillation is promptly done.

Closed-chest defibrillation is usually done by applying electrodes over the base and apex of the heart; an alternate method consists of placing one large electrode posteriorly near the vertebral column and a smaller one anteriorly near the cardiac apex (Fig. 19-4). Defibrillation is best done with a direct current, about 400 J.

With open-chest defibrillation, the electrodes are applied directly to the heart and an appropriate impulse delivered. Unless a serious biochemical abnormality is present, such as hypokalemia or digitalis intoxication, the usual cause of failure to defibrillate is either an anoxic or an acidotic myocardium, or ineffective transmission of an electrical impulse through the myocardium. Vigorous cardiac massage should precede defibrillation to oxygenate the myocardium sufficiently. Correction of acidosis with bicarbonate can be confirmed by blood-gas determinations. Intramyocardial injection of epinephrine may stimulate myocardial tone but should not be done until correction of anoxia and acidosis has been confirmed.

When the electric shock is applied through the electrodes compressing the heart, the myocardium should be observed closely. Adequate transmission of a current through the myocardium will stop all fibrillatory activity, though it may recur within a few seconds. If the fibrillatory activity was not momentarily stopped, enough current was not transmitted, from either inadequate voltage, inadequate electrodes, or inadequate application of the electrodes to the heart. Unless a myocardial infarction has occurred, it should be possible to defibrillate the majority of fibrillating hearts, though the ensuing cardiac arrest may be refractory to therapy. This concept is important to be certain that an inadequate technique of defibrillation, often from a faulty defibrillator, is not erroneously diagnosed as refractory cardiac arrest.

Fifty-three of 125 patients with 173 episodes of ventricular fibrillation survived to leave the hospital. The most significant factor influencing survival was the institution of defibrillation within 1 min of onset of fibrillation or ability to defibrillate with less than five shocks.

Therapy Following Cardiac Resuscitation. Following restoration of an adequate heart beat and blood pressure, the critical question is the extent of injury to the central nervous system. Significant brain injury is usually indicated by continuing coma. A detailed neurologic evaluation to elicit specific normal and abnormal reflexes should be done promptly. Permanent brain injury is frequent after more than 5 min of cardiac arrest, even though experimentally cerebral neurons can tolerate nearly 20 min of normothermic ischemic anoxia.

Mild hypothermia should be started soon with a water mattress, lowering body temperature to near 34°C if feasible. Abundant experimental data indicate that this mild degree of hypothermia significantly enhances recovery from cerebral injury. The hypothermia should be instituted promptly because a fever of 39 to 40°C often develops within 2 to 4 h.

Massive intravenous steroid therapy is usually given for 24 to 48 h to minimize cerebral edema. The efficacy is difficult to measure.

Continuous oscilloscopic monitoring of the cardiac rhythm is essential; arrhythmias are common, and fibrillation may recur. Intravenous infusion of lidocaine or procainamide is useful for suppressing arrhythmias. Adequacy of cardiac output and ventilation should be monitored by periodic blood-gas determination of arterial and central venous blood. Fluid therapy requires special care, for an adequate blood volume is needed for cardiac and renal function, but excessive fluids may intensify cerebral edema.

PROGNOSIS. If serious cardiac or cerebral injury is not present following resuscitation, prognosis is excellent. This fact is the basis for the enthusiastic development of widespread training in cardiopulmonary resuscitation by all physicians, paramedical personnel, and laypeople, for most effective resuscitation is accomplished when begun within 1 to 2 min after onset of cardiac arrest.

Careful study of patients who survive cardiac arrest subsequently discharged from the hospital has found a sobering recurrence of cardiac arrest within 1 to 3 years, a frequency of 30 to 40 percent or higher. Myerburg analyzed 61 survivors of prehospital cardiac arrest. There were 24 late deaths (39 percent), 16 of which were due to recurrent arrest. Ten percent of these occurred within the first year after discharge from the hospital, with a subsequent frequency near 5 percent per year for the next 3 years. Wilber and Ruskin reviewed experiences with electrophysiologic testing in 166 survivors of out-of-hospital cardiac arrest. Ventricular arrhythmias could be suppressed with therapy in 75 percent of the group. Re-

current cardiac arrest occurred at a frequency of about 6 percent per year in those responding to treatment but was much higher, near 30 percent, in those not responding. Roy and Josephson reported similar findings. Arrhythmias could be induced with programmed ventricular stimulation in 61 percent of the group. Survival was significantly greater in patients in whom medical or surgical therapy could prevent the induction of a sustained arrhythmia.

MITRAL STENOSIS

HISTORICAL DATA. A valiant effort to treat mitral stenosis by excising a portion of the valve with a valvulotome was made by Cutler and Levine in 1923, but the resulting mitral insufficiency caused a prohibitive operative mortality. Souttar, in England, performed a digital commissurotomy in one patient in 1925. Thereafter surgical efforts virtually ceased for over 20 years until 1948–1949 when Harken and Bailey independently demonstrated the value of digital commissurotomy. These early commissurotomies, often limited in extent, frequently produced striking clinical improvement, even though mitral stenosis often recurred within 5 years. A transventricular mitral dilator developed around 1957 produced a more extensive commissurotomy and was widely adopted. Subsequently the increasing safety of cardiopulmonary bypass made commissurotomy under direct vision the procedure of choice.

ETIOLOGY. All evidence indicates that mitral stenosis is almost always due to rheumatic fever, even though a definite history of rheumatic fever can be obtained in only about 50 percent of patients. Congenital mitral stenosis is very rare, less than 300 cases having been reported. After the initial episode of rheumatic fever, symptoms of mitral stenosis may not appear for 10 or more years but may develop as soon as 3 years in some patients and as late as 25 years in others. Selzer and Cohn suggested that scarring of the mitral valve from rheumatic fever produces turbulent flow of blood that in turn causes progressive scarring and contraction over many years. This would explain the appearance of severe mitral stenosis 20 to 30 years after the last known bout of rheumatic fever.

PATHOLOGY. Although rheumatic fever produces a pancarditis, involving pericardium, myocardium, and endocardium, serious permanent injury results primarily from the endocarditis. Permanent myocardial injury following recovery from acute myocarditis is uncommon; it is seldom of clinical significance but an occasional patient is seen with significant myocardial dysfunction. Endocarditis produces ulceration of the endocardium along the edges of the valve leaflets where they normally appose in systole. Tiny, 1- to 2-mm nodules of fibrin and platelets accumulate and may coalesce to fusion of the leaflets at the commissures. A more serious injury evolves from extensive valvulitis with fibrosis and contraction of the body of the leaflets, compounded in subsequent years with calcification and decreasing leaflet mobility. Inflammation of the chordae tendineae similarly leads to fibrosis with contraction, thickening, and fusion. With severe disease the chordae contract and pull the valve leaflets down to fuse with the tips of the papillary muscles.

In many patients mitral stenosis gradually increases in severity over many years, at times more than 20. Previously these progressive changes were considered due to clinically silent episodes of rheumatic fever. The now accepted hypothesis is that the changes are hemodynamic in origin, resulting from turbulent flow of blood through the scarred mitral orifice.

The possibilities of surgical correction vary greatly with the extent of the valve injury. When simple fusion of the commissures is the only lesion, mitral commissurotomy is highly successful. If the chordae tendineae have contracted and fused to make the leaflets immobile, commissurotomy may be only moderately effective and perhaps impossible. With extensive fibrosis and rigidity of the leaflets, valve replacement is often necessary. How often this is required varies with the type of patient operated on. When operation is performed "early" in the course of the disease (before extensive fibrosis and contraction have occurred), valvular reconstruction, rather than replacement, is possible in the majority of patients, i.e., 85 to 90 percent.

PATHOPHYSIOLOGY. A normal mitral valve has a cross-sectional area between 4 and 6 cm^2. Reduction of the cross-sectional area to 2 to 2.5 cm^2 constitutes the mildest form of mitral stenosis. Typical auscultatory findings are present, but the patient is usually asymptomatic (Class I). Further reduction to the range of 1.5 to 2.0 cm^2 produces some symptoms (Class II disability); these are more severe with a cross-sectional area in the range of 1 to 1.5 cm^2. Patients with a cross-sectional area of less than 1 cm^2 are usually seriously disabled (Class IV). A valve area near 0.6 cm^2 is said to be the minimal size compatible with life.

Three significant physiologic events result from mitral stenosis—increase in left atrial pressure, decrease in cardiac output, and increase in pulmonary vascular resistance. Increase in left atrial pressure (normally less than 12 mmHg) is the immediate consequence of mitral stenosis. The degree of elevation of left atrial pressure varies with three factors: (1) the cross-sectional area of the mitral orifice, (2) cardiac output, and (3) cardiac rate. These three factors represent physical laws determining pressure-flow relations through a stenotic orifice, namely, cross-sectional area of orifice, total volume of flow, and duration of time during which flow occurs. When left atrial pressure rises to exceed oncotic pressure of plasma (25 to 30 mmHg), transudation of fluid across the pulmonary capillaries will occur. The result of this transudation depends upon the capacity of the pulmonary lymphatics to transport the additional fluid. When the fluid load exceeds the capacity of the lymphatic circulation, pulmonary edema results. Left atrial pressure and concomitant pulmonary symptoms vary with the degree of mitral stenosis, the cardiac output as influenced by exercise or emotion, and the length of diastole determined by cardiac rate.

As the oncotic pressure of plasma is 24 to 30 mmHg,

about that of a column of blood 12 to 14 in. high, pulmonary congestion in the upright position may be much greater in the lower lobes of the lung than in the upper, for the average thorax is about 20 in. high. A patient with only basilar rales in the upright position may develop extensive pulmonary congestion when supine, with cough, dyspnea, or frank pulmonary edema. This explains paroxysmal nocturnal dyspnea.

The cardiac output is fixed at a low level by the rigid stenotic orifice. With exercise, cardiac output cannot be increased significantly, and dyspnea results. The general fatigue and limitation of physical activity with mitral stenosis is a clinical reflection of this physiologic inability to increase cardiac output.

The degree to which pulmonary vascular resistance increases with mitral stenosis varies greatly among different patients. The cause of this variation is unknown. Some, with severe mitral stenosis, have little change, while in others vascular resistance increases to levels fifteen to twenty times greater than normal. This increased resistance is primarily a result of vasoconstriction in the pulmonary arterioles, ultimately intensified by hypertrophy of the media and intima. In far advanced cases recurrent pulmonary emboli may create additional obstruction, but this is uncommon. In the vast majority of patients, the increased vascular resistance either decreases greatly or disappears following surgical correction, a course that is very different from that seen with pulmonary hypertension from congenital heart disease.

Two other serious disabilities that appear with chronic mitral stenosis are atrial fibrillation and systemic embolization. Atrial fibrillation is the ultimate consequence of the atrial hypertrophy produced by chronic left atrial hypertension. Fibrillation produces some decrease in cardiac output and also is often a prelude to more serious arrhythmias. The most serious consequence is the development of thrombi, usually in the ineffectively contracting left atrial appendage. The frequency of thrombi varies with both the duration of mitral stenosis and the presence of atrial fibrillation. Ultimately thrombi develop in 15 to 20 percent of patients, after which episodes of arterial embolism appear with increasing frequency. Before either anticoagulant therapy or operation was possible, cerebral embolism caused death in 20 to 25 percent of patients dying from mitral stenosis.

CLINICAL MANIFESTATIONS. Symptoms. The most important symptom is *dyspnea*. This appears whenever mean left atrial pressure exceeds 30 mmHg long enough to produce significant transudation of fluid into the pulmonary capillaries. Characteristically, it first appears with extreme exertion and subsequently, with more severe stenosis, occurs with lesser degrees of exertion. It may also appear with emotion or other circumstances that increase cardiac output.

Several other symptoms subsequently appear, all developing as a result of recurrent pulmonary congestion. A chronic *cough*, worse in the evenings in the recumbent position, is frequent, reflecting basilar congestion. *Orthopnea* and *paroxysmal nocturnal dyspnea* similarly reflect the influence of the upright position on the localization of pulmonary congestion. In the upright position, congestion may be limited to the lower lobes but becomes more diffuse in the supine position. Mobilization of peripheral edema from the lower extremities when the patient is supine intensifies the degree of pulmonary congestion. *Hemoptysis* is a frequent symptom, varying from expectoration of blood-tinged sputum to massive amounts of bright red blood, in unusual circumstances exceeding 1 L. Such severe hemoptysis, although an alarming symptom, usually subsides spontaneously. Rarely, an emergency mitral valvotomy is required. Episodes of *pulmonary edema* occur when pulmonary congestion greatly exceeds the capacity of the pulmonary lymphatics. In contrast to hemoptysis, pulmonary edema may be fatal unless quickly and effectively treated.

Eventually failure of the right side of the heart appears, manifested by venous distention, hepatic enlargement, and peripheral edema. This may be intensified by the development of either pulmonary hypertension or tricuspid insufficiency. Atrial fibrillation develops eventually in most patients. Initially it may be transient, but ultimately in most patients chronic atrial fibrillation is the most common rhythm.

Arterial embolism is a constant threat, especially with atrial fibrillation, although emboli can occur with a sinus rhythm. Emboli evolve from stasis in the dilated left atrium, especially in the atrial appendage. Rarely, large thrombi 5 to 10 cm in diameter may fill much of the left atrium and partly obstruct the ostia of the pulmonary veins.

Angina pectoris develops in about 10 percent of patients. The basic cause is unclear, for it is usually not due to associated coronary atherosclerosis. Possible mechanisms include a low cardiac output, impaired blood flow during diastole because of tachycardia, and recurrent small emboli to the coronary arteries.

Physical Examination. A patient with chronic, severe mitral stenosis may be thin and frail, with the muscular wasting characteristic of a chronic illness. Dilated neck veins are visible if congestive failure is present. Rubor and/or cyanosis are often seen over the fingers or lips. These signs reflect a chronic severe restriction in cardiac output, resulting in blood flowing slowly through peripheral capillary beds. Rales are frequently audible over the lung bases.

Often with pure mitral stenosis, the cardiac size is normal, and the apical impulse is normal or decreased in intensity. A forceful, heaving left ventricular impulse immediately suggests that another disease, such as mitral insufficiency or aortic valvular disease, is present. With increased pulmonary vascular resistance, palpation of the left parasternal area may find a "lift," resulting from contraction of a hypertrophied right ventricle. The pulse rhythm may be regular but is usually atrial fibrillation.

The three significant auscultatory findings with mitral stenosis are the diastolic rumble, an opening snap, and an increased first sound. The apical diastolic rumble, at times sharply localized to an area at the apex only 2 to 3 cm in diameter, is the hallmark of mitral stenosis. It may be of grade I or II intensity in some patients, while in

others it is unusually loud with a palpable thrill. The intensity of the murmur, however, does not correlate with the severity of the stenosis. Rarely "silent" mitral stenosis is present without an audible murmur. This results from a calcified, fibrosed valve with little mobility. The increased first sound, the origin of which is not certain, is another distinctive feature and is often the first auscultatory abnormality detected. The opening snap, closely following the second sound, is the third distinctive feature. In many patients careful auscultation can immediately establish the diagnosis of mitral stenosis by finding the triad of an opening snap, followed by a diastolic rumble, and an accentuated first sound.

A short apical systolic murmur may be heard in patients with pure mitral stenosis without any associated mitral insufficiency. Loud pansystolic murmurs, however, which are transmitted to the axilla usually indicate associated mitral insufficiency. A systolic murmur from tricuspid insufficiency may be confused with one arising from mitral insufficiency. The systolic murmur of tricuspid insufficiency, although audible at the apex with hypertrophy of the right ventricle, is usually heard equally well near the sternum and may be accentuated with deep inspiration.

Laboratory Studies. The initial change in mitral stenosis is dilatation of the left atrium (Fig. 19-5). Echocardiography is the simplest and most precise method for making this determination. Once it has been determined that the left atrium is enlarged, there is little correlation between the actual size of the left atrium and the severity of the mitral stenosis. Left atrial enlargement can also be detected with a lateral chest radiograph exposed during oral administration of barium to outline the esophagus. Characteristically, the middle third of the esophagus is displaced backward to form a slight concave curve. With additional degrees of enlargement, the dilated left atrium may be visible as a double shadow in the posteroanterior radiograph, forming a separate dense shadow behind the normal shadow of the right atrium. The left border of the cardiac shadow also shows characteristic changes with mitral stenosis, for the normal concavity between the shadow of the aortic knob and the left ventricle becomes obliterated as both the left atrium and the pulmonary artery enlarge to produce a "straight" left heart border. The overall cardiac size may be normal, but lateral views can demonstrate enlargement of the right ventricle when pulmonary vascular resistance has increased. Calcification of the mitral valve is visible with chronic disease in older patients.

Engorged pulmonary veins can be unusually prominent, often with a greater degree of dilatation in the veins to the upper lobes. With pulmonary hypertension the pulmonary arteries are also enlarged. With chronic, severe left atrial hypertension, dilated pulmonary lymphatics become visible as transverse lines across the lower lung fields, "Kerley lines," indicating significant left atrial hypertension.

The electrocardiogram is not diagnostic but often shows T-wave abnormalities characteristic of left atrial enlargement; atrial fibrillation is the most common ar-

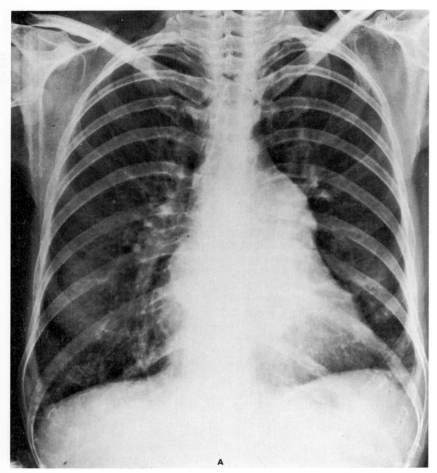

Fig. 19-5. *A*. Chest radiograph of a patient with mitral stenosis showing a heart of normal size. The prominent pulmonary artery along the left cardiac border is characteristic of this condition. The enlarged left atrium can be seen as a double density behind the shadow normally formed by the right atrium.

rhythmia seen. If pulmonary hypertension is present, signs of right ventricular hypertrophy are also evident.

2-D echocardiography, however, has been a major advance in noninvasive diagnostic therapy. It can estimate the degree of stenosis and also leaflet mobility. It is of particular value in doubtful cases. Some clinics no longer employ catheterization, simply proceeding from the findings with echocardiography to operation.

Cardiac catheterization can evaluate mitral stenosis precisely, as well as detect the presence of additional valvular disease, such as mitral insufficiency or aortic valvular disease. Left atrial pressure may be estimated from the pulmonary capillary "wedge" pressure. The preferred technique is to enter the left atrium directly with a catheter, usually by puncture of the atrial septum. The left atrial pressure in isolated mitral stenosis is increased from the normal range of 5 to 10 mmHg to levels of 20 to 30 mmHg with severe stenosis, producing a diastolic pressure gradient between the left atrium and ventricle of 10 to 20 mmHg. The most precise measurement of the severity of stenosis is done by calculating the cross-sectional area of the mitral valve, determined by the pressure gradient and the cardiac output. Angiography may demonstrate rigidity and limited mobility of the valve

leaflets but is not of great diagnostic value. It is of particular value, however, in determining the presence of mitral insufficiency by noting the reflux of dye after injection into the left ventricle. Coronary arteriography is an important part of the evaluation of cardiac catheterization, especially in patients over forty years of age in whom coronary atherosclerosis may be present.

TREATMENT. Operation should be routinely considered for hemodynamically significant mitral stenosis, even though symptoms are minimal. The risk is small, about 1 percent, the possibility of reconstruction rather than replacement very good (over 90 percent), and the slight but definite hazard of cerebral embolism is always present, especially once atrial fibrillation has developed. If peripheral embolism has occurred, operation should be performed as soon as the patient has recovered from the embolic episode, for sooner or later emboli almost always recur. Until operation is performed, continuous anticoagulant therapy should be employed.

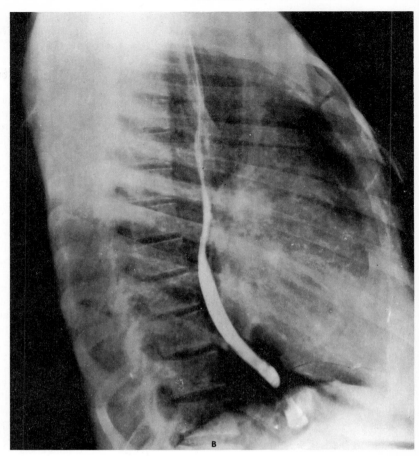

Fig. 19-5. *B.* Lateral radiograph of the same patient shows enlargement of the left atrium, producing a concave displacement of the esophagus, which has been filled with barium.

Even though early operation is the preferred approach, it is important to remember that mitral stenosis can almost always be successfully operated upon, no matter how far advanced the disease or how severe the pulmonary hypertension. The immediate risk of operation is increased with far advanced disease (5 to 7 percent), but surviving patients nearly always show remarkable improvement with a significant decrease, or complete disappearance, of pulmonary hypertension. This improvement is related to the fact that mitral stenosis is a unique condition that keeps blood from entering the left ventricle; so in contrast to other valvular diseases, the left ventricle has not been injured from long-standing hemodynamic stresses.

General Considerations. Since 1971 at New York University virtually all mitral valve operations have been performed with cardiopulmonary bypass, abandoning the "closed" commissurotomy performed blindly with the index finger introduced through the left atrial appendage. The risk of operation is very small, less than 1 percent. The hazard of emboli from thrombi in the atrium or calcium in the mitral valve is significantly less than with closed commissurotomy. Of even greater importance,

however, is that much more effective commissurotomy can be performed, for a high percentage of patients require more than simple commissurotomy to totally correct the stenosis. This includes separation of fused chordae, splitting of papillary muscles, debridement of calcium, and often correction of minimal to moderate associated mitral insufficiency with the Carpentier reconstruction techniques.

With the recent interest in catheter balloon valvuloplasty, these considerations are especially pertinent because balloon valvuloplasty has all the limitations of the old "closed" commissurotomy.

Technique of Open Mitral Commissurotomy. A median sternotomy incision is usually employed. This permits ready access to all cardiac structures, including palpation of the tricuspid valve, which is frequently diseased in severely ill patients. The standard cardiopulmonary bypass technique is used, with a perfusate temperature of 25 to 30 degrees. The heart is arrested with the cold blood hyperkalemic technique. Topical hypothermia is also used, keeping myocardial temperature below 15°C. The left atrium is incised in the interatrial groove anterior to the point of entry of the right pulmonary veins. By extending the atriotomy beneath the superior vena cava superiorly and the inferior vena cava inferiorly, adequate

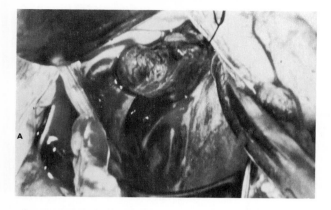

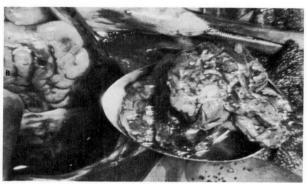

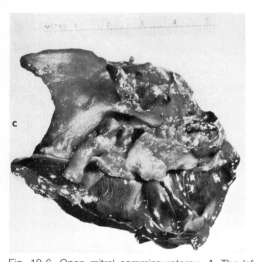

Fig. 19-6. Open mitral commissurotomy. *A.* The left atrium has been incised and the edges retracted. A small thrombus is present in the midportion of the field, demonstrating the pathologic condition that frequently causes cerebral embolism with mitral stenosis. *B.* Large clot found within the left atrium. With cardiopulmonary bypass functioning, the left atrium has been opened widely. The laminated clot is being removed with a large spoon. A clamp occluding the ascending aorta to avoid embolization of clot is visible at the top of the illustration. *C.* Large laminated clot removed at operation from a patient with mitral stenosis. The inability to detect the presence of such a clot before operation is the most cogent reason that all mitral commissurotomies should be performed with a pump-oxygenator as a "standby," to be employed if such a clot is found.

exposure of the mitral valve can be obtained. The Carpentier self-retaining retractor has been routinely used for the past 5 years and provides far better exposure than that previously obtained with other methods.

Any thrombi in the atrium or atrial appendage are carefully removed (Fig. 19-6). The atrial appendage is subsequently routinely excluded from the atrial cavity by closure of the orifice from within the atrium (Fig. 19-7A). This technique has been employed for over a decade without significant injury to other structures, especially the circumflex coronary artery.

The fused commissures of the mitral valve are best exposed by inserting traction sutures into the aortic and mural leaflets. By applying *horizontal,* not vertical, traction on the two leaflets, the fused commissures can be clearly visualized and carefully incised with a knife. As the commissure is incised, the chordae arising from the underlying papillary muscle can be seen and identified (Fig. 19-8). The commissurotomy is carefully performed throughout the length of the fused commissure, stopping where the normal commissural leaflet is found 3 to 4 mm from the mitral annulus.

Division of any chordae is carefully avoided. In at least 30 percent of patients there is significant fusion and contraction of the chordae beneath the commissures, often virtually approximating the fused commissures to the underlying papillary muscles. In such instances the papillary muscle is carefully incised for 10 to 15 mm to provide adequate mobility to the mobilized chordae. This greatly increases the efficacy of the commissurotomy and is one of the key advantages of the open procedure.

Opening the fused commissures sufficiently to correct the stenosis without producing significant mitral insufficiency is the key consideration with each operation. After the commissurotomy is completed, the presence of insufficiency can be assessed by a variety of methods. We currently prefer the method popularized by Carpentier, distending the left ventricular cavity with fluid injected through a bulb syringe and noting the apposition of the leaflets. Though subjective, it is simple and has been reasonably reliable. The ability to correct focal insufficiency by a variety of the Carpentier techniques of mitral reconstruction has greatly facilitated the performance of "radical" commissurotomy.

An alternate method, used for several years, is more cumbersome but probably more precise. If a small catheter is placed in the ascending aorta and fluid injected, currently cold blood cardioplegia, distention of the ventricle can be done and regurgitation assessed. The technique is no longer used primarily because the bulb syringe technique is simpler and about as reliable.

A final routine check for mitral insufficiency is performed near the end of bypass with the heart closed, filled with blood, and beating. A finger can be introduced into the left atrium and the functioning mitral valve palpated while the ventricle is ejecting blood with a systolic pressure of 80 to 100 mm.

Following bypass, adequate correction of the mitral stenosis should be routinely confirmed by measuring both left atrial and ventricular pressure by needle puncture,

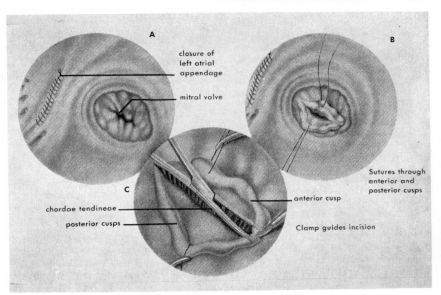

Fig. 19-7. *A.* Closure of left atrial appendage. *B.* Exposure of mitral valve with horizontal traction on sutures. *C.* Right-angle clamp guides incision.

confirming elimination or marked reduction of the end-diastolic pressure gradient. This is an important checkpoint, apparently neglected in many reports of operative technique; with fibrosis and stiff mitral leaflets an opening that seems adequate may still be functionally obstructive because of impaired mobility. If a significant residual gradient is present, 5 to 7 mm, a decision must be made as to whether the gradient can be reduced by additional surgical maneuvers, or whether it should be accepted or the valve replaced. A significant residual gradient is usually associated with recurrent symptoms from progressive stenosis within a few years.

Following operation, convalescence is usually short and benign. If atrial fibrillation has been present for only a few months, cardioversion may be effective. If atrial fibrillation has been chronic, with significant hypertrophy

of left atrial musculature, it is often not successful. The frequency of persistent atrial fibrillation is a strong reason for routine closure of the atrial appendage at the time of operation.

Technique of Mitral Valve Replacement. The initial approach is identical to that used for mitral commissurotomy, described in the preceding section. A sternotomy incision is preferable. Mitral replacement, rather than commissurotomy or reconstruction, is usually necessary if both insufficiency and stenosis are present. The most common pathologic condition requiring replacement is extensive calcification of the valve with stiffening and fibrosis (Fig. 19-9). Calcification limited to the commissures, however, does not preclude effective commissurotomy.

The valve is excised by incising it a few millimeters from the annulus with a circumferential incision. Underlying papillary muscles are divided near their apices. Usually some chordae can be preserved to the annulus of the mural leaflet, but unusual efforts are not made to accomplish this, for the physiologic importance of preserv-

Fig. 19-8. *A.* Separation of fused chordae tendinae with incision into papillary muscle. *B.* Deeper incision into papillary muscle when valve leaflets are fused to underlying papillary muscle.

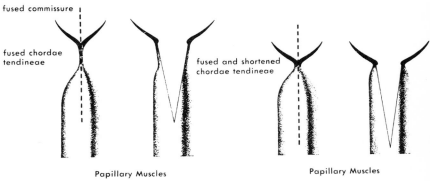

A   *B*

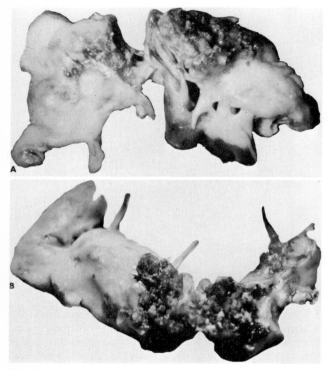

Fig. 19-9. *A.* Excised mitral valve with severe calcification. When such calcification is present, satisfactory function can rarely be restored to the valve. *B.* Calcified mitral valve removed from another patient in whom prosthetic replacement of the mitral valve was necessary.

ing mural leaflet chordae is uncertain. The choice between a porcine (Fig. 19-10) or a metallic prosthesis is discussed in the subsequent section. An identical technique is used for insertion (Fig. 19-11).

The prosthetic valve is inserted with a series of 12 to 18 pledgeted mattress sutures of polyester fabric (currently ticron) (Fig. 19-12). How often pledgeted sutures are needed is uncertain as interrupted sutures or a continuous suture have been effectively used by others in some patients; pledgeted mattress sutures have been employed at NYU routinely for over 15 years because the technique is simple and significant periprosthetic leak is virtually unknown. Care is taken to insert the sutures in the annulus of the mitral valve but no deeper in order to avoid injury to adjacent structures, especially the circumflex coronary artery or the conduction bundle. Throughout the insertion of the prosthetic valve, care is taken to avoid undue traction on the mitral annulus that may inadvertently tear the annulus from the underlying ventricular muscle and result in subsequent rupture of the left ventricle, discussed in a subsequent section.

Following closure of the atriotomy a small catheter is left across the prosthetic valve, fibrillation is induced, and the aorta is unclamped. Air is removed by a variety of maneuvers, including venting of the aorta through a 3- to 4-mm incision and partially cross-clamping the aorta at the time of defibrillation. A left ventricular vent is not used because of the hazard of rupture of the left ventricle during subsequent manipulation of the heart to remove the vent.

Rupture of the left ventricle is a rare but highly lethal complication following insertion. A prospective study of techniques to avoid this complication revealed that routine preservation of a few chordae to the annulus of the mural leaflet, in combination with other techniques, has been associated with absence of this complication for over 5 years, a marked contrast to preceding experiences. Whether preservation of chordae prevents this complication or not cannot be proved, but certainly it is strongly recommended until a better explanation is available.

Convalescence is usually benign except in Class IV patients with long-standing congestive failure who are catabolic with the myriads of complications from malnutrition. These patients require intense care for days or weeks, with particular attention to precise caloric and protein intake, recorded on a daily basis. This often entails a combination of tube feeding and hyperalimentation because some chronically ill emaciated patients are simply unable to eat an adequate amount in the first days or weeks following operation.

Antibiotics are routinely given during operation at measured intervals to maintain a bactericidal level of the antibiotic appropriate for the organisms presently existing in the hospital environment. These are stopped 2 to 3 days following operation, usually when intracardiac lines have been removed. Anticoagulation with sodium warfarin is started about 3 days following operation, subsequently maintained with a prothrombin time near 20 s. This is significantly less than a greater degree of anticoagulation popularly recommended but has been used for over a decade with satisfactory protection from thromboembolism, but a far lower frequency of hemorrhage from anticoagulation. Warfarin is stopped after 3 months in patients with porcine prostheses unless there is chronic atrial fibrillation or a large left atrium. In such patients it may be continued indefinitely. If warfarin is stopped, an antiplatelet agent, usually aspirin, is given for the next year. Warfarin is continued permanently, of course, in patients with metallic prostheses.

Most patients improve promptly after operation, obtaining the full therapeutic benefit within 3 to 6 months. During this time, careful attention to sodium intake and body weight is necessary, for renal excretion of sodium may remain impaired for weeks or months.

Prosthetic Valves. An ideal prosthetic valve does not exist. The two basic valves available are metallic prostheses and the tissue prostheses. Both have advantages and disadvantages. The caged ball valve prosthesis, originally used by Starr in 1961 and subsequently undergoing numerous modifications, remains one of the best metallic prostheses, using the model 6120 with the silastic ball, which has undergone few changes since it was developed in 1966. The other popular valve is a disc valve, so-called low-profile, though the physiologic benefits of the low profile have never been proved. It does have the advan-

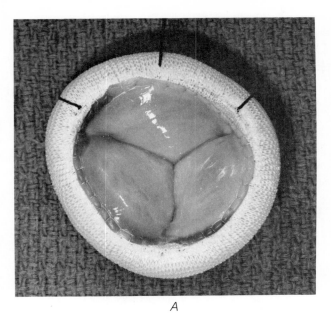

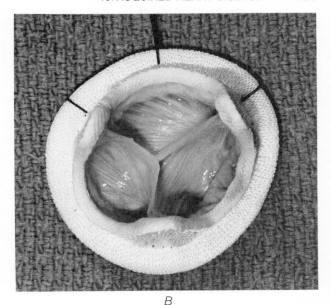

A

B

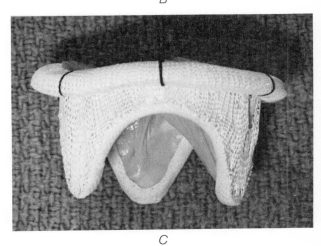

C

Fig. 19-10. Mitral valve prostheses. Carpentier-Edwards porcine prosthesis. *A.* Atrial view; *B.* Ventricular view; *C.* Side view.

tage of a larger cross-sectional area. The one with the longest experience is the Bjork-Shiley disc valve introduced in the late 1960s and subsequently widely used (Fig. 19-13). Several other disc valves exist, the most recent being the St. Jude prosthesis, which has now been in use for over 5 years. All metallic prostheses require permanent anticoagulation and hence have the lifelong hazard of both thromboembolism and hemorrhage from anticoagulants.

Different types of tissue valves have been studied for over two decades because tissue valves have a far lower frequency of thromboembolism. Valves studied include fascia lata valves, dura mater valves, homograft valves, and heterograft valves. All these failed, usually within 1 to 4 years, because of fibrosis and insufficiency, with the sole exception of the antibiotic preserved aortic homograft valve. All others failed, usually within 1 to 4 years, because of fibrosis and insufficiency, until the gluteraldehyde preserved porcine valve was developed, principally by Carpentier in Paris and Hancock in the United States in the mid-1970s (Fig. 19-14). A pericardial heterograft valve was also developed, primarily by Ionescu in England, and has been widely used, though currently is less popular because of a seemingly higher late failure rate.

Patients with a sinus rhythm without extensive cardiac enlargement often do not require anticoagulants for more than 3 months after operation. The principal concern is durability. At least 95 percent of valves perform well for at least 5 years, but after 7 to 8 years there is an exponential rise in valve failure, totaling near 20 percent within a decade. Significant 15-year data are not yet available but the overall course strongly suggests that all tissue valves will ultimately require replacement unless fundamental changes in their method of preparation can be found.

The key question is whether a patient should have a metal valve with permanent anticoagulation but reasonably certain durability or a porcine valve, perhaps not requiring anticoagulation but with the likelihood of eventual replacement, especially after 8 to 10 years.

At NYU, porcine prostheses have been widely used for nearly a decade. Experiences with over 1500 such prostheses were reported in 1986. At present, the advantages and disadvantages of both types of prostheses should be carefully explained to the patient, who ultimately makes the final decision. This is an important concept because of the increasing legal importance of "informed consent." A recommendation by the surgeon should, of course, be given to the patient, which, in our experience, will be accepted in about 80 percent of patients. The remaining

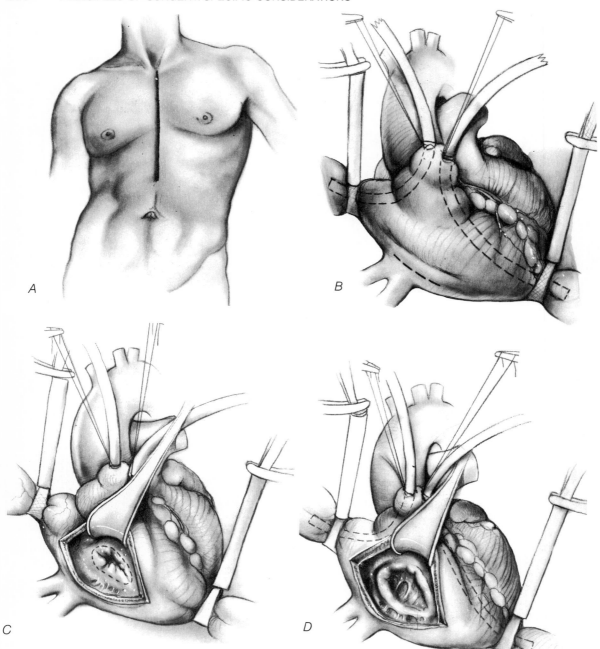

Fig. 19-11. Insertion of mitral valve prosthesis. *A.* A median sternotomy is the preferred incision, providing ready access to all areas of the heart. *B.* Cannulae are introduced through the atrial wall into the venae cavae. Normally these are not snared with encircling tapes unless a patent foramen ovale is encountered which causes aspiration of air from the opened left atrium into the right atrium. *C.* The mitral valve is exposed with an incision in the left atrium anterior to the point of entry of the right pulmonary veins. Exposure is facilitated by intermittent occlusion of the aorta, which will arrest and stop the heart, and also decrease the amount of blood in the operative field. *D.* The mitral valve with the papillary muscles is completely excised, leaving a small rim of annulus. The cavity of the left ventricle is carefully inspected and a prosthesis of appropriate size

chosen, making certain that the cage of the prosthesis can be readily accommodated in the ventricular cavity. *E.* A Carpentier-Edwards porcine prosthesis is preferred. It is inserted with 12 to 15 mattress sutures of #0 Dacron. Often the mattress sutures are buttressed with Teflon felt on the ventricular surface (not shown). *F.* Following insertion of the valve, a Foley catheter is placed across the valve to keep the valve incompetent and avoid air embolism. *G.* Final view of the valve in position before closure of the atriotomy. *H.* The atriotomy incision is closed around the Foley catheter, after which the heart is allowed to fill with blood and displace air. Subsequently the Foley catheter is removed, which permits the left ventricle to contract normally. (Figure continued on next page.)

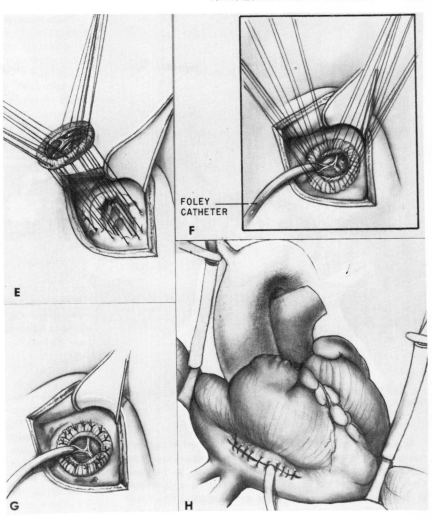

FOLEY CATHETER

Fig. 19-11 *E,F,G,H.* Continued.

20 percent vary widely. Some patients prefer a tissue prosthesis to avoid anticoagulants while others strongly prefer a metallic prosthesis with permanent anticoagulation to minimize the risk of a repeat operation. The surgical recommendation is based upon several factors, especially the intelligence and reliability of patients and their ready access to reliable medical care. This varies widely with socioeconomic circumstances. If a patient can take sodium warfarin satisfactorily, a metallic prosthesis is recommended for the majority of patients under sixty years of age. In older patients with the higher frequency of hypertension and stroke, a porcine prosthesis is usually recommended, carefully explaining the durability considerations.

Porcine prostheses are unsatisfactory in children because of the rapid development of calcification. In children, metallic prostheses are virtually the only choice available except for the antibiotic preserved aortic homograft. Although procurement of adequate homograft tissue is very difficult in most parts of the world, outstanding results have been reported from New Zealand and Australia, with excellent function in such valves for well over a decade.

PROGNOSIS. Following Commissurotomy. Following an adequate mitral commissurotomy that does not produce insufficiency, long-term prognosis is very good. As the valve is not normal, long-term function will probably be determined by the degree of fibrosis in the leaflets and the chordae. If these fibrotic changes are extensive enough to produce significant turbulent flow of blood, eventual stiffening and calcification of the leaflets is probable. However, if disease is predominantly in the commissures, excellent long-term function may be expected.

In our experience, operative mortality was 1.7 percent, long-term mortality 2.5 percent. Postoperative emboli occurred in 3 percent, often in association with failure to obliterate the left atrial appendage. Five years following operation, 87 percent of patients who had no residual valve dysfunction after operation remained free of any complications.

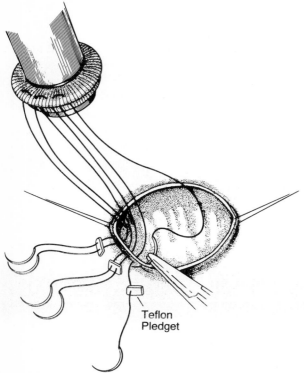

Fig. 19-12. Technique for suturing a mitral valve prosthesis with Dacron pledgets seated above the mitral annulus.

In a report by Halseth et al. only 11 percent of patients required valve replacement at operation. Operative mortality was 1.5 percent; 10-year survival was 81 percent. Only 7 percent of 191 patients required valve replacement in the next several years. In the series reported by Cohn et al. of 120 patients there were no operative deaths and five late deaths from noncardiac causes. Actuarial projections at 10 years found a survival rate near 95 percent, 91 percent freedom from emboli, 84 percent freedom from reoperation.

Fig. 19-13. Bjork-Shiley tilting disc valve.

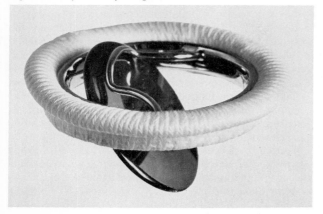

These experiences are particularly significant because during the 1950s and 1960s a recurrence rate as high as 30 to 40 percent within 5 years after operation was reported following commissurotomy, clearly in retrospect owing to an ineffective commissurotomy. Unwarranted pessimism was expressed at that time about the durability of commissurotomy, simply because residual stenosis remained following operation.

These considerations are especially pertinent now because of the recent interest in percutaneous balloon mitral valvuloplasty. The effective mitral valve area has been increased from 0.8 to 1.7 cm², but some regurgitation resulted in 43 percent of patients. The noninvasive features make balloon valvuloplasty a serious consideration in patients who are poor candidates for operation because of other diseases such as stroke or advanced age. The data do not support, however, that this procedure is more than a palliative one, with results similar to those obtained with digital commissurotomy in the early 1950s. Far better results can be obtained in good-risk patients with an open operative technique.

Following Valve Replacement. If valve replacement is necessary, long-term results are not nearly as satisfactory as those following commissurotomy. Five-year survival is near 80 percent, 10 years 60 percent. A major factor in determining 5-year survival is the severity of left ventricular failure before operation. Patients in Class II or early Class III have a 5-year survival about 90 percent while those near Class IV are about 60 percent. These data clearly indicate the importance of preoperative irreversible injury to the ventricle and, accordingly, the need for earlier operation. The frequency of emboli has decreased markedly since 1973.

In 1985 Starr summarized his 25 years of experience with over 2000 ball valve prostheses, 34 percent of which were mitral valve replacements. In 1979 Bjork described his experiences with 1800 Bjork-Shiley valves. The 5-year survival after mitral replacement was 66 percent. Frequency of thromboembolism was 4 percent per patient year and frequency of thrombosis of the prosthesis was 1 percent per year.

Edmonds et al. summarized overall reported experiences with thromboembolic complications of different types of valve prostheses. The major problem with tissue prostheses is durability with the estimated failure rate by 10 years of at least 20 percent. Oyer et al. reported a study of over 1400 patients who received Hancock prostheses. The probability of freedom from tissue failure 5 years following operation was 95 percent. At NYU 1643 porcine prostheses in 1492 patients were inserted; 556 patients have isolated mitral replacement. Freedom from late cardiac death was about 85 percent at 5 years.

When either type of prosthetic valve replacement is done, metallic or porcine, there is a small but permanent risk of endocarditis, ranging between 1 and 2 percent per patient per year. Prophylactic antibiotics should be routinely used when episodes of transient bacteremia can be anticipated, such as dental extraction or cystoscopy.

MITRAL INSUFFICIENCY

Prosthetic replacement of the mitral valve is often necessary with rheumatic mitral insufficiency, especially if valvular calcification and fibrosis are severe. If the aortic leaflet of the mitral valve is relatively free of disease, some patients may be treated with annuloplasty. Long-term results following annuloplasty in selected cases have been reported by Reed et al.

Over the past 15 years, Carpentier has serially reported impressive results with a complex mitral valve reconstruction, including excision of part of the diseased mural leaflet and reconstruction of the annulus with a prosthetic ring. Additional technical maneuvers, applicable for specific pathologic problems, include shortening of elongated chordae, attachment of flail chordae to adjacent structures of transposition of chordae. This technique has been used at NYU since 1980 in nearly 200 selected patients with excellent results to date. Long-term data are not available, but in all likelihood the Carpentier technique may be used in the majority of patients with nonrheumatic mitral insufficiency resulting from ruptured chordae tendineae, mitral prolapse, or coronary disease, because inflammatory changes do not destroy the mobility of the leaflets.

ETIOLOGY. In the United States mitral insufficiency from rheumatic fever has steadily decreased in frequency, now representing less than one-half of patients seen. The most common cause is mitral valve prolapse, often complicated by rupture of chordae tendineae. Ischemic papillary muscle disease complicating extensive occlusive disease of the coronary arteries has become an increasingly common cause. Bacterial endocarditis remains an infrequent but important cause.

It is now known that some degree of prolapse of the mitral valve is surprisingly frequent, detectable in as many as 5 percent of the normal population. In the majority of patients, the hemodynamic disturbance is minimal. In chronic cases, however, severe changes evolve with dense extensive calcification, progressive elongation of chordae, and increasing asymmetric dilatation of the annulus of the mitral valve.

PATHOLOGIC ANATOMY. The basic changes with rheumatic fever were described in the preceding section on Mitral Stenosis. Insufficiency develops from fibrosis and contraction of the mitral leaflets, usually combined with calcification restricting mobility. Fibrosis and contraction of chordae tendineae are important contributory factors. These changes are usually gradually progressive because of the turbulent flow of blood.

Carpentier, in a study of over 50 rheumatic hearts, carefully delineated the additional pathologic changes that evolve and augment the insufficiency. These are predominantly progressive elongation of chordae (as much as 5 to 10 mm) and asymmetric dilatation of the mitral annulus, as dilatation predominantly occurs in the posteromedial portion of the annulus of the mural leaflet, not involving the annulus of the aortic leaflet at all, as it is part of the basic fibrous skeleton of the heart.

PATHOPHYSIOLOGY. The basic physiologic change is elevation of left atrial pressure as blood regurgitates through the incompetent mitral valve during ventricular systole. The ventricular pressure spike is commonly to levels of 30 to 40 mmHg, but levels as high as 80 to 90 mmHg have been recorded. In diastole the left atrial pressure drops sharply to approach the left ventricular diastolic pressure, although a small gradient usually remains because of the large blood flow through the mitral valve during diastole. Mean left atrial pressure is usually 15 to 25 mmHg. The mitral regurgitation produces enlargement of the left atrium, although for unknown reasons the degree of left atrial enlargement varies greatly among different patients and is not proportional to the degree of regurgitation. In some patients with significant regurgitation only slight left atrial enlargement is present, while in others giant left atria evolve, enlarging to contact the right chest wall. In contrast to mitral stenosis, pulmonary vascular changes appear rather late in the course of the disease, perhaps as a result of a large left atrium absorbing much of the kinetic energy of the regurgitating blood without sustained elevation of left atrial pressure. Fortunately, the dilated left ventricle with mitral insufficiency may function adequately for surprisingly long periods of time, maintaining the left ventricular diastolic pressure near the normal range of 8 to 12 mmHg until eventually left ventricular failure appears.

As there is little stasis of blood in the left atrium, in contrast to mitral stenosis, left atrial thrombosis and arterial embolism are much less frequent than with mitral stenosis.

Physical Examination. The two characteristic features of mitral insufficiency are the apical systolic murmur and the increased force of the apical impulse. The systolic murmur is heard best at the apex, which is often displaced downward and to the left from enlargement of the left ventricle. It is well transmitted to the axilla. The quality is of a harsh, blowing type. With severe insufficiency, the murmur is pansystolic, appearing immediately after the first sound and continuing until the second sound. The intensity of the murmur does not correlate with the severity of the regurgitation, but the pansystolic characteristic does. Murmurs not extending completely through systole are seen with less serious degrees of regurgitation. The systolic murmur is a highly characteristic feature of mitral insufficiency and is absent only in most unusual circumstances. A diastolic murmur is usually present in addition, resulting from increased flow across the mitral valve as a result of blood regurgitated into the atrium during systole. The absence of an opening snap and the normal quality of the first heart sound both suggest that the diastolic murmur is due to increased flow of blood rather than anatomic mitral stenosis.

CLINICAL MANIFESTATIONS. Symptoms. Patients with mild mitral insufficiency are usually asymptomatic. The diagnosis is usually made after discovery of an apical systolic murmur. In former years, mitral valve prolapse was confused with rheumatic mitral insufficiency. The development of echocardiography has greatly simplified the differential diagnosis.

With significant mitral insufficiency, the most common

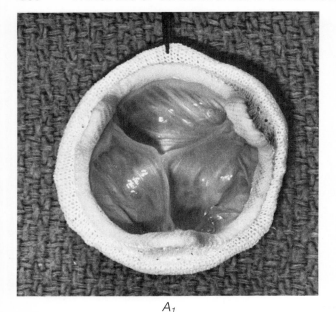

A₁

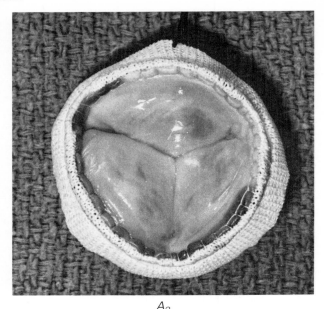

A₂

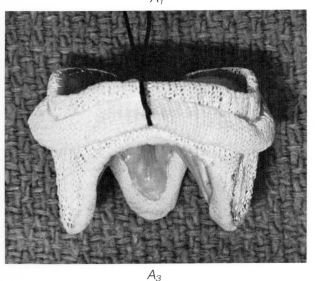

A₃

Fig. 19-14. *A.* Carpentier-Edwards porcine aortic valve prosthesis. *A₁.* Aortic view; *A₂.* Ventricular view; *A₃.* Side view. *B.* Ionescu bovine pericardial prosthesis. *B₁.* Aortic view; *B₂.* Ventricular view; *B₃.* Side view.

symptoms are fatigue, dyspnea on exertion, and palpitation. A most important point is that these symptoms may remain mild despite impressive physical findings of mitral insufficiency with progressive cardiac enlargement. Eventually, left ventricular failure evolves with a rise in end-diastolic pressure and progressive pulmonary congestion. Respiratory symptoms become prominent with exertional dyspnea, cough, and paroxysmal nocturnal dyspnea.

The apical impulse is usually forceful and prolonged, occupying an area of 3 to 4 cm^2. The first heart sound is usually normal, though it may be confused with the early onset of the systolic murmur.

LABORATORY EXAMINATIONS. The chest x-ray shows enlargement of both the left ventricle and the left atrium

(Fig. 19-15). In some patients, massive enlargement of the left atrium occurs with the wall of the atrium extending to the right chest wall and producing a grotesque deformity. The electrocardiogram does not contribute materially to the diagnosis. It may be normal with significant disease. In about 50 percent of patients, left ventricular hypertrophy can be recognized. 2-D echocardiography combined with Doppler flow studies can reasonably approximate the degree of regurgitation, though the method is far from quantitatively reliable.

The most precise studies are obtained by cardiac catheterization and cineangiography, noting reflux of dye into the left atrium when injected into the left ventricle. With minimal or severe insufficiency the dye studies are quite satisfactory, but with intermediate forms of insufficiency, the method is only reasonably good but thus far the best one available. Left atrial pressure tracings show a prominent V wave from regurgitation of blood during systole.

TREATMENT. Indications for Operation. Symptoms of fatigue and dyspnea may remain only moderately severe for a long time despite progressive deterioration in cardiac function, as evidenced by progressive left ventricular enlargement. Selecting the proper time for operation is best done from laboratory evaluation, not from severity of symptoms. A fall in an ejection fraction with exercise, measured with radionuclide studies, is currently the best measurement of early onset of serious impairment in ventricular function. This change may well antedate visible enlargement of the left ventricle on the chest x-ray. Operation at this earlier stage will avoid the late onset of cardiac failure 3 to 5 years following valve replacement, apparently from preoperative irreversible ventricular dysfunction.

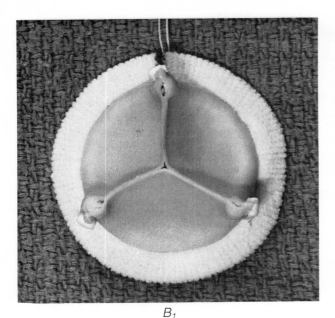

B_1

Fig. 19-14 B_1,B_2,B_3. Continued.

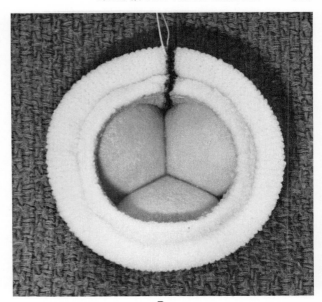

B_2

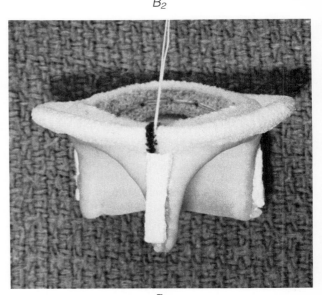

B_3

Replacement versus Reconstruction. Over the past two decades, the majority of patients have been treated with mitral valve replacement. Repair has been employed for some patients with isolated ruptured chordae of the mural leaflet, using the technique developed by McGoon. Reed and Claus successfully used a measured asymmetric annuloplasty for insufficiency in children and adults in whom annular dilatation was prominent. Carpentier, in Paris, France, however, for over 15 years has evaluated methods for mitral valve reconstruction, serially developing several techniques over this time. His overall experiences with over 2000 patients were summarized in 1983. Well over one-half of Carpentier's extensive experience has been with patients with rheumatic valvular disease. A question exists about the applicability of these techniques to nonrheumatic causes of mitral insufficiency, now constituting the majority of cases in this country. Since 1980, we have employed the Carpentier reconstructive techniques, with excellent results to date. The best results have been in patients with prolapse and ruptured chordae, with only one known late recurrence. Similar encouraging results have been reported by Cosgrove et al. If experiences by others in the future are similar, reconstruction, rather than replacement, may become the most commonly performed operation for nonrheumatic mitral insufficiency.

In 1980 Reed summarized experiences with 198 patients. Results were quite good, with a late mortality of only 9 percent, a low frequency of thromboembolism, and only 8 percent of patients requiring repeat operation. This operation is particularly attractive in children, avoiding the use of the Carpentier rigid annuloplasty ring. Chaval et al. described excellent results with reconstruction in 89 children, 84 of whom had rheumatic valve disease. Ten years following operation 90 percent of patients were alive, 98 percent free from thromboemboli, and 78 percent did not require reoperation.

LATE RESULTS. Late results following prosthetic valve replacement were discussed in the preceding section on Mitral Stenosis. Following successful mitral valve reconstruction, significant long-term results are not available from reports in this country except for repair of ruptured chordae. A 1986 study by Orzalak et al. assessed 131 patients who had repair of rupture chordae tendineae of the mitral valve. Mitral valve annuloplasty was performed in addition to leaflet repair in 88 percent of patients. The probability of the patient's requiring a repeat operation was near 10 percent at 5 years, rising to about 25 percent at 10 years. Recurrent rupture of chordae did not occur, a curious phenomenon noted by others.

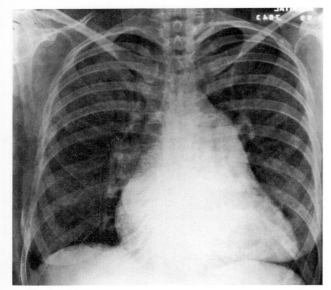

Fig. 19-15. Chest radiograph of a patient with mitral insufficiency. The distinctive features include an enlarged cardiac shadow with a prominent pulmonary artery. The shadow of the left atrium is visible in the right border of the cardiac shadow behind the shadow of the right atrium. The pulmonary vascular markings are prominent.

Carpentier has reported excellent long-term results at both 5 and 10 years following reconstruction. Thromboembolism after the first few months following reconstruction has been gratifyingly low, well under 1 percent per patient year. Recurrent insufficiency requiring repeat operation has occurred in a small percentage of patients each year. The majority of Carpentier's patients had rheumatic mitral insufficiency. Even better long-term results may be obtained when reconstruction has been successfully accomplished in nonrheumatic patients, especially if operation is performed before severe injury to the left ventricle has occurred.

AORTIC STENOSIS

HISTORICAL DATA. Effective surgical treatment of aortic valve disease first became possible in 1960–1961 with the development of satisfactory prosthetic valves by Starr and Edwards and by Harken and associates. Earlier attempts to correct aortic valvular disease by cusp replacement with prosthetic cusps of Teflon cloth or by extensive debridement of calcific material from calcified valve cusps initially gave satisfactory results in some patients, but a high failure rate within 1 to 2 years led to abandonment of these techniques as soon as a satisfactory prosthetic valve became available.

Several modifications of metallic prostheses have been evaluated, but only two basic designs have proved durable, the original ball valve prosthesis and the tilting disc prosthesis. Currently, the durability of these two prostheses is excellent but the major limitation of all metallic prosthetic valves has been thromboembolism, partly controlled with permanent anticoagulation. Despite careful

anticoagulation, some thromboembolic events occur with a frequency of at least 1 to 2 percent per year.

With the significant hazard of thromboembolism, there has been a long and continued investigation of tissue prostheses that often do not require permanent anticoagulation and have a much lower frequency of thromboembolism. One of the most durable has been the homograft aortic valve, first investigated by Barratt-Boyes in 1962 and still used in their institution, using the technique of antibiotic preservation developed in 1968. Currently, about 80 percent of these prostheses are functioning well 10 years following operation.

Several other tissues were evaluated and subsequently discarded because of lack of durability, including autologous fascia lata; allograft dura mater valves; and formaldehyde preserved porcine valves. Subsequently, the gluteraldehyde preserved porcine valve was introduced by Carpentier in 1968 and has subsequently become the most widely used tissue prosthesis. Bovine pericardium, gluteraldehyde treated, was developed by Ionescu but has not been as popular as the porcine valve. At present, 5-year durability with porcine valves is near 95 percent but decreases to about 80 percent at 10 years, with a sharp rise in frequency of failure rate between the eighth and tenth years. Fifteen year data are not available, but the outlook is not encouraging.

ETIOLOGY. About one-half of patients operated upon will be found to have calcification of a congenitally malformed valve, usually a bicuspid valve. Usually, there is a history of negligible disability for decades until calcification has made the valve rigid, with the time interval varying widely from the fourth or even the seventh or eighth decade. In about one-third of patients rheumatic fever is apparently the basic cause.

The third major cause, increasing in frequency with aging of the population, seems to be simply acquired calcific aortic stenosis, a process of diffuse calcification developing in cusps that are neither congenitally malformed nor show any signs of previous inflammation. It is probably similar to calcification that sporadically develops in other soft tissues with aging but is seen more frequently in patients in their seventh and eighth decades.

PATHOLOGY. The pathologic features of diseased aortic valves reviewed at operation in 374 patients were described by Subramanian. A calcified congenital bicuspid valve represented about 46 percent of the cases. The bicuspid valve was fibrosed with deposits of calcium throughout the valve substance as well as on the aortic wall immediately above and the ventricular wall immediately below. Rheumatic aortic stenosis was present in about 35 percent of cases, with the basic findings of fusion of the commissures with supraimposed calcification. In about 10 percent of patients, the disease process was apparently "acquired aortic stenosis," consisting of three leaflets of equal size without significant commissural fusion but dense infiltration of the base of the cusps, rather than the free margins, with calcium.

In older patients coronary atherosclerosis is found in a significant percentage of patients, at least 30 to 50 percent. The frequency is such that routine coronary angiography should be performed upon patients over 40 years of age before operation. With rheumatic aortic disease, mitral stenosis or insufficiency is found in a high percentage of patients. This is as expected, as the aortic valve and the mitral valve are contiguous structures.

A normal aortic valve has a cross-sectional area of 2.5 to 3.5 cm depending upon body size. Moderately severe stenosis is present when the valve orifice has narrowed to about 1.0 cm; 0.8 cm is an approximate area where operation is usually indicated because of pathophysiologic abnormalities. This is a changing field, however, so operation at an earlier time may be recommended in the future because of persistent left ventricular dysfunction following operation in a significant percentage of patients. Cross-sectional areas as low as 0.4 to 0.6 cm^2 may be found in advanced disease, often with a systolic gradient of 100 mm or greater across the valve. Usually, at catheterization a gradient of at least 50 mm is found with significant stenosis.

The increased workload on the myocardium imposed by the stenosis results in progressive concentric ventricular hypertrophy but little dilatation. For this reason heart size may appear almost normal on the chest x-ray. The left ventricular diastolic pressure becomes elevated above the upper limit of normal of 12 mm as the left ventricle gradually fails. Left atrial pressure is not elevated until left ventricular failure develops, explaining the late onset of symptoms.

Myocardial ischemia, manifested as angina pectoris, is a common symptom. This apparently results from the combination of two factors, the increased left ventricular work and myocardial hypertrophy as well as the decreased cardiac output. This factor is apparently responsible for the well-known tendency of aortic stenosis to result in "sudden death" with very few premonitory symptoms.

CLINICAL MANIFESTATIONS. Symptoms. Characteristically, there is a long asymptomatic period, sometimes for 10 to 20 years. Classical physical findings may be present with slight dyspnea on exertion as the only symptom. Three symptoms are characteristic, any or all of which may be present: angina pectoris, syncope, or dyspnea. Sudden death, which accounts for 15 to 20 percent of fatalities from aortic stenosis, becomes much more of a threat once these symptoms are present. Syncope develops in about one-third of patients. This apparently is from decreased cerebral blood flow. In some patients, it may result after minimal effort, with little warning. In a small percentage of patients it may result from a conduction abnormality, apparently an intermittent heart block from involvement of the atrioventricular node by calcium spicules arising from the stenotic valve.

Angina pectoris develops in 30 to 40 percent of patients, a manifestation of myocardial ischemia. Probably these episodes are associated with "silent" episodes of muscle necrosis because some patients with surprisingly few symptoms are found to have large amounts of myocardium replaced by scar tissue.

The average life expectancy once angina or syncope has appeared is about 3 years.

Left ventricular failure is an even more ominous finding, as the life expectancy is slightly more than a year. Atrial fibrillation, a consequence of prolonged elevation of left atrial pressure, is similarly a grave event, as it indicates an advanced stage of left ventricular failure unless mitral valve disease is present.

The cardiac size is not increased, for the principal change in the left ventricle is concentric hypertrophy, not dilatation. The apical impulse has been described as a "prolonged heave," not a "forceful thrust," as is found with ventricular dilatation from aortic or mitral insufficiency. The peripheral pulse, similarly, is slow and prolonged, well illustrated with a pulse tracing recorded by arterial puncture as a dome-shaped peak in systole, contrasting sharply with the sharp systolic upstroke seen with aortic insufficiency.

LABORATORY STUDIES. The heart size is usually normal on x-ray. Calcification of the aortic valve is usually visible in patients over thirty-five years of age.

The electrocardiogram is not reliable because of the wide variation. In some patients left ventricular hypertrophy is evident, but in some seriously ill patients with severe aortic stenosis the electrocardiogram is virtually normal. The echocardiogram may supply supportive information by noting the increased thickness of the left ventricular wall and also confirming the presence of calcification in the aortic valve. Conduction abnormalities are frequent, apparently from spicules of calcium projecting into the conduction bundle located just beneath the base of the noncoronary sinus. Some patients develop complete heart block.

Cardiac catheterization readily confirms the diagnosis, both measuring the gradient and permitting calculation of the cross-sectional area of the valve. Gradients exceeding 50 mm are usually found with significant stenosis. A cross-sectional area near 0.8 to 1.0 cm^2 is considered the range at which operation should be routinely recommended, though this concept has frequently changed toward more liberal indications for operation as results with aortic valve replacement have improved. With the current interest in balloon valvuloplasty concepts as to what represents critical aortic stenosis will change even further. Probably the best method of following asymptomatic patients and determining the time for operation is evaluation of ventricular function with radionuclide studies once or twice a year, recommending operation when there is a decrease in ejection fraction with exercise, contrary to the normal response.

At catheterization coronary arteriography should be routinely done, for associated coronary disease is found in at least 30 to 50 percent of patients studied, the frequency increasing with the age of the patient studied. Concomitant mitral valve disease and left ventricular function can also be evaluated at catheterization. In some patients with a broad thick chest and distant heart sounds because of emphysematous lungs, the physical findings are deceptively minimal, with a faint unimpressive systolic murmur being the only initial abnormality found on physical examination. In such patients, echocardiography is helpful in deciding whether catheterization should be

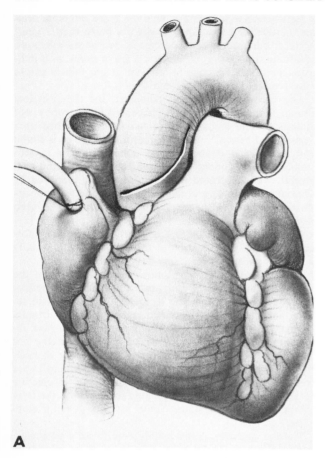

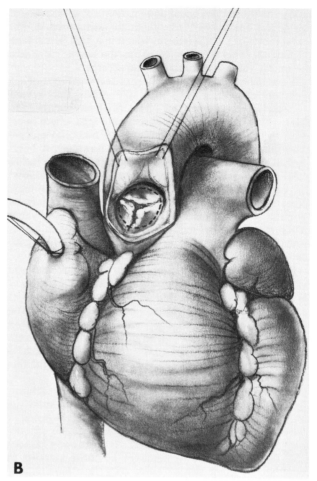

Fig. 19-16. Insertion of aortic valve prosthesis. *A.* Cardiopulmonary bypass is instituted following cannulation of the right atrium with a single large cannula. Usually the ascending aorta is cannulated for arterial return (not shown). The aorta is opened with an oblique incision, initially begun about a centimeter above the right coronary artery. *B.* The heart is arrested with the cold blood potassium technique. Coronary perfusion is no longer employed. The aortic valve is then excised, with care to avoid the loss of any calcific fragments into the ventricle that might subsequently embolize. *C.* The Carpentier porcine prosthesis, which is normally used. *D.* Valve sutured in position. *E.* Final position of the valve. Care is taken, as the valve is tied in position, to seat the valve well below the coronary ostia, actually farther below than is shown here. *F.* The aortotomy is closed with a continuous synthetic suture.

done, for a benign aortic systolic murmur becomes increasingly common in older age groups.

TREATMENT. Indications for Operation. In asymptomatic patients, the finding at catheterization of an aortic cross-sectional area of 0.8 cm is clearly an indication for operation. Sudden death remains a small but definite hazard in such patients, so operation should be clearly urged despite the well-being of the patient. In the presence of any of the classic three symptoms, angina, syncope, or dyspnea, operation should similarly be strongly recommended, especially if catheterization demonstrates an aortic valve area near 1.0 cm^2 or less. The frequency of sudden death increases sharply in symptomatic patients.

Technique of Operation (Fig. 19-16). The operative technique is a standard one, using a median sternotomy, cardiopulmonary bypass with hyperkalemic cardioplegia induced with cold blood. If aortic insufficiency is not present, cardiac arrest may be induced by clamping the aorta and infusing cold blood directly into the aortic root. Otherwise, the aorta is clamped and opened, following which cold blood is directly infused into the coronary ostia through a hand-held metallic or silastic coronary cannula. With direct ostial infusion, pressure and flow should be monitored, for excessive flows can induce myocardial edema. Once the heart has arrested, the calculated orifice pressure should be in the range of 50 to

60 mm, usually corresponding with a flow rate near 200 mL/min in a normal left coronary ostium and near 100/min in a right coronary. The flow rates, of course, vary with the size of the coronary arteries. A large amount of cold blood is used, serially monitoring the different areas of the myocardium to be certain that all areas are cooled below 15°C, requiring 1500 to 2000 mL of blood in some patients. Measuring myocardial temperature in at least four zones of the heart with a needle thermistor confirms equal infusion of cold blood. Subsequently, topical hypothermia is routinely employed with

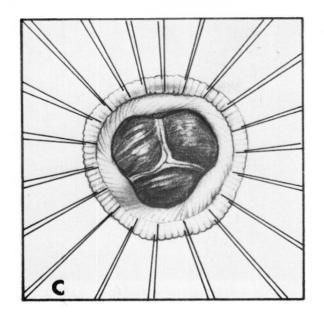

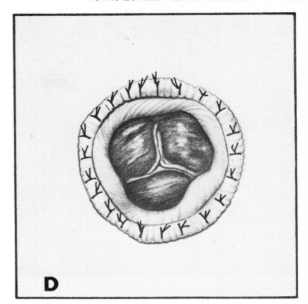

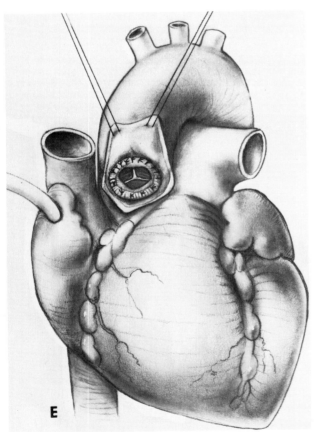

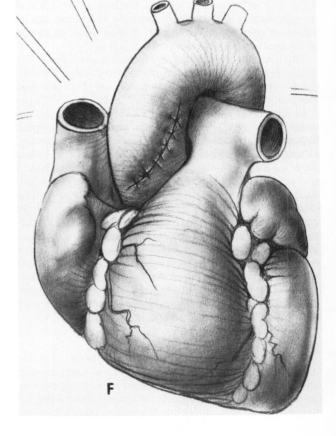

Fig. 19-16 *C,D,E,F.* Continued.

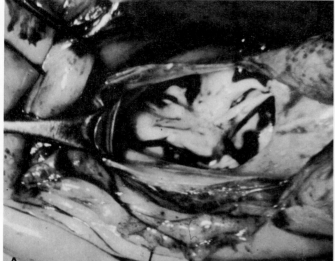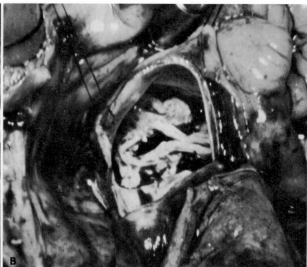

Fig. 19-17. *A.* Stenotic aortic valve exposed during cardiopulmonary bypass through a transverse aortotomy. The valve orifice has been almost obliterated by calcification and apposition of the cusps. *B.* Calcified aortic valve in another patient exposed through a transverse aortotomy. Fusion has produced a small eccentric rigid ostium that is both stenotic and insufficient.

Fig. 19-18. Calcified fragments removed with rongeurs from a patient with severe aortic stenosis. The multiplicity of such fragments emphasizes the grave risk of embolization of calcified material during aortic valve replacement with reduction of severe or fatal neurologic injury. Careful packing of the ventricle with gauze before removal of the calcified valve is essential.

large volumes of a cold electrolyte solution, both filling the pericardium and subsequently wrapping the heart in a laparotomy pad and using a constant infusion of cold fluid. The effectiveness of this method of myocardial preservation is extraordinary because the heart can be safely arrested for 3 h or longer, though this long period of time is seldom necessary.

This form of myocardial preservation provides a dry quiet operative field that has made aortic valve replacement a procedure with a remarkably low mortality and morbidity.

In almost all patients, aortic valve replacement is required (Fig. 19-17). A few elderly patients with a small hypoplastic annulus have been treated by debridement, as long as this does not produce insufficiency. This procedure had a disappointing frequency of recurrence within 3 to 5 years and should be considered a palliative procedure used only when special circumstances indicate prosthetic replacement would be hazardous or unsatisfactory. Great care is taken at operation to avoid losing any calcific fragments detached during removal of the valve that could subsequently be embolized (Fig. 19-18). A gauze pack is routinely placed in the ventricle before removal of the valve is begun. A number of maneuvers during the procedure (frequent removal of the pack, lavage of the ventricle, and keeping the ventricular cavity dry with a vent inserted through the left atrium across the mitral valve) make it possible to avoid emboli in the vast majority of patients.

The choice of a metallic or porcine prosthetic valve was discussed in the section on Mitral Valve Replacement, emphasizing that the surgeon should make a recommendation based upon the specific characteristics of the patient but also emphasizing that the patient should have the final decision. At NYU either the Bjork disc prosthesis or the Starr-Edwards ball valve prosthesis has been used, though recently a small number of the St. Jude metallic

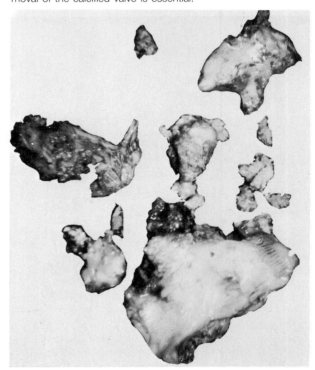

prostheses have been inserted. A larger cross-sectional area with less hemolysis can be obtained with a disc prosthesis than with a ball valve but has the hazard of the rare but catastrophic thrombosis of the prosthesis, virtually unknown with a ball valve prosthesis. A 23-mm Bjork prosthesis, with a cross-sectional area of 250 mm^2, is suitable for the majority of patients, using the 21-mm size for those with a small stature.

With tissue prostheses, the Carpentier porcine prosthesis is currently the most popular. There is less flexibility of valve size with porcine prostheses. A 23-mm valve is satisfactory for most patients under 140 lb, but a larger size is needed otherwise. The 21 mm is too small for all but patients of small stature. A pledgeted mattress suture technique is used routinely, probably unnecessary in many patients, but it clearly virtually eliminates the hazard of periprosthetic leaks (see Fig. 19-12).

The left ventricular-aortic systolic gradient is routinely measured following bypass. Depending upon the cardiac output, a gradient is rarely larger than 10 to 20 mm if a prosthesis of adequate size has been chosen.

Associated coronary disease is present in a large percentage of patients and is usually routinely bypassed at the time of operation.

POSTOPERATIVE CARE. Postoperative care is usually uneventful. Arrhythmias are among the more frequent complications, so 24-h monitoring of the cardiac rhythm with an oscilloscope is routinely done for 2 to 3 days. Pacemaker wires are routinely left in the right ventricle and atrium for 4 to 5 days.

Anticoagulant therapy is started 2 to 3 days following operation, keeping the prothrombin time near 20 s. The anticoagulation program routinely used for tissue valves and metallic valves is discussed under Mitral Valve Replacement.

Except for patients with serious preoperative ventricular dysfunction, patients become asymptomatic with a normal range of physical activity within 2 to 3 months following operation. Permanent periodic medical supervision, however, should be done for all patients because of the problems inherent with any prosthetic valve. Thromboembolism, anticoagulant hemorrhage, and endocarditis are the three principal complications of any patient with a prosthetic valve that requires periodic monitoring. With current prostheses and good anticoagulant therapy, thromboembolism occurs with a frequency of 1 to 2 percent per year in most reports, but fortunately most of these are small. Bloomfield reported an analysis of 540 patients with a disc or a porcine prosthesis inserted, finding no significant difference in the frequency of thromboembolism in patients with different prostheses. Endocarditis remains a grave hazard in any patient if a transient bacteremia occurs, such as a dental extraction or a cystoscopy.

Patients with significant cardiac enlargement and decreased ventricular function following operation should be monitored closely. How carefully this should be done is yet unclear because there remains a significant frequency of sudden death within the first 3 to 5 years following operation. A sobering point is the fact that there is a *greater* risk of death within the first 1 to 2 years following leaving the hospital than from the operation itself.

PROGNOSIS. The operative mortality from aortic valve replacement is at a remarkably low level, usually between 1 and 2 percent for uncomplicated patients, and seldom exceeding 10 percent, even with far advanced complex problems. Christakis et al. reported an analysis of over 40 variables influencing operative results. Operative death was usually a result of operative hemorrhage, or subsequent arrhythmias. Heart block has become uncommon.

Five-year survival in the usual patient is now near 85 to 90 percent. With severe impairment of ventricular function before operation, however, 5-year survival is much smaller, in the range of 60 to 70 percent, emphasizing the need for prompt operation in asymptomatic patients when signs of impaired ventricular function are found with laboratory studies.

Mortality in the first 5 years after operation is due to cardiac causes in at least 50 percent of cases; a significant number of deaths occur suddenly. This fact emphasizes that most patients are currently operated upon after significant permanent ventricular injury has occurred.

In the past 1 to 2 years there has been considerable interest in percutaneous balloon valvuloplasty as a palliative procedure. At present, all physiologic data would indicate that balloon valvuloplasty should be restricted to high-risk elderly patients in whom short-term palliation seems the best immediate goal. Its application to good-risk patients, knowing the excellent results with prosthetic replacement, would seem unwarranted, especially because of the insidious development of permanent injury to the left ventricle in patients who have few symptoms.

AORTIC INSUFFICIENCY

ETIOLOGY AND PATHOLOGY. A variety of diseases can produce aortic insufficiency. Inflammatory disease is a frequent cause. At present, perhaps the most common is bacterial endocarditis that has produced destruction or perforation of a valve cusp. Rheumatic fever was formerly the most common inflammatory disease but is steadily declining in frequency in the United States (Fig. 19-19). Syphilis is now a rarity.

Annular ectasia is an unusual type of collagen disease seen with increasing frequency as the average age of the population increases. This is seen in the most extreme form with the classic Marfan's syndrome with extensive cystic medial necrosis in the aorta, most probably in the ascending aorta. The aortic root gradually enlarges, starting in the sinuses of Valsalva and progressing to a discrete aneurysm in the ascending aorta. The pathology is unusual as the dilatation decreases and almost stops at the level of the innominate artery. The size and shape of the aneurysm is quite characteristic, resembling a truncated cone with the narrow apex near the level of the innominate artery. Aortic insufficiency results from dilatation of the aortic ring.

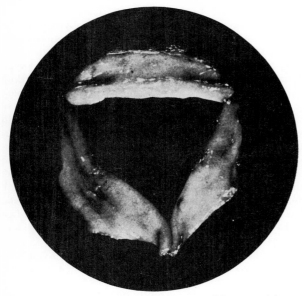

Fig. 19-19. Three aortic valve cusps removed from an eighteen-year-old boy with rheumatic aortic insufficiency. The contracted free margins of each cusp are clearly shown, illustrating the mechanism of production of aortic insufficiency from contracture and retraction of the free margins of the aortic valve cusps.

In less severe forms, there is simply a localized aneurysm in the ascending aorta with or without aortic insufficiency and no other signs of connective tissue disease; histologic examination of the excised aneurysm usually finds the characteristic cystic medial necrosis. Atherosclerotic aneurysms produce insufficiency by dilatation of the ring, though the histologic disease in the aorta is principally in the intima and media, contrasting markedly to that with cystic medial necrosis.

Another variant of collagen disease is the so-called floppy valve, a type of myxomatous degeneration of the valve that becomes elongated and sags into the ventricular lumen, often with no other histologic abnormality. The gross appearance suggests a variant of the more common mitral valve prolapse.

A dissecting aneurysm produces insufficiency by dissection of the aortic wall with detachment and prolapse of the valve cusps, usually the noncoronary. Congenital aortic insufficiency is rarely present at birth but may develop in older patients if stiffening and calcification of the malformed valve produces an insufficient rather than a stenotic valve.

The cardiac response to blood regurgitating into the left ventricle in diastole is an increase in left ventricular stroke volume, accomplished by dilatation of the heart. This results in gradual dilatation of the left ventricle, producing some of the largest hearts seen in clinical cardiology in neglected cases, with an apex of the left ventricle that extends almost to the chest wall and a cardiac weight approaching 1000 g. This cardiac response is quite different from that with aortic stenosis, where concentric muscular hypertrophy with little dilatation is the predominant change.

PATHOPHYSIOLOGY. Surprisingly large volumes of blood regurgitate into the ventricle with severe aortic insufficiency. This may be two or three times greater than the normal stroke volume of 60 to 75 mL. The compensatory ability of the heart is remarkable, as this increased workload may be tolerated for 10 to 15 years or longer. There is little elevation in left ventricular diastolic pressure until cardiac failure develops. There is no increase in left atrial pressure or pulmonary congestion until the onset of cardiac failure, so symptoms of pulmonary congestion appear only with advanced disease, completely contrasting to their early appearance with mitral stenosis. As severe cardiac failure progresses, left ventricular end-diastolic pressure rises to 20 to 30 mm. At this time, the clinical findings of insufficiency may actually decrease because the volume of blood regurgitating during diastole is less.

With marked dilatation of the left ventricle some mitral insufficiency may develop from dilatation of the annulus of the mitral valve. When a rheumatic history is present, it is difficult, or impossible, to determine from angiography whether the mitral insufficiency represents simple dilatation or rheumatic valvulitis. Mitral insufficiency resulting from simple dilatation of the mitral ring usually regresses satisfactorily following replacement of the aortic valve.

CLINICAL MANIFESTATIONS. Symptoms. There is naturally a wide variability in the rate of progression of symptoms, depending upon the degree of insufficiency. A symptom-free period of 8 to 10 years is common, but once symptoms appear, death has usually occurred in the past within 4 or 5 years. In general, citing statistics from the presurgical era, about 40 percent of patients died within 10 years, another 50 percent within 20 years. The terminal illness is usually progressive cardiac failure, as sudden death is much less common than with aortic stenosis.

Palpitation is one of the earliest, nonspecific symptoms, apparently arising from forceful contraction of the dilated left ventricle. Angina pectoris is a common symptom with advanced disease, usually with severe aortic incompetence in which the regurgitant flow is more than 50 percent of forward flow. Dyspnea with exertion appears fairly early during the progression of the disease and gradually increases in severity.

Physical Examination. Palpation readily discloses a prominent cardiac impulse, located downward and to the left of the normal location. The hallmark of aortic insufficiency is a high-pitched decrescendo diastolic murmur along the left sternal border, starting immediately after the second sound. The length of the murmur corresponds somewhat with the severity of the insufficiency. If the murmur is loudest to the right of the sternum, dilatation of the aortic ring, as in Marfan's syndrome, is likely. An ejection systolic murmur of moderate intensity is also frequent.

Examination of the peripheral arterial circulation usually finds several abnormalities. The pulse pressure is increased, partly from an increase in systolic pressure but principally from a decrease in diastolic pressure below the normal range near 80 mm. The diastolic pressure may be as low as 40 mm, but true diastolic pressure, measured by direct arterial puncture, is never less than 30 to 35 mmHg, even though on auscultation a diastolic pressure of 0 may be obtained from dilatation of peripheral arteries. The exact level of diastolic pressure does not closely correlate with the severity of the aortic insufficiency because of the influence of peripheral resistance. With vasodilatation, diastolic pressure may be low without marked regurgitation while conversely, with severe vasoconstriction, diastolic pressure may be elevated but severe regurgitation present.

Peripheral pulses are usually visible, forceful, and bounding. "Pistol shot" sounds are readily heard with the stethoscope over peripheral arteries. A wide variety of other auscultatory phenomena have been described, some over a century ago, all of which indicate vasodilatation and a hyperactive peripheral circulation.

LABORATORY STUDIES AND DIAGNOSIS. The chest x-ray shows enlargement of the left ventricle with the apex displaced downward and to the left. As the normal cardiothoracic ratio is 0.5 or less, asymptomatic patients may be periodically followed with biannual x-rays, as long as the heart size is normal. The size of the left ventricle can be evaluated more precisely with 2-D echocardiography. The electrocardiogram is normal early in the disease, but with cardiac enlargement signs of left ventricular hypertrophy become prominent. The cardiac rhythm usually remains sinus. Atrial fibrillation is uncommon before advanced disease is present and has an ominous prognosis unless it arises from another cause. Its presence from aortic insufficiency indicates an elevation of left ventricular end-diastolic pressure long enough to produce left atrial hypertrophy. Findings on cardiac catheterization are usually normal except for the visible reflux of dye from the aortic root into the ventricle with angiography. With cardiac failure, left ventricular end-diastolic pressure rises above the normal limit of 12 mm. Values of 15 to 20 are common with early cardiac decompensation.

It has long been recognized that postponing operation until symptoms are disabling is not satisfactory, for some patients with early onset of symptoms already have substantial enlargement of the left ventricle and die from cardiac failure in the next 3 to 5 years despite correction of the insufficiency. Hence, clinical investigation for some time has sought a laboratory measurement that would identify the proper time for operation. Simply using changes in the cardiothoracic ratio is also unsatisfactory, for cardiac enlargement to a cardiothoracic ratio of 0.6 or greater indicates advanced disease.

At present, demonstrating a fall in ejection fraction with exercise with radionuclide studies seems one of the best indicators that operation should be performed in asymptomatic patients. The reliability of this "early warning" signs is not yet proved by 5- to 10-year postoperative data because the key question is whether a significant number of patients will continue to die from left ventricular dysfunction in the first 5 years after operation. This has certainly been true in past years when less sensitive criteria were used. Henry assessed echocardio-

graphic findings in this regard, and recommended operation when end-systolic dimension had enlarged to 55 mm.

TREATMENT. The principal decision with treatment is deciding when to operate. In some patients who are still alive despite advanced left ventricular dysfunction, with an end-diastolic pressure of 30 mm or above, uncertainty exists about how much improvement can be expected from aortic valve replacement, as it often appears that the principal symptoms are advanced left ventricular dysfunction (or "myopathy"). Available studies do not permit a precise decision in this regard. In even the most advanced cases, valve replacement can usually be performed with an operative risk less than 10 percent. As death is virtually a certainty unless operation is done, operation is rarely contraindicated on the basis of left ventricular dysfunction, carefully explaining to the patient and the family beforehand that the degree of improvement following operation may be limited and cannot be known with any certainty for at least 6 to 12 months following operation.

The operative technique, choice of valve, postoperative care, and prognosis are very similar to those discussed in the section on Aortic Stenosis.

TRICUSPID STENOSIS AND INSUFFICIENCY

ETIOLOGY. Organic disease of the tricuspid valve is almost always due to rheumatic fever. With the exception of septic endocarditis, usually in drug addicts, it virtually never occurs as an isolated lesion, but only in association with extensive disease of the mitral valve. With mitral disease the frequency of associated tricuspid disease is near 10 to 15 percent, although an incidence as high as 30 percent has been reported. Rarely, blunt trauma produces rupture of a papillary muscle or chordae with resulting tricuspid insufficiency.

Tricuspid insufficiency is the more common lesion encountered; pure stenosis is infrequent, as stenotic lesions usually have concomitant insufficiency. Functional tricuspid insufficiency is much more common than insufficiency from organic disease. It develops from dilatation of the tricuspid annulus and right ventricle as a result of pulmonary hypertension and right ventricular failure. These abnormalities, in turn, result from left ventricular failure and chronic elevation of left atrial pressure.

PATHOLOGY. With tricuspid stenosis the pathologic changes are similar to those found with the more familiar mitral stenosis. There is fusion of the commissures to form a small central opening 1 to 1.5 cm in diameter. As right atrial pressure is normally only 4 to 5 mmHg, significant tricuspid stenosis may be present with a valve orifice considerably larger than that seen with mitral stenosis.

Tricuspid insufficiency results from fibrosis and contraction of the valve leaflets, often in association with shortening and fusion of chordae tendineae. Calcification is rare. With dilation of the tricuspid annulus the valve leaflets appear stretched but otherwise are pliable and seemingly normal even though serious regurgitation is present. Apparently the dilatation and deformity of the annulus are irreversible. Valves with functional tricuspid insufficiency usually do not regain competency, even though the mitral valve disease is corrected and pulmonary artery systolic pressure returns to normal.

PATHOPHYSIOLOGY. With tricuspid stenosis the mean right atrial pressure is elevated to 10 to 20 mmHg. The higher pressures are found with a tricuspid valve orifice smaller than 1.5 cm^2 and a mean diastolic gradient between the atrium and ventricle of 5 to 15 mmHg. A gradient above 5 mm represents significant tricuspid stenosis. When mean right atrial pressure remains above 10 to 15 mmHg, edema and ascites usually appear.

A moderate degree of tricuspid insufficiency may be tolerated, with little adverse influence on the circulation except for a decrease in cardiac output. This is in striking contrast to mitral insufficiency, where the regurgitating blood and elevation of left atrial pressure produces pulmonary congestion. The unusual patient with isolated tricuspid insufficiency produced by a traumatic injury may do well for years, as the only physiologic disturbance is elevation of venous pressure and a decrease in cardiac output. The purest example of the surprising tolerance for tricuspid insufficiency is seen in the drug addict with septic endocarditis who has been treated by total excision of the tricuspid valve. Some, but not all, patients tolerate absence of the tricuspid valve with total tricuspid insufficiency for months or years.

CLINICAL MANIFESTATIONS. The symptoms and signs of tricuspid valve disease are similar to those of right heart failure resulting from mitral valve disease. These all result from chronic elevation of right atrial pressure above 5 to 10 mm. The most familiar ones are edema, ascites, and hepatomegaly. Characteristic murmurs are present and may be associated with hepatic pulsations. As similar findings result from right heart failure without tricuspid disease, the concomitant presence of tricuspid disease in the patient in heart failure with mitral valve disease may be easily overlooked.

Physical Examination. The characteristic murmur of tricuspid stenosis is best heard as a diastolic murmur at the lower end of the sternum. It is a low-pitched murmur of medium intensity and can easily be overlooked, as it is well localized at the lower end of the sternum. During inspiration the intensity of the murmur increases as the volume of blood returning to the heart is temporarily increased by an increase in intrathoracic negative pressure. Tricuspid insufficiency produces a prominent systolic murmur at the lower end of the sternum and also at the cardiac apex, where it may be confused with the systolic murmur of mitral insufficiency. The murmur is often seen in association with an enlarged pulsating liver and prominent engorged peripheral veins. A prominent jugular pulse, especially when the cardiac rhythm is sinus, may be the best clue to unsuspected tricuspid disease.

LABORATORY STUDIES. The x-ray will show enlargement of the right atrium and right ventricle. Prominent P waves may be visible on the electrocardiogram if a sinus rhythm is present. Echocardiography will confirm enlargement of the right atrium and ventricle and may be helpful with Doppler studies in recognizing tricuspid in-

sufficiency. Cardiac catheterization and angiography are required to confirm the diagnosis. Tricuspid stenosis can be confirmed by demonstrating a diastolic gradient between the atrium and ventricle above 4 to 5 mm. As the gradient is small, precise measurements are essential. Cineangiography is the best method for detecting insufficiency but is not always satisfactory because the catheter through which the dye is injected is lying across the tricuspid orifice and may deform the valve leaflets.

Carpentier has cautioned that palpation at the time of operation may be unreliable. If the blood volume and cardiac output are adequate, palpation has been quite reliable in our experience. It should be emphasized that the regurgitant jet is quite different from that present with mitral disease, as the pressures are lower. The jet is of lower volume and much more diffuse.

TREATMENT. Usually the surgical decision about tricuspid insufficiency is a tentative one until the valve is examined at operation. Mild degrees of tricuspid insufficiency are usually left alone, especially in the absence of pulmonary hypertension. The degree of hypertrophy of the right atrial wall is a helpful guide, as the absence of significant right atrial hypertrophy indicates that chronic severe elevation of right atrial pressure has not been present.

With significant tricuspid insufficiency, annuloplasty or tricuspid replacement should usually be done. Precise data confirming the importance of correcting the tricuspid disease in association with mitral valvular disease are virtually impossible to obtain because the hemodynamic changes following correction of the mitral disease far overshadow those of tricuspid disease. However, the significant improvement in cardiac output in the rare patient with isolated tricuspid insufficiency following trauma is the best example of the magnitude of benefit that may be achieved.

In the majority of patients seen clinically, tricuspid disease is due to dilatation of the annulus, as evidenced not only by the large annulus but also by the absence of fibrotic changes in the leaflets. Usually, the leaflets appear entirely normal. Virtually all such patients can be treated by an annuloplasty. For over a decade at NYU a simple posterior leaflet annuloplasty as described by Boyd from our institution in 1974 has been quite satisfactory. The Carpentier ring annuloplasty is a bit more complicated with slight risk of heart block. Excellent results have been reported by Carpentier et al. and by Kirklin et al. The DeVega annuloplasty (a purse-string suture technique) has been widely used, but at least two groups have described a significant late failure rate. In our experience, the posterior leaflet annuloplasty is simpler and safer in the absence of significant leaflet disease or pulmonary hypertension.

In the minority of patients with tricuspid stenosis from commissural fusion, a commissurotomy may be performed. This may often be combined with annuloplasty.

Valve replacement is seldom necessary except in patients with significant pulmonary hypertension and leaflet disease precluding annuloplasty. In a 1986 report of experiences with 151 valve replacements and 63 valve repairs, the prosthetic valve subsequently had to be replaced in 20

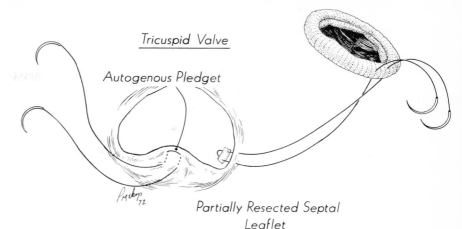

Tricuspid Valve

Autogenous Pledget

Partially Resected Septal
Leaflet

Fig. 19-20. Technique for suturing the tricuspid valve prosthesis with Dacron pledgets seated below the tricuspid annulus. The pledgets are used in all areas except the area of the partially resected septal leaflet, which is used as an autogenous pledget to avoid the conduction bundle and the production of heart block.

patients, principally because of progressive thrombosis. These included both ball valves and disc valves. Significant 10-year durability data with porcine prostheses are not yet available, though durability should be higher than the 85 to 90 percent 10-year durability with mitral or aortic porcine prostheses, where higher pressures are present.

Barratt-Boyes et al. preferred an aortic or pulmonary homograft valve, citing experiences with 75 patients, 70 percent of whom were free of valve dysfunction 8 years following operation.

The ball valve prosthesis was initially widely used for tricuspid replacement, but reports of late disastrous thrombotic encapsulation of the cage and ball led to a search for a better prosthesis. The Bjork disc prosthesis has been the preferred mechanical low-profile prosthesis, but the frequency of thrombotic occlusion seems even higher than with the ball valve. At present, any type of prosthesis may ultimately require reoperation, either for thrombosis with a mechanical prosthesis or for biologic deterioration with a porcine prosthesis.

When the prosthetic valve is inserted, particular care is required along the septal leaflet where the conduction bundle is located between the coronary sinus and the ventricular septum. In this area sutures should be placed through the base of the septal leaflet to avoid injury to the conduction bundle (Fig. 19-20). Nevertheless, a heart block may develop sometime after operation, probably a result of an inflammatory reaction stimulated by the prosthetic valve ring.

In the unfortunate patient with septic tricuspid endocarditis, almost always a drug addict, Arbulu demonstrated that total excision of the tricuspid valve *without replacement* could be tolerated. This approach permitted removal of all infected tissue without insertion of a foreign body, increasing the likelihood of cure of the endocarditis with antibiotics. Of the 50 long-term survivors, 11

subsequently required prosthetic replacement. The 15-year survival in this group was near 63 percent, and the majority of late deaths was due to recurrent drug addiction. Stern and Frater questioned this approach, stating that there was little proof that insertion of a prosthetic valve was associated with an immediate high frequency of recurrent endocarditis if the proper antibiotic was given for the infectious organism present.

Operative risk for isolated tricuspid disease is very small, 1 to 2 percent. In previous years, the reported mortality for patients undergoing tricuspid surgery in conjunction with aortic or mitral surgery was high, 25 to 40 percent, primarily because the presence of tricuspid disease represented far advanced cardiac failure. An additional cause of high mortality was probably inadequate myocardial preservation of the hypertrophied right ventricle. With present techniques, however, tricuspid surgery seems to add little increased risk to concomitant aortic or mitral surgery.

PROGNOSIS. Starr reported that 5-year survival was 59 percent, 10-year survival 36 percent with mechanical prostheses, and virtually identical with repair techniques, indicating that long-term prognosis is principally determined by residual myocardial function. Peterffy described hemodynamic findings months or years following tricuspid valve replacement or repair. Higher pressures were found in patients with a tricuspid replacement with a disc prosthesis; postoperative right atrial pressure averaged 11 mm, rising to 17 with exercise. With repair, lower pressures were found, 7 mm at rest, 14 with exercise.

MULTIVALVULAR HEART DISEASE

With rheumatic heart disease, more than one cardiac valve is frequently involved. Prominent signs of disease in one valve can readily mask disease in others. Echocardiography is a valuable noninvasive technique for suggesting that multivalvular disease is present. An important principle at cardiac catheterization with cineangiography is to evaluate all cardiac valves with a combined right and left heart catheterization. With present operative techniques, usually disease in all involved valves can be corrected at operation. Tricuspid disease is one of the most difficult to recognize. This is one of the great advantages of the sternotomy incision, routinely palpating the tricuspid valve with a finger introduced into the right atrial cavity before bypass is started.

MITRAL STENOSIS AND AORTIC STENOSIS. In this type of multivalvular disease the clinical signs of mitral stenosis with pulmonary congestion overshadow those of aortic stenosis because the volume of blood entering the left ventricle is restricted by the stenotic mitral valve. An aortic valve gradient of only 20 to 30 mm may be present if cardiac output is low, but calculation of the cross-sectional area of the aortic valve will precisely diagnose the degree of stenosis. If uncertainty remains, the valve can be examined directly at operation.

MITRAL STENOSIS AND AORTIC INSUFFICIENCY. If aortic insufficiency is prominent, mitral stenosis can easily be overlooked because the classic diastolic rumble of mitral stenosis is overshadowed by the prominent aortic murmurs. Precise cardiac catheterization should make the diagnosis. If there is any uncertainty at operation, the mitral valve should be explored by incising the left atrium.

A difficult clinical problem exists with severe mitral stenosis and minimal to moderate aortic insufficiency. The reduced flow through the mitral valve minimizes the effect of the aortic insufficiency, which may become more troublesome following correction of the mitral stenosis. A final decision must often be made at operation, noting the degree of left ventricular hypertrophy that is present.

MITRAL STENOSIS AND TRICUSPID DISEASE. Tricuspid disease is virtually always associated with severe mitral disease. As physical findings may not be prominent, the *routine palpation of the tricuspid valve* at the time of any mitral valve operation is most important.

AORTIC DISEASE AND FUNCTIONAL MITRAL INSUFFICIENCY. With dilatation of the left ventricle from cardiac failure from aortic insufficiency, dilatation of the mitral annulus can produce functional mitral insufficiency without intrinsic valvular disease. A final decision must usually be made at operation, opening the left atrium and inspecting the mitral valve. Preoperative angiography unfortunately is often indeterminate about the importance of "moderate" mitral insufficiency. With the reliability of the mitral valve reconstructive techniques, especially the annuloplasty ring, significant mitral insufficiency can usually be corrected by reconstruction rather than concomitant mitral valve replacement. Prosthetic valve replacement is probably only necessary in the rare instance of severe leaflet disease, a decision easily made when the valve is inspected at operation.

TRIVALVULAR DISEASE. Severe trivalvular disease is now a rarity because of the decreasing frequency of rheumatic fever. In some patients with advanced heart failure and pulmonary hypertension from aortic and mitral disease, significant tricuspid insufficiency is present from dilatation of the annulus. In such patients tricuspid annuloplasty is usually successful. Replacement of all three

cardiac valves with mechanical prostheses is now seldom necessary.

CARDIAC TRAUMA

Penetrating Trauma

In 1896, Rehn first successfully sutured a stab wound of the heart, but for decades this remained an isolated historic achievement. The hazards of thoracotomy were the principal reason that the 1943 contribution of Blalock and Ravitch, when they introduced pericardial aspiration as a method of treatment for tamponade following penetrating injuries of the heart, was such a significant one. They recognized that many patients survived because the development of tamponade prevented exsanguination. Aspiration remained a definitive and reasonably effective form of therapy for tamponade for over 25 years, but with further advances in therapy has been almost completely replaced for the past two decades with prompt thoracotomy. Aspiration is now used primarily for resuscitation as a lifesaving method of treatment. Removal of as little as 15 to 20 mL of blood by subxyphoid aspiration may abort impending cardiac arrest.

ETIOLOGY AND PATHOLOGY. The two life-threatening problems are tamponade and hemorrhage. Tamponade develops rapidly as the normal pericardium can accommodate only 100 to 250 mL of blood. Small wounds, such as those from an icepick or a knife, often produce tamponade because the laceration in the pericardium is small. Larger wounds, produced by bullets or large knives, threaten immediate death from exsanguination as blood can be expelled through the pericardial laceration into the pleural cavity. The right ventricle, which constitutes most of the anterior portion of the heart, is the cardiac chamber most frequently injured.

TREATMENT. The dominant problem may be hemorrhage, tamponade, or both. The patient should obviously be taken to the operating room as quickly as possible, which will vary with the circumstances and the hospital environment. As stated by Kirklin and Barratt Boyes, "No more than 5 min need elapse between admission and the patient's transfer to the operating table." Rapid transfusion of fluids, intubation, and immediate transportation to the operating room are the key principles in treatment.

Emergency room thoracotomy is frequently done in some institutions, including Bellevue Hospital. It may be lifesaving in some patients with agonal respirations or cardiac arrest but is probably futile with established cardiac arrest and dilated pupils indicating brain injury. After emergency thoracotomy temporary hemostasis may permit restoration of cardiac function long enough for transportation to the operating room. Ivatory reported experiences with emergency room thoracotomy in 22 patients without detectable vital signs. Cardiac function was restored in 16 of these, eight of whom eventually recovered without objective neurologic injury.

An emergency unsterile thoracotomy can be quickly done in less than 1 to 2 min by a trained surgeon. With the patient in a slight left anterolateral position, a curved skin incision is made beneath the left nipple to parallel the intercostal spaces. The fourth or fifth intercostal space should be entered, as the pectoralis major arises from the third to the fifth ribs and causes troublesome bleeding with a higher incision. Once the pleural space is entered, the intercostal incision can be quickly completed with scissors, or the fingers separating the ribs, carrying the incision anteriorly beyond the angle of the rib, almost to the sternum. Unless the incision is long enough, exposure is seriously hampered. Subsequent wound infection following an unsterile thoracotomy is surprisingly rare, less than 5 percent.

The key to cardiac tamponade, the other major life-threatening problem, is simply considering the diagnosis in any patient with hypotension and a penetrating thoracic wound. The classic triad emphasized by Beck decades ago was the combination of hypotension, elevated venous pressure, and a small quiet heart. Only a few conditions, such as cardiac failure or pulmonary embolism, produce the combination of hypotension and elevated venous pressure. When the diagnosis is first suspected, pericardial aspiration, or subxyphoid exploration, should be promptly done. A most dramatic experience is to remove as little as 10 to 15 mL of blood from the pericardium of a moribund patient with an imperceptible blood pressure and be rewarded with a prompt rise in blood pressure to 70 to 80 mm and a return of consciousness. Isaacs demonstrated the exponential rise in intrapericardial pressure as fluid is added. Elevation of intrapericardial pressure above 15 to 17 mm virtually stopped cardiac output unless venous pressure was elevated by infusion of fluids.

In some patients with severe tamponade, an unusual degree of restlessness is present with the patient wildly rolling about. This contrasts strikingly with the usual quiet apathetic state of patients in hemorrhagic shock. This may be due to severe cerebral anoxia, resulting from the combination of arterial hypotension and venous hypertension.

Operative Therapy. In the operating room a median sternotomy is the preferred incision, as it provides ready access to all chambers of the heart. An anterior thoracotomy can be made more rapidly but does not give good exposure of the right heart.

When circumstances permit, a pump oxygenator, or a simpler apparatus for autotransfusion of blood, should be available. This is not often needed, as most cardiac injuries permitting survival long enough to reach the operating room can be controlled by digital pressure and suturing.

Ventricular lacerations can usually be controlled by digital pressure and then sutured with continuous or interrupted mattress sutures. Atrial lacerations may be initially controlled with tangential application of vascular or wide Allis clamps.

Following control of the cardiac laceration, a search should routinely be made for other intrathoracic injuries. Laceration of the internal mammary artery is a common associated injury. Injuries to intracardiac structures, such as a cardiac valve or the ventricular septum, rarely occur but can be treated at a later time.

Following repair of the cardiac laceration and correction of hypovolemia, recovery is uneventful in most patients. Wound infection, pericarditis, or recurrent bleeding are all uncommon.

Blunt Trauma

Blunt cardiac trauma usually results from automobile accidents, such as a "steering wheel" injury or some similar form of severe blunt injury to the chest wall. Probably 900,000 cases of cardiac trauma occur annually in the United States. Many of these are instantaneously fatal. The direct injury may cause an underlying cardiac contusion. Alternately, when the heart is suddenly compressed, intracardiac pressure apparently becomes high enough to rupture different cardiac structures, such as the ventricular septum, the chordae of the mitral or tricuspid valves, or the free cardiac wall. Injuries of this severity are usually fatal. Only rarely is a patient seen with a laceration of a tricuspid valve or the ventricular septum.

The myocardial contusion varies from simple subepicardial hemorrhage to a full-thickness myocardial contusion, which rarely progresses to an infarction.

The clinical picture is that of pericarditis with a pericardial effusion and chest pain. The classic picture of a myocardial infarction or cardiac failure is uncommon.

The electrocardiogram is a nonspecific diagnostic guide, as false-positive and false-negative results are common. The best diagnostic evaluation is done by a combination of serial measurement of myocardial enzymes, combined with 2-D echocardiography. Frazee et al. summarized experiences with 291 patients with thoracic trauma. Twenty percent of the group (58) had elevated cardiac enzymes (CPK-MB) within 24 h. Of this group, 60 percent were classified as simply "cardiac concussion," as the 2-D echocardiogram was normal. The remaining 40 percent were diagnosed as cardiac contusion, as abnormalities were visible on the echocardiogram. Patients with an abnormal echocardiogram were treated like patients with a subendocardial myocardial infarction, as arrhythmias frequently occurred in this group. The majority recovered within a short period of time.

Cardiac injury almost never produces permanent cardiac disability. From a physiologic standpoint, serious cardiac disability does not occur until more than 30 to 50 percent of the myocardium has been lost. An injury severe enough to produce irreversible loss of myocardium of this extent is almost always fatal.

Foreign Bodies

The report by Harken in 1946 is a classic. It describes the successful removal of 56 intramyocardial foreign bodies during World War II without a single death. About two-thirds of the removed foreign bodies had bacteria on culture.

In general, foreign bodies greater than 1 cm usually cause complications, such as pericardial effusion or pericarditis, but smaller foreign bodies are well tolerated. In 1966, Bland and Beebe reported a 20-year follow-up of 40 patients from World War II who had small foreign bodies in the heart. Although major complications did not occur, most patients had a permanent emotional disability, apparently from anxiety associated with the uncertain prognosis of a foreign body in the heart. The difficulty with removing small asymptomatic foreign bodies was emphasized in the report; elective removal was attempted in eight patients, but successfully completed in only three.

Harrison and Sabiston described the intraoperative use of echocardiography with a hand-held probe. After palpation of the heart failed to reveal the location of the bullet, echocardiography identified the fragment, over 1 cm beneath the epicardial surface and about 3 cm from the entrance site. Precise location permitted the performance of a limited ventriculotomy with successful removal of the bullet.

The safety of cardiopulmonary bypass, combined with the use of echocardiography, would suggest that all intramyocardial foreign bodies should be surgically removed. Foreign bodies that are within the cardiac cavities, usually dislodged from a complication of intravascular catheters, can be removed with a percutaneous catheter method. Uflacker et al. reported the successful percutaneous removal of a foreign body in 20 patients.

CARDIAC TUMORS

Metastatic neoplasms are the most common cardiac neoplasms, occurring in 4 to 12 percent of the autopsies performed on patients with neoplastic disease. The most frequent primary cardiac tumor is *myxoma,* comprising 50 to 60 percent of all primary cardiac neoplasms. *Sarcomas* are found in 20 to 25 percent of cases, and *rhabdomyomas* in 10 to 15 percent. Benign but extremely rare neoplasms include fibromas, angiomas, lipomas, teratomas, and cysts.

The clinical significance of cardiac tumors is similar to that of many other cardiac lesions in that accurate diagnosis and successful treatment first became possible with the development of extracorporeal circulation. Before 1950 cardiac tumors were usually first diagnosed at autopsy. Several excellent reviews have previously summarized the pathologic findings and clinical features. A classic analysis was published by Yater in 1931, and a detailed French monograph was published by Mahaim in 1945. In 1949 Whorton described the clinical findings in 100 sarcomas of the heart, and in 1951 Prichard reviewed 150 lesions, most of which were metastatic in origin.

In 1953 Steinberg et al. reported the diagnosis of an atrial myxoma in three patients by angiocardiography. The first successful removal of an atrial myxoma was performed by Crafoord in 1954, using extracorporeal circulation. Other successful reports quickly followed, and in 1967 Thomas et al. stated that there had been 126 attempted excisions of atrial myxomas, either planned or inadvertent, 85 of which had been successful.

The use of echocardiography, first reported in 1968, was a major diagnostic advance. 2-D echocardiography is now the keystone of diagnostic studies. Fyke reported 30 cardiac tumors seen following the introduction of 2-D echocardiography. Twenty-five were operated on based solely on the echocardiographic examination.

Myxoma

Sixty to seventy-five percent of cardiac myxomas develop in the left atrium, almost always from the atrial septum near the fossa ovalis. Most other myxomas develop in the right atrium. Less than 20 have been found in either the right or left ventricle. The curious predilection for a myxoma to develop from the rim of the fossa ovalis in the left atrium has been studied by several observers, but a satisfactory explanation has not been found.

Myxomas are apparently true neoplasms, although their similarity to an organized atrial thrombus led to considerable debate at one time about whether they represented a true neoplasm or not. Their occurrence in the absence of other organic heart disease, histochemical studies demonstrating mucopolysaccharide and glycoprotein, and a distinct histologic appearance all indicate that myxomas are true neoplasms. In 1976 Dang and Hurley reported 19 recurrences of a myxoma following surgical excision in 16 patients, conclusively establishing the low-grade malignant potential of the tumor.

PATHOLOGY. The tumors are usually polypoid, projecting into the atrial cavity from a 1- to 2-cm stalk attached to the atrial septum. The maximum size ranges from 0.5 to greater than 10.0 cm. Only the superficial layer of the septum is involved; invasion of the septum does not occur. Some myxomas grow slowly, for a few patients have had symptoms for many years. There is no tendency to invade other areas of the heart; distant metastases have rarely been reported. The friable consistency of a myxoma is of particular significance, for fatal emboli have occurred following digital manipulation of the tumor at operation.

Histologically, a myxoma is covered with endothelium and composed of a myxomatous stroma with large stellate cells mixed with fusiform or multinucleated cells. Mitoses are infrequent. Lymphocytes and plasmacytes are regularly found. Hemosiderin, a result of hemorrhage into the tumor, is also common.

PATHOPHYSIOLOGY. A myxoma may cause no difficulty until it grows large enough to obstruct the flow of blood through either the mitral or tricuspid valve, or fragments to produce peripheral emboli. The frequency of embolization, estimated to occur in 40 to 50 percent of patients, is not surprising, for an astonishing degree of to-and-fro motion of a myxoma, swinging on a small pedicle with each cardiac contraction, may be seen with echocardiography or angiography. Intermittent acute obstruction of the mitral orifice has been reported to produce syncope or even sudden death. Some myxomas produced generalized symptoms resembling an autoimmune disorder, including fever, weight loss, clubbing, myalgia, and arthralgia. Possibly such patients have an immune reaction to the neoplasm.

CLINICAL MANIFESTATIONS. Symptoms may be those of mitral valve obstruction, resembling mitral stenosis, except for acute exacerbations, presumably due to transient lodging of the myxoma in the mitral orifice; peripheral embolization; or generalized autoimmune symptoms described in the previous section. The diagnosis is made in many patients following an embolic episode, either from histologic examination of the surgically removed embolus or as a result of subsequent diagnostic studies to determine the reason for embolism. The precision and reliability of 2-D echocardiography has greatly simplified diagnosis. Angiography is optional unless additional disease is suspected. Computerized axial tomography has been reported to be helpful with small tumors.

Abnormalities are usually found on examination of the heart and also on the electrocardiogram, but these are not diagnostic.

TREATMENT. Operation should be performed as soon as possible after the diagnosis has been established because a disabling or fatal cerebral embolus is an ever-present hazard.

A sternotomy incision is used. Once extracorporeal circulation has been established, ventricular fibrillation is induced and the aorta clamped to avoid embolism. Palpation is avoided. The right atrium is opened and the fossa ovalis incised to expose the stalk of the myxoma. The left atrium is then opened in the interatrial groove. With the myxoma visualized, the segment of atrial septum from which the tumor arises is excised, after which the myxoma is removed through the incision in the left atrium (Fig. 19-21). The defect in the atrial septum is closed with a small patch. The technique is simple and permits exploration of both atria and ventricles.

A few cases of recurrent myxoma have been reported, some of which have been successfully operated upon. Initially these were thought to represent inadequate excision of the site of origin, but some have recurred at more remote sites in the atrium, indicating the multipotential source of these unusual neoplasms. Hence, it seems prudent to perform periodic echocardiography routinely for 1 to 2 years following operation.

Larrieu et al. described experiences with 18 myxomas in a series of 25 cardiac tumors over a period of 24 years. Fyke et al. treated 21 patients with mitral myxoma in the first 7 years following the introduction of 2-D echocardiography. Kirklin-Barrat Boyce summarized reports of 202 surgically removed myxomas, with 10 operative deaths (5 percent); 160 were in the left atrium, 33 in the right, 2 in both atria, 3 in the right ventricle, and 4 in the left ventricle.

Metastatic Neoplasms

Cardiac metastases have been found in 4 to 12 percent of autopsies performed for neoplastic disease. Although they have occurred from primary neoplasms developing in almost every known site of the body, the most frequent have been carcinoma of the lung or breast, melanoma, and lymphoma. Cardiac metastases involving only the heart are very unusual. Similarly, a solitary cardiac metastasis is infrequent; usually there are multiple areas of

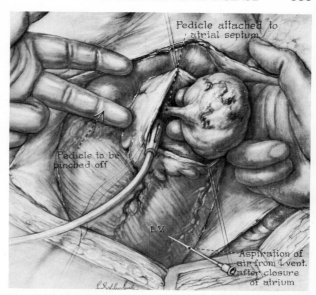

Fig. 19-21. Pedunculated atrial myxoma removed at operation in 1957. The patient has remained free of cardiac symptoms since that time. (From: *Bahnson HT, Spencer FC, Andrus EC: Diagnosis and treatment of intracavitary myxomas of the heart. Ann Surg 145:915, 1957, by permission of Lippincott, Philadelphia.*)

involvement. Cardiac involvement is particularly common with leukemia or lymphoma, developing in 25 to 40 percent of patients. All areas of the heart are involved with equal frequency except the cardiac valves, perhaps as a result of the absence of lymphatics in valves.

The diagnosis of a primary cardiac malignant tumor can be suspected in a patient in whom an unexplained hemorrhagic pericardial effusion develops, especially in association with a bizarre cardiac shadow on the radiograph. Echocardiography should confirm the presence of an abdominal cardiac mass. Thoracotomy is usually required to establish the diagnosis. Only rarely is effective therapy possible.

Rhabdomyoma

A cardiac rhabdomyoma is probably not a true tumor but a hamartoma, representing a focal arrest and maturation of cardiac muscle. The nodules have also been termed *nodular glycogenic degeneration*, being interpreted as a manifestation of glycogen storage disease. About one-half of the patients have tuberous sclerosis of the brain. On histologic examination cells with large vacuoles are found in which the nuclei appear suspended by threads of cytoplasm, giving origin to the term ''spider cell.''

Although rhabdomyoma is said to be the most common cardiac tumor in children, it is a rare lesion. Reece et al. indicated that only about 110 cases have been reported in the literature prior to 1984.

The cardiac lesions may be solitary or multiple nodules or may present a diffuse infiltration of the cardiac muscle. The lesions do not grow.

Most cases have been recognized in infancy. The average age was 5 months. The disease is apparently fatal, for older children and adults with such tumors are not seen. Whether the death is from the tumor or from associated disease is uncertain.

Symptoms may result from obstruction of a ventricular chamber or from arrhythmias such as recurrent ventricular tachycardia. Complete excision has been accomplished in a few patients. If tuberous sclerosis of the brain is not present, it appears that a rare infant may be successfully operated upon and cured of potentially fatal arrhythmias.

Miscellaneous Tumors

Unusual benign lesions of the heart include fibromas, lipomas, angiomas, teratomas, and cysts. Fewer than 50 examples of each of these types of lesions have been reported. Fibromas have been found most frequently in the left ventricle, often as 2- to 5-cm nodules within the muscle. Sudden death, probably from a cardiac arrhythmia, has been reported with such tumors and may be the reason that only 18 percent of the reported tumors have been found in adults.

Lipomas are usually asymptomatic tumors found projecting from the epicardial or endocardial surface of the heart in older patients. Only about 30 such cases have been reported. Angiomas are commonly small, focal vascular malformations of no clinical significance, except for four that have been found associated with a heart block. Pericardial teratomas and bronchogenic cysts are rare lesions that may cause symptoms from compression of the right atrium and obstruction of venous return. About 30 such patients have been reported in the surgical literature, most of them children. Some of the larger cysts, up to 10 cm in diameter, may produce grotesque deformities from extensive invagination of the right atrial wall. Myxomas are by far the most common benign tumor in adults, but are seldom found in children.

CORONARY ARTERY DISEASE

HISTORICAL DATA. Starting in the late 1930s, different investigators attempted to increase the blood supply of the ischemic heart by developing collateral circulation with vascular adhesions. Beck was the leading investigator, trying different methods for many years, but ultimately all failed. Probably the fundamental biologic reason for failure is the natural tendency for vascular adhesions to progressively fibrose and become more avascular with time.

A separate ingenious concept arose in 1946 when Vineberg developed implantation of the internal mammary artery into a tunnel in the myocardium. This was applied clinically by Vineberg in 1950 and continued for many years. For unknown reasons, the artery remains patent in well over 90 percent of patients, but the amount of flow through the patent artery is distressingly small, often as little as 5 to 10 mL/min. An occasional patient has been reported in whom the implanted artery was of substantial benefit, carrying as much as 50 mL of blood per minute, but these fortunate results were infrequent. For this reason, the procedure has been virtually abandoned.

Attempts at endarterectomy without bypass grafting have been made sporadically since 1956, but late patency rates were prohibitively low, probably from late cicatrial contractions of collagen in the arterial wall. In recent years some groups have reinvestigated the concept of the combination of endarterectomy with bypass.

In 1986, over 200,000 bypass procedures were performed in the United States. It is estimated that at least 6 million patients in this country have known coronary artery disease.

The development of the bypass operation for coronary occlusive disease between 1967 and 1968 was a dramatic milestone. For the first time it was possible to increase immediately the blood flow to the myocardium. Most of the basic clinical investigations evolved from studies in three centers in the United States during this time. Favalaro et al. from the Cleveland Clinic began using longer and longer segments of saphenous vein to bypass occlusive disease in the right coronary artery, eventually interposing grafts between the aorta proximally and the termination of the right coronary distally. Johnson et al., in 1969, showed that similar grafts could be effectively used for the left coronary artery. This was a quantum achievement. Previously, direct operative procedures upon the left coronary artery had a prohibitive mortality. Green, following extensive experimental studies by others, anastomosed the left internal mammary artery to the anterior descending, using an operative microscope. The internal mammary was not widely used for over a decade but since 1980 has been widely adopted and is now used in the majority of bypass operations. This change resulted from 10-year angiographic studies that found excellent patency rates of internal mammary grafts (>90 percent) but disappointing deterioration in vein grafts between 5 and 10 years after operation with less than 50 percent satisfactory patency.

ETIOLOGY AND PATHOGENESIS. Atherosclerosis is the fundamental cause. It is a common disease in the Caucasian male throughout the world, involving males about four times as frequently as females. The frequency varies widely throughout the world, being less common in populations where the average blood cholesterol is less than 200. The frequency is the lowest in Japan, where the average blood cholesterol is near 160 mg/100 mL. The United States has the second highest frequency in the world.

The basic lesion is a segmental atherosclerotic plaque, often localized within the first 5 cm of the origin of the coronary artery from the aorta. Involvement of small distal vessels is usually less extensive; arterioles and intramyocardial vessels are usually free of disease. This segmental localization makes bypass grafts possible. Among the three major coronary arteries, the proximal anterior descending is often occluded, with the distal half of the artery remaining patent. The right coronary is often occluded throughout its course, but almost always the posterior descending and left atrial-ventricular groove branches are patent. The circumflex is often diseased proximally, but one or more distal marginal branches are patent.

The popular terminology, single, double, or triple vessel disease, refers, of course, to the number of coronary arteries involved. In over 50 percent of patients, "triple" vessel disease is present.

CLINICAL MANIFESTATIONS. The myocardial ischemia produced by coronary disease can produce several serious events: angina pectoris, myocardial infarction, or sudden death. Angina is the most frequent symptom, but unfortunately myocardial infarction or sudden death may appear without warning.

Angina pectoris, the most common manifestation, is demonstrated by periodic discomfort, usually substernal, typically appearing with exertion, after eating, or with extreme emotion. Characteristically these symptoms subside within 3 to 5 min, or may be dramatically relieved by sublingual nitroglycerin. In about 25 percent of patients, the symptoms are not typical and may radiate to bizarre areas, such as the teeth, the shoulder, or the epigastrium. Establishing a diagnosis of angina in these patients is difficult, perhaps impossible without diagnostic studies. Physical examination is usually normal. Differential diagnosis includes anxiety states, musculoskeletal disorders, and reflux esophagitis.

The risk of sudden death varies with the extent of disease and the degree of impairment of ventricular function. It ranges from 2 percent to as high as 10 percent. Death apparently results from ventricular fibrillation, for postmortem examination may not find any acute change.

Myocardial infarction is the most common serious complication. At least 2 million infarcts occur in the United States annually. With modern therapy, mortality is near 10 to 15 percent. Most deaths occur in the first 30 to 60 min after the onset of symptoms, before the patient ever reaches a hospital. With modern treatment in coronary care units, the fatality rate is small.

In a small percentage of patients congestive heart failure eventually develops, resulting from multiple infarctions that ultimately destroy over 40 percent of the left ventricular muscle mass. Often the origin is puzzling. Some patients have had angina for years, with one or more infarctions, but others have been almost asymptomatic for over a decade after a small infarction first established the presence of coronary disease. Despite the paucity of symptoms, ischemic infarction of muscle apparently steadily but "silently" progressed. The frequency, diagnosis, and treatment of so-called silent ischemia is currently one of the most active areas in cardiology (1987). Other patients, by contrast, undergo rapid destruction of ventricular function within 2 to 3 years. Multiple tiny emboli from an ulcerated atherosclerotic plaque may be one possible mechanism.

With chronic congestive failure, manifested by a right atrial pressure above 10 to 15 mmHg, the outlook is ominous, for there is insufficient left ventricular muscle to provide adequate cardiac output. Most patients die within 1 to 2 years. Bypass grafting may be futile in such circumstances unless there is a large ventricular aneurysm present that can be excised. Cardiac transplantation is now being used with increasing frequency in this group of patients with far advanced disease.

LABORATORY STUDIES. The chest x-ray is usually normal, and the electrocardiogram is normal at rest in about 70 percent of patients. The simplest and most widely used study is the stress test with the exercise electrocardiogram, noting electrocardiographic signs of ischemia during graded amounts of exercise. More complex studies include radionuclide imaging with thallium or radionuclide angiography, noting changes in ejection fraction with exercise. A decrease in ejection fraction with exercise is a characteristic finding with significant coronary disease.

Coronary arteriography (Fig. 19-22) remains the cornerstone of evaluation, for it outlines both the location and severity of the disease and the degree of impairment of ventricular function. The number of vessels diseased, the location of proximal stenoses, and the ventricular function as measured by ejection fraction are the three most important prognostic indicators of the severity and prognosis with coronary disease.

"Angiographically significant" stenosis is considered present when the diameter is reduced by more than 70 percent, corresponding to a reduction in cross-sectional area greater than 90 percent; some groups use a more liberal indication, considering a reduction in diameter of 50 percent (equivalent to a 75 percent reduction in cross-sectional area) as significant.

Ventricular function is usually expressed as ejection fraction, considering the range of 0.50 to 0.70 as normal; 0.30 to 0.50 moderately depressed; and below 0.30, especially below 0.20, as severely depressed. An ejection fraction below 0.30 is usually associated with intermittent or chronic congestive heart failure. The long-term course of coronary disease is a balance between two opposing factors, the rate of progression of the atherosclerotic stenoses as balanced by the rate of development of collateral circulation. The ventricular function probably reflects the ability of the heart to develop sufficient collateral circulation to compensate for the arterial stenoses present. This ability to develop collateral circulation varies widely; some patients with extensive triple vessel disease have normal ventricular function while others with less severe disease have marked impairment.

When a ventriculogram is evaluated, the contraction of individual segments of ventricular wall is separately analyzed, i.e., regional wall motion. Segmental wall motion is classified as normal, hypokinetic (impaired), akinetic (little or no visible contraction), or dyskinetic (paradoxical contraction, as with a left ventricular aneurysm).

Although angiography and ventriculography are the most precise methods for evaluating coronary disease, several limitations of the technique should also be emphasized, for erroneous decisions can easily be made.

An angiogram indicates the severity and complexity of the disease but is seldom, if ever, a reliable guide to state that a patient is "inoperable" because of the diffuse dis-

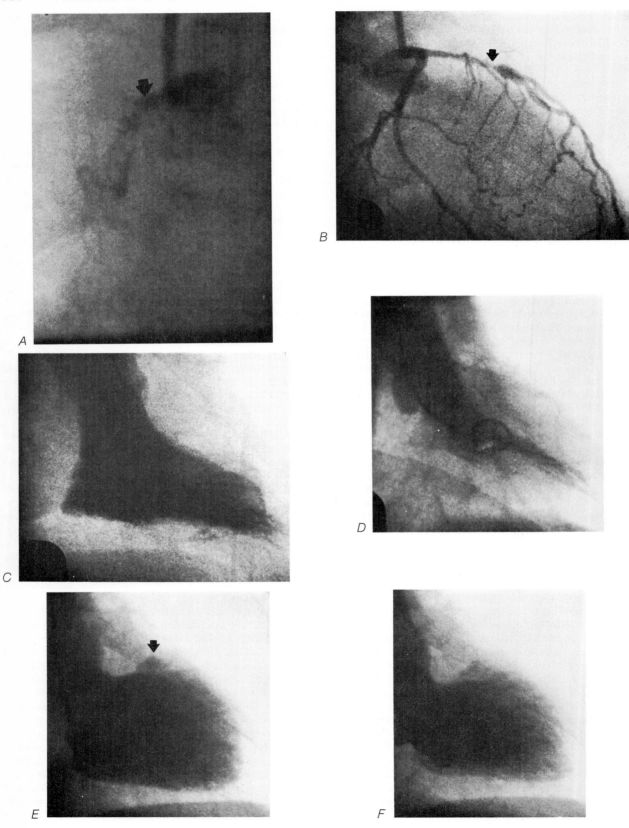

ease present and the small size of the vessels. With the ability to graft vessels as small as 1 mm, combined with endarterectomy when necessary, bypass grafts can virtually always be inserted even though the degree of improvement may be only moderate.

It is also a serious error to conclude from the ventriculogram that a diseased artery supplying an akinetic or dyskinetic area should not be bypassed because that segment of the ventricle is "scar." At operation such areas virtually always contain a significant percentage of viable muscle, estimated to range from 40 to 80 percent. Often improved contractility can be seen following bypass.

The ventriculogram should not be used to conclude that a patient is "inoperable" because of severe impairment of ventricular function, though ejection fraction may be less than 20 percent and end-diastolic pressure above 30 mm. This represents an advanced stage of disease with a grim prognosis, but criteria for operation depend upon the clinical condition of the patient, whether congestive failure is intermittent or chronic, and whether chronic right heart failure is present, reflected by a right atrial pressure near 15 mm or higher, and hepatomegaly.

CORONARY BYPASS. Indications. The clinical status of the patient with coronary disease is usually in one of five groups: asymptomatic, stable angina of varying severity, unstable angina, acute myocardial infarction, and postinfarction angina.

Asymptomatic: Angiographically Significant Coronary Disease with Little or No Angina. This type of patient is the most common clinical problem. The three major types of therapy available are medical (drug) therapy, bypass surgery, or angioplasty. Angioplasty has been applied with steadily increasing frequency for isolated stenotic lesions and by some groups for multiple stenoses. The role of angioplasty will probably not be clearly defined for at least another 5 years. In one series, angioplasty was initially successful in 70 percent of patients, without any deaths, but 33 percent of the successfully dilated patients required either subsequent repeat dilatation or bypass surgery. With significant occlusive disease in the left main coronary, there is virtually uniform agreement that such patients should be operated upon promptly, even if totally asymptomatic.

Stable Angina of Varying Severity. There is uniform agreement that severe angina not responding to drug therapy should be operated upon. The majority of patients have

Fig. 19-22. *A.* Right coronary artery, left anterior oblique projection. There is total obstruction of the vessel immediately distal to its aortic origin *(arrow).* A network of collateral vessels on the anterior surface of the right atrium and the right ventricle is apparent. *B.* Left coronary artery, right anterior oblique projection. There is severe narrowing of the left anterior descending coronary artery *(arrow)* distal to the origin of the second septal branch. *C.* Left ventricle in right anterior oblique projection in diastole. There is a normal contour of the chamber. *D.* Same ventricle in systole showing excellent contraction of all areas of the ventricle. *E.* Left ventricle in diastole, right anterior oblique projection. There is increased rounding of the ventricle and bulging of the anterolateral wall. A localized bulge on the superior portion of the anterolateral wall is evident *(arrow).* *F.* The same ventricle in systole. The degree of left ventricular contraction is generally markedly impaired.

extensive disease with little angina. Data increasingly indicate that the presence and severity of angina per se is an unreliable guide for deciding upon operation.

One of the most important studies was done by the European Coronary Surgery Study group in the 1970s. This found that 5-year survival with triple vessel disease was near 90 percent with bypass as compared with near 80 percent with medical therapy. The most extensive study was done by the Coronary Artery Surgery Study (CASS), a multicenter study among 15 institutions between 1974 and 1979, during which over 24,000 patients were entered into the registry. Over 75 percent of patients in the study had a normal ejection fraction (greater than 0.50). Patients with triple vessel disease, good ventricular function, and mild angina did equally well with medical or surgical therapy, as 5-year survival in either group was above 90 percent. These data were initially widely heralded as showing that bypass was "unnecessary," overlooking the disconcerting fact that medical therapy was continued only as long as angina remained stable. In this favorable group, however, 38 percent of patients "crossed over" to surgical therapy within 5 years, indicating the relentless progression of the disease. At present, medical therapy is adequate with good ventricular function only if angina is not progressive.

With triple vessel disease and impaired ventricular function (ejection fraction less than 0.50), results are much better with bypass, as 7-year survival is 84 percent compared with 70 percent with medical therapy.

With single vessel disease, initial treatment with medical therapy or angioplasty is usually satisfactory. However, the outstanding results with internal mammary bypass grafting, an operative risk less than 1 percent, and a 10-year patency rate greater than 90 percent certainly indicate that surgical therapy may be used if either of the other two methods is unsatisfactory. With double vessel disease, intermediate in severity between single and triple vessel disease, bypass is usually not performed in stable patients with satisfactory ventricular function, but multiple factors enter into the decision with individual patients.

Unstable Angina. "Acute coronary insufficiency" exists when angina is persistent and does not respond to therapy with nitroglycerin and other nitrates. It apparently is an acute physiologic state in which the blood flow to a segment of myocardium is seriously jeopardized but necrosis has not yet occurred. It probably arises from a sudden decrease in regional blood flow. Virtually everyone agrees that the condition is a medical emergency. The patient should be promptly hospitalized in a coronary care unit. If collateral blood flow increases and compensates for the ischemia, manifested by subsidence of the angina, recovery is prompt. Otherwise, acute infarction or death can occur.

Most patients respond to acute medical therapy. Those who do not should be operated upon promptly. In patients who recover, coronary angiography should be done soon to decide if elective bypass should be performed, for such patients have a significant frequency of infarction or death within 1 to 2 years after the event.

Acute Infarction. The best therapy for an acute myocardial infarction is one of the most rapidly changing areas in cardiology. Data now are convincing that the infarction is produced by an acute thrombosis in a major artery in the majority of patients. The immediate intravenous administration of a thrombolytic agent, usually streptokinase, is becoming increasingly popular after a study of several thousand uncontrolled patients found a definite decrease in mortality when streptokinase was administered in the first 4 to 6 h after onset of symptoms, with the best results occurring when administration was within 1 to 2 h. In the United States a national study is still evaluating the effectiveness of tissue plasminogen activator (TPA), a far more effective thrombolytic drug.

A more complex form of therapy is the intracoronary administration of the thrombolytic agent in the catheterization laboratory. This may be combined with angioplasty. After thrombolytic therapy has reopened a thrombosed vessel precipitating an acute infarction, the residual stenosis may be treated by angioplasty, bypass, or drug therapy. Thrombolytic therapy, combined with angioplasty, is a simpler and safer procedure than emergency coronary bypass and can be applied more quickly for most patients.

A certain degree of irreversible necrosis develops between 30 and 60 min following occlusion of the coronary artery. Infarction continues to evolve for several hours, probably in the marginal zones of the initial complete infarction. This is probably the basis for the benefit from immediate revascularization, similar to removal of an acute arterial occlusion in other areas of the body. A very short time exists during which therapy may be effective.

When a massive infarction produces cardiogenic shock, mortality remains high, well above 50 percent. Most of these patients have triple vessel disease with a preexisting significant impairment of ventricular function. Probably the best approach for these patients is immediate bypass, perhaps preceded by intraaortic balloon support. Significant data are not yet available.

Postinfarction Angina. Patients recovering from myocardial infarction who develop recurrent angina can be safely operated upon promptly. With present techniques of cardioplegia, the risk of operation seems unrelated to the time lapsing since the initial infarction.

Contraindications. The only absolute contraindication at the author's institution is chronic congestive failure with pulmonary hypertension, a right atrial pressure above 15 mm, and hepatomegaly. The unfortunate patient in this group usually has already necrosed the majority of the left ventricular muscle, so cardiac transplantation is the only therapy likely to be helpful.

Intermittent congestive failure, manifested by intermittent episodes of pulmonary edema, is not a *contraindication* to operation but actually a strong *indication for immediate operation.* This indicates a serious degree of myocardial ischemia that can easily progress to an irreversible stage or death. The intermittent episodes probably evolve from an acute ischemic episode that elevates end-diastolic pressure sufficiently to produce pulmonary edema. Such patients have been regularly operated upon with continuing good long-term results.

A severe depression of ejection fraction to the range of 0.20 to 0.25, or lower, is still erroneously considered a contraindication to bypass, though contrary experiences have been published by several groups. The erroneous concept probably arose from previous experiences with ineffective myocardial preservation that produced some degree of infarction during operation. Jones et al. reported experiences with 188 patients with an ejection fraction below 0.35, about 24 percent of whom had ejection fraction lower than 0.20. Operative mortality was only 2.1 percent.

Pigott and Kouchoukos reported results for 192 patients with an ejection fraction less than 35 percent. Seventy-seven were operated upon; 115 were treated medically. Seven-year actuarial survival was 63 percent in the surgical group, 34 percent in the medical group. Recurrent infarction developed in 19 percent of the medical group as compared with 7 percent of the surgical group.

Operative Technique. At the author's institution all procedures are performed with extracorporeal circulation at a flow rate near 2.3 L/m²/min and a perfusate temperature of 25 to 30°C. The heart is arrested with the cold blood potassium technique. Cold blood is infused at an aortic root pressure of 80 to 100 mmHg to permit adequate perfusion beyond the occluded vessels. This is confirmed by measuring regional myocardial temperatures in at least four regions of the myocardium, and continuing infusion of cold blood until the "warmest" zone has cooled below 15°C. This can usually be done with 1500 mL but may at times require 2000 or 2500 mL. Topical hypothermia is then employed to prevent rewarming, both by pericardial lavage and by a continuous pericardial infusion of cold electrolyte. Blood is reinfused into the aorta usually after each anastomosis, certainly after every 20 to 30 min. The left heart is decompressed, either by emptying the right heart with a large lumen cannula or with a catheter introduced through a pulmonary vein. Particular attention is given to periodic monitoring of right heart temperatures to be certain that reflux of blood from the cavae does not warm the right ventricle and septum. With this technique, the heart can be arrested for well over 2 h, even though this is rarely necessary. There is ample time for grafting all diseased vessels.

Saphenous veins of appropriate size (greater than 3.5 mm) are removed from the lower extremity, using the lesser saphenous or the cephalic veins if adequate saphenous veins are not available. The left internal mammary artery is routinely used in the vast majority of patients (Fig. 19-23). In recent years, following the lead of others, bilateral mammary grafting has been employed with increasing frequency, usually in healthy patients under fifty-five years of age. With the heart arrested and cooled, bypass grafts are attached to all diseased coronary arteries, making a short arteriotomy and attaching the vein end to side with a continuous suture of 7-0 polypropylene. Three- to four-power optical magnification is routinely used. Internal mammary anastomoses are done with 8-0 polypropylene. Cold blood is routinely infused down each graft after it is constructed. When the aorta is unclamped, warm blood is perfused down the grafts until these are attached to the aorta. This is probably superfluous in

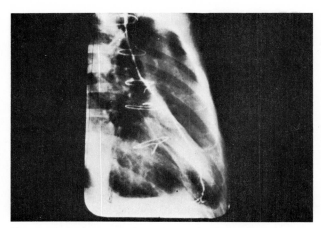

Fig. 19-23. Angiogram performed several months after left internal mammary–left anterior descending coronary bypass, showing a good flow from the internal mammary artery into the anterior descending coronary and its branches.

many patients but seems quite important when serious ischemia is present, especially with left main coronary disease.

An alternative is to attach several grafts to the aorta proximally before bypass is started and then serially construct the distal anastomoses. This is a simpler and more expeditious method, though it requires more judgment about the exact length of grafts and has less freedom of choice once the aorta is clamped and the heart emptied. The usual number of anastomoses constructed varies between three and six. As many as nine to ten anastomoses have been constructed in a few patients with no measurable increase in operative mortality.

Following bypass, flow rates are measured through the grafts with a flowmeter, finding a mean flow between 50 and 80 mL/min in most vessels with an adequate runoff.

Postoperative Management. Postoperative care is usually uncomplicated. The patients remain in a cardiac recovery unit for 12 to 18 h, after which the further care is routine. Initially, adequacy of blood volume and cardiac output are periodically monitored by measurement of left atrial pressure with a catheter inserted at the time of operation and a Swan-Ganz catheter in the pulmonary artery. Minor atrial arrhythmias are fairly common and easily treated with appropriate medication. A mild pericardiotomy syndrome, manifested by fever, a pericardial friction rub, pleural effusion, and a normal white blood cell count, is fairly common and usually responds promptly to therapy with ibuprofen. Prednisone is seldom necessary. Most uncomplicated patients are discharged from the hospital in 7 to 9 days.

Normal sedentary activity is gradually resumed over the next 2 to 3 months. After 3 months have passed, the ejection fraction should probably be routinely measured with exercise before vigorous physical exercise is permitted. If significant arrhythmias were present preoperatively, these must be carefully monitored indefinitely because these are often not improved with bypass and are a fairly common cause of late death. In patients with nor-

mal ventricular function beforehand, after 3 months a full return to normal physical activity, with participation in physically active sports, is routinely recommended.

Results. Operative Risk and Major Complications. Operative risk is very small, near 1 percent for the usual patient. Similar low-risk results have been reported by many experienced cardiac surgical groups throughout the world. Moderate impairment of ventricular function does not increase operative risk, though with severe impairment of ventricular function, an ejection fraction less than 0.30, the risk is probably near 3 to 4 percent.

With an uncomplicated operation, electrocardiographic signs of myocardial infarction develop in less than 5 percent of patients. With enzymatic studies, a somewhat higher frequency may be found, though inconsistencies often exist between the electrocardiographic findings and the enzymatic changes. It is rare for enzymatic changes to represent a significant physiologic problem if the patient is asymptomatic without significant changes on the electrocardiogram. A very minimal elevation of myocardial enzymes indicates the absence of any injury, but the significance of a moderate elevation is uncertain.

Operative risk rises somewhat with age, though patients in their seventh or eighth decade are readily operated upon if angina is crippling and cerebral function is satisfactory.

The most serious complication with operation is stroke, a frequency of 1 to 2 percent, more commonly seen in patients in the sixth, seventh, or eighth decades. The exact cause of stroke is usually impossible to determine. The four most common probable causes are atherosclerotic disease in the carotid arteries or the aortic arch, or emboli of thrombotic material or air from the heart. Usually the stroke, fortunately infrequent, is both unexpected and cannot be explained.

We no longer believe that asymptomatic carotid disease is a significant cause of perioperative stroke. Carotid artery disease is surgically treated only in the patient with acute ischemic symptoms such as transient ischemic attacks. Unless acute ischemic symptoms are present, we are not aware of any data that show a benefit from performing carotid endarterectomy either before or concurrently with coronary bypass.

Considerable attention has been focused upon unrecognized atherosclerotic disease in the aortic arch as a source of emboli, especially in older patients. In patients over seventy years of age, a special aortic arch cannula is now routinely used, placing the tip beyond the orifice of the left subclavian artery to avoid dislodgment of atherosclerotic material from the transverse arch by the jet of blood emerging from the perfusion cannula. This cannula is routinely used in all patients with any suspected disease in the transverse aortic arch. In patients with palpable disease of the aortic arch, the aortic arch is also surgically explored, using the technique of circulatory arrest at a perfusate temperature below 18°C. The arch can be readily explored through an appropriately placed 5- to 6-cm aortotomy and any loose atherosclerotic debris removed. This has been done in at least 100 patients, finding intimal ulcerations with loose debris in perhaps 40 to 50 percent of this group. The exploration is clearly safe, with the strong impression that significant protection from stroke results.

Relief of Angina. The immediate relief of angina is the most dramatic aspect of bypass. Angina is either completely relieved or markedly decreased in at least 90 to 95 percent of patients if complete revascularization is done. Persistent angina almost always indicates that either a graft has become occluded or a significant stenosis was not bypassed.

Improvement in Ventricular Function. With former techniques, significant improvement in impaired ventricular function could not be demonstrated. With present techniques of myocardial preservation, the abnormal responses to exercise existing before operation, principally a fall in ejection fraction, are often abolished following complete revascularization. This is also usually associated with an improvement in regional wall motion abnormalities.

Vein Graft Patency. With a proper operative technique, combined with the preoperative use of dipyridamole and aspirin, patency a month following operation should be in the range of 90 to 95 percent. Current data are limited because angiograms are now seldom performed in the immediate postoperative period. In the first 5 years after operation, patency decreases slowly, about 2 to 3 percent per year, so 5-year patency is in the range of 75 to 80 percent. Occlusion of a graft during this time is probably due to the anastomotic technique, trauma to the vein graft at the time of operation, or, rarely, postoperative adhesions.

In the period 5 to 10 years after operation, there is an alarming increase of atherosclerotic disease in the vein grafts, as a result of which vein graft patency at 10 years is probably no better than 50 percent, and significant atherosclerosis is present in many of the grafts remaining patent. For unknown reasons, a small number of grafts, near 20 percent, remain in excellent condition more than 10 years after operation.

For this reason, in the past few years use of the internal mammary artery has increased markedly including the more frequent use of bilateral and sequential mammary grafts.

Progression of Atherosclerosis. All angiographic studies have reported a serious frequency of progressive atherosclerosis in the coronary arteries, ranging from 5 to 10 percent per year. Progressive disease was observed in between 65 and 70 percent of patients treated either medically or surgically.

National studies demonstrated that reduction in total plasma cholesterol and low-density lipoprotein cholesterol, often with an elevation in the high-density lipoprotein, resulted in significant improvement and a 2 percent reduction in coronary risk for each 1 percent reduction in plasma cholesterol levels.

Recurrent Angina. Angina gradually recurs following operation, at a rate of 3 to 5 percent per year. When significant angina recurs, angiography should be promptly done. In the majority of patients, recurrent angina is due to one of two causes, progressive stenosis or occlusion of a bypass graft or progressive stenosis in a previously un-

grafted artery. Either situation can be treated with repeat bypass grafting.

Arrhythmias and Sudden Death. Arrhythmias are usually little improved in patients with significant preoperative myocardial scarring. In some patients with virtually normal ventricular function, arrhythmias may be improved because ischemia was apparently the basic cause. Effective treatment of arrhythmias associated with ventricular scars remains unsatisfactory. The more frequent use of 24-h electrocardiographic monitoring may be helpful in developing more effective antiarrhythmic therapy. Electrophysiologic studies have been of benefit in some patients with recurrent arrhythmias. Patients with recurrent ventricular tachycardia have been effectively treated by electrically locating and then ablating one or more irritable foci.

Sudden death remains a grim possibility in any patient with coronary artery disease. Over 300 patients per year were studied following emergency resuscitation from cardiac arrest on the streets of Seattle. Over 75 percent of the patients had coronary disease, but less than one-half had a significant recent infarction.

The influence of medical and surgical treatment on "sudden death" was reported from results with over 13,000 patients in the CASS. Over a period of 4.6 years, sudden death occurred in 452 patients (3.4 percent of the group). This occurred in 6 percent of the medically treated patients but only 2 percent of the surgically treated patients.

Longevity. The influence of coronary bypass on longevity, of course, depends upon the status of the disease process in the patient operated upon. The CASS data indicate that bypass had little influence on 5-year longevity when performed upon patients with triple vessel disease, little angina, and good ventricular function. Nearly 40 percent of the unusually good risk group developed angina within 5 years and were operated upon. The data were even more convincing for similar patients with single or double vessel disease. For most other categories of patients, which represent a high percentage of all patients with coronary disease, bypass surgery clearly significantly improved longevity. These include patients with left main disease, triple vessel disease with impaired ventricular function, triple vessel disease with severe proximal stenoses or severe angina, and patients with a previous history of severe arrhythmias or "sudden death." In our experiences with 1100 patients operated upon between 1968 and 1975 the 5-year survival rate, including operative deaths, was 88 percent with only 49 cardiac deaths occurring after discharge from the hospital in the entire group. After the patients left the hospital, the average mortality was 1.5 percent per year for the next 5 years, a rate almost identical to that of a matched group of similar age and sex.

The similarity of survival (Fig. 19-24) between the two groups strongly indicated the significant influence of bypass on longevity. This is particularly true because the patients operated upon were usually in a high-risk category with severe angina not responding to medical therapy. Loop et al. noted a 5-year survival among different

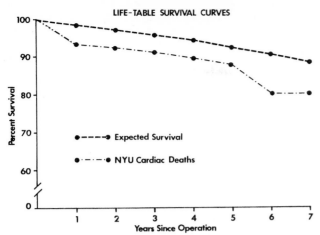

Fig. 19-24. Life table survival curves comparing patients undergoing coronary artery bypass with matched age group.

groups of 90 to 93 percent. Kirklin et al. reported a 5-year survival following triple bypass of 89 percent, and 88 percent following two vessel disease. Most reports show little influence of extent of disease (double or triple vessel disease) on 5-year survival, in marked contrast to that regularly found in medically treated patients.

A 10-year survival of 75 to 88 percent in several thousand patients was reported by Cosgrove et al. for different groups. The 10-year survival varied between 84 percent with a normal ventricle and 54 percent with severe impairment.

Late death, like recurrent angina, is usually found to result from stenosis of a previously inserted bypass graft or progressive disease in an ungrafted vessel. The rare occurrence of death in patients with three functioning grafts, usually from an arrhythmia, also indicates the influence of bypass on longevity. The major factor determining longevity seems to be the adequacy of revascularization of all major coronary arteries.

FUTURE CONSIDERATIONS. Multiple Internal Mammary Anastomoses. Since the 1984 report by Grondin documented the alarming deterioration of vein grafts between 5 and 10 years following operation, while mammary arteries remained patent without change in 90 to 95 percent of patients, a wider application of mammary grafting has been reported by several groups. In brief, certain facts are well established with internal mammary grafting.

1. The 10-year patency rate is near 95 percent, with no signs of deterioration after the first few postoperative months. The mammary artery seems to be relatively immune to atherosclerosis.
2. A patent mammary artery can enlarge substantially over a number of years, perhaps responding to a decrease in peripheral resistance in the coronary vascular bed as atherosclerosis occludes adjacent vessels. This striking ability to enlarge with time indicates the possibilities with multiple anastomoses constructed from a single mammary artery.
3. In retrospect, the concern in the 1970s about the mammary artery was probably due to improper surgical technique, as the vessel is unusually fragile.

4. Data now indicate that bilateral mammary grafts can be performed without significant morbidity. In several significant reports Lytle et al. described experiences with bilateral mammary grafting in 500 patients with little increase in morbidity.

Loop et al. compared longevity in patients who received one mammary graft as compared with those in whom only vein grafts were used. The series included 2306 internal mammary grafts and 3625 vein grafts. There was a statistically significant difference in survival at 10 years, gradually becoming apparent 5 years after operation.

Scanty data are available concerning "free" grafts of mammary artery, in which the artery is divided and reimplanted into the aorta, identical to the method used with a saphenous vein graft. Such "free" grafts no longer function as a pedicle. Loop reported reasonably good results in over 50 such patients operated upon under specific circumstances over a period of years, but no series has yet appeared in which such grafts were used routinely. If excellent results similar to those obtained with mammary pedicle grafts can be obtained with "free" grafts, an even wider use of the mammary artery is possible.

Silent Ischemia. Better therapy is clearly needed to prevent the development of extensive ventricular injury from coronary disease, the so-called "bad" left ventricle with an ejection fraction 0.20 to 0.25 or lower. Such patients are seen too often. The disconcerting fact is that such patients have often had "good" medical management since their coronary disease was first recognized years before, and have had neither recurrent major infarctions nor severe angina. Despite periodic medical observation and therapy, the disease has "silently" progressed. Some method other than severity of angina needs to be used to detect such patients and have bypass performed earlier. Some form of periodic stress testing, perhaps at least annually in patients with known coronary disease, seems to be necessary. One of the most definitive studies at present is a measurement of change in ejection fraction with exercise, especially in comparison with studies done in previous years.

LEFT VENTRICULAR ANEURYSM

HISTORICAL DATA. Safe excision of a ventricular aneurysm was not possible on a routine basis until the development of a pump oxygenator. Cooley, in 1958, is credited with one of the first reports of successful excision of an aneurysm with cardiopulmonary bypass. In the next few years, excision became a standard procedure in most cardiac clinics. Effler reported in 1965 that 61 such patients had been operated upon at the Cleveland Clinic. Series of more than 100 such aneurysms are now frequently reported.

ETIOLOGY, PATHOLOGY, AND PATHOGENESIS. A left ventricular aneurysm develops over a period of 4 to 8 weeks or longer in 10 to 15 percent of patients following a myocardial infarction (Fig. 19-25). It results when a severe transmural infarction destroys virtually all muscular fibers in the area of the infarction, which are subse-

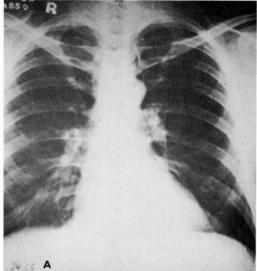

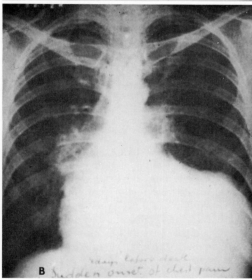

Fig. 19-25. Ventricular aneurysm. *A.* Chest radiograph showing a heart of normal size 2 days following an acute myocardial infarction. *B.* Chest radiograph showing cardiac enlargement from a large left ventricular aneurysm which progressively enlarged before a fatal episode of cardiac arrhythmia.

quently replaced by fibrous tissue. It probably does not occur more frequently following a transmural infarction because collateral circulation is sufficient to maintain viability of a variable number of muscle fibers in the zone of the infarct.

The classic aneurysm is simply an avascular scar 4 to 6 mm thick that bulges outward when the remaining left ventricular muscle contracts in systole. Hence, the term, "paradoxical contraction," more commonly termed "dyskinesis," as opposed to *hypokinesis* (impaired contractility) or *akinesis* (absence of contractility). Mural thrombi are found attached to the ventricular surface of the scar in over one-half of patients, but arterial emboli

are rare. The aneurysm usually enlarges a moderate degree and then becomes stationary; progressive enlargement and rupture, as usually occurs with atherosclerotic aortic aneurysms, is rare. Spotty calcification eventually develops in the aneurysmal wall in chronic cases. Over 80 percent of aneurysms are in the anterolateral portion of the left ventricle, evolving after occlusion of the anterior descending coronary. Lateral or posterior aneurysms are uncommon.

A "false" aneurysm is rare. It is a hematoma that is formed after rupture of a myocardial infarction has been temporarily supported by adjacent fibrous tissue. Excision should be done promptly, for such aneurysms soon expand and rupture.

In 30 to 40 percent of cases, significant coronary disease is limited to the anterior descending coronary, which is either completely occluded or severely stenosed. Multivessel disease is present in the other patients. Small aneurysms (less than 5 cm diameter) have negligible physiologic significance except possibly as a site of arrhythmias. Larger aneurysms decrease ventricular function apparently by dissipating energy of ventricular contraction with the ineffective paradoxical expansion of the wall of the aneurysm during systole. Possibly, the altered geometry of the left ventricular cavity is also significant, though this is difficult to measure. With larger aneurysms, the left ventricular volume is increased and left ventricular hypertrophy develops. The decrease in effective ventricular contraction eventually results in cardiac failure and angina, though angina may be due to the accompanying coronary disease as well. Arrhythmias are prominent in 10 to 15 percent of patients.

As the physiologic burden from an aneurysm is related to its size, the magnitude of improvement following operation is somewhat related to the size of the aneurysm. For this reason, it is doubtful that an aneurysm is ever large enough to be truly "inoperable" simply because of size. If a patient is alive with a large aneurysm, removal of the aneurysm should improve function of the remaining ventricular fibers if these are not harmed at the time of operation from either excessive resection of ventricular wall or inadequate myocardial preservation.

As the development of an aneurysm depends upon almost total destruction of muscle fibers, a true aneurysm, composed of akinetic scar, must be distinguished from a scar that results from an infarction that may be akinetic but whose wall is composed of varying proportions of fibrous tissue and viable muscle fibers. Excision of such akinetic scars has been investigated in some detail in the past but has not been found clinically beneficial.

Because of the wide spectrum between a ventricular "scar" and a true "aneurysm," accurate data to define natural history are almost impossible to obtain. The natural history of a patient with a ventricular aneurysm will, of course, be determined by at least three factors: the size of the aneurysm, the residual coronary disease, and the function of the remaining viable muscle. Five-year survival with an untreated aneurysm has ranged from as low as 10 percent to as high as 70 percent among different reports. Brusche et al. reported that 5-year survival in a patient with an akinetic segment was 70 percent; with a dyskinetic segment and good residual ventricular function, 54 percent; with a dyskinetic segment and poor ventricular function, 36 percent.

CLINICAL MANIFESTATIONS. Dyspnea or angina, either alone or in combination, are the two most common symptoms. Arrhythmias are prominent in a minority of patients. Abnormalities on physical examination are usually not diagnostic. The apical impulse may be forceful and diffuse with a "double impulse."

The chest x-ray may show a localized enlargement in the anteroapical area of the left ventricle. Electrocardiographic changes usually show only the signs of the previous infarction. Most diagnostic information comes from the left ventricular angiogram, outlining an akinetic area bulging paradoxically during systole. Often a clear differentiation cannot be made between an akinetic scar and a true aneurysm, with the final decision being made at the time of operation. If a discrete scar is found at operation, containing few or no muscle fibers, resection is indicated. If a diffuse bulging is present without discrete borders and obviously containing a moderate amount of muscle tissue, resection is probably contraindicated.

TREATMENT. Operation is indicated for symptomatic aneurysms larger than 5 to 6 cm. A moderate asymptomatic aneurysm may be simply observed. The operative procedure includes excision of the aneurysm and bypass grafting of the diseased coronary arteries. Grafting of the diseased anterior descending coronary, which often supplies principally ventricular scar, is of questionable value, though at NYU it has usually been grafted because of the possibility that improved blood supply to the ventricular septum might benefit ventricular arrhythmias.

In general, the aneurysm is not manipulated until the heart has been fibrillated or the aorta clamped to prevent dislodgment of mural thrombi. Once the heart is arrested or fibrillated, the heart is mobilized by freeing the aneurysm from the pericardial adhesions, often by simply incising the wall of the aneurysm and leaving part of the wall attached to the pericardium. After the heart is mobilized completely, a *subtotal* excision of the aneurysm is performed, dividing the wall of the aneurysm about 2 cm from its junction with left ventricular muscle. The *subtotal* concept is a crucial one, as the suture line closing the ventriculotomy is subsequently inserted through scar rather than through viable muscle surrounding the aneurysm. This precaution also avoids any excessive reduction in size of the ventricular cavity (Fig. 19-26). In all likelihood, operative deaths from excision of huge aneurysms probably result from excessive excision of the wall of the aneurysm with injury of the surrounding viable ventricular muscle.

The wall of the aneurysm usually includes the area of the anterior descending coronary, with the scar extending into the ventricular septum. Bypass grafting of the anterior descending in such instances is of uncertain significance, as the muscle supplied by the anterior descending has been infarcted. If significant tributaries to the ventricular septum are patent, the artery should be preserved and a bypass graft attached.

Usually, the extent of the endocardial scar is greater than that of the aneurysm. Because of the hazard of malignant ventricular arrhythmias, a localized excision of the subendocardial scar for one or more centimeters around the periphery of the aneurysm seems worthwhile, as this is easily done without significant injury to functioning ventricular muscle. Electrophysiologic studies have found that trigger zones for arrhythmias are usually located in the scar within 1 to 3 cm of the border of the aneurysm. When preoperative ventricular arrhythmias are prominent, electrophysiologic mapping to locate and excise the irritable foci should be done at the time of operation.

The opening following excision of the aneurysm is closed in an axis that conforms best to that of the residual ventricular fibers. Two or three rows of continuous synthetic sutures are used, occasionally reinforced with Teflon felt if the tissues are friable. Recurrence of an aneurysm is virtually unknown.

Technique of Operation. A sternotomy incision is employed. With huge aneurysms, an additional lateral thoracotomy is occasionally necessary. Pericardial adhesions may be severe. Dissection of these adhesions to mobilize the heart is best postponed until bypass is started. With bypass functioning, the perfusate is cooled, the aorta clamped, and the heart arrested with the cold blood potassium technique.

If concomitant coronary bypass grafting is to be done, the bypass grafts should be attached first to permit intermittent infusion of the cardioplegic solution through the grafts to provide additional myocardial protection. Attachment of all grafts may not be possible until the heart is mobilized and the aneurysm excised.

With the heart arrested and collapsed, pericardial adhesions may be divided and the aneurysm opened. With a huge aneurysm and dense adhesions, after the aneurysm has been opened and the origin from the wall of the left ventricle identified, the aneurysm can simply be divided a short distance from the pericardial adhesions, leaving this part of the aneurysmal wall in situ and thus avoiding troublesome bleeding.

RESULTS. Prognosis is determined principally by the residual ventricular function, which, in turn, is influenced by the size of the aneurysm and the severity of the coronary disease. In general, if angina was the prominent symptom before operation, 5-year survival is 60 percent or better, while if congestive heart failure was the principal indication for operation, 5-year survival is much less, near 30 percent.

Most patients are significantly improved following operation, manifested by relief of angina and improvement in ventricular function. With hemodynamic studies, significant improvement in ventricular function can be demonstrated in some patients, while others show very little change. Improvement in ejection fraction generally occurred when more than 24 cm^2 of aneurysmal wall were resected.

Olearchyk et al. described experiences with 244 cases with a 5-year survival near 70 percent. Dobell et al. in a series of 67 patients found a 5-year survival of 84 percent

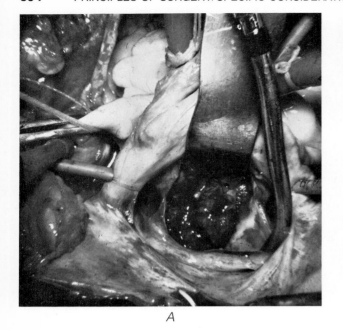

A

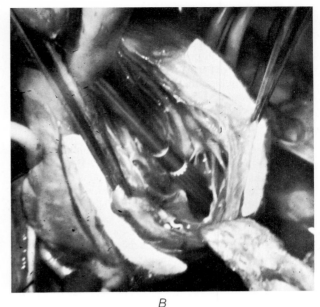

B

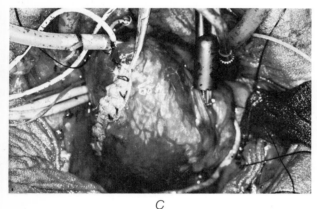

C

Fig. 19-26. *A.* Photograph of left ventricular aneurysm involving the posterior part of the left ventricle, an unusual location. *B.* The aneurysm has been excised, and the interior of the left ventricle is being inspected. The suction tip is within the ostium of the mitral valve, showing the proximity of the aneurysm to the mitral valve. The unusual occurrence of these aneurysms may be related to the fact that myocardial infarction in this area is often fatal because of concomitant mitral insufficiency. *C.* Completed repair of the aneurysm with a long suture line buttressed with Teflon felt. A coronary bypass graft is visible at the top of the field which was inserted into a branch of the circumflex coronary artery.

when angina was the prominent symptom, 53 percent if congestive failure were significant.

Akins et al. in a series of 100 ventricular aneurysms reported a 2 percent operative mortality and a 6-year survival of 77 percent.

PERICARDITIS

Acute Pyogenic Pericarditis

Pyogenic pericarditis has become a rare disease. It more commonly occurs in infants and children, often with a lack of resistance to infection because of a systemic disease. Hier et al. in 1985 stated that only about 200 cases had been reported in the Western literature in the previous 25 years. The diagnosis, once suspected, can be easily confirmed by echocardiography and pericardial aspiration. In virtually all series the most common organisms have been *Haemophilus influenzae* and the *Staphy-*

lococcus. If subxyphoid drainage is not satisfactory, as indicated by continuing sepsis or signs of tamponade, pericardiectomy is safe and effective. Morgan et al. described experiences with 15 children. The causative organism was *H. influenzae* in seven, *Staphylococcus* in three, other organisms in five. Treatment with pericardiocentesis was satisfactory in four; subxyphoid drainage was effective in one; while the others required pericardiectomy, after which all patients recovered without complications or recurrent symptoms.

Chronic Constrictive Pericarditis

HISTORICAL DATA. The first pericardiectomy in the United States was performed by Churchill in 1929. For the next two decades, operations were often limited in scope, apparently because of uncertainty as to how much of the constricted pericardium should be removed. In 1949, Holman concluded that constriction of the caval orifices was important in the pathogenesis and adopted a median sternotomy approach for its surgical correction. Subsequently, in 1952, Isaacs demonstrated that the fundamental pathophysiologic change was constriction of the ventricles, with resulting impairment of distensibility in diastole. These classic experiments led to the modern operation, a radical removal of the constricting scar from both ventricles, with secondary emphasis on removal over the atria and vena cavae.

ETIOLOGY. In the majority of patients, the cause is unknown, probably the end stage of an undiagnosed viral pericarditis. Tuberculosis is a rarity. In recent years, intensive radiation has become a significant cause in some series. Constrictive pericarditis rarely develops after an open heart operation. Kutcher et al. reported 11 cases following over 5000 open heart procedures. Cameron et al. described 11 percent of 95 cases related to postcardiac surgical problems.

PATHOLOGY AND PATHOPHYSIOLOGY. The pericardial cavity is obliterated by fusion of the parietal pericardium to the epicardium, forming dense scar tissue that encases and constricts the heart. In chronic cases, areas of calcification develop, adding an additional element of constriction.

The physiologic handicap is limitation of diastolic filling of the ventricles. This results in a decrease in cardiac output from a decrease in stroke volume. The right ventricular diastolic pressure is increased with a corresponding increase in right atrial and central venous pressure, ranging from 10 to 30 mmHg. The venous hypertension produces hepatomegaly, ascites, peripheral edema, and a generalized increase in blood volume.

CLINICAL MANIFESTATIONS. The disease is a slowly progressive one with increasing ascites and edema. Fatiguability and dyspnea on exertion are common, but dyspnea at rest is unusual. The ascites is often severe, as a result of which the diagnosis is easily confused with cirrhosis.

Hepatomegaly and ascites are often the most prominent physical abnormalities. Peripheral edema is moderate in some patients, severe in others. These findings are manifestations of advanced congestive failure from any form of heart disease. With constrictive pericarditis, however, the usual cardiac findings are a heart of normal size without murmurs or abnormal sounds. Atrial fibrillation is present in about one-third of the patients, and a pleural effusion is common in more severe cases. A paradoxical pulse is found in a small percentage of patients.

Chronic Constrictive Pericarditis

LABORATORY FINDINGS. Venous pressure is elevated, often to 15 to 20 mmHg or higher. The electrocardiogram, though not diagnostic, is usually abnormal with a low voltage and inverted T waves. The chest x-ray usually shows a heart of normal size, but pericardial calcification may be seen in a significant percentage of cases, often being the first clue to the diagnosis. CT may demonstrate a thickened pericardium.

Findings on cardiac catheterization are highly characteristic. There is elevation of the right ventricular diastolic pressure with a change in contour, showing an early filling with a subsequent plateau, the "square root" sign. Also, there is "equalization" of pressures in the different cardiac chambers as right atrial pressure, right ventricular diastolic pressure, pulmonary artery diastolic pressure, and pulmonary wedge pressure are similar. The one condition that cannot be excluded with certainty is a restrictive cardiomyopathy.

TREATMENT. Once the diagnosis has been made, pericardiectomy should be done promptly because the disease relentlessly progresses. Operation can be done through a sternotomy incision or a long left anterolateral thoracotomy. The constricting pericardium should be removed from all surfaces of the ventricle, mobilizing the heart to where it can be held freely upward in the hand. Removal over the atria and the cavae is somewhat optional, although this is usually done as well. The heart-lung machine is usually kept on a standby basis in the event of significant hemorrhage. If this occurs, the patient can be heparinized, the blood aspirated and returned to the patient until the laceration is repaired. The pericardium is removed bilaterally from the pulmonary veins on the right to the pulmonary veins on the left. Both phrenic nerves are mobilized and protected. Particular care is taken to remove pericardium over the pulmonary artery where residual constriction can seriously impair the operative result.

As the constricting scar develops from organization of an exudate between the pericardium and epicardium, the plane of dissection may often be external to the epicardium, which will greatly decrease operative hemorrhage. If the epicardium is thickened, it must be removed from the underlying myocardium, though this is tedious and results in diffuse bleeding.

Intracardiac pressures should be measured by direct needle puncture before and following pericardiectomy. Often with a complete pericardiectomy, the characteristic pressure abnormalities are either eliminated or greatly improved. If significant abnormalities remain, the operative field should be carefully checked for any residual sites of constriction. In all likelihood the slow recovery over many months in the past was simply a result of inadequate pericardiectomy, *not* underlying "ventricular atrophy."

RESULTS. Following a radical pericardiectomy that corrects the hemodynamic abnormalities, patients improve promptly with a massive diuresis. The risk of operation varies with the age of the patient and the severity of the disease; it is usually well under 5 percent. A good result can be anticipated, well over 90 percent.

Cameron et al. reported experiences with treatment of 95 patients. Thirty-one percent of cases resulted from radiotherapy. This group had the highest operative mortality, 21 percent.

HEART BLOCK AND PACEMAKERS

Alfred T. Culliford and Frank C. Spencer

Initially pacemakers were used for complete heart block, either resulting from operations or developing in older patients. Now pacemakers are used for a wide variety of arrhythmias, including the "sick sinus syndrome," an alternating bradycardia and tachycardia, and arrhythmias associated with varying degrees of atrioventricular (AV) block.

Approximately 120,000 implants are performed annually in the United States. The chief indications for permanent pacing were sick sinus syndrome (48 percent) and impairment of conduction in the atrioventricular node and HIS-Purkinge system (42 percent).

Heart Block

ETIOLOGY. Acquired heart block in the elderly, now termed "Lev's disease," appears to be a primary disease, a fibrosis of the conduction system without other significant cardiac disease. Another cause is calcification of cardiac valves involving the conduction system. Heart block from myocardial infarction is usually temporary, becoming permanent in only about 5 percent of patients.

Congenital heart block has been reported with increasing frequency. A recent report on 599 infants and children found the greatest risk of death in early infancy. After the first year of life, the outlook was much improved. Children with complete block and additional cardiac disease, however, had a 28 percent mortality. In small premature neonates with congenital complete heart block, permanent pacemakers have been implanted with good long-term results, indicating the refinements in design and size currently available.

Besley et al. reported experiences with implantation of pacemakers in 13 young adults with an average follow-up of 4 years. The authors questioned the concept that congenital heart block in older patients is usually a benign condition.

PATHOLOGY AND PATHOPHYSIOLOGY. In normal cardiac conduction, the cardiac impulse arises in the sinoatrial node near the junction of the superior vena cava with the right atrium. The impulse is propagated through the right atrial wall via internodal pathways to the AV node, lying medial to the ostium of the coronary sinus. From this node it travels along the bundle of HIS near the annulus of the tricuspid valve to pass through the central fibrous body of the ventricular septum near the junction of the muscular and membranous components. Here the bundle divides into right and left bundles, which, in turn, travel to their respective ventricles. The most common surgical trauma producing complete heart block occurs during repair of a ventricular septal defect or an ostium primum defect. It rarely may follow prosthetic replacement of the aortic, mitral, or tricuspid valve, either by direct injury or from traction and subsequent fibrosis. Injuries of the right or left conduction bundle per se are apparently not of great clinical significance.

Heart block seriously impairs cardiac output in several ways. The resulting bradycardia, varying from 25 to 60 beats/min depending upon the idioventricular response, decreases coronary and cerebral circulation. Refractory congestive failure may exist even with rates as high as 45 beats/min. There is intolerance to exercise and even symptoms of cerebral vascular insufficiency with syncope and convulsions.

Clinical symptoms attributed to first-degree heart block (PR interval 0.2 s) are rare. With second-degree heart block (intermittent lack of AV conduction) symptoms become apparent if the bradycardia is severe or persistent. In third-degree heart block (complete lack of AV conduction) bradycardia is persistent and symptoms are quite common.

With complete AV disassociation, there may be periods of transient ventricular asystole with syncope, convulsions, and even death. Equally disastrous in some patients, rather than cardiac arrest, are bouts of ventricular tachycardia or fibrillation, as ventricular "escape" mechanisms result from absence of normal AV conduction. With lesser degrees of heart block, the cardiac rate may be normal most of the time but abruptly change into complete AV disassociation with its attendant complications. Any such episode may be followed by recovery or may result in death. Intermittent attacks of syncope and convulsions with heart block were designated the Stokes-Adams syndrome. Some patients never develop these symptoms but become disabled with cardiac failure.

CLINICAL MANIFESTATIONS. Although some patients may be asymptomatic with a rate as low as 35 beats/min, most have symptoms with a rate less than 45. Episodic Stokes-Adams attacks are the most frequent disability; between attacks the patient feels well. During these episodes, syncope appears abruptly, often with convulsions. The 12-month mortality rate for patients with Stokes-Adams attack who are not paced is 25 to 50 percent.

In milder forms, recurrent syncope may be the only symptom. Differential diagnosis must consider heart block, aortic stenosis, simple syncope, carotid sinus syndrome, epilepsy, or occlusive arterial disease of the cerebral circulation. The diagnosis can be quickly established with the electrocardiogram.

With intermittent heart block, or a "sick sinus syndrome" (tachy-bradyarrhythmia), a 24-h Holter monitoring may be necessary to make the diagnosis. This test is now performed with increasing frequency because certain cardiac arrhythmias can only be recognized by this form of continuous monitoring. Between intermittent episodes, there may be no findings whatever.

Certain electrocardiographic abnormalities suggest the diagnosis. These include trifascicular block, degrees of block less than complete AV disassociation, and the Mobitz type II block. These often signify impending AV disassociation.

As mentioned above, some patients become disabled from progressive heart failure related to inadequate cardiac output. Dramatic improvement, with prompt diuresis, often follows insertion of a pacemaker.

Pacemakers

HISTORICAL DATA. The entire field of pacemakers has expanded to a surprising degree since Bigelow and Callaghan in 1950–1951 developed an electric pacemaker that would increase the rate of the hypothermic heart. In 1952, Zoll convincingly demonstrated clinical possibilities by restarting the hearts of terminal patients with complete heart block, using electrical stimulation through the chest wall with a 60-cycle alternating current–powered Grass stimulator. Surgical interest was heightened with the development of open heart surgery and the unfortunate production of heart block during repair of congenital cardiac lesions. Lillihei demonstrated that direct cardiac pacing could be performed with an electrode implanted in the ventricle, although long-term stimulation with such electrodes ultimately failed, often due to infection. A completely implantable permanent pacemaker was described by Senning in 1959 and by Chardack in 1960. A remarkable clinical discovery was made by Furman and Schwedel in 1959, who found that the heart could be permanently paced with a transvenous catheter wedged into the endocardial surface of the right ventricle. They reported that one could safely leave a catheter in the superior vena cava across the tricuspid valve and permanently positioned in the right ventricle. Once the safety of the technique was established, the transvenous method quickly became the procedure of choice, with far less morbidity and mortality than the previous transthoracic approach.

Other investigators making significant contributions after 1960 include Frank, Kantrowitz, Escher, and Parsonnet. By 1978, Tyers estimated that 100,000 pacemakers were implanted each year for a wide variety of arrhythmias.

Several major technical developments have evolved, rendering pacemaker implantation a safe and predictable form of therapy. Early pacemakers were in epoxy, which permitted some transmission of body fluids. This accounted for the early depletion of the energy cells. Hermetic sealing has gradually been adopted since 1970, virtually avoiding permeation of body fluids. Tyers deserves credit for this important concept. It is estimated that as many as 40,000 early pacemaker recalls were necessary because of the premature power cell failure from penetration of body fluids. Fortunately, this is now almost never seen.

Another major development was the introduction of the lithium-polymer iodine cell in 1968, developed and refined by the Catalyst Research-Wilson Greatbatch Corporation. Over 200,000 of these had been implanted by 1978 without a single proved battery failure. Lithium batteries, a large variety of which have subsequently been developed, have much greater longevity than the zinc–mercuric oxide batteries originally used. Early pacemakers often failed within 2 to 3 years, perhaps sooner, because of permeation of body fluids. With refined lithium-iodine cells, 5 years of pacing is virtually a certainty, and the probability of 10 years of effective pacing is estimated to be greater than 90 percent.

PHYSIOLOGY OF CARDIAC PACEMAKERS. The electrical resistance of the normal heart is 300 to 500 Ω, while the fibrillating threshold to electrical stimulation is at least ten times greater. The efficacy of cardiac pacing depends upon the ability of the heart to respond to short bursts (2 ms) of electric current, ideally less than 1.5 to 2 mA. This amount of current is effective if delivered directly to the heart, but much larger currents are necessary to pace the ventricle through the intact chest wall.

The site of cardiac pacing, the right or left ventricle, apparently is of little significance. The electrode size,

configuration, and material are all important. There is a direct linear relationship between stimulation threshold and electrode surface area, the lowest threshold being associated with the smallest surface area. The optimal surface area for an electrode is about 12 mm^2. The energy capacity of a pacemaker is usually expressed as microjoules. One microjoule is one-millionth of the energy expended by a current of 1 A flowing for 1 s through a resistance of 1 Ω. Energy output in different pacemakers varies from 10 to 150 μJ, depending upon several factors. Other characteristics of the pacemakers include a voltage ranging from 2.5 to 7.5 V, delivering 3.5 to 15 mA, and pulse duration ranging from 0.15 to 1.5 ms.

When a pacemaker is implanted, it is crucial to determine the pacing threshold, measuring this in both milliamperes and volts. Threshold determination is particularly important with intravenous implantations in order to ensure that the catheter in the right ventricle is in the proper position. With satisfactory location of an electrode, a threshold of 0.4 to 0.8 mA at 0.2 to 0.4 V and a pulse width of 1 ms should be obtained.

After implantation, the threshold rises rapidly twofold to threefold in the next 2 to 4 weeks, stabilizing after about 1 month. Hence, the pulse generator output is adjusted in anticipation of this rise in threshold. An excessive rise in threshold may occur from infection or fibrosis, with resultant loss of pacing, termed "exit block." Special high-output pacemaker generators, stimulating up to 10 V, may be used in patients in whom previous pacemakers have failed because of exit block.

Ventricular pacing may be done with unipolar or bipolar leads. In the bipolar system, both the positive and negative electrodes are in contact with the endocardium. With epicardial implantation, both electrodes must be attached. If unipolar pacing, which is the most common, is used, the top of the electrode is the stimulating pole. Most efficient stimulation results from cathodal stimulation. The only particular advantage of bipolar stimulation is that the sensitivity to external magnetic interference is much less.

METHODS OF PACING. Initial pacemakers stimulated the ventricle at a fixed rate. These fixed-rate asynchronous units had numerous disadvantages, including the possible production of ventricular fibrillation by competition with the patient's own rhythm. Fixed-rate pacemakers have been supplanted by demand pacemakers, usually triggered from a ventricular electrode. These are of two types, the R-wave-inhibited type and the R-wave-triggered pacemaker. A more complex type is the atrioventricular pacemaker, requiring an electrode in the right atrium as well as in the ventricle (Fig. 19-27A and B). The resulting pacing may be through the atrium, or it may be atrioventricular synchronous pacing, stimulating first the atrium, then after an appropriate delay, the ventricle (Fig. 19-28). All of these have the advantage of coordinating with the patient's own cardiac rhythm and supplying an "atrial kick" when the atrioventricular sequential pacing is employed. Finally, the development of programmable pacemakers in the last 5 years permits adjustment of rate, pulse amplitude, and duration, which greatly enhances the function of pacemakers in different circum-

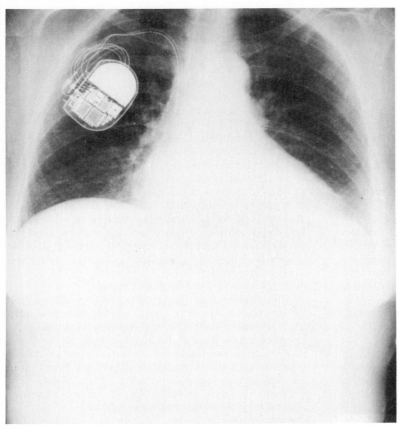

A

Fig. 19-27. *A* and *B*. AP and lateral chest x-ray of patient who developed complete heart block following aortic valve replacement, septal myotomy and myomectomy, ventricular aneurysm resection, and coronary artery bypass grafting. Dual chamber pacing was employed to optimize cardiac output.

stances. Undoubtedly, the entire field will continue to evolve rapidly as new benefits from different types of pacing are found.

With the growing complexity of the mode of pacing, location, and function of cardiac electrodes and with the multiplicity of terms introduced by trade companies, the Pacemaker Study Group of the American Heart Association introduced a simple generic three-letter identification code to identify the chamber paced, the chamber sensed, and the mode of generator function (Table 19-1, Fig. 19-29).

Initial pacemakers were heavy and bulky, a nuisance for adults but a serious problem for children, with the danger of erosion of the overlying skin. Developments in printed electric circuits and semiconductors have led to a progressive decrease in size. In 1978 Culliford et al. reported a technique of implantation in premature infants. In a 1981 review, Young surveyed the status of pacemakers in children, reviewing over 10 reports describing experiences with 448 implantations. The small pacemakers weigh only 50 g with a 20- to 25-mL volume, as compared with older units of 160 to 200 g and 160- to 200-mL volume.

Nuclear Pacemakers. Smyth et al. reported experiences with isotopic pacemakers in 59 patients. Details of nuclear-powered pacemakers are presented in his report.

Tyers and Brownlee raised issues about nuclear pacemakers, which are usually powered by plutonium 238. The basic concern is the long-term effect of radiation on the patient. The amount of radiation is very small in a nuclear pacemaker, but the effects of radiation on the induction of thyroid cancer were not known for over 20 years. Also bone marrow is susceptible to induction of leukemia by radiation. In addition, there is the real risk of environmental contamination. A sobering point is that if one of these units were lost in the ocean, 98 percent of the original 3100 microcuries of plutonium 238 would still be present more than 800 years later. The basic advantage, of course, is that these pacemakers should certainly function for 10 years, possibly indefinitely, and so the probability of battery change is remote. Because of the hazards, however, nuclear pacers are not recommended for younger patients.

IMPLANTATION OF PACEMAKERS. Medical therapy for chronic heart block has virtually disappeared with the development of effective pacemakers. Several years ago, in one group of 100 patients treated before pacemakers were available, 30 percent were dead in 6 months and 75

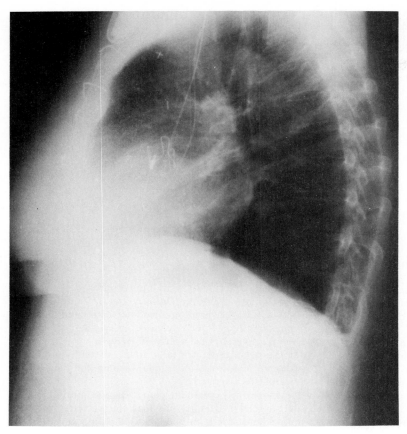

B

Fig. 19-27 *B*. Continued.

percent within 5 years. Hence, pacemakers are now employed promptly for bradycardias, even when they are asymptomatic, and are also widely used for several other arrhythmias. For transitory heart block following myocardial infarction, temporary pacing with a catheter electrode introduced through a peripheral vein and advanced into the right ventricle is usually effective. The block disappears in 90 to 95 percent of patients. Heart block following intracardiac operations is common, almost always subsiding in the next several days. A routine in the majority of cardiac centers is to leave pacing wires in the atrium and ventricle before the chest is closed, removing these several days later. Usually the wires can be used to pace the heart with an external generator for as long as 2 to 3 weeks.

The vast majority of pacemakers are inserted by the transvenous route because of the low morbidity. In order of preference, the cephalic vein, the external jugular vein, or the internal jugular vein may be used. In 1980, Brodman and Furman described a 12-year experience with 1800 patients, in 90 of whom the use of the internal jugular vein was necessary after finding that both the cephalic and external jugular veins were unsatisfactory.

Once the vein has been surgically exposed, the transvenous endocardial electrode can be advanced into the right ventricle, guided under fluoroscopic control, and wedged in an appropriate area. As mentioned earlier, determination of threshold is crucial in securing proper positioning of the catheter. Once the catheter has been positioned, the pacemaker is implanted in a subcutaneous pocket over the chest wall. Morbidity with the transvenous technique is small. Migration of the catheter from improper fixation is the most common complication. Perforation of the ventricle can occur with resultant diaphragmatic pacing or even tamponade. Infection or venous thrombosis is surprisingly rare.

Direct surgical approaches employ one of three routes: short left intercostal, subxiphoid, or left subcostal incision. Morbidity is definitely greater with a direct surgical approach than with a transvenous approach. However, with the development of the sutureless myocardial electrode, a "screw-in" electrode 6 mm in length, morbidity is much less than it used to be. Once the electrode is secured, the frequency of electrode complication is significantly less than with the transvenous approach, though the morbidity from the surgical procedure generally outweighs the advantages. Most would agree that the direct approach should be employed primarily for patients in whom the transvenous route has not been satisfactory because of pulmonary hypertension, dilated right atrium or ventricle, endocardial fibrosis, or tricuspid regurgitation.

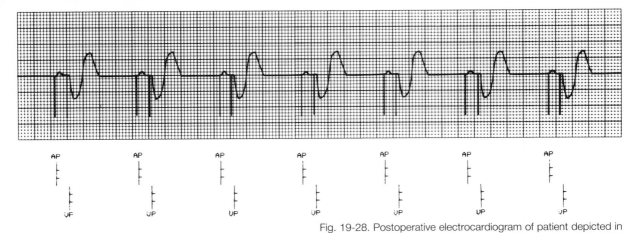

Fig. 19-28. Postoperative electrocardiogram of patient depicted in Fig. 19-27 with AV sequential pacemaker functioning. AP = atrial pace, VP = ventricular pace.

As mentioned earlier, the pacemakers are usually of the "demand" variety, with a basic rate between 70 and 80 beats/min, varying with the patient's own rhythm. The recent development of programmable pacemakers permits the subsequent alteration of pacing rate, pulse width, and amplitude. Also, the mode of pacing can be changed if conditions change.

Recovery following operation is usually uneventful. Antibiotics are given for 3 to 4 days. Difficulties with the subcutaneous implantation of the generator are infrequent, especially with the small generators now available and with meticulous surgical technique at the time of implantation.

Following discharge from the hospital, the patient should be seen in 2 to 3 weeks, because a rise in pacing threshold will occur. After this, the patient should be followed at 3-month intervals indefinitely.

Telephone electrocardiographic surveillance has been a significant advance in periodically evaluating patients over a large geographic distance. Convincing data from several sources indicate that this type of periodic monitoring is mandatory for good care. A typical report from

Table 19-1. THREE-LETTER IDENTIFICATION CODE

1st letter	*2d letter*	*3d letter*
Chamber paced	*Chamber sensed*	*Mode of response*
V—Ventricle		I—Inhibited
A—Atrium		T—Triggered
D—Double chamber		O—Not applicable

First letter: The paced chamber is identified by V for ventricle, A for atrium, or D for double—both atrium and ventricle.
Second letter: The sensed chamber, if either, is again V for ventricle, A for atrium.
Third letter: The mode of response, if any, is either:
  I for inhibited, a pacemaker whose output is blocked by a sensed signal, or
  T for triggered, a unit whose output is discharged by a sensed signal.
  O indicates that a specific comment is not applicable.

Rubin et al. described telephonic surveillance over a period of 3 years in 216 patients, finding 82 complications, 60 of which were asymptomatic. They estimated that telephonic surveillance may have decreased the death rate in pacemaker patients by nearly 50 percent.

As the pulse generator fails, there is usually a gradual slowing of the rate, giving ample warning that the generator should be changed.

Patients with permanent pacemakers requiring subsequent surgical procedures in which electrocautery is to be employed are at risk for pacemaker malfunction. Electromagnetic fields as high as 60 V/m are commonly induced with electrocautery, which far exceeds the energy level required to activate the sensing circuit in most pacemakers (usually in the area of 0.1 V/m). As a result, the intense signal may inhibit the pulse generator in a pacemaker-dependent patient or may damage the circuitry or reset programmable units. A variety of arrhythmias have been observed: ventricular asystole, multiple premature ventricular contractions, ventricular tachycardia, and fibrillation. In patients for whom electrocautery cannot be avoided, brief bursts of bipolar cautery should be used because it minimizes the ambient electrical field around the probe. The program for programmable units should be available in the operating room and a thorough preoperative evaluation of the patient may indicate the advisability of a backup temporary transvenous wire in patients who are totally pacemaker-dependent. Awareness of the adverse effects electrocautery may have on paced patients will provide enhanced interoperative and postoperative monitoring. The importance of these potentially serious and lethal complications is reinforced when one considers that many of the over 500,000 individuals in the United States who now have permanent pacemakers will require elective or emergency surgical care in the future.

AUTOMATIC IMPLANTABLE DIFIBRILLATORS. In 1980, Mirowski reported on the successful termination of malignant ventricular arrhythmias with an automatic implantable defibrillator. Although this form of therapy is still in the early stages of development, a 1984 report

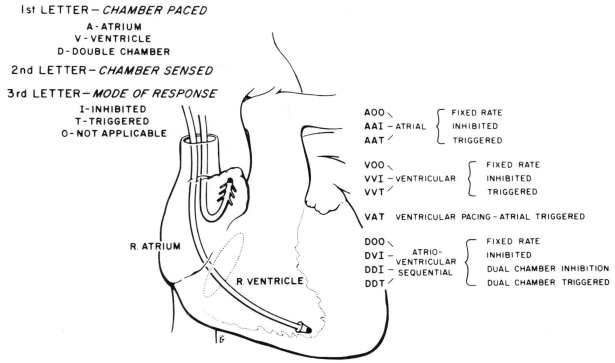

1st LETTER — *CHAMBER PACED*
  A - ATRIUM
  V - VENTRICLE
  D - DOUBLE CHAMBER

2nd LETTER — *CHAMBER SENSED*

3rd LETTER — *MODE OF RESPONSE*
  I - INHIBITED
  T - TRIGGERED
  O - NOT APPLICABLE

AOO ╲
AAI — ATRIAL   { FIXED RATE
AAT ╱   INHIBITED
                   TRIGGERED

VOO ╲
VVI — VENTRICULAR { FIXED RATE
VVT ╱   INHIBITED
                    TRIGGERED

VAT VENTRICULAR PACING - ATRIAL TRIGGERED

DOO ╲
DVI — ATRIO-   { FIXED RATE
DDI — VENTRICULAR   INHIBITED
DDT ╱ SEQUENTIAL   DUAL CHAMBER INHIBITION
                      DUAL CHAMBER TRIGGERED

R. ATRIUM

R. VENTRICLE

Fig. 19-29. Three-letter identification code presently in international use. *(Reprinted courtesy of the American Heart Association.)*

showed apparent early success for 78 consecutive patients with ventricular tachycardia and fibrillation refractory to antiarrhythmic drugs who received implantable automatic internal cardioverter-defibrillator devices.

Others have combined endocardial resection, intraoperative electrophysiologic studies, and implantation of these devices. Twelve such patients were reported by Watkins in 1984. The survival period has been 32 months thus far, with 2 deaths occurring that were not attributable to cardiac causes. The device had been noted to be repetitively successful in terminating fatal ventricular arrhythmias in these patients.

As increasing numbers of patients survive the "sudden cardiac death syndrome" because of prompt treatment and the growing popular awareness of resuscitative techniques, this form of therapy should prove promising for patients failing pharmacologic management of malignant arrhythmias if continued clinical experience and technological advances support the thus far favorable, but limited, clinical observations.

ASSISTED CIRCULATION AND ARTIFICIAL HEARTS

Assisted Circulation

Temporary assisted circulation is a valuable clinical modality when a transient cardiac injury is present, as opposed to a permanent injury such as extensive myocardial infarction. The usual indication for assisted circulation occurs following a cardiac operation when myocardial function is significantly depressed, usually manifested by a cardiac index less than 2.0 L/m^2/min. In such instances, assisting the circulation for 24 to 48 h or longer may permit spontaneous improvement in cardiac function, probably from resolution of myocardial edema. The improvement in function is probably accomplished by maintaining adequate perfusion while decreasing the work of the myocardium, hence the term "assisted circulation."

As the concept of temporary assisted circulation is based upon the ability of the heart to spontaneously recover from an existing injury, assisted circulation is seldom effective if required for more than 2 to 3 days, as such patients usually have irreversible myocardial infarction.

Because of the vascular circulation in the heart, the subendocardial area is the most vulnerable, as it is the farthest removed from the coronary arteries on the epicardial surface. With severe myocardial edema from any cause, subendocardial necrosis can result, probably from constriction and compression of terminal coronary arterioles, perhaps analogous to the compartmental syndromes that may occur in the leg after a crush injury, when edema progresses to such an extent that circulation is stopped and tissue necrosis occurs.

The concept of assisting the failing heart by pumping part or all of the circulation through a heart-lung machine has been investigated since the onset of extracorporeal circulation around 1955. It was quickly observed by several groups that a heart unable to maintain circulation after operation with extracorporeal circulation could be supported with a heart-lung machine for 1 to 2 h and then function satisfactorily, apparently recovering from a transient injury. From these observations, the concept of "assisted circulation" was born, supporting the circulation for days, until spontaneous recovery of cardiac function occurred.

If severe myocardial edema is present, the prompt use of assisted circulation may permit full recovery because the edema resolves without the development of extensive necrosis. Delayed use of assisted circulation may permit some patients to spontaneously recover, but others will progress to infarction. Belatedly trying assisted circulation with these patients will inevitably result in a higher mortality because irreversible necrosis is present.

INTRAAORTIC BALLOON PUMPING. Intraaortic balloon pumping is the most effective clinical technique for assisted circulation. This was developed primarily through the efforts of Austen and his associates. A balloon catheter is inserted into a peripheral artery, usually the femoral, and advanced into the thoracic aorta. The safest method for insertion is by direct arteriotomy, but percutaneous insertion of a balloon can be done in urgent problems, initiating balloon pumping much more rapidly. The percutaneous method has more complications, however, especially in females with small femoral arteries.

With electronic synchronization, the balloon is alternately inflated during diastole and deflated during systole. When functioning properly, cardiac index is increased about 0.5 to 0.7 L/min. The pump can be used for several days with minimal morbidity. The blood platelet count usually decreases, probably from trauma from inflation of the balloon. This may be treated with platelet transfusions.

Ischemia of the extremity in which the balloon catheter has been inserted is the most common complication. With large femoral arteries this is unusual. In patients with small or diseased femoral arteries, however, insertion of a balloon may be catastrophic, resulting in either gangrene of the extremity or death. Viability of the extremity must be confirmed by frequent examination of the extremity for the first few hours after the balloon has been inserted. Viability, of course, depends upon continued flow of blood to the extremity around the catheter lying within the artery. If the artery is occluding the lumen, either because of the small size of the artery or because of an atherosclerotic plaque, the same severe ischemia exists as that produced by acute arterial occlusion from an embolus.

At NYU the balloon pump is used promptly if the cardiac index remains below 2 L despite other forms of therapy. It seems lifesaving in postoperative patients, where transient injury may regress after 2 to 4 days. In the last 2 to 3 years, the frequency of use of a balloon has decreased markedly, probably because of the concurrent improvement in the effectiveness of techniques of myocardial preservation.

In one other group, 188 patients were discharged from the hospital following support. The average period of support in these patients was about 60 h. Patients who achieved a cardiac index greater than 2 L were successfully weaned from the pump, while those whose cardiac index remained below the 2.0-L level had a mortality well above 50 percent. In another report only 35 percent of the group ultimately survived hospitalization. Three patients developed the grim complication of paraplegia.

LEFT HEART BYPASS. Dennis demonstrated the benefits of assisted circulation with left heart bypass in experimental studies, withdrawing blood from the atrium and infusing it into a peripheral artery. Difficulties with closed chest cannulation of the left atrium, however, prevented clinical application of the procedure. In the early 1960s Spencer used left heart bypass in a small group of patients by performing a thoracotomy, directly cannulating the left atrium, and employing left heart bypass for 3 to 4 h. Longer periods, however, were impractical.

Clinical use of the technique for patients in cardiogenic shock is under active investigation, though significant data are not yet available. Litwak devised a new type of left heart bypass, to be used in patients who could not be weaned from the heart-lung machine following operation. Silastic cannulae were left in the left atrium and femoral artery and brought through the chest wall before the incision was closed. Pumping was done with a roller pump with silastic tubing, infusing enough heparin to keep the activated clotting time near 150 s. The technique produced significant platelet destruction but otherwise was well tolerated.

With some modifications the Litwak technique was adopted at New York University. Flow rates up to 3500 mL/min could be obtained. Support was used for periods ranging from 16 to 70 h. In 1983 Rose et al. summarized total experiences at NYU with a series of 35 patients. Seventeen patients survived to have the device removed, four of whom died in the next 2 to 4 months. Three of the deaths were from sepsis. Of 13 long-term survivors, five had mild to moderate cardiac symptoms and eight were asymptomatic. The data fully indicate the value of assisted circulation because the device clearly permitted recovery of a heart whose function was temporarily decreased to a near lethal degree.

OTHER FORMS OF LEFT HEART BYPASS. Left heart–aortic bypass with a roller pump has the advantage of ease of applicability and simplicity, but it is moderately traumatic, is nonpulsatile, and is not coordinated with the patient's own cardiac contractions, as is electronically done with intraaortic balloon pumping. Much effort has accordingly been expended to develop physiologically more efficient forms of left heart assist that would effectively support the circulation for weeks or months.

Pierce et al. described experiences with 30 patients over a period of 6 years. Subsequent to 1979, survival increased to about 50 percent, partly because of use of the left atrium rather than the left ventricle for cannulation. Seven patients remained well 5 to 36 months after discharge from the hospital. The Pierce Donachy pump is currently one of the most effective temporary left heart pumps. It is expensive and somewhat difficult to insert but can clearly function satisfactorily for weeks without significant blood trauma. It seems to be a potentially ideal bridge for transplantation. Park and Magovern reported the use of a centrifugal pump in 41 patients, not all of whom required anticoagulation. Schoen et al. reported experiences with diaphragm pumps for temporary circulatory assistance.

Artificial Hearts

Attempts to develop an artificial heart have continued for decades, with a large interdisciplinary program coordinated by the National Heart and Lung Institute. The group headed by Kolff has the longest continued studies of different forms of artificial hearts, with impressive results in calves that survived with an artificial heart for many months. These studies led to the first clinical trial of an artificial heart at Salt Lake City, Utah, in December 1982. The patient survived slightly more than 100 days. Several patients have been successfully operated on, but subsequent thromboembolism was crippling.

The major obstacle is the lack of an artificial substance that resembles a normal intima in the bloodstream. All existing substances result in a surface aggregation of platelets and institution of the thrombotic process. Hence, thromboembolism is a serious or prohibitive risk unless anticoagulation is used, which, in turn, causes problems from bleeding.

Among the several artificial hearts currently under study, the Jarvik-7 model is the most popular. The cumbersome pneumatic-driven pumps, requiring tubes through the chest wall, have been a serious handicap. At present, the best use of heart pumps seems to be as a bridge until clinical transplantation can be done, for results with transplantation are far better. In the future, some type of electrically powered artificial heart seems far preferable to the pneumatic-powered devices.

Griffith et al. in 1987 reported experiences with the Jarvik-7 total artificial heart in six moribund patients, using this as a bridge to transplantation. Four patients were currently well, subsequently having the device removed and a successful transplant performed. In these six patients, total mechanical support was used for a total of 52 days with excellent function of the artificial heart.

Bibliography

Introduction; Clinical Manifestations

Arciniegas E: *Pediatric Cardiac Surgery.* Chicago, Year Book Medical Publishers, 1985.

Gibbon JH Jr, Sabiston DC Jr, Spencer FC: *Surgery of the Chest,* 3d ed. Philadelphia, Saunders, 1976.

Kirklin JW, Barratt-Boyes BG: *Cardiac Surgery.* New York, Wiley, 1986.

Perloff JK: *The Clinical Recognition of Congenital Heart Disease,* 3d ed. Philadelphia, Saunders, 1987.

Smith P: Several consequences of cardiopulmonary bypass. *Lancet* 1:823, 1986.

Sotaniemi KA: Five-year neurological and EEG outcome after open heart surgery. *J Neurol Neurosurg Psychiatry* 48:569, 1985.

Stark J, de Leval M (eds): *Surgery for Congenital Heart Defects.* London, Grune and Stratton, 1983.

Starr A: Presidential address: The thoracic surgical industrial complex. *Ann Thorac Surg* 42:124, 1986.

Extracorporeal Circulation

Bartlett RH, Gazzaniga AB, et al: Extracorporeal membrane oxygenation (ECMO) in neonatal respiratory failure. 100 cases. *Ann Surg* 204(3):236.

Boyd AD, Tremblay RE, et al: Estimation of cardiac output soon after intracardiac surgery with cardiopulmonary bypass. *Ann Surg* 150:613, 1959.

Brantigan CO, Grow JB: Cricothyroidotomy: Elective use in respiratory problems requiring tracheostomy. *J Thorac Cardiovasc Surg* 71:72, 1976.

Buckberg GD: Studies of control reperfusion after ischemia. *J Thorac Cardiovasc Surg* 92(suppl):483, 1986.

DeWall RA, Warden HE, et al: The helix reservoir pump-oxygenator. *Surg Gynecol Obstet* 104:699, 1957.

Esposito R, Culliford A, et al: What is the relationship between plasma heparin concentration and (ACT) activated clotting time? Presented at the 1982 meeting of the American Association for Thoracic Surgery, Phoenix.

Gibbon JH Jr: Application of a mechanical heart and lung apparatus to cardiac surgery. *Minn Med* 37:171, 1954.

Jones RE, Donald DE, et al: Apparatus of the Gibbon type for mechanical bypass of the heart and lungs: Preliminary report. *Proc Staff Meetings Mayo Clin* 30:105, 1955.

Proceedings of Cardioplegia: The First Quarter Century. An International Symposium on Myocardial Protection, London, 1980.

Spencer FC, Benson DW, et al: Use of a mechanical respirator in the management of respiratory insufficiency following trauma or operation for cardiac or pulmonary disease. *J Thorac Cardiovasc Surg* 38:758, 1959.

Stephen Thomas J (ed): *Manual of Cardiac Anesthesia.* New York, Churchill, Livingstone, 1984.

Cardiac Arrest and Ventricular Fibrillation

Cobb LA, Werner JA, Trobaugh GB: Sudden cardiac death. I. A decade's experience with out-of-hospital resuscitation. *Mod Concepts Cardiovasc Dis* 49:31, 1980.

Cobb LA, Werner JA, Trobaugh GB: Sudden cardiac death. II. Outcome of resuscitation; management, and future directions. *Mod Concepts Cardiovasc Dis* 49:37, 1980.

Del Guercio LRM, Feins NR, et al: Comparison of blood flow during external and internal cardiac massage in man. *Circulation* 31(suppl I):I171, 1965.

Dunn HM, McComb JM, et al: Survival to leave hospital from ventricular fibrillation. *Am Heart J* 112:745, 1986.

Geehr EC, Lewis FR, Auerbach PS: Failure of open-heart massage to improve survival after prehospital non-traumatic cardiac arrest. *N Engl J Med* 314:1189, 1986.

Hughes WG, Ruedy JR: Should calcium be used in cardiac arrest? *Am J Med* 81(2):285, 1986.

Joseph WL, Maloney JV Jr: Extracorporeal circulation as an adjunct to resuscitation of the heart. *JAMA* 193:683, 1965.

Jude JR, Elam JO: *Fundamentals of Cardiopulmonary Resuscitation.* Philadelphia, Davis, 1965.

Koehler RC, Chandra N, et al: Augmentation of cerebral perfusion by simultaneous chest compression and lung inflation with abdominal binding after cardiac arrest in dogs. *Circulation* 67(2):266, 1983.

Kouwenhoven WB, Jude JR, Knickerbocker GG: Closed chest cardiac massage. *JAMA* 137:1064, 1960.

Kouwenhoven WB, Milnor WR, et al: Closed chest defibrillation of the heart. *Surgery* 42:550, 1957.

Myerburg RJ, Kessler KM, et al: Long-term survival after pre-hospital cardiac arrest: Analysis of outcome during an eight year study. *Circulation* 70(4):538, 1984.

Roy D, Waxman HL, et al: Clinical characteristics and long-term follow-up in 119 survivors of cardiac arrest: Relation to inducibility at electrophysiologic testing. *Am J Cardiol* 52(8):969, 1983.

Rudikoff MT, Maughan WL, et al: Mechanisms of blood flow during cardiopulmonary resuscitation. *Circulation* 61(2):345, 1980.

Safar P: Cerebral resuscitation after cardiac arrest: A review. *Circulation* 74(6, 2):IV138, 1986.

Sanders AB, Kern KB, et al: Improved resuscitation from cardiac arrest with open-chest massage. *Ann Emerg Med* 13:672, 1984.

Sanders AB, Kern MD, et al: Correspondence: More on open-chest cardiac massage after cardiac arrest. *N Engl J Med* 315:968, 1986.

Spencer FC, Bahnson HT: Treatment of cardiac arrest, in Benson CD, et al (eds): *Pediatric Surgery*. Chicago, Year Book Medical Publishers, 1962, vol I, p 522.

Surawicz B: Ventricular fibrillation. *J Am Coll Cardiol* 5(suppl 6):43B, 1985.

Wilber DJ, Garan H, Ruskin JN: Electrophysiologic testing in survivors of cardiac arrest. *Circulation* 75(suppl III):146, 1987.

Williams GR, Spencer FC: The clinical use of hypothermia following cardiac arrest. *Ann Surg* 148:462, 1958.

Zimmerman JM, Spencer FC: The influence of hypothermia on cerebral injury resulting from circulatory occlusion. *Surg Forum* 9:216, 1958.

Mitral Stenosis and Insufficiency

Chauvaud S, Perier P, et al: Long-term results of valve repair in children with acquired mitral valve incompetence. *Circulation* 74:1104, 1986.

Cobanoglu A, Grunkemeier GL, et al: Mitral replacement: Clinical experience with a ball-valve prosthesis. Twenty-five years later. *Ann Surg* 202:376, 1985.

Cohn LH, Allred EN, et al: Long-term results of open mitral valve reconstruction for mitral stenosis. *Am J Cardiol* 55:731, 1985.

Ferrazzi P, McGiffin DC, et al: Have the results of mitral valve replacement improved? *J Thorac Cardiovasc Surg* 92:186, 1986.

Halseth W, Elliott D, et al: Open mitral commissurotomy: A modern re-evaluation. *J Thorac Cardiovasc Surg* 80:842, 1980.

Hetzer R, Bougioukas G, et al: Mitral valve replacement with preservation of papillary muscles and chordae tendineae—revival of a seemingly forgotten concept. I. Preliminary clinical report. *J Thorac Cardiovasc Surg* 31:291, 1983.

Higgs LM, Glancy DL, et al: Mitral restenosis: An uncommon cause of recurrent symptoms following mitral commissurotomy. *Am J Cardiol* 26:34, 1970.

Isom OW, Spencer FC, et al: Long-term results in 1375 patients undergoing valve replacement with the Starr-Edwards cloth-covered steel ball valve prosthesis. *Ann Surg* 186:310, 1977.

Kirklin JW, Barratt-Boyes BG: *Cardiac Surgery*. New York, Wiley, 1986.

McGoon DC: Repair of mitral insufficiency due to ruptured chordae tendineae. *J Thorac Cardiovasc Surg* 39:357, 1960.

McKay RG, Lock JE, et al: Balloon dilation of mitral stenosis in adult patients: Postmortem and percutaneous mitral valvuloplasty studies. *J Am Coll Cardiol* 9:723, 1987.

Miller DC, Oyer PE, et al: Ten to fifteen year reassessment of the performance characteristics of the Starr Edwards model 6120 mitral valve prosthesis. *J Thorac Cardiovasc Surg* 85:1, 1983.

O'Brien MF, Stafford EG, et al: Aortic valve replacement with cryopreserved homograft valves and with antibiotic 4°C stored valves: A comparative follow-up study. Presented at the 67th Annual Meeting of the American Association for Thoracic Surgery, 1987.

Oyer P, Miller D, et al: Clinical durability of the Hancock porcine bioprosthetic valve. *J Thorac Cardiovasc Surg* 80:824, 1980.

Palacios I, Block PC, et al: Percutaneous balloon valvotomy for patients with severe mitral stenosis. *Circulation* 75:778, 1987.

Reed GE, Pooley R, Moggio R: Durability of measured mitral annuloplasty. Seventeen-year study. *J Thorac Cardiovasc Surg* 79:321, 1980.

Selzer A, Cohn KE: Natural history of mitral stenosis: A review. *Circulation* 45:878, 1972.

Souttar PW: The surgical treatment of mitral stenosis. *Br Med J* 2:603, 1925.

Spencer FC, Colvin SB, et al: Experiences with the Carpentier techniques of mitral valve reconstruction in 103 patients (1980–1985). *J Thorac Cardiovasc Surg* 90:341, 1985.

Spencer FC, Galloway AC, Colvin SB: A clinical evaluation of the hypothesis that rupture of the left ventricle following mitral valve replacement can be prevented by preservation of the chordae of the mural leaflet. *Ann Surg* 202:673, 1985.

Spencer FC, Baumann FG, et al: Experiences with 1643 porcine prosthetic valves in 1492 patients. *Ann Surg* 203:691, 1986.

Starr A, Edwards ML: Mitral replacement: Clinical experience with a ball valve prosthesis. *Ann Surg* 154:726, 1961.

Teply J, Grunkemeier G, et al: The ultimate prognosis after valve replacement: An assessment at twenty years. *Ann Thorac Surg* 32:111, 1981.

Aortic Stenosis and Insufficiency

Arciniegas E: *Pediatric Cardiac Surgery*. Chicago, Year Book Medical Publishers, 1985.

Bloomfield P, Kitchin AH, et al: A prospective evaluation of the Bjork-Shiley, Hancock, and Carpentier-Edwards heart valve prostheses. *Circulation.* 73:1213, 1986.

Christakis GT, Weisel RD, et al: Can the results of contemporary aortic valve replacement be improved? *J Thorac Cardiovasc Surg* 92:37, 1986.

Isner JM, Salem DN, et al: Treatment of calcific aortic stenosis by balloon valvuloplasty. *Am J Cardiol* 59:313, 1987.

Kirklin JW, Barratt-Boyes BG: *Cardiac Surgery*. New York, Wiley, 1986.

Lombard JT, Selzer A: Valvular aortic stenosis. A clinical and hemodynamic profile of patients. *Ann Intern Med* 106:292, 1987.

Meurs AA, Grundemann AM, et al: Early and 8 year results of aortic valve replacement: A clinical study of 232 patients. *Eur Heart J* 6:870, 1985.

O'Brien MF, Stafford EG, et al: Aortic valve replacement with cryopreserved homograft valves and with antibiotic 4°C stored valves: A comparative follow-up study. Presented at the Annual Meeting of the American Association for Thoracic Surgery, April 1987.

Olson LJ, Subramanian R, Edwards WD: Surgical pathology of pure aortic insufficiency: A study of 225 cases. *Mayo Clin Proc* 59:835, 1984.

Perloff JK: *The Clinical Recognition of Congenital Heart Disease,* 3rd ed. Philadelphia, Saunders, 1987.

Schneider JF, Wilson M, Gallant TE: Percutaneous balloon aortic valvuloplasty for aortic stenosis in elderly patients at high risk for surgery. *Ann Intern Med* 106:696, 1987.

Stark J, de Leval M (eds): *Surgery for Congenital Heart Defects.* London, Grune and Stratton, 1983.

Subramanian R, Olson LJ, Edwards WD: Surgical pathology of pure aortic stenosis: A study of 374 cases. *Mayo Clin Proc* 59:683, 1984.

Tricuspid Stenosis and Insufficiency

Arbulu A, Thoms NW, Wilson RF: Valvulectomy without prosthetic replacement: A lifesaving operation for tricuspid *Pseudomonas* endocarditis. *J Thorac Cardiovasc Surg* 64:103, 1972.

Arbulu A, Asfaw I: Tricuspid valvulectomy without prosthetic replacement. Ten years of clinical experience. *J Thorac Cardiovasc Surg* 82:684, 1981.

Boyd AD, Engelman RH, et al: Tricuspid annuloplasty. *J Thorac Cardiovasc Surg* 68:344, 1974.

Carpentier A, Chauvaud S, et al: Reconstructive surgery of mitral valve incompetence. Ten-year appraisal. *J Thorac Cardiovasc Surg* 79:338, 1980.

Cobanoglu A, Starr A: Tricuspid valve surgery: Indications, methods, and results. *Cardiovasc Clin* 16:375, 1986.

Isom OW, Spencer FC, et al: Long-term results in 1375 patients undergoing valve replacement with the Starr-Edwards cloth-covered steel ball valve prosthesis. *Ann Surg* 186:310, 1977.

Peterffy A: Surgical management of tricuspid valvular disease. Ten years' experience of 141 consecutive patients. *Scand J Thorac Cardiovasc Surg* 26(suppl):1, 1980.

Peterffy A, Jonasson R, Henze A: Haemodynamic changes after tricuspid valve surgery. A recatheterization study in forty-five patients. *Scand J Thorac Cardiovasc Surg* 15:161, 1981.

Robin E, Thoms NW, et al: Hemodynamic consequences of total removal of the tricuspid valve without prosthetic replacement. *Am J Cardiol* 35:481, 1981.

Spencer FC, Shabetai R, Adolph R: Successful replacement of the tricuspid valve 10 years after traumatic incompetence. *Am J Cardiol* 18:916, 1966.

Stern HJ, Sisto DA, et al: Immediate tricuspid valve replacement for endocarditis. Indications and results. *J Thorac Cardiovasc Surg* 91:163, 1986.

Thorburn CW, Morgan JJ, et al: Long-term results of tricuspid valve replacement and the problem of prosthetic valve thrombosis. *Am J Cardiol* 51:1128, 1983.

Wellens F, Jacques G: Tricuspid valve replacement. *Cardiovasc Clin* 17:111, 1987.

Multivalvular Heart Disease

Bonchek LI, Starr A: Ball valve prostheses: Current appraisal of late results. *Am J Cardiol* 35:843, 1975.

Kirklin JW, Barratt-Boyes BG: *Cardiac Surgery.* New York, Wiley, 1986.

Spencer FC, Baumann FG, et al: Experiences with 1643 porcine prosthetic valves in 1492 patients. *Ann Surg* 203:691, 1986.

Cardiac Trauma

Blalock A, Ravitch MM: A consideration of the nonoperative treatment of cardiac tamponade resulting from wounds to the heart. *Surgery* 14:157, 1943.

Bland EF, Beebe GW: Missiles in the heart: A 20-year follow-up report of World War II cases. *N Engl J Med* 274:1039, 1966.

Estrera AS, Schreiber JT: Management of acute cardiac trauma. *Cardiol Clin* 2:239, 1984.

Evans J, Gray L, et al: Principles for the management of penetrating cardiac wounds. *Ann Surg* 189:777, 1979.

Frazee RC, Mucha P Jr, et al: Objective evaluation of blunt cardiac trauma. *J Trauma* 26:510, 1986.

Gay W: Blunt trauma to the heart and great vessels. *Surgery* 91:507, 1982.

Harken DE: Foreign bodies in and in relation to the heart and thoracic vessels. *Surg Gynecol Obstet* 83:117, 1946.

Holdeger WF, Lyons C, Edwards WS: Indications for removal of intracardiac foreign bodies. *Ann Surg* 163:249, 1966.

Isaacs JP: Sixty penetrating wounds to the heart: Clinical and experimental observations. *Surgery* 45:696, 1959.

Ivatury R, Shah P, et al: Emergency room thoracotomy for the resuscitation of patients with ''fatal'' penetrating injuries of the heart. *Ann Thorac Surg* 32:377, 1981.

Marshall WG Jr, Bell JL, Kouchoukos NT: Penetrating cardiac trauma. *J Trauma* 24:147, 1984.

Reid CL, Kawanishi DT, et al: Chest trauma: Evaluation by two-dimensional echocardiography. *Am Heart J* 113:971, 1987.

Spencer FC: Treatment of chest injuries. *Curr Probl Surg* January 1964.

Spencer FC, Kennedy JH: War wounds of the heart. *J Thorac Cardiovasc Surg* 33:361, 1957.

Sugg WL, Ecker RR, et al: Penetrating wounds of the heart: An analysis of 459 cases. *J Thorac Cardiovasc Surg* 56:531, 1968.

Tenzer ML: The spectrum of myocardial contusion: A review. *J Trauma* 25:620, 1985.

Cardiac Tumors

Attar S, Lee Y, et al: Cardiac myxoma. *Ann Thorac Surg* 29:397, 1980.

Bahnson HT, Spencer FC, Andrus EC: Diagnosis and treatment of intracavitary myxomas of the heart. *Ann Surg* 145:915, 1957.

Calhoun T, Terry E, et al: Myocardial fibroma or fibrous hamartoma. *Ann Thorac Surg* 32:406, 1981.

Chan HSL, Sonley MJ, et al: Primary and secondary tumors of childhood involving the heart, pericardium, and great vessels. A report of 75 cases and review of the literature. *Cancer* 56:825, 1985.

Crafoord C: Case report. *Int Symp Cardiovasc Surg Henry Ford Hosp* p 202, 1955.

Fyke FE, Seward JB, et al: Primary cardiac tumors: Experience with 30 consecutive patients since the introduction of two-dimensional echocardiography. *J Am Coll Cardiol* 5(6):1465, 1985.

Gassman HS, Meadows R, Baker LA: Metastatic tumors of the heart. *Am J Med* 19:357, 1955.

Geha AS, Weidman WH, et al: Intramural ventricular cardiac fibroma: Successful removal in two cases and review of the literature. *Circulation* 36:427, 1967.

Hanfling S: Metastatic cancer to the heart. *Circulation* 22:474, 1960.

Larrieu A, Jamieson W, et al: Primary cardiac tumors. Experience with 25 cases. *J Thorac Cardiovasc Surg* 83:339, 1982.

Mahaim I: *Les tumors et les polypes du coeur: Étude anatomo-clinique.* Paris, Masson et Cie, 1945.

Prichard RW: Tumors of the heart. *Arch Pathol* 21:98, 1951.

Reece IJ, Cooley DA, et al: Cardiac tumors: Clinical spectrum and prognosis of lesions other than classical benign myxoma in 20 patients. *J Thorac Cardiovasc Surg* 88:439, 1984.

Spencer FC: The heart, in Nealon TF (ed): *Management of the Patient with Cancer.* Philadelphia, Saunders, 1965, p 537.

Whorton CM: Primary malignant tumors of the heart. *Cancer* 2:245, 1949.

Yater WM: Tumors of the heart and pericardium. *Arch Intern Med* 48:627, 1931.

Coronary Artery Disease

Amsterdam EA, Martschinske R, et al: Symptomatic and silent myocardial ischemia during exercise testing in coronary artery disease. *Am J Cardiol* 58:43B, 1986.

Barner HB, Standeven JW, Reese J: Twelve-year experience with internal mammary artery for coronary artery bypass. *J Thorac Cardiovasc Surg* 90:668, 1985.

Cameron A, Kemp HG Jr, Green GE: Bypass surgery with the internal mammary artery graft: 15 year follow-up. *Circulation* 74:III30, 1986.

Catinella FP, Cunningham JN Jr, et al: Cold blood should not be used for vein preparation prior to coronary bypass grafting. *J Thorac Cardiovasc Surg* 82:904, 1981.

Chesebro JH, Clements IP, et al: A platelet-inhibitor-drug trial in coronary-artery bypass operations. *N Engl J Med* 307:73, 1982.

Cobb LA, Werner JA, Trobaugh GB: Sudden cardiac death. I. A decade's experience with out-of-hospital resuscitation. *Mod Concepts Cardiovasc Dis* 49:31, 1980.

Cobb LA, Werner JA, Trobaugh GB: Sudden cardiac death. II. Outcome of resuscitation; management, and future directions. *Mod Concepts Cardiovasc Dis* 49:37, 1980.

Cosgrove DM, Loop FD, et al: Determinants of 10-year survival after primary myocardial revascularization. *Ann Surg* 202:480, 1985.

Culliford AT, Colvin SB, et al: The atherosclerotic ascending aorta and transverse arch: A new technique to prevent cerebral injury during bypass: Experience with 13 patients. *Ann Thorac Surg* 41:27, 1986.

Cunningham JN Jr, Adams PX, et al: Preservation of ATP, ultrastructure, and ventricular function after aortic cross-clamping and reperfusion. Clinical use of blood potassium cardioplegia. *J Thorac Cardiovasc Surg* 78:708, 1979.

Cunningham JN Jr, Catinella FP, Spencer FC: Blood cardioplegia—clinical and experimental results, in Engleman RE, Levitsky S (eds): *A Handbook of Clinical Cardioplegia.* Mt Kisco, NY, Futura, 1982, chap 17.

Dilley RB, Cannon JA, et al: The treatment of coronary occlusive disease by endarterectomy. *J Thorac Cardiovasc Surg* 50:511, 1965.

European Coronary Surgery Study Group: Prospective randomized study of coronary artery bypass surgery in stable angina pectoris. Second interim report. *Lancet* 491, Sept 6, 1980.

Falcone C, deServi S, et al: Clinical significance of exercise-induced silent myocardial ischemia in patients with coronary artery disease. *J Am Coll Cardiol* 9:295, 1987.

Frick MH, Valle M, Harjola PT: Progression of coronary artery disease in randomized medical and surgical patients over a 5-year angiographic follow-up. *Am J Cardiol* 52:681, 1983.

Galbut DL, Traad EA, et al: Twelve-year experience with bilateral internal mammary artery grafts. *Ann Thorac Surg* 40:264, 1985.

Green GE, Spencer FC, et al: Arterial and venous microsurgical bypass grafts for coronary artery disease. *J Thorac Cardiovasc Surg* 60:491, 1970.

Grondin CM, Campeau L, et al: Comparison of late changes in internal mammary artery and saphenous vein grafts in two consecutive series of patients 10 years after operation. *Circulation* 70:1208, 1984.

Holmes DR Jr, Davis KB, et al: The effect of medical and surgical treatment on subsequent sudden cardiac death in patients with coronary artery diease: A report from the coronary artery surgery study. *Circulation* 73:1254, 1986.

Huddleston CB, Stoney WS, et al: Internal mammary artery grafts: Technical factors influencing patency. *Ann Thorac Surg* 42:543, 1986.

Isom OW, Spencer FC, et al: Does coronary bypass increase longevity? *J Thorac Cardiovasc Surg* 75(1):28, 1978.

Isom OW, Spencer FC, et al: Long-term survival following coronary bypass surgery in patients with significant impairment of left ventricular function. *Circulation* 51–52(suppl 1):141, 1975.

Johnson WD, Flemma RJ, et al: Extended treatment of severe coronary artery disease: A total surgical approach. *Ann Surg* 170:460, 1969.

Johnson WD, Brenowitz JB, Gessert R: Long term results of total coronary artery reconstruction. Presented at the American Association for Thoracic Surgery meeting, April 1987.

Kaiser GC: CABG: Lessons for the randomized trials. *Ann Thorac Surg* 43:3, 1986.

Kennedy JW, Killip T, et al: The clinical spectrum of coronary artery disease and its surgical and medical management, 1974–1979. The coronary artery surgery study. *Circulation* 66:III16, 1982.

Levy RI: Cholesterol and coronary artery disease. What do clinicians do now? *Am J Med* 80:18, 1986.

Loop FD, Lytle BW, et al: Free (aorto-coronary) internal mammary artery graft. Late results. *J Thorac Cardiovasc Surg* 92:827, 1986.

Loop FD, Lytle BW, et al: Influence of the internal-mammary-artery graft on 10-year survival and other cardiac events. *N Engl J Med* 314:1, 1986.

Mock M, Ringqvist I, et al: The survival of medically treated patients in the coronary artery surgery study (CASS) registry. *Circulation* 66:562, 1982.

Orszulak TA, Schaff HV, et al: Initial experience with sequential internal mammary artery bypass grafts to the left anterior descending and left anterior descending diagonal coronary arteries. *Mayo Clin Proc* 61:3, 1986.

Pigott JD, Kouchoukos NT, et al: Late results of surgical and medical therapy for patients with coronary artery disease and depressed left ventricular function. *J Am Coll Cardiol* 5:1036, 1985.

Rankin JS, Newman GE, et al: Clinical and angiographic assessment of complex mammary artery bypass grafting. *J Thorac Cardiovasc Surg* 92:832, 1986.

Reeder GS, Vlietstra RE, et al: Comparison of angioplasty and bypass surgery in multivessel coronary artery disease. *Int J Cardiol* 10:213, 1986.

Ringqvist I, Fisher LD, et al: Prognostic values of angiographic indices of coronary artery disease from the coronary artery surgery study (CASS). *J Clin Invest* 71:1854, 1983.

Russo P, Orszulak TA, et al: Use of internal mammary artery

grafts for multiple coronary artery bypasses. *Circulation* 74:III48, 1986.

Sauvage LR, Wu HD, et al: Healing basis and surgical techniques for complete revascularization of the left ventricle using only the internal mammary arteries. *Ann Thorac Surg* 42:449, 1986.

Spencer FC: Binocular loupes (microtelescopes) for coronary artery surgery. *J Thorac Cardiovasc Surg* 62:163, 1971.

Spencer FC: Surgical procedures for coronary atherosclerosis. *Prog Cardiovasc Dis* 14:399, 1972.

Spencer FC: The influence of coronary bypass on ventricular function, consensus meeting on coronary artery bypass surgery, medical and scientific aspects. National Institute of Health, Bethesda, MD, December 1980.

Spencer FC: The internal mammary artery: The ideal coronary bypass graft? *N Engl J Med* 314:50, 1986.

Spencer FC, Green GE, et al: Surgical therapy for coronary artery disease. *Curr Probl Surg* September 1970.

Spencer FC, Green GE, et al: Coronary artery bypass grafts for congestive heart failure. A report of experiences with 40 patients. *J Thorac Cardiovasc Surg* 62:529, 1971.

Spencer FC, Yong NK, Prachuabmoh K: Internal mammary-coronary artery anastomoses performed during cardiopulmonary bypass. *Cardiovasc Surg* 5:292, 1964.

Stoney WS, Alford WC Jr, et al: The fate of arm veins used for aorta-coronary bypass grafts. *J Thorac Cardiovasc Surg* 88:522, 1984.

Tector AJ: Fifteen years' experience with the internal mammary artery graft. *Ann Thorac Surg* 42:S22, 1986.

Vineberg AM: Technical considerations for the combined operation of left internal mammary artery or right and left internal mammary implantations with epicardiectomy and free omental graft. *J Thorac Cardiovasc Surg* 53:837, 1967.

Ventricular Aneurysm

Akins CW: Resection of left ventricular aneurysm during hypothermic fibrillatory arrest without aortic occlusion. *J Thorac Cardiovasc Surg* 91:610, 1986.

Bruschke AV, Proudfit WL, Sones FM: Progress study of 590 consecutive non-surgical cases of coronary disease followed by 5–9 years. Ventriculographic and other correlations. *Circulation* 47:1154, 1973.

Faxon DP, Myers WO, et al: The influence of surgery on the natural history of angiographically documented left ventricular aneurysm: The coronary artery surgery study. *Circulation* 74:110, 1986.

Froehlich RT, Falsetti HL, et al: Prospective study of surgery for left ventricular aneurysm. *Am J Cardiol* 45:923, 1980.

Gay W: Management of ventricular aneurysms following myocardial infarction. *World J Surg* 2:743, 1978.

Jatene AD: Left ventricular aneurysmectomy resection or reconstruction. *J Thorac Cardiovasc Surg* 89:321, 1985.

Josephson M, Harken A, Horowitz L: Long-term results of endocardial resection for sustained ventricular tachycardia in coronary disease patients. *Am Heart J* 104:51, 1982.

Kirklin JW, Barratt-Boyes BG: *Cardiac Surgery*. New York, Wiley, 1986.

Loop F, Cosgrove D: Results of ventricular aneurysmectomy. *Am J Surg* 141:684, 1981.

Novick RJ, Stefaniszyn HJ, et al: Surgery for postinfarction left ventricular aneurysm: Prognosis and long-term follow-up. *Can J Surg* 27:161, 1984.

Olearchyk AS, Lemole GM, Spagna PM: Left ventricular aneurysm. Ten years' experience in surgical treatment of 244

cases. Improved clinical status, hemodynamics, and long-term longevity. *J Thorac Cardiovasc Surg* 88:544, 1986.

Pericarditis

Culliford A, Lipton M, Spencer F: Operation for chronic constrictive pericarditis: Do the surgical approach and degree of pericardial resection influence the outcome significantly? *Ann Thorac Surg* 29:146, 1980.

Hier-Madsen K, Saunamaki KI, et al: Purulent pericarditis in children. Review and case report. *Scand J Thorac Cardiovasc Surg* 19:185, 1985.

Kutcher MA, King SB 3rd, et al: Constrictive pericarditis as a complication of cardiac surgery: Recognition of an entity. *Am J Cardiol* 50:742, 1982.

McCaughan BC, Schaff HV, et al: Early and late results of pericardiectomy for constrictive pericarditis. *J Thorac Cardiovasc Surg* 89:340, 1985.

Miller J, Mansour K, Hatcher C: Pericardiectomy: Current indications, concepts, and results in a university center. *Ann Thorac Surg* 34:40, 1982.

Morgan RJ, Stephenson LW, et al: Surgical treatment of purulent pericarditis in children. *J Thorac Cardiovasc Surg* 85:527, 1983.

Nishimura RA, Connolly DC, et al: Constrictive pericarditis: Assessment of current diagnostic procedures. *Mayo Clin Proc* 60:397, 1985.

Seifert FC, Miller DC, et al: Surgical treatment of constrictive pericarditis: Analysis of outcome and diagnostic error. *Circulation* 72:II264, 1985.

Heart Block and Pacemakers

Besley D, McWilliams G, et al: Long-term follow-up of young adults following permanent pacemaker placement for complete heart block. *Am Heart J* 103:332, 1982.

Brodman R, Furman S: Pacemaker implantation through the internal jugular vein. *Ann Thorac Surg* 29:63, 1980.

Carver J, Spitzer S, Mason D: Current concepts in pacing. *Geriatrics* 36:105, 1981.

Chardack WM, Gage AA, et al: The long-term treatment of heart block. *Prog Cardiovasc Dis* 9:105, 1966.

Culliford A, Isom O, Doyle E: Pacemaker implantation in the extremely young. A safe and cosmetic approach. *J Thorac Cardiovasc Surg* 75:763, 1978.

Furman S, Escher DJ, et al: Implanted transvenous pacemakers: Equipment, technic and clinical experience. *Ann Surg* 164:465, 1966.

Griffin JC, Mason JW, et al: The treatment of ventricular tachycardia using an automatic tachycardia terminating pacemaker. *PACE* 4:582, 1981.

Levine PA, Balady GJ, et al: Electrocautery and pacemakers: Management of the paced patient subject to electrocautery. *Ann Thorac Surg* 41:313, 1986.

Reid PR, Griffith LS, et al: Implantable cardioverter-defibrillator: Patient selection and implantation protocol. *PACE* 7(II):1338, 1984.

Watkins L, Mirowski M, et al: Automatic defibrillation in man: The initial surgical experience, *J Thorac Cardiovasc Surg* 82:492, 1981.

Assisted Circulation and Artificial Hearts

Amsterdam E, Awan N, et al: Intra-aortic balloon counterpulsation: Rationale, application and results, in Rackley C (ed): *Critical Care Cardiology*. Philadelphia, Davis, 1981.

Axelrod HI, Galloway AC, et al: Percutaneous cardiopulmonary bypass with a synchronous pulsatile pump combines effective unloading with ease of application. *J Thorac Cardiovasc Surg* 93:358, 1987.

Bregman D: Mechanical support of the circulation. *Cleveland Clin Q* 48:181, 1981.

Bregman D, Casarella W: Percutaneous intraaortic balloon pumping: Initial clinical experience. *Ann Thorac Surg* 29:133, 1980.

Gaines WE, Pierce WS, et al: The Pennsylvania State University paracorporeal ventricular assist pump: Optimal methods of use. *World J Surg* 9:47, 1985.

Glassman E, Engelman RM, et al: Method of closed-chest cannulation of left atrium for left atrial-femoral artery bypass. *J Thorac Cardiovasc Surg* 69:283, 1975.

Griffith BP, Hardesty RL, et al: Temporary use of the Jarvik-7 total artificial heart before transplantation. *N Engl J Med* 316:130, 1987.

Joyce LD, DeVries WC, et al: Response of the human body to the first permanent implant of the Jarvik-7 total artificial heart. *Trans Am Soc Artif Intern Organs* 29:81, 1983.

Kolff J, Beeb GM: Artificial heart and left ventricular assist devices. *Surg Clin North Am* 65:661, 1985.

Levinson MM, Smith RG, et al: Thromboembolic complications of the Jarvik-7 total artificial heart: Case report. *Artif Organs* 10:236, 1986.

Macoviak J, Stephenson L, et al: The intraaortic balloon pump: An analysis of five years' experience. *Ann Thorac Surg* 29:451, 1980.

Pae WE Jr, Pierce WS, et al: Long-term results of ventricular assist pumping in postcardiotomy cardiogenic shock. *J Thorac Cardiovasc Surg* 93:434, 1987.

Park SB, Liebler GA, et al: Mechanical support of the failing heart. *Ann Thorac Surg* 42:627, 1986.

Pennock JL, Pierce WS, et al: Survival and complications following ventricular assist pumping for cardiogenic shock. *Ann Surg* 198:469, 1983.

Pierce WS: The implantable ventricular assist pump. *J Thorac Cardiovasc Surg* 87:811, 1984.

Pierce WS: The artificial heart—1986: Partial fulfillment of a promise. *ASAIO-Trans* 32:5, 1986.

Pierce W, Myers J, et al: Approaches to the artificial heart. *Surgery* 90:137, 1981.

Rose D, Colvin S, et al: Long-term survival with partial left heart bypass following perioperative myocardial infarction and shock. *J Thorac Cardiovasc Surg* 83:483, 1982.

Rose DM, Colvin SB, et al: Late functional and hemodynamic V status of surviving patients following insertion of the left heart assist device. *J Thorac Cardiovasc Surg* 86:639, 1983.

Schoen FJ, Palmer DC, et al: Clinical temporary ventricular assist. Pathologic findings and their implications in a multi-institutional study of 41 patients. *J Thorac Cardiovasc Surg* 92:1071, 1986.

Spencer FC, Eiseman B, et al: Assisted circulation for cardiac failure following intracardiac surgery with cardiopulmonary bypass. *J Thorac Cardiovasc Surg* 49:56, 1964.

Sturm J, McGee M, et al: Treatment of postoperative low output syndrome with intraaortic balloon pumping: Experience with 419 patients. *Am J Cardiol* 45:1033, 1980.

Van Citters RL, Bauer CB, et al: Artificial heart and assist devices: Directions, needs, costs, societal and ethical issues. *Artif Organs* 9:375, 1985.

Chapter 20

Diseases of Great Vessels

Frank C. Spencer

ANEURYSMS OF THE THORACIC AORTA

Aneurysms of the thoracic aorta may be classified in five groups, varying with the anatomic location: (1) ascending aorta; (2) transverse aortic arch; (3) traumatic, usually occurring distal to the left subclavian artery; (4) descending thoracic aorta; and (5) thoracoabdominal. The etiology, disability, and surgical approach all vary with these different types.

GENERAL CONSIDERATIONS. The most frequent causes of a thoracic aneurysm are atherosclerosis, aortic dissection, or a collagen degenerative disease, the prototype of which is Marfan's syndrome. "Annulo-ectasia" is a popular descriptive term for the common condition of idiopathic dilatation of the aortic annulus, producing aortic insufficiency in association with a localized aneurysm in the ascending aorta. This is probably a localized form of collagen degenerative disease, for it does not develop in other areas of the body. Trauma is an important but infrequent cause of aneurysms in specific locations. Syphilis at one time was a frequent cause but is now very rare. Infrequently, a thoracic aneurysm results from some type of granulomatous disease of unknown etiology.

Dissecting aneurysms are considered in a subsequent section, for the aortic dissection involves a large part or all of the thoracic aorta.

Pathology. The four major types of aneurysm, considered serially in the subsequent sections, are: aneurysms of the ascending aorta, transverse aortic arch, descending thoracic aorta, and thoracoabdominal aneurysms. Aneurysms may be conveniently grouped by their anatomical location, for each type has specific characteristics and requires a form of treatment specific for that anatomical area.

Aneurysms of the ascending aorta are the most frequent, representing over 40 percent of aneurysms in large series. Perhaps this is because the ascending segment is the widest part. The descending thoracic aorta is involved in about 35 percent, the transverse arch and the thoracoabdominal areas in about 10 percent each.

In all areas the natural history is that of progressive enlargement with eventual rupture. Posttraumatic aneurysms are distinctive for their very slow growth, for a few instances of such aneurysms existing for 10 to 20 years before enlarging have been reported. In the vast majority of patients, the aneurysm steadily enlarges until rupture occurs. In a large series reported by Pickerstaff et al., the 1-year survival was about 60 percent, the 5-year survival near 20 percent. McNamara et al. summarized observations with 260 patients with thoracic aneurysms, 126 of whom were treated surgically. Five-year survival in nonsurgically treated patients was only 21 percent. The prognosis for the thoracic aneurysm is somewhat worse than that with an abdominal aneurysm.

Clinical Manifestations. The majority of aneurysms are asymptomatic until significant enlargement has occurred. Pain may infrequently occur, but the majority are accidentally discovered during a routine chest x-ray. Large aneurysms in the transverse aortic arch create symptoms from compression of adjacent structures such as the trachea or superior vena cava. Syphilitic aneurysms were well known for their tendency to invade bone, producing back pain from erosion of the thoracic spine, but this seldom occurs with other aneurysms. Usually, there are no physical abnormalities or any hemodynamic disturbances. Hence, the principal indication for treatment is to prevent death from rupture.

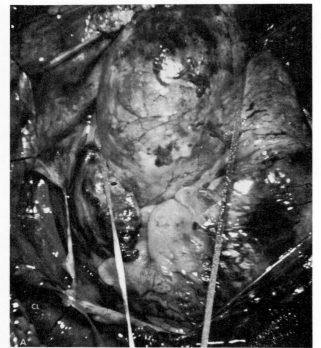

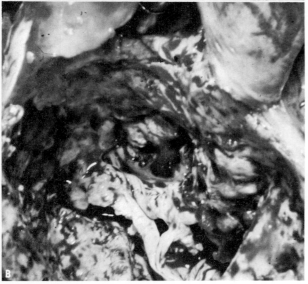

Fig. 20-1. Operative photograph of a patient with a large aneurysm of the ascending aorta. *A.* The aneurysm in the proximal aorta has been isolated and the aorta elevated by encircling umbilical tapes. *B.* Once the aorta has been incised, the incompetent aortic valve is exposed. The aortic insufficiency was produced by dilatation of the aortic annulus.

Once an abnormal shadow has been recognized on the chest x-ray, diagnosis can be readily established with an aortogram or computed tomography (CT). Unless the aneurysm is quite small, all should be treated promptly by excision. If serious complicating diseases, such as age, previous strokes, or heart disease, significantly increase operative risk, they may be observed for a few months or a year, with periodic sonograms or CTs to determine if enlargement is occurring. Once significant enlargement has been demonstrated, operation should be done promptly.

Treatment. The basic steps of treatment are to open the aneurysm, remove the contents and the diseased intima, insert a prosthetic graft (usually Dacron), and then wrap the wall of the aneurysm about the graft. The exact approach varies with different areas and is described in each section. This "inclusion" technique was an important contribution by Rudolf Matas in New Orleans in 1902 but was forgotten until the late 1950s, when it was reinstituted by DeBakey and Cooley and quickly adopted by others.

Aneurysms of the Ascending Aorta

Aneurysms localized to the ascending aorta are often due to a degenerative connective tissue disease of the media of the aortic wall. The origin is usually unknown. This is seen typically as one manifestation of a generalized disorder in Marfan's syndrome or as an isolated disease in Erdheim's cystic medial necrosis. The histologic abnormality described as "cystic medial necrosis" is now recognized as a nonspecific abnormality occurring in several diseases. Atherosclerotic aneurysms are seldom limited to the ascending aorta. Dissecting aneurysms, discussed in the next section, usually begin in the ascending aorta and extend distally. The dissection may stop near the origin of the innominate artery (DeBakey Type II) or may extend throughout the entire thoracic aorta (DeBakey Type I). Syphilis is now an infrequent cause. In the series of 90 patients reported by Miller et al., an unknown degenerative disease of connective tissue was the cause in 60 cases, aortic dissection in 12, syphilis in 10, and atherosclerosis in 8.

PATHOLOGY. As an aneurysm develops in the proximal ascending aorta, dilatation of the annulus of the aortic valve occurs, stretching the cusps of the aortic valve apart and producing aortic insufficiency (Fig. 20-1). Cardiac failure from the resulting aortic insufficiency is often the significant clinical problem rather than enlargement of the aneurysm with compression of adjacent structures or rupture. In the past, saccular syphilitic aneurysms enlarged to massive proportions, eroding through the sternum (Fig. 20-2), but these aneurysms are now rare. Once significant aortic insufficiency has developed, progression is rapid, with death from cardiac failure in 1 to 2 years unless operation is performed. Before surgical therapy was available, most patients with Marfan's syndrome died in the third decade from dissecting aneurysms or aortic insufficiency. Gott et al., based on experience with 50 patients with Marfan's syndrome, concluded that elective operation should be done when the diameter of the aortic root enlarged to 6 cm.

CLINICAL MANIFESTATIONS. Patients are often asymptomatic when the diagnosis is made following recognition of dilatation of the ascending aorta on a chest radiograph performed for other purposes. Frequently, the first symptom is due to congestive heart failure from aortic insuffi-

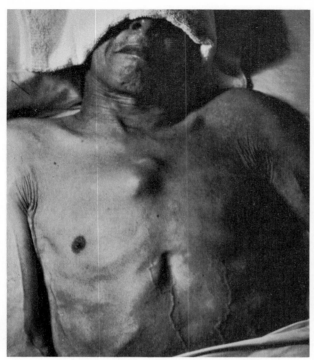

Fig. 20-2. Patient with a large syphilitic aneurysm eroding through the sternum and projecting beneath the skin. Fortunately such lesions are now rare. An attempt at operative extirpation of the lesion was unsuccessful because of hemorrhage.

ciency. Rarely, expanding saccular aneurysms are seen with symptoms from compression of the superior vena cava or the trachea. Physical examination usually finds no abnormalities except those of aortic insufficiency, the diastolic murmur and the wide pulse pressure.

DIAGNOSTIC FINDINGS. The diagnosis can be suspected from the radiographic findings of dilatation of the ascending aorta. Aortography or a CT scan confirms the diagnosis. The aortographic demonstration of a fusiform aneurysm in the proximal ascending aorta, tapering to an aorta of near-normal diameter at the level of the innominate artery, is virtually diagnostic of cystic medial necrosis (Fig. 20-3).

TREATMENT. Because of the progressive nature of the aortic insufficiency, operation should be performed as soon as possible after the diagnosis is made. As with aortic insufficiency from other causes, postponing operation because of the absence of symptoms while progressive enlargement of the left ventricle occurs is a serious error because the likelihood of sudden death from irreversible ventricular injury is greatly increased in the first few years following operation.

Operation is performed with cardiopulmonary bypass, excising the ascending aorta and replacing it with a woven Dacron graft. Concomitant valve replacement is performed if aortic insufficiency is present.

If aortic valve disease is present but the aortic annulus is not significantly dilated, the aortic valve can be re-

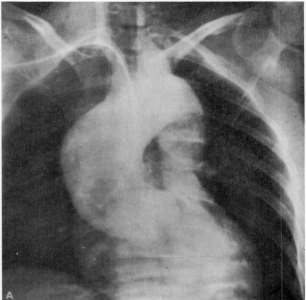

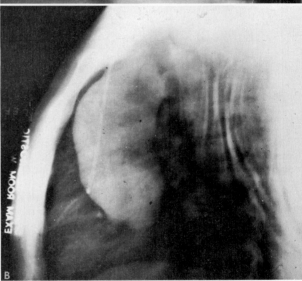

Fig. 20-3. *A.* Posteroanterior view of a thoracic aortogram showing a large aneurysm in the ascending aorta, stopping near the innominate artery. Resection of the aneurysm was successfully performed. The patient was well 15 years following operation. *B.* Lateral view of a thoracic aortogram in the same patient.

placed and the prosthetic valve inserted a few millimeters above the site of origin of the coronary arteries, leaving the coronary arteries in their normal anatomical location. However, if the aortic annulus is significantly dilated, this should be excised also because of the frequency of recurrent aneurysms in this area. This necessitates replantation of the ostia of the coronary arteries. The decision can usually be readily made at operation, for with significant dilatation of the aortic annulus, the ostia of the coronary arteries are displaced more than 1 cm from the aortic ring.

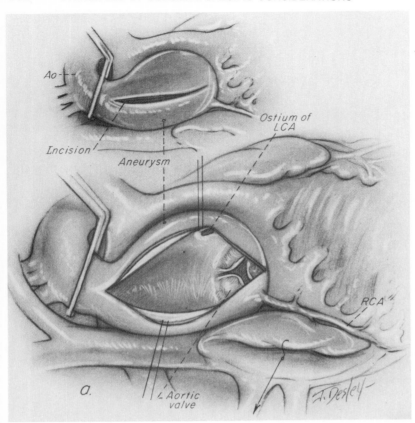

Fig. 20-4. Replacement of aortic valve and ascending aorta using the inclusion technique. *A.* After CPB is established the aortic clamp is placed and the aneurysm is opened longitudinally *(inset).* The ostia of the left and right coronary arteries are identified, usually displaced somewhat downstream to their normal position. The cold cardioplegic solution is given. *B.* After the aortic valve is excised, the Dacron graft with the attached Bjork-Shiley valve is sutured into place. A hole has been cut in the graft preparatory to suturing this around the ostium of the left coronary artery. *C.* The anastomosis is begun between the graft and the aortic wall around coronary ostium. *D.* Interrupted everting mattress sutures are used, supported by felt strips on the aortic side. *E.* The anastomosis is partially complete. *F.* The anterior row of sutures has been placed. *G.* After felt strips are placed around the aorta, the distal anastomosis is begun with a continuous everting mattress suture. *H.* The distal anastomosis has been completed. The clamp is removed, and the suture lines are inspected for leakage. (From: *Kirklin JW, Barratt-Boyes BG: Cardiac surgery, in Aortic Valve Disease. New York, Wiley, 1986, chap 12, pp 390–392, with permission.*)

This type of reconstruction is termed the "conduit" operation, consisting of replacement of the aortic valve, replantation of the coronary ostia, and replacement of the ascending aorta with prosthetic graft (Fig. 20-4).

The composite operation can be safely performed with excellent results. Kouchoukos et al. reported experiences with 125 patients operated upon over a period of 10 years with an operative mortality of 5 percent. Average follow-up was 55 months with an actuarial survival at 7 years between 65 and 70 percent. In 1985, Cabral et al. reported experiences with 100 patients operated upon over a period of 7 years with an operative mortality of 4 percent and a late mortality of 8 percent during a follow-up period averaging about 3 years. Grey and Cooley described experiences with 140 patients, using the composite repair in 89 of the group and a separate graft-valve repair in 51. In the series reported by Moreno-Cabral et al. 85 percent required concomitant aortic valve replacement.

How often the composite operation should be used as opposed to separate graft-valve replacement varies markedly among different institutions. The long-term durability of the composite operation is yet unknown, for pseudoaneurysms have developed at the site of replantation of the coronary ostia in a few patients.

Aneurysms of the Transverse Aortic Arch

Aneurysms of the transverse aortic arch are almost always due to atherosclerosis. They usually occur in pa-

tients over sixty years of age with associated coronary and cerebral vascular disease. Diagnosis is usually confirmed with aortography and CT to differentiate the aneurysm from a malignant mediastinal tumor. The degree of involvement of the great vessels arising from the aortic arch can also be determined.

TREATMENT. The operative procedure is a complex one involving myocardial protection while the coronary circulation is interrupted, maintenance of blood flow to arteries to the brain, and perfusion of the body distal to the left subclavian artery (Fig. 20-5). Until the concept of

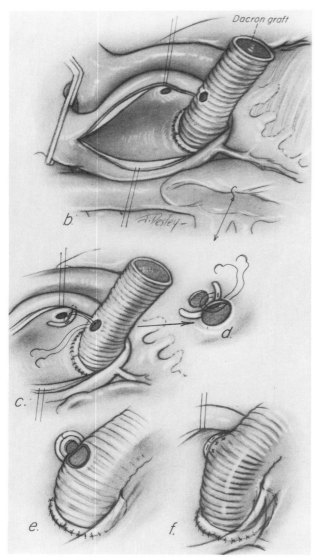

Fig. 20-4 *B,C,D,E,F.* Continued.

combining cardiopulmonary bypass with hypothermia and circulatory arrest was introduced, these aneurysms had the highest operative mortality of any aortic aneurysms, approaching 75 to 80 percent. The demonstration that the brain could tolerate circulatory arrest for 45 min if the brain temperature was carefully lowered to 15 to 17°C formed the basis for the modern approach. Griepp et al. applied the concept for arch aneurysms, reporting a series of 14 patients with an ischemia time near 42 min. Among 10 patients operated upon electively, only one died.

Crawford et al. described experiences with 67 patients, treating aneurysms located in the distal arch by simple proximal and distal clamping, while the hypothermic circulatory arrest technique was used in 27 extensive aneurysms with 26 survivors. Sweeney and Cooley concluded that higher temperatures were safer for short periods and were accompanied by less bleeding. Most groups, including ourselves, have found a brain temperature near 15°C safer, providing time for a more precise reconstruction.

Aneurysms distal to the innominate artery may be safely treated by a short period of cross-clamping and excision. Cooley et al. described experiences with 32 patients treated with this technique, with an average cross-clamp time of 27 min. The mortality was 6 percent but the occurrence of paraplegia in three patients, all of whom were clamped more than 30 min, is alarming.

More recently Frist et al. proposed reconsidering the old technique of cerebral perfusion, describing experiences with 10 patients with eight survivors and no postoperative strokes. This approach should be considered if a cerebral ischemia time exceeding 45 min is anticipated.

Traumatic Thoracic Aneurysms

ETIOLOGY AND PATHOLOGY. Traumatic aneurysms almost invariably arise from transection of the thoracic aorta due to closed-chest trauma. The majority result from horizontal deceleration injuries, typically steering wheel trauma in an automobile accident. McCollum et al. in 1979 described five different forms of trauma. Out of a group of 50 patients, 35 were injured in an automobile accident, 6 were hurt in crushing injuries, and 4 were injured in falls from a height. Traumatic rupture and traumatic thoracic aneurysms have a common etiology but a different clinical course. Traumatic aneurysms evolve in those few patients fortunate enough not to succumb from exsanguinating hemorrhage in the weeks following injury. If a patient survives longer than 6 to 8 weeks following injury, the risk of acute rupture is small. In a review of the English and French literature between 1950 and 1965, Bennett and Cherry found rupture occurring 9 times in a total of 105 aneurysms. The usual course is one of progressive enlargement with compression of adjacent structures.

Most aneurysms arise just distal to the left subclavian artery, opposite the point of insertion of the ligamentum arteriosum. Fortunately, involvement of the aortic arch or the ascending aorta is rare. Although a huge aneurysm filling most of the hemithorax is occasionally seen, the point of origin is invariably near the ligamentum arteriosum. Reconstruction can usually be done with a short prosthetic graft. Direct anastomosis is seldom possible.

CLINICAL MANIFESTATIONS. Unlike most aneurysms from other causes, traumatic thoracic aneurysms enlarge slowly and in some patients remain stationary for 10 to 20 years; the diagnosis is made in retrospect while evaluating an asymptomatic patient with a history of closed-chest trauma 10 to 20 years before. In the series of McCollum et al., time intervals between trauma and operation varied from 3 months to 32 years, with an average near 12 years for the 50 patients. In 25 patients, the interval was greater than 10 years and in 6 greater than 20 years.

As the aneurysm enlarges, compression of the left recurrent laryngeal nerve, the left main bronchus, and the esophagus occurs. Symptoms usually announce enlargement well before rupture occurs. This small risk of rup-

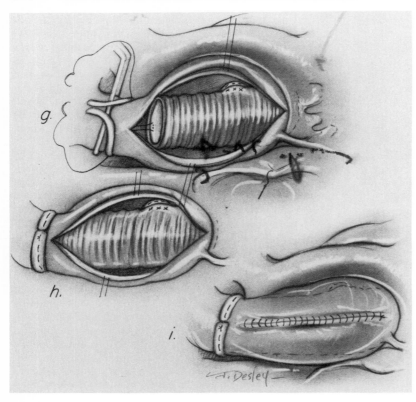

Fig. 20-4 *G,H,I.* Continued.

ture contrasts with the majority of aneurysms from other causes, where the threat of rupture constitutes the major reason for recommending excision before symptoms develop.

In the McCollum series, pain was the most common symptom, occurring in 24 percent of patients. Hoarseness from recurrent laryngeal involvement was present in 14 percent, dyspnea in 8 percent; 28 percent were asymptomatic. Usually there are no abnormalities on physical examination unless compression of the left main bronchus has occurred. No murmurs can be heard.

DIAGNOSTIC FINDINGS. The chest radiograph usually shows an ovoid density near the left subclavian artery. If the aneurysm has been present for several years, calcification is often visible in the wall. Exact dimensions may be outlined by a CT scan. Aortography is needed to confirm the diagnosis as well as the degree of involvement of adjacent structures (Fig. 20-6).

TREATMENT. The problem of management of acute rupture of the thoracic aorta, with the risk of exsanguinating hemorrhage, is discussed in the section Wounds of the Great Vessels. Elective excision is recommended for the majority of patients. An asymptomatic aneurysm first recognized over a decade after injury presents a choice between periodic observation and elective excision. Operative risk is small but not insignificant, and so several factors must be evaluated in making a recommendation for an individual patient. The probability of eventual enlargement requiring operation is the major consideration, as well as the small risk of rupture. I am not aware of an

autopsy report of a traumatic aneurysm that remained asymptomatic throughout the patient's lifetime.

Technique of Operation. (See Descending Thoracic Aneurysm.)

Aneurysms of the Descending Thoracic Aorta

ETIOLOGY AND INCIDENCE. Aneurysms in the descending thoracic aorta may result from atherosclerosis, syphilis, trauma, or a dissection of the aortic wall. Most are due to atherosclerosis and are exceeded only by abdominal aneurysms in frequency of occurrence. They are most common in men in the fifth to the seventh decades. Saccular aneurysms from syphilis, once very common, are now rare. Dissecting aneurysms and traumatic aneurysms are considered in the accompanying sections.

The majority of atherosclerotic aneurysms are located in the proximal part of the descending thoracic aorta, beginning distal to the left subclavian artery. They extend for varying distances and often can involve the entire descending thoracic aorta. They are generally fusiform (Fig. 20-7), rather than saccular.

Thoracic aneurysms enlarge and rupture at a rate greater than abdominal aneurysms. Bickerstaff described the natural history of 72 patients observed over a period of 30 years. The descending aorta was involved in 27. In the overall group, rupture occurred in 53 patients (74 percent). Thirty-seven of these had no prior diagnosis of aneurysms; in 16 others the mean interval between diagnosis and rupture was 2 years. Actuarial 5-year survival for

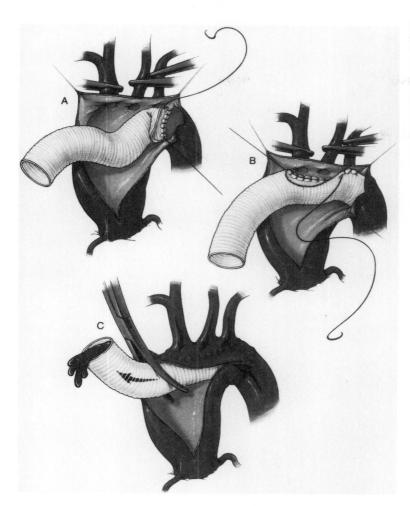

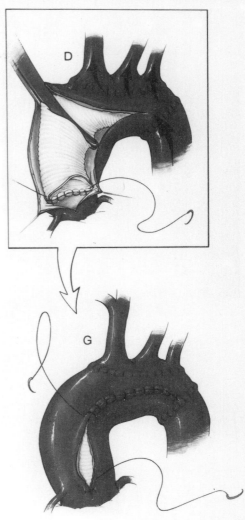

Fig. 20-5. Technique of graft inclusion and direct brachiocephalic arterial reattachment. *A.* With the head of the operating table down, the brachiocephalic arteries are clamped. With perfusion just to fill the aorta, the aneurysm is incised. The distal anastomosis is made between the graft and the normal upper descending thoracic aorta using #000 or #0000 prolene sutures. *B.* Anastomotic leakage is checked by clamping the graft and temporarily increasing perfusion. An oval opening is made with the graft under tension and sutured around the brachiocephalic artery origins. *C.* The head is lowered, the free end of the graft is elevated and filled with blood, and the clamps are removed from the brachiocephalic vessels to expel air. *D.* The graft is clamped proximal to the brachiocephalic arteries, full perfusion is resumed, and rewarming is started. Proximal anastomosis is performed depending on the extent of involvement. When uninvolved, the proximal graft is sutured to the ascending aorta. *G.* In either situation, air is removed by filling the heart and graft with blood as the anastomosis is completed and the aneurysmal wall is sutured around the graft. (From: *Crawford ES, Crawford JL: Diseases of the Aorta. Baltimore, Williams & Wilkins, 1984, pp 24–25, with permission.*)

all patients was 13 percent, for patients without dissection, 20 percent. Similar statistics have been cited by McNamara et al.

CLINICAL MANIFESTATIONS. Most patients are asymptomatic. The diagnosis is made after the accidental finding of an asymptomatic mass on a chest x-ray. In symptomatic patients, most symptoms result from an aneurysm enlarging and compressing the left main bronchus with resulting cough and dyspnea. Erosion into a bronchus or pulmonary parenchyma can produce hemoptysis. Enlarging aneurysms near the left recurrent laryngeal nerve where it encircles the ligamentum arteriosum will paralyze the vocal cord and produce hoarseness.

Physical examination is usually normal. Rarely a bruit is audible in the left paravertebral area. Peripheral pulses are normal unless compression of the origin of the left subclavian artery produces hypotension in the left arm.

DIAGNOSTIC FINDINGS. The diagnosis usually can be suspected from the appearance of a mass in the region of

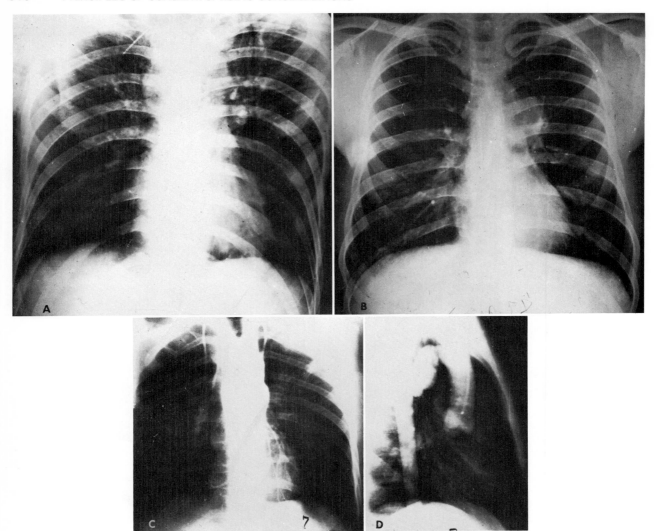

Fig. 20-6. *A.* Chest radiograph following an automobile accident, demonstrating widening of the mediastinum with subcutaneous emphysema. Traumatic rupture of the aorta was not recognized at this time. *B.* Chest radiograph 5 months after the injury demonstrated a left upper mediastinal mass. *C.* Posteroanterior view of an aortogram demonstrating a localized thoracic aneurysm. This lesion was excised successfully. *D.* Lateral view of an aortogram in the same patient. *E.* Chest radiograph in a different patient 2 years after an automobile accident demonstrated an asymptomatic mass in the upper mediastinum. *F.* Aortography demonstrated a saccular thoracic aneurysm, which was subsequently resected successfully. *G.* Aortogram in the same patient as in *F.* This film demonstrated the size and extent of the aneurysm as additional contrast material flowed freely within the lesion.

the aorta on the chest radiograph. The differential diagnosis includes bronchogenic carcinoma, metastatic carcinoma, or mediastinal tumors. Laminar calcification may be visible in the wall of the aorta.

CT is a valuable noninvasive technique to determine the size of an aneurysm. It is especially useful to periodically evaluate small aneurysms for enlargement. Aortography may be used to confirm the diagnosis and to delineate the precise extent of the aneurysm. Concomitant atherosclerotic disease in the coronary, renal, and carotid arteries frequently occurs. Hence, preoperative evaluation should carefully investigate these organ systems, often performing coronary arteriography, perhaps carotid arteriography or simpler noninvasive carotid studies.

TREATMENT. In most patients once the diagnosis of a discrete aneurysm has been made, excision should be recommended. Only with small aneurysms associated with significant coronary or cerebral vascular disease is a nonoperative policy of observation with frequent chest radiographs indicated.

The technique of operation is detailed in Fig. 20-8. A left posterolateral thoracotomy through an appropriate interspace, usually the fourth, fifth, or sixth, is made. Initially, the aorta is mobilized and encircled proximal and distal to the aneurysm. With proximal aneurysms involving the left subclavian artery, the aorta is encircled between the left carotid and left subclavian arteries. This is facilitated by opening the pericardium and dissecting the

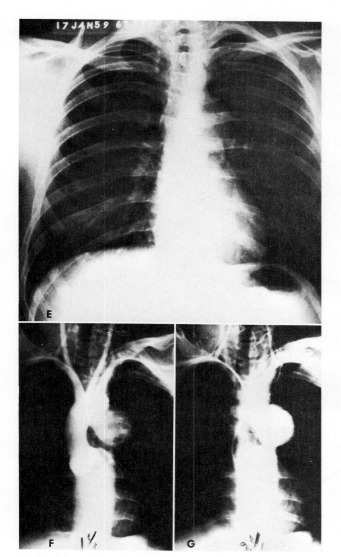

Fig. 20-6 *E,F,G.* Continued.

Somatosensory potential monitoring to evaluate spinal cord function while the aorta was occluded has been routinely used with the majority of operations performed upon the thoracic aorta at our hospital in recent years. Laboratory and clinical data indicate that paraplegia usually results from spinal cord ischemia when thoracic aneurysms do not extend below the diaphragm, while with thoracoabdominal aneurysms, direct interruption of critical blood supply to the spinal cord is a major factor. The inability of temporary bypass to protect from paraplegia over the past two decades has been principally due to an *inadequate flow through the shunt with inadequate distal perfusion pressure.* To date, in aneurysms not extending below the diaphragm, maintaining a distal aortic perfusion pressure above 60 mmHg by providing adequate flow of blood through the temporary bypass has been associated with preservation of sensory potentials during operation and absence of paraplegia, even with occlusion of the thoracic aorta for longer than 60 min. The exact flow rate needed cannot be predicted precisely in advance. Flow rates as high as 4 or more L/min have been needed in some patients. Distal aortic pressure, rather than flow rate, is the key requirement in order to perfuse the spinal cord through collateral circulation. Vascular resistance through collateral circulation is greater than the resistance present when spinal cord blood flow is through normal channels.

Published data do not show a significant reduction in the frequency of paraplegia when conventional temporary bypass is used. Livesay and Cooley reported experiences with 360 thoracic aneurysms employing some form of shunt or bypass in 97 of the group. Paraplegia occurred in 6.5 percent and was not decreased by temporary shunts. Paraplegia occurred principally with extensive aneurysms and with cross-clamp times exceeding 30 min. With thoracoabdominal aneurysms requiring excision of the segment of aorta between T10 and L2, paraplegia occurred in 15 to 20 percent of patients in the series reported by Crawford et al.

The surgical technique is a standard one. Initial dissection is limited to isolating the aorta proximally and distally sufficiently to permit the application of vascular clamps. The aorta is then opened widely, removing the thrombi from the lumen and any gross areas of calcification or degeneration in the intima. Most of the intima and all of the media are carefully preserved. Ostia of bleeding intercostal vessels are directly sutured. A standard woven Dacron graft is then inserted by end-to-end anastomosis (Fig. 20-9), after which the wall of the aneurysmal sac can be sutured around the prosthetic graft to supplement hemostasis.

Operative risk is usually less than 5 percent in elective operations unless serious concomitant coronary artery disease is present. Long-term prognosis is principally determined by the concomitant presence of coronary and cerebral atherosclerosis.

Thoracoabdominal Aneurysms

Thoracoabdominal aneurysms are rare, occurring in older patients with extensive atherosclerosis. Excision is

intrapericardial portion of the aortic arch. The vagus nerve and recurrent laryngeal nerve should be mobilized and protected.

A partial bypass is routinely used at NYU to protect from paraplegia. For the past several years a femoral artery–femoral vein bypass with a pump oxygenator has been used for most patients but with proximal aneurysms, the traditional left atrial–femoral bypass is often used as larger cannulae can be used and a higher flow rate obtained if necessary. A Gott heparinized shunt was used for several years, but this form of shunting is now considered unsatisfactory.

The principal hazards with clamping of the thoracic aorta are paraplegia and renal failure from the distal ischemia produced. Theoretically, this should be preventable by some form of partial bypass, perfusing the distal aorta during this time. Most types of temporary bypass require total body heparinization with subsequent increase in operative hemorrhage.

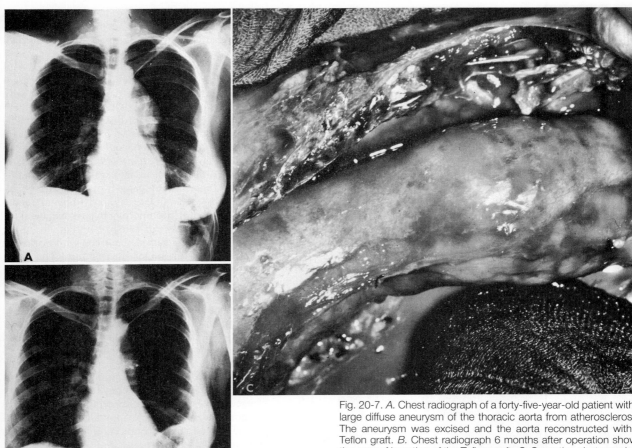

Fig. 20-7. *A.* Chest radiograph of a forty-five-year-old patient with a large diffuse aneurysm of the thoracic aorta from atherosclerosis. The aneurysm was excised and the aorta reconstructed with a Teflon graft. *B.* Chest radiograph 6 months after operation shows the area of insertion of the Teflon graft. *C.* Operative photograph of atherosclerotic aneurysm demonstrated in the chest radiograph seen in *A.*

a complicated surgical procedure, involving restoration of blood flow to the celiac, superior mesenteric, and renal arteries. The diagnosis is often initially made after a chest x-ray shows enlargement of the aorta near the diaphragm. Even with large thoracoabdominal aneurysms, the abdominal component usually cannot be palpated because it is concealed in the upper abdomen by the stomach and pancreas. A diagnosis can be made precisely, however, by aortography and CT.

Early experiences with these complex aneurysms were summarized by DeBakey in 1965. A multiple bypass technique was used, attaching a graft from the thoracic aorta above to the abdominal aorta below (Fig. 20-10). From this initial graft branch grafts were serially attached to the celiac, superior mesenteric, and renal arteries. Operative mortality remained at least 50 percent with this complex procedure.

Subsequently, a major advance was developed by Crawford with the intralumenal technique, simply inserting the graft inside the sac of the aneurysm with appropri-

ate side-to-side anastomoses between the graft and the ostia of the different arteries. In 1978, Crawford et al. summarized experiences with 82 patients, 77 of whom survived operation. In 1986, Crawford et al. summarized their very large experience with 605 such operations. About 70 percent of the patients were symptomatic; rupture had occurred in 4 percent of the group. Operative mortality was about 9 percent.

Crawford et al. reported significant observations of the natural history of the disease, describing observations upon 94 patients observed over a period of 25 years in whom operation was not performed for a variety of reasons. Only 24 percent of the group were alive 2 years after a decision was made that operation would not be performed; half of the deaths were due to rupture. By contrast, among 604 patients treated surgically, nearly 60 percent were alive 5 years following operation.

Operations upon the segment of aorta between the tenth thoracic and the second lumbar vertebra have the highest associated frequency of paraplegia, ranging between 20 and 40 percent. Crawford has found that the frequency could be significantly decreased by reattaching large lumbar vessels to the aortic graft at the time of oper-

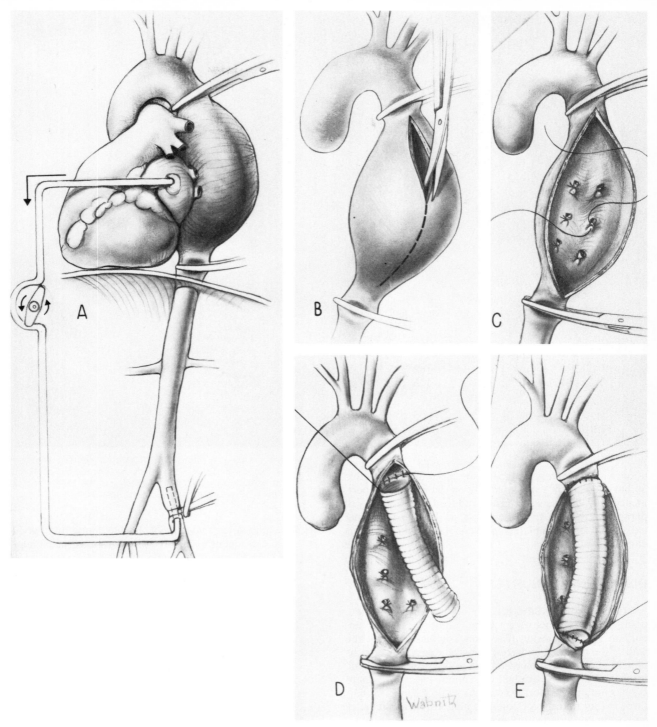

Fig. 20-8. Procedure for excision of an aneurysm of the thoracic aorta. *A.* An aneurysm of the thoracic aorta. Initial dissection is limited to isolation of the aorta proximal and distal to the aneurysm. Left atriofemoral bypass is then instituted at a flow rate near 2 L/min. (See text for other methods of shunting.) Pressures should be monitored in the aorta and also in the femoral artery to ensure adequacy of perfusion of the arterial circulation proximal and distal to the aneurysm. *B.* Aneurysm is widely opened, removing only the inner lining to avoid excessive bleeding where the aneurysm may be adherent to the vertebral column and lung. *C.* Bleeding intercostal arteries may be oversewed from within the lumen of the aneurysm. *D.* A woven Dacron prosthesis is used for reconstruction of the aorta, employing a continuous suture for the anastomosis. *E.* Following completion of the anastomosis the adventitial sac remaining from the aneurysm can be used to surround the graft (not illustrated).

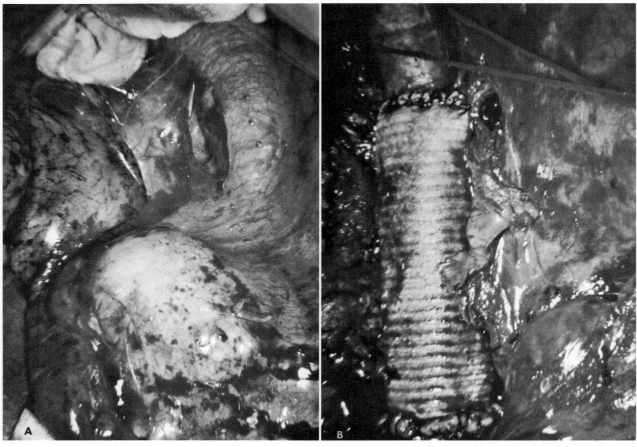

Fig. 20-9. *A.* Operative photograph of saccular syphilitic aneurysm of distal thoracic aorta. *B.* Teflon graft used to restore continuity following excision of a syphilitic aneurysm of the lower thoracic aorta. This graft was used in the patient seen in *A.*

ation with a patch graft technique, a technique that this author described experimentally in laboratory experiments in 1958. This significantly reduced the frequency of paraplegia to near 15 percent, but to date *no technique* exists that can completely prevent paraplegia with this complex problem.

DISSECTING ANEURYSMS

ETIOLOGY AND INCIDENCE. The term "dissecting aneurysm" is a misnomer because the condition is not an aneurysm but an "aortic dissection," a dissection of the wall of the aorta. A localized aneurysm develops months or years later in an area where the aortic wall has become weakened from the original dissection, but a true aneurysm is not present during acute dissection. The disease is three to four times more common in males than in females and occurs predominantly in older patients, those beyond the fifth decade. However, it occurs in every age group, the youngest person being only 14 months of age.

It results from a combination of hypertension and a disease of the media of the aorta of unknown type. Roberts has emphasized that a history of hypertension may be obtainable in only 60 to 75 percent of patients, but hypertrophy of the left ventricle characteristic of hypertension

is present in at least 90 percent. He has found that hypertension is frequently the precipitating factor in patients with Marfan's syndrome who develop dissection, and predicted that proper control of hypertension would virtually eliminate the disease. This prediction well emphasizes the importance of control of hypertension in long-term therapy.

The disease in the media is of unknown type, with no consistent histologic abnormality. Cystic medial necrosis, a histologic abnormality, has been widely described with Marfan's syndrome but is best considered a marker of a connective tissue abnormality, not a disease entity.

Patients with Marfan's syndrome usually develop a progressive fusiform aneurysm in the ascending aorta which eventually ruptures or dissects. There is a greater frequency of dissection in patients with coarctation or congenitally bicuspid aortic valve. Whether this is related to turbulent flow of blood producing these abnormalities or to associated connective tissue defects in the media is uncertain. Disease of the media of the aorta must be a major factor in etiology because there are an estimated 20 million patients with hypertension in the United States,

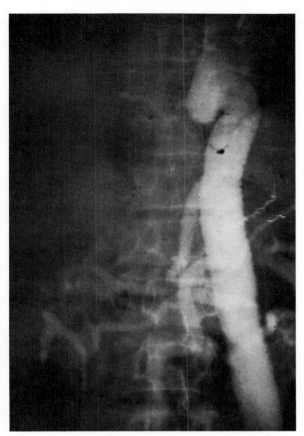

Fig. 20-10. Angiogram of Dacron graft 1 year after excision of thoracoabdominal aneurysm. The graft was inserted between the thoracic aorta, as an end-to-side anastomosis, and the abdominal aorta, not shown in this illustration. Side branches to the superior mesenteric artery, celiac artery, and right and left renal arteries are individually visible.

but only about 2000 dissecting aneurysms are reported each year.

It should be emphasized that the disease is *not due* to atherosclerosis. Atherosclerosis is a disease of the intima, occurring more frequently in the terminal abdominal aorta. Aortic dissection is a disease of the media, almost always occurring in the thoracic aorta. The frequency of occurrence of aortic dissection in older age groups led to confusion with atherosclerosis. The distinction between the two diseases is most important in evaluating prognosis and planning long-term therapy.

Experimentally, a dissecting aneurysm can be produced in young rats with a diet containing 50 percent sweet peas, which causes a distinct abnormality of connective tissue, known as *lathyrism*. The abnormal chemical agent that weakens the cross-linking of collagen is a beta-amino nitrile. To date, this experimental observation has had little clinical significance except to confirm the probable pathogenesis of aortic dissection.

Wilson and Hutchins reviewed 204 patients undergoing autopsy. The most common associated conditions were hypertension, Marfan's syndrome, and inflammatory in-

juries of the aortic media. No common pathogenetic mechanism was found.

PATHOLOGY. The two major pathologic abnormalities are a transverse tear of the intima and media, usually involving about half the circumference of the aorta, which permits blood to enter the media. The aortic wall then progressively separates (''dissects'') with an inner true lumen and an outer false lumen composed of the outer half of the media and the adventitia. In the detailed analysis published by Roberts, the intimal tear was located in the ascending aorta in about 70 percent of patients, in the aortic arch in 10 percent, in the upper descending thoracic aorta near the ligamentum arteriosum in 20 percent, and in the abdominal aorta in about 2 percent. In the experience of Miller et al. with 125 patients, the intimal tear was in the ascending aorta in 30 percent. In a few patients, no tear in the intima can be found at autopsy, a fact that leads to the theory that dissection of the aorta is the primary process with ''rupture of the vasovasorum'' and secondary rupture into the aortic lumen. Almost all clinical data make this hypothesis unlikely.

Once the dissection begins, it usually extends rapidly through the thoracic and abdominal aorta into the peripheral arteries. Four types of dissection, proposed by DeBakey as Types A, B, C, and D, depending upon both the site of origin and the extent of distal dissection, are shown in Fig. 20-11. Roberts has estimated that the entire aorta will dissect within minutes unless some structural abnormality that has disrupted continuity of the aortic wall, such as atherosclerosis or coarctation, halts the dissection. In over 50 percent of patients, the dissection process extends into a peripheral artery. If this theory is correct, younger patients with less atherosclerosis would more frequently have dissection of the entire aorta. A ''reentry'' tear can be identified in about 10 percent of patients, located in the aorta in about half and a peripheral artery in the others.

As dissection progresses, branch vessels are sheared off, either becoming obliterated or establishing a communication with the false lumen occluded by the dissection. Proximally, the coronary arteries may be involved. Frequently one or more aortic valve cusps are detached and prolapse into the lumen, creating aortic insufficiency. Distally, any artery may be involved; carotid artery involvement may produce neurologic injury. Obstruction of the subclavian arteries produces differences in blood pressure between the two arms. Dissection of intercostal arteries may cause spinal cord injury with paraplegia. In one series, 6 of 125 patients had paraplegia on admission. Dissection of renal arteries may produce renal insufficiency. In the extremities, acute obstruction of the iliac or femoral arteries may cause claudication or even gangrene.

The dissection may terminate fatally at any time by rupture of the false lumen with exsanguination. Rupture into the pericardial cavity is the most common, probably because the adventitia is thin over the intrapericardial ascending aorta. Rupture into the left pleural cavity or the retroperitoneal tissues is less common.

The grim mortality is documented in virtually every

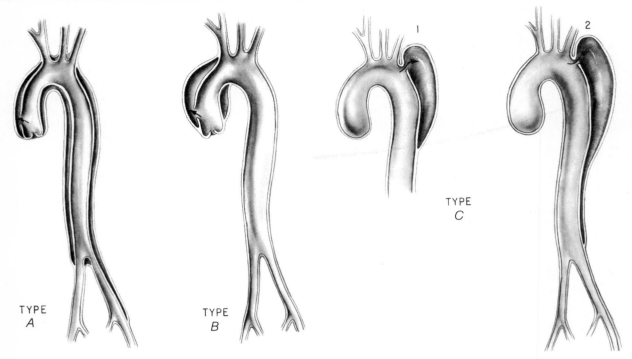

TYPE
A

TYPE
B

TYPE
C

Fig. 20-11. Different types of aortic dissection. *A.* Dissecting aneurysm that begins in the ascending aorta near the aortic valve and extends throughout the aorta down to the external iliac arteries. Unfortunately, this is a common type of dissecting aneurysm. *B.* Dissecting aneurysm limited to the ascending aorta. This is commonly seen in the Marfan syndrome. *C*1. Dissecting aneurysm beginning distal to the left subclavian artery. The localized nature of this aneurysm makes it readily accessible to surgical excision. *C*2. Dissecting aneurysm arising distal to the left subclavian artery but extending into the abdominal aorta. Only partial excision of the area of dissection is possible.

report, with 30 to 50 percent of patients dying within 24 h, 50 to 75 percent within 1 to 2 weeks, and 90 percent of untreated patients within 1 to 3 months. In the classic review of 425 cases by Hirst et al., 74 percent died within 2 weeks and 91 percent within 6 months.

Mortality is much higher with dissection originating in the ascending aorta, almost surely due to the thin adventitia over the intrapericardial aorta. In a group of 62 patients reported by Lindsay and Hurst, almost all of 40 patients whose dissection began in the ascending aorta died within 3 weeks. Only 8 percent of these patients lived 1 month.

This high mortality is the reason emergency operation has been progressively adopted in the last few years for dissections involving the ascending aorta.

In the few patients who survive an aortic dissection, endothelial lining of the false lumen develops, termed a *healed dissecting aneurysm*. This occurs in about 20 percent of patients. Such patients have a so-called double-barreled aorta, with a wide variety of bizarre circulatory patterns. For example, one renal artery may arise from the "false" lumen and the other from the true lumen (Fig. 20-12), or alternatively both renal arteries can arise from the false lumen. In other patients, one iliac artery may originate from the false lumen, the other from the true lumen. In most patients the false lumen gradually becomes aneurysmal and ruptures, especially if significant hypertension is present.

CLINICAL MANIFESTATIONS. The abrupt onset of excruciating pain, almost immediately reaching its peak intensity, is very characteristic of a dissecting aneurysm. A myocardial infarction, by contrast, may gradually develop pain of increasing severity over several minutes.

Sutton et al. reported that chest pain occurred in nearly 80 percent of 113 patients. Usually this was in the anterior chest. Back pain occurred with dissection of the proximal descending aorta in about a third of patients, indicating that absence of back pain did not exclude the dissection of the thoracic aorta. Another significant characteristic of the pain is its tendency to migrate into different areas as dissection extends distally. As might be predicted from the wide variation in the extent of the dissection process, many pain syndromes may occur. Pain may radiate to the neck, the arm, the epigastrium, or the leg. Seldom is pain completely absent, probably in no more than 10 percent of patients.

Syncope occurs in 10 to 20 percent, and some neurologic symptoms are present in 20 to 40 percent. These may result from ischemia of the brain, spinal cord, or a peripheral nerve, depending upon whether a carotid artery, an intercostal artery, or a peripheral artery has been compromised. A stroke develops in about 10 percent of patients, paraplegia in 3 to 5 percent.

Hypertension, often of severe degree, is present in 75 to 85 percent of patients. A frequent clinical picture is that of an acutely ill patient who is hypertensive, pale,

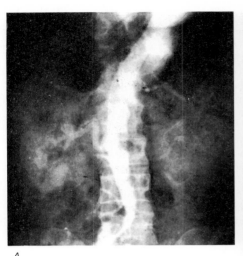

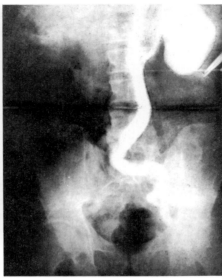

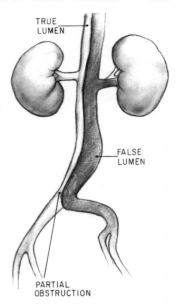

TRUE LUMEN

FALSE LUMEN

PARTIAL OBSTRUCTION

A

B

Fig. 20-12. *A.* Aortogram showing an unusual pattern of aortic dissection in which dissection extended from the thoracic aorta into the abdominal aorta, creating two lumens, with the right renal artery arising from one and the left renal artery from the other. Focal stenosis of the right common iliac artery is seen at the lower part of the field producing intermittent claudication, which was the presenting complaint of the patient. *B.* Aortogram performed by a different root opacifies the left kidney and the left common iliac artery. The condition of the dissected aorta is illustrated in the accompanying drawing. Circulation was reestablished by excising the septum between the two channels at the aortic bifurcation. (From: *Gryboski W, Spencer FC: Intermittent claudication caused by a dissecting aneurysm of the aorta. South Med J 58:593, 1965, with permission.*)

and sweaty from severe vasoconstriction. An aortic diastolic murmur appears in 20 to 30 percent of patients and is of great diagnostic significance, as it originates from detachment of an aortic valve cusp. Unequal carotid or subclavian pulses may be found, caused by unequal compression of these vessels. A variety of neurologic abnormalities may be detected, the most common being either a monoplegia or paraplegia.

DIAGNOSTIC FINDINGS. On the chest radiograph a widened mediastinum or a left pleural effusion from extravasation of blood is frequently seen. In some patients, however, the radiograph may be completely normal. The electrocardiogram is of particular value in distinguishing dissecting aneurysm from myocardial infarction, but there are no characteristic features of aortic dissection. The most common abnormality is left ventricular hypertrophy from the antecedent hypertension.

CT is a valuable noninvasive technique that may establish the diagnosis promptly and quickly in many patients. 2-D echocardiography may also be diagnostic, actually demonstrating the intimal flap. Aortography is the most definitive diagnostic procedure, outlining the double lumen. In some patients, the diagnosis cannot be made by any other technique, as there are no abnormal physical

findings and the only symptom is a history of severe back pain.

The importance of immediate aortography or CT in any patient with unexplained sustained severe chest pain cannot be overemphasized. The history of pain may be the *only* abnormality detected. Occasionally a patient is seen a few days or weeks after an acute dissection with no symptoms and no abnormality on physical examination, electrocardiogram, or chest x-ray. Such patients often exsanguinate without any preliminary warning symptoms.

TREATMENT. Modern surgical treatment evolved from the work of DeBakey and Cooley, who reported in 1955 successful excision and grafting of a dissecting aneurysm in the thoracic aorta. Another key concept in treatment, developing from the work of Wheat and colleagues, is the importance of immediate drug therapy both to control the hypertension and to decrease forceful contractility of the left ventricle (dP/dt). Drug therapy should be started as soon as the diagnosis is suspected, preferably in the emergency room, because it may stop the dissection process and prevent exsanguination. Wheat and associates discovered the importance of drug therapy following their ingenious evaluation of observations from the poultry industry that the high fatality rate from spontaneous dissecting aneurysm in certain flocks of turkeys could be dramatically reduced by adding a small amount of reserpine to the turkey food. An intravenous infusion of sodium nitroprusside is usually done, preferably combined with immediate administration of a beta-blocking drug, such as propanolol.

Dissections of the ascending aorta are usually promptly operated upon, generally as an emergency. Both Najafi and Miller have performed emergency operations for over a decade. Ergin and Griepp analyzed 93 publications and recommended immediate operation for both Type A and Type B dissections.

The principal objective at operation is to excise the ascending aorta, as neither excision of the intimal tear nor obliteration of the distal false lumen influences prognosis. In the Miller series of 125 patients, the intimal tear was not excised in 22 percent of patients. Aortic valve replacement was rarely necessary (11 percent); it was sufficient simply to resuspend the aortic cusp, a technique reported by this author in 1962.

With dissections of the descending thoracic aorta many groups use drug therapy initially, as the risk of acute rupture is substantially less. Operation is promptly performed if signs of continued dissection are present, such as continued pain or enlargement of the mediastinal hematoma, or signs of proximal aortic dissection, such as the appearance of an aortic diastolic murmur or a pericardial effusion. With an aggressive policy of emergency operation on all patients the mortality is presently 22 percent with ascending dissections, 14 percent with descending dissections. Wolff et al. reported immediate operation for acute ascending aortic dissection in 48 patients with 6 deaths and overall good results. The incompetent aortic valve was resuspended in 32 of the group; 8 patients required aortic valve replacement as well because of inherent valvular disease. Most patients in recent years with ascending aortic dissections have been operated upon promptly, excising the ascending aorta and restoring continuity with a woven Dacron prosthesis (Figs. 20-13 and 20-14). With descending aortic dissections, drug therapy has been employed initially, reserving operations for patients in whom the dissection process was not controlled.

Several groups, including ours at NYU, have adopted this technique of performance of the distal aortic anastomosis with the "open" technique during a brief period of circulatory arrest. This permits the performance of a more precise anastomosis and also avoids the possible injury of the dissected aorta from application of a vascular clamp. Once the distal anastomosis has been accomplished, the prosthetic graft can be occluded and flow to the brain restored while the proximal anastomosis is performed.

The main cause of operative death is hemorrhage from the suture lines. Performing the distal anastomosis with an "open" technique during circulatory arrest permits precise inclusion of all layers of the dissected aorta with less risk of hemorrhage. At NYU the proximal anastomosis is usually performed with a continuous suture of 4-0 prolene, avoiding undue tension on the suture line which can lacerate the friable intima. An alternative method is to reconstitute the dissected aorta between two strips of Teflon felt, one placed within the lumen and the other around the adventitia, after which the graft is sutured to this reconstructed aorta.

PROGNOSIS. Permanent therapy is necessary because aortic dissection is an acute event in a patient with hypertension and a chronic degenerative disease of the media of the aorta. The false lumen remaining beyond the site of aortic reconstruction may gradually enlarge and become aneurysmal in the first few years following operation. Patients over sixty years of age are also in the age group where atherosclerotic disease of the coronary and cerebral circulations is common. In the series of Miller et al., excluding operative deaths, 5-year survival was 76 percent, 10-year survival 37 percent. Sixty-one percent of late deaths were related to cardiac or cerebral causes.

Control of hypertension is most imortant, as this lessens the frequency of aneurysmal dilatation of the remaining dissected aorta. More than one fatal aortic rupture has resulted from inadvertent cessation of antihypertensive therapy years after recovery from emergent surgical treatment of aortic dissection. These guidelines are especially important in patients with dissections of the descending thoracic aorta, treated initially with drug therapy. They should be carefully observed at 3- to 6-month intervals for development of an aneurysm, as this occurs in at least 25 to 30 percent of such patients. With the present availability of CT and sonography, precise periodic evaluation of the size of the dissected aorta can easily be done.

WOUNDS OF THE GREAT VESSELS

Penetrating Injuries

With penetrating chest wounds, injuries of the heart or great vessels are a frequent cause of death. The two immediate threats to life are cardiac arrest from exsanguination or tamponade. Tamponade is discussed in Chap. 19.

With injuries of the aorta or vena cava, only a few patients are alive when first seen in a hospital emergency room. They are usually in profound shock with signs of massive intrathoracic bleeding. Unless an operating room is immediately available, immediate thoracotomy may offer the only chance for survival. "Slash" thoracotomy with limited aseptic technique has been employed at Bellevue Hospital for several years, occasionally resuscitating a moribund patient. Infection following such a thoracotomy is surprisingly rare. Once hemorrhage has been controlled, the patient can be transferred to the operating room for definitive surgical exploration and repair.

When threatened exsanguination does not mandate immediate thoracotomy, aortography should be seriously considered in any patient with a possible injury of the great vessels from a penetrating wound of the mediastinum. The development of frequent use of aortography is of the major advances in therapy of thoracic trauma of the past decade. Indications should be liberal because some grave injuries may not be recognizable by other methods until serious complications develop.

Aortography helps choose between a sternotomy and a thoracotomy. Median sternotomy, combined with extension into the neck if necessary, provides the best combined exposure of the heart and great vessels. Exposure of the left subclavian artery, however, is limited and may require a lateral thoracotomy, converting the sternotomy to a T incision. This extensive incision in the thoracic cage may require ventilatory support for several days afterward; so it should be avoided if a simpler approach is possible. If aortography indicates that injury of the left

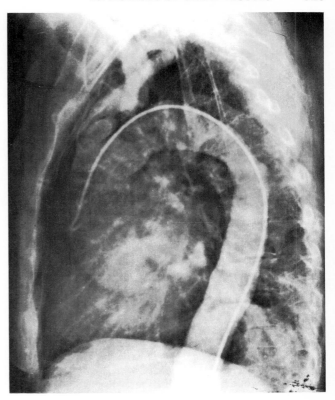

Fig. 20-13. *Opposite.* Thoracic aortogram, performed with a catheter introduced retrograde through the femoral artery, showing a dissecting aneurysm arising distal to the left subclavian artery. The outer channel is faintly visualized as a double density beyond the left subclavian artery. *Lower left.* Operative photograph of dissecting aneurysm arising distal to the left subclavian artery. A clamp is visible on the aorta proximal to the left subclavian artery, which has been encircled with an umbilical tape. The vagus nerve is visible proximally. Laminated clot was found in the lumen of the aneurysm. *Lower right.* Dacron graft inserted to restore aortic continuity following excision of the aneurysm.

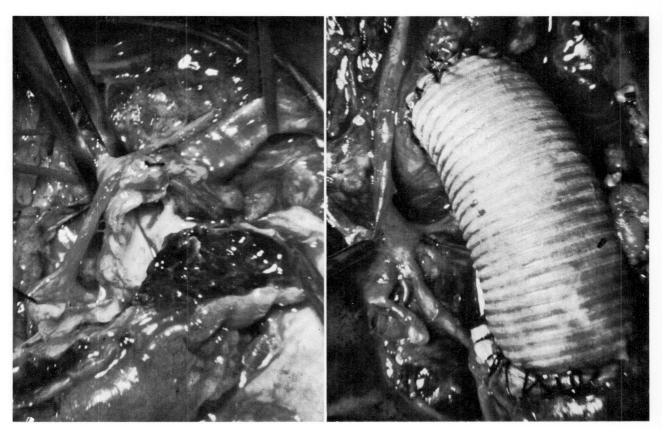

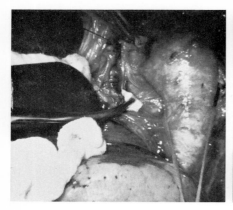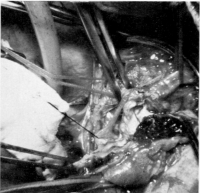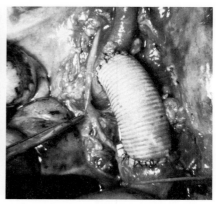

Fig. 20-14. *Left.* Operative photograph of dissecting aneurysm of upper thoracic aorta, starting a few days before operation. The hematoma in the aortic wall is visible. *Center.* With a functioning left atrial bypass, the aorta has been occluded and the aneurysm incised. A tape encircles the left subclavian artery. The vagus nerve with the recurrent nerve encircling the aorta is visible. The aneurysm began in the classic location, just beyond the left subclavian artery. A large thrombus is present in the aortic wall. *Right.* Aortic reconstruction was accomplished with a short woven Dacron graft. The proximal anastomosis is immediately beyond the left subclavian artery.

subclavian artery is the only injury, a left anterior thoracotomy in the third interspace is a better incision.

Richardson described experiences with 76 gunshot wounds of the mediastinum. Immediate operation was performed for 33 patients in *unstable* condition, with 12 deaths. Forty-three patients in *stable* condition had several diagnostic studies, including angiography, after which 27 were operated upon, 11 of whom had injuries to the great vessels. There were three deaths in this group, all from delayed complications (7 percent). In 1985, Zakharia et al. described experiences with nearly 2000 thoracic battle wounds. Over 1400 thoracotomies were performed. Cardiac injuries occurred in 225 patients, great vessel wounds in 54, with an 87 percent survival in those with vessel injuries.

Nonpenetrating Injuries

The possibility of traumatic laceration of the aorta has emerged in the past two decades as one of the most important diagnostic considerations in treating blunt injuries, especially those following an automobile accident. Parmley et al.; they emphasized that between 10 and 20 percent of patients lived longer than 30 min after injury before exsanguination. The frequency of aortic laceration increases with the severity of the trauma; it is a common finding after severe trauma that produces instant death. It is estimated that 10 to 15 percent of patients seen alive following severe blunt trauma will have an aortic laceration. Liberal use of aortography with *all* severe chest injuries is the best diagnostic approach, because *no single* clinical finding can diagnose or exclude significant vascular injuries.

Passaro and Pace in 1959 are credited with the first successful repair of a traumatic aortic laceration. In 1961 the author reported 15 patients with traumatic injuries and reviewed published experiences of others, finding virtually no successful reports of surgical repairs except the one case reported by Passaro.

ETIOLOGY AND PATHOLOGY. Rupture of the aorta usually results from a deceleration-type injury, typically an automobile accident. In the vast majority of patients, the laceration occurs just distal to the left subclavian artery. Apparently the descending thoracic aorta and the aortic arch decelerate at different rates because of differences in anatomic structure, producing a transverse tear near the site of insertion of the ligamentum arteriosum. The tear may involve part or all of the layers of the aortic wall, varying from laceration of the intima to transection of the aorta with retraction of the two ends (Fig. 20-15). Usually the injury is a partial laceration with formation of a localized hematoma. Aortic dissection following trauma is rare.

Fatal hemorrhage is prevented in some patients by the adventitia, which has been reported to constitute 60 percent of the tensile strength of the aortic wall. It is quite astonishing at operation to find the transected edges of the intima retracted for 1 to 2 cm, with exsanguination temporarily prevented by the adventitia.

The extensive 1981 review by Fisher and associates summarized available information. They found that aortic and great vessel laceration constituted the most common site of vascular injury after blunt chest trauma, citing 54 cases of their own and 456 cases previously reported by others. The second most common injury was an innominate artery laceration (26 cases). Injuries of the right carotid or right subclavian are virtually unknown; only 4 cases of laceration of the common carotid artery could be found. There were 13 injuries of the subclavian, virtually all of which involved the left subclavian. Multiple vascular lacerations were found in only 3 percent of cases. Lacerations of the aorta in other areas are very rare, with only isolated reports of injury of the ascending aorta or laceration near the diaphragm.

In surviving patients, a mediastinal hematoma forms and produces widening of the mediastinal shadow, easily recognized on the chest x-ray. This is the *key to the diagnosis.* Several radiographic abnormalities have been de-

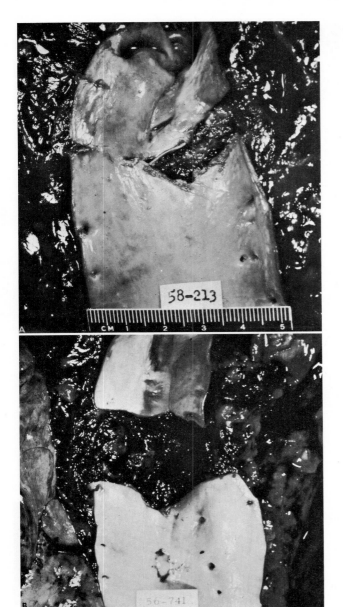

Fig. 20-15. *A.* Translated aorta found at autopsy when the patient was exsanguinated 24 h following injury. The patient had only minor chest pain before the terminal event. The sharp, transverse laceration of the aorta is the usual finding, resulting from the deceleration forces at the time of injury. *B.* Partial transection of the aorta found at autopsy when the patient was suddenly exsanguinated 3 weeks following an automobile accident. An aortic lesion had not been previously suspected.

small group of patients, less than 10 percent, have been reported who had aortic laceration but did not have significant mediastinal widening.

In surviving patients first seen in the hospital emergency department, there is a grave risk of imminent rupture, as about 40 percent of such patients exsanguinate within the next 48 h. The statistical risk of fatal rupture within the first 5 days after hospital admission is shown in Fig. 20-16. The risk decreases sharply after 2 weeks. Surviving patients gradually developed a false aneurysm, described earlier in this chapter under Traumatic Thoracic Aneurysms. Although traumatic aneurysms enlarge slowly, there is a small but ever-present hazard of rupture; about 20 percent of patients with false aneurysms seen more than 10 years after injury die from rupture within the next 5 years.

CLINICAL MANIFESTATIONS. Usually there are no symptoms or signs to indicate that an aortic injury is present. Dyspnea and chest pain are usually present, but these result from the almost universally present rib fractures. A hemothorax, with varying degrees of shock, is also common. A murmur has seldom been heard. Rarely, signs of acute obstruction of the aorta, apparently from prolapse of a segment of intima into the lumen, are present.

DIAGNOSTIC FINDINGS. As the history and the physical examination provide virtually no clues to the diagnosis, the chest x-ray is most important. Widening of the mediastinum (Fig. 20-17) is present in 80 to 90 percent of patients. It may result from causes other than rupture of the aorta, hence, aortography is necessary for the definitive diagnosis (Fig. 20-18). As emphasized earlier, an aortogram should be performed in the majority of patients with severe chest trauma, regardless of clinical findings.

TREATMENT. Thoracotomy should be performed as soon as possible after the diagnosis has been established. Akins et al. provide evidence that prompt operation would seem wiser in most instances.

The surgical approach is through a left posterolateral thoracotomy in the fourth intercostal space. At NYU a femoral-femoral bypass with a pump oxygenator and cannulae in a femoral artery and vein is routinely used. The use of a shunt or a bypass during operation, as opposed to the simpler clamp and repair technique, varies widely among different institutions. In a careful survey of published reports by others, Pate found that 8 of 30 patients treated by simply clamping and rapid suture repair developed paraplegia (20 percent). Among 68 patients who had either a shunt or a bypass, only 4 developed papaplegia, a frequency of 6 percent. The key point with femoral-femoral bypass is to use a flow rate high enough to keep the distal aortic pressure above 60 mmHg. Certainly, if the repair could be accomplished predictably within less than 30 min the risk of paraplegia would seem small, but attempting repair of an acute aortic laceration without distal circulation is a serious "gamble."

Once the left chest has been opened, the hematoma overlying the thoracic aorta should not be disturbed until proximal aortic control has been obtained. This is best done by opening the pericardium and encircling the aorta

scribed, but simply recognizing a wide mediastinal shadow is by far the most significant. Several mathematical indices were analyzed, but all were found inferior to the subjective impression of *mediastinal widening*. The critical measurement separating positive from negative cases was a mediastinal width of 8.0 cm.

No single finding either diagnoses or excludes aortic laceration. This can only be done with aortography. A

Mode of Death	No. of Patients
Other subsystem trauma	13
Multiple	8
Head injury	3
Hemorrhagic shock during thoracotomy	2
Acute cardiac failure	4
Diffuse mediastinal and chest wall hemorrhage after repair	2
Total	19

Fig. 20-16. Mode of death after repair of acute traumatic aortic transection (UAB; 1967–July 1984; n = 47, 13 deaths and GLH; 1965–November 1984; n = 32, 6 deaths). (From: *Kirklin JW, Barratt-Boyes BG: Cardiac Surgery. New York, Wiley, chap 53, p 1459, with permission.*)

distal or proximal to the left common carotid artery. Slight manipulation of the mediastinal hematoma may result in abrupt rupture and massive hemorrhage. Surgical repair usually requires the insertion of a short Dacron graft, though some groups have reported repair by direct suture.

Overall mortality with traumatic injuries ranges between 15 and 25 percent, usually because of associated injuries. In the series of 79 patients reported by Kirklin-Barratt-Boyes, mortality was 24 percent and paraplegia developed in 16 percent.

OBSTRUCTION OF THE SUPERIOR VENA CAVA

Obstruction of the superior vena cava produces an unusual but distinctive clinical syndrome that can be easily recognized once the diagnosis is considered. Diagnostic errors are common, primarily because of the infrequent occurrence of the disease and because of lack of familiarity with the distinctive clinical features. The 1981 report by Parish emphasized that the diagnosis can be made on physical examination in most patients.

Fig. 20-17. Chest radiograph of a patient with traumatic rupture of the thoracic aorta, illustrating the characteristic widening of the mediastinum. When this is observed following a chest injury, emergency aortography should be performed to establish the diagnosis of rupture of the thoracic aorta.

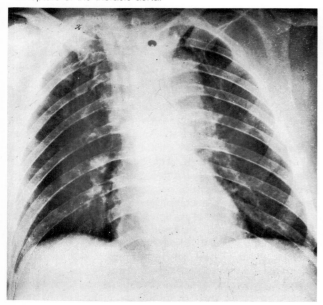

Fig. 20-18. Aortogram demonstrating traumatic rupture of the thoracic aorta distal to the left subclavian artery. The point of rupture can be seen as an irregular border of the thoracic aorta, in association with localized bulging. This angiogram represents the *first* instance in which emergency aortography was employed to establish firmly the diagnosis of traumatic rupture of the aorta. (From: *Spencer FC, Guerin PF, et al: A report of 15 patients with traumatic rupture of the thoracic aorta. J Thorac Cardiovasc Surg 41:1, 1961, with permission.*)

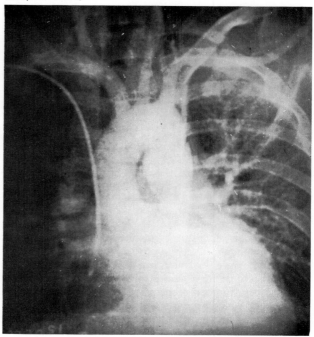

Several excellent reviews of this subject have been published in the last three decades, all finding that a malignant tumor is the most frequent cause. An extensive review made by McIntire and Sykes is a fundamental reference. Effler and Groves reported 64 patients, 48 of whom had a malignant neoplasm. Panker and Maddison summarized reports totaling 438 cases, only 15 percent of which were from benign causes. Mahajan reviewed published reports of benign causes of superior vena cava obstruction, a total of only 16 cases. Lochridge et al. described 66 cases seen in the previous 10 years; 64 were malignant.

ETIOLOGY. Over 90 percent of patients have obstruction from a malignant process. The percentage has apparently risen in recent years, especially since obstruction from expanding aortic aneurysms has decreased. The most common neoplasm is a bronchogenic carcinoma invading the mediastinum. Less frequent lesions are primary mediastinal tumors such as thymoma or lymphoma. Metastatic neoplasms are unusual.

Obstruction from a chronic fibrosing mediastinitis, usually of unknown cause, is infrequent. It is the only condition in which a long-term cure is possible. The etiology in most patients is unknown, although the disorder has been recognized for decades. The Parish report includes three cases resulting from the use of central venous catheters.

PATHOPHYSIOLOGY. With obstruction of the superior vena cava there is an increase in venous pressure to levels between 20 and 50 mmHg. The degree of increase in venous pressure varies with both the rate of development of the obstruction and the site of obstruction. Obstruction between the azygos vein and right atrium is less disabling than at other sites because the azygos vein can provide collateral venous decompression. The usual patient will have obstruction of the vena cava above the level of the azygos. Doty, in a 1982 detailed article, cited a venographic report by Dyet, who found that about 40 percent of patients have displacement but incomplete obstruction by tumor, about 20 percent have obstruction between the azygos vein and the heart, and about 40 percent have obstruction of the superior vena cava above the azygos, the usual finding in patients with disabling symptoms.

Acute obstruction of the vena cava, as during a thoracic operation, can produce fatal cerebral edema within a few minutes. This also occurred with early experiences in infants with the Glenn operation of anastomosis of the superior vena cava to the right pulmonary artery. At the opposite extreme are instances where superior vena cava obstruction develops slowly, permitting time for the development of collateral circulation, as a result of which symptoms are mild.

CLINICAL MANIFESTATIONS. With mild obstruction, frequent symptoms are headache, swelling of the eyelids, puffiness of the face, or enlargement of the neck. The severity is related to posture. Patients quickly find that symptoms increase if they bend over or lie down. With acute obstruction, resulting from hemorrhage into a rapidly growing neoplasm, more serious symptoms of cerebral congestion appear, including drowsiness and blurring of vision. Edema of the vocal cords produces hoarseness or dyspnea from laryngeal obstruction. As the majority of cases are due to a rapidly growing bronchogenic carcinoma, pulmonary symptoms such as cough and hemoptysis are also often present. In most patients death results within a few months.

In the minority of patients in whom obstruction results from a benign process, usually fibrosing mediastinitis, collateral circulation generally enlarges sufficiently to where little disability is present. Prominent features include dilated veins with edema and cyanosis, the degree varying with the degree of stasis. Venous hypertension is obvious from prominence and distention of veins in the arms and face. Effler and Groves described 16 patients with obstruction from a benign process, all of whom eventually developed sufficient collateral circulation to have minimal symptoms. No fatalities occurred as a result of chronic venous obstruction. We observed one patient over a period of 30 years in whom the superior vena cava became obstructed following an intracardiac operation for correction of anomalous pulmonary veins entering the superior vena cava. Venous hypertension initially was severe, above 35 mmHg, producing a bilateral chylothorax controlled by ligation of the thoracic duct. The child was almost six years of age at this time. Within a few months, however, all symptoms subsided, and the patient, now a young married woman with children, has no limitation of physical activities.

DIAGNOSTIC STUDIES. Although the clinical picture is characteristic when fully developed, early manifestations such as swelling of the eyes or headache may be confused with angioneurotic edema, congestive heart failure, or constrictive pericarditis. Elevation of venous pressure, usually between 20 and 50 mmHg, is diagnostic. Venography readily outlines the location and extent of the obstruction, although the elevated venous pressure may result in bleeding. Often venography is omitted if the diagnosis of a malignant process is obvious. The usual consideration is to determine the type of malignancy present by an appropriate biopsy. Thoracotomy is usually avoided if malignancy is present. Doty has emphasized that morbidity from a thoracic operation is less if a sternotomy is employed, because venous collateral circulation is interrupted to a lesser degree than with a lateral thoracotomy.

TREATMENT. With a malignant process, involvement of the superior vena cava almost precludes surgical resection. Isolated exceptions are rare.

The standard therapy is intensive radiation therapy, often in combination with diuretics and chemotherapy. The degree of improvement in symptoms varies with the type of neoplasm, but the majority improve rapidly, within a few weeks, probably from diminution in edema associated with a growing neoplasm. Death from the neoplasm, however, is virtually inevitable within the next several months, with rare survivors to 2 years.

With benign obstructions, as the report of Effler and Groves indicates, there is no urgency in performing an operation if symptoms are mild. In all likelihood these symptoms will improve, or subside completely, as collateral circulation develops.

Little et al. reviewed 42 patients with malignant superior vena cava obstruction. Thirty-three of the patients underwent radiotherapy; in all of these the obstruction clinically resolved within 14 days. Median survival of the entire group was only 5 months, emphasizing again the grim prognosis.

A number of ingenious attempts have been made to reconstruct an obstructed superior vena cava, although the clinical need for superior vena cava reconstruction is uncommon. Prosthetic grafts to date have been almost uniformly unsuccessful. The most favorable graft is a composite one of autogenous veins. Good results in three patients lasting for several years were reported by Hanlon and Danis. A collective review of surgical approaches was published by Gomes and Hufnagel. The best technique appears to be that reported by Doty and Baker, which consists of constructing a spiral vein graft by comparing the diameters of the innominate vein and saphenous vein, followed by appropriate mathematical calculations and construction of a composite vein over a stent. Doty summarized his experiences with 10 patients, 4 with benign disease. All grafts remained patent up to 18 months. The 4 patients with benign disease remained asymptomatic 3 months to 6 years after operation, while all with malignancy died within 21 months.

The graft sizes ranged from 9 to 13 mm and could be constructed from a segment of saphenous vein obtained from the thigh within about 30 min. This technique seems clearly superior to prosthetic materials. Unless the saphenous veins are not available, there would seem to be little indication to employ prosthetic materials. The only indication for the operation, however, seems to be the unusual patient with a benign process in whom collateral circulation is inadequate to relieve symptoms.

Rarely, a localized granuloma may compress and thrombose the vena cava. Patency can be restored by opening the vein and removing the thrombus. Three such patients were reported by Pate and Hammon, but the paucity of reports since that time suggests that thrombectomy is not usually feasible.

Bibliography

Aneurysms of the Ascending Aorta

Akins C, Buckley M, et al: Myocardial protection with hypothermia and potassium cardioplegia during operation for ascending aortic aneurysms. *J Thorac Cardiovasc Surg* 79:700, 1980.

Bahnson HT, Spencer FC: Excision of aneurysm of the ascending aorta with prosthetic replacement during cardiopulmonary bypass. *Ann Surg* 151:879, 1960.

Cabrol C, Pavie A, et al: Long-term results with total replacement of the ascending aorta and re-implantation of the coronary arteries. *J Thorac Cardiovasc Surg* 91:17, 1986.

Cooley DA: *Surgical Treatment of Aortic Aneurysms.* Philadelphia, Saunders, 1986.

Crawford ES, Crawford JL: *Diseases of the Aorta.* Baltimore, Williams & Wilkins, 1984.

Culliford AT, Cyaliotis B, et al: Aneurysms of the ascending aorta and transverse arch: Surgical experience in 80 patients. *J Thorac Cardiovasc Surg* 83:701, 1982.

Gott VL, Pyeritz RE, et al: Surgical treatment of aneurysms of the ascending aorta in the Marfan syndrome. Results of composite-graft repair in 50 patients. *N Engl J Med* 314:1070, 1986.

Grey DP, Ott DA, Cooley DA: Surgical treatment of aneurysm of the ascending aorta with aortic insufficiency. A selective approach. *J Thorac Cardiovasc Surg* 86:864, 1983.

Kouchoukos NT, Marshall WG Jr, Wedige-Stecher TA: Eleven-year experience with composite graft replacement of the ascending aorta and aortic valve. *J Thorac Cardiovasc Surg* 92:691, 1986.

Liddicott JE, Bekassy SM, et al: Ascending aortic aneurysms: Review of 100 consecutive cases. *Circulation* 51–52(suppl. 1):202, 1975.

McDonald G, Schaff H, et al: Surgical management of patients with the Marfan syndrome and dilatation of the ascending aorta. *J Thorac Cardiovasc Surg* 81:180, 1981.

Miller D, Stinson E, et al: Concomitant resection of ascending aortic aneurysm and replacement of the aortic valve. Operative and long-term results with "conventional" techniques in ninety patients. *J Thorac Cardiovasc Surg* 79:388, 1980.

Moreno-Cabral CE, Miller DC, et al: Degenerative and atherosclerotic aneurysms of the thoracic aorta. Determinants of early and late surgical outcome. *J Thorac Cardiovasc Surg* 88:1020, 1984.

Pressler V, McNamara JJ: Aneurysm of the thoracic aorta. Review of 260 cases. *J Thorac Cardiovasc Surg* 89:50, 1985.

Spencer FC, Blake HA: A report of the successful surgical treatment of aortic regurgitation from a dissecting aortic aneurysm in a patient with the Marfan syndrome. *J Thorac Cardiovasc Surg* 44:238, 1962.

Aneurysms of the Transverse Aortic Arch

Crawford E, Saleh S: Transverse aortic arch aneurysm: Improved results of treatment employing new modifications of aortic reconstruction and hypothermic cerebral circulatory arrest. *Ann Surg* 194:180, 1981.

Crawford ES, Snyder DM: Treatment of aneurysms of the aortic arch. A progress report. *J Thorac Cardiovasc Surg* 85:237, 1983.

Crawford ES, Crawford JL: *Diseases of the Aorta.* Baltimore, Williams & Wilkins, 1984.

Ergin M, Griepp R: Progress in treatment of aneurysms of the aortic arch. *World J Surg* 4:535, 1980.

Frist WH, Baldwin JC, et al: A reconsideration of cerebral perfusion in aortic arch replacement. *Ann Thorac Surg* 42:273, 1986.

Kay GL, Cooley DA, et al: Surgical repair of aneurysms involving the distal aortic arch. *J Thorac Cardiovasc Surg* 91:397, 1986.

Livesay JJ, Cooley DA, et al: Surgical experience in descending thoracic aneurysmectomy with and without adjuncts to avoid ischemia. *Ann Thorac Surg* 39:37, 1985.

Sweeney MS, Cooley DA, et al: Hypothermic circulatory arrest for cardiovascular lesions: Technical considerations and results. *Ann Thorac Surg* 40:498, 1985.

Traumatic Thoracic Aneurysms

Bennett DE, Cherry JK: The natural history of traumatic aneurysms of the aorta. *Surgery* 61:516, 1967.

McCollum C, Graham J, et al: Chronic traumatic aneurysms of the thoracic aorta: An analysis of 50 patients. *J Trauma* 19:248, 1979.

Spencer FC, Guerin PF, et al: A report of fifteen patients with traumatic rupture of the thoracic aorta. *J Thorac Cardiovasc Surg* 41:1, 1961.

Aneurysms of the Descending Thoracic Aorta

Bahnson HT: Definitive treatment of saccular aneurysms of the aorta with excision of the sac and aortic suture. *Surg Gynecol Obstet* 96:382, 1953.

Bickerstaff LK, Pairolero PC, et al: Thoracic aortic aneurysms: A population-based study. *Surgery* 92:1103, 1982.

Crawford ES, Snyder DM, et al: Progress in treatment of thoracoabdominal and abdominal aortic aneurysms involving celiac, superior mesenteric, and renal arteries. *Ann Surg* 188:404, 1978.

Crawford ES, Crawford JL, et al: Thoracoabdominal aortic aneurysms: Preoperative and intraoperative factors determining immediate and long-term results of operations in 605 patients. *J Vasc Surg* 3:389, 1986.

Culliford A, Ayvaliotis B, et al: Aneurysms of the descending aorta: Surgical experiences in 48 patients. *J Thorac Cardiovasc Surg* 85:98, 1983.

Cunningham JN Jr, Laschinger JC, et al: Measurement of spinal cord ischemia during operations upon the thoracic aorta: Initial clinical experience. *Ann Surg* 196:285, 1982.

DeBakey ME, Cooley DA, et al: Aneurysms of the thoracic aorta. Analysis of 179 patients treated by resection. *J Thorac Surg* 36:393, 1958.

Krieger KH, Spencer FC: Is paraplegia after repair of coarctation of the aorta due principally to distal hypotension during aortic cross-clamping? *Surgery* 97:2, 1985.

Laschinger JC, Cunningham JN Jr, et al: Monitoring of somatosensory evoked potentials during surgical procedures on the thoracoabdominal aorta. I. Relationship of aortic crossclamp duration, changes in somatosensory evoked potentials, and incidence of neurologic dysfunction. *J Thorac Cardiovasc Surg* 94:260, 1987.

Laschinger JC, Cunningham JN Jr, et al: Monitoring of somatosensory evoked potentials during surgical procedures on the thoracoabdominal aorta. II. Use of somatosensory evoked potentials to assess adequacy of distal aortic bypass and perfusion after thoracic aortic cross-clamping. *J Thorac Cardiovasc Surg* 94:266, 1987.

Laschinger JC, Cunningham JN Jr, et al: Monitoring of somatosensory evoked potentials during surgical procedures on the thoracoabdominal aorta. III. Intraoperative identification of vessels critical to spinal cord blood supply. *J Thorac Cardiovasc Surg* 94:271, 1987.

Laschinger JC, Cunningham JN Jr, et al: Monitoring of somatosensory evoked potentials during surgical procedures on the thoracoabdominal aorta. IV. Clinical observations and results. *J Thorac Cardiovasc Surg* 94:275, 1987.

Livesay JJ, Cooley DA, et al: Surgical experience in descending thoracic aneurysmectomy with and without adjuncts to avoid ischemia. *Ann Thorac Surg* 39:37, 1985.

Pressler V, McNamara JJ: Aneurysms of the thoracic aorta. Review of 260 cases. *J Thorac Cardiovasc Surg* 89:50, 1985.

Spencer FC, Zimmerman JM: The influence of ligation of intercostal arteries on paraplegia in dogs. *Surg Forum* 9:340, 1959.

Vasko JS, Spencer FC, Bahnson HT: Aneurysm of the aorta treated by excision: Review of 237 cases followed up to seven years. *Am J Surg* 105:793, 1963.

Thoracoabdominal Aneurysms

Crawford ES, Crawford JL, et al: Thoracoabdominal aortic aneurysms: Preoperative and intraoperative factors determining immediate and long-term results of operations in 605 patients. *J Vasc Surg* 3:389, 1986.

Crawford ES, DeNatale RW: Thoracoabdominal aortic aneurysm: Observations regarding the natural course of the disease. *J Vasc Surg* 3:578, 1986.

Crawford ES, Snyder D, et al: Progress in treatment of thoracoabdominal and abdominal aortic aneurysms involving celiac, superior mesenteric, and renal arteries. *Ann Surg* 188:404, 1978.

DeBakey ME, Crawford ES, et al: Surgical considerations in the treatment of aneurysms of the thoraco-abdominal aorta. *Ann Surg* 162:650, 1965.

Spencer FC, Zimmerman JM: The influence of ligation of intercostal arteries on paraplegia in dogs. *Surg Forum* 9:340, 1959.

Dissecting Aneurysms

Dalen J, Pape L, et al: Dissection of the aorta: Pathogenesis, diagnostic, and treatment. *Prog Cardiovasc Dis* 23:237, 1980.

DeBakey ME, Henly WS, et al: Surgical management of dissecting aneurysms of the aorta. *J Thorac Cardiovasc Surg* 49:130, 1965.

Ergin MA, Galla JD, et al: Acute dissections of the aorta. Current surgical treatment. *Surg Clin North Am* 65:721, 1985.

Gryboski W, Spencer FC: Intermittent claudication caused by a dissecting aneurysm of the aorta. *South Med J* 58:593, 1965.

Hirst AE, Johns VJ, Kime SW: Dissecting aneurysm of the aorta: A review of 505 cases. *Medicine (Baltimore)* 37:217, 1958.

Lindsay J, Hurst JW: Clinical features and prognosis in dissecting aneurysm of the aorta. *Circulation* 35:880, 1967.

Miller D, Stinson E, et al: Operative treatment of aortic dissections. Experience with 125 patients over a sixteen-year period. *J Thorac Cardiovasc Surg* 78:365, 1979.

Miller D, Stinson E, Shumway N: Realistic expectations of surgical treatment of aortic dissections: The Stanford experience. *World J Surg* 4:571, 1980.

Najafi H, Dye WS, et al: Acute aortic regurgitation secondary to aortic dissection: Surgical management without valve replacement. *Ann Thorac Surg* 14:474, 1972.

Roberts W: Aortic dissection: Anatomy, consequences, and causes. *Am Heart J* 101:195, 1981.

Spencer FC, Blake HA: A report of the successful surgical treatment of aortic regurgitation from a dissecting aortic aneurysm in a patient with the Marfan syndrome. *J Thorac Cardiovasc Surg* 44:238, 1962.

Sutton M, Oldershaw P, et al: Dissection of the thoracic aorta. A comparison between medical and surgical treatment. *J Cardiovasc Surg* 22:195, 1981.

Sweeney MS, Cooley DA, et al: Hypothermic circulatory arrest for cardiovascular lesions: Technical considerations and results. *Ann Thorac Surg* 40:498, 1985.

Wheat M: Acute dissecting aneurysms of the aorta: Diagnosis and treatment—1979. *Am Heart J* 99:373, 1980.

Wheat M: Current status of medical therapy of acute dissecting aneurysms of the aorta. *World J Surg* 4:563, 1980.

Wilson SK, Hutchins GM: Aortic dissecting aneurysms: Causative factors in 204 subjects. *Arch Pathol Lab Med* 106:175, 1982.

Wolfe WG, Oldham HN, et al: Surgical treatment of acute ascending aortic dissection. *Ann Surg* 197:738, 1983.

Wounds of the Great Vessels

Akins C, Buckley M, et al: Acute traumatic disruption of the thoracic aorta: A ten-year experience. *Ann Thorac Surg* 31:305, 1981.

Bennett DE, Cherry DK: The natural history of traumatic aneurysms of the aorta. *Surgery* 61:516, 1967.

Blake HA, Inmon TW, Spencer FC: Emergency use of antegrade aortography in diagnosis of acute aortic rupture. *Ann Surg* 152:954, 1960.

Brawley RK, Murray GF, et al: Management of wounds of the innominate, subclavian, and axillary blood vessels. *Surg Gynecol Obstet* 131:1130, 1970.

Burney RE, Gundry SR, et al: Comparison of mediastinal width, mediastinal-thoracic and -cardiac ratios, and "mediastinal widening" in detection of traumatic aortic rupture. *Ann Emerg Med* 12:668, 1983.

Kirklin JW, Barratt-Boyes BG: *Cardiac Surgery*. New York, Wiley, 1986.

Magilligan D, Davila J: Innominate artery disruption due to blunt trauma. *Arch Surg* 114:307, 1979.

Parmley LF, Mattingly TW, Manion WC: Penetrating wounds to the heart and aorta. *Circulation* 17:953, 1958.

Parmley LF, Mattingly TW, et al: Non-penetrating traumatic injury of the aorta. *Circulation* 17:1086, 1958.

Pate JW: Traumatic rupture of the aorta: Emergency operation. *Ann Thorac Surg* 39:531, 1985.

Rich N, Spencer F: *Vascular Trauma*. Philadelphia, Saunders, 1978, p 427.

Richardson JD, Flint LM, et al: Management of transmediastinal gunshot wounds. *Surgery* 90:671, 1981.

Robbs J, Baker L, et al: Cervicomediastinal arterial injuries. A surgical challenge. *Arch Surg* 116:663, 1981.

Saylam A, Melo J, et al: Early surgical repair in traumatic rupture of the thoracic aorta. *J Cardiovasc Surg* 21:295, 1980.

Spencer FC, Guerin PF, et al: A report of 15 patients with traumatic rupture of the thoracic aorta. *J Thorac Cardiovasc Surg* 41:1, 1961.

Williams S, Burney RE, et al: Indications for aortography. Radiography after blunt chest trauma: A reassessment of the radiographic findings associated with traumatic rupture of the aorta. *Invest Radiol* 18:230, 1983.

Zakharia AT: Cardiovascular and thoracic battle injuries in the Lebanon war. Analysis of 3,000 personal cases. *J Thorac Cardiovasc Surg* 89:723, 1985.

Obstruction of the Superior Vena Cava

Doty D: Bypass of superior vena cava. Six years' experience with spiral vein graft for obstruction of superior vena cava due to benign and malignant disease. *J Thorac Cardiovasc Surg* 83:326, 1982.

Effler DB, Groves LK: Superior vena caval obstruction. *J Thorac Cardiovasc Surg* 43:574, 1962.

Gomes MN, Hufnagel CA: Superior vena cava obstruction: Review of literature and report of two cases due to benign intrathoracic tumors. *Ann Thorac Surg* 20:344, 1975.

Hanlon CR, Danis RK: Superior vena caval obstruction: Indications for diagnostic thoracotomy. *Ann Surg* 161:771, 1965.

Little AG, Golomb HM, et al: Malignant superior vena cava obstruction reconsidered: The role of diagnostic surgical intervention. *Ann Thorac Surg* 40:285, 1985.

Lochridge S, Knibbe W, Doty D: Obstruction of the superior vena cava. *Surgery* 85:14, 1979.

Parish J, Marschke R, et al: Etiologic considerations in superior vena cava syndrome. *Mayo Clin Proc* 36:407, 1981.

Pate JW, Hammon J: Superior vena cava syndrome due to histoplasmosis in children. *Ann Surg* 161:778, 1965.

Chapter 21

Peripheral Arterial Disease

Anthony M. Imparato and Thomas S. Riles

It is difficult for a student of medicine at this time to realize that most of the vascular operations commonly performed today have evolved during the past 40 years, although sporadic attempts to perform arterial surgery are documented in the early history of surgery. In part, progress awaited the development of modern techniques of anesthesia and asepsis that have occurred since 1900. Nevertheless Eck performed the first successful blood vessel anastomosis, anastomosing the portal vein to the inferior vena cava in dogs in 1877; Matas performed endoaneurysmorrhaphy in 1888; and Murphy performed the first end-to-end arterial anastomosis in human beings following excision of an arteriovenous fistula in the thigh in 1897. Thereafter, a series of advances, including substitution of autologous vein for artery (Goyanes, 1906; Bernheim, 1915) and the epochal work of Carrel in 1912, laid the groundwork for direct arterial surgery. The explosive development of direct arterial surgery occurred after 1950, starting with the successful treatment of ischemic arterial disease by endarterectomy (dos Santos, 1947), venous substitution for occluded arteries (Kunlin, 1951), successful excision of an abdominal aneurysm with replacement by an aortic homograft (Dubost, 1952), and development of a cloth material to replace blood vessels (Voorhees and Blakemore, 1952). Carotid and renal arterial reconstructions were first done successfully between 1955 and 1960.

The development of practical and reliable arteriographic techniques and the availability of heparin and antimicrobial and antibiotic substances made possible the emergence of the modern era of vascular surgery, the history of which is beautifully documented by Charles G.

Rob in *The Classics of Vascular Surgery,* a collection of copies of the original papers that chronicles this progress.

CONGENITAL ARTERIOVENOUS FISTULAS

ETIOLOGY AND PATHOLOGY. Congenital arteriovenous fistulas, though rare, constitute one manifestation of a number of more commonly related abnormalities of differentiation of the anlage of the vascular system. These vary in appearance from simple port-wine stain to the massively hypertrophied extremity that contains multiple recognizable elements, including capillary, arterial, and venous channels, dilated and visible in and through the skin with or without multiple abnormal arteriovenous communications. When arteriovenous fistulas are part of the lesion, most often there are multiple vascular elements within it. In the absence of arteriovenous communications, there is more apt to be a preponderance of one element over another such that there may be only capillary hemangiomata in the skin or there may be a great number of markedly dilated venous channels presenting as localized or diffuse cavernomatous venous malformations.

Vascular lesions associated with congenital arteriovenous malformations most commonly occur in the extremities, which may be hypertrophied, and involve not only the skin and subcutaneous tissue but the muscles and bone as well. The lesions tend to become more prominent with the growth of the individual. Visibly dilated venous channels may dilate progressively. Ulceration and bleeding may supervene. Uncontrolled bleeding may lead to amputation of the extremity. Rarely, ischemic pain and even digital gangrene may develop as a result of shunting of blood through the fistulas.

CLINICAL MANIFESTATIONS. The presenting complaint may vary, but not infrequently it relates to a mother's awareness that the extremity of one of her young children is larger than the other and perhaps few or many dilated veins may have been noticed over the extremity. At the other end of the spectrum of complaints is the patient who is now in adult life, has known of a vascular malformation for many years, and has been ''shopping around'' for someone to get rid of it. Occasionally a patient will present with marked facial deformity with marked asymmetry, obviously dilated venous channels on the face and neck, strawberrylike or mulberrylike protrusions from the skin, and similar discoloration and tumefaction of the mucous membranes of the mouth and pharynx. On occasion nothing will have been noticed in even a pubertal child until a minor injury calls attention to the extremity, which is then found to be warmer and larger than its counterpart and exhibits some dilated blood vessels, raising the suspicion of either a soft tissue or bone infection. On rare occasions the patient will become aware of a thrill or an audible bruit.

The physical examination is quite variable and depends upon the location and components of the malformation. Since those associated with arteriovenous fistulas usually contain multiple components, there may be a spectrum of abnormalities that might include enlargement of the extremity, port-wine staining of a portion of the skin, mulberrylike protrusions in other areas, markedly dilated venous channels visible in the skin, and a spongy lobulated appearance of portions of the extremity or occasionally only of a digit. The hallmark of the complex congenital arteriovenous fistula is the palpation of a thrill and the auscultation of a bruit. The bruit may be heard in a sharply localized area or diffusely throughout the extremity. On rare occasions the physical findings are subtle and may simply mimic a very early acute deep venous occlusion with some swelling of an extremity, some discoloration, and some barely visible dilated veins. Here too auscultation for a bruit will establish the diagnosis.

Arteriography is required to confirm the diagnosis, which becomes apparent from the characteristic appearance of abnormally dilated arteries feeding into abnormally dilated veins directly (Fig. 21-1). Frequently the precise site of communication between the arterial and venous system is not delineated, but its location can be approximated. Almost invariably in the congenital variety the communications are numerous.

Congenital arteriovenous communications within the central nervous system constitute a subject quite apart from those occurring in the integument. Suffice it to say that such abnormalities are encountered in relation both to the spinal cord and to the brain.

TREATMENT. The keynote to treatment is conservatism. Since congenital arteriovenous fistulas seldom result in cardiac difficulties, the decision to treat malformations on the surface of the body need only be based upon whether a lesion threatens to ulcerate and bleed, whether the hemihypertrophy of the extremity may lead to serious orthopaedic problems, or whether the deformity is so cosmetically repulsive that the patient must have help. Only rarely is a congenital arteriovenous fistula treatable either by localized interruption of arteriovenous communications or by en bloc resection of the sites of communication and their neighboring abnormal blood vessels. More often the extensive involvement of the skin, subcutaneous tissue, muscle, and bone makes it impossible for en bloc resection to be performed. In most instances, therefore, the lesion must be considered incurable, although excellent palliation can be afforded by setting limited goals. There are times when resection of markedly dilated subcutaneous venous channels may help to protect the nourishment of the skin. There are other times when ligation of multiple small branches leading into the malformation may help to shrink it and improve the nourishment of the skin. It is certain, however, that ligation of the major artery leading into the area, be it the femoral, the popliteal, or one of the major tibials in the lower extremity or a counterpart in the upper extremity or in the head and neck, should not be performed, since this not infrequently either results in gangrene distal to the ligature of the major artery or destroys accessibility to the arteriovenous communications themselves. When accessibility is destroyed, the possibility of performing a technique that is now receiving wide attention and achieving quite satisfactory results is destroyed. This technique is

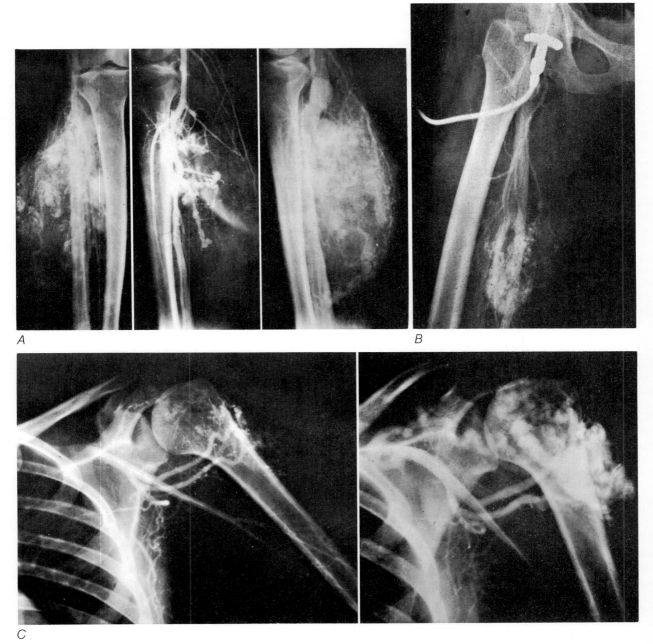

Fig. 21-1. Series of angiograms demonstrating congenital arteriovenous fistulas. *A.* This series of three views shows a popliteal arteriogram in the same patient. The first view is a posteroanterior view that demonstrates the great degree of enlargement of the calf. The next two views are early and late exposures in the arterial phase in a lateral projection. The extensive staining in the late arterial phase is highly suggestive of congenital arteriovenous fistulas. *B.* Arteriogram in the thigh area of a second patient. Note the diffuse staining produced by injection into the profunda femoris vessel. *C.* These two views demonstrate early and late arteriograms in the shoulder area. In this patient the fistulas originate from the circumflex humeral vessels.

the percutaneous passage of catheters to the areas of the malformation with occlusion of the arteriovenous communications employing particulate matter, such as microspheres, Gelfoam, or glues. Repeated treatments may be given over a period of time, during which portions of the malformation may be obliterated, stability can be established, and the procedure repeated on subsequent occasions. With this technique it is possible to embolize into the hypertrophied arterial branches feeding directly into the malformation. The only danger of the technique lies in pursuing the obliteration too aggressively and precipitating infarction. This is a particularly dangerous complication because not only is tissue lost but also uncontrollable hemorrhage from tissues adjacent to the infant may result. The catheter technique has been successfully applied to malformations of the pelvis and buttock, which were of quite difficult access, as well as to malformations of the head, neck, extremities, and even the brain.

Increasingly favorable experiences with this intraarterial embolization have been reported. Combinations of Gelfoam, pellets, and autologous muscle have been injected by the Seldinger technique. Inoperable lesions may be treated by embolization alone, while extensive lesions may be managed by embolization followed by excision.

ARTERIAL TRAUMA

HISTORICAL DATA. The feasibility of routinely repairing injured limb arteries in military casualities was first demonstrated in the Korean conflict in 1952; earlier attempts in World War II were generally unsuccessful. Several factors contributed to this improvement in results: (1) the prompt evacuation of the wounded by helicopter so that definitive treatment could be started within 2 to 4 h of injury, (2) the realization that extensive debridement of traumatic wounds, together with antibiotic administration and secondary closure controlled infection, and (3) the familiarity of surgeons with new vascular surgical techniques and instruments. Following this war experience, injured extremity arteries encountered in civilians have been almost routinely repaired to avoid the approximately 50 percent incidence of gangrene associated with ligation of major extremity arteries.

PATHOLOGY. Most arterial injuries result from penetrating wounds that partly or completely disrupt the wall of the vessel. Nonpenetrating injuries, usually associated with fractures of adjacent bones, occur less frequently but have a more serious prognosis.

With lacerations or transections, the extent of injury varies with the type of trauma. With clean incised wounds, such as those made by a knife or an icepick, injury to the arterial wall is minimal and repair may require no more than simple suture. By contrast, trauma from high velocity missiles will disrupt the intima and media for a distance beyond the actual laceration and require wider debridement at the time of surgical repair, often necessitating insertion of a conduit to bridge the defect.

Extensive communicated fractures may be associated with either contusion of the artery, leading to thrombosis, or to spasm. Arterial spasm alone, though an infrequent response to injury, may precipitate thrombosis.

Arterial contusion from a blunt injury may result in multiple areas of fragmentation of the arterial wall with intramural hemorrhage or detachment of the intima with prolapse into the lumen. This results in luminal obstruction that can be detected only by arteriotomy and inspection. When contusion is misdiagnosed as spasm, the delay in treatment with persistence of ischemia can result in

gangrene. Volkmann is ischemic contracture of the muscles of the forearm is often due to untreated spasm or contusion of the brachial artery accompanying supracondylar fracture of the humerus.

PATHOPHYSIOLOGY. The consequences of ischemia following an arterial injury vary with the tolerance of different tissues for anoxia. In the extremity the peripheral nerves are the most sensitive. Paralysis and anesthesia quickly develop when arterial blood flow is seriously decreased. Striated muscle is almost equally sensitive and will usually become necrotic if arterial blood flow is decreased to such a degree that anesthesia and paralysis are present. Skin, tendon, and bone all have a greater tolerance for anoxia and may survive an ischemic injury which has produced irreversible extensive muscle necrosis. This is seen in an extremity in which an arterial repair is performed several hours after injury. The skin may appear viable, but the extremity is anesthetic and paralyzed, and after a period of time will be found to have widespread necrosis of the muscles.

Striated muscle will tolerate ischemia 6 to 8 h. Every effort should be made to complete arterial repair within 6 h after injury if anesthesia *or* paralysis is present, indicating a severe degree of ischemia. A definite time limit does not exist, however, beyond which arterial repair is futile, for the importance of the time interval varies with the collateral circulation. The collateral circulation, in turn, varies with the artery injured, with the degree of soft tissue injury which has interrupted collateral circulation, with associated shock, and with ambient temperature. In some patients with little disturbance of collateral circulation, arterial repair may be successfully performed 12 to 15 h after injury.

CLINICAL MANIFESTATIONS. Shock, present in over 50 percent of patients with an arterial injury, is usually due to either hemorrhage from the injured artery or associated injuries. The degree of shock varies with the severity of the blood loss or the severity of other injuries. When profound, the severe associated peripheral vasoconstriction may conceal the presence of an arterial injury until blood pressure has been restored to near normal levels.

With blunt trauma, multiple organ injuries are commonly present. These include skull fractures, rib fractures, or blunt abdominal injuries. Careful assessment of each injury, with subsequent assignment of priorities in therapy, is a critical part of initial evaluation of the patient.

In the injured extremity, fractures and nerve injuries are commonly present either with penetrating wounds or following blunt trauma. The presence of a fracture or extensive soft tissue injury greatly influences the prognosis of an arterial injury. For example, in one series of arterial injuries the presence of a fracture of a femur in association with an injury of the femoral artery raised the incidence of gangrene from 11 to 55 percent.

In the extremity, the arterial injury frequently produces the five abnormal findings associated with acute ischemia, conveniently remembered as five p's: *p*ain, *p*aralysis, *p*aresthesia or anesthesia, loss of *p*ulses, and *p*allor. Of these five, the neurologic findings, paralysis and paresthesia, are the most important, because loss of neurologic function indicates a degree of tissue ischemia that will progress to gangrene unless arterial blood flow is improved. Absence of a pulse in the presence of a normal pulse in the contralateral extremity immediately suggests an arterial injury. In the presence of shock, evaluation of peripheral pulses may be difficult until blood volume is restored. The presence of a peripheral pulse does not exclude an arterial injury since a tangential laceration of the wall of an artery sealed by a blood clot preserves some flow through the arterial lumen.

With penetrating wounds, bright red bleeding, even in small amounts, immediately suggests arterial injury. Contained bleeding may produce a tense hematoma palpable around the wound, without external evidence of bleeding. A systolic bruit or rarely a continuous bruit may indicate that an acute arteriovenous fistula has been produced.

An arterial injury can be present with virtually no abnormalities in the extremity and so a penetrating injury near a major artery should alert to the possibility of an arterial injury that may result in exsanguinating secondary hemorrhage, the occurrence of a false aneurysm, or an arteriovenous fistula in the area where the hematoma formed around the lacerated artery.

With any suspicion of arterial injury, as occurs with diminished or absent pulses or with signs of ischemia, an arteriogram should be performed and is of particular value in determining whether the abnormalities are due to arterial injury or to angulation of the artery at the fracture site.

TREATMENT. Preoperative Considerations. Control of bleeding is the most urgent immediate problem and can usually be accomplished by direct digital pressure on the bleeding site or by tightly packing the wound with gauze and applying a pressure dressing. A large amount of packing may be required, for the efficacy of the packing depends upon compression of the artery between the overlying skin and the underlying bone. Tourniquets are best avoided for most injuries. When used they must be carefully padded to avoid the risk of permanent injury to peripheral nerves.

Shock should be treated by the rapid infusion of fluids (500 mL every 5 to 10 min) until the systolic blood pressure rises to 80 mmHg, after which additional fluids can be infused more gradually. Usually 1000 to 2000 mL of fluid will be required. Blood is preferable, but until the necessary cross-matching has been done, crystalloids, plasma, or dextran may be used.

Antibiotic therapy should be started promptly and appropriate prophylactic therapy for tetanus begun. Sympathetic blocks and systemic anticoagulant therapy have no significant role in preoperative care.

Operative Technique. An important basic tenet regarding arterial trauma is that almost all injuries can be repaired successfully with available surgical techniques. The prognosis then becomes a question of whether the repair was performed before irreversible muscle necrosis developed and how well the bone and associated soft tissue trauma can be managed. The only special instruments required are atraumatic vascular clamps and arterial su-

tures, usually of synthetic fiber (Dacron, polypropylene) fashioned to be monofilamentous, sizes 4-0 to 7-0, with swaged needles. The surgical incisions should be placed to expose the artery proximal and distal to the site of injury, and then the hematoma surrounding the injury can be widely opened and the artery mobilized. When soft tissue trauma is extensive and it is anticipated that arterial anastomosis will be delayed, insertion of a temporary bypass shunt between the proximal and distal ends of the artery to maintain distal flow is recommended to maintain tissue viability while other pressing problems are attended to. When there is associated bone trauma with comminuted displaced fracture fragments, stabilization of the fracture either by internal or external fixation may facilitate the arterial repair and prevent its disruption. Most injuries are best treated by excision of 2 to 4 mm of the injured arterial wall followed by end-to-end anastomosis, avoiding tangential repairs that often result in constriction and subsequent thrombosis. With transection of an artery, retraction of the two ends of the vessel may result in the erroneous impression that a segment of artery has been destroyed. In most instances mobilization of the two ends and application of gentle traction on the ends of the artery with vascular clamps will demonstrate that direct anastomosis can be performed, since 1 to 2 cm of a peripheral artery can be excised and the vessel ends still be approximated. In two series of civilian injuries reported by Patman et al. and by Morris et al., primary repair was possible in 85 to 90 percent of patients. Before the anastomosis is performed, the degree of back-bleeding from the distal artery should be noted and any blood clots removed with a catheter. The anastomosis should be performed with 4-0 or 6-0 arterial sutures using a continuous suture interrupted in two or three areas to avoid a purse-string effect. Individual sutures should be 1 to 1.5 mm in depth and a similar distance apart for large arteries such as the aorta or iliac arteries, but considerably closer for smaller vessels. With arteries smaller than the superficial femoral, interrupted or horizontal mattress sutures may be employed. Either a continuous over-and-over suture or an everting suture is satisfactory (Fig. 21-2).

When direct anastomosis cannot be performed because of loss of 2 cm or more of artery, an autogenous vein is the preferable graft, reversing the ends of the vein which is usually the saphenous. If for some reason a vein cannot be utilized, a graft of Goretex is preferable. If a prosthetic graft is used, the diameter rarely should be more than 6 mm.

When all the major venous structures in an extremity have also been interrupted, failure to restore some venous return results in a higher incidence of failure of arterial reconstruction than if vein continuity is established. In some instances the venous repair will undergo thrombosis and subsequent recanalization, thus restoring the effectiveness of the venous repair.

With contaminated wounds, the best protection from infection following adequate debridement and arterial reconstruction is approximation of the adjacent muscles over the arterial repair, leaving the remaining wound

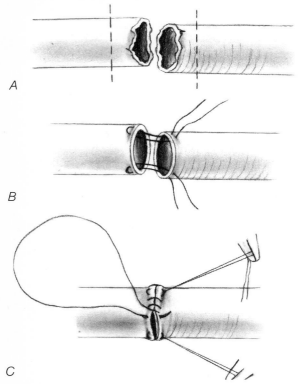

Fig. 21-2. *A.* Repair of traumatic transection of a peripheral artery. Initially the edges of the injured artery are debrided, removing 1 to 2 mm of normal arterial wall, especially if the injury is from a high-velocity missile that traumatizes adjacent segments of arterial wall. *B.* Initially the two ends of the artery are aligned with mattress sutures of 4-0 or 5-0 synthetic, monofilament material placed about 180° apart. *C.* Anastomosis is then performed with a continuous suture of the same material, usually as a simple over-and-over suture. Alternatively, an everting suture can be employed. With small vessels, simple interrupted or horizontal mattress sutures can be used to lessen the risk of constriction of the lumen.

open, to be closed by secondary sutures 4 to 7 days later. On occasion the aid of the plastic surgeon may be needed to effect the mobilization of musculocutaneous flaps or even the transfer of free flaps with their own blood supply that may have to be based upon neighboring arteries to achieve protective coverage of repaired arteries.

Ligation of an injured artery should be performed only for minor arteries such as the radial or ulnar, neither of which is essential for limb survival provided that one remains uninjured and its patency has been demonstrated by an Allen test. Back-bleeding is an inadequate guide to the safety of ligation of major arteries since it indicates only that some collateral circulation is present but does not guarantee that collateral flow will be sufficient to prevent gangrene. In the Korean conflict, good or fair back-bleeding was recorded in 9 of 20 arterial ligations performed in one group of patients, all of which resulted in gangrene. Arterial spasm alone, an unusual manifestation of injury, may be treated by the topical application of 2 to 5% papaverine or by the gentle perfusion of the artery

with dilute papaverine solution (0.5 mg/cc of saline). Another technique, reported by Mustard and Bull, is the forceful dilation of the area of spasm by the injection of saline solution into the lumen of the artery mindful of the fact that too forceful dilation may produce intimal disruption and possibly thrombosis. The importance of differentiating spasm from contusion with disruption of the wall of the artery has been mentioned previously. Unless the area of constriction can be satisfactorily corrected, it should be excised and continuity reestablished by direct anastomosis or a vascular graft.

Postoperative Care. Anticoagulant therapy is not recommended routinely after arterial repair, for it provides little protection from thrombosis but does increase the risk of bleeding into the wound. Sympathetic blocks are similarly of little value. The most important consideration following operation is to detect peripheral pulses, which indicate satisfactory restoration of arterial flow. If pulses cannot be detected or if previously palpable pulses disappear, an arteriogram should be performed or the site of anastomosis should be reexplored. The important principle to reemphasize is that with modern vascular techniques a traumatic injury of a normal artery can almost always be successfully repaired.

When a limb artery is repaired hours after injury, ischemic swelling may occur in the muscles in their fascia-enclosed compartments and progress to such an extent that ischemic necrosis results. Prompt fasciotomies over the muscle compartments, decompressing the edematous, turgid muscles, may be of great value.

When arterial repair is delayed several hours peripheral pulses may be restored, but the extremity remains paralyzed and anesthetic. The skin may be viable, but the underlying muscles may be infarcted. Such patients must be carefully observed, because extensive muscle necrosis will result in serious toxic manifestations, with high fever, myoglobinuria, hyperkalemia, and occasionally renal insufficiency. A decision to amputate such extremities as a life-saving measure, as opposed to widespread debridement of the necrotic muscles, is a difficult one to make, and each case must be evaluated carefully; in some the extremity may be salvaged following extensive debridement of necrotic muscles, with preservation of a useful, though impaired, extremity.

The development of a postoperative infection around the site of arterial repair is a grave complication, because frequently the anastomosis will disrupt and life-threatening hemorrhage occur. The infection should be treated promptly by widespread drainage and additional debridement. If infection involves the arterial reconstruction, ligation of the artery is usually required to prevent fatal hemorrhage. Occasionally bypass grafts may be inserted through channels circumventing the area of infection, anastomoses being performed between the artery proximal and distal to the point of injury. Despite massive contamination, the policy of widespread debridement, followed by secondary wound closure, almost always prevents postoperative wound infections.

PROGNOSIS. Emphasizing early repair of arterial injuries of the extremities, a number of series report minimal amputation rates (3 to 4 percent) with excellent long-term patencies in the range of 85 percent even if vein graft replacement of a segment was used. The immediate maintenance of viability is the critical goal; if ischemia develops later, secondary reconstructions are often feasible.

Popliteal Artery Entrapment Syndrome

Popliteal artery entrapment syndrome consists of intermittent claudication caused by an abnormal relation of that artery to the muscles, usually the medial head of the gastrocnemius, resulting in ischemia of the leg at an unusually early age.

HISTORICAL DATA. In 1879, a medical student named Stuart recognized an anatomic abnormality associated with a thrombosed aneurysm of the popliteal artery which led to amputation of the extremity. A number of reports, beginning with Hamming in 1959, documented approximately 60 similar cases. Inshua in 1970 was able to classify the anatomic abnormalities of the structures in the popliteal fossa which led to the development of the syndrome.

ETIOLOGY AND PATHOLOGY. Normally the popliteal artery enters the popliteal fossa through the arch of the adductor magnus muscle and passes along a longitudinal plane accompanied by the popliteal and tibial veins. The artery exits dorsal to the popliteus muscle, having passed approximately midway between the lateral and medial heads of the gastrocnemius muscle, and divides into its branches at the terminal portion of the popliteal fossa. As a consequence of developmental abnormalities, the popliteal artery may be severely compressed by portions of the medial head of the gastrocnemius muscle, at times continuously and at other times only during tensing of that muscle. As repeated trauma to the vessel ensues, typical arteriosclerotic changes appear, with irreversible stenosis and thrombosis. On occasion, poststenotic dilatation and aneurysm formation may be seen.

CLINICAL MANIFESTATION. Almost all patients experience either gradual or sudden onset of progressive intermittent claudication of the leg and sometimes of the foot; the remaining few present with acute ischemia of the leg. Ischemic gangrene has been encountered very rarely. The symptoms are usually unilateral but may be bilateral.

On physical examination there are the usual findings of popliteal arterial stenosis or occlusion with diminished or absent popliteal, dorsalis pedis, and posterior tibial pulses. On occasion all pulses appear to be normal but can be made to disappear on dorsiflexion of the foot, and a pulsatile mass may be noted in the fossa.

DIAGNOSIS. It is essential to establish the diagnosis early, since correction of the abnormality may prevent irreversible changes that might then require more complex arterial reconstructions. Any individual in the preatherosclerotic age group who presents with typical ischemic intermittent claudication or who is found to have a pulsatile popliteal mass should be suspected of having popliteal artery entrapment syndrome. The physical findings may be minimal or nil; therefore, angiographic studies are essential to making the diagnosis.

Angiography may demonstrate stenosis, occlusion, or poststenotic dilatation of that artery. Occasionally there may be no visible abnormalities on the angiographic study until the foot is passively dorsiflexed, after which stenosis of the popliteal artery may be seen.

The differential diagnosis requires exclusion of all other causes of popliteal artery occlusion, including thromboangiitis obliterans, embolic occlusion, cystic degeneration of the popliteal artery, atherosclerosis obliterans, as well as other trauma to the vessel.

TREATMENT. Surgical correction is required. The type of surgical procedure which should be performed depends entirely upon the condition of the popliteal artery. When the popliteal artery has had no permanent structural changes, various types of myotomy procedures which can be determined only at the operating table may prove to be curative. In instances in which structural changes have already occurred, in addition to the correction of the anatomic abnormalities, replacement of the artery with vein may be required to restore flow. The results in these young people, who ordinarily have normal arteries above and below the site of compression, are excellent. In most instances the reported case histories indicate that unilateral correction is sufficient, but it is essential that both limbs be studied, since bilateral corrections may be necessary.

PROGNOSIS. The prognosis for immediate restoration of flow to the extremity is excellent. The long-term prognosis will depend upon the material employed to reconstruct occluded arteries. It would appear desirable to avoid the use of plastic prostheses and employ autologous tissue for the arterial reconstructions.

Anterior Compartment Syndrome

The anterior tibial compartment syndrome is a progressive neuromuscular disability related to pressure from tissue fluid within the closed anterior tibial compartment.

ETIOLOGY. Any condition which increases the presence of fluid or compromises the outflow of fluid from this closed space may result in augmented pressure and clinical consequences. The swelling continues until the intracompartmental pressure exceeds arterial pressure. The critical structures coursing through the closed compartment and subjected to the effects of the intracompartmental pressure include the tibial artery, the anterior tibial nerve, and the anterior tibial, extensor digitorum longus, peroneus tertius, and extensor hallucis longus muscles. The unyielding walls of the compartment are composed of the tibia, the interosseous membrane, and the anterior crural fascia.

In some cases, there is a readily demonstrable arterial lesion; the syndrome has been associated with arterial trauma, arterial embolism, and acute arterial thrombosis. It has also been a complication of femoropopliteal bypass procedures and also of cardiopulmonary bypass. In a second group of patients, the syndrome is caused by severe exertion, and there is no proved anatomic lesion.

CLINICAL MANIFESTATIONS. In young patients with idiopathic anterior tibial syndrome, a history of marked exertion should be investigated. Characteristically, in most cases, the pain is the first and dominant symptom. Initially, it begins as a dull ache which soon becomes severe and is primarily located over the anterior compartment, where palpation may elicit tenderness. Motion of the leg or foot increases the severity of pain. Subsequently, erythema of the skin over the anterior compartment becomes apparent, and there is measurable increase in the size of the calf. As the syndrome progresses, these signs become more apparent. The dorsalis pedis pulse may be normal, diminished, or absent. Actually, its absence is a late sign and occasionally follows the loss of motor power of the muscles of the anterior compartment. The anterior tibial muscle and the extensor hallucis longus usually become paralyzed first, whereas the extensor digitorum longus loses its function later and is usually the first to return after release of pressure. Loss of the extensor digitorum brevis is an ominous sign. Loss of sensation is confined to the area served by the deep peroneal nerve.

The syndrome must be differentiated from a common condition known as "shin splints." The pain in the latter condition is usually over bone and can be relieved by rest, elevation, and application of cold. There is no associated marked swelling and muscle paresis with shin splints. Other conditions to be differentiated include cellulitis, thrombophlebitis, and stress fractures of the tibia.

TREATMENT. This is directed at decompressing the anterior tibial compartment and should be performed early to avoid anoxic necrosis of the muscle mass. Treatment can be effected with fasciotomy. The skin is incised lateral to the tibial crest over the midportion of the anterior tibial muscle, and the incision is carried through subcutaneous tissue and the fascia. Muscle bellies are then allowed to bulge. The skin may be closed over the bulging muscle or can be left open for secondary closure. A variation of the procedure employs two small incisions, one in the craniad and the other in the caudad portion of the anterior compartment. The fascia is then incised blindly between these two small incisions. An additional maneuver is to divide *between the tibia and fibula* the uppermost inch or two of the ligament over which the anterior tibial artery crosses to pass from the popliteal fossa to the anterior tibial compartment.

PROGNOSIS. If decompression is performed before muscle necrosis is present, return of function is complete. Thus, in many instances, fasciotomy is indicated prior to total disappearance of the pedal pulse. If fasciotomy is delayed until muscle necrosis occurs or neurologic findings are advanced, total recovery of function is not to be anticipated, and rehabilitation is required.

Traumatic Arteriovenous Fistulas

HISTORICAL DATA. That an arteriovenous fistula is a communication between an artery and a vein was first recognized by William Hunter in 1764. Previously the lesion had not been distinguished from a traumatic aneurysm. In a careful description of two patients in whom fistulas developed following phlebotomy, he described

the typical clinical findings of a thrill, continuous murmur, dilated artery proximal to the fistula, and dilated pulsating veins. The abnormal physiology of an arteriovenous fistula was carefully analyzed in a scholarly monograph published by Holman in 1937. Attempted therapy by proximal ligation of the involved artery, which was frequently effective for traumatic aneurysms, was often disastrous for arteriovenous fistulas, because gangrene resulted. The gangrene developed because blood flowing through collateral circulation around the ligated artery would flow through the fistula instead of into the distal extremity.

Matas in 1888 established effective therapy with his technique of endoaneurysmorrhaphy. Directly incising the fistulous sac, followed by suture of the communication between the artery and the vein, was more effective than indirect therapy of proximal and distal ligation of the involved artery and vein.

Although the collateral circulation which develops with an arteriovenous fistula made it possible to treat such fistulas by excision without gangrene resulting, intermittent claudication that results from interruption of the artery was frequently permanent. Consequently, after World War II, reconstruction of the injured artery became the preferable form of treatment.

ETIOLOGY AND PATHOLOGY. An arteriovenous fistula usually results from a penetrating injury that simultaneously injures an artery and an adjacent vein, permitting blood to flow directly from the injured artery into the vein. A fistula may be established immediately at the time of operation, in which case there is little external loss of blood, or it may become apparent days or weeks following injury as clot surrounding the lacerated artery and vein is liquefied.

Unusual forms of arteriovenous fistulas have been reported following different surgical operations. Injury of the iliac artery and vein is a well-recognized, fortunately rare complication of removal of an intervertebral disc. Arteriovenous fistulas have been reported following thyroidectomy, nephrectomy, or even thoracentesis, in all instances representing a concomitant injury of an artery and a vein, sometimes due to simultaneous ligation of artery and vein by the same ligature.

PATHOPHYSIOLOGY. A series of anatomic and physiologic changes begins to evolve when an arteriovenous fistula is produced (Fig. 21-3). The immediate effects are a decrease in blood flow to tissues distal to the lesion and an increase in venous pressure. The peripheral vascular resistance is lowered to that of the venous system as a result of blood bypassing the arteriolar vascular bed resulting in systolic and diastolic blood pressure, an increase in heart rate, and an increase in cardiac output.

In the ensuing days, several compensatory events occur as a result of the decrease in peripheral vascular resistance: The blood volume is increased, systolic blood pressure increases with a corresponding widening of pulse pressure, and a decrease in pulse rate occurs. Locally there is the progressive development of extensive collateral circulation around the fistula, within a few weeks the blood flow to the distal extremity may ap-

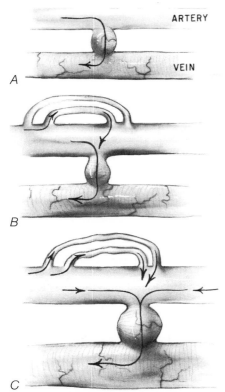

ARTERY

VEIN

A

B

C

Fig. 21-3. *A.* Immediately following the development of an arteriovenous fistula there is shunting of blood from the artery through the fistula into the vein, from which it returns to the heart. This results in a decrease in peripheral vascular resistance, a fall in diastolic blood pressure, and an increase in heart rate. The venous pressure rises in the involved vein. Peripheral blood flow is decreased in the involved artery distal to the fistula. *B.* After several weeks, collateral circulation enlarges around the fistula because of the decreased vascular resistance at the site of the fistula. As the collateral circulation develops, the involved artery and vein also dilate, increasing the amount of blood flowing through the fistula. *C.* After several years, extensive dilatation may develop about a fistula with marked enlargement of collateral circulation. In addition there is enlargement of the artery immediately distal to the fistula, through which blood flows in a retrograde fashion through the fistula toward the heart. The vein may enlarge to marked proportions, creating varicosities in the extremity. Ultimately such progressive dilatation after a period of years may result in congestive heart failure from the increased cardiac output.

proach normal limits. There is a progressive dilation of the "fistulous circuit," including the heart, the arteries leading to the fistula, the fistula itself, and the venous channels leading from the fistula to the heart.

In subsequent months or years, additional changes evolve. The artery both proximal and distal to the fistula may dilate in response to the marked increase in flow through the fistula. The involved veins progressively dilate with marked tortuosity; external rupture with hemorrhage, however, is very rare. Chronic venous congestion may develop in the extremity, causing skin ulcerations resembling those from varicose veins, and bleeding from the ulcerated areas may become a major problem. In

growing children, there may be hypertrophy of the involved limb from increased growth of the bones and soft tissues. With large fistulas, involving vessels as large as the iliac artery and vein, continued dilation of the heart eventually terminates in heart failure. This, however, is an unusual complication with the majority of arteriovenous fistulas, because the volume of blood shunted is not enough to produce heart failure. Only with large arteries and veins do cardiac symptoms appear.

Two rare complications with arteriovenous fistulas are bacterial endarteritis in the fistula and spontaneous closure. Bacterial endarteritis has been reported in only a few patients and is similar to bacterial endocarditis. Usually with intensive chemotherapy the infection can be controlled or eliminated, after which surgical excision of the fistula should be promptly carried out. A fistula may close spontaneously, occasionally after it has been present for several months. Shumacker reported eight such experiences in 245 patients.

CLINICAL MANIFESTATIONS. A penetrating injury producing an arteriovenous fistula often causes surprisingly few symptoms. External loss of blood can be small, and few disturbances of peripheral circulation develop. Subsequently the patient may be entirely asymptomatic. There is usually awareness of a soft mass in the area of the fistula, which transmits a buzzing sensation when the fingers are placed over it. The patient is rarely totally unaware of the presence of a fistula, the first manifestation of which may be acute congestive heart failure that can be expected to promptly improve with surgical correction of the fistula.

In some patients the venous hypertension produces varices with peripheral pigmentation and ulceration. Surgical mishaps have resulted from unwise attempts to remove such varices without recognizing their origin.

On physical examination, a soft, diffuse mass is usually palpable and often visible. Dilated veins may surround the area. On palpation a thrill is usually felt, maximal in systole. Auscultation reveals a continuous murmur, loudest in systole, which has been described as a "machinery" murmur, emphasizing the rhythmic rise and fall in intensity and pitch during systole and diastole. It is similar to the murmur of a patent ductus arteriosus. Detection of this classic finding establishes the diagnosis and differentiates the lesion from an arterial aneurysm.

Another significant finding is the demonstration of slowing of the pulse when the fistula is obliterated by digital compression, as evidenced by disappearance of the murmur. The slowing of the pulse results from the increase in peripheral vascular resistance when the fistula is digitally occluded causing the blood pressure to rise with reflex slowing of the heart rate. The bradycardia results from a neurogenic reflex mediated through pressure-sensitive receptors in the great vessels and carotid sinuses; it can be blocked by atropine.

Usually there are no signs of arterial insufficiency in the extremity. With large fistulas, the pulse pressure is increased, both from an elevation of systolic pressure and a decrease in diastolic pressure. If cardiac enlargement has occurred, a systolic murmur may be audible at the apex of the heart. Usually cardiac failure is found only with fistulas between large vessels, such as the aorta and the vena cava, or when the fistula has been present for many years, allowing time for progressive enlargement of the fistulous opening. In World War II cardiac failure was rarely seen in a collected series of 593 patients treated surgically.

The physical findings are usually sufficient to establish the diagnosis, but if uncertainty exists, an arteriogram readily demonstrates the rapid opacification of adjacent veins and the greatly increased collateral circulation. As the veins fill rapidly, the exact site of the fistula may be obscured unless serial angiograms are obtained. A common problem in differential diagnosis in the cervical area is with a venous "hum," an auscultatory curiosity resulting from flow of blood in the jugular veins. The murmur of a venous hum promptly disappears when intrathoracic pressure is raised by forced expiration against a closed glottis, as well as by light digital compression of the vein to stop venous flow.

TREATMENT. Formerly treatment of traumatic arteriovenous fistula was delayed for 2 to 4 months to permit the development of collateral circulation in order for the extremity to survive following ligation of the involved artery. Although gangrene virtually never occurred following ligation, claudication frequently resulted, often in as many as 50 percent of patients, despite the abundant collateral circulation. Currently, the majority of patients are treated by division of the fistula and reconstruction of the involved artery, and preferably the injured vein as well. Excision is performed only for fistulas involving small vessels not essential to normal circulation of the extremity, such as the radial or ulnar arteries. Most fistulas are treated at the time of the arterial injury if the proper diagnosis is made. Otherwise operation is performed within 2 or 3 weeks, after the immediate effects of the injury on the soft tissues have subsided and the likelihood of infection occurring from the original injury has decreased significantly. Arteriovenous fistulas have been occluded by glues and coils inserted under radiographic control.

Operative Technique. The incision should be placed so as to permit exposure of the artery and vein proximal and distal to the fistula before the fistula is dissected. Once these vessels are isolated and temporarily occluded, the fistulous sac can be incised and the opening directly isolated. Although a large aneurysmal sac may be present, the basic lesion is usually an incomplete laceration of the arterial wall, involving only a short length of artery. A long segment of artery may be incorporated in the wall of the aneurysmal sac, however, and it must be freed and mobilized to perform arterial repair. Once the involved vessels have been mobilized, most of the remaining sac may be left, for complete excision is difficult and of little benefit.

In many patients the artery can be repaired by direct anastomosis. In a group of 29 aneurysms and arteriovenous fistulas resulting from civilian injuries, all were treated by end-to-end arterial anastomosis. In a series of 134 patients with fistulas, an anastomosis was performed in 61, a vessel graft in 23, a lateral repair in 4, and simple division of the fistula in 10.

Repair of the involved vein is indicated if the vein is a large one, such as an iliac or common femoral vein. Permanent edema has been frequent following ligation of such large veins. Repair can often be done by lateral suture.

PROGNOSIS. Convalescence following operation is usually uneventful, and long-term results are excellent if arterial continuity is preserved. Hughes and Jahnke published a 5-year follow-up of 148 such lesions treated during the Korean conflict with satisfactory results in the majority of patients.

THORACIC OUTLET SYNDROMES

A variety of physical abnormalities have been recognized which constrict or compress the brachial plexus, the subclavian artery, or the subclavian vein near the first rib and clavicle. Several descriptive terms have been employed, indicating the causative mechanism thought to be present. These include cervical rib, scalenus anticus syndrome, costoclavicular syndrome, and hyperabduction syndrome. The disability is dependent upon which of the major neural or vascular structures is compressed. Regardless of the specific mechanism involved, all such abnormalities may be conveniently grouped together as neurovascular compression syndromes occurring near the thoracic outlet.

HISTORICAL DATA. Cervical ribs have been reported as anatomic curiosities for hundreds of years. They occur in about 0.5 percent of the normal population. Murphy in 1905 described a successful operation upon a patient whose subclavian artery was compressed by a cervical rib. By 1916 Halsted was able to find reports of more than 500 cases of symptoms from a cervical rib. Attention was focused on the scalenus anticus muscle in 1927 when Adson and Coffey observed constriction of the subclavian artery by a scalenus anticus muscle and subsequently proposed that compression by an abnormal scalenus anticus muscle created a syndrome identical to that caused by cervical rib. They also emphasized the role of the scalenus anticus muscle in producing symptoms from a cervical rib, the two structures jointly compressing the brachial plexus between them.

Subsequently the frequency of compression between the clavicle and first rib was recognized and the mechanisms well defined in 1943 by the report of Falconer and Weddell, who named this type of compression the *costoclavicular syndrome*. A short time later, in 1945, Wright observed patients in whom vascular symptoms resulted from hyperabduction and introduced the term *hyperabduction syndrome*.

Some degree of compression of the subclavian artery may be demonstrated in a high percentage of normal individuals in whom no symptoms whatever are present, but it formerly was thought that compression syndromes producing significant disability were rare. Since the publication by Roos of a simplified transaxillary approach to relieve compression syndromes at the thoracic outlet and since the introduction of peripheral nerve conduction velocity determinations, the conditions have been recognized with increasing frequency. It has even been suggested that for certain patients who have thoracic outlet syndromes a diagnosis of angina pectoris is erroneously made. Further experience will be needed to determine the exact frequency of these disorders. The aforementioned transaxillary approach to resection of the first rib may help define the frequency of the condition more exactly since this approach permits a clear view of the structures, both normal and abnormal, that produce compression syndromes.

REGIONAL ANATOMY. The subclavian artery leaves the thorax by passing over the first rib between the scalenus anticus muscle anteriorly and the brachial plexus and scalenus medius posteriorly. It then passes under the clavicle and subclavius muscle to enter the axilla beneath the pectoralis minor muscle. The subclavian vein has an almost identical course except that it passes anterior to the scalenus anticus muscle and has an intimate relationship to the head of the clavicle and the most medial portion of the first rib. The route of the brachial plexus nearly parallels that of the subclavian artery in the neck, lying posterolaterally between it and the scalenus posterior muscle.

A potential area of compression exists in the interscalene triangle between the scalenus anticus anteriorly, the scalenus medius posteriorly, and the first rib inferiorly. Only slightly distal to this area, in the narrow space between the clavicle and the first rib, is another potential site of compression. In the axilla, where the pectoralis minor tendon attaches to the coracoid process, an area of potential obstruction of the axillary artery exists where it travels around the coracoid process. During hyperabduction the axillary vessels and brachial plexus are bent at an angle of approximately 90° in this area.

When a cervical rib persists, there may be in addition either a bony or a ligamentous structure, originating on the lowermost cervical vertebra, coursing in, passing under the brachial plexus and subclavian artery, and attaching to the first rib.

ETIOLOGY. Although cervical ribs are found in about 0.5 percent of the normal population, only about 10 percent of these produce symptoms. Asymptomatic anomalies of the first rib are also frequently seen. Thus, additional factors other than the presence of a cervical rib or anomalous first rib must contribute to the compression syndromes. Symptoms are very rare in children and most frequently are seen in thin women in the third and fourth decades. An unusually well-developed musculature seems also to predispose to compression. A congenital variation in the anatomy of the head and neck has been suggested as a predisposing factor, a familiar type of patient being a thin woman with a long, narrow neck. The onset of symptoms in the second and third decade could be due to gradual descent of the shoulder girdle, perhaps from atrophy of the regional musculature.

Local anatomic variations are probably of particular significance. The width of the first rib in individuals in whom we have resected this structure has appeared to be unusually great. The width of the scalene anticus muscle at its insertion into the first rib varies greatly. A wide scalenus anticus muscle, which narrows the space in the interscalene triangle, has often been found at operation in symptomatic patients. Interdigitations of scalene muscles forming slings under the brachial plexus and axillary arteries have been encountered. Cervical ribs vary from short and rudimentary to completely formed and articulating anteriorly with the first rib. Some incomplete ribs are connected by fascial bands to the first rib that compress the brachial plexus. Fractures of the clavicle or first rib may subsequently produce a large bony callus, especially if there is poor alignment of the ends of the fractured bone.

CLINICAL MANIFESTATIONS. Disability from compression may be produced in several ways and depends upon which portions of the neurovascular bundle are involved. Compression of the brachial plexus usually causes pain, paresthesia, and a feeling of numbness. Often these symptoms are greatest in the C_8–T_1 distribution, because the ulnar nerve is derived from this most caudad portion of the plexus which rides over the first rib. Compression of the upper portion of the plexus may also occur, resulting in pain referred to the entire arm and shoulder and occasionally to the neck and cheek. Muscular weakness or paralysis, or atrophy of muscles are less frequent and appear only in far advanced cases. Vascular symptoms may be intermittent from compression or temporary occlusion of the subclavian artery, producing claudication with exercise, pallor, or a sensation of coldness, numbness, or paresthesia. In chronic cases, a different and more serious mechanism evolves, for intermittent compression and trauma of the subclavian arteries produce atheromatous changes in the artery and, rarely, a poststenotic aneurysm. From either arterial abnormality, emboli may be dislodged into the peripheral circulation and produce ischemia in the hand, sometimes with focal areas of gangrene requiring amputation of digits. Thrombosis of the subclavian artery may eventually result.

A third group of vascular symptoms consists of intermittent episodes of vasoconstriction, similar to those seen in Raynaud's disease. Unilateral Raynaud's phenomenon, though rare, almost always suggests a focal disturbance in the blood supply to the involved extremity due to a local lesion such as a cervical rib. A possible explanation for this infrequent occurrence has been proposed by Telford and Mottershead, who, on anatomic dissection, found that in 10 to 15 percent of patients the sympathetic innervation of the extremity traveled in a separate cord not incorporated in the main trunks of the brachial plexus. This isolated filament of fibers presumably would be more prone to direct compression and irritation. Finally, intermittent compression of the subclavian vein may cause signs of venous hypertension in the upper extremity with edema and the development of varicosities. The so-called effort thrombosis, a condition of acute thrombosis of the subclavian vein, may be a result of a thoracic outlet compression syndrome of the axillary vein with intimal damage.

The symptomatology of the thoracic outlet syndrome depends on whether nerves, blood vessels, or both are compressed. Usually compression of one of these dominates the clinical picture. Symptoms of nerve compression manifested by pain and paresthesia are present in almost all patients, the pain usually being of insidious

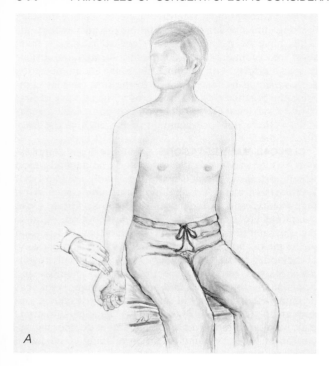

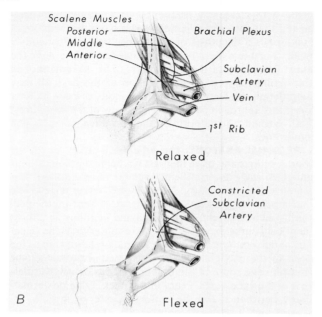

Fig. 21-4. Technique of performance of the Adson maneuver for obstruction of the subclavian artery by the scalenus anticus muscle. *A.* The patient should be seated with his elbows at his sides and his neck extended. During deep inspiration his chin is turned to the affected side, while the intensity of the radial pulse is palpated. All these positions increase the tension on the scalenus anticus muscle. *B.* Course of the brachial plexus and subclavian artery between the scalenus anticus and medius muscles. A localized dilatation of the subclavian artery distal to the scalenus anticus is illustrated. Immediately distal to the scalenus anticus and medius muscles is another potential area of constriction, between the clavicle and the first rib. When the scalenus anticus muscle is relaxed, there is minimal compression of the subclavian artery. With tension on the scalenus anticus muscle, compression of the subclavian artery results in decrease in the radial pulse, in some patients resulting in disappearance of the pulse. A bruit may become audible in the supraclavicular area as the scalenus anticus muscle is progressively stretched to compress the subclavian artery.

onset, commonly involving the neck, shoulder, arm, and hand with occasional radiation to the anterior chest or parascapular area. Paresthesia in a specific nerve distribution occur in most patients, the ulnar nerve being involved in 90 percent.

Symptoms of arterial compression were observed less frequently, in about one-quarter of patients. Raynaud's phenomenon and symptoms of venous compression are even less common.

Physical Examination. Objective physical signs are more common in patients with vascular compression than in those with neural disorders. In only about 20 percent of patients with nerve compression are objective signs of decreased sensation found; some of these show additional muscle weakness or even atrophy. In the presence of neurologic symptoms at least one of the vascular compression signs can be expected, consisting essentially of loss of radial pulse with either Adson's test, hyperabduction, or hyperextension. In Adson's test, the patient sits with his hands on his knees, inspires deeply, extends his head backward, and turns his chin toward the affected side. Deep inspiration, extension of the neck, and turning of the head all tense the scalene anticus muscle and may decrease or obliterate the radial pulse (Fig. 21-4). Simultaneous auscultation of the supraclavicular space for bruit should be performed. In certain patients, a bruit will appear as the head is turned, reach a peak intensity, and cease as compression is increased to the point of obliterating the radial pulse. In other patients turning the head to the opposite side may demonstrate compression more effectively. The possibility of compression of the neurovascular bundle between the first rib and the clavicle also may be tested by displacing the shoulders backward and

downward. The test is considered positive if the radial pulse is obliterated. The hyperabduction maneuver is performed by fully abducting the arm above the head and noting the effect upon the radial pulse.

In evaluating the maneuvers to detect neurovascular compression, it is important to remember that they are positive in a high percentage of normal individuals. This is particularly true of the costoclavicular compression or the hyperabduction test. A positive result, therefore, does not in itself establish a thoracic outlet syndrome; absence of any positive findings, however, suggests some other diagnosis.

The signs of arterial compression may be evident by direct physical examination. There may be differences in the qualities of the pulses between the two arms when the subclavian, brachial, radial, and ulnar arteries are compared. A localized supraclavicular bruit may be present. On occasion a particularly wide pulse, denoting a subclavian or axillary aneurysm, is palpable, usually in the infraclavicular area. With mild forms of ischemia there may be only pallor on elevation while in the more severe forms, especially with embolization, there may be atrophy of the skin, brittle nails, or even focal ulceration. In approximately 5 percent of patients frank Raynaud's phenomenon can be induced by application of cold to the extremity. In the approximately 10 percent of patients, signs of venous obstruction, i.e., edema and venous distention, are apparent.

LABORATORY STUDIES. Chest and cervical spine radiographs may demonstrate bony abnormalities, either as cervical ribs, bifid first ribs, fusion of the first and second ribs, or clavicular deformities either congenital or traumatic.

For diagnosing arterial abnormalities, arteriography may be especially useful in demonstrating intimal irregularities, stenoses, or aneurysms of the subclavian artery. The arteriographic studies are of no value where there is no evidence of arterial compression or occlusion. Venographic studies are useful in patients with signs of venous compression, especially in establishing a differential diagnosis between thoracic outlet compression and other entities which mimic the condition.

The determination of nerve conduction velocities through the thoracic outlet as well as electromyographic determinations have been used to attempt to establish objective criteria for diagnosing neural compression. By applying electrical stimulation to various of the distal components of the brachial plexus and measuring conduction velocities to pinpoint areas of abnormal conduction, it is possible to evaluate sites of involvement of various neural structures. Where atypical thoracic outlet neural compression syndromes are present, other nerves such as the median and the musculocutaneous can be similarly studied. Differential diagnoses between compression at the thoracic outlet, at the carpal tunnel at the wrist, and at the pronator level are possible. When this is combined with carefully performed electromyographic studies, very specific diagnoses are possible.

TREATMENT. The treatment can be divided into that for the arterial, venous, and neurologic compressions. Treatment of the arterial compression depends upon the specific entity produced: embolization, stenosis and thrombosis, aneurysm formation, or intermittent vasospasm (Raynaud's). Occlusion of the subclavian artery, if not associated with severe ischemia, may require no therapy except an exercise program to promote development of collateral circulation. With atherosclerotic plaques or aneurysms of the subclavian artery, frequently associated with embolic episodes, therapy usually involves resection of the first rib, preferably by the transaxillary approach, as well as removing the source of emboli. The presence of a thrombus in an aneurysm or ulceration in an atherosclerotic plaque requires resection of the involved artery through an additional supraclavicular incision that may require resection of the medial half of the clavicle if an aneurysm associated with a cervical rib is present, and replacement, preferably with autologous tissue; composite grafts of saphenous veins have been useful. On occasion direct exposure of the arteries in the arm or forearm is necessary to remove emboli.

The venous occlusions are more difficult to treat, because the compressing mechanism may not be apparent from either physical examination or laboratory studies. It appears clear from results of transaxillary resection of the first rib that the most proximal part of the vein can be decompressed by this procedure, but the roles of the clavicle, the pectoralis minor, and clavipectoral fascia in producing compression cannot be evaluated by this approach. Resection of the medial half of the clavicle may be required for complete decompression of the vein. Those patients with effort thrombosis seen within the first day or two of its occurrence should be considered for combined surgical procedures of venous thrombectomy and relief of the compressing mechanism. Anticoagulation therapy should then be used, perhaps for as long as 1 year.

The management of the neural compression syndromes generally involves a conservative, nonsurgical approach. An exercise program designed to strengthen the muscles of the shoulder girdle and lessen the tendency of the shoulder to droop has been of value in some patients with mild to moderate symptoms. A series of such exercises is carefully described by Allen et al. As an example of this approach, less than half of a group of 300 patients with thoracic outlet syndromes required surgical intervention. The selection of patients for operation should depend upon the severity of the symptoms, failure to respond to a nonsurgical program, and the specificity of the diagnosis.

Operative Technique. It is important to include the entire extremity in the sterile operative field, permitting manipulation of the extremity in order to define the most likely area of compression. Whether or not a cervical rib is present, the transaxillary approach is favored for the decompression for its simplicity, the clarity with which the compression mechanisms can be diagnosed, the excellent cosmetic result, and the ease with which cervical ribs together with the first rib can be excised. If vasomotor symptoms are prominent, sympathectomy can be performed through the same transaxillary approach, exposing the third and second thoracic ganglia as well as the lower third of the stellate ganglion; this includes the first thoracic ganglion but avoids the production of Horner's syndrome. If removal of the second and third intercostal nerves with their ganglia is thought necessary, since 10 to 15 percent of the sympathetic ganglia to the upper extremity are contained in these nerves, it can be carried out.

The transaxillary approach is performed by making an incision in the lowermost portion of the axilla from the pectoralis major anteriorly to the latissimus dorsi posteriorly (Fig. 21-5). The incision is deepened to the muscles of the chest wall, the serratus anterior and the intercostal muscles coming into view. The dissection is continued upward, avoiding the intercostobrachial nerve, with the arm hyperabducted to raise the neurovascular bundle off the first rib. By gentle dissection, it is possible to outline the scalene muscles and identify the attachment of the cervical rib to the first rib if one is present. The scalene muscles are transected and permitted to retract, and the muscles along the inferior border of the first rib are simi-

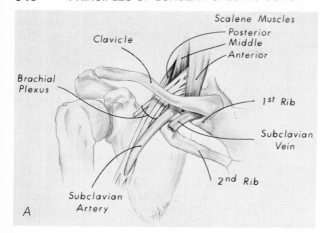

A

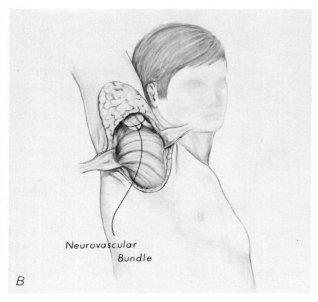

B

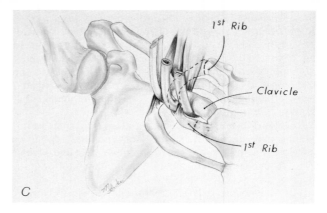

C

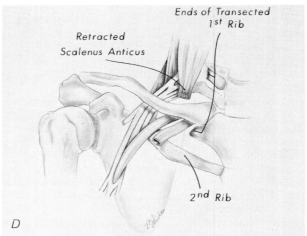

D

Fig. 21-5. Technique of transaxillary resection of the first rib. *A.* The critical relations of the first rib, clavicle, scalene muscles, and neurovascular structures are shown. The lowermost portion of the brachial plexus, which gives rise to the ulnar nerve, is in contact with the first rib and explains the most characteristic neurologic symptoms usually involving the ulnar aspect of the forearm and fourth and fifth fingers. *B.* Operative incision below the axillary hairline with hyperabduction of the arm which raises the neurovascular bundle out of the operative field. *C.* Effect of hyperabduction in exposing the first rib and scalene muscles, retracting the neurovascular bundle. *D.* Effect of first rib resection, which requires cutting all three scalene muscles, in relieving the compression of artery, vein, and brachial plexus.

larly incised. The first rib and cervical rib usually can be removed in their entirety, including periosteum, from the costochondral junction anteriorly to the posterior angle of the rib. The parietal pleura lies deep to the dissection; care must be taken to avoid puncturing it. If the pleura is punctured, the wound is closed around a catheter in the axilla while the anesthetist expands the lung. This usually suffices to correct the pneumothorax. On occasion it has been necessary to aspirate air from the pleural cavity in the early postoperative period. If resection of the second or third portions of the axillary artery is required due to the presence of an aneurysm associated with a cervical rib or due to marked arterial degeneration posterior to the anterior scalene muscle, a second incision is required, usually in the supraclavicular area, sometimes in association with a resection of the medial half of the clavicle.

If a sympathectomy is indicated, the parietal pleura is stripped from the chest wall attachments and the sympathetic chain exposed, dissected free, and excised.

The postoperative course is usually benign, with the patient ready for discharge by the third postoperative day.

Other approaches have been described for excising the first rib. The posterior approach has been advocated by many but is an operation of greater magnitude. The anterior transthoracic approach has been proposed by others for more extensive exposure. Although most agree that the supraclavicular approach is probably archaic, since it does not permit thorough exploration of the area and easy excision of the first rib (now of paramount importance in treatment), it has been proposed as the first approach to perform scalenectomy, reserving the transaxillary approach for failures of the more simple procedures.

The surgical approach for venous compression is more complex than simply performing transaxillary decompression. With the transaxillary approach it is possible to sever constricting bands which appear to be extensions of the manubrial insertion of the sternocleidomastoid muscles. The head of the clavicle may participate prominently in the compression, so that on occasion it has been necessary to resect the medial half of the clavicle. Upon completion of the external decompression of the vein, an operative venogram is recommended both to confirm the adequacy of the decompression and to detect intrinsic abnormalities of vein, such as webs which may occur at the junction of the subclavian vein with the internal jugular. This latter abnormality may require venotomy and excision of the web with subsequent closure of the subclavian vein.

PROGNOSIS. The prognosis is dependent upon the specific syndrome present. The arterial compression syndromes can be quite satisfactorily relieved and arterial reconstructions performed with a high degree of precision. In our experience it has been possible to stop embolic episodes and restore circulation to the upper extremity by standard arterial reconstructive procedures. Patients with Raynaud's phenomenon and cervical rib in whom associated sympathectomies have been performed have variable results. Although immediate effects of sympathectomy have been excellent, relapses have occurred quite abruptly as early as 6 months following operation.

The venous compression disorders also have given variable results. It is not clear at present whether thrombectomy, with or without relief of the venous compression mechanism, is any better than prolonged anticoagulant therapy. Those patients with chronic venous occlusions of the subclavian and axillary veins who have been followed for years have shown remarkable recovery, with subsidence of edema coincident with the appearance of a prominent venous pattern on the chest wall and little or no resulting disability.

The results of operations performed for neurologic syndromes have been most difficult to evaluate. While some patients have experienced dramatic improvement, others have had no benefit. Still others have had relapses after initial improvement. Roos has reported from a wide experience with transaxillary resection of the first rib that 80 to 90 percent of those with predominantly neurologic symptoms obtained complete relief, while approximately 50 percent of those with predominantly vascular symptoms became free of symptoms.

MANIFESTATIONS OF ARTERIAL OCCLUSIVE DISEASE

Acute Arterial Occlusion

Recognition of acute arterial occlusion is vital, since it may progress to ischemic necrosis within hours. A thrombus propagates distally as well as proximally to the point where it lodges, occluding collateral channels, thereby worsening the ischemia.

Acute occlusion usually appears without specific symptoms. Prompt diagnosis is essential for successful therapy, because within 4 to 8 h after acute occlusion ischemic necrosis in the involved muscles may become irreversible. An additional feature in the pathogenesis of acute arterial occlusion that emphasizes the time factor is the tendency for thrombi to develop in the arteries distal to the point of occlusion where the flow of blood is either decreased or stagnant. This development, superimposed upon the acute obstruction, makes surgical therapy to restore circulation much more difficult. With persisting ischemia, thrombosis finally develops in the venous system as well, making surgical therapy impossible.

The usual causes of acute arterial occlusion are embolism, trauma, or thrombosis. Thrombosis of a previously undiagnosed aneurysm, such as a popliteal aneurysm, is a less frequent cause. Each of these is discussed in subsequent sections. Embolism is noteworthy in that it often appears without any previous signs of underlying disease as an acute catastrophe involving an extremity. In many it is the first symptom of serious underlying heart disease: mitral stenosis, atrial fibrillation, or myocardial infarction. Arterial trauma, when occurring as an isolated injury, may be easily recognized. When complicated with associated fractures or head injuries, the diagnosis may be difficult.

FIVE P's. For emphasis the five prominent features of acute arterial occlusion may be summarized as five p's as discussed above, under Arterial Trauma: *p*ain, *p*aralysis, *p*aresthesia, *p*allor, and absence of *p*ulses.

Pain present in 75 to 80 percent of patients with acute arterial occlusion heralds the onset of ischemia. It is absent in some patients, apparently because of the prompt onset of complete anesthesia. In others, when collateral circulation minimizes the degree of ischemia produced, pain may be minimal.

Paralysis and paresthesia (or anesthesia) are most important in evaluating the severity of ischemia. The importance of these features is based on the fact that the peripheral nerve endings are the most sensitive tissues to anoxia in the extremity. A familiar illustration of the sensitivity of sensory nerve endings to anoxia is the common experience of one's foot "going to sleep" while one sits with the extremity flexed in an unusual position. The sensitivity of striated muscles to anoxia is almost as great as that of nerve endings. Hence, an extremity with paralysis and paresthesia will almost surely develop gangrene, while, conversely, if motor and sensory function are intact even though signs of ischemia are present, gangrene probably will not occur. The neurologic findings then are an important clue both to the need for prompt therapy and for the evaluation of the effectiveness of therapy in relieving ischemia. Recognition that a paralyzed anesthetic extremity will develop gangrene in most patients within 6 to 8 h after onset emphasizes the urgency for immediate treatment.

Pallor is also an important sign, representing varying degrees of decreased circulation. Associated with visible pallor may be the sensation of coldness.

Absence of pulses confirms the diagnosis and localizes

the point of occlusion. With uncertainty, as in an edematous extremity, an oscillometer or a Doppler device may be of some value in confirming the absence of pulses. When palpation is indeterminate, the presence of neurologic symptoms indicates the urgency for deciding whether arterial occlusion is present. A frequent example seen is a patient with a swollen extremity with a fracture of the femur in whom swelling of the extremity may make palpation of the pulses difficult. To determine whether an associated injury of the femoral artery is present may require arteriography. If neurologic symptoms are present, angiography should be performed on an emergency basis.

Chronic Arterial Occlusion

The picture of chronic progressive ischemia is typically and most often seen with atherosclerosis involving the abdominal aorta and its branches to the lower extremities, including the iliac, femoral, and popliteal arteries. The course may be gradual and progressive or it may be accelerated with acute episodes due to segmental arterial thrombosis or minor traumatic injuries to the toes resulting in gangrene. Diabetic patients in general tend to have more distal arterial involvement of the popliteal and tibial arteries. Their clinical syndromes are further modified by the not infrequent presence of diabetic neuropathy and by their characteristic susceptibility to necrotizing infections.

Atherosclerotic disease of the arteries to the lower extremities may be divided into three large groups, dependent upon the level of involvement. These are aortoiliac, femoropopliteal, and tibioperoneal. There are distinctive clinical features about each of the categories, although more than one area is involved in at least one-third of patients seen. Aortoiliac disease in the fourth, fifth, and sixth decades is characterized by relatively mild atherosclerosis with aortic occlusion from superimposed thrombosis, while in the seventh and eighth decades atherosclerosis is severe and thrombosis is relatively limited. Isolated femoropopliteal disease is especially frequent in cigarette smokers, while isolated tibioperoneal disease occurs predominantly in diabetics. No matter where the obstruction is located, the physiologic deficit is decreased blood flow to the lower extremities, with symptoms ranging from intermittent claudication to gangrene. Tissue necrosis is more prone to occur with more distal arterial disease because potential for the development of collateral circulation is less.

HISTORY. A detailed history and physical examination are often sufficient to establish the diagnosis of extremity ischemia and to suggest the underlying mechanisms leading to its occurrence. Pain is the key symptom resulting from the ischemia of arterial occlusion. Careful documentation of its mode of onset, its location and distribution, and its character and duration serves as the basis for all additional investigations. When arterial occlusion develops over longer periods of time, ischemia may be subtle and may not become manifest until there are demands for blood beyond basal requirements, such as with exercise.

Pain is experienced during exertion and gradually disappears within minutes upon cessation of activity. This represents the characteristic symptom of *intermittent claudication,* the most common complaint produced by limb ischemia. The areas that are felt to be painful are usually those requiring the largest amount of blood during exertion, e.g., muscle groups. Claudication is a highly specific symptom, virtually diagnostic of chronic arterial insufficiency. For varying periods of time the only measure of progression of arterial insufficiency may be the worsening of claudication with progressively smaller amounts of exercise being required to produce the symptom.

Chronic arterial occlusion may progress, and intermittent pain involving muscle groups may be supplanted by continuous *pain at rest* referred to the sites most distal to the arterial occlusion, viz., toes, feet, fingers, hands. The large muscle groups that are the first to express the ischemic state are almost never the site of rest pain in chronic arterial occlusions. Ischemic rest pain is distinguishable by history from other types of foot or hand pain because pain is worsened by elevation of the extremity, even if only to the supine position, and is relieved by placing the extremity in the dependent position. Patients with pain related to diabetic neuropathy or other painful foot conditions report no such positional dependence.

In the upper extremity, although atherosclerosis that progresses to rest pain and gangrene is unusual, other types of lesions, either embolic or vasospastic, may do so. Claudication of the arm with exercise may be moderately disabling, but more serious symptoms are uncommon. Rest pain and tissue necrosis when present usually denote digital vessel occlusion either due to embolization from proximal lesions or end-stage Raynaud's phenomenon.

Other aspects of history that are critically important in determining treatment and prognosis include smoking, diabetes, cardiac disorders, trauma, familial disease, and occupational history, as well as drug therapy.

PHYSICAL EXAMINATION. Physical examination is of paramount importance in assessing the presence and severity of vascular disease. The color, temperature, and pulse pattern of the extremities involved frequently permits estimation of the level of arterial occlusion, the severity of ischemia, and the abruptness of the onset. Acute arterial occlusion characteristically produces marked color and temperature differences; chronic occlusion may produce no visible changes but only a difference in palpable pulses early in the course of disease. When acute occlusion progresses to gangrene it is manifest frequently as ''wet'' gangrene, with blebs, bullae, and violaceous discoloration. When chronic occlusion progresses gradually to severe ischemia, characteristic changes associated with atrophy appear and progress to localized tissue necrosis. The final stage is usually the mumification characteristic of dry gangrene, which starts peripherally in the toes and extends proximally to involve the entire foot and leg. Palpation of peripheral pulses is a most important feature of the examination. In the lower extremity, the femoral, popliteal, posterior tibial, and dorsalis pedis pulses should be noted. It is important to remember that the common femoral artery extends only about 5 cm below the inguinal ligament before bifurcating into the profunda femoris and superficial femoral arteries. In the upper extremity the brachial, radial, and ulnar pulses should be noted. In many patients it is possible to feel the digital pulses at the bases of the phalanges. The integrity of the palmar arterial arches can be tested by the performance of the Allen test. This is done by having the patient make a tight fist, then occluding the radial and ulnar arteries at the wrist and having the patient slowly open the hand. With the hand in a relaxed position, the integrity of the radial artery in the hand is determined by releasing radial compression and noting the return of color. The maneuver is repeated releasing the ulnar artery while the radial remains compressed. The ability to determine definitely the presence or absence of a peripheral pulse is one of the most essential features of an adequate evaluation of the peripheral circulation.

With chronic ischemia, characteristic nutritional changes develop in the feet. These include the loss of hair from the toes, the development of brittle, opaque nails, the appearance of atrophy and rubor in the skin, and atrophy of muscles of the feet with increasing prominence of the interosseous spaces. Hence, a simple glance at a foot can determine the presence or absence of serious vascular disease. The importance of this evaluation is emphasized by the fact that gangrene seldom appears in an extremity with chronic vascular disease until these stigmata of chronic ischemia have appeared.

Characteristic color changes also appear with advanced arterial insufficiency, consisting of a purplish rubor in dependency, changing to pallor when the extremity is elevated. The colors are quite different from the chronic congested extremity with venous insufficiency.

The location of ulcerations offers a major clue to cause, for ulceration from venous insufficiency is virtually unknown below the level of the malleolus. By contrast, most ulcers from arterial insufficiency begin over the toes, corresponding to the most distal parts of the arterial tree. Ischemic ulcers on occasion develop on the leg or about the ankle without involvement of the toes, perhaps as a result of local tissue infarction, especially after localized trauma, or from arterioarterial embolization.

Palpation of the extremity for temperature and moisture may provide useful information, especially with vasospastic conditions with increased sympathetic tone, where the cool, sweaty extremity affords an important clue to the diagnosis.

Auscultation is of value for certain disorders, particularly arteriovenous fistulas, where detection of the classic continuous murmur quickly establishes the diagnosis. With localized stenotic lesions in peripheral arteries, usually from atherosclerotic plaques, a systolic bruit may be heard, promptly confirming the presence of arterial stenosis.

Estimation of venous filling time is of some value in the diagnosis of arterial insufficiency, but the test is of no value where incompetent valves are present in the venous system. In the absence of varicosities, the test is performed by elevation of the extremities until collapse of the veins has occurred. The extremities are then quickly lowered, and the time required for the veins to fill, usually on the dorsum of the foot or hand, is noted. Normally venous filling will occur within 10 to 15 s. Prolonged filling frequently denotes arterial insufficiency. Venous filling times of longer than 1 min denote a very high degree of arterial compromise.

The general physical examination is important to determine whether there are any underlying or associated disorders and whether there are additional areas of arterial involvement detectable by finding absent pulses elsewhere or bruits over arteries such as the carotids. It is vital to know about the presence of aneurysms in the abdomen, groin, or thorax. Examination of the heart is essential to determine whether there are valvular lesions, rhythm disorders, or congenital lesions that might serve as the nidus for thromboemboli.

General Laboratory Examinations

In arterial occlusive disease the diagnosis is almost always made by the history and the physical examination. Noninvasive studies using ultrasound, plethysmography, x-ray and magnetic resonance have been useful in confirming the diagnosis and differentiating arterial disease from other clinical syndromes. Angiography continues to be the most important laboratory technique. A high quality study is essential to planning surgical therapy.

Doppler Ultrasound. Doppler ultrasound is based on the shift in ultrasound frequency (called the "Doppler effect") that arises if an ultrasound beam is transmitted to and reflected from moving blood cells. The frequency shift is proportional to the velocity of the blood flow. It may be analyzed audibly by listening to the intensity, pitch, and phasicity of the sound or may be recorded graphically either as a simple wave form or as a complete sound spectrum analysis. A common application of Doppler ultrasound is to determine systolic arterial pressure. The probe is used as a sensitive stethoscope over an artery distal to a pressure cuff. Inflation of the cuff to a suprasystolic level will result in cessation of blood flow and hence, disappearance of the Doppler signal. Pressures obtained by this method are generally compared to the pressure in the arm or unaffected extremity and reported as a ratio of the normal systolic pressure. (If arm pressure is equal to 120 mmHg and dorsalis pedis pressure is equal to 40 mmHg, the ankle/arm index is 0.33.) In patients without arterial disease, the ankle/arm pressure ratio is 1 or higher. In claudication, it is generally between 1 and 0.5 and with more advanced degrees of ischemia is generally less than 0.5. Diabetics may have high indices due to calcification of the arterial wall. When doubt exists about the diagnosis, stress testing is helpful. This may be accomplished by treadmill exercise or by the reactive hyperemia test with a thigh tourniquet. The drop in pressure and the recovery time are proportional to the extent of the arterial occlusive disease. Segmental pressures are obtained by application of cuffs at different levels of the leg. The pressure gradients between the levels provide information about location of the disease.

B-Scan Ultrasound. B-Scan ultrasound can be used for visualization of blood vessels, either as a static or as a real-time echo. The main application is for visualization of aortic aneurysms. The value in the diagnosis of occlusive disease is limited when the vessel wall is extensively calcified. A highly valuable application is in combination with Doppler ultrasound, where the B-Scan is used as a guide for precise placement of the Doppler sample.

Plethysmography. Plethysmography records changes in volume of a limb, digit, or eye to each myocardial contraction. It has applications in peripheral arterial, cerebrovascular, and venous disease. Instrumentation includes strain gauge, photo, impedance, ocular, and air plethysmography. The latter comprises pulse volume recording (PVR) and phleorheography (PRG). Plethysmography can be used for analysis of the pulse waveform and for determination of arterial pressures as well as arterial and venous blood flow.

Arteriography. The most important laboratory examination is selective arteriography to outline the location and extent of arterial obstruction. Selection of the appropriate method of examination varies with the disease present, for virtually every artery in the body can now be successfully outlined by appropriate catheter angiography. Percutaneous introduction of the arterial catheter is the most frequently employed technique. Newer digital subtraction techniques have had some application in special situations. Utilizing a series of radiographic images recorded on a magnetic tape, nonvascular shadows can be subtracted from the image containing the contrast medium. This technique enhances the outline of the artery. Reasonably good views of the arteries can be obtained with less dye and smaller catheters, although resolution may be inferior to conventional arteriography. Also, overlapping images of multiple arteries may interfere with accurate interpretation.

ARTERIAL EMBOLISM

It has been long recognized that the majority of arterial emboli originate in the heart. The embolus originated in the heart in 86 percent of 426 emboli reported by Darling and associates and in 91 percent of 214 emboli reported by Cranley et al. In the past few years there has been increasing recognition of emboli which originate in atherosclerotic arteries, either fragments of a plaque or thrombi adherent to the surface of an ulcerated plaque which subsequently dislodge. For simplicity in presentation, emboli arising from the heart, constituting the majority of emboli seen, are referred to as *cardioarterial embolization*. As a separate entity, the frequency of which is yet unknown, emboli arising from an atherosclerotic artery and lodging in the distal branches are referred to as *arterioarterial emboli*.

Cardioarterial Embolization

HISTORICAL CONSIDERATIONS. Emboli have been long recognized as a cause of acute arterial occlusion resulting in gangrene. Several unsuccessful embolectomies were attempted near the end of the nineteenth century, but the first successful embolectomy is credited to Lahey in 1911. For many years embolectomies performed within 4 to 6 h after lodging of the embolus were successful, while those performed later had a progressively higher failure rate. Less than 15 years ago a serious proposal was made that emboli that had lodged more than 12 h earlier should not be operated upon. It is now well established that such a viewpoint is erroneous. The difficulties with late operation upon still viable extremities have been found due to inadequate removal of distal thrombi. With the combination of operative angiography and the balloon catheter developed by Fogarty et al. in 1963, viability can be preserved in well over 90 percent of patients operated upon if operation is performed before the muscles become necrotic, regardless of whether the embolus lodged 3 h or 3 days beforehand.

INCIDENCE AND ETIOLOGY. In about 90 percent of patients with lower extremity emboli, the embolus originates in the heart from one of three causes: mitral stenosis, atrial fibrillation, or myocardial infarction. In some patients it is the first sign of previously unrecognized heart disease. Hence, an embolus, though a serious or even catastrophic event, is best regarded as a manifestation of serious heart disease that must be treated separately.

With mitral stenosis emboli originate from thrombi that have formed in the left atrium because of restriction of blood flow through the stenotic mitral valve. Most such patients also have atrial fibrillation with impaired contractility of the atrium. Atrial fibrillation from atherosclerosis without mitral stenosis can occur and becomes increasingly frequent in older patients. Emboli have been recognized to occur following the spontaneous or induced conversion of fibrillation to sinus rhythm, probably because the contractions of the atrial appendage expel thrombi that have accumulated during the impaired contractility from fibrillation. Emboli following a myocardial infarction originate from mural thrombi forming over the endocardial surfaces of the infarcts. Their frequency is greatest in the first 2 to 3 weeks following infarction and in some patients are the first sign of myocardial infarction.

An unusual cause of peripheral embolization is the so-called paradoxic embolus, when a thrombus arising in the venous circulation passes through a congenital atrial or ventricular septal defect and lodges in a peripheral artery. Other unusual causes include bacterial endocarditis, mural thrombi in subclavian or popliteal aneurysms, and atrial myxoma. In 4 to 5 percent of patients, despite the most diligent search, the source is never found.

PATHOLOGY. Most emboli ejected from the heart, 70 percent of the 426 emboli reported by Darling, lodge in the arteries of the lower extremities. Unfortunately 20 to 25 percent lodge in the cerebral circulation, usually intracranially, and are surgically inaccessible. Five to ten percent lodge in visceral arteries, the superior mesenteric or renal, and an unknown number lodge in silent areas of the circulation, such as the spleen, for which clinical signs are obscure.

Emboli usually lodge at bifurcations of major arteries where the diameter abruptly narrows. Common sites are the bifurcation of the abdominal aorta, the common iliac artery, the common femoral artery, and the popliteal arteries (Fig. 21-6). In the upper extremities similar patterns are found, including the distal subclavian artery and the bifurcation of the common brachial. The severity of the ischemia produced is due both to the abrupt occlusion and the fact that the site of occlusion involves two major arteries, whereas an occlusion either immediately proximal or distal to a site of bifurcation would permit collateral circulation through the bifurcation.

PATHOPHYSIOLOGY. The result of arterial embolization is the immediate onset of severe ischemia of the tissues normally supplied by the occluded artery. Depending upon the artery involved, if untreated, gangrene occurs in about 50 percent of patients. The prominent early symptoms of pain, paralysis, and paresthesia all result from the great sensitivity of peripheral nerves to oxygen deprivation. Striated muscle is secondary only to peripheral nerves in susceptibility to anoxia. Necrosis may appear within 4 to 6 h after onset of ischemia but varies with a number of factors. These include the size of the artery occluded, the collateral circulation around the site of occlusion, blood pressure, and temperature. If collateral circulation is well developed, necrosis may not appear for 8 to 12 h; occasionally moderate ischemia is present but necrosis does not develop. The fact that muscle necrosis often begins within 4 to 6 h is the reason that surgical embolectomy is successful within 4 to 6 h but considerably less effective after longer periods of time.

Sluggish flow of blood in arteries distal to the embolus results in secondary thrombosis usually in continuity with the original embolism within the distal arterial tree (Fig. 21-7). Secondary thrombi further occlude major collateral channels and intensify the ischemia. Effective therapy becomes more difficult because not only the primary embolus but also the secondary thrombus must be removed. Eventually the progressive circulatory stasis is further complicated by extensive venous thrombosis.

CLINICAL MANIFESTATIONS. The five p's, discussed earlier under Acute Arterial Occlusion, pain, paralysis, paresthesia, absent pulses, and pallor, describe the principal clinical features of arterial embolism. The onset is abrupt in most cases, gradual in a few. In 75 to 80 percent of patients there is severe and unremitting pain, usually referred to the most peripheral portions of the limb. The color may be extreme pallor or mottling from alternate areas of pallor and cyanosis. Sensory disturbances vary from anesthesia to paresthesia. Paralysis may be a feature; complete paralysis and anesthesia mask the true nature of the disorder, diverting the physician into investigations for neurologic disease while muscle necrosis is occurring.

The neurologic symptoms are the crucial prognostic signs. If motor and sensory functions are intact, the extremity will survive even though chronic ischemia may persist.

Physical Examination. The extremity is often pale and cold with collapsed peripheral veins. With less severe

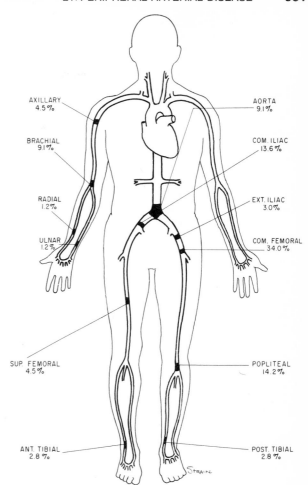

Fig. 21-6. Frequency of involvement of different peripheral arteries by arterial emboli. In the majority of patients arteries in the lower extremity are involved. *(Redrawn from Haimovici H: Peripheral arterial embolism. Angiology 1:20, 1950, with permission.)*

degrees of ischemia there may be cyanosis instead of pallor. A temperature level may be detected that coincides with the level at which the color changes. The arterial pulse is absent at the site of occlusion, frequently with accentuation of the pulse immediately proximal to this point. Sensory impairment varies from hypesthesia to anesthesia, and motor disturbances from weakness to paralysis.

The level of occlusion can often be estimated from the color, temperature level, and pulse findings. Ordinarily acute ischemia develops one joint below the site of occlusion. An iliac embolus produces ischemia at the level of the hip joint, while a common femoral embolus produces ischemia distal to the knee. The extent of ischemia varies with the effectiveness of collateral circulation. Muscle turgor in the ischemic limb is most important. Shortly after the onset of ischemia, the muscles are soft. With continuing ischemia, edema appears, progresses to necrosis, and finally to rigor mortis. Early ischemic edema

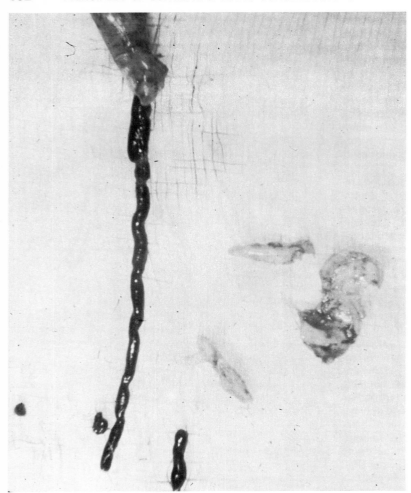 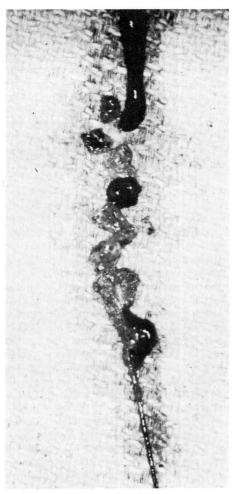

Fig. 21-7. Embolic material and secondary clot. The embolic material that was deposited in the heart chambers during active blood flow is gray to salmon-colored, of firm consistency, and unattached to the arterial wall. It is composed mainly of fibrin and degenerated platelets. The gelatinous clot that appears homogeneous is a secondary stasis clot and was formed when blood flow ceased. It contains all the blood elements and is dark red in color.

creates a "doughy" sensation on palpation. The importance of this physical finding is the fact that as long as the muscles are soft to palpation, the extremity can be salvaged with effective embolectomy and thrombectomy, regardless of how long the embolus has been present. Conversely, the presence of stiff muscles warns that necrosis has occurred. This is most clearly apparent in the leg where the muscle tone of the gastrocnemius and soleus group can be easily evaluated. Some limbs with early muscle necrosis can be salvaged by embolectomy and thrombectomy, combined with extensive fasciotomy and later debridement of localized muscle necrosis, but failure is frequent.

An additional important aspect of physical examination is the cardiac examination for underlying heart disease. The cardiac rhythm, murmurs, or friction rubs may provide clues to atrial fibrillation, mitral stenosis, or acute myocardial infarction. Examination of other peripheral arteries for pulses and bruits provides additional clues to underlying cardiac or arterial disease.

LABORATORY STUDIES. A critical decision to be made when the patient is first encountered is whether an angio-gram should be performed. The diagnosis of acute arterial occlusion can be readily made from the history and physical findings. An electrocardiogram and a chest radiograph should both be done to evaluate the presence of heart disease. If performance of angiography delays surgical therapy beyond the 4- to 6-h "golden period" of therapy, it should be omitted. Intraoperative angiography is one alternative. Angiography is particularly useful where the site of the embolus is uncertain and in distinguishing between arterial embolism and arterial thrombosis superimposed upon an atherosclerotic plaque.

DIAGNOSIS. The condition most easily confused with an arterial embolus is acute thrombosis of an artery previously diseased with atherosclerosis. The importance of differentiating the two conditions is to determine the method of surgical therapy, for a more extensive operative procedure is required with thrombosis. Certain clinical findings suggest thrombosis rather than embolism. Atherosclerosis is usually seen in older age groups, and often symptoms of chronic ischemia, such as claudication, have been present for some time. The involved extremity may show signs of chronic ischemia, such as loss of hair from the toes and atrophy of the skin and nails. The absence of heart disease, which could cause an arterial embolus, further supports the diagnosis of thrombosis. At times differential diagnosis is difficult or even impossible, because an embolus may occur in an older patient with atrial fibrillation who also has claudication from femoral atherosclerosis. In this case, an arteriogram is of great value. With atherosclerosis and secondary arterial thrombosis, diffuse changes of atherosclerosis can be seen throughout the peripheral arteries, often with the development of prominent collateral circulation. By contrast, with embolism, where the distal arteries are usually normal except at the site of occlusion, collateral vessels may not be apparent.

Rarely, acute extensive thrombophlebitis may be confused with acute arterial occlusion. Thrombophlebitis may be associated with extensive vasospasm, causing pain and peripheral vasoconstriction with diminished pulses. A bluish extremity, termed *phlegmasia cerulea dolens,* is also characteristic of venous thrombosis. With arterial embolism, edema appears only after extensive gangrene has developed.

Even more rarely, acute dissecting aneurysm of the thoracic aorta with obliteration of peripheral pulses may suggest multiple peripheral emboli. A dissecting aneurysm can be suspected because of pain in the chest or back, often with a left pleural effusion.

TREATMENT. Indications for Operation. Because patients with arterial emboli usually have serious heart disease, the operative procedure must be planned with regard to the influence of anesthesia and operation on the heart disease. This is particularly critical when the embolus has resulted from a myocardial infarction. With modern vascular techniques, however, embolectomy can be performed in most patients with minimal trauma, often with local anesthesia. Hence, a decision not to operate because of heart disease should be made only if death is imminent. The reason for this is that failure to remove a peripheral embolus, which subsequently produces gangrene, of necessity requires a major amputation, a much greater surgical stress than simple embolectomy.

As emphasized in this chapter, the urgency for performing arterial embolectomy can be simply estimated from the presence of paralysis and anesthesia. When these are present, muscle necrosis often occurs within 4 to 6 h. If they are absent, a more conservative approach may be undertaken. However, their absence does not guarantee that claudication will not subsequently develop in the extremity with resumption of normal physical activity.

An unusual indication for nonsurgical therapy occurs with a migrating embolus. An embolus may lodge in a proximal artery, such as the common femoral, then frag-ment spontaneously within a few hours and migrate distad. Such patients may on occasion recover completely, but most remain with significant residual occlusion of peripheral arteries. Peripheral pulses should be unequivocally present before simple observation is continued for a long period of time.

Preoperative Therapy. The prompt intravenous administration of heparin to inhibit the development of thrombi distal to the embolus is the most important therapeutic measure in the treatment of an arterial embolus. Heparin, 5000 to 10,000 units, is given intravenously by continuous drip or repeated at 3- to 6-h intervals, depending upon the clotting time, if embolectomy is delayed. Lumbar sympathetic blocks are of dubious value and cannot be safely performed in the presence of systemic anticoagulation. Other measures to influence collateral circulation, such as orally administered vasodilator drugs, are of little value. Intraarterial administration of drugs such as reserpine and tolazoline (Priscoline) sometimes dramatically improves the appearance of acutely ischemic extremities by eliminating functional arterial resistance to flow.

A program for administering extremely large doses of heparin to promote lysis of thrombi and thereby improve the chances of operative success has been proposed by Blaisdell et al., who recommend that 30,000 units of heparin be administered intravenously as a bolus followed by doses of 2000 to 3000 units per hour by continuous I.V. drip. If clinical improvement occurs, operation is deferred. If no clinical improvement is observed, operative intervention is carried out. This requires close observation by highly experienced teams well versed in recognizing the sometimes subtle changes that denote either worsening or improvement of ischemia.

Operative Technique. For operations on the extremities, local anesthesia can be used in seriously ill patients. Frequently the operative incisions are short since the Fogarty balloon catheter has permitted removal of propagated clot both distal and proximal to emboli, making possible performance of the entire operative procedure through limited surgical incisions. Frequently, it is possible to perform the entire embolectomy and thrombectomy through incision in the upper thigh over the common femoral artery. With emboli at the common femoral bifurcation, it is possible to remove thrombi from the arterial tree down to the ankle through the same incision. Rarely is it necessary to enter the peritoneal cavity for aortoiliac embolectomy. This should be avoided when possible, for these patients are usually quite ill from their cardiac disease.

In general, surgical incisions are placed directly over the uppermost level of arterial occlusion unless the aortoiliac system is involved, in which case incisions are placed over both common femoral arteries. Once the artery has been isolated proximal to distal to the embolus, 5000 units of heparin should be given intravenously. A transverse or a longitudinal arteriotomy is then made in the artery immediately proximal to its bifurcation, where the embolus is usually lodged. The embolus characteristically "pops" out as soon as the lumen is entered and can be recognized by its gray appearance and nonadherence to the arterial wall. Hence, removal is a simple procedure, but removal of thrombi that have formed distad or even proximally may be unusually complex. Fogarty balloon catheters have virtually eliminated the need to make multiple incisions along the course of the arterial tree for the laborious retrograde washing out of thrombi. The preferred technique is to pass the catheter into the distal artery as far as possible, inflate the balloon, and withdraw it in its inflated state. Comparison of the length of the catheter inserted with the length of the extremity indicates how far the catheter has been advanced. Passage of catheters into the aorta for the removal of aortoiliac thrombi is similarly performed. Occasionally it is impossible to pass the balloon catheter into various distal branches, either the anterior and posterior tibial in the calf or the radial and ulnar in the forearm. In such instances separate incisions are made over these vessels, followed by separate introduction of the catheter into each branch. Dale has used polyethylene catheters to aspirate clot. With these techniques, retrograde flushing of the artery through a distal incision is rarely necessary.

As indicated, the most crucial aspect of the operation is determining the completeness of removal of propagated thrombi. Back-bleeding is a notoriously unreliable indicator. Back-bleeding can occur through the nearest arterial branch, while the major artery distad is still occluded. Failure to remove all residual thrombus usually results in reocclusion. The operative procedure should be continued until, by an appropriate combination of techniques, all pulses are restored at the ankle or wrist, or an operative arteriogram has demonstrated that the arteries are patent. On occasion, restoration of a pulse can be misleading, and bounding pulses may be felt in an artery partly reopened but with persisting distal obstruction. For this reason operative angiography is often critical to success.

If severe ischemic injury has been present beforehand, wide fasciotomy of the fascial envelope containing the major muscles may help preserve limb viability, especially if embolectomy has been delayed beyond the golden first 4 to 6 h and increased muscle turgor was palpable before operation.

Postoperative Care. The most important aspect of postoperative care is to be certain that peripheral circulation is adequate. A palpable pulse is the best clinical sign. This should be identified immediately after operation and its presence periodically confirmed by palpation. Pulses which are difficult to feel can be checked with the Doppler instrument, which permits not only auscultation over pedal arteries but also measurement of pressures within those vessels. Disappearance of a previously palpable pulse or a change in Doppler measurements associated with unsatisfactory appearance of the extremity is an indication for either arteriography or immediate reoperation.

The persistence of paralysis and anesthesia following operation is ominous; gangrene is almost a certainty. Conversely, restoration of normal neurologic function indicates adequate circulation for muscle viability. This is particularly reassuring either when pulses cannot be restored or palpation is inconclusive because of edema and swelling.

The mode of heparin administration in the postoperative period is critical, since fresh surgical wounds are subject to hemorrhage, while delay of anticoagulation may predispose to further embolization. Some surgeons give no heparin for 6 h postoperatively and then administer it by intermittent intravenous injection in doses of 5000 units every 4 to 6 h. Oral therapy with coumadin derivatives is begun after 3 to 4 days and continued as long as the patient is at risk. Salzman et al. have reported that continuously administered intravenous heparin, avoiding peak effects which reach infinity during the intermittent administration, is associated with a lesser incidence of hemorrhage. Thrombolysis may accompany heparin administration, especially when porous knitted vascular prostheses are employed. The importance of prompt and continuous anticoagulant therapy cannot be overemphasized, for the arterial embolus is only a symptom of serious heart disease. Recurrence of embolization, each incident associated with a 25 to 30 percent likelihood of lodging in the brain, is distressingly common unless the heart disease is effectively treated. Patients with intractable atrial fibrillation should be maintained on permanent anticoagulant therapy. Those with mitral stenosis should have a mitral valvulotomy performed soon. Those with myocardial infarction should receive anticoagulants for several weeks, by which time the endocardial surface of the infarct will have healed and the likelihood of embolism is small.

Antibiotic therapy generally is started at the time of operation and continued for 2 to 4 days postoperatively.

PROGNOSIS. The most important feature influencing survival of the extremity following embolectomy is the time elapsing between the occurrence of embolization and successful restoration of flow at operation. As mentioned repeatedly, removal within 4 to 6 h after onset is almost always associated with an excellent prognosis, having the two great advantages of avoiding muscle necrosis and limiting secondary thrombus formation beyond the site of embolism. In both of the large series reported by Darling et al. and Cranley et al., excellent results were obtained in 85 to 95 percent of patients. With more than 6 h elapsed between embolization and embolectomy, unsuccessful results were more common. These particularly occur with inexperienced vascular surgeons and limited facilities. The crucial concept is that as long as the calf muscles are "soft" before operation, indicating that muscle necrosis has not occurred, salvage of the extremity should approach 95 percent or higher, regardless of the duration of ischemia. In delayed cases, achieving this goal taxes the resources, skills, and ingenuity of the vascular surgeon to the utmost, for thrombi may have accumulated from the aortic bifurcation to the posterior tibial artery at the ankle and complete removal requires a combination of careful surgical exploration, frequently multiple incisions, and serial operative angiography. If muscle necrosis is present before operation, indicated by a rigid calf muscle, possibilities of limb salvage are small, and the possibility of precipitating fatal myoglobinuria may constitute a contraindication to surgical restoration of flow. Rarely, a functional extremity may be salvaged in which virtually all the calf muscles are lost from necrosis but a viable foot is preserved.

The crucial long-term feature determining prognosis is the ability to prevent further emboli. Without adequate prophylactic anticoagulation, recurrence is dismally inevitable, eventually terminating with fatal or crippling cerebral thrombosis. Vigilance to prevent emboli can be relaxed only when a myocardial infarction has healed or mitral stenosis has been treated by valvulotomy.

In any large series of patients with arterial embolism, death occurs in 25 to 30 percent of patients during that hospitalization. This is almost always due to the underlying heart disease causing the embolus, indicating the gravity of the basic illness. In some instances death is due to either inadequate management of the embolic episode, with the complications of sepsis from gangrene, or to recurrent embolism to the brain or viscera, a result of inadequate anticoagulant therapy.

Arterioarterial Embolization

HISTORICAL CONSIDERATIONS. In the past decade there has been increasing awareness of the existence of arterioarterial embolism and its role in producing previously unexplained ischemic syndromes. With cerebrovascular insufficiency, the ophthalmologic visualization of minute particles of atherosclerotic plaque or platelet fibrin emboli in the retina, in association with an ulcerated atherosclerotic plaque at the bifurcation of the carotid artery, suggested the source of the minute emboli. In the lower extremities, sudden onset of toe and foot ischemia with little or no impairment of peripheral pulses (the "blue toe" syndrome) led to the finding that minute emboli were the mechanism, having originated in aortic or iliac atherosclerotic plaques. The finding of peripheral emboli beyond aneurysms has been described periodically. Miles et al. have cited observations suggesting that small emboli in the coronary circulation could come from ulcerated plaques, producing diffuse myocardial scarring from myriads of tiny emboli.

PATHOGENESIS. The basic process seems to be ulceration of an atherosclerotic plaque with discharge of minute fragments of atherosclerotic debris into the circulation. The ulcerated surface may become covered by platelets and fibrin which in turn are intermittently dislodged. How often these are subsequently resorbed is not known. The embolic may arise from an atherosclerotic artery near the end organ where the emboli lodge or they may originate some distance away, a condition occasionally seen when emboli in the toes apparently originate from plaques in the abdominal or thoracic aorta. Repeated embolic episodes are frequent, at times with almost complete recovery from ischemia between each episode; in other patients progressively greater degrees of ischemia occur, ultimately terminating in necrosis.

CLINICAL FINDINGS. As noted briefly above, a most striking syndrome occurs with emboli from the distal thoracic aorta, the "blue toe" syndrome. There is severe ischemia of the toes and feet, bilaterally, in association with renal failure. Before the pathogenesis was understood, the diagnosis remained an enigma, for pulses often remained palpable even while distal ischemia progressed to gangrene. There is a wide range in severity, from complete clearing of ischemia to progressive occlusion and gangrene. Similar embolization from the infrarenal aorta or iliac arteries also produces blue toes without renal failure.

Similar episodes occur in the cerebrovascular circulation with any combination of neurologic symptoms from the most transient, fleeting symptoms to complete stroke with cerebral infarction. In the upper extremity the subclavian artery is most frequently involved, with repeated attacks simulating Raynaud's phenomenon.

DIAGNOSIS. The diagnosis can be suspected from the combined findings of severe ischemia of a digit with palpable pulses. Determining the source of the emboli is crucial, for many can be corrected surgically, often by simple endarterectomy. Hence, detailed angiographic studies are necessary. The source of the embolus can be estimated by noting the peripheral circulation in other areas, where previous emboli may have lodged. For example, involvement of branches of the profunda femoris artery indicate emboli arising proximal to this level. Concomitant involvement of renal artery branches suggests that the emboli originated in the thoracic aorta. Similarly, in the upper extremity emboli may arise from the subclavian artery or, alternatively, from lesions located far distad, such as small aneurysms in the palm of the hand. These diagnostic possibilities can be resolved only by precise, extensive angiography.

TREATMENT. When the atherosclerotic plaque can be related to the pattern of distal embolization (Fig. 21-8), arterial reconstruction of the atherosclerotic segment by either endarterectomy or replacement with a prosthetic graft has prevented further embolism. In the carotid system, there is now extensive experience with arterial reconstruction to prevent recurrent ischemic episodes, so-called transient ischemic attacks (TIA). The operation is effective and durable. Similar procedures have been performed in the subclavian artery to prevent TIA in the upper extremity. In the lower extremity experience is still limited, but good results in a series of 10 cases operated upon at New York University have confirmed both the validity of the concept and the surgical approach.

In theory, emboli from platelet or fibrin aggregates should be inhibited or prevented by anticoagulants, but their effectiveness is as yet uncertain. Paradoxically, anticoagulant therapy might prevent healing of an ulcerated plaque and thereby increase the tendency to embolization. This may explain the infrequent clinical puzzle of an embolus developing *after* heparin therapy has been started.

ACUTE ARTERIAL THROMBOSIS

ETIOLOGY AND PATHOLOGY. Acute arterial thrombosis usually occurs in an artery previously narrowed by ath-

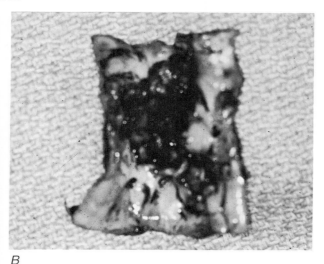

B

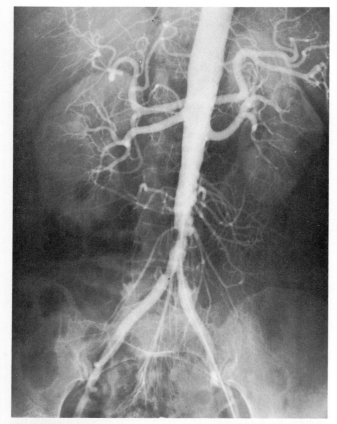

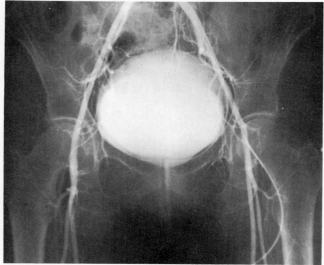

A

Fig. 21-8. Arterioarterial embolization, also known as atheroembolization, in a patient in whom marked ischemia of the toes developed in the presence of palpable pedal pulses. Several attacks occurred with progressive ischemia. *A.* Angiograms showing infrarenal abdominal aortic plaques. Occlusion of small calf arteries without involvement of renal arteries suggested that this infrarenal plaque was the source of emboli. *B.* Aortic plaque removed by endarterectomy. There was no recurrence of embolization at the tenth year follow-up.

Unusual causes of arterial thrombosis are cervical ribs or repeated occupational trauma, such as from operation of pneumatic tools, the vibrations of which locally injure the arterial wall and produce thrombosis. Very rarely arterial thrombosis develops within a normal artery. This can happen with debilitating infections, especially in infants, usually with diarrhea and dehydration. It may also occur with primary hematologic disorders, such as polycythemia vera.

Iatrogenic thrombosis has become much more common due to percutaneous introduction of catheters for cardiac catheterization or selective angiography. Thrombosis develops from detachment of a flap of intima from the arterial wall with subsequent formation of an occluding thrombus. Acute lower extremity arterial thrombosis has also been seen following long periods of immobilization such as long automobile or plane trips. The condition is similar to acute venous thrombosis, which occurs more commonly.

CLINICAL MANIFESTATIONS. When thrombosis occurs suddenly, the findings are similar to those occurring with arterial trauma or embolism: pain, absence of pulses, paresthesia, and paralysis.

A critical differential diagnosis is between arterial embolus and arterial thrombosis, a distinction that cannot always be made with accuracy, although several clues are helpful. A history of claudication in the involved extremity indicates chronic arterial disease. Similarly, examination of the extremity may show the stigmata of chronic arterial insufficiency, including absence of hair and

erosclerosis. In some patients the process of occlusion is gradual; no acute symptoms appear, but chronic arterial insufficiency slowly becomes more severe. In others, however, sudden thrombosis precipitates acute symptoms, closely mimicking arterial embolization.

trophic changes in the skin and nails. Significant findings may also be present in the contralateral, asymptomatic extremity. Differentiation between the two conditions is important, because although operation is necessary with either if circulation is impaired to such an extent that gangrene is imminent, the type of operative procedure for each condition varies greatly. Restoration of blood flow in an extremity with chronic occlusive disease, with an arterial thrombosis superimposed upon an artery previously narrowed by atherosclerosis, is much more difficult than the performance of simple embolectomy upon an artery with no intrinsic vascular disease. Additionally, patients with emboli require long-term anticoagulant therapy. Patients with arterial thrombosis should have an arteriogram before operation to assess the extent of occlusive disease and to evaluate the patency of the vascular bed beyond the point of occlusion in order to determine where a bypass graft can be inserted distad.

TREATMENT. Operative correction of the arterial occlusion requires both removal of the thrombus and correction of the atherosclerotic stenosis. The operative techniques are described in detail in the section Chronic Arterial Occlusion. Usually either the atherosclerotic narrowing is removed directly with an endarterectomy or a bypass graft is inserted around the area of obstruction.

ATHEROSCLEROTIC OCCLUSIVE DISEASE

Occlusive Disease of the Lower Extremity

AORTOILIAC DISEASE

Recognition of the ischemic syndrome produced by atherosclerotic disease of the bifurcation of the abdominal aorta is credited to Leriche, who described in the early 1940s the clinical characteristics of occlusion of the abdominal aorta, i.e., claudication, sexual impotence in the male, and absence of gangrene. The development of angiography, pioneered by dos Santos, greatly facilitated diagnosis.

PATHOLOGY. Some degree of atherosclerosis is almost universally seen at autopsy in the abdominal aortas of patients over sixty years of age, but symptoms from decrease in blood flow do not occur unless the cross-sectional area of the aorta has been narrowed by as much as 90 percent. There may be only fibrointimal thickening or typical atherosclerotic plaques with ulceration and superimposed thrombosis or embolization of portions of atherosclerotic plaques. As in other arteries, the disease often begins at bifurcations where flow patterns conducive to intimal thickening occur. Involvement is often greatest at the aortic, the iliac, and the common femoral bifurcations. It may extend proximally in the abdominal aorta up to the level of the renal arteries, but occlusion proximal to the renal arteries is rare.

Patients are occasionally seen in the fifth and sixth decades with thrombosis of the abdominal aorta but only mild atherosclerosis of the common iliac arteries. The thrombus often propagates up to the level of the renal arteries, rarely occluding one renal artery, and extends up to near the superior mesenteric artery. These patients contrast to a curious degree with patients in the seventh and eighth decades who may have unusually severe atherosclerosis but without thrombosis and total occlusion, despite advanced stenosis. This variation with age suggests that some unrecognized factor leading to hypercoagulability in the younger group may precipitate the thrombotic process.

Fortunately clinically significant atherosclerosis of the abdominal aorta is virtually always segmental. Proximally it stops at the level of the renal arteries; distad the profunda femoris artery is almost always patent, though not infrequently involved with correctable stenotic lesions even in the presence of a totally occluded superficial femoral artery (Fig. 21-9). Reconstruction can be done in most of the patients, directing flow distad into the patent profunda femoris artery, which, however, may require either bypass or endarterectomy to serve as a suitable outflow tract. If the superficial femoral artery is also occluded, additional reconstruction is usually not required unless tissue necrosis is present. Otherwise, simple aortoiliac or aortoprofunda femoris reconstruction will suffice to relieve claudication.

A separate therapeutic consideration is the 10 percent of persons with aortoiliac occlusive disease who have small aneurysms as well. This group must be treated by aortic graft replacement of the aneurysmal segment, for aneurysmal dilation may continue following endarterectomy or simple bypass procedures.

Concomitant coronary or cerebral atherosclerosis occurs frequently. This has led to an increased interest in overcoming the effects of aortoiliac occlusions without invading the abdominal cavity, through the performance of so-called extraanatomical bypass grafts, popularized by Blaisdell et al. In these procedures one or both axillary arteries serve as the takeoff vessels for grafts leading to the groin. To overcome unilateral iliac arterial occlusions, cross-femoral grafts also have been used successfully.

In addition, patients with detectable involvement of cerebral or coronary arteries are evaluated for possible angiographic studies of those arteries and for possible cerebrovascular or coronary arterial reconstructive procedures as well.

PATHOPHYSIOLOGY. The slow progression of aortoiliac occlusive disease usually is associated with the development of collateral flow through the lumbar arteries, anastomosing distad with the branches of the gluteal arteries and the profunda femoris arteries sufficient to prevent ischemia at rest, symptoms of claudication appearing only with exercise. Sexual impotence is frequent because of decreased blood flow through the hypogastric arteries. Since blood flow is adequate at rest, the extremities remain well nourished. Only with additional occlusions in the superficial femoral, profunda femoris, or popliteal and tibial arteries do nutritional changes with ulceration and gangrene appear.

Rapidly developing occlusion of the aorta before collateral circulation develops may result in severe ischemic

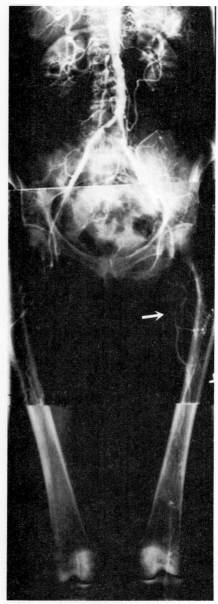

Fig. 21-9. Angiogram illustrating that the profunda femoris artery is usually patent in the presence of aortoiliac occlusive disease. Advanced lesions may be present, however, requiring surgical correction to render the profunda femoris suitable for an outflow tract. Arrow points to patent mid-profunda femoris artery.

nonoccluding or even nonstenosing atherosclerotic plaques that give rise to emboli. These emboli may occlude pedal or digital arteries, resulting in the so-called blue or purple toe syndrome (see discussion under Arterioarterial Embolization).

CLINICAL MANIFESTATIONS. The classic symptoms are intermittent claudication involving calf, thigh, and buttock and sexual impotence of varying severity in males. Claudication may be symmetric or asymmetric, depending upon the pattern of involvement of the iliac arteries, and may vary in severity from difficulty after walking three to four blocks to inability to walk, even indoors. Rest pain, ulceration, or gangrene are rare with chronic aortoiliac occlusion, and, when present, almost always indicate additional distal disease, particularly in diabetics where associated occlusions of the tibial arteries are common.

Symptoms may remain stable for years or even improve with exercise as collateral vessels enlarge. Conversely, symptoms may worsen with progression of distal atherosclerosis, sometimes dramatically, with hypotension secondary to myocardial infarction or cardiac arrhythmias, or to administration of drugs that diminish ventricular systolic thrust, such as propanolol. Impotence is a complex syndrome which may arise from multiple causes. Its presence or absence cannot be relied upon to diagnose aortoiliac disease. Although it may improve after successful arterial reconstruction, the outcome in any particular patient is unpredictable.

Physical Examination. The principal finding is diminution or absence of the femoral pulses, combined with absence of popliteal and pedal pulses. Pulsations in the abdominal aorta may be palpable if occlusion is limited to near the aortic bifurcation, but these are absent if the abdominal aorta is occluded up to the renal arteries. A systolic bruit denoting stenosis is often audible over the aorta or iliac arteries. It does not correlate, however, with the degree of stenosis. Nutrition in the extremities is usually normal. With signs of chronic ischemia, such as absence of hair, brittle nails, or rubor, additional atherosclerotic disease in the femoral or popliteal arteries is probably present.

Occasionally patients are seen with aortoiliac disease with acute episodes of severe ischemia of the toes or feet, often with cyanosis and rest pain. The diagnosis may be especially puzzling if the aortoiliac obstruction is not severe. Occasionally pedal pulses are palpable. The syndrome arises from arterioarterial embolization of fragments of atherosclerotic plaques or minute thrombi dislodged from the surface of such plaques. The diagnosis may be suspected if a localized bruit in the abdomen or groin is found.

As multiple areas of atherosclerosis are frequent, particular care should be taken to search for bruits over the carotid or subclavian arteries, as well as to note the adequacy of pulses in the upper extremities.

LABORATORY STUDIES. With the exception of patients experiencing arterioarterial embolization, the diagnosis usually can be established by the history and physical examination. Radiographs often show calcification in the

changes in the legs, even though no additional disease is present distad. In some extreme cases, thrombosis of an atherosclerotic aorta may propagate up to the level of the renal arteries, rarely occluding one renal artery and extending up to near the superior mesenteric artery.

Yet another manifestation of aortoiliac occlusive disease may be necrotic toe and foot lesions secondary to embolization of minute particles (atheroemboli) from the aorta or iliac arteries. These may occur in the presence of

wall of the aorta, but as the calcification is most marked in the media, it does not correlate with the degree of flow obstruction. An unsuspected abdominal aortic aneurysm, however, may be outlined by the calcification within its wall. Noninvasive tests may document reduced blood flow to the lower extremities, confirming the physical findings. These studies are most useful when the vessels are not completely occluded. With stenosis, the patient may have pulses at rest, but after a period of exercise, these values are markedly reduced. Demonstration of this change may be helpful in distinguishing between symptoms due to vascular disease and those due to neurogenic disease. Aortography is performed if surgical reconstruction is being considered. It delineates the proximal extent of the occlusion and, more importantly, may outline the patent arteries beyond the obstruction, especially the profunda femoris vessels that determine the feasibility of revascularization.

MEDICAL MANAGEMENT. The need for surgical reconstruction depends upon the severity of the symptoms and the age of the patient. Intermittent claudication in most instances denotes mild ischemia even in the presence of extensive arterial occlusions and, of itself, is only a relative and weak indication for surgical intervention. In 80 percent of patients affected, the course is relatively benign. Two-thirds of all patients affected can be managed successfully without operative intervention. Few patients fail to improve on a program of active and vigorous leg exercises and cessation of smoking; even in young patients whose livelihood may depend upon walking ability, rarely is operation needed until a 6-month to a 1-year trial of medical therapy has been attempted. By contrast, a retired patient of seventy with angina pectoris and claudication does not require operation. The presence of trophic changes in the feet, rubor, absence of hair, and brittle nails is a useful guide to the risk of gangrene, for gangrene is rare except with acute arterial occlusion as long as trophic changes are absent. Claudicators progress to gangrene at the rate of 2.3 percent per year. These usually are the patients with the most severe claudication and the most marked involvement of the tibial arteries, in whom surgical reconstructions either cannot be done or, if done at higher levels, do not result in control of the necrotizing ischemia. Thus, prophylactic intervention in claudicators probably does not avert the appearance of gangrene at a later date (see Table 21-1).

If operation is not recommended, daily exercise to the point of claudication should be encouraged, for this may enhance collateral circulation, as manifested by gradual increase in walking tolerance. If walking is not feasible, a similar exercise can be performed indoors by having the patient raise himself on his toes and then rock back on his heels, repeating the sequence rapidly until calf cramps occur. Following a rest period the exercise is repeated, as often as twenty or more times daily.

Abstinence from tobacco in any form is mandatory. There is reasonable statistical evidence that claudication improves when smoking is stopped and that the risk of gangrene is greater in patients who smoke. The precise mechanism is unknown, but tobacco is a potent vasocon-

Table 21-1. FATE OF 104 CLAUDICATORS*

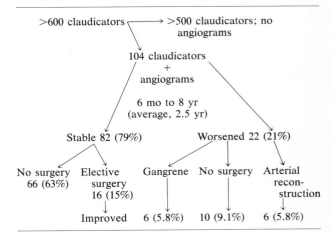

* These patients had arteriograms and were followed for 6 months to 8 years (average, 2.5 years) in an attempt at nonsurgical management.
SOURCE: From Imparato AM, Kim GE, Crowley JG: 1975, with permission.

strictor. Robichek et al. have reported that continued smoking after arterial reconstructions results in premature failures. Drug therapy with vasodilators may be tried, but unfortunately few patients have had any improvement in claudication. Alcohol, orally administered, is employed for its peripheral vasodilator effect.

With severe ischemia, one of the most crucial points in management is educating the patient to protect the feet from any form of trauma, be it thermal, mechanical, or inflicted by trimming of calluses, corns, or toenails. A familiar tragedy is that a trauma that would be minor in a foot with normal circulation will produce gangrene of a toe in a severely ischemic foot that not only fails to heal but may gradually progress upward to result in a low thigh amputation. Infection associated with unguis incarnatus or dermatophytosis similarly may cause decompensation of the circulation with gangrene, probably from an increase in local tissue metabolism.

Therapy directed toward lowering blood lipid concentrations by diet, drugs, or even surgical procedures remains of uncertain benefit. Anticoagulant therapy with heparin or warfarin sodium has not been helpful. The recent exciting discovery that acetylsalicylic acid in small doses strikingly alters platelet aggregation and may thereby prevent intravascular thrombosis is now undergoing clinical evaluation and holds considerable therapeutic promise.

SURGICAL TREATMENT. Operations that have been used to relieve the symptoms of aortoiliac occlusion include (a) direct aortic reconstruction, either by bypass or endarterectomy, (b) indirect revascularization or extraanatomic bypass, or (c) balloon dilatation of stenotic lesions using percutaneous catheters. Occasionally lumbar sympathectomy, either by operation or by phenol injection, has been used to promote peripheral vasodilatation. These will be discussed under the section Femoropopliteal Occlusive Disease.

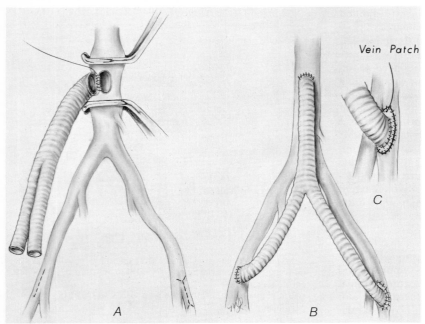

Fig. 21-10. Bypass graft of abdominal aorta. Dissection and exposure are similar to that for endarterectomy procedures. *A.* The proximal anastomosis is performed either end-to-side or end-to-end to the aorta proximal to the point of obstruction. End-to-end aortic anastomosis is preferred by many to lessen the risk of distal embolization. Knitted Dacron is preferred. *B.* The distal anastomoses are performed as end-to-side anastomoses either to the iliac artery proximal to the inguinal ligament or to the common femoral artery at the point of origin of the profunda femoris artery, depending upon the degree of atherosclerotic involvement of the external iliac artery. Anastomoses distal to the inguinal ligament are avoided whenever possible to avoid trauma to the prosthesis passing under the inguinal ligament and to lessen the risk of infection posed by having a plastic prosthesis in the groin. *C.* A vein roof patch may be employed to facilitate suture of the prosthesis to small arteries.

An operation on the abdominal aorta is a major procedure that is associated with a 2 to 10 percent risk of complication depending on the degree of associated medical problems. Complications may stem from associated vascular disease (coronary, carotid, renal, and lower extremity occlusive disease), from failure of other organs (pulmonary and renal), or from perioperative events (bleeding, thrombosis, and infection). Because of these risks, any elective procedure should be carefully planned and discussed with the patient to be certain that the operative risk is matched by the anticipated improvement. Many will refuse operation unless for limb salvage when informed of the risk and reassured about the relatively benign prognosis of intermittent claudication.

Preoperative evaluation should include a thorough history, physical examination, and appropriate diagnostic studies to evaluate the heart, lungs, kidneys, and peripheral vessels. Determination of the left ventricular ejection fraction is particularly useful in evaluating cardiac risk. An angiogram visualizing the aorta from the level of the renal arteries to the arch vessels of the feet is preferred, not only for planning the surgical procedure but also for anticipating possible lower extremity complications. At the time of the operation the blood pressure, cardiac rhythm, urinary output, and intracardiac pressures should be continuously monitored. Careful thought must also be given to the infusion of fluids and blood products.

A number of factors may influence the choice between bypass and endarterectomy for aortic reconstruction. Bypass with a prosthesis is technically less demanding and therefore, for most surgeons, can be performed with less blood loss and operating time. The late complications of infection of the prosthesis, anastomotic aneurysms, and aortoenteric fistulas must be considered because they are all potentially lethal. Endarterectomy leaving only autologous tissue has as good patency rates as bypass, and it is free of the complications associated with plastic prostheses. This operation is especially suited for good risk patients with long life expectancies.

Bypass Grafting (Figs. 21-10 and 21-11). Although bypass may be performed to the iliac vessels, the operation most customarily performed is an aortobifemoral procedure, circumventing occlusive disease in the external iliac and common femoral arteries. Antibiotics are given during the course of the operation. The femoral arteries are exposed from the inguinal ligament distally to the profunda femoris arteries. The latter may require extensive dissection to reach a relatively atherosclerotic free segment. A separate incision is made in the abdomen to expose the infrarenal aorta.

A variety of prosthetic grafts with varying permeabilities is now available. Dacron woven prostheses are less permeable to blood but tend to form a gelatinous neointima that has the potential of embolizing. Knitted grafts are more porous, requiring preclotting, but in time be-

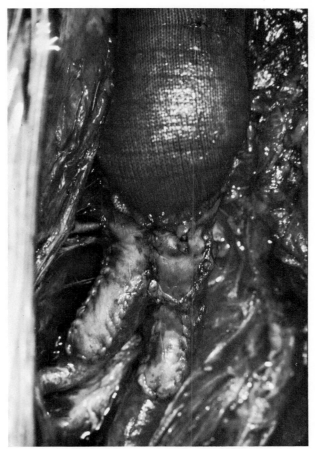

Fig. 21-11. Interposition of vein roof patches over the profunda femoris and superficial femoral arteries facilitates suture of plastic prostheses to the common femoral artery in aortofemoral bypass procedures.

come better incorporated into the surrounding tissues. Over a period of time postoperatively, knitted prostheses have shown a tendency to dilate and collect gelatinous thrombus along the inner wall, losing the original advantage of neointimal incorporation. New woven velous grafts may combine the advantages of both in maintaining diameter and adherent neointima.

After heparinizing the patient, the aorta is clamped and either an end-to-end or an end-to-side anastomosis is constructed using 3-0 or 4-0 nonabsorbable suture. The limbs of the bifurcated graft are then tunneled retroperitoneally, posterior to the ureters and mesosigmoid colon, under the inguinal ligaments to the groin wounds. End-to-side anastomoses are then made to the femoral arteries. A variety of adjunctive techniques, such as local endarterectomy or vein patch angioplasty, may be used if there is extensive atherosclerotic disease of the femoral vessels. After restoring blood flow, intraoperative angiograms are recommended since the potential for technical imperfections, especially at the distal anastomoses, can lead to early and disastrous reocclusions.

Thromboendarterectomy (Fig. 21-12). An alternative procedure that has been used to disobliterate occlusive atherosclerotic disease from the level of the renal arteries to the mid profunda femoris arteries is thromboendarterectomy. It avoids the often precarious complications associated with plastic prostheses and is most useful when the procedure can be limited to the aorta and common iliac arteries. It requires particular skill and expertise for successful performance, is more time consuming when the external iliac and femoral vessels are included in the procedure, but requires later operation for reocclusion, false aneurysm, or infection less frequently than bypass procedures.

A crucial decision about the extent of the endarterectomy performed depends on the distribution of the atherosclerotic process. In some instances termination of significant occlusive atherosclerosis just distal to the bifurcation of the common iliac arteries requires only aortobilateral common iliac endarterectomy. In other cases extensive involvement of the external iliac and common femoral arteries mandates extension to include groin vessels.

The aorta proximally and the external and hypogastric arteries distad are encircled with plastic tapes. The lumbar and inferior mesenteric arteries are similarly exposed. Fifty milligrams of heparin is then given by intravenous injection before occlusive clamps are applied to avoid thrombus formation during the periods of stasis. External iliac clamps are applied before clamping the abdominal aorta to protect from distal embolization. Incisions are made over the distal common iliac arteries, and cleavage planes between the plaques and media are developed. A longitudinal incision is made into the aorta above the level of the inferior mesenteric artery and an appropriate cleavage plane near the junction of the arterial intima and media identified. Using various techniques, including arterial strippers, the core of atherosclerotic material is freed proximally. Usually by blunt dissection the aortic and iliac cores can be mobilized and removed in one piece. A critical aspect of the operative procedure distad is careful inspection of the intima of the proximal external iliac artery to eliminate ledges of thickened intima by suturing. The caliber of the external iliac arteries may be measured with catheters. A diameter smaller than #16 Foley catheter often indicates the necessity of extending the endarterectomy to the common femoral arteries. In the hypogastric arteries, endarterectomy is limited to removal of the occluding material near the ostia, for distal dissection of this artery is usually technically unsatisfactory.

The aortotomy incision is closed with a simple continuous suture of 4-0 or 5-0 monofilament nonabsorbable suture. The iliac arteriotomies may be closed similarly or with a patch graft of either autologous saphenous vein or a prosthetic patch of knitted Dacron. The choice depends upon both the diameter of the artery and the rigidity of the wall. After the incisions are sutured, the occluding clamps are sequentially removed to permit flushing initially into the hypogastric arteries and subsequently into the external iliacs. Strong femoral pulses should be palpa-

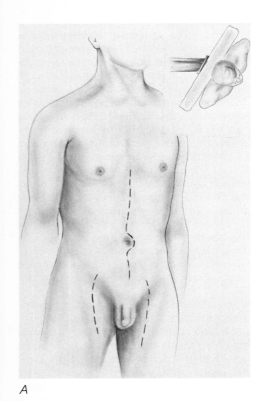

A

Fig. 21-12. Endarterectomy for atherosclerotic obstruction of the aortoiliac segments. *A.* A midline incision from xiphoid process to pubic symphysis is employed. Rotation of the operating table 30 to 40° to the right side facilitates retraction of the intestines. The thighs should be included in the operative field to permit exposure of the bifurcation of the common femoral arteries. *B.* The intestines are either encased in a plastic bag or covered with moist pads. The retroperitoneal tissues are incised exposing the aorta up to the left renal vein. *C.* The arteriotomy incisions are shown placed according to the distribution of the disease. *D.* Endarterectomy strippers may be used to separate the atherosclerotic cores in the iliac arteries. *E.* Following endarterectomy the distal intima is carefully attached to the arterial wall with vertically oriented interrupted sutures to prevent its dissection when circulation is reestablished. *F.* The multiple arteriotomies are either closed by direct suture or with roof patches of autologous vein or Dacron if the vessels are narrow.

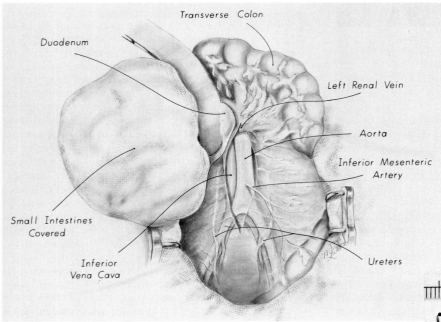

Transverse Colon

Duodenum

Left Renal Vein

Aorta

Inferior Mesenteric Artery

Small Intestines Covered

Inferior Vena Cava

Ureters

B

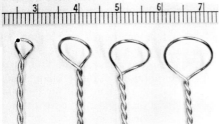

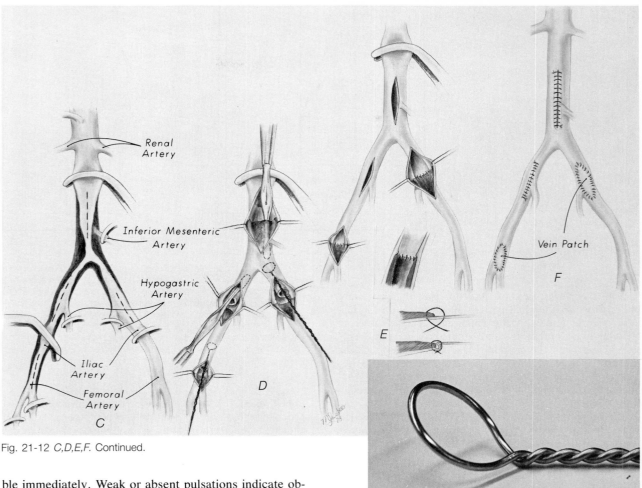

Fig. 21-12 *C,D,E,F.* Continued.

ble immediately. Weak or absent pulsations indicate obstruction from either retained plaques or stenotic suture lines, in which case the arteriotomy should be promptly reopened and the obstruction corrected. In such circumstances operative angiography is definitely needed, although completion arteriography is becoming more frequently employed.

Once blood flow is restored, heparin may be neutralized with protamine, giving 1 to 1.5 mg for each milligram of heparin used. Often, unless bleeding appears to be excessive, heparin is not neutralized by protamine administration. The posterior peritoneum is sutured over the reconstructed aorta (Fig. 21-12). A concomitant bilateral lumbar sympathectomy is a simple adjunct to the reconstructive procedure but not clearly beneficial. Many uncontrolled data, attesting to higher patency rates, are available regarding the beneficial effects of sympathectomy performed with arterial reconstruction. In our own series, sympathectomy has been performed on only rare occasions in association with arterial reconstruction, with no apparent effect on patency. When it is performed, the sympathetic chain can be identified by palpation as cord-like nodular structures parallel to the aorta on the left and just under the lateral border of the vena cava on the right.

Results and Prognoses. Immediate results of aortoiliac reconstructions are excellent. Nearly 100 percent patency rates can be achieved by meticulous technique and proper selection of operative procedures. The immediate functional results are predictable from the angiographic patterns of arterial involvement and the preoperative status of the patients (Fig. 21-13). Claudication is almost always relieved. If tissue loss with gangrene is present, however, additional reconstructive procedures in the distal arterial tree are needed in about 50 percent of the patients.

Following aortoiliac reconstruction, long-term patency rates range from 70 to 90 percent. The greatest risk for occlusion of the graft is recurrent stenosis from progressive fibrosis and narrowing of the arterial lumen at the distal anastomoses. Other late complications include false aneurysms at the proximal as well as the distal suture lines. Infection occurs in 1 to 2 percent of patients. The most devastating complication of aortoiliac bypass is aortoenteric fistula. These patients present with gastrointestinal bleeding usually into the third portion of the duodenum from the aortic suture line.

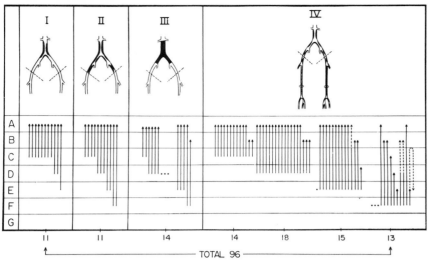

Fig. 21-13. Preoperative angiographic studies provide an excellent index of functional results that can be achieved by aortoiliacfemoral reconstructions. Functional categories *A* to *D* are increasing severities of claudication, while *E* and *F* represent rest pain and gangrene respectively. Even in the presence of disseminated distal occlusive lesions and ischemic lesions, aortoiliac reconstructions to the profunda femoris artery resulted in marked improvement. (From: *Imparato AM et al: Results in 96 aorto-iliac reconstructive procedures. Surgery 68:610, 1970, with permission.*)

It is clear from the data available that the procedure chosen for an individual patient must vary with the disease present and with the experience of the surgeon. Whichever technique is used, immediate patency rates should approach 100 percent. False aneurysms following the use of bypass grafts have greatly decreased in frequency with the use of synthetic sutures and the avoidance of excessive tension on the suture line, although they still occur too frequently. False aneurysms generally do not occur following endarterectomy, and infection with endarterectomy in which autologous tissue only is used, is rare. The principal cause of late death after operation is coronary arterial disease.

It is hoped that with recent advances in diagnosis and treatment of coronary artery disease, perioperative and postoperative deaths from myocardial infarction will be reduced. In recent years we have used the radioactive thallium cardiac function test to identify patients with the most severe coronary disease. Individuals with low left-ventricular ejection fractions are frequently subjected to coronary angiography. With this information, patients may be advised to (a) have coronary bypass surgery prior to undergoing aortic reconstruction, (b) have intensive medical therapy prior to aortic surgery, or (c) not undergo aortic reconstruction.

Extraanatomic Bypass Grafts. A number of factors have led to a growing interest in the use of extraanatomic bypass grafts to overcome the effects of aortoiliac occlusions. The magnitude of the direct aortic operation makes it less suitable for aged, debilitated patients and has led to the development of the axillofemoral and femorofemoral bypass grafts. The early success rate of extraanatomic grafts has made them useful in patients in whom early death from coronary or other vascular disease is quite high. Late graft failure, anastomotic aneurysms, and axillary artery thrombosis have made these procedures less applicable in patients who are good operative risks and have long life expectancies.

When the angiogram has shown the occlusive process to be limited to a single iliac or common femoral artery, a procedure that can be performed with minimal risk and excellent long-term results is a femoral-cross-femoral bypass. This can be done under regional or even local anesthesia. After exposing both groins, a tunnel is made in the subcutaneous tissue connecting the groin incisions. A Dacron or a PTFE (polytetrafluoroethylene) graft is placed through the tunnel. End-to-side anastomoses are made to each femoral artery. Adjunctive procedures such as endarterectomy or vein patch angioplasty may be necessary depending on the extent of disease in the femoral vessels.

If the aorta and/or both iliac vessels are stenotic, it is necessary to find another inflow vessel for the reconstruction since the pressure will be reduced in both femoral arteries. In this situation, the axillary artery is used as the inflow source.

After suitable outflow tracts have been prepared, either unilaterally or bilaterally as the degree of ischemia of the extremities dictates, the axillary artery is exposed in the infraclavicular region. Care must be taken to select axillary arteries that are fully patent. Comparisons of bilateral upper extremity blood pressures are mandatory, since the relatively high incidence of subclavian arterial lesions, usually on the left side, may lead to graft failure. If a blood pressure differential exists or if supraclavicular bruits are heard, arch aortography is indicated. We now favor the right axillary artery, since the innominate, right subclavian complex seems to be involved less often by advanced atherosclerosis. An incision is made over the coracoid process parallel to the clavicle, exposing the pectoralis major muscle, which is divided in the direction of its fibers, exposing the tendon of the pectoralis minor muscle. This is severed from its attachment to the coracoid process, exposing the axillary artery surrounded by the brachial plexus. The artery is dissected free of these nerves, sometimes producing transient, partial brachial plexus neuropathies. The subscapular artery serves as a useful landmark and is usually though not invariably preserved. A curved tunneler is used to create a subcutaneous tunnel between the infraclavicular incision and the groin incision. When indicated, a suprapubic tunnel is made to connect groin incisions, thereby permitting an additional femorofemoral bypass graft. This latter addition to unilateral axillofemoral grafts is said by some to have a higher late patency rate than the unilateral axillofemoral alone or than bilateral separate axillofemoral grafts.

When doing extraanatomic bypass grafting, it is advisable to check the condition of the entire system with operative angiograms, since there are many pitfalls to the procedure. These include not only the usual problems with operations on atherosclerotic arteries but also accumulations of clot within the prosthesis caused by leakage of tissue thromboplastins and blood from the subcutaneous tunnel into the prosthesis. There are now series that suggest that the immediate and long-term patency rates for axillofemoral grafts are comparable to those for aortofemoral grafts; operative mortality is lower. They are subject to the same complications (such as false aneurysms and infection) as other prostheses anastomosed in the groin.

Balloon Angioplasty. Selected, usually short segmental areas of stenosis or even total occlusion of the common and external iliac arteries lend themselves to percutaneous passage of balloon catheters (Grüntzig) for the purpose of dilating those vessels if stenotic or restoring a lumen if totally occluded. In approximately 10 percent of patients, serious local complications occur and can include rupture of the vessel with retroperitoneal hemorrhage or total occlusion of a previously stenotic vessel, necessitating emergency surgical intervention. In carefully selected patients employing precisely the same indications for other types of surgical intervention, balloon dilation can produce dramatic improvement both radiographically and clinically and therefore is a technique that must be considered in the management of patients with aortoiliac occlusive disease. The technique may be helpful in dealing with multilevel occlusions, especially those in which localized hemodynamically significant lesions of the iliac arteries occur in association with extensive occlusive lesions of the femoral and popliteal in which the aortoiliac inflow lesions can be dilated with a balloon and the occlusive lesions in the thigh and calf are treated by conventional surgical techniques.

FEMOROPOPLITEAL OCCLUSIVE DISEASE

PATHOLOGY. The most common site for atherosclerotic occlusion in the lower extremities is the distal superficial femoral artery within the adductor canal. This may be related to the anatomic relationship between the distal femoral artery and adductor magnus tendon as the artery traverses the adductor foramen to enter the popliteal fossa. Occlusion extends gradually proximally in the superficial femoral artery until it is occluded at its origin from the common femoral. Occlusion of the profunda femoris artery is infrequent, however. Hence, atherosclerotic occlusion of the superficial femoral artery alone usually produces claudication but no more serious circulatory impairment.

The importance of the profunda femoris artery in arterial reconstructions of the aortoiliac system has been realized for many years, and correction of ostial stenoses, incident to femoral popliteal reconstructions, has been routinely performed by some. Recently Martin emphasized its importance as a valuable contributor of blood to the extremity in the presence of superficial femoral arterial occlusions, suggesting that the profunda femoris ostium be enlarged even in the absence of high-grade stenosis. Few direct measurements of flow have been made before and after this reconstruction.

When more extensive occlusive disease develops, usually from occlusion of the popliteal artery or its branches, the anterior and posterior tibial arteries, more serious circulatory insufficiency appears. With occlusion of this extent, ulceration and gangrene are common. Such diffuse patterns of atherosclerosis are particularly common in diabetic patients.

CLINICAL MANIFESTATIONS. Segmental occlusion of the superficial femoral artery produces claudication in the calf with moderate exercise, but no symptoms at rest. Physical examination finds a normal femoral pulse but absent popliteal and pedal pulses. Rarely pedal pulses are present at rest but disappear with exercise. The nutrition of the foot is normal. If additional occlusive disease is present beyond the femoral artery, claudication is more severe, perhaps associated with ischemic rest pain and trophic changes in the foot, and ulceration and gangrene ultimately ensue. Fortunately, the rate of progression of atherosclerotic occlusion is slow in many patients, and the risk of gangrene developing within 5 years in an extremity with claudication as the only symptom is only about 5 percent.

LABORATORY STUDIES. Arteriography is required to determine the segmental nature of the occlusive disease and the consequent possibilities of arterial reconstruction. Adequate visualization of the popliteal artery and its branches is essential (Fig. 21-14). With current techniques, revascularization procedures extended to the popliteal artery are quite satisfactory if the anterior or posterior tibial branches are patent. The peroneal artery, which does not directly contribute to the formation of the pedal arch, is less satisfactory. If all three branches are occluded, under special circumstances, reconstructive procedures may be to blind popliteal segments or extended down to the pedal arches of the foot. This is discussed under Tibioperoneal Arterial Disease. Noninvasive studies of the extremity in patients with localized superficial femoral arterial occlusions are of limited value in planning operative intervention and determining prog-

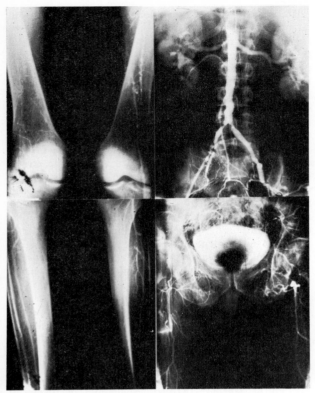

Fig. 21-14. Representative angiographic study required to evaluate patients for arterial reconstruction for claudication. Only in this manner can the inflow and outflow tracts be critically evaluated and arterial reconstructions planned.

nosis, although they are of considerable value in following the postoperative course of such patients and may detect the early signs of threatened graft failure.

TREATMENT. If claudication is the only symptom, operation is an elective decision, determined from the age and occupation of the patient. As the risk of gangrene with claudication alone is small, this alone does not constitute a clear-cut indication for operation. When trophic changes appear in the feet, operation is indicated because of the risk of gangrene. Care to avoid trauma to the foot, described in the section Aortoiliac Disease, is similarly applicable. The patient must avoid even minor trauma or exposure to extremes of heat or cold. Recommendations similar to those made for aortic occlusive disease regarding tobacco, alcohol, exercise, and vasodilatory drugs are applicable. In patients able to walk at least one city block, or 300 feet, a vigorous exercise program of walking at least 1 mile daily has resulted in marked improvement in claudication in at least 50 percent of patients within 6 to 12 months.

Direct Arterial Reconstruction. The basic principle of arterial reconstruction is that there must be both adequate inflow and adequate outflow of blood from the area of reconstruction. Early operative failures are almost always due either to obvious technical faults or to inadequate inflow or outflow.

A variety of techniques and materials have been used to reconstruct the superficial femoral and popliteal arteries. Bypass grafting has been performed using autologous vein (reversed saphenous, nonreversed in situ saphenous, femoral, brachial or cephalic), homograft vein (saphenous or umbilical), bovine arterial grafts, and prosthetic grafts (Dacron and PTFE). Endarterectomy of the superficial femoral and popliteal arteries has also been performed. Autologous reversed saphenous vein bypass has been the most frequently performed operation over the past three decades and remains the standard by which all other operations must be compared. Prosthetic grafts in general have decreased long-term patency rates and therefore are reserved for those situations in which autologous tissue cannot be used. Failure of prosthetic grafts has been related to kinking across joints, fibrointimal proliferation at distal suture lines, and dilatation of the grafts with the development of gelatinous thrombus in the lumen.

Both Wylie and Imparato described similar 5-year results following either endarterectomy or vein bypass. We compared three different techniques—venous bypass, long endarterectomy procedures with a venous roof patch, and endarterectomy performed through multiple arteriotomies with multiple vein roof patches—and found almost identical results 5 to 7 years later. Late failures were due to progressive distal atherosclerosis in one-third, to intimal proliferation in the areas of arterial reconstruction in another third, and to undetermined causes in the remainder.

Bypass Grafting. The technique of bypass grafting is illustrated in Fig. 21-15. It is particularly attractive because of its simplicity and ease of performance. The precision required for obtaining nearly 100 percent immediate patency can best be evaluated by operative angiography. Relatively small imperfections in the anastomotic suture lines or within the body of the graft can lead to deposition of platelet-fibrin aggregates with occlusion within a few hours.

The saphenous vein is carefully removed from the inguinal ligament to the knee, reversed to permit blood to flow in the direction of the venous valves, and then attached with end-to-side anastomoses to the femoral and popliteal arteries proximal and distal to the obstruction. If the vein is small, an alternative technique of leaving the vein in its bed in the nonreversed position has been successfully used. With this in situ method, the valves of the vein are disrupted by passage of an instrument along the course of the vein. Care also must be taken to interrupt the tributaries of the vein, otherwise arteriovenous fistulas will form once the bypass is completed. There are reports of in situ grafts with veins as small as 2 mm in diameter. This technique is particularly useful for long bypasses to the tibial or peroneal arteries since it allows the surgeon to use long, narrow veins and also to have more compatible vessels for suturing at both the proximal and distal anastomoses. The vein should be at least 4 to 5 mm in diameter.

Endarterectomy. Since its introduction over 35 years ago, between 1951 and 1953, endarterectomy has been

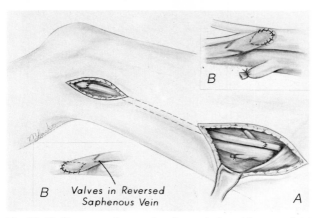

Fig. 21-15. Bypass graft procedure for occlusion of the superficial femoral artery. *A.* Incisions employed for exposure of the major vessels. A proximal incision is made over the saphenous vein from just below the inguinal ligament to the apex of Scarpa's triangle, avoiding undermining of adjacent skin flaps which might result in ischemic necrosis. The distal incision is made on the medial aspect of the popliteal fossa to expose the popliteal artery. The adductor magnus tendon, the site often of most severe superficial femoral arterial involvement, is shown. It is frequently cut to facilitate passing the vein graft from adductor canal to popliteal fossa. *B.* Completed bypass graft of the reversed saphenous vein. The anastomoses are performed end-to-side to the common femoral and popliteal arteries. The vein is brought either subcutaneously or through the subsartorial canal. Inserts show details of the bevel created in the vein bypass and reversal of the valves. An alternative technique is to leave the saphenous vein in its usual location, without reversal, destroying the valves, accomplishing an in situ nonreversed bypass graft.

modified several times. A completely open technique that involved incising the artery throughout its length, removing the atherosclerotic core, and suturing the long arteriotomy had a very high failure rate. Similarly, closed techniques with mechanical strippers often failed, usually due to leaving loose fragments of intima or atherosclerotic plaque in the lumen. Closure of the long arteriotomy with a vein roof patch, developed by Edwards et al., gave significantly better results. A subsequent modification was the use of multiple vein roof patches to close multiple arteriotomies used for semiclosed endarterectomy. This technique is illustrated in Fig. 21-16. Operative angiography is essential to be certain that atherosclerotic debris has been entirely removed from the lumen.

TIBIOPERONEAL ARTERIAL DISEASE

PATHOLOGY. Occlusive disease of the tibial arteries occurs most commonly in patients with diabetes mellitus, in patients with Buerger's disease, and in some instances of arterioarterial embolism.

In the diabetic patient for unknown reasons there are different patterns of disease that can be recognized. All tibial arteries as well as the pedal arches may be occluded. In such instances surgical reconstruction is impossible. In other patients one or more of the tibial arteries may be entirely patent, or there may be proximal occlusion with patent vessels starting at the level of the

malleoli. With this pattern of involvement, arterial reconstruction is possible if grafts are extended to the ankles. In some diabetic patients there is additional disease in the aortoiliac or femoral areas that must be dealt with.

CLINICAL MANIFESTATIONS. Tibial arterial occlusions may merely produce claudication of the foot or, more often, advanced ischemia. Diabetic neuropathy may be difficult to differentiate from ischemic rest pain. Characteristically, ischemic pain is relieved by placing the foot in a dependent position, while that of diabetic neuropathy is not. A frequent problem in the diabetic patient is ulceration on the plantar surface of the foot, secondary to pressure associated with diabetic neuropathy. A more serious problem is a spreading necrotizing infection, with absent pedal pulses. Because of associated ischemia the infection is often refractory to both antibiotic therapy and surgical debridement unless revascularization can be done. This type of progressive, refractory infection may lead to amputation before tissue ischemia per se has caused widespread necrosis. Infection undoubtedly increases the metabolic requirements of the tissue and thereby accentuates the degree of ischemia. A third type of terminal event in the ischemic diabetic foot is soft tissue atrophy to a severe degree, terminating with progressive, ischemic dry gangrene of the toes and foot.

LABORATORY STUDIES. Precise angiography is essential to determine the adequacy of the proximal circulation in the aorta and iliac arteries, as well as in the distal arterial tree, especially the small arteries of the ankle and foot. Significant advances in the technique of angiography have permitted excellent delineation of small arterial branches in these areas. Such studies may be done by direct needle puncture of the femoral artery, followed by injection of a large bolus (50 mL) of contrast medium with serial films made over a long period of time (Fig. 21-17). An alternative technique is to produce ischemic vasodilation by temporary arterial occlusion with an inflated blood pressure cuff for 5 min or longer, injecting the dye immediately after deflation of the cuff. This almost invariably produces excellent opacification of distal vessels.

TREATMENT. Unless the extremity is in jeopardy, arterial reconstructions into the tibial arteries are avoided because of the unpredictable outcome in any particular patient. When a reconstruction fails, amputation is usually necessary because the trauma of surgical dissection usually impairs collateral circulation to a significant degree. If operation is not considered indicated, treatment is primarily directed at careful avoidance of foot trauma, as emphasized in the preceding sections.

Surgical reconstruction is most successful if it is to a tibial artery that communicates with a patent pedal arch. Bypasses to peroneal arteries or incomplete tibial vessels are associated with a high incidence of early and late graft failure. In some cases when the pedal arch is thrombosed, even a patent reconstruction may not relieve the ischemia of the distal foot. In these difficult situations, desperate attempts to perform vascular reconstruction may compromise the inevitable amputation. In particular, nonhealing wounds may lead to a below-knee amputation where a transmetatarsal procedure would have suc-

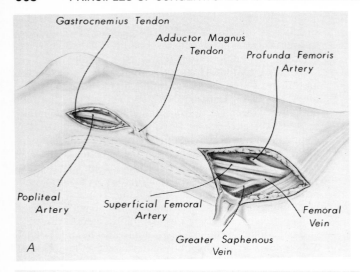

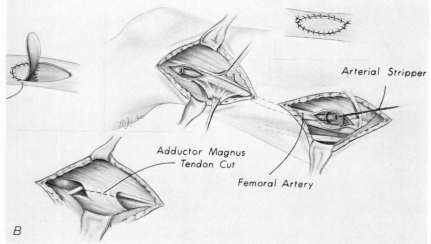

ceeded, or an above-knee amputation may become necessary where a below-knee would have succeeded.

When a necrotizing infection is present, characteristically extending as a necrotic phlegmon rather than as an abscess and requiring debridement as opposed to drainage, therapy is almost hopeless without arterial reconstruction. A combined approach of debridement of all infected tissue followed by revascularization into the distal tibial and malleolar vessels has been successful. As a practical guideline, if more than one-half of the sole of the foot has been destroyed, the limb will never be suitable for weight bearing, despite effective arterial reconstruction; so amputation is the primary choice. In all such difficult problems intensive antibiotic therapy for the specific organism involved is essential.

Direct Arterial Reconstruction. Direct arterial reconstructions to the tibial arteries have been successfully performed employing reversed autologous saphenous vein, in situ saphenous vein, and even Goretex. The critical distal anastomoses can be made to accessible portions of the tibial arteries in the calf and ankle to as low as the

Fig. 21-16. *A.* Femoral popliteal endarterectomy performed by exposing the femoral artery proximally and the popliteal artery distad. *B.* An endarterectomy stripper is used to detach atherosclerotic material via a plane in the media or between media and adventitia. Cutting the adductor magnus tendon facilitates passage of the arterial stripper. The distal intima in the popliteal artery is carefully sutured to prevent detachment and dissection of this free edge when circulation is restored. Arteriotomies are closed with autologous vein roof patches. Angiographic studies are performed to ensure that all debris has been removed, since even minute fragments left behind may result in immediate rethrombosis. Alternative techniques include exposing the entire femoral artery, opening it longitudinally in its entirety and suturing a long roof patch for closure, utilizing CO_2 intramural injection to accomplish endarterectomy, or utilizing a vibrating ring endarterectomy stripper.

level of the malleoli (Fig. 21-18). Combinations of endarterectomy and bypass procedures are possible to the level of the upper third of the calf; in our experience endarterectomy is impossible below that level.

Late results are gratifying when performed for impending limb loss, with limb salvage rates of greater than 50 percent being achieved to as late as the tenth year of

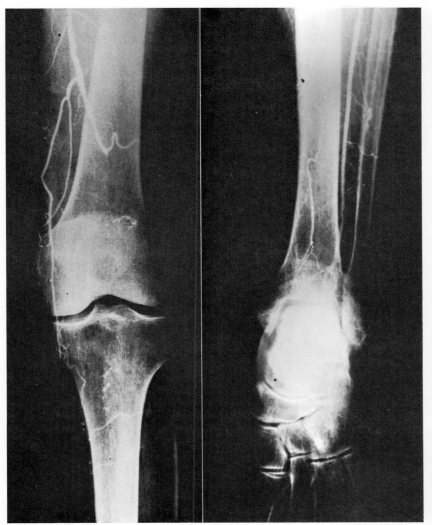
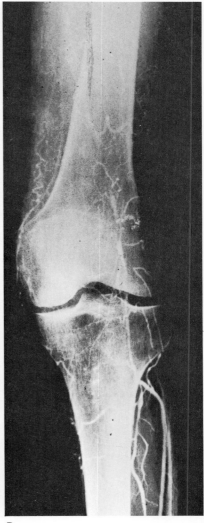

A   *B*

Fig. 21-17. Preoperative angiographic studies in the presence of tibial disease. *A.* Angiographic studies routinely performed showing poor visualization of tibial arteries. *B.* Angiogram in the same patient obtained 6 weeks later, when an ischemic lesion developed in the foot, showing patency of the anterior tibial artery. This degree of opacification was obtained using the ischemic hyperemia technique described in the text.

follow-up, although late patency rates of bypass grafts of tibial arteries may be no more than 10 percent by the tenth year.

The details of surgical technique are critically important and require the use of optical magnification, very fine suture material, and immediate intraoperative angiography upon completion of anastomoses to correct any minor imperfections that result from the surgical manipulations.

Prognosis. As mentioned earlier, arterial reconstructions in this area are performed only when ulceration and gangrene threaten amputation. Arterial reconstruction is initially successful in about 85 percent of patients, both with reconstruction at the proximal tibioperoneal level and with reconstruction extending down to the malleolus. Immediate failures are almost always due to technical errors or inadequate outflow tracts. Failures occur if the dorsal arch at the ankle is not complete. When the reconstruction is initially successful, limb salvage is excellent, for the necrotic tissue can be debrided and the wound subsequently closed by skin grafting. If the arterial reconstruction fails before complete healing is obtained, however, amputation is usually required.

If healing is complete and the arterial reconstruction subsequently becomes occluded, a significant percentage of patients remain with a viable functional extremity. Some reconstructions into the proximal tibial arteries so far have remained patent for as long as 10 years with limb salvage exceeding 50 percent. Fewer data are available for bypass grafts extending down to the ankle, but the failure rate within 2 years after operation seems to exceed 50 percent, while some reconstructions are still patent up to 7 years.

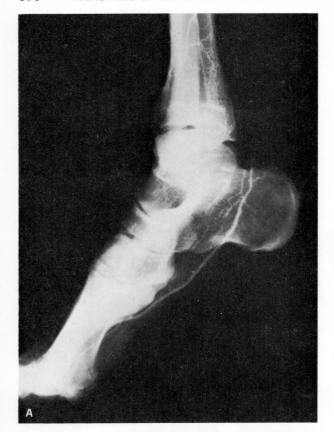

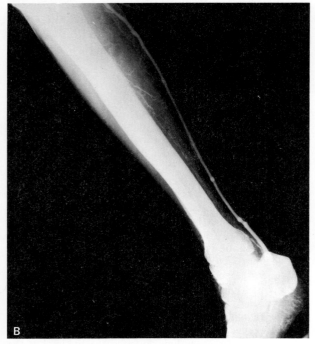

Fig. 21-18. *A.* Operative prereconstruction angiogram showing pedal arch. *B.* Postreconstruction operative angiogram showing reversed autologous saphenous vein bypass graft to the posterior tibial artery at malleolar level.

GENERAL CONSIDERATIONS

COMPLICATIONS OF ARTERIAL RECONSTRUCTIONS.
The most common complication after arterial reconstruction is graft thrombosis. In the early postoperative period, reoperation is usually worthwhile since minor technical errors can result in rapid aggregation of platelets and graft thrombosis. Careful intraoperative analysis using angiography as well as visual inspection of the suture lines often reveals the site of failure. With appropriate corrective action, most grafts can be salvaged. For late graft failures, angiography is essential to planning therapy. Reports of successful treatment with thrombolytic agents and, in some cases, balloon angioplasty have been encouraging. In very late graft failures, decisions to perform reoperation must follow the same criteria used for the original procedure. It has frequently been observed that among patients operated for threatened limb loss, only half go on to require secondary reconstructions if the initial graft fails. Frequently these patients presented initially with a nonhealing ulcer or infections secondary to trauma. If the wounds heal during the period of graft patency, it does not necessarily follow that the wounds will reappear with graft occlusion. Also, in some instances the graft has given the patient time to develop new collateral circulation that then can sustain the limb after the occlusion.

Infected Prosthesis. The large number of patients now alive with artificial, plastic blood vessel replacements has introduced a numerically significant new pathologic entity, viz., the infected plastic prosthesis. Plastic blood vessel substitutes, especially if placed in the groins, are subject to infection that usually cannot be eradicated unless the plastic material is removed from the infected area. Axillofemoral bypass grafts have been employed to permit removal of infected intraabdominal grafts. Infections in the groin, in the presence of noninfected intraabdominal arteries, have been treated by performing iliac to superficial femoral or popliteal bypass grafts, avoiding the infected groin by leading the graft through the obturator foramen to the posteromedial aspect of the thigh or to the medial aspect of the popliteal fossa, thus permitting the radical debridement of infected tissue and grafts from the groins. These have been highly successful when properly planned in association with prolonged antibiotic therapy. These procedures are indicated at a stage when infection may appear relatively innocuous. Injection of a radiopaque contrast medium into the sinuses has been helpful in delineating the true nature and extent of the problem. Aggressive and extensive surgical procedures are required to prevent exsanguinating hemorrhage from breakdown of suture lines secondary to the local infection. Although obturator bypass grafts have been successful in dealing with infections in the groins, removal of aortic prosthesis with end closure of the infrarenal aorta has resulted frequently in subsequent rupture of the aorta.

Lumbar Sympathectomy. Lumbar sympathectomy is often tried in desperation as an alternative to amputation when arterial reconstruction cannot be performed. It also may be combined with reconstruction, although its value in this case cannot be determined. As an isolated procedure, improvement can be significant in 20 to 60 percent of patients in this group. Occasionally a brilliant result occurs, consisting of relief of rest pain and marked increase in temperature of the foot. Unfortunately it has not been possible to predict which patients with impending limb loss would respond favorably. Therefore, in our series all patients, whether diabetic or not, whose conditions were considered inoperable from the point of view of arterial reconstruction on the basis of angiographic studies had lumbar sympathectomies. Some 60 percent responded favorably for longer than 6 months, while 40 percent came to early amputation within 2 months. Extensive gangrene of the forefoot was an unfavorable prognostic sign.

The technique of performing sympathectomy with a percutaneous injection of phenol in the region of the lumbar ganglia has proven to be equally effective and much less hazardous for the patient with lower extremity ischemia. We have used this technique exclusively for the past 5 years when a sympathetic ablation is desired.

Amputation. (See Also Chap. 44.) Some important guidelines should be emphasized when amputation threatens because of progressive ulceration of the foot. First, an arterial reconstructive procedure may be successful if only one major arterial branch is patent, such as a branch of the popliteal artery, the anterior tibial, the posterior tibial, or even the peroneal artery. Second, a foot will remain useful for weight bearing as long as the posterior half, including the heel, is intact. If more than 50 percent of the sole has been lost, however, the foot is probably useless for weight bearing even if arterial reconstruction is successful. With these two guidelines, angiograms should be seriously considered for virtually all patients in whom amputation is being considered. Of 100 patients threatened by amputation, either because of rest pain (38 percent) or ulceration with gangrene (62 percent), arterial reconstructive procedures were performed in 73 and lumbar sympathectomy in 13. The leg was salvaged in 64, and a minor amputation was possible in 10 others.

Both morbidity and mortality are surprisingly high in patients requiring amputation for peripheral vascular disease. Mortality is related to the advanced age in many and to the rate of severe coronary occlusive disease among patients exceeding 50 percent. Morbidity is primarily related to failure of wound healing from improper selection of the site of amputation. In general, as long as gangrene is limited to a toe, the amputation should be delayed and the ischemic toe permitted to mummify and undergo virtual autoamputation. Delay permits growth of collateral circulation in the more proximal tissues so that wound healing may occur if the toe is allowed to gradually separate over a period of weeks; a definite amputation often results in failure and extension of the wound onto the foot. A transmetatarsal amputation may be effective in some diabetic patients when infection superimposed upon a gangrenous toe requires operation. This is successful if pedal pulses are palpable but ineffective if gangrene has extended into the forefoot. Foot amputations proximal to the transmetatarsal level are generally unsatisfactory for weight bearing except for Syme's amputation, which is almost never successful in the presence of peripheral vascular disease.

Below-knee amputations can be successfully performed in a high percentage of patients, even in the absence of a popliteal pulse. Preservation of the knee joint greatly facilitates the wearing of a prosthesis. Guidelines are still being sought to determine the likelihood of wound healing if a below-knee amputation is performed in the absence of a popliteal pulse. The degree of skin bleeding is one of the most useful guidelines, though not infallible, that has yet appeared. Preoperatively, segmental Doppler pressure determinations and radioactive xenon uptake studies have been employed to predict the healing of amputations both at the below-knee level and at the metatarsal level. A below-knee amputation is a significant benefit to the patient if successful but is detrimental if the wound fails to heal and a subsequent above-knee amputation must be performed.

THE DIABETIC FOOT

The foot of the diabetic patient has distinct characteristics and can quickly progress to threaten limb and life. The diabetic has an extraordinary susceptibility to infection. After a seemingly trivial injury, within hours or days a virulent necrotizing infection can appear that rapidly spreads along musculofascial planes. It characteristically begins in an interdigital space, spreads along the plantar fascia, and may continue along tendon sheaths into the muscles of the leg. Frequently the infecting organism is gas producing and may be of the clostridial group. A life-threatening infection quickly evolves. These infections often occur with patent major arteries and seemingly are not closely related to local ischemia.

A second peculiarity of the diabetic is diabetic neuropathy. Characteristically this appears as hypalgesia or true anesthesia of some portion of the sole of the foot, subsequently complicated by trophic ulcers. These also are unrelated to ischemia and often develop with strongly palpable pedal pulses. The trophic ulcer, anesthetic and painless initially, then becomes a portal of entry for necrotizing infection.

In the diabetic foot the arterial occlusive disease typically involves the popliteal artery and its branches down to the pedal arches. The process may be diffuse, or one or more arteries may be spared. Arteries proximal to the popliteal may be normal or may show a typical "nondiabetic" pattern of atherosclerosis. The microangiopathy that is present in diabetics and appears to play a major role in the lesions that develop in the kidney and in the retina of the eye does not appear to play such a role in the ischemic conditions that afflict the foot. If the macroangiopathy can be corrected by revascularization procedures performed to the pedal arteries if necessary, the most severe degrees of ischemia can be reversed. Whether microangiopathy plays a role in the susceptibility to infection is not clear, although radical debridement without correction of the angiopathy in the presence of patent or restored major arteries results in control of the infection.

CLINICAL MANAGEMENT. Infection. In some instances a rampant uncontrolled infection with clostridia may necessitate immediate open amputation through the midcalf or midthigh to prevent death from septic shock. If patients are seen earlier, immediate widespread incision and drainage with debridement of infected tissue may prevent amputation. At an earlier stage, when infection is the dominant process without extensive tissue necrosis, localized debridement combined with intensive antibiotic therapy may be successful. A basic guideline is that all necrotic tissue must be extensively debrided, because simple drainage is hopelessly inadequate in the presence of extensive tissue necrosis, as is radical debridement alone because of the underlying tissue ischemia. In such instances the combination of radical debridement with arterial reconstruction down to the ankle may permit salvage of the extremity.

Gangrene. If gangrene of a toe is present and not complicated by infection, a much more leisurely approach is indicated, quite in contrast to the urgency of therapy if spreading infection is present. Localized dry gangrene of a toe is best treated by postponing operation, often permitting autoamputation over a period of weeks, during which time the development of collateral circulation may permit wound healing to occur. In all likelihood such instances of gangrene of a digit represent occlusion of a critical digital vessel. This may be followed by the development of enough collateral circulation to salvage the foot, but such circulation requires time to develop.

Trophic Ulcers. A trophic ulcer can be readily recognized by several characteristics. It is usually a sharply demarcated, punched out area on the sole of the foot overlying a pressure point, usually the metatarsal heads. A location over the first or third metatarsal head is particularly common. Often the ulcers are completely anesthetic and hence relatively free of pain until secondary infection develops. Similarly, the pedal pulses may be entirely normal.

Treatment in the majority of patients consists of local cleansing, protection from trauma, and most important of all, avoidance of weight bearing. Reconstruction of shoes to distribute weight differently is often effective. Special types of shoes, such as those lined with lamb's wool, are useful. Effective therapy requires long-term careful periodic observation to readjust the weight-bearing characteristics of the foot so that pressure on the area of ulceration is avoided. Any superimposed infection requires antibiotics and local debridement. As most patients do not have any vascular occlusion, arterial reconstruction is not needed.

Occlusive Disease of the Upper Extremity

Upper extremity ischemia can result from a variety of conditions, often complex and difficult to diagnose, unlike lower extremity ischemia where arteriosclerosis and embolic occlusions are the major etiologic conditions. Severe ischemia is more apt to present as focal gangrene of the fingers rather than threatened loss of the entire extremity. The ischemia is less apt to be associated with surgically correctable causes and may require extensive investigation to determine cause and treatment.

PATHOLOGY. The upper extremity is singularly free of occlusive atherosclerotic disease, although atherosclerosis is occasionally encountered in a particularly severe form in young patients with presenile arteriosclerosis. Major arterial occlusions result from emboli originating in the heart, from thoracic outlet compression, from vascular trauma associated with fractures of long bones, and from thrombotic occlusions following the introduction of catheters into upper extremity arteries. These conditions account for most of the surgical interventions required upon upper extremity arteries. Occlusions of aortic arch vessels caused by arteritis or atherosclerosis occasionally warrant intervention to relieve upper extremity ischemia. A host of conditions, including scleroderma, lupus erythematosus, mixed connective tissue diseases, and allergic necrotizing arteritis, affect the small arteries and arterioles of the hands. Occupational injury in workers who use vibrating tools or who inflict trauma upon the hypothenar eminences with the use of hammers, constitutes another group of etiologic factors. Vasospastic disorders presenting with Raynaud's phenomenon constitute a group of disorders peculiar to the upper extremity. A partial listing of conditions that may be associated with upper extremity ischemia is shown in Table 21-2.

PATHOPHYSIOLOGY. Stenosis in major arteries becomes hemodynamically significant only after the cross-sectional area of the artery has been reduced by 75 percent or more, corresponding to a 50 percent or greater reduction in diameter. The compensatory mechanisms in the upper extremity consist of opening and enlargement of collateral channels with dilatation of arterioles. These effectively reduce peripheral resistance distal to a stenotic or occluded artery and are very efficient. Consequently, isolated chronic obstructions and occlusions of the subclavian, axillary, brachial, or even radial or ulnar arteries are well tolerated. Peripheral pulses may be palpable and the extremity may remain symptom-free unless increased metabolic demands are created by exercise, or vasospasm related to the exposure to cold ensues. Acute occlusions of these major arteries may produce more pronounced ischemia because collateral channels may not have time to enlarge, and thrombi may propagate proximal and distal to areas of acute occlusion obstructing collateral channels. Emboli tend to lodge at bifurcations, thereby obstructing main channels as well as collateral channels. Consequently, distal pressures are often reduced, resting flow may be severely diminished, and arterial pulses may disappear. Compensatory mechanisms in the upper extremity are sufficiently active that recovery from even acute arterial occlusions may be quite prompt; improvement in distal flow may occur within relatively few hours as evidenced by the return of palpable pulses.

Vasomotor tone, controlled by the influence of the sympathetic nervous system on the arteriolar bed, can be dramatically affected by exposure to cold, emotional stimuli, and respiratory reflexes. These effects are most impressive in patients afflicted with Raynaud's phenomenon.

Table 21-2. CAUSES OF UPPER EXTREMITY
ISCHEMIA

I. Major arterial occlusions
  A. Arteriosclerosis
    1. Atherosclerosis (aortic arch vessels)
    2. Aneurysms (subclavian)
    3. Embolization
      a. Cardiac
      b. Arterioarterial
  B. Trauma
    1. Blunt and penetrating injuries
    2. Iatrogenic
      a. Arteriography, cardiac catheterization, arterial
        monitoring
      b. Dialysis shunts, occlusions of axillofemoral
        arterial bypasses
    3. Parenteral drug abuse
  C. Thoracic outlet compression (arterial)
  D. Arteritis
    1. Giant cell arteritis and Takayasu's syndrome
    2. Buerger's disease
II. "Small" vessel occlusions and vasospasm
  A. Autoimmune diseases
    1. Scleroderma
    2. Lupus erythematosus
    3. Rheumatoid arthritis
    4. Mixed connective tissue disorders
    5. Polyarteritis
    6. Allergic
  B. Blood dyscrasias
    1. Cryoglobulinemia
    2. Cold agglutinins
    3. Polycythemia
  C. Trauma
    1. Vibrating tools
    2. Hypothenar hammer syndrome
    3. Frostbite
    4. Radiation injury
    5. Electrical burns
  D. Drug poisoning
    1. Ergot
  E. Uremia
    1. Arteriopathy

CLINICAL MANIFESTATIONS. The clinical manifestations of upper extremity ischemia are determined by the site of arterial occlusion, by the rapidity with which it occurs, and by the mechanism responsible, be it spasm, embolic occlusion, or chronic long-standing or intermittent obstruction. A common clinical entity of acute ischemia is seen in the patient who is subjected to cardiac catheterization through a brachial artery that then becomes occluded. There may be blanching, relatively mild numbness with some easy fatigability of the hand when performing repetitive motions, and absent pulses at the wrist, all of which may appear immediately following occlusion. Within 12 to 24 h there may be a return of a weak radial or ulnar pulse with reappearance of normal color and warm skin. Ischemia may be apparent only when comparing the two extremities raised overhead. Over a period of days or weeks, except under unusual exertion of the hand and forearm or by the use of sophisticated noninvasive testing of segmental pressure or digital pulse volume recordings, all signs of ischemia may have disappeared. On the other hand, embolic occlusion may result in progressive ischemia of the entire hand and forearm. In instances of chronic long-standing ischemia, abnormalities may be detected only by careful noninvasive testing or by arteriographic survey, and hand and forearm claudication be minimal.

Occlusion of more distal vessels, as in the hand, due either to microembolization or various types of arteritis, may result in a mottled appearance of the fingertips. This may progress to gangrene with severe pain, even in the presence of palpable pulses at the wrist.

Vasospasm can be quite dramatic; a pink, warm hand may suddenly become ashen or cyanotic and mottled in its entirety, or there may be blanching of single digits that on recovery may pass through a phase of hyperemia before normal color returns.

DIAGNOSIS. The diagnosis of upper extremity ischemia requires a careful history to determine if the ischemia is due primarily to chronic occlusion, to acute occlusion, to intermittent occlusion, or to vasospasm. The circumstances leading to the ischemia must be elicited. An occupational history and a history of drug ingestion must be taken. The physical examination must include a record of the appearance of the extremity and the pulse pattern, including the presence or absence of digital pulses. Palpation of the supraclavicular region may detect the presence of a subclavian artery aneurysm, and palpation of the infraclavicular area may reveal prominent pulsation produced by poststenotic dilatation associated with a cervical rib. Auscultation in this area for bruit must be performed, not only in the neutral resting posture, but also during the shoulder girdle maneuvers. The Allen test is used to determine the patency of the palmar arches. (See the section Thoracic Outlet Syndromes.)

Segmental pressure measurements may define the site of occlusion. Digital pressure measurements or plethysmographic studies combined with physical examination of arm and forearm arteries may help differentiate hand and digital vessel occlusions from vasospastic phenomena and more proximal occlusions. By recording digital pulse volumes and determining digital pulse contours plethysmographically following exposure to heat, cold, or emotional stress, vasomotor tone may be defined. The most definitive examination is angiography. This is done by passing a catheter to the level of the aortic arch through the femoral artery to permit radiographic visualization of the entire upper extremity from the origin of the major vessels to the digital tufts. Complete angiography helps to differentiate between the four major causes of upper extremity ischemia: thrombus, embolus, and vasospastic or arteriopathic disorders. When the occlusive process is predominantly in the arteries of the hand and digits, one must carefully review the angiographic studies for a site from which microemboli might have originated. The major systemic conditions that must be searched for include scleroderma and the CRST syndrome, which includes digital skin binding, telangiectasias, digital calcinosis, and Raynaud's phenomenon. The antinuclear antibody should be measured; Coombs' test coupled with serum complement should be performed; LE cells should be looked for, and SLE antibody against native DNA should be investigated. Mixed connective tissue disease can be detected by an abnormality in circulating antinuclear antibody directed against acid nuclear proteins.

SURGICAL TREATMENT. Severe hand ischemia associated with occlusive lesions of the subclavian, brachial, or antecubital arteries is the prime indication for arterial reconstruction surgery in the upper extremity. Digital arterial occlusions without proximal major arterial occlusions are not amenable to surgical intervention. The specific surgical procedures to be performed on the arterial system depend on the mechanism of occlusion and its site. Proximal reconstructive procedures are best performed using autologous tissue. Vein patches are used to close arteriotomies of arteries that are frequently smaller than those encountered in the lower extremities.

Lesions of the innominate and subclavian arteries are often amenable to bypass procedures with plastic arterial prostheses anastomosing the proximal end to the ascending aorta and the distal end to the most proximal portion of the axillary artery. The brachial and antecubital arteries are best managed either by autologous vein bypass procedures, or, where iatrogenic injury has occurred, by thrombectomy and venous patch angioplasty. Although the forearm arteries are amenable to disobliteration of embolic occlusions, it is unusual for there to be a need to perform direct arterial reconstructions on those vessels. Operations on the palmar arteries, except for small aneurysms that may have been the origin of emboli, are rarely necessary. Digital arterial reconstructions are employed for occlusion induced by acute trauma.

Sympathectomy may be of value in vasospastic disorders and will be discussed under Raynaud's Disease. Combinations of thoracic outlet decompression and arterial reconstruction are discussed under Thoracic Outlet Syndromes.

PROGNOSIS. The prognosis for a patient with a major arterial occlusion of the upper extremity, acute or chronic, is generally excellent. Recovery from an acute occlusion is generally satisfactory even without surgical intervention. When surgical intervention is required, complete or nearly complete restoration of flow is usually achieved. The vasospastic disorders infrequently require surgical intervention on the arterial system, except when small-vessel occlusions are secondary to atheroembolization, as from the subclavian artery at the thoracic outlet or from the innominate or left subclavian arteries at their origins from the aortic arch. Medical therapy is usually satisfactory in the vasospastic disorders unless the underlying metabolic disorder is rapidly progressive, in which case, digital gangrene often leads to multiple amputations. The results of sympathectomy are variable and unpredictable.

Extracranial Occlusive Cerebrovascular Disease

HISTORICAL CONSIDERATIONS. One of the most astonishing historical facts of twentieth century medicine relates to the belated recognition 35 years ago that the majority of ischemic strokes are due to occlusive atherosclerotic disease of the extracranial arteries in the neck, not to intravascular arterial occlusions. The earliest recorded recognition of this possible relationship was made by Wepfer in 1658, rediscovered by Savory in 1856, and again by Hung in 1914. The latter described the postmortem findings of infarction of a cerebral hemisphere in a patient with patent territorial (middle cerebral) arteries but a thrombosed extracranial internal carotid artery. This fact was considered to be a curiosity for almost four more decades, because of both the unavailability of techniques for studying afflicted patients in vivo and the practice of performing incomplete postmortem examinations in order to preserve the cervical carotid arteries for the injection of embalming fluid. The intracranial arteries were examined, as were the origins of the great vessels from the aortic arch, but the critical carotid bifurcation in the neck was left untouched.

The development of safe techniques for cerebral angiography, combined with careful clinical pathologic studies of the type of vascular disease in large numbers of patients with strokes, led to recognition of the frequency with which stroke syndromes were due to extracranial vascular disease. Classic studies were reported by Fischer between 1951 and 1954 and by Hutchinson and Yates in 1956.

The report of Eastcott, Pickering, and Rob documenting the successful operation for carotid bifurcation disease stimulated wide interest in the surgical management of this condition, although three groups, including Carre et al., Stuly et al., and DeBakey, claimed priority in having performed earlier operations. The first significant series in the United States was reported by Lyons and Galbraith in 1957. It was soon established that the operation of endarterectomy for carotid bifurcation atherosclerotic lesions could be performed in large numbers of afflicted individuals with a high degree of safety, in spite of the unmatched sensitivity of the brain to ischemia, and that long-term patency could be expected. The effect of the surgical approach on the natural history of stroke syndromes continues to be the subject of disagreement.

ETIOLOGY AND PATHOLOGY. Although the term *stroke* encompasses a variety of clinical situations in which major neurologic deficits occur because of involvement of the brain, the term *ischemia stroke* refers to cerebral infarction occurring as a result of impairment of regional blood flow. Atherosclerosis is the basis for this in the vast majority of patients. Smaller percentages of ischemic strokes are (1) secondary to cerebral embolization of thrombi that originate in the heart, (2) due to fibromuscular hyperplasia, (3) associated with obliterative ateritis of the great vessels as they originate from the aortic arch (see Aortic Arch Occlusive Disease, in Chap. 20), (4) due to blunt or penetrating trauma, (5) secondary to forceful hyperextension of the neck resulting in dissection and tearing of the carotid intima, and (6) due to dissecting thoracic aortic aneurysms which involve the carotid arteries.

A clinical pathologic correlation between the appearance of surgically removed plaques and the specific syndromes presented by patients operated on at New York University confirmed the early findings of Millard Fisher,

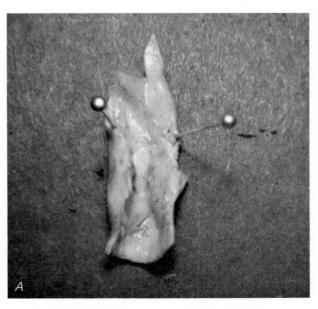

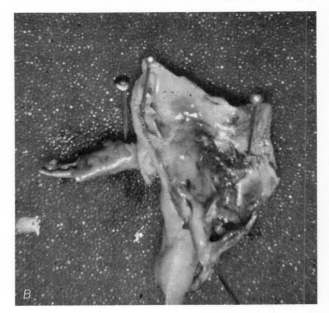

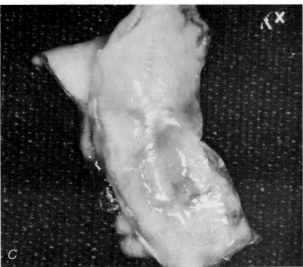

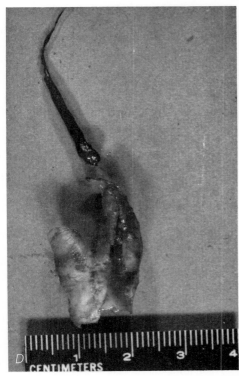

Fig. 21-19. Carotid plaque dynamics in the pathogenesis of stroke syndromes are suggested by the variation in appearance of lesions surgically removed. *A.* Smooth fibrous plaque producing marked stenosis and decreased blood flow. *B.* Ulcerated plaque giving rise to embolization. *C.* Hemorrhage into the wall of a plaque that can result in sudden stenosis or ulceration and subsequent ulceration and embolization. *D.* Total occlusion of an internal carotid artery secondary to thrombosis.

showing that patients with generalized symptoms of cerebral ischemia had major stenotic fibrotic lesions that had smooth surfaces, while those with focal symptoms were found to have plaques with either frank ulcerations or cul de sacs that were thought to be craters created when portions of the plaques broke away as emboli. Intramural hemorrhage was the most common single, pathologic finding and could be responsible for fragmentation of plaques, development of sudden stenosis, breakdown of the plaque, and subsequent thrombosis.

If patients with stroke syndromes are studied with four-vessel angiography, opacifying both carotid and both vertebral arteries from their origins to their points of entry into the skull, significant extracranial occlusive disease will be found in about 75 percent of the group. The segmental localization is impressive. In the carotid artery, almost all plaques are found at the carotid bifurcation, starting in the distal centimeter of the common carotid and involving the proximal external carotid and the proximal 1 to 2 cm of the internal carotid (Fig. 21-19). Fortu-

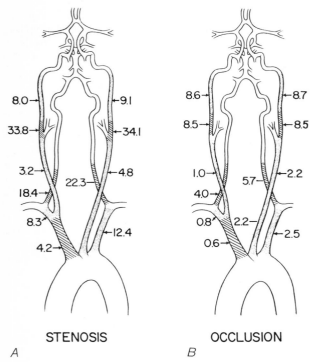

STENOSIS   OCCLUSION

A   *B*

Fig. 21-20. Frequency distribution of lesions according to anatomic locations and stenosis versus occlusion. The predominance of stenotic lesions over occlusions favors embolization as a common mechanism for the production of cerebral ischemia. The predominance of extracranial lesions renders surgical intervention feasible.

nately for surgical reconstruction, and also a striking example of segmental localization of atherosclerosis, the internal carotid beyond the first 1 to 2 cm is usually uninvolved to beyond its point of entry into the skull. The next area of predilection for plaques is at the so-called carotid siphon where the internal carotid artery curves to issue from under the dura. Because of the freedom from involvement of this portion, arterial reconstruction almost always can be done if the internal carotid is not thrombosed. Disease in the middle cerebral artery is rare. In the vertebral-basilar system, plaques are usually at the origin of the vertebrals from the subclavian, and disease of the vertebral beyond its origin is unusual. In the basilar artery localized atherosclerosis is more common. Within the thorax, the great vessels are infrequently diseased. Lesions are multiple in more than 50 percent of patients (Fig. 21-20).

Soon after the recognition of the frequency of extracranial vascular disease, it became apparent that simple reduction in cerebral blood flow from extracranial arterial stenosis and occlusions was not an adequate explanation for many of the neurologic syndromes encountered, and it now seems clear that arterioarterial embolization of fragments of plaque or platelet-fibrin aggregates is probably the most frequent mechanism of neurologic injury (Fig. 21-20). Ophthalmologic visualization of these foreign bodies suddenly appearing in the retina during transient ischemic attacks was one of the first clues to the mechanism of the syndrome. The second method for production

of symptoms is the obvious one of decrease in flow from marked stenosis or occlusion. Because of abundant collateral circulation in the brain through the circle of Willis, major arteries may become narrowed or occluded without any symptoms whatever unless multiple areas are diseased. As with stenotic lesions in the vascular system elsewhere there is little decrease in blood flow until the cross-sectional area of a vessel is narrowed by more than 75 percent. If collateral circulation is adequate, even multiple complete occlusions may be harmless. Routine postmortem studies by Martin and associates of a large group of patients dying from different causes demonstrated that in as many as 40 percent of the patients at least one of the four major extracranial arteries was significantly narrowed or occluded, even though there were no neurologic symptoms before death.

The atherosclerotic plaques removed from the vessels of symptomatic patients have varied greatly in composition and appearance. Some were principally fibrotic, with smooth internal surfaces; others showed advanced degenerative changes, with intramural hemorrhage and little stenosis, but with ulceration of the intimal surface. Plaques with a smooth intimal surface are probably harmless until the cross-sectional area of the artery is reduced to a marked degree. An ulcerated plaque, however, even though the lumen is compromised little, may cause serious or even catastrophic injury from repeated embolization or from thrombosis of the artery.

CLINICAL MANIFESTATIONS. A great variety of clinical syndromes result from the different patterns of occlusive disease in the carotid, vertebral, and subclavian arteries. These will be only briefly summarized here, for they are described in considerable detail in Millikan's excellent paper. The classic stroke from unilateral carotid disease is ipsilateral blindness and contralateral hemiplegia. The presence of aphasia depends upon involvement of the dominant cerebral hemisphere. At the other extreme are the most fleeting focal neurologic defects such as a transient monoplegia, transient hemiplegia, or transient ipsilateral blindness, viz., amaurosis fugax. These episodes, clearing within minutes to hours after an abrupt onset, are termed *transient ischemic attacks* (TIA). Between such episodes the patient may be completely well, but unfortunately such attacks often precede a catastrophic stroke. One retrospective study of patients with severe strokes found that almost 75 percent had such premonitory symptoms in the weeks or months before the stroke appeared.

Between these two extremes, TIA on the one hand and the massive stroke on the other, a wide variety of motor and sensory syndromes of varying severity and duration is seen. Various attempts at simple classification of these syndromes, such as RIND (reversible ischemic neurologic deficit), threatened stroke, stroke in evolution, and completed stroke, have been only partially successful and have led to some confusion, since not all reports use the same criteria for arriving at a classification. Their unilateral localization is strongly suggestive of carotid artery disease. They may be precipitated by hypotension, hypoxia, or changes in position or posture, or they may be unrelated to any known cause.

With disease of the vertebral-basilar system, a number

of brainstem symptoms occur. In contrast to carotid disease, the symptoms are often bilateral, involving either both arms or both legs, but may alternate in severity from one side of the body to the other. Tinnitus, dizziness, vertigo, diplopia, and dysarthria are also common. One type of characteristic syndrome is the so-called drop attack, in which the patient may literally fall to the ground with little or no warning, with or without loss of consciousness, and recover equally rapidly with only residual dizziness or mild ataxia.

Disease of the subclavian artery proximal to the origin of one of the vertebral arteries, more commonly the left, produces the so-called subclavian steal syndrome. The proximal obstruction in the subclavian artery decreases the pressure in that artery at the point of origin of the vertebral artery; this results in an actual reversal of flow in the vertebral artery, with blood draining out of the basilar artery into the arm. Although this phenomenon is seen frequently on angiographic studies, production of symptoms from ischemia of the brainstem by exercising the arm is uncommon.

Physical Examination. Examination is directed primarily at determining the presence of any neurologic deficit as well as the pattern of arterial involvement. Palpation of the carotid pulses is useful only for the rare instance of intrathoracic occlusion of the common carotid artery. Palpation for the internal carotid pulse in the pharynx posterior to the tonsillar pillars is no longer advised. Separate palpation of the external and internal carotid arteries is impossible because of their location next to one another. Hence, the carotid pulses are normal on palpation in almost all patients with occlusive disease at the carotid bifurcation. Auscultation over the carotid bifurcation for a bruit is essential because a bruit is audible just anterior to the sternocleidomastoid muscle near the level of the angle of the mandible in a significant number of patients with stenosis. Auscultation in the supraclavicular fossae may reveal bruits from subclavian-vertebral disease. When bruits are detected, they must be differentiated from murmurs of cardiac valvular lesions, such as aortic stenosis, that are transmitted along the great vessels into the neck. If occlusive disease of a subclavian artery is present, the blood pressures will be significantly different in the two arms.

A number of noninvasive techniques are useful for evaluating the condition of the carotid bifurcations not only in patients with bruits but also as screening techniques in otherwise healthy individuals. The most useful of these are duplex scanning, oculoplethysmography, and B-mode ultrasound imaging.

DIAGNOSIS. The differential diagnosis of cerebrovascular insufficiency syndromes is extremely complex and involves exclusion of a variety of intracranial lesions in addition to generalized conditions that can effect cerebral hypoxia. The latter include myocardial infarction, cardiac arrhythmias, Adams-Stokes-syndrome, Menière's disease, and a number of metabolic disorders, such as diabetic ketosis and hypoglycemia.

The diagnosis of ischemic stroke syndromes ultimately depends upon angiographic delineation of the intra- and extracranial cerebral arteries (Fig. 21-21). The greatest

risks related to angiography generally are assumed by the patients most seriously afflicted with arterial disease, particularly those who have already developed serious neurologic deficits. The overall risk of stroke or death incident to cerebral angiography is about 0.5 to 1 percent. Less serious complications, such as hematomas and temporary or permanent loss of arterial pulses distal to puncture sites, occur with greater frequency.

Patients with amaurosis fugax, transient paralysis or weakness of the extremity, weakness of facial muscles, and transient disorders of speech all require more extensive investigation to rule out nonischemic causes, but the ultimate study in these patients is cerebral angiography to delineate the aortic arch and its major branches to their intracranial terminations.

Timing of the angiographic study may be critical. Those patients with transient neurologic deficits may have their studies performed as soon as possible; patients who have suffered profound and extensive neurologic insult, especially if associated with altered consciousness, should have radiographic studies postponed, because if these are performed during the first week of illness, the complication rate is excessive.

The finding of asymptomatic bruits on routine physical examination introduces the need to make difficult decisions. The study by Thompson, in which patients with asymptomatic bruits were shown to have "significant" lesions by angiography and appeared to be protected from future stroke by operative intervention, suggests a more aggressive attitude. A number of other studies, however, suggest that patients with carotid bruits may not be at great risk of stroke during the performance of unrelated operative procedures that are considered to increase stroke risk. Indeed, those who suffered strokes during major operations were those who did not have bruits, raising a number of questions relating to how best to identify stroke-prone individuals and the factors that precipitate cerebral infarction. At the other end of the spectrum are patients with asymptomatic carotid stenoses, discovered either during screening noninvasive studies or investigation of carotid bruits. Computed tomography of the brain has revealed that a number of these patients have suffered silent cerebral infarcts and that this group should have angiographic studies.

The attitude of the authors of this chapter toward asymptomatic bruits, in the face of conflicting data, is to study angiographically those patients who appear to have hemodynamically significant lesions when tested by oculoplethysmography or by duplex scan and who are physiologically fit and thought to have long life expectancies. Operations are offered to patients who have 70 percent stenosis or lesions with irregular contour. Prior to a major intraabdominal or intrathoracic procedure, these patients are studied routinely by duplex scanning of the carotid arteries.

TREATMENT. General Considerations. The Joint Study of Extracranial Arterial Occlusion as a Cause of Stroke clearly shows that to be effective, surgical treatment must be performed before major neurologic deficits are produced from cerebral infarction. Operations are generally performed on patients who have had transient ischemic

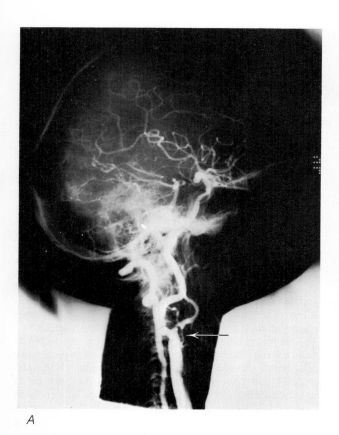

A

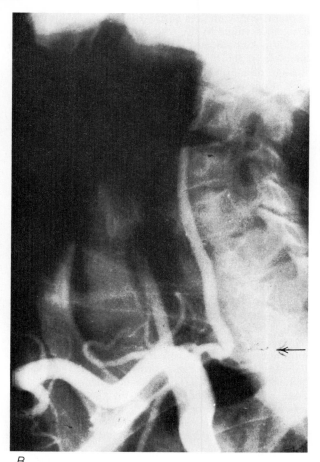

B

Fig. 21-21. Angiographic studies of the cerebral circulation for stroke syndromes should outline the major extracranial as well as the intracranial arteries. This facilitates planning operative procedures and aids in making differential diagnoses of the various causes of stroke syndromes. Cervical carotid and vertebral arteries are outlined by retrograde right brachial arterial injection. *A.* Arrow points to significant lesion in the internal and external carotids. *B.* Arrow points to typical stenotic lesion at the origin of the vertebral with an associated kink.

attacks and carotid lesions that produce 50 to 70 percent stenosis or have irregular contours. Operation upon patients with acute strokes has been associated with a high mortality, considerably higher than that for patients treated medically. Recently, however, this conclusion has been challenged, and certain patients with acute strokes have been successfully operated upon with marked neurologic improvement. Thromboendarterectomy for totally occluded internal carotid arteries in patients with acute neurologic deficits, a procedure previously considered unsafe because of the occurrence of intracerebral hemorrhage resulting from restoration of arterial perfusion through areas of infarcted cerebrum, is now judged feasible by some and has been shown to reverse relatively severe neurologic deficits.

As the prevalence of arterioarterial embolization in the production of stroke syndromes has become clear, there has been renewed interest in altering the coagulability of the blood. Heparin, as therapy for transient cerebral ischemic episodes of increasing frequency, does not appear to decrease the incidence of stroke in patients with high-grade carotid stenoses. Oral anticoagulants may decrease the incidence of TIAs, but not of completed strokes, and are associated with a considerable risk of hemorrhage. The striking finding of the influence of acetylsalicylic acid

on platelet aggregation may be of considerable therapeutic significance. Clinical trials employing aspirin and other antiplatelet drugs have also failed to yield clear-cut results about protection from stroke. One study reported by Bousser, considered definitive, suffers from protocol defects shared by other studies. Angiographic studies to define the presence of extracranial arterial lesions were not performed. The entire spectrum of ischemic cerebral disease was not studied. Only selected and clearly defined clinical categories were included, and patients with tight carotid stenoses were excluded.

An additional question has been raised regarding the universal use of anticoagulant and antiplatelet drugs in patients who exhibit intraplaque hemorrhage resulting in significant stenosis and ulceration. It has been suggested that antithrombotic agents might aggravate such hemorrhages.

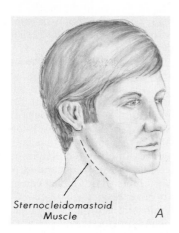

Sternocleidomastoid Muscle

A

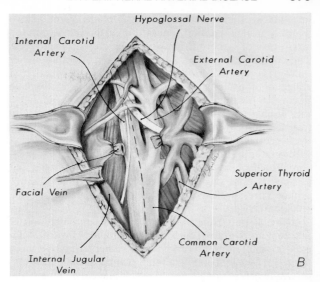

Internal Carotid Artery

Hypoglossal Nerve

External Carotid Artery

Facial Vein

Superior Thyroid Artery

Internal Jugular Vein

Common Carotid Artery

B

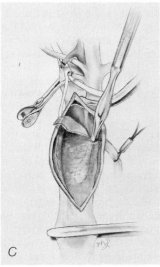

C

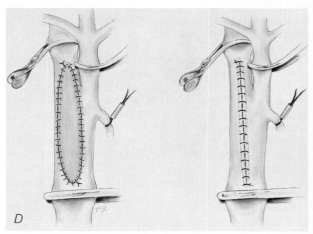

D

Fig. 21-22. Technique of carotid endarterectomy. *A*. A skin incision is made anterior to the sternocleidomastoid muscle. *B*. The carotid artery branches are widely mobilized. The internal carotid artery is clamped before widely mobilizing the frequently thrombus-containing bulb, thereby protecting the brain from embolization, which may occur during the dissection. The vagus and hypoglossal nerves are carefully protected. Mobilization of the hypoglossal is facilitated by dividing the sternocleidomastoid artery and vein. A longitudinal arteriotomy is made extending above and below the plaque at the carotid bifurcation. *C*. After division of the intima above the plaque, the plaque can be easily dissected from the underlying media or from the adventitia. The distal intima is carefully inspected and sutured if necessary. *D*. The arteriotomy is either closed primarily with 5-0 Tevdek, or a vein roof patch fashioned from autologous saphenous vein is used to avoid producing stenosis. The technique for restoring flow after completion of the closure is crucial to avoid embolization to the brain. The internal carotid clamp is temporarily removed and reapplied. The common and external carotid clamps are removed, and after 1 or 2 min of flushing of the carotid bulb the internal carotid clamp is removed.

Atherosclerotic Disease of the Internal Carotid Artery. Atherosclerosis of the origin of the internal carotid artery is the most common form of extracranial vascular disease. Involvement is limited to the first 1 to 2 cm of the origin of the internal carotid and hence is ideal for surgical correction (Fig. 21-21).

When complete occlusion develops in the carotid artery, an organized thrombus develops above the atherosclerotic plaque and extends superiorly into the intracranial internal carotid, making successful operation impossible. In approximately 10 percent of patients with complete occlusion, the thrombus has not propagated more than 2 to 3 cm, and surgical removal is still possible.

The ideal patient for operation is one with TIAs who has been shown to have significant carotid bifurcation disease producing either hemodynamically significant stenosis or marked irregularity of the contour of the arteries at the carotid bulb, without any permanent neurologic abnormality. In such patients operation can be performed with a variety of anesthetic techniques. Mortality and major neurologic complications are in the range of 1 to 4 percent, the risk factors having been defined by a number of authors. Details of the operation are shown in Fig. 21-22.

The hazards of operation are greater and the likelihood of benefit much less when a stroke has occurred. If the internal carotid has become totally occluded, producing a major neurologic deficit, operation performed within 6 h after onset of symptoms may produce dramatic recovery. The operative mortality, however, is considerably higher than with elective operations, especially with altered states of consciousness. If operation is delayed much beyond 6 h after the onset of symptoms, reopening a totally obstructed carotid artery may be followed first by transient improvement, then worsening of symptoms and even death from hemorrhage into the area of infarction precipitated by the restoration of arterial perfusion pressure. It has been suggested by Warren and Triedman that this catastrophe might be prevented by careful avoidance of blood pressure elevation during operation and for some weeks afterward.

If the acute stroke has resulted from embolization of atheromatous debris or platelet aggregates, with occlusion of small intracerebral vessels, emergency operation upon the nonstenosing ulcerated plaque at the carotid bifurcation is not immediately helpful, and carotid clamping might worsen the neurologic deficit. At a later time such patients should be considered for operation to prevent future embolization if the permanent neurologic deficit is not severe.

In patients with chronic strokes in whom acute injury weeks or months earlier produced a permanent neurologic deficit indicative of total hemispheric infarction, operation is of little value. If, however, the neurologic deficit does not indicate total hemispheric dysfunction, operation to prevent additional injury from repeated embolization has been of value. A challenging group consists of asymptomatic patients with loud bruits. Thompson et al. have reported a lowered stroke incidence in such patients if angiographic studies revealed significant carotid lesions.

Following endarterectomy of the stenotic carotid artery, the likelihood of long-term patency of the reconstructed artery is excellent. Early occlusion is due to neointimal hyperplasia; occlusion occurring years postoperatively is due to atherosclerosis.

The effect of prophylactic carotid endarterectomy in altering the incidence of mortality in future stroke has been analyzed in detail by the Joint Study. Although the results of the study were not completely definitive, certain facts emerged. The natural history of the disease definitely can be changed if the operative mortality and stroke rate can be kept at low levels (1 to 5 percent). Those patients with the most severe and extensive involvement, that is to say, those with bilateral carotid lesions or with stenosis opposite complete occlusion, who survive operations enjoy the greatest protection from future stroke and from death from stroke. Strokes in the neurologic area corresponding to the surgically repaired artery are markedly reduced.

In our own series of nearly 2500 carotid operations performed in conscious patients, the perioperative stroke rate has been 2.5 percent, varying from 1.1 percent in patients who were neurologically intact and had bilaterally patent arteries, to 7.7 percent in patients who had contralateral carotid stenosis and failed to tolerate carotid clamping, requiring temporary shunts. Late follow up, indicates a reduction in stroke rate. This reduction in stroke rate is reported to range from 30 to 300 percent for 5 years.

Subclavian-Vertebral Disease. Stenosis involving only the vertebral artery is infrequent. It is physiologically significant only when bilateral or if one vertebral is congenitally hypoplastic or absent. The disease is frequently limited to the site of origin of the vertebral from the subclavian. The atherosclerotic plaques in this area usually have a smooth intimal surface, in contrast to the frequency of ulcerated plaques in the carotid artery. On occasion, however, ulcerated plaques at the origin of the vertebral arteries have been encountered and are thought to have been the source of emboli that produce focal brainstem neurologic deficits. In addition, there are frequently tortuous kinks in the first few centimeters of the vertebral artery that can be shown to result in total occlusion when the head is turned to one side. Symptoms are probably due to decreased flow through the basivertebral system, although embolization cannot be entirely excluded. Concomitant disease in the basilar artery is frequent.

Atherosclerotic stenosis or occlusion of the subclavian artery proximal to the site of origin of the vertebral artery produces the clinical picture termed the *subclavian steal syndrome* and on occasion, embolization to the brainstem arteries. The former abnormality was well defined by Reivich et al. in 1961, following an angiographic description in 1960 by Contorni of retrograde flow in the involved vertebral artery. The reduction in pressure in the subclavian artery beyond the stenosis results in retrograde flow from the brainstem down the vertebral artery to the arm, hence the term "subclavian steal." The clinical picture is that of ischemic neurologic symptoms in association with mild ischemia in the involved arm. Diagnosis can be easily made by finding a decreased pulse and blood pressure in the symptomatic arm, often in association with a localized bruit in the supraclavicular space. Serial angiograms after injection of contrast media into the opposite brachial artery or the ascending aorta will demonstrate reversal of flow in the involved vertebral artery by initially opacifying the opposite vertebral artery in a normal fashion, followed by retrograde opacification of the involved vertebral. Although this phenomenon is not infrequent on angiographic examination, clinical symptoms are not common, perhaps because collateral circulation in the brain can readily compensate for the amount of blood diverted away from the brain by the retrograde vertebral flow.

Operations upon the vertebral artery usually can be performed without thoracotomy. Surgical exposure of the subclavian-vertebral junction is obtained through a transverse supraclavicular incision that divides the clavicular head of the sternocleidomastoid muscle and the underlying scalenus anticus muscle. If the stenosing plaque has a smooth intimal surface, endarterectomy may not be necessary. The artery can be simply widened with a patch angioplasty with autologous saphenous vein. If the vertebral artery is significantly tortuous and redundant, predisposing to kinking, plication can be performed. In 120 arterial reconstructions of vertebral arteries performed by the authors, only 1 postoperative stroke was encountered. Late follow-up, without a comparable control series, reveals a remarkably low stroke rate of about 1 percent per patient follow-up year and normal survival for the age group involved.

Operations for the subclavian steal syndrome are seldom necessary. When done, a transthoracic approach to the subclavian artery can be avoided by employing a bypass graft from the ipsilateral common carotid artery to the distal subclavian artery. This is physiologically possible because the common carotid is large enough to deliver sufficient blood to supply both the brain and the upper extremity. On occasion, when the common carotid or innominate arteries are markedly stenotic and not suitable, axilloaxillary bypass grafting has been useful. Reimplantation of the distal end of the transected subclavian artery to the side of the common carotid is also described.

Aortic Arch Occlusive Disease. Occlusive disease of the major branches of the aortic arch was described as a clinical syndrome by Savory in 1854; it is due to atherosclerosis in this country. In the Orient it occurs in young women, is due to an arteritis, and is known by the eponym "Takayasu's disease," named for the ophthalmologist who described it. Syphilitic arteritis, formerly a common cause, is now most unusual.

Although symptoms are apt to be mild due to the very proximal location of the occlusive process, permitting many pathways for collateral circulation, ischemic symptoms of the upper extremities or the brain can occur. Unless severe ischemic symptoms appear or symptoms that threaten brain function occur, surgical intervention is not indicated. Operative intervention, of necessity, must be via thoracotomy with the use of multiple bypass grafts from the ascending aorta proximally to the carotid or subclavian arteries distally since endarterectomy procedures are usually not possible. Thoracotomy may be avoided in those instances in which one of the arch vessels is spared and a cervical carotid-subclavian bypass can be performed. The theoretic objection that siphoning of blood from a normal artery to a diseased artery may produce a steal syndrome has not been manifest. In one large series, operative mortality was 5 percent, and successful revascularization was achieved in the majority of patients.

ANEURYSMS

Aneurysm can be defined as the inappropriate dilation of an artery. This dilation can involve the entire circumference of the artery and results in a *fusiform* appearance of the artery. It can also be focal, causing a bubblelike projection of the arterial wall and producing a *saccular* appearance. The so-called dissecting aneurysm of the aorta is a misnomer because the primary process is a longitudinal splitting of the layers of the arterial wall, which often results in fusiform and sometimes in saccular dilation of the artery. Fusiform aneurysms are usually secondary to arteriosclerosis and are infrequently due to dis-

section secondary to medial necrosis, as in Marfan's syndrome. Saccular aneurysms may be due to a variety of causes, including trauma, infection, and fibromuscular hyperplasia. Fusiform aneurysms require prosthetic replacement to restore or to maintain arterial continuity; saccular aneurysms may be treated by resection and angioplastic closure of the involved artery.

Aneurysms can further be classified as *true aneurysms* when all the layers of the arterial wall contribute to the dilation and as *false aneurysms* when only a fibrous sac exists. The fibrous sac results from a tangential hole in an artery and the organization of a contained hematoma.

Several milestones in vascular surgery evolved as a consequence of the treatment of aneurysms. In the second century A.D., Antyllus treated an arterial aneurysm by ligature immediately above and below the lesion, followed by incision of the aneurysm, evacuation of the clot, and exteriorization of the cavity. John Hunter, in 1786, electively ligated a femoral artery proximal to a popliteal aneurysm to minimize blood loss during subsequent attempts at extirpation. The anatomic term *Hunter's canal* originated from this surgical episode. In 1888 Rudolph Matas described his operation of endoaneurysmorrhaphy, in which the aneurysm is widely opened and the communications with the parent artery are sutured. This imaginative approach promptly became the standard treatment and was modified little during the next 55 years. Subsequently, as techniques of vascular reconstruction developed and prosthetic conduits became available, modern procedures evolved.

Abdominal Aortic Aneurysms

HISTORICAL DATA. The modern era of treatment of abdominal aneurysms began with the first successful excision of an abdominal aneurysm and replacement with an aortic homograft by Dubost in 1951. Previous therapeutic efforts, such as wiring to promote clotting and wrapping or coating with plastics, and other techniques to include thrombosis, are principally of historic interest. Techniques to promote thrombosis of the aneurysm have been reintroduced, combined with extraanatomic bypass procedures to maintain flow to the lower extremities in poorrisk patients.

INCIDENCE. Abdominal aneurysms, the most common of the arteriosclerotic aneurysms, are increasing in frequency as a consequence of our aging population. Men are affected more frequently than women, in a ratio approximating 10:1.

ETIOLOGY AND PATHOLOGY. The vast majority of abdominal aneurysms are arteriosclerotic in origin, with their pathogenesis probably different from occlusive atherosclerosis. Aneurysms result from degenerative changes in the media, while atherosclerotic occlusion results from a proliferative reaction in the media causing narrowing of the arterial lumen. The distribution of the two processes is different, the atherosclerotic occlusive process involving the aorta at sites of bifurcations, attachments, tapers, and curvatures, while aneurysmal disease has its own characteristic patterns of involvement.

The authors have never seen an abdominal aneurysm arising below the renal arteries from any cause except arteriosclerosis, although they have been reported from syphilis, trauma, Marfan's syndrome, and bacterial endocarditis.

The anatomic location of abdominal aneurysms makes them accessible to surgical therapy, for a graft can be inserted proximally from the abdominal aorta below the renal arteries to the common iliac arteries distad. The size of abdominal aneurysms varies greatly, small ones 2 to 3 cm in diameter being detected accidentally by aortography, sonography, or computed tomography (CT) of the abdomen, while others may enlarge to a diameter of 10 to 15 cm before being discovered accidentally by palpation. The usual course of untreated aneurysms was well documented in the classic report by Estes in 1950. Without treatment there is a 20 percent chance of rupture within 1 year after diagnosis and a 50 percent chance within 4 or 5 years. Complications seldom arise from expanding aneurysms until rupture occurs. Erosion of bone, so common in syphilitic aneurysms, virtually never occurs with arteriosclerotic aneurysms. There is usually no impairment of peripheral circulation unless distal embolization from the shaggy laminated thrombus lining the lumen occurs.

Although aneurysms frequently originate within 1 to 2 cm of the origin of the renal arteries, actual involvement of the origin of the renal arteries in the aneurysm, necessitating reconstruction of the renal arteries during surgical excision, is unusual. In a series of over 170 abdominal aneurysms at the Johns Hopkins Hospital, only 3 aneurysms involving the renal arteries were found.

Adherence to neighboring structures, with the exception of the inferior vena cava and the iliac veins, is unusual unless the lesion is classified as an "inflammatory aneurysm." In this situation there is an intensive adventitial fibroplastic reaction frequently extending from the common iliacs to the origin of the renal arteries. The 3rd and 4th portions of the duodenum and the ureters become firmly attached, making their separation particularly hazardous. Involvement of the renal arteries by this reaction simulates a suprarenal aneurysm when in reality the true aneurysm begins below the level of the renals. Preoperatively the true anatomic involvement is suggested by the CT scan of the abdominal aorta and can be confirmed by aortography to include lateral views.

An abdominal aneurysm is often associated with generalized atherosclerosis. In a series of 1400 patients, some signs of coronary artery disease were present in 30 percent of the patients, and 40 percent of the patients had some increase in systolic blood pressure. Associated occlusive disease of the carotid arteries was found in 7 percent, of the renal arteries in 2 percent, and of the iliac arteries in 16 percent of the patients. Concomitant clinically significant aneurysms were found in the thoracic aorta in 4 percent, in the femoral artery in 3 percent, and in the popliteal artery in 2 percent of the group.

CLINICAL MANIFESTATIONS. Symptoms. Most patients are unaware of their abdominal aneurysms until a mass is discovered by the patient or the physician. The importance of careful deep palpation of the abdomen, outlining the abdominal aorta when possible, is obvious. Occasionally, low back pain caused by an abdominal aneurysm may be diagnosed erroneously as due to an orthopaedic condition. The pain apparently arises from tension on retroperitoneal tissues from the aneurysm; erosion of bone almost never occurs. Virtually any intraabdominal condition may be simulated by an abdominal aortic aneurysm, including renal colic, acute appendicitis, diverticulitis, peptic ulcer, pancreatitis, or cholecystitis. Rarely, there is gastrointestinal bleeding from erosion into the duodenum as the presenting manifestation. With beginning leakage of the aneurysm or frank rupture momentarily contained retroperitoneally, acute abdominal conditions such as perforated ulcer, hemorrhagic pancreatitis, or generalized peritonitis may be simulated.

Sometimes, sudden vascular collapse with shock is the first indication. Most patients, however, have some premonitory symptoms prior to rupture. The absence of signs preceding fatal rupture is a strong reason for removing most abdominal aneurysms as soon as the diagnosis is made, even though the condition is asymptomatic. Symptoms from an aneurysm are an urgent indication for operation and are sometimes called a *syndrome of impending rupture*.

Physical Examination. An abdominal aneurysm larger than 5 cm in diameter can be diagnosed with reasonable certainty. Once the patient has relaxed the muscles of the abdominal wall, careful deep palpation can usually outline the abdominal aorta near the bifurcation, generally slightly inferior to the umbilicus. The aorta may be traced proximally into the upper abdomen, where it is concealed beneath the pancreas and transverse colon. A normal aorta is seldom over an inch in diameter. Careful palpation can usually distinguish the lateral walls of the aorta and hence provide an estimate of the width. Finding a pulsating mass greater than an inch in diameter should raise the suspicion that an aneurysm is present.

Confusion may arise in thin females with diastasis of the rectus muscles in whom the aortic pulsations are abnormally prominent. This is particularly true if an increased pulse pressure is present. Such patients may come to the physician because of concern over the prominent pulsations, and vague tenderness may be elicited in palpating the aorta. Almost always careful palpation will demonstrate that the aorta is of normal diameter but when palpation is uncertain, an echogram or CT of the abdomen may be required to exclude the presence of a small aneurysm. In the majority of patients palpation either establishes or excludes the diagnosis.

Peripheral pulses should be carefully examined, for associated occlusive vascular disease may be present due to embolization from the aneurysm or occlusive atherosclerosis. The presence of a bruit over the bifurcation of the carotid arteries is particularly significant, because an asymptomatic stenosis of a carotid artery can significantly increase the risk of hypotension occurring during operation.

Laboratory Studies. A radiograph of the abdomen, including anteroposterior and lateral views, will establish the diagnosis in many patients by demonstrating calcifica-

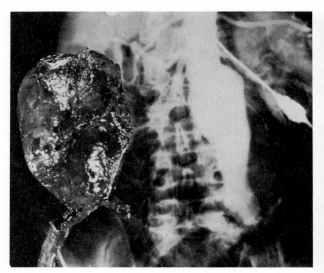

A

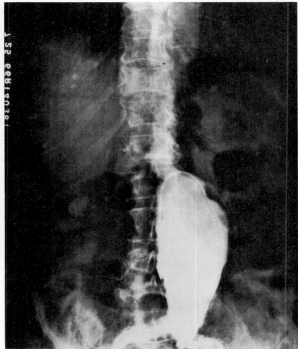

B

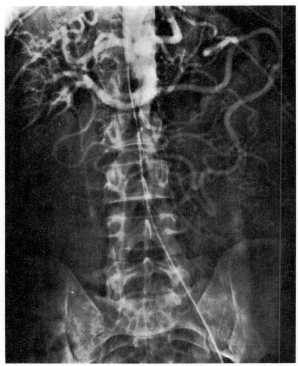

C

Fig. 21-23. *A.* Aortogram showing abdominal aneurysm in the distal aorta. Superimposed on the film is a photograph of a lesion excised at operation, indicating the large laminated clot filling the aneurysm. *(Courtesy of Dr. Henry T. Bahnson, Department of Surgery, University of Pittsburgh.) B.* Anteroposterior lumbar aortogram performed by percutaneous introduction of an arterial catheter, illustrating a large abdominal aneurysm arising in the lower abdominal aorta. Linear calcification of the lower thoracic and upper abdominal aorta is also visible. *C.* Abdominal aortogram in a patient with atherosclerotic occlusion of the abdominal aorta that has extended up to the level of the renal arteries. The superior mesenteric artery is visible as well as the right renal artery. Extensive collateral circulation has developed, particularly in the left flank.

tion in the wall of the aneurysm. The lateral view is particularly helpful, since it permits visualization of the usually thin calcific rim of the aneurysm wall, which may be obscured by the shadows of the vertebral bodies in the frontal projections. An estimate of the size of the aneurysm is obtainable by measuring the distance from the anterior border of the vertebral bodies to the calcium in the anterior wall of the aneurysm and making the appropriate correction for the usual 20 percent magnification produced by the diverging x-rays. The uppermost extent of the aneurysm can often be determined from this view. If combined with left lateral views of the chest it permits recognition of upper abdominal and thoracoabdominal aneurysms. A rapid-sequence excretory urogram may also be useful in detecting renal involvement. The use of ultrasound and especially CT helps to delineate aneurysms more accurately and helps to establish the true size of the aneurysm. This is especially important with aneurysms 4 to 6 cm in diameter where knowledge of true size may be critical in establishing the need for operation.

Aortography (Fig. 21-23) is used infrequently by us because of the small but definite risk it entails and because the diagnosis can usually be established by other means. In addition, a laminated thrombus within the aneurysm may mark the true size of the lesion. Formerly, it was thought that in order to establish relationship of the renal arteries to the aneurysm, aortography was essential, but accumulated experience has found renal artery involvement in only about 1 percent of patients, and CT may provide this information. Nevertheless, some highly experienced vascular groups insist upon performing angiographic studies on all abdominal aortic aneurysm patients to delineate associated vascular lesions. It has not been shown that this has resulted in either increased survival or decreased morbidity, but angiography does result in a higher incidence of incidental operations on the renal and mesenteric arteries.

Our own preference is to perform aortography only for specific indications, avoiding it in the majority of patients. These indications include uncertainty of diagnosis in the presence of small aneurysms (Fig. 21-23), the suspicion of an extensive lesion involving the upper abdominal and thoracic aorta as well, the presence of lower extremity arterial occlusions manifested by absent pulses or to define the extent of the lesion if the existence of an inflammatory aneurysm is suspected. Markedly depressed renal function or uncontrolled hypertension, though somewhat increasing the risk of aortography, are additional indications for this diagnostic procedure.

TREATMENT. Indications for Operation. Aneurysms smaller than 5 cm in diameter can be relatively safely observed unless they expand or become symptomatic. An asymptomatic aneurysm measuring at least 5 to 6 cm in diameter constitutes an indication for operation unless there are other conditions that either markedly increase the operative risk or promise to markedly shorten life expectancy. Asymptomatic aneurysms smaller than 5 to 6 cm are usually considered to carry a very small risk of rupture, while those 5 to 6 cm and larger carry at least a 20 percent yearly risk of rupture. There is very little correlation between the size of the asymptomatic aneurysms beyond 5 to 6 cm, the absence of symptoms, and the tendency to rupture, although the peak incidence of rupture has been reported to occur in 7 cm aneurysms. Operative mortality with a ruptured aneurysm is nearly ten times greater than that for elective excision.

On the other hand, when the aneurysm becomes painful, operation ceases to be elective, for pain often denotes either rupture or impending rupture. The pain may be located in the back, the flank, or the abdominal region and may vary in both intensity and character, simulating many other intraabdominal and musculoskeletal conditions. Abdominal tenderness should increase the suspicion of impending or frank rupture. In such situations the indications for operation are extended to include conditions that might otherwise preclude an elective operation.

Preoperative evaluation to estimate surgical risk, which can then be compared to the risk of rupture of the aneurysm, is critical. Operative mortality for elective aneurysm operations is most often related to acute myocardial infarction. Although many different criteria have been described to determine cardiac risk, we have found estimation of the left ventricular ejection fraction the single most useful parameter. When that fraction is below 35 percent, the risk that the patient will suffer an acute myocardial infarction is 85 percent. Such patients are evaluated with coronary angiography with a view to performing myocardial revascularization prior to or simultaneously with abdominal aortic aneurysm repair. Patients with ejection fractions between 35 and 50 percent, who would experience a 20 percent risk of acute myocardial infarction, are individually evaluated regarding the severity of angina pectoris and the persistence of ischemic ECG changes. This is done to help determine the need for coronary angiography. Those with ejection fractions greater than 50 percent have minimal cardiac risk.

Some surgeons routinely perform coronary angiography prior to abdominal aortic operations and are guided by the distribution and extent of the coronary atherosclerosis in determining which condition should be corrected first. This probably results in too many prophylactic coronary artery operations and has led to aneurysm rupture during the recovery phase from the prophylactic coronary operation.

Excretory urography and especially creatinine clearance studies have been useful. Clearances greater than 30 mL/min usually indicate that there is sufficient renal function for the patient to undergo operation. When lesser levels of clearance are encountered, renal angiography is performed to detect possibly correctable renal lesions.

Duplex scanning of the carotid arteries may be performed to detect flow-impeding lesions that are sometimes corrected prior to the aneurysm operation. Pulmonary function, coagulation, and platelet studies are also valuable in planning operations.

Technique of Operation for Abdominal Aneurysms. The operative procedure for excision of abdominal aneurysms is illustrated in Fig. 21-24. In addition to the obvious risk of hemorrhage, which is avoidable with careful technique, there are several common hazards. These include infection, renal failure, declamping shock, peripheral embolization to lower extremity arteries, and ischemic necrosis of the colon. Infection of a plastic prosthesis is an ever-present and serious complication. It may be prevented by meticulous aseptic technique and by the administration of large doses of antibiotics, preoperatively, during the operation, and for about 5 days postoperatively. Irreversible renal failure has virtually been eliminated (except in the presence of ruptured aneurysm) by careful attention to renal function during the entire operative procedure, especially during the phase of aortic clamping. Normal quarter-hourly urine output is achieved by carefully maintaining normal cardiodynamics and state of hydrations, replacing lost blood promptly, and administering electrolyte solutions to compensate for the known fluid shifts that occur intraoperatively. Diuretics are administered only to evaluate the function of the kidneys if anuria is encountered; fluid boluses or low molecular-weight dextran may be used to expand circulating volume rapidly. An intrapulmonary catheter of the Swan-Ganz type is an invaluable aid in determining normal cardiodynamics and states of hydration.

Declamping hypotension is related to several factors, such as duration of aortic occlusion, adequacy of blood volume, and degree of collateral circulation to the lower extremities. While the aorta is occluded, the lower extremities are relatively ischemic, as a result of which there is pooling of blood in dilated vessels and accumulation of ischemic products of metabolism. If the aorta is unclamped suddenly when ischemia has been severe, profound hypotension, cardiac arrhythmias, and even cardiac arrest can occur. Such problems can be almost completely avoided by different techniques. Hypotension is uncommon if the aorta is occluded for less than 1 h. After longer periods, gradual restoration of the circulation is useful. An effective approach is as follows: Once the proximal aortic anastomosis and one iliac anastomosis have been completed and the system has been flushed antegrade and retrograde to clear clot and atheromatous debris, flow is restored to the ipsilateral hypogastric artery, permitting gradual reopening of the circulation. When adjustment has occurred, the ipsilateral external iliac artery is similarly unclamped while anastomoses are performed on the contralateral side, and the same sequence is repeated. In a series of 750 aortic aneurysm operations reported by Imparato et al., declamping shock did not occur with this technique, vasopressors were not needed, and sodium bicarbonate was not required.

Distal embolization of atherosclerotic or thrombotic debris can be particularly hazardous, varying with the friability of the contents of the aneurysm. The following guidelines are useful: The external and internal iliac arteries are mobilized and occluded before the aorta is clamped proximally. At this time 5000 units of heparin is given intravenously. Subsequently, as the individual iliac anastomoses are completed, retrograde flushing of the iliac arteries is allowed to occur. If this cannot be accomplished, a rubber catheter is passed into the external iliac arteries in order to gently pry apart the walls that may have been deformed by application of arterial clamps. Fogarty catheters are not routinely passed into the distal arteries because, if aneurysmal disease is present in the femoral and popliteal arteries or if there is atherosclerosis, a thrombus or plaque may be dislodged. The selective iliac "flush" technique described above has been very effective. Finally, at the conclusion of the operation, the peripheral pulses are examined to be certain that they are the same as before operation.

Ischemic injury of the colon can be avoided by dissecting within the wall of the aneurysm rather than outside it and ligating the inferior mesenteric artery at its origin, carefully avoiding injury to any collateral vessels in the mesentery of the left colon. The technique of removing only the inner portion of the aneurysm, leaving the adventitial sheath, facilitates dissection, avoids injury to adjacent structures such as the vena cava, and provides a soft-tissue covering of the prosthesis to prevent subsequent erosion of the duodenum or other structures. When the inferior mesenteric artery has been ligated, at least one hypogastric artery must be preserved to maintain collateral circulation to the colon through the middle hemorrhoidal arteries. If one or both hypogastric arteries have been ligated, either transplanting to the aortic prosthesis a button of aneurysm wall containing the inferior mesenteric artery or bypassing from the prosthesis to the infe-

rior mesenteric artery should be performed. With these guidelines, significant ischemic injury of the colon is very rare, occurring probably only when atherosclerosis has compromised the collateral circulation. If ischemic injury is suspected, however, then a "second-look" laparotomy procedure 24 h later is indicated to detect irreversible colon ischemia before bowel perforation and peritonitis occur.

An alternative technique to abdominal aortic aneurysm operation has been a retroperitoneal approach that avoids manipulation of the abdominal viscera. Postoperative recovery is said to be smoother by avoiding the problems of prolonged intestinal atony. For patients who present with apparently prohibitive risks for intraabdominal operations, Leather et al. have described a procedure in which the common iliac arteries are ligated through small groin incisions, thereby promoting thrombosis of the aneurysm. Flow to the lower extremities is maintained by performing axillofemoral, femorofemoral bypasses with plastic prostheses. On occasion it is necessary to occlude lumbar arteries by injecting various types of glues through catheters passed by way of the brachial arteries into the aneurysm itself. It has recently been reported that aneurysms so treated can still rupture unless the infrarenal aorta has also been ligated, thereby decreasing the usefulness of the procedure.

Postoperative Complications. The operative mortality for elective excision of an abdominal aneurysm approaches 2 percent. It varies with the age of the patient and the degree of associated coronary atherosclerosis. Atelectasis, pneumonia, and cardiac arrhythmias are relatively common. Fluid balance must be carefully monitored to avoid congestive heart failure. Nasogastric intubation is required for 4 to 5 days, and if bowel function has not resumed, mechanical intestinal obstruction, which can usually be managed by intestinal intubation, should be suspected. The occurrence of bowel movements during the first 24 to 72 h should raise the suspicion of ischemic colitis, often detectable by the testing of stool for blood. Renal function is estimated from the volume of urinary output and changes in blood chemistry in order to detect the rare instance of progressive renal failure that may be due to a variety of causes, one being embolization to renal arteries during the operative procedure. Lower extremity ischemia associated with loss of previously palpable pedal pulses demands prompt reoperation to remove embolic material originating in the operative site from limb arteries.

With careful management recovery from most elective aneurysm operations is relatively uneventful.

PROGNOSIS. The reported 5-year survival following resection of abdominal aneurysms has varied from 30 to 60 percent. Fatalities are usually due to cardiac or cerebral complications of atherosclerosis. Complications from the prosthetic graft are unusual. The most frequent of these is development of a false aneurysm, often at the proximal suture line, with subsequent rupture or erosion into the duodenum. The possibility of this can be minimized by suturing the prosthesis to the immediate infrarenal aorta that is usually not aneurysmal and covering

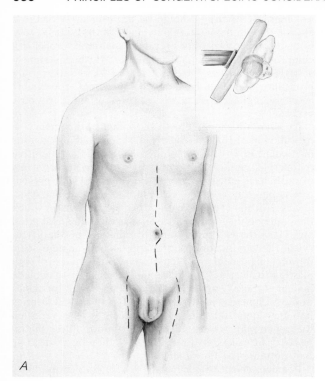

A

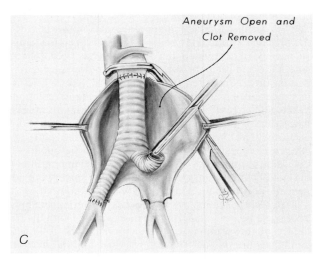

Aneurysm Open and
Clot Removed

C

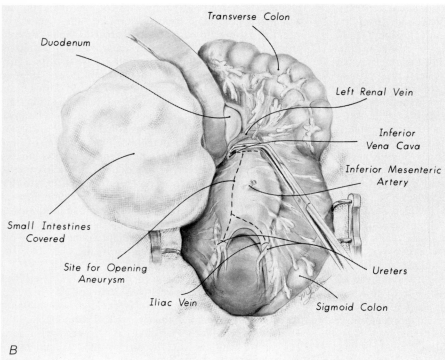

Transverse Colon

Duodenum

Left Renal Vein

Inferior
Vena Cava

Inferior Mesenteric
Artery

Small Intestines
Covered

Site for Opening
Aneurysm

Ureters

Iliac Vein

Sigmoid Colon

B

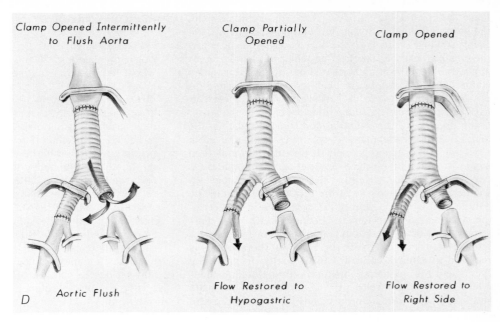

Clamp Opened Intermittently to Flush Aorta

Clamp Partially Opened

Clamp Opened

D   Aortic Flush

Flow Restored to Hypogastric

Flow Restored to Right Side

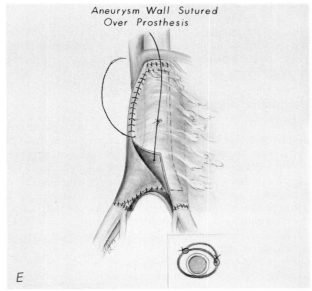

Aneurysm Wall Sutured Over Prosthesis

E

Fig. 21-24. Procedure for substituting aortoiliac bifurcation prosthesis for abdominal aortic aneurysm. *A.* A midline incision extending from xiphoid process to pubic symphysis is usually employed. Insert shows rotation of the table to the patient's right side, which facilitates retraction of the small bowel. *B.* Surgical exposure of vital structures and lines of incision of the aneurysm are shown. *C.* Endarterectomy of the aneurysm wall is performed; the lumbar arteries transfixed with sutures and the prosthesis in place are shown. *D.* Technique for preventing embolization of atherosclerotic debris to the lower extremities and gradually restoring lower extremity circulation to avoid declamping shock. (1) Aorta is flushed through one open limb of the prosthesis. (2) Flow gradually restored to one hypogastric artery and, when the blood pressure has been stabilized, to the ipsilateral external iliac artery. (3) The sequence is repeated on the opposite side. *E.* The remains of the aneurysm wall and the base of the left colon mesentery are carefully sutured over the prosthesis and suture lines to prevent adherence of the bowel and to bolster the suture lines to prevent aorticointestinal fistulas. [From: *Imparato AM et al: Avoidance of shock and peripheral embolism during surgery of the abdominal aorta. Surgery 73(1):68, 1973, with permission.*]

the graft with the adventitia of the aneurysm, thereby separating the prosthetic graft from the intestine. Sexual dysfunction consisting of retrograde ejaculation or impotence occurs in 25 to 50 percent of male patients.

RUPTURED ABDOMINAL ANEURYSM

CLINICAL MANIFESTATIONS. A ruptured abdominal aneurysm is a grave surgical emergency whose onset is characterized by acute vascular collapse, usually with abdominal or flank pain. With collapse, the diagnosis initially may be uncertain, unless a pulsating mass is palpated. A frequent erroneous diagnosis is renal colic or massive myocardial or pulmonary infarction. The diagno-

sis usually can be established by careful, deep palpation of the abdomen that should outline a pulsating, ill-defined mass in the epigastrium or flank.

TREATMENT. Operation should be performed as quickly as possible, infusing 500 to 1000 mL of fluid every few minutes until serious hypotension has been corrected. A midline incision is preferred. Proximal control of the aorta generally can be obtained by isolating the aorta above the stomach just below the diaphragm. This should be done initially, because once the posterior peritoneum is incised and the hematoma surrounding the ruptured aneurysm evacuated, massive hemorrhage can occur with exsanguination. The aorta can be safely clamped below the diaphragm for 20 to 30 min without serious ischemic injury to the intestines or liver. Once it has been clamped, the ruptured aneurysm can be widely incised, intraabdominal clots evacuated, and the proximal aorta below the renal arteries isolated, after which a clamp can be applied to the infrarenal aorta and the previously applied clamp below the diaphragm released. When possible, to prevent embolization to the lower extremities, the external iliac arteries are occluded prior to clamping the aorta. If the urgency of the situation does not permit this, the femoral arteries are manually compressed in the groin while the aortic clamp is applied. Reconstruction is then similar to that with elective excision of an abdominal aneurysm, although excision of the wall of the aneurysm should be limited because of the serious condition of the patient. On occasion, the infradiaphragmatic portion of the aorta cannot be clamped, because of either the massive amount of retroperitoneal hematoma or free rupture into the peritoneal cavity. In this case, left thoracotomy is required to achieve control. Consequently, in preparing the patient for emergency operation for abdominal aneurysm, the chest as well as the abdomen must be made surgically accessible. Unfortunately, despite successful removal of the aneurysm, death results in 30 to 50 percent of patients.

The unheralded rupture of asymptomatic aneurysms, with resulting high fatality rates, is the most urgent reason for recommending routine operation of abdominal aneurysms as soon as the diagnosis of a clinically significant aneurysm is made.

Peripheral Aneurysms

If traumatic and congenital malformations, considered in different chapters, are excluded, almost all peripheral aneurysms result from arteriosclerosis, for syphilitic aneurysms are now seldom seen. Mycotic aneurysms associated with bacterial endocarditis are now usually associated with intravenously administered drugs in drug abusers. The majority of peripheral arteriosclerotic aneurysms are in the popliteal artery. Infrequent sites include the femoral, carotid, or subclavian arteries. Each of these is considered separately.

Peripheral aneurysms usually occur in men in the fifth to seventh decades, often with hypertension and signs of atherosclerosis in other organs. Multiple aneurysms are frequent. In contrast to abdominal or thoracic aneurysms, where rupture is the greatest threat, peripheral aneurysms infrequently rupture but cause disability due to distal embolization or thrombosis, with subsequent ischemia and gangrene of extremities.

Peripheral aneurysms are readily amenable to successful therapy if operated upon electively before embolization with irreversible occlusion of outflow vessels and acute ischemia develop in the extremity. Tortuosity of the involved artery sometimes makes it possible to mobilize the artery proximal and distal to the aneurysm and reestablish continuity following excision by end-to-end anastomosis. Continuity can also be established preferably with saphenous vein, but if this is not possible, a knitted Dacron prosthesis or PTFE is preferred.

POPLITEAL ANEURYSM

Popliteal aneurysms are usually arteriosclerotic, occurring in men in the sixth and seventh decades of life, half of whom may be hyperactive. They occur bilaterally in at least 25 percent of patients afflicted. Their detection raises the suspicion that other arteriosclerotic aneurysms are present, and these must be searched for in the abdomen, groins, and thorax.

Though often small (3 to 4 cm) and asymptomatic, they pose a grave threat to the viability of the affected extremity due to their tendency to embolize to tibial arteries or to thrombose. Once either complication has occurred, retrieval is virtually impossible.

CLINICAL MANIFESTATIONS. Finding of a pulsating mass behind the knee is characteristic enough to permit an accurate diagnosis. Rarely, the aneurysm may enlarge sufficiently to cause local pain and tenderness. Rupture is unusual. In some instances the presenting manifestation may be acute ischemia of the extremity, and the aneurysm is discovered at operation for acute popliteal occlusion.

If the aneurysm is thrombosed, pulsations may be absent, and a mass may or may not be felt. Differential diagnosis must include other cystic tumors about the knee joint, such as Baker's cyst, as well as other causes of tibial arterial occlusion, such as emboli, Buerger's disease, and diabetes mellitus. The presence or absence of pedal pulses should be carefully noted.

Calcification in the wall of the aneurysm is often visible on a radiograph. The diagnosis can be confirmed by CT and by arteriography, although much of the cavity of the aneurysm may be filled with thrombus (Fig. 21-25).

TREATMENT. Because of the hazards of thrombosis, embolization, and gangrene, operation should be performed as soon as possible after the diagnosis is made even though the aneurysm is small, asymptomatic, and seemingly stable. A retrospective study of gangrene and amputation from popliteal aneurysms that have embolized found no warning signs that such a catastrophe was imminent, although the absence or disappearance of one or both pedal pulses in the presence of a pulsating aneurysm usually signifies that distal embolization has occurred and that acute ischemia will occur very shortly.

Operative Technique. With the patient in a prone position, an incision across the popliteal crease readily exposes the artery proximal and distal to the aneurysm. A transverse incision in the line of the popliteal crease, with extension vertically downward on the medial aspect of the upper calf and upward along the posterolateral aspect of the thigh, has also been used. An alternative exposure is particularly useful when the femoral artery needs to be exposed for some distance from the popliteal. With the patient supine, an incision is made on the medial aspect of the lower thigh and extended across the knee joint into the upper calf, transecting the muscles inserting into the upper medial tibial plateau as well as the head of the gastrocnemius tendon. Transection of these muscles provides unusually wide exposure and has not resulted in any late impairment of function of the extremity.

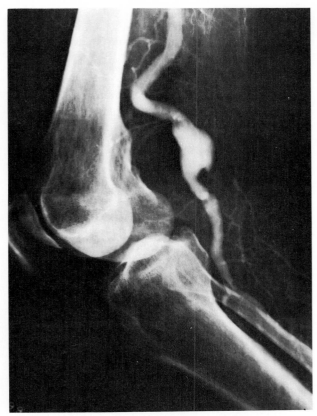

Fig. 21-25. Femoral angiogram indicating the presence of a popliteal aneurysm. Characteristic tortuosity of the involved artery is present. Such tortuosity sometimes makes it possible to establish continuity by direct anastomosis following excision of the aneurysm.

Once the artery has been isolated distal to the aneurysm, vascular clamps are applied and the aneurysm widely opened. Any laminated thrombus is removed, as well as the inner lining of the wall of the aneurysm, preserving the adventitial sheath. The origins of the geniculate branches of the popliteal artery are sutured from within the lumen. This technique preserves branches of the popliteal vein that are usually stretched over the wall of the aneurysm, and also the collateral circulation is less disturbed. A small amount of heparin should be given systemically before the application of clamps.

If the aneurysm is small and the popliteal artery tortuous, an end-to-end anastomosis is sometimes possible. Most patients, however, require a short graft, preferably a reversed autologous saphenous vein. Short grafts of knitted Dacron have also been satisfactory.

Although variations in the suitability of vein grafts in different reports are as low as 43 percent in some, it has been our experience that a vein substitution for the popliteal aneurysm can be achieved in approximately 85 to 90 percent of the patients.

Acute Ischemia. When operation is required because thrombosis has produced severe ischemia with impending gangrene, a different approach is needed, and restoration of flow is difficult and uncertain. Simple excision of the aneurysm, of course, is futile with the obstructed distal circulation. The major consideration is removal of these distal thrombi, which usually have become intimately adherent to the tibial arterial walls, followed by restoration of arterial continuity across the occluded aneurysm, as in elective procedures. Operative incision and exposure should be planned to permit precise cannulation of the anterior and posterior tibial arteries with balloon-tipped catheters to remove propagated thrombus. Retrograde flushing with saline solution from the posterior and anterior tibial arteries is much less satisfactory than the Fogarty catheter technique. Operative angiography should be available to be certain that all thrombi have been removed. In many patients the distal thrombi have become adherent to the arterial wall and resist removal. If thrombi are not completely removed, as confirmed by angiography, rethrombosis terminating in gangrene and amputation is almost a certainty.

FEMORAL ANEURYSM

INCIDENCE AND PATHOLOGY. Although considerably less often encountered than popliteal aneurysms, femoral aneurysms occur in the same population group with the same predisposing factors, exposing patients to the same dangers of embolization, thrombosis, and lower extremity ischemia with a rare incidence of rupture. Their location is in the common femoral or superficial femoral artery, with equal incidence, while approximately half the afflicted patients have involvement of both areas. Involvement of the profunda femoris is extremely rare. The false anastomotic aneurysm associated with aortofemoral artificial prostheses will be discussed under Traumatic Aneurysms.

CLINICAL MANIFESTATIONS. Symptoms usually consist of an awareness of a pulsating mass in the upper thigh until thrombosis or embolization produces ischemic symptoms in the extremity. The diagnosis can often be easily made on physical examination, outlining the pulsating mass in the femoral artery. A radiograph may show calcification in the wall of the aneurysm. Arteriography is useful to delineate the relationship of the aneurysm to the profunda femoris artery, as well as to define the patency of the distal circulation.

TREATMENT. Surgical correction should be performed promptly, unless coexisting cerebral or coronary artery disease makes the risk of operation prohibitive. If operation is postponed because of concomitant disease, such decisions should be made with the full realization that a subsequent amputation because of gangrene may entail an even greater operative risk to the patient.

At operation the arteries can be mobilized proximal and distal to the point of aneurysm and the aneurysm excised. Vascular continuity may be restored with either a saphenous vein graft or an 8-mm knitted Dacron or Goretex prosthesis. Patency of the profunda femoris artery should be maintained by using a Y-bifurcation graft if necessary. Complications following operation are unusual unless peripheral arterial occlusion has already produced severe

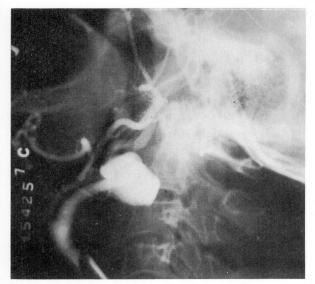

Fig. 21-26. Carotid arteriogram illustrating saccular aneurysm of the internal carotid artery. The internal carotid proximal and distal to the aneurysm is opacified.

ischemic signs. In most patients following operation the prognosis is determined by the coexisting atherosclerotic disease, rather than the femoral aneurysm.

CAROTID ARTERY ANEURYSM

INCIDENCE AND PATHOLOGY. The infrequent occurrence of carotid aneurysms has been documented by several reports. Over a period of time during which 2300 operations for aneurysms had been performed, seven carotid artery aneurysms were noted.

Most carotid aneurysms result from arteriosclerosis and involve either the common carotid artery at the bulb or the extracranial internal carotid artery. Unusual causes include trauma, bacterial infection, or cystic medial necrosis. The main hazard from an aneurysm is embolization of thrombotic material into the cerebral circulation with production of cerebral infarcts. Infrequently, such aneurysms may enlarge and rupture.

CLINICAL MANIFESTATIONS. Patients are usually seen because of a mass in the neck. Pulsations are often prominent and provide an easy clue to the diagnosis. A more difficult problem arises if pulsations are absent, because of laminated thrombus occupying most of the cavity of the aneurysm. Arteriography is the most definitive laboratory technique, establishing the diagnosis and also defining the relationship of the common and internal carotid arteries to the aneurysm (Fig. 21-26). The differential diagnosis should include prominent pulsations from buckling of the carotid artery, a condition seen in hypertensive women, and other solid tumors of the neck, such as a lymph node or a carotid body tumor.

TREATMENT. Because of the constant risk from cerebral infarction, the aneurysm should be excised as soon as possible. The major consideration in planning operation is protection of the brain from ischemic injury while the carotid artery is occluded during excision. In one report, 12 patients were described in whom the aneurysm was excised without any protection of the brain from ischemia. Six of the twelve had a transient neurologic injury, while four developed a permanent neurologic deficit.

The safest surgical technique is excision of the aneurysm under local or regional block anesthesia, keeping the patient awake to assess constantly the tolerance of the brain for temporary occlusion of the carotid artery. If ischemic symptoms develop, an internal shunt may be utilized to maintain cerebral blood flow. Even with a large aneurysm, regional block anesthesia is adequate. On occasion, dislocation of the mandible at the temporomandibular joint is necessary to achieve adequate exposure.

Experiences indicate that in over one-half of the patients there is sufficient tortuosity and elongation of the carotid artery proximal and distal to the site of involvement of the aneurysm to permit mobilization of the ends of the carotid artery and direct anastomosis, although a vein graft may be needed to bridge the gap (Fig. 21-27). Following excision of the aneurysm with reconstruction of the carotid artery, convalescence has usually been uncomplicated, and long-term results are excellent. The most severe complications of the operative procedure are related to proximity of the aneurysm to major cranial nerves VII to XII. Especially with unusually large internal carotid aneurysms, multiple peripheral nerve palsies resulting in marked deviation of the tongue, hoarseness, facial palsies, and difficulty in swallowing should be expected. Even with dislocation of the mandible at the temporomandibular joint, exposure may still be quite limited, and the nerve palsies are to be expected. Recovery from these usually occurs within 6 to 12 months. Even in the absence of transection of these nerves, recovery may be incomplete.

SUBCLAVIAN ANEURYSMS

The majority of subclavian aneurysms develop as secondary complications of a cervical rib and are discussed in the section Thoracic Outlet Syndromes. The extremely rare subclavian aneurysm that results from arteriosclerosis is similar to other peripheral arteriosclerosis aneurysms; it occurs in older men, often with arteriosclerotic aneurysms elsewhere. The diagnosis is usually readily made from physical examination. The most important differential diagnosis is from the frequently seen tortuosity of the innominate and subclavian arteries that occurs in hypertensive patients. Careful examination of the bulge will differentiate a true aneurysm from a tortuous vessel. If aneurysm cannot be excluded, an arteriogram should be done. Excision with reconstruction of the involved artery can be easily performed.

Visceral Aneurysms

SPLENIC ARTERY ANEURYSM

Significant aneurysms of the splenic artery are uncommon. Because of their rarity and unusual manifestations,

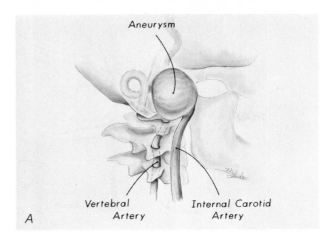

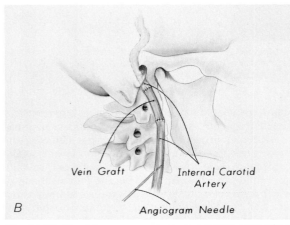

Fig. 21-27. Carotid aneurysmectomy is possible even when the internal carotid artery is involved in its upper extracranial portion, since the artery can be exposed through lateral neck incisions to the base of the skull. *A.* Internal carotid aneurysm. *B.* Replacement with vein graft. (From: *Sanoudos GM et al: Internal carotid aneurysm. Am Surg 39:118, 1973, with permission.*)

several detailed reviews have been published. In 1953 Owens and Coffey reported six patients and found a total of 198 cases in previous reports. Of historical interest is the fact that President Garfield in 1881 died from a traumatic aneurysm of the splenic artery 2 months after being shot by an assassin.

INCIDENCE AND PATHOLOGY. A report of unusual interest is that of Bedford and Lodge in 1960 who published findings from 250 consecutive postmortem examinations in older patients. Routine dissection of the splenic artery found 26 aneurysms, an incidence of nearly 10 percent. All had been asymptomatic. Their size was small, ranging from a few millimeters to as large as 2.5 cm: most were close to 1 cm in diameter. In the 204 cases reviewed by Owens and Coffey, the average diameter was 3 cm. This great discrepancy between the high autopsy incidence and the rarity of clinically symptomatic aneurysms indicates that small aneurysms are probably of no clinical significance and are usually overlooked.

These aneurysms, like other arteriosclerotic aneu-

rysms, occur in older patients with an average age near fifty. Surprisingly, though, the aneurysms are more frequent in women, in contrast to the overwhelming predominance of the usual arteriosclerotic aneurysm in men. In the Owens and Coffey series, 127 patients were women and 63 were men. Bedford and Lodge noted that the aneurysms tended to develop at bifurcations of the splenic artery and suggested that degeneration of the media, as well as atherosclerosis, might be a predisposing factor.

The aneurysms are usually single and in the main trunk of the splenic artery. Rupture is more likely to occur during pregnancy. The actual risk of rupture is uncertain, for many are recognized only after rupture. Rupture is obviously a grave event, for of 131 symptomatic patients reported by Owens and Coffey 94 died from rupture and only 7 from other causes. In 37 female patients, rupture occurred during late pregnancy.

CLINICAL MANIFESTATIONS. Pain in the epigastrium or left flank is the most frequent symptom, occurring in 93 of 131 symptomatic patients in the Owens series. Other symptoms are nonspecific gastrointestinal symptoms, usually interpreted as due to peptic ulcer. These include nausea, vomiting, dyspepsia, and constipation or diarrhea. Gastrointestinal hemorrhage has occurred in about one-third of patients. For unknown reasons gastrointestinal symptoms may exist for months or years before the diagnosis is made. This may be fortuitous.

Often rupture is the first sign of the aneurysm, as it was in 46 percent of the patients in one series. A "double" rupture is a significant clinical sequence, recognized in about one-half of patients. The first rupture is hemorrhage into the lesser omental sac; this ceases temporarily but is followed in 1 to 2 days by secondary hemorrhage and exsanguination.

With the small size of the splenic aneurysms, physical abnormalities are usually not found. For unknown reasons, moderate splenomegaly has been reported in 40 to 50 percent of patients. However, a mass has been palpated in only 20 percent, and pulsations or a bruit in 10 percent. Radiographic identification of a mass with calcium in the walls suggestive of an aneurysm has been reported in 15 percent of the group.

TREATMENT. Obviously symptomatic aneurysms should be excised as soon as the diagnosis is made, usually with concomitant splenectomy. The widespread use of aortography for investigating many abdominal conditions has disclosed aneurysms smaller than 1 cm that are asymptomatic. Their treatment is uncertain because of the rarity of rupture. On the other hand, it is disquieting to note that rupture without preceding symptoms is the first event in one-half of the patients with ruptured splenic aneurysms. From data available, surgical treatment does not seem indicated for asymptomatic aneurysms smaller than 1 cm, but those greater than 3 cm should be excised. Further data are needed to be certain of these guidelines.

RENAL ARTERY ANEURYSM

INCIDENCE AND PATHOLOGY. Aneurysms of the renal artery are similar to aneurysms of the splenic artery in

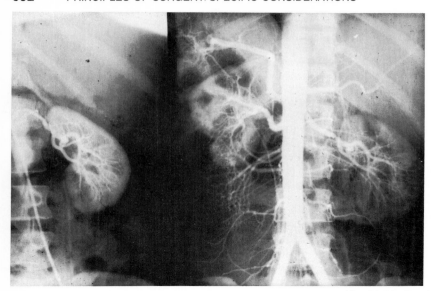

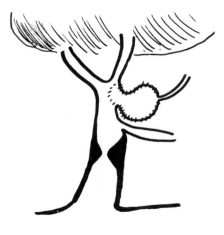

Fig. 21-28. Renal artery aneurysms are frequently saccular, as shown in the angiographic study, and may be associated with arterial hypertension.

that recognition has greatly increased with the use of angiography. The widespread use of renal angiography to investigate patients with hypertension has been chiefly responsible for the increasing recognition of renal aneurysms. Apparently, about 1 percent of hypertensive patients will be found on angiography to have a small aneurysm of one renal artery.

These aneurysms are equally common in males and females, usually in the fifth and sixth decades, but they have been found in all age groups, even in patients as young as nine months. Anatomically they may be saccular or fusiform. Unusual varieties include false aneurysm from trauma, dissecting aneurysm, or arteriovenous fistula. The saccular aneurysm is apparently congenital, arising from a defect in elastic tissue of the wall of the artery, often near a bifurcation. It varies from 1 to 3 cm in size and often develops extensive eccentric calcification, a so-called signet ring on the radiograph. It is infrequently associated with hypertension and rarely ruptures. The fusiform aneurysm develops distal to an area of constriction of the renal artery and is basically a poststenotic aneurysm similar to that seen in other parts of the arterial circulation. Because of the proximal stenosis, it is frequently seen with hypertension.

The aneurysms occur with frequency in either renal artery, usually in the main renal artery or one of its branches. An intrarenal location is uncommon. In one report, 92 aneurysms were in the main renal artery, 44 were in an extrarenal branch, and 15 were intrarenal.

Rupture has been reported in at least 24 patients, with a fatal outcome in 20. Eight of these episodes occurred during pregnancy. Rupture has been recognized rarely in a calcified aneurysm.

CLINICAL MANIFESTATIONS. Abdominal or flank pain has occurred in about 50 percent of the patients but is probably unrelated to the aneurysm. Investigation of the symptom subsequently led to finding the aneurysm. Hematuria, gross or microscopic, has also been reported

in 30 to 40 percent of patients. As expected, hypertension has been frequently seen with poststenotic aneurysms and has been improved or cured in over one-half of these after operation. By contrast, hypertension in one series was present in only 7 of 12 with a saccular aneurysm and improved after operation in only 1 of the 7. A mechanism by which a saccular aneurysm can produce hypertension is not clear except for the rather nebulous possibility of compression or distortion of the renal artery. The association may simply be fortuitous.

There are usually no abnormalities on physical examination. Occasionally a localized bruit is audible. Radiographic examination may show signet ring calcification which must be differentiated from calcification of mesenteric lymph nodes or calcification of other visceral arteries. The intravenous pyelogram is abnormal in about one-half of the patients because of ischemia, infarction, or localized pressure defects. Aortography is essential to establish the diagnosis and define the precise location (Fig. 21-28). As mentioned earlier, most aneurysms have been found during aortography performed for other purposes.

TREATMENT. Prompt operation is indicated whenever an aneurysm is found during investigation of a patient for hypertension. With poststenotic aneurysms the aneurysm can be excised and the renal artery reconstructed, with an excellent likelihood of improving the hypertension. With a saccular aneurysm and hypertension, operation is probably indicated to reconstruct the renal artery, although the prognosis for improving the hypertension is less favorable. In the 17 patients reported by Smith, 5 had successful operations, while 12 with small aneurysms of questionable significance had been followed without operation for an average of 3 years without complications. The ''bench'' technique, in which the kidney is removed from its bed by transecting the main arteries and veins and leaving the ureter intact, performing microsurgical arterial repair on branch arteries, and then reattaching the main vessels to the iliac vessels, has permitted removal of branch artery aneurysms without sacrifice of kidneys. In a patient with a small calcified aneurysm without symptoms or hypertension, there probably is little indication for operation, for the risk of rupture is almost negligible. With larger aneurysms, certainly with symptoms present, operation should be performed.

ETIOLOGY AND PATHOLOGY. A traumatic aneurysm is produced from a tangential laceration of the wall of an artery. Usually continuity of flow through the lacerated artery is maintained. By contrast, injuries that transect an artery often require immediate treatment because of hemorrhage or ischemia in the affected limb and consequently seldom evolve into an aneurysm.

Following the laceration, blood extravasates into adjacent soft tissues to form a hematoma that compresses and seals the point of injury. If the artery is confined within a small space surrounded by fascia, the hematoma may be small enough to escape recognition. Both the patient and the physician are unaware that an arterial injury has occurred. After days or weeks, the blood clot gradually liquefies; then the firm, immobile mass surrounding the artery begins to pulsate. A descriptive term for these lesions is "pulsating hematoma." With the appearance of pulsation, the aneurysm begins to enlarge. This is ominous, for enlargement is progressive and relentless, destroying nerves, even eroding bone, and eventually terminating in rupture and death.

Traumatic aneurysms are often termed false aneurysms, as distinguished from true aneurysms (see the discussion under Aneurysms, above), for the wall is composed of fibrous tissue rather than components of normal arterial wall, as with arteriosclerotic or syphilitic aneurysms.

As the hematoma enlarges in a recent wound, the tissues are firm, tender, perhaps warm. These findings of redness, tenderness, and heat are, of course, the usual characteristics of an abscess. Occasional vivid reports appear in the surgical literature in which an unsuspecting physician widely incised such a red, tender mass to drain an abscess, with resultant violent hemorrhage.

A similar therapeutic catastrophe occasionally occurs when a traumatic aneurysm stabilizes for years and is subsequently confused with a neoplasm. If the previous history of trauma is not available, the differential diagnosis is difficult, for the aneurysm is partly filled with clot and closely resembles a solid tumor. Attempted biopsy of such lesions, with frightening consequences, has been reported.

Usually there is no disability from a traumatic aneurysm except for the local mass until it enlarges to compress adjacent nerves, causing pain, paresthesia, and eventually paralysis. The peripheral arterial circulation is usually normal. Peripheral embolization of thrombi from the aneurysm is unusual except for the rare aneurysm of the subclavian artery following trauma. Here, intermittent compression by the clavicle may dislodge emboli.

Ischemic symptoms in the arm may dominate the clinical picture, requiring arteriography to disclose small traumatic aneurysms.

CLINICAL MANIFESTATIONS. A localized mass is often the only finding. As it enlarges, there is pain or paralysis from compression of nerves. On physical examination the borders of the mass are ill defined because the hematoma surrounding the aneurysm is beneath the deep fascia. Pulsations may or may not be present, depending upon the amount of thrombus in the lumen. A systolic bruit is frequently audible. Peripheral pulsations are normal.

If the mass pulsates, the diagnosis is reasonably certain from the physical findings. Otherwise arteriography is required to differentiate it from a neoplasm or a cyst. On arteriography the full size is not disclosed, as much of the cavity is filled with thrombus.

TREATMENT. Operation should be performed as soon as the diagnosis has been established because of the inevitable outcome of enlargement and rupture. If neurologic symptoms are present, operation should be done urgently, within hours, to prevent irreversible pressure injury of crucial nerves. At operation the incision should be placed to permit exposure of the uninvolved artery proximal and distal to the aneurysm. With these vessels temporarily occluded, the aneurysm can be widely incised, clots evacuated, and the point of origin from the artery identified. Dissection around the aneurysm before it is opened should be avoided; it is unnecessary, complicated, and often dangerous.

With unusually large aneurysms, it is important to remember that there is only one small opening in the wall of the aneurysm, the tangential laceration of the arterial wall from which the aneurysm began. Hence, if the aneurysm is inadvertently entered, this small opening can be digitally occluded to control bleeding while further exposure is obtained.

Once the aneurysm has been opened and the inner contents removed, the site of communication with the parent artery can be mobilized and the injured area excised. Complete excision of the wall of the aneurysm is unnecessary and should be avoided because of the surrounding dense fibrotic reaction. Once the involved artery has been mobilized, arterial continuity can usually be restored by end-to-end anastomosis or by insertion of a short graft, preferably autologous vein. Ligation should be performed only for small arteries, such as the radial, not essential to normal circulation. Convalescence after operation is usually uneventful and long-term results excellent. Hughes and Jahnke reported continuing good results 5 years after surgical treatment of 67 traumatic aneurysms during the Korean conflict.

ANASTOMOTIC FALSE ANEURYSM

False aneurysm can occur at any arterial suture line but is most frequently encountered where plastic prostheses have been sutured to host arteries, usually in the groin, at the terminal ends of bypass grafts. The longest interval between the original operation and the appearance of false aneurysms in the authors' experience has been 20 years. The incidence was estimated at 2 to 25 percent when suture material such as silk was used. Since the introduction of Prolene and other synthetics, the incidence has decreased.

CLINICAL MANIFESTATIONS. Thrombosis and rupture are the two major complications encountered with false aneurysms. Neighboring structures such as the duodenum may become adherent to an infrarenal aortic suture line and result in an aortoduodenal fistula from rupture, manifest by massive upper gastrointestinal hemorrhage, of a false aneurysm. The clinical presentation depends upon the location of the anastomotic false aneurysm and varies from the presence of a gradually enlarging pulsatile mass to the appearance of acute ischemia of a limb due to thrombosis of, or embolization from, the aneurysm. The patient may present in shock due to the intraabdominal rupture of an iliac or aortic false aneurysm.

TREATMENT. Treatment is surgical and varies according to the location of the aneurysm. The most commonly encountered groin aneurysm can usually be managed by resection of the terminal inch or two of the old prosthesis together with the false aneurysm wall, preserving the posterior wall of the common femoral artery together with the ostia of the profunda femoris artery and the superficial femoral, if it is patent. A segment of new prosthesis is anastomosed to bridge the gap. Immediate results are excellent but recurrences occur.

Mycotic Aneurysm

Mycotic aneurysm is an aneurysm resulting from the introduction of bacteria into the arterial wall. This can be caused by embolization of septic emboli from bacterial endocarditis, from contiguous infection, and from direct trauma to arteries with nonsterile needles, particularly in intravenous drug abusers. The term "infected aneurysm" is preferable for secondary infection of an already existing aneurysm. Since the advent of antibiotics, septic aneurysms resulting from bacterial endocarditis have decreased in incidence and the types of bacteria associated with them has changed from a predominance of *Streptococcus* and *Staphylococcus* to a wider spectrum of bacteria, including enteric organisms and fungi.

CLINICAL MANIFESTATIONS. These vary with the location of the aneurysm, which may remain totally undetected until rupture and shock occur. When a superficial vessel is involved, there may be a tender pulsatile mass with local signs of infection, at times associated with systemic signs of sepsis.

TREATMENT. The underlying condition requires antibiotic therapy. The aneurysm is excised; the involved artery is ligated proximally and distally. Arterial continuity may have to be re-established through extraanatomic routes, preferably with autologous tissue. Many technically complex surgical problems are associated with treatment of mycotic aneurysms. The prognosis for limb survival and patient survival is uncertain. Those mycotic aneurysms encountered in intravenous drug abusers are associated with high rates of recurrence since the original drug addiction is difficult to eliminate and repeated needle trauma persists.

BUERGER'S DISEASE

HISTORICAL DATA. The entity referred to as Buerger's disease was first described by Winiwarter in 1879 and elaborated upon by Buerger in 1908 and again in 1924. The descriptive term *thromboangiitis obliterans* (TAO) emphasizes the inflammatory reaction in the arterial wall, with involvement of the neighboring vein and nerve, terminating in thrombosis of the artery. In 1960 doubt was cast upon the specificity of the pathologic findings when Wessler et al. pointed out that arterial occlusion from any cause, be it atherosclerosis or even embolic occlusion, may result in a similar type of angiitis, indistinguishable from what was usually considered to be specific for TAO. The relatively widespread use of arteriography has shown that many cases of so-called Buerger's disease probably represented presenile atherosclerosis occurring in the third, fourth, and fifth decades of life.

INCIDENCE AND ETIOLOGY. In our experience, we have made the diagnosis in fewer than 0.25 percent of all our patients with occlusive arterial disease of the extremities. The disease is found most frequently in men between twenty and forty years of age, is uncommon in women, who compose only 5 to 10 percent of patients with Buerger's disease, and is also rare in blacks. Initially it was felt that the disease was much more common in the Jewish race; subsequent statistical studies have shown that this frequency has been greatly exaggerated and the incidence is only slightly greater if at all.

Heavy tobacco smoking, usually 20 or more cigarettes per day, has been almost universally associated with this disease. The tobacco habit is firmly entrenched in these individuals in spite of obvious remissions that occur upon cessation of smoking. DeBakey and Cohen analyzed 936 patients and found that only 10 percent successfully stopped smoking over a 10-year period.

Although the correlation between Buerger's disease and smoking is strong, the mechanisms involved are not clear. Either there is a particular response to tobacco (since there are so many more smokers than patients with Buerger's disease), or, as in the Orient, particular brands of cigarettes are associated with the disease. This has never been noted in the West. It has recently been suggested that there is an association with rickettsial disease.

PATHOLOGY. The gross features of Buerger's disease are characteristic of an inflammatory process. The diseased artery is usually surrounded by a dense fibrotic reaction, often incorporating the adjacent vein, less often the neighboring nerve. Although this is usually considered to be characteristic of thromboangiitis obliterans, it also occurs occasionally with atherosclerosis obliterans and very frequently in association with aneurysmal disease.

The distribution of arterial involvement is different from that of atherosclerosis in that smaller, more peripheral arteries, usually in segmental distribution, are involved. In the lower extremities the disease generally occurs beyond the popliteal arteries, starting in tibial vessels extending into the vessels of the foot, in a fashion similar to the typical arterial involvement in the diabetic. In the upper extremities, where atherosclerotic and diabetic involvement are extremely rare, TAO is manifested by arterial involvement usually distal to the forearm in about 30 percent of these patients. The visceral and cardiac circulations can be involved, but this occurs rarely.

Early in the course of Buerger's disease, there is involvement of superficial veins, producing the characteristic migratory, recurrent superficial phlebitis, while the larger and deeper veins (such as femoral and iliac) are rarely affected.

Although some doubt has been raised about the specificity of the histologic findings, most observers consider them to be characteristic. Precise retrospective diagnoses have been made on the basis of histologic examination of amputated extremities.

Microscopic examination of small thrombosed arteries shows extensive proliferation of intimal cells and fibroblasts throughout all segments of the arterial wall, with preservation of the basic architecture of the artery. Lipid deposition and calcification, frequently seen in atherosclerosis, are absent. Inflammatory cells, usually lymphocytes, are observed, while giant cells, whose presence was noted originally by Buerger, generally are absent. Necrosis of the arterial wall is very unusual, as is abscess formation. The thrombus in the arterial wall shows an unusual degree of fibroblastic activity with endothelial proliferation, suggesting the presence of a primary antigen in the blood. Spaces within the thrombus, interpreted as partial though functionally ineffectual recanalization, are common but not particularly characteristic of Buerger's disease, since this is seen with all thrombotic occlusions.

Involvement of the neighboring vein and nerve by the inflammatory and fibrotic reactions completes the histologic appearance of the lesions.

Periods of exacerbation of the acute process may be manifested by acute superficial phlebitis, with eventual progression of arterial occlusions and ischemia counterbalanced by remissions, during which collateral circulation becomes effective in younger patients. The ultimate severity and extent of the extremity ischemia are determined by the frequency and duration of the acute attacks and the length of the quiescent periods. The cycles can usually be broken by cessation of smoking.

DeBakey and Cohen studied this progression in a group of 936 patients followed during a 10-year period after diagnosis and noted a three times higher mortality rate (10 percent), predominantly from cardiovascular disease, than in a control population. Postmortem examination revealed the familiar pattern of atherosclerotic disease in coronary and cerebral vessels, rather than the characteristic histologic pattern of thromboangiitis obliterans found in upper and lower extremity vessels. The limb amputation rate was 20 to 30 percent in 10 years, with an additional 40 percent showing some progression of ischemia but not requiring amputation.

CLINICAL MANIFESTATIONS. There may be a phase of recurrent migratory superficial phlebitis involving superficial veins of the feet, which may occur over a period of years before there is any suspicion of arterial involvement. Invariably the patient is a cigarette smoker, and with continued smoking intermittent claudication appears as the first manifestation of ischemia. Reflecting the peripheral involvement of pedal arteries, pain while walking is usually referred to the arch of the foot, somewhat less often to the calf of the leg, but almost never to the thigh or buttock unless there is associated atherosclerosis obliterans. Upper extremity claudication is rare, probably a reflection of the distribution of arterial involvement, which is usually distal to the wrist. Progression of ischemia is similar to that in all chronic progressive arterial occlusions, in which the initial pain induced by exercise progresses to rest pain, postural color changes, trophic changes, and eventually ulceration and gangrene of one or more digits and finally of an entire foot or hand, necessitating major amputations. Patients with Buerger's disease may eventually require quadruple extremity amputations.

One variant of the typical syndrome is first manifest by painful vesicles of the pulp of fingers with surrounding intensive hyperemia and hypersensitivity, recurring as acute attacks over 2- to 4-year intervals, associated with progressive claudication of the feet and calves. The prognosis appeared to be worsened not only by continued smoking but by smoking certain types of cigarettes.

Pain in Buerger's disease, as in other ischemic conditions of the extremities, is common and may result from phlebitis, ischemic neuritis, or progressive skin and muscle ischemia manifested by the typical ischemic rest pain. This is unremitting and prevents patients from sleeping but is somewhat ameliorated by placing the affected limb in the dependent position. There may be blanching on elevation and rubor on dependence, as well as marked blanching on exposure to cold.

Physical Examination. The most frequent finding is absence of the posterior tibial and dorsalis pedis pulses in the feet. Often the popliteal pulse is palpable, especially in the early stages of the disease. Absence of the posterior tibial pulse is highly suggestive of the diagnosis, especially when bilateral. In the upper extremity, the radial pulse may be congenitally absent in 5 to 10 percent of patients, but absence of both pulses again is very suggestive of the disease. Signs of chronic tissue ischemia include loss of hair from the digits, atrophy of the skin, brittle nails, and rubor on dependency. In more advanced cases there may be ulceration or gangrene in the digits, often beginning near the nail and involving only the distal portion of the digit. With more extensive disease, gangrene extends into the foot. In the upper extremity, fortunately, extension of gangrene beyond the fingers is rare, and amputation of the hand is almost never necessary.

Edema is seen with advanced ischemia, resulting from keeping the extremity in a dependent position to relieve rest pain. Superficial phlebitis involving segments of superficial veins is frequent, but rarely is phlebitis found in the large veins, such as the femoral or iliac. Accordingly, edema on the basis of phlebitis is unusual.

Laboratory Studies. The most significant laboratory examination is arteriography. The arteriographic findings, as emphasized by McKusick et al., are frequently characteristic. Typically, the contours of the large arteries are smooth, without the characteristic irregularities seen in atherosclerosis. In arteries the caliber of the tibials, there are abrupt areas of occlusion, frequently surrounded by extensive collateral circulation that evolves over many years, is unusually tortuous, and has been termed "tree root" or "spiderlike." A "corkscrew" deformity also has been noted in peripheral arteries, probably representing partial recanalization of arteries previously occluded by thrombi. The combination of extensive occlusive disease in tibial arteries with larger vessels that remain smooth and normal in appearance, especially in association with extensive collateral circulation, is highly characteristic of Buerger's disease and is most useful in differentiating it from atherosclerosis.

DIAGNOSIS. Buerger's disease can be differentiated from atherosclerosis without undue difficulty. Other entities with occlusive disease of tibial arteries, however, closely resemble Buerger's disease. These include diabetes mellitus, popliteal aneurysms, repeated episodes of arterioarterial embolization from proximal atherosclerotic plaques, and different collagen disorders. Patients with any of these may have palpable popliteal pulses, absent pedal pulses, and severe ischemia in the digits. In most of these, however, the upper extremities are not involved. Positive factors supporting the diagnosis of Buerger's disease are its onset in men between the ages of twenty and forty years, a history of migratory phlebitis, strong dependence upon tobacco, usually cigarettes, and associated involvement of the upper extremities. The occurrence of elevated titers to rickettsia has also been suggested as a diagnostic as well as an etiologic factor in the evolution of the disease.

Factors suggesting that the disease is not Buerger's disease include diabetes mellitus, palpable popliteal or abdominal aneurysms, audible bruit over a major artery, high blood cholesterol, calcification of peripheral arteries, and onset after forty years of age.

Usually the diagnosis can be made from the history and physical examination. Angiographic studies are needed for confirmation and to define the possibilities of arterial reconstruction. Final proof of the diagnosis may require gross and microscopic examination of the diseased arteries.

TREATMENT. The most important aspect of treatment is to have the patient forego the use of tobacco in any form. Simply decreasing the frequency of cigarette smoking is ineffective. The great difficulty in getting the patient to stop smoking cannot be overemphasized, for the pernicious addiction to smoking in this disease closely resembles the tenacity of heroin addiction. In most teaching institutions there are one or more pathetic individuals who have undergone amputation of both legs and most of the fingers of each hand but who are trying to get someone to light a cigarette for them.

Sympathectomy may be performed but its benefit is difficult to measure because of the episodic characteristics of Buerger's disease. Perhaps 50 percent of patients significantly benefit from the procedure. Vasodilating drugs may be tried but are of questionable value.

Education regarding foot care similar to that described for the atherosclerotic patient is very important since often gangrene is precipitated by minor trauma to the foot, such as unwise trimming of a callus or wearing tight shoes.

Arteriography should be performed to confirm the diagnosis and exclude other forms of smaller arterial occlusions that may require surgical therapy. If a popliteal pulse is absent, it may indicate the possibility of performing local direct arterial reconstruction.

Occasionally patients with Buerger's disease develop atherosclerotic obstruction of major arteries that are surgically accessible to reconstruction. Such a combination of arterial disease is suggested if the popliteal pulse is absent. In these patients arterial reconstruction may be successfully done upon the atherosclerotic disease, with marked circulatory improvement. Direct surgical approach to the vessels primarily involved by Buerger's disease, however, is usually not possible.

A conservative approach is indicated when amputation is required in these younger patients in the twenty- to forty-year-old age group, since the episodic nature of the disease indicates that conservatism may be rewarded by subsidence of the acute episodes with subsequent partial revascularization by the growth of collateral circulation. As long as gangrene is confined to a toe, amputation should be postponed as long as possible unless rest pain or infection cannot be controlled otherwise.

Once gangrene has involved the foot extensively, there is little point in delaying amputation, because a functional foot can rarely be obtained if the point of amputation is more proximal than the base of the metatarsal bones. Often a below-knee amputation can be performed, rather than an above-knee, because of the lack of involvement of the femoral and popliteal arteries.

Long-term anticoagulant therapy has not been of measurable benefit. Therapy with adrenal steroids, so effective for many inflammatory conditions, has similarly not been of consistent value and may aggravate the intimal changes in the tibial arteries.

PROGNOSIS. The variability of long-term survival data is probably related to the difficulty in establishing the specific diagnosis of Buerger's disease. The risk of amputation within 10 years after onset of symptoms is probably near 20 percent, although this varies with the continued use of tobacco as well as the degree to which the ischemic foot is carefully protected. In the few patients who stop smoking completely, progression of the disease may be greatly restricted. A marked advance in therapy would be the discovery of a method by which abstinence from tobacco could be achieved uniformly in this unfortunate group of individuals.

VASOSPASTIC DISORDERS

Raynaud's Disease

The syndrome described by Maurice Raynaud in 1862, now termed *Raynaud's phenomenon,* consists of recurrent episodes of vasoconstriction in the upper extremities, initiated by exposure to cold or emotional stress. Three sequential phases classically occur: pallor, cyanosis, and rubor. It is now recognized that Raynaud's phenomenon may exist as a primary disorder, termed *Raynaud's disease,* or may be a secondary manifestation of a more serious vascular disease, often not evident for some years after the initial appearance of the recurrent color changes. The more common disorders associated with Raynaud's phenomenon include Buerger's disease (thromboangiitis obliterans), scleroderma, cervical rib or other thoracic outlet syndrome, and atherosclerosis. It occasionally results from recurrent minor trauma, such as from the use of mechanical vibrating tools. Rarely, other collagen diseases, such as periarteritis nodosa or disseminated lupus erythematosus, are found. Hence, in the evaluation of a patient the critical decision is to determine whether the disease is primary Raynaud's disease or a secondary manifestation of a more serious disorder. Some suspect that it is always secondary to some other underlying disorder.

ETIOLOGY. The cause of primary Raynaud's disease is unknown. It is much more frequent in women, with a ratio of about 5:1, and appears in over 90 percent of patients before forty years of age. In men, it is usually much less severe in intensity. DeTakats and Fowler observed abnormal electroencephalograms in some patients, suggesting a primary disease in the midbrain, but the existence of a primary neurologic disease has not been established.

PATHOLOGY. The clinical picture of Raynaud's phenomenon is related to the anatomy and physiology of the arteriolar circulation in the dermis. The arterioles penetrate the dermis at right angles with an irregular reticulate pattern and arborize into a capillary network. Some fluctuation in vasomotor tone, as with pallor or blushing, is a normal physiologic variation. In Raynaud's disease, vasospasm occurs with such severity that dermal circulation momentarily ceases, with the production of severe pallor. If the vasospasm is less severe, with slowing but not cessation of the dermal circulation, cyanosis appears, a result of sluggish flow of blood with an increase in the percentage of reduced hemoglobin in the capillaries. When the vasospasm subsides, a reactive hyperemia with vasodilation develops, probably from the accumulation of tissue metabolites during the anoxic period, producing an unusual redness or rubor.

The basis for the increased tendency of the dermal arterioles to vasoconstriction is unknown. It may be a sensitivity in the arterioles themselves, or possibly may result from hyperactivity of the sympathetic nervous system. Initially the arterioles are normal on histologic examination. With chronic disease, there is progressive hypertrophy of the arteriolar walls and ultimate occlusion. Detailed histologic observation of early phases of Raynaud's disease are not available, because tissue biopsies are seldom performed at this time.

In the majority of patients the episodes of vasoconstriction are precipitated by exposure to cold. In about 25 percent of patients intense emotion, as well as cold, may be the initiating factor. Only rarely is emotion alone the significant stimulus without an abnormal sensitivity to cold.

In most patients the upper extremities are symmetrically involved. Unilateral involvement by Raynaud's phenomenon almost always denotes a proximal mechanical cause, either occlusion of one of the major proximal arteries, recurrent embolization, or neurovascular compression. In 10 to 15 percent of patients the legs are involved as well as the arms.

With repeated episodes of vasoconstriction and ischemia, trophic changes gradually appear. These include atrophy of the skin with loss of elasticity and hair. The term *sclerodactylia* has been applied to this appearance, since it resembles the changes found in scleroderma in other organs. However, long-term studies have demonstrated conclusively that the presence of sclerodactylia in the fingers does not indicate that generalized scleroderma will appear in the future. Focal areas of ulceration develop and leave characteristic scars with healing. Recurrent superficial infections, such as paronychia, may occur. In the more extreme forms of ischemia, gangrene may require amputation of one or more digits, but fortunately gangrene almost never progresses to involve the hands.

CLINICAL MANIFESTATIONS. The patient is usually a young woman who has noted that episodes of cold precipitate vasoconstriction with a repetitive sequence of pallor, cyanosis, and rubor. Several variations in the color phenomena may occur with less severe disease. For example, there may be only cyanosis followed by rubor or only episodes of mild cyanosis.

In addition to the color changes, the patient may have paresthesia and localized pain in the digits. If infection or ulceration is present, pain is more severe. Except for the discomfort in the hands, the patients usually have no other symptoms.

Physical Examination. In the early phases, the extremities may be entirely normal with peripheral pulses of equal volume. The best index to its severity is the extent of trophic changes in the fingers, manifested by atrophy of the skin and nails with loss of hair over the terminal phalanges. In more advanced stages, signs of chronic ischemia are obvious, with punctate scars from healed ulcerations, chronic rubor, and absence of radial or ulnar pulses.

Arteriography is of value in establishing the diagnosis by revealing the absence of occlusive arterial disease and the presence of terminal arterial vasospasm. The most critical examination is demonstration of the vasoconstrictor response to cold. Induction of the characteristic pallor-cyanosis-rubor sequence in both hands following exposure to cold establishes the diagnosis, although it does not differentiate between primary and secondary Raynaud's phenomenon. An electroencephalogram might be obtained to pursue the observation that abnormal electroencephalographic tracings are present in some patients.

Once the presence of Raynaud's phenomenon has been confirmed, the principal question is whether the vasomotor changes are primary or secondary to some other vascular disease. The possibility of early scleroderma can be evaluated by study of the motility of the esophagus and small bowel. Other blood tests to screen for collagen disorders, such as lupus, should be done. The presence of cervical ribs can be easily determined by radiographs of the cervical spine and thorax. Other compression syndromes of the subclavian artery can be detected by performing the maneuvers described under Thoracic Outlet Syndromes. Complete angiographic studies to opacify the arterial circulation from the aortic arch to the small arteries of the hand should be done to exclude the possibility of proximal atherosclerotic plaques producing distal emboli. Occasionally skin and lymph node biopsies are useful.

An important principle in diagnosis is continued observation of the patient over a period of several years. Even after a thorough examination has failed to detect any underlying disease, a disease may appear later. Indeed, patients should be followed indefinitely with this fact in mind.

TREATMENT. In the majority of patients disability is mild. Avoiding cold or other stimuli which precipitate vasoconstriction is adequate. Moving to a warm climate may be considered, but this does not eliminate the attacks. Tobacco certainly should be avoided because of its potent vasoconstrictor action, but this alone does not abolish the syndrome. Various vasodilator drugs have been repeatedly tried, but none has been of consistent benefit. Methyldopa was the earliest effective medication. Intraarterial reserpine often produced dramatic responses of vasodilatation followed by prolonged periods of freedom from recurrent attacks, but its production has been discontinued. Orally administered calcium channel blockers have become the drugs of choice and offer the promise of reasonably good control. Uncontrolled observations show beneficial effects of prostaglandin E, administered intravenously to patients with severe ischemic changes in the fingers and hands. In addition to the healing of ulcerated lesions, improvement in digital blood flow and skin temperature was also reported. The validity of the findings has been questioned, however, because of the failure to observe a control series.

Although cervical dorsal sympathectomy with removal of the first, second, and third thoracic ganglia, preserving the cervical portion of the stellate ganglion to avoid Horner's syndrome, can give excellent immediate results in patients before the advent of the ulceration, relapses are common. DeTakats and Fowler tabulated reports from different groups, including 40 cases of their own, and found that in 424 sympathectomies 55 percent improved. For this reason, sympathectomy is usually employed only when symptoms are severe and other therapy is ineffective. More radical sympathectomies have not given any better results. Proximally all of the stellate ganglion has been removed, producing Horner's syndrome; distad the fourth thoracic ganglion has been included. Another technical modification has been to include the second and third intercostal nerves with the third ganglion because of the demonstration by Skoog that 10 to 15 percent of sympathetic ganglia to the upper extremity are contained in these two intercostal ganglia. Also there has been considerable discussion about differences in preganglionic and postganglionic sympathectomy. None of these variations has been found significant, however, and the conservative sympathectomy involving the first, second, and third

thoracic ganglia is usually performed. Severe trophic changes before operation are unfortunately often associated with a poor result. Patients with scleroderma also obtain little benefit.

Operative Technique. At least four different surgical techniques have been employed at different times for sympathectomy. Originally most were done through a posterior approach, with the patient in a prone position and an incision similar to that for a thoracoplasty. The sympathetic chain was exposed by resecting a short segment of the second or third rib, followed by an extrapleural dissection to isolate the sympathetic chain. In large, muscular individuals this approach is quite difficult and provides only limited exposure. It has been virtually abandoned.

A second technique, a supraclavicular approach, provides excellent exposure in patients of small stature with long thin necks. However, in those with short, thick necks, significant trauma to the brachial plexus, resulting in a painful neuritis, may complicate the postoperative course. An excellent description of the technique was published by Nanson.

Ideal exposure can be obtained by an anterior transthoracic incision, opening the hemithorax in the third or fourth intercostal space. This, of necessity, involves a major thoracotomy, though a simple one. It has been favored by Palumbo, who also emphasized that removal of the lower one-third of the stellate ganglion would adequately sympathectomize the extremity without producing Horner's syndrome.

In recent years the transaxillary approach has become preferred. This is done through a short incision in the axilla, followed by resection of a short segment of the second or third rib and exposure of the sympathetic chain. Good technical descriptions have been published by Roos and by Kirtley et al. The thoracotomy is of much less magnitude than that through the anterior approach, and the incision is in an inconspicuous location.

PROGNOSIS. The prognosis in most patients with primary Raynaud's disease is good, with the exception of the discomfort associated with the abnormal sensitivity to cold. Even in the more advanced forms, tissue loss seldom exceeds the loss of one or more digits. More serious systemic vascular disease does not develop, and although symptoms may continue for many years, there is no known impairment of longevity or health.

On the other hand, patients with secondary Raynaud's phenomenon afflicted with severe collagen disorders frequently progress to loss of tissue, often with amputations of portions of the fingers. This group requires unceasing care of the hands with careful attention to aggressive local treatment of minor injuries and infections.

Uncommon Vasomotor Diseases

Rare, unusual vasomotor diseases include livedo reticularis and acrocyanosis, which primarily result from vasoconstriction, and erythromelalgia, apparently a result of vasodilatation. The disability with these disorders is usually episodic and mild. Their clinical significance lies primarily in differentiating them from more serious underlying disease, such as Buerger's disease, scleroderma, or disseminated lupus erythematosus. Only salient clinical features of these bizarre diseases will be presented here.

LIVEDO RETICULARIS

This unusual vasomotor condition is characterized by a persistent mottled reddish blue discoloration of the skin of the extremities. It is more prominent in the legs and feet than in the hands or arms and only infrequently involves the trunk. Although the severity varies with temperature, becoming worse on exposure to cold, it never entirely disappears spontaneously.

ETIOLOGY AND PATHOLOGY. The cause is unknown, although miscellaneous associated vascular diseases such as hypertension or emotional disorders have been found in different patients.

The pathophysiologic feature apparently is a stenosis of the arterioles that pierce the cutis at right angles and arborize into the peripheral capillaries of the skin. The obstruction of the arterioles, either spastic or organic, therefore affects the peripheral capillary arborizations and accounts for the peculiar reticular nature of the discoloration.

The pathologic change in the arterioles varies from no visible abnormality to proliferation of the intima, in some patients progressing to complete occlusion. With severe organic obstruction, focal ulceration of the skin, usually over the lower legs, may occur.

CLINICAL MANIFESTATIONS. Patients with livedo reticularis complain of the persistent reddish blue mottling over the legs and feet, varying somewhat with temperature. Often the cosmetic appearance is the only concern of the patient. In some there are localized symptoms of coldness, numbness, dull aching, and paresthesia. With severe forms and localized tissue ischemia, there may be pain from local ulceration. These symptoms are more prone to appear during the winter in association with cold temperatures.

The diagnosis is usually made from physical examination, with observation of the persistent blotchy discoloration, and a history of prolonged persistence in association with some variation with environmental temperature. Peripheral pulsations are normal, and trophic changes are not present in the digits. Only with more extreme forms are ischemic ulcers present over the lower legs. These usually heal after a short period of time.

TREATMENT. In most patients no treatment is necessary except reassurance regarding the benign nature of the condition. Gangrene rarely occurs. Avoiding extremes of cold is beneficial in some patients. Vasodilating agents may be tried, but none has been found of consistent benefit. Sympathectomy should be employed if the disability is severe enough to produce local ulceration. After sympathectomy the discoloration may decrease in extent and remain pink rather than blue. In most patients the disorder is a permanent one, remaining as a moderate cosmetic disturbance, but fortunately with no other disability.

ACROCYANOSIS

Acrocyanosis is a disorder characterized by persistent but painless cold and cyanosis of the hands and feet. The cause and the pathologic and pathophysiologic features are virtually unknown, for the disease consists primarily of persistent color changes. Usually it is confused with Raynaud's phenomenon because of the prominent localized cyanosis. Detailed investigation of the pathophysiologic features by Lewis and Landis concluded that the fundamental disorder was a localized abnormality in vasomotor tone in the circulation of the hands and feet. Apparently the basic physiologic condition is a slow rate of blood flow through the skin, the result of chronic arteriolar constriction, which results in a high percentage of reduced hemoglobin in the blood in the capillaries and production of the cyanotic color. Endocrine dysfunction has been found in some patients, but no consistent pattern has been established.

Usually the disorder is found in a young woman who has noted persistent coldness and blueness of the fingers and hands for many years, often with symptoms of less severity in the toes and feet. The abnormalities are more prominent in cold weather, but the extremities are never completely normal. With heat the color may change from deep purple to red, but there are no episodes of blanching, such as occurs with Raynaud's phenomenon. The peripheral pulses are normal, and there are no trophic changes indicative of chronic tissue ischemia, such as atrophy of the skin, sclerosis, or ulceration.

The principal differential diagnosis is from Raynaud's disease because of the prominent color changes in both disorders. The absence of pallor, as well as the absence of signs of chronic ischemia, are the most useful features. Similarly, the constant presence of the color changes in acrocyanosis, as opposed to the intermittent episodic occurrence in Raynaud's disease, is characteristic.

Usually reassurance is the only treatment needed, with the avoidance of cold temperatures when possible. Sympathectomy can be employed with reasonably good results if the disability is more serious. Prognosis is excellent, with tissue loss virtually never occurring. Usually the color changes remain for many years or permanently.

ERYTHROMELALGIA

This rare disorder is characterized by red, warm, painful extremities. The clinical characteristics were described by S. Weir Mitchell in 1872, and the disorder was named by him in 1878. The cause of the primary disease is unknown. Similar phenomena, so-called secondary erythromelalgia, can occur as a result of hypertension or polycythemia vera.

The basic abnormality is an unusual sensitivity to warmth, for skin temperatures of 32 to 36°C, which produce no effects in normal individuals, will regularly induce the painful burning sensation. The exact temperature at which the distress can be produced varies with different patients but may be a precise one for any individual patient. It was termed by Lewis a "critical point." The increase in temperature is usually a result of vasodilatation with increase in blood flow. The exact basis for the spontaneous vasodilatation with the rise in temperature and the burning sensation is not known.

The disease is equally prevalent in men and women, usually of middle age. The distress may be greater in the summer months, but only a general relationship to extremes of heat or cold may be present. The patient soon learns that exposing the extremities to cold, such as by immersing them in ice water, may abort an attack.

Physical examination usually reveals no abnormalities of the peripheral arteries. The diagnosis is usually established by demonstration of a close relationship between the symptoms and skin temperature. This may be induced by direct application of heat, noting the skin temperature at which distress appears. Erythromelalgia should be differentiated from the painful red but cold extremities that occur with Buerger's disease and also with peripheral neuritis.

Aside from the troublesome symptoms, the disorder is a benign one. Avoiding extremes of heat is one of the most useful therapeutic measures. Acetylsalicylic acid, 0.65 g, has been found beneficial in many patients, although the mode of action is uncertain. A trial of therapy with vasoconstrictor drugs, such as ephedrine, should be employed, but consistent value from one drug has not been found. The disorder is usually a permanent one, but no permanent disability results.

FROSTBITE

Several forms of cold injury have been described, usually varying with the environmental conditions under which exposure occurs. These different syndromes include acute pernio (chilblains), chronic pernio, trench foot, immersion foot, and frostbite. Acute and chronic pernio are focal injuries of the skin and subcutaneous tissue resulting from exposure to cold of moderate intensity, representing an increased susceptibility to cold injury in a particular individual. The disorder is seldom a surgical problem, because the lesions are focal, superficial ones that heal readily. Trench foot and immersion foot are primarily military injuries produced by prolonged exposure to cold in damp surroundings, often with temperatures well above freezing, but in circumstances where there is an element of prolonged immobility. Immersion foot is probably simply the seagoing counterpart of trench foot. Such injuries are rarely seen in civilian practice. For practical purposes frostbite is the type of injury usually encountered and will be discussed in detail. The tissue response in the other disorders mentioned, however, is a similar type of response to cold, modified somewhat with the environmental conditions.

ETIOLOGY. Frostbite results when tissues are exposed to cold for varying periods of time. The severity varies both with the temperature and the duration of exposure. It has been demonstrated experimentally that freezing begins in mammalian tissues when the temperature in the deeper parts reaches 10°C and that −5°C is the lowest temperature to which cells may be slowly frozen and still survive. Frostbite injury usually results from exposure

over a period of several hours. In the Korean conflict, 90 percent of the cases occurred at temperatures near −7°C after exposure for 7 to 18 h. A different form of frostbite is produced by acute exposures to below zero temperatures, commonly occurring in airplanes at high altitudes and hence termed "high altitude" frostbite. In such injuries the exposed part is acutely frozen with deposition of ice crystals in the tissues. This unusual form of injury is different from the usual case of frostbite, where a "slow freeze" results.

Several factors influence the injurious effect of cold. Two of the most significant ones are humidity and the presence of wind, both of which accelerate the withdrawal of heat from body tissues. Immobility or occlusive vascular disease also are significant factors, both influencing the rate of peripheral blood flow. Acclimatization has been demonstrated in some persons repeatedly exposed to cold, such as those who live in northern latitudes, and probably is a localized vasomotor adaptation. By contrast, extremities previously injured by cold may remain permanently susceptible to future cold injury, perhaps from an intensified vasoconstrictor response.

PATHOLOGY. The degrees of severity of a frostbite injury have been conventionally grouped into four clinical types analogous to the classification of burn injury. First degree injury consists of edema and redness of the affected part without necrosis; formation of blisters represents a second-degree injury; necrosis of the skin constitutes a third-degree injury; in a fourth-degree injury gangrene of the extremity develops, requiring amputation.

As frostbite occurs, the injured tissue becomes numb and moderately stiff without extensive discomfort. With subsequent rewarming the tissues become reddened, hot, and edematous. At this time blisters erupt and gangrene gradually appears in the more seriously injured tissues. Edema increases to a maximum within 24 to 48 h and then gradually is resorbed as gangrenous tissue begins to demarcate. The extent of gangrene is difficult to estimate initially and requires observations for as long as 30 days or more. Fortunately the degree of gangrene is often much less than that initially feared, because the skin may be gangrenous but the underlying tissue viable. For this reason amputation is delayed until the extent of gangrene is definitely known.

Following recovery of the extremity, there is frequently a permanent increase in vasoconstrictor tone resulting in hyperhidrosis and an abnormal sensitivity to cold. Pain and paresthesia are also common, perhaps as residuals from ischemic neuritis.

It is uncertain whether the fundamental injury from cold results from direct freezing with disruption of cell membranes or whether the injury is primarily an ischemic necrosis from widespread thrombosis of arterioles and capillaries. Certainly vascular occlusion is a prominent feature, whether it is a primary or a secondary event. With exposure to cold, there is severe vasoconstriction, decreasing the rate of blood flow in the chilled extremity, with resulting stasis, sludging of blood, and eventual widespread thrombosis. In clinical experiments, immersion of the arm for 2 h in water at 13°C decreases blood flow to about 3 percent of normal, while immersion of a finger in water at 7°C stops blood flow altogether. In addition to sludging and capillary thrombosis, there is an increase in capillary permeability, resulting in the formation of edema when blood flow is increased after rewarming.

On histologic examination of the injured tissues, edema, infiltration of inflammatory cells, and deposition of fibrin are prominent findings. Widespread thrombosis of small vessels is frequently seen. In addition, focal areas of necrosis may be evident in skin, muscle, and other tissues.

CLINICAL MANIFESTATIONS. Frequently, the patient is unaware that frostbite is occurring. The usual injury occurs with exposure to near freezing temperatures for several hours, often combined with wind, high humidity, damp or wet shoes, or immobility from tightly constricting shoes or confinement in a cramped position. All these factors influence the rate of heat transfer between the extremity and the environment. Initially there may be mild discomfort, but as the extremity becomes numb and somewhat stiff, frequently discomfort is minimal.

When rewarmed, the extremity quickly becomes red, edematous, hot, and painful. This is due to vasodilatation and widespread extravasation of fluid through the walls of capillaries whose permeability has been increased from injury. Edema reaches its peak intensity within 48 h and then gradually subsides over several days. Gangrene gradually becomes evident and slowly demarcates over a period of many days. An ominous sign, indicating that gangrene will develop, is the persistence of coldness and numbness in an area while surrounding tissues become edematous, hot, and painful. The persistent coldness and numbness indicate cessation of all circulation with the certain outcome of ischemic necrosis.

TREATMENT. Frostbite seldom occurs during exposure to cold if proper precautions are taken. This includes wearing dry, insulated, loosely fitting clothing and carefully avoiding long periods of immobility of the exposed extremities. Most cases of clinical frostbite occur in circumstances where exposure to cold inadvertently occurs for long periods of time because of coma from injury, alcohol, or other factors.

Rapid warming of the injured tissue is the most important aspect of treatment. Several studies have clearly demonstrated the advantages of the rapid-rewarming method over any other. The frozen tissue should be placed in warm water, with a temperature in the range of 40 to 44°C. Complete rewarming usually requires about 20 min. Higher temperatures are more injurious than beneficial. A frostbitten part should never be exposed to hot water, an open fire, or excessive dry heat, as in an oven, for the loss of sensitivity in the frozen area makes it especially vulnerable to injury. Warming in water is much more rapid than application of warm blankets, which require three or four times as long as the immersion method.

Following rewarming, the injured extremity should be elevated to minimize formation of edema and carefully protected in a sterile environment. Usually it is left exposed but surrounded by a protective cradle. Blisters are opened only when necessary to remove necrotic skin.

Antibiotic therapy and tetanus antiserum are routinely given to lessen the risk of infection. Demarcation of gangrenous areas should be carefully observed, often for several weeks, before amputation is performed. Often a gangrenous area which initially appears to involve the foot will gradually regress with the separation of superficial areas of gangrenous skin, ultimately with the loss of one or more digits but preservation of the foot.

Angiography of the frostbite patient can define the extent of organic vascular stenosis and the degree of functional vasospasm, thus aiding the choice of therapy. The use of other fast-acting vasodilators such as papaverine might be appropriate.

Both experimental and clinical experiences indicate a beneficial effect from sympathectomy, especially when employed in the first few days after frostbite has occurred. Shumacker and Kilman reported 66 sympathectomies in 38 patients, 24 of which were performed soon after injury. Their experience indicated that sympathectomy should be performed for injuries severe enough to produce necrosis of tissue, both to minimize the extent of necrosis and to prevent the usual late vasomotor sequelae. Golding et al. found in experimental and clinical studies (68 patients) that the proper time for sympathectomy was between 36 and 72 h after injury. Earlier sympathectomies accelerated the rate of edema formation, while sympathectomies performed following the peak intensity of edema seemed to hasten absorption of edema and minimize eventual tissue necrosis. Sympathectomy is also beneficial in alleviating the late sequelae from cold injury, i.e., paresthesia, coldness, and hyperhidrosis.

If vascular injury is the primary event, therapeutic measures to decrease vasoconstriction or blood clotting, such as sympathectomy or the administration of heparin, should be of routine benefit. The theoretic benefit from sympathectomy is the release of vasospasm, which may precipitate thrombosis in injured capillaries and arterioles. Heparin and dextran have also been given in attempts to lessen the degree of small vessel thrombosis that is such a prominent feature on histologic examination of the injured tissues. Although theoretically plausible, consistent benefit has not been demonstrated from the routine use of either heparin or dextran.

PROGNOSIS. Following recovery from injury, all studies have found a significant percentage of residual disability in the extremity. Simeone evaluated 1061 limbs 4 months after frostbite while the patients were still in the hospital and found painful feet and hyperhidrosis the most common complaints. Ervasti described similar sequelae in 812 cases of frostbite 5 to 18 years after injury. Orr and Fainer reported that gangrene occurred in only 6 percent of 1880 cases from the Korean conflict, but some disability remained in 10 to 20 percent of patients.

Bibliography

Occlusive Disease: General

Collins GJ Jr: Vascular occlusive disorders. Medical and surgical management. Mt Kisco, NY, Futura Publishing, 1981.

Dale WA: The beginnings of vascular surgery. *Surgery* 76:849, 1974.

Goldenfarb PB, Cathey MH, Cooper GR: The determination of ADP induced platelet aggregation in normal men. *Atherosclerosis* 12:335, 1970.

Greenhalgh RM, Rosengarten DS, Mervart I: Serum lipids and lipo proteins in peripheral vascular disease. *Lancet* 2:947, 1971.

Hardy JD, Conn JH, Fain WR: Nonatherosclerotic occlusive lesions of small arteries. *Surgery* 57:1, 1965.

Honour AJ, Pickering GW, Sheppard BL: Ultrastructure and behavior of platelet thrombi in injured arteries. *Br J Exp Pathol* 52:482, 1971.

Lassen NA, Holstein P: Use of radioisotopes in assessment of distal blood flow and distal blood pressure in arterial insufficiency. *Surg Clin North Am* 54(1):39, 1974.

Rob CG: *The Classics of Vascular Surgery*, in Reemtsma K (ed): *The Classics of Surgery Library, Classics in Vascular Surgery*. Medford, NJ, Apollo, 1982.

Rutherford RB: *Vascular Surgery*. Philadelphia, Saunders, 1977.

Salzman EW: The limitations of heparin therapy after arterial reconstructions. *Surgery* 57:131, 1965.

Schatz IJ: Classification of primary hyperlipidemia. *JAMA* 210:701, 1969.

Schnetzer GW: Platelets and thrombogenesis: Current concepts. *Am Heart J* 83:552, 1972.

Scott HW Jr: Metabolic surgery for hyperlipidemia and atherosclerosis. *Am J Surg* 123:3, 1972.

Stanley JC, Gewertz BL, et al: Arterial fibrodysplasia: Histopathologic character and current etiologic concepts. *Arch Surg* 110:561, 1975.

Thompson JE, et al: Peripheral-arterial surgery. *N Engl J Med* 302:491, 1980.

Manifestations of Chronic Arterial Occlusion

Bernstein EF: *Noninvasive Diagnostic Techniques in Vascular Disease*. St Louis, Mosby, 1982.

Boyd AM: The natural course of arteriosclerosis of the lower extremities. *Angiology* 11:10, 1960.

Cronenweth JL, Warner KG, et al: Intermittent claudication: Current results of nonoperative management. *Arch Surg* 119:430, 1984.

Ekroth R, Dahilof AG, et al: Physical training of patients with intermittent claudication: Indications, methods, and results. *Surgery* 84:640, 1978.

Goldenfarb PB, Cathey MH, Cooper GR: The determination of ADP induced platelet aggregation in normal men. *Atherosclerosis* 12:335, 1970.

Goodreau JJ, Creasy JK, et al: Rational approach to the differentiation of vascular and neurogenic claudication. *Surgery* 84:749, 1978.

Imparato AM, Kim GE, et al: Intermittent claudication: Its natural course. *Surgery* 78:795, 1975.

Karayannacos PE, Yahson D, Vasko JS: Narrow lumbar spine canal with vascular syndromes. *Arch Surg* 111:803, 1976.

Mannick JA: Current concepts in diagnostic methods. Evaluation of chronic lower-extremity ischemia. *N Engl J Med* 309:841, 1983.

Lassen NA, Holstein P: Use of radioisotopes in assessment of distal blood flow and distal blood pressure in arterial insufficiency. *Surg Clin North Am* 54:39, 1974.

Strandness DE: Evaluation of the patient for vascular surgery. *Surg Clin North Am* 54:13, 1974.

Taylor LM Jr, Porter JM: Drug treatment of claudication: Hemorrheologic agents and antiserotonin drugs. *J Vasc Surg* 3:374, 1986.

Yao JST, Bergan JJ: Application of ultrasound to arterial and venous diagnosis. *Surg Clin North Am* 54:25, 1974.

Aortoiliac Occlusive Disease

Brewster DC, Darling RC: Optimal methods of aortoiliac reconstruction. *Surgery* 84:739, 1978.

Flanigan DP, Ryan TJ, et al: Aortofemoral or femoropopliteal revascularization? A prospective evaluation of the papaverine test. *J Vasc Surg* 1:215, 1984.

Garrett HE, Crawford ES, et al: Surgical considerations in the treatment of aorto-iliac occlusive disease. *Surg Clin North Am* 46:949, 1966.

Guida PM, Moore SW: Obturator bypass techniques. *Surg Gynecol Obstet* 128:1307, 1969.

Imparato AM, Sanoudos G, et al: Results in 96 aortoiliac reconstructive procedures: Preoperative angiographic and functional classifications used as prognostic guides. *Surgery* 68:610, 1970.

Inihara T: Endarterectomy for occlusive disease of the aortoiliac and common femoral arteries: Evaluation of results of the eversion technique endarterectomy. *Am J Surg* 124:235, 1972.

Jones AF, Kempezinski RF: Aortofemoral bypass grafting: A reappraisal. *Arch Surg* 116:301, 1981.

Kwaan JHM, Molen RV, et al: Peripheral embolism resulting from unsuspected atheromatous aortic plaques. *Surgery* 78:583, 1975.

LoGerfo FW, Johnson WC, et al: Comparison of the late patency rates of axillobilateral femoral and axillounilateral femoral grafts. *Surgery* 81:33, 1977.

Lorentsen E, Hael BL, Hal R: Evaluation of the functional importance of atherosclerotic obliterations in the aorto-iliac artery by pressure-flow measurements. *Acta Med Scand* 191:399, 1972.

Lowenstein MH, Machleder HI: Sexual function after aortoiliac surgery. *Ann Surg* 191:787, 1975.

Mannick JA, Williams LE, Nabseth DC: The late results of axillofemoral grafts. *Surgery* 68:1038, 1970.

Martinez BD, Hertzer NR, et al: Influence of distal arterial occlusive disease on prognosis following aortobifemoral bypass. *J Vasc Surg* 88:795, 1980.

May AG, Van de Berg L, et al: Critical arterial stenosis. *Surgery* 54:250, 1963.

Nash RL, Menzoian JO, et al: The multidisciplinary approach to vasculogenic impotence. *Surgery* 89:124, 1981.

Ray LI, O'Connor JB, et al: Axillofemoral bypass: A critical reappraisal of its role in the management of aortoiliac occlusive disease. *Am J Surg* 138:117, 1979.

Sethi GK, Scott SM, Takaro T: Multiple-plane angiography for more precise evaluation of aortoiliac disease. *Surgery* 78:15, 1975.

Szilagyi DE, Smith RF, et al: Infection in arterial reconstruction with synthetic grafts. *Ann Surg* 176:321, 1972.

Szilagyi DE, Smith RF, et al: Anastomotic aneurysms after vascular reconstruction: Problems of incidence, etiology, and treatment. *Surgery* 78:800, 1975.

Szilagyi DE, Elliott JP Jr, et al: A thirty-year survey of the reconstructive surgical treatment of aortoiliac occlusive disease. *J Vasc Surg* 3:421, 1986.

Ward RE, Holcroft JW, et al: New concepts in the use of axillofemoral bypass grafts. *Arch Surg* 118:573, 1983.

Transluminal Arterial Balloon Dilatation (Balloon Angioplasty)

Alpert JR, Ring EJ, et al: Balloon dilatation of iliac stenosis with distal arterial surgery. *Arch Surg* 115:715, 1980.

Borozan PG, Schuler JJ, et al: Long-term hemodynamic evaluation of lower extremity percutaneous transluminal angioplasty. *J Vasc Surg* 2:785, 1985.

Colapinto RF, et al: Percutaneous transluminal angioplasty of peripheral vascular disease: A two year experience. *Cardiovasc Intervent Radiol* 3:213, 1980.

Gallino A, Mahler F, et al: Percutaneous transluminal angioplasty of the arteries of the lower limbs. *Circulation* 70:619, 1984.

Gewertz BL, Ball DG, Zareus C: Limb salvage in poor risk patients using transluminal angioplasty. *Arch Surg* 118:1209, 1983.

Kumpe DA, et al: Percutaneous transluminal angioplasty in the selected management of proximal arterial occlusive disease of the lower extremities: A preliminary report. *Surgery* 87:488, 1980.

Martin EC, Fankuchen EL, et al: Angioplasty for femoral artery occlusion: Comparison with surgery. *Am J Rad* 137:915, 1981.

Potter CT, Judkins MP: Transluminal treatment of arteriosclerotic obstruction: Description of a new technique and a preliminary report of its application. *Circulation* 30:654, 1964.

Rush DS, Gewertz BL, Lu C-t: Limb salvage in poor-risk patients using transluminal angioplasty. *Arch Surg* 118:1209, 1983.

Zarins CK, Lu C-t, et al: Limb salvage by percutaneous transluminal recanulization of the occluded superficial femoral artery. *Surgery* 87:701, 1980.

Femoropopliteal Occlusive Disease

Allan JS, Taylor GW: The relationship between blood flow and failure of femoropopliteal reconstructive arterial surgery. *Br J Surg* 59:549, 1972.

Brief DK, Brener BJ, et al: Crossover femoropopliteal grafts followed up five years or more. An analysis. *Arch Surg* 110:1294, 1975.

Cranley JJ, Hafner CD: Newer prosthetic material compared with autogenous saphenous vein for occlusive arterial disease of the lower extremity. *Surgery* 89:2, 1981.

Cutler BS, Thompson JE, et al: Autologous saphenous vein femoropopliteal bypass: Analysis of 298 cases. *Surgery* 79:324, 1976.

Dale WA: Autogenous vein grafts for femoropopliteal arterial repair. *Surg Gynecol Obstet* 123:1282, 1966.

DeWeese JA, Rob CG: Autogenous venous bypass grafts five years later. *Ann Surg* 174:346, 1971.

Evans LE, Webster MW, et al: Expanded polytetrafluoroethylene femoropopliteal grafts: Forty-eight month follow-up. *Surgery* 89:16, 1981.

Imparato AM, Bracco A, Kim GE: Comparisons of three technics for femoral-popliteal arterial reconstructions. *Ann Surg* 177:375, 1973.

Koontz TJ, Stausel HC Jr: Factors influencing patency of the autogenous vein femoropopliteal by-pass graft: An analysis of 74 cases. *Surgery* 71:753, 1972.

Leather RP, Shah DM, et al: Instrumental evolution of the valve incision method of in situ saphenous vein bypass. *J Vasc Surg* 1:113, 1984.

Mannick JA: Femoro-popliteal and femoro-tibial reconstructions. *Surg Clin North Am* 59:581, 1979.

Martin P, Jamieson C: The rationale for and measurement after profundaplasty. *Surg Clin North Am* 54:95, 1974.

Plecha FR, Plecha FM: Femorofemoral bypass grafts: Ten year experience. *J Vasc Surg* 1:555, 1984.

Plecha FR, Pories WJ: Intraoperative angiography in the immediate assessment of arterial reconstruction. *Arch Surg* 105:902, 1972.

Poliwoda H: Treatment of acute and chronic arterial occlusions with streptokinase. *Aust Ann Med* 19(suppl 1):25, 1970.

Reichle FA, Rankin KP, Tyson RR: Long-term results of 474 arterial reconstructions for severely ischemic limbs: A fourteen year follow-up. *Surgery* 85:93, 1979.

Rosenberg N, Thompson JE, et al: The modified bovine arterial graft. *Arch Surg* 111:222, 1976.

Sawyer PN, Kaplitt MJ, et al: Analysis of peripheral gas endarterectomy in 127 patients. *Arch Surg* 97:859, 1968.

Shah DM, Buckbinder D: Modified technique to produce valvular incompetence in in situ saphenous vein arterial bypass. *Arch Surg* 116:356, 1981.

Szilagyi DE, Smith RF, et al: Long-term behavior of a dacron arterial substitute: Clinical, roentgenologic and histologic correlations. *Ann Surg* 162:453, 1965.

Szilagyi DE, Smith RF, et al: Autogenous vein grafting in femoral popliteal atherosclerosis: The limits of its effectiveness. *Surgery* 86:836, 1979.

Towne JB, Bernhard VM, et al: Profundaplasty in perspective: Limitations in the long-term management of limb ischemia. *Surgery* 90:1037, 1981.

Veith FJ, Gupta SK, et al: Six-year prospective multicenter randomized comparison of autologous saphenous vein and expanded polytetrafluoroethylene grafts in infrainguinal arterial reconstructions. *J Vasc Surg* 3:104, 1986.

Vollmar J, Frede M, Laubach K: Principles of reconstructive procedures for chronic femoro-popliteal occlusions: A report of 546 operations. *Ann Surg* 168:215, 1968.

Walker PM, Imparato AM, Riles TS: Long-term results in superficial femoral artery endarterectomy. *Surgery* 89:23, 1981.

Weisel RD, Johnson KW, et al: Comparison of conduits for leg revascularization. *Surgery* 89:8, 1981.

Tibioperoneal Occlusive Disease

Edwards WH, Mucherin JL Jr: The role of graft materials in femorotibial bypass grafts. *Ann Surg* 191:721, 1980.

Flinn WR, Flanigan DP, et al: Sequential femoral-tibial by-pass for severe limb ischemia. *Surgery* 88:357, 1980.

Imparato AM, Kim GE, Chu DS: Surgical exposure for reconstruction of the proximal part of the tibial artery. *Surg Gynecol Obstet* 136:453, 1973.

Imparato AM, Kim GE, et al: Angiographic criteria for successful tibial arterial reconstructions. *Surgery* 74:830, 1973.

Imparato AM, Kim GE, et al: The results of tibial artery reconstruction procedures. *Surg Gynecol Obstet* 138:33, 1974.

Kahn SP, Lindenauer M, et al: Femorotibial vein bypass. *Arch Surg* 107:309, 1973.

Reichle FA, Martinson MW, Kevin PR: Infrapopliteal arterial reconstruction in the severely ischemic lower limb. A comparison of long term results of peroneal and tibial bypasses. *Ann Surg* 191:59, 1980.

Reichle FA, Tyson RR: Comparison of long-term results of 364 femoropopliteal or femorotibial bypasses for revascularization of severely ischemic lower extremities. *Ann Surg* 182:449, 1975.

Occlusive Disease of the Upper Extremity

Machleder HI (ed): *Vascular Disorders of the Upper Extremity.* Mt Kisco, NY, Futura, 1983.

Porter JM, Rivers SP, et al: Evaluation and management of patients with Raynaud's syndrome. *Am J Surg* 142:183, 1981.

Robbs JV, Human RR, Rajaruthnam P: Operative treatment of nonspecific aortoarteritis (Takayusu's arteritis). *J Vasc Surg* 3:605, 1986.

Whitehouse WM Jr, Zelenoc GB, et al: Arterial bypass grafts for upper extremity ischemia. *J Vasc Surg* 3:569, 1986.

Zelenock B, Cronenwett JL, et al: Brachiocephalic arterial occlusions and stenoses. Manifestations and management of complex lesions. *Arch Surg* 120:370, 1985.

Lumbar Sympathectomy

Berardi RS, Siroospour D: Lumbar sympathectomy in the treatment of peripheral vascular occlusive disease: Ten year study. *Am J Surg* 130:309, 1975.

Collins GJ Jr, Rich NM, et al: Clinical results of lumbar sympathectomy. *Ann Surg* 47:31, 1981.

Cross FW, Cotton LT: Chemical lumbar sympathectomy for ischemic rest pain. A randomized, prospective controlled clinical trial. *Am J Surg* 150:341, 1985.

Grover-Johnson N, Baumann FG, et al: Effect of surgical lumbar sympathectomy of innervation of arterioles in the lower limb of patients with diabetes. *Surg Gynecol Obstet* 153:39, 1981.

Kim GE, Ibrahim IM, Imparato AM: Lumbar sympathectomy in end stage arterial occlusive disease. *Ann Surg* 183:157, 1976.

Plecha FR: A new criterion for predicting response to lumbar sympathectomy in patients with severe arteriosclerotic occlusive disease. *Surgery* 88:375, 1980.

Raskin NH, Levinson SA, et al: Post-sympathectomy neuralgia: Amelioration with diphenylhydantoin and carbamazepine. *Am J Surg* 128:75, 1974.

Walker PM, Johnson KW: Predicting the success of a sympathectomy: A prospective study using discriminant function and multiple regression analysis. *Surgery* 87:216, 1980.

Key JA, Mackay IM, Johnson KW: Phenol sympathectomy for vascular occlusive disease. *Surg Gynecol Obstet* 146:741, 1978.

Wright CJ, Cousins MJ: Blood flow distribution in the human leg following epidural sympathetic blockage. *Arch Surg* 105:334, 1972.

Complications of Vascular Reconstructions

Baumann FG, Imparato AM, Kim GE: The evolution of early fibromuscular lesions hemodynamically induced in the dog renal artery: 1. Light and transmission electron microscopy. *Circ Res* 39:809, 1976.

Beebe HG, Clark WF, DeWeese JA: Atherosclerotic change occurring in an autogenous venous arterial graft. *Arch Surg* 101:85, 1970.

Bunt TJ: Synthetic vascular graft infections. I. Graft infections. *Surgery* 93:703, 1984.

Bunt TJ: Synthetic vascular graft infections. II. Graft-enteric erosions and graft-enteric fistulas. *Surgery* 94:1, 1983.

Graor RA, Risius B, et al: Local thrombolysis in the treatment of thrombosed arteries, bypass grafts, and arteriovenous fistulas. *J Vasc Surg* 2:406, 1985.

Hamaker WR, Doyle WF, et al: Subintimal obliterative prolifera-

tion in saphenous vein grafts. A cause of early failure of aorta to coronary artery by-pass grafts. *Ann Thorac Surg* 13:488, 1972.

Imparato AM, Baumann FG, et al: Electron microscopic studies of experimentally produced fibromuscular arterial lesions. *Surg Gynecol Obstet* 68:682, 1976.

Imparato AM, Bracco A, Hammond R: The effect of intimal and neo-intimal fibromuscular fibroplasia on arterial reconstructions. *J Cardiovasc Surg (Torino)* Special Issue, 488, 1975.

Reilly LM, Altman H, et al: Late results following surgical management of vascular graft infection. *J Vasc Surg* 1:36, 1984.

The Diabetic Foot

Barker WF: Peripheral vascular disease in diabetes: Diagnosis and management. *Med Clin North Am* 55:1045, 1971.

Friedman SA, Friedberg P, Colton J: Vasomotor tone in diabetic neuropathy. *Ann Intern Med* 77:353, 1972.

LeFrock JL, Joseph WS: Lower extremity infections in diabetics. *Infect Surg* 135, 1986.

Levin MD, O'Neal LW: *The Diabetic Foot.* St Louis, Mosby, 1973.

Amputations

Barnes RW, Sharick GD, Slaymaker EE: An index of healing in below-knee amputation: Leg blood pressure by Doppler ultrasound. *Surgery* 79:13, 1976.

Beradi RS, Keenin Y: Amputations in peripheral vascular occlusive disease. *Am J Surg* 135:231, 1978.

Bone GE, Pomajzl MJ: Toe blood pressure by photoplethysmography: An index of healing in forefoot amputation. *Surgery* 72:569, 1981.

Cohen SO, Goldman LD, et al: The deleterious effect of immediate postoperative prosthesis in below-knee amputation for ischemic disease. *Surgery* 76:992, 1974.

Delancy JP: The use of radionuclides in the study of limb blood flow, in Bernstein EE (ed): *Noninvasive Diagnostic Techniques in Vascular Surgery.* St Louis, Mosby, 1982, chap 14, p 148.

Denaro JA, Weinstein G, et al: Evaluation of peripheral vascular disease using radioactive xenon. *Rev Surg* 32:65, 1975.

Hicks L, McClelland RN: Below-knee amputations for vascular insufficiency. *Am Surg* 46:239, 1980.

Hunsaker RH, Schwartz JA, et al: Dry ice cryomputation: A twelve-year experience. *J Vasc Surg* 2:812, 1985.

Kelly JP, James JM: Criteria for determining the proper level of amputation in occlusive vascular disease: A review of 323 amputations. *J Bone Joint Surg [Am]* 39A:883, 1957.

Kim GE, Imparato AM, et al: Lower limb amputation for occlusive vascular disease. *Am Surg* 42:598, 1976.

Lim RC, Schecter WP: Transmetatarsal amputation. *Arch Surg* 112:1366, 1977.

McIntyre KE Jr, Bailey SA, et al: Guillotine amputation in the treatment of nonsalvageable lower extremity infections. *Arch Surg* 119:450, 1984.

Moore WS: Amputation level determination using isotope clearance technique, in Bernstein EE (ed): *Noninvasive Diagnostic Techniques in Vascular Surgery.* St Louis, Mosby, 1982, chap 40, p 385.

Pollock SB Jr, Ernst CB: Use of Doppler pressure measurements in predicting success in amputation of the leg. *Am J Surg* 139:303, 1980.

Robinson K: Long posterior flap myoplastic below-knee amputation in ischemic disease. *Lancet* 1:183, 1972.

Rush DS, Huston CC, et al: Operative and late mortality rates of above-knee and below-knee amputations. *Am Surg* 47:36, 1981.

Sizer JS, Wheelock FC Jr: Digital amputations in diabetic patients. *Surgery* 72:980, 1972.

Wagner FW Jr: The syme amputation, in *American Academy of Orthopaedic Surgeons: Atlas of Limb Prosthetics. Surgical and Prosthetic Principles*. St Louis, Mosby, 1981, pp 326–340.

Arterial Embolism

Billig DM, Hallman GL, Cooley DA: Arterial embolism. *Arch Surg* 95:1, 1967.

Blaisdell FW, Graziano CT, Effency DJ: In vivo assessment of anticoagulation. *Surgery* 82:827, 1977.

Blaisdell FW, Steele M, Allen RE: Management of acute lower extremity arterial ischemia due to embolism and thrombosis. *Surgery* 84:822, 1978.

Cranley JJ, Krause RJ, et al: Peripheral arterial embolism: Changing concepts. *Surgery* 55:57, 1964.

Crawford ES, DeBakey ME: The retrograde flush procedure in embolectomy and thrombectomy. *Surgery* 40:737, 1956.

Darling RC, Austen WG, Linton RR: Arterial embolism. *Surg Gynecol Obstet* 124:106, 1967.

Fisher DR Jr, Clagett GP, et al: Dilemmas in dealing with the blue toe syndrome: Aortic versus peripheral source. *Am J Surg* 148:836, 1984.

Fisher ER, Hellstrom HR, Myers JD: Disseminated atheromatous emboli. *Am J Med* 29:176, 1960.

Flory CM: Arterial occlusions produced by emboli from eroded aortic atheromatous plaques. *Am J Pathol* 21:549, 1945.

Fogarty TJ, Cranley JJ, et al: A method for extraction of arterial emboli and thrombi. *Surg Gynecol Obstet* 116:241, 1963.

Haimovici H: Peripheral arterial embolism. *Angiology* 1:20, 1950.

Kassirer JP: Atheroembolic renal disease. *N Engl J Med* 280:817, 1969.

Miles RM, Dale D, Booth JL: The dynamics of peripheral arterial embolism. *Ann Surg* 167:801, 1968.

Spencer FC, Eiseman B: Delayed arterial embolectomy: A new concept. *Surgery* 55:64, 1964.

Tawes RL Jr, Harris EJ, et al: Arterial thromboembolism. A 20-year perspective. *Arch Surg* 120:595, 1985.

Buerger's Disease

Hill GL: A rational basis for management of patients with the Buerger syndrome. *Br J Surg* 61:476, 1974.

Kjeldsen K, Mozes M: Buerger's disease in Israel: Investigations on carboxyhemoglobin and serum cholesterol levels after smoking. *Acta Chir Scand* 135:495, 1969.

McKusick VA, Harris WS, Ottesen OE: The Buerger syndrome in the United States: Arteriographic observations, with special reference to involvement of the upper extremities and the differentiation from atherosclerosis and embolism. *Bull Johns Hopkins Hosp* 110:145, 1962.

McKusick VA, Harris WS, et al: Buerger's disease: A distinct clinical and pathologic entity. *JAMA* 181:5, 1962.

McPherson JR, Guergels JL, Gifford RW Jr: Thromboangiitis obliterans and arteriosclerosis obliterans: Clinical and prognostic differences. *Ann Intern Med* 59:288, 1963.

Silbert S: The etiology of thromboangiitis obliterans. *JAMA* 129:5, 1945.

Walker DH, Mattern WD: Rickettsial vasculitis. *Am Heart J* 100:896, 1980.

Wessler S: Buerger's disease revisited. *Surg Clin North Am* 49:703, 1969.

Wessler S, Si-Chun M, et al: Critical evaluation of thromboangiitis obliterans: Case against Buerger's disease. *N Engl J Med* 262:1149, 1960.

Arterial Trauma

Hughes CW, Cohen A: The repair of injured blood vessels. *Surg Clin North Am* 38:1529, 1958.

Liekweg WG, et al: Management of penetrating carotid arterial injury. *Ann Surg* 188:587, 1978.

Miller HH, Welch CS: Quantitative studies on time factor in arterial injuries. *Ann Surg* 130:428, 1949.

Morris GC Jr, Beall AC Jr, et al: Surgical experience with 220 acute arterial injuries in civilian practice. *Am J Surg* 99:775, 1960.

Mustard WT, Bull CA: A reliable method for relief of traumatic vascular spasm. *Ann Surg* 155:339, 1962.

Patman RD, Poulos E, Shires GT: The management of civilian arterial injuries. *Surg Gynecol Obstet* 118:725, 1964.

Rich NM, Hobson RW, Fedde W: Vascular trauma secondary to diagnostic and therapeutic procedures. *Am J Surg* 128:715, 1974.

Spencer FC: Vascular injury and arteriovenous fistula, in *Lewis-Walters Practice of Surgery*. Hagerstown, MD, WF Prior, 1965, vol XI, chap 8.

Spencer FC, Grewe RV: The management of arterial injuries in battle casualties. *Ann Surg* 141:304, 1955.

Popliteal Artery Entrapment Syndrome

Albertazzi VJ, Elliott TE, Kennedy JA: Popliteal artery entrapment. *Angiology* 20:119, 1969.

Brightmore TGJ, Smellie WAB: Popliteal artery entrapment. *Br J Surg* 58:481, 1971.

Hamming JJ: Intermittent claudication at an early age, due to an anomalous course of the popliteal artery. *Angiology* 10:369, 1959.

Harris JD, Jepson RP: Entrapment of the popliteal artery. *Surgery* 69:246, 1971.

Inshua JA, Young JR, Humphries AW: Popliteal artery entrapment syndrome. *Arch Surg* 101:771, 1970.

Stuart ATP: Note on variation in the course of the popliteal artery. *J Anat Physiol* XIII:162, 1879.

Anterior Compartment Syndrome

Carter AB, Richards RL, Zachary RB: The anterior tibial syndrome. *Lancet* 2:928, 1949.

Getzen LC, Carr JE III: Etiology of anterior tibial compartment syndrome. *Surg Gynecol Obstet* 125:347, 1967.

Hayden JW: Compartment syndromes. Early recognition and treatment. *Postgrad Med* 74:191, 1983.

Mavor GE: The anterior tibial syndrome. *J Bone Joint Surg [Br]* 38B:513, 1956.

Moretz WH: The anterior compartment (anterior tibial) ischemia syndrome. *Ann Surg* 19:728, 1953.

Rollins DL, Bernhard VM, Towne JB: Fasciotomy. An appraisal of controversial issues. *Arch Surg* 116:1747, 1981.

Traumatic Arteriovenous Fistulas

Creech O Jr, Gantt J, Wren H: Traumatic arteriovenous fistula at unusual sites. *Ann Surg* 161:908, 1965.

Hughes CW, Jahnke EJ Jr: The surgery of traumatic arteriovenous fistulas and aneurysms: A five-year follow up study of 215 lesions. *Ann Surg* 148:790, 1958.

Shumacker HB Jr: Arterial aneurysms and arteriovenous fistulas: Report on spontaneous cures, in Elkin DC, DeBakey ME (eds): *Vascular Surgery*. Washington, D.C. Office of the Surgeon General, U.S. Public Health Service, 1955.

Spencer FC: Vascular injury and arteriovenous fistula, in *Lewis-Walters Practice of Surgery*. Hagerstown, MD, WF Prior, 1965, vol XI, chap 8.

Congenital Arteriovenous Fistulas

Cross FS, Glover DM, et al: Congenital arteriovenous aneurysms. *Ann Surg* 148:649, 1958.

Fry WJ: Surgical considerations in congenital arteriovenous fistula. *Surg Clin North Am* 54(1):165, 1974.

Olcott C, Newton TH, et al: Intra-arterial embolization in the management of arteriovenous malformations. *Surgery* 79:3, 1976.

Robertson DJ: Congenital arteriovenous fistulae of the extremities: Hunterian Lecture. *Ann R Coll Surg Engl* 18:73, 1956.

Rosenfeld L: Experiences with vascular abnormalities about the parotid gland and upper neck. *Arch Surg* 79:553, 1959.

Spencer FC: Vascular injury and arteriovenous fistula, in *Lewis-Walters Practice of Surgery*. Hagerstown, MD, WF Prior, 1965, vol XI, chap 8.

Szilagyi ED, Smith RF, et al: Congenital arteriovenous anomalies of the limbs. *Arch Surg* 111:423, 1976.

Tice DA, Clauss RH, et al: Congenital arteriovenous fistulae of the extremities: Observations concerning treatment. *Arch Surg* 86:460, 1963.

Thoracic Outlet Syndromes

Adams JT, DeWeese JA: Effort thrombosis of the axillary and subclavian veins. *J Trauma* 11:923, 1971.

Adson AW: Surgical treatment for symptoms produced by cervical ribs and the scalenus anticus muscle. *Surg Gynecol Obstet* 85:687, 1947.

Beyer JA, Wright IS: The hyperabduction syndrome: With special reference to its relationship to Raynaud's syndrome. *Circulation* 4:161, 1951.

Dale WA: Thoracic outlet compression syndrome. Critique in 1982. *Arch Surg* 117:1437, 1982.

Falconer MA, Weddell G: Costoclavicular compression of the subclavian artery and vein: Relation to the scalenus anticus syndrome. *Lancet* 2:539, 1943.

Jochamisen PR, Hartfall WG: Per axillary upper extremity sympathectomy: Technique reviewed and clinical experience. *Surgery* 71:686, 1972.

Kirtley JA, Riddell DH, et al: Cervico-sympathectomy in neurovascular abnormalities of the upper extremities: Experiences in 76 patients with 104 sympathectomies. *Ann Surg* 165:869, 1967.

Lord JW Jr, Rosati LM: Neurovascular compression syndromes of the upper extremity. *Ciba Found Clin Symp* 10:35, 1958.

Nanson EM: The anterior approach to upper dorsal sympathectomy. *Surg Gynecol Obstet* 104:118, 1957.

Patman RD, Thompson JE, Persson A: Management of post-traumatic pain syndromes: Report of 113 cases. *Ann Surg* 177:780, 1973.

Pollak EW: Surgical anatomy of the thoracic outlet syndrome. *Surg Gynecol Obstet* 150:97, 1980.

Roos DB: Transaxillary first rib resection for thoracic outlet syndrome: Indications and techniques. *Contemp Surg* 26:55, 1985.

Roos DB: The place for scalenectomy and first-rib resection in thoracic outlet syndrome. *Surgery* 92:1077, 1982.

Roos DB: Thoracic outlet and carpal tunnel syndromes, in Rutherford RB (ed): *Vascular Surgery*. Philadelphia, Saunders, 1984, chap 70.

Ross JP: The vascular complications of cervical rib. *Ann Surg* 150:340, 1959.

Sanders RJ, Raymer S: The supraclavicular approach to scalenectomy and first rib resection: Description of a technique. *J Vasc Surg* 2:751, 1985.

Scher LA, Veith FJ, et al: Vascular complications of thoracic outlet syndrome. *J Vasc Surg* 3:565, 1986.

Telford ED, Mottershead S: Pressure at the cervicobrachial junction: An operative and anatomical study. *J Bone Joint Surg [Br]* 30B:249, 1948.

Urschel HD, Paulson DL, McNamara JJ: Thoracic outlet syndrome. *Ann Thorac Surg* 6:1, 1968.

Extracranial Occlusive Cerebrovascular Disease

Baker WH, Littooy FN, et al: Carotid endarterectomy without a shunt: The control series. *J Vasc Surg* 1:50, 1984.

Baker DJ, Gluecklich B, et al: An evaluation of electroencephalographic monitoring for carotid study. *Surgery* 78(6):787, 1975.

Ball JB Jr, Lukin RR, et al: Complications of intravenous digital subtraction angiography. *Arch Neurol* 42:969, 1985.

Barner HB, Kaiser GC, Willman VL: Hemodynamics of carotid-subclavian bypass. *Arch Surg* 103:248, 1971.

Barnes RW, Nix ML, et al: Late outcome of untreated asymptomatic carotid disease following cardiovascular operations. *J Vasc Surg* 2:843, 1985.

Berkoff HA, Tunipseed WD: Patient selection and results of simultaneous coronary and carotid artery procedures. *Ann Thorac Surg* 38:172, 1984.

Bogousslavsky J, Hachiniski SC, et al: Cardiac and arterial lesions in carotid transient ischemic attacks. *Arch Neurol* 43:223, 1986.

Bousser MG, Eschwege E, et al: AICLA controlled trial of aspirin, dipyridamole in secondary prevention of athero-thrombotic cerebral ischemia. *Stroke* 14:5, 1983.

Brewster DC, Moncure AC, et al: Innominate artery lesions: Problems encountered and lessons learned. *J Vasc Surg* 2:99, 1985.

Cebul RD, Ginsberg MD: Noninvasive neurovascular tests for carotid artery disease. *Ann Intern Med* 97:867, 1982.

Cervantes FD, Schneiderman LJ: Anticoagulants in cerebrovascular disease. A critical review of studies. *Arch Intern Med* 135:875, 1975.

Clagett PG, Rabinowitz M, et al: Morphogenesis and clinicopathologic characteristics of recurrent carotid disease. *J Vasc Surg* 3:10, 1986.

Collins GJ, Rich NM, et al: Fibromuscular dysplasia of the internal carotid arteries. *Ann Surg* 194:89, 1981.

Cote R, Barnett HJ, Taylor DW: Internal carotid occlusion: A prospective study. *Stroke* 14:898, 1983.

Croft RJ, Ellam LD, Harrison MJ: Accuracy of carotid angiography in the assessment of atheroma of the internal carotid artery. *Lancet* 1:997, 1980.

Dent TL, Thompson NW, Fry WJ: Carotid body tumors. *Surgery* 80:365, 1976.

Ehrenfeld WK, Wylie EJ: Spontaneous dissection of the internal carotid artery. *Arch Surg* 111:1294, 1976.

Eikelboom BC, Riles TS, et al: Inaccuracy of angiography in the diagnosis of carotid ulceration. *Stroke* 14:882, 1983.

EC-IC Bypass Study Group: Failure of extracranial-intracranial arterial bypass to reduce the risk of ischemic stroke: Results of an international randomized trial by the EC-IC bypass study group. *N Engl J Med* 313:1191, 1985.

Ferguson GG: Carotid endarterectomy: To shunt or not to shunt. *Arch Neurol* 43:615, 1986.

Fields WM: Selection of stroke patients for arterial reconstructions. *Am J Surg* 125:527, 1973.

Fields WS, Lemak NA, et al: Controlled trial of aspirin in cerebral ischemia. *Stroke* 8:53, 1977.

Fisher DF, Clagett PG, et al: Mandibular subluxation for high carotid exposure. *J Vasc Surg* 1:727, 1984.

Ford JJ, Baker WH, Ehrenhaft JL: Carotid endarterectomy for nonhemispheric transient ischemic attacks. *Arch Surg* 110:1314, 1975.

Giordano JM, Trout HH III, et al: Timing carotid endarterectomy after stroke. *J Vasc Surg* 2:250, 1985.

Glover JL, Bendick PJ, et al: Duplex ultrasonagraphy, digital subtraction angiography and conventional angiography in assessing carotid atherosclerosis. *Arch Surg* 119:664, 1984.

Goldstone J, Effeney DJ: The role of carotid endarterectomy in the treatment of acute neurologic deficits. *Prog Cardiovasc Dis* 22:415, 1980.

Green RM, Messick WJ, et al: Benefits, shortcomings, and costs of EEG monitoring. *Ann Surg* 201:785, 1985.

Halstuk KS, Baker WH, Littoog FN: External carotid endarterectomy. *J Vasc Surg* 1:398, 1984.

Hart R, Hindman B: Mechanisms of perioperative cerebral infarction. *Stroke* 13:766, 1982.

Hays RJ, Levinson SA, Wylie EJ: Intraoperative measurement of carotid back pressure as a guide to operative management for carotid endarterectomy. *Surgery* 72:953, 1972.

Hertzer NR, Beven EG, et al: Early patency of the carotid artery after endarterectomy: Digital subtraction angiography after two hundred sixty-two operations. *Surgery* 92:1049, 1982.

Hirsh J: Progress review: The relationship between dose of aspirin, side effects and antithrombotic effectiveness. *Stroke* 16:1, 1985.

Hugenholz H, Elgie RG: Carotid thrombo-endarterectomy: A reappraisal. Criteria for patient selection. *J Neurosurg* 53:776, 1980.

Humphries AW, Young JR, et al: Relief of vertebrobasilar symptoms by carotid endarterectomy. *Surgery* 57:48, 1965.

Hunter GC, Sieffert G, et al: The accuracy of carotid back pressure as an index for shunt requirements. *Stroke* 13:319, 1982.

Imparato AM: The carotid bifurcation plaque—a model for the study of atherosclerosis. *J Vasc Surg* 3:249, 1986.

Imparato AM: The "major" and "minor" carotid artery in arterial reconstruction. *Stroke* IX:15, 1974.

Imparato AM: Vertebral arterial reconstruction: A nineteen year experience. *J Vasc Surg* 2:626, 1985.

Imparato AM, Baumann G, et al: The significance of gross hemorrhage in carotid plaques. *Ann Surg* 197:195, 1983.

Imparato AM, Bracco A, et al: The hypoglossal nerve in carotid arterial reconstructions. *Stroke* 3:576, 1972.

Imparato AM, Ramirez A, et al: Cerebral protection in carotid surgery. *Arch Surg* 117:1073, 1982.

Imparato AM, Riles TS, Gorstein F: The carotid bifurcation

plaque: Pathologic findings associated with cerebral ischemia. *Stroke* 10:238, 1979.

Imparato AM, Riles TS, et al: The management of TIA and acute strokes after carotid endarterectomy, in *Complications in Vascular Surgery.* New York, Grune & Stratton, 1985, chap 43, p 725.

Imparato AM, Riles TS, et al: Controversies in surgery: Anesthetic management in carotid surgery. *Aust NZ J Surg* 55:315, 1985.

Jacobs NM, Grant EG, et al: The role of duplex carotid sonography, digital subtraction angiography, and arteriography in the evaluation of transient ischemic attack and the asymptomatic carotid bruit. *Med Clin North Am* 68:1423, 1984.

Jacobson JH, Mozersky DJ, et al: Axillary-axillary bypass for the subclavian steal syndrome. *Arch Surg* 106:24, 1973.

Joint Study of Extracranial Arterial Occlusion as a Cause of Stroke:

    I. Fields WS, North RR, et al: Organization of study and survey of patient population. *JAMA* 203:955, 1968.

    II. Hass WK, Fields WS, et al: Arteriography, techniques, sites and complications. *JAMA* 203:961, 1968.

    III. Bauer RB, Meyer JS, et al: Progress report of controlled long term survival in patients with and without operation. *JAMA* 208:509, 1969.

    IV. Blaisdell WF, Clauss RH, et al: A review of surgical considerations. *JAMA* 209:1889, 1969.

    V. Fields WS, Maslenikov V, et al: Progress report of prognosis following surgery or non surgical treatment for transient cerebral ischemic attacks and cervical carotid lesions. *JAMA* 211:1993, 1970.

Killen DA, Foster JH, et al: The subclavian steal syndrome. *J Thorac Cardiovasc Surg* 51:539, 1966.

Kollarits CR, Lubow M, Hissong SL: Retinal strokes: I. Incidence of carotid atheromata. *JAMA* 222:1275, 1972.

Lazar ML, Clark K: Microsurgical cerebral revascularization: Concepts and practice. *Surg Neurol* 1:355, 1973.

Levin SM, Sondheimer FD, Lewis JM: The contralateral diseased but asymptomatic carotid artery: To operate or not? An update. *Am J Surg* 140:203, 1980.

Lusby RJ, Ferrel LD, et al: Carotid plaque hemorrhage: Its role in production of cerebral ischemia. *Arch Surg* 117:1479, 1982.

Meyer FB, Sundt TM, et al: Emergency carotid endarterectomy for patients with acute carotid occlusion and profound neurologic deficits. *Ann Surg* 203:82, 1986.

McCullough JL, Mentzer RM Jr, et al: Carotid endarterectomy after a completed stroke: Reduction in long-term neurologic deterioration. *J Vasc Surg* 2:7, 1985.

Millikan CH: Transient cerebral ischemia: Definition and natural history. *Prog Cardiovasc Dis* 22:303, 1980.

Mohr JP: Lacunes. *Stroke* 13:3, 1982.

Najafi H, Javid H, et al: Emergency carotid thromboendarterectomy: Surgical indication and results. *Arch Surg* 103:610, 1971.

O'Donnel TF, Erdoes L, et al: Correlation of B-mode ultrasound imaging and arteriography with pathologic findings at carotid endarterectomy. *Arch Surg* 120:443, 1985.

Posner MP, Riles TS, et al: Axillo-axillary bypass for symptomatic stenosis of the subclavian artery. *Am J Surg* 145:644, 1983.

Putnam SF, Adams HP Jr: Usefulness of heparin in initial management of patients with recent transient ischemic attacks. *Arch Neurol* 42:960, 1985.

Quinones-Baldrich WJ: Moore WS: Asymptomatic carotid stenosis: Rationale for management. *Arch Neurol* 42:378, 1985.

Reivich M, Holling E, et al: Reversal of blood flow through the vertebral artery and its effect on cerebral circulation. *N Engl J Med* 265:878, 1961.

Rhodes LE, Stanley JC, et al: Aneurysms of extracranial carotid arteries. *Arch Surg* 111:339, 1976.

Riles TS, Imparato AM, Kopelman I: Carotid artery stenosis with contralateral occlusion: Long-term results in fifty-four patients. *Surgery* 87:363, 1980.

Riles TS, Kopelman I, Imparato AM: Myocardial infarction following carotid endarterectomy. *Surgery* 85:249, 1979.

Roederer GO, Langlois YE, et al: The natural history of carotid arterial disease in asymptomatic patients with cervical bruits. *Stroke* 15:605, 1984.

Rosenthal JJ, Gaspar MR, Movius HR: Intraoperative arteriography in carotid thromboendarterectomy. *Arch Surg* 106:806, 1973.

Ross RS, McKusick VA: Aortic arch syndrome. *Arch Intern Med* 92:701, 1953.

Schmidley JW, Caronna JJ: Transient cerebral ischemia: Pathophysiology. *Prog Cardiovasc Dis* 22:325, 1980.

Sobel M, Imparato AM, et al: Contralateral neurologic symptoms after carotid surgery. *J Vasc Surg* 3:623, 1986.

Steed DL, Peitzman AB, et al: Causes of stroke in carotid endarterectomy. *Surg* 92:634, 1982.

Thompson JE: Complications of carotid endarterectomy and their prevention. *World J Surg* 3:155, 1979.

Thompson JE: History of carotid artery surgery. *Surg Clin North Am* 66:225, 1986.

Thompson JE, Patman RD, Persson AV: Management of asymptomatic carotid bruits. *Am Surg* 42:77, 1976.

Thompson JE, et al: Carotid surgery for cerebrovascular insufficiency. *Curr Probl Surg* 15:1, 1981.

Towne JB, Bernhard VM: Neurologic deficit following carotid endarterectomy. *Surg Gynecol Obstet* 154:849, 1982.

Walker PM, Paley D, et al: What determines the symptoms associated with subclavian artery occlusive disease? *J Vasc Surg* 2:154, 1985.

Warlow C: Carotid endarterectomy: Does it work? *Stroke* 15:1068, 1984.

Weinstein GS, Imparato AM: Clinicopathologic correlation in postendarterectomy recurrent stenosis. *J Vasc Surg* 3:657, 1986.

Weksler BB, Lewin M: Anticoagulation in cerebral ischemia. *Stroke* 14:658, 1983.

Wells CE: Role of stroke in dementia. *Stroke* 9:1, 1978.

Whisnant JP, Sandok BA, Sundt TM: Carotid endarterectomy for unilateral carotid system transient cerebral ischemia. *Mayo Clin Proc* 58:171, 1983.

Wylie EJ, Hein MF, Adams JE: Intracranial hemorrhage following surgical revascularization for treatment of acute strokes. *J Neurosurg* 21:212, 1964.

Yatsu FM, Fields WS: Asymptomatic carotid bruit: Stenosis or ulceration. A conservative approach. *Arch Neurol* 42:383, 1985.

Zarins CK, Giddens DP, et al: Carotid bifurcation atherosclerosis: Quantitative correlation of plaque localization with flow velocity profiles and wall shear stress. *Circ Res* 53:502, 1983.

Abdominal Aneurysms

Adar R, Rabbi I, et al: Left renal vein division in abdominal aortic aneurysm operations. Effect of renal function. *Arch Surg* 120:1033, 1985.

Bergan JJ, Yao JST: *Aneurysms, Diagnosis and Treatment.* New York, Grune & Stratton, 1982.

Bernstein EF, Chan EL: Abdominal aortic aneurysm in high risk patients. Outcome of selective management based on size and expansion rate. *Ann Surg* 200:255, 1984.

Bernstein EF, Dilley RB, et al: Growth rates of small abdominal aortic aneurysms. *Surgery* 80:765, 1986.

Boucher CA, Brewster DC, et al: Determination of cardiac risk by dipyridamole-thallium imaging before peripheral vascular surgery. *N Engl J Med* 312:389, 1985.

Brenner DJ, Darling RD, et al: Major venous anomalies complicating abdominal aortic surgery. *Arch Surg* 108:159, 1974.

Brewster DC, Retana A, et al: Angiography in the management of aneurysms of the abdominal aorta: Its value and safety. *N Engl J Med* 292:(16):822, 1975.

Brown OW, Hollier LH, et al: Abdominal aortic aneurysm and coronary artery disease. A reassessment. *Arch Surg* 116:1484, 1981.

Bunt TJ, Wilson TG: Infected abdominal aortic aneurysm. *South Med J* 78:419, 1985.

Bush HL Jr, Huse JB, et al: Prevention of renal insufficiency after abdominal aortic aneurysm resection by optimal volume loading. *Arch Surg* 116:1517, 1981.

Connelly TL, McKinnon W, et al: Abdominal aortic surgery and horseshoe kidney. *Arch Surg* 115:1459, 1980.

Couch NP, O'Mahoney J, et al: The place of abdominal aortography in abdominal aortic aneurysm resection. *Arch Surg* 118:1029, 1983.

Crawford ES, Saleh SA, et al: Infrarenal abdominal aortic aneurysm: Factors influencing survival after operation performed over a 25-year period. *Ann Surg* 193:699, 1981.

Crawford ES, Crawford JL, et al: Thoraco-abdominal aortic aneurysms: Preoperative intraoperative factors determining immediate and long-term results of operation in 605 patients. *J Vasc Surg* 3:389, 1986.

Crawford JL, Stowe CL, et al: Inflammatory aneurysms of the aorta. *J Vasc Surg* 2:113, 1985.

Creech O Jr: Endo-aneurysmorrhaphy and treatment of aortic aneurysm. *Ann Surg* 164:935, 1966.

Darling R, Messina C, et al: Autopsy study of unoperated abdominal aortic aneurysm—the case for early resection. *Circulation* 56 (suppl 2):161, 1977.

Dean RH, Keyser JF III, et al: Aortic and renal disease. Factors affecting the value of combined procedures. *Ann Surg* 200:336, 1984.

DeBakey MR, Crawford ES, et al: Aneurysm of abdominal aorta: Analysis of results of graft replacement therapy one to eleven years after operation. *Ann Surg* 160:622, 1964.

Dent TL, Lindenauer M, et al: Multiple arteriosclerotic arterial aneurysms. *Arch Surg* 105:338, 1972.

Ernst CB: Prevention of intestinal ischemia following abdominal aortic reconstruction. *Surgery* 93:102, 1982.

Estes JE Jr: Abdominal aortic aneurysm: A study of one hundred and two cases. *Circulation* 2:258, 1950.

Flanigan D, Quinn T, Kraft R: Selective management of high risk patients with abdominal aortic aneurysms. *Surg Gynecol Obstet* 150:171, 1980.

Gaspar MR: Role of arteriography in the evaluation of aortic aneurysms: The case against, in Bergan JJ, Yao JST (eds): *Aneurysms, Diagnosis and Treatment.* New York, Grune & Stratton, 1982, p 243.

Gomes AS, Baker JD, et al: Acute renal dysfunction after major arteriography. *AJR* 145:1249, 1985.

Graham LM, Zelenock GB, et al: Clinical significance of arteriosclerotic femoral artery aneurysms. *Arch Surg* 115:502, 1980.

Grindlinger GA, Vegas AM, et al: Volume loading and vasodilators in abdominal aortic aneurysmectomy. *Am J Surg* 139:480, 1980.

Hardy JD, Timmis HH: Abdominal aortic aneurysms: Special problems. *Ann Surg* 173:945, 1971.

Hertzer NR, Beven EG, et al: Coronary artery disease in peripheral vascular patients. A classification of 1000 coronary angiograms and results of surgical management. *Ann Surg* 199:223, 1984.

Hiatt JCG, Wiley FB, et al: Determinants of failure of the treatment of ruptured abdominal aortic aneurysm. *Arch Surg* 118:1264, 1984.

Hicks G, Eastland M, et al: Survival improvement following aortic aneurysm resection. *Ann Surg* 181:863, 1975.

Hollier LH, Stanson AW, et al: Arteriomegaly: Classification and morbid implications of diffuse aneurysmal disease. *Surg* 93:700, 1983.

Imparato AM: Abdominal aortic surgery: Prevention of lower limb ischemia. *Surgery* 93:112, 1983.

Imparato AM, Berman IR, et al: Avoidance of shock and peripheral embolism during surgery of the abdominal aorta. *Surgery* 73:68, 1973.

Inahara T, Geary GL, et al: The contrary position to the nonresective treatment of abdominal aortic aneurysm. *J Vasc Surg* 2:42, 1985.

Jarrett F, Darling CR, et al: Experience with infected aneurysms of the abdominal aorta. *Arch Surg* 110:1381, 1975.

Karmody AM, Leather RP, et al: The current position of nonresective treatment for abdominal aortic aneurysm. *Surgery* 94:591, 1983.

Kim GE, Imparato AM, et al: Dilatation of synthetic grafts and junctional aneurysms. *Arch Surg* 114:1296, 1979.

Knight DG, Lane B, et al: Dynamic preoperative assessment of cardiac reserve in elective aortic surgery. *Br J Surg* 70:362, 1983.

Laetir GM, Crawford ES, et al: Progress in the treatment of ruptured abdominal aortic aneurysm. *World J Surg* 4:653, 1980.

Lawrence RJ, Ferguson MD, et al: Spinal ischemia following abdominal aortic surgery. *Ann Surg* 181:267, 1975.

Leather RP, Shah D, et al: Nonresective treatment of abdominal aortic aneurysm. Use of acute thrombosis and axillo-femoral by-pass. *Arch Surg* 114:1402, 1979.

Lobbato VJ, Rothenberg RE, et al: Coexistence of abdominal aortic aneurysm and carcinoma of the colon: A dilemma. *J Vasc Surg* 2:724, 1985.

McAuley CE, Steed DL, Webster MW: Bacterial presence in aortic thrombus at elective aneurysm resection: Is it clinically significant? *Am J Surg* 147:322, 1984.

Mehrez IO, Nabseth DC, et al: Paraplegia following resection of abdominal aortic aneurysm. *Ann Surg* 156:890, 1962.

Morgan RJ, Abbott WM: Safe management of patients with simultaneously occurring prostatism and abdominal aortic aneurysm. *Am J Surg* 143:319, 1982.

Pairolero PC, Gilmore JC, et al: Isolated iliac artery aneurysms. *Surgery* 93:688, 1983.

Pairolero PC, Walls JT, et al: Subclavian artery aneurysms. *Surgery* 90:757, 1981.

Pasternack PF, Imparato AM, et al: The value of radionuclide angiography as a predictor of perioperative myocardial infarction in patients undergoing abdominal aortic aneurysm resection. *J Vasc Surg* 1:320, 1984.

Pennell RC, Hollier LH, et al: Inflammatory abdominal aortic aneurysms: A 30 year review. *J Vasc Surg* 2:859, 1985.

Porter JM, McGregor F, et al: Renal function following abdominal aortic aneurysmectomy. *Surg Gynecol Obstet* 123:819, 1966.

Rob C: Extraperitoneal approach to the abdominal aorta. *Surgery* 53:87, 1963.

Sethi GK, Hughes RK, Takaro T: Dissecting aortic aneurysms. *Ann Thorac Surg* 18:301, 1974.

Stanley JC, Fry WJ: Pathogenesis and clinical significance of splenic artery aneurysms. *Surgery* 76:898, 1974.

Stanley JC, Thompson NW, Fry WJ: Splanchnic artery aneurysms. *Arch Surg* 101:689, 1970.

Stowe CL, Safi JJ, et al: Inflammatory aneurysms of the aorta. *J Vasc Surg* 2:113, 1985.

String ST: Cholelithiasis and aortic reconstruction. *J Vasc Surg* 1:664, 1985.

Sweeney MS, Gadacz TR: Primary aortoduodenal fistula: Manifestation, diagnosis and treatment. *Surgery* 96:492, 1984.

Szilagyi DE, Elliot JP, Smith RF: Clinical fate of the patient with asymptomatic abdominal aortic aneurysm and unfit for surgical therapy. *Arch Surg* 104:600, 1972.

Szilagyi DE, Hageman JH, et al: Spinal cord damage in surgery of the abdominal aorta. *Surgery* 83:38, 1978.

Szilagyi DE, Smith RF, et al: Contribution of abdominal aortic aneurysmectomy to prolongation of life. *Ann Surg* 164:678, 1966.

Thompson JE, Hollier LH, et al: Surgical management of abdominal aortic aneurysms: Factors influencing mortality and morbidity—a 20 year experience. *Ann Surg* 181:654, 1975.

Trastek VF, Pairolero PC, et al: Splenic artery aneurysms. *Surgery* 91:694, 1982.

Whittemore AD, Clowes AW, et al: Aortic aneurysm repair. Reduced operative mortality associated with maintenance of optimal cardiac performance. *Ann Surg* 192:414, 1980.

Peripheral Aneurysms: General

Howell JF, Crawford ES, et al: Surgical treatment of peripheral arteriosclerotic aneurysm. *Surg Clin North Am* 46:979, 1966.

Popliteal Aneurysm

Alpert J: Aneurysms of the popliteal artery. *J Med Soc NJ* 67:791, 1970.

Anton GE, Hertzer NR, et al: Surgical management of popliteal aneurysms. *J Vasc Surg* 3:125, 1986.

Edmunds LH, Darling RC, Linton RR: Surgical management of popliteal aneurysm. *Circulation* 32:517, 1965.

Gifford RW Jr, Hines EA Jr, Janes JM: Analysis and follow-up study of 100 popliteal aneurysms. *Surgery* 33:284, 1953.

Hunter JA, Julian OC, et al: Arteriosclerotic aneurysms of the popliteal artery. *J Cardiovasc Surg* 2:404, 1961.

Femoral Aneurysm

Crawford ES, Edwards WH, et al: Peripheral arteriosclerotic aneurysm. *J Am Geriatr Soc* 9:1, 1961.

Papas G, Janes JM, et al: Femoral aneurysms: Review of surgical management. *JAMA* 190:489, 1964.

Stoney RJ, Albo RJ, Wylie EJ: False aneurysms occurring after arterial grafting operations. *Am J Surg* 110:153, 1965.

Tolstedt GE, Radke HN, Bell JW: Late sequela of arteriosclerotic femoral aneurysms. *Angiology* 12:601, 1961.

Carotid Artery Aneurysm

Beall AC Jr, Crawford ES, et al: Extracranial aneurysms of the carotid artery: Report of seven cases. *Postgrad Med* 32:93, 1962.

Kianouri M: Extracranial carotid aneurysms. *Ann Surg* 165:152, 1967.

Sanoudos GM, Ramp J, Imparato AM: Internal carotid aneurysm. *Am Surg* 39:118, 1973.

Spencer FC: Aneurysm of the common carotid artery treated by excision and primary anastomosis. *Ann Surg* 145:254, 1957.

Subclavian Aneurysm

Howell JF, Crawford ES, et al: Surgical treatment of peripheral arteriosclerotic aneurysm. *Surg Clin North Am* 46:979, 1966.

Splenic Artery Aneurysm

Bedford PD, Lodge B: Aneurysm of the splenic artery. *Gut* 1:312, 1960.

Owens JC, Coffey RJ: Aneurysm of the splenic artery, including a report of 6 additional cases. *Int Abstr Surg* 97:313, 1953.

Renal Artery Aneurysm

Cerny JC, Chang C, Fry WJ: Renal artery aneurysms. *Arch Surg* 96:653, 1968.

Garritano AP: Aneurysm of the renal artery. *Am J Surg* 94:638, 1957.

Poutasse EF: Renal artery aneurysm: Report of 12 cases, two treated by excision of the aneurysm and repair of renal artery. *J Urol* 77:697, 1957.

Traumatic Aneurysm

Crawford ES, DeBakey ME, Cooley DA: Surgical considerations of peripheral arterial aneurysms. *Arch Surg* 78:226, 1959.

Dickinson EH, Hood RH, Spencer FC: Traumatic aneurysm of the innominate artery. *US Armed Forces Med J* 3:1871, 1952.

Hughes CW, Jahnke EJ Jr: The surgery of traumatic arteriovenous fistulas and aneurysms: A five year follow-up study of lesions. *Ann Surg* 148:790, 1958.

Raynaud's Disease

Burton EE Jr, et al: Raynaud's phenomenon: Treatment with intraarterial reserpine. *Cutis (NY),* 9:464, 1972.

DeTakats G, Fowler EF: The neurogenic factor in Raynaud's phenomenon. *Surgery* 51:9, 1962.

Farmer RG, Gifford RW Jr, Hines EA Jr: Raynaud's disease with sclerodactylia: A follow-up study of seventy-one patients. *Circulation* 23:13, 1961.

Gifford RW Jr, Hines EA Jr, Craig WMcK: Sympathectomy for Raynaud's phenomenon: Follow-up study of 70 women with Raynaud's disease and 54 women with secondary Raynaud's phenomenon. *Circulation* 17:5, 1958.

Harris RW, Andros G, et al: Large-vessel arterial occlusive disease in symptomatic upper extremity. *Arch Surg* 119:1277, 1984.

Kirtley JA, Riddell DH, et al: Cervicothoracic sympathectomy in neurovascular abnormalities of the upper extremities: Experiences in 76 patients with 104 sympathectomies. *Ann Surg* 165:869, 1967.

Palumbo LT: Anterior transthoracic approach for upper thoracic sympathectomy. *Arch Surg* 72:659, 1956.

Porter JM, Bardana EJ, Baur GM: The clinical significance of Raynaud's syndrome. *Surgery* 80:756, 1976.

Porter JM, et al: Evaluation and management of patients with Raynaud's syndrome. *Am J Surg* 142:183, 1981.

Smith CR, Rodeheffer FJ: Treatment of Raynaud's phenomenon with calcium channel blockers. *Am J Med* 78:(suppl 2B):39, 1985.

Taylor LM Jr, Baur GM, Porter JM: Finger gangrene caused by small artery occlusive disease. *Ann Surg* 193:453, 1981.

Varadi DP, Lawrence AM: Suppression of Raynaud's phenomenon by methyldopa. *Ann Intern Med* 124:13, 1969.

Willerson JT, Decker JL: Raynaud's disease and phenomenon, a medical approach. *Am Heart J* 82:572, 1971.

Uncommon Vasomotor Diseases

Estes JE: Vasoconstrictive and vasodilative syndromes of the extremities. *Mod Concepts Cardiovasc Dis* 25:355, 1956.

Lewis T, Landis EM: Observations upon the vascular mechanism in acrocyanosis. *Heart* 15:229, 1930.

Frostbite

Couch NP, Sullivan J, Crane C: Predictive accuracy of renal vein renin activity in surgery of renovascular hypertension. *Surgery* 79:70, 1976.

Ervasti E: Frostbites of the extremities and their sequelae: A clinical study. *Acta Chir Scand* 299:1, 1962.

Golding MR, Martinez A, et al: The role of sympathectomy in frostbite, with a review of 68 cases. *Surgery* 57:774, 1965.

Mundth ED, Long DM, Brown RB: Treatment of experimental frostbite with low molecular weight dextran. *J Trauma* 4:246, 1964.

Penn I, Schwartz SI: Evaluation of low molecular weight dextran in the treatment of frostbite. *J Trauma* 4:784, 1964.

Shumacker HB Jr, Kilman JW: Sympathectomy in the treatment of frostbite. *Arch Surg* 89:575, 1964.

Simeone FA: A preliminary follow-up report in cases of cold injury from World War II, in Ferrer MI (ed): *Cold Injury. Trans 4th Conf Josiah Macy Jr Found NY* 1956, pp 197–223.

Snider RL, Porter JM: Treatment of experimental frostbite with intra-arterial sympathetic blocking drugs. *Surgery* 77(4):557, 1975.

Chapter 22

Venous and Lymphatic Disease

Lazar J. Greenfield

VENOUS DISEASE

Functional Anatomy of the Veins

Evolution in human beings to an upright position imposed a significant work load on the venous system. Since the systemic veins contain approximately two-thirds of the circulating blood volume under relatively low pressure, movement from the lower extremities must overcome gravity and intraabdominal pressure to return blood to the right ventricle. The left ventricle provides the initial force called *vis a tergo,* which is reduced through the capillary bed to a pressure of about 15 mmHg in the venules. In addition, the calf muscles provide an important pump function as they compress deep veins within an unyielding fascial compartment. Proximal flow is assured by the presence of the delicate but strong venous valves, which prevent reflux distally. Perforating or communicating veins connect the superficial venous system with the deep and direct flow internally from the superficial veins in all areas of the lower extremity except the foot, where the opposite occurs (Fig. 22-1). Each valve is based within a dilated sinus of the vein, which keeps the valve cusps away from the walls and promotes rapid closure when flow ceases. Numbers of valves increase with distance from the heart while the vena cava and common iliac veins are valveless. Valves are the focal point of most of the pathology of venous thrombosis since their sinuses are where the initial thrombus forms and the loss of valvular function after recanalization of a thrombus produces venous insufficiency.

The structure of veins also is related to their functional requirements, with the unsupported superficial vein walls containing more smooth muscle while the deep veins are thin-walled and lacking in significant smooth muscle. In some areas such as the calf, there are spindle-shaped sinusoids that can become sites of venous stasis when the patient is at bed rest, facilitating the development of venous thrombosis.

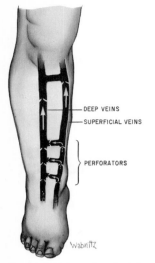

DEEP VEINS

SUPERFICIAL VEINS

PERFORATORS

Wabritz

Fig. 22-1. Schematic orientation of venous valves and flow of blood in the superficial, deep, and perforating veins of the lower leg.

The major superficial veins of the lower extremity are the greater and lesser saphenous veins and their tributaries. The deep veins follow the course of the major arteries and share their names. In the lower leg the veins are paired and join at the knee to form the popliteal vein, which continues through the adductor hiatus to become the superficial femoral vein. The latter is joined by the deep femoral vein in the upper thigh to become the common femoral vein, which becomes the external iliac vein as it enters the pelvis beneath the inguinal ligament. The perforating veins are so named because they penetrate the fascia of the lower leg to connect the superficial and deep systems. The perforators adjacent to the medial malleolus are often responsible for the development of stasis ulcers at that level when they become incompetent.

Respiration and exercise have significant effects on normal venous flow. During inspiration, diaphragmatic descent increases intraabdominal pressure, transiently decreasing venous return. During expiration, abdominal pressure falls and the distally trapped blood accelerates flow cephalad. During exercise, the calf muscle pump reduces venous pressure in the deep veins by emptying them and when the muscle relaxes, the superficial veins drain into the deep system rapidly. The ability to move large volumes of blood during the hyperemia of exercise prevents edema formation by maintaining a normal pressure gradient across the capillary bed.

Etiology of Deep Vein Thrombosis

Development of a thrombus within a vein may be considered functionally as an exaggeration of the normal process of hemostasis. When disruption of normal endothelium occurs, subendothelial structures trigger a reaction in platelets, coagulation proteins, and adjacent endothelial cells that results in a hemostatic plug. Soon fibrin is deposited and within 24 h the platelet plug is replaced by fibrin which allows the vessel to heal. The occurrence

of this process in a nontraumatized vein was recognized by Virchow who, in 1856, introduced the term thrombosis and postulated three possible mechanisms: stasis, endothelial damage, and hypercoagulability.

STASIS. In the surgical patient, stasis is the most important factor in the development of deep vein thrombosis (DVT), especially when there is prolonged immobilization in bed. When contrast medium is injected in the veins of the lower extremities of a bedridden patient, it may remain in venous valve sinuses for as long as an hour, confirming the pooling effect in the soleal veins. This is the favored location for the formation of a nidus of thrombus that then promotes successive layering of platelets, fibrin, and leukocytes to produce an organized thrombus. This process can begin under general anesthesia in the operating room but usually requires other contributing factors such as shock, infection, trauma, or congestive heart failure. Aging, obesity, pregnancy, and malignancy are also important added risk factors.

ENDOTHELIAL DAMAGE. Endothelial injury can occur in collapsed vessels when the intimal walls are in contact, and further injury can be demonstrated after hypoxemia that occurs when there is venous stasis. Similarly, leukocyte adherence to endothelial intracellular junctions can be demonstrated in areas of stasis after trauma at a remote site. In spite of these changes, however, routine histological examination of veins containing thrombus usually fails to show an inflammatory response consistent with vessel wall injury.

HYPERCOAGULABILITY. Patients who present at an early age with spontaneous venous thrombosis, who have a strong family history of DVT, or who develop recurrent venous thromboembolism are usually considered "prethrombotic" or "hypercoagulable." They deserve careful study for associated disorders as described by Shattil and listed in Table 22-1.

Idiopathic DVT may also be the first clue to occult malignancy. The association between venous thrombosis and cancer was first suggested by Trousseau and often has been confirmed in postmortem studies. In a recent series reported by Aderka et al., 34 percent of otherwise healthy patients with idiopathic DVT were found to have a malignancy diagnosed an average of 24 months later. Increased likelihood of cancer in these patients was associated with age over sixty-five, anemia, and eosinophilia. The earliest onset malignancies were found within one year and tended to occur in the pelvic organs and breast. Prolonged follow-up is appropriate, however, since some malignancies did not appear until after 5 years, which also suggests coincidence rather than a direct relationship. There is a direct relationship between the use of oral contraceptive anovulatory agents and thrombotic disorders that occur 3 to 6 times more frequently in those women.

The most common transient hypercoagulable states are associated with recent trauma, major surgical procedures and sepsis. In addition to the possible roles of stasis and increased circulating procoagulant factors, the fibrinolytic system is inhibited after surgery and trauma and there is less lytic activity in the veins of the lower extremity than in those of the upper extremity.

Table 22-1. CONDITIONS ASSOCIATED WITH
RECURRENT VENOUS THROMBOEMBOLISM

Accelerated or inappropriate hemostatic plug formation

Endothelial cell damage
    Atherosclerosis and hypercholesterolemia
    Homocystinuria
    Vasculitis and the lupus anticoagulant
Inappropriate platelet plug formation
    Essential thrombocythemia
    Paroxysmal nocturnal hemoglobinuria
    Heparin-associated thrombocytopenia
Inappropriate fibrin plug formation
    Disseminated intravascular coagulation
    Infusion of prothrombin complex concentrates

Defects in the mechanism limiting hemostatic plug size

Stasis
    Previous deep vein thrombosis
    Congestive heart failure
    Hyperviscosity syndrome: polycythemia; serum
    hyperviscosity
Antithrombin III deficiency
Protein C deficiency
Defective lysis of fibrin plugs
Dysfibrinogenemia
    Decreased plasminogen activator activity
    Decreased plasminogen activity

SOURCE: Shattil SJ: Diagnosis and treatment of recurrent venous thromboembolism. *Med Clin North Am* 68:577–601, 1984.

Pathophysiology

A propagating thrombus may become attached to the opposite wall, causing interruption of flow, retrograde thrombosis, and signs of venous stasis in the extremity (Fig. 22-2). Subsequent formation of edema within the confines of the deep muscular fascia may produce pain and/or limited dorsiflexion of the foot (Homans's sign). The latter sign as originally described by Homans is only an indication of muscular irritability and its use far exceeds its reliability. More commonly, in about 60 percent of patients the thrombus propagates without interrupting flow and develops a long floating "tail" that is more susceptible to breaking loose from its tenuous anchor within the valvular sinus. It is the latter sequence of events that is the most dangerous aspect of the disorder, because major pulmonary embolism can and does occur without premonitory signs or symptoms at its point of origin.

The site of venous obstruction determines the level at which swelling is observed clinically. Swelling at the thigh level always implies obstruction at the level of the iliofemoral system, whereas swelling of the calf or foot suggests obstruction at the femoropopliteal level (Fig. 22-3). Autopsies suggest that it is more common for thrombi to originate in the veins of the soleus and then propagate proximally, but there is evidence that primary thrombosis of the femoral and iliac venous tributaries occurs as well.

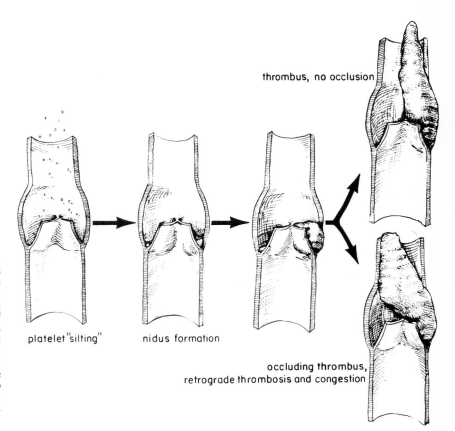

Fig. 22-2. The evolution of venous thrombosis begins with stagnant flow that permits silting of platelets and possibly hypoxemic injury to valvular sinus endothelium. The resulting nidus of thrombus releases thrombin that aggregates more platelets in a cycle of thrombus propagation. As the thrombus grows, it may extend into the lumen without occlusion or may occlude the vein with retrograde thrombosis and venous hypertension. [From: *Greenfield LJ: Acute venous thrombosis and pulmonary embolism, in Hardy JD (ed): Hardy's Textbook of Surgery. Philadelphia, Lippincott, 1983, with permission.*]

platelet "silting"

nidus formation

thrombus, no occlusion

occluding thrombus,
retrograde thrombosis and congestion

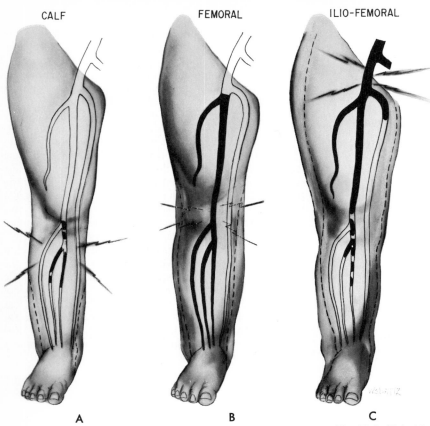

CALF FEMORAL ILIO-FEMORAL

A B C

Fig. 22-3. Clinical features of venous thrombosis. *A.* When thrombosis is localized to veins of the calf and the popliteal vein, there is minimal swelling at the level of the ankle. Calf pain and tenderness are usually present. *B.* When there is thrombosis of the femoral vein and associated thrombosis of the calf veins, swelling is usually present and extends to just above the level of the knee. Popliteal tenderness and calf tenderness may be present. *C.* In iliofemoral venous thrombosis, there is thrombosis of the iliac and proximal femoral vein, and frequently the calf veins also are involved. Edema is present from the foot to the inguinal ligament. There is usually tenderness in the groin as well as popliteal and calf tenderness.

Resolution of deep vein thrombosis with recanalization will alter the competence of the valves within the veins and can result in the postthrombotic syndrome, which will be discussed.

Diagnosis

CLINICAL MANIFESTATIONS. Major venous thrombosis involving the deep venous system of the thigh and pelvis produces a characteristic clinical picture of pain, extensive pitting edema, and blanching that has been termed *phlegmasia alba dolens* or "milk leg." Association with pregnancy may be related to hormonal effects on blood, relaxation of vessel walls, or mechanical compression of the left iliac vein at the pelvic brim, resulting in the term "milk leg of pregnancy." It was originally believed that the blanching was due to spasm and compromise of arterial flow, but efforts to achieve sympatholysis are ill-advised because it is the subcutaneous edema that is responsible for the blanching. In addition to pregnancy, other mechanical factors that can affect the left iliac vein include compression from the right iliac artery or an overdistended bladder, and congenital webs within the vein. These factors are responsible for the observed 4:1 preponderance of left versus right iliac vein involvement.

As venous thrombosis progresses, impeding most of the venous return from the extremity, there is danger of limb loss from cessation of arterial flow. This clinical picture differs from alba dolens, with more congestion producing *phlegmasia cerulea dolens,* which is characterized by loss of sensory and motor function. Venous gangrene is likely unless an aggressive approach is utilized to remove the thrombus and restore blood flow. A variant of this disorder occurs peripherally in the leg and is associated with concurrent malignant disease and a high mortality rate.

Fortunately, these major complications occur in less than 10 percent of patients with venous thrombosis. Only 40 percent of patients with venous thrombosis have any clinical signs of the disorder. In addition, false-positive clinical signs occur in up to 30 percent of patients studied. Because of this there has been a great deal of interest in the development of screening tests that can reveal thrombi before they become evident clinically. Contrast venography provides direct evidence of both occlusive and nonocclusive thrombi, but it is an invasive procedure and usually requires moving the patient to a radiographic suite. Ideally, the screening test would be accurate, noninvasive, and able to be performed at the bedside. Although the ideal has not yet been achieved, there are a number of tests that have proved useful.

RADIOACTIVE-LABELED FIBRINOGEN. In 1957, Ambrus et al. showed that radioactive thrombi resulted from injection of radiolabeled fibrinogen and thrombin into an occluded vessel, and in 1960, Hobbs and Davies demonstrated preferential uptake of ^{131}I-labeled fibrinogen in formation of a thrombus. Clinical application of this finding required simplification of the test by development of portable scintillation counters for bedside use. After iodine blockage of the thyroid gland, the counts are obtained from marked locations on the lower extremities and expressed as a percentage of the radioactivity measured by counting over the heart. An increase of 20 percent or more in one area indicates the presence of an underlying thrombus. The test permits sequential scanning of the extremities over a period of days and is most sensitive to thrombi forming in the veins of the calves shortly after an operative procedure. It does not permit detection of thrombi in pelvic veins, and it cannot be used in an extremity in which there is a healing wound, fracture, cellulitis, arthritis, edema, ulceration, or superficial thrombophlebitis. It is also contraindicated in patients under thirty years of age and in women of childbearing age. Apart from these conditions it is quite accurate, however, and has a 90 percent positive correlation with contrast venograms. A negative correlation usually is explained by cessation of active thrombosis and failure to incorporate the tagged fibrinogen, making the test most useful clinically in discriminating between old and new venous thrombi.

ULTRASOUND. The Doppler ultrasound probe can be used to advantage to detect major venous thrombi with a high degree of accuracy, but it is a subjective form of testing dependent on the examiner's experience. The principle is based on the change in flow signal produced by intraluminal thrombi. The examination begins at the ankle with identification of the posterior tibial vein signal adjacent to the artery. The flow signal should be altered by distal and proximal compression, producing augmentation and interruption of flow, respectively, which can also be produced by the Valsalva maneuver. The same maneuvers are repeated over the superficial and deep femoral veins and can be done over the popliteal vein as well (Fig. 22-4). Failure of augmentation of flow on compression below the probe or release of interruption of flow above the probe suggests a venous thrombus. The sensitivity of the test exceeds 90 percent, but the specificity is 5 to 10 percent lower because of the possibility of other mechanical problems (e.g., Baker's cyst, hematoma) interfering with venous flow. A negative Doppler ultrasound examination is reassuring, but a positive or equivocal test should be confirmed by contrast venography. A negative test in the leg is not reassuring when thromboembolism is suspected, because the thrombus may have been evacuated from the extremity.

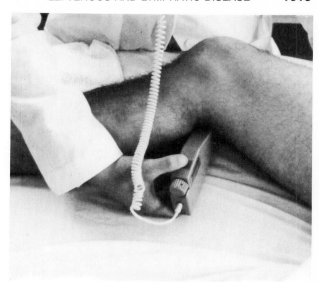

Fig. 22-4. The Doppler probe can be used at the bedside to assess flow in all the venous tributaries of the leg. Distal and proximal compression produce alterations in flow that are attenuated or absent when a thrombus is present.

The addition of real-time B-mode imaging to Doppler measurement in a portable duplex device offers a new approach to detection and characterization of venous thrombi. To date, however, the echographic imaging has been limited to the extremities.

IMPEDANCE PLETHYSMOGRAPHY. The impedance method measures the volume of the extremity to temporary occlusion of the venous system. The diagnosis of venous thrombosis depends on the changes in venous capacitance and rate of emptying after release of the occlusion. A proximal thigh cuff is inflated to 50 mmHg or until maximum filling has occurred by plateau of the electrical signal. The cuff is then rapidly deflated, allowing rapid outflow and reduction of volume in a normal limb (Fig. 22-5). Prolongation of the outflow wave suggests major venous thrombosis with 95 percent accuracy and is much more reliable than any voluntary technique of venous occlusion. The deficiency of this technique, as with all noninvasive methods, is the lack of detection of calf vein thrombosis or old postthrombotic sequelae. The strain gauge plethysmograph can be used in a similar fashion.

VENOGRAPHY. The injection of contrast material for direct visualization of the venous system of the extremity is the most accurate method of confirming the diagnosis of venous thrombosis and the extent of involvement. Injection is usually made into the foot while the superficial veins are occluded by tourniquet, and a supplemental injection into the femoral veins may be required to visualize the iliofemoral system (Fig. 22-6). Potential false-positive examinations may result from external compression of a vein or washout of the contrast material from venous flow from collateral veins. The procedure can also be performed with isotope injection using a gamma scintillation counter to record flow of the isotope. Delayed imaging of

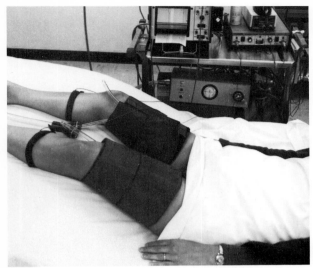

Fig. 22-5. The plethysmograph measures the volume change in the lower extremity following temporary occlusion of venous return by pneumatic cuffs. When the cuff pressure is released, there is rapid outflow of blood and reduction in limb volume unless proximal venous thrombosis is present. Both strain gauge (shown) and impedance sensors may be used for the volume recordings.

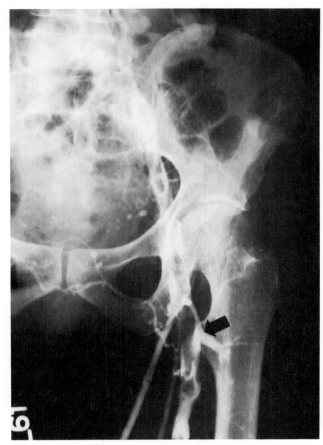

Fig. 22-6. Contrast venogram demonstrating a thrombus within the femoral vein. It is outlined by the contrast material which indicates that it is free-floating at that level. [From: *Greenfield LJ: Complications of venous thrombosis and pulmonary embolism, in Greenfield LJ (ed): Complications in Surgery and Trauma. Philadelphia, Lippincott, 1984, with permission.*]

persistent ''hot spots'' may also reflect isotope retention at the sites of thrombus formation (Fig. 22-7). A perfusion lung scan can also be obtained for baseline comparison and for detection of silent embolism. There is less definition of deep vein thrombi with this technique than with contrast venography, but it is a valuable technique for sequential study of patients and avoids the potential thrombogenesis associated with the injection of contrast medium.

Prophylaxis

Theoretically, it should be possible to prevent formation of venous thrombi either by eliminating or reducing venous stasis or by altering blood coagulability. The belief that early ambulation prevents stasis and reduces the formation of thrombi has been controversial, and studies using tagged fibrinogen have not supported this assumption. One possible explanation for this is that early ambulation often involves having the patient walk to a nearby chair and sit, whereupon the legs are subjected to even more stasis.

There has been more benefit from the prophylactic use of anticoagulant drugs. There are good data to support the use of preoperative oral anticoagulant therapy with warfarin derivatives in high-risk patients. Unfortunately, this procedure increases the risk of hemorrhage, and because of the added difficulties of laboratory control of prothrombin time, there has not been widespread acceptance of this approach. It remains, however, the recommendation of a national task force on prophylaxis for patients undergoing surgery for fractured hips as reported by Hyers, Hull, and Weg. They also recommend adjusted-dose heparin to prolong the APTT to the upper normal range for patients having elective hip surgery. The administration of dextran, which produces a variety of effects on platelets and clotting factors, has been demonstrated to reduce the incidence of detectable thrombi. However, it too can produce hemorrhagic problems as well as allergic reactions and, in older patients, congestive heart failure.

There has been much wider acceptance of the administration of heparin prior to and following surgery in low (''mini'') doses that do not alter the laboratory clotting profile. Generally, a 5000-unit dose is given subcutaneously 2 h preoperatively and then every 12 h postoperatively for 6 days. This provides protection for most high-risk groups with the exception of those undergoing orthopedic or urological procedures. The beneficial effect may be due to the enhancement of heparin cofactor (antithrombin III), a natural inhibitor of activated factor X. Although some studies have failed to show a protective effect, Kakkar et al. in a randomized series of 4121 patients showed that heparin protected against fatal pulmonary embolism as well as deep venous thrombosis.

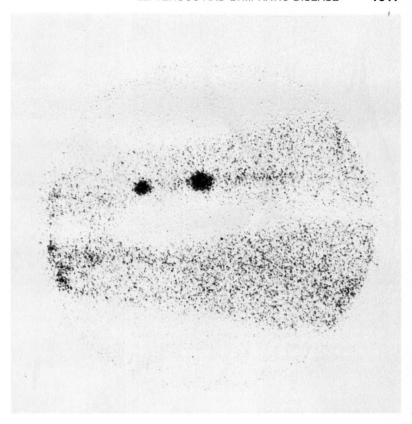

Fig. 22-7. Isotope scan following the injection of macroaggregated albumin ^{131}I showing an acute thrombus in the popliteal vein.

Intermittent pneumatic leg compression prevents stasis and increases fibrinolytic activity with virtually no side effects. The pneumatic boots can be applied in the operating room to minimize the risk of venous thrombosis beginning under general anesthesia. It is recommended for groups in which low-dose heparin is either contraindicated or ineffective, but should not be used in patients with peripheral arterial insufficiency.

Medical Treatment

The approach to management of the patient with deep venous thrombosis is based on three objectives: minimizing the risk of pulmonary embolism, limiting further thrombosis, and facilitating resolution of existing thrombi to avoid the postthrombotic syndrome.

Initially, the patient is anticoagulated and placed at bed rest with the foot of the bed elevated 8 to 10 in. Generally, pain, swelling, and tenderness resolve over a 5- to 7-day period, at which time ambulation can be permitted with elastic stocking support. Standing still and sitting should be prohibited to avoid increased venous pressure and stasis.

ANTICOAGULATION. The foundation of therapy for deep venous thrombosis is adequate anticoagulation, initially with heparin and then with coumarin derivatives for prolonged protection against recurrent thrombosis. Unless there are specific contraindications, heparin should be administered in an initial dose of 100 to 150 units/kg intravenously. Heparin is an acid mucopolysaccharide that neutralizes thrombin, inhibits thromboplastin, and reduces the platelet release reaction. It may be administered by continuous or intermittent intravenous doses regulated by whole blood clotting time or activated partial thromboplastin time. Bleeding complications can be minimized by doses of heparin that prolong the laboratory clotting determinations by about twice the normal time with no loss of effectiveness. Continuous intravenous infusion regulated by an infusion pump seems to minimize the total dose required for control and is associated with a lower incidence of complications.

Oral administration of anticoagulants is begun shortly after initiation of heparin therapy, because several days are usually required to bring the prothrombin time within the therapeutic range of 1.4 times the control value. The coumarin derivatives block the synthesis of several clotting factors, and prolongation of the prothrombin time beyond the level suggested is associated with a higher incidence of bleeding complications. Fortunately, administration of vitamin K usually can restore the prothrombin time rapidly. After an episode of acute deep venous thrombosis, anticoagulation therapy should be maintained for a minimum of 3 months; some investigators favor 6 months for treatment of thrombi in the larger veins. Many drugs interact with coumarin derivatives (e.g., barbiturates), and therefore it is essential to establish a routine for regular monitoring of prothrombin time after the patient leaves the hospital.

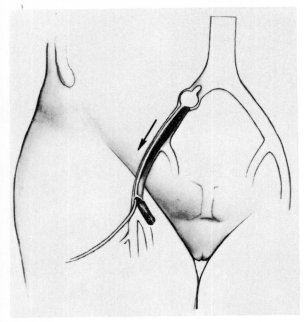

Fig. 22-8. Venous thrombectomy using a Fogarty catheter to extract the proximal thrombus. Increased intraabdominal pressure by the Valsalva maneuver minimizes the risk of embolism. *(Courtesy of C. Rob and R. Smith.)*

FIBRINOLYSIS. There has been great interest in the use of fibrinolytic agents to activate the intrinsic plasmin system. Both streptokinase and urokinase have been used and found to be effective, although they are associated with a relatively high incidence of hemorrhagic complications as reported by Common et al. These agents have no advantage over heparin in the treatment of recurrent venous thrombosis or thrombosis that has existed for over 72 h, and they are contraindicated in postoperative or posttraumatic patients.

In a prospective study of 29 patients with major DVT (thrombosis involving the popliteal veins, with or without calf veins), Kakkar and Lawrence compared hemodynamic and clinical results in patients receiving 5-day treatment with heparin or streptokinase, followed by a 6-month course of coumadin. Overall, at 2-year follow-up they found over half of the limbs with evidence of the postthrombotic syndrome. Clinically, 14 percent of patients had no symptoms, 20 percent had severe symptoms, and the remainder demonstrated mild to moderate changes. No difference was seen between patients receiving heparin or streptokinase. Although a drug to restore venous patency and preserve valve function has not yet been found, other thrombolytic drugs such as tissue plasminogen activator (TPA) are currently under investigation and may provide better alternatives to treatment.

Surgical Approaches

OPERATIVE THROMBECTOMY. The direct surgical approach to remove thrombi from the deep veins of the leg utilizes the common femoral vein and is facilitated by the use of a Fogarty venous balloon catheter and an elastic wrap for milking the extremity (Fig. 22-8). Although the operative results are impressive, venograms obtained prior to discharge from the hospital show iliac occlusion in the majority of patients, and there does not seem to be any lesser incidence of the postthrombotic syndrome. Consequently, the procedure is usually reserved for limb salvage in the presence of phlegmasia cerulea dolens and impending venous gangrene.

In considering the reasons why the procedure has not lived up to expectation, there may be an explanation other than rethrombosis. It is customary to assume that the iliac system has been cleared if there is brisk retrograde blood flow after a proximal thrombus has been removed. This can be misleading if the common iliac vein remains obstructed and the retrograde flow is from the internal iliac vein. Conversely, poor retrograde flow may be seen when an iliac vein valve is intact despite removal of all proximal thrombus. Therefore, intraoperative venography should be performed in all cases. After completion of the thrombectomy, a small catheter may be left in a branch of the saphenous vein for postoperative regional heparin administration and postoperative venography.

In recent reports, an attempt has also been made to prevent rethrombosis after thrombectomy by creation of a peripheral arteriovenous fistula using the saphenous vein or one of its branches. The fistula is either allowed to close or is ligated after 2 to 3 months. Early results in 57 patients reported by Einarsson et al. showed patency of the iliofemoral segment by venography in 61 percent, and 75 percent had a good clinical result. Measurement by venous function, however, using plethysmography and foot volumetry showed normal results in only 29 percent.

VENA CAVAL INTERRUPTION. Adequate anticoagulation is usually effective in managing deep venous thrombosis, but if recurrent pulmonary embolism occurs during anticoagulant therapy or if there is a contraindication to anticoagulation, a surgical approach is necessary. Vena caval interruption is also indicated when a complication of anticoagulation forces is to be discontinued, as prophylaxis against recurrence of embolism after pulmonary embolectomy and in some high-risk patients who could not tolerate even a small embolic recurrence.

Early surgical efforts to prevent recurrence of pulmonary embolism were directed to the common femoral vein, which was ligated bilaterally. This resulted in a high incidence of sequelae due to stasis in the lower extremity and an unacceptable rate of pulmonary embolism. The next approach used was ligation of the inferior vena cava below the renal veins, which added the adverse effect of a sudden reduction in cardiac output under general anesthesia. This effect, coupled with stasis sequelae and recurrent embolism through dilated collateral veins, led to efforts to compartmentalize the vena cava by means of sutures, staples, and external clips in order to provide filtration without occlusion (Fig. 22-9).

Because these procedures required general anesthesia and laparotomy, the next logical step was to devise a transvenous approach that could be performed under

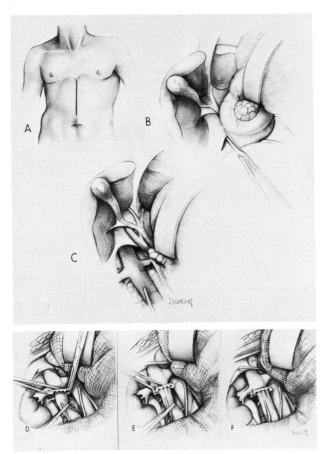

Fig. 22-9. Partial interruption of inferior vena cava using a serrated clip. *A*. Transperitoneal approach is preferred to permit high interruption of vena cava and concomitant ligation of the left spermatic or ovarian veins. *B*. Kocher maneuver. *C*. Vena cava cleared immediately below renal veins. *D*. Clip applied. *E*. Clip closed. *F*. Final position of clip in the immediate infrarenal region to prevent cul-de-sac. (From: *Adams JT, DeWeese JA: Surg Gynecol Obstet 123:1087, 1966, with permission.*)

local anesthesia. The Mobin–Uddin ''umbrella'' unit was inserted from the jugular vein and positioned under fluoroscopic control below the renal veins, where it usually produced (in 70 percent of cases) thrombosis of the vena cava and occasionally detached, resulting in fatal embolism.

The Greenfield cone-shaped filter was developed to maintain patency after trapping emboli. This is possible because of the unique geometry of the cone that collects emboli in its apex and retains perimeter flow. Preservation of flow avoids stasis and facilitates lysis of the embolus (Fig. 22-10). It can be inserted from either the jugular vein, left axillary vein, or the femoral vein, the latter insertion being reserved for inadequate size or technical problems with the jugular vein, or open wound of the neck. The rate of recurrent embolism with this device has been 5 to 6 percent over 12 years of follow-up. Its long-term patency rate of 95 percent allows it to be placed above the renal veins when necessary for embolism control, such as when there is a thrombus within the renal veins or vena cava. Another device, the Hunter balloon, occludes the vena cava after it is positioned below the renal veins and contributes to stasis sequelae.

The indications for insertion of a vena caval filter are listed in Table 22-2 and will be reviewed in the section on pulmonary thromboembolism.

OTHER TYPES OF VENOUS THROMBOSIS

Superficial Thrombophlebitis

The term thrombophlebitis should be restricted to the disorder of the superficial veins characterized by a local inflammatory process that is usually aseptic (Fig. 22-11). The cause of thrombophlebitis in the upper limb is usually acidic fluid infusion or prolonged cannulation. In the lower extremities it is usually associated with varicose veins and may coexist with deep vein thrombosis. Its association with the injection of contrast material can be

Fig. 22-10. The Greenfield filter is made of stainless steel and shaped in a cone to preserve perimeter flow after an embolus is trapped in its apex. Preservation of flow provides continued filtration, minimizes stasis sequelae, and facilitates lyses of trapped thrombus. The recurved hooks provide secure fixation in the vena cava.

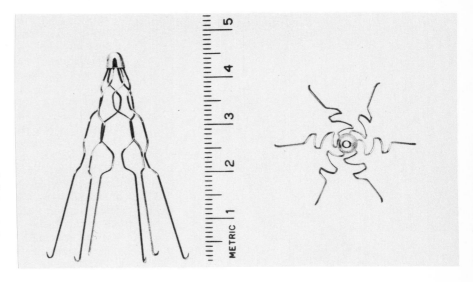

Table 22-2. INDICATIONS FOR INSERTION OF A
VENA CAVAL FILTER

1. Recurrent thromboembolism in spite of adequate anticoagulation
2. Documented thromboembolism in a patient who has a contraindication to anticoagulation
3. Complication of anticoagulation that forces therapy to be discontinued
4. Chronic pulmonary embolism with associated pulmonary hypertension and cor pulmonale (class V)
5. Immediately following pulmonary embolectomy
6. Relative indications—patient with more than 50% of the pulmonary vascular bed occluded (class III) who cannot tolerate any additional embolism; patient with a large free-floating iliofemoral thrombus on venogram

minimized by washout of the contrast material with heparinized saline.

Thrombophlebitis Migrans

Thrombophlebitis migrans, a condition of recurrent episodes of superficial thrombophlebitis, has been associated with visceral malignancy, systemic collagen vascular disease, and blood dyscrasias. Involvement of the deep veins and the visceral veins has also been described.

Subclavian Vein Thrombosis

Thrombosis of the subclavian vein is most likely to be secondary to an indwelling catheter and can occur in the pediatric age group. It may also occur as a primary event in a young athletic person (effort thrombosis), presumably as a result of injury or compression at the thoracic inlet. If seen within 48 h of onset, it is possible to use thrombolytic drugs followed by a venogram to define a potentially correctable abnormality. If seen later, it usually responds to elevation of the limb and anticoagulation, although some venous insufficiency and discomfort with exercise may persist.

Inferior Vena Caval Thrombosis

Thrombosis of the inferior vena cava can result from tumor invasion or propagating thrombus from the iliac veins. More commonly, however, it results from ligation, plication, or insertion of partially occluding caval devices. Any caval filtration device can become totally occluded by a trapped massive thrombus, causing sudden reduction in venous return and cardiac output. In the patient with known prior pulmonary embolism it is a grave error to ascribe the resulting hypotension to recurrent embolism and treat the patient with vasopressor agents. In this situation the cause of the hypotension is functional hypovolemia which can readily be confirmed by measurement of central venous pressure. Thrombosis of the renal vein can result from extension of vena caval thrombosis but is most likely to occur in association with the nephrotic syndrome. It can be a source of thromboembolism and has been treated successfully by suprarenal placement of the Greenfield filter.

Visceral Venous Thrombosis

Portal vein thrombosis can occur in the neonate, usually secondary to propagating septic thrombophlebitis of the umbilical vein. Collateral development leads to the occurrence of esophageal varices. In the adult, thrombosis of the portal, hepatic, splenic, or superior mesenteric vein can occur spontaneously but usually is associated with hepatic cirrhosis. Thrombosis of mesenteric or omental veins can simulate an acute condition of the abdomen but usually results in prolonged ileus rather than intestinal infarction.

Hepatic vein thrombosis (Budd–Chiari syndrome) usually produces massive hepatomegaly, ascites, and liver failure. It can occur in association with a congenital web, endophlebitis, or polycythemia vera. Although some success has been reported using a direct approach to the congenital webs, the usual treatment is a side-to-side portacaval shunt to allow decompression of the liver.

The development of pelvic sepsis after abortion, tubal infection, or puerperal sepsis can lead to septic thrombophlebitis of the pelvic veins and septic thromboembolism. Ligation of the ovarian vein and vena cava has been the traditional treatment, but the emphasis should be on drainage or excision of the abscesses and appropriate antibiotic therapy. It is also appropriate to use the Greenfield filter in this situation because it is inert stainless steel and avoids the development of an intraluminal abscess that can occur after ligation of the vena cava as demonstrated experimentally by Peyton, Hylemon, et al. in 1983.

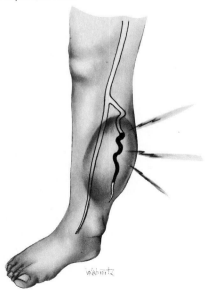

Fig. 22-11. Clinical presentation of superficial venous thrombosis. There is usually redness, tenderness, and swelling surrounding a palpable thrombosed superficial vein.

PULMONARY THROMBOEMBOLISM

The clinical significance of major pulmonary embolism can be appreciated by referring to the annual mortality attributed to it, which has been estimated to be 90,000 deaths in the United States alone. It is estimated that 5 of every 1000 adults undergoing major surgery will die from massive pulmonary embolism. Because it represents the most important complication of deep vein thrombosis, it is of particular concern to surgeons whose patients are prone to develop deep vein thrombosis in the immediate postoperative period.

Just as with deep vein thrombosis, our understanding of the pathophysiology of pulmonary embolism dates back to Virchow, who first recognized the association between the two findings. It also became obvious in the early reports by pathologists that pulmonary embolism could be well tolerated by some patients who then died of other causes. In fact, the full spectrum of the disorder ranges from asymptomatic minor embolism to sudden death from massive embolism.

Diagnosis

CLINICAL MANIFESTATIONS. The signs and symptoms of an embolic episode obviously depend primarily on the quantity of embolus involved and, to a lesser extent, on the cardiopulmonary status of the patient. In the classic presentation, the patient suddenly develops chest pain, cough, dyspnea, techypnea, and marked anxiety. Although hemoptysis has traditionally been associated with pulmonary embolism, it is actually an uncommon sign, and when present it usually occurs late in the course of the disease and represents pulmonary infarction. Objectively, the patient with major embolism usually shows tachycardia, an increased pulmonary second sound, cyanosis, prominent jugular veins, and varying degrees of collapse. Less commonly, there may be wheezing, a pleural friction rub, splinting of the chest wall, rales, low-grade fever, ventricular gallop, and wide splitting of the pulmonic second sound. The incidence of these findings found in the Urokinase Pulmonary Embolism Trial is shown in Table 22-3.

The differential diagnosis includes esophageal perforation, pneumonia, septic shock, and myocardial infarction. Since all these entities are life-threatening, it is manda-tory that an orderly approach be formulated to confirm or reject the working diagnosis. Laboratory studies in general are not very helpful in the differential diagnosis, although a white blood cell count of less than 15,000/mm^3 may be suggestive when a pulmonary infiltrate is present to help rule out pneumonitis. The following examinations are particularly useful in the evaluation of suspected major embolism.

ELECTROCARDIOGRAPHY. The most common electrocardiographic change associated with pulmonary embolism is nonspecific ST and T wave changes (66 percent of patients). More specific signs of right ventricular overload such as the often quoted S_1, Q_3, T_3 pattern are seldom seen. Consequently, the primary value of the electrocardiogram is to exclude the presence of a myocardial infarction. The finding of a myocardial infarction does not exclude the diagnosis of pulmonary embolism, and in some cases a lung scan or pulmonary angiogram may be required to clarify the problem.

CHEST RADIOGRAPHY. Although the chest radiograph may suggest the diagnosis of pulmonary embolism because of central vascular enlargement, asymmetry of the vascular markings with segmental or lobar ischemia (Westermark's sign), or pleural effusion, these signs are nonspecific. The chest radiograph then serves to exclude other diagnostic possibilities such as pneumonia, pneumothorax, esophageal perforation, or congestive heart failure. It is also critical in the interpretation of a lung scan, because any radiographic density or evidence of chronic lung disease makes a perfusion defect less likely to represent pulmonary embolism. Any pulmonary vascular or cardiac disease also reduces the applicability of lung scanning to the diagnosis.

ARTERIAL BLOOD GASES. The widespread availability of blood gas and pH determinations has improved the assessment of all critically ill patients and provides important support for the diagnosis of pulmonary embolism. Hypoxemia with Pa_{O_2} of less than 60 mmHg is found in the majority of patients and is felt to be due to shunting by overperfusion of nonembolized lung and a widened alveolar-arterial oxygen gradient due to reduced cardiac output. The reduction in arterial P_{CO_2} that follows major embolism is the most discriminating finding, because hypoxemia is present in several disorders likely to be misdiagnosed as massive embolism (e.g., septic shock). If hypoxemia and hypocarbia are not present, the diagnosis of major embolism in the severely ill patient is unlikely, and an alternative diagnosis should be sought.

CENTRAL VENOUS PRESSURE. In the patient with systemic hypotension, central venous pressure can supply valuable information, and the line provides access for administration of drugs and fluids as well. Low central venous pressure virtually excludes pulmonary embolism as the primary cause of the hypotension because massive embolism almost always is accompanied by right ventricular overload and elevated right atrial pressures. Elevated right ventricular filling pressures may be transient, however, as hemodynamic accommodation occurs, and in subacute or chronic embolism the central venous pressure may be normal.

Table 22-3. CLINICAL MANIFESTATIONS OF MAJOR PULMONARY EMBOLISM

Symptoms	Incidence, %	Signs	Incidence, %
Dyspnea	80	Tachypnea	88
Apprehension	60	Tachycardia	63
Pleural pain	60	Accentuated P_2	60
Cough	50	Rales	51
Hemoptysis	27	S_3 or S_4	47
Syncope	22	Pleural rub	17

Data from the Urokinase Pulmonary Embolism Trial: A National Cooperative Study. *Circulation* 2(suppl):47, 1973.

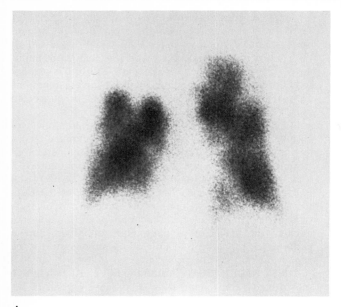

A

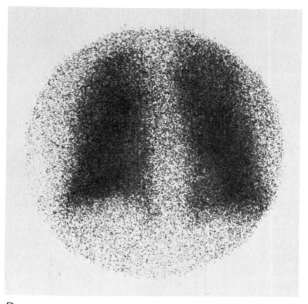

B

Fig. 22-12. *A.* A radionuclide perfusion scan following intravenous injection of macroaggregated albumin tagged ^{99m}Tc showing filling defects in the right lung. *B.* A ventilation scan performed with^{133}Xe showing normal ventilation. These findings suggest the diagnosis of pulmonary embolism.

Fig. 22-13. A selective pulmonary angiogram demonstrating absence of filling of left pulmonary arterial branches due to a large embolus obstructing the left main pulmonary artery.

LUNG SCAN. The availability and widespread usage of lung photoscanning have led to overemphasis on this test and a tendency to overdiagnose pulmonary embolism. In a nonhypotensive patient with a normal chest radiograph, the lung scan is a valuable screening test that has increasing validity as the size of the perfusion defect approaches lobar distribution (Fig. 22-12). Smaller peripheral perfusion defects are much more difficult to interpret because pneumonitis, atelectasis, or other ventilation abnormalities alter pulmonary perusion. A normal lung scan, on the other hand, usually excludes the diagnosis of pulmonary embolism. Adding a ventilation scan for combined ventilation-perfusion imaging increases the accuracy of the diagnosis of thromboembolism, provided that there are at least two moderate-sized areas or one large area of ventilation-perfusion mismatch. The assumption that the underperfused regions of the lung after embolism will remain normally ventilated, producing the mismatch in the scans, is clouded by the known physiologic effect of bronchoconstriction produced by embolism. When the additional variable of wide variance in scan interpretation among observers is considered, the diagnosis is much more reliable when it is based on arteriography.

PULMONARY ARTERIOGRAPHY. Selective pulmonary arteriography is the most accurate method of confirming the presence, size, and distribution of pulmonary emboli. The procedure is invasive, requiring passage of a cardiac catheter into the pulmonary artery for injection of a bolus of contrast medium. A rapid film changer produces a series of radiographs that outline areas of decreased perfusion and usually show filling defects or the rounded trailing edge of impacted emboli (Fig. 22-13). Straight cutoffs of the smaller pulmonary arteries are more difficult to interpret, particularly if there is associated chronic lung dis-

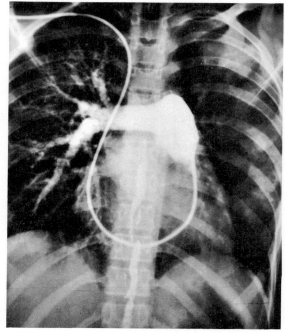

ease that tends to obliterate pulmonary vessels. The procedure can be performed with low risk, although pulmonary hypertensive and cardiac patients are at highest risk for this type of study, which usually carries a 0.3 to 0.5 percent mortality rate. Avoidance of injection of contrast medium into the main pulmonary artery minimizes the complications and mortality rates. Additional useful information is obtained prior to contrast injection by measurement of pulmonary arterial pressures. A normal pulmonary angiogram excludes the diagnosis of pulmonary embolism in acutely ill patients.

Pathophysiology

Although deep vein thrombosis precedes pulmonary embolism, less than 33 percent of patients with documented pulmonary embolism show clinical signs of venous thrombosis. Despite this, it is estimated that 85 to 90 percent of all pulmonary emboli originate from the veins of the lower extremity, and the remainder arise from the right side of the heart or other veins. In addition, the emboli from a recent thrombus tend to be multiple, fragmenting either in the right side of the heart or during impaction into the pulmonary vascular bed. Older thrombi, however, contain laminated fibrin layers that make them more solid and more difficult to lyse.

Once the embolus has lodged and interrupted pulmonary blood flow, the ratio of regional ventilation to perfusion increases, and the lung responds by bronchoconstriction to reduce wasted ventilation. This response is mediated by a local reduction in CO_2 output, since it can be prevented by ventilation with increased concentration of CO_2. Some experimental studies also suggest a generalized neural reflex vasoconstriction, but even if this occurs in human beings, it is not likely to be as significant a factor in survival as the mechanical effect of major vascular occlusion. Similarly, the effects of vasoactive humoral agents can be demonstrated in animals. There is evidence that serotonin is elaborated from platelets adherent to the embolus, which also contributes to the bronchoconstriction. The ability of heparin to inhibit the release of serotonin adds further justification to the early use of this drug. Other vasoactive agents such as histamine and prostaglandins may play a role in human beings, but the net effect is a reduction in size of peripheral airways, reduced lung volume, and reduced static pulmonary compliance.

The hypoxemia that characterizes major embolism is thought to be due to a ventilation-perfusion imbalance secondary to the ventilation changes described above, although the findings in some patients resemble true arteriovenous shunting. Such shunting is anatomically possible if there is an unobliterated foramen ovale that opens in the presence of elevated right atrial pressures. Such an opening can allow passage of a venous embolus into the systemic circulation; it then is termed *paradoxical embolism*. Although there may be some improvement in Pa_{O_2} after supplemental oxygen is administered, the effects usually are minimal. The return of pulmonary blood flow

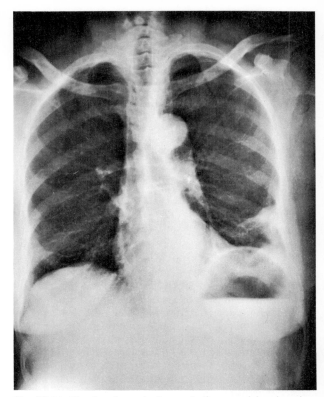

Fig. 22-14. Chest radiograph demonstrating a peripheral wedge-shaped area of infarction on the left side.

effected by embolectomy restores respiratory gas exchange, but the ischemia may result in loss of capillary integrity, causing interstitial pulmonary edema or overt pulmonary hemorrhage.

Pulmonary infarction as a consequence of embolism is relatively rare and is associated clinically with problems of poor systemic perfusion such as shock and congestive heart failure. In these patients the symptoms include pleuritic chest pain, dyspnea, cough, and hemoptysis. The signs include fever, tachycardia, splinting, and occasionally friction rub. There is usually prominent leukocytosis, an elevated lactic dehydrogenase level, and bilirubinemia. A wedge-shaped density usually is seen on chest radiography (Fig. 22-14).

The pulmonary vascular and cardiac effects of embolism are a direct consequence of the degree of filling of the pulmonary vascular bed. Occlusion of more than 30 percent of the vascular tree is required to begin to elevate mean pulmonary artery (PA) pressure, and usually more than 50 percent occlusion is required to reduce systemic pressure. The degree of pulmonary hypertension produced is proportional to the extent of angiographic vascular occlusion, but in a previously normal patient the limit of pressure elevation observed is approximately 40 mmHg mean.

The fate of pulmonary emboli in patients is not easy to predict, although a great deal of experimental work in animals has been reported. Injection of autologous thrombi into the pulmonary circulation of dogs is followed by relatively rapid recovery of pulmonary function and objective evidence of lysis over a period of weeks. Activation of plasminogen to plasmin, which is found in high concentration in the pulmonary circulation, promotes this fibrinolytic effect. The resolution of aged thrombi proceeds more slowly and is hampered further by impaction of the embolus and isolation from pulmonary blood flow. Consequently, resolution after massive embolism in patients is unpredictable and often incomplete. It is not unusual to find residual fibrin strands or webs in the pulmonary arteries at autopsy as remnants of prior embolism.

Management

ANTICOAGULATION. The hemodynamic variables mentioned above provide a means of classification of patients that employs five grades of severity and is a useful guide to therapy and prognosis (Table 22-4). The minor degrees of embolism (classes I and II) can usually be managed by anticoagulants alone with a satisfactory outcome (Fig. 22-15). Heparin is selected for initial treatment in a dose designed to prolong the partial thromboplastin time to at least twice normal. At this dosage of approximately 150 units/kg, there is adequate protection against further attachment of thrombus and platelets to the embolus. Heparin should be administered intravenously by pump-regulated continuous infusion. Conti, Daschbach, and Blaisdell have advocated higher doses of heparin to prolong the activated clotting time to 150 to 190 s with no increase in bleeding complications and improved control of recurrent embolism. However, heparin control of recurrent embolism is imperfect and recurrence was reported in 16 percent of patients by Wilson, Bynum, and Parkay, with a bleeding complication rate of 27 percent. In spite of this, heparin remains the initial treatment of choice and most clinicians also begin oral anticoagulation therapy to allow several days' overlap of the drugs as prothrombin time is extended into the therapeutic range.

THROMBOLYTIC THERAPY. Thrombolytic therapy has been advocated for the treatment of both deep vein thrombosis and pulmonary embolism. Two plasminogen activators, streptokinase and urokinase, are available for this and can be effective as documented in two large clinical trials (Urokinase Pulmonary Embolism Trial). The drugs are administered by intravenous infusion after a loading dose, and beneficial effects in thromboembolism usually can be seen in 12 to 24 h. Present laboratory tests to confirm the presence of a lytic state following streptokinase or urokinase administration have not proved useful in predicting the therapeutic response to these drugs or in preventing hemorrhagic complications. There were hemorrhagic side effects judged to be significant in 30 percent of the patients treated with both drugs, half of whom required transfusion. In addition to bleeding complications, the use of streptokinase for embolism has been associated with allergic reactions, fever, and the adult respiratory distress syndrome as reported by Martin et al. Also, in the first phase of the study, there was no significant difference between urokinase and heparin treatment in terms of the recurrence rate of embolism or mortality rate at 2 weeks.

More recently, recombinant human tissue–type plasminogen activator (rt-PA) has become available as a relatively clot-specific thrombolytic agent. In a series of 36 patients with documented pulmonary embolism by angiography, peripheral infusion of 50 mg over 2 h improved the angiographic score by 21 percent and an additional 40 mg over 6 h improved the average score by 49 percent as reported by Goldhaber et al. Since patients with hypotension were excluded, the initial pulmonary arterial pressure was only moderately evaluated to 22 mmHg and declined to 17 mmHg after infusion. Significant groin hematomas were seen in five patients, hematuria in two patients, and periodontal oozing in three patients. Two patients had major hemorrhage requiring operative treatment that in one case required relief of pericardial tamponade 8 days after coronary artery bypass. One patient had recurrent embolism and died for a mortality rate of 3

Table 22-4. CLASSIFICATION OF PULMONARY THROMBOEMBOLISM

Class	Symptoms	Arterial gases	% PA occlusion	Hemodynamics
I	None	Normal	<20	Normal
II	Anxiety, hyperventilation	Pa_{O_2} <80 mmHg Pa_{CO_2} <35 mmHg	20–30	Tachycardia
III	Dyspnea, collapse	Pa_{O_2} <65 mmHg Pa_{CO_2} <30 mmHg	30–50	CVP elevated, $\overline{PA}$ > 20 mmHg
IV	Shock, dyspnea	Pa_{O_2} <50 mmHg Pa_{CO_2} <30 mmHg	>50	CVP elevated, $\overline{PA}$ > 25 mmHg BP < 100 mmHg
V	Dyspnea, syncope	Pa_{O_2} <50 mmHg Pa_{CO_2} 30–40 mmHg	>50	CVP elevated, $\overline{PA}$ > 40 mmHg CO low, no shock

CVP = central venous pressure
PA = pulmonary artery
$\overline{PA}$ = mean pulmonary artery pressure

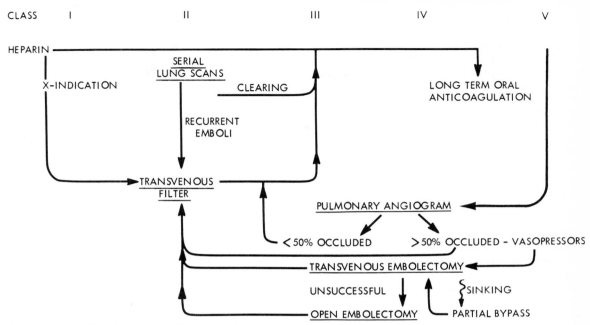

Fig. 22-15. Management algorithm for patients with documented pulmonary embolism stratified by class (see Table 22-4). Treatment is based on anticoagulation as shown for each class. In major embolism (classes III and IV), the findings at angiography and hemodynamic status influence the choice of procedures undertaken. [From: *Greenfield LJ: Acute venous thrombosis and pulmonary embolism, in Hardy JD (ed): Hardy's Textbook of Surgery. Philadelphia, Lippincott, 1983, with permission.*]

percent and a morbidity rate of 33 percent in these patients with submassive embolism. In spite of hope that this agent would be specific for thrombus fibrin, plasma fibrinogen declined 55 percent in patients who received 2-chain rt-PA and 34 percent in those who received 1-chain rt-PA.

The advantage of thrombolytic therapy may well be to improve the ultimate resolution of major thromboembolism as demonstrated by Sharma, Burleson, and Sasakara. Their follow-up studies in patients treated with urokinase or streptokinase showed a better restoration of pulmonary-capillary blood volume and diffusing capacity at 2 weeks than in patients treated with heparin and anticoagulants alone. The reason for the continued improvement that was seen at 1 year was not clear but was felt to be related either to more complete early resolution of the embolic condition, allowing more effective natural lytic processes, or to more complete clearance of peripheral venous thrombi, preventing silent recurrent embolism. Therefore, the patient who is not in shock and who has no clear contraindication to the use of thrombolytic therapy would probably benefit from its use.

VENA CAVAL INTERRUPTION. In some patients, anticoagulants cannot be used because of associated problems (e.g., peptic ulcer disease), and management must be directed toward a mechanical means of protection against recurrent embolism as outlined previously (Table 22-2). Other patients, in whom anticoagulation appears to be

adequate, sustain recurrent embolism and become candidates for surgical intervention. The third indication is when there has been a complication of anticoagulant therapy forcing it to be discontinued and leaving the patient with untreated DVT. Another indication for a vena caval filter is protection against recurrent embolism in a patient who has sustained massive pulmonary embolism requiring open or catheter embolectomy. In these patients, in spite of a satisfactory embolectomy of the pulmonary circulation, the original focus of venous thrombosis remains untreated, and recurrent embolism is likely.

There are two additional relative indications for a vena caval filter in a patient with active or recent deep vein thrombosis. One is the high-risk patient over 40 years of age who is obese and has a serious associated medical illness (e.g., heart disease), malignant disease, or a history of previous embolism and who undergoes a major abdominal or vascular procedure. The final relative indication is the patient in whom 40 to 50 percent of the vascular bed has been occluded (class III) and who would most likely not be able to tolerate additional emboli, particularly if there is associated cardiac or pulmonary disease.

PULMONARY EMBOLECTOMY. In patients who sustain massive embolism (classes III and IV), management must be a coordinated and rapidly responsive effort, since survival may be only a matter of minutes. As indicated earlier, it is critical to document the diagnosis of massive pulmonary embolism by pulmonary arteriography because the clinical diagnosis, regardless of "classic" appearance, often is in error. The initial approach to patients who have either transient collapse (class III) or persistent systemic hypotension (class IV) should include full heparinization and administration of inotropic drugs if necessary to support the circulation while the diagnosis is confirmed. Isoproterenol (4 mg in 1000 mL of 5% dextrose in water) is useful initially because of its bronchodilating and vasodilating effects as well as its positive inotropic cardiac effect. It may provoke arrhythmias, however, and necessitate use of dopamine. In the class II patient who responds to heparin and does not require vasopressors for systemic pressure or urine output, careful monitoring is essential to determine whether anticoagulation alone will control the disorder (Fig. 22-15). In most circumstances the spontaneous lysis of pulmonary emboli will proceed over a period of days and can be documented by serial lung scans performed at weekly intervals. The rate of clearing may be prolonged for weeks, particularly after a sizable embolism, and may be incomplete, as indicated previously. The latter condition has been observed in association with persistent pulmonary hypertension even after additional lytic drugs (e.g., urokinase) were administered. Lytic agents, however, may become a useful adjunct in management in the future.

The direct surgical approach to pulmonary embolism can be traced back to Trendelenburg (1908), who demonstrated the feasibility of pulmonary embolectomy experimentally but had no successes clinically. It remained for his pupil Kirschner (1924) to confirm the possibility of embolectomy by a successful clinical outcome. Because this procedure was attempted without circulatory support using a direct approach to the pulmonary artery at thoracotomy, the number of survivors was very small, and the first successful case in the United States was not reported until 1958 by Steenburg. A modification of this technique using hypothermia to occlude the circulation temporarily was reported by Allison et al. in 1960. The very high mortality rate associated with the Trendelenburg procedure prompted Gibbon to consider the use of extracorporeal circulation to bypass the impacted pulmonary circulation. However, the first successful open embolectomy during cardiopulmonary bypass was not reported by Sharp until 1962. Since then partial bypass support has also been utilized for the patient in shock. Local anesthesia is used, and the femoral artery and vein are cannulated for venoarterial bypass. The equipment is fully portable (Fig. 22-16), and patients can be supported during pulmonary arteriography and then transported to the operating room, where they can tolerate general anesthesia and sternotomy much better while being maintained on partial cardiopulmonary bypass. Once the mediastinum is opened, the partial bypass can be converted to total bypass by insertion of a superior vena caval catheter; the pulmonary emboli are then removed through a pulmonary arteriotomy.

Open pulmonary embolectomy still carries a mortality rate in the range of 50 percent, however, and uncontrollable pulmonary hemorrhage may follow open restoration of pulmonary perfusion. Consequently, an alternative approach utilizing local anesthesia has been suggested by Greenfield et al. for transvenous removal of pulmonary emboli. A cup device attached to a steerable catheter is inserted in either the jugular or the femoral vein, and the cup is positioned under fluoroscopy adjacent to the embolus seen on arteriography (Fig. 22-17). The position is

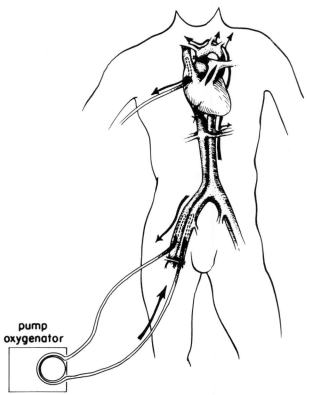

pump oxygenator

Fig. 22-16. The patient who sustains massive pulmonary embolism with shock (class IV) and fails to respond to resuscitation must be supported by partial bypass and considered for open pulmonary embolectomy. The femoral artery and vein can be cannulated under local anesthesia as shown. The patient will then tolerate a general anesthetic and sternotomy, at which time a cannula can be inserted into the superior vena cava for total cardiopulmonary bypass. The main pulmonary artery is opened and the emboli are extracted by forceps and suction. [From: *Greenfield LJ: Complications of venous thrombosis and pulmonary embolism, in Greenfield LJ (ed): Complications in Surgery and Trauma. Philadelphia, Lippincott, 1984, with permission.*]

verified by injection of contrast medium through the catheter. Then syringe suction is applied to aspirate the embolus into the cup, where it is held by suction vacuum as the catheter and captured embolus are withdrawn. Clinical experience with the technique in 29 patients showed that emboli could be extracted in 26 of them (90 percent) with an overall survival of 76 percent. Emboli could not be removed when they had been impacted for more than 72 h or if the patient suffered cardiac arrest at the time of angiography, in which case open embolectomy was required. Placement of a Greenfield vena caval filter after removal of sufficient emboli to produce near normal hemodynamics protected the patients from recurrent embolism.

PULMONARY HYPERTENSION AND THROMBOEMBOLISM

Pulmonary emboli may accumulate gradually over a prolonged period if they fail to undergo lysis and obliter-

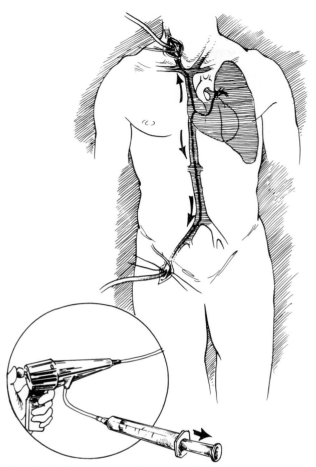

Fig. 22-17. Transvenous pulmonary embolectomy can be performed under local anesthesia via the jugular or femoral vein. The cup-catheter is positioned under fluoroscopy adjacent to the embolus and syringe suction is applied to capture the embolus within the cup. While suction is maintained, the catheter and trailing embolus are withdrawn through the venotomy. Multiple passages allow clearing of the vascular bed and restoration of cardiac output. [From: Greenfield LJ: *Complications of venous thrombosis and pulmonary embolism, in Greenfield LJ (ed): Complications in Surgery and Trauma. Philadelphia, Lippincott, 1984, with permission.*]

ate the pulmonary vascular bed. The clinical picture in this case is one of chronic cor pulmonale because significant pulmonary hypertension results from changes in the pulmonary vascular bed (class V). The presentation may be subtle with only dyspnea or syncope on exertion, but there is a loud P_2 and right-sided strain on the electrocardiogram. The sequence may also occur unaccompanied by significant respiratory symptoms, and this may explain the etiology in some of the patients considered to have primary pulmonary hypertension. When the diagnosis is made, there is very limited life expectancy, but the patient may benefit from a vena caval procedure to prevent further embolism even if the disorder is primary pulmonary hypertension as reported by Greenfield, Scher, and Elkins. The rationale for this is that they will ultimately

develop right heart failure, predisposing to pulmonary embolism that is lethal even if small. When acute cardiopulmonary decompensation occurs in these patients after embolism, they are not good candidates for embolectomy because of fixation of the older thrombi to the pulmonary arterial wall. They should be classified separately (class V) and managed by long-term anticoagulation therapy, or in some cases should be considered for heart-lung transplantation.

Recurrent thromboembolism may lead to progressive obliteration of the pulmonary vascular bed if the thrombi fail to undergo lysis. The resultant pulmonary hypertension produces exertional dyspnea and signs of right heart strain with cor pulmonale. With further progression of right heart overload tricuspid insufficiency may develop. This disorder may be difficult to distinguish from primary pulmonary hypertension, although the latter is more likely to be found in women under 20 years of age without a history of deep vein thrombosis. Severe pulmonary hypertension is a serious problem and usually limits the life expectancy to less than 2 years from diagnosis.

Open thrombectomy for chronic occlusion was first performed by Allison et al. in 1958 and remains a possibility for improving pulmonary blood flow. To be eligible for this procedure the occlusion must involve the proximal portion of the pulmonary arterial tree and the distal bed must be patent. The physiologic basis for continued distal patency after proximal occlusion is bronchial arterial collateral flow. The procedure also has a significant mortality, reported at 38 percent by Cabrol et al. in a series of 16 patients. For the majority of patients with severe pulmonary hypertension, however, the outlook is poor unless they receive maximum protection from recurrent embolism, which in our experience has required both anticoagulation therapy and vena caval filter placement.

VARICOSE VEINS

The prevalence of varicose veins in adults increases with age and is generally greater in women. It increases with increasing parity, is directly related to body mass, and has an inconsistent relationship with occupations that require prolonged standing. There is also a striking geographical variation in occurrence that is not well understood, although there appears to be a relationship with low-fiber diets and prolonged sitting as reported by Beaglehole.

Diagnosis

It is important to distinguish between primary varicose veins and the more serious condition of varicosities secondary to underlying deep venous disease. The latter situation is usually associated with stasis dermatitis or ulceration. In primary varicosities there is often a family history and a favorable outcome to medical or surgical treatment. The etiology is unknown, but the more widely accepted hypotheses attribute the disorder to either primary valvular weakness or weakness of the vein walls

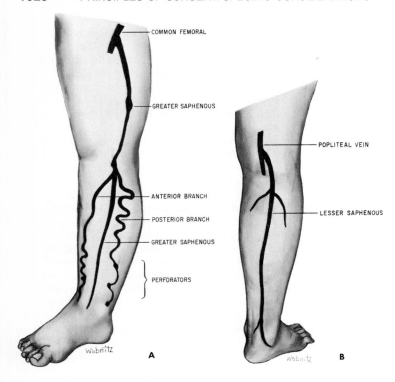

COMMON FEMORAL

GREATER SAPHENOUS

ANTERIOR BRANCH

POSTERIOR BRANCH

GREATER SAPHENOUS

PERFORATORS

POPLITEAL VEIN

LESSER SAPHENOUS

A

B

Fig. 22-18. *A.* The usual course of the greater saphenous vein and its major branches in the lower leg, emphasizing the fact that branch varicosities are the ones usually seen. Perforating veins, posterior and superior to medial malleoli, are indicated. *B.* The usual course of the lesser saphenous vein is shown in the lower leg.

allowing valvular distraction and incompetence. The theory of arteriovenous communication producing high pressure and flow is less well substantiated. There is rarely an association of varicosities with congenital or acquired arteriovenous fistulas. In the Klippel–Trenaunay syndrome, varicose veins develop in the leg in childhood and there is limb hypertrophy. Pelvic visceral varicosities with hemorrhagic complications also may develop. Servelle advises operative treatment in childhood to avoid limb length abnormality and has occasionally found compressive bands over major veins.

Varicose veins are the most common vascular disorder affecting human beings, who are unique among animals in this susceptibility. The term varicose means dilated and the characteristic enlarged and tortuous superficial veins can be diagnosed by inspection of standing patients. The usual distribution of varices is below the knee in branches of the greater saphenous system (Fig. 22-18). In the absence of postthrombotic sequelae, varicose veins are best evaluated by Doppler ultrasound and venous reflux plethysmography. If the abnormalities found are limited to the superficial veins, the condition is probably primary, whereas the finding of deep or perforator venous disease suggests that the varicosities are secondary and no benefit can be expected from their excision. These patients require lifelong elastic stocking support and may require operative treatment for local complications of their venous insufficiency.

The symptoms associated with varicose veins are nonspecific aching and heaviness of the legs that can be attributed to the congestion and pooling of blood in the enlarged superficial venous system. The symptoms are worsened by prolonged sitting and standing and relieved by elevation of the legs above the level of the heart. The use of calf-length elastic stocking support in the range of 20 to 30 mmHg usually suffices to provide relief. Although mild edema may occur from varicosities alone, it usually reflects additional incompetence of the deep or perforating venous system and may require stronger elastic stocking support. Obviously, the differential diagnosis for any patient presenting with bilateral lower-extremity edema also includes cardiac and renal disease, which should be investigated.

Night cramping of the legs is secondary to muscle spasms and is not usually due to venous disease. Arterial insufficiency should be excluded, but it may not be possible to identify a specific etiology. Some patients obtain relief by performing calf-stretching exercises prior to retiring and others may be helped by the administration of quinine sulfate, which reduces muscular irritability.

Treatment

The majority of patients can be managed by conservative methods, but if these fail to control symptoms or if additional complications of venous stasis develop, such as dermatitis, bleeding, thrombosis, or superficial ulceration, the patient may become a candidate for more aggressive management. Cosmetic concern or ill-defined pain patterns are less reliably improved by operation.

The two methods of treatment currently employed are ablative surgery and injection sclerotherapy, the latter being more popular in European countries than in this country. The objective of ablation is to redirect venous

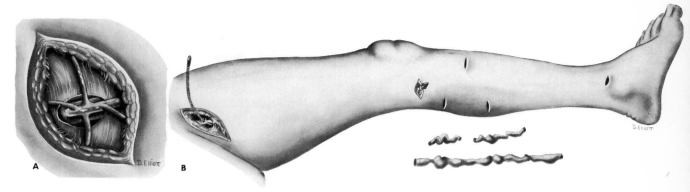

Fig. 22-19. Operative approach for ligation and stripping of the saphenous vein. *A.* The groin incision, showing the junction of the greater saphenous and femoral veins. Note four major branches of the saphenous vein that require ligation and division. *B.* A counterincision at the knee or ankle permits stripping of the saphenous vein. Additional incisions permit removal of branch varicose veins.

return through veins with intact valves and to improve appearance by removal or ligation of the varicosities (Fig. 22-19). The traditional procedure includes stripping of the long saphenous vein from ankle to groin by avulsion from its bed. More recently, Ludbrook and others have pointed out that it is advisable to save the normal portion of the saphenous vein below the knee to avoid the complications of its removal at that level and to allow it to be used for arterial bypass at a future time.

Injection sclerotherapy is designed to destroy the endothelium of the vein and promote its obliteration by scar. If pressure is not applied to the vein after injection of the sclerosant, a thrombus will form and later recanalize, leading not only to recurrence but occasionally to worsening of the problem. The technique for injection involves placement of the needle and syringe with the patient standing followed by elevation of the leg, injection of the agent, and bandage compression of the area for 2 to 3 weeks. Efforts are made to sclerose veins in proximity to perforating veins, which can be palpated as fascial defects, in order to reduce the chances of recurrence. Comparison of these techniques has shown that the results are comparable short-term but that surgical treatment clearly produces the best results after 3 to 5 years of observation as reported by Hobbs. Sclerotherapy also can produce allergic reactions, deep vein thrombosis, and inflammatory reaction with possible skin slough if the sclerosant escapes from the vein. It is useful primarily for management of smaller varicose veins and for recurrent or persistent varicosities after operative treatment.

CHRONIC VENOUS INSUFFICIENCY

In spite of optimal anticoagulation and bed rest for patients with acute deep vein thrombosis, approximately 50 percent will develop the postthrombotic syndrome as a reflection of chronic venous insufficiency. The underlying pathology consists of recanalization of the deep veins

with persistent deformity and incompetence of the valves. The result is a long column of blood unrestrained by valvular support that transmits pressures of over 100 mmHg to the venules, promoting both fluid and protein loss into the tissues. The perivascular fibrinous deposits remain in place because of inadequate fibrinolysis as demonstrated by Browse and interfere with oxygenation and metabolism of the tissues. The result is thickening and liposclerosis of the subcutaneous tissues to produce the characteristic ''brawny'' edema, which is relatively nonpitting. The loss of red cells results in hemosiderin deposits to produce the characteristic pigmentation. When the distal perforating veins become incompetent there is additional pressure, with skin atrophy leading ultimately to necrosis and chronic stasis ulceration (Fig. 22-20). There is often an associated dermatitis that may be due to various salves and ointments used to treat the condition. Dryness and scaling with pruritus also occur, and with constant scratching, secondary infection and cellulitis may result.

In contrast to normal patients who reduce their distal venous pressure with exercise, patients with the postthrombotic syndrome gain no benefit from their muscle pump (Fig. 22-21). If there has been failure of recanalization with persistent obstruction, the increase in blood flow with exercise may increase venous hypertension to produce ischemic pain referred to as ''venous claudica-

Fig. 22-20. Extensive chronic venous ulcers of the lower leg.

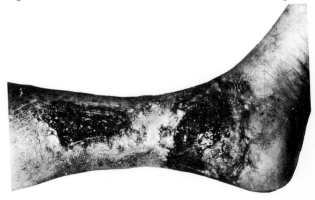

AMBULATORY VENOUS PRESSURE CHANGES

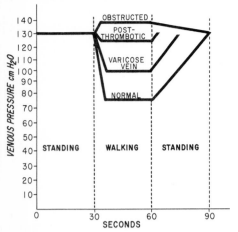

Fig. 22-21. Direct measurement of the responses in venous pressure in the superficial veins at the ankle with exercise. In the standing position, venous pressure is slightly higher than hydrostatic pressure in a column extending from ankle to heart. This pressure is approximately the same for normal persons and for those with venous insufficiency or chronically obstructed veins in which collaterals have formed. With walking, however, normal persons demonstrate a rapid decrease in venous pressure and a slow return to normal when exercise stops; patients with varicose veins show a lesser decrease in pressure with walking but a more prompt return to normal following cessation of exercise; patients with postthrombotic veins demonstrate little if any decrease in venous pressure with walking and a rapid return to normal; patients with obstructed veins show an increase in pressure with walking and a slow return to normal.

tion." This may become disabling and lead to consideration of venous bypass procedures to be described.

Diagnosis

Prior to the development of current techniques of noninvasive testing for venous disease, the methods of evaluation depended on physical examination while different sites were compressed. These tests are still useful if a noninvasive vascular laboratory is not available.

CLINICAL COMPRESSION TESTS. In the Trendelenburg test the limb is elevated to evacuate the veins; then pressure by hand or tourniquet is applied to the saphenofemoral junction (Fig. 22-22). With the patient standing, the lower leg is observed for the rate of filling of the varicosities. Gradual filling occurs in normal patients when the perforating veins are competent. Rapid filling occurs if

Fig. 22-22. The four possible results of the Trendelenburg compression test. The patient has been lying down with leg elevated; he then stands up with compression over the saphenofemoral junction. A. Negative-negative response in which there is gradual filling of veins from below over a 30-sec period and there is continued slow filling after release of hand. B. Negative-positive response. On standing, there is gradual filling of the distal veins; on release of compression there is rapid retrograde filling of the saphenous vein. C. Positive-negative response. With the hand in place, filling of superficial varicosities through incompetent perforators occurs; with release of compression there is further slow filling of the veins. D. Positive-positive response. On standing with the hand in place, there is filling of varices through incompetent perforators. On release of compression there is additional rapid filling of the saphenous vein.

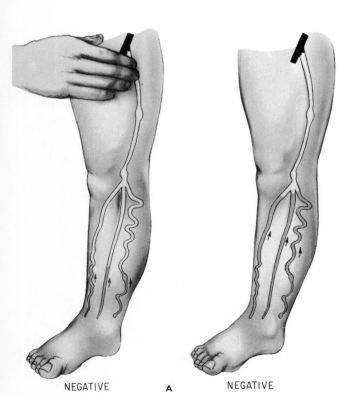

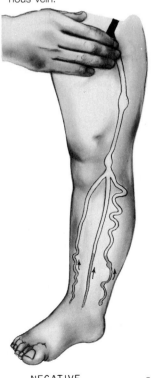

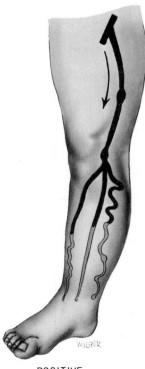

NEGATIVE   **A**   NEGATIVE   NEGATIVE   **B**   POSITIVE

the perforators are incompetent. The second phase of the test consists of release of the pressure to see if the upper thigh varices fill rapidly, indicating incompetence of the saphenofemoral valve.

In the Perthes test a tourniquet is placed around the upper leg and the patient is instructed to walk. If the varicose veins disappear, the deep venous system is patent and the perforating veins are competent. If pain occurs with walking, the deep system is obstructed and the superficial system represents the major source of venous outflow. Obviously, it would be a serious error to excise superficial veins under these circumstances. Sequential tourniquets also may be used to define and isolate areas of incompetent perforating veins (Ochsner–Mahorner test).

LABORATORY MEASUREMENTS. Direct measurement of venous pressure by needle and strain gauge provides the most accurate assessment of venous hemodynamics, but it is invasive and cumbersome to use. It has, however, served to validate the noninvasive tests to be described.

Doppler Examination. A directional Doppler can be used at the bedside to determine venous patency and valvular competence. Reflux retrograde flow can be observed at the femoral level during Valsalva maneuver or at the popliteal level with the patient standing and the calf alternately compressed and released (Fig. 22-4). A similar maneuver should be used when listening over perforating veins.

Plethysmography. The strain gauge plethysmograph measures venous capacity and outflow making it more valuable for acute thrombosis than for chronic changes where it may be normal or indicate persistent obstruction. The photoplethysmograph (PPG) uses infrared light to measure subcutaneous vascular volume and can provide a reliable index of valvular incompetence. The venous refilling time, after calf muscle exercise empties the veins, will be shortened considerably in the presence of valvular incompetence. Although the technique is primarily qualitative, Norris et al. have developed an in vivo calibration technique to provide quantitative information that correlates well with ambulatory venous pressure measured directly.

Duplex Scanning. The most promising of the newer diagnostic techniques is the combination of ultrasound duplex scanning using a B-mode imager with a pulsed Doppler instrument to provide both imaging and flow patterns. Thrombi can be visualized within the veins and flow observed if the vein remains patent. Normal veins can be compressed by the scanner head over the vessel while thrombosed veins are incompressible. Venous valves can also be visualized and their competence assessed under a variety of flow alterations as demonstrated by Kohler and Strandness.

Supportive Therapy

Perhaps the most important aspect of patient management is the education of the patient to emphasize the im-

Fig. 22-22 *C,D.* Continued.

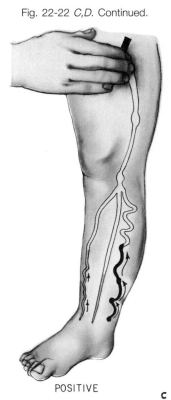
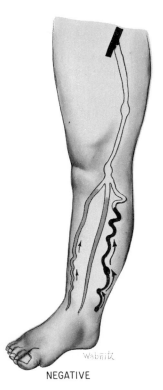
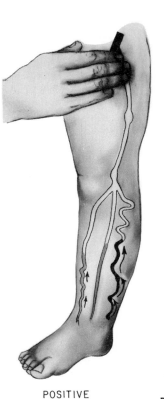
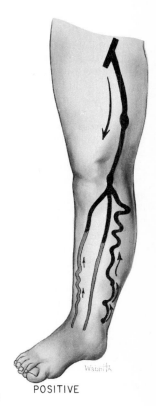

POSITIVE   NEGATIVE   **C**   POSITIVE   **D**   POSITIVE

portance of elastic stocking support, frequent elevation of the legs above the level of the heart, and the avoidance of prolonged sitting and standing. Frequent follow-up examinations are essential not only to assess compliance with the prescribed regimen but also to detect early recurrent thrombosis. Patient compliance can be improved by including other family members in the discussion and by the use of calf-length elastic stockings, which are easier to manage than full-length hose and less likely to produce a tourniquet effect at the knee. The patient should acquire two sets of pressure gradient stockings so that a clean pair is always available.

Operative Management

The development of a stasis ulcer requires immediate efforts to promote healing by frequent cleansing, bed rest, foot elevation, and the use of paste boots or elastic sealed dressings. The use of local medications should be avoided to minimize allergic reactions. Patients who fail to heal after prolonged outpatient care will require hospitalization and may need skin grafts for larger ulcers.

PERFORATOR VEIN LIGATION. Permanent healing of chronic stasis ulcers that recur after skin grafting is not likely unless the perforating veins responsible for the ulcer are identified and ligated. The typical location for these is posterior and superior to the medial malleolus as described by Dodd and Cockett. However, ligation of the perforator vessels still leads to recurrent ulceration in 15 percent of patients despite vigorous medical therapy, including support stockings, leg elevation, wound care, and patient education. The patients in whom medical and routine surgical therapy fail may be considered for attempted reconstruction of their venous systems.

VENOUS RECONSTRUCTION. The present attitude of most surgeons toward venous reconstruction is critical and pessimistic as reviewed by Bernstein in 1986. The venous system, unlike the arterial system, tends to recanalize, thus making it more difficult to quantitate the obstruction and identify the patient who may benefit from venous reconstruction. Dale estimated that the percentage of patients with chronic venous insufficiency who could benefit from reconstruction was 1 to 2 percent of that population. Surgical reconstruction can be divided into two categories: bypassing obstructive disease and restoring valvular competence. To evaluate patients, it is necessary to obtain both ascending and descending venograms.

The most widely accepted procedure for venous reconstruction is the saphenous vein cross-over graft, first described by Palma and Esperon in 1958. The procedure consists of isolating the normal contralateral saphenous vein and dividing it distally. The vein is then tunneled suprapubically and anastomosed to the contralateral femoral vein, distal to its obstruction. In 1982, Dale described 59 patients who had the Palma bypass with excellent results in 63 percent, good results in 17 percent, and a failure rate of 20 percent. Husni in 1981 and Smith and Trimble in 1977 had reported similar results. The saphenous

vein cross-over graft has generally been accepted as useful; however, the natural history of iliac vein occlusion is recanalization, and very few patients with iliofemoral thrombosis became candidates for surgery.

Use of the saphenous vein for popliteal-to-femoral vein bypass was described by Warren and Thayer in 1954, with good clinical results in 10 of 14 patients. The saphenous vein is dissected free below the knee and anastomosed to the popliteal vein, which is obstructed proximally. Husni has popularized this procedure and has reported the outcome in 27 patients, with a good result in 63 percent. Dale reported good results in 10 patients (60 percent), and Smith and Trimble, in a collected series of 59 patients, reported good results in 76 percent. However, with rich collateral veins in the thigh, identifying the patient with an obstructed superficial femoral vein who may benefit from the saphenous-to-popliteal vein bypass is difficult. Kistner and Sparkuhl, on the other hand, recognized that patients with superficial femoral vein incompetence and symptoms of thrombotic syndrome could benefit from superficial femoral vein ligation. They ligated the superficial femoral vein of five patients and had good results in four.

Methods of reconstruction for venous incompetence of the iliofemoral system include valvuloplasty as described by Kistner, venous segment transfer as described by Kistner and Sparkuhl, and valve autotransplantation as described by Taheri et al.

Valvuloplasty. In 1980, Kistner, after studying 200 limbs with ascending and descending venography, found 28 that could be treated by valve repair, and 72 percent had an excellent result. In this procedure, floppy incompetent valves are tethered against the vein wall or shortened using interrupted 8-0 monofilament suture (Fig. 22-23). After DVT, most patients have scarred and thickened valves that do not lend themselves to this type of reconstruction. Since Kistner routinely combined valvuloplasty with saphenous vein stripping and perforator ligation, the results have been difficult to interpret, but they have found good to excellent results in 80 percent of cases as reported by Ferris and Kistner.

Vein Segment Transfer. In 1979, Kistner and Sparkuhl described six patients who had vein segment transfer. Of these patients, one had venous occlusion and the other five had good results 1 year postoperatively. In this procedure, competent valves are identified in the saphenous vein, superficial femoral vein, and profundus system. The vessel with the incompetent valve identified by descending venography is divided and anastomosed distal to the portion of the system with a competent valve (Fig. 22-24). This renders the previously incompetent system competent and, when combined with saphenous vein stripping and perforator ligation, improves the clinical and venographic results.

Autologous Vein Transplantation. The third reconstructive procedure for iliofemoral incompetence consists of autologous vein valve transplantation. This was developed by Taheri and coworkers and consists of harvesting a segment of brachial vein with a competent valve from

Valve Repair II

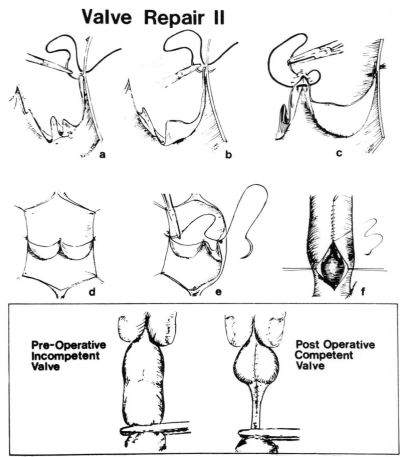

Fig. 22-23. The highest valve in the superficial femoral vein may be eligible for direct repair using the technique proposed by Kistner. A longitudinal venotomy exposes the valve cusps which are repaired by suture plication as shown *(A–E)*. After closure of the vein *(F)*, restored competence of the valve can be demonstrated by milking it proximally. [From: *Bergan J, Yao J (eds): Operative Techniques in Vascular Surgery. Orlando, FL, Grune and Stratton, 1980, with permission.*]

the arm and interposing it into the femoral system just below the origin of the superficial femoral vein or more distally at or above the popliteal vein. In 1986, the investigators described 66 patients, with good results in 78 percent. In this series 31 patients had postoperative venograms, and 28 had valvular competence. This procedure is still considered experimental and is awaiting long-term confirmation. Bergan and colleagues have pointed out that for venous valve surgery to be successful, it usually must be accompanied by saphenous vein stripping and perforator ligation. They reported a series of 12 patients who had only venous valve reconstruction without the more distal stripping and perforator ligation. These patients had good results initially; however, at 1 year, nine of the limbs had reverted to their preoperative condition owing to recurrent symptoms and delayed venous refill time. The difficulty in identifying patients who could

benefit from these procedures was put into perspective by Dale who, after 2 years of investigating, failed to identify a group of patients who would benefit from venous valve transplantation or valvuloplasty.

Husni found that venous reconstruction fails in three situations: when the bypass graft is too small in caliber; when venous hypertension is mild to moderate, that is, less than 80 percent of the standing venous pressure; and when a thrombectomy or endophlebectomy has to be performed before anastomosis. In these patients who are at high risk for failure, he has recommended a distal arteriovenous fistula. The use of arteriovenous fistulas after iliofemoral thrombectomy or reconstruction of the venous system is controversial. Most of the experience has been accumulated in Europe where it is believed to reduce the incidence of early rethrombosis. The two most commonly used sites are the femoral triangle and the ankle. After surgery on the iliofemoral system, an H-shaped fistula can be established easily by anastomosing a branch of the saphenous vein end-to-side to the proximal portion of the superficial femoral artery. At the ankle, the posterior tibial artery may be anastomosed to the posterior tibial vein or the greater saphenous vein. Two problems have led to the reluctance of some surgeons to adopt this procedure:

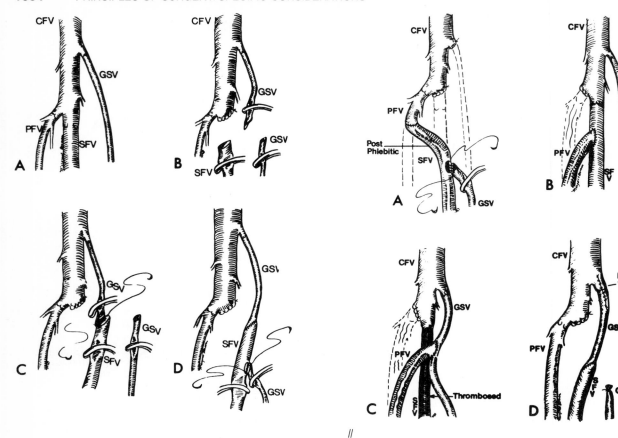

Fig. 22-24. I. An alternative technique for restoring valvular competence is to use the existing competent greater saphenous vein (GSV) as a new conduit for the incompetent superficial femoral vein (SFV) by dividing the veins at the level of the proposed anastomosis (A,B), connecting the SFV to the GSV (C) and then reimplanting the distal GSV into the SFV (D).

II. Where the SFV shows postphlebitic stenosis, it may be preferable to attach it to a competent profunda femoral vein (PFV) and add the inflow from the GSV (A). Where the PFV is incompetent, it can be connected to a competent SFV (B) or to the GSV to bypass an obstructed SFV (C). The transposition procedure can also be used in conjunction with valvuloplasty (D) when both techniques are required for restoring valvular competence. [From: *Bergan J, Yao J (eds): Operative Techniques in Vascular Surgery. Orlando, FL, Grune and Stratton, 1980, with permission.*]

the fear of damaging functioning valves distal to the fistula and the requirement for a second operation to close the fistula. Fistulas are usually closed 3 to 4 months postoperatively, and problems with incompetent valves distal to the fistula have not been reported. In 1981, Kroener and Bernstein reported on the effects of arteriovenous fistulas in dogs. They found a marked increase in the success of venous reconstructive procedures when a fistula was used, and no damage to the venous valves was noted when the fistula was taken down after 5 weeks. Two steps during primary venous reconstruction simplify closing the fistula later. The fistula is made distal to the venous reconstruction, thus avoiding damage to this area at reoperation, and a ligature is wrapped around the fistula and left in the subcutaneous tissue where it can be found under local anesthesia.

It seems reasonable to use the arteriovenous fistula in venous procedures that have been compromised, such as an iliofemoral thrombectomy, when the system has not been effectively cleared, or in a cross-over vein graft where the saphenous vein is of marginal size, since venous dilatation will occur proximal to the fistula. Smith has recommended that the fistula not be used if the ankle-arm index is less than 0.75 to avoid distal arterial problems in the same limb, and that the fistula should not exceed 4 mm in diameter to avoid distal venous hyperten-

sion, valvular damage, and significant effects on cardiac hemodynamics.

It has been noted in the past that the majority of iliofemoral thromboses occur on the left side. This is attributed to the right iliac artery compressing the left iliac vein as it crosses the fifth lumbar vertebra. Various autopsy series and operative studies have documented the presence of left iliac vein webs and scarring in patients who have had iliofemoral thrombosis. There was early interest in this problem by Calnan et al. in 1964 and Cockett and Thomas in 1965 who advocated surgical correction of these lesions. Dale reviewed eight such patients identified by venography and subsequently operated on four, trimming out anterior webs or scar tissue and using a venous patch for closure. Two of the patients had excellent results, but in one edema developed later, and a fourth patient had a complicated postoperative course, complaining of excruciating pain and postoperative swelling. Dale currently recommends operations only for the patient whose symptoms are severe and who will accept the operation knowing that the results are not predictable. Smith and Trimble have followed 30 patients with this problem and have operated on 14, with an 85 percent postoperative improvement rate. Cockett and Thomas, on the other hand, found the results unsatisfactory, and after operating on 30 patients using several different methods, they recommended abandoning the procedure.

VENOUS TRAUMA

Venous injuries of the extremities are usually associated with arterial injuries because of their anatomical proximity. In this situation, application of a tourniquet not only renders the limb ischemic but also can increase blood loss from the venous injury. Since the venous system is under relatively low pressure, direct pressure applied to the wound suffices for control. Direct ligation of injured superficial veins is appropriate treatment except when they are the sole remaining venous drainage of the extremity which mandates their repair.

Treatment of injuries of the deep veins changed dramatically as a result of the military experience in Southeast Asia as reported by Rich et al. It was well demonstrated that ligation of major extremity veins resulted in higher rates of disability and limb loss than when the veins were repaired or replaced by autogenous vein segments. The concept of primary repair of venous injuries by suture vein patch or vein graft interposition has been extended to civilian injuries by Agarwal et al. with favorable results. These repairs have not been associated with increased complications such as thrombophlebitis or pulmonary embolism as was originally of concern. Although injuries to the inferior vena cava are unusual, the morbidity and mortality rates are high, especially for the retrohepatic vena cava. Kudsk, Bongard, and Lim have reported their experience in 70 patients with both penetrating and blunt trauma, resulting in 55 percent survivors. They emphasized the importance of adequate resuscitation and the significance of associated injuries. Malt, Remonsnyder, and Harris showed that venous repair is also essential for the success of upper extremity replantation after nearly complete or complete traumatic amputation.

Iatrogenic vascular trauma has increased in frequency with the proliferation of invasive diagnostic and therapeutic puncture and biopsy techniques. The subclavian vein is particularly vulnerable to injury and thrombosis because of its use for venous access and placement of long-term catheters. Placement of these catheters also increases the risk of sepsis and the possibility of catheter breakage with embolization. A technique for retrieval of a catheter fragment in the subclavian vein by Fogarty catheter was reported by Mathur et al.

Use of a temporary arteriovenous fistula distal to the repair of a traumatic venous injury of the lower extremity in eight patients was reported by Richardson et al. in 1986. The posterior tibial artery and vein were utilized and the external shunt allowed infusion of heparin and access for postoperative venograms. In six patients the shunt functioned for an average of 10 days and all patients with functioning shunts for 72 h or longer had patent venous repairs without subsequent edema.

LYMPHATICS AND LYMPHEDEMA

Developmental Anatomy and Function

The exact origin of lymphatic vessels is a matter of disagreement among embryologists. The original theory of Sabin traced the origin from the venous system while Huntington and McClure suggested that lymphatics form by fusion of mesenchymal spaces or clefts. The latter has been labeled the centripetal theory. By the sixth week of gestation, there are paired lymph sacs in the neck and lumbar areas and at the eighth week, there is a retroperitoneal lymph sac with a developing cisterna chyli. These systems develop communicating channels that ultimately form the thoracic duct by merger of the right lymphatic duct with the left across the fourth to sixth thoracic vertebrae to drain into the left subclavian vein. Smaller lymphatic ducts persist that drain into the right subclavian vein.

Developmental arrest or abnormalities may result in primary hypoplasia or absence of ducts and lymph nodes. Abnormal growth of jugular lymph sacs can produce unilocular or multilocular lymph cysts termed cystic hygromas. In addition to the neck, these cysts may be found in the axilla, mediastinum, retroperitoneum, or intestinal mesentery. Hyperplastic changes may also occur to produce lymphangiomas with or without other vascular malformations.

The function of the lymphatic system begins with lymphatic capillaries that collect fluid and protein from the extravascular spaces. In addition to the protein that cannot be reabsorbed by the venules, red cells, bacteria, and other larger particles can only be evacuated through the lymphatics. This unique permeability is facilitated by the absence of a basement membrane beneath the lymphatic endothelial cells. The lymphatic capillaries are found beneath the epidermis in the superficial dermis. These vessels drain into valved channels in the deep dermis and subdermal tissues, forming larger channels that follow the vascular pathways superficial to the deep fascia. Although lymphatics can be found in the intermuscular fascia, they are absent in muscles, tendon, cartilage, brain, and cornea.

Lymph is transported by afferent vessels to regional lymph nodes that vary in size according to their function and activity. Within the medullary sinuses of the node, circulating lymphocytes are replaced and initial contact of foreign material with the immune system is made. Efferent lymph leaves the node via hilar channels that are less numerous than the afferent channels that enter the convex side of the node. In addition to direct thoracic duct drainage into the subclavian vein, there are other lymphovenous communications within nodes and in peripheral vessels. Central lymphatic flow is promoted by the lymphatic valves, muscular contractions in larger ducts, respiration, arterial pulsation, and external massage.

Classification

The original classification of Allen was into two types, one where there was no known cause and one secondary to a known disease or disorder. The primary lymphedemas were called *congenital* when present at birth and *praecox* when there was onset in childhood. When the onset was delayed into later life, Kinmonth added the term *tarda*. With the advent of lymphography it became possible to classify the primary lymphedemas structurally into *hyperplasias* and *hypoplasias*. The present classification as proposed by Kinmonth is as follows:

1. Primary lymphedema
   a. Primary hypoplastic
      (1) Distal hypoplasia or aplasia
      (2) Proximal hypoplasia
      (3) Proximal and distal hypoplasia
   b. Primary hyperplastic
      (1) Bilateral hyperplasia
      (2) Megalymphatic
2. Secondary lymphedema
   a. Malignancy
   b. Radiation
   c. Trauma or surgical excision
   d. Inflammation or parasitic invasion
   e. Paralysis

The primary lymphedemas are hypoplastic in 92 percent of cases. Their subgroups are defined by lymphography and behave differently. Those with distal hypoplasia have a mild, nonprogressive form of the disorder provided that their proximal pathways are normal. Most of these patients are women and notice the onset after puberty. In proximal hypoplasia, the lymphedema is more extensive, involving the entire extremity, and it occurs equally among males and females. The combination of proximal and distal hypoplasia shows features of both groups and tends to be progressive.

The primary hyperplastic lymphedemas are uncommon (8 percent) and those with bilateral hyperplasia can usually be recognized by diffuse capillary angiomata on the lateral sides of the feet. Lymphography shows dilated lymphatics with normal valves in contrast to the findings in the megalymphatic group where no valves can be seen. In this latter group, chylous reflux may produce chylometrorrhea, skin vesicles, or chyluria.

The most common cause of secondary lymphedema in this country is malignant disease metastatic to lymph nodes. Surgical removal of nodes, especially when combined with radiation therapy that produces lymphatic fibrosis, is another common cause. In tropical and subtropical countries, filariasis is the most common cause of secondary lymphedema, producing the typical appearance of elephantiasis. Other infective and chemical agents such as silica can enter the lymphatic system via barefoot walking and cause fibrosis of lymphatics and lymph nodes.

Diagnosis

Lymphedema occurs as the result of an abnormality of the lymphatic system, and the term should be restricted to situations where other causes of edema have been excluded or a specific lymphatic abnormality has been demonstrated. The presence of bilateral dependent "pitting" edema usually indicates a renal or cardiac etiology. Other generalized hypoproteinemias may be seen in malnutrition, cirrhosis, and protein-losing enteropathy, or they may be idiopathic. Allergies or hereditary causes are unusual. In unilateral edema, venous disease is the most likely etiology and can be recognized by the examinations described in the previous section.

CLINICAL MANIFESTATIONS. The patient with lymphedema complains of swelling and fatigue. Limb size increases during the day and decreases at night but is never normal. It is important to determine whether there is a family history of primary lymphedema and whether the patient has visited any countries where filariasis is endemic. The presence of weight loss and diarrhea suggests small bowel lymphangiectasia. On examination, lymphedema is characteristically firm and rubbery but nonpitting. Lymph vesicles may be present containing fluid of high protein concentration. Complications of lymphedema such as infection, cellulitis, erythema, and hyperkeratosis may be present. It is important to document limb size to identify isolated limb gigantism and the Klippel–Trenaunay syndrome which may have hypoplastic lymphatics in addition to venous abnormalities, capillary nevus, and limb elongation. The patient should be examined for upper extremity and genital lymphedema, hydroceles, and amelogenesis imperfecta.

LYMPHATIC VISUALIZATION. Lymphatics can be visualized by dye injection in the extremities and mesentery, and also by ingestion of cream or milk to visualize intestinal lacteals and major ducts.

Dye Infection. A highly diffusible dye such as patent blue as introduced by Hudack and McMaster or sky blue dye as recommended by Butcher and Hoover can be injected in 0.2-mL amounts subcutaneously into each interdigital web. Massage of the skin and movement of the joints will usually define a network of fine intradermal lymphatics (Fig. 22-25). If the collecting vessels are obstructed or inadequate, the dye will diffuse through the dermal lymphatics to produce a marbled appearance called "dermal backflow."

Radiologic Lymphography. The technique of lymphography was developed by Kinmonth, who demonstrated that it was possible to cannulate the lymphatics visualized by dye injection and then inject contrast medium (Lipiodol). This is a meticulous and tedious procedure that may require general anesthesia as originally proposed by Kinmonth. If the lymphatics in the foot are not usable, it is possible either to cannulate lymphatics adjacent to groin nodes or to inject the node directly. With adequate visual-

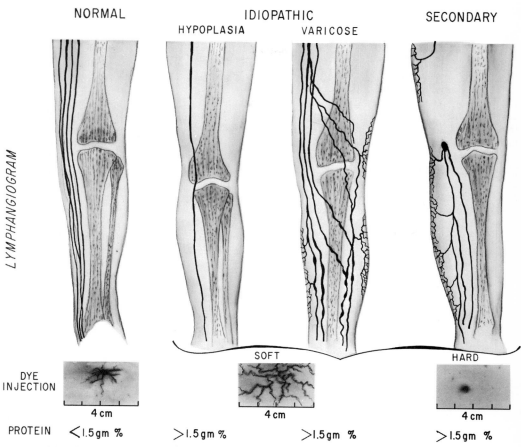

Fig. 22-25. Schematic illustration of the diagnostic procedures for lymphedema: dye injections, lymphangiograms, and protein analysis.

ization, the lymphatics in the extremity will be identified, often as parallel tracks that are of uniform size and bifurcate as they proceed proximally in contrast to the venous system (Fig. 22-25). Normally, there is some dilatation at the level of the valves.

Radionuclide Lymphatic Clearance. Radionuclide scanning using human serum albumin labeled with radioactive iodine or technetium 99m colloid has been used to monitor lymphatic clearance by serial scanning. Although the technique is simpler than standard lymphography, it has major disadvantages due to haziness of the scan, radiation dosage, and distribution of the radionuclide into the extracellular fluid, making calculations of clearance dependent on leg volume.

ANALYSIS OF TISSUE FLUID. Tissue fluid or lymph can be aspirated or collected from a tube in the subcutaneous tissues but contributes little to the diagnosis of lymphedema. Characteristically, lymphedema fluid has a protein content of more than 1.5 g/dL in contrast to edema fluid from venous hypertension, which is usually less. Also, the ratio of albumin to globulin is higher in lymphedema fluid than in plasma, which is helpful in the presence of an inflammatory exudate where the protein content is high but the albumin to globulin ratio is normal.

Management

SUPPORTIVE TREATMENT. There are significant anatomic and physiologic limitations to the treatment of lymphedema. From the standpoint of physiology, the removal of fluid is not as effective as in edema of other causes because of the residual protein in lymphedema. In addition, from an anatomical standpoint, the development of fibrosis produces irreversible changes in the subcutaneous tissues. Therefore, the options are limited and the primary objectives remain for control of edema, maintenance of healthy skin, and avoidance of the complications of cellulitis and lymphangitis.

The initial objective of control of edema can be approached by elevation and the use of sequential pneumatic compression boots to massage the leg. These treatments can be done at home with equipment rented for this purpose. Once the leg has reached optimal size, the patient should be fitted with firm elastic stockings as described earlier for venous insufficiency. The stockings should be removed at night and the foot of the bed elevated to maintain the pressure gradient from leg to right atrium.

The onset of redness, pain, and swelling usually signifies early cellulitis or lymphangitis which can be recognized by red streaking up the leg. The usual causative organism is either staphylococcus or beta-hemolytic streptococcus which must be treated vigorously, usually with intravenous antibiotics. In the absence of treatment, the infection may obliterate more lymphatics and produce constitutional signs of fever, malaise, nausea, and vomiting. Another frequent complication is eczema, which will usually respond to hydrocortisone cream. Antifungal agents may be necessary, both topically and systemically, for chronic infections, particularly between the toes. In contrast to the stasis edema of venous insufficiency, ulceration is unusual, although fissures and lymph fistulas may develop and require surgical excision.

The secondary lymphedemas may lend themselves to treatment of the underlying disorder such as using diethylcarbamazine for filariasis or appropriate antibiotics for tuberculosis or lymphogranuloma venereum. In rare cases of long-standing secondary lymphedema such as in the arm following radical mastectomy, a lymphangiosarcoma may develop appearing as a raised blue or reddish nodule. Satellite tumors and early metastases may develop if it is not recognized and widely excised.

OPERATIVE TREATMENT. Only 15 percent of patients with primary lymphedema become candidates for operative treatment, which usually is directed to reducing leg size. The indications for operation are related to functional rather than cosmetic improvement since the appearance of the extremity even after a successful procedure will still be abnormal and show extensive scarring. The best results are obtained when the bulk of the extremity has severely impaired movement or when there have been recurrent attacks of cellulitis. Although some efforts have been made to develop techniques to improve lymphatic drainage, most of the established procedures consist of excisional operations.

Three of the excisional procedures were based on the incorrect assumption that the deep fascia acted as a barrier to lymphatic drainage, and the efforts of Kondoleon, Sistrunk, and Thompson to excise fascia and/or insert a dermal flap into muscle proved ineffective in improving lymphatic drainage. The original procedure devised by Charles consisting of wide excision of lymphedematous tissue followed by skin grafting is still useful when the overlying skin is in poor condition as in elephantiasis. The procedure used more often, however, is Kinmonth's modification of Homan's procedure where skin flaps are raised to allow excision of the underlying subcutaneous tissues.

The most logical albeit technically demanding approach has been directed to establishing lymphaticovenous anastomoses. Initial efforts in this area were made by Nielubowicz et al. who divided a lymph node, removing the pulp under magnification, and then sutured the node capsule with its afferent lymphatics into a vein. This procedure is more suitable for secondary lymphedema than primary where the disorder lies in the lymphatic channels themselves. Another promising technique of direct lymphovenous connection was developed by Cordeiro and modified by Degni, who used a special needle for insertion of lymphatic vessels directly into veins and fixed them there by a single suture. Using this technique, Fox, Montorsi, and Romagnoli treated 8 secondary and 12 primary lymphedema patients followed for up to 4 years. Good results were obtained in 2 of 4 postmastectomy lymphedemas with poor results in the 2 patients who had postoperative lymphangitis. Nine of 11 patients with primary lymphedemas had good functional results allowing the patients to resume normal activity. The authors recommend long-term preoperative anti-inflammatory and antimicrobial therapy to avoid postoperative lymphangitis.

It is obviously difficult to evaluate the results of such procedures when combined with resectional operations and in the absence of postoperative lymphography to demonstrate patency of the anastomoses. However, the deleterious effects of lymphangiographic contrast on lymphatics were well demonstrated by O'Brien et al., who measured limb volume after lymphangiography in 100 patients and found that 32 percent had a significant increase in leg volume and 19 percent developed lymphangitis. Therefore, it seems advisable to use lymphangiography only for diagnostic studies and not for pre- or postoperative evaluation until safer contrast material becomes available. Further efforts to combine resectional operations with microlymphovenous anastomoses as reported by O'Brien and Shafiroff may offer some brighter prospects for improvement of these debilitating disorders.

Bibliography

Venous Disease

Aderka D, Brown A, et al: Idiopathic deep vein thrombosis in an apparently healthy patient as a premonitory sign of occult cancer. *Cancer* 57:1846, 1986.

Ambrus JS, Ambrus CM, et al: Clinical and experimental studies of fibrinolytic enzymes. *Ann NY Acad Sci* 68:97, 1957.

Common HH, Seaman AJ, et al: Deep vein thrombosis treated with streptokinase or heparin: Follow-up of a randomized study. *Angiology* 27:645, 1976.

Einarsson E, Albrechtsson U, et al: Follow-up evaluation of venous morphologic factors and function after thrombectomy and temporary arteriovenous fistula in thrombosis of iliofemoral vein. *Surg Gynecol Obstet* 163:111, 1986.

Hobbs JT, Davies JWL: Detection of venous thrombosis with ^{131}I-labelled fibrinogen in the rabbit. *Lancet* 2:134, 1960.

Homans J: Diseases of the veins. *N Engl J Med* 231:51, 1944.

Hyers TM, Hull RD, et al: Antithrombotic therapy for venous thromboembolic disease. *Chest* 89(suppl):265, 1986.

Kakkar VV, Carrigan TP, et al: Efficacy of low doses of heparin in prevention of deep vein thrombosis after major surgery: A double blind, randomized trial. *Lancet* 2:101, 1972.

Kakkar VV, Lawrence D: Hemodynamic and clinical assessment after therapy for acute deep vein thrombosis. A prospective study. *Am J Surg* 150:54, 1985.

Peyton JWR, Hylemon MB, et al: Comparison of Greenfield filter and vena caval ligation for experimental septic thromboembolism. *Surgery* 93(4):533, 1983.

Shattil SJ: Diagnosis and treatment of recurrent venous thromboembolism. *Med Clin North Am* 68:577, 1984.

Virchow R: *Gesamelte Abhandlungen zur wissenschaftlichen Medizin*. Frankfurt, Merdinger Sohn, p 219, 1856.

Pulmonary Thromboembolism

Allison PR, Dunhill MS, et al: Pulmonary embolism. *Thorax* 15:273, 1960.

Cabrol C, Cabrol A, et al: Surgical correction of chronic postembolic obstruction of the pulmonary arteries. *J Thorac Cardiovasc Surg* 76:620, 1978.

Conti S, Daschbach M, et al: Comparison of high-dose versus conventional-dose heparin therapy for deep vein thrombosis. *Surgery* 92:972, 1982.

Goldhaber SZ, Vaughan DE, et al: Acute pulmonary embolism treated with tissue plasminogen activator. *Lancet* 2:886, 1986.

Greenfield LJ: Pulmonary embolism: Diagnosis and management. *Curr Probl Surg* 13:1, 1976.

Greenfield LJ: Intraluminal techniques for vena caval interruption and pulmonary embolectomy. *World J Surg* 3:4559, 1978.

Greenfield LJ, Bruce TA, et al: Transvenous pulmonary embolectomy by catheter device. *Ann Surg* 174:881, 1971.

Greenfield LJ, Scher LA, et al: KMA-Greenfield^R filter placement for chronic pulmonary hypertension. *Ann Surg* 189:560, 1979.

Martin TR, Sandblom RI, et al: Adult respiratory distress syndrome following thrombolytic therapy for pulmonary embolism. *Chest* 1:151, 1973.

Sharma GVRK, Burleson VA, et al: Effect of thrombolytic therapy on pulmonary capillary blood volume in patients with pulmonary embolism. *N Engl J Med* 303:842, 1980.

Steenburg RW, Warren R, et al: A new look at pulmonary embolectomy. *Surg Gynecol Obstet* 107:214, 1958.

Urokinase Pulmonary Embolism Trial: A National Cooperative Study. *Circulation* 2(suppl):47, 1973.

Wilson JE III, Bynum LJ, et al: Heparin therapy in venous thromboembolism. *Am J Med* 70:808, 1981.

Varicose Veins and Chronic Venous Insufficiency

Beaglehole R: Epidemiology of varicose veins. *World J Surg* 10:898, 1986.

Bergan JJ, Flin WR, et al: Venous reconstruction surgery. *Surg Clin North Am* 62:399, 1982.

Bernstein EF: Future prospects in the treatment of venous disease. *World J Surg* 10:959, 1986.

Browse ML, Burnard KG: The postphlebitic syndrome: A new look, in Bergon JJ, Yao JST (eds): *Venous Problems*. Chicago, Year Book Medical Publications, 1978.

Calnan JS, Kountz S, et al: Venous obstruction in the aetiology of lympyoedema praecox. *Br Med J* 2:221, 1964.

Cockett FB, Thomas ML: The iliac compression syndrome. *Br J Surg* 52:816, 1965.

Dale WA: Reconstructive venous surgery. *Arch Surg* 114:1312, 1979.

Dale WA: Venous bypass surgery. *Surg Clin North Am* 62:391, 1982.

Hobbs JT: Surgery and sclerotherapy in the treatment of varicose veins: A random trial. *Arch Surg* 109:793, 1974.

Husni EA: Reconstruction of veins: The need for objectivity. *J Cardiovasc Surg* 24:525, 1983.

Keister HW, Bowers RF: Results obtained by superficial femoral vein ligation. *Surgery* 47:224, 1960.

Kistner RL: Surgical repair of the incompetent femoral vein valve. *Arch Surg* 110:1336, 1975.

Kistner RL: Primary venous valve incompetence of the leg. *Am J Surg* 140:218, 1980.

Kistner RL, Sparkuhl RD: Surgery in acute and chronic venous disease. *Surgery* 85:31, 1979.

Kohler TR, Strandness DE Jr: Noninvasive testing for the evaluation of chronic venous disease. *World J Surg* 10:903, 1986.

Kroener JM, Bernstein EF: Valve competence following experimental venous valve autotransplantation. *Arch Surg* 110:1467, 1981.

Ludbrook J: Primary great saphenous varicose veins revisited. *World J Surg* 10:954, 1986.

Norris CS, Beyran A, et al: Quantitative photoplethysmography in chronic venous insufficiency: A new method of noninvasive estimation of ambulatory venous pressure. *Surgery* 94:758, 1983.

Palma EC, Esperon R: Vein transplants and grafts in the surgical treatment of the postphlebitic syndrome. *J Cardiovasc Surg* 1:94, 1960.

Servelle M: Klippel and Trenaunay's syndrome: 768 operated cases. *Ann Surg* 201:365, 1985.

Smith DE: Surgical management of obstructive venous disease of the lower extremity, in Rutherford RB (ed): *Vascular Surgery*. 2d ed, Philadelphia, Saunders, 1984, pp 1412–1433.

Smith DE, Trimble C: Surgical management of obstructive venous disease of the lower extremity, in Rutherford RB (ed): *Vascular Surgery*. Philadelphia, Saunders, 1977, pp 1247–1268.

Taheri SA, Heffener R, et al: Vein valve transplantation. *Contemp Surg* 22:17, 1983.

Taheri SA, Heffener R, et al: Five years' experience with vein valve transplant. *World J Surg* 10:935, 1986.

Taheri SA, Lazar L, et al: Vein valve transplantation. *Surgery* 1:29, 1982.

Warren R, Thayer TR: Transplantation of the saphenous vein for postphlebitic stasis. *Surgery* 35:867, 1954.

Venous Trauma

Agarwal N, Shah PM, et al: Experience with 115 civilian venous injuries. *J Trauma* 22:827, 1982.

Kudsk KA, Bongard F, et al: Determinants of survival after vena caval injury: Analysis of a 14-year experience. *Arch Surg* 119:1009, 1984.

Malt RA, Remonsnyder JP, et al: Long-term utility of replanted arms. *Ann Surg* 176:334, 1972.

Mathur AP, Pochaczevsky R, et al: Fogarty balloon catheter for removal of catheter fragment in subclavian vein. *JAMA* 217:481, 1971.

Rich NM, Hobson RW II, et al: Repair of lower extremity venous trauma: A more aggressive approach required. *J Trauma* 14:639, 1974.

Richardson JB, Jurkovich GJ, et al: A temporary arteriovenous shunt (Scribner) in the management of traumatic venous injuries of the lower extremity. *J Trauma* 26:503, 1986.

Lymphatics and Lymphedema

Allen EV: Lymphedema of the extremities. Classification, etiology and differential diagnosis: Study of 300 cases. *Arch Intern Med* 54:606, 1934.

Cordeiro AK: Novas tecnias de anastomose linfovenoa para

tratamento cirurgico de linfedma de nembros inferiores e linfedma de membro superior pos mastectomia. *Maternidade Infuncia* 34:211, 1975.

Degni M: New technique of lymphatic-venous anastomosis for the treatment of lymphedema. *Vasa* 3:479, 1974.

Huntington GS, McClure CFW: The anatomy and development of the jugular lymph sacs in the domestic cat. *Am J Anat* 10:177, 1910.

Kinmonth JB: *The Lymphatics. Diseases, Lymphography and Surgery*. London, Arnold, 1972.

Nielubowicz J, Olszewski W: Surgical lymphaticovenous shunts in patients with secondary lymphedema. *Br J Surg* 55:440, 1968.

O'Brien BM, Das SK, et al: Effect of lymphangiography on lymphedema. *Plast Reconstr Surg* 68:922, 1981.

O'Brien BM, Shafiroff BB: Microlymphaticovenous and resectional surgery in obstructive lymphedema. *World J Surg* 3:3, 1979.

Sabin FR: On the origin of the lymphatic system from the veins and the development of lymph hearts and thoracic duct in the pig. *Am J Anat* 1:367, 1902.

Chapter 23

Surgically Correctable Hypertension

William J. Fry and Richard E. Fry

Elevated blood pressure, especially elevated diastolic pressure, is a too frequent cause of devastating illness and death. In 1981 the American Heart, Lung and Blood Institute released these statistics: One of six Americans, or 35,000,000 people, has definite high blood pressure. Of these individuals, 18,000,000 are aware of their disease; 12,000,000 receive treatment, but only 5,000,000 are adequately treated. Further estimates show that death from myocardial infarction and stroke would be decreased 20 percent if hypertension could be recognized early and appropriately treated.

The ravages of untreated hypertension significantly reduce life expectancy because of secondary involvement of the heart, brain, and kidneys. Insurance tables show that a male with a blood pressure of 150/100 has a risk of death two to three times greater than one with a blood pressure of 110/70. Even modest increase in the diastolic pressure above 82 mmHg can be correlated with a higher mortality, especially of women in the fifteen- to forty year-old age group (Table 23-1). Optimal control of the blood pressure is often difficult. Numerous medications may be necessary, and problems with drug side effects and patient compliance make proper treatment difficult. Palliation is the rule, and the opportunity for cure is seen in those patients with surgically correctable lesions, 5 to 15 percent of the total hypertensive population.

PHYSIOLOGY AND PATHOPHYSIOLOGY

Systolic and diastolic blood pressure are reflections of the peak left ventricular pressure and the static tone of the capacitance vessels during ventricular relaxation. The "normal" values are by age: adults, less than 140/90; adolescents, 100/75; children, 85/55; and infants, 70/45. These values are not absolute, as the aforementioned risk of death with a diastolic pressure greater than 82 attests.

The blood pressure is affected by cardiac output, peripheral resistance, and blood volume. Blood viscosity and vessel compliance have a lesser influence. Increased intravascular volume and red-cell mass as seen in polycythemia rubra vera can cause hypertension, while decreased intravascular volume secondary to hemorrhage will lower the blood pressure. *Cardiac output,* the volume of blood pumped per unit of time by the heart, has great effect on the blood pressure. Hyperdynamic states such as thyrotoxicosis may increase the blood pressure, while ischemic myocardial disease can lead to pump failure and hypotension. *Peripheral vascular resistance,* or the resistance to flow at the arteriolar level, has marked influence on the blood pressure and can vary greatly in response to blood volume changes and circulating vasoactive substances.

Right atrial stretch receptors and carotid and aortic arch baroreceptors modulate the blood pressure through sympathetic and parasympathetic neural signals. These areas are responsible for regulation and maintenance of blood pressure through their influence on cardiac performance and total peripheral resistance. Neural mechanisms may have a role in essential hypertension by the establishment of a higher "set point."

Humoral mechanisms specifically affect the blood pressure. Catecholamines increase small vessel tone; steroids and mineralocorticoids increase total body water and sodium, and potentiate the vasoconstrictive effect of norepinephrine and epinephrine. Angiotensin II, produced by renal ischemia, increases the blood pressure through a combination of its powerful vasoactive properties and its stimulation of aldosterone secretion which expands intravascular volume. Recently, atriopeptides stored in granules within the wall of the atrium have been

Table 23-1. VARIATIONS IN MORTALITY AMONG WOMEN ACCORDING TO SYSTOLIC AND DIASTOLIC PRESSURES. RATIOS OF ACTUAL TO EXPECTED MORTALITY—STANDARD FEMALE RISKS—100 PERCENT

| Systolic blood pressure, mmHg | Diastolic blood pressure, mmHg | Mortality ratio %* Issue age | | |
		15–39	*40–69*	*All ages*
128–137	<83	137	93	97
	83–87	147	92	98
	88–92	179	88	93
	93–97	209	92	110
138–147	<83	161	125	128
	83–87	162	150	151
	88–92	150	170	168
	93–97	(394)	168	170
	94–102	(826)	171	220
148–157	<88	—	117	90
	88–92	(301)	219	214
	93–97	—	140	140
	98–102	—	214	183
158–167	<88	—	138	138
	88–92	—	129	127
	93–97	—	179	182
	98–102	—	(246)	(250)

* Where the number of policies terminated by death is 10 to 34, the mortality ratio is enclosed in parentheses. A dash indicates fewer than 10 policies terminated by death.
SOURCE: Lew EA: High blood pressure, other risk factors and longevity: The insurance viewpoint, in JH Laragh (ed): *Hypertension Manual.* New York, Yorke Medical Books, 1974, p 43.

defined. These may contribute to systemic pressure by their natriuretic, diuretic, and antihypertensive effects.

CLINICAL MANIFESTATIONS

Hypertension is an insidious disease. Symptoms such as headache and epistaxis may accompany severe elevation of blood pressure but are nonspecific. Often a patient will realize the presence of hypertension only after hospitalization for myocardial infarction or stroke. Cardiovascular, cerebrovascular, and renovascular disease are the symptoms commonly caused by hypertension. Cardiac effects are secondary to left ventricular hypertrophy. There is an increased distance between the nutrient capillaries in ventricular hypertrophy that effectively compromises nutrient blood flow. The blood supply to the heart may be further compromised by atherosclerotic coronary artery disease. Accelerated atherosclerosis leads to peripheral and splanchnic vascular disease. Cerebrovascular atherosclerosis increases risk of stroke, while chronic hypertension compromises renal function through nephrosclerosis. Malignant hypertension is accompanied by encephalopathy, retinal and cerebral hemorrhage. All of these processes, working in concert or alone, subject the afflicted individual to an increased mortality.

SURGICAL HYPERTENSION AND RATIONALE FOR OPERATIVE THERAPY

Surgically correctable hypertension accounts for 5 to 15 percent of the total spectrum of this disease. A list of these types may be seen in Table 23-2. All these conditions involve a circulating substance producing increased blood pressure. They differ only in the site of origin and whether the release of the substance is due to a parenchymal disorder such as pheochromocytoma, or due to altered blood flow as in renal artery occlusive disease. The place of surgery in the treatment of "essential" disease is of historical and research interest, but at this time no techniques have been devised that consistently lower blood pressure in those without obvious reasons for operative therapy.

Operative therapy, when appropriate, should be employed rather than instituting or continuing medical therapy. Medical therapy is often ineffective. The myriad medications with their adverse reactions, coupled with poor control of the hypertensive state, are usually not effective. Lowering the blood pressure will do little to ameliorate the ravages of Cushing's disease or to prevent the parenchymal deterioration of renal occlusive disease. Operative therapy offers an opportunity for complete cure rather than palliation.

Table 23-2. SURGICALLY CORRECTABLE FORMS OF HYPERTENSION

Renovascular hypertension
Primary hyperaldosteronism
Hyperadrenocorticism
Pheochromocytoma
Coarctation of the aorta
Unilateral renal parenchymal disease

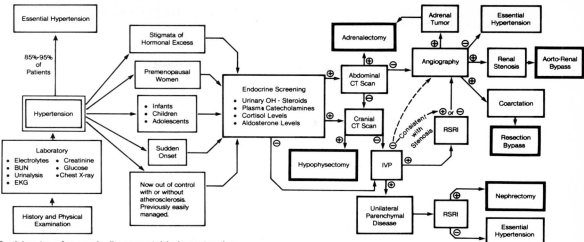

Fig. 23-1. Decision tree for surgically correctable hypertension.

PATIENT EVALUATION AND WORK-UP

Because most patients will have essential hypertension, screening all hypertensives for a surgical lesion may be unproductive and expensive. An algorithm for evaluating the hypertensive patient is shown in Fig. 23-1. A thorough history and physical examination can effectively lead to appropriate evaluation. An operative lesion should be suspected in patients who exhibit (1) sudden onset of severe or malignant hypertension; (2) easily controlled disease, with or without atherosclerosis, that becomes labile or difficult to treat; or (3) signs of hormonal excess. It should also be suspected when hypertension is present in adolescents or children or in premenopausal women. Patients who fall into these categories are more likely to have a surgically correctable lesion. Special attention to the details of the ocular funduscopic examination can help in grading the severity and chronicity of "newly discovered" hypertension. Physical findings such as peripheral edema, pulmonary rales/rhonci, and the presence of a third heart sound may suggest more severe or long-standing hypertension. Basic laboratory studies such as serum electrolytes, blood urea nitrogen (BUN), creatinine, and fasting serum glucose may lead to further endocrine or renal work-up. Electrocardiogram and chest x-ray can document the presence of left ventricular hypertrophy or rib notching. Urinalysis, creatinine clearance, and 24-h protein excretion further evaluate renal function and suggest nephropathy, either hypertensive or inflammatory. These screening examinations should lead to basic endocrine screening and then to the more definitive intravenous pyelogram, CT scanning, and angiographic studies. Information obtained from these tests will direct the clinician to appropriate operative therapy. The specific place and nature of these studies will be discussed later in the chapter.

PHEOCHROMOCYTOMA

Pheochromocytoma is a rare tumor of the adrenal medulla that exhibits a striking variety of presentation, making diagnosis difficult. Afflicted patients can present with a paroxysmal or sustained hypertension associated with sweating, headache, encephalopathy, and cardiac failure, among other symptoms. Pheochromocytomas are found in only 0.1 to 0.6 percent of all patients with hypertension. The severe nature of the disease and the high mortality rate in the untreated dictate early diagnosis and removal of the tumor. Eleven to twenty-three percent of all tumors are found to be malignant; the malignant form of the disease is not easily distinguished from benign, except in locally aggressive or metastatic tumors. The adrenal gland is the site of origin in 87 percent of all cases, the remainder being extraadrenal. Approximately 10 to 15 percent are bilateral and are usually associated with neurofibromatosis, the multiple endocrine adenomatosis (MEA) type II syndrome, and rarely, the von Hippel-Lindau syndrome. Medullary tumors produce both epinephrine and norepinephrine, while extraadrenal sites usually produce nearly pure norepinephrine.

Once a pheochromocytoma is suspected, the screening tests of urinary catecholamine excretion and serum levels should be obtained for normal values (Table 23-3). A recent study has shown increased accuracy of diagnosis using plasma catechol levels rather than urinary levels or levels of catechol metabolites. When chemical evidence is obtained, localization of the tumor may be determined using intravenous pyelogram (IVP), CT scanning, angiography, or venous sampling techniques. Intravenous pyelogram is accurate only 50 percent of the time and has been supplanted by newer methods. CT scanning is a

Table 23-3. NORMAL VALUES FOR URINARY CATECHOLAMINES

Catecholamines	$<100\ \mu g/24\ h$
VMA	$<6.8\ mg/24\ h$
Metanephrine	$<1.3\ mg/24\ h$
Epinephrine	$<25\ mg/24\ h$
Norepinephrine	$<160\ mg/24\ h$

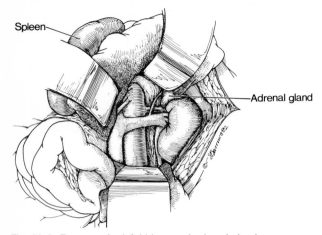

Fig. 23-2. Exposure for left kidney and adrenal gland.

screening procedure of choice and has excellent specificity and sensitivity in identifying adrenal masses. Tumors and normal adrenal glands may be hard to define if there is a paucity of retroperitoneal fat. If a tumor is located and elevated serum catecholamines are present, the diagnosis is complete. Scintigraphic methods using ^{131}I-metaiodobenzylguanidine have been shown to accurately locate pheochromocytomas in 90 percent of patients studied. This method can be useful when a biochemically proved tumor cannot be localized. Angiography and venous sampling techniques should be reserved for those patients with tumors difficult to locate. Transcatheter brush biopsy of inferior vena caval tumor thrombi is a newer technique, but has limited applicability at this time. Transabdominal adrenalectomy with examination of both glands is a preferred surgical approach (Fig. 23-2). The surgeon must also inspect the paraspinous area, bladder, and the organ of Zuckerkandl to rule out the presence of extramedullary tumors. The extent of resection will be dictated by the size of the tumor, the amount of local invasion, and the presence of metastases.

The perioperative treatment plays a major role in the care of the patient with pheochromocytoma. All patients will be relatively hypovolemic, requiring adequate volume replacement. Fluid and cardiac status should be adequately monitored and maintained with pulmonary artery wedge catheterization or at least a central venous line. Use of phenoxybenzamine and nitroprusside can aid in controlling blood pressure during operation, while lidocaine should be available for arrhythmias. After removal of the tumor, hypotension secondary to vasodilatation and hypovolemia are not infrequent. Monitoring of the blood pressure in the intensive care unit with the use of volume replacement and vasopressors, if necessary, is mandatory. Results of benign tumor resection are excellent, with a normal life expectancy. A malignant tumor carries a poor prognosis of 44 percent 5-year survival rate and a 19 percent 5-year disease-free interval. Extra-adrenal lesions have an even poorer outcome because they frequently indicate inoperable tumor and rapid metastases. (See Chap. 37.)

PRIMARY HYPERALDOSTERONISM

Increased primary aldosterone secretion by the zona glomerulosa of the adrenal cortex is associated with hypokalemia, hypernatremia, hypervolemia, and increased blood pressure. Clinically, the patient will exhibit signs of muscle weakness, headache, and malaise. Most patients are women in the thirty- to fifty-year-old age group. Laboratory examination demonstrates increased urinary potassium excretion, increased serum sodium and increased bicarbonate levels. Low plasma renin levels after sodium restriction and furosemide with upright posture is a helpful diagnostic test. The absence of aldosterone suppression after saline loading also aids in diagnosis. The combination of low plasma renins and high serum aldosterone levels gives 95 percent accuracy in diagnosing hyperaldosteronism. CT scanning should be used initially for tumor localization, with angiography and adrenal vein sampling reserved for ambiguous cases. Renal angiography should be strongly considered when the tumor is not easily found. An arterial lesion can be ruled out and a tumor may often be detected. Adrenal venography may be helpful in localizing some tumors when CT scanning and arteriography are not diagnostic.

The decision to employ operative therapy is based on the cause of the increased aldosterone. The anterior abdominal approach is preferred, although flank and posterior approaches are also used (Fig. 23-3). Excision of aldosterone-producing adenomas gives excellent cure rates ranging from 60 to 90 percent. Patients with diffuse cortical hyperplasia do not respond as well to adrenalectomy. If spironolactone can decrease blood pressure effectively preoperatively, the response to operation is generally good. If there is no response, medical treatment may be

Fig. 23-3. Exposure for right kidney and adrenal gland.

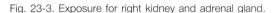

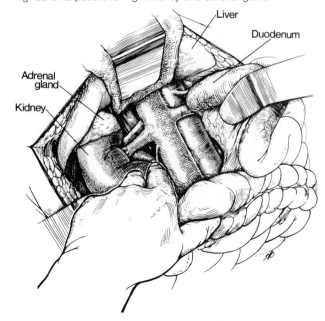

indicated. In cases of adrenal hyperplasia, bilateral adrenalectomy may be considered to alleviate symptoms.

HYPERADRENOCORTICISM

In his book, *The Pituitary Body* (1912), Harvey Cushing described a patient with hypertension, truncal obesity, striae, amenorrhea, and hirsutism. Although the pituitary was thought to be the primary cause of disease, reference was made to planned operative exploration of the adrenal glands. After further investigation, "Cushing's disease" was fully described and more clearly elucidated in 1932. Other causes of adrenal excess are possible, but the classic symptoms are due to an increase in circulating glucocorticoids. Women thirty to fifty years of age are most commonly affected. The cause of the disease may originate in the adrenal gland itself, in the pituitary gland, or from other tumors, the so-called "ectopic ACTH syndrome."

DIAGNOSIS. A more complete explanation of Cushing's disease and its diagnosis is given in Chap. 37. For screening purposes, increased urinary 17-hydroxysteroid levels and loss of diurnal variations in serum cortisol levels are enough to establish a diagnosis of hyperadrenocorticism. Pituitary or adrenal disease can be differentiated by ACTH levels and their response to dexamethasone suppression (see Chap. 37). Abdominal or cranial CT scan and adrenal vein sampling may help in anatomic location. Scintillation scanning of the adrenal with ^{131}I-6 beta-idiomethyl-19-norcholesterol can help localize adrenal or abdominal lesions suspected from biochemical tests. It should be reserved for those patients in whom CT scanning does not localize the lesion. Sella turcica films are not accurate, and the absence of abnormality does not rule out pituitary adenoma.

THERAPY. Surgical therapy should be tailored to the type of lesion, and every effort should be made to locate the tumor before proceeding with adrenal excision. Ectopic and adrenal lesions account for 20 to 25 percent of cases of hyperadrenocorticism and are best treated by excision of the tumor. Bilateral adrenal hyperplasia is usually caused by pituitary tumors. Those patients with moderate symptoms may be effectively treated with pituitary irradiation or transsphenoidal hypophysectomy. If gross sellar enlargement is evident, transsphenoidal ablation may be indicated.

If evaluation of the patient indicates unilateral adrenal enlargement, adenoma or carcinoma is probable. Total or partial adrenalectomy affords excellent cure rates in adenoma. Both glands should be examined at operation, as 10 percent of cases involves both adrenals. Adrenal carcinoma requires extensive dissection with wide excision of the tumor. Cure rates are poor, with most patients surviving only 3 years after diagnosis. Serum cortisol levels should be followed after operation, as these may rise with recurrence. All patients undergoing adrenal surgery for Cushing's disease should be prepared preoperatively with intravenous steroids and followed carefully in the postoperative period for signs of corticosteroid insufficiency.

Ortho para-DDD, a DDT congener, and the agent mitotane have been shown to cause regression in adrenal carcinoma. Use of this drug may provide prolonged remission in patients with metastatic or unresectable tumor.

Ectopic ACTH Syndrome

Several nonadrenal tumors are capable of producing ACTH or ACTH-like substances. Usually this occurs in patients with metastatic malignant tumors. Oat cell tumors of the lung, pancreatic carcinoma, and thymic tumors are the most common cause of this disease. Because of advanced malignancy, classic stigmata are not always present. Tumor removal is preferred; however, extensive tumor growth often makes this impossible. Some palliation may be offered with appropriate chemotherapy.

COARCTATION OF THE AORTA

Congenital narrowing of the aorta, either proximally or distally to the ductus arteriosus, is a frequent cause of hypertension in infants and children. The aortic narrowing and increased resistance to blood flow may contribute to the increased blood pressure, along with decreased renal artery perfusion with secondary hyperreninemia and angiotensin II formation. The entire thoracic and abdominal aorta can be involved, as well as intestinal and renal vessels. Patients with neurofibromatosis and hypertension have an increased incidence of upper thoracic and abdominal coarctation.

Diagnosis is most easily made by comparing blood pressure in the upper and lower extremities. A difference of 20 to 40 mmHg should be seen. Older children and adults may exhibit overdevelopment of the upper body and underdevelopment of the lower limb. Systolic precordial murmurs, left ventricular hypertrophy on ECG, notching of the ribs, and a "3 sign" on chest x-ray are also suggestive of coarctation of the aorta. Arteriographic appearance is diagnostic and helps with operative planning.

Surgical resection with primary anastomosis or graft interposition is the treatment of choice. Use of the left subclavian artery as a "patch graft" is also effective. Untreated patients have a mortality of approximately 60 percent. Most patients should be operated upon between six and sixteen years of age. Early intervention may be necessary if cardiac decompensation supervenes or if medical treatment is not effective. If performed in the optimal age range, a 95 percent cure rate can be seen, with an operative mortality of approximately 1 to 3 percent. When patient age increases, operative mortality increases, since the operation becomes technically more difficult. The cure rate also declines because the hypertension tends to become "fixed" by the long-standing coarctation. (See Chap. 19.)

RENOVASCULAR HYPERTENSION

Renovascular hypertension may be defined as elevation in the diastolic and systolic pressure associated with

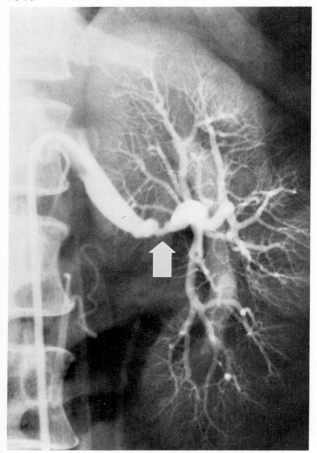

Fig. 23-4. Radiographic appearance of fibromuscular artery disease.

renal artery occlusive disease. There must be attendant dampening and reduction in total renal blood flow, causing the juxtaglomerular apparatus to secrete renin. The pathophysiology of renovascular hypertension was clarified by Goldblatt in the 1930s when he produced hypertension in laboratory animals by constriction of the renal artery. Shortly after that, the renoangiotensin system was delineated by Page, Helmer, and Menendez. The first arteriographic demonstration of an occluding lesion to the kidney was demonstrated by John Sid dos Santos. He attempted an endarterectomy of this vessel; it failed and the patient was cured with a nephrectomy. For several years nephrectomy was performed for hypertension in association with small kidneys, and when there was lack of good function on excretory pyelogram. This frequently resulted in failure to relieve hypertension.

It was not until the advent of arteriography and new techniques in vascular surgery that the observations by DeCamp, Morris, DeBakey, and the Cleveland Clinic group spearheaded by Harriet Dustan proved that normal blood pressure could be restored in hypertensive patients with careful technical reconstruction of a stenotic lesion in the renal artery. These pioneers not only demonstrated

the feasibility of making the correct diagnosis but showed that, with refined techniques in reconstructive vascular surgery, predictable and long-term amelioration of hypertension could be achieved.

ETIOLOGY. Atherosclerosis accounts for over 80 percent of the occluding lesions seen in the renal artery, associated with attendant hypertension (Fig. 23-18*A*). This is primarily a disease afflicting males between the ages of fifty-five and seventy-five.

Fibrodysplasia accounts for approximately 18 percent of the occluding lesions seen in the renal artery (Fig. 23-4). It is primarily a disease of young people, being the most common etiologic factor in children and young women of the childbearing age group. Fibrodysplasia may take many forms, the most common of which is the medial fibrodysplasia. The classification of this disease process is outlined in Fig. 23-5. Histologically, the vasa vasora are always occluded in this disease, which may account for the overgrowth of collagen tissue. This may lend credence to the theory that this is primarily a disease of trauma or stretching of the renal artery. The right renal artery is affected 85 percent of the time. The right kidney is the most mobile kidney and is stretched repeatedly during pregnancy. Aneurysms are often associated with medial fibrodysplasia, being a secondary consequence of this process. This predisposition in the female may be secondary to the continual stretching of the renal arteries secondary to pregnancy, and/or may be associated with estrogens that are known to cause medial degeneration of the vessel walls. The condition is associated with thrombosis, accounting for the vasa vasora occlusions.

The fibrodysplastic lesions seen in children have so far

Fig. 23-5. Classification of fibromuscular renal artery disease.

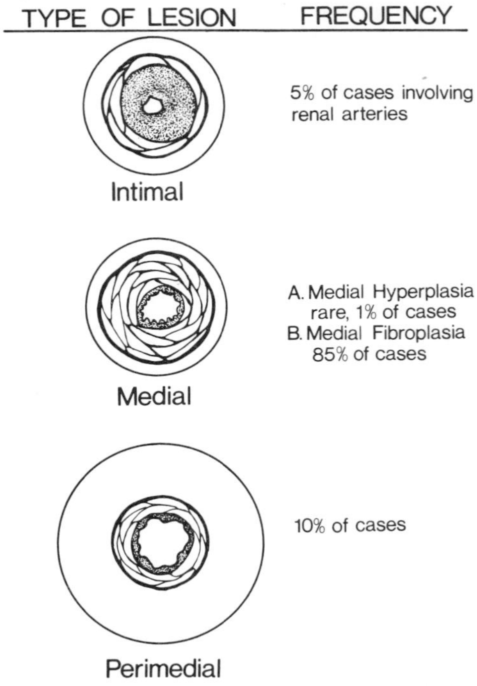

TYPE OF LESION	FREQUENCY
Intimal	5% of cases involving renal arteries
Medial	A. Medial Hyperplasia rare, 1% of cases B. Medial Fibroplasia 85% of cases
Perimedial	10% of cases

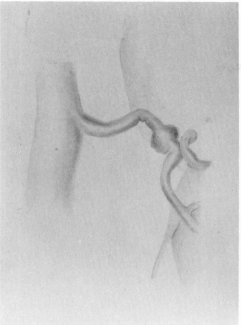
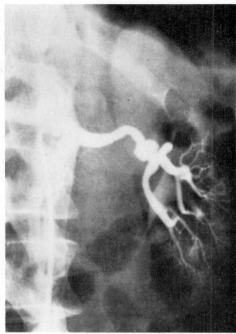

Fig. 23-6. Arteriogram and artist's concept of a solitary renal artery aneurysm.

defied any consistent delineation of etiology. The lesions most commonly seen in children are intimal hyperplasia and medial dysplasia. There is no question that upon occasion this disease progresses, and at least 15 percent of our patients have shown progression or formation of new lesions in 5- and 10-year follow-ups. Medial fibrodysplastic lesions may lend themselves to dilation, either directly or with a Gruntzig catheter. Intimal lesions and perimedial lesions do not lend themselves to dilation.

Trauma is an increasingly common etiologic factor in renovascular occlusive disease. Partial disruption of the renal artery may occur with severe trauma, producing a significant flow pressure gradient. The ability to delineate these problems early is paramount, as the attendant scarring around the renal hilus makes later reconstructive angioplasty exceedingly difficult. Fractures of the kidney may partially devascularize segments of the kidney that, if not recognized, may later produce hypertension.

Aneurysms of the renal arteries in and of themselves do not cause hypertension (Fig. 23-6). They are often associated with medial fibrodysplastic disease or severe atherosclerosis which may cause a secondary narrowing of the renal artery. Upon occasion, renal artery aneurysms will be the source of thrombus which may embolize distally into the renal parenchyma, causing ischemia and secondary hypertension.

Embolus is an uncommon but well-recognized cause of renovascular hypertension, with most emboli originating in the heart, though some originate from atherosclerotic aortic disease.

Dissections of the renal artery may be secondary to trauma, aortic dissections that extend into the renal ar-

tery, or fibrodysplastic disease. Dissections of the renal artery may pose problems in operative repair. With care, in most instances adequate revascularization can be accomplished.

Coarctation of the aorta, either classic or abdominal aortic coarctation, may produce a reduction in flow and pressure to the kidney, activating the release of renin. An abdominal aortic coarctation is depicted in Fig. 23-7.

Other, more obscure causes are vasculitis and collagen disease, rarely cysts or neoplasms of the kidney, and acquired or congenital arteriovenous fistulae within the kidney or the renal vessels.

Renin is produced when there is a reduction in flow and pressure to the renal parenchyma. This activates the juxtaglomerular cells to produce excessive amounts of renin that then sets up the production of angiotensin (Fig. 23-8). The use of angiotensin II antagonists (such as captopril) has been shown to be effective in the diagnosis and treatment of renovascular hypertension. Captopril has renal toxicity and may cause renal artery thrombosis. For these reasons, it should not be used as definitive therapy for renovascular hypertension.

CLINICAL MANIFESTATIONS. The clinical manifestations of renovascular hypertension are not clear. One must have a high index of suspicion in order to make this diagnosis. Renovascular hypertension is one of the most common causes of hypertension in the child. It is usually sustained and severe in nature, not easily controlled by medication. The sudden onset of hypertension in an adult should always alert the clinician to the possibility of renal artery occlusive disease. This is particularly true in women of the childbearing age. In those persons with ath-

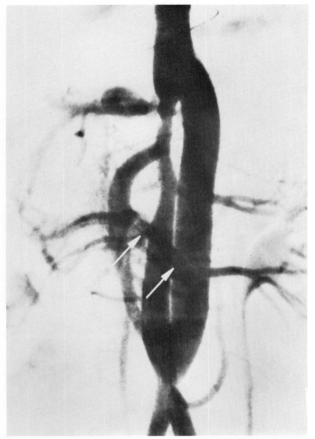

Fig. 23-7. Coarctation of the abdominal aorta after reconstruction. Arrows at repaired renal artery and bypass graft.

erosclerosis, it should likewise be remembered that sudden onset of hypertension may be related to occlusive disease involving the renal artery. The hallmark of renovascular hypertension is a sustained elevation of the diastolic blood pressure that is not readily controlled with

Fig. 23-8. Renin-angiotensin cascade.

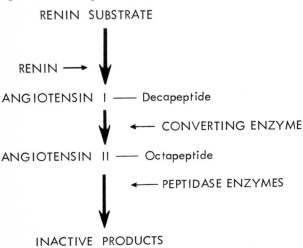

the usual forms of therapy. Easily controlled hypertension is not likely to have occlusive disease of the renal artery as its source. We always hold the child, the adolescent, the young female, and the atherosclerotic male in high suspicion of having occlusive disease of the renal artery when they present with hypertension.

Routine laboratory determinations are mentioned to emphasize the electrolyte derangement as outlined earlier, particularly in aldosterone-producing adenomas of the adrenal gland. An additional emphasis is important, as most hypertensive patients are treated with diuretics and electrolyte imbalance may be common.

Physical examination may or may not be helpful in making the diagnosis of renal artery occlusive disease. It certainly will delineate those patients with coarctation of the aorta as exemplified by reduced femoral pulses, and perhaps an attendant bruit over either the thoracic or abdominal aorta. Bruits over the kidney are common in patients with renovascular occlusive disease, but because of obesity they may be difficult to hear. It must be remembered that bruits may emanate from other vessels and may be confusing, particularly in the atherosclerotic patient. Auscultation of the back in the area of the costovertebral angle on occasion may be helpful in the delineation of a bruit. It is particularly noteworthy that in the atherosclerotic age group there may be other disease, especially of the subclavian vessels, that may not allow the diagnosis of hypertension to be made with one blood pressure determination. Blood pressure taken in both arms is mandatory whenever elevation of the blood pressure is suspected.

LABORATORY EVALUATION. The extent of laboratory evaluation of the hypertensive patient needed to make the diagnosis of renovascular occlusive disease is debated among the experts. There is no question but that in those clinics where an aggressive approach is taken, many more patients with renovascular occlusive disease are seen than in those where little attention is paid to extensive clinical and laboratory evaluation of the hypertensive patient.

Intravenous Pyelography. The intravenous pyelogram is not a good screening procedure for patients with suspected renovascular hypertension. It is least accurate in the child and most accurate in the atherosclerotic adult. There is a 75 percent false-negative rate in children and a 20 to 28 percent false-negative rate in the atherosclerotic adult. Classic findings upon intravenous pyelography—delayed opacification of the collecting system, reduction in size of the affected kidney, and ureteral notching—are the hallmarks of the radiologic diagnosis of renovascular occlusive disease as an etiologic factor in hypertension. We feel very strongly that intravenous pyelography should be done as a screening procedure on those patients suspected of having renovascular hypertension to make sure there are no intrinsic lesions in the kidney, such as ureteropelvic obstructive disease, neoplasm, pyelonephritis, cysts, or other parenchymal lesions associated with hypertension.

Renin Assays. Renin assay studies may be very helpful in the localization and delineation of severity of the renovascular occlusive disease. Before the advent of convert-

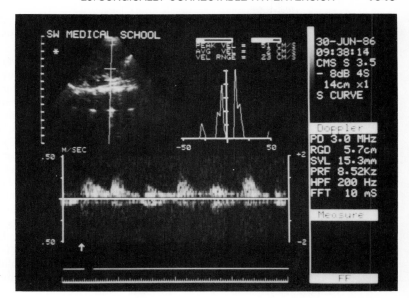

Fig. 23-9. B-mode ultrasonic/coupled Doppler wave-form of stenotic renal artery.

ing enzyme inhibitors (captopril, enalapril), the determination of peripheral venous renin and systemic renins are difficult. Blocking agents such as propranolol depress the output of renin, and to obtain accurate and meaningful renin determinations patients required cessation of medication and a strong natriuresis. This essentially eliminated many patients from study as the risk of hypertensive crisis with cessation of medication was high. It has been shown by several authors that the administration of a converting enzyme inhibitor produces an excess amount of renin in patients with occlusive renovascular disease. This is in spite of the fact that the patient may be on large doses of beta blocking agents such as propranolol. Preliminary work shows that peripheral renin determinations followed by the administration of 25 mg of captopril will produce a marked rise in systemic renin at 1 h. This has made elective renal vein renin determinations more accurate. They now may be done without cessation of therapy and reveal marked differences in the involved kidney vs. the normal kidney. In a study by Thibonnier, 19 patients were shown to have positive differential renin studies after the administration of captopril. All these patients were shown to have renal artery stenosis on arteriography and ultimately underwent successful renal revascularization. The utilization of renal systemic renin indices in conjunction with the captopril test is helpful. This test allows delineation of bilateral disease, comparing one kidney with the other, and demonstrating depression of renin production in the involved kidney. Use of converting enzyme inhibition in the determination of renal systemic index allows accurate prediction of success in operative therapy. The renal systemic renin index (RSRI) is outlined in the formula:

$$RSRI = \frac{\text{individual renal renin activity} - \text{systemic renin activity}}{\text{systemic renin activity}}$$

If the value of the affected kidney is >0.48 with the contralateral kidney ≤0.31, the chance for cure or improvement is high.

Noninvasive Techniques. The advent of the range-gated Doppler ultrasound has enabled accurate visualization and waveform analysis of the renal artery (Fig. 23-9). Strandness and his colleagues have demonstrated the applicability of this technique in the diagnosis of renovascular occlusive disease. These methods are very accurate and can show changes in the flow patterns in the main renal artery and in the kidney itself.

Arteriography. Arteriography remains the only accurate method of diagnosis of occlusive vascular disease involving the kidney. There is real hope that the computer-augmented venous arteriogram may be helpful, as it is much less invasive and may be performed on an outpatient basis. At the present time, 80 percent of the studies done utilizing this technique are accurate and helpful in the diagnosis of occlusive vascular disease of the kidney. Because of various problems with technique, 20 percent of the examinations are not of sufficient quality to make an accurate diagnosis. The drawbacks of digital venous arteriogram are (1) the inability to achieve multiple views of the renal artery, (2) overlap of the renal vessels by the mesenteric vasculature, and (3) poor definition of the intrarenal vessels. Because of these shortcomings, routine use of intravenous digital renal arteriography has been abandoned in our clinic. Use of the duplex scanning techniques coupled with the measurement of systemic renins with converting enzyme inhibition has obviated the need for an invasive screening technique.

The use of intraarterial digital arteriography is helpful because it allows use of small amounts of contrast material and does allow for multiple views of the renal artery. Small-vessel definition is inferior to standard angiography, but it is much better than that seen with the intravenous digital studies. It is also an exceedingly safe tech-

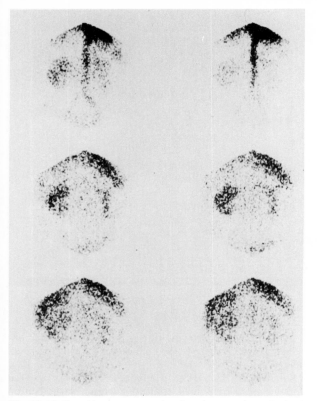

Fig. 23-10. Renal isotope scan showing decreased uptake in the left kidney.

nique, especially when it is combined with the new nonionic contrast material.

The intraarterial injection of contrast material and the selective renal artery injection of contrast material remain the mainstay of the diagnosis of renovascular occlusive disease. This allows for multiple projections to make sure that no lesion is left unrecognized. One may accurately measure the extent of the lesion and the reduction in cross-sectional area, and thus determine the significance of lesions encountered.

We have found that the visualization of collateral vessels around an occluding lesion is an important prognostic sign. This finding reinforces the significance given to an occluding lesion in the renal artery. We, along with others, have noted that there is a relative reduction in renin production as determined by renal vein renin sampling when there are multiple collaterals around a renal artery occluding lesion. It is important to remember this point, as it is one of the main associated factors in false-negative renin determinations.

Split-Renal Function Studies. These are utilized by a small number of clinics throughout the United States. The kidneys seldom vary significantly in their excretive ability to handle water, sodium, or creatinine. The functionally ischemic kidney conserves and reabsorbs sodium and water. This, then, shows a relative concentration of solutes such as creatinine.

These characteristics of the ischemic kidney have led to the description of several function tests that have been utilized in the diagnosis of renovascular hypertension. The Howard test measures urine volume and sodium concentration, as well as creatinine concentration. The involved kidney should have at least a 50 percent reduction in urine volume and 15 percent reduction in serum sodium concentration, with an attendant 15 percent increase in creatinine concentration over the so-called "normal" kidney. The Rappaport test utilizes the sodium-creatinine ratios from each kidney. The tubular rejection fraction ratio is obtained by multiplying the sodium-creatinine ratio on the left by that on the right. A ratio of less than 0.6 indicates significant left renal artery stenosis, and a ratio of more than 1.6 implicates the right renal artery. The test is felt to be negative when the values are between these two levels. The Stamey test utilizes osmotic diuresis or the intravenous infusion of urea. Para-aminohippurate, a solute excreted by the kidney but not reabsorbed by the tubules, is added to the infusion. The Stamey test is positive if there is a two-thirds reduction in urine volume and a 100 percent increase of para-aminohippurate concentration on the affected side. As a side benefit, the Stamey test also determines effective renal plasma flow in each kidney. This adds some credence to the test, as it delineates renal function.

Most clinics do not utilize renal function tests for several reasons. As can be appreciated, ureteral catheters must be placed in each ureter in order to allow individual collections. The introduction of infection and bleeding as a result of the trauma of the inlying catheters imputes a significant morbidity to these procedures. When this fact is combined with the fact that these tests are not as accurate as renal vein renin determinations, and are virtually useless in segmental renal artery lesions and in patients with bilateral disease, the importance of this series of tests is diminished.

Renal Scan. Radioisotope renal scanning allows surgeons to evaluate blood flow to the kidney (Fig. 23-10). Most renal scans depend on renal function. Information obtained by renal scans may be inaccurate if active parenchymal disease exists in conjunction with occlusive vascular disease. The ability to differentiate between primary renal artery occlusive disease and diffuse intraparenchymal disease on a renal scan is difficult. Because of these drawbacks the renal scan is used infrequently as a routine test in patients with renal artery occlusive disease.

Renal Biopsy. Percutaneous renal biopsy may be helpful, on occasion, in the preoperative evaluation of those patients demonstrating significant renal artery occlusive disease. The demonstration of an increased number of granules in the juxtaglomerular cells, with the maintenance of normal glomeruli, may be helpful in predicting the result with revascularization of the kidney. The morbidity associated with percutaneous renal biopsy in the form of bleeding and the production of arteriovenous fistulae has precluded it as a consistently useful modality in the preoperative evaluation of patients for renovascular reconstruction.

TREATMENT. The prognosis in operative therapy after the diagnosis is made depends upon the expertise of the surgeon, the durability of graft material used, and the extent of the secondary ravages of hypertension in the patient.

The refinement of vascular reconstructive techniques has contributed to more effective arterial reconstruction. The morbidity and mortality of the operative procedure are negligible. The utilization of autogenous tissue has assured accurate renal artery anastomoses. There is some excessive growth of scar tissue at the interface between Dacron prostheses and host artery, causing a higher incidence of late failure, but the Dacron prosthesis has proved to be a durable substance in the reconstruction of renal arteries in those adults with suitably sized vessels. PTFE prostheses are also suitable conduits for aortorenal bypass. Their drawback is the same as outlined for Dacron with the exception that these grafts tend to have a higher incidence of intimal proliferation at the graft artery interface. We believe that because of these drawbacks, aspirin therapy should be started the day before operation if one anticipates the use of Dacron or PTFE graft. This may prevent the deposition of platelets at the graft-artery interface, reducing the amount of platelet growth factor and its effect on intimal proliferation at this site. The use of aspirin in the postoperative period appears to be the most effective therapy at this time to reduce intimal proliferation and therefore the chance of recurrent stenosis.

The controversy over medical therapy versus operative therapy continues. Dean has demonstrated that renovascular lesions continue to progress even under optimal therapy, thus contributing to the potential loss of renal function. No accelerated atherosclerosis has been demonstrated in the renal architecture after successful renal artery revascularization. While the Mayo Clinic series was not done by the double-blind method, it would seem to indicate that medical therapy for patients with hypertension secondary to renal artery occlusive disease has a much higher mortality rate than does long-term follow-up of patients treated with operative therapy.

New drug therapy for renovascular hypertension is not without some drawbacks. The advent of the converting enzyme inhibitors such as captopril has brought hope that renovascular hypertension could be treated medically. This is possible in some patients, but there are problems with membranous glomerulopathy associated with long-term drug therapy. Proteinuria and, at times, irreversible renal damage may occur while taking this drug, making it hazardous without careful patient monitoring. In addition, a marked reduction in vascular outflow resistance at the arteriolar level within the kidney can cause stasis and thrombosis distal to a critical renal artery stenosis. This has been reported on many occasions, and we have seen five patients in whom this has occurred with an attendant marked reduction in renal function and mass.

There is no question that renal artery reconstruction in the child is a durable procedure that produces a positive effect, with blood pressure reduction over a long period of time. The same is true with the treatment of fibrodysplastic disease in the young female. There is some debate as to the routine recommendation of operative therapy for the atherosclerotic patient. It would appear that the patient with minimal generalized disease and focal extensive disease involving the ostia of the renal artery benefits most from revascularization of occluding lesions. In the patient with severe generalized atherosclerosis, as manifested by involvement of other organs such as heart and brain, the chance for salutary results is somewhat less; in this group of patients, operation should be reserved for those with uncontrollable hypertension and/or failing renal function secondary to progressive renal artery occlusive disease.

Preoperative Preparation. Past recommendations that most major antihypertensive drugs be stopped at varying times prior to operation are difficult to reconcile. There were isolated reports of death secondary to anesthesia superimposed on a patient taking propranolol. As we have reviewed these incidents, it becomes clear that all these patients were hypovolemic at the time of induction of anesthesia. There is no question but that the beta blockade incurred by the use of propranolol, combined with the alpha blockade induced by anesthesia superimposed on a hypovolemic patient, is dangerous. On the other hand, the authors have observed many problems with uncontrollable hypertension in the preoperative period after important drug therapy is stopped. This is particularly true of the patient with renovascular hypertension where control is often difficult and where sudden changes in blood pressure not only add an extra burden to the heart but place the patient in jeopardy for intracranial bleeding or acute renal failure.

With the recognition that most problems are secondary to hypovolemia and that the correction of this state is critical in the preoperative period, the authors have found it perfectly safe to continue all antihypertensive therapy in the preoperative and perioperative periods.

By definition, the average patient with hypertension is hypovolemic. When drug therapy utilizing a diuretic is superimposed upon this state, patients present themselves in need of volume replacement prior to operation. Cognizance of this fact in treating the young patient with an otherwise normal heart is important. Routinely, these patients are hydrated in the 18 to 24 h preoperatively, with particular attention being paid to potassium replacement. The hypokalemia exhibited by these patients is again usually secondary to the diuretic therapy. Great care must be taken when hydration is accomplished in these patients to prevent excessive elevation of blood pressure. It may be necessary on occasion to control blood pressure during this period of time with vasodilating drugs such as intravenous sodium nitroprusside.

The patient with myocardial disease poses a somewhat different problem than does the young patient with hypertension. Prolonged hypertension causing left ventricular hypertrophy and superimposed coronary artery occlusive disease requires careful monitoring prior to increasing the patient's total blood volume. This requires the placement of a Swan-Ganz catheter, with determination of the patient's cardiac output and total peripheral resistance, as well as of the pulmonary capillary wedge pressure. Most

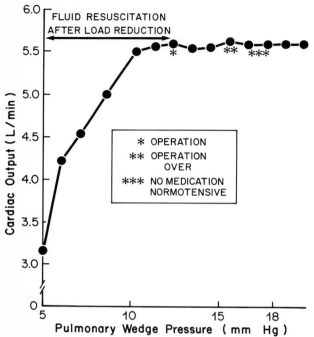

Fig. 23-11. Improvement in cardiac performance seen with volume loading and afterload reduction in a patient with renovascular hypertension.

patients will have a reduced cardiac output initially, and with the judicious use of fluid replacement and with reduction of the afterload, when appropriate, with a vasodilating drug such as nitroprusside, the optimal cardiac function can be achieved (Fig. 23-11).

It is important to point out that in those patients with severe myocardial disease, reducing the afterload may not be sufficient to achieve optimal cardiac function. It may be necessary to utilize digitalis therapy in order to optimize the patient's cardiac function. The utilization of this technique allows the establishment of a Starling function curve for each individual patient, giving the ability to determine the optimal amount of fluid needed to maintain this state. With the utilization of the Swan-Ganz catheter, the monitoring of the pulmonary capillary wedge pressure is possible in the operating room to maintain optimization of cardiac function. The authors have found this technique exceedingly helpful in the atherosclerotic patient and have been able to operate upon poor-risk patients without difficulty.

Recent data from our laboratory indicate a marked shift of blood flow away from the endocardial area of the left ventricle in the hypertensive patient. Judicial monitoring, fluid replacement, and the reduction of afterload have been shown experimentally to help optimize myocardial blood flow by stabilizing cardiac function. Intravenous nitroglycerin helps to stabilize myocardial blood flow. Low-dose nitroglycerin should always be used in conjunction with other vasodilators when unloading the heart. This may help to prevent a "steal" phenomenon from occurring that may further deprive the myocardium of adequate blood flow.

Operative Therapy. Several techniques for renal revascularization have been developed through the years. The bypass technique has achieved the greatest popularity because of the facility with which it can be done and the excellent long-term results. Endarterectomy, particularly championed by Wylie, has achieved some popularity. This outstanding technique unfortunately is not useful in patients with fibrodysplasia or in patients who have soft, ulcerating occlusive disease, as sometimes seen in association with aortic aneurysmal formation.

The authors have long favored the use of an autogenous saphenous vein sutured end-to-side to the aorta and end-to-end to the renal artery as the procedure of choice for arterial reconstruction of the renal artery. This technique allows for tailoring of the graft to the distal renal artery and is useful for revascularizing when several branches are involved. This procedure requires meticulous technique and careful exposure of the renal vasculature. It is felt very strongly that end-to-side distal bypass is inappropriate, as this forms two parallel conduits of blood flow. The host renal artery invariably thromboses, and upon occasion this thrombus will propagate over the anastomosis of the bypass graft, causing a secondary occlusion. We have seen several renal infarctions secondary to this process. The flow patterns of the end-to-end anastomosis and the facility that it allows in reimplantation of various branches make end-to-end anastomosis the preferred technique.

The exposure is best accomplished through a long, transverse, upper abdominal incision. This allows elevation of the colon and duodenum on the right and of the colon, spleen, pancreas, and stomach on the left, affording extensive exposure of the entire kidney and its vasculature, as well as of the aorta (Figs. 23-2 and 23-3). With the dislocation of the bowel out of the abdominal cavity, there is no restriction in the operative exposure of these areas. It allows for careful dissection of the entire renal vasculature when necessary, including the second and third branchings of the renal artery. Since exposure and control are the sine qua non of this operation, the technique cannot be overemphasized. The approach through the midline, elevating the pancreas and duodenum off the aorta, is unnecessarily restrictive to the operative therapy of these patients.

Following adequate exposure of the renal artery and its branches, the lateral side of the aorta is dissected free so that a partially occluding clamp can be applied. If the aorta is not suitable, either the hepatic or splenic arteries may be used as inflow sources. The vein graft is sutured to the side of the aorta after it is widely spatulated (Fig. 23-12). On the right side the graft can be placed either posterior or anterior to the cava. The authors generally prefer retrocaval placement of the graft as it seems to lie better in this position than it does anterior to the cava. The patient is then totally heparinized (150 units/kg of body weight), and the proximal renal artery is clamped and divided. A small Heifitz clip is placed on the distal renal artery to prevent backbleeding. The proximal renal artery is ligated. Attention is then directed to the distal renal artery, which is spatulated widely so that the vein graft can be sutured end-to-end with an eccentric anasto-

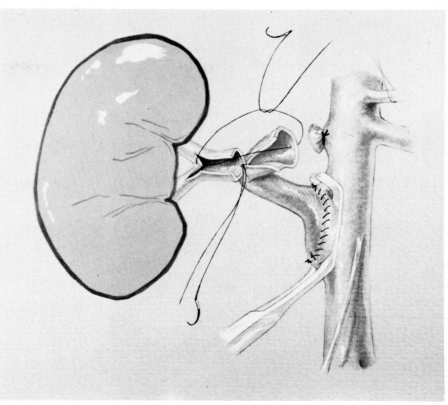

Fig. 23-12. Aortorenal bypass illustrating anastomotic technique.

mosis measuring approximately three times greater in diameter than the vessel itself. The authors have found that this prevents postoperative stenosis at the suture line, as it allows for any cicatrix formation to occur without compromising the lumen of the vessel. Utilizing this technique, early and late suture line strictures have not been a problem. Following the completion of the anastomosis, as illustrated in Fig. 23-13, the distal clamp on the renal artery is removed, the heparin is reversed, and the partially occluding clamp on the aorta is slowly released. Great attention must be paid to hemostasis, as invariably there are small collaterals that will be interrupted in the dissection of the renal artery which may bleed in the postoperative period. Any question arising in the arterial reconstruction must be clarified by a completion arteriogram. This can easily be done on the operating table by gently occluding the graft and injecting a small amount of contrast material to demonstrate the distal anastomosis.

Occasionally, there are patients for whom, because the saphenous vein is not available or because of the size of the renal artery, Dacron prosthetic material may be chosen as a conduit. Generally, we have reserved this material for patients in the atherosclerotic age group and have utilized the same technique as outlined with the vein graft. It must be pointed out that the prosthetic graft should be carefully covered with retroperitoneal tissue interposed between the prosthesis and the duodenum in order to ensure that an aortoduodenal fistula does not occur. There have been several reports in the literature of

this happening as a sequela of this operative procedure. The Dacron prosthesis is generally more difficult to tailor to the distal anastomosis and should be reserved for renal arteries which are 5 mm in diameter or larger. The authors have not used the PTFE grafts for aortorenal bypass, and generally do not recommend their use because of the high incidence of early thrombosis and intimal hyperplasia at the suture line between the host and prosthetic material.

Wylie et al. have championed the use of autologous arterial grafts, particularly in children. They utilize the internal iliac artery. This is a very suitable graft that is generally readily accessible; however, several things must be kept in mind if it is to be used routinely. In fibrodysplastic disease, particularly in children, it is not uncommon to have generalized involvement, including the internal iliac artery. Utilizing both internal iliac arteries would not seem prudent, particularly in the male. Wylie et al. have recommended utilization of the common iliac artery with its bifurcation into the internal and external iliac artery as a method of revascularizing both renal arteries at the same time. They have utilized a plastic prosthesis to replace the common iliac–external iliac arterial system. This has some drawbacks in that the prosthetic material may become inadequate for supply to the lower extremity as the child grows, and a chance for prosthetic infection is always present.

The only instances of significant vein graft dilatation have occurred when the saphenous vein has been used in

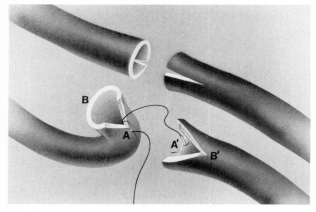

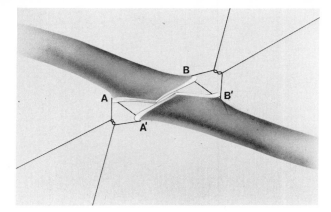

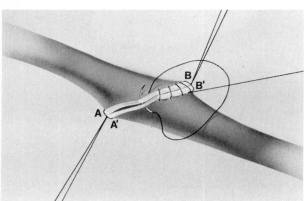

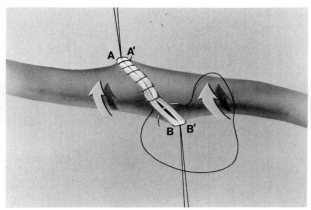

Fig. 23-13. End-to-end spatulated arterial anastomosis using two-point transfixion.

children. Dilatation is seen in approximately 15 percent of the cases. It has not required graft excision; however, these patients must be watched closely. There is some indication that the harvesting and care of the vein are partially responsible for degeneration, but this is not completely substantiated. Because of the incidence of aneurysmal dilation in the autogenous saphenous vein used in children, we would recommend the use of autologous artery whenever possible. Since there have been no aneurysmal changes in vein grafts used in adult patients, we feel that autogenous saphenous vein is the preferable conduit to use in renal arterial reconstruction. Whenever possible the saphenous vein should be harvested at the ankle. This has two advantages. The veins appear thicker; we have seen little in the way of aneurysmal dilatation in veins harvested from this area. In most instances harvesting the vein at the ankle preserves the rest of the saphenous vein for future need.

Transaortic endarterectomy in atheromatous occlusive disease of the renal artery has proved to be a good technique for disobliteration in certain select patients with renal artery occlusive disease. As mentioned before, patients with a soft, ragged aortic intima do not lend themselves well to endarterectomy. This technique is particularly useful in patients who have multiple renal arteries affected by atherosclerosis, allowing a one-stage operative procedure with a relatively short clamp time. Figure

23-14 illustrates five partially occluded renal arteries. Exposure of the aorta is carried out utilizing the same technique as previously described for exposure of the left renal artery. By extending the dissection, the entire abdominal aorta with all its branches may be exposed. Following exposure of the entire upper abdominal aorta, the patient is heparinized, and a clamp is applied to the supraceliac aorta. Following this, the aorta is opened through the midline between the renal arteries, and the incision is carried off to the left superior mesenteric artery (Fig. 23-15).

It is important to note that the renal arteries must be dissected free on both sides prior to opening the aorta. The endarterectomy of the aorta is started superiorly and carried distally to the point of the renal artery ostia. At this point the assistant gently inverts the renal artery so that the entire plaque can be removed; by this technique one can see whether there is feathering of the plaque so that there is no question of a distal intimal flap. Following the removal of the atheromatous material from the aorta and the renal arteries, the endarterectomy is terminated below the renal arteries; the flap may be tacked at this point if necessary (Fig. 23-16). The aortotomy is then closed utilizing a running arterial suture. The clamps are slowly removed, allowing blood flow in the aorta and the

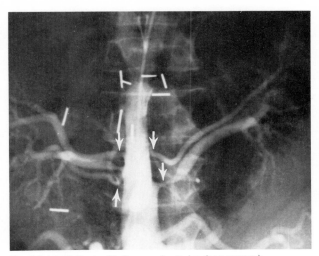

Fig. 23-14. Patient with five renal arteries (see arrows).

visceral and renal arteries. At the completion of the procedure an arteriogram must be done in order to determine good flow to both renal arteries and to rule out any chance for an intimal flap. This is best done by reapplying the clamps and injecting a small amount of contrast material into the aorta in order to visualize both renal arteries. If a small intimal flap is evident it can be dealt with by a separate arteriotomy in the renal artery with or without the utilization of a venous patch graft. When the operative ultrasound is available, it may obviate the need for postoperative angiogram. It has been shown to be exceedingly accurate and when it becomes generally available may replace the need for angiography. Utilizing this technique, Wylie and associates have reported excellent results, substantiated in a limited series by the authors.

The technique of ex vivo repair of renal artery lesions has been championed by Belzer. His reports indicate that, in certain well-selected cases, this technique is very helpful. It should be reserved for lesions that involve mul-

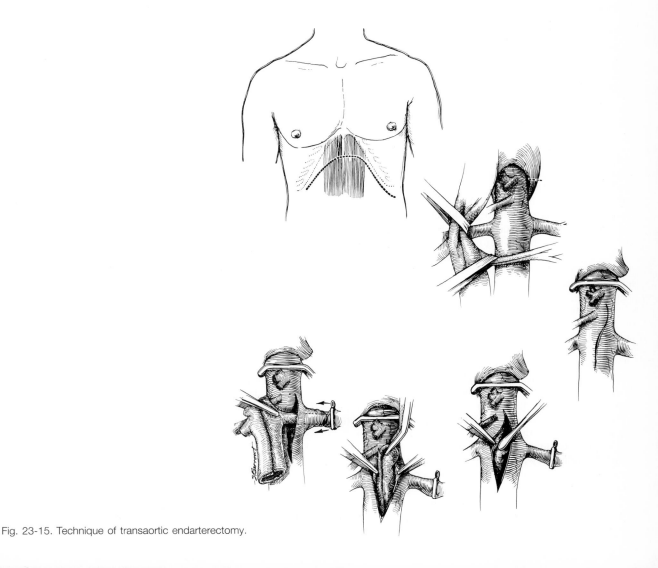

Fig. 23-15. Technique of transaortic endarterectomy.

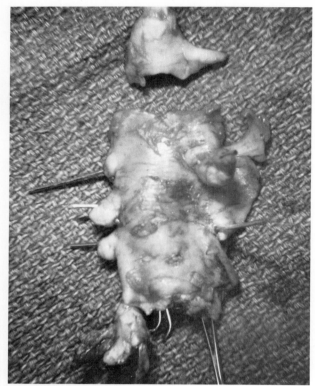

Fig. 23-16. Endarterectomy specimen of lesion seen in Fig. 23-14. Probes are in the renal artery orifices.

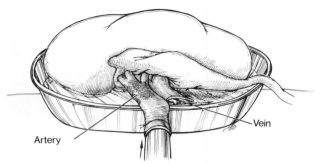

Fig. 23-17. Kidney prepared for ex vivo repair.

tiple branches such as fibrodysplastic disease; aneurysm where multiple branches are involved; renal artery dissections; or those lesions, previously revascularized, with problems such as secondary stenosis. Reoperation on the renal artery is particularly difficult as the renal vein invariably becomes adherent to the renal artery, and it is difficult to dissect free without a great deal of blood loss. The ability to take the kidney out of the abdomen and perfuse it in a bloodless field allows an accurate, safe technique for renal revascularization in the difficult lesion.

The kidney is removed from the abdomen by dividing the renal artery and vein; the renal artery is then perfused with cold Locke's solution at 4°C. This washes all the blood from the renal vasculature and cools the kidney. It allows the surgeon adequate time to carefully dissect out the renal vasculature. Repair can then be instituted (Fig. 23-17). Multiple renal artery lesions can be repaired by utilizing the internal iliac artery or by fashioning multiple branches off an autogenous saphenous vein. Following the completion of the multiple distal anastomoses, the kidney may be implanted back into the original bed or may be moved down into the pelvis, anastomosing the renal artery to the internal iliac artery and renal vein to the iliac vein, a technique similar to that of a renal transplant. If great care is taken in dissecting out the ureter to preserve its blood supply, it is not necessary to reimplant the ureter. We routinely leave the ureter intact and, in

most instances, have reanastomosed the renal vein and utilized the graft, either autogenous saphenous vein or internal iliac graft anastomosis to the side of the aorta. This is feasible and seems to cut down the number of anastomoses and any potential problems with a pelvic kidney.

The problems attendant on the use of this technique are important to recognize. Removal of the kidney from the abdomen completely interrupts all arterial collaterals. Therefore, it is incumbent upon the surgeon to make sure that the anastomoses are technically perfect and that blood flow is reestablished to the kidney at the time of reimplantation. This is best done with a completion arteriogram. If the kidney is placed back in its original bed, it is important to fix it to Gerota's fascia so that it will not rotate on its axis and cause kinking of the renal artery bypass graft.

Belzer has reported outstanding results with this technique; when it is used for the indications outlined, it extends the ability of the vascular surgeon to salvage kidneys with extensive renovascular disease.

Nephrectomy. Nephrectomy is seldom indicated in the treatment of renovascular hypertension because the goal is to preserve renal mass whenever possible. The removal of thrombus from a renal artery where there has been an extensive infarction is contraindicated. This requires a nephrectomy, as the chance for reestablishing significant renal function is negligible (Fig. 23-18*A*, *B*, *C*). Multiple areas of infarction secondary to emboli from a renal artery aneurysm, or from ulcerative aortic disease, are best treated by a nephrectomy unless the contralateral kidney is severely diseased. Severe intraparenchymal occlusive disease, of either an atherosclerotic or a fibrodysplastic nature, does not lend itself to revascularization and is best treated by nephrectomy. This assumes a relatively normal contralateral kidney.

RESULTS. The effectiveness of operative therapy for renal artery occlusive disease is determined by reduction of blood pressure over a long period of time. Over 50 patients in the pediatric age group have been followed by the authors. It has been particularly gratifying to see this group of patients maintain normal pressures through follow-up as long as 18 years. In this series of patients, 85 percent have been cured and are off all medication. Twelve percent are improved, requiring only minimal medication in the form of a diuretic to maintain normal

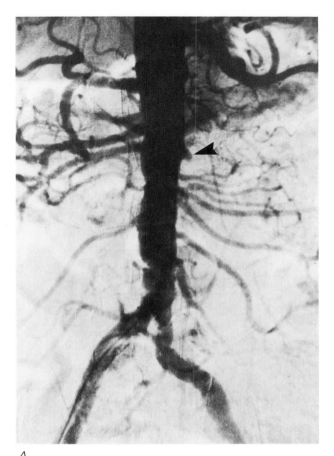

A

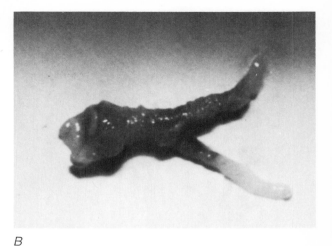

B

C

Fig. 23-18. *A.* Flush aortogram showing occluded left renal artery with distal vessel reconstitution (arrow). *B.* Extensive thrombus taken from the occluded renal artery seen in the previous arteriogram. *C.* Isotope washout curve of left kidney (bottom curve), showing minimal function after technically successful revascularization.

blood pressure. Of the entire group of children treated, only one patient has had no salutary result from the operative procedure. The latter patient has a diffuse vasculitis involving both renal arteries and the interrenal branches.

Fibrodysplastic disease in the adult, primarily in female patients, has been followed in a series of 144 patients for a minimum of 5 years to a maximum of 21 years. A sustained 55 percent cure rate and a 39 percent improved rate have been noted, giving a total of 94 percent positive results with only a 6 percent failure rate.

Atherosclerosis as a cause of renovascular occlusive disease is difficult to categorize. It is best categorized as *focal* and *diffuse* disease. Focal disease does not have any associated atherosclerotic or aneurysmal involvement of the cerebral, coronary, visceral, or lower extremity vessels. In this group of patients, followed for a minimum of 5 years, the long-term records reveal 91 percent good results with only 9 percent failure. This group generally does well, with a 12 percent attrition rate, secondary to

other manifestations of atherosclerosis, over a 5-year period.

Generalized atherosclerosis with overt generalized disease has been a problem in both medical and surgical therapy. The authors have examined a series of 58 patients who fall into this category and were operated upon for renal revascularization. The results were outstanding, with a cure or improved rate of 93 percent. There is a consistent 15 percent renal function improvement rate in this series of patients. The long-term mortality rate of this group is higher than that of any other group because of established generalized atherosclerotic disease. The most common cause of demise is myocardial infarction. In view of these results, the authors have taken a more liberal attitude in recommending operative therapy in this group of patients. Concomitant operative procedures significantly increase the operative mortality of these patients. When aortic grafting for aneurysmal or occlusive disease is performed concomitantly with renal revascularization, great care must be taken in assessing the myocardial reserve of the patient. Extreme care must be taken in monitoring and maintaining optimal cardiac function in the preoperative, perioperative, and postoperative periods.

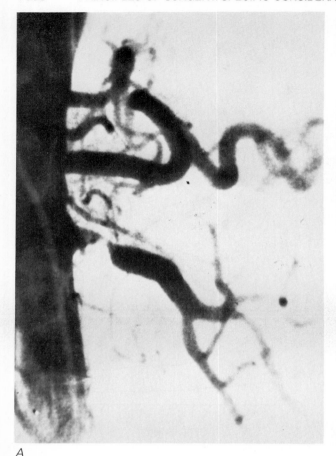

A

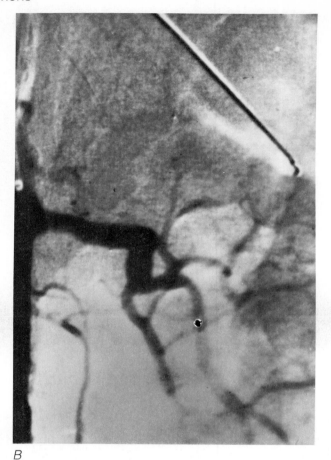

B

Fig. 23-19. *A.* Stenotic atherosclerotic renal artery lesion before balloon angioplasty. *B.* After the procedure.

The utilization of long-term medical therapy for the patient with overt renovascular occlusive disease carries a relatively high mortality, as reported by several authors. Dean has reported a rather alarming progression of atherosclerotic occlusive disease in the renal arteries in those patients treated with a careful medical program. It would seem that this form of therapy is not as good an alternative as arterial reconstruction.

The use of balloon angioplasty to dilate lesions of the renal artery has achieved great popularity (Fig. 23-19*A*, *B*). The longest mean follow-up is approaching 2 years. The cure or improvement rate is generally between 10 and 15 percent lower than that achieved by careful surgical repair. Although the technique has the attractive features of a less invasive procedure and a shorter hospital stay, complications occur. A 5 to 10 percent morbidity rate has been reported, including perforation of the renal artery (Fig. 23-20), thrombosis of the renal artery, distal embolization, disruption of aortic or renal artery atheromata, inability to pass the guidewire through the stenosing lesion, femoral artery thrombosis, and hematoma. It would seem currently that this is an alternative that may supplant surgical therapy in selected fibromuscular or atheromatous lesions involving the midrenal artery. Ostial atheromas and complex fibromuscular lesions are often not suitable for balloon angioplasty.

Bibliography

Endocrine Disease and Hypertension

Bravo EL, Gifford RW: Pheochromocytoma: Diagnosis, localization and management. *N Engl J Med* 311:1298, 1984.

Carpenter PC: Cushing's syndrome: Update of diagnosis and management. *Mayo Clin Proc* 61:49, 1986.

Guerin CK, Wahner HW, et al: Computed tomographic scanning vs. radioisotope imaging in adrenocortical diagnosis. *Am J Med* 75:653, 1983.

Mackett MCT, Crane MG, Smith LL: Surgical treatment of aldosterone-producing adrenal adenomas: A review of 16 patients. *Am J Surg* 142:89, 1981.

Schteingart DE, Motazedi A, et al: Treatment of adrenal carcinomas. *Arch Surg* 117:1142, 1982.

Sisson JC, Shapiro B, et al: Locating pheochromocytomas by scintigraphy using ^{131}I-metaiodobenzylguanidine. *Ca-A* 34:86, 1984.

vanHeerden JA, Scheps SG, et al: Pheochromocytoma: Current status and changing trends. *Surgery* 91:367, 1982.

Coarctation of the Aorta

Dean RH, Scott HW: Subisthmic aortic coarctations, in Dean RH, O'Neill JA (eds): *Vascular Disorders of Childhood.* Philadelphia, Lea & Febiger, 1983.

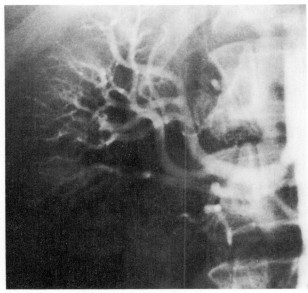

A

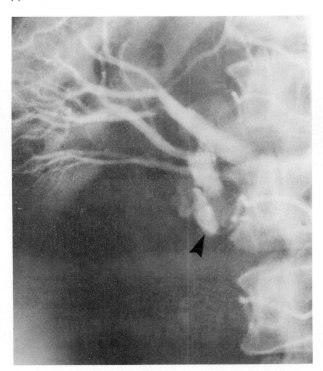

B

Fig. 23-20. *A.* Arteriogram of right renal artery stenosis at ostium. *B.* Perforation of right renal artery after attempted balloon angioplasty (extravasation at arrow).

Marol BJ, Humphries JO, et al: Prognosis of surgically corrected coarctation of the aorta. A twenty-year post-operative appraisal. *Circulation* 47:119, 1973.

Petracek MR, Hammon JW: Thoracic-aortic (isthmic) coarctation, in Dean RH, O'Neill JA (eds): *Vascular Disorders of Childhood.* Philadelphia, Lea & Febiger, 1983.

Schumacker HB Jr, King H, et al: Coarctation of the aorta. *Curr Probl Surg* February 1968.

Renovascular Hypertension

Cohn JN, Franciosa JA: Vasodilator therapy of cardiac failure, part I. *N Engl J Med* 297:27, 1977.

Cohn JN, Franciosa JA: Vasodilator therapy of cardiac failure, part II. *N Engl J Med* 297:254, 1977.

Dean RH, Kiefer RW, et al: Renovascular hypertension: Anatomic and renal function changes during drug therapy. *Arch Surg* 16:1408, 1981.

Dean RH, Krueger TC, et al: Operative management of renovascular hypertension. Results after followup of 15–23 years. *J Vasc Surg* 1:234, 1984.

Dean RH, Lawson JD, et al: Revascularization of the poorly functioning kidney. *Surgery* 85:44, 1979.

Kohler TR, Zierler RE, et al: Noninvasive diagnosis of renal artery stenosis by ultrasonic duplex scanning. *J Vasc Surg* 4:450, 1986.

Kuhlmann U, Greminger P, et al: Long-term experience and percutaneous transluminal dilatation of renal artery stenosis. *Am J Med* 79:692, 1985.

Moncure AC, Brewster DC, Darling RC: Use of splenic and hepatic arteries for renal revascularization. *J Vasc Surg* 3:196, 1986.

Pickering TG, Sos TA, Laragh JH: The role of balloon dilatation in the treatment of renovascular hypertension. *Am J Med* 77 (suppl):61, 1984.

Stanley JC, Ernest CB, Fry WJ: *Renovascular Hypertension.* New York, Saunders, 1984.

Stanley JC, Fry WJ: Pediatric renal artery occlusive disease and renovascular hypertension: Etiology, diagnosis and operative treatment. *Arch Surg* 116:669, 1981.

Stanley JC, Rhodes EL, et al: Renal artery aneurysms: Significance of macroaneurysms exclusive of dissections and fibrodysplastic mural dilations. *Arch Surg* 110:1327, 1975.

Stanley JC, Whitehouse WM, et al: Reoperation for complications of renal artery reconstructive surgery undertaken for treatment of renovascular hypertension. *J Vasc Surg* 2:133, 1985.

Stoney RJ, DeLuccia N, et al: Aorto-renal arterial autografts. Long-term assessment. *Arch Surg* 116:416, 1981.

Stoney RJ, Silane M, Salvatierra O: Ex vivo renal artery reconstruction. *Arch Surg* 113:1272, 1978.

Stuart MT, Smith RB, et al: Concomitant renal revascularization of patients undergoing aortic surgery. *J Vasc Surg* 2:400, 1985.

Textor SC, Gephardt GN, et al: Membranous glomerulopathy associated with captopril therapy. *Am J Med* 74:705, 1983.

Textor SC, Tarazir C, et al: Regulation of renal hemodynamics and glomerular filtration of patients with renovascular hypertension during converting enzyme inhibition with captopril. *Am J Med* 76 (suppl):29, 1984.

Thibonnier M, Joseph A, et al: Improved diagnosis of unilateral renal artery lesions after captopril administration. *JAMA* 251:56, 1984.

Ying CY, Tifft CP, et al: Renal revascularization in the azotemic hypertensive patient resistant to therapy. *N Engl J Med* 311:1070, 1984.

Chapter 24

Manifestations of Gastrointestinal Disease

Seymour I. Schwartz

Symptoms represent subjective manifestations of disturbance in function and are not specific for a disease but rather for a pathophysiologic state. In the gastrointestinal tract, the following changes in physiologic function may be implicated: altered secretion, altered motility, inadequate digestion, inadequate absorption, obstruction. The resultant symptoms of gastrointestinal disease include abdominal pain, dysphagia, anorexia, nausea and vomiting, bloating or distention, constipation, and diarrhea.

Signs of gastrointestinal disease are objective demonstrations of a pathologic process. These include tenderness, abdominal wall rigidity, palpable masses, altered bowel sounds, evidence of gastrointestinal bleeding, poor nutrition, jaundice, and stigmata of hepatic dysfunction.

PAIN

Pain (from the Latin *poena,* penalty, punishment, torment) is the predominant sensory experience by which humans judge the existence of disease within themselves. Most diseases of the abdominal viscera are associated with pain at some time during their course. Indeed, the correct diagnosis of acute abdominal disorders (the "acute abdomen") usually amounts to the correct identification of the cause of the abdominal pain.

Although there is not yet unequivocal proof that each peripheral nerve fiber is devoted to but one type of sensory modality—pain, touch, cold, or warmth—most physiologists now subscribe to the *specificity theory,* which holds that pain is a separate sensory modality with its own specific neural apparatus. In 1965 Melzack and Wall proposed the *gate-control theory.* They disagreed with the proposal that sensation is achieved by a fixed direct-line communication from skin to brain. Their contribution was the suggestion that the amount and quality of perceived pain are determined by many physiologic and psychologic variables. Modulation of nociceptive impulses occurs at the dorsal horn and at various levels of the ascending afferent systems. The gate-control theory has been the basis for methods of pain-inhibiting electrical stimulation. With transcutaneous nerve stimulation (TNS), electrodes are placed on the surface overlying the painful area, and nonpain fibers are activated.

Appropriate stimuli initiate impulses in skin, muscle, or viscera. These sensory impulses are transmitted to the posterior horn of the spinal cord in the primary sensory neuron that has its cell body in the dorsal root ganglion. The secondary sensory neuron in the posterior horn transmits the impulses in the contralateral spinothalamic tract to the posterolateral nucleus of the thalamus. The

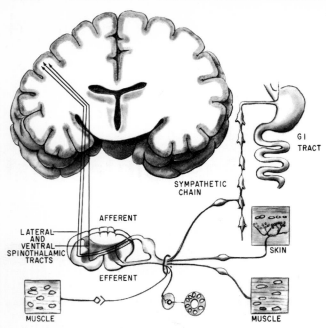

Fig. 24-1. Schematic representation of pathways involved in abdominal pain.

tertiary sensory neuron transmits the impulses from the thalamus to the postcentral gyrus of the cerebral cortex (Fig. 24-1).

Three kinds of pain have been designated: superficial, or cutaneous pain; deep pain from muscles, tendons, joints, and fascia; and visceral pain. The first two may be combined as somatic pain. Knowledge of visceral pain has lagged, in part because of the difficulty of the laboratory investigation.

PAIN PATHWAYS. Until well into the twentieth century, the viscera were thought to be completely insensitive. The first important observer of visceral sensation was William Harvey in the seventeenth century. When the young son of Count Montgomery sustained a chest wound which on healing left the heart exposed, Harvey observed that touching the heart caused not the slightest sensation. After the discovery of local anesthesia, Lennander found that human abdominal viscera are insensitive to cutting, crushing, and even burning. He categorically stated in 1901 that the viscera are wholly insensitive and that only traction or irritation of the parietal peritoneum could cause abdominal pain. The record was set straight in 1911 by Hurst, who demonstrated that distention of any hollow viscus is painful. Ryle amplified this by emphasizing that contraction of smooth muscle of hollow viscera is a physiologic stimulus adequate to cause pain.

The current and preferable terminology uses the term *visceral afferents* to denote all afferent fibers from the viscera including those that give rise to visceral reflexes as well as those that subserve pain. The terms *autonomic, sympathetic,* and *parasympathetic* are reserved for the visceral *efferent* fibers.

Pain impulses from the abdominal cavity reach the central nervous system by three routes: from the viscera via visceral afferents that travel with (1) the sympathetic and (2) the parasympathetic nerves, and from the parietal peritoneum, body wall, diaphragm, and root of mesenteries via somatic afferents that travel in (3) the segmental spinal nerves or phrenic nerves. Primary sensory neurons for pain, both visceral and somatic, are mostly small (1 to 2 μm), unmyelinated fibers but with some small (3 to 4 μm), myelinated fibers (Gasser classes C and A delta, or groups IV and III in Lloyd's terminology).

The route of a typical afferent from an abdominal viscus is as follows: the axons of nerve endings in the wall of the viscus follow the artery to the aorta and then through the collateral sympathetic ganglion without synapsing. They then enter the splanchnic nerve, traverse the paravertebral sympathetic ganglion, again without synapsing, and join the spinal nerve via the white ramus communicans. The cell body of this primary visceral afferent neuron is located in the spinal ganglion from which central processes are sent to the dorsal horn of the spinal cord via the dorsal root.

The central processes of the primary sensory neuron synapse with at least three distinct spinal tracts: (1) secondary pain neurons whose axons ascend for two or three segments and then cross in the anterior commissure to the anterolateral spinothalamic tract, (2) secondary sensory neurons whose processes ascend the posterior columns, and (3) many small neurons in the substantia gelatinosa that contribute to the tract of Lissauer. As the secondary sensory neurons ascend, collaterals are given off to the reticular substance forming the core of the brainstem and to the hypothalamus. The role of these extraspinothalamic pathways is uncertain—they may be alternative pain pathways, may inhibit central pain responses, or may be involved in the affective aspects of pain. Sensory tracts synapse in the thalamus with tertiary neurons that project to the cortex. The cortical areas involved with pain are not completely known. Stimulation of various areas of the postcentral gyrus in the conscious human being produces contralateral paresthesia of small areas of the body, but even total hemispherectomy does not consistently abolish pain, though localization is defective. The functions of the thalamus in human beings, in contrast to animals, are largely expressed through the cortex. But one function that may have been retained in the evolutionary process is the expression of the affective aspects of sensation. Affectivity—pleasantness and unpleasantness—is considered a primitive function that has remained at the thalamic level despite development of the cerebral cortex.

Though the thalamus and frontal cortex are the principal areas of the brain involved with pain, they cannot be considered as *the* brain centers, since the hypothalamus, the limbic system, the brainstem reticular formation, and the parietal cortex are also involved in pain reception. Opiate receptors exist in the brainstem and spinal cord, and naturally occurring opiates are found in the brain and pituitary. These are collectively called *endorphins.* Pain relief from low-frequency electrical stimulation exerts its effect by increasing these endorphin levels, an effect that can be blocked by the opiate antagonist, naloxone.

Abdominal Pain

PATHOPHYSIOLOGY

Three distinct types of pain are involved in the general symptom complex of abdominal pain: visceral pain, (deep) somatic pain, and referred pain.

VISCERAL PAIN. True visceral pain, or splanchnic pain, arises in abdominal organs invested with visceral peritoneum via impulses conducted to the spinal cord over visceral afferent nerve fibers. As noted above, the viscera are normally insensitive to stimuli that produce pain when applied to the skin. Adequate stimuli for visceral pain are those arising from their own environment—pathologic conditions of the viscera. Stimuli that produce pain include increased tension in the wall of hollow viscera from either distention or spastic contraction, stretching of the capsules of solid viscera, ischemia, and certain chemicals. The threshold for pain is lowered by inflammation and by ischemia, so that normal muscular contractions that would ordinarily not be felt may produce pain.

The role of chemical substances in visceral pain is not clear. Experimentally, pain can be produced by the intra-arterial injection of acid, alkaline, or hypertonic solutions: lactate, potassium ions, or bradykinin. Potassium that is released from cells by injury or ischemia has long been known as a pain-producing agent, and it has been suggested that the release of intracellular potassium ions may be the actual physiologic stimulus for pain. Some pain receptors have been classified as chemoceptors, and the pain of ischemia has been attributed to increasing concentrations of hydrogen ions. The pain of inflammation is thought to be caused by the accrual of algesic bradykinin peptides that activate pain receptors more or less selectively. The bradykinin effect is facilitated in the presence of prostaglandins, and it is this mechanism that is inhibited by aspirin.

Visceral pain tends to be rather diffuse and poorly localized, has a high threshold, and exhibits an exceedingly slow rate of adaptation. The high threshold and poor localization are probably in part attributable to the relatively sparse distribution of sensory endings in the viscera. The pain is felt by the patient to be "deep" in those cutaneous areas or zones that correspond roughly to the segmental distribution of somatic sensory fibers that take origin from the same segments of the cord as the visceral afferent fibers from the viscus in question.

With severe visceral or deep somatic pain, concomitant responses, presumably due to autonomic reflexes, may be prominent. These include sweating; nausea, sometimes with vomiting; tachycardia or bradycardia; fall in blood pressure; cutaneous hyperalgesia, hyperesthesia, or tenderness; and involuntary spastic contractions of abdominal wall musculature. The muscular rigidity accompanying severe pain is most marked when the body wall is involved by the pain-inciting lesion, e.g., the boardlike rigidity associated with perforated peptic ulcer. The distribution is regional rather than segmental and thus involves sustained reflexes in several segmental nerves. Maintained muscular rigidity may of itself become painful, so that on occasion the deep muscular tenderness outlasts and outweighs the original visceral pain.

SOMATIC PAIN. Pain arising in the abdominal wall, particularly the parietal peritoneum, root of the mesenteries, and respiratory diaphragm, is mediated by somatic afferents in segmental spinal nerves. Pain from parietal structures is for the most part sharper and brighter than visceral pain; it is well localized close to the site of stimulation; and when the source is on one side of the midline, the pain is also lateralized. Acute appendicitis is a common visceral disease that well illustrates typical visceral and somatic abdominal pain. The visceral pain of early appendicitis is perceived diffusely and dully in the periumbilical and lower epigastric regions, and there is little or no rigidity of the abdominal musculature. Later, when parietal peritoneum becomes involved in the inflammatory process, the somatic component of pain is more severe and sharply localized in the right lower quadrant. There is also cutaneous hyperesthesia, tenderness, and muscular rigidity in the right lower quadrant.

REFERRED PAIN. Visceral disease may give rise to pain localized to more superficial areas of the body, often at a considerable distance from the diseased viscus. The reference is usually dermatomic, but on occasion pain may be referred to the scar of a previous surgical operation, trauma, or localized pathologic process. This is called *habit reference* and implies that pain perception is influenced by the individual's prior pain experience.

The currently accepted reasoning for the dermatomic reference of visceral pain is the *convergence-projection* hypothesis. Since the pain fibers in the posterior roots greatly outnumber the fibers in the spinothalamic tracts, several pain fibers must converge on one tract fiber. This same convergence may occur at thalmaic or cortical levels as well. When afferents from the skin and viscera converge on the same neuron at some point in the pain pathway, the resulting impulses, on projection to the brain, are interpreted as coming from the skin, an interpretation learned from previous experiences in which the same tract fiber was stimulated by cutaneous afferents.

CLINICAL CONSIDERATIONS

ETIOLOGY. Abdominal pain may be caused by a great variety of gastrointestinal and intraperitoneal diseases, and, because of overlapping nerve distribution, the pain may be secondary to extraperitoneal disorders. Pain of intraabdominal origin (Table 24-1) may emanate from the peritoneum, hollow intestinal viscera, solid viscera, mesentery, or pelvic organs and may be caused by inflammation, mechanical processes such as obstruction or acute distention, and vascular disturbances.

The extraperitoneal causes of abdominal pain are outlined in Table 24-2. Most of the intrathoracic diseases that

Table 24-1. GASTROINTESTINAL AND INTRAPERITONEAL CAUSES OF ABDOMINAL PAIN

I. Inflammation
  A. Peritoneum
    1. Chemical and nonbacterial peritonitis—perforated peptic ulcer, gallbladder, ruptured ovarian cyst, mittelschmerz
    2. Bacterial peritonitis
      a. Primary peritonitis—pneumococcal, streptococcal, tuberculous
      b. Perforated hollow viscus—stomach, intestine, biliary tract
  B. Hollow intestinal organs
    1. Appendicitis
    2. Cholecystitis
    3. Peptic ulceration
    4. Gastroenteritis
    5. Regional enteritis
    6. Meckel's diverticulitis
    7. Colitis—ulcerative, bacterial, amebic
    8. Diverticulitis
  C. Solid viscera
    1. Pancreatitis
    2. Hepatitis
    3. Hepatic abscess
    4. Splenic abscess
  D. Mesentery
    1. Lymphadenitis
  E. Pelvic organs
    1. Pelvic inflammatory disease
    2. Tuboovarian abscess
    3. Endometritis

II. Mechanical (obstruction, acute distention)
  A. Hollow intestinal organs
    1. Intestinal obstruction—adhesions, hernia, tumor, volvulus, intussusception
    2. Biliary obstruction—calculi, tumor, choledochal cyst, hematobilia
  B. Solid viscera
    1. Acute splenomegaly
    2. Acute hepatomegaly—cardiac failure, Budd-Chiari syndrome
  C. Mesentery
    1. Omental torsion
  D. Pelvic organs
    1. Ovarian cyst
    2. Torsion or degeneration of fibroid
    3. Ectopic pregnancy
III. Vascular
  A. Intraperitoneal bleeding
    1. Ruptured liver
    2. Ruptured spleen
    3. Ruptured mesentery
    4. Ruptured ectopic pregnancy
    5. Ruptured aortic, splenic, or hepatic aneurysm
  B. Ischemia
    1. Mesenteric thrombosis
    2. Hepatic infarction—toxemia, purpura
    3. Splenic infarction
    4. Omental ischemia
IV. Miscellaneous
  A. Endometriosis

cause abdominal pain are confused with upper abdominal disorders, since their segmental distribution is similar. The intraspinal diseases have pain patterns similar to the referred pain from abdominal pathologic conditions, but they are usually not accompanied by tenderness or muscular rigidity. Inflammation of peripheral nerves, as in the case of herpes zoster, may be accompanied by tenderness and pain before the lesion becomes apparent. The pain usually has a distribution similar to that associated with myocardial infarction or biliary tract disease.

CLINICAL EVALUATION. Since pain is the subjective reaction to a stimulus that initiates transmission along nerve pathways to cortical centers, the patient's response is dependent upon both physical and psychologic factors. Physical requirements for response to pain include the patient's consciousness to permit perception, and integrity of the entire avenue along which impulses are transmitted to the brain. With repeated stimulation, the cortical threshold becomes lowered, and resistance is reduced along nerve pathways, which results in hypersensitivity and "facilitated pain." Hyperthyroidism, hyperadrenalism, and the menopausal syndrome are all associated with increased response to pain, while hypothyroidism is usually accompanied by an increased pain threshold. Sensitivity alters with age, increasing from infancy to adult life and then gradually diminishing in the elderly patient.

The physical responses to painful stimuli are also variable. While superficial pain is frequently associated with diffuse sympathetic nervous system stimulation and outpouring of epinephrine as part of a defense reaction, severe deep pain is more often accompanied by bradycardia, hypotension, nausea and vomiting, sweating, and, at times, syncope. Continued pain may cause a decrease in

Table 24-2. EXTRAPERITONEAL CAUSES OF ABDOMINAL PAIN

Cardiopulmonary
  Pneumonia
  Empyema
  Myocardial ischemia
  Active rheumatic heart disease
Blood
  Leukemia
  Sickle cell crisis
Neurogenic
  Spinal cord tumors
  Osteomyelitis of spine
  Tabes dorsalis
  Herpes zoster
  Abdominal epilepsy
Genitourinary
  Nephritis
  Pyelitis
  Perinephric abscesses
  Ureteral obstruction (calculi, tumors)
  Prostatitis
  Seminal vesiculitis
  Epidydimitis

Vascular
  Dissection, rupture, or expansion of aortic aneurysm
  Periarteritis
Metabolic
  Uremia
  Diabetic acidosis
  Porphyria
  Addisonian crisis
Toxins
  Bacterial (tetanus)
  Insect bites
  Venoms
  Drugs
  Lead poisoning
Abdominal wall
  Intramuscular hematoma
Psychogenic

renal blood flow, renal clearance, and oliguria. Cardiac arrhythmias may also occur, and, in the extreme case, neurogenic shock may result.

History. In eliciting a description of pain, the character, severity, location, timing, and factors that either augment or reduce the pain should all be defined. Certain pathologic states are associated with characteristic pain patterns. Colic—biliary, ureteral, or intestinal—is intermittent, frequently occurring in waves, and is described as cramping, or the patient may use the very term "colicky." Pain of a penetrating ulcer is "burning," while pain accompanying expansion of an abdominal aneurysm is "boring and pounding," and the pain accompanying pleuritis or perforation of a viscus has been described as "knifelike."

The severity of the pain is an expression of the intensity of stimuli plus the patient's physical and emotional response. Colicky pain related to acute distention of the biliary tract, intestine, or ureters, and pain of neurologic origin such as herpes and tabes all have an extremely high intensity. Pain evoked by inflammatory stimuli is less marked. In patients with peritonitis, the degree of pain and muscular rigidity generally parallel each other. Severe pain may be manifested by physical responses, to which previous reference has been made.

In general, abdominal pains that persist for 6 h are caused by conditions of surgical significance. However, it is rare for any pain to be absolutely constant. The pain resulting from distention of hollow viscera is generally intermittent, while the pain of peritonitis is most frequently continuous. Pain that awakens the patient from sleep is usually characteristic of organic disease. Ulcer pain frequently occurs at night or prior to a meal, whereas gallbladder pain may be stimulated by eating. Peptic ulcer pain also has a seasonal variation, occurring more frequently in the spring and fall. In addition to the effect of digestion of food on the pain, the effects of position, motion, and respiration have diagnostic importance.

The location of pain should include a description of original situation, any shifting, and radiation. The initial location may better define the visceral involvement, since once peritonitis occurs, pain becomes diffuse. Because of variation in location of the organs and the pathologic processes, as well as the vagueness of visceral pain, it is difficult to totally exclude diseases on the basis of location, but certain relationships generally pertain (Fig. 24-2). Visceral intestinal pain is usually experienced in the midportion of the abdomen. Duodenal pain is felt in the epigastrium, while the pain of the remainder of the small intestine is characteristically referred to the region of the umbilicus. Pain originating in the large bowel is less well localized and frequently experienced in the hypogastrium. Sigmoid dilatation may result in suprapubic or presacral pain.

The patient's age represents a factor that focuses attention on certain processes. Acute colicky pain in a child under two is suggestive of intussusception, whereas peptic ulcer is extremely uncommon in the young age group. Appendicitis is most frequently a disease of the young adolescent, cholecystitis is more commonly seen in the middle-age group, while diverticulitis rarely occurs before the age of thirty-five.

Vomiting is indicative of severe irritation of the peritoneum, stretching of the mesentery, obstruction, or absorbed toxins. The exact timing of vomiting in relation to the onset of pain is pertinent. Pain almost always precedes vomiting by several hours in patients with appendicitis. Vomiting may also occur early in relation to the onset of pain in patients with peritonitis and biliary or ureteral colic. With intestinal obstruction, the interval between the onset of pain and vomiting provides some indication of the level of obstruction. Frequent vomiting is indicative of intestinal obstruction, while a clear emesis may accompany biliary obstruction or diseases with pyloric obstruction.

An evaluation of bowel habits is particularly pertinent in patients with colonic obstruction, and a menstrual history is imperative in women with lower abdominal or pelvic pain. Past history should be complete and include pertinent medical illnesses, previous surgical treatment, trauma, and drugs.

Physical Examination. Pain itself evokes physical changes which may be manifested on examination. Hyperalgesia may occur at the site of the original stimulus or in the area of referred pain. Muscle contraction may be a consequence of deep pain, or the muscle spasm itself may be responsible for pain. The autonomic responses to pain include pallor, sweating, nausea, vomiting, bradycardia, hypotension, and syncope. Regard for the patient's general appearance includes the attitude in bed, tissue turgor, respiratory rate, and temperature. Restricted motion in bed suggests peritonitis, whereas writhing is more frequently an accompaniment of biliary or ureteral colic.

The abdomen should be examined in a routine manner with inspection, auscultation, percussion, and palpation performed sequentially. On inspection, restricted motion of the abdominal wall during respiration suggests diffuse peritonitis. Maintenance of the hip in a position of flexion is suggestive of a psoas abscess, appendicitis, or a pelvic abscess. Auscultation for bowel sounds may reveal the borborygmi associated with mechanical intestinal obstruction, while an absence of bowel sounds is suggestive of diffuse peritonitis. Percussion is performed for the detection of free peritoneal fluid, distention, and the absence of liver dullness associated with a perforated viscus. Palpation should always begin away from the area of pain and include all possible sites for hernia. Superficial palpation may demonstrate hyperesthesia locally or in a segmental area of referred pain. Deep palpation may detect a mass. Muscle rigidity is a relative term, and its evaluation is dependent on the patient's cooperation. Pelvic and rectal examination are integral procedures for the evaluation of the acute surgical abdomen, as is a thorough examination of the chest for cardiac and pulmonary disease.

Laboratory Procedures. The hemogram with specific interest in the white blood cell count to define the presence of an inflammatory process and a hematocrit reading to determine if there is hemoconcentration or anemia should be routine. Urinalysis is directed toward evaluating dia-

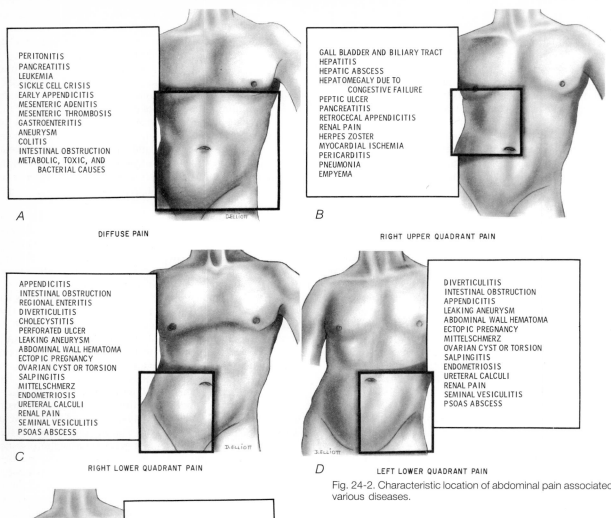

A   DIFFUSE PAIN

PERITONITIS
PANCREATITIS
LEUKEMIA
SICKLE CELL CRISIS
EARLY APPENDICITIS
MESENTERIC ADENITIS
MESENTERIC THROMBOSIS
GASTROENTERITIS
ANEURYSM
COLITIS
INTESTINAL OBSTRUCTION
METABOLIC, TOXIC, AND
    BACTERIAL CAUSES

B   RIGHT UPPER QUADRANT PAIN

GALL BLADDER AND BILIARY TRACT
HEPATITIS
HEPATIC ABSCESS
HEPATOMEGALY DUE TO
    CONGESTIVE FAILURE
PEPTIC ULCER
PANCREATITIS
RETROCECAL APPENDICITIS
RENAL PAIN
HERPES ZOSTER
MYOCARDIAL ISCHEMIA
PERICARDITIS
PNEUMONIA
EMPYEMA

C   RIGHT LOWER QUADRANT PAIN

APPENDICITIS
INTESTINAL OBSTRUCTION
REGIONAL ENTERITIS
DIVERTICULITIS
CHOLECYSTITIS
PERFORATED ULCER
LEAKING ANEURYSM
ABDOMINAL WALL HEMATOMA
ECTOPIC PREGNANCY
OVARIAN CYST OR TORSION
SALPINGITIS
MITTELSCHMERZ
ENDOMETRIOSIS
URETERAL CALCULI
RENAL PAIN
SEMINAL VESICULITIS
PSOAS ABSCESS

D   LEFT LOWER QUADRANT PAIN

DIVERTICULITIS
INTESTINAL OBSTRUCTION
APPENDICITIS
LEAKING ANEURYSM
ABDOMINAL WALL HEMATOMA
ECTOPIC PREGNANCY
MITTELSCHMERZ
OVARIAN CYST OR TORSION
SALPINGITIS
ENDOMETRIOSIS
URETERAL CALCULI
RENAL PAIN
SEMINAL VESICULITIS
PSOAS ABSCESS

Fig. 24-2. Characteristic location of abdominal pain associated with various diseases.

E   LEFT UPPER QUADRANT PAIN

GASTRITIS
PANCREATITIS
SPLENIC ENLARGEMENT, RUPTURE,
    INFARCTION, ANEURYSM
RENAL PAIN
HERPES ZOSTER
MYOCARDIAL ISCHEMIA
PNEUMONIA
EMPYEMA

betes, porphyria, the presence of infection, or red cells associated with calculi. An elevated serum amylase level is most frequently associated with acute pancreatitis but does occur with a variety of other intraabdominal processes including perforated viscera, cholecystitis, choled-

ocholithiasis, and intraabdominal bleeding. A sickle cell preparation may be called for in blacks. Emergency radiographic studies include supine films and upright or lateral decubitus films to determine the presence of air within the intestinal lumen or free within the peritoneal cavity. A chest x-ray is particularly applicable in patients over forty with upper abdominal pain, as is an electrocardiogram to rule out myocardial ischemia, which may mimic cholecystitis. The determination of the presence of free blood or significant amounts of peritoneal fluid may be accomplished by paracentesis with microscopic examination of the specimen or, in the case of lower abdominal or pelvic pain, culdocentesis and culdoscopy. It is to be emphasized that laparotomy may constitute an important tool in the diagnoisis of acute abdominal pain.

INTRACTABLE PAIN

The control of pain associated with diseases that cannot be satisfactorily treated is one of the most challenging and often frustrating problems the clinician has to face. Examples are unresectable carcinoma of the pancreas and chronic pancreatitis. Opiate analgesics if given in sufficient dosage can usually control abdominal pain, but at the risk of addiction and negating the patient's ability to function as an effective person. This is probably the best therapy, however, for a patient with incurable disease and a life expectancy of a few weeks or months. It should not be used in patients with severe pain from nonmalignant causes with an unpredictable life expectancy.

Neurosurgical intervention on the pain pathways, though disappointing at times, is the treatment of choice for intractable pain in properly selected patients. Narcotic addiction prior to surgery usually compromises the result, as an addicted patient continues to be addicted even though pain is relieved by the procedure.

Splanchnicectomy and celiac ganglionectomy can effectively control abdominal pain if somatically innervated structures are not involved in the pain-producing process. When both visceral and somatic pain fibers are involved, posterior rhizotomy or tract interruption is indicated. The spinothalamic tracts are usually interrupted, either by surgical incision or injection of sclerosing chemicals, in the spinal cord a few segments above the segments where the noxious impulses are entering. The interruption has also been done at medullary or mesencephalic levels. After anterolateral chordotomy, pain and temperature sensation are lost, while proprioception and touch are virtually unimpaired. Paresthesia often replaces pain in the anesthetic areas, and in a significant number of patients, after about 1 year, the paresthesia becomes disagreeable and painful. For this reason, root or tract interruption is most useful in patients with intractable pain and a life expectancy of a year or so.

For patients with pain arising from areas too great to be controlled by peripheral interventions, prefrontal lobotomy may be considered. Such lesions do not abolish pain but diminish the reaction to pain. The price paid for such relief, however, includes inability to experience pleasure, as well; i.e., there is a flattening of all affect and the development of a more or less apathetic state.

It is obvious from the above that there is a need for a means to relieve intractable pain that would be nonaddicting, would not affect the patient's personality or mind, and would not destroy normal neural tissue. A dorsal column stimulator is now commercially available. Impulses arising from electrostimulation of descending dorsal column fibers are used to inhibit, in accordance with the gate-control theory, prolonged small-fiber afterdischarge that is uniquely related to pain. Electrodes are implanted four to eight segments above the pain input. The external transmitter is controlled by the patient. There is a buzzing or tingling sensation below the site of the stimulator, but pain is usually controlled without significant alteration of normal sensory function. Transcutaneous electrical stimulation has been used effectively to control postoperative pain.

DYSPHAGIA

Dysphagia refers to a difficulty in swallowing and is related to either a functional alteration in the mechanism of deglutition or physical encroachment upon the lumen of the esophagus. The term *odynophagia* is used when swallowing is painful.

ACT OF SWALLOWING. This is classically divided into three stages. In the first stage the bolus of food or liquid is voluntarily moved into the pharynx by contraction of the mylohyoid muscle. In the second stage, the material is transported through the pharynx by waves of contractions that are involuntary, or reflex. This reflex is initiated by a stimulus from the base of the tongue, soft palate, uvula, and posterior pharyngeal wall and travels up the glossopharyngeal nerve, the second division of the trigeminal nerve, and the superior laryngeal nerve. The impulses terminate in the medulla and initiate a series of efferent stimuli that coordinate contraction of the pharyngeal constrictors. Elevation of the soft palate closes off the nasopharynx, and contraction of the suprahyoid muscles elevates the larynx and trachea. Ventilation is inhibited, and the respiratory tract is completely sealed off by approximation of the vocal cords and posterior displacement of the epiglottis. The terminal phase of the second stage is relaxation of the cricopharyngeus muscles, permitting the bolus to enter the upper esophagus.

The third stage of deglutition transports the bolus through the esophagus into the stomach. Waves of positive pressure sweep down the body of the esophagus in an orderly fashion, and the wave of pressure may reach an intensity of 50 to 100 cmH$_2$O. This wave is effected by a reflex arc, the afferent impulses of which are carried through the glossopharyngeal nerve and the efferent impulses transported by the vagi. Auerbach's plexuses within the wall of the esophagus are also involved. When distention by a solid bolus of food occurs, secondary peristaltic contractions result in that segment. Nonperistaltic tertiary esophageal contractions are seen in the lower esophagus of normal people after the age of forty. They are important considerations in the differential diagnosis of esophageal varices.

Transport of the bolus through the esophagus is dependent upon the pressure gradient produced by the primary peristaltic contraction plus, in the case of liquids, the effect of gravity. The final phase of deglutition is the propulsion of the bolus from the esophagus into the stomach. This is dependent upon relaxation of the inferior esophageal sphincter, which reacts reflexly and autonomously in response to pressure or peristalsis in the lower esophagus.

ETIOLOGY. Dysphagia may be due to oropharyngeal or esophageal causes. The former includes disorders of the mouth, upper respiratory tract, and pharynx. Any painful lesion of the mouth or tongue, including pharyngitis, retropharyngeal abscess, or oral carcinoma, may be implicated. Acute thyroiditis is usually accompanied by pharyngeal dysphagia. Neuromuscular disturbances that may affect deglutition include poliomyelitis, syringomyelia, glossopharyngeal neuritis, and myasthenia. Alteration of the muscle itself, as is seen in amyloidosis and scleroderma, also results in dysphagia, which may be either oropharyngeal or esophageal in location.

Esophageal dysphagia is related to a great variety of

Table 24-3. CAUSES OF ESOPHAGEAL DYSPHAGIA

Cause	Predominant sex	Age incidence		Salient historical and related characteristics
		10–45	45 and over	
Carcinoma	Male	Rare	Common	Duration of symptoms less than 2 years; painful swallowing occurs early, dysphagia later.
Peptic esophagitis	Male	Common	Common	Heartburn for years, often preceding dysphagia; odynophagia later.
Achalasia	Male-female	Common	Common	Liquids, especially cold, cause dysphagia early; regurgitation easy; odynophagia mild and late.
Contractile ring	Male	Rare	Common	Brief, intermittent attacks of dysphagia with no interval symptoms.
Diffuse spasm	Male	Rare	Rare	Affects elderly persons; multiple ringlike contractions along esophageal tube.
Zenker's diverticulum	Male	Rare	Rare	Sticking feeling in neck, gurgling on swallowing; occasional regurgitation of decayed food.
Scleroderma	Female	Common	Rare	Skin changes; Raynaud's disease.
Paraesophageal hiatal hernia	Female	Rare	Rare	Attacks of substernal pressure, pain, dysphagia, and belching during meals.
Extrinsic masses		Common	Rare	Symptoms of primary disorder.

SOURCE: After Ingelfinger, *Med Sci,* Apr. 10, 1960, pp 451–470, with permission.

causes, which are listed in Table 24-3. The level at which the patient localizes a sticking sensation usually corresponds well to the level of the responsible lesion. Dysphagia may be caused by disturbance in esophageal motility with either hypomotility or hypermotility implicated (see Chap. 25). The passage of fluid through the esophagus may also be impaired by encroachment upon the lumen. In the proximal esophagus, Zenker's pharyngoesophageal diverticulum, obstructing bands, and hypertrophic spurs of the anterior cervical vertebrae may be implicated. Dysphagia in the region of the cervical esophagus may also be due to esophageal carcinoma, cervical lymphadenopathy, stenosis secondary to ingestion of a caustic substance, or pressure from an enlarged thyroid. In the middle third of the esophagus, carcinoma, stenosis, esophagitis, and traction diverticulum may all be causes. In addition, a wide variety of mediastinal inflammatory malignant lesions may encroach upon the lumen. Vascular lesions such as enlargement of the left atrium, aneurysm in the arch of the aorta, and anomalous right subclavian artery are rare causes of dysphagia in this region. In the lower third of the esophagus, primary carcinoma and carcinoma of the stomach with craniad extension represent common causes, particularly in the older age group. Other lower esophageal causes of dysphagia include reflux esophagitis, achalasia, contractile rings, and epiphrenic diverticula.

Dysphagia is a relatively common manifestation of emotional diseases. Inability to swallow accompanies anxiety states, conversion hysteria, and anorexia nervosa.

CLINICAL EVALUATION. History should include a precise description of the symptom with particular reference to the duration, location, and timing in relation to ingestion of food. True dysphagia occurs within 15 min of swallowing. The patient can usually pinpoint the site of obstruction. The determination of the amount of weight loss and the presence of associated vomiting are important. Physical examination is directed toward the detection of cervical nodes suggesting mediastinal or esophageal lesions, enlargement of the esophagus, and stigmata of scleroderma. Barium study of the esophagus is frequently diagnostic, and the use of cineradiography and/or manometric motility studies is particularly applicable in determining disorders of motility. In the case of intrinsic esophageal lesions, the ultimate diagnostic study is esophagoscopy with biopsy.

ANOREXIA

Anorexia is the absence of the desire to eat and can be related to a variety of organic and psychologic disturbances. Since appetite is essentially a central phenomenon, anorexia is dependent upon central effects producing a loss of appetite. Animal experiments have demonstrated a feeding center in the lateral hypothalamus and a satiety center in the medial hypothalamus. In most instances, gastric hypofunction, mucosal pallor, and decrease in gastric motility and secretion have been associated with anorexia, but the stomach itself plays a minor role. Anorexia may also occur when both the secretory and motor activity of the stomach and gastrointestinal tract are increased. Visceral stimuli are generally carried to the midbrain via the vagus, pelvic, and sympathetic nerves, but combined sympathetic and parasympathetic denervation may not alter appetite or preclude the possibility of anorexia. The absence of precise pathophysiologic explanation and the protean disorders associated with the symptom of anorexia make it of little diagnostic significance. Among the organic diseases associated with anorexia are inflammatory processes within the intestinal tract; carcinoma of the stomach, pancreas, and liver; hepatitis and alcoholism; advanced renal disease with uremia; congestive heart failure; and certain endocrine disorders such as panhypopituitarism, adrenal cortical insufficiency, and hyperparathyroidism. Many, if not most, drugs can cause anorexia; there is no medication that consistently increases appetite.

NAUSEA AND VOMITING

Nausea and vomiting may occur separately but are closely allied. Nausea usually refers to the feeling of an imminent desire to vomit. Vomiting may be defined as the forceful expulsion of gastrointestinal contents through the mouth. In most instances, nausea precedes vomiting.

In spite of the frequency and great clinical importance of vomiting, the nervous mechanism of the act and the physical and chemical stimuli are not well understood. Most physiologists have agreed to the existence of a vomiting center and to its location in the reticular core of the medulla oblongata. There are actually two medullary centers concerned with emesis: (1) a sensory "chemoreceptive trigger zone" and (2) an integrated center that is concerned directly with the production of vomiting. The former is implicated in drug-induced emesis and also in the vomiting associated with uremia, infections, and radiation sickness.

Afferent pathways to the vomiting center emanate from almost all sites in the body. Impulses from the gastrointestinal system pass through the emetic center by way of afferent fibers in both the vagal and sympathetic nerves. Although neither vagotomy nor sympathectomy alone abolishes the vomiting of peritonitis, the vagus is considered the more important afferent pathway from this stimulus. The vomiting induced by intestinal distention is dependent upon afferent impulses transmitted in the sympathetic nerves, as evidenced by the fact that denervation of the mesenteric pedicle prevents vomiting associated with distention of that segment. Distention of the gallbladder and extrahepatic biliary tract also causes vomiting that may be obviated by a combination of vagotomy and splanchnicectomy. Pyloric pouch distention vomiting is abolished by vagotomy alone. However, it is known that vomiting may be a consequence of surgical vagotomy and that the higher the vagotomy, the more frequent the incidence of vomiting. In this circumstance, the vomiting is related to esophageal stasis with regurgitation of esophageal contents into the pharynx and subsequent pharyngeal irritation.

The act of vomiting is primarily a motor function involving the respiratory and somatic muscular systems in addition to the gastrointestinal tract. Vomiting occurs in the normal fashion following total denervation of the intestine. The efferent neuropathways involve the phrenic nerves to the diaphragm, spinal nerves to the abdominal and intercostal muscles, and efferent visceral fibers along the vagus and sympathetic nerves to the intestine and muscles of the pharynx and larynx. The act of vomiting depends upon the coordinated closure of the glottis, contraction and fixation of the diaphragm in the inspiratory position, closure of the pylorus, and relaxation of the rest of the stomach including the cardia. Relaxation of the upper half of the stomach and the esophageal cardia is followed by peristaltic contractions passing from the midstomach to the incisura angularis. Contraction at the incisura persists and prevents the contents of the stomach from passing into the gastric antrum. This is followed by forceful contraction of the abdominal, diaphragmatic, and intercostal muscles, which transmit a pressure to the stomach and cause regurgitation. Reverse peristalsis in the stomach plays no major role in the mechanism of vomiting. Reverse peristalsis of the small intestine frequently occurs and results in the passage of intestinal contents into the stomach and the presence of bile in the vomitus after repeated retching. This type of intestinal activity, however, has been shown to occur normally in the duodenum and does not contribute to the act of vomiting. Vomiting is frequently associated with autonomic activity, including pallor, sweating, increased salivation, and cardiovascular changes which include irregularity, ectopic beats, heart block, and, rarely, arrest.

All organic diseases of the alimentary tract and its appendages, as well as diseases of almost every organ of the body, have been associated with vomiting. Derangements of the autonomic nervous system, psychogenic disturbances, and the ingestion of noxious materials may also cause vomiting. A broad spectrum of drugs is considered as emetic agents. These include morphine, cardiac glycosides, quinine and quinidine, veratrine alkaloids, pilocarpine, Pituitrin, Pitocin, acetylcholine, ergot alkaloids, atropine, tartar emetic, ipecac, zinc sulfate, and bacterial endotoxins. With each of these causes of vomiting any combination of three major factors may be involved: impulses arising from the gastrointestinal tract, central or cerebral impulses, and chemical materials transported in the blood.

The vomiting associated with shock and severe pain may be related to a reduced blood supply in the cerebral medullary centers or vasoconstriction in the splanchnic areas. Reduction of oxygen supply to the vomiting center has been implicated in the vomiting associated with anemia, vascular occlusion, and increased intracranial pressure. Migraine may also induce vomiting by an effective increase in intracranial pressure with interference of blood supply to the cerebromedullary center. Emetic drugs act in one of two ways, either directly on the cerebrum, hypothalamus, or brainstem or by their irritative effect on the gastric and intestinal mucosa. These two factors may also be involved in vomiting induced by spoiled or contaminated food and the vomiting following the ingestion of alcohol. The vomiting associated with diabetic acidosis, uremia, and Addisonian crisis has been related to changes in electrolytes and, more specifically, acidosis and hyperkalemia affecting the emesis center. An augmented irritability of the emesis center is postulated as playing a significant role in the vomiting of thyrotoxicosis.

The gastrointestinal pathophysiologic processes leading to vomiting are many and varied. Obstruction to passage of food at any level will eventually be accompanied by vomiting. The higher the obstruction, the more rapid the onset of vomiting. The rapidity is also related to the acuteness of onset, since a gradual obstruction is attended by compensation with stretching of muscle fibers and hypertrophy. Inflammatory diseases and malignant tumors of the stomach are frequent causes of vomiting and are usually preceded by anorexia and nausea. In the child under three months of age, vomiting of clear, non-bile-stained materials is highly suggestive of hypertrophic pyloric stenosis. Acute inflammatory diseases of the intestine and pelvic organs are associated with nausea and vomiting through visceral reflexes; the more common disorders include appendicitis, cholecystitis, hepatitis, pancreatitis, and salpingitis.

The pattern of vomiting is of clinical significance. Vomiting without antecedent nausea suggests a central nervous system lesion with increased intracranial pressure, such as hemorrhage or brain tumor. In these cases, vomiting is usually sudden in onset and often projectile. Projectile vomiting is also characteristic of hypertrophic pyloric stenosis. Emesis that follows and relieves epigastric pain is usually associated with intragastric lesions or pyloric spasm. Vomiting that immediately follows eating is noted with toxic causes, such as uremia and hyperemesis gravidarum, gastritis, high intestinal obstruction, and gastric neoplasms. Vomiting of large amounts of digested food at 12- to 48-h intervals is suggestive of chronic pyloric obstruction. Vomiting of feculent material is associated with gastrocolic fistula. Continued retching and vomiting, especially in alcoholics, may lacerate the gastroesophageal mucosa and result in the Mallory-Weiss syndrome with severe bleeding and, at times, exsanguination. An extension of this process is the spontaneous rupture of the esophagus which occurs more frequently in vomiting by the patient with a full stomach (Boerhaave's syndrome).

CONSEQUENCES OF VOMITING. Depending upon its intensity and duration, vomiting may produce hypovolemia, hypokalemia, alteration in the acid-base balance, and the consequences of starvation. Vomitus, without admixture of ingested food, is isoosmotic with the extracellular fluid. The electrolyte composition is extremely variable and dependent upon the extent of hydrogen ion excretion.

When hydrogen ion is excreted into the gastric juice, there is a shift of bicarbonate ion into the plasma, and, to maintain electric neutrality of the blood, chloride is excreted into the gastric juice. Concentration of bicarbonate in the plasma is augmented by the loss of chloride and excessive sodium in the vomitus. In general, an inverse relation exists between the concentration of hydrogen ion and sodium ion in the vomitus. Even in the achlorhydric state, when vomiting results in a depletion of sodium chloride and potassium chloride, chloride is excreted in excess of the physiologic proportions existent in plasma, i.e., 145 meq of sodium and 100 meq of chloride. As the plasma bicarbonate rises, the body compensates by increasing renal excretion of bicarbonate and reducing the rate and depth of respiration to decrease the respiratory loss of $HHCO_3$ to maintain the acid/base ratio. These compensatory features may maintain the normal blood pH, while the urine is alkaline because of excretion of

bicarbonate. Determination of plasma electrolytes is only partly informative, since it is dependent upon the relative loss of electrolytes and water and also upon the solutions ingested.

With continued vomiting, the plasma and extracellular potassium concentration becomes reduced as a result of the increased quantities of potassium excreted in the urine in exchange for sodium, which in turn is related to the lack of availability of hydrogen ions depleted by loss in the vomitus. Adrenal cortical stimulation intensifies the potassium loss and potentiates the absorption of bicarbonate by the renal tubular cell. The extracellular and subsequently intracellular potassium concentrations become reduced, sodium cations shift into the cell, and, in order to conserve sodium, an acid urine is formed in the face of generalized alkalosis. This intensifies the alkalosis and sets up a vicious cycle which includes shift of more potassium out of the cell in exchange for sodium.

The fluid loss results in reduction in the circulating blood volume, and in time the consequences of starvation such as cellular breakdown of protein and increased renal load of nitrogenous waste products cause a rise in the BUN (blood urea nitrogen) level. Fat stores are utilized. Ketone bodies are formed, and since they require sodium for excretion, this further depletes the body stores of sodium.

Therapy should be instituted early, correcting relatively minor defects, since advanced deficiencies are critical and difficult to reverse. Drugs used to treat vomiting include anticholinergics, antihistamines, phenothiazine derivatives, and orthopramides.

CONSTIPATION AND DIARRHEA

Alteration in bowel habits may be related to the type of food ingested, psychologic disorders, or lesions in the gastrointestinal tract.

INTESTINAL TRANSIT. The rate of gastric emptying varies with the amount and quality of food and the emotional state of the individual. Generally, the healthy stomach is emptied within 3 to 4 h, and passage through the duodenum and jejunum is rapid. Digested food usually begins to traverse the ileocolic sphincter in 2 to 3 h and completes its passage into the cecum in 9 h. Some delay occurs almost constantly in the distal ileum, where "segmentation" of a radiopaque bolus can be noted. The contents of the small intestine travel at an average rate of 1 in./min, or 22 ft in 4 h.

The chyme that enters the cecum is semiliquid in consistency. Most of the absorption of water that occurs in the large intestine takes place in the cecum and ascending colon. The intensity and frequency of muscular contractions increase from the duodenum to the rectum. Mass peristalsis carries the bolus from the hepatic flexure onward. These waves occur at varying times but are known to be frequent after meals, the so-called "gastrocolic reflex." Although some food products are evacuated within 24 h of ingestion, the major portion requires several days for disposition.

Normally, the fecal bolus does not pass beyond the sigmoid into the rectum until defecation is about to occur. The passage into the rectum is brought about by powerful peristaltic waves with concomitant relaxation of the smooth musculature at the rectosigmoid junction. Distention of the rectum initiates afferent nervous impulses conducted via hypogastric and pelvic nerves to the sacral cord, whence efferent impulses are discharged. The process of defecation may be entirely involuntary but is usually assisted by voluntary contractions of the muscles of the abdomen and diaphragm and voluntary relaxation of the external anal sphincter. The intraluminal pressure is increased, forcing the stool through the relaxed internal sphincter and the voluntarily relaxed external sphincter. The entire colon, distal to the splenic flexure, is usually emptied at one time.

Although intestinal motility continues after transection of the nerves, under normal conditions the vagi, splanchnics, and pelvic nerves do play a significant role. Parasympathetic efferent supply to the small intestine and proximal colon courses over the vagi, while the remainder of the colon innervation is carried over the lower sacral segment via the pelvic nerves. Splanchnic nerves supply sympathetic innervation. The intrinsic myenteric reflexes are the prime movers, but motility is augmented by parasympathetic stimulation, while sympathetic stimulation results in inhibition of tone. Sympathetic stimulation explains the reflex ileus that is known to accompany retroperitoneal trauma or dissection.

The external anal sphincter, a voluntary muscle, receives nerve fibers from the gray matter of the conus terminalis, where the reflex is located. Transection of the cord in this region does not affect reflex contraction. If the lower segment of the cord is destroyed, the external sphincter becomes relaxed and no longer contracts. If the afferent nerves are destroyed, the fecal bolus may accumulate without sensation. It has been suggested that the medullary center may be implicated in the act of defecation, since a central nervous system influence is capable of causing either diarrhea or constipation.

In addition to neurogenic factors, chemicals also influence defecation. Acetylcholine-like drugs increase the tone and activity of the intestine. Pilocarpine causes smooth muscle contraction, while neostigmine and Mecholyl inhibit the destruction of cholinesterase and produce intestinal activity. Serotonin also alters intestinal motility with resultant increased activity. Guanethidine causes increased motility by its inhibitory effect on the sympathetic nerves, and reserpine acts by its effect on serotonin release. Vasopressin strongly induces motility in the entire intestine. Potassium is implicated in intestinal motility, since the function of the muscle cell is dependent upon its potassium level. Drugs may also delay the passage of intestinal contents. Morphine and codeine decrease the propulsive motility by resulting in a marked increase in tone. Atropine decreases motility by paralyzing the parasympathetic nerve endings.

Constipation

Constipation may be defined as an abnormal retention of fecal matter or undue delay in discharge when com-

pared with the patient's usual bowel habits. The term is used in a variety of ways. It may refer to the fact that the stool occurs with relative infrequency, that the stool is insufficient in quantity, or that it is abnormally hard and dry.

ETIOLOGY. Constipation may be due to psychologic factors, dietary constituents, laxatives and drugs, neurogenic causes, decreased skeletomuscular power, and mechanical factors that are either intrinsic or extrinsic to the gastrointestinal tract.

Psychogenic constipation may be related to improper training, and the symptom frequently dates from early childhood. The end result may be a functional megacolon, which is considered to be more common than Hirschsprung's disease. *Dietary factors* include a lack of bulky foods and the use of laxatives that lead to overstimulation of the bowel with eventual fatigue. Drugs with constipating effects have been referred to in the section Intestinal Transit.

Decreased muscular power in the skeletal muscles of the diaphragm, abdominal wall, and pelvic floor may all cause constipation. Weakness of the diaphragm may be associated with a variety of chronic pulmonary diseases, while weakness of the abdominal wall may occur in pregnancy, in the presence of large, rapidly expanding intraabdominal masses, and in patients with marked ascites. Weakness of the pelvic floor is usually a consequence of pregnancy. The role of *atony of the intestinal muscle* is difficult to evaluate and may be of minimal importance. Hypokalemia results in ileus based on this cause. Collagen and endocrine disorders are thought to be associated with intestinal atony. *Neurogenic causes* include tabes dorsalis, multiple sclerosis, spinal cord tumors, and trauma. These lesions may result in deficient reflex activity or may directly destroy or depress the autonomic innervation of the intestine. In Hirschsprung's disease the neurologic deficit in the myenteric and submucosal plexuses interrupts the peristaltic action to that segment. *Factors intrinsic to the gastrointestinal tract* that contribute to the symptom of constipation include tumors, fecal impactions, intussusception, and volvulus. The mechanical factor is also implicated at the anal sphincter, when spasm and the voluntary avoidance of defecation because of pain occur in patients with hemorrhoids, fissures, or proctitis. *Extrinsic causes* consist of large intraabdominal masses such as ovarian cysts, fibroids, pregnancy, and obstructing adhesions.

ASSOCIATED SYMPTOMS AND EFFECTS. Obstipation, which is defined as the absence of passage of both flatus and feces, is suggestive of mechanical obstruction. Reflex symptoms accompanying constipation include back and hip pain, headache, and, occasionally, tachycardia. So-called intestinal toxemia in patients with chronic constipation remains unproved but probably occurs. Fecal accumulations within the rectum may reach large size and contribute to the formation of anal lesions such as hemorrhoids, fissures, and ulcers. Constipation also has a significant role in the development of colonic diverticula and sigmoid volvulus.

CLINICAL EVALUATION. The history should include complete elaboration of bowel habits and also the patient's dietary intake. Direct questioning concerning the color, consistency, and caliber of the stool, the presence of melena or unaltered blood, mucus, or undigested fats or foods, and the occurrence of tenesmus is indicated. Although abdominal examination may reveal a mass, the rectal is usually the most rewarding aspect of the physical examination. Proctosigmoidoscopy may define the presence of inflammation, tumors, or the melanosis coli of patients who take laxatives chronically. Radiographic examination with a barium enema is indicated in all patients with prolonged constipation.

Diarrhea

Diarrhea refers to an excessively rapid evacuation of excessively fluid stool. It may be acute, in which case it is usually related to dietary, toxic, or infectious causes. When diarrhea is chronic or recurrent, it is more likely a manifestation of gastrointestinal disease.

ETIOLOGY. Even when discussion is limited to chronic diarrhea, classification is at best imperfect. Table 24-4 lists some of the causes of diarrhea that are of interest to surgeons.

PATHOPHYSIOLOGY. The conventional view has been that increased intestinal motor activity producing rapid intestinal transit is responsible for diarrhea. Evidence has now accumulated that the pathophysiologic mechanism for diarrhea is primarily an abnormality of intestinal water and electrolyte transport. Distention of the bowel by this increased fluid stimulates propulsive contractions. Hypermotility then is a secondary phenomenon, not primary, in most types of diarrhea.

There are four principal pathophysiologic mechanisms involved in the production of diarrhea: (1) excessive intestinal secretion ("secretory" diarrhea), (2) the presence in the bowel lumen of increased amounts of poorly absorbable, osmotically active substances ("osmotic" diarrhea), (3) inhibition or absence of a normal active ion transport process, and (4) deranged bowel motility. These mechanisms are by no means mutually exclusive, and more than one mechanism is usually involved in any patient with diarrhea.

Active ion secretion by the small intestine is the most important factor in *secretory diarrhea*. In some syndromes, decreased absorption also plays a role. Cholera has been the most extensively studied of the secretory diarrheas. The toxins of *Vibrio cholerae* activate adenylate cyclase in the basolateral membrane of the mucosal cells, which in turn causes a rise in intracellular cyclic AMP concentration. Cyclic AMP causes chloride and bicarbonate to be actively secreted into the lumen. Water is transported passively in response to osmotic gradients.

Table 24-4. CAUSES OF DIARRHEA

Functional enterocolonic disease	Gastrojejunocolic fistula
Mucous colitis	Inadvertent gastroileostomy
Organic colonic disease	Postvagotomy diarrhea
Ulcerative colitis	Disorders of the solid viscera
Crohn's colitis	Pancreatic insufficiency
Diverticulitis	Biliary fistula
Neoplastic lesions	Watery diarrhea syndrome (VIPoma)
Polyposis	Enteric infections
Villous adenoma	Salmonella
Carcinoma	Shigella
Fecal impaction	Pseudomembranous colitis
Lymphogranuloma venereum	Parasitic infestations
Endometriosis	Amebiasis
Toxic colitis	Leishmaniasis
Arsenic	Ascaris
Mercury	Liver flukes
Alcohol	Schistosomiasis
Small intestinal disease	Trichinella
Crohn's disease	Metabolic disorders
Tuberculous enteritis	Thyroid
Malabsorption due to disease	Thyrotoxicosis
Sprue	Medullary carcinoma—calcitonin
Carcinoid	Hyperparathyroidism
Intestinal lipodystrophy	Uremia
Malabsorption due to mechanical defects	Diabetes mellitus
Short gut syndrome	Addison's disease
Blind loop syndrome	Drugs
Fistulas	Cathartics
Gastric factors	Sympatholytic
Hyperchlorhydria	Propranolol
Zollinger-Ellison syndrome	Parasympathomimetic
Postsurgical problems	Urecholine
Dumping syndrome	Neostigmine
Afferent loop syndrome	Acetylcholine

Characteristic features of secretory diarrhea are (1) the diarrhea is usually voluminous, (2) the osmolality of the stool fluid is isotonic, and (3) the diarrhea usually persists even when the patient fasts.

Osmotic diarrhea results when poorly absorbable solutes accumulate in the bowel lumen. These osmotically active substances result from (1) incomplete digestion of ingested food; (2) failure to absorb a dietary nonelectrolyte that is normally handled by a special transport mechanism, e.g., glucose; and (3) ingestion of poorly absorbable solutes, e.g., the magnesium ion in laxatives. Characteristic features of osmotic diarrhea are (1) the diarrhea stops when the patient fasts or stops ingesting the poorly absorbable solute; (2) the osmolality of fecal fluid is greater than the sum of the concentrations of normal electrolytes.

Malabsorption of a normal ion is an infrequent cause of chronic diarrhea. The best-studied example is congenital chloridorrhea. Passive absorption or secretion down electrochemical gradients is normal, but these patients are unable to actively absorb chloride ion against a gradient. Characteristic features are (1) the diarrhea disappears or is greatly improved on fasting, (2) the osmolality of the fecal fluid is normal; and (3) the ionic composition of the fecal fluid is abnormal, reflecting malabsorption of a specific ion.

Deranged bowel motility is the least understood of the pathophysiologic mechanisms of diarrhea. It is difficult to separate abnormal motility that is secondary to stimulation by distention, as occurs in secretory and osmotic diarrhea, from primary intestinal motility abnormalities. Examples of syndromes in which primary motor abnormalities are thought to play a major role include the diarrheal phase of irritable colon syndrome, diabetic enteropathy, and scleroderma.

CONSEQUENCES OF DIARRHEA. The consequences are dependent upon the intensity and duration of the symptom. Severe or prolonged diarrhea may result in dehydration, electrolyte loss, and acidosis. The fecal sodium and chloride concentrations are usually lower than the plasma levels, whereas the potassium and bicarbonate levels are higher. The villous adenoma excretes a fluid that is particularly high in potassium, with concentrations many times that of plasma.

Acidosis may result because of a high bicarbonate content in the stool or may be related to the production of acid due to starvation or to the dehydration compromising renal function. Dehydration and acidosis accelerate the body depletion of potassium by a shift of the cation out of the cell in exchange for sodium and hydrogen ions. These factors coupled with the large amount of potassium lost in the stool because of excretion into the intestine in exchange for sodium absorption from the lower small intestine and colon may result in significant hypokalemia.

Plasma or electrolyte determinations do not represent a guide to the severity of volume loss, since this reflection is dependent upon the relative tonicity of the stool with respect to extracellular fluid and the amount of fluid lost. In the absence of associated bleeding, the hematocrit is the better index of the severity of dehydration.

CLINICAL EVALUATION. History. Direct questioning should elicit the duration of diarrhea, the time of day during which diarrhea occurs, the patient's description of the stool, the presence of accompanying pain or urge to defecate, and the presence of other manifestations of gastrointestinal disease such as anorexia, nausea, and vomiting. A family or community history of similar episodes suggests an infectious basis. Diarrhea that alternates with constipation occurs with colon lesions such as carcinoma, diverticulitis, partial intestinal obstruction, and chronic constipation treated with laxatives. Recurrent episodes of diarrhea are characteristic of ulcerative colitis, psychogenic causes, and amebic colitis. Ulcerative colitis may be associated with red stools, while the patient may recognize infestation by the presence of the offending organism in the stool. Large, pale, bulky stools suggest pancreatic deficiency. Large amounts of mucus in the stool are seen in patients with mucous colitis, ulcerative colitis, carcinoma of the colon, and villous adenoma.

Pain is frequently present with ulcerative colitis and diverticulitis, and also may be noted when diarrhea is due to carcinoma. Tenesmus commonly accompanies ulcerative colitis, carcinoma of the rectum, and lymphogranuloma venereum. Anorexia, nausea, and/or vomiting are more characteristic symptoms of intestinal malignancy, ulcerative colitis, and severe bacillary or amebic dysentery.

Physical Examination. *Fever* may be present with a variety of inflammatory processes and occurs more rarely as an accompaniment of neoplastic disease, with the exception of lymphoma. Arthritis is particularly common in ulcerative colitis, regional enteritis, and lipodystrophy. This also applies to other hypersensitivity reactions such as iritis and erythema nodosum. A palpable *abdominal mass* should be sought. In the left lower quadrant, this may suggest sigmoid carcinoma or diverticulitis with inflammatory obstruction. Granulomas of regional enteritis, amebic infection, and tuberculosis may all cause palpable masses. *Tenderness* suggests regional enteritis, diverticulitis, or intraabdominal inflammatory processes. *Digital examination* of the rectum may define the presence of lymphogranuloma venereum, carcinoma, granulomas, ulcerative colitis, diffuse polyposis, or a fecal impaction. *Proctosigmoidoscopy* should represent an integral part of the examination of the patient with diarrhea. A friable rectal mucosa may suggest ulcerative colitis or amebiasis. The overwhelming majority of patients with ulcerative colitis have lesions which may be visualized by this technique. Malignant lesions, polyps, and villous adenomas can usually be defined by proctosigmoidoscopy.

Stool. The stool should be evaluated for consistency and the presence of mucus and occult and unaltered blood. Fatty stools suggest pancreatic insufficiency or malabsorption. Carcinoma and diverticulitis may be associated with bloody stools. Microscopic examination for ova and parasites is particularly pertinent to the diagnosis of infestations.

Radiologic Studies. Abdominal films may demonstrate intestinal obstruction, a mass, or calculi associated with chronic pancreatitis. Barium enema is an essential part of the examination and is frequently diagnostic for ulcerative colitis, tumors, and diverticulitis. Reflux into the terminal ileum may define the presence of regional enteritis or tuberculous enteritis. In rare instances, regurgitation of barium into the jejunum or stomach will demonstrate a fistula. The upper gastrointestinal series is also of importance, particularly in determining the presence of gastrocolic fistula, blind loop syndrome, and iatrogenic gastroileostomy. The barium meal may be utilized as a method of determining intestinal transit time in patients with massive resection. Primary malabsorption syndromes may be associated with a small bowel pattern which is quite characteristic. Pancreatography may be indicated.

Laparotomy. In some cases, laparotomy should be considered a diagnostic procedure. Small bowel biopsy is indicated in the differential diagnosis of malabsorption syndrome, regional enteritis, Whipple's disease, lymphomas, and tumors of the small intestine.

INTESTINAL OBSTRUCTION

Intestinal obstruction exists when there is interference with the normal aboral progression of intestinal contents. The term *mechanical intestinal obstruction* is used if an actual physical barrier blocks the intestinal lumen. The term *ileus,* though properly a synonym for intestinal obstruction from whatever cause, by common usage now connotes failure of downward progress of bowel contents because of disordered propulsive motility of the bowel.

Gastric outlet obstruction is discussed in Chap. 26, esophageal obstruction in Chap. 25, and mesenteric vascular obstruction in Chap. 35. Discussion of specific entites causing intestinal obstruction in infancy and childhood will be found in Chap. 39.

Mechanical Obstruction

ETIOLOGY. The causes of mechanical obstruction may be classified according to the manner in which the obstruction is produced: (1) by obturation of the lumen, as in gallstone ileus, (2) by encroachment on the lumen by intrinsic disease of the bowel wall, as in regional enteritis or carcinoma, or (3) by lesions extrinsic to bowel such as an adhesive band (Table 24-5).

Classification of intestinal obstruction on clinical and pathologic grounds is also necessary. In *simple mechanical obstruction* the lumen is obstructed, but the blood supply is intact. If mesenteric vessels are occluded, then *strangulated obstruction* exists. *Closed-loop obstruction* results when both limbs of the loop are obstructed so that neither aboral progression nor regurgitation is possible. Obstruction is further delineated by classification as partial or complete, acute or chronic, high or low, small intestinal or colonic.

INCIDENCE. Probably about 20 percent of surgical admissions for acute abdominal conditions are for intestinal

Table 24-5. MECHANISMS OF INTESTINAL OBSTRUCTIONS

Mechanical obstruction of the lumen
  Obturation of the lumen
    Meconium
    Intussusception
    Gallstones
    Impactions—fecal, barium, bezoar, worms
  Lesions of bowel
    Congenital
      Atresia and stenosis
      Imperforate anus
      Duplications
      Meckel's diverticulum
    Traumatic
    Inflammatory
      Regional enteritis
      Diverticulitis
      Chronic ulcerative colitis
    Neoplastic
    Miscellaneous
      K^+-induced stricture
      Radiation stricture
      Endometriosis
  Lesions extrinsic to bowel
    Adhesive band constriction or angulation by adhesion
    Hernia and wound dehiscence
    Extrinsic masses
      Annular pancreas
      Anomalous vessels
      Abscesses and hematomas
      Neoplasms
  Volvulus
Inadequate propulsive motility
  Neuromuscular defects
    Megacolon
    Paralytic ileus
      Abdominal causes
        Intestinal distention
        Peritonitis
        Retroperitoneal lesions
      Systemic causes
        Electrolyte imbalance
        Toxemias
    Spastic ileus
  Vascular occlusion
    Arterial
    Venous

obstruction. Adhesive bands are now the most frequent cause of obstruction for all age groups combined. Strangulated groin hernia, formerly the most common cause, is now in second place, with neoplasm of the bowel in third place. In some recently reported series, neoplasm has taken over second place, with hernia now in third. These three etiologic agents account for more than 80 percent of all intestinal obstruction.

The order of frequency differs for different age groups. Hernia is by far the most common cause of obstruction in childhood. Colorectal carcinoma and diverticulitis coli are prominent etiologic agents in the older age group, and these lesions are becoming more prominent in the overall picture as more of the population is living into the geriatric age, where these lesions prevail.

The mortality rate from intestinal obstruction was over 50 percent in the United States in the early part of this century. The mortality rate is now under 10 percent. The factors principally responsible for the reduction are (1) recognition of the role of fluid and electrolyte therapy, (2) gastrointestinal decompression by intubation, and (3) antibiotics.

Though the mortality rate is now but one-fifth of the rate in the early twentieth century, it is still distressingly and needlessly high. This death rate could be appreciably lowered if patients with hernias were urged to have their hernias repaired, since herniorrhaphy can now be done with only about a 0.1 to 0.2 percent mortality even in the presence of other chronic systemic disease. A further lowering of the death rate could be attained if a larger percentage of patients could be operated upon before a simple mechanical obstruction has progressed to strangulated obstruction with its greatly increased morbidity and mortality.

PATHOPHYSIOLOGY. Though simple mechanical obstruction, strangulated obstruction, and ileus have much in common, there are important differences in pathophysiology and management. Also, colon obstruction differs in some aspects from small bowel obstruction.

Simple Mechanical Obstruction of the Small Intestine. The principal physiologic derangements of the mechanically obstructed intestine with intact blood supply are accumulation of fluid and gas above the point of obstruction and altered bowel motility, which lead also to systemic derangements.

Fluid and Electrolyte Losses. Death from intestinal obstruction was for many years attributed to "toxins" that were absorbed from the intestine. In 1912 Hartwell and Hoguet were able to prolong the life of dogs with high intestinal obstruction by the daily parenteral administration of physiologic saline solution. Gamble later demonstrated that the "toxic" factor in simple mechanical obstruction was actually the loss of fluid and electrolytes from the body by vomiting and by sequestering in the obstructed bowel.

Accumulation of large quantities of fluid and gas within the lumen of the bowel above an obstruction is striking and progressive. The net movement of a substance across the intestinal mucosa is equal to the difference between the unidirectional flux from intestinal lumen to blood (absorption) and the opposite flux from blood to lumen (secretion). Accumulation of fluid within the bowel—a negative net flux—will result if the flux from lumen to blood (absorption) is decreased or if the flux from blood to lumen (secretion) is increased. After 48 h of obstruction, the rate of entry of water into the intestinal lumen increases as a consequence of blood to lumen flux. The findings for sodium and potassium are parallel.

Davenport has reported that normal fluxes occurred in the direction of blood to lumen, but fluxes from lumen to blood were depressed or abolished in an obstructed ileal segment. As a result, water, sodium, and chloride (and presumably other ions) moved into the obstructed intestinal segment but not out of it, distending it with fluid having approximately the electrolyte composition of plasma.

Wright et al. studied net flux in patients with mature ileostomies. Closed loops were produced by proximal and distal obstructing balloons inserted through the ileostomy. Absorption of a test solution was found to increase at moderate elevations of pressure, but fell below normal at pressures three or four times normal. Conversely, secretion of fluid into the lumen increased progressively as pressure rose. They concluded that increased secretion is the primary cause of fluid loss and distention in intestinal obstruction, with decreased absorption playing a lesser role. Prostaglandin release in response to bowel distention is thought to be the mechanism by which secretion into obstructed loops is increased.

The bowel immediately above the obstruction is the most affected initially. It becomes distended with fluids and electrolytes, and circulation is impaired. With increasing intraluminal pressure the fluid is dispersed orad until it reaches bowel that is still capable of absorbing. When obstruction has been present for a long time, the proximal portions of the intestine also lose their ability to handle fluid and electrolytes, and the entire bowel proximal to the obstruction becomes distended.

A second route of fluid and electrolyte loss is into the wall of the involved bowel, accounting for the boggy edematous appearance of the bowel often seen at operation. Some of this fluid exudes from the serosal surface of the bowel, resulting in free peritoneal fluid. The extent of fluid and electrolyte loss into the bowel wall and peritoneal cavity depends on the extent of bowel involved in venous congestion and edema, and the length of time before the obstruction is relieved.

The most obvious route of fluid and electrolyte loss is by vomiting—or gastrointestinal tube after treatment is initiated. The aggregate of these losses (1) into the bowel lumen, (2) into the edematous bowel wall, (3) as free peritoneal fluid, and (4) by vomiting or nasogastric suction, rapidly depletes the extracellular fluid space, leading progressively to hemoconcentration, hypovolemia, renal insufficiency, shock, and death unless treatment is prompt and resolute. The blood chemistry values to be expected in intestinal obstruction will be found below under Clinical Manifestations.

Intestinal Gas. Much of the distention of the bowel above a mechanical obstruction can be accounted for by the fluid sequestered within the lumen. Intestinal gas is also responsible for distention.

The approximate composition of small intestine gas (Table 24-6) shows that the basic composition is that of

Table 24-6. INTESTINAL GAS

	Percent
Nitrogen	70
Oxygen	12
Carbon dioxide	8
Hydrogen sulfide	5
Ammonia and amines	4
Hydrogen	1

swallowed air to which small amounts of gases not found in the atmosphere have been added.

Gases are absorbed from the intestine at rates that are directly related to the partial pressure of the particular gas in the intestine, in the plasma, and in the air breathed. Thus with nitrogen there is little diffusion, since the partial pressures of the gas are virtually the same in intestine, plasma, and air. On the other hand carbon dioxide diffuses very rapidly, because the partial pressure of carbon dioxide is high in the intestine, intermediate in plasma, and very low in air. For this reason, though carbon dioxide is produced in large amounts in the intestine, it contributes little to gaseous distention because of its rapid diffusibility.

Bowel Motility. With obstruction of the lumen, peristalsis increases in an "attempt" to overcome the obstruction. After a short time, continuous peristalsis above the obstruction gives way to regularly recurring bursts of peristaltic activity interspersed with quiescent periods. The duration of the quiescent period is related to the level of the obstruction in the gastrointestinal tract—it is 3 to 5 min with high obstruction, 10 to 15 min with lower ileal obstruction. These muscular contractions may be of sufficient magnitude to traumatize the bowel and contribute to the swelling and edema of the bowel wall. As bowel above the obstruction distends, bowel below the obstruction becomes progressively more quiet. This results from an inhibitory reflex initiated by distention of the bowel above.

Strangulated Obstruction. Occlusion of the blood supply to a segment of bowel in addition to obstruction of the lumen is usually referred to as strangulated obstruction. Interference with the mesenteric blood supply is the most serious complication of intestinal obstruction. This frequently occurs secondary to adhesive band obstruction, hernia, and volvulus.

The accumulation of fluid and gas in obstructed loops and the altered motility seen in simple mechanical obstruction are rapidly overshadowed by the consequences of blockage of venous outflow from the strangulated segment—extravasation of bloody fluid into the bowel and bowel wall.

In addition to the loss of blood and plasma-like fluid, the gangrenous bowel leaks toxic materials (not to be confused with the pre-Gamble "toxins") into the peritoneal cavity. These have been variously identified as exotoxins or endotoxins, or toxic hemin breakdown products.

The pathophysiology of the strangulated loop is related to several factors: (1) that the contents of an obstructed bowel are toxic; (2) that bacteria are necessary for the production of this toxin; (3) that neither living tissue nor mucous membrane, nor any of the secretions of the mucous membrane, are necessary for the formation of the toxin; (4) that the toxin does not pass through normal mucosa; (5) that absorption of the toxin is more important than its production, as the toxin is physiologically lost if it exists within a loop and is never absorbed; (6) that circulatory damage aids absorption; and (7) that symptoms may be correlated with the toxin formed in the obstructed intestine.

Closed-Loop Obstruction. When both afferent and efferent limbs of a loop of bowel are obstructed, closed-loop intestinal obstruction exists. This is a clinically dangerous form of obstruction because of the propensity for rapid progression to strangulation of the blood supply before the usual manifestations of intestinal obstruction become obvious. Interference with blood supply may occur either from the same mechanism that produced obstruction of the intestine—twist of the bowel on the mesentery, extrinsic band—or from distention of the obstructed loop. The secretory pressure in the closed loop quite rapidly reaches a level sufficient to interfere with venous return from the loop. Widespread distention of the intestine usually does not occur, and so neither does abdominal distention.

Colon Obstruction. The effects on the patient with colon obstruction are usually less dramatic than the effects of small bowel obstruction. First, colon obstruction, with the exception of volvulus, usually does not strangulate. Second, because the colon is principally a storage organ with relatively minor absorptive and secretory functions, fluid and electrolyte sequestration progresses more slowly. Systemic derangements therefrom are of less magnitude and urgency than in small bowel obstruction.

Progressive distention is the most dangerous aspect of nonstrangulated colon obstruction. If the ileocecal valve is incompetent, then partial decompression of the obstructed colon may occur by reflux into the ileum. But if the ileocecal valve is competent, then the colon becomes essentially a closed loop—closed below by the obstructing lesion and above by the competent valve. If the obstruction is not relieved, distention progressing to rupture of the colon threatens. The cecum is the usual site of rupture, because it is the segment of the colon with the largest diameter. According to the law of Laplace, the pressure required to stretch the walls of a hollow viscus decreases in inverse proportion to the radius of curvature. Applying this law to the colon, given an equal pressure throughout the colon, we find that the greatest distention will occur in the portion of the colon with the largest radius (Fig. 24-3).

CLINICAL MANIFESTATIONS. The initial symptoms of simple mechanical intestinal obstruction are abdominal pain, vomiting, and failure to pass gas or feces by rectum. Abdominal distention is a later symptom.

As the bowel obstructs, severe *cramping pain* is felt synchronously with hyperperistalsis. Initially, the waves of cramps are unremitting, but after a short time attacks of pain alternate with quiescent periods during which the patient may feel quite well. The pain is diffuse, poorly localized, and is felt across the upper abdomen in high obstruction, at the level of the umbilicus in low ileal obstruction, in the lower abdomen in colon obstruction, and in the perineum as well as the abdomen in rectosigmoid obstruction. The period between attacks of pain is short with high intestinal obstruction (4 or 5 min) and is longer the lower the obstruction (15 to 20 min). When obstruction is not relieved, the characteristic colicky pain may cease (as distention becomes extreme) and be replaced by a steady generalized abdominal discomfort. There is no real pain in adynamic ileus, just a steady generalized ab-

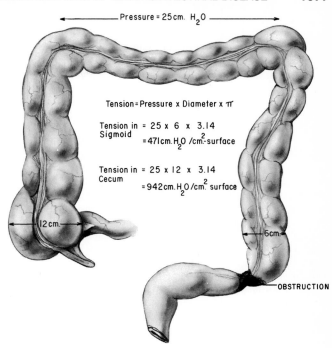

Fig. 24-3. Physics of cecal rupture in colon obstruction.

dominal discomfort similar to that seen in neglected simple mechanical obstruction. Steady severe pain with no quiescent periods is usually indicative of strangulation.

Vomiting, like pain, usually occurs almost immediately after obstruction of the bowel. This early vomiting is "reflex" vomiting and is followed by a variable quiescent period before vomiting resumes. The quiet interval is short in high obstruction but may even be a day or two with low small bowel obstruction. The vomitus associated with low obstruction frequently becomes thick, dark, and malodorous (i.e., feculent) from stagnation and bacterial action but is not actually regurgitated feces. With high obstruction, vomiting is more frequent and copious and may effectively decompress the obstructed bowel. With low small bowel obstruction, vomiting is less frequent and less productive; little decompression of bowel occurs, because of the excessive length of bowel that the regurgitated material must traverse and because segmentation of the boggy loops prevents regurgitation. Reflex vomiting is unusual in colon obstruction. Thus, vomiting does not occur in most cases until retrograde distention involves the small bowel. When the ileocecal valve is competent, small bowel distention and vomiting may not occur in colonic obstruction.

Failure to pass gas or feces (obstipation) through the rectum is a valuable diagnostic symptom. Gas and feces distal to the obstruction may pass through the rectum after obstruction occurs, however, particularly if the obstruction is high in the jejunum. Cramping pain followed shortly by explosive diarrhea often indicates partial intestinal obstruction.

Abdominal distention is the result of fairly long-standing obstruction. There may be no generalized distention with high small bowel obstruction.

Physical examination of a patient with simple mechanical obstruction within the first 24 h may yield surprisingly few abnormal findings except during periods of colicky pain. Vital signs are essentially normal, and dehydration and distention are not yet marked. Strangulated obstruction is likely if the patient appears seriously ill during this early period. *Palpation* during colic usually demonstrates muscle guarding; between attacks of pain only slight tenderness remains. A mass or localized area of tenderness usually indicates strangulation. *Auscultation* is of great value: in simple mechanical obstruction the abdomen is quiet except during attacks of colic, at which time the sounds become loud, high-pitched, and metallic and occur in bursts or rushes; in paralytic ileus an occasional isolated bowel sound is heard; gangrenous bowel produces complete silence. By the second or third day of obstruction serious illness is obvious. Dehydration and distention are marked, and vital signs are increasingly abnormal, though frank shock does not occur until very late in simple obstruction.

Laboratory Findings. The loss of large amounts of essentially isotonic extracellular fluid into the intestine is principally responsible for the laboratory findings in simple mechanical obstruction. The body responds to this sudden volume decrease by antidiuresis and renal sodium retention. In the early phases, in which the effects are predominantly those of extracellular fluid loss, the hematocrit rises roughly in proportion to the fluid loss. There is little change in the concentration of sodium, potassium, and chloride in the plasma. Acid-base changes, as manifested by the pH and carbon dioxide level, are slight. The markedly reduced urine flow is reflected in a somewhat elevated BUN level. The dehydration and antidiuresis is often so marked that patients may not be able to produce a urine specimen until after intravenous fluid therapy has been started. Urinary specific gravity of 1.025 to 1.030 is the rule; mild proteinuria or acetonuria may also be present.

In the untreated patient, sodium-free water, derived from catabolism of cells and oxidation of fat, tends to restore the acute loss of extracellular fluid volume but at the expense of plasma osmolality. Thus, there is a gradual reduction of the plasma sodium and chloride concentration. Urine volume gradually increases, though not to normal, with excretion of potassium, including the potassium freed by cellular catabolism. The previously noted progressive increase in the hematocrit is halted or actually reversed by the ingress of endogenous water. Acid-base effects are determined by the nature of the fluid lost. Metabolic acidosis due to the combined effects of dehydration, starvation, ketosis, and loss of alkaline secretions is most common. Metabolic alkalosis is infrequent and is principally due to loss of highly acid gastric juice. With great distention of the abdomen, the diaphragm may be sufficiently elevated to embarrass respiration, resulting in carbon dioxide retention and respiratory acidosis.

The white blood cell count is useful in differentiating between different types of obstruction. In general, simple mechanical obstruction calls forth only modest numbers of leukocytes—white blood cell counts often to 15,000/mm^3 with some shift to the left. White blood cell counts of 15,000 to 25,000/mm^3 and marked polymorphonuclear predominance with many immature forms strongly suggest that the obstruction is strangulated, but this is not a sensitive indicator. Very high white cell counts, such as 40,000 to 60,000/mm^3, suggest primary mesenteric vascular occlusion.

Serum amylase level elevations may occur in intestinal obstruction and compromise the differential diagnostic value of the test. Amylase gains entry to the blood by regurgitation from the pancreas because of back pressure in the duodenum, or by peritoneal absorption after leakage from dying bowel. Recently a prospective evaluation of the classic signs of vascular compromise were evaluated. No preoperative clinical parameter, including the presence of continuous abdominal pain, fever, peritoneal signs, leukocytosis, acidosis, hyperamylasemia, or any combination of these were sensitive indicators. The preoperative assessment of the presence or absence of strangulation was correct in only 70 percent of cases.

Radiologic Findings. When properly done, this is the most important diagnostic procedure. The films must be of good technical quality—not the type that are made in the emergency room by a substitute technician with a portable x-ray machine.

X-rays should be made as early in the hospitalization as the patient's condition permits—usually within the first hour. Plain films of the abdomen (without contrast medium) in the supine and upright positions, and posteroanterior and lateral views of the chest are obtained. If the patient is too weak to remain in the sitting position for the 15 min that is necessary to demonstrate air under the diaphragm (best seen on the posteroanterior chest film), then a left lateral decubitus film may be substituted.

The diagnostic features that enable one to distinguish in the majority of cases between simple mechanical obstruction and paralytic ileus are summarized in Table 24-7. Representative films of the three types of obstruction are shown in Fig. 24-4.

Gas-fluid levels are among the important criteria in the x-ray diagnosis of intestinal obstruction. Gas is normally visible in the colon and stomach on plain films of the abdomen in normal adults. Small bowel gas may be visible in infants and occasionally in apparently normal adults. The transit time of swallowed air is normally so rapid that there is an insufficient amount in any one place to show on the x-ray. But if the normal aboral progression of intestinal content is interfered with, then gas collects along with retained fluid and produces gas-fluid levels that are best seen on the upright film of the abdomen. Though gas-fluid levels are highly suggestive of intestinal obstruction (including ileus), they may be seen in other conditions such as extreme aerophagia, gastroenteritis, severe constipation, and sprue.

Barium enema is indicated when the clinical picture and plain films suggest colon obstruction, to give information on the type and location of the obstruction. Barium enema is often helpful also when the distribution of

Table 24-7. RADIOLOGIC SIGNS IN INTESTINAL OBSTRUCTION

Sign	Simple mechanical obstruction (see Fig. 24-4A, B)	Adynamic ileus (see Fig. 24-4C)
Gas in intestine	Large bow-shaped loops in ladder pattern	Copious gas diffusely through intestine
Gas in colon	Less than normal	Increased, scattered through colon
Fluid levels in intestine	Definite	Often very large throughout
Tumor	None	None
Peritoneal exudate	None	Present with peritonitis; otherwise absent
Diaphragm	Somewhat elevated; free motion	Elevated; diminished motion

SOURCE: From Eisenberg RL: *Gastrointestinal Radiology.* Philadelphia, Lippincott, 1983, with permission.

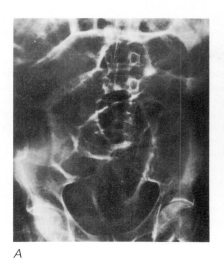
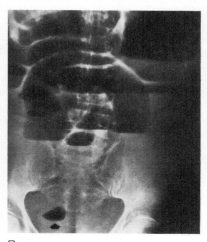
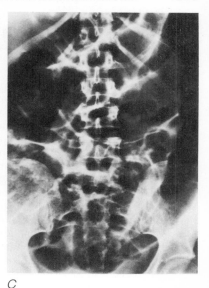

A   *B*

C

Fig. 24-4. *A.* Supine and *B.* upright views demonstrate large amounts of gas in dilated loops of small bowel, but only a single, small collection of gas (arrow) in the colon. *C.* Large amounts of gas and fluid are retained in loops of dilated small and large bowel. The entire small and large bowel appears almost uniformly dilated, with no demonstrable point of obstruction. (From: *Eisenberg RL: Gastrointestinal Radiology. Philadelphia, Lippincott, 1983, p 420, Fig. 33-10, with permission.*)

Fig. 24-5. The antegrade administration of barium demonstrates the precise site of small bowel obstruction. A radiolucent gallstone (arrow) is causing the distal ileal obstruction. (From: *Eisenberg RL: Gastrointestinal Radiology. Philadelphia, Lippincott, 1983, p 420, Fig. 33-13, with permission.*)

gas is not clear on the plain films. Barium enema may be used therapeutically for attempted reduction of nonstrangulated intussusception in children. The dangers of barium enema in obstruction are the possibility of perforating an inflammatory lesion such as diverticulitis or appendicitis and, second, changing a partial colon obstruction to a complete one by forcing barium up past a partially obstructing lesion to form an obstructing concentration of inspissated barium.

Intravenous urography may be indicated to look for ureteral calculi, which often produce marked paralytic ileus.

The principal indication for administration of contrast medium above an obstruction is to differentiate postoperative ileus from mechanical obstruction (Fig. 24-5). The actual point of obstruction rarely can be demonstrated because of dilution of the contrast medium, but if some medium is seen to go through the gastrointestinal tract, the diagnosis of ileus is strengthened. Some surgeons are loath to give barium above an obstruction and prefer to use a liquid medium such as Gastrografin. There is, however, little evidence that small amounts of barium are harmful in small bowel obstruction.

MANAGEMENT. The principles of treatment are fluid and electrolyte therapy, decompression of the bowel, and timed surgical intervention.

Essentially all patients with mechanical intestinal obstruction except those in the immediate postoperative period should be operated upon. The decision to be made is *when* to operate—selection of the optimal time for the individual patient.

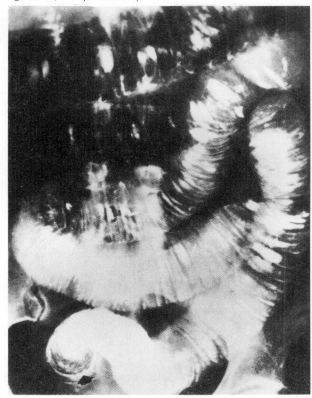

Patients with simple mechanical obstruction who can be operated upon within the first 24 h of the disease do not need extensive preoperative preparation, because water and salt depletion and distention are usually not serious at this stage. After the history and physical examination have established the presumptive diagnosis, laboratory studies should be done, intravenous repletion initiated, decompression started with a nasogastric sump tube in the stomach, and abdominal and chest x-ray films taken on the way to the operating room. This whole process should take less than 2 h. The mortality rate is less than 1 percent for patients with simple mechanical obstruction who are operated upon within the first 24 h.

If the obstruction has been present for more than 24 h when the patient is first seen, depletion and distention may be so severe that if strangulation or closed-loop obstruction seems unlikely, the patient's best interests are served by a period of preparation before the obstruction is surgically relieved. In general, the longer the obstruction has existed, the longer it will take to get the patient ready for surgical treatment. Patients with moderate derangements, particularly hypokalemia, usually require 6 to 12 h; in those with severe problems, up to 24 h may be necessary, mainly because of the hazard of giving intravenous potassium ion faster than it can equilibrate.

With the possible exception of patients with early simple mechanical obstruction, all patients with intestinal obstruction should have a plastic venous catheter threaded into the superior vena cava for frequent measurements of the central venous pressure (CVP), as well as for rapid administration of fluid, and an indwelling catheter inserted into the bladder for accurate continual measurement of the urinary output.

The initial hematocrit reading may be used to estimate the extent of extracellular fluid loss, and thus the volume necessary for restoration of this static debt. For example, if the hematocrit has risen to 55 percent, this indicates a loss of approximately 40 percent of the plasma and extracellular fluid volume.

If acid gastric juice loss is prominent, then normal saline solution is used; otherwise lactated Ringer's solution and 5% dextrose in water in about equal proportions are preferred to replace the lost fluid and to cover maintenance fluid needs. Potassium chloride also will be necessary but should not be given until a good urinary output is established. Antibiotics should also be given in generous dosage and may be added to the intravenous fluids. The choice of antibiotics is a matter of individual preference: the authors currently use ampicillin-gentamycin-clindamycin, or metronidazole with a third-generation cephalosporin.

The rate of fluid administration is best controlled by monitoring the CVP. Fluids may be given rapidly as long as the CVP remains below 10 to 12 cmH$_2$O. The end point of volume replacement is indicated by a sudden rise in the CVP. Other guides are return of skin turgor and the hourly rate of urine production.

The goal in terms of electrolyte concentration and acid-base balance is restoration of these to, or close to, the normal range by the time the volume deficit has been repaired. This is usually possible in patients with reasonably normal renal and pulmonary functions.

When the possibility of strangulation exists, preoperative treatment to fluid-electrolyte normality is not possible or advisable. This is an emergency situation requiring vigorous preparation with fluids and electrolytes, massive antibiotics, nasogastric suction, and an operation at the earliest possible moment to remove the cause of the strangulation and/or nonviable bowel. Despite application of these principles, the mortality rate in strangulated obstruction is still about 25 percent.

Intubation. Tubes for gastrointestinal aspiration, available in bewildering variety, are basically of but two types: "short" tubes for gastric aspiration and "long" tubes for aspiration of the small intestine. The Levin tube, for nasogastric intubation, is preferred by many surgeons for preoperative gastrointestinal decompression in patients with obstruction. Complete decompression of the gastrointestinal tract is not accomplished, since only the intestinal gas and fluid from the upper intestine that regurgitates into the stomach is removed. The stomach is completely emptied, however, which prevents any possible aspiration during anesthesia, and progression of intestinal distention is halted, since all swallowed air is removed. Nasogastric tubes with a double lumen, one for aspiration plus a small second channel to allow ingress of air into the stomach—the sump tube—perform much more efficiently than the old single-lumen tubes.

Long intestinal tubes, of which the Miller-Abbott tube is the prototype, have a lumen for aspiration plus a mercury-containing balloon or small bag at or near the distal end. When inflated in the intestine, the balloon is carried distad by peristalsis. The purpose of the mercury is to aid in getting the tube through the pylorus. After the tube is passed into the stomach, the patient lies on his right side with feet slightly elevated, so that gravity will help pull the tip of the tube through the pylorus.

There is now good evidence that the use of suction as definitive therapy (except as noted below) should be condemned—temporizing may lead to death from strangulated obstruction. The principal indications now for primary intubation therapy are obstruction in the immediate postoperative period, partial small bowel obstruction, or obstruction due to inflammation that is expected to subside under conservative therapy. Some surgeons prefer to use a long intestinal tube for preoperative gastrointestinal decompression in patients with obstruction, feeling that decompression of the intestine per se is sufficiently important to warrant the extra time and trouble necessary to pass an intestinal tube as compared to the Levin nasogastric tube. Emptying of the stomach is inadequate with the long tube, however, and a second short tube is required for this purpose.

Operation. Proper timing of the operation for intestinal obstruction is essential. There are four types of obstruction in which the operation should be done as an emergency as soon as possible after admission: strangulation, closed-loop obstruction, colon obstruction, and early simple mechanical obstruction.

The principal hazard to life in strangulation is septic

shock from transperitoneal absorption of toxins spilled from dying bowel. In closed-loop obstruction, which cannot be decompressed by intubation, the hazard is that the loop will strangulate, and it must be treated with the same urgency as strangulation.

In colon obstruction, which also cannot be decompressed by tube, a competent ileocecal valve preventing regurgitation into the ileum converts the colon into a closed loop. Since fluid and electrolyte abnormalities progress slowly in colon obstruction, a brief period of hydration while laboratory studies are being done is all that is necessary before operation. And, as noted above, when patients with simple mechanical obstruction get to the surgeon early in the course of their disease, immediate surgical procedures may be carried out with essentially no mortality. Thus only in *late* simple mechanical obstruction of the small intestine does extensive preparation for operation take priority over immediate operation.

Anesthesia. General anesthesia is safest for the patient and the method of choice from the point of view of both surgeon and anesthesiologist. Endotracheal intubation, at times performed initially under local anesthesia, is particularly indicated to prevent aspiration of regurgitated gastric content. The surgeon should not be tempted to use local anesthesia for abdominal exploration on the assumption that local anesthesia is easier on the poor-risk patient than general anesthesia—it is not. Local anesthesia should be used only when the surgeon knows the cause of the obstruction and plans a limited procedure only, such as cecostomy.

Surgical Procedures. Surgical procedures for the relief of intestinal obstruction may be divided into five categories:

1. Procedures not requiring opening of bowel—lysis of adhesions, manipulation-reduction of intussusception, reduction of incarcerated hernia
2. Enterotomy for removal of obturation obstruction—gallstone, bezoars
3. Resection of the obstructing lesion or strangulated bowel with primary anastomosis
4. Short-circuiting anastomosis around an obstruction
5. Formation of a cutaneous stoma proximal to the obstruction—cecostomy, transverse colostomy (Figs. 24-6 and 24-7).

On opening the peritoneum, the presence or absence of free peritoneal fluid should be noted, as well as the appearance of the fluid. Bloody fluid denotes strangulation, whereas clear straw-colored fluid is found with simple obstruction. The point of obstruction is usually best found by starting in the right lower quadrant. If the cecum is grossly distended, the obstruction is in the colon. If collapsed small bowel is found, then this is followed back to the point of obstruction, thus avoiding evisceration of the proximal distended loops.

The surgeon is sometimes faced with the difficult decision of whether to resect or to replace in the abdomen a loop of intestine of questionable viability. Before release the strangulated loop of viable bowel has a dull purple-red appearance and is devoid of motion. After release there is a dramatic color change to bright red in the obviously viable loop as well as a return of peristalsis. Conversely,

in obviously dead bowel there is no color change and no motion after release of the strangulating obstruction. The loop that only partially pinks up and has little or no motion is the problem. It is usually best to wrap the questionable segment in moist laparotomy pads and leave it completely undisturbed for 10 min by the clock. If the circulation is obviously better at the end of this time, the loop is replaced in the abdomen. If the viability of the segment is still in doubt, resection should be done. Fluorescein staining and Doppler evaluations have been used to distinguish between viable and dead bowel, but results are not consistent. If a very long segment of bowel is involved, requiring a very extensive resection, then an attempt should be made to restore flow in the larger vessels supplying the segment. Even if this is unsuccessful, one should probably accept the risk of replacing nonviable bowel rather than make an intestinal cripple. The patient is observed very closely; if evidence of progressive toxicity develops, reoperation and resection are done. In any event, reexploration and reevaluation of the status of the bowel about 24 h later may be advisable.

Decompression of grossly distended intestine during the operative procedure is sometimes necessary, particularly in late simple mechanical obstruction. Operative decompression is still a contentious point. There is no doubt that the operation is facilitated: the site of obstruction is more easily found, the uncontrolled eventration of distended loops through the incision is avoided, the bowel can be returned to the peritoneal cavity without the kinks that may cause segmentation and postoperative obstruction, and closure of the incision is possible without a struggle. Relief of distention also improves the blood supply to the intestine, and peristalsis returns sooner. It is also probable that removal of toxic bowel content is worthwhile. Whereas the normal mucosa is impermeable to these toxins, permeability is affected by impairment of the blood supply, and absorption may occur in compromised bowel.

Operative aspiration can be done in a variety of ways. Multiple needle aspirations are ineffective and definitely increase the morbidity: studies have shown a wound infection rate of 20 percent versus a rate of 4 percent in a comparable group of patients without needle aspiration. Decompression with an ordinary suction tip through multiple enterotomies, though effective, is similarly attended by an increased infection rate, plus the risk of small bowel fistula. An effective, safe method of decompression is by passage of a tube from above downward, so that the entire gastrointestinal tract proximal to the obstruction is decompressed. A firm tube with generous lumen (Baker tube) is introduced through a proximal jejunostomy. It may be preferable to pass the tube transnasally or through a gastrostomy and thread it into the small intestine. The tube is advanced by manipulation through the intact bowel until the entire length of involved bowel down to the obstructed segment is pleated on the long tube. The tube is secured in that position for postoperative decompression.

Postoperative Care. The principles of postoperative care are the same as for the preoperative preparation of the

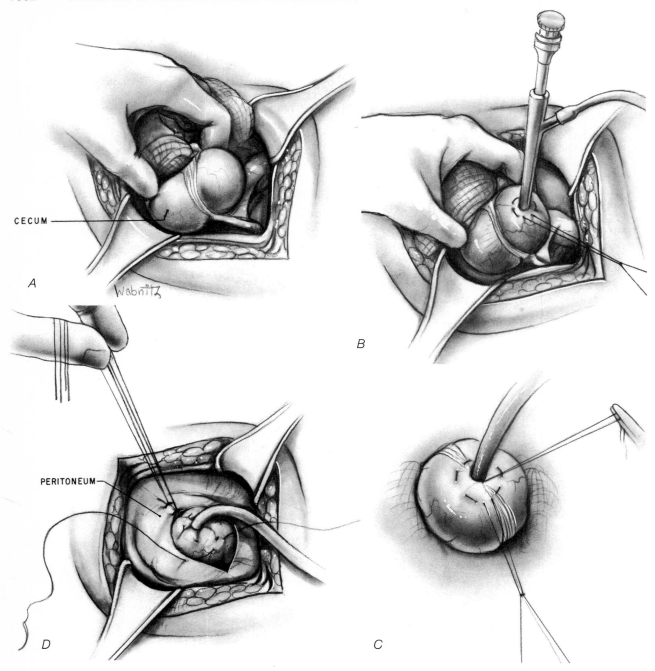

CECUM

A

Wabnitz

B

PERITONEUM

D

C

Fig. 24-6. Tube cecostomy. *A.* A McBurney incision is made in the right lower quadrant, the lateral peritoneal attachment of the cecum is divided, and the cecum is delivered into the wound, using a dry sponge. *B.* The distended cecum is held by the assistant, using gauze sponges, while the surgeon decompresses the cecum with a large trocar connected to suction. If distention is not great, this step may be omitted. *C.* A large rubber tube is then placed in the cecum by enlarging the opening made by the trocar, and the tube is secured in place with two concentric purse-string sutures. *D.* The peritoneum is sutured circumferentially to the cecum. Fascia is approximated; skin and subcutaneous tissues are packed open. The tube is connected to straight drainage.

patient with obstruction—fluids and electrolytes, antibiotics, and gastrointestinal decompression.

Fluid and electrolyte management is more difficult in the postoperative intestinal obstruction patient than in the usual postoperative abdominal surgical patient because of the large third space of sequestered, isotonic fluid. There is continued loss in the immediate postoperative period into the sequestered fluid space. This loss slows in rate, however, and is reversed in direction after a variable pe-

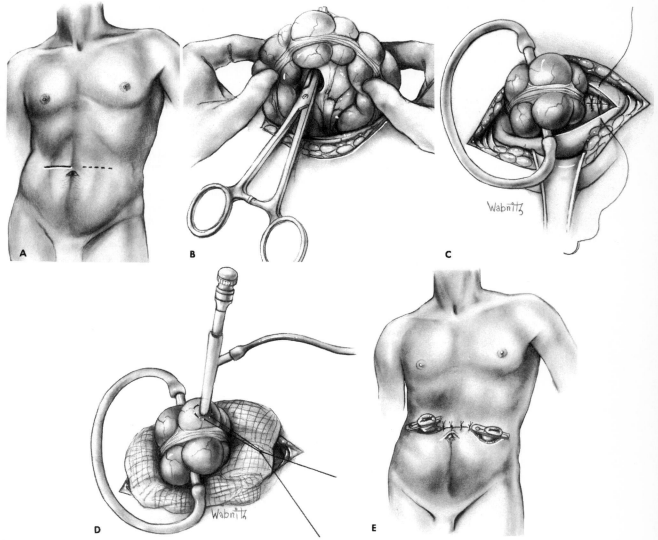

Fig. 24-7. Transverse loop colostomy. *A.* A short transverse incision is made about midway between costal margin and umbilicus. Choice of right or left depends on the type of definitive surgical treatment planned for the future. *B.* After freeing the omentum, an opening is made in an avascular area of the transverse mesocolon close to the bowel. *The middle colic artery must be avoided. C.* A glass rod is inserted through the mesentery and secured in place by rubber tubing. The incision is closed in layers about the colon loop. No sutures are placed in the colon. *D.* If colon distention is extreme, trocar decompression may be done immediately after closing the incision. Otherwise the colostomy is opened with cautery about 24 to 36 h after operation. *E.* Double-barrel colostomy may be performed initially using deMartel's clamps. A small catheter can be inserted into the proximal limb to achieve immediate decompression.

riod, usually about the third postoperative day. This large autoinfusion, as fluid is picked up by the vascular compartment from the sequestered fluid, must be allowed for in planning the daily ration of intravenous fluid therapy, lest the patient be watered into congestive failure. Serum sodium and potassium levels must be watched very closely and kept in the normal range. A deficit of either or both of these ions is associated with prolonged paralysis of the gastrointestinal tract.

Decompression of the gastrointestinal tract is also harder to handle than in the usual postoperative patient, because restoration of normal propulsive intestinal motility is usually significantly delayed after release of intestinal obstruction. Whereas bowel function usually resumes on about the third day after abdominal operation, after intestinal obstruction it is often 5 or 6 days before gastrointestinal decompression can be discontinued. After 2 or 3 days of suction drainage it is often advisable to discontinue the suction and vent the intestinal tube to straight drainage only, to minimize fluid and electrolyte losses. This also obviates the problem of bleeding from ''tube ulcers'' that form when the mucosa is suctioned into the side vents.

Ileus

Ileus may be divided into three groups: *adynamic, or inhibition, ileus,* in which there is diminished or absent motility because of inhibition of the neuromuscular apparatus; *spastic ileus,* in which the bowel musculature remains tightly contracted without coordinated propulsive motility; and the *ileus of vascular occlusion,* in which the bowel wall is incapable of coordinated motility, because it is dying from ischemia.

Spastic ileus, an uncommon form caused by uncoordinated hyperactivity of the intestine, is seen in heavy-metal poisoning, in porphyria, and sometimes in uremia. Therapy of the intestinal manifestations is usually not indicated—therapy should be aimed at the underlying disorder.

Adynamic ileus of some degree is extremely common, since it occurs after every abdominal operation. The rate of recovery of motor function is different in different segments of the gastrointestinal tract: small bowel motility returns within 24 h and gastric motility within 48 h, but colonic inertia persists for 3 to 5 days. Oral intake usually can be resumed on the third or fourth postoperative day. Only when postoperative ileus persists does it become a clinical problem. Common causes of serious degrees of inhibition ileus are many and varied and include intraperitoneal inflammations such as acute appendicitis or acute pancreatitis; retroperitoneal pathologic conditions such as ureteral colic, retroperitoneal hematoma, or fracture of the spine; thoracic lesions such as basal pneumonia or fractured ribs; and systemic causes such as severe toxemia, hyponatremia, hypokalemia, or hypomagnesemia. Several drugs have also been implicated. These include: morphine, propantheline, antacids, anticoagulants, phenothiazines, and ganglionic blocking agents.

Overactivity of the sympathetic system appears to be the common denominator in inhibition ileus associated with many of the lesions listed above; alterations in the composition of the internal environment also play an important role.

Centrally induced inhibition of motility is virtually exclusively dependent on the hormonal component of the sympathoadrenal system. Pseudoobstruction of the colon may develop as a result of inhibition of the sacral parasympathetic nerves.

CLINICAL MANIFESTATIONS. The primary disease causing the ileus may predominate in the clinical picture, or conversely, in some cases, abdominal findings may so predominate that the primary process is overlooked. In postoperative ileus, the division between physiologic ileus and the undue abnormal prolongation of bowel hypofunction is blurred. Instead of passing flatus and becoming hungry on about the third day, as expected following abdominal operation, the patient is noted to be distended and disinterested in food and surroundings. Examination confirms that there is generalized abdominal distention with tympany and scattered, occasional bowel sounds.

Assistance from the laboratory is needed mainly in evaluating some of the causes of ileus, such as acute anemia, sepsis, hyponatremia, hypokalemia, and hypoosmolarity.

As outlined above (Table 24-7 and Fig. 24-4), x-ray can often help in the differential diagnosis between postoperative adynamic ileus and postoperative mechanical obstruction. If the plain films are inconclusive, contrast medium is given by mouth or through a gastrointestinal tube. In inhibition ileus, some medium should reach the cecum in about 4 h, whereas a stationary column of medium for 3 or 4 h indicates complete obstruction of the small intestine.

Adynamic ileus characteristically involves both the small and large bowel to a greater or lesser degree. Occasionally, there is marked distention confined largely to the colon without evidence of mechanical obstruction of the bowel itself or interference with its blood supply—this is known as pseudoobstruction of the colon or Ogilvie's syndrome. Barium enema is indicated to rule out organic obstruction. Cecal perforation may occur even though mechanical intestinal obstruction is absent.

TREATMENT. The treatment of ileus is essentially the treatment of the primary lesion. Postoperative ileus is caused in the vast majority of patients either by focal inflammation—leaking anastomosis, abscess following contamination—or by gross fluid-electrolyte derangements. When these problems are promptly eradicated, the ileus will take care of itself.

Treatment of the distention is best done by passage of a long tube. Unfortunately it is much more difficult to pass than in mechanical obstruction because of the difference in motility of the intestine. If the long tube will not pass the pylorus, then gastric suction should be used and will prevent further distention.

Nonoperative methods of increasing gastrointestinal motility continue to be evaluated. Gastrointestinal pacing by means of an electrode in the tip of the nasogastric tube through which physiologic electric currents are delivered appears to be of little value. Similarly, injections of D-pantothenyl alcohol (a component of coenzyme A that is necessary for the production of acetylcholine) have been shown to be ineffective in postoperative ileus.

Vasopressin, which causes contraction of smooth muscle, and parasympathomimetic drugs such as neostigmine or Urecholine will often increase intestinal motility but are not safe to use, because perforation of the bowel can result if there is mechanical obstruction. Metoclopramide, a dopamine antagonist derived from procainamide, enhances gastrointestinal motility without causing spasm, and has been used extensively in Europe for postoperative ileus. No convincing advantage over placebo can be shown in double-blind studies, however.

Rarely, paralytic ileus does not respond to conservative measures—the obstruction does not relent, and operation must be considered. In most such cases, mechanical obstruction will be found. If no mechanical factors are found, a long tube should be manipulated by the surgeon well down into the small bowel. If the ileocecal valve is competent and marked colon distention is present, then cecostomy should be added. The ileus will be made worse by the operation but can now be managed with adequate decompression. Nonobstructive colon dilation is best managed by colonoscopy.

Pseudoobstruction

Recently a group of patients has been identified that has manifestations of bowel obstruction but no organic lesion. Although the entire gastrointestinal tract is involved, the disorder usually presents with symptoms and signs related to the small intestine. The symptoms are generally intermittent and extend over years. Vomiting that relieves the abdominal pain is characteristic. Distention may be marked. The pseudoobstruction may be caused by an hereditary hollow visceral myopathy. Diabetes mellitus, hypothyroidism, pheochromocytosis, hypoparathyroidism, dermatomyositis, lupus erythematosus, myotonic dystrophy, parkinsonism, multiple sclerosis, and amyloidosis have been associated causes. Esophageal manometry is useful for screening and the mecholyl test is positive for patients who have pseudoobstruction. Treatment of underlying diabetes, collagen vascular disease, or amyloidosis does not relieve the pseudoobstruction.

GASTROINTESTINAL BLEEDING: HEMATEMESIS, MELENA, AND RECTAL BLEEDING

Bleeding may be a manifestation of a variety of diseases along the entire length of the gastrointestinal tract from the oropharynx to the anus. Bleeding represents the initial symptom of gastrointestinal disease in more than one-third of these patients, and in 70 percent there is no history of a previous bleeding episode.

DEFINITIONS. *Hematemesis* refers to the vomiting of blood that is either fresh and unaltered or digested by gastric secretion. It is a manifestation of a bleeding site located between the oropharynx and the ligament of Treitz and may be accompanied by simultaneous melena. The character of the specimen depends on the site of bleeding, the rate of hemorrhage, and the rate of gastric emptying. The presence of blood clots reflects massive bleeding, while a coffee-ground vomitus usually indicates a slower bleeding rate with retention in the stomach and alteration of the blood to form acid hematin.

Melena is usually defined as the passage of a black, tarry stool. Only 50 mL of blood is necessary to produce this sign, and, following the cessation of a bleeding of 1000 mL, the finding may persist for as long as 5 days. A guaiac-positive stool, indicative of occult blood, may persist for 3 weeks following hematemesis or melena. In general, blood from the distal colon is red and not thoroughly mixed with the stool, whereas blood from the upper gastrointestinal tract produces a tarry stool. However, massive bleeding from the upper gastrointestinal tract may be associated with red or currant jelly clots if the bleeding is rapid and gastrointestinal motility is increased. Red or black stools may also result from the ingestion of food dye substances and iron. The tarry color, which accom-

panies upper gastrointestinal bleeding, is attributable to the production of acid hematin by action of gastric acid on the hemoglobin or the production of sulfide from heme by the action of hydrogen sulfide on the iron in the heme molecule. Melena without hematemesis generally indicates a lesion distal to the pylorus but has been associated with bleeding varices and gastritis.

CONSEQUENCES OF GASTROINTESTINAL BLEEDING. Hypotension and shock are dependent upon the rate of the bleeding and the patient's response to the blood loss. It is difficult to estimate the amount of blood loss in either the vomitus or stool, because both specimens contain a mixture of multiple components. The hematocrit and hemoglobin levels are unreliable until equilibration occurs, i.e., 6 to 48 h subsequent to the bleeding, and estimations of blood volume have also proved unreliable, since the error associated with the technique is great and the range of normals for a given physical state is wide. Shortly after bleeding has begun, a vasovagal reaction is associated with bradycardia, whereas with the passage of time the heart rate increases and the cardiac output decreases. The clinical picture of shock may reflect a coronary occlusion or myocardial ischemia precipitated by hemorrhage rather than the consequences of massive blood loss per se. Another consequence of hypotension is reduced renal blood flow, resulting in either oliguria or anuria.

Azotemia, which is characteristically associated with bleeding esophagogastric varices, also occurs in patients with other types of massive hemorrhage. BUN levels of 30 mg/dL or more occur in two-thirds of patients with bleeding varices, and an elevation of 50 mg/dL or more occurs in one-fifth of the cases. Following cessation of the bleeding, normal levels are usually achieved within 3 days. Azotemia usually does not occur with hemorrhage originating in the colon, and since it is dependent upon bacterial action, normal BUN levels may be associated with upper gastrointestinal tract bleeding in patients on antibiotics that sterilize the intestinal flora. The level to which the BUN rises parallels the extent of gastrointestinal bleeding, but it may be potentiated by shock, impairment of renal function, and increased catabolism. In the presence of blood in the intestinal tract renal function can be evaluated by clearance studies.

Upper Gastrointestinal Tract Bleeding

ETIOLOGY. Although a great variety of lesions above the ligament of Treitz have been implicated in the cause of upper gastrointestinal tract hemorrhage, in the vast majority it is due to peptic ulceration, acute mucosal lesions—gastritis and erosions—esophagogastric varices, reflux esophagitis, or gastric neoplasms (Table 24-8).

Peptic ulceration represents the most common cause and accounts for one-half to two-thirds of the cases. Hemorrhage from a duodenal ulcer occurs four times more frequently than from a gastric ulcer, but since this represents the relative incidence of the two lesions, the two types have an equal tendency to bleed. Massive bleeding occurs in 10 to 15 percent of ulcer patients with

Table 24-8. ETIOLOGY OF UPPER GASTROINTESTINAL TRACT BLEEDING IN 14,265 CASES

Author	Year	Number of cases	Peptic ulcer, %	Acute mucosal lesions, %	Esophageal varices, %	Reflex esophagitis, %	Gastric cancer, %	Other, %	Undetermined, %
Ferguson	1962	1124	62	4	7	1	4	1	20
Hirschowitz	1963	216	58	22	1	1	1	5	12
Dorsey	1965	405	68	2	2	3		5	20
Jones	1970	4131	58	26	3	2	3	6	3
Katz	1970	800	24	33	17			10	16
Palmer	1970	1400	45	12	19	8		11	7
Schiff	1970	640	53	1	13	2	2	8	21
Halmagyi	1970	199	65	1	7	6	1	15	5
Preston	1970	535	50	2	30			7	17
Schiller	1970	2149	45	3	2		2	22	26
Foster	1971	296	67	13	9		3	4	4
Crook	1972	880	50	19	11	3	2	5	4
Himal	1978	964	62	16	7			3	11
Dronfield	1982	526	49	5	2	6	3	8	27
Average			52	14	8	2	2	8	14

hemorrhage and is the first symptom in 16 percent of the patients who bleed. The bleeding is generally caused by the inflammatory process eroding into the regional artery. In the case of duodenal ulcers, the gastroduodenal artery is involved, while the left and right gastric arteries and their branches are most frequently involved with gastric ulcers. Most bleeding ulcers are chronic lesions, and the adjacent arteries suffer from local inflammatory changes. Since hemostasis is dependent upon the retraction of the walls of the vessel, persistent bleeding is more likely to occur with chronic lesions and in older patients with atherosclerotic vessels.

Peptic ulceration of the stomal mucosa at the site of a gastroenterostomy is to be considered in any patient who has had previous gastric surgical treatment. It is a more frequent occurrence when less than two-thirds of the stomach has been removed and an accompanying vagotomy has not been performed, especially if there is retained antrum.

The next most common cause of gross upper gastrointestinal tract hemorrhage after peptic ulcer is a diverse group of lesions that can best be collectively termed *acute mucosal lesions* until they are clearly delineated and separated into entities. The reported incidence (Table 24-8) ranges from 1 to 33 percent. The true incidence will not be known until endoscopy is universally applied early in the course of upper gastrointestinal tract hemorrhage. Pathologically, these lesions are sometimes single but more often multiple, or the mucosa may be diffusely involved in hemorrhagic necrosis. The process usually does not extend through the muscularis mucosae, and therefore the lesions are technically *erosions,* not true ulcers. In contradistinction to chronic benign ulcers, which are characteristically located in the antrum or on the lesser curvature, acute erosive lesions are found in the body and fundus of the stomach, sparing the antrum, and on the greater curvature as often as on the lesser curvature. "Tube ulcers," related to suction-drawing mucosa into the apertures of the nasogastric tube, may cause bleeding.

"Stress ulceration" is a much abused term, which, if used at all, should be confined to the acute gastroduodenal lesions that occur secondary to shock and sepsis following operation, trauma, or burns. McClelland et al. have shown in patients with trauma and hemorrhagic shock that gastric secretion is not increased but that splanchnic blood flow is significantly decreased. They conclude that "ischemic damage to the superficial gastric mucosa may induce stress ulceration." Sepsis also plays a prominent role. Upper gastrointestinal tract bleeding has been noted in approximately one-third of surgical patients with septicemia; coagulation abnormalities that attend sepsis have been implicated.

Probably closely related to stress erosion is the acute ulceration or erosion of the stomach and duodenum that occurs in burn patients. Such lesions are usually referred to as *Curling's ulcers,* after the man who described them in 1842. Curling's ulcers occur in about 12 percent of patients hospitalized for burns. The incidence increases with burn size—up to a 40 percent incidence in burns of 70 percent or more of the body surface. Sepsis is an additive stress. In two-thirds of patients with Curling's ulcer the presenting clinical sign is bleeding, and in 45 percent such bleeding is massive. Though there are many similarities between stress erosions and Curling's ulcers, their distribution is somewhat different: Curling's ulcers are about evenly divided between single and multiple, and between stomach and duodenum.

Another eponymic ulcer that is probably closely related to stress erosion is the *Cushing ulcer.* In 1932, Harvey Cushing described a variety of esophagogastroduodenal lesions in nine patients following craniotomy. Since then the belief has persisted that dysfunction in specific areas of the brain leads to gastrointestinal ulceration. In many of these patients, the etiologic factors are probably the same as for patients after any major operation, but there is some evidence that significant gastric hypersecretion may occur after certain intracranial operations or trauma.

Adrenal corticosteroids, given in large doses for prolonged periods, frequently lead to gastroduodenal erosions or ulcers, or to activation of preexisting quiescent peptic ulcers. Patients receiving steroids for rheumatoid arthritis or lupus erythematosus are more prone to this complication than patients with asthma or inflammatory bowel disease. Despite the fact that steroids do not increase the gastric acid output, antacid therapy is often efficacious. The distribution of "steroid ulcers" is much the same as that of postoperative "stress ulcers."

Aspirin and alcohol are the major offenders in a large group of ingested agents that may produce erosive, hemorrhagic gastritis and duodenitis. The incidence with which this lesion is diagnosed is directly related to the degree to which early endoscopic examination is employed. Alcohol is a known gastric secretagogue, but aspirin and similar agents are not; the latter presumably act by increasing back-diffusion of HCl through the gastric mucosa. The hemorrhage is generally mild to moderate but is sometimes massive. Since the gastric mucosa normally renews itself every 48 to 72 h, the process is self-limited if symptoms can be controlled until mucosal regeneration occurs. Emergency operation for exsanguinating hemorrhage is sometimes necessary.

Esophagogastric varices constitute the most common cause of bleeding in patients with cirrhosis or extrahepatic obstruction of the portal vein. These account for approximately 10 percent of all cases of upper gastrointestinal tract bleeding, but the incidence varies widely, being significantly higher in hospitals with a large indigent population. Bleeding varices constitute 95 percent of the cases of massive hematemesis in the child, and they are usually associated with extrahepatic obstruction of the portal vein. In cirrhotic patients, varices are the cause of bleeding in 53 percent of the cases, while gastritis is implicated in 22 percent and duodenal and gastric ulcers in 20 percent. Correlation of the lesions and severity of bleeding reveals that in the majority of cases (70 percent) patients with bleeding from varices have severe hemorrhage while 84 percent of patients with bleeding from gastritis demonstrate mild to moderate blood loss. The precipitation of the bleeding episode has been ascribed to two major factors: increased pressure within the varix and ulceration secondary to esophagitis. Although esophagogastric varices are almost always associated with portal hypertension, the diagnosis has been established in occasional patients with normal portal pressures. The veins responsible for the bleeding are usually opened laterally by transmural erosion, and any hemostasis that occurs is dependent upon occlusion of the opening by a thrombus. The bleeding is nearly always associated with hematemesis and is generally very profuse.

Hiatal hernia frequently may be associated with occult bleeding but is usually not a cause of gross upper gastrointestinal tract hemorrhage, accounting for approximately 2 percent of the cases. The bleeding in the sliding hernia is related to *reflux peptic esophagitis*. Bleeding is more commonly seen with paraesophageal hernias and is thought to be caused by the retention of acid contents within the incarcerated gastric pouch or congestion of the vascular supply of the herniated portion of the stomach.

A variety of miscellaneous lesions account for up to 8 percent of occasional upper gastrointestinal tract bleeding, while in 16 percent the diagnosis is never determined. Neoplasms are not commonly implicated, and there is evidence that the incidence of carcinoma of the stomach is decreasing in the United States. Bleeding associated with *gastric carcinoma* is caused by erosion of the tumor into underlying vessels. It is usually mild to moderate, but if a large vessel is involved, massive bleeding can occur. Massive hemorrhage may be the initial symptom in a patient with gastric carcinoma. Other tumors occur less frequently. Leiomyoma and leiomyosarcoma of the stomach or esophagus may be manifested by profuse bleeding, usually in men in the third decade of life. Leukemia with intestinal infiltrates may cause significant gastrointestinal bleeding. Also, polyps, either single, familial, or associated with the Peutz-Jeghers syndrome, are included as neoplastic lesions with a bleeding potential.

Vascular lesions, including angiomas, hereditary hemorrhagic telangiectasia (Rendu-Osler-Weber syndrome), and vasculitis, have all been reported as etiologic factors in upper gastrointestinal tract bleeding. Spontaneous rupture of aortic, hepatic arterial, and splenic arterial aneurysms into the gastrointestinal tract may produce alarming bleeding. Characteristically, aortoenteric fistula is manifested by moderate bleeding that stops for a variable period of time only to recur as massive bleeding.

Inflammation of the mucosa with erosion of small or large vessels may accompany prolapsing gastric mucosa and duodenal diverticula. Prolapsing gastric mucosa, which is usually not considered a common source of bleeding, may be accompanied by moderate blood loss. Similarly, although duodenal diverticula are generally considered to be asymptomatic, massive hemorrhage has accompanied ulceration of this lesion. Hepatic trauma with development of a central or subcapsular hematoma that discharges into the biliary tree is responsible for the development of the syndrome known as *hematobilia,* which can represent a cause of moderate or massive bleeding. Hematobilia can also occur with cholecystitis, cholelithiasis, and passage of stones. The interval between trauma and the bleeding manifestation is variable. Another traumatic cause of upper gastrointestinal tract bleeding is the Mallory-Weiss syndrome, which consists of linear tears of the esophagogastric junction induced by severe vomiting, usually in alcoholic patients.

DIAGNOSIS. History and Physical Examination. The patient's own account of the amount of bleeding is frequently misleading. Vomiting of large amounts of blood is most suggestive of bleeding ulcer or esophagogastric varices. A history of active ulcer symptoms preceding the hemorrhage with cessation of the pain at the onset of bleeding suggests that the bleeding is originating from a peptic ulcer. Twenty percent of patients with bleeding have no previous history of ulcer. Although there is an increased incidence of the ulcer diathesis in cirrhotic patients, esophagogastric varices represent the most common cause of bleeding in these patients and account for over 50 percent of the bleeding episodes. Violent retching and vomiting in alcoholics or pregnant women is characteristic of Mallory-Weiss syndrome. The history should include questions directed toward the recent ingestion of drugs implicated as causes of gastrointestinal bleeding, particularly salicylates, phenylbutazone (Butazolidin), alcohol, anticoagulants, and steroids. A history regarding the bleeding tendency during childhood, in early adulthood, and in other members of the family focuses on the possibility of hematologic disorders. Previous gastric surgical treatment such as gastroenterostomy or partial gastrectomy directs one's thinking toward the possibility of a marginal ulcer. Heartburn, epigastric substernal pain accentuated by the recumbent position and the ingestion of large meals, suggests the presence of a hiatal hernia. A recent history of upper abdominal or chest trauma is most compatible with a diagnosis of hematobilia, particularly when the bleeding is accompanied by jaundice and intermittent colicky pain.

Examination of the patient with upper gastrointestinal tract bleeding is directed at uncovering stigmata of the various diseases considered in the etiology. The skin and mucous membranes should be examined for icterus, spider angiomas, liver palms, and decreased hair over the extremities, all suggestive of hepatic disease. The mucous membrane should be investigated for melanin spots of the Peutz-Jeghers syndrome. Hereditary telangiectasia lesions are most common on the lips, tongue, and ears. Lymphadenopathy, particularly in the left supraclavicular region, may suggest a malignant intraabdominal process. Abdominal palpation more commonly reveals tenderness when the bleeding is related to ulcer or gastritis, whereas a palpable liver, particularly when accompanied by splenomegaly and abdominal veins that fill in a centrifugal pattern from the umbilicus, is more indicative of bleeding varices. Examination should always include aspiration via nasogastric tube in order to determine presence of blood at this level and the extent of bleeding at the time of examination.

Special Diagnostic Procedures. The extent of anemia may be assessed by the hematocrit level. It should be appreciated that, with acute blood loss, the initial level may be normal, since the hematocrit reduction does not occur for 4 to 6 h, during which time equilibration occurs. Repeat hematocrit readings taken at 4- to 6-h intervals are more meaningful. Leukocytosis, with levels of 25,000/mm^3, may accompany acute hemorrhage, but more marked increases are suggestive of leukemia. Both the neutrophils and platelets may be reduced in the case of hypersplenism secondary to primary hepatic disease, suggesting bleeding from esophagogastric varices.

Clinical chemistries are directed toward evaluating the extent of bleeding and, particularly, determining the presence of hepatocellular dysfunction. None of the tests define the site of bleeding. A rise in the BUN level parallels the extent of hemorrhage and is related to the absorption of blood products from the gastrointestinal tract, possible associated reduction in renal flow secondary to shock or dehydration, and, at times, the presence of preexisting renal disease. In the presence of marked hepatic dysfunction, the BUN level may not be elevated, since the liver is unable to synthesize urea. In this circumstance, the blood ammonia level is frequently elevated with bleeding varices, since it is related to the extent of portal collateralization and reduced hepatic function. The validity of this test, however, is not uniform. Normal values may be present in patients with variceal bleeding.

Determination of the blood clotting factors is of great importance, particularly in patients bleeding from stress ulceration. Reduced platelet adhesiveness, thrombocytopenia, prolonged prothrombin time, and other clotting defects are common in such patients. The bleeding often stops, obviating emergency operation, following the administration of fresh platelet infusions, vitamin K, and fresh-frozen plasma.

Rarely, bleeding is so rapid that immediate operation without preoperative diagnostic procedures is necessary to save life. More commonly, transfusions can easily allow time for diagnosis and preparation; further, many patients stop bleeding soon after admission. As the above tests are being done, the patient should be rapidly transfused to circulatory normality, with vital signs, central venous pressure, and urinary output as guides. The stomach should be completely evacuated using iced Ringer's lavage through a nasogastric tube; an Ewald tube may be advisable initially if many large clots are present.

Endoscopy is the first special diagnostic procedure to be considered; it is virtually mandatory if the bleeding is thought to be from esophagogastric varices or from an acute mucosal lesion. Esophagoscopy defines the bleeding point in the case of varices, since liver function tests, manometry, barium x-ray, and isotopic studies merely indicate the presence of portal hypertension or varices but do not determine if these lesions are actually bleeding. The reported esophagoscopic accident rate is 0.25 percent, and an experienced endoscopist is required. A 33 percent disagreement rate between two experienced endoscopists evaluating a given group of patients is reported. This is related to the difficulty in differentiating varices from mucosal folds. Gastroduodenoscopy with fiberoptic instruments is particularly valuable in revealing acute gastritis, erosions, and small superficial ulcers that are not demonstrable on upper gastrointestinal tract x-ray.

Radiologic Studies. Radionuclide imaging is emerging as an accurate, safe, minimally invasive method of detecting gastrointestinal bleeding (Fig. 24-8). ^{99m}Tc sulfur colloid has been widely used but has the disadvantages that the intense uptake by the liver and spleen compromises its value in upper gastrointestinal bleeding, and the rapid clearance of the colloid from the blood limits its use to those patients who are bleeding at the time of the injection. ^{99m}Tc-labeled erythrocytes have the advantage that imaging can be continued for up to 24 h. This is a significant advantage since most gastrointestinal bleeders do not bleed continuously. In accuracy and sensitivity the method is at least as good as, and perhaps better than, selective angiography. A disadvantage is that it cannot pinpoint the bleeding site as well as angiography. Radionuclide imaging should be utilized (if available) prior to angiography. Angiography will be unproductive if the technetium scan is negative.

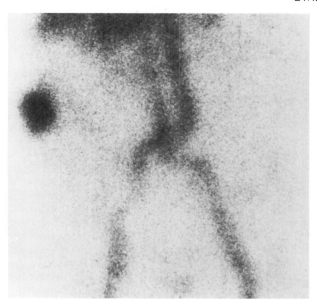

Fig. 24-8. ^{99m}Tc-labeled erythrocyte scan. Fifteen-minute film demonstrating a bleeding site in the right upper quadrant. The diagnosis of bleeding duodenal ulcer was established.

Selective arteriography of the celiac and superior mesenteric arteries and their branches is a relatively safe and accurate method of identifying active bleeding points in the upper gastrointestinal tract (Fig. 24-9). Angiography is usually done after endoscopy and radionuclide imaging. In any event, it must come before the upper gastrointestinal barium x-rays, which will obscure the field. Although bleeding at the rate of 1 to 2 mL/min can be detected experimentally, bleeding must be at the rate of 3 to 5 mL/min for accurate clinical angiographic diagnosis. The diagnostic accuracy of angiography in visualizing actively bleeding arterial lesions is about 90 percent; the accuracy in variceal bleeding, using the venous phase of the angiogram, is only about 20 percent.

In addition to diagnosis, selective arterial catheterization can be used for therapy of gastrointestinal bleeding. After the bleeding point is identified, a small therapeutic catheter is guided into the artery supplying the bleeding area, and vasoconstrictive agents, usually vasopressin at the rate of 0.1 to 0.2 units/min, are infused. Several comparative studies of systemic intravenous vasopressin versus regional arterial vasopressin have not shown any advantage for the more difficult and dangerous arterial route. The selective angiographic catheter may also be used to decrease the blood flow to a vascular bed by transcatheter embolization. Gelfoam soaked in contrast medium is the most frequently used material, but a great variety of materials can be used, including bits of autologous muscle, tiny detachable balloons, mini-coiled springs, and liquid acrylic monomers that instantly solidify on contacting blood. The occlusion is sometimes compromised by the opening up of collateral flow. The principal risk is that the blood supply will be so reduced that infarction occurs.

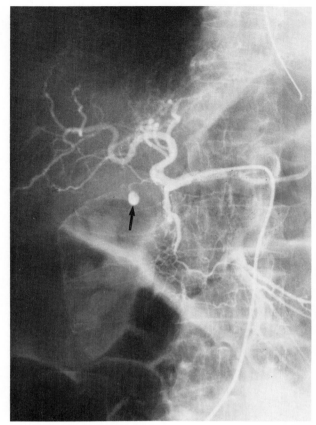

Fig. 24-9. Selective angiography in upper gastrointestinal bleeding. Dye injection into the common hepatic artery has outlined a bleeding duodenal ulcer (arrow). Later films showed a persistent puddling of contrast medium in the duodenum after all intravascular contrast had disappeared.

An upper gastrointestinal tract series, the cornerstone of morphologic radiographic diagnosis, should be done next, if endoscopy and arteriography have not revealed the bleeding site. As with endoscopy, the stomach should be evacuated of clots prior to the examination. In the case of bleeding ulcer, delaying for several days after hemorrhage has ceased does not increase the accuracy of diagnosis. The question of safety in the patient with bleeding has been raised, since the routine gastrointestinal series involves compression that may be attended by increasing hemorrhage. The Hampton technique for demonstration of bleeding ulcers obviates the use of palpation or compression and is attended by a diagnostic accuracy of 86 percent for demonstration of ulcers. The diagnostic accuracy in the case of bleeding varices is approximately 50 percent. Both the Valsalva and Müller maneuvers may occasionally show varices when other methods fail. Radiographs have proved of little value in the diagnosis of gastritis, with a yield of approximately 25 percent.

Percutaneous splenoportography affords a high yield for the diagnosis of esophageal varices but is rarely performed on an emergency basis. Before carrying out this procedure, a platelet count greater than 50,000/mm^3 and a prothrombin time greater than 35 percent of normal should be demonstrated. Splenic pulp manometry has been applied as an emergency test in the differential diagnosis of upper gastrointestinal tract bleeding. A 90 percent accuracy has been reported, but there is a zone of splenic pulp pressures that cannot differentiate variceal bleeding from other causes.

Balloon tamponade has been used as a diagnostic-therapeutic measure. However, varices are controlled even temporarily in only 65 to 75 percent of patients, and a peptic ulcer may coincidentally stop bleeding after a gastric balloon is inflated.

In some instances, an operation is performed on a patient with massive upper gastrointestinal tract bleeding in whom a diagnosis has not been established preoperatively. Laparotomy is to be considered as an important diagnostic tool. Once the peritoneal cavity has been opened, inspection of the liver may reveal cirrhosis, and distention of the omental vessels may suggest portal hypertension. In most cases, however, a determination of the source of bleeding requires a long gastrotomy that permits visualization of the gastric mucosa and the proximal portions of the duodenum. An attempt should be made to identify duodenal ulcer or a gastric lesion, and if these are not apparent, traction on the lower end of the nasogastric tube that is brought out through the gastrotomy will often expose the cardiac end of the stomach and distal esophagus to inspection. Intraoperative esophagogastroscopy by the usual route also may be helpful. Occasionally, in the absence of a preoperative diagnosis, no site of bleeding will be found at operation. In this situation, some surgeons do a vagotomy and drainage procedure; others simply close and hope that if bleeding recurs, the diagnosis can be made at that time and specific therapy instituted. The "blind" gastric resection that was formerly done in this situation has fallen into disfavor.

Lower Gastrointestinal Tract Bleeding

Bleeding distal to the ligament of Treitz is manifested by the passage of tarry stools or unaltered blood (hemochezia) and is characteristically unaccompanied by hematemesis. It is usually moderate or mild but may be massive.

ETIOLOGY. A great variety of lesions extending from the ligament of Treitz to the anus may be implicated as causes of lower gastrointestinal tract bleeding (Table 24-9).

Jejunal and Ileal Bleeding. Meckel's diverticulitis, intussusception, and regional enteritis represent the most common causes. Meckel's diverticulitis with associated bleeding occurs most frequently in children, and the bleeding episode is related to gastric mucosa within the diverticulum stimulating ulceration of the adjacent ileum. Ileocecal intussusception is also a lesion of childhood, occurring most commonly before the age of two and attended by a characteristic currant jelly stool. The cause of this mechanical process in childhood is usually undetermined, while ileocecal intussusception in the adult is usually secondary to an intestinal polyp or tumor. Regional enteritis is accompanied by severe melena in approximately 5 percent of the cases, while some rectal bleeding is a common symptom in about 20 percent of the patients with this disease. Although tumors of the small intestine are rare, approximately half are accompanied by bleeding. The neoplasms include leiomyomas, polyps, either single or multiple (familial polyposis), and the polyps of the Peutz-Jegher syndrome. Carcinomas, sarcomas, and leukemias have all been reported to be associated with bleeding, whereas bleeding is an uncommon manifestation of a carcinoid tumor. Hemangiomas, hereditary telangiectasis, microaneurysms of blood vessels within the wall of the intestine, mesenteric thrombosis, drug reactions, and blood dyscrasias all represent rare causes of small intestinal bleeding.

Colonic Bleeding. The common causes include carcinoma, diverticula, vascular ectasias, colitis, and polyps (Table 24-9). Although carcinoma represents the most common cause of rectal bleeding, the bleeding associated with this lesion is rarely massive. Carcinoma of the right colon, particularly of the cecum, is usually accompanied by melena that may be so subtle that it is not considered until anemia has become established. Diverticulosis presents the most common cause of *massive* rectal bleeding.

Table 24-9. CAUSES OF LOWER GASTROINTESTINAL BLEEDING BY AGE GROUP, IN ORDER OF FREQUENCY*

Infants and children	Adolescents and young adults	Adults to 60 years	Adults over 60 years
Meckel's diverticulum	Meckel's diverticulum	Diverticulosis	Vascular ectasias
Polyps	Inflammatory bowel	Inflammatory bowel	Diverticulosis
Ulcerative colitis	disease	disease	Malignancy
Duplications	Polyps	Polyps	Polyps
		Malignancy	
		Congenital arteriovenous malformations	

* Less frequent causes not specific for any age group.
   Infectious diarrheas (amebiasis, shigellosis), ischemic colitis, drug-induced cecal ulceration (e.g., vincristine), vascular lesions, vascular tumors, varices, coagulopathies.
SOURCE: From Boley SJ, Brandt LS, Frank MS: 1981, with permission.

This is related to erosion of vessels within the neck of the diverticulum. In contrast, the bleeding that accompanies diverticulitis is mild to moderate and is caused by a superficial erosion of smaller vessels on the surface of the mucosa. Although the bleeding that accompanies ulcerative colitis is usually mild to moderate, massive hemorrhage may occur. Polyps that may be single or multiple and may be located in any segment of the colon represent a relatively frequent source of rectal bleeding. Rarer causes include cecal ulceration, sarcomas, lymphomas, leukemia, hematologic disorders, and impairment of the vascular supply due to mesenteric thrombosis, ischemic colitis, or secondary to aortic resection with interruption of a functionally important inferior mesenteric artery.

Prior to angiography, bleeding lesions of the right colon were thought to be rare, but in the past decade many reports have emphasized that the right colon is a common site of bleeding. Diverticula were thought to be the responsible lesion. Boley and associates have shown that vascular ectasias are probably responsible for much of the right colon bleeding; they suggest that ectasias may be the commonest cause of major lower intestinal bleeding in the elderly. They present evidence that these vascular ectasias (1) are degenerative lesions of aging and are not congenital or neoplastic; (2) occur in patients over sixty years of age; (3) are not associated with angiomatous lesions of the skin or other viscera; (4) occur in the cecum and proximal ascending colon; (5) are small, usually less than 5 mm in diameter; (6) can be diagnosed only by angiography; and (7) usually cannot be identified by the surgeon at operation or by the pathologist using standard techniques—injecting-clearing techniques must be used.

Rectal and Anal Bleeding. This is usually manifested by unaltered blood on the surface of the stool. The causes include hemorrhoids, fissures, and proctitis. It is to be emphasized that the presence of hemorrhoids in a patient with rectal bleeding should not preclude investigation of other possible sources, particularly carcinoma.

DIAGNOSIS. A precise description of the bleeding episode and the nature of the stool is indicated. The question of familial polyposis and drug ingestion should be investigated. Physical examination includes a search for skin and mucosal lesions of hemorrhagic telangiectasia (Rendu-Osler-Weber syndrome) or the Peutz-Jegher syndrome. Abdominal palpation may reveal a mass, tumor, or intussusception, the last frequently accompanied by absence of bowel sounds in the right lower quadrant. Rectal examination may be diagnostic for tumor, polyps, or anal lesions. Proctosigmoidoscopy should be done early in the hospital course. Colonoscopy may be helpful if the patient is not bleeding actively at the time of the examination. With active massive bleeding, colonoscopy is useless.

As with upper gastrointestinal bleeding, radionuclide imaging using ^{99m}Tc-labeled erythrocytes is supplanting angiography as the procedure that follows endoscopy. Bleeding at a rate of 1 mL/min can be detected by this technique.

Selective angiography is still the most accurate method of diagnosis, provided there is active bleeding at the rate of at least 2 or 3 mL/min at the time of the examination. The small intestine and right half of the colon are examined by catheterization of branches of the superior mesenteric artery. Examination of the left colon is sometimes more difficult, since the inferior mesenteric artery may be more difficult to catheterize. As with upper gastrointestinal tract bleeding, regional infusion of vasoconstrictive agents via a catheter in the artery supplying the bleeding site is often an effective method of controlling bleeding.

Barium contrast studies, if needed, should follow angiography so that the contrast material does not obscure the angiographer's field. Barium enema studies, including air contrast, represent a reliable, accurate method of diagnosing colon lesions but yield no information as to whether or not the lesions visualized are responsible for the bleeding. Gastrointestinal series with small bowel follow-through is less productive in the case of lesions of the small intestine. Every effort should be made to demonstrate the bleeding site prior to operation, since diagnosis at the operating table is often not possible.

JAUNDICE

The term *jaundice* is derived from the French word meaning "yellow" and refers to the presence of an excess of bile pigments in the tissues and the serum. It is the presenting sign of a number of hepatic and nonhepatic diseases. The differential diagnosis and management are dependent upon an appreciation of the normal and abnormal variants of bile pigment metabolism. A flow sheet analysis of hyperbilirubinemia is presented in Table 24-10.

NORMAL BILE PIGMENT METABOLISM. The bile pigment bilirubin (Fig. 24-10) is a tetrapyrrole which is formed to the greatest extent from hemoglobin and, to a lesser extent, from myoglobin breakdown and hepatic synthesis itself. When the red blood cell is destroyed by the reticuloendothelial system, either at the end of its natural life span or prematurely, the iron and globin are removed, and the heme ring is opened and transformed into biliverdin, which is green. The latter is reduced to become bilirubin, which is yellow. The bilirubin combines with albumin to form a relatively stable protein-pigment complex and is transported as such to the hepatic parenchymal cell. This complex, which is referred to as *indirect-reacting* bilirubin, since it gives the van den Bergh diazo reaction only after treatment with alcohol and other substances that split the protein bond, is poorly soluble in water and is not excreted in the urine.

In the hepatic parenchymal cell the albumin is removed, and the bilirubin is conjugated with glucuronic acid to form a diglucuronide, which is water-soluble and is excreted into the bile canaliculi. This substance gives an immediate diazo reaction, is therefore termed *direct-reacting,* and is readily passed into the urine. Normally there is less than 1.2 mg of direct-reacting serum bilirubin and less than 0.3 mg of indirect-reacting serum bilirubin per dL of serum.

The conjugated bilirubin, which is excreted via the bile

Table 24-10. ANALYSIS OF A CASE OF HYPERBILIRUBINEMIA

Fractionate serum bilirubin and measure urine bilirubin and urobilinogen to determine whether:

I. Unconjugated hyperbilirubinemia

Determine mechanism on basis of age, clinical features, and laboratory findings:

A. Production of bilirubin beyond excretory capacity. Evidence of:

   1. Hemolysis

      a. Extracorpuscular
         (1) Immune body reactions
            (a) Transfusion reactions
            (b) Erythroblastosis
         (2) Infections and chemicals
         (3) Physical agents
         (4) Secondary hemolysis in pregnancy

      b. Intracorpuscular
         (1) Congenital hemolytic jaundice
         (2) Sickle cell anemia
         (3) Mediterranean anemia

   2. No hemolysis

      a. Pulmonary infarction
      b. Transfusion of aged red blood cells
      c. Hematomas
      d. "Shunt" hyperbilirubinemia

B. Deficient hepatic uptake of bilirubin:

   1. ? Gilbert's disease (normal biopsy, low-grade hyperbilirubinemia)
   2. ? Acquired liver disease

C. Deficient conjugation of bilirubin:

   1. Physiologic jaundice of newborn
   2. Crigler-Najjar syndrome (transferase deficiency)

      a. Inadequate bilirubin glucuronide synthesis

   3. Inhibition of glucuronyl transferase

      a. Large doses of vitamin K analogs in premature infants
      b. Increase level of pregnanediol
      c. Breast milk containing pregnane-3-(*a*), 20-(*β*)-diol
      d. Novobiocin

   4. Competitive inhibition

      a. Drugs detoxified as glucuronides

II. Conjugated hyperbilirubinemia

Determine mechanism on basis of age, clinical features, and laboratory findings:

A. Defect in bilirubin excretion
Confirm with serum alkaline phosphatase (elevated), cephalin flocculation (normal). In absence of rapid subsidence, exploratory surgery is desirable to differentiate:

1. Extrahepatic biliary obstruction
Identify by radiologic means and/or direct inspection during surgical intervention.
    a. Calculus
    b. Stricture
    c. Neoplasm

2. Intrahepatic biliary obstruction
Confirm absence of extrahepatic biliary obstruction with operative or T-tube cholangiography. Identify localization of lesion by surgical biopsy.
    a. Lesion of bile canaliculi   (1) Drugs   (2) Viruses
    b. Lesion of bile ductules   (1) Drugs   (2) Viruses
    c. Lesion of bile ducts   (1) Drugs   (2) Viruses

B. Deficient liver cell secretion of bilirubin
May need to differentiate from excretory defect by surgical exploration, cholangiography, or biopsy:

1. Persistence of excretory defect in immature liver after development of adequate glucuronide-synthesizing capacity
2. Dubin-Johnson syndrome (biopsy showing characteristic pigment)
3. Rotor syndrome (absence of characteristic pigment)

III. Combined unconjugated and conjugated hyperbilirubinemia

Determine mechanism on basis of clinical features and laboratory findings:

A. Familial defect or immature liver reflected in partial deficiency of glucuronide formation or excretion

B. Acquired liver cell damage
Confirm with liver function tests and determine primary abnormality:

1. Deficient hepatic uptake of bilirubin
2. Deficient conjugation of bilirubin
3. Deficient secretion or excretion of conjugated bilirubin

C. Hemolysis with secondary liver damage.
Demonstrate presence of hemolysis:

1. Hepatic damage secondary to shock
2. Hepatic damage secondary to hemolysis

D. Biliary obstruction with secondary liver damage:

1. Bile stasis with secondary injury
2. Ascending cholangitis

SOURCE: Leevy CM: *Evaluation of Liver Function in Clinical Practice.* Indianapolis, The Lilly Research Laboratories, 1965, with permission.

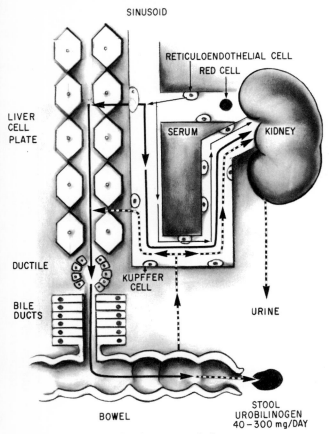

Fig. 24-10. Normal bile pigment metabolism.

into the intestine, is acted upon by bacteria and undergoes a series of reductive reactions leading to the formation of two groups of compounds, the colorless urobilinogens and the colored urobilin. The normal daily fecal excretion ranges between 40 and 300 mg with an average of 100 to 200 mg. In children the values are lower, and in newborn infants, because of the absence of bacterial flora, urobilinogen may be absent. A reduction in enteric bacteria is also responsible for the reduced pigment excretion that accompanies the use of intestinal antibiotics. Some of the urobilinogen is resorbed by way of the portal venous system and returns to the liver, where it is either removed or, to a small extent, excreted in the urine.

ABNORMAL BILE PIGMENT METABOLISM. No classification of jaundice is totally satisfactory. The classification most widely used distinguishes between hemolytic, obstructive, and hepatocellular jaundice. However, it is more reasonable to categorize (1) those disease states in which the bile flow is unimpeded and (2) those types that are associated with an impairment of the bile flow (Fig. 24-11).

Normal Bile Excretion. The overproduction of bile pigment from excessive hemolysis creates a situation in which the normal liver is confronted with more pigment than it is able to remove. This occurs in the physiologic jaundice of infancy and all pathologic hemolytic states. However, the reserve capacity of the liver is great, and even when the bilirubin production is increased six times, there is only a 2- to 3-mg rise in the serum bilirubin level per dL. In this situation, the increase in serum bilirubin is in the unconjugated indirect-reacting pigment. No bilirubin appears in the urine, but there is an increase in the fecal and urinary urobilinogen. An excess of bilirubin production also occurs in *shunt hyperbilirubinemia,* in which indirect-reacting bilirubin accumulates in the absence of any reduction in red cell life span.

Constitutional defects of liver function may also cause hyperbilirubinemia without impairment of bile flow. In Gilbert's disease, there is a defect in the bilirubin transport into the liver cell, while in the Crigler-Najjar syndrome the defect is an inability of the liver to conjugate the bilirubin with glucuronic acid. In these states, the elevation of bile pigment is in the indirect-reacting fraction. All other hepatic function tests are normal, and no histologic abnormalities are noted. With all of the above-mentioned diseases, the bilirubin pigment is attached to the albumin and cannot be excreted by the kidney, thus prompting the term *acholuric jaundice.*

Impaired Bile Excretion. All other lesions are associated with an accumulation of conjugated bilirubin in the blood and impaired excretion. The bilirubin pigment, which is water-soluble, is readily excreted into the urine, which becomes brown. Obstructive jaundice may be intrahepatic or extrahepatic.

Intrahepatic Obstructive Jaundice. In the Dubin-Johnson syndrome, which is associated with the appearance of iron-free pigment in the hepatic cells and normal liver function, the hepatic excretion of the conjugated bilirubin is impaired. Intrahepatic cholestasis has also been related to a variety of drugs and hepatocellular diseases. Methyltestosterone and norethandrolone damage the microvilli of the bile canaliculi and may cause jaundice. The phenothiazine drugs, such as chlorpromazine, may evoke a hypersensitivity reaction in a small percentage of patients and result in cholangiolitic hepatitis and intrahepatic cholestasis. A lesion along the excretory path within the liver is believed to cause the obstructive jaundice associated with primary biliary cirrhosis.

The jaundice from hepatocellular degeneration, such as occurs in hepatitis and cirrhosis, is associated with morphologic changes in the parenchymal cells and abnormal liver function tests. With these diseases, a Kupffer cell liver block has been proposed to result in regurgitation of bilirubin from the bile canaliculi into the tissue spaces. This defect, coupled with the reduction in the ability of the liver cell to convert the bilirubin protein to the bilirubin glucuronide, causes a rise in both bilirubin and its conjugates. In contrast to the pure obstructive jaundice, urinary urobilinogen may be increased, since the parenchyma is no longer capable of clearing the serum urobilinogen entering from the intestinal tract. However, the excretion of bile may be so suppressed that virtually no bilirubin reaches the intestine; under these conditions the stools are clay-colored, and the production and resorption of the bilirubin from the intestine is diminished, in

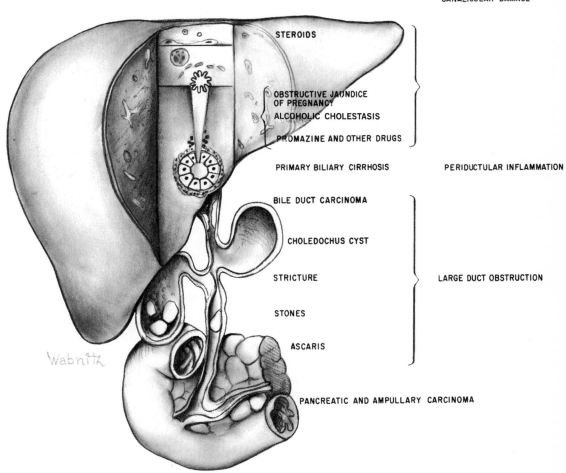

CAUSE OF
JAUNDICE

POSTULATED
DEFECT

HEMOLYSIS

SHUNT
HYPERBILIRUBINEMIA
GILBERT

NEONATE, CRIGLER - NAJJAR

DUBIN-JOHNSON
HYPERBILIRUBINEMIA

EXCESS BILIRUBIN PRODUCTION
BILIRUBIN TRANSPORT
BILIRUBIN CONJUGATION

CONJUGATION TRANSPORT

CANALICULAR DAMAGE

STEROIDS

OBSTRUCTIVE JAUNDICE
OF PREGNANCY
ALCOHOLIC CHOLESTASIS

PROMAZINE AND OTHER DRUGS

PRIMARY BILIARY CIRRHOSIS

PERIDUCTULAR INFLAMMATION

BILE DUCT CARCINOMA

CHOLEDOCHUS CYST

STRICTURE

STONES

ASCARIS

LARGE DUCT OBSTRUCTION

PANCREATIC AND AMPULLARY CARCINOMA

Wabnitz

Fig. 24-11. Abnormal bile pigment metabolism.

which case the urine urobilinogen falls to a low level. In rare instances of intrahepatic bile duct atresia absolute obstruction of the bile conduits within the liver results in jaundice.

Extrahepatic Cholestasis. This is caused by an anatomic obstacle to the flow of bile from the liver to the intestine. The obstacle may be situated anywhere from the junction of the right and left hepatic ducts to the termination of the common bile duct in the duodenum. Atresia, stricture, choledocholithiasis, tumors of the bile duct and pancreas, choledochal cysts, and parasites have all been implicated.

Obstruction of the extrahepatic ducts results in an increase in the serum bilirubin, particularly the direct-reacting type, the appearance of bile in the urine, and the passage of clay-colored stools. When the total bilirubin level is above 3 mg/dL, the increases in both the direct- and indirect-reacting fractions parallel one another. With complete and persistent obstruction, the serum bilirubin may plateau. If the obstruction is fluctuating, the levels will change.

EVALUATION AND MANAGEMENT OF THE PATIENT WITH JAUNDICE. For a discussion of neonatal jaundice and biliary atresia see Chap. 31.

Jaundice is apparent when the serum bilirubin level exceeds 2 mg/dL. Tissues rich in elastic fibers have a particular affinity for bilirubin, thus accounting for the earlier appearance and greater intensity in the sclerae and in the skin of the face and upper trunk. Jaundice is not a mere reflection of yellow light through the skin from underlying interstitial fluid but rather a deposition in the tissue fibers and cells. Tissues stain more readily with direct bilirubin than with the indirect-reacting fraction. There is a failure to stain in areas of marked edema and vitiligo.

The diagnosis of jaundice attempts to define the precise cause and is also directed toward the division into surgically correctable lesions, on the one hand, and other types in which surgical intervention is not indicated.

History. Jaundice secondary to obstruction of the extrahepatic ducts usually starts insidiously and becomes progressively more pronounced. Gastrointestinal disturbances are uncommon, with the exception of those related to biliary calculi. Although, classically, carcinoma of the head of the pancreas is painless, some 20 to 30 percent of these patients do complain of deep epigastric distress or backache. Extrahepatic obstruction associated with ascending cholangitis is accompanied by spiking fevers and abdominal pain. A history of pruritus preceding the onset of jaundice occurs frequently with both extrahepatic biliary obstruction and intrahepatic obstruction secondary to primary cholangiolitis or primary biliary cirrhosis. A detailed family history and history of drug ingestion are imperative before subjecting a patient to surgical treatment, since both constitutional deficiencies and drug-induced jaundice result in a defect in excretion of bile. Loss of appetite, fever, and change of smoking habits are particularly suggestive of hepatitis, and history should be taken of possible contact with persons with known cases and of injections in the previous 6 months. Inquiry into chronic alcohol ingestion is important to rule out jaundice associated with cirrhosis.

Physical Examination. Physical examination also contributes to the diagnosis. Inspection of the skin may reveal a rash, typical of drug reactions, spider angiomas of cirrhosis, or excoriations suggestive of pruritus. Anemia and splenomegaly may be present with hemolytic jaundice. Hepatomegaly and hepatic tenderness are predominant findings with viral hepatitis. A palpable gallbladder in a patient with extrahepatic obstruction occurs more frequently when the obstruction is related to malignancy distal to the cystic duct entrance into the common duct, and less commonly when obstruction is due to biliary calculi. This axiom, known as Courvoisier's law, however, is not universal. Careful search for extrahepatic neoplasm should be made, and the stigmata of portal hypertension including prominent abdominal wall veins and ascites should be investigated.

Laboratory Studies. Hemolytic jaundice is accompanied by anemia and an increased reticulocyte count. Smears for sickle cells, spherocytes, and target cells should be made. The white blood cell count is usually not elevated in viral hepatitis, while it is frequently markedly increased with extrahepatic obstruction and accompanying ascending cholangitis. Stools should be studied for pigment and the presence or absence of guaiac, indicative of

bleeding. With carcinoma of the pancreas, approximately one-third of the patients have guaiac-positive stools; this occurs more frequently in patients with obstructive jaundice secondary to carcinoma of the ampulla of Vater.

The so-called liver function tests are directed toward assessing the degree of functional impairment of the liver and differentiating between "medical" and "surgical" jaundice. The extreme functional reserve of the liver occasionally produces normal results in the face of significant lesions, and none of the tests provides a pathologic diagnosis. Tests should be performed to determine exposure to hepatitis.

Serum bilirubin is normally present in concentrations up to 1.5 mg/dL and, as previously mentioned, appears both in water-insoluble unconjugated form, which gives the indirect van den Bergh reaction, and the water-soluble conjugated form, which reacts directly. Up to 1.2 mg/dL of unconjugated bilirubin is present in the normal serum. Increases in this fraction accompany hemolytic processes such as physiologic jaundice of the newborn, erythroblastosis, and hereditary and acquired hemolytic crises. This fraction is also elevated in the Crigler-Najjar syndrome and in Gilbert's disease. In patients with jaundice secondary to obstruction of the flow of bile or hepatocellular degeneration, the determination of the direct fraction is a more sensitive index of impairment than the total serum bilirubin.

Normally no bilirubin is present in the urine, and bilirubinuria does not accompany hemolytic jaundice or jaundice related to deficiency in the glucuronal transferase system, since the unconjugated fraction, which is increased in these situations, cannot be excreted by the kidney. An elevation in the direct-reacting bilirubin level is associated with bilirubinuria. The production of foam by shaking the urine suggests the elevation. Increased direct-reacting serum bilirubin may not appear in the urine of patients with severe renal failure.

Enzyme studies are also applicable to the differential diagnosis of jaundice. A markedly elevated serum alkaline phosphatase level is usually associated with obstructive jaundice of either extrahepatic or intrahepatic origin. Elevations in SGOT and SGPT are indicative of hepatocellular disease. Gamma glutamyl transpeptidase (GGTP) is elevated in alcoholic liver disease but more markedly increased in patients with extrahepatic cholestasis.

Other laboratory findings, such as a reduction in serum albumin and a reduction in the esterified fraction of the cholesterol, and abnormal turbidity studies are altered with hepatocellular disease. Removal of foreign dye from the liver is dependent upon hepatic blood flow, hepatocellular function, and biliary excretion. The response of prothrombin time to injection of parenteral vitamin K is helpful in establishing a differential diagnosis between hepatocellular and obstructive jaundice. An increase in the prothrombin time within 48 h of parenteral administration suggests the diagnosis of obstructive jaundice, while a lack of response is more compatible with hepatocellular disease.

Other Diagnostic Procedures. *Radiologic Studies.* An x-ray of the abdomen is indicated, since 20 percent of gallstones are radiopaque (see Chap. 31). Oral cholecys-

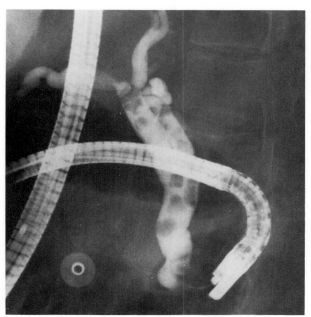

Fig. 24-12. Endoscopic retrograde cholangiopancreatogram (ERCP) showing multiple stones in a dilated common bile duct and in the cystic duct remnant.

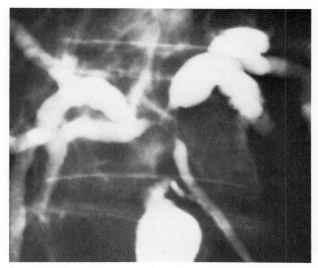

Fig. 24-13. Percutaneous transhepatic cholangiogram defining intrahepatic ductal dilatation. There is almost complete obstruction at the confluence of the right and left hepatic ducts due to carcinoma (Klatskin tumor). Note that there is radiopaque substance in the common duct and gallbladder.

tography is rarely effective if the serum bilirubin level is above 1.8 mg/dL, while the intravenous studies are unrewarding if the serum bilirubin level exceeds 3.5 mg/dL. The upper gastrointestinal series may define a widened "C loop," suggestive of carcinoma of the pancreas.

Recent advances that have contributed significantly in the differential diagnosis of jaundice include endoscopic retrograde cholangiopancreatography (ERCP), percutaneous transhepatic cholangiography (PTC) with the skinny Chiba needle, ultrasonography, computed tomography (CT), and radionuclide scanning. In experienced hands 90 to 95 percent success rates for ERCP (Fig. 24-12) definition of the extrahepatic biliary system have been reported, but in most institutions the yield is less than 65 percent. Cholangitis and pancreatitis are uncommon complications. The technique is uniquely suited to the evaluation of sclerosing cholangitis and carcinoma of the ampulla of Vater, in which case biopsy can establish the diagnosis. In a randomized trial comparing PTC with ERCP for bile duct visualization in deeply jaundiced patients, PTC (see Fig. 24-13) was demonstrated to be the procedure of choice when cholestasis had a surgical cause. PTC was successful in 95 percent of cases with extrahepatic cholestasis and in 25 percent of patients with intrahepatic cholestasis, while ERCP was successful in 62 percent of patients with extrahepatic and 76 percent with intrahepatic cholestasis. In the patient with extrahepatic obstructive jaundice, provision for early operation should be made if bile peritonitis, an uncommon complication, occurs. ERCP is preferred when coagulation defects preclude PTC.

Compound B scanning provides echographic patterns in patients who are deeply jaundiced and whose ducts cannot be visualized with contrast media. Dilated ducts,

calculi, and tumors can be defined by serial laminographic scans. Equipment capable of defining gray scale has increased the sensitivity of this technique (Fig. 24-14). CT employing the body scanner also will demonstrate dilatation of intrahepatic and/or extrahepatic portions of the biliary tract (Fig. 24-15). The ^{99m}Tc-pyridoxylideneglutamate biliary scan is a safe, noninvasive means of distinguishing between jaundice due to hepatobiliary disease and that due to partial or complete extrahepatic biliary duct obstruction. It is applicable even if the bilirubin is elevated to the 20 mg/dL level.

Liver Biopsy. Percutaneous needle biopsy of the liver may, on one hand, prevent procrastination of surgical intervention and progressive parenchymal damage in patients with extrahepatic biliary obstruction; on the other hand, it may preclude laparotomy in patients with severe hepatocellular disease. Patients should be screened for deficiency in the clotting mechanism, and the risk is small. Characteristic lesions of viral hepatitis, cholangiolitic hepatitis, and bile laking suggestive of extrahepatic biliary obstruction can be defined by this technique.

Laparotomy. This is considered an important tool in the diagnostic armamentarium. Laparotomy for obstructive jaundice is never urgent unless there is an acute suppurative cholangitis. Surgical intervention is indicated when other diagnostic procedures have raised a suspicion of extrahepatic obstruction and when the danger of operating on a patient with possible hepatocellular jaundice is considered minimal. An approach to the diagnosis of jaundice in a patient potentially requiring surgical management is shown in Fig. 24-16.

Algorithm for Diagnosis (Fig. 24-16). Given a patient in whom there is a high index of suspicion that jaundice is related to extrahepatic ductal obstruction, the initial investigative procedure, based on yield and cost effectiveness, should be ultrasonography. This will determine if

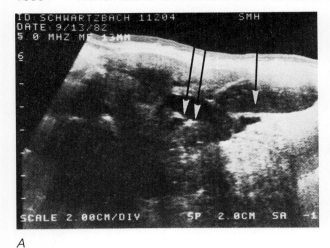

A

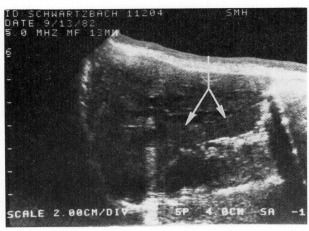

B

Fig. 24-14. Ultrasound of patient with carcinoma of the pancreas causing obstruction of the common bile duct and dilatation of the gallbladder and intrahepatic ducts. *A.* Single arrow points to dilated gallbladder, double arrow to dilated common duct. *B.* Arrow points to dilated intrahepatic duct.

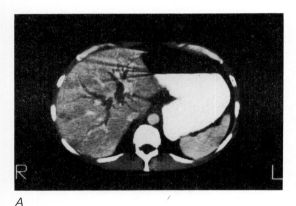

A

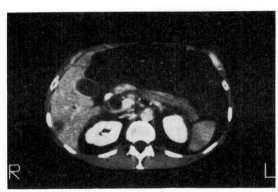

B

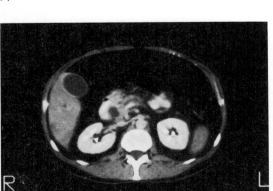

C

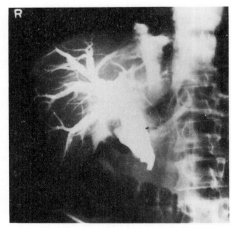

D

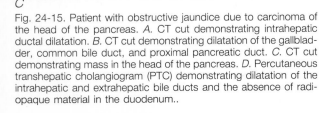

Fig. 24-15. Patient with obstructive jaundice due to carcinoma of the head of the pancreas. *A.* CT cut demonstrating intrahepatic ductal dilatation. *B.* CT cut demonstrating dilatation of the gallbladder, common bile duct, and proximal pancreatic duct. *C.* CT cut demonstrating mass in the head of the pancreas. *D.* Percutaneous transhepatic cholangiogram (PTC) demonstrating dilatation of the intrahepatic and extrahepatic bile ducts and the absence of radiopaque material in the duodenum..

Determine Presence or Absence of Intra-and/or Extrahepatic Ductal Obstruction

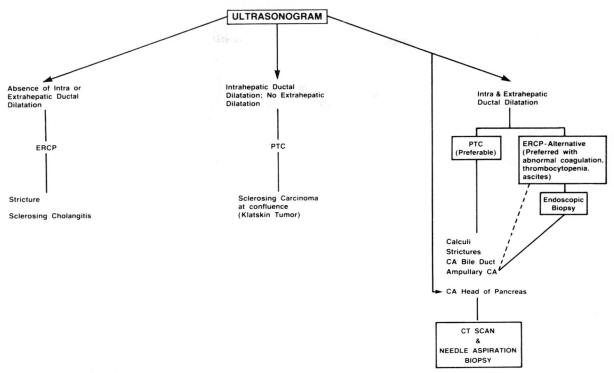

Fig. 24-16. Algorithm for the diagnosis of obstructive jaundice.

intrahepatic ductal dilatation and/or dilatation of the extrahepatic ducts and gallbladder is present. Once ductal dilatation is defined, a PTC should be performed to localize the level of obstruction. If obstruction is present at the confluence of the hepatic ducts, the common hepatic duct, or proximal common duct, no further diagnostic procedure is necessary. If the obstruction is located at the distal common duct, a CT scan may be indicated to define the presence of a mass in the head of the pancreas and the resectability of such a lesion. If no mass is present, ERCP can be performed to determine if an ampullary lesion is present. In most instances upper gastrointestinal series adds little to the diagnosis. This also applies to the liver spleen scan.

Bibliography

Pain

Carlsson CA, Pellettieri L: A clinical view on pain physiology. *Acta Chir Scand* 148:305, 1982.

Cope Z: *The Early Diagnosis of Acute Abdomen,* 15th ed. London, Oxford University Press, 1979.

Long DM: Electrical stimulation for the control of pain. *Arch Surg* 112:884, 1977.

Melzack R, Wall PD: Pain mechanisms: A new theory. *Science* 150:971, 1965.

Nathan PW: Pain. *Br Med Bull* 33:149, 1977.

Pflug AE, Bonica JJ: Physiopathology and control of postoperative pain. *Arch Surg* 112:773, 1977.

Sherman JE, Liebeskind JC: An endorphrinergic, centrifugal substrate of pain modulation. Recent findings, current concepts and complexities, in Bonica JJ (ed): *Pain.* New York, Raven, 1980, p 191.

White JC, Smithwick RH, Simeone FA: *The Autonomic Nervous System: Anatomy, Physiology, Surgical Application,* 3d ed. New York, Macmillan, 1952.

Zimmermann M: Peripheral and central nervous mechanisms of nociception, pain and pain therapy: Facts and hypotheses, in Bonica JJ, Liebeskind JC, Albe-Fessard DG (eds): *Advances in Pain Research and Therapy.* New York, Raven, 1979, vol 3, p 3.

Dysphagia

Davenport HW: *Physiology of the Digestive Tract,* 4th ed. Chicago, Year Book Medical Publishers, 1977.

Grant AK, Skyring A (eds): *Clinical Diagnosis of Gastrointestinal Disease.* Oxford, Blackwell Scientific Publications, 1981.

Greenberger NJ: *Gastrointestinal Disorders: A Pathophysiological Approach,* 2d ed. Chicago, Year Book Medical Publishers, 1981.

Sleisenger MH, Fortran JS: *Gastrointestinal Disease,* 2d ed. Philadelphia, Saunders, 1978.

Anorexia, Nausea, and Vomiting

Davenport HW: *Physiology of the Digestive Tract,* 4th ed. Chicago, Year Book Medical Publishers, 1977.

Grant AK, Skyring A (eds): *Clinical Diagnosis of Gastrointestinal Disease.* Oxford, Blackwell Scientific Publications, 1981.

Greenberger NJ: *Gastrointestinal Disorders: A Pathophysiological Approach,* 2d ed. Chicago, Year Book Medical Publishers, 1981.

Hawkins C: Anorexia and loss of weight. *Br Med J* 2:1373, 1976.

McGuigan JE: Anorexia, nausea and vomiting, in MacBryde CM, Blacklow RS (eds): *Signs and Symptoms,* 5th ed. Philadelphia, Lippincott, 1970.

Constipation and Diarrhea

Davenport HW: *Physiology of the Digestive Tract,* 4th ed. Chicago, Year Book Medical Publishers, 1977.

Dobbins JW, Binder HJ: Pathophysiology of diarrhea: Alterations in fluid and electrolyte transport. *Clin Gastroenterol* 10:605, 1981.

Fingl E, Preston JW: Antidiarrheal agents and laxatives: Changing concepts. *Clin Gastroenterol* 8:161, 1979.

Jaffe BM, Condon S: Prostaglandins E and F in endocrine diarrheagenic syndromes. *Ann Surg* 184:516, 1976.

McJunkin B, Fromm H, et al: Factors in the Mechanism of diarrhea in bile acid malabsorption: Fecal pH—a key determinant. *Gastroenterology* 80:1454, 1981.

Summers RW: Role of motility in infectious diarrhea. *Gastroenterology* 80:1070, 1981.

Intestinal Obstruction

Adams JT: Adynamic ileus of the colon; An indication for cecostomy. *Arch Surg* 109:503, 1974.

Baker JW: Selective usage of the original and modified Baker intestinal tube. *Surg Gynecol Obstet* 149:577, 1979.

Barnett WO, Petro AB, Williamson JW: A current appraisal of problems with gangrenous bowel. *Ann Surg* 183:653, 1976.

Berardi RS: Collective review: Anomalies of midgut rotation in the adult. *Surg Gynecol Obstet* 151:131, 1980.

Berardi RS: Collective review: Paraduodenal hernias. *Surg Gynecol Obstet* 152:99, 1981.

Bizer LS, Liebling RW, et al: Small bowel obstruction: The role of nonoperative treatment in simple intestinal obstruction and predictive criteria for strangulation obstruction. *Surgery* 89:407, 1981.

Boley SJ, Agrawal GP, et al: Pathophysiologic effects of bowel distention on intestinal blood flow. *Am J Surg* 117:228, 1969.

Boley SJ, Sprayregan S, et al: Initial results from an aggressive roentgenological and surgical approach to acute mesenteric ischemia. *Surgery* 82:848, 1977.

Bulkley GB, Zuidema GD, et al: Intraoperative determination of small intestinal viability following ischemic injury. A prospective, controlled trial of two adjuvant methods (Doppler and fluorescein) compared with standard clinical judgment. *Ann Surg* 193:628, 1981.

Davidson ED, Hersh T, et al: The effects of metoclopramide on postoperative ileus. *Ann Surg* 190:27, 1979.

Frimann-Dahl J: *Roentgen Examinations in Acute Abdominal Disease,* 3d ed. Springfield, Ill, Charles C Thomas, 1974.

Gammill SL, Nice CM Jr: Air fluid levels: Their occurrence in normal patients and their role in the analysis of ileus. *Surgery* 71:771, 1972.

Graber JN, Schultz WJ, et al: Relationship of duration of postoperative ileus to extent and site of operative dissection. *Surgery* 92:87, 1982.

Hofstetter SR: Acute adhesive obstruction of the small intestine. *Surg Gynecol Obstet* 152:141, 1981.

Kvist E: Gallstone ileus; a retrospective study. *Acta Chir Scand* 145:101, 1979.

Landman MD, Longmire WP Jr: Neural and hormonal influences of peritonitis on paralytic ileus. *Am Surg* 33:756, 1967.

Levitt MD: Intestinal gas production—recent advances in flatology. *N Engl J Med* 302:1474, 1980.

Levitt MD, Bond JH, Levitt DG: Gastrointestinal gas, in Johnson LR (ed): *Physiology of the Gastrointestinal Tract.* New York, Raven, 1981.

Miller RE, Brahme F: Large amounts of orally administered barium for obstruction of the small intestine. *Surg Gynecol Obstet* 129:1185, 1969.

Nachlas MM, Younis MT, et al: Gastrointestinal motility studies as a guide to postoperative management. *Ann Surg* 175:510, 1972.

Nadrowski L: Paralytic ileus: Recent advances in pathophysiology and treatment. *Curr Surg* 40:260, 1983.

Öhman U: Studies on small intestinal obstruction, I-VI. *Acta Chir Scand* 141:413, 417, 536, 545, 763, 771, 1975.

Osteen RT, Guyton S, et al: Malignant intestinal obstruction. *Surgery* 87:611, 1980.

Politzer J-P, Devroede G, et al: The genesis of bowel sounds: Influence of viscus and gastrointestinal content. *Gastroenterology* 71:282, 1976.

Quatromoni JC, Rosoff L Sr, et al: Early postoperative small bowel obstruction. *Ann Surg* 191:72, 1980.

Sarr MG, Bulkley GB, Zuidema GD: Preoperative recognition of intestinal strangulation obstruction. *Am J Surg* 145:176, 1983.

Shields R: The absorption and secretion of fluid and electrolytes by the obstructed bowel. *Br J Surg* 52:774, 1965.

Smith J, Kelly KA, Weinshilboum RM: Pathophysiology of postoperative ileus. *Arch Surg* 112:203, 1977.

Smith JA, Forward AD, et al: Metronidazole and tobramycin in intra-abdominal sepsis. *Surg Gynecol Obstet* 155:235, 1982.

Snape WJ Jr: Pseudo-obstruction and other obstructive disorders. *Clin Gastroenterol* 11:593, 1982.

Stewardson RH, Bombeck CT, Nyhus LM: Critical operative management of small bowel obstruction. *Ann Surg* 187:189, 1978.

Sykes PA, Boulter KH, Schofield PF: The microflora of the obstructed bowel. *Br J Surg* 63:721, 1976.

Tinker MA, Teicher I, Burdman D: Cellulose granulomas and their relationship to intestinal obstruction. *Am J Surg* 133:134, 1977.

Villar HV, Norton LW: Massive cecal dilation: Pseudoobstruction versus cecal volvulus. *Am J Surg* 137:170: 1979.

Wangensteen OH: Understanding the bowel obstruction problem. *Am J Surg* 135:131, 1978.

Weigelt JA, Snyder WH III, Norman JL: Complications and results of 160 Baker tube plications. *Am J Surg* 140:810, 1980.

Wickstrom P, Haglin JJ, Hitchcock CR: Intraoperative decompression of the obstructed small bowel. *Surgery* 73:212, 1973.

Wolff LH, Wolff WA, Wolff LH Jr: A re-evaluation of tube cecostomy. *Surg Gynecol Obstet* 151:257, 1980.

Wright HK, O'Brien JJ, Tilson MD: Water absorption in experimental closed segment obstruction of the ileum in man. *Am J Surg* 121:96, 1971.

Gastrointestinal Bleeding

Athanasoulis CA: Therapeutic applications of angiography. *N Engl J Med* 302:1117, 1174, 1980.

Atkenson RJ, Nyhus LM: Gastric lavage for hemorrhage in the upper part of the gastrointestinal tract. *Surg Gynecol Obstet* 146:797, 1978.

Boley SJ, Brandt LJ, Frank MS: Severe lower intestinal bleeding: Diagnosis and treatment. *Clin Gastroenterol.* 10:65, 1981.

Boley SJ, Sammartano R, et al: On the nature and etiology of vascular ectasias of the colon: Degenerative lesions of aging. *Gastroenterology* 72:650, 1977.

Bounous G: Acute necrosis of the intestinal mucosa. *Gastroenterology* 82:1457, 1982.

Bowden TA Jr, Hooks VH III, Mansberger AR Jr: Intraoperative gastrointestinal endoscopy. *Ann Surg* 191:680, 1980.

Colacchio TA, Forde KA, et al: Impact of modern diagnostic methods on the management of active rectal bleeding. *Am J Surg* 143:607, 1982.

Dent TL: Collective review: Evaluation of the bleeding patient. *Surg Gynecol Obstet* 151:817, 1980.

Donaldson RM Jr: Assessing the usefulness of diagnostic procedures. *Gastroenterology* 72:762, 1977.

Dronfield MW, Langman MJS, et al: Outcome of endoscopy and barium radiography for acute upper gastrointestinal bleeding: Controlled trial in 1037 patients. *Br Med J* 284:545, 1982.

Dykes PW, Keighley MRB (eds): *Gastrointestinal Hemorrhage.* Bristol, Wright, PSG, 1981.

Eisenberg RL: *Diagnostic Imaging in Internal Medicine.* New York, McGraw-Hill, 1985.

Eisenberg RL: *Diagnostic Imaging in Surgery.* New York, McGraw-Hill, 1987.

Giacchino JL, Geis WP, et al: Changing perspectives in massive lower intestinal hemorrhage. *Surgery* 86:368, 1979.

Hastings PR, Skillman JJ, et al: Antacid titration in the prevention of acute gastrointestinal bleeding: A controlled, randomized trial in 100 critically ill patients. *N Engl J Med* 298:1041, 1978.

Himal HS, Perrault C, Mzabi R: Upper gastrointestinal hemorrhage: Aggressive management decreases mortality. *Surgery* 84:448, 1978.

Johnson WC, Nabseth DC, et al: Bleeding esophageal varices. Treatment with vasopressin, transhepatic embolization and selective splenorenal shunting. *Ann Surg* 195:393, 1982.

Kivilaakso E, Silen W: Pathogenesis of experimental gastric-mucosal injury. *N Engl J Med* 301:364, 1979.

McKusick KA, Froelich J, et al: ^{99m}Tc red blood cells for detection of gastrointestinal bleeding: Experience with 80 patients. *Am J Roentgen* 137:1113, 1981.

Meyers MA, Alonso DR, et al: Pathogenesis of bleeding colonic diverticulosis. *Gastroenterology* 71:577, 1976.

Michel L, Serrano A, Malt RA: Mallory-Weiss syndrome. Evolution of diagnostic and therapeutic patterns over two decades. *Ann Surg* 192:716, 1980.

Milliser RV, Greenberg SR, Neiman BH: Exsanguinating stercoral ulceration. *Am J Dig Dis* 15:485, 1970.

Nance FC, Kaufman HJ, Batson RC: The role of the microbial flora in acute gastric stress ulceration. *Surgery* 72:68, 1972.

Nath RL, Sequeira JC, et al: Lower gastrointestinal bleeding: Diagnostic approach and management conclusions. *Am J Surg* 141:478, 1981.

Odonkor P, Mowat C, Himal HS: Prevention of sepsis-induced gastric lesions in dogs by cimetidine via inhibition of gastric secretion and by prostaglandin via cytoprotection. *Gastroenterology* 80:375, 1981.

O'Donnell TF Jr, Gembarowitz RM, et al: The economic impact of acute variceal bleeding: Cost-effectiveness implications for medical and surgical therapy. *Surgery* 88:693, 1980.

Orloff MJ, Bell RH Jr, et al: Long-term results of emergency portacaval shunt for bleeding esophageal varices in unselected patients with alcoholic cirrhosis. *Ann Surg* 192:325, 1980.

Peterson WL, Barnett CC, et al: Routine early endoscopy in upper-gastrointestinal-tract bleeding. A randomized, controlled trial. *N Engl J Med* 304:925, 1981.

Pruitt BA, Foley FD, Moncrief JA: Curling's ulcer: A clinical-pathological study of 323 cases. *Ann Surg* 172:523, 1970.

Robert A: Cytoprotection by prostaglandins. *Gastroenterology* 77:761, 1979.

Schiff L: Hematemesis and melena, in MacBryde CM (ed): *Signs and Symptoms,* 5th ed. Philadelphia, Lippincott, 1970.

Smith JL, Graham DY: Variceal hemorrhage: A critical evaluation of survival analysis. *Gastroenterology* 82:968, 1982.

Storey DW, Bown SG, et al: Endoscopic prediction of recurrent bleeding in peptic ulcers. *N Engl J Med* 305:915, 1981.

Stothert JC Jr, Simonowitz DA, et al: Randomized prospective evaluation of cimetidine and antacid control of gastric pH in the critically ill. *Ann Surg* 192:169, 1980.

Sutherland D, Frech RS, et al: The bleeding cecal ulcer: Pathogenesis, angiographic diagnosis, and nonoperative control. *Surgery* 71:290, 1972.

Villar HV, Fender HR, et al: Emergency diagnosis of upper gastrointestinal bleedings by fiberoptic endoscopy. *Ann Surg* 185:367, 1977.

Webb WA, McDaniel L, et al: Endoscopic evaluation of 125 cases of upper gastrointestinal bleeding. *Ann Surg* 193:624, 1981.

Winzelberg GG, Froelich JW, et al: Radionuclide localization of lower gastrointestinal hemorrhage. *Radiology* 139:465, 1981.

Zinner MJ, Zuidema GD, et al: The prevention of upper gastrointestinal tract bleeding in patients in an intensive care unit. *Surg Gynecol Obstet* 153:214, 1981.

Jaundice

Boucher IAD: Diagnosis of jaundice. *Br Med J* 283:1281, 1981.

Cooperberg P, Golding RH: Advances in ultrasonography of the gallbladder and biliary tract. *Radiol Clin North Am* 20:611, 1982.

Elias E, Hamlyn AN, et al: A randomized trial of percutaneous transhepatic cholangiography with the Chiba needle versus endoscopic retrograde cholangiography for bile duct visualization in jaundice. *Gastroenterology* 71:439, 1976.

Havrilla TR, Hagga JR, et al: Computed tomography and obstructive biliary disease. *Am J Roentgen* 128:765, 1977.

Jander HP, Galbraith J, Aldrete JS: Percutaneous transhepatic cholangiography using the Chiba needle: Comparison with retrograde pancreatocholecystography. *South Med J* 73:415, 1980.

Levitt RG, Sagel SS, et al: Accuracy of computed tomography of the liver and biliary tract. *Radiology* 124:123, 1977.

Popper H, Schaffner F: *Liver: Structure and Function.* New York, McGraw-Hill, 1957.

Schwartz SI: *Surgical Diseases of the Liver.* New York, McGraw-Hill, 1964.

Sivaprasad R, Gopalaswamy N: Jaundice: An internist's perspective. *Radiol Clin North Am* 18:179, 1980.

Vennes JA, Bond JH: Approach to the jaundiced patient. *Gastroenterol* 84:1615, 1983.

Williams JAR, Baker RJ, et al: Role of biliary scanning in the investigation of the surgically jaundiced patient. *Surg Gynecol Obstet* 144:525, 1977.

Chapter 25

Esophagus and Diaphragmatic Hernias

Peter C. Pairolero, Victor F. Trastek, and W. Spencer Payne

Surgery of the esophagus is primarily a development of the twentieth century, and its major advances have paralleled those of thoracic surgery. Operations on the esophagus were carried out in earlier years, but they were concerned mainly with removal of foreign bodies or with local excision of malignant lesions or diverticula of the cervical esophagus. Transabdominal procedures for the relief of esophageal achalasia were done in the early 1900s, as were staged reconstructive operations for corrosive stricture and malignant lesions; but only later, after the development of techniques permitting intrathoracic operations, was the thoracic portion of this organ approached with confidence. The first successful one-stage transpleural esophagogastrectomy for carcinoma was performed in 1933 by Ohsawa. Marshall was the first to perform this operation successfully in the United States, in 1937. Thereafter, advances in all aspects of thoracic surgery came rapidly, and as a result the esophagus became accessible to the surgeon's knife. The reductions in surgical morbidity and mortality were not matched at first, however, by similar advances in the understanding of the function of the esophagus. Largely as a result of studies of esophageal motility carried out by Ingelfinger and by Code and Schlegel, the surgical approach to esophageal lesions now rests on sounder physiologic grounds.

ANATOMY

The esophagus is a long muscular tube, extending downward from the pharynx at the C_6 level and terminating in a region commonly referred to as the "cardia," whose definition is highly variable (Fig. 25-1). In its course between these two points, it occupies in the neck a

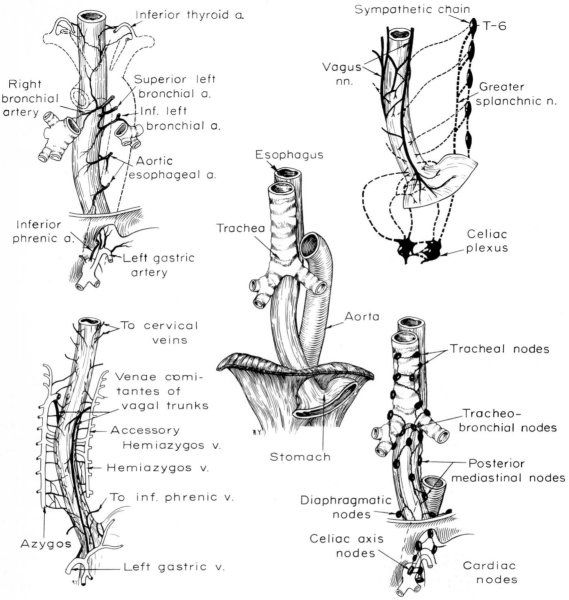

Fig. 25-1. Anatomy of the human esophagus. *Upper left:* Arterial supply. *Lower left:* Venous drainage. *Upper right:* Innervation. *Lower right:* Lymphatic system. [From: *Ellis FH Jr, in Davis L (ed): Christopher's Textbook of Surgery, 8th ed. Philadelphia, Saunders, 1964, p 591, with permission.*]

midline position immediately behind the trachea. In the thorax it inclines posteriorly behind the great vessels, curving slightly to the left to pass behind the left main bronchus, whence it inclines slightly to the right as it continues in the posterior mediastinum. It again deviates to the left behind the pericardial sac, where it runs anterior to the thoracic aorta, crossing it to the left of the midline. It reaches the abdomen through the esophageal hiatus, a noose of diaphragmatic muscle composed chiefly of the right crus of the diaphragm. An esophageal segment of variable length usually occupies an intraabdominal location before joining the stomach at the point referred to as the *cardia.* In general, this term applies to a vague region including the lower esophagus, the esophagogastric junc-

tion, and the upper portion of the stomach. Identification of the esophagogastric junction by reference to the mucosal lining is also difficult. From a practical standpoint, the junction can best be described as that point where the esophageal tube meets the gastric pouch.

There are important supporting structures in the region of the diaphragm and the esophagogastric junction. The anatomy of the diaphragmatic crura varies. The muscle fibers that form the crura arise from the lateral aspects of the second, third, and fourth lumbar vertebrae and pass superiorly and anteriorly past the aorta to form the margins of the esophageal hiatus, inserting into the central tendon of the diaphragm.

Many variations may be seen. In the most common, the right crus contributes all the fibers that form the esophageal hiatus and is reinforced by muscle from the left side. The second most common type is quite similar, but a slip of muscle from the left crus passes behind the esophagus to form part of the right margin of the hiatus. These two variations account for four-fifths of the known instances. The phrenoesophageal membrane or ligament, another important anatomic structure, was described by Laimer in 1883. Composed of mature collagenous fibers, this structure is a continuation of the transversalis fascia of the abdominal parietes and inserts onto the circumference of the lower thoracic esophagus 2 to 3 cm above the true esophagogastric junction. A contribution to this structure is provided by fascia arising from the upper surface of the diaphragm. Further support is given by the pleura above and the peritoneal reflection below. The fibers themselves fan out and insert into the lower esophagus over a relatively wide zone (Fig. 25-2A).

The blood supply of the esophagus is provided in its cervical portion by the inferior thyroid arteries and in its thoracic portion by the aorta itself and by esophageal branches of the bronchial arteries. Supplemental vessels come from arteries on the abdominal side of the diaphragm as well as branches from intercostal arteries. The venous drainage is more complex. Subepithelial and subvenous channels course longitudinally to empty above into the hypopharyngeal and below into the gastric veins. These channels also penetrate the esophageal muscle, from which they receive branches, and leave the esophagus to form a periesophageal plexus, the longest trunks of which accompany the vagus nerves. Drainage from the cervical portion of the esophagus empties ultimately into the inferior thyroid and vertebral veins, drainage from the thoracic portion into the azygos and hemiazygos veins, and from the abdominal portion into the left gastric vein.

The lymphatic vessels run longitudinally in the wall of the esophagus before penetrating the muscle layers to reach regional lymph nodes. Thus malignant lesions of the middle or upper esophagus may metastasize first to the cervical nodes, and lesions of the lower esophagus to gastric and celiac nodes. On leaving the esophagus, however, the lymphatic channels go to the nearest group of nodes, which within the thorax are usually identified by their location as tracheal, tracheobronchial, posterior mediastinal, or diaphragmatic.

The esophagus receives both vagal and sympathetic nerves, its upper portion being supplied by the recurrent nerves, by branches from the IXth and Xth cranial nerves and the cranial root of the XIth, and by sympathetic nerves. The vagal trunks send branches to the remaining voluntary muscles, and the parasympathetic preganglionic fibers to the smooth muscles. The vagus nerves lie on either side of the esophagus through most of its course, forming a plexus about it. At the hiatus, however, two major trunks emerge, the left one coming to lie anteriorly and the right one posteriorly. The vagal plexuses

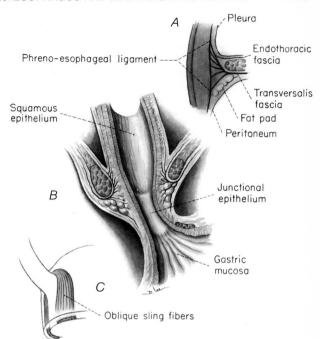

Fig. 25-2. Gross anatomy of region of esophagogastric junction area. *A.* Details of origin and insertion of phrenoesophageal membrane or ligament. *B.* Cross section of distal esophagus and proximal stomach. *C.* Oblique gastric sling fibers.

are joined by mediastinal branches of the thoracic sympathetic chain of the splanchnic nerves. The lower end of the esophagus and the esophagogastric junction zone also receive sympathetic branches from the periarterial plexus along the left gastric and left inferior phrenic arteries.

The esophageal wall is composed of an inner circular layer of muscle and an outer longitudinal layer without a surrounding serosal covering. Striated muscle fibers make a considerable contribution to the outer longitudinal coat in the upper portion of the esophagus, whereas smooth muscle predominates in the lower portion. Measurements of the thickness of the muscle layers of the distal esophageal wall have demonstrated a subtle increase in the segment that corresponds to the physiologic gastroesophageal sphincter. Also, an area of thickened muscle known as the gastric sling fibers of Willis can be demonstrated partially encircling the proximal part of the stomach at the esophagogastric junction area (Fig. 25-2B).

There is a prominent submucosa containing mucous glands, blood vessels, Meissner's plexus of nerves, and a rich network of lymphatic vessels. The mucosal lining is characteristically made up of squamous epithelium, although ectopic islands of gastric mucosa have been identified, particularly in the proximal portions of the esophagus. The distal 1 or 2 cm of the esophageal lumen is lined by columnar epithelium, the columnar-squamous junction lying not at the true esophagogastric junction but within the lower esophagus (Fig. 25-2).

PHYSIOLOGY AND PHYSIOLOGIC TESTS

The esophagus provides a channel by which ingested material is conveyed from the pharynx to the stomach. At either end of the tube are regulatory mechanisms that assist in this function. Current knowledge of the physiology of the esophagus has been gained by the use of special recording techniques to detect and record intraesophageal pressures. In routine tests, three or four pressure-detecting units (fine water-filled and perfused polyvinylchloride tubes attached to strain-gauge manometers) are positioned at various points in the esophagus. Some prefer to use a terminal balloon-covered transducer in addition to the tubes with lateral openings at 5-cm intervals (Fig. 25-3). The infusion of distilled water at a constant rate through the open-tipped tubes provides accurate pressure recordings while the balloon-covered transducer provides higher sensitivity in study of sphincter function. Measurements are made with the esophagus at rest and after swallowing, the resting pressures being measured while the units are being withdrawn in stepwise fashion from the stomach into the esophagus prior to the recording of deglutition pressures (Fig. 25-4).

At the upper end of the esophagus there is a zone, about 3 cm long, of increased pressure that relaxes promptly with swallowing and contracts thereafter as a wave of high pressure passes through it (Fig. 25-4). Contractions of this *upper esophageal sphincter* (UES) are in peristaltic sequence with those of the pharynx above and the esophagus below, and the primary peristaltic wave of

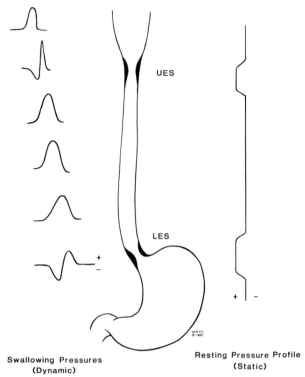

Swallowing Pressures (Dynamic)

Resting Pressure Profile (Static)

Fig. 25-4. Simplified representation demonstrating normal physiologic manometric pressures in pharynx, upper esophageal sphincter (UES) esophagus, and lower esophageal sphincter (LES). On right, static or resting high-pressure zones of LES and UES are defined, as pressure-sensing catheter is withdrawn from stomach below to pharynx above. On left are shown normal sequential swallowing pressure events from pharynx downward. Note that these dynamic events are peristaltic, with both upper and lower sphincters showing relaxation prior to contraction and return to resting tone.

Fig. 25-3. Balloon-covered differential transformer and cluster of three polyvinylchloride tubes used in measurement of esophageal and sphincteric pressures. Each tube has side opening (arrow) 5 cm from opening in next tube, is infused with water at rate of 1.4 mL/min by individual pump, and is attached to pressure-sensitive recording device. At Mayo Clinic, balloon-covered pressure transformer is routinely included as highly sensitive additional means of studying sphincter function. (From: *Code CF, Kelley ML Jr, et al: Gastroenterology 43:521, 1962, with permission.*)

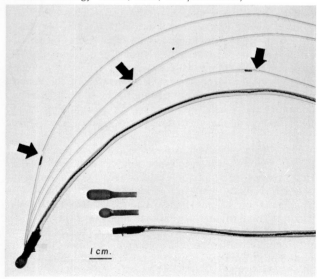

l cm.

the esophagus is thus initiated. The sphincter relaxes to allow the wave to pass and then closes more tightly before returning to a lower, but elevated, resting tone. This wave of positive pressure sweeps in an orderly peristaltic fashion down the body of the esophagus, reaching an intensity of 50 to 100 cmH$_2$O and being somewhat more forceful in the lower esophagus than above. The resting pressures in the body of the esophagus are normally less than atmospheric, because of negative intrathoracic pressure.

There is also a *lower esophageal sphincter* (LES)—a zone of increased pressure at the lower end of the esophagus, somewhat longer (3 to 5 cm long) than that at the upper end, which can be detected by withdrawing the recording units from the stomach into the esophagus (Fig. 25-4). It is located in the region of the hiatus; and in response to a swallowing effort, relaxation of this zone of increased pressure can be identified, along with the immediately following sphincteric contraction in sequence with the peristaltic wave from the esophagus above (Fig. 25-4).

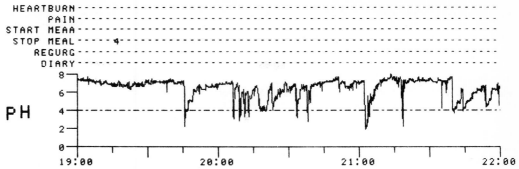

Fig. 25-5. Portion of 24-h pH monitor demonstrating frequent episodes of lower esophageal pH below 4 in a young patient with severe gastroesophageal reflux symptoms.

Measurements of the adaptive response of the LES to graded increases in intragastric pressure provide information pertinent to LES function. This sphincteric response is reflex in nature and is eliminated by vagotomy or atropine. In such a study, with the distal perfused pressure-sensing catheter in the stomach and the next in the higher-pressure zone of the sphincter, intragastric pressure is raised by either abdominal compression or the Valsalva maneuver. The ratio of simultaneous pressure recordings of the two sites provides an index to sphincter function. A ratio of increased sphincter pressure to increased intragastric pressure is usually 1.5, and a ratio less than 1 is considered abnormal. The placement of a third pressure-sensing catheter above the sphincter provides additional information regarding competence. If there is little or no rise in sphincter pressure, there is free transmission of intragastric pressure into the esophagus—the so-called common cavity effect.

The most sensitive objective test of gastroesophageal reflux is the *acid (pH) reflux test,* introduced by Tuttle and Grossman. The acid reflux test is performed by placing 300 mL of 0.1N HCl in the stomach. A pH electrode is placed 5 cm proximal to the manometrically defined LES. While a variety of maneuvers to increase intragastric pressure are performed, esophageal pH is monitored. A decrease in pH to less than 4 is considered positive evidence of gastroesophageal reflux. Johnson and DeMeester have further modified the technique by recording pH changes and correlating these with the patient's symptoms over a 24-h period (Fig. 25-5). The final record is analyzed in terms of the percent of time that pH is less than 4 while the patient is upright and recumbent. Additionally, the number of single reflux episodes and of those greater than 5 min duration are scored. Although not widely utilized clinically, this test provides detailed information not otherwise obtainable.

The *acid-clearing test* is used in patients with documented evidence of gastroesophageal reflux to measure the efficiency of the esophagus to clear instilled HCl by dry swallowing. Essentially, it provides an indirect index of the time refluxed gastric secretions are in contact with esophageal mucosa. A close correlation exists between evidence of esophagitis and a positive result on the clear-

ing test. It is performed by placing a pH probe 5 cm above the LES and instilling 15 mL of 0.1N HCl 10 cm above the electrode. Normally, the esophagus is able to clear the acid from the distal esophagus with 10 dry swallows.

The *acid perfusion test* was developed by Bernstein and Baker as a provocative test for symptomatic reflux esophagitis, and as a means of reproducing esophageal pain to differentiate it from pain of other causes. The test is performed by introducing, via a tube placed at mid-esophagus, a continuous infusion of saline solution, which is alternated at 15- to 20-min intervals with a solution of 0.1N HCl. The results are negative if HCl produces no symptoms and saline reproduces symptoms, or if the pain elicited by infusion is different from spontaneous symptoms. The test is of limited use because of a high incidence of both false-negative and false-positive results.

Helm and associates noted a *galvanometric difference* in the electrical potential of gastric and esophageal mucosa and used this to identify the squamocolumnar junction. An electrode drawn from the stomach through the esophagus will show a 25-mV decrease in potential difference (PD) as it passes from gastric onto esophageal mucosa. While not a critical piece of information, it can be useful in orienting mucosa to manometric events.

Despite extensive knowledge regarding the effects of various hormones, drugs, foods, and other chemicals on lower-esophageal sphincter pressure, there has been only one *pharmacologic test* of esophageal function, and it has largely fallen into disuse. Kramer and Ingelfinger described the increased sensitivity and marked contractile response of the achalasic esophagus to parasympathomimetic drugs, a reaction indicative of denervation as defined by Cannon's law. The test is subjectively unpleasant, and it has been largely replaced by standard manometric studies.

Various safe, noninvasive *radioactive scanning techniques* for studying not only reflux, but the events of esophageal and gastric emptying after the ingestion of labeled liquids or solids, are in the developmental stage.

Although *radiography and endoscopy* are essential in the study of esophageal disease, except possibly for cine radiography, they provide no direct assessment of esophageal function. In addition to the usually ingested liquid radiopaque media, the mixture of barium with solid foods (the so-called barium sandwich) for fluoroscopic examination can provide functional information not defined by other tests and thereby lend objective credence to otherwise unexplained esophageal symptoms.

The details of esophageal innervation remain to be clarified, but esophageal peristalsis seems to be under vagal control, because division of these nerves produces simultaneous low pressures in the body of the esophagus after deglutition. The inferior esophageal sphincter, however, continues to relax with swallowing even after complete denervation, suggesting a certain degree of autonomy.

In spite of the clear demonstration of a physiologic sphincter at the lower end of the esophagus, there remains considerable controversy concerning the exact mechanism by which gastroesophageal reflux is prevented under normal circumstances. Factors that have been suggested as important include the diaphragm, a valve-flap mechanism, the gastric sling fibers and oblique angle of entry, and the mucosal rosette. There is substantial evidence to suggest that the first three are not involved in gastroesophageal competence and that the main antireflux mechanisms, acting together, are the musculature of the intrinsic sphincter and the prominent folds of epithelial gastric lining at the cardia. Studies by Goyal indicate that the LES is controlled by neural, hormonal, myogenic, and mechanical influences.

In the past some observers believed that the basal sphincter pressure was maintained by continuous vagal tone and that sphincter relaxation was a result of a decrease of tonic vagal activity. However, it is now held that both relaxation and contraction of the LES are due to the vagal transmission of active inhibitory or excitatory impulses but that neither acts as the major determinant of basal LES pressure. The role of sympathetic innervation on the LES is less well understood. Stimulation of alpha-adrenergic receptors causes the LES to contract, and stimulation of beta-adrenergic receptors causes it to relax. It is further hypothesized that sympathetic nerves act to modulate vagal activity on the LES. The fact that complete pharmacologic denervation of the LES does not influence basal sphincter pressure suggests that basal sphincter pressure is not due to tonic autonomic neural activity but that it may be due to tonic myogenic activity of the LES muscle itself. Many hormones, drugs, and various chemicals have been known to modify basal pressure of the LES (Table 25-1). It has been held that circulating gastrin is the major determinant of basal LES pressure and that this effect is modulated by interaction of secretin. However, recent studies do not support these views but suggest that the changes previously observed were obtainable only in response to unphysiologically high levels of these hormones. Other hormones such as prostaglandins, histamine, and serotonin produce less clear or more variable effects on LES pressure, depending on experimental conditions.

Thus, at this time it appears that the basal LES pressure is due to background basal tone provided by intrinsic myogenic activity of the sphincter muscle itself and that this tone is modulated by a variety of excitatory and inhibitory neurohormonal influences. The sphincter relaxation is chiefly due to neural activity mediated by inhibitory vagal and extravagal pathways.

Table 25-1. REGULATION OF LES PRESSURE

	Increase	*Decrease*
Hormones	Gastrin	Secretin
	Motilin	Cholecystokinin
	Substance P	Gastric inhibitory
	Vasopressin	polypeptides
	Glucagon	Vasoactive
		intestinal
		polypeptides
		Progestational
		agents
Drugs	α-Adrenergic	α-Adrenergic
	agonist	antagonist
	Norepinephrine	Phentolamine
	Phenylephrine	β-Adrenergic
	Cholinergic	agonist
	Bethanechol	Isoproterenol
	Methacholine	Anticholinergic
	Anticholinesterase	Atropine
	Edrophonium	Theophylline
	Betazole	
	Metoclopramide	
Miscellaneous	Prostaglandin $F_{2\alpha}$	Prostaglandins E_1,
	Protein meal	E_2, A_2
	Gastric	Nicotine
	alkalinization	Ethanol
		Fat meal
		Chocolate
		Gastric
		acidification

SOURCE: Data from Castell DO: The lower esophageal sphincter: Physiologic and clinical aspects. *Ann Intern Med* 83:390, 1975.

Loss of the LES basal tone can occur as a consequence of pregnancy (because of elevated levels of progesterone and estrogen), excessive ingestion of alcohol, smoking, and use of drugs that especially inhibit the LES (atropine, nitrites, beta-adrenergic agents, etc.). The LES basal tone can be enhanced by neutralization of gastric acid and by administration of drugs such as bethanecol or metoclopramide.

When the LES is challenged by an increase in intragastric pressure, its resting tone increases. This response is due to a vagus-mediated neural reflex that can be blocked by atropine or vagotomy, as shown by Cohen and Lipshutz. The ability to increase the LES pressure so that it is greater than the rise in intragastric pressure is one of the essential features of the competent LES and the basis of the test alluded to above.

FUNCTIONAL DISTURBANCES OF THE ESOPHAGUS

The development of techniques for physiologic evaluation of esophageal function has permitted the classification of esophageal motor disorders in two main categories: (1) those characterized by disturbances of the esophagus and lower sphincter, such as esophageal achalasia and diffuse spasm of the esophagus; and (2) those characterized by failure of the normal gastroesophageal competence mechanism, which leads to gastro-esophageal reflux and its complications. Although the causes of these conditions remain in doubt, their clinical and physiologic manifestations are well known, so surgical treatment can be undertaken on sound grounds in properly selected patients.

Motility Disturbances

ACHALASIA

Achalasia of the esophagus, or "cardiospasm," as it is more commonly but inaccurately known, has been recognized by the medical profession for more than 300 years. As early as 1674, Thomas Willis in his *Pharmaceutice Rationalis* described the symptoms of this condition and advised forceful dilation as treatment. It is a condition in which peristalsis is absent from the body of the esophagus and the inferior esophageal sphincter fails to relax in response to swallowing.

The causes of the condition are unknown, although a variety have been suggested, including inherent weakness of the esophagus, spasm of the esophagus, mechanical factors such as external compression or trauma, and congenital factors. Most students of the subject now agree that the disease has a neurogenic basis, and pathologic evidence supporting this belief is provided by degeneration or absence of the ganglion cells of Auerbach's plexus in the esophagus of many patients with the disease, a finding first reported by Rake in 1926. Subsequent studies have shown that the changes occur throughout the thoracic esophagus, particularly in the body of the organ, but one-third of the patients are unaffected.

Fig. 25-6. Achalasia of esophagus, radiographs illustrating varying degrees of esophageal dilatation and tortuosity. Effects are absent or mild in 20 percent of patients, moderate in 45 percent, and marked or advanced in 35 percent. All have absent peristalsis and nonrelaxing lower esophageal sphincter.

The reason for these nerve-cell changes remains obscure; infections due to bacteria or viruses, infestations by parasites, and vitamin deficiencies all have been incriminated. That the primary site of the disorder may be in the extraesophageal nerve supply—either the vagus nerve itself or its central nuclei—has been suggested by pathologic studies of biopsy and autopsy material and by experiments involving the selective destruction of the motor nuclei of the vagus nerve in the medulla of the cat and the dog.

CLINICAL MANIFESTATIONS. Whatever the cause of the disease, its clinical manifestations are now well recognized. It occurs with equal frequency in men and in women, and although it may appear at any age, it is more frequently seen in persons between the ages of thirty and fifty years. The earliest and most constant symptom is obstruction to swallowing, which at first may be intermittent. However, as the condition progresses, difficulty is experienced with all efforts to swallow. As a rule, the patient experiences more difficulty with cold than with warm foods, and solids may at first seem to pass more easily than liquids. Pain is rare and is more likely to occur in the early stages of the disease than later; it becomes less noticeable as the esophagus dilates. Regurgitation of ingested food and liquids is a common symptom and may occur particularly at night when the patient is recumbent, leading to aspiration and the development of pulmonary complications. Carcinoma of the esophagus occurs approximately seven times as often in patients with esophageal achalasia as in the general population.

Radiographic studies are helpful in the diagnosis of the disease, because even in its early stages evidence of obstruction at the cardia and slight dilatation of the esophagus may be noted. As the disease progresses, the classic radiographic signs develop (Fig. 25-6), the esophagus becoming dilated and its lower portion projecting beaklike into the distal narrowed segment with very little, if

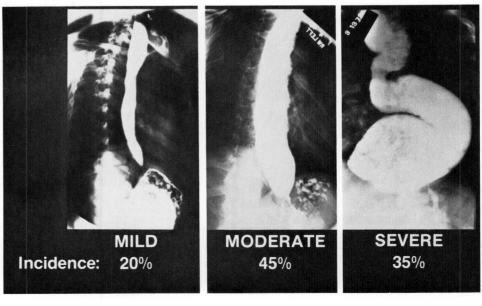

MILD
Incidence: 20%

MODERATE
45%

SEVERE
35%

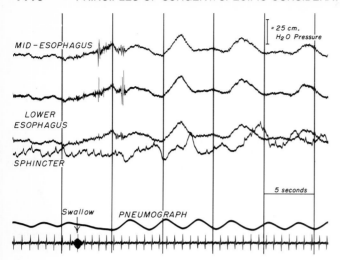

Fig. 25-7. Achalasia of esophagus: response to deglutition. In response to swallowing, feeble simultaneous contractions occur in body of esophagus, with failure of sphincteric relaxation. (From: *Ellis FH Jr, Payne WS: Adv Surg 1:179, 1965. Copyright 1965 by Year Book Medical Publishers, Inc. Used by permission.*)

any, barium present in the stomach. In some cases, the esophagus may reach huge proportions, so that it may be seen on the ordinary thoracic radiograph. Differentiation between early stages of esophageal achalasia and benign stricture or carcinoma of the cardia may be difficult, and esophagoscopy may be required for diagnosis.

Fig. 25-8. Method of performing hydrostatic dilation. *A.* Passage of #41 French olive-tipped bougie into stomach. *B.* Passage of #50 to #60 French sound guided by flexible wire spiral. *C.* Passage of hydrostatic dilator into esophagogastric junction. *D.* Distention of dilator. (From: *Olsen AM, Harrington SW, et al: J Thorac Surg 22:164, 1951, with permission.*)

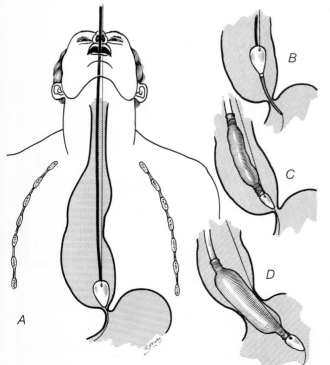

PHYSIOLOGIC STUDIES. Confirmation of the clinical diagnosis can be provided by studies of esophageal motility. Such studies demonstrate that the pressure in the body of the esophagus is higher than normal, often equaling atmospheric pressure, presumably because of esophageal dilatation with retention of food and fluid. In response to a swallowing effort, feeble, simultaneous, repetitive contractions occur throughout the esophagus, but there is no coordinated peristaltic wave (Fig. 25-7). Although relaxation of the UES occurs normally, in the majority of cases the lower sphincter fails to relax after swallowing. Cohen and Lipshutz, using perfused catheters, demonstrated that the LES pressure at rest is increased in patients with achalasia to approximately twice that seen in normal subjects. Furthermore, when the sphincter occasionally does relax during swallowing, the relaxation is incomplete. In some patients with achalasia, contractions of the esophagus and the sphincter may be vigorous and simultaneous, and the term *vigorous achalasia* has been applied to this subgroup.

TREATMENT. Current knowledge does not permit restoration of the disordered esophageal motility to normal. Effective therapy, therefore, can be directed only to relief of the distal esophageal obstruction. Because diet and drugs are ineffective, this must be accomplished either by forceful dilation of the esophagus or by surgical means.

Mechanical, pneumatic, and hydrostatic dilation have been used with success. At the Mayo Clinic, hydrostatic dilation (Fig. 25-8) has been used extensively in the past and has been found to be a useful technique. Okike and associates reported good to excellent results in 65 percent of patients observed for an average of 9½ years (Table 25-2). The method is not without risk; an esophageal perforation occurred in about 2 percent of cases. Forceful dilatation has been done with a pneumatic balloon catheter, inflating the balloon to a 35-mm diameter at approximately 300 torr. This has been performed at the Mayo Clinic in approximately 50 patients; three perforations have occurred. Currently pneumatic dilatation seems most appropriate for those patients who are poor surgical

Table 25-2. COMPARISON OF TWO METHODS USED IN TREATING ACHALASIA AT THE MAYO CLINIC, 1949 THROUGH 1975

Factors	Dilation (N = 431)		Esophagomyotomy (N = 468)	
Result, %				
Excellent	28	65*	50	85*
Good	37		35	
Fair	16		9	
Poor	19		6	
Follow-up, years	1–18		1–17	
No. patients	311		456	
Percent	72		97	
Age, years	1–85		4–81	

* Significantly different ($p < 0.001$)
SOURCE: Okike N, Payne WS, et al: *Ann Thorac Surg* 28:119, 1979.

risks or who have recurrent achalasia following a modified Heller myotomy.

Limitations of medical therapy, including the use of forceful dilation, have led to surgical efforts to relieve the symptoms of esophageal achalasia. The techniques have included excisional or bypassing procedures and denervation procedures. The latter were ineffective, and the uniform development of severe reflux esophagitis after any procedure that destroys or bypasses the inferior esophageal sphincter has rightly led to their abandonment.

Current surgical therapy stems historically from the double cardiomyotomy first proposed by Heller in 1913. It has been modified by a number of surgeons in subsequent years. The simplest and most effective modification involves an incision through the muscle layers of the distal esophagus, through a thoracic approach. The mucosa is exposed to free completely the narrowed distal esophageal segment of its circular musculature, but the incision is extended onto the stomach only far enough to ensure completeness of this portion of the procedure (Fig. 25-9). Generally, 1 cm onto the stomach is adequate. The most proximal portion of the stomach can be recognized by multiple transverse mucosal veins. Damage to the vagus nerves and the supporting structures about the hiatus is avoided. An operation carried out in the manner described, without ancillary procedures, should relieve the distal esophageal obstruction in almost every patient and should rarely lead to esophageal reflux. Okike and associates, reviewing the Mayo Clinic experience from 1949 to 1976, reported that 94 percent of 468 patients treated in this fashion were benefited by the operation, and approximately 85 percent had excellent or good results (Table 25-2). More recent reviews of other series confirm our favorable experience with surgical treatment of achalasia.

Because of the superior results obtainable by a properly performed esophagomyotomy, operation is replacing all other forms of treatment for achalasia. Forceful dilation should be used only for selected patients whose general condition precludes a major operation or for patients who decline to undergo operation. Thus, myotomy should be offered to all but extremely high-risk patients.

The late results of a properly performed esophagomyotomy are so satisfactory that it is neither necessary nor advisable to consider the performance of ancillary esophageal procedures at the time of myotomy. Indeed, Peyton et al., Mansour et al., Menguy, and others have reported the performance of an antireflux procedure at operation on all achalasia patients without a pre-existent sliding esophageal hiatal hernia. Not only does this unnecessarily complicate the surgical approach, it is an overreaction to the 3 percent incidence of incompetence after myotomy alone. Further, the failure rate of antireflux procedures exceeds the failure rate they are designed to prevent. Fewer than 6 percent of patients have poor results requiring reoperation for any cause. Indeed, the majority of patients requiring reoperation for achalasia require treatment for persistent obstruction at the distal esophagus because of persistent achalasia, not because of stricture or esophagitis. In the majority of patients requiring reoperation, the previous myotomy is found to have healed; and the patients respond rather well to performance of a properly designed remyotomy with attention to the details outlined. Only rarely is it necessary to perform esophagogastrectomy. If esophagogastrectomy is required, an antireflux procedure is generally necessary; care, however, must be taken to avoid a 360° fundoplication as this will almost certainly obstruct the amotile esophagus.

DIFFUSE SPASM

The causes of the hypermotility disorders are also unknown, although they too may be related to abnormalities affecting the vagus supply to the organ. Diffuse spasm of the esophagus, hypertensive gastroesophageal sphincter, and the hypercontracting lower esophageal sphincter are the conditions under discussion, and there is little evidence that they may be precursors of esophageal achalasia.

MANIFESTATIONS. Differentiation of these conditions from esophageal achalasia can usually be made on clinical grounds. Pain and dysphagia are the predominant symptoms, pain being more pronounced and dysphagia occurring intermittently or not at all. The pain may manifest only as a sensation of discomfort under the lower half of the sternum, or it may be severe and colicky, with extension through to the back or into the neck, shoulders, or arms, resembling cardiac pain. It may be provoked by eating, or it may come on spontaneously, even awakening the patient at night. Patients so afflicted tend to be highstrung and nervous, and the diagnosis of psychoneurosis may be entertained. The symptoms are intermittent and are more likely to be troublesome than incapacitating; even during an attack, the patient seldom appears to be seriously ill.

Radiologic abnormalities of the esophagus occur in fewer than half the cases. When present, however, they may be striking, with a range from simple narrowing to segmental spasm finally to extreme changes, including

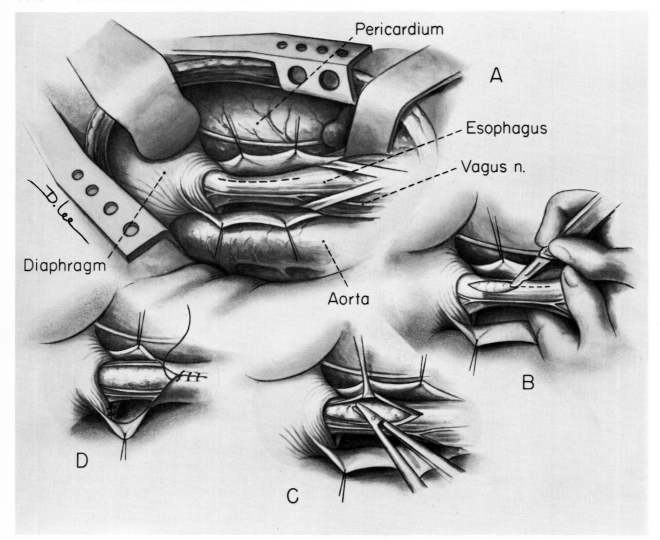

Fig. 25-9. Modified Heller esophagomyotomy for achalasia of esophagus. *A.* Transthoracic exposure of distal esophagus for esophagomyotomy. Esophagus has been mobilized and elevated from its bed by Penrose drain. Intended incision is indicated by dashed line. *B.* Beginning incision. *C.* Dissection of mucosa from muscularis. *D.* Restoration of esophagogastric junction to intraabdominal position, with suture narrowing of esophageal hiatus if necessary. (From: *Ellis FH Jr, Kiser JC, et al: Ann Surg 166:640, 1967, with permission.*)

pseudodiverticulosis (Fig. 25-10). A small diaphragmatic hernia is frequently present, and an epiphrenic diverticulum commonly coexists. A localized area of obstruction may be detectable in patients with hypertensive gastroesophageal sphincter as well as in those with hypercontracting LES.

DIAGNOSIS. Because esophageal radiographs may appear normal in patients with these disorders, and clinical history may be rather nonspecific, the diagnosis usually rests on the results of esophageal-motility studies. In patients with diffuse spasm, there is a specific abnormal pattern of the deglutitive pressures. A primary peristaltic wave can be recognized over the upper half of the esophagus, but in the lower third to two-thirds it is replaced by simultaneous, repetitive, and occasionally prolonged pressure increases of considerable magnitude (Fig. 25-11). Evidence of hiatal herniation is common. In most patients, however, there is no evidence of abnormality of the two sphincters unless there is a hypertension or hypercontraction of the LES, in which case resting pressures in that region are excessive and relaxation may be poor or pressures excessive as the swallowing peristalsis passes through the sphincter. Occasionally these sphincteric changes are the only manifestations of disease.

TREATMENT. The use of an extended esophagomyotomy for the treatment of patients with "diffuse nodular myomatosis of the esophagus" was suggested in 1950 by Lortat-Jacob. Although physiologic studies were not made in his patients, many probably had forms of esophageal hypermotility disturbances. A similar approach was

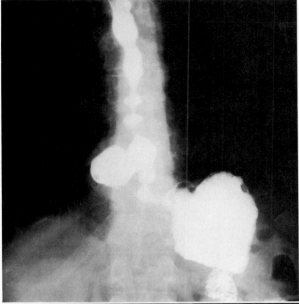

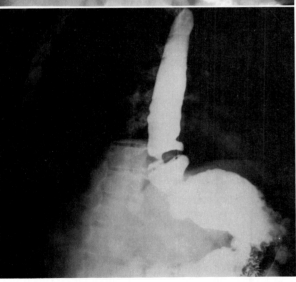

Fig. 25-10. Hypermotility disturbances: esophageal radiographs from two cases. *Top:* Diffuse spasm of esophagus with epiphrenic diverticulum and small hiatal hernia. *Bottom:* Hypertensive gastroesophageal sphincter with small hiatal hernia. (From: *Ellis FH Jr, Payne WS: Adv Surg 1:179, 1965. Copyright 1965 by Year Book Medical Publishers, Inc. Used by permission.*)

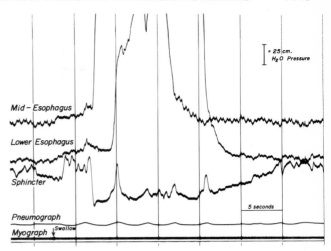

Fig. 25-11. Diffuse spasm: motility in esophagus and sphincter. Note giant repetitive contractions. Sphincter relaxes normally. Peristalsis, although usually absent, is present in this case. (From: *Ellis FH Jr, Code CF, Olsen AM: Surgery 48:155, 1960, with permission.*)

initiated independently at the Mayo Clinic in 1956 in order to control the severe symptoms of hypermotility disturbance of the esophagus in carefully selected patients.

In many respects, the technique of the operation resembles that used for achalasia of the esophagus. However, the proximal limit of the esophageal muscular incision varies, depending on the preoperative estimate of the extent of the disease as defined by esophageal motility studies. It may occasionally extend as high as the aortic arch or above (Fig. 25-12). If esophageal motility demon-

strates a hypertensive LES, the myotomy must be carried down onto the stomach as it is for achalasia. If the LES is normal, the myotomy can stop on the distal esophagus. Surgical repair of an associated diaphragmatic hernia is essential. Henderson and associates have stressed the need for an antireflux procedure at operation on all patients with diffuse spasm, and extension of the myotomy from the stomach to 10 cm above the aortic end. Flye and Sealy have reported similar good results with long esophagomyotomy, reserving antireflux operations for patients with manifest hernia or incompetence. Surgical treatment is less effective than for achalasia; only 78 percent of these patients so treated are benefited. Leonardi and associates reported a 91 percent improvement rate in 11 patients when a more proximal myotomy was done to save a sphincter that was not manometrically affected as shown in Fig. 25-12.

Patients therefore should be selected carefully for this operation, the ideal candidate being an emotionally stable person with serious disability from the disease but without evidence of associated gastrointestinal problems. There should be demonstrable evidence of the severity of the disease in the form of a markedly abnormal esophageal motility pattern, ideally associated with radiographic evidence of esophageal spasm.

Disturbances of Gastroesophageal Competence (Gastroesophageal Reflux and Its Complications)

While it is clear that the loss of gastroesophageal competence is the cause for gastroesophageal reflux and its complications, the precise mechanism of competence is still debated. It is generally conceded that there is normally a high-pressure zone (HPZ) 3 to 5 cm long, of 10 to 20 mmHg, which is largely responsible for maintaining a

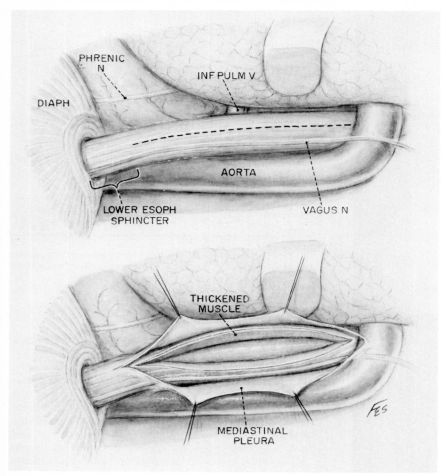

Fig. 25-12. Long esophagomyotomy for diffuse spasm of esophagus. Note that incision extends to aortic arch and spares lower esophageal sphincter. This technique is applicable in diffuse spasm when lower esophageal sphincter is demonstrated manometrically to be normal and only the body of esophagus is affected by motility disturbances.

protective pressure barrier between the stomach and the esophagus to prevent reflux. This barrier relaxes with swallowing to provide unimpeded transport of a bolus, and promptly returns to its resting tone. By mechanisms poorly understood, the intensity of this HPZ increases with intraabdominal and intragastric pressure, effecting an antireflux barrier responsive to changing conditions. Physiologists classically have held that the HPZ is equivalent to LES, but more recently this has been challenged by DeMeester and associates. They conceived that the HPZ was entirely an artifact of esophageal environment and not entirely a result of active motor tone of the sphincter (Fig. 25-13). In brief, they held that the HPZ resulted from exposure of a segment of distal esophagus to intraabdominal positive pressure. Regardless of the merit of these controversies, Cohen and Harris succeeded, by study of the length and magnitude of this HPZ among patients with and without hiatal hernias, in distinguishing those with reflux from those without. Subsequently Olsen and Harrington, Schlegel, and Payne, by the criterion of a hypotensive LES, were able to select a group of patients without hiatal hernia who had significant reflux. In clinical practice, however, it has generally not been possible to select patients for treatment of reflux

on the basis of objective measurement of HPZ. This is not only because there is considerable pressure overlap between refluxers and nonrefluxers in many cases, but mainly because the decision to treat is not whether a given patient is refluxing, but what and how severe are the subjective and objective complications attributable to reflux.

While the majority of patients with clinically significant gastroesophageal reflux have an associated sliding esophageal hiatal hernia, the converse is not true. Indeed, the vast majority of patients with hiatal hernia do not have significant reflux, and the hernia per se does not present a clinical problem.

Sometimes systemic collagen disease involves the esophagus. Scleroderma is probably the most common disease that gives rise to motor failure of the distal esophagus. On manometric study there is a loss of both esophageal peristalsis and sphincter tone. This permits free re-

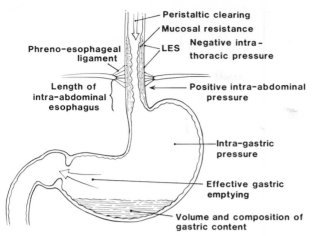

Fig. 25-13. Factors that affect gastroesophageal competence or permit gastroesophageal reflux and its complications. These include esophageal peristalsis with its clearing action, intrinsic lower-esophageal-sphincter tone, intraabdominal position of part of esophagus, site of phrenoesophageal ligament insertions, intraabdominal and intrathoracic pressures, intragastric pressure, effective gastric emptying, and concentration and composition of digestive secretions (acid-bile-pancreatic) present in stomach and available for reflux into esophagus.

flux of gastric contents without a clearing mechanism and results in a particularly virulent form of reflux esophagitis.

Other causes of gastroesophageal reflux include operations that destroy or bypass the normal lower esophageal competence mechanism. These include poorly executed myotomies, resections of the esophagogastric junction, and various types of cardioplasties.

Gastroesophageal reflux may also occur in the presence of a normal competence mechanism, when gastric emptying is impaired by gastric-outlet obstruction or failure of gastric motility.

Almost all of the subjective and objective complications of gastroesophageal reflux (Table 25-3) result from the acute sensitivity of esophageal mucosa to a variety of digestive secretions. While acid peptic secretions are generally implicated, bile and pancreatic secretions, irrespective of pH, are equally irritating and corrosive. The

Table 25-3. COMPLICATIONS OF
GASTROESOPHAGEAL REFLUX

Intractable subjective distress
Esophagitis
Bleeding
Stenosis of esophagus
  Reversible
  Irreversible
Shortening of esophagus
  Reversible
  Irreversible
Esophageal-ulcer penetration or perforation
Columnar epithelial-lined lower esophagus (Barrett esophagus)
Motility disturbances of esophagus

severity of complications is related to the type and concentration of secretions refluxed and their contact time with esophageal mucosa.

SYMPTOMS. Heartburn is the classic symptom of gastroesophageal reflux. It is described as a burning retrosternal distress beginning in the epigastrum and extending for varying distances toward the neck. There may be, at times, actual regurgitation of bitter, sour liquid into the mouth, which may cause gagging or retching. Reflux symptoms are usually precipitated by a full stomach or by postural changes such as leaning over, lifting, or recumbency. Nocturnal distress is common, the patients awakening one or more times during sleep with heartburn, regurgitation, or actual respiratory aspiration with cough and choking. Often it is possible to control such symptoms with topical antacids, weight reduction, slant bed, cimetidine, and metoclopramide. When symptoms become intractable to medical management and the patient's ability to function is seriously impaired by symptoms of reflux, surgical restoration of competence is indicated, irrespective of the degree of objective esophagitis or other complications of reflux.

ESOPHAGITIS AND BLEEDING

Esophagitis is an objective finding and not a symptom. It can be suspected from history or esophageal x-rays, but endoscopy is required for diagnosis. It is defined as an objective change in the esophageal mucosa as a consequence of corrosive injury. Objective esophagitis does not necessarily correlate with either the duration or severity of its symptoms, though there is a general parallel. In some patients with intractable subjective distress, no objective endoscopic mucosal change is evident, but mucosal biopsy will demonstrate occult histologic changes. Diffuse distal esophageal erythema is one of the earliest gross signs of esophagitis. This may progress to linear rows of discrete superficial ulcers and subsequently to their coalescence, giving the appearance of linear streaks of ulceration and friable mucosa. Eventually this can lead to an extensive loss of normal epithelium in the distal esophagus or a deep solitary ulcer. When esophagitis becomes severe, patients often complain of painful swallowing (*odynophagia*). With deep penetrating ulceration, there is often an intractable constant pain radiating to the thoracic spine. Although the esophagus may have a hemorrhagic appearance and there may be chronic blood loss from ulcerative esophagitis, massive upper gastroesophageal bleeding is uncommon. Bleeding, when present, is probably more often attributable to an associated hiatal hernia with gastric erosions in the intrathoracic loculus of the stomach or where the stomach is impinged upon by the hiatus. Severe esophagitis is not often reversible by medical means and usually requires an antireflux operation for its control.

STENOSIS OF THE ESOPHAGUS

As consequences of chronic recurrent corrosive injury, varying degrees of transmural inflammation, muscle contracture, and collagen deposition can occur in the wall of

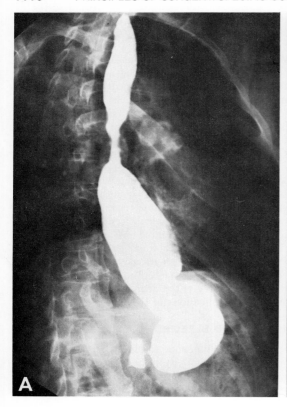
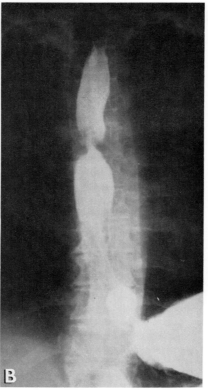

Fig. 25-14. *A.* Esophagus of patient who had esophageal hiatal hernia with reflux esophagitis, shortened esophagus, and stricture. Esophagogastric junction is at midthoracic level, with stricture (several centimeters long) above. Typical esophageal peristalsis extended up to, but not beyond, midthoracic esophagogastric junction. Most of stomach had been pulled up into chest as consequence of acquired shortening of esophagus. *B.* Barrett esophagus. Small diaphragmatic hernia (sliding type) and midesophageal stricture. Tubular structure between stricture and stomach is columnar epithelial-lined esophagus with typical esophageal motility. (From: *Burgess JN, Payne WS, et al: Mayo Clin Proc, 46:728, 1971, with permission.*)

the esophagus. Classically this occurs in the lower few centimeters of the esophagus at the esophagogastric junction. In patients with protracted emesis or with protracted nasogastric intubation, long-tapered stenoses affecting the lower half of the esophagus are seen. These stenoses represent a tissue response to corrosive injury. The vast majority of stenotic lesions are amenable to simple dilation therapy, and symptoms of dysphagia are relieved thereby. Stenosis of the esophagus is an important complication of gastroesophageal reflux; and if it recurs or if symptoms of reflux persist after dilation, an antireflux operation is indicated. Surgical treatment is the most definitive means of preventing progressive and irreversible esophageal injury.

On rare occasions, reflux esophagitis and stenosis progress to such a severe panmural stage that an actual irreversible stricture is formed. If such a stricture cannot be dilated to a #50 French size with use of a swallowed thread or an endoscopically placed wire as a guide, stricture resection is the only method for restoring unobstructed swallowing. This rare late manifestation of reflux esophagitis poses special problems in surgical management to ensure that reflux, esophagitis, and stenosis do not recur after surgical relief of the stricture.

SHORTENED ESOPHAGUS

Just as stenosis of the esophagus is the result of annular contraction of the esophagus due to corrosive injury, so shortening occurs as the result of linear contracture (Fig. 25-14*A*). Whereas stenosis often accompanies shortening, shortened esophagus is occasionally seen without significant stenosis; and, of course, stenosis is usually seen without shortened esophagus. The vast majority of patients in whom a shortened esophagus is suspected on the basis of x-rays or endoscopic findings do not prove to have the condition when surgically explored. In such cases surgical mobilization usually permits the esophagogastric junction to be reduced below the diaphragm for the performance of one of the antireflux procedures. Under rare circumstances, however, the esophagus is so permanently fibrosed and shortened that one must consider a Collis gastroplasty to effectively lengthen the esophagus so that an antireflux procedure can be done below the diaphragm. In rare cases shortening is so marked that even this cannot be accomplished, and more complex surgical maneuvers are required.

While shortening is an important complication to be aware of in surgical management of gastroesophageal reflux, the symptoms in some patients have ceased entirely or are controllable medically. Thus, as an isolated finding without symptoms, shortening is not an indication for surgical treatment.

COLUMNAR EPITHELIAL-LINED LOWER ESOPHAGUS (BARRETT ESOPHAGUS)

As a consequence of the corrosive injury and destruction when the squamous epithelial lining of the lower esophagus has been damaged or destroyed by the corrosive effect of gastroesophageal reflux, replacement of normal epithelium with columnar epithelium occurs in some patients. It is as yet uncertain whether this is the result of metaplasia or cephalad growth of columnar epithelium from the gastric cardia. The abnormal esophageal lining may extend to the level of the aortic arch or higher (Fig. 25-14B). There is often a stenosis of the esophagus at the new squamocolumnar junction and evidence of esophagitis in the squamous epithelial-lined portion above the stricture. The columnar epithelium is largely mucus-producing, with only sparse parietal cells. Rarely, there is a deep, solitary, benign ulcer in the columnar epithelial-lined portion of the lower esophagus. This is referred to as a Barrett ulcer.

The risk of an adenocarcinoma developing in patients with Barrett esophagus is greater than in the general population, but the critical study of a large group of patients with Barrett esophagus to determine the incidence of subsequent malignancy has not been done. At the present time, prophylactic resection is not indicated. Correction of reflux does not prevent subsequent malignant transformation and does not usually cause regression of the abnormal columnar epithelial lining.

Operation is recommended to control intractable symptomatic reflux and stenosis. Standard antireflux procedures usually suffice. Most stenoses are readily dilatable prior to repair. Resection is generally indicated only when cancer is diagnosed or suspected. Many patients with Barrett esophagus are largely asymptomatic at diagnosis. In the absence of other reflux complications, these fortunates do not require specific treatment but do need careful follow-up for early detection of esophageal malignancy.

ESOPHAGEAL-ULCER PENETRATION AND PERFORATION

Esophageal perforation is a rare spontaneous complication of gastroesophageal reflux and esophagitis, yet among patients with postemetic rupture of the distal esophagus a high percentage have preexisting diaphragmatic hernia, esophagitis, and ulceration. The majority of instrumental perforations occur during attempts to dilate benign stenoses of the distal esophagus or to biopsy blindly beyond a stenotic lesion. Penetrating ulcers rarely produce a spontaneous rupture into the mediastinum or pleural spaces. They are more prone to produce intractable penetrating back pain, odynophagia, and bleeding.

MOTILITY DISTURBANCES

Various nonspecific motility disturbances may accompany reflux esophagitis. These may range from increased irritability, with occasional episodes of simultaneous nonperistaltic contraction, to diminution or even complete loss of lower-sphincter tone and contractility of the body of the esophagus. High-amplitude peristaltic contractions may be seen with distal stenotic obstruction, and with time these may give way to fatigue with complete loss of motor activity. Generally, the motility disorders of reflux esophagitis and its complications are reversible by surgical correction of reflux or obstruction.

CONTRACTION RINGS OF LOWER ESOPHAGUS

A ringlike constriction at the squamocolumnar junction, demonstrated radiographically by Schatzki and Gary in patients with diaphragmatic hernia, is now generally recognized as a minor complication of gastroesophageal reflux. It is an organic lesion consisting of a dense annular connective band in the submucosa at the squamocolumnar junction. The degree of impingement of the esophageal lumen varies greatly, and some patients are totally asymptomatic. The symptoms of esophageal obstruction (*dysphagia*) begin to occur with increasing frequency as ring diameter becomes less than 15 mm. Antecedent history of heartburn is frequent, and some patients experience recurrence of gastroesophageal reflux symptoms after the ring is dilated. In the majority, dilation relieves dysphagia, and reflux symptoms are mild and controllable. On rare occasions the mucosal ring will require surgical excision or disruption at the time of hiatal hernia repair and performance of an antireflux procedure.

RESPIRATORY ASPIRATION

Contamination of the upper and lower respiratory tracts by spontaneous gastroesophageal reflux of stomach contents is a generally accepted complication of gastroesophageal incompetence. Upper respiratory infections, sore throat, hoarseness, cough, choking, asthma, fever, pneumonitis, bronchiectasis, and lung abscess are recognized results of aspiration. What is unclear and difficult to document is the incidence of these complications. Some patients give a clear sequential clinical history of recurrent heartburn followed immediately by choking and coughing with recurrent episodes of fever, asthma, or pneumonitis. Others present with a respiratory problem, and the esophageal aspect is otherwise minor or asymptomatic. The 24-h acid-reflux test has the potential of sorting and relating respiratory events objectively to episodes of gastroesophageal reflux and directing therapy appropriately toward antireflux measures. In most cases, however, respiratory aspiration is just one of several well-defined subjective and objective complications of gastroesophageal reflux, and surgical indications are clear.

INDICATIONS FOR SURGICAL TREATMENT

The indications for surgical treatment of gastroesophageal reflux depend on objective assessment of severity and intractability of complications listed in Table 25-3. Although it is essential to correlate the occurrence of complications with that of gastroesophageal reflux as effect and cause, surgery is not indicated for gastroesophageal incompetence alone. Finally, before resorting to operation, it should be established that symptoms and complications cannot be controlled by simpler means.

Since the anatomic repair of esophageal hiatal hernia is an integral part of restoration of gastroesophageal competence and an essential feature of most of the antireflux operations, the details of surgical techniques appear in the succeeding section on esophageal hiatal hernia.

DIAPHRAGMATIC HERNIAS

A variety of acquired and congenital herniations occur through the diaphragm. All are associated with protrusion of abdominal viscera from the high-pressure abdomen into the low-pressure thorax. Like most abdominal hernias, diaphragmatic hernias carry a high risk of volvulus, obstruction, and strangulation of herniated hollow viscera. An exception is the pure sliding esophageal hernia, wherein the only clinical implication is that associated with gastroesophageal reflux and its complications. Another exception is the congenital posterolateral or Bochdalek hernia, in which the threat is not just herniation of viscera, but more importantly the high incidence of associated congenital anomalies, especially a life-threatening congenital dysfunction of the lungs. With these two ex-

ceptions, all the hernias of the diaphragm carry the pure risk of any abdominal hernia and require simple reduction and anatomic repair for management.

Development Anatomy

The diaphragm has a highly complex origin. The classic concept of formation was suggested in 1905 by Broman, who demonstrated that the diaphragm receives contributions from the septum transversum, the mesentery of the esophagus, the pleuroperitoneal membranes, and the musculature of the chest wall. There are two paired (pleuroperitoneal membranes, chest wall musculature) and two unpaired (septum transversum, mesentery) components (Fig. 25-15).

The septum transversum develops during the fourth week of gestation and initially appears as a thick, incomplete partition between the pericardial and peritoneal cavities. Originally, the septum is located opposite the anlage of the cervical vertebrae, but with growth, the septum

Fig. 25-15. Development of diaphragm as viewed from below. *A.* Lateral view of embryo at end of fifth week of gestation (dotted line indicates the level of section B). *B.* Transverse section showing unfused pleuroperitoneal membranes. *C.* Similar section at end of eighth week, showing fusion of pleuroperitoneal membranes. *D.* Transverse section through a 12-week-old embryo, demonstrating ingrowth of chest wall musculature into diaphragm. *E.* View of diaphragm of newborn, indicating probable embryologic origin of its components. (From: *Moore KL: The Developing Human: Clinically Oriented Embryology,* 2d ed. Philadelphia, Saunders, 1977, with permission.)

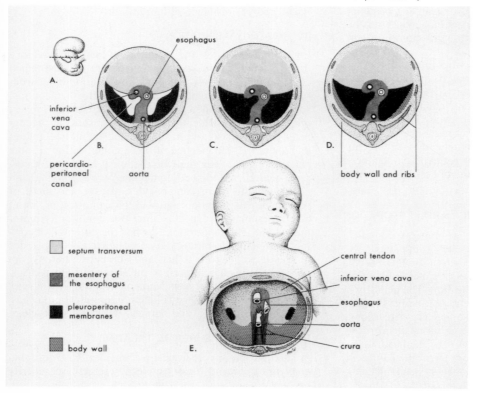

becomes displaced caudally to reach the level of the first lumbar vertebra. Eventually, it fuses dorsally with the ventral mesentery to the esophagus and with the pleuroperitoneal membranes. In the adult, the septum transversum forms the central tendon of the diaphragm. The dorsal mesentery of the esophagus also appears during the fourth week of gestation and constitutes the median portion of the diaphragm dorsal to the septum transversum. In the adult, this mesentery forms the crura of the diaphragm, including the esophageal hiatus and aortic hiatus. During the fifth week of gestation, the pleuroperitoneal membranes first appear along the lateral body wall and extend medially, where they fuse with the dorsal mesentery of the esophagus and the dorsal portion of the septum transversum, thereby completing the partition between the thoracic and abdominal cavities by the eighth week of gestation. Although the pleuroperitoneal membranes may form large portions of the primitive diaphragm, they represent relatively small, intermediate portions of the adult diaphragm. Finally, with further development of the lung, the pleural cavities enlarge and burrow into the lateral body walls where chest wall musculature is split off, forming the peripheral muscular portion of the diaphragm. Failure of any component to develop or to fuse with adjacent structures may result in congenital continuity of the pleural and peritoneal cavities.

Because the diaphragm is formed from the fusion of several components, a number of developmental defects occur, resulting in herniation of abdominal structures into the thorax. A hernial sac may or may not be present. Two fundamental types of defects may occur:

1. Complete or partial absence of the diaphragm. Failure of one or more of the diaphragmatic components to develop or failure of the components to join one another results in a communication between the thorax and the abdomen. No hernial sac is present because the diaphragm never formed. To this group of defects belong absence of the diaphragm, hernia into the pericardium, and herniation through the foramen of Bochdalek.
2. Failure of complete muscularization. In this group of defects, normal fusion of the diaphragmatic components occurs, but the muscular tissue fails to spread over the entire diaphragm. The portion of the diaphragm unsupported by muscle eventually bulges into the thoracic cavity, forming a hernial sac. This thin, bulging membrane may or may not rupture. To this group of defects belong all hernias of the foramen of Morgagni, eventration, and herniation through the foramen of Bochdalek.

Classifying diaphragmatic defects embryologically is not convenient clinically because the hernial sac is not easily detected. Moreover, absence of the sac does not necessarily mean that one was not present initially. A more practical classification incorporates morphology and anatomic location (Table 25-4).

Esophageal Hiatal Hernia

Esophageal hiatal hernias are not only the most common hernias of the diaphragm but also are among the more common abnormalities affecting the upper gastrointestinal tract.

Table 25-4. CLASSIFICATION OF CONGENITAL DIAPHRAGMATIC DEFECTS

Absent diaphragm
Diaphragmatic hernia
    Posterolateral (Bochdalek)
    Anterior (Morgagni)
    Paraesophageal
Eventration

There are two main types of esophageal hiatal hernias: the sliding hernia and the paraesophageal hernia (Fig. 25-16). A third type might well be described as a combination of these two pure types and carries the potential risks of both (Fig. 25-17).

The most common is the *sliding hernia,* in which there is axial displacement of the esophagogastric junction through the esophageal hiatus into the chest. Although such hernias are known to move in and out of the thorax with changes in intrathoracic and intraabdominal pressures, the term "sliding" is applied not because of this behavior but because the hernia has a partial parietal peritoneal sac, whose posterior wall is formed by the stomach.

In the *paraesophageal hiatal hernia,* the esophagogastric junction keeps to its normal position below the diaphragm, but the fundus and successively greater portions of the greater curvature of the stomach roll into the thorax through the esophageal hiatus alongside the esophagus. In its ultimate form the paraesophageal hiatal hernia presents with totally intrathoracic upside-down stomach (Fig. 25-18).

Esophageal hiatal hernia is relatively common, occurring in five individuals per 1000 population. Less than 5 percent ever develop any symptom or complication requiring surgical intervention.

SLIDING ESOPHAGEAL HIATAL HERNIA

This hernia accounts for 90 percent of the esophageal hiatal hernias. It is of clinical significance only because of its very high coincidence with gastroesophageal reflux. A causal relationship has long been sought but has been largely elusive. DeMeester and associates believed that the presence or absence of reflux with hiatal hernia is largely explainable by the absence or presence of a segment of distal esophagus exposed to normal positive intraabdominal pressure. Thus, vagaries in the level of phrenoesophageal ligamentous insertion into the esophagus may explain why some patients with hiatal hernia have competence and others do not. Other investigators have speculated on which comes first, reflux or hernia, or whether there is such a thing as primary sphincter failure in some individuals. Irrespective of the theoretical aspects, current operations for the control of gastroesophageal reflux depend on anatomic repair of the sliding esophageal hernia and reduction by 2 cm or more of the tubular distal esophagus below the diaphragm, as well as an anatomic valvuloplasty.

BASIC SURGICAL PROCEDURES. The primary goal of surgical treatment for sliding esophageal hernia is restora-

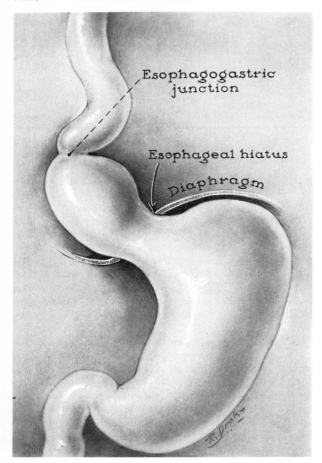

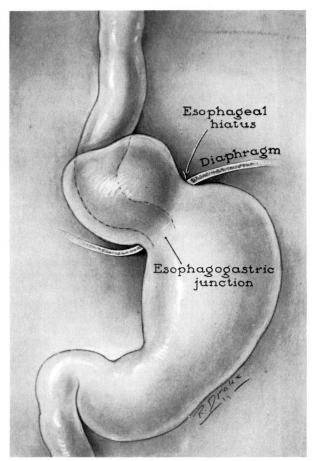

Fig. 25-16. Two chief varieties of esophageal hiatal hernia. *Left:* Sliding esophageal hiatal hernia. *Right:* Paraesophageal hiatal hernia. (From: *Mobley JE, Christensen NA: Gastroenterology 30:1, 1956. By permission of Williams & Wilkins Company.*)

tion of gastroesophageal competence. Because restoration of normal anatomy has been found to be inadequate for restoration of normal pressures to the hypotensive sphincter, "antireflux" operations have been devised to accomplish this end more effectively. Typical of these are the operations associated with the names Belsey, Nissen, and Hill. All are variations of a basic "wrap-around" procedure, and their success in preventing reflux makes it unnecessary, if not irrational, to perform concomitant vagotomy and pyloroplasty unless there is an active duodenal ulcer. The routine use of these additional procedures is also discouraged because of their disagreeable side effects.

Belsey's operation (Fig. 25-19) is a transthoracic procedure that creates a segment of intraabdominal esophagus held in place by a buttress of plicated stomach that surrounds approximately 280° of the distal esophagus. Long-term results indicate that the procedure is successful in relieving symptoms in 85 percent of patients and that the recurrence rate varies between 10 and 15 percent, depending on the length of follow-up.

Nissen's fundoplication can be performed either transabdominally or transthoracically (Fig. 25-20). This operation, which totally surrounds the distal esophagus with

the adjacent gastric fundus, also produces good clinical results and a low recurrence rate. A worldwide survey of the results of the Nissen operation indicated an overall success rate of 96 percent, failures being usually the result of either recurrent hernia or postoperative reflux. Some dissatisfaction with this procedure has been expressed by Woodward and associates, who found an unacceptably high rate of dysphagia and the so-called "gas-bloat syndrome"—complications that should be minimal or absent if, during operation, one uses an indwelling nasogastric tube of ample caliber to prevent excessive narrowing of the distal esophagus. Long-term follow-up, furthermore, has shown that these symptoms, when they do occur, become less severe as time goes on. Some believe that the gas-bloat syndrome is due to accidental injury to vagus nerves and note relief with gastric drainage procedures such as pyloroplasty.

Hill's operation (Fig. 25-21) is basically a posterior gastropexy performed transabdominally, but incorporating plicating sutures to narrow the esophagogastric junction.

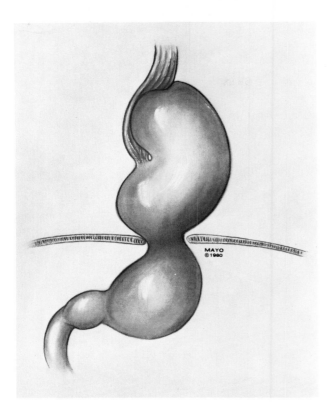

Fig. 25-17. Combined sliding and paraesophageal hiatal hernia. Esophagogastric junction is displaced above diaphragm (sliding component), and greater curvature of stomach has rolled into chest through esophageal hiatus. Hiatus impinges on stomach, producing hour-glass deformity. [From: *Payne WS, in Nyhus LM, Baker RJ (eds): Mastery of Surgery. Boston, Little, Brown, 1984, with permission.*]

He reported 149 cases in which this technique was employed during an 8-year period. There were no deaths and no anatomic recurrences in the follow-up period, and 97 percent of the patients were improved.

In addition to these gratifying clinical and radiologic results, physiologic studies of postoperative sphincteric function are encouraging. Not only is the amplitude of the lower esophageal sphincteric pressure more than doubled, but also the high-pressure zone is lengthened and the normal neural and hormonal response at the sphincter is restored. Now both experimental and clinical evidence suggest that the 360° wrap afforded by the Nissen fundoplication is the most effective of the three antireflux procedures in restoring lower esophageal sphincter pressure and preventing reflux.

Not all surgeons have obtained satisfactory results with these basic antireflux procedures. Therefore, Pearson and his colleagues have encouraged the use of a Collis gastroplasty with a Belsey-type 280° fundoplication. Henderson and Marryatt and Orringer and associates favored the Collis gastroplasty with a 360° Nissen-type fundoplication. Payne utilized an uncut Collis gastroplasty with either Nissen fundoplication if esophageal peristalsis is present or Belsey-type fundoplication if it is not. Csendes and Larrain favor the performance of a parietal cell vagotomy as a technical aid in effecting a Hill-type repair. Obviously there is not universal agreement on the type of repair to be used.

Technique. The surgical technique of left transthoracic modified (uncut) Collis gastroplasty with Nissen fundoplication performed at the Mayo Clinic is illustrated in Fig. 25-22.

Intraoperative esophageal manometry before and after repair has shown that the procedure restores a high-pressure zone 20 to 40 mmHg in magnitude and 3 to 4 cm in length that corresponds with the region of the fundoplication below the level of the diaphragm.

Piehler and associates recently reported the Mayo Clinic's experience with the uncut Collis–Nissen fundoplication. In a review of 136 patients, there was no operative mortality. Over 90 percent of these patients were improved at 3 years, and 84 percent had good to excellent results. These data support the continued use of the uncut Collis–Nissen operation. Obviously, the perfect operation for gastroesophageal reflux has yet to be devised and continued small modification will no doubt be required in the future. Periodic objective assessment of results is essential in guiding intelligent and rational changes.

MANAGEMENT OF UNUSUAL REFLUX PROBLEMS. A shortened esophagus poses a special problem for surgical correction of gastroesophageal reflux, since it makes reduction of the herniated stomach below the diaphragm infeasible. When the shortening is no greater than 5 to 6 cm, the cut Collis gastroplasty has been an effective means of creating a tubular extension of esophagus made up of lesser curvature of the stomach (Fig. 25-23). One of the standard antireflux procedures, Nissen or Belsey, may then be applied to the distal end below the diaphragm. When shortening is more extensive and the esophagogastric junction is fixed at the carinal or aortic level, one may elect vagotomy, antrectomy, and a long limb (45-cm) Roux en Y gastric drainage procedure (Fig. 25-24); alternatively, bowel interposition or modified Ivor-Lewis resection may be considered.

Esophageal strictures that cannot be dilated are rare, but they too pose a special problem. Whereas resection and reanastomosis is a simple technical feat, recurrence is almost certain. "Inkwelling" of the anastomosis is not reliable in preventing reflux. Intrathoracic Nissen fundoplication is hazardous. Antrectomy with the Roux en Y gastric drainage procedure is a reliable alternative, and bowel interposition another. Woodward and associates have championed the Thal procedure, but this has been met with less than universal enthusiasm by others. The stomach is increasingly being employed as the favored organ for esophageal replacement. When it is placed totally in the thorax and anastomosed high to the esophagus without redundancy—and this disposition is accompanied by pyloroplasty or pyloromyotomy—it usually provides comfortable digestion without reflux problems. This modification of the Ivor-Lewis procedure awaits long-term follow-up in patients with benign disease.

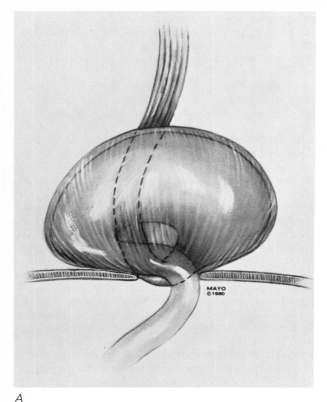

A

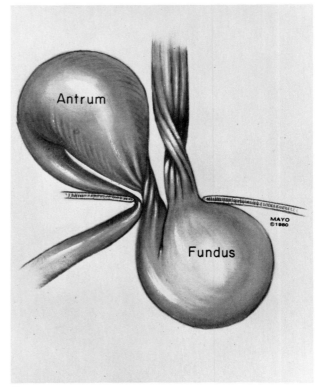

B

Fig. 25-18. *A*. Totally intrathoracic upside-down stomach, or advanced paraesophageal hiatal hernia. *B*. Gastric volvulus is a major complication of totally intrathoracic upside-down stomach. Note that fundus of stomach has fallen below diaphragm, with antrum remaining above diaphragm. This produces twisted obstruction at midstomach and lower esophagus. [From: *Payne WS, in Nyhus LM, Baker RJ (eds): Mastery of Surgery. Boston, Little, Brown, 1984, with permission.*]

PARAESOPHAGEAL HIATAL HERNIA

The pure paraesophageal hiatal hernia is a rare entity. It usually presents as a combined sliding and paraesophageal hernia. Even when the paraesophageal hiatal hernia has advanced to the stage of total intrathoracic upside-down stomach (Fig. 25-18), it has a sliding component as well in most cases. By this, it is implied that the distal esophagus and esophagogastric junction are not well tethered below the diaphragm and that the esophagogastric junction is displaced along with the rolling paraesophageal herniation of the stomach. The observation that most paraesophageal hernias are combined hernias has special implications in treatment to be discussed.

When a paraesophageal hernia of any size presents in pure form, the symptoms and complications result from the anatomic defect and not from any physiologic derangement of gastroesophageal competence. The most common complication—irrespective of the size of the paraesophageal hernia—is chronic, recurrent, asymptomatic occult gastrointestinal blood-loss anemia. Collis has alluded to the occurrence of anemia with hiatal hernia, but more recent studies clearly implicate the paraesophageal component in the genesis of most. A riding ulcer or gastritis where the hiatus impinges on herniated stomach can be demonstrated in some patients. Others appear to bleed from transient erosions secondary to stasis within the suprahiatal loculus of stomach. Classically, such stasis is evident on chest x-ray as a globular shadow with an air-fluid level superimposed on the cardiac silhouette. When blood-loss anemia occurs in patients with pure or combined paraesophageal hernia and more usual causes for gastrointestinal blood loss can be excluded, surgical correction of the anatomic hernia is usually curative.

The second most frequent complication of paraesophageal hernia is gastric volvulus (Fig. 25-18*B*). This is seen almost exclusively with massive paraesophageal hernia, wherein most or all of the stomach comes to reside in a huge parietal peritoneal sac in the chest behind the heart. Various mechanisms and twisting deformities have been described, the most common being that in which the fundus of the totally intrathoracic stomach descends through the hiatus to the abdomen, leaving the antrum in the chest. This produces complete angulation obstruction of the distal esophagus, and two closed-loop segments of the stomach: the fundus below the diaphragm and antrum above, with duodenum obstructed as it passes through the crowded hiatus. Although detorsion and return of the

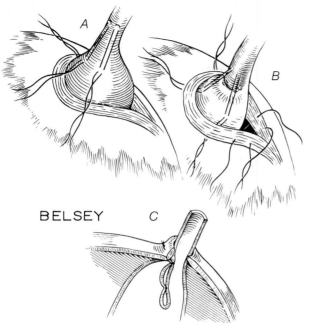

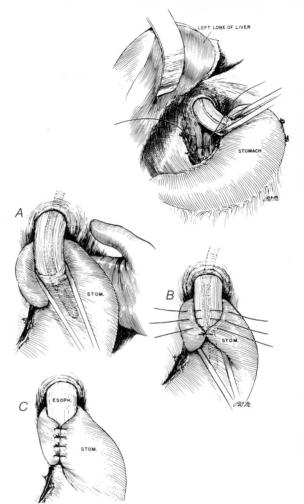

Fig. 25-19. Belsey Mark IV transthoracic repair of sliding esophageal hiatal hernia. Exposure is gained through left thoracotomy incision. After complete mobilization of cardia, lower 4 cm of esophagus is cleared of connective tissue. *A.* Mattress sutures are placed between gastric fundus and muscular layers of esophagus, 1 to 2 cm above and below esophagogastric junction. *B.* After these mattress sutures are tied, a second row of mattress sutures is placed to imbricate additional fundus onto lower esophagus. Note that these sutures pass through hiatus and out through the tendinous portion of diaphragm. Before these sutures are tied, crural sutures are placed to narrow esophageal hiatus. *C.* Completed repair after reduction of hernia and tying of sutures to maintain reconstruction. Previously placed crural sutures have been tied behind esophagus to narrow hiatus (not shown).

Fig. 25-20. Transabdominal Nissen fundoplication. *Above:* Abdominal exposure and mobilization of distal esophagus and upper stomach in preparation for carrying out fundoplication. *A.* Mobilized fundus is displaced behind esophagus by surgeon's right hand. *B.* Placement of sutures to encircle distal esophagus with generous portion of fundus. Note indwelling #40 French gastric tube. *C.* Completed procedure. (From: *Ellis FH Jr: Surg Clin North Am, 51: 575, 1971, with permission.*)

entire stomach to the chest may occur spontaneously, or be effected by nasogastric tube decompression, unrelieved volvulus can progress to gastric strangulation infarction. Gastric volvulus thus is a life-threatening complication of the large paraesophageal hernia. Volvulus may be a chronic recurring problem, alone or in combination with chronic blood-loss anemia.

Because of the high incidence of both bleeding and volvulus in the massive paraesophageal hernias, surgical repair is generally indicated even in the absence of symptoms or complications. The smaller paraesophageal hernias and lesser combined sliding and paraesophageal hernias are repaired only when complicated or symptomatic.

The classic method for repair of pure paraesophageal hiatal hernia differs from that described for sliding esophageal hernia. Since the lower esophageal sphincter functions normally, the esophagogastric junction is not disturbed. Rather, the herniated stomach is reduced, the hernia sac is excised, and the widened hiatus is narrowed by placing sutures in the crura, anterior to the esophagus, as in the technique described by Hill and Tobias.

Recent reviews, however, suggest that the problem is more complex. Simple anatomic repair is followed by a significant incidence of recurrence of anatomic hernia and by organoaxial and other gastric volvuluses, as well as by late occurrence of gastroesophageal reflux. Both the Toronto and Mayo groups have espoused the addition of antireflux measures to anatomic repair, and Geha has suggested gastropexy by temporary gastrostomy tube placement following anatomic repair. Whatever the final answer to this vexing problem, it probably will take into account the extreme rarity of pure paraesophageal hiatal hernia and will always include, in repair of the combined hernias, antireflux features that also fix the mobile stomach so it cannot undergo volvulus.

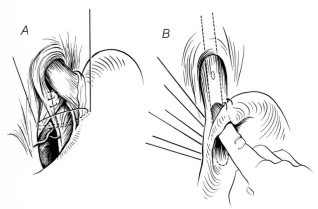

Fig. 25-21. Hill's transabdominal repair of sliding esophageal hiatal hernia. *A.* Reduced esophagogastric junction; crural sutures narrowing hiatus are in place behind esophagus. Single suture is shown incorporating gastrohepatic omentum along lesser curvature of stomach and preaortic fascia. Care is taken in placing sutures to avoid injury to adjacent vagal nerve trunks. Two or three additional sutures are similarly placed on lesser curvature, anchoring stomach posteriorly (posterior gastropexy). *B.* When these sutures are tied, gastric sling fibers should be sufficiently shortened to permit distal phalanx of index finger to invaginate snugly into terminal esophageal lumen alongside Levin tube. Angle of His is further accentuated by placement of sutures between gastric fundus and terminal esophagus. [From: *Payne WS, Ellis FH Jr, in Ellis FH Jr (ed): Lewis-Walters' Practice of Surgery, vol 5, Thoracic Surgery, chap 15, p 1. New York, Harper & Row, 1971, with permission.*]

Posterolateral (Foramen of Bochdalek) Hernia (See also Chapter 39)

Congenital hernias through the posterolateral aspect of the diaphragm are the most frequent diaphragmatic hernias in infants. This hernia was first described by Bochdalek in 1848. These hernias often present as a respiratory emergency at or shortly after birth, depending on the amount of herniated abdominal viscera present in the thorax. Rarely, such defects remain undetected until later childhood (Fig. 25-25) or adult life.

Gastrointestinal rather than respiratory symptoms predominate in older children and adults. Abdominal pain is present in approximately half of these patients. Vomiting, dyspnea, and chest pain occur occasionally. Obstruction is rare.

Foramen of Morgagni Hernias

Although it has been called *anterior diaphragmatic parasternal,* or *retrosternal hernia,* this type is best known by the eponym, foramen of Morgagni hernia (Fig. 25-26). A foramen of Morgagni hernia occurs through the sternocostal hiatus, which is a small triangular area of the diaphragm located on either side of the xyphoid process. Embryologically, the hiatus represents the junction of the septum transversus and the components of the chest wall. Although the hiatus normally permits passage of only vessels, it is a potential site for herniation of abdominal contents. Actual herniation may be the result of trauma

and is almost exclusively seen in adults. Seventy percent of patients are females with ages ranging from 3 months to 78 years. Ninety percent of the hernias occur through a diaphragmatic defect in the right parasternal area. Eight percent are bilateral, and 2 percent occur on the left. A hernial sac is always formed. The abdominal organs found in these hernias in their order of decreasing frequency are omentum, colon, stomach, liver, and small bowel.

Most patients with hernias of the foramen of Morgagni are asymptomatic. Only about one-third have symptoms that could be related to the hernia. These are predominantly gastrointestinal symptoms, with upper abdominal or subcostal discomfort, fullness, cramping, and occasionally vomiting. A few patients have histories suggestive of partial obstruction of the large bowel. Serious complications are rarely encountered, and emergency operations are rarely required. When these hernias occur in infancy and childhood, they may manifest with severe cardiorespiratory symptoms, similar to those associated with hernia of the foramen of Bochdalek. Occasionally, an adult patient with a large hernia of the foramen of Morgagni will present with respiratory distress related to the hernia.

The diagnosis of hernia of the foramen of Morgagni is often obvious on standard x-rays of the thorax, especially when gas-containing bowel is present in the hernial mass. The x-ray reveals a rounded shadow of variable size in the right cardiophrenic angle (Fig. 25-27*A* and *B*). Lateral views of the thorax show the lesion anteriorly very near the anterior chest wall (Fig. 25-27*B*). The demonstration of colon (Fig. 25-27*C*) within this mass or of angulation of the transverse colon toward the defect after a barium enema provides evidence for diagnosis. Radiographic examination of the upper gastrointestinal tract is usually diagnostically less rewarding. A CT scan may be diagnostic (Fig. 25-27*D*).

Occasionally, a definitive diagnosis cannot be established before surgical exploration, and other conditions, such as pleuropericardial cyst, pleural or pulmonary neoplasms, and mediastinal and diaphragmatic tumors, are considered in the differential diagnosis.

TREATMENT. Surgical repair is mandatory for all hernias of the foramen of Morgagni. Although a transabdominal approach provides the advantages of greater ease of exposure and repair of the defect, its use should be restricted to those instances in which a preoperative diagnosis is established. An upper abdominal incision provides easy access to either a right- or left-sided hernia or to bilateral hernias. When a definite preoperative diagnosis cannot be established and operation is performed for an indeterminate thoracic mass, a transthoracic operation is indicated. This approach, although technically more difficult for repairing the hernia, affords a better opportunity to diagnose and treat an intrathoracic lesion.

The hernia is reduced, the sac is excised, and the defect is closed. Repair is effected by approximating the posterior margin of the defect to the musculoskeletal chest wall anteriorly with interrupted nonabsorbable suture material. Operative morbidity and mortality rates are negligible.

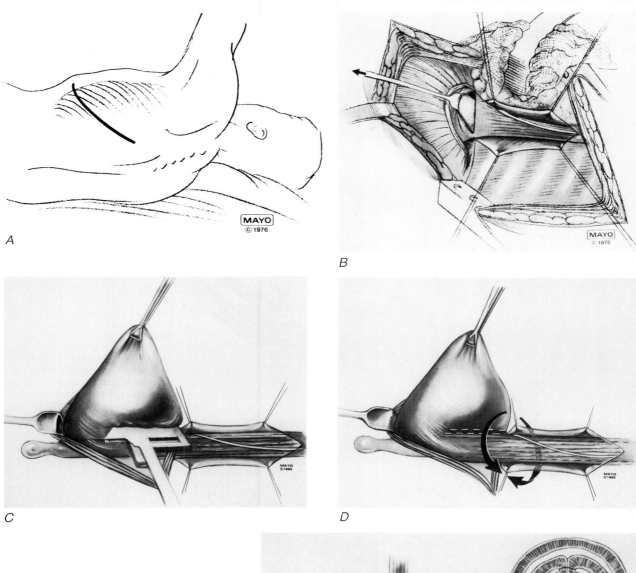

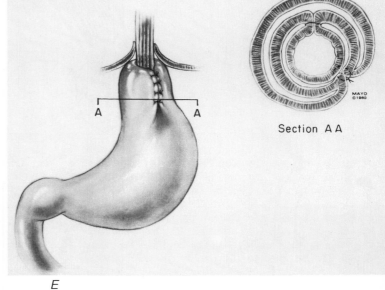

Fig. 25-22. *A.* Placement of incision. *B.* Ventral application of traction through hiatus. *C.* Placement of stapling device. *D.* Tubular extension of esophagus created by stapling. *E.* Completed fundoplication. [From: *Piehler JM, Payne WS, et al: The uncut Collis–Nissen procedure for esophageal hiatal hernia and its complications, in Farnell MB, McIlrath DC (eds): Problems in General Surgery. New Approaches to Old Problems. Philadelphia, Lippincott, vol 1, pp 1–14, 1984, with permission.*]

Section A A

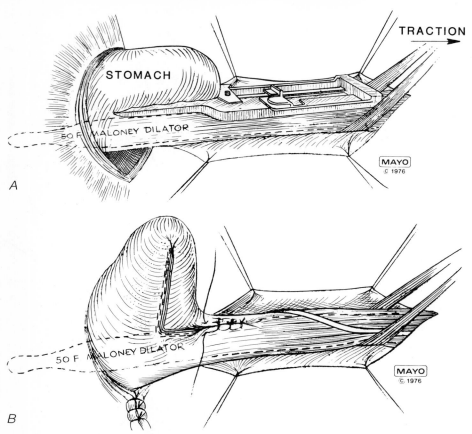

Fig. 25-23. Collis gastroplasty for shortened esophagus. After left thoracotomy, phrenoesophageal attachments have been taken down and multiple short gastric vessels have been interrupted through hiatus. *A.* With #50 French Maloney dilator in place, GIA stapling device is applied to stomach at angle of His, parallel to lesser curvature and Maloney dilator. Activation of instrument creates stapled cut-tubular extension of esophagus made up of lesser curvature of stomach. *B.* Staples are buried beneath a row of sutures. Either 280 or 360° fundoplication can be effected (not shown). Esophageal lengthening procedure permits reduction of valvuloplasty below diaphragm. [From: *Payne WS, in Jackson JW (ed): Operative Surgery: Cardiothoracic Surgery, 3d ed. London, Butterworth, 1978, p 438, with permission.*]

Fig. 25-24. Operative procedures for management of short-esophagus diaphragmatic hernia with stricture. *Left:* Esophagogastrectomy with Roux en Y esophagojejunostomy. *Center:* Esophagogastrectomy with colon interposition and pyloroplasty. *Right:* Gastric tube of Gavriliu.

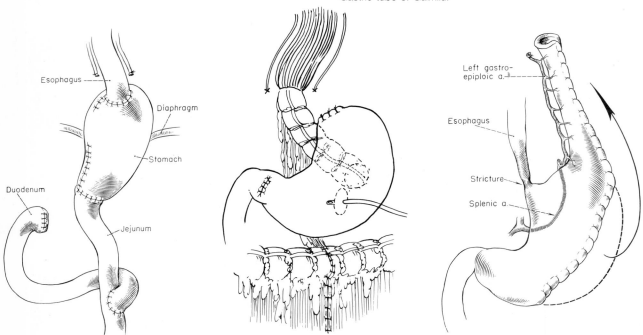

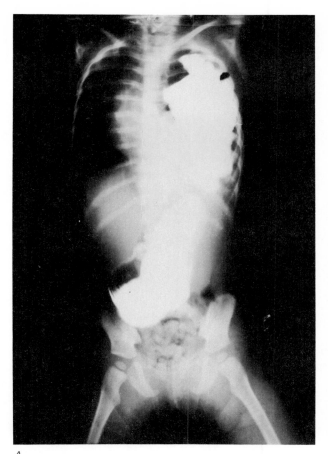

A

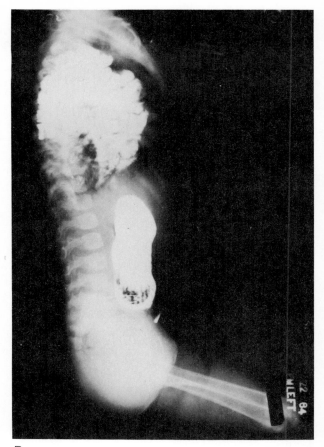

B

Fig. 25-25. Roentgenogram of 18-month-old girl with hernia of left foramen of Bochdalek without sac. Contrast material was used to delineate findings on plain chest roentgenograms, as no respiratory distress was present. *A.* Posteroanterior projection demonstrating abdominal viscera nearly filling left thoracic cavity. Mediastinum has shifted to right. *B.* Lateral projection delineating individual loops of intestine in thoracic cavity. Abdomen is scaphoid. (From: *Whittaker LD, Lynn HB, et al: Hernias of the foramen of Bochdalek in children. Mayo Clin Proc 43:580, 1968, with permission.*)

Fig. 25-26. Bilateral foramen of Morgagni hernia as seen at operation from abdominal approach. (From: *Comer TP, Clagett OT: J Thorac Surg 52:461, 1966, with permission.*)

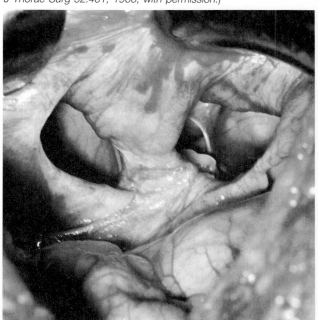

Eventration of the Diaphragm

Complete or partial unilateral elevation of the diaphragm is commonly referred to as eventration. Eventration differs from true diaphragmatic hernias in that there is no localized diaphragmatic defect with discrete margins through which abdominal contents may protrude. Instead, there is a diffuse or localized bulging of the diaphragm itself (Fig. 25-28). In eventration there must be a third layer representing the diaphragm interposed between the pleural and peritoneal layers; this middle layer may consist of only a thin fibrous sheet with scattered atrophic muscle cells. It may be impossible, without resorting to histologic examination, to distinguish eventration from hernias of the foramen of Bochdalek.

Both acquired and congenital factors have been implicated in the genesis of eventration. Acquired eventration implies paralysis of the phrenic nerve subsequent to dis-

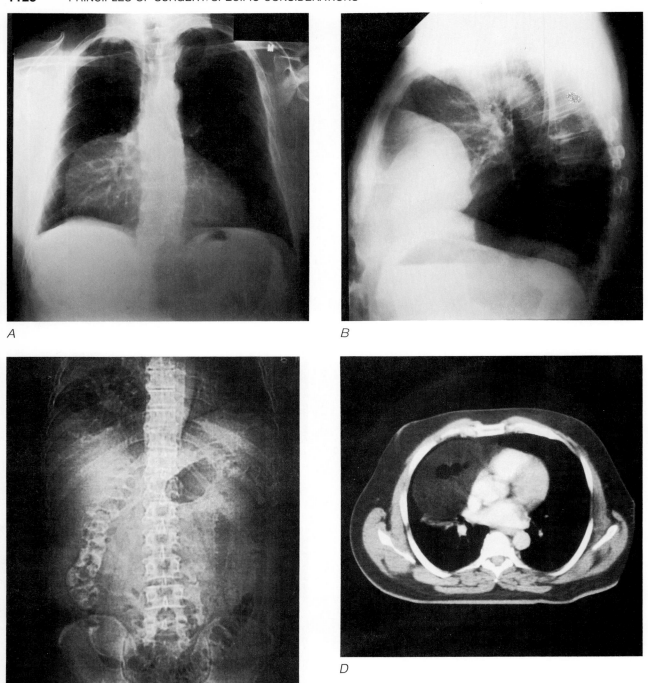

A

B

C

D

Fig. 25-27. Typical right-sided hernia of foramen of Morgagni. *A.* Anteroposterior projection. *B.* Lateral projection. *C.* Anteroposterior projection demonstrates loop of transverse colon in right-sided foraminal hernia. *D.* Computed tomogram demonstrating omentum and colon in chest.

ease or injury. Infections, neoplasms, poisons, surgical and accidental trauma, including injury to the phrenic nerve at the time of birth, are frequently implicated and may result in either temporary or permanent nerve paral-

ysis, followed by elevation of the hemidiaphragm. Congenital eventration, however, implies anomalous development of the diaphragm in that there is a failure of normal ingrowth of striated muscle into part or all of the

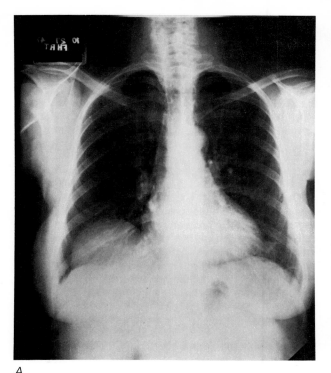

A

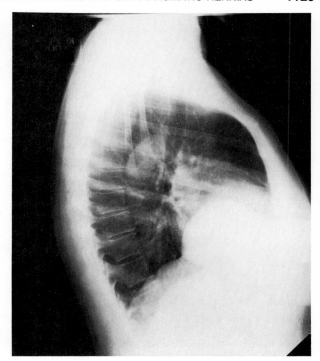

B

Fig. 25-28. *A.* Posteroanterior chest roentgenogram demonstrating localized eventration of right diaphragm. *B.* Lateral projection. (From: *Neuman HW, Ellis FH Jr, Andersen HS: Eventration of the diaphragm. Proc Staff Meet Mayo Clin 30:310, 1955, with permission.*)

diaphragm. Congenital eventration is associated with an intact phrenic nerve that may or may not result in diaphragmatic contraction in response to nerve stimulation, depending on the amount of muscle present. Partial or complete inversion of the stomach and intestinal malrotation usually accompanies congenital eventration. Transposition of abdominal organs, megacolon, and hypospadias also have been reported.

Eventration occurs at any age, most commonly on the left, with a male to female ratio of approximately 2:1. Most patients with eventration are asymptomatic, the condition being detected on routine chest x-ray. In the newborn, serious respiratory difficulties are frequently encountered, similar to those of massive congenital diaphragmatic hernias already described. In the adult patient, when decreased cardiopulmonary reserve develops in combination with intraabdominal pressure secondary to obesity, digestive and respiratory symptoms related to eventration may appear for the first time. Digestive symptoms often are vague. Occasionally, palpitations or arrhythmias are encountered. Hemodynamics rarely are affected by mediastinal shift and vascular angulation.

Radiography of the chest is necessary for diagnosis. Ideally, the elevated hemidiaphragm will be visualized high in the thorax. This is in distinction to the picture seen in diaphragmatic hernia in which the diaphragm is located normally with intestines above.

TREATMENT. Prompt emergency surgical repair is indicated in the newborn who is dyspneic and cyanotic. In older children and adults in whom symptoms are disabling, elective surgical repair is indicated. Surgical treatment is directed toward restoration of the diaphragm to its normal position. Such procedures help stabilize the mediastinum and permit more normal pulmonary ventilation. The procedure most frequently used is diaphragmatic plication (Fig. 25-29). In the infant, the transabdominal approach is preferred for the same reasons indicated for the repair of hernias of the foramen of Bochdalek. In adults, the thoracic approach gives better exposure and greater ease of repair. When viscera are adherent to the undersurface of the diaphragm, a thoracoabdominal incision may be advantageous. Because of possible injury to the phrenic nerve, especially in congenital eventration, excision of the diaphragm is rarely performed.

In patients of any age, and particularly in those in whom surgical treatment is contraindicated, symptomatic palliation is indicated. These measures include restriction of activities, weight reduction, and avoidance of abdominal distention, lifting, or straining.

Rupture of the Diaphragm

Loss of continuity of the diaphragm with herniation of the abdominal viscera into the thorax may result from major trauma. Both blunt and penetrating injuries to chest or abdomen have been implicated. Rupture rarely follows disruption of surgical incisions in the diaphragm. Disrup-

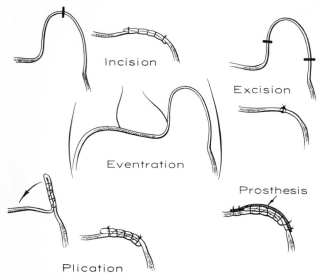

Fig. 25-29. Diaphragmatic eventration and operative procedures available for its correction. [From: *Ellis FH Jr, in Nyhus LM, Harkins HN (eds): Hernia. Philadelphia, Lippincott, 1964, p 554, with permission.*]

tion of the diaphragm also may occur as a consequence of some acute inflammatory process, such as subphrenic abscess or empyema. Valsalva maneuvers during extreme or trivial exertion also have been implicated. These so-called spontaneous ruptures of the normal diaphragm have occurred after heavy lifting, twisting, and coughing.

The precise incidence of traumatic diaphragmatic hernias is not known. Most war injuries have been associated with penetrating missile injuries, while most civilian injuries in the past have been due to blunt trauma related to traffic accidents.

Although rupture may occur in any portion of the diaphragm, including the normal hiatus, most (60 percent) are crescentic lacerations that affect the tendinous dome of the left diaphragm. Rupture of the left side is reported to be about eight times as common as rupture of the right.

Blunt trauma, producing a sudden increase in intraabdominal pressure relative to intrathoracic pressure, results in a pressure gradient across the diaphragm sufficient to rupture it. The right diaphragm may be less vulnerable because it is protected in part by the liver, and a more even distribution of pressure forces is created over the entire hemidiaphragm. While this explanation is helpful in appreciating left-sided predominance in blunt trauma, the high incidence (60 percent) of left diaphragmatic injury in penetrating trauma is less easily explained. Bekassy and associates studied the pressure required to rupture the right and left diaphragmatic leaves in fresh autopsy material. They reported a difference in the pressure required, with the left diaphragm disrupting at significantly lower pressures than the right. Hill emphasized that the diaphragmatic crura are solid structures that can withstand trauma well and are rarely injured. The strength of the esophageal hiatus with restraining phrenoesophageal membranes is not as great as the strength of

the crura of the remainder of the fibromuscular diaphragm, so herniation through the esophageal hiatus may result from severe compression of the abdomen.

Not all diaphragmatic disruptions are associated with herniation. Although the normal pressure gradients across the diaphragm are responsible for the herniation, the size of the defect and the bulk and physical characteristics of the abdominal viscera adjacent to the defect determine whether herniation will occur. In one study only about 1 percent of the patients with penetrating wounds of the diaphragm actually had herniation of viscera into the chest. In another series some complication of the herniation was the chief clinical manifestation.

The manifestations of traumatic diaphragmatic disruption and herniation, other than those of associated injury, are related to the effects on the herniated viscera and the effect of herniated viscera on cardiorespiratory dynamics. Incarceration, obstruction, and strangulation are the chief effects of herniation on abdominal viscera. Rupture of the diaphragm per se may partially or completely interrupt phrenic innervation. Herniation of viscera into the thorax also can result in the compression of a considerable volume of lung parenchyma. In addition, paradoxic movement of abdominal viscera in and out of the chest, with or without phrenic nerve paralysis, may interfere significantly with alveolar ventilation. Compression of lung tissue increases right-to-left shunting of blood with resultant hypoxemia, while ineffective alveolar ventilation leads to respiratory acidosis. With extensive herniation, mediastinal displacement to the contralateral side results in further embarrassment of respiration and interference with venous return to the heart. Cardiac function may be suppressed by tamponade because of visceral herniation into the pericardial sac. The manifestations of all these aberrations may be further compounded by blood loss, visceral ruptures, fluid sequestration, sepsis, and injuries to other parts of the body.

The diagnosis of traumatic rupture of the diaphragm may be difficult during the early period after the injury, especially when clinical features are dominated by associated injuries. Significant associated multiple organ injury is the case more often than not. Rib, extremity, pelvic, and skull fractures dominate the list of bony injuries, while injuries to the spleen, liver, stomach, and bowel head the list of associated organ injuries. While a preoperative diagnosis can be made during the early postinjury period on the basis of obvious herniated abdominal viscera in the thorax, often definitive diagnosis of diaphragmatic injury or hernia is made coincident to surgical exploration for associated organ injury. Physical findings are notoriously nonspecific and misleading, and radiographic alterations are all too often subtle, nonspecific, or absent even in retrospect. According to the review of Drews and associates, the radiographic signs suggestive or diagnostic of diaphragmatic injury are diaphragmatic elevation (with or without pleural effusion), atelectasis with silhouetting of the ipsilateral diaphragm, and evidence of an air-filled or solid viscus above the diaphragm. Carter and Brewer emphasized that the presence of an air bubble above the diaphragm is suggestive of a diaphrag-

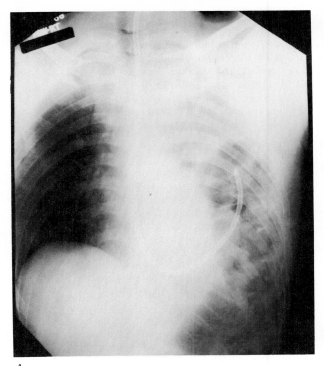

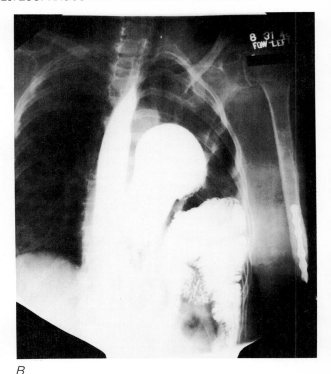

A

B

Fig. 25-30. Large traumatic diaphragmatic hernia with abdominal viscera filling left thorax. *A.* Use of gastric tube confirms nature of gas-containing structure in left side of chest. *B.* Contrast material demonstrates presence of stomach and small intestine in thorax. (From: *Bernatz PE, Burnside AF Jr, Clagett OT: Problem of the ruptured diaphragm. JAMA 168:877, 1958, with permission.*)

matic hernia and that the passage of a nasogastric tube into the stomach or the visualization of a thin contrast medium in the stomach, small intestine, or colon confirms the diagnosis of intrathoracic viscera (Fig. 25-30). For suspected right-sided herniations, CT scan, liver scan, or selective angiography may confirm the presence of a hernia.

The following guidelines suggested by Drews and associates are pertinent to the diagnosis and management of acute diaphragmatic injuries.

1. Any injury involving the area from the fourth intercostal space to the level of the umbilicus should be considered as potentially involving the diaphragm.
2. Careful evaluation of the plain chest x-ray is crucial. If it is abnormal and an operation is not immediately contemplated for other reasons, an appropriate contrast study should be done to help determine if the diaphragm is intact.
3. Even in the absence of other operative indications, acute diaphragmatic disruption should be promptly repaired by the use of interrupted nonabsorbable sutures.
4. Abdominal exploration is mandatory in the acute injury, and careful examination of the entire diaphragm must be part of any abdominal exploration after trauma.
5. Upper gastrointestinal contrast studies should always be done before hospital discharge after recovery from massive thoracoabdominal trauma involving the diaphragm. Occasionally, a barium enema x-ray study is indicated.

Many diaphragmatic ruptures may remain occult or asymptomatic for months or years. Most patients who present late, however, have symptoms of acute gastrointestinal obstruction.

TREATMENT. Acute diaphragmatic injuries should be explored and repaired by the abdominal approach, while chronic herniations are best managed transthoracically. The high incidence of associated concomitant injury to stomach, spleen, liver, bowel, and other abdominal viscera makes laparotomy more appropriate for the acutely injured patient. A separate thoracotomy or thoracoabdominal incision should be considered in the acutely injured patient if there is a concomitant critical thoracic injury. The late repair of diaphragmatic hernias almost always necessitates thoracotomy for the lysis of adhesions between herniated viscera and intrathoracic structures. When obstruction or strangulation is associated with chronic hernia, combined thoracic and abdominal exposure is often indicated.

All traumatic diaphragmatic disruptions should be repaired. Interrupted figure-of-eight stitches of nonabsorbable suture material are generally recommended for repair. Suture imbrication of the torn leaves is advised by many. On rare occasions, prosthetic material has been required to bridge defects or to reinforce suture line repair.

The results of the repair of diaphragmatic disruptions are almost universally favorable. The overall morbidity (60 to 80 percent) and mortality (18 percent) have remained unchanged in recent decades. The two most important factors contributing to poor results are the number and severity of associated injuries and the delay both in the recognition of the diaphragmatic injury and in the treatment before the development of related complications.

OROPHARYNGEAL DYSPHAGIA

Swallowing begins in the mouth and ends at the esophagogastric junction. Normally it progresses rapidly as an uninterrupted sequential event from oral to pharyngeal to esophageal phases. Poorly definable dysfunctions of the oral and pharyngeal phases occur as the consequences of primary motor and sensory neurologic deficits and certain neuromuscular and muscular diseases. Although paralysis of the tongue, palate, or vocal cords often is demonstrable on examination, subtle defects in airway closure or impairments of laryngeal excursion and of pharyngeal function with swallowing often escape definition. Of major importance in this group of patients with oropharyngeal dysphagia are those whose condition is largely or exclusively due to cricopharyngeal dysfunction and is potentially reversible (Table 25-5).

Although medical management has succeeded in certain cases of neuromuscular disease, by and large it has been disappointing; so cricopharyngeal myotomy has been tried in refractory cases. The results of myotomy in many of these conditions have been quite variable. The chief problem (alluded to above) appears to be proper selection of patients—presumably just those in whom the problem is largely or exclusively cricopharyngeal. Manometry has been largely disappointing in selection of patients for operation. While incomplete relaxation, hypertension, and premature contractions of the UES have been described, study findings are more often normal or show only weak pharyngeal contractions. Hurwitz and Duranceau, in a collective review, found good results in only 64 percent of patients treated by cricopharyngeal myotomy. Until better selection becomes possible, treatment should be restricted to those in whom voluntary tongue, laryngeal, and pharyngeal movement is intact and pharyngeal sensation is present.

Table 25-5. ETIOLOGY OF OROPHARYNGEAL DYSPHAGIA ASSOCIATED WITH DYSFUNCTION OF THE UPPER ESOPHAGEAL SPHINCTER

CNS disease
    Cerebrovascular accident
    Parkinson's disease
    Bulbar poliomyelitis
    Multiple sclerosis
    Amyotrophic lateral sclerosis
Muscular disease
    Muscular dystrophy (motonic, oculopharyngeal)
    Inflammatory (dermatomyositis, polymyositis)
    Metabolic myopathy (thyrotoxicosis, hypothyroidism)
    Myasthenia gravis
Miscellaneous
    Radical oropharyngeal surgery
    Cricopharyngeal "spasm" (globus)
    Premature contraction (pharyngoesophageal diverticulum)

It is important to appreciate that the above comments apply only to patients with cricopharyngeal dysphagia secondary to neuromuscular disorders or radical surgery. Patients with pharyngoesophageal diverticulum do not have demonstrable etiologic neuromuscular disease; and though UES dysfunction is implicated, the late results of treatment are infinitely superior. The technique for cricopharyngeal myotomy is described under Diverticula.

DIVERTICULA

Diverticula of the esophagus are among the more common lesions that cause esophageal dysfunction. They may have serious consequences if neglected, but current techniques of management offer a particularly rewarding opportunity for effective surgical treatment.

Typical diverticula of the esophagus are thought to be acquired lesions, resulting either from protrusion of mucosa through a defect in the esophageal musculature *(pulsion diverticula)* or from the traction effect of adjacent, chronically inflamed, granulomatous parabronchial lymph nodes *(traction diverticula)*. Such acquired lesions should be clearly differentiated from the rare congenital diverticulum of the esophagus and the occasional duplication, enterogenous cyst, or neoplasm that may have a fistulous communication with the esophageal lumen.

Pharyngoesophageal Diverticulum

NATURE AND PRESENTATION. The most common diverticulum of the esophagus arises at the pharyngoesophageal junction. Typically, it is located posteriorly in the midline, protruding between the oblique fibers of the inferior pharyngeal constrictors just above the transverse fibers of the cricopharyngeus. Although the lesion was first described in 1769 by the English surgeon Ludlow, Zenker's name has become intimately associated with it as a result of his studies on 27 collected cases in 1874.

Pharyngoesophageal diverticulum is definitely an acquired abnormality, since it rarely is encountered before thirty years of age and usually occurs after fifty. Esophageal motility studies in patients with pharyngoesophageal diverticulum have demonstrated premature contraction of the cricopharyngeus muscle during swallowing. This occurs frequently enough so that its partial obstructive effects are implicated in the development of the diverticulum. Because of the recurrent pressures involved and the effect of gravity and peristalsis, a globular dependent sac filled with ingested material gradually develops, insinuating itself posteriorly between the esophagus and the cervical vertebrae. In more advanced stages it may descend into the mediastinum. There has been a high association with esophageal conditions, particularly hiatal hernia. Gastroesophageal reflux symptoms, however, are extremely rare.

Since the mouth of the diverticulum is located above the upper esophageal sphincter, there is no barrier to prevent spontaneous pharyngeal reflux and aspiration. Particularly in the sleeping or obtunded patient, this may result in recurrent episodes of airway contamination and aspiration pneumonitis.

A sensation of high cervical obstruction to swallowing is the most common symptom. The patients complain of a noisy, gurgling sound in their throats with drinking and the regurgitation of portions of recent meals into the mouth. This food is undigested, but it may have an offensive odor due to decomposition. Frequently such regurgitation is associated with paroxysms of coughing, which may occur either immediately after meals or on reclining and may even awaken the patient from sleep.

The patient with a neglected pharyngoesophageal diverticulum may find eating to be a slow and laborious process, with dysphagia and interruptions by episodes of regurgitation and cough. In the extreme case, fatigue, malnutrition, hoarseness, and suppurative lung disease may further complicate the clinical course. Occasionally, patients with pharyngoesophageal diverticula are unaware of the abnormality until they experience some complication. An infrequent complication of a chronically neglected diverticulum is the development of squamous cell carcinoma. In a recent review of 1249 patients seen at the Mayo Clinic during a 50-year period, squamous cell carcinoma occurred in 0.4 percent of the patients.

The diagnosis may be strongly suspected from the patient's history, but it can be firmly established only by radiographic examination of the esophagus with contrast medium (Fig. 25-31). Esophagoscopy usually is not necessary. Esophageal motility studies and pH reflux testing are of more theoretical interest than aid in making the diagnosis unless other distal esophageal or gastric abnormalities are suspected.

TREATMENT. In general, any diverticulum arising in the pharyngoesophageal region and producing symptoms warrants surgical treatment. In a given patient, the minimal surgical risks of intervention must be weighed against the severity of symptoms and the risk of present or potential complications arising from the diverticulum or in consequence of associated hypoxic episodes from aspiration.

Currently, most patients with pharyngoesophageal diverticulum seek medical assistance before complications become severe, and little or no preoperative preparation is required. If dehydration is present, it should be corrected prior to operation. When aspiration pneumonitis or lung abscess has complicated a diverticulum, attempts should be made to resolve acute sepsis before proceeding with operation. Usually, however, it is necessary to correct the esophageal problem before the pulmonary process will improve. We also feel that malnutrition should not delay operation, since treatment restores swallowing within 24 h, and oral intake can be supplemented parenterally if necessary. Perforation of the diverticulum is a surgical emergency.

Preoperatively, a liquid diet is provided the evening prior to operation. Endotracheal anesthesia is routinely employed; prior to tracheal intubation, the reverse Trendelenburg position minimizes the risk of aspiration from the diverticulum. After intubation, rapid sealing of the airway with a cuffed balloon prevents intraoperative respiratory contamination by diverticular contents.

One-Stage Diverticulectomy with Myotomy. Although a wide variety of ingenious surgical procedures have been devised and may continue to be used in the treatment of

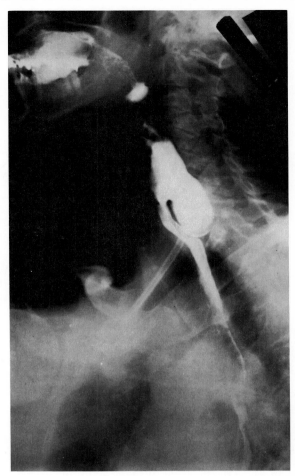

Fig. 25-31. Pharyngoesophageal diverticulum demonstrated radiographically. Note that main lumen is angulated and compressed by this moderate-sized diverticulum. (From: *Payne WS, Clagett OT: Curr Probl Surg April 1965, p 1. Copyright 1965 by Year Book Medical Publishers, Inc. Used by permission.*)

this condition, one-stage diverticulectomy with concomitant esophageal myotomy is the most definitive method of treatment. In our experience, dependable results with myotomy alone are confined to cases of small diverticula, which are less amenable to surgical excision. Therefore, we prefer diverticulectomy with myotomy for the larger diverticula (Fig. 25-32) and myotomy for the smaller diverticula (Fig. 25-33).

The right-handed surgeon will find a left cervical incision provides excellent exposure. Both the horizontal and oblique lower cervical incision have been used. After the incision has been deepened, exposure of the retropharyngeal space and the diverticulum is obtained by retracting the sternocleidomastoid muscle and the carotid sheath and its contents laterally, the thyroid gland and larynx medially, and the omohyoid muscle inferiorly. The apex of the diverticulum is grasped with an Allis forceps and elevated into the wound. The diverticulum must be thoroughly dissected, so that the neck of the mucosal sac and the surrounding ring of the muscular defect are clearly defined.

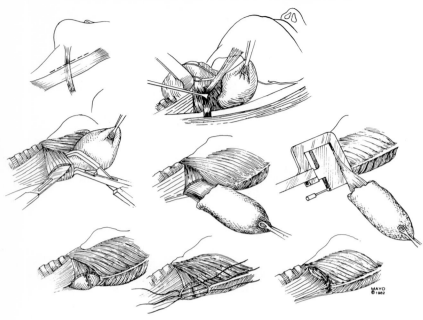

Fig. 25-32. The technique of transcervical pharyngoesophageal diverticulectomy with cricopharyngeal myotomy. Steps shown from top left to bottom right. Top row: The approximate location of the oblique skin incision (dotted line) is along the anterior border of the left sternocleidomastoid muscle. The location of the neck of the diverticulum is just cephalad to the omohyoid muscle. Middle row: After the connective tissue has been freed circumferentially from the neck of the diverticulum, the diverticulum is retracted in a cephalad direction and the plane between the cricopharyngeus muscle in the mucosa is developed with right-angle forceps. This myotomy is carried in the vertical posterior plane for 3 cm, completely dividing the cricopharyngeal muscle. With a #28 French esophageal stethoscope in the lumen of the esophagus, the sac is gently retracted and the TA 30 stapling device is applied across the neck of the diverticulum at right angles to the long axis of the pharynx and esophagus. Staples are fired and the amputation of the sac is completed, being careful not to encroach on the lumen. Bottom row: The completed myotomy and closure of the diverticulectomy. Sutures are placed in a transverse fashion of the muscularis layer covering the mucosal staple line. Penrose or suction-type drains are brought out from the retropharyngeal space below the incision. The incision is closed in the usual fashion with absorbable subcuticular suture. [From: *Payne WS, Reynolds RR: Surgical treatment of pharyngoesophageal diverticulum (Zenker's diverticulum). Surg Rounds 5:18, 1982, with permission.*]

Once the diverticulum is free circumferentially, it is retracted in a cephalad direction. A plane is developed between the cricopharyngeus muscle and the esophageal mucosa at the neck of the diverticulum. The myotomy is carried out for a distance of 3 cm onto the esophagus in the posterior vertical midline. Although the sac can be amputated using a "clamp and sew" technique, we currently prefer a stapling device for transection and closure. The stapling device is applied to the neck of the sac at right angles to the long axis of the pharynx and esophagus. With a #28 French esophageal stethoscope in the lumen of the esophagus, the staples are fired and amputation of the sac is completed, taking care not to encroach on the lumen of the esophagus. When the diverticulum is completely excised and the mucosa satisfactorily approximated, the muscular and fascial layers of the hypopharynx are closed over the repair in a transverse direction. Two small Penrose rubber drains or a suction type of catheter are placed near the site of repair in the prevertebral space and brought to the outside through the lower end of the incision prior to closure.

In Welsh and Payne's 1973 review of 809 consecutive one-stage diverticulotomy operations performed during a 27-year period, the surgical mortality was 1.4 percent. Esophagocutaneous fistulas developed postoperatively in 2.5 percent, but all closed spontaneously in a matter of days. There were no instances of serious mediastinal infection. Unilateral paralysis of the vocal cords was noted postoperatively in 2.8 percent of patients; in only three was this paralysis permanent. Late symptoms or radiologic evidence of recurrence of the diverticulum developed in 7 percent of patients; 93 percent of those followed 5 to 14 years had highly satisfactory results. Addition of cricopharyngeal myotomy to diverticulectomy, a development of the past decade, has not brought significant improvement in overall results, though postoperative leak has been obviated and symptoms from recurrent diverticula minimized. In the Mayo Clinic's recent experience, radiographic evidence of recurrent phrenoesophageal diverticulum occurred in 2.6 percent of the cases. Symptoms of recurrence were usually high cervical esophageal obstruction with retention and regurgitation of undigested food. A third of the patients had aspiration. Reoperation with diverticulectomy and myotomy was usually curative.

Cricopharyngeal Myotomy Alone (Fig. 25-33). Cross and associates suggested the use of a myotomy as an adjunct to one-stage diverticulectomy to prevent recurrence. Belsey used myotomy with diverticulopexy. Sutherland re-

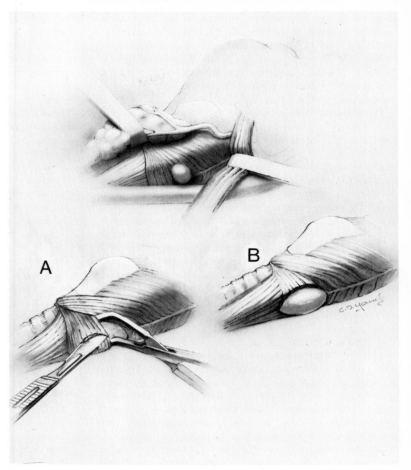

Fig. 25-33. Cricopharyngeal myotomy. This is indicated for smaller diverticula not amenable to diverticulectomy. Surgical exposure of small diverticulum and cricopharyngeus is best obtained below omohyoid. *A.* Right-angled forceps is used to develop a dissection plane below neck of small diverticulum between esophageal mucosa and muscle. *B.* Vertical extramucosal myotomy, 3 to 4 cm long, is effected; and mucosa is allowed to pout through incision. Drainage and closure are provided as with diverticulectomy. [From: *Payne WS, in Shields TW (ed): General Thoracic Surgery, 2d ed. Philadelphia, Lea & Febiger, 1983, p 864, with permission.*]

ported use of cricopharyngeal myotomy as the sole means of treating pharyngoesophageal diverticulum.

Myotomy alone is certainly an effective means of dealing with smaller diverticula, not only because it reduces the tone of the partially obstructing sphincter, but also because it eliminates the distal support of the diverticular neck and obliterates the septating spur. Dohlman and Mattsson have accomplished this same reentry effect by an endoscopic diathermic division of the spur formed by the diverticular esophageal wall.

In regard to the technique of cricopharyngeal myotomy, surgical exposure is accomplished as described for diverticulectomy (Fig. 25-33). After the diverticulum is freed to its neck, the transverse fibers of the cricopharyngeal muscle bordering the inferior margin of the neck of the diverticulum are easily identified and incised verti-

cally. The incision is carried down to mucosa and is extended caudad onto the esophagus in the posterior midline with the length of the incision averaging about 3 cm. After the myotomy, the esophageal and cricopharyngeal muscles are dissected for half the circumference of the mucosal tube to allow the mucosa to protrude freely through the incision. The cervical wound is then closed, with drainage.

Epiphrenic Diverticulum

Probably no other benign lesion affecting the esophagus has been so poorly understood for so long as the epiphrenic diverticulum. Unfortunately, lack of basic knowledge concerning pathogenesis has all too often resulted in poor surgical results. Current surgical methods can provide a safe and rational management in most cases.

NATURE AND PRESENTATION. This diverticulum also is an acquired abnormality, occurring chiefly in adult patients. As its name implies, the epiphrenic diverticulum usually occurs in the lower thoracic esophagus—typically within 10 cm of the cardia—but it may be at higher levels in the thoracic zone. Its pathologic anatomy is almost identical to that of pulsion diverticula in the pharyngoesophageal region, in that the diverticulum is essentially a herniated sac of mucosa and submucosa protruding through the usual supporting sheath of esophageal musculature. The sac may be covered by thin bands of attenuated muscle, which are often not discernible except on microscopic study.

The association of epiphrenic diverticula with motility disturbances and esophageal hiatial hernia was first appreciated by Vinson in 1934. Others since have noted the incidence of associated abnormal esophageal and diaphragmatic conditions. These and other data suggest that the majority of pulsion diverticula of the lower esophagus develop as the result of a variety of esophageal conditions. Debas and associates, in a review of 65 symptomatic Mayo Clinic patients undergoing manometric as well as radiographic and endoscopic investigation, found that 50 had esophageal motility disturbances, usually diffuse spasm or achalasia. Among the 15 with normal peristalsis, it was usual to find esophageal hiatal hernia, esophagitis, or stricture. In only 2 of these 65 cases were no associated esophageal abnormalities detectable, leaving the diverticulum probably the sole cause of the symptoms.

Habein and associates, in a study of 149 patients with epiphrenic diverticulum, estimated that only 15 to 20 percent of such lesions produce definite symptoms. Thus the majority of epiphrenic diverticula are either asymptomatic or so mildly symptomatic that they do not pose a surgical problem. Symptoms, when present, are those of esophageal obstruction, retention, and regurgitation. Tracheobronchial aspiration and suppurative pneumonitis do occur, though less commonly than with pharyngoesophageal diverticula. Regurgitated matter is characteristically bland, containing undigested food and saliva. In some situations it may be difficult to differentiate these symptoms from those caused by related underlying esophageal motor disorders.

The symptoms of epiphrenic diverticulum are often less definite than those of pharyngoesophageal diverticulum and may be only suggestive of the diagnosis. Radiographic examination of the esophagus with contrast medium is the best way to determine the presence and location of this pulsion diverticulum and associated conditions (Fig. 25-10, *top*). Esophagoscopy is not required to establish a diagnosis but should be performed to seek out and define associated esophageal disease, especially stenoses or filling defects. Studies of esophageal motility are essential in planning surgical management of epiphrenic diverticulum.

TREATMENT. The management of epiphrenic diverticulum is surgical, and an operation is indicated in patients with progressive symptoms. Progressive enlargement of an epiphrenic diverticulum is a relative indication for surgical intervention. Diverticulectomy should also be considered when an operation is indicated for an associated esophageal condition. A diverticulum causing few or no symptoms does not warrant surgical intervention if more serious associated conditions can be excluded.

Technique. The chief preoperative considerations in treatment for epiphrenic diverticulum are precise definition of all associated esophageal conditions and a specific plan to deal with each in a definitive manner. Preoperative attempts to empty the esophagus or diverticulum are not ordinarily required or indicated; a liquid diet a few days prior to operation usually suffices. At the time of operation, tracheal intubation with the patient awake under topical anesthesia is prudent. After the airway is sealed with a balloon-cuffed endotracheal tube, general anesthesia is induced.

Left thoracotomy (Fig. 25-34) should be used almost routinely in the surgical treatment of epiphrenic diverticulum, since this incision provides the necessary exposure for excision of the diverticulum and, more importantly, is usually required to correct frequently associated esophageal and diaphragmatic conditions. Furthermore, the results of diverticulectomy are more satisfactory if a long, extramucosal esophagomyotomy is performed routinely. If there is an associated diaphragmatic hernia that needs repair following diverticulectomy and myotomy, a nonobstructive antireflux procedure such as the Belsey Mark IV is advised.

RESULTS. The significance of the present concept of the surgical treatment of pulsion diverticula of the lower esophageal region is clearly apparent on review of the Mayo Clinic experience from 1944 through 1976. Early in this experience, diverticulectomy and correction of associated diaphragmatic hernia were done without concomitant esophagomyotomy. Of 29 patients so treated, 7 had significant postoperative complications—including 4 recurrent epiphrenic diverticula. Later, esophagomyotomy was performed routinely with diverticulectomy; and of the 29 patients so treated, only 1 had a postoperative complication.

Parabronchial or Midesophageal Diverticulum

Granulomatous infections of mediastinal lymph nodes may cause traction diverticula. Although they occur typically in relation to subcarinal and parabronchial lymph nodes in the middle third of the esophagus, they can be at any level. Generally these minute triangular esophageal deformities are of little or no clinical significance except as indications of a previous, often healed infection; they produce no esophageal symptoms and require no treatment. When symptoms are present, they are usually attributable to some other, unrelated process.

If symptoms occur, the usual studies should be carried out to determine the cause and rule out other conditions. These include radiographic examination, endoscopy, and motility studies. When active infection is suspected, appropriate skin tests and microbiologic studies are indicated.

Interest in traction diverticula thus is focused chiefly on distinguishing them from more serious conditions. Rarely, however, such a diverticulum may be the site of serious complications. These include obstruction to swallowing, esophagitis, hemorrhage, perforation, empyema,

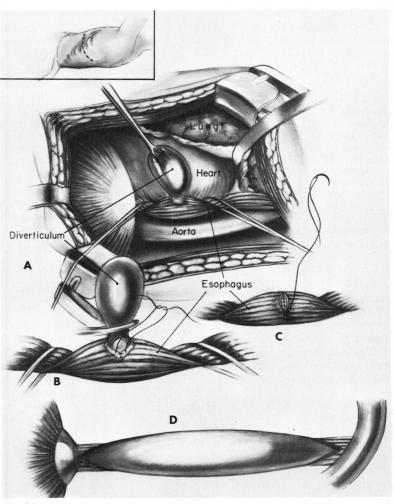

Fig. 25-34. Surgical management of pulsion diverticula of lower esophagus. *Inset:* Placement of left posterolateral thoracotomy incision. *A.* Exposure of diverticulum obtained when chest is entered through bed of left eighth rib. Esophagus has been delivered from its mediastinal bed, tapes have been passed around esophagus, and esophagus has been rotated to bring diverticulum into view. Neck of mucosal diverticulum has been dissected, exposing defect in esophageal muscular wall. *B.* "Cut-and-sew" technique of diverticulectomy. Amputation and closure are effected in transverse axis. Mucosal sutures are tied with knots within esophageal lumen. *C.* Closure of esophageal musculature over mucosal suture line. *D.* Site of diverticular incision has been rotated back to right and is not visible. A long esophagomyotomy, extending from esophagogastric junction to aortic arch, has been performed. Musculature of esophagus has been freed from approximately 50 percent of circumference of esophageal mucosal tube to allow mucosa to bulge through muscular incision. Frequently associated sliding esophageal hiatal hernia is shown. When present, it too should be repaired at time of operation. (From: *Payne WS, Olsen AM: The Esophagus. Philadelphia, Lea & Febiger, 1974, p 220, with permission.*)

pericarditis, or fistula formation with the tracheobronchial tree.

Usually the symptomatic traction diverticulum can be managed by simple excision. Fistulas between the esophagus and lower respiratory tract respond to excision and closure of the communication with interposition of normal tissues to prevent recurrence. Perforation with empyema or pericarditis often requires specific antibiotic treatment as well as surgical drainage and temporary diversion of the esophagus.

BENIGN CYSTS AND TUMORS

Benign cysts and tumors of the esophagus are uncommon and amount to less than 10 percent of esophageal neoplasms. They are of clinical concern, not only because they must be distinguished from more serious conditions but also because on occasion they can produce significant clinical symptoms and even threaten life. More than half of the 246 benign esophageal tumors and cysts seen at the Mayo Clinic were surgically or endoscopically removed; the rest were encountered at autopsy (Table 25-6).

Leiomyomas are the most common benign tumors. Those less than 5 cm in diameter are rarely symptomatic.

Table 25-6. BENIGN TUMORS AND CYSTS OF ESOPHAGUS SEEN AT THE MAYO CLINIC

Type	Total	Type	Total
Leiomyoma	145	Myxofibroma	2
Cyst	55	Fibrolipoma	2
Polyp	12	Neurofibroma	2
Papilloma	5	Fibroma	1
Lipoma	5	Lymphangioma	1
Hemangioma	4	Mucocele	1
Adenoma	3	Duplication	1
Granular cell		Chondroma	1
myoblastoma	3		
Indeterminate	3		

Most leiomyomas occur in the lower half of the esophagus, and the majority of these are extramucosal and can be treated by simple enucleation. Radiographic examination often suggests the diagnosis (Fig. 25-35). Those encountered in the region of the esophagogastric junction tend to be large, circumferential, obstructive lesions and often require esophagogastrectomy for successful removal. Reconstruction requires special attention with regard to unobstructed restoration of esophagogastric continuity, provision against consequences of concomitant vagotomy, and prevention of subsequent gastroesophageal reflux and its complications.

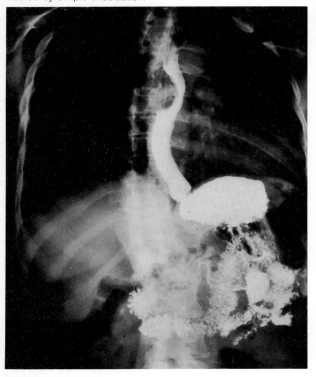

Fig. 25-35. Radiograph of esophagus, demonstrating extramucosal filling defect that proved to be a leiomyoma that could be treated by simple enucleation.

Cysts are the second most common benign lesions of the esophagus. In infants and children they more commonly cause symptoms through compression of the adjacent esophagus or tracheobronchial tree. Most can be removed successfully by enucleation. Complete reduplication is extremely rare; but it is seen, and often features a lining of esophageal, gastric, or small-intestinal epithelium.

Various polypoid intraesophageal tumors have been described, including mucosal polyps, chondromas, lipomas, fibrolipomas, and myxofibromas. Some pedunculated polypoid benign tumors have produced huge esophageal filling defects. Others are more cigar-shaped and have actually been long enough to protrude from the mouth when regurgitated. The smaller lesions can be managed by endoscopic snare; others require esophagotomy for removal.

MALIGNANT TUMORS

INCIDENCE AND ETIOLOGY. Carcinoma of the esophagus is predominantly a disease of males (male-to-female ratio, 3:1) between the ages of fifty and seventy years. The incidence varies widely throughout the world, being notably high in China, Japan, Scotland, Russia, and the Scandinavian countries. In South Africa incidence is especially high among the native Bantu. Although the basic cause of the disease is unknown, dietary and alcoholic habits, as well as tobacco use, have been implicated. A particularly high incidence has been noted among patients with achalasia and corrosive esophagitis. Joske and Benedict found an unusually high incidence of cancer of the cervical esophagus in patients with Plummer–Vinson (Paterson–Kelly) syndrome. Other conditions and disorders associated with a high incidence of esophageal carcinoma include lye burns, diverticula of the esophagus, the columnar epithelial-lined lower esophagus of Barrett, and the syndrome known as *tylosis palmaris et plantaris.*

PATHOLOGY. Although nearly all malignant tumors arising in the body of the esophagus are squamous-cell carcinomas, most of those involving the esophagogastric junction are adenocarcinomas of gastric origin. Figure 25-36 shows the approximate anatomic location and distribution by histopathologic type of the usual esophageal cancers. It should be noted that almost as many tumors affected the cardia as affected the entire cervical and thoracic zones of the esophagus combined.

The remainder of the malignant tumors of the esophagus are rare sarcomas, mostly leiomyosarcomas. These are predominantly extramucosal; but in contrast to the benign leiomyomas, they tend to ulcerate and calcify. Carcinosarcoma, adenoid cystic carcinoma, and small cell carcinoma have been reported. There have also been rare reports of primary malignant melanomas of the esophagus. Nearly all these malignant melanomas were associated with melanosis and had a poor prognosis.

Some carcinomas develop as bulky, fungating, obstructive growths and others as superficially ulcerated, surface-spreading tumors producing little obstruction. All

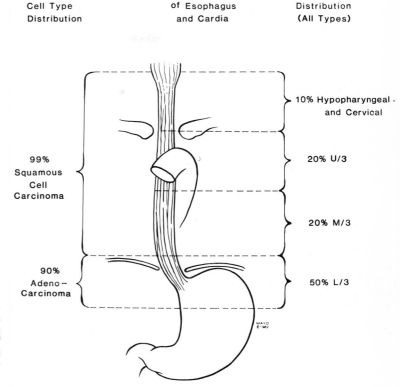

Cell Type Distribution	Carcinoma of Esophagus and Cardia	Distribution (All Types)

99% Squamous Cell Carcinoma

90% Adeno- Carcinoma

10% Hypopharyngeal and Cervical

20% U/3

20% M/3

50% L/3

Fig. 25-36. Approximate anatomic distribution of primary carcinomas of esophagus and cardia is shown on right. On left is distribution of the two most common cell types of primary carcinoma. Note that nearly half of carcinomas occur in lower third (L/3) or cardia, and that these are predominantly adenocarcinomas of gastric epithelial origin.

these tumors spread via lymphatic vessels, by direct extension from the esophagus, and by vascular invasion. Tumors of the cervical esophagus disseminate through the lymphatic vessels to cervical nodes, particularly the anterior jugular and supraclavicular nodes. Those arising in the thoracic esophagus spread early to local mediastinal (peritracheal and esophageal) glands as well as supraclavicular and, occasionally, subdiaphragmatic nodes. In contrast, lesions of the gastroesophageal junction spread most frequently to the celiac axis and superior gastric lesser curvature lymph nodes. Occasionally, they may involve middle and superior mediastinal lymph nodes. Neoplasms in any location can metastasize through the bloodstream to the liver, lung, or bone. Reports from China clearly define premalignant esophageal epithelial changes, with atypia progressing to in situ, early invasive, and more massive squamous cell cancers. Evolution from asymptomatic abnormal cytology to dysphagia has been estimated to take about 3 years. Dysphagia usually occurs when about half to two-thirds of the circumference of the esophagus is involved by gross tumor.

MANIFESTATIONS AND DIAGNOSIS. The earliest and almost constant feature of carcinoma of the esophagus is progressive dysphagia. Initially, it is noted with ingestion of solid foods, but ultimately the swallowing of even liquids and saliva becomes difficult. The inevitable consequence is inanition. As obstructive symptoms progress, aspiration pneumonitis is not infrequent. Painful swallowing is especially suggestive of malignancy. Occult mild anemia is common, but massive bleeding is not.

The diagnosis of carcinoma of the esophagus can be made with a high degree of accuracy by the usual radiographic examination of the esophagus and stomach. This usually demonstrates an irregular, ragged mucosal pattern with annular luminal narrowing. Unlike the more chronic benign obstructive lesions, carcinoma usually is not associated with marked proximal dilatation of the esophagus.

Esophagoscopy should be performed in all instances of suspected esophageal cancer—regardless of the interpretation of the radiograph—both to establish a tissue diagnosis and to determine accurately the upper limit of the lesion. When a lesion involves the mid or upper esophagus, it is usually desirable to perform bronchoscopy to detect malignant involvement of the adjacent tracheobronchial tree. Cytologic study of smears made from suggestive lesions is a valuable diagnostic adjunct. Occasionally, study of esophageal motility may suggest malignant involvement, but this technique is of greater assistance in defining one of the more common motility disturbances as a cause for dysphagia. The role of routine computerized tomography (CT) is controversial. Although helpful if distant metastasis to the liver or lung is suspected, the ability of CT to accurately determine the extent of local invasion or metastatic involvement of lymph nodes is less precise and most often the resectability of a tumor can only be

Table 25-7. POSTSURGICAL TNM
CLASSIFICATION FOR ESOPHAGEAL
CARCINOMA

T Classification
    T0 = no evidence of tumor
    T1 = tumor invasion of the mucosa or
        submucosa but not the muscle wall
    T2 = tumor invasion of the muscle wall
    T3 = tumor invasion beyond the muscle wall

N Classification
    N0 = no lymph-node metastasis
    N1 = unilateral regional lymph-node metastasis
    N2 = bilateral regional lymph-node metastasis
    N3 = extensive multiple regional lymph-node metastasis

M Classification
    M0 = no evidence of distant metastasis
    M1 = distant metastasis present

determined at the time of operation. The role of magnetic resonance (MR) scanning is being evaluated. Occasionally surgical exploration is required to establish the presence or absence of malignant growth when clinical manifestations are suggestive but results of diagnostic studies are not definitive.

A report from the Honan province of China indicates that the application of special cytologic screening techniques to a high-risk population permits detection of carcinoma of the esophagus before symptoms develop and at a stage when nearly all cases are resectable, with more than a 90 percent chance of 5-year survival.

TREATMENT. There are only two methods of treatment proved to benefit patients with carcinoma of the esophagus: surgical resection and irradiation. Neither of these methods is new; hence it is not surprising that there has been no recent notable improvement in survival statistics among patients with esophageal cancer in the stage usually encountered. Survival is clearly stage-dependent. Most patients present with advanced disease (Stage III) including full-thickness wall invasion and lymph-node metastases. The TNM staging system (Tables 25-7, 25-8) is currently the only accurate way to predict the survival of subgroups of patients with esophageal carcinoma. Staging also allows more meaningful comparison of the different forms of treatment.

Table 25-8. POSTSURGICAL STAGING FOR
ESOPHAGEAL CARCINOMA

Stage I
    T1 N0 M0

Stage II
    T2 N0 M0

Stage III
    T3 N0 M0
    Any T, any N, M0

Stage IV
    Any T, any N, M1

Irradiation. Squamous cell carcinoma of the esophagus is a radiosensitive and theoretically radiocurable tumor. In contrast, radiation therapy for adenocarcinoma of the gastroesophageal junction is much less effective. Unfortunately, although the primary lesion may be controlled, failures result from the presence of tumor outside the irradiated field, and few permanent cures are obtainable. Pearson, the strongest proponent, reported 17 percent 5-year survival in patients who completed radiation therapy of 5000 to 6000 rad; but nearly half of his patients were unable to complete therapy. Extensive review of reports published in a recent 25-year period suggests 6 percent overall 5-year survival after radiotherapy alone.

Radical radiation therapy is not without risk. Radiation pneumonitis, local tumor recurrence, postradiation stricture, functional dysphagia, tracheoesophageal fistula, perforation, spinal-cord injury, pericardial effusion, and constrictive pericarditis are among the more serious complications—any one of which is likely to occur in half of those treated.

Preoperative radiation in lesser doses of 2000 to 5000 rad and surgical resection at varying intervals after its completion have produced favorable results reported by the originators of these techniques, but not duplicated by others. At best, preoperative radiation appears to improve the resectability rate modestly without affecting survival.

Palliative low-dose radiotherapy (2000 to 3000 rad), judiciously applied, may alleviate distressing symptoms such as pain, dysphagia, and bleeding with minimal risk of morbidity.

Chemotherapy. Chemotherapy alone has had little demonstrable effect in palliating patients with either squamous cell carcinoma or adenocarcinoma of the esophagus. Because of the belief that this disease is often systemic at the time of diagnosis, combined modality treatment using chemotherapy, radiation therapy, and resection in a staged regimen has gained popularity. Recent studies have been encouraging but it is too early to make any long-term predictions.

Surgery. Surgical treatment, too, suffers from being a local form of therapy, but it is more effective in controlling local disease and restoring function. Although it is not without risk (mortality is currently reported at 2 to 6 percent), more than 90 percent of those surviving resection experience unobstructed swallowing throughout their subsequent course. In a recent review of 100 patients with carcinoma of the esophagus and cardia who underwent Ivor Lewis esophagogastrectomy at the Mayo Clinic, 5-year survival for patients with Stage I neoplasm was 85.7 percent; Stage II neoplasm 34.1 percent; and Stage III neoplasm 15.2 percent. Overall 5-year survival for the entire 100 patients including operative mortality (3 percent) and death from all causes was 22.7 percent (Fig. 25-37). Cell type, sex, and location of primary tumor did not have an effect on survival. Metastatic lymph-node involvement uniformly adversely influenced survival.

In the past, a large number of ingenious surgical procedures were developed to effect tumor ablation and esophageal reconstruction. Some were elaborate multistaged

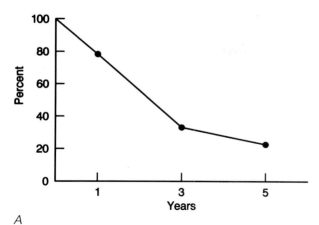

A

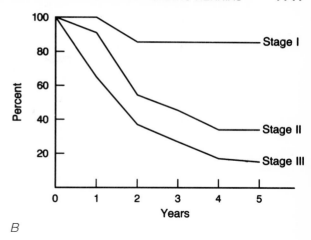

B

Fig. 25-37. Survival following resection of esophageal carcinoma. *A.* Overall probability of survival (death from all causes of 100 patients with carcinoma of the esophagus after Ivor Lewis esophagogastrectomy). Zero time on abscissa represents day of operation. *B.* Probability of survival (death from all causes of 100 patients with carcinoma of the esophagus by postsurgical TNM classification). Zero time on abscissa represents day of operation. (From: *King RM, Pairolero PC, et al: Ivor Lewis esophagogastrectomy for carcinoma of the esophagus: Early and late functional results. Ann Thorac Surg 44:119, 1987, with permission.*)

operations and many interfered seriously with eating and digestive comfort, even if the tumor was permanently eradicated. Today every effort is made to minimize the duration of the treatment period, utilizing one-stage pro-

cedures that provide restoration of function with minimal permanent disability.

In most cases—whether the primary lesion is high in the cervical esophagus, at the esophagogastric junction, or in between—the stomach can be effectively mobilized and advanced cephalad at one operation to replace the resected esophagus (Fig. 25-38). Indeed, stomach perfused by right gastric and right gastroepiploic vessels can be made to reach and serve reliably as high as the hyoid bone when placed in the posterior mediastinal bed of the resected esophagus, or as high as the cricoid when passed substernally. Since vagotomy necessarily accompanies

Fig. 25-38. Esophageal reconstruction utilizing stomach. *Above:* Mobilized stomach nourished by distal vascular pedicles of right gastric and right gastroepiploic vessels. Left gastric and short gastric vessels have been interrupted and esophagogastric junction has been divided and closed. Since vagotomy has been effected, a pyloroplasty (or pyloromyotomy) has been performed. *Below left:* Posterior mediastinal passage of vascularized stomach through esophageal hiatus to neck for anastomosis to pharynx or cervical esophagus. *Right:* Substernal or anterior mediastinal tunnel permits passage of stomach to neck for anastomosis to cervical esophagus. Either route can be utilized when colon is interposed between neck and stomach to replace or bypass entire thoracic esophagus.

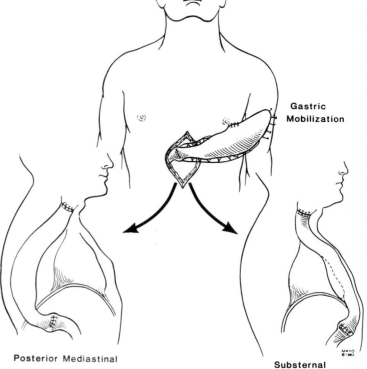

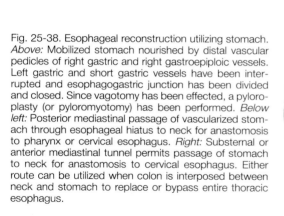

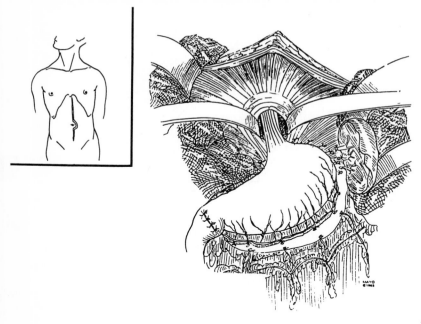

Fig. 25-39. Ivor Lewis esophagogastrectomy-laparotomy. Stomach is prepared for transposition into the chest by preserving right gastric and right gastroepiploic vessels. Pyloromyotomy or pyloroplasty is routinely performed. *Insert:* Upper midline incision from xiphoid to just below umbilicus. (From: *Payne WS, Trastek VF, et al: Current techniques for the surgical management of malignant lesions of the thoracic esophagus and cardia. Mayo Clin Proc 61:564, July 1986, with permission.*)

esophageal resection, pyloroplasty or pyloromyotomy should routinely accompany this use of stomach in esophageal reconstruction.

Generally, both gastroesophageal reflux and gastric dumping are infrequent sequelae of esophagogastrostomy when anastomosis is effected at the carinal level or above, provided the entire stomach lies intrathoracically without redundancy.

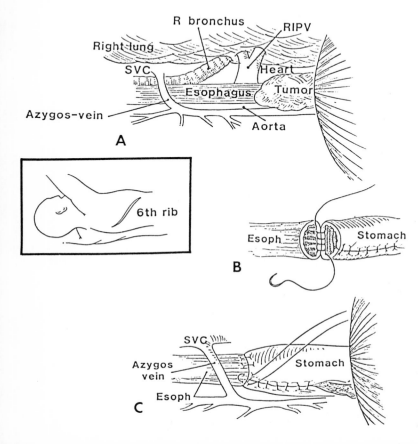

Fig. 25-40. Ivor Lewis esophagogastrectomy-right thoracotomy. *A.* Tumor and esophagus are freed to a level above the azygos vein. *B.* An end-to-end anastomosis is performed over #50 French dilator. *C.* Completed anastomosis. *Insert:* Chest is entered through fifth interspace. (From: *Payne WS, Trastek VF, et al: Current techniques for the surgical management of malignant lesions of the thoracic esophagus and cardia. Mayo Clin Proc 61:564, July 1986, with permission.*)

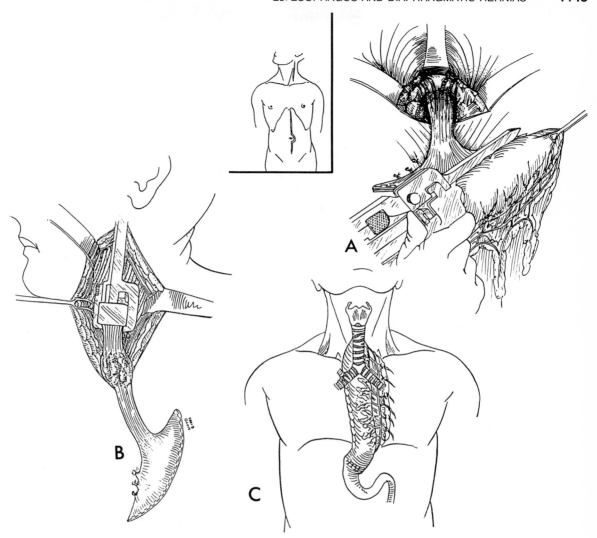

Fig. 25-41. Transhiatal esophagectomy. *Insert:* The neck and abdomen are prepared simultaneously. The midline incision and preparation of the stomach are the same as for the Ivor Lewis esophagogastrectomy (Fig. 25-39). *A.* The stomach is transected just distal to the gastroesophageal junction using the stapling device. *B.* The esophagus is mobilized bluntly from the mediastinum and transposed into the neck, carefully preserving the recurrent nerve. The cervical esophagus is divided using the stapling device. *C.* The stomach is passed through the posterior mediastinal bed, and the anastomosis is constructed at the cervical region over a #50 French dilator. (From: *Payne WS, Trastek VF, et al: Current techniques for the surgical management of malignant lesions of the thoracic esophagus and cardia. Mayo Clin Proc 61:564, July 1986, with permission.*)

Technical Options. The details of the resection and reconstruction vary with individual lesions, surgeons, and surgical intent. Currently the two most commonly performed procedures at the Mayo Clinic are the Ivor Lewis esophagogastrectomy for cardiac and intrathoracic locations (Figs. 25-39, 25-40) and the transhiatal esophagogastrectomy with cervical anastomosis without thoracotomy for a variety of esophageal lesions (Fig. 25-41). Total gastrectomy with Roux en Y reconstruction is reserved for the gastric lesions that extend up to but are not actually invading the distal esophagus. The left transthoracic esophagogastrectomy with esophagogastrostomy in the left chest for more distal esophageal and gastroesophageal lesions is used only in selected cases. Functional results are enhanced by an anastomotic stoma that accepts a #50 French bougie coupled with invagination into the stomach.

In current practice, colon interposition is largely reserved for those patients in whom disease or previous surgery makes the stomach unsuitable for esophageal replacement (Fig. 25-42). Both the right and left colon and iso- and antiperistaltic segments of the colon have been employed to reach as high as the pharynx. The colon can be passed either substernally or through the posterior mediastinal bed of the resected esophagus. Either the middle colic or inferior mesenteric vessels can serve as blood supply. To improve survival of the colon transposed into the neck, a second blood supply can be con-

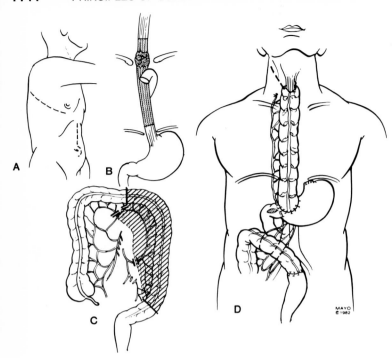

Fig. 25-42. Substernal colon interposition following total esophagectomy for carcinoma. *A* and *B*. At initial operation, esophagus is removed through right thoracotomy and a feeding gastrostomy tube inserted with establishment of proximal cervical esophageal stoma. *C* and *D*. At second operation, left colon is mobilized on vascular pedicle and brought through gastrohepatic omentum. Colon is advanced cephalad through substernal tunnel to neck for anastomosis to cervical esophagus. End-to-side cologastrostomy is effected in abdomen with pyloroplasty or pyloromyotomy. Colonic continuity is restored by colocolostomy.

structed by attaching a colic artery and vein to neck vessels using microvascular techniques.

With colon interposition it is essential that a generous tunnel be provided to minimize vascular compression. If the colon is placed in a substernal position, resection of a portion of the manubrium, clavicle, and first or second costochondral arch is frequently required. The colon must also be straight from proximal anastomosis to cologastrostomy. When the entire stomach needs to be removed with the esophagus, a long-limb Roux en Y is attached to the abdominal end of the colon interposition to prevent severe bile reflux up to the colon into the mouth (Fig. 25-43).

Decision to Operate and Selection of Techniques. Surgery provides such satisfactory local control of disease, with restoration of swallowing, that many surgeons feel

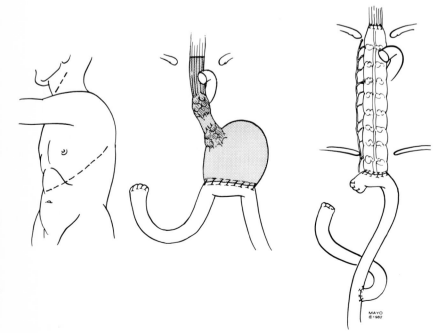

Fig. 25-43. Interposition of colon for esophagus and stomach (latter being unsuitable for interposition because of previous surgery), with long-limb Roux en Y required to prevent bile reflux.

that it should be employed whenever technically feasible. Others cite a median survival of 2 months in patients with known unresectable disease or liver metastases and favor a less aggressive approach. The ability of endoscopic laser therapy to open an obstructed esophagus with minimal morbidity and mortality has made it a primary approach in the palliation of many of these patients. A Celestin or similar palliative tube inserted at the time of abdominal exploration provides a reasonable lumen for unobstructed swallowing in most patients. There is also renewed interest in the palliative transoral endoscopic placement of plastic tubes for inoperable carcinomas. With either method of placement, palliative intubation is restricted to lesions below the cervical esophagus. It may provide satisfactory palliation in cases of acquired malignant tracheoesophageal fistula. Although substernal gastric bypass was initially suggested as a palliative method of management for this type of fistula, a recent review by Orringer has shown a high complication rate, and he no longer recommends this procedure as a palliative maneuver.

Feeding gastrostomy provides no palliation for esophageal obstruction and should be employed only in maintaining nutrition during outpatient radiotherapy, as a temporary measure between stages of esophageal reconstruction, or as an expedient when esophageal obstruction cannot be palliated and parenteral support is impractical. Transendoscopic placement of a gastrostomy tube has been an attractive alternative to surgical placement in selected patients, permitting them to leave the hospital. For others, repeated esophageal dilation treatment can provide reasonable palliation of dysphagia, if they live near the care center.

Unresolved is the management of cervical esophageal and hypopharyngeal cancers. Radiotherapy has surpassed surgery in effecting cure and has the added virtue of preserving voice and laryngeal function if the tumor is locally controlled. Unfortunately, cure and control are not often achieved by this means, and neither esophageal nor laryngeal function is ultimately preserved: the surgeon is often required to perform laryngopharyngoesophagectomy for recurrent or persistent cancer in a heavily radiated field. Reconstruction poses special considerations to restore function (Fig. 25-44).

DeSanto and Carpenter have reviewed the Mayo experience with various reconstructions, which include cervical flaps of the Wookey type, Bakamjian deltopectoral flaps, colon tissue, and gastric interposition of Akiyama. More recently, free transfer of a segment of jejunum has been employed with microvascular anastomosis to cervical vessels. The major problem of hypopharyngeal and cervical esophageal cancer rests not so much with the reconstruction techniques, but with the primary disease and its advanced stage at diagnosis. This, of course, is true for all esophageal cancers.

That cure of early cancer can be achieved frequently with currently available treatment modalities is evident from the Chinese reports of the results in early cancer detected by cytologic screening of a high-risk population. The resectability rate of 170 early esophageal cancers was 100 percent and the 5-year survival was 90 percent.

Postoperative Care. Care following any of the surgical procedures for esophageal cancer is similar to that following any major gastrointestinal and thoracic procedure. Fluid and electrolyte balance, chest physiotherapy, nasogastric intubation, and early ambulation are essential features. Chest tubes, placed at operation, can be removed when drainage ceases. Oral feeding is resumed with the clinical return of gastrointestinal activity, provided contrast radiography demonstrates the absence of anastomotic leak. In nutritionally depleted patients, parenteral alimentation is begun the day after surgery and continued until oral intake is well established. Total hospitalization averages 10 to 12 days.

ESOPHAGEAL PERFORATION

Irrespective of cause, esophageal perforation or rupture may initiate a virulent periesophageal infection. Prompt recognition and proper treatment may avert death or obviate a prolonged and difficult convalescence. In spite of all efforts, esophageal perforation continues to be associated with high mortality and morbidity.

INCIDENCE. Most esophageal perforations today occur after some form of esophageal instrumentation. The number of such perforations appears to have increased over the past 40 years as a result of the greater use of esophagoscopy, gastroscopy, esophageal dilation, and even simple esophageal intubation for diagnosis or treatment.

Of equal interest are those less frequently encountered instances of noninstrumental perforation, which occur as the result of accidental ingestion of foreign bodies or as a consequence of the strain of emesis with or without predisposing esophageal disease. Various other conditions also have been implicated in the noninstrumental perforation of the esophagus, including "stress" associated with neurologic disease or following operations or burns remote from the esophagus. Infrequently, the esophagus may be perforated as the result of either penetrating or nonpenetrating external trauma.

ETIOLOGY. The wall of the esophagus can be breached in a number of ways by either an instrument or a foreign body: (1) simple penetration of the entire wall, (2) simple splitting or rupture of it by strain exceeding its circumferential tensile strength, (3) breaking down of the wall by a localized inflammatory process resulting from mucosal tears, and (4) perforation developing from pressure necrosis or devascularization.

Perforation by instrument or foreign body can occur at any level of the esophagus; however, the sites of normal narrowing are the ones most frequently involved. The greatest narrowing is at the esophageal introitus, and it accounts for the high incidence of perforations seen in this region. Impingement of the rigid scope on bodies of hyperextended cervical vertebrae may crush the mucosa, particularly in the presence of hypertrophic bony spurs.

The second most common site for instrumental or foreign-body perforations has been the lower esophagus, immediately above the point where the organ narrows to pass through the diaphragmatic hiatus. The increased occurrence of disease and frequent need for endoscopic

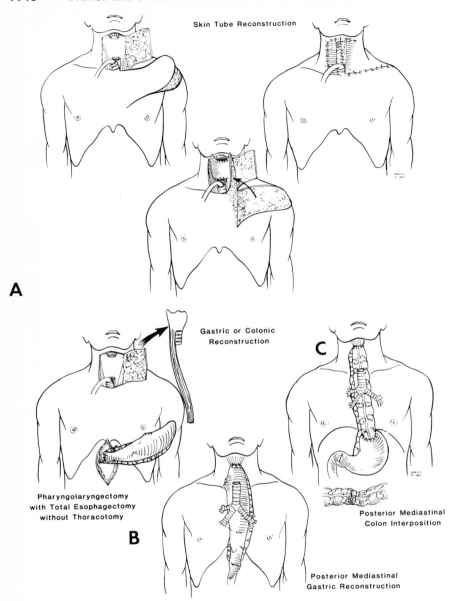

Skin Tube Reconstruction

A

Gastric or Colonic Reconstruction

Pharyngolaryngectomy with Total Esophagectomy without Thoracotomy

B

Free Segment of Jejunum (with Microvascular Anastomosis)

Posterior Mediastinal Gastric Reconstruction

C

Posterior Mediastinal Colon Interposition

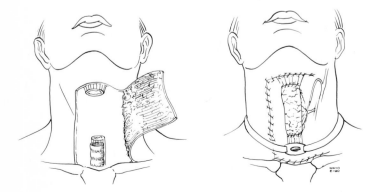

Fig. 25-44. Hypopharyngeal and cervical esophageal cancers pose special reconstruction problems following cervical laryngopharyngoesophagectomy and tracheostomy. Four methods are currently available to effect this reconstruction: *A.* Bakamjian deltopectoral skin-tube reconstruction of pharyngoesophageal continuity. *B.* Posterior mediastinal passage of vascularized pedicle of stomach to neck for anastomosis to pharynx after total esophagectomy. *C.* Posterior mediastinal passage of vascularized colon for interposition between pharynx and stomach. *D.* Free transfer of short segment of jejunum between pharynx and low cortical esophagus with microvascular anastomosis of jejunal vessels to external carotid artery branch and jugular vein.

manipulations in this region contribute further to the incidence of perforation at this level. Perforations of the middle third and abdominal part of the esophagus occur infrequently.

The mechanism of postemetic perforation of the lower esophagus has attracted considerable interest. Mackler showed that inflation of the fresh human cadaveric esophagus resulted in simple longitudinal splitting when the pressure exceeded its circumferential tensile strength. In 95 percent of the 65 specimens studied, such tears occurred in the distal portion of the esophagus. Duval, as reported by Kinsella and coworkers, demonstrated that the rapidity of the increase in pressure rather than the amount of pressure per se may be a critical factor in such injuries. The fact that most postemetic perforations occur in adults rather than in children may be explainable by the higher incidence of predisposing factors in adults and especially by the fact that the strength of the esophagus is thirteen times greater in infants (less than one year old) and four times greater in children (less than twelve years old) than it is in adults.

PATHOPHYSIOLOGY. The consequences of esophageal perforation are due to contamination of periesophageal spaces by corrosive digestive fluids, foods, and bacteria, which leads to a diffuse cellulitis with localized or extensive suppuration.

Anatomic considerations are important, both in the evolution of signs and symptoms and in treatment. The majority of cervical esophageal perforations are posterior and result in suppuration first in the retrovesical space and then extending along fascial planes into the mediastinum.

Perforations of the anterior wall of the cervical esophagus and those involving the lateral pharyngeal spaces and pyriform fossae enter the pretracheal space. The pretracheal space communicates with the mediastinum via the fascial attachment to the pericardium. The manifestations of perforation depend on the relation of the esophagus to the contiguous spaces. The upper two-thirds of the thoracic esophagus is in proximity to the right pleural cavity. The lowest third of the esophagus lies adjacent to the left pleural space. In rare cases, the intraabdominal or subphrenic esophagus may be perforated, leading to peritonitis and intraabdominal abscess.

Although the perforation need not be extensive or impressive to produce marked local or systemic reaction, the consequent sequestration of body fluids in the adjacent spaces may add hypovolemia to bacteremic shock. In addition, the accumulation of fluid and leakage of free air from the perforated hollow viscus may significantly interfere with normal cardiorespiratory dynamics.

MANIFESTATIONS AND DIAGNOSIS. The diagnosis of esophageal perforation depends on suspicious awareness of the possibility as well as on knowledge of the circumstances in which it may occur, the patient's symptoms, the presence of physical signs, and demonstration of the perforation and its secondary manifestations by radiography.

Although the symptoms of perforation depend to a large degree on its site and the extent of inflammatory

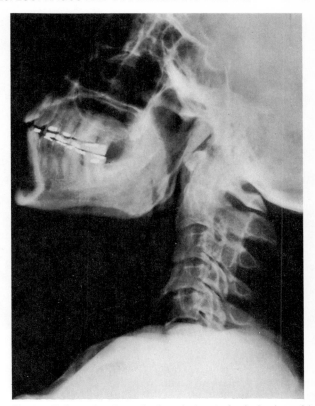

Fig. 25-45. Lateral radiograph of cervical part of spinal column 2 h after instrumental perforation of cervical part of esophagus. Note anterior displacement of trachea by anterior bulging of retrovisceral space, emphysema in tissue planes, and hypertrophic bony spurs on lower cervical vertebrae. [From: *Ellis FH Jr, Payne WS, in Artz CP, Hardy JD (eds): Complications in Surgery and Their Management, 2d ed. Philadelphia, Saunders, 1967, with permission.*]

reaction, the most frequent early complaints are pain, fever, and dysphagia. Dyspnea is usually related to pleural-space involvement, with or without pneumothorax. Cervical tenderness is an early and constant feature of cervical esophageal perforation. Cervical crepitation may be minimal but is an almost constant finding.

The physical findings with thoracic esophageal perforation are usually limited to the thorax. Cervical crepitation may be a feature, but there is usually no cervical tenderness. Auscultation over the heart may elicit signs of mediastinal emphysema (Hamman's sign). With thoracic and subphrenic esophageal perforations, cardiorespiratory embarrassment attended by shock and cyanosis is more commonly seen early, but it may develop at a late stage.

Radiographic studies are of great assistance in diagnosis. Anteroposterior and lateral views of the cervical part of the spinal column often demonstrate pathognomonic signs of cervical perforation (Fig. 25-45). Anterior displacement of the trachea, widening of the retrovisceral space, air in tissue spaces, and occasionally widening of the superior mediastinum are seen. Widening of the superior mediastinum is a common sign in perforation of the cervical or upper thoracic part of the esophagus. Media-

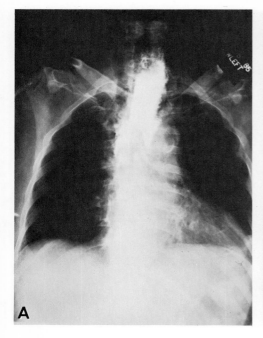

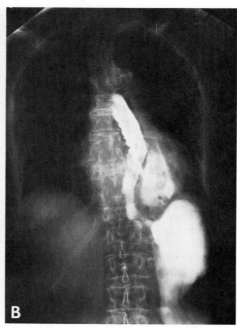

Fig. 25-46. Esophageal perforation. *A.* Extravasation of ingested contrast medium into neck and superior mediastinum, pathognomonic of cervical esophageal perforation. Note failure of distal part of esophagus to fill. [From: *Ellis FH Jr, Payne WS, in Artz CP, Hardy JD (eds): Complications in Surgery and Their Management, 2d ed. Philadelphia, Saunders, 1967, with permission.*] *B.* Postemetic perforation of distal esophagus. Note extravasation of contrast medium into left chest.

stinal emphysema and pleural effusion, with or without pneumothorax, may be present with thoracic or subphrenic esophageal injuries. Studies with opaque medium are indicated to localize the site or sites of perforation and to detect associated abnormalities (Fig. 25-46). The medium should be nonirritating and, preferably, absorbable. Endoscopic procedures are rarely indicated in diagnosis of esophageal perforations, except when a foreign body is present.

TREATMENT. Although there is wide agreement that most perforations of the esophagus are best treated by immediate surgical exploration, repair, and drainage, this is not universally accepted or always feasible. Parenteral antibiotic therapy plus parenteral fluid and electrolyte correction and cardiorespiratory support are appropriate for all patients with esophageal injury.

Confined thoracic esophageal leaks—those demonstrable as local extravasation of contrast media confined to the mediastinum, without pleural contamination and with little or no associated systemic evidence of sepsis—usually will resolve with antibiotics and parenteral alimentation and nothing by mouth.

Surgical Exploration and Management. Simple surgical exploration and drainage of the retrovisceral space—or, on rare occasions, of the pretracheal space—is the treatment of choice for cervical esophageal perforations (Fig. 25-47). Suppuration extending as low as the fourth thoracic vertebra can be evacuated effectively by this route. The usually encountered early cervical perforation may be small, and the inflammatory reaction may be slight; but major lacerations, when present, require suture closure, with drainage of considerable retrovisceral and mediastinal collections.

Instrumental and other perforations of the thoracic and subphrenic parts of the esophagus are often large and require surgical exploration, repair, and drainage. The upper two-thirds of the esophagus is best approached transpleurally by a right midthoracotomy and the lower third by a lower left thoracotomy. The rare subphrenic lacerations are best explored transabdominally. Gastric decompression, either by nasogastric tube or by gastrostomy, is indicated. On occasion, resection of the perforated region and associated esophageal lesion is required.

Late localized cervical and mediastinal abscesses are uncommon complications after adequate early surgical treatment of perforations. When present, they can be drained either by cervical mediastinotomy or transthoracically. As a rule, the late development of empyema after thoracic esophageal perforation can be prevented by early and adequate closed intercostal-tube drainage of the pleural space. When empyema occurs, it usually responds to appropriate open or closed drainage; if it does not, thoracotomy may be required for pulmonary decortication.

Esophagopleural or esophagocutaneous fistulas may occur as a complication of any esophageal perforation. If the esophagus is not obstructed distad and good drainage is provided, such fistulas invariably close with time, provided that there is no undrained local infection, foreign body, malignant change, or epithelialization of the tract. In management of an esophageal fistula, it is best to seek

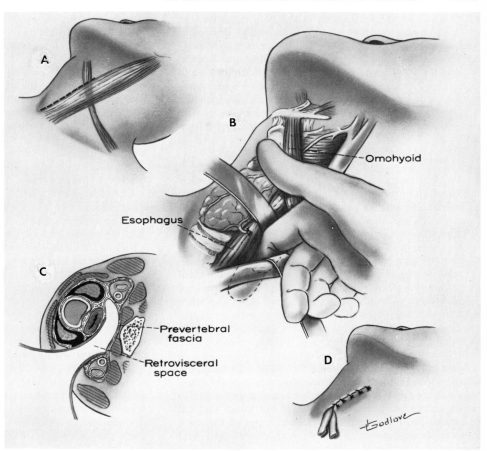

Fig. 25-47. Cervical mediastinotomy. *A.* Access to retrovisceral-prevertebral space is gained through low cervical incision. *B.* Retraction of sternomastoid muscle and cephalic vessels laterally and trachea and thyroid medially gives access to prevertebral (retrovisceral) space. *C.* Gross section of space to be opened in neck. *D.* Posterior collections as low as fourth thoracic vertebra are adequately drained via small rubber drains through this incision. (From: *Payne WS, Larson RH: Surg Clin North Am 49:999, 1969, with permission of Saunders.*)

out and treat for any factors that may contribute to chronicity. Generally it is wise during the healing stage of chronic fistulas to carry out repeated esophageal dilation over a previously swallowed thread, even if no obstruction is demonstrated. With healing, cicatricial narrowing may occur after any perforation; but it is uncommon.

Nutrition is extremely important in the healing of perforations and closure of fistulas. Parenteral alimentation today provides complete nutritional support, which can be maintained indefinitely; but it is usually not required for periods greater than 3 to 4 weeks. If a chronic cutaneous fistula is well drained, oral feedings usually can be resumed despite some nutritional loss through the tract.

RESULTS. The results of the surgical treatment of esophageal perforation depend not only on the cause, site, and severity of the reaction but also, to a large extent, on the lapse of time between perforation and treatment and on the type of treatment.

For perforation of the cervical esophagus, regardless of cause, the results of treatment have been excellent with early cervical exploration and drainage. Even in major cervical injury with marked contamination and delayed treatment, the results of surgical management have been generally satisfactory. However, the incidence of complications, secondary procedures, prolonged hospitalization, and late sequelae has been greater in the group treated initially by medical means only. Mortality from cervical perforation is confined almost exclusively to that subgroup, which further emphasizes the wisdom of early surgical treatment of cervical esophageal perforation.

The results of treatment for perforations of the thoracic and subphrenic esophagus have been less satisfactory. Delay of diagnosis and treatment beyond 18 h appears to be a major factor contributing to morbidity and mortality. Recent reports of series of thoracic esophageal perforations mention mortality in excess of 60 percent with the usual surgical methods in late perforation and between 10 and 30 percent with early treatment.

Differing Opinions

Not all surgeons agree with the operative management outlined. There are instances of cervical and of thoracic esophageal perforation (usually instrumental) in which—

given a late and benign course or the patient's refusal of other methods—success may be obtained by nonoperative management (parenteral alimentation and antibiotics and intercostal tube drainage, etc.). Neuhof and Jemerin in 1943 reported 60 percent survival after surgical drainage alone, but 16 percent after conservative nonsurgical management. A decade later, Seybold and coworkers and Weisel and Raine reported greatly reduced mortality with early suture closure and drainage of esophageal perforation.

Other Methods

The high mortality associated with late diagnosis and treatment of intrathoracic esophageal perforations has led to the development of several other methods of management, which are applicable under various circumstances.

There has been great enthusiasm for reinforcing the suture repair of esophageal tears. Thal has employed gastric fundus as a reinforcing buttress patch; others, pedicles of diaphragm (Rao and associates), pericardium (Millard), intercostal muscle (Dooling and Zick), parietal pleura (Grillo and Wilkins), or latissimus dorsi and other muscle pedicles (Pairolero). Variations on the esophageal exclusion described by Johnson and associates include the partial exclusion and diversion techniques of Urschel and coworkers and of Menguy.

Most current reviews continue to show high mortality when esophageal resective procedures and primary anastomoses are performed in the presence of a recent perforation. It may be preferable to carry out initial surgical resection—with esophageal diversion or one of the complete or partial diversions described above—and deal with reconstruction at a later date.

CONCLUSION. It is impossible, of course, to prescribe a technique applicable to all thoracic esophageal perforations or even those of a given variety. It is essential, however, to have a clear understanding of the clinical problems and the multiple techniques available for rational management of individual patients.

CORROSIVE ESOPHAGITIS (See also Chapter 39)

The ingestion of strong acid or alkali causes a severe inflammatory reaction of the affected mucosa, known as *corrosive esophagitis*. Lye, a strong cleaning agent containing sodium hydroxide and sodium carbonate, is most commonly responsible for such injuries, although various other fluids, including mineral acids, strong bases, phenol, and organic solvents, can produce similar effects. The nature and concentration of the agent ingested determine the degree and extent of the injury, which may involve limited areas of the mouth or esophagus, the entire esophagus, or even the stomach.

PATHOLOGY. The pathologic changes after ingestion of lye are classified in much the same way as thermal burns of the skin. They have been shown experimentally to consist of edema and congestion of the submucosal layer, with associated inflammation and thrombosis of its vessels. Sloughing of the superficial layers occurs, with varying degrees of liquefaction necrosis of the muscularis, followed by fibrosis and delayed reepithelialization. In severe cases the entire mucous membrane of the upper portion of the alimentary tract may slough, and subsequent development of an esophageal stricture is inevitable. Kirsh and Ritter have noted that lye of extremely high concentration in liquid form has become widely available for home use in the past decade. This has markedly altered the extent and severity of injuries following ingestion. Indeed, full-thickness esophageal and gastric necrosis is being seen with increasing frequency. Some of the ingested nonviscous strong acids may miraculously spare the esophagus on their way to causing severe gastric antral burns.

CLINICAL MANIFESTATIONS. During the acute phase of the reaction, burns of the lips, tongue, mouth, and pharynx are apparent. Hoarseness, stridor, and aphonia suggest laryngeal edema or actual epiglottic or laryngeal destruction. Pain in the involved region is common, and there may be associated vomiting. Painful dysphagia is prominent during the acute phase, which lasts from several days to several weeks. As the chronic phase develops, dysphagia due to stricture formation may become the predominant symptom. Gastric injury may be manifested by bleeding or antral obstruction. Clinical signs of perforation of esophagus or stomach, or both, may be apparent and should be sought.

TREATMENT. In view of the instantaneous nature of corrosive injury, it is not reasonable to attempt dilution or neutralization. The immediate effort should be directed to detection and management of attendant airway obstruction and blood-volume depletion. Intravenous fluids and antibiotics are administered promptly, and oral intake is prohibited. The severity of oral burns may be marked, and not necessarily proportional to the severity of esophageal or gastric injury. Early endoscopy and water-soluble contrast radiography of the esophagus and stomach should be performed. The esophagoscope is passed to the first burned area, not beyond. Kirsh and Ritter emphasized the importance of defining, early, the type of corrosive ingested; and they have provided criteria for diagnosing the full-thickness injuries that are more commonly incurred with the liquid corrosives. For injuries of that nature, successful management requires early esophagectomy or total esophagogastrectomy.

Under usual circumstances, however, injury is confined to the mucosa. As soon as patients can swallow their saliva, they are instructed to swallow a thread as a guide for subsequent endoscopy and dilation therapy. Steroids are of questionable efficacy in preventing stricture formation, and they may mask more serious mediastinal, peritoneal, or pulmonary complications. Bouginage, performed early, increases the risk of perforation; so it is not started until acute inflammation has largely subsided, as determined by repeated endoscopy.

Stricture formation is rare if the treatment outlined is initiated promptly. However, should esophagoscopy reveal evidence of stricture formation, dilation of the strictured zone by bouginage over the swallowed thread may be begun within a few weeks of the injury. Some patients may need dilation periodically for a long while, even a year or more. When patients are seen in the chronic phase of the disease and a string has not been ingested previously, it may be necessary to perform gastrostomy for feeding purposes and also for retrograde dilation of the esophageal stricture.

In a small percentage of cases it may become apparent that repeated dilation cannot maintain a satisfactory esophageal lumen. Then extensive reconstructive operative procedures are required to establish a satisfactory, functioning esophageal substitute. Many procedures have been devised, including use of skin-lined tubes and segments of intestine or stomach, as reported by Yudin; the Russian surgeons have had extensive experience with these. Currently preferred is total bypass of the strictured esophagus by a segment of right or left colon interposed substernally between the pharynx and stomach. For lesser degrees of stricture, the lesion may be approached transthoracically and either resected or bypassed with a segment of jejunum or colon. Reconstruction by free transfer of autogenous jejunum with microvascular anastomosis is becoming an important addition to the management of some of these more localized strictures.

MISCELLANEOUS ESOPHAGEAL LESIONS

Plummer–Vinson (Paterson–Kelly) Syndrome

In 1919, Paterson and Kelly independently described a clinical state with which the names of Plummer and Vinson later became associated in the United States. The typical patient is a middle-aged, edentulous woman with atrophic oral mucosa, spoon-shaped fingers and brittle nails, and a long-standing history of anemia and dysphagia. Because of the common finding of iron-deficiency anemia, the term *sideropenic dysphagia* has been used by some to describe the condition, which is more common in the Scandinavian countries than in the United States.

The dysphagia is explained by endoscopic and radiographic demonstration of a fibrous web partially obstructing the esophageal lumen in an eccentric fashion a few millimeters below the cricopharyngeus muscle. A dietary deficiency has been established as the cause, and the condition responds well to iron therapy and forceful dilation of the web.

In approximately 10 percent of cases, a malignant lesion of the oral cavity, hypopharynx, or esophagus develops. The syndrome covers a broad range of clinical entities, and not all patients exhibit hypochromic anemia, nor do they necessarily show evidence of malnutrition. Conversely, not all patients with the other clinical features of the Plummer–Vinson syndrome are found to have esophageal webs. And furthermore, some upper-esophageal webs in younger patients who lack the clinical stigmata of the classic syndrome may have a congenital basis.

Mallory–Weiss Syndrome

In 1929, Mallory and Weiss reported 15 cases of gastrointestinal bleeding after repeated emesis. Linear tears in the mucosa of the esophagogastric junction were demonstrated at postmortem examination in some of these patients. In subsequent years the condition has been noted

more commonly, and it should be considered in differential diagnosis of unexplained hematemesis.

The mechanism of the development of the lacerations is similar to that involved in the development of spontaneous rupture of the esophagus—namely, an explosive vomiting effort against a closed cardia or esophagus. A history of prolonged retching or vomiting, often but not always associated with alcoholism, is characteristic. Early diagnosis can be facilitated by radiographic studies to exclude the possibility of other lesions and by endoscopy to identify the site of bleeding.

Bleeding may cease with conservative management, but surgical exploration may be required if it persists. The upper end of the stomach should be exposed through a long gastrotomy, and after manual evacuation of clots and insertion of proper retractors for exposure, the lacerated areas should be repaired with sutures. Prompt arrest of bleeding by this technique can be expected.

Acquired Fistula

Occasionally, a fistulous communication requiring treatment may develop between the esophagus and the lower part of the respiratory tract. Other potential sites of fistulous communication include the aorta, the vena cava, and the heart. The commonest cause of acquired fistula is malignancy, and in the course of incurable carcinoma of the esophagus, the lungs, or the neck structures, such fistula usually is a preterminal event.

Typically, a fistula between the esophagus and the tracheobronchial tree produces cough on eating or drinking, although it may present more subtly, with pulmonary symptoms alone. The basic features of surgical treatment include division of the fistulous tract and suture closure of the defect in the esophagus and respiratory tree, with interposition of viable tissue to prevent recurrence. Additionally, distal esophageal obstruction should be corrected.

The management of congenital tracheoesophageal fistula with and without atresia is discussed in the chapter dealing with pediatric surgery.

Bibliography

General Texts

Brewer LA III: History of surgery of the esophagus. *Am J Surg* 139:730, 1980.

Payne WS, Olsen AM: *The Esophagus.* Philadelphia, Lea & Febiger, 1974.

Postlethwait RW: *Surgery of the Esophagus.* New York, Appleton-Century-Crofts, 1979.

Smith RA, Smith RE: *Surgery of the Oesophagus.* London, Butterworth, 1972.

Anatomy

Carey JM, Hollinshead WH: An anatomic study of the esophageal hiatus. *Surg Gynecol Obstet* 100:196, 1955.

Hayward J: Phreno-oesophageal ligament in hiatal hernia repair. *Thorax* 16:41, 1961.

Higgs B, Shorter RG, Ellis FH Jr: A study of the anatomy of the human esophagus with special reference to the gastroesophageal sphincter. *J Surg Res* 5:503, 1965.

Payne WS: The role of esophageal blood supply, in *Cancer of the Esophagus in 1984: 135 Questions.* Compiled by Giuli R, First Polydisciplinary International Congress of the International Organization for Statistical Studies on Diseases of the Esophagus. Paris, edited and published by Maloine SA, 1984, pp 222–225.

Pera C, Suñer M, Capdevila J: Anatomical demonstration of the lower oesophageal sphincter: A biometrical analysis of 300 specimens (abstract). *Bull Soc Int Chir* 34:285, 1975.

Thomas DM, Langford RM, et al: The anatomical basis for gastric mobilization in total oesophagectomy. *Br J Surg* 66:230, 1979.

Physiology and Physiologic Tests

Bernstein LM, Baker LA: A clinical test for esophagitis. *Gastroenterology* 34:760, 1958.

Bombeck CT, Dillard DH, Nyhus LM: Muscular anatomy of the gastroesophageal junction and role of phrenoesophageal ligament: Autopsy study of sphincter mechanism. *Ann Surg* 164:643, 1966.

Castell DO, Harris LD: Hormonal control of gastroesophageal-sphincter strength. *N Engl J Med* 282:886, 1970.

Castell DO, Levine SM: Lower esophageal sphincter response to gastric alkalinization: A new mechanism for treatment of heartburn with antacids. *Ann Intern Med* 74:223, 1971.

Code CF, Creamer B, et al: *An Atlas of Esophageal Motility in Health and Disease.* Springfield, IL, Charles C Thomas, 1958.

Cohen S, Lipshutz W: Hormonal regulation of human lower esophageal sphincter competence: Interaction of gastrin and secretin. *J Clin Invest* 50:449, 1971.

Earlam R: *Clinical Tests for Oesophageal Function.* New York, Grune & Stratton, 1975.

Henderson RD: *Motor Disorders of the Esophagus.* Baltimore, Williams & Wilkins, 1976.

Ingelfinger FJ: Esophageal motility. *Physiol Rev* 38:533, 1958.

Jahadi MR, Chandler JP: Detecting gastroesophageal reflux by pH recording and acid reflux test. *Am J Surg* 38:281, 1972.

Johnson LF, DeMeester TR: Twenty-four-hour pH monitoring of the distal esophagus: A quantitative measure of gastroesophageal reflux. *Am J Gastroenterol* 62:325, 1974.

O'Sullivan GC, DeMeester TR, et al: Interaction of lower esophageal sphincter pressure and length of sphincter in the abdomen as determinants of gastroesophageal competence. *Am J Surg* 143:40, 1982.

Sarna SK, Daniel EE, Waterfall WE: Myogenic and neural control systems for esophageal motility. *Gastroenterology* 73:1345, 1977.

Skinner DB, Belsey RHR, et al (eds): *Gastroesophageal Reflux and Hiatal Hernia.* Boston, Little, Brown, 1972.

Skinner DB, Booth DJ: Assessment of distal esophageal function in patients with hiatal hernia and/or gastroesophageal reflux. *Ann Surg* 172:627, 1970.

Snape WJ Jr, Cohen S: Hormonal control of esophageal function. *Arch Intern Med* 136:538, 1976.

Functional Disturbances of the Esophagus

Motility Disturbances

Arvanitakis C: Achalasia of the esophagus: A reappraisal of esophagomyotomy vs forceful pneumatic dilation. *Am J Dig Dis* 20:841, 1975.

Barker JR, Franklin RH: Heller's operation for achalasia of the cardia: A study of the early and late results. *Br J Surg* 58:466, 1971.

Cohen S, Lipshutz W: Lower esophageal sphincter dysfunction in achalasia. *Gastroenterology* 61:814, 1971.

Creamer B, Donoghue FE, Code CF: Pattern of esophageal motility in diffuse spasm. *Gastroenterology* 34:787, 1958.

Csendes A, Velasco N, et al: A prospective randomized study comparing forceful dilatation and esophagomyotomy in patients with achalasia of the esophagus. *Gastroenterology* 80:789, 1981.

Ellis FH Jr: Surgical management of esophageal motility disturbances. *Am J Surg* 139:752, 1980.

Flye MW, Sealy WC: Diffuse spasm of the esophagus. *Ann Thorac Surg* 19:677, 1975.

Heller E: Extramuköse Cardioplastik beim chronischen Cardiospasmus mit Dilatation des Oesophagus. *Mitt Grengeb Med Chir* 27:141, 1913.

Henderson RD, Ho CS, Davidson JW: Primary disordered motor activity of the esophagus (diffuse spasm): Diagnosis and treatment. *Ann Thorac Surg* 18:327, 1974.

Leonardi HK, Crozier RE, Ellis FH Jr: Reoperation for complications of the Nissen fundoplication. *J Thorac Cardiovasc Surg* 81:50, 1981.

Mansour KA, Symbas PN, et al: A combined surgical approach in the management of achalasia of the esophagus. *Am Surg* 42:192, 1976.

Menguy R: Management of achalasia by transabdominal cardiomyotomy and fundoplication. *Surg Gynecol Obstet* 133:482, 1971.

Nelems JMB, Cooper JD, Pearson FG: Treatment of achalasia: Esophagomyotomy with antireflux procedure. *Can J Surg* 23:588, 1980.

Okike N, Payne WS, et al: Esophagomyotomy versus forceful dilation for achalasia of the esophagus: Results in 899 patients. *Ann Thorac Surg* 28:119, 1979.

Patrick DL, Payne WS, et al: Reoperation for achalasia of the esophagus. *Arch Surg* 103:122, 1971.

Peyton MD, Greenfield LJ, Elkins RC: Combined myotomy and hiatal herniorrhaphy: A new approach to achalasia. *Am J Surg* 128:786, 1974.

Vantrappen G, Hellemans J: Treatment of achalasia and related motor disorders. *Gastroenterology* 79:144, 1980.

Disturbances of Gastroesophageal Competence

Barrett NR: Chronic peptic ulcer of the oesophagus and "oesophagitis." *Br J Surg* 38:175, 1950.

Behar J, Biancani P, Sheahan DG: Evaluation of esophageal tests in the diagnosis of reflux esophagitis. *Gastroenterology* 71:9, 1976.

Borrie J, Goldwater L: Columnar cell-lined esophagus: Assessment of etiology and treatment; A 22-year experience. *J Thorac Cardiovasc Surg* 71:825, 1976.

Brand DL, Ylvisaker JT, et al: Regression of columnar esophageal (Barrett's) epithelium after anti-reflux surgery. *N Engl J Med* 302:844, 1980.

Burgess JN, Payne WS, et al: Barrett esophagus: The columnar-epithelial-lined lower esophagus. *Mayo Clin Proc* 46:728, 1971.

Cameron AJ, Ott BJ, Payne WS: The incidence of adenocarcinoma in columnar-lined (Barrett's) esophagus. *N Engl J Med* 313:857, 1985.

Henderson RD, Pearson FG: Surgical management of esophageal scleroderma. *J Thorac Cardiovasc Surg* 66:686, 1973.

Lam CR, Taber RE, Arciniegas E: The nature and surgical treatment of lower esophageal ring (Schatzki's ring). *J Thorac Cardiovasc Surg* 63:34, 1972.

Orringer MB: Respiratory symptoms and esophageal reflux. *Chest* 76:618, 1979. (Editorial.)

Orringer MB, Dabich L, et al: Gastroesophageal reflux in esophageal schleroderma: Diagnosis and implications. *Ann Thorac Surg* 22:120, 1976.

Ottinger LW, Wilkins EW Jr: Late results in patients with Schatzki rings undergoing destruction of the ring and hiatus herniorrhaphy. *Am J Surg* 139:591, 1980.

Payne WS, McAfee MK, et al: Adenocarcinoma of the columnar epithelial-lined lower esophagus of Barrett, in Delarue NC, Wilkins EW, Wong J (eds): *International Trends in General Thoracic Surgery,* vol V, *Esophageal Carcinoma.* St. Louis, Mosby. (In press.)

Schatzki R, Gary JE: Dysphagia due to a diaphragm-like localized narrowing in the lower esophagus ("lower esophageal ring"). *Am J Roentgen* 70:911, 1953.

Diaphragmatic Hernias

Esophageal Hiatal Hernia

Behar J, Sheahan DG, et al: Medical and surgical management of reflux esophagitis: A 38-month report on a prospective clinical trial. *N Engl J Med* 293:263, 1975.

Belsey R: Reconstruction of the esophagus with left colon. *J Thorac Cardiovasc Surg* 49:33, 1965.

Bushkin FL, Neustein CL, et al: Nissen fundoplication for reflux peptic esophagitis. *Ann Surg* 185:672, 1977.

DeMeester TR, Johnson LF, Kent AH: Evaluation of current operations for the prevention of gastroesophageal reflux. *Ann Surg* 180:511, 1974.

Demos NJ: A simplified, improved technique for the Collis gastroplasty for dilatable esophageal strictures. *Surg Gynecol Obstet* 142:591, 1976.

Demos NJ: Correction of paraesophageal hiatal hernia. *NY State J Med* 77:1281, 1977.

Ellis FH Jr: Controversies regarding the management of hiatus hernia. *Am J Surg* 139:782, 1980.

Fonkalsrud EW, Ament ME, et al: Gastroesophageal fundoplication for the management of reflux in infants and children. *J Thorac Cardiovasc Surg* 76:655, 1978.

Gavriliu D: État actuel du procédé de reconstruction de l'oesophage par tube gastrique (138 malades opérés). *Ann Chir* 19:219, 1965.

Glasgow JC, Cannon JP, Elkins RC: Colon interposition for benign esophageal disease. *Am J Surg* 137:175, 1979.

Hawe A, Payne WS, et al: Adenocarcinoma in the columnar epithelial lined lower (Barrett) oesophagus. *Thorax* 28:511, 1973.

Hiebert CA, O'Mara CS: The Belsey operation for hiatal hernia: A twenty year experience. *Am J Surg* 137:532, 1979.

Hill LD: An effective operation for hiatal hernia: An eight year appraisal. *Ann Surg* 166:681, 1967.

Hill LD: Incarcerated paraesophageal hernia: A surgical emergency. *Am J Surg* 126:286, 1973.

Jolley SG, Herbst JJ, et al: Surgery in children with gastroesophageal reflux and respiratory symptoms. *J Pediatr* 96:194, 1980.

Leonardi HK, Crozier RE, Ellis FH Jr: Reoperation for complications of the Nissen fundoplication. *J Thorac Cardiovasc Surg* 81:50, 1981.

Mansour KA, Burton HG, et al: Complications of intrathoracic Nissen fundoplication. *Ann Thorac Surg* 32:173, 1981.

Nissen R: Eine Einfache Operation zur Beeinflussung der Refluxoesophagitis. *Schweiz Med Wochenschr* 86:590, 1956.

Orringer MB, Orringer JS, et al: Combined Collis gastroplasty—fundoplication operations for scleroderma reflux esophagitis. *Surgery* 90:624, 1981.

Orringer MB, Skinner DB, Belsey RHR: Long-term results of the Mark IV operation for hiatal hernia and analyses of recurrences and their treatment. *J Thorac Cardiovasc Surg* 63:25, 1972.

Orringer MB, Sloan H: Complications and failings of the combined Collis-Belsey operation. *J Thorac Cardiovasc Surg* 74:726, 1977.

Payne WS: Surgical treatment of paraesophageal hiatal hernia, in Nyhus LM, Baker RJ (eds): *Mastery of Surgery.* Boston, Little, Brown, 1984.

Payne WS: Prevention and treatment of biliary-pancreatic reflux esophagitis. *Surg Clin North Am* 63:851, August 1983.

Payne WS: Surgical management of reflux-induced oesophageal stenoses: Results in 101 patients. *Br J Surg* 71:971, December 1984.

Payne WS: Paraesophageal hiatal hernia, in Nyhus LM, Baker RJ (eds): *Mastery of Surgery.* Boston, Little, Brown, 1984, pp 329–337.

Payne WS: Reflux oesophagitis with stricture: Alternative methods of management, in Dudley H, Carter DC, Jackson JW, Cooper DKC (eds): *Operative Surgery.* London, Butterworth, 1986, pp 314–325.

Payne WS, Andersen HA, Ellis FH Jr: Reappraisal of esophagogastrectomy and antral excision in the treatment of short esophagus. *Surgery* 55:344, 1964.

Pearson FG, Langer B, Henderson RD: Gastroplasty and Belsey hiatus hernia repair: An operation for the management of peptic stricture with acquired short esophagus. *J Thorac Cardiovasc Surg* 61:50, 1971.

Piehler JM, Payne WS, et al: The uncut Collis-Nissen procedure for esophageal hiatal hernia and its complications. *Probl Gen Surg* 1:1, 1984.

Pridie RB: Incidence and coincidence of hiatus hernia. *Gut* 7:188, 1966.

Richardson JD, Larson GM, Polk HC Jr: Intrathoracic fundoplication for shortened esophagus: Treacherous solution to a challenging problem. *Am J Surg* 143:29, 1982.

Skinner DB: Esophageal reconstruction. *Am J Surg* 139:810, 1980.

Urschel HC Jr, Razzuk MA: "Collis-Belsey" fundoplication for uncomplicated hiatal hernia and gastroesophageal reflux. *Ann Thorac Surg* 27:564, 1979.

Miscellaneous Diaphragmatic Conditions

Beck WC, Motsay DS: Eventration of diaphragm. *Arch Surg* 65:557, 1952.

Bekassy SM, Dave KS, et al: "Spontaneous" and traumatic rupture of the diaphragm: Long-term results. *Ann Surg* 177:320, 1973.

Broman I: Über die Entwickelung und Bedeutung der Mesenterien und der Korperhohlen bei den Wirbeltieren. *Ergeb Anat Entwicklngsgesch* 15:332, 1905.

Carter R, Brewer LA III: Strangulating diaphragmatic hernia. *Ann Thorac Surg* 12:281, 1971.

Chin EF, Duchesne ER: The parasternal defect. *Thorax* 10:214, 1955.

Comer TP, Clagett OT: Surgical treatment of hernia of the foramen of Morgagni. *J Thorac Cardiovasc Surg* 52:461, 1966.

Drews JA, et al: Acute diaphragmatic injuries. *Ann Thorac Surg* 16:67, 1973.

Hill LD: Injuries of the diaphragm following blunt trauma. *Surg Clin North Am* 52:611, 1972.

Pairolero PC, Payne WS: Diaphragm, in Goldsmith HS: *Practice of Surgery*. Hagerstown, Harper & Row, 1980.

Shoemaker R, Palmer G, et al: Aggressive treatment of acquired phrenic nerve paralysis in infants and small children. *Ann Thorac Surg* 32:251, 1981.

Wilson RF: Discussion. *Ann Thorac Surg* 16:77, 1973.

Oropharyngeal Dysphagia

Black RJ: Cricopharyngeal myotomy. *J Otolaryng* 10:145, 1981.

Duranceau A, Forand MD, Fauteux JP: Surgery in oculopharyngeal muscular dystrophy. *Am J Surg* 139:33, 1980.

Ellis FH Jr, Crozier RE: Cervical esophageal dysphagia: Indications for and results of cricopharyngeal myotomy. *Ann Surg* 194:279, 1981.

Orringer MB: Extended cervical esophagomyotomy for cricopharyngeal dysfunction. *J Thorac Cardiovasc Surg* 80:669, 1980.

Palmer ED: Disorders of the cricopharyngeus muscle: A review. *Gastroenterology* 71:510, 1976.

Diverticula

Allen TH, Clagett OT: Changing concepts in the surgical treatment of pulsion diverticula of the lower esophagus. *J Thorac Cardiovasc Surg* 50:455, 1965.

Debas HT, Payne WS, et al: Physiopathology of lower esophageal diverticulum and its implications for treatment. *Surg Gynecol Obstet* 151:593, 1980.

Habein HC Jr, Moersch HJ, Kirklin JW: Diverticula of the lower part of the esophagus: A clinical study of 149 nonsurgical cases. *Arch Intern Med* 97:768, 1956.

Huang B, Payne WS, Cameron AJ: Surgical management for recurrent pharyngoesophageal (Zenker's) diverticulum. *Ann Thorac Surg* 37:189, March 1984.

Huang BS, Unni KK, Payne WS: Long-term survival following diverticulectomy for cancer in pharyngoesophageal (Zenker's) diverticulum. *Ann Thorac Surg* 38(3):207, September 1984.

Payne WS, Pairolero PC, Piehler JM: The management of Zenker's diverticulum: Diverticulectomy, in Kittle CF (ed): *Current Controversies in Thoracic Surgery*. Philadelphia, Saunders, 1986, pp 3–9.

Payne WS, Reynolds RR: Surgical treatment of pharyngoesophageal diverticulum (Zenker's diverticulum). *Surg Rounds* 5(6):18, June 1982.

Payne WS, Trastek VF: The role of stapling devices in the treatment of pharyngoesophageal (Zenker's) diverticulum, in Ravitch MM, Steichen FM (eds): *Principles and Practices of Surgical Stapling*. Chicago, Year Book Medical Publishers, 1987, pp 79–98.

Welsh GF, Payne WS: The present status of one-stage pharyngoesophageal diverticulectomy. *Surg Clin North Am* 53:953, 1973.

Benign Cysts and Tumors

Bernatz PE, Smith JL, et al: Benign, pedunculated intraluminal tumors of the esophagus. *J Thorac Surg* 35:503, 1958.

Schmidt HW, Clagett OT, Harrison EG Jr: Benign tumors and cysts of the esophagus. *J Thorac Cardiovasc Surg* 41:717, 1961.

Malignant Tumors

Akiyama H, Hiyama M, Miyazono H: Total esophageal reconstruction after extraction of the esophagus. *Ann Surg* 182:547, 1975.

Akiyama H, Tsurumaru M, et al: Principles of surgical treatment for carcinoma of the esophagus: Analysis of lymph node involvement. *Ann Surg* 194(4):438, 1981.

Bakamjian VY: Total reconstruction of pharynx with medially based deltopectoral skin flap. *NY State J Med* 68:2771, 1968.

Beahrs OH, Myers MA (eds): *Manual for Staging of Cancer*. American Joint Committee on Cancer Staging. Lippincott Medical, 1983.

Belsey RHR: Palliative management of esophageal carcinoma. *Am J Surg* 139:789, 1980.

Cameron AJ, Ott BJ, Payne WS: The incidence of adenocarcinoma in columnar-lined (Barrett's) esophagus. *N Engl J Med* 313:857, 1985.

Chang TS, Hwang OL, Wang-Wei: Reconstruction of esophageal defects with microsurgically revascularized jejunal segments: A report of 13 cases. *J Microsurg* 2:83, 1980.

Cooper JD, Jamieson WRE, et al: The palliative value of surgical resection for carcinoma of the esophagus. *Can J Surg* 24:145, 1981.

DeSanto LW, Carpenter RJ: Reconstruction of the pharynx and upper esophagus after resection for cancer. *Head Neck Surg* 2:369, 1980.

DiCostanzo DP, Urmacher C: Primary malignant melanoma of the esophagus. *Am J Surg Pathol* 11(1):46, 1987.

Drucker MH, Mansour KA, et al: Esophageal carcinoma: An aggressive approach. *Ann Thorac Surg* 28:133, 1979.

Earlam R, Cunha-Melo JR: Oesophageal squamous cell carcinoma: I. A critical review of surgery. *Br J Surg* 67:381, 1980.

Ellis FH Jr: Esophagogastrectomy for carcinoma: Technical considerations based on anatomic location of lesion. *Surg Clin North Am* 60:265, April 1980.

Ellis FH Jr, Gibb P, Watkins E Jr: Esophagogastrectomy: A safe, widely applicable, and expeditious form of palliation for patients with carcinoma of the esophagus and cardia. *Ann Surg* 198(4):531, 1983.

Ellis FH Jr, Salzman FA: Carcinoma of the esophagus: Surgery versus radiotherapy. *Postgrad Med* 61:167, 1977.

Gatzinsky P, Berglin E, et al: Resectional operations and long-term results in carcinoma of the esophagus. *J Thorac Cardiovasc Surg* 89:71, 1985.

Gluckman JL, McDonough J, et al: The free jejunal graft in head and neck reconstruction. *Laryngoscope* 91:1887, 1981.

Goldberg SJ, King KH: Endoscopic Nd:YAG laser coagulation as palliative therapy for obstructing esophageal carcinoma. *Am J Gastroenterol* 81(8):629, 1986.

Goldfaden D, Orringer MB, et al: Adenocarcinoma of the distal esophagus and gastric cardia: Comparison of results of transhiatal esophagectomy and thoracoabdominal esophagogastrectomy. *J Thorac Cardiovasc Surg* 91:242, 1986.

Guojun H, Lingfang S, et al: Diagnosis and surgical treatment of early esophageal carcinoma. *Chin Med J* 94:229, April 1981.

Harrison DFN: Surgical repair in hypopharyngeal and cervical esophageal cancer: Analysis of 162 patients. *Ann Otol Rhinol Laryng* 90:372, 1981.

Harrison DFN, Thompson AE, Buchanan G: Radical resection for cancer of the hypopharynx and cervical oesophagus with repair by stomach transposition. *Br J Surg* 68:781, 1981.

Hawe A, Payne WS, et al: Adenocarcinoma in the columnar epithelial lined lower (Barrett) oesophagus. *Thorax* 28:511, 1973.

Keagy BA, Murray GF, et al: Esophagogastrectomy as palliative treatment for esophageal carcinoma: Results obtained in the setting of a thoracic surgery residency program. *Ann Thorac Surg* 38(6):611, 1984.

King RM, Pairolero PC, et al: Ivor Lewis esophagogastrectomy for carcinoma of the esophagus: Early and late functional results. *Ann Thorac Surg.* (In press.)

Kiviranta UK: Corrosion carcinoma of the esophagus: 381 cases of corrosion and nine cases of corrosion carcinoma. *Acta Otolaryng (Stockh)* 42:89, 1952.

Lea JW, Prager RL, Bender HW Jr: The questionable role of computed tomography in preoperative staging of esophageal cancer. *Ann Thorac Surg* 38(5):479, 1984.

Lewis I: The surgical treatment of carcinoma of the oesophagus: With special reference to a new operation for growths of the middle third. *Br J Surg* 34:18, 1946.

Marcial–Rojas RA, Vallecioool LA: Primary adenoidcystic carcinoma of the esophagus: Report of one case and review of the literature. *Arch Otolaryng* 70:197, 1959.

Marks RD Jr, Scruggs HJ, Wallace KM: Preoperative radiation therapy for carcinoma of the esophagus. *Cancer* 38:84, 1976.

Meyers WC, Seigler HF, et al: Postoperative function of "free" jejunal transplants for replacement of the cervical esophagus. *Ann Surg* 192:439, 1980.

Miller JI, McIntyre B, Hatcher CR: Combined treatment approach in surgical management of carcinoma of the esophagus: A preliminary report. *Ann Thorac Surg* 40(3):289, 1985.

Molina JE, Lawton BR, et al: Esophagogastrectomy for adenocarcinoma of the cardia: Ten years' experience and current approach. *Ann Surg* 195:146, 1982.

Nakamura T, Nagamachi Y: Long loop Roux–Y esophagojejunostomy following total gastrectomy. *Gastroenterol Jpn* 13:415, 1978.

Ong GB: Resection and reconstruction of the oesophagus in oesophageal cancer. *J Jpn Assoc Thorac Surg* 22:769, 1974.

Orringer MB: Substernal gastric bypass of the excluded esophagus—results of an ill-advised operation. *Surgery* 96:(3):467, 1984.

Orringer MB: Transhiatal esophagectomy without thoracotomy for carcinoma of the thoracic esophagus. *Ann Surg* 200(3): 282, 1984.

Payne WS, Bernatz PE: One-stage resection and reconstruction for carcinoma of the esophagogastric junction, in Varco RL, Delaney JP (eds): *Controversy in Surgery.* Philadelphia, Saunders, 1976.

Payne WS, Fisher J: Esophageal reconstruction: Free jejunal transfer or circulatory augmentation of pedicled intestinal interpositions using microvascular surgery. *International Trends in General Thoracic Surgery,* vol 5, 1986.

Payne WS, Trastek VF, et al: Current techniques for the surgical management of malignant lesions of the thoracic esophagus and cardia. *Mayo Clin Proc* 61:564–572, 1986.

Shields TW, Rosen ST, et al: Multimodality approach to treatment of carcinoma of the esophagus. *Arch Surg* 119:558, 1984.

Skinner DB: En bloc resection for neoplasms of the esophagus and cardia. *J Thorac Cardiovasc Surg* 85:59, 1983.

Skinner DB, DeMeester TR: Permanent extracorporeal esophagogastric tube for esophageal replacement. *Ann Thorac Surg* 22:107, 1976.

Steiger Z, Franklin R, et al: Eradication and palliation of squamous cell carcinoma of the esophagus with chemotherapy, radiotherapy, and surgical therapy. *J Thorac Cardiovasc Surg* 82:713, 1981.

Talbert JL, Cantrell JR: Clinical and pathologic characteristics of carcinosarcoma of the esophagus. *J Thorac Cardiovasc Surg* 45:1, 1963.

West PN, Marbarger JP, et al: Esophagogastrostomy with the EEA stapler. *Ann Surg* 193:76, 1981.

Wilkins EW Jr: Long-segment colon substitution for the esophagus. *Ann Surg* 192:722, 1980.

Wookey H: Cited by Bakamjian VY, Total reconstruction of pharynx with medially based deltopectoral skin flap. *NY State J Med* 68:2771, 1968.

Wychulis AR, Gunnlaugsson GH, Clagett OT: Carcinoma occurring in pharyngoesophageal diverticulum: Report of three cases. *Surgery* 66:979, 1969.

Esophageal Perforation

Bradley SL, Pairolero PC, et al: Spontaneous rupture of the esophagus. *Arch Surg* 116:755, 1981.

Cameron JL, Kieffer RF, et al: Selective nonoperative management of contained intrathoracic esophageal disruptions. *Ann Thorac Surg* 27:404, 1979.

Finley RJ, Pearson FG, et al: The management of nonmalignant intrathoracic esophageal perforations. *Ann Thorac Surg* 30:575, 1980.

Grillo HC, Wilkins EW Jr: Esophageal repair following late diagnosis of intrathoracic perforation. *Ann Thorac Surg* 20:387, 1975.

Michel L, Grillo HC, Malt RA: Operative and nonoperative management of esophageal perforations. *Ann Surg* 194:57, 1981.

Michel L, Grillo HC, Malt RA: Esophageal perforation. *Ann Thorac Surg* 33:203, 1982.

Pairolero PC, Payne WS: Esophageal perforation, in English GM (ed): *Otolaryngology.* Hagerstown, Harper & Row, 1981.

Payne WS, Larson RH: Acute mediastinitis. *Surg Clin North Am* 49:999, 1969.

Sarr MG, Pemberton JH, Payne WS: Management of instrumental perforations of the esophagus. *J Thorac Cardiovasc Surg* 84:211, August 1982.

Schwartz ML, McQuarrie DG: Surgical management of esophageal perforation. *Surg Gynecol Obstet* 151:668, 1980.

Skinner DB, Little AG, DeMeester TR: Management of esophageal perforation. *Am J Surg* 139:760, 1980.

Worman LW, Hurley JD, et al: Rupture of the esophagus from external blunt trauma. *Arch Surg* 85:333, 1962.

Wychulis AR, Fontana RS, Payne WS: Instrumental perforations of the esophagus. *Dis Chest* 55:184, 1969.

Wychulis AR, Fontana RS, Payne WS: Noninstrumental perforations of the esophagus. *Dis Chest* 55:190, 1969.

Corrosive Esophagitis

Buntain WL, Payne WS, Lynn HB: Esophageal reconstruction for benign disease: A long-term appraisal. *Am Surg* 46:67, 1980.

Campbell GS, Burnett HF, et al: Treatment of corrosive burns of the esophagus. *Arch Surg* 112:495, 1977.

Kirsh MM, Ritter F: Caustic ingestion and subsequent damage to the oropharyngeal and digestive passages. *Ann Thorac Surg* 21:74, 1976.

Yudin SS: The surgical construction of 80 cases of artificial esophagus. *Surg Gynecol Obstet* 78:561, 1944.

Miscellaneous Esophageal Lesions

Adler RH: Congenital esophageal webs. *J Thorac Cardiovasc Surg* 45:175, 1963.

Hastings PR, Peters KW, Cohn I Jr: Mallory-Weiss syndrome: Review of 69 cases. *Am J Surg* 142:560, 1981.

Mallory GK, Weiss S: Hemorrhages from lacerations of the cardiac orifice of the stomach due to vomiting. *Am J Med Sci* 178:506, 1929.

Chapter 26

Stomach

Frank G. Moody, James M. McGreevy, and Thomas A. Miller

ANATOMY

FUNCTIONAL RELATIONSHIPS. The stomach is an expanded segment of the foregut responsible for the initial breakdown and predigestion of a meal. Its location in the upper abdomen beneath the left hemidiaphragm allows for free expansion of its thin-walled distensible fundus, which receives and stores solid foods that pass into it from the esophagus above. The thicker-walled, more muscular distal portion of the stomach, the antrum, grinds and mixes the food and then forces it back into the fundus for further reduction in size and predigestion. Small particles move forward into the duodenum where they are further processed by intestinal secretions. The distal stomach is delineated by a thick band of circular smooth muscle, the pyloric sphincter. This sphincter prevents duodenogastric reflux and assists in gastric emptying by relaxing during antral propulsive contractions.

The fundus is lined by a highly specialized epithelium that secretes hydrochloric acid, pepsin, and intrinsic factor. The mucosa of the antrum participates in the process of gastric acid secretion by releasing the secretagogue, gastrin, into the circulation. This event is mediated by vagal release of acetylcholine and is modulated by the pH of the antral lumen. The stomach, therefore, can be considered as two organs: its proximal portion is designed for storage and digestion, and its distal part is adapted to the role of mixing and evacuation.

Of importance to the functional activity of the stomach in disease is its relationship to other intraabdominal organs. The most important adjacent organs are the pancreas and the liver, which lie dorsad and ventrad, respectively, and the spleen, which lies directly to the left of the stomach's greater curve (Fig. 26-1). Inflammation of the pancreas may delay gastric emptying, while enlargement by neoplasm may cause a sense of fullness or even obstruction to the gastric outlet. Liver or splenic enlargement may also interfere with the storage capacity of the stomach by infringing on its lumen. The transverse colon, which lies caudad, may also interfere with gastric function by direct neoplastic extension. More commonly, however, the stomach affects adjacent organs by penetration from peptic ulceration of either the stomach or duodenum. Another closely related structure is the biliary tree. It runs posterior to the first part of the duodenum only a few centimeters from the gastric outlet and is vulnerable to injury not only from peptic ulcer of the duodenum but from attempts at treatment by gastrectomy.

BLOOD SUPPLY AND LYMPHATICS. The stomach has a blood supply so extensive and interconnected that three of its four major nutrient arteries can be ablated without incurring necrosis or even significant dysfunction. A submucosal plexus of arterioles provides for rapid healing of wounds and a low incidence of anastomotic disruption after operative manipulation. Because of this vascular anatomy, mucosal lesions may bleed extensively, even when small or superficial. The major arterial supply to the

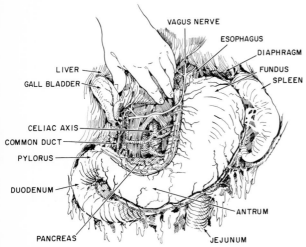

Fig. 26-1. Position of the stomach relative to the other principal organs of the upper abdomen.

stomach is shown in Fig. 26-2. The lesser curve of the stomach is supplied primarily by the left gastric artery, which arises from the celiac axis. The right gastric artery, arising from the ascending hepatic artery, is usually a small vessel that provides branches to the first part of the

Fig. 26-2. Blood supply to the stomach. Legend: F—fundus; C—cardia; P—pylorus; S—spleen; A—aorta; E—esophageal arteries; SP—splenic artery; LG—left gastric artery; CH—common hepatic artery; RG—right gastric artery; GD—gastroduodenal artery; PD—pancreaticoduodenal artery; RGE—right gastroepiploic artery; LGE—left gastroepiploic artery; SG—short gastric arteries. *(Courtesy of KR Larsen, PhD.)*

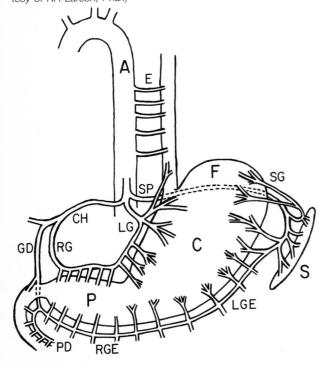

duodenum and the pylorus. Right and left gastroepiploic arteries arise from the gastroduodenal and splenic arteries, respectively. They form an arcade along the greater curve, the right providing blood to the antrum and the left supplying the lower portion of the fundus. The short gastric arteries arising from the splenic artery are small and relatively insignificant in terms of the amount of blood that they deliver to the most proximal portion of the body of the stomach.

The lymphatic drainage of the stomach follows the distribution of the blood supply. An understanding of lymphatic channels and their nodal communications is important to the assessment of tumor spread from gastric cancer. These routes of flow are shown schematically in Fig. 26-3. Lymph from the upper lesser curvature of the stomach drains into the left gastric and paracardial nodes (Region I). The antral segment on the lesser curve (Region II) drains into the right suprapancreatic nodes. Lymph from Region III, high on the greater curvature, flows into the left gastroepiploic and splenic nodes, while the distribution of flow along the right gastroepiploic enters nodes at the base of the vascular pedicle serving this area (Region IV). Knowledge of these areas is of practical importance when operating for cure of gastric cancer. Unfortunately, the routes of metastatic spread in this disease are unpredictable. Therefore, removal of lymph nodes is more important for ascertaining prognosis than for gaining a cure.

INNERVATION. Motor aspects as well as secretory aspects of gastric function are controlled by the autonomic nervous system. The vagus nerves provide a predominant part of this innervation. The major branches of the vagi are shown schematically in Fig. 26-4. Each vagus has a single branch within the abdomen: the hepatic arising from the left anterior vagus, and the celiac from the right posterior vagus. The axial orientation of the vagi relates to the rotation of the stomach to the left as the lengthened foregut returns to the celomic cavity from the yolk sac during gestation. Each vagus terminates in the anterior and posterior nerves of Laterjet, respectively. Small branches course along the smaller blood vessels as they enter the gastric wall along its lesser curve. Knowledge of the anatomy of these nerves has resulted in a new technique, highly selective vagotomy, for treatment of peptic ulcer. In this procedure, the antral branches called the "crow's-foot" are preserved, while the more proximal branches are divided as they enter the stomach. The left anterior vagus will often divide into two or three branches before passing through the esophageal hiatus. The right posterior vagus may occasionally give off a small branch that courses to the left behind the esophagus to join the cardia. This branch has been termed the "criminal nerve of Grassi" in recognition of its important role in the etiology of recurrent ulcer when it is left undivided.

The splanchnic innervation to the stomach is less distinct than that of vagal origin. It has been demonstrated that some of the vagal fibers are adrenergic as well as cholinergic. The majority of sympathetic innervations, however, appear to be adrenergic. They accompany the gastrosplenic artery and its branches, which is appropriate for their function of control of blood flow and muscu-

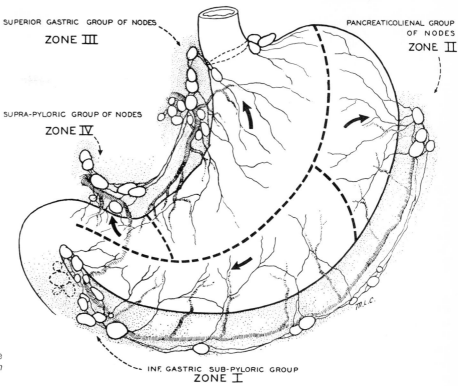

SUPERIOR GASTRIC GROUP OF NODES
ZONE III

PANCREATICOLIENAL GROUP
OF NODES
ZONE II

SUPRA-PYLORIC GROUP OF NODES
ZONE IV

INF. GASTRIC SUB-PYLORIC GROUP
ZONE I

Fig. 26-3. Lymphatic drainage of the stomach. (From: *Coller FA, et al: Arch Surg 43:751, 1941, with permission.*)

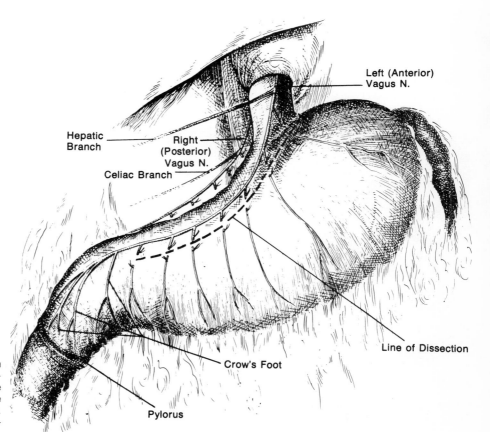

Left (Anterior) Vagus N.

Hepatic Branch

Right (Posterior) Vagus N.

Celiac Branch

Line of Dissection

Crow's Foot

Pylorus

Fig. 26-4. Diagram of the distribution of the vagus nerve within the abdomen. It also shows where the branches of the nerve of Laterjet are divided for a parietal cell vagotomy. (From: *Moody FG: Mt Kisco, NY: Futura, 1:1–15, 1980.*)

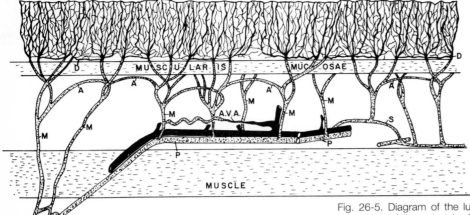

Fig. 26-5. Diagram of the lush mucosal capillary network of the stomach and the network of relatively large caliber arterioles that exist in the submucosa. Legend: D—anastomosing channels; A—anastomosis; M—mucosal arteries; AVA—arteriovenous anastomosis; P—submucous plexus; S—subsidiary anastomosing channels. (From: *Barlow TE, et al: Surg Gynecol Obstet 93:668, 1951, with permission.*)

lar function rather than secretory events within the mucosa. There is, in general, a paucity of knowledge about the precise role that local sympathetic nerves play in gastric function.

MORPHOLOGY. The gastric wall consists of an external serosa that covers an inner oblique, a middle circular, and an outer longitudinal layer of smooth muscle. The submucosa and mucosa provide a continuous inner integument that is separated by a thin sheet of smooth muscle, the muscularis mucosa (Fig. 26-5). A prominent characteristic of the mucosa is a rich mucosal capillary network that

Fig. 26-6. Fundic gastric mucosa illustrating multiple gastric pits (P), some of which are filled with secretion (S). "Cobblestone" appearance of the epithelium is suggested *(arrows)* (×400). *(Courtesy of CA Zalewsky, PhD.)*

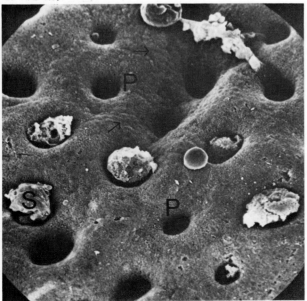

is derived from small arteries that originate in the submucosa. Arteriovenous shunts are rarely seen within the gastric wall.

The mucosal lining of the gastric antrum (distal one-third) is distinctly different from that of the gastric fundus (proximal two-thirds). The latter has an elaborate network of deep glands, four or five of which join an indentation within the mucosal surface called a *pit* or *foveolus*. Individual pits are seen along with the cells that line the interfoveolar area in a scanning electron micrograph in Fig. 26-6. The gastric glands consist of six major cell types: surface, mucous neck, progenitor, chief, parietal, and endocrine cells (Fig. 26-7). The surface epithelial cells are distinguished by abundant mucous granules within their apical surface. These cells are designed to protect the epithelium from ingestants and the injurious effects of gastric acid. They are also the likely source of a sodium-rich alkaline secretion. The mucous neck cells line the entrance to gastric glands. They may serve the purpose of partially buffering nascent acid as it enters the gastric pits. Cells at the base of the gastric pits serve as stem or progenitor cells for the development of new surface cells and also the cells of the gastric glands. Knowledge of the function of the parietal cells distributed within the gastric glands is more secure than that of surface cells, for it has been proved that they are the site of secretion of hydrochloric acid. The characteristics of a resting and secreting cell are shown in Fig. 26-8*A* and *B*. Chief cells are the source of pepsinogen, a proteolytic enzyme that is converted to its active form, pepsin, at a pH below 2.5. A variety of endocrine cells exist within the gastric gland. Some secrete gastrin or serotonin, while the function of the others has not as yet been elucidated.

The antral mucosa is less specialized than that within the fundic area. In fact, by light microscopy, one can only identify surface epithelial cells and mucous neck cells. There are no parietal or chief cells. Gastrin-producing

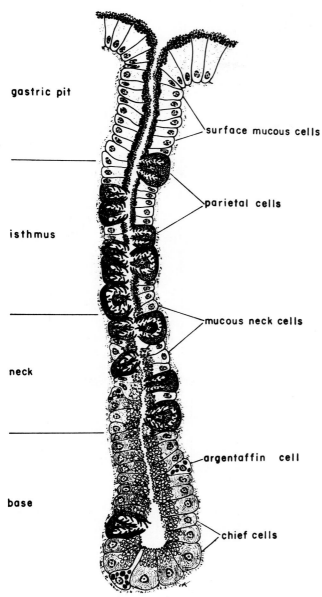

gastric pit

surface mucous cells

parietal cells

isthmus

mucous neck cells

neck

argentaffin cell

base

chief cells

Fig. 26-7. Diagram of a single gastric gland of the bat. Between five and seven of these units open into the base of a single gastric pit (foveolus). (From: *Ito S, et al: J Cell Biol 16:543, 1963, with permission.*)

cells (G-cells), however, can be identified by radioimmunofluorescence.

SPHINCTERS. The entrance of ingestants into the stomach is controlled by a highly specialized 5-cm area of smooth muscle, termed the *lower esophageal sphincter.* This sphincter, which presents a high-pressure zone between the esophagus and stomach, relaxes to allow the passage of foodstuffs. It then contracts to prevent the regurgitation of gastric contents into the esophagus. This sphincter is important because it protects the esophageal mucosa from corrosion by gastric acid.

The lower esophageal sphincter does not have a physical correlate, i.e., an identifiable mound of smooth muscle that can be easily felt and even seen when cut in cross section. By contrast, the pyloric sphincter, which prevents (or minimizes) duodenogastric reflux, is both anatomic and physiologic. It also serves as a metering point for the movement of food particles into the duodenum. Particles that are more than 2 mm in size are rejected and forced back into the body of the stomach for further trituration and preliminary digestion.

PHYSIOLOGY

STORAGE. The major function of the stomach is to prepare ingested food for digestion and absorption as it descends through the small intestine. The process of early digestion requires that solid foodstuffs be stored for a prolonged period of time (4 hours) as they undergo reduction in size and preliminary breakdown into basic metabolic constituents. Once the meal has been processed to an appropriate particulate size and chemical composition, it is delivered intermittently to the duodenum for further digestion.

The storage function of the stomach is greatly enhanced by the process of receptive relaxation. This is an event whereby the upper portion of the stomach relaxes as the intake of food is anticipated. Solid food settles and layers within the greater curvature of the fundic area of the stomach. Liquids pass rapidly from the stomach along its lesser curve (the magenstrasse), thereby leaving the solid mass quite undisturbed. Processing of the food mass is initiated by a skimming from the outermost layers of the gastric bolus. Salivary digestion occurs within its middle and gastric digestion at its periphery. Food particles are reduced in size by a grinding action of the antrum as well as digestion and dilution by the gastric secretions. The storage function of the stomach is enhanced by the antrum and pylorus, which constantly return material to the proximal stomach until it is ready for delivery to the duodenum. A surprising aspect of this very active mechanical process is that it proceeds for several hours after a solid meal without sensation of its occurrence.

Satiety is a feeling of gratification after eating. Morbidly obese individuals do not experience this feeling until they have consumed more food (calories) than they need. Appetite control is based upon genetic, cultural, psychological, environmental, and physical factors, all of which play a role in how much one eats. The pathophysiologic consequence of abnormalities of this appetite control mechanism is obesity more often than malnutrition.

DIGESTION. Gastric digestion involves the breakdown of foodstuffs into fine particles. Starches undergo enzymatic breakdown as long as the pH within the center of the gastric bolus remains favorable for the activity of salivary alpha-amylase (pH > 5). Peptic digestion within the stomach is primarily designed to reduce the size of meat particles and initiate the dispersion of fats, proteins, and carbohydrates by breaking down cell walls. The gastric mucosa also secretes a lipase that assists in the early

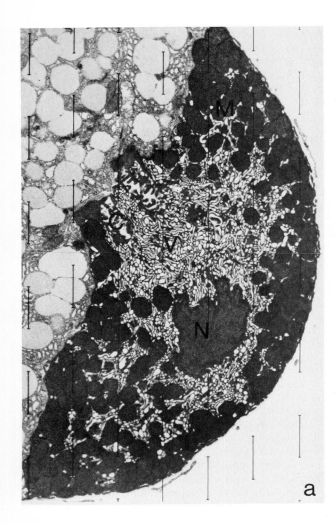

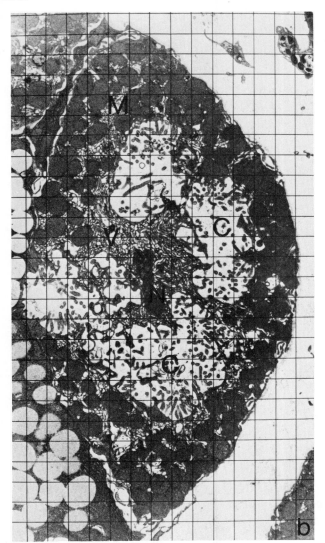

Fig. 26-8. *A.* Resting, unstimulated parietal cell in which the cytoplasm is occupied primarily by tubulovesicles (V) and peripheral mitochondria (M). Apical canaliculi (C) and nucleus (N) are present. A stereometric grid to measure membrane density covers the cell (×9500). *B.* Histamine-stimulated parietal cell with extensive development of canaliculi (C). Remaining tubulovesicles (V) surround the nucleus (N), and mitochondria (M) occupy the periphery. A stereometric grid to measure membrane density covers the cell (×9000). *(Courtesy of CA Zalewsky PhD.)*

phase of fat digestion. The majority of digestion occurs within the duodenum and upper small bowel. The stomach is merely responsible for improving the efficiency of the process.

Gastric Acid Secretion. Acid-peptic disease of the esophagus, stomach, and duodenum represents one of the most common pathologic entities of the foregut. While gastric acid is usually not the single or even the predominant causative factor in peptic diseases, it is a critical component in their genesis. The dictum "no acid, no ulcer" has gained general support since the discovery by Beaumont (1833) that the stomach could secrete hydrochloric acid. Furthermore, all therapies for gastric and duodenal ulcer are based on control of intraluminal pH by either neutralization or inhibition of acid secretion.

It is convenient to consider the secretion of gastric acid in terms of its neurohumoral control. There is only a low rate of acid secretion during the interdigestive period when the stomach is at rest (2 to 3 meq/h). The sight and smell of food and its ingestion lead to a brisk secretion of hydrochloric acid. This activity is initiated by stimuli that pass from the cerebral cortex to the vagal centers within the hypothalamus. Action potentials descend the vagi and release acetylcholine within the enteric plexuses and their nerve endings in the gastric wall. Acetylcholine in turn leads to the release of gastrin from the antral mucosa and the secretion of acid and pepsinogen from the fundic mucosa. Gastrin is also a stimulant of acid secretion, and its action is greatly enhanced by the vagal release of acetylcholine. Histamine also participates in the acid secretory event and may, in fact, be a critical modulator of the process.

The gastrointestinal hormone, gastrin, is a polypeptide that has been well studied during the past decade since its isolation and purification by Gregory and Tracy. Numerous clinicians and scientists have made important contributions to our understanding of how this hormone might carry out its important activities within the gastrointestinal tract. Foremost among these is the late Morton Grossman who, over a 30-year period, stimulated numerous collaborators to find out how gastrin might contribute to acid secretion in the normal state and in disease. Unfortunately, the answer is still not known. It is to the credit of Yalow and Berson, and their collaborators, that the technique of radioimmunoassay has allowed a reasonably full description of its biologic function.

The vagal release of gastrin is enhanced by antral distension and contact of its mucosa with proteins. The ingestion of a meal is associated with a cumulative release of gastrin that provides for a constant flow of acid secretion during gastric digestion. This gastrin release is facilitated as long as the intraluminal pH is high. Conversely, gastrin release is attenuated by a low pH on the antral mucosal surface. This negative feedback mechanism provides the principal control for the rate of acid secretion. Furthermore, it offers a check on the indiscriminate secretion of acid during the interdigestive period. The process described above is called the "cephalogastric" phase of acid secretion.

The duodenum and intestines also play a role in controlling acid secretion. Acidification of the duodenum leads to the release of secretin. Secretin inhibits both gastrin release and the secretion of gastric acid. Gastrin, which is also present within the mucosa of the duodenum and upper intestine, may be the source of the small stimulus for acid secretion that occurs as the products of a meal move through the intestinal tract. The intestinal phase of gastric secretion accounts for about 5 percent of the cumulative acid secretory response during the ingestion of a meal.

Parietal Cell Function. The parietal cell (Fig. 26-8*A* and *B*) is the putative site of hydrochloric acid secretion. In the resting state, its cytoplasm consists of numerous mitochondria and tubulovesicles. With stimulation, there is a remarkable elaboration of membrane into an intracellular canaliculus. This is the presumed site of the transfer of hydrogen ions (H^+) to the luminal side of the plasma membrane into the tubule of the gastric gland. How this occurs is not completely known. A current scheme involves the translocation of a proton (H^+) at some site on the membrane in exchange for a potassium ion (K^+). This H^+ for K^+ exchange requires energy provided by oxidative phosphorylation. The hydrolysis of ATP derived from this process is facilitated by a specific enzyme, adenosine triphosphatase (ATPase). There is speculation that the Cl^- in this process is provided by its own translocation process. The extraordinary aspect of gastric acid secretion is that it moves H^+ against a millionfold chemical gradient (10^{-7} in the blood to 10^{-1} in gastric juice).

The parietal cell will secrete acid in response to acetyl-

choline, gastrin, and histamine. Acid secretion can be inhibited by a class of agents (cimetidine) that block histamine receptors on the parietal cell (H_2, as opposed to the heart and lung histamine receptors called H_1). Recently, an inhibitor (omeprazole) of the hydrogen-potassium ATPase has been discovered that may have clinical value because of its specificity. Prostaglandins are also potent inhibitors of acid secretion that are being evaluated for their clinical usefulness. Anticholinergics in high doses are partial antagonists of the secretory process, but their pronounced effects on delaying gastric emptying preclude their value as antisecretory agents. Vagotomy profoundly diminishes the response of the parietal cell to gastrin and histamine, an effect that has contributed to its effectiveness as a therapy for peptic ulcer.

Surface Cell Function. The surface epithelial cells line the outermost layer of the gastric epithelium and thereby are exposed to the contents of the gastric lumen. They are relatively impervious to H^+ ions and are protected from mechanical injury by a thin layer of mucus. This mucus layer is renewed constantly by a large number of mucus granules stored beneath the apical plasma membrane. Surface cells also produce a sodium-rich alkaline (bicarbonate) secretion that may play an important role in reducing the pH at the apical surface. This is a new concept that has not yet assumed clinical relevance because of the low rate of alkaline secretion. It is important to recognize that a break in the barrier to H^+ ions may render the epithelium of the stomach susceptible to acute erosive gastritis.

Gastric Analysis. There are a variety of ways to assess the acid secretory capacity of the stomach. The most accurate is to aspirate gastric contents under controlled conditions through a nasogastric tube. It is best to have the patient lying in a semirecumbent position on the left side. The study is commenced by aspirating the stomach of its contents and then instilling and immediately recovering 50 mL of normal saline. Complete recovery reveals appropriate tube placement. Aspirations are then done by hand syringe every 5 min for 1 h. The aspirates are pooled in 15-min aliquots. At the end of the final aspirate, the stomach is stimulated to secrete by the intravenous administration of histalog in a dose of 2 μg/kg, or pentagastrin in a dose of 6 μg/kg. Aspiration is continued as described above, with four 15-min collections obtained over a 1-h period. The volume of the collections is measured, and an aliquot is titrated electrometrically to determine its content of H^+. The rate of secretion is then expressed as the number of milliequivalents produced per hour during the basal or prestimulatory phase and during maximal and peak output. Maximal acid output (MAO) is obtained by averaging the output of the two final 15-min periods. Peak output is the highest rate of secretion obtained during a 15-min period after stimulation. Basal acid output (BAO) is normally 2 to 3 meq/h; secretory output (MAO) is in the range of 10 to 15 meq/h. Patients with duodenal ulcer have higher values, while those with gastric ulcer may have lower values. However, there is remarkable overlap between either condition and the normal. Another role for gastric analysis is its use as a screen for the Zollinger-Ellison (ZE) syndrome. In this illness characterized by flagrant ulcer disease, basal acid outputs may be in excess of 50 meq/h.

Pepsinogen. The role of pepsinogen in gastroduodenal disease has not been well defined. Pepsinogen, a proenzyme, does not assume its proteolytic activity until activated by a pH below 2.5. Pepsin, the activated enzyme, can digest food and devitalized tissue but has virtually no effect on healthy, well-nourished cells. Its role, therefore, in the pathogenesis of peptic ulcer is obscure. The well-circumscribed, clean nature of a peptic ulcer bed, however, is likely a consequence of its activity. Pepsinogen is stored within chief cells in the form of granules whose release is under vagal control. It is interesting that so little is known about a substance that assumes illusionary importance by the terms "peptic ulcer" and "dyspepsia."

GASTRIC EMPTYING. Control Mechanisms. Gastric emptying is modulated by a highly integrated process that includes mechanical, chemical, and neurohumoral mechanisms. Solids are preprocessed in the stomach over a period of hours during which they are reduced in size and dispersed within the gastric juice for efficient digestion. In addition, the osmolality of the chyme is reduced by dilution. The latter function is important in the prevention of the dumping syndrome. Dumping occurs when an osmotic load is delivered to the intestine, causing an influx of water, intestinal distention, and rapid transit of the predigested meal. This leads to light-headedness, sweating, tachycardia, crampy abdominal pain, and diarrhea. It is, therefore, logical that one of the important control mechanisms should include osmoreceptors within the duodenum.

An understanding of the neurohumoral control of gastric emptying is currently incomplete. The observation that truncal vagotomy does not predictably lead to delayed gastric emptying has lead to ambiguity about the role of the autonomic nervous system. In fact, vagotomy may hasten the transit of liquids when a pyloroplasty or gastroenterostomy has been performed. The antrum appears to be the key component in propulsion from the stomach, and its activity is clearly under vagal control. Apparently the myenteric plexuses that are a component of the enteric nervous system can continue to function in response to intraluminal stimulation of food even in the absence of central vagal innervation. Furthermore, denervation causes an increase in serum gastrin as a consequence of loss of antral acidification. Possibly the law of Cannon, in which denervated receptors become more sensitive to chemical stimuli, is at work in this situation, whereby the gastrin receptors that stimulate gastric smooth muscle contractions may be rendered supersensitive to a point of compensating for the loss of centrally mediated vagal release of acetylcholine.

What is known is as follows: Anticipation of a meal leads to vagally mediated gastrin release, gastric acid secretion, receptive relaxation of the proximal stomach, rhythmic antral contractions, and coordinated relaxation of the pyloric sphincter. Ingestion of the meal accentuates all these responses. Emptying of liquids is continuous and relatively rapid, depending on the osmolarity. Solids must

be reduced to a few millimeters in diameter before antral discharge occurs.

Gastric motor function is related in some way to the electromyographic activity within its smooth muscle. The stomach has a pacemaker high on the greater curve that likely initiates contractions in the area by phasic spike potentials that entrain a series of action potentials toward the pylorus (Fig. 26-9). The precise role of the myoelectric entrainment is not understood, nor is it a critical phenomenon since division of the stomach does not interfere with aboral electrical activity or gastric emptying.

Fats delay gastric emptying by an unknown mechanism. Gastric lipase may be responsible in that it is slow to reduce the droplet size of fats. It is also possible that the antral or duodenal mucosa may have a chemical sensor for specific fatty acids. Finally, lipid-related cholecystokinin release may affect gastric emptying by retarding emptying.

Gastric Emptying Studies. There are a variety of ways to assess gastric emptying. The simplest is to instill a known volume of saline into the stomach and attempt to recover it at a fixed time. Lewis recommends instillation at 750 mL into the unoperated stomach. Gastric aspiration at 30 min with returns of less than 200 mL indicates normal pyloric function. Pyloric dysfunction or obstruction usually yields greater than 400 mL. This saline load test can provide a qualitative view of the stomach's capacity to empty a liquid meal. A barium radiograph can also provide some information on adequacy of emptying and may reveal pathology that might contribute to a delay such as pyloric obstruction. Computerized radionuclide scans have provided a quantitative way to measure the emptying rate of liquids as well as solids. Radiolabeled technetium is used to monitor the rate of liquid emptying. The solid phase is measured with radioactive chicken livers. An example of the appearance of such a study is shown in Fig. 26-10. These studies are particularly helpful in patients who have gastric atony from vagal denervation, diabetes, or other associated illness.

OTHER GASTRIC FUNCTIONS. The stomach plays an important role in hematopoiesis through its production of intrinsic factor by the parietal cell. Intrinsic factor is essential for the ileal absorption of vitamin B_{12}. Of added, but not critical, importance is a relationship between acid secretion and iron absorption by the duodenum, a relationship that involves the important role of acid in proteolysis and breakdown of animal cells.

Gastric acidification is also important in maintaining sterility of the foregut. Only a few unusual fusiform bacillae can withstand the challenges of a low gastric pH. It is known that the upper gastrointestinal tract is rapidly colonized by enteric bacteria when the stomach is rendered achlorhydric by medical or surgical means.

Immunologic Sensing. It is reasonable to assume that the gastric mucosa is involved in the detection of harmful ingestants. It is well suited for this purpose with its ability to protect its surface by rapid mucus release, creating an unstirred layer that may form a first line of defense against harmful macromolecules. If potentially dangerous substances (with chemical or oncological portend) should

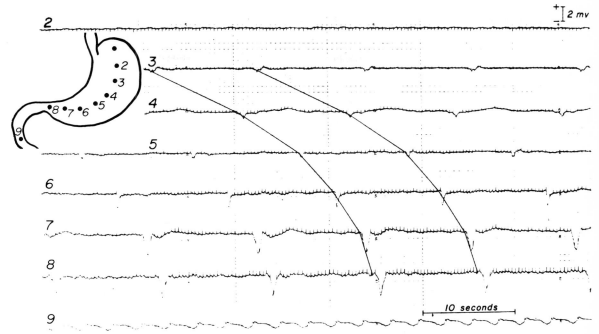

Fig. 26-9. Illustration of electrical activity measured at different sites on the stomach. The recordings demonstrate the distal migration of myoelectric complexes from the gastric pacemaker. (From: *Kelly KA, et al: Am J Physiol 217:465, 1969, with permission.*)

Fig. 26-10. A normal solid-phase gastric emptying study using 100 μC technetium sulfur colloid. Gamma camera images were made at *A*, immediately after ingestion of the radioactive meal; *B*, after 15 min; *C*, after 30 min; *D*, after 45 min; *E*, after 60 min; and *F*, after 90 min. The sequential pictures show more activity in the small bowel and less in the stomach. *(Courtesy of P Christian.)*

permeate the mucosa, they immediately encounter the lamina propria and its army of mast cells and free-floating macrophages and lymphocytes. The role of the gastric mucosa in immunosurveillance has not yet been elucidated.

Heat Exchange. The stomach with its lush mucosal microcirculation is an excellent heat exchanger. This is an important function, for it ensures the intraluminal contents a relatively stable thermal environment for their

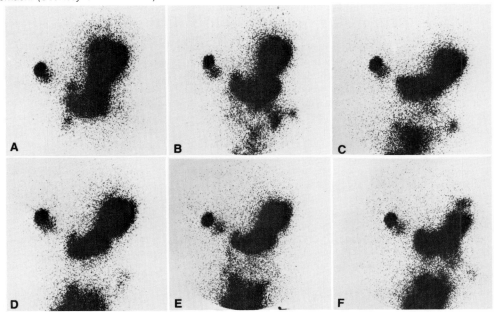

enzymatic digestion. Furthermore, the mechanism offers protection against cooling of adjacent viscera or significant changes in core temperature.

GASTRIC DYSFUNCTION

SYMPTOMS. Anorexia. Lack of appetite, or anorexia, is a common symptom that everyone has from time to time, especially during a viral illness. In fact, it is so frequently associated with psychologic stress that it may initially be overlooked as an early sign of a serious illness. For example, most patients with cancer of the gastrointestinal tract will recall that they were anorectic during the early phase of their illness. Anorexia is usually the reason for weight loss in neoplastic as well as other diseases within the gastrointestinal tract.

Nausea and Vomiting. The gastrointestinal tract is capable of protecting itself from harmful ingestants by a forceful evacuation of its contents through the mouth. Vomiting is a complex process. After a deep breath, the glottis is closed. The stomach then evacuates its contents by retropulsion. The reversed movement of gastrointestinal contents is assisted by a tightening of the muscles of the abdomen and thorax, a decrease in acid secretion, and an autonomic response that includes sweating, pallor, and tachycardia. Nausea is a sensation of impending emesis and may be of central or peripheral origin. It is not always accompanied by vomiting. In fact, many patients with vaguely defined gastrointestinal disease will complain of nausea. It is a symptom that accompanies low-grade visceral pain such as might occur in gallstone disease, mild pancreatitis, peptic ulcer, or the early phase of acute appendicitis.

The vomiting of "intestinal origin" is often associated with other signs such as abdominal distention or emesis of blood (varices, gastritis, or peptic ulcer) or intestinal contents. The character of the vomitus may be helpful in establishing a diagnosis. Lack of bile suggests a point of obstruction above the papilla of Vater. Feculent vomiting is associated with low small bowel obstruction, its brown color and foul odor being a result of bacterial overgrowth by enteric organisms. Obstruction at this level is usually accompanied by generalized abdominal distention, in contrast to chronic pyloric obstruction in which there is distention of the mid and left upper abdomen from a fluid- and air-filled stomach.

Pain. The mucosa of the stomach is devoid of pain endings. This explains in part the relatively painless nature of erosive gastritis, gastric cancer, and even peptic ulcer disease of the stomach. Acute gastric distention may also be a relatively pain-free event, especially in the postoperative period. Acid-peptic disease of the duodenum, however, has a very characteristic pain pattern depending upon the depth of ulceration. Early superficial ulceration is usually associated with a gnawing sensation within the midepigastrium. When acid is unbuffered, such as might occur in the early morning hours, the pain is sharp and more intense. A characteristic of duodenal ulcer pain is that it disappears as soon as an antacid or other neutralizing substance is ingested. Gastric ulcer pain is more

subtle and diffuse in nature, often coming on during or after eating, rather than before. The sudden onset of severe, unrelenting, generalized abdominal pain is a sign of ulcer perforation. This, of course, is a catastrophic event that requires immediate surgical attention.

Regurgitation. The reflux of gastric contents into the esophagus may be associated with three complaints: (1) heartburn, (2) expectoration of gastric chyme, and (3) cough from aspiration. Heartburn is a sensation of mild to moderate substernal discomfort. It is an annoying, diffuse, burning pain that is usually well tolerated by the patient. Not only acid but also alkaline regurgitation can cause this symptom, which may be associated with inflammation within the esophageal mucosa. A severe subxiphoid or substernal pain exacerbated by feeding (odynophagia) is a sign of esophageal ulceration. Difficulty in swallowing (dysphagia) accompanies esophageal obstruction from peptic stricture, esophagogastric cancer, or a primary motor disturbance such as achalasia or esophageal spasm.

Regurgitation is a sign of loss of the high-pressure zone that normally exists between the stomach and esophagus. Recall that the pressure within the body of the esophagus reflects intrathoracic pressure, and therefore is subatmospheric (-5 to -10 mmHg). Gastric pressures are positive, 5 to 10 mmHg. The pressures within the lower esophageal segment (LES) must, therefore, be in excess of 15 mmHg in order to prevent reflux. Factors that control the pressure within the LES are not completely known, but they include vagal release of acetylcholine, intraabdominal pressure, intragastric pressure, and ill-defined humoral mechanisms, which may include cyclic nucleotides and prostaglandins. Pharmacologic doses of acetylcholine, metoclopromide, gastrin, and calcium blocking agents can reconstitute low esophageal sphincter pressures. The LES can also be repaired operatively by wrapping the upper part of the stomach around the lower end of the esophagus (Nissen fundoplication).

SIGNS. Bleeding. Upper gastrointestinal bleeding demands a thorough evaluation of the alimentary tract. Hematemesis (vomiting of blood) may be a dramatic, exsanguinating event, or it may be a manifestation of a minor bleed from gastritis or peptic ulcer. The nature of the vomitus may provide a clue to the rate and site of bleeding. Coffee-ground emesis (acid-hematin) is usually a sign of peptic ulcer. Bright-red emesis may be from an esophageal varix, a gastric mucosal tear, gastritis, or a peptic ulcer. Gastric or duodenal bleeding can occur without hematemesis. In this instance the stool is usually black. More rapid bleeding, however, can result in bright-red stools. Newer technology now permits rapid identification and control of the offending lesion. This is accomplished by upper gastrointestinal endoscopy whereby the esophagus, stomach, and duodenum can be safely and quickly inspected. Bleeding sites can be controlled by electrocoagulation or photocoagulation, and biopsies of suspicious lesions can be obtained for histologic examination.

Weight Loss. Gastric disease, especially neoplasia, is usually accompanied by gradual loss of weight. Benign gastric ulcer is associated with weight loss as a consequence of the avoidance of food which might induce abdominal pain. Duodenal ulcer is usually accompanied by weight gain in response to pain control by the ingestion of milk and other alkalinizing foods.

Gastric Distention. Acute gastric dilatation provokes an intense autonomic response that includes pallor, rapid respirations, bradycardia, and hypotension. This is a dramatic and serious complication that may follow any operation within the abdomen. It can easily be diagnosed by inspection and percussion of the abdomen which reveals a markedly distended stomach. Once recognized, the problem is easily remedied, by the passage of a nasogastric tube and gastric aspiration.

Abdominal Tenderness. Peptic ulcer disease may be accompanied by tenderness on deep palpation within the midepigastrium. This is a common sign when an active ulcer is present within the duodenum; gastric ulcers, except when they penetrate through the gastric wall, are usually nontender. Gastric neoplasms are also not associated with discomfort on palpation. Perforated ulcers are usually accompanied by marked, generalized tenderness in response to the intense chemical peritonitis that accompanies the leak of gastric acid into the abdominal cavity.

Palpable Tumor. Gastric neoplasms of the distal stomach may present as a palpable mass within the epigastrium or left upper abdomen. Gastric tumors can usually be distinguished from mass lesions that arise within the pancreas, since they are more anterior and often movable. Liver tumors are even more superficial and usually will descend with deep inspiration. Neoplasms of the proximal stomach are hidden from detection by physical examination by the left hemithorax.

DIAGNOSIS. Radiography. Visualization of the upper gastrointestinal tract by barium radiography has provided a safe, convenient, reliable way to detect gastric and duodenal disease. Unfortunately, over half of the acute lesions of the duodenum and almost all superficial erosions of the stomach go undetected by this type of examination. It still remains, however, a starting point for patients with chronic symptoms of upper gastrointestinal disease. A normal upper gastrointestinal barium series is shown in Fig. 26-11. Multiple views are required to gain a full view of the stomach and duodenal bulb.

Endoscopy. Patients who present with the signs and symptoms of upper gastrointestinal hemorrhage are usually subjected to endoscopy early in their hospital course, especially when the bleeding is massive or persistent. Endoscopy for chronic symptoms is also a routine procedure that can be done on an ambulatory basis with high yield and little risk or discomfort to the patient. Most gastroenterologists, and an increasing number of general surgeons, are proficient at the technique of upper gastrointestinal endoscopy. An advantage of the technique is the opportunity it provides to obtain photographs and biopsies of suspicious lesions.

POSTGASTRECTOMY SYNDROMES. Operations upon the stomach that include resection, pyloric ablation (pyloroplasty) or bypass (gastroenterostomy), and total gastric vagotomy may be accompanied by unpleasant side effects. For convenience, they have been termed

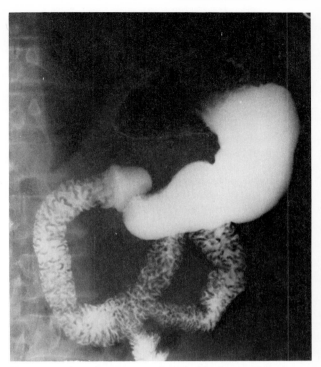

Fig. 26-11. Normal upper gastrointestinal barium radiograph.

"postgastrectomy syndromes" (Table 26-1). They occur to varying degrees in about 20 percent of patients in the early months after stomach surgery. With time and attention to diet, the symptoms disappear in the majority of patients. About 5 percent of patients, however, remain symptomatic for the remainder of their lives, and 1 percent become permanently disabled to a point of being considered "gastric cripples." It is for this reason that lesser procedures such as proximal gastric vagotomy without drainage have replaced the more extensive 75 percent gastric resection or pyloroplasty and truncal vagotomy for the treatment of acid-peptic disease of the duodenum.

Surprisingly, total gastrectomy with esophagojejunal reconstruction is fairly well tolerated by patients who require it for gastric cancer or the Zollinger-Ellison syndrome. They usually remain on the slender side but have few gastrointestinal complaints if they eat several small meals a day. It is essential that they receive injections of vitamin B_{12} on a monthly basis, since they cannot absorb

Table 26-1. POSTGASTRECTOMY SYNDROMES

Small capacity
Dumping
Bile gastritis
Afferent loop
Efferent loop
Postvagotomy diarrhea
Anemia
Metabolic bone disease

it from the gut in the absence of intrinsic factor that formerly came from the parietal cells.

The dumping syndrome, characterized by light-headedness, diaphoresis, palpitations, crampy abdominal pain, and diarrhea, is a consequence of the rapid movement of gastric contents into the upper intestinal tract. It usually is related to the ingestion of a high-carbohydrate meal. Pyloric bypass or ablation appears to be the main contributor to this syndrome. Vagotomy and the type of gastric reconstruction do not appear to be important variables in its frequency. The mystery is why it occurs as a chronic symptom so infrequently.

Extensive gastrectomy is accompanied by early satiety, a symptom called the *small-capacity syndrome*. This is a serious problem, since it can lead to profound weight loss and malnutrition.

Truncal vagotomy requires an accompanying drainage procedure (pyloroplasty or gastroenterostomy); otherwise gastric stasis may lead to nausea, vomiting, or gastric ulceration. The extragastric vagal denervation associated with this procedure may also contribute to gallstone formation and incapacitating, explosive diarrhea.

Bile gastritis has been recognized as a consequence of gastrectomy in recent years. It is an entity that is characterized by vague symptoms of low-grade epigastric pain, chronic nausea, and bilious vomiting. Barium examination of the stomach is usually nonrevealing. Erosive gastritis may be seen during endoscopic examination of the gastric mucosa. Biopsy often reveals round cell infiltration and edema, especially at the site of mucosal lesions. Unfortunately, patients without gastrointestinal complaints may have similar findings. The strongest evidence that bile may be involved in the syndrome relates to the observation that approximately half of individuals who undergo biliary diversion by Roux en Y gastrojejunostomy will gain symptomatic relief.

The afferent loop syndrome is a clearly defined entity that is characterized by bilious vomiting after distal gastric resection and gastrojejunal anastomosis (Billroth II). The patient will complain of a severe midepigastric pain after eating which is relieved by the emesis of a large volume of bile. Its pathogenesis relates to an obstruction at the junction of the afferent limb coming from the duodenum to the gastric remnant. Food usually has already passed from the stomach into the efferent limb; therefore, it is not mixed with the emesis, as is the case when the efferent loop is obstructed. These conditions are mechanical in nature, as a consequence of either recurrent ulcer or a technical error at the time of reconstruction. Their correction requires reoperation.

Acid-reducing procedures of all types can be accompanied by an iron deficiency or even macrocytic anemia. Bile gastritis and duodenal bypass may increase the frequency and severity of hematologic disturbances. Also of concern is an increased incidence of cancer in the gastric remnant after acid reduction procedures for duodenal ulcer. Little attention has been given to the pathogenesis of this unusual but serious complication.

Diarrhea is one of the most common and distressing complaints after gastric surgery. In a small number of patients it contributes to profound, life-threatening malnutrition. In most patients, however, avoidance of foods that contribute to dumping provides a return to a normal bowel habit. Postvagotomy diarrhea is explosive and unpredictable, a most undesirable sequela that has no therapy except antimotility drug control. Occasionally, gastric surgery will unmask nontropical sprue or a lactase deficiency. These conditions can be diagnosed by small bowel mucosal biopsy, with specific histochemical staining for the presence or absence of lactase.

Recurrent ulcer is a disappointing postgastrectomy sequela. Some patients may present with multiple symptoms including dumping, bilious vomiting, and pain from recurrent ulcer. This presents a quandary in diagnosis and management. Most students of the postgastrectomy syndromes are ultraconservative in offering patients further reconstructive surgery, since the results are modest even in the hands of those skilled in the management of such complex problems.

GASTRIC DISEASE

Peptic Ulcer—Duodenum

Peptic ulcer disease of the duodenum is one of the most common illnesses of the foregut. The stomach's complicity relates to the presumed role of gastric acid secretion in ulcerogenesis. While it is true that achlorhydric patients rarely develop peptic ulcers and that most patients with hyperchlorhydria from gastrinoma (Zollinger-Ellison syndrome) have severe ulcer disease, patients with more common forms of duodenal ulcer may not have hypersecretion of acid. It is for this reason that the role of acid in ulcerogenesis is ambiguous and to this day subject to challenge.

PATHOPHYSIOLOGY. Chronic duodenal ulceration is almost never of neoplastic origin except in rare instances of duodenal cancer. Acute ulcers may occur in a setting of extreme psychological or physical stress. The etiology of acute and chronic ulceration is multivariate. It involves aggressive factors, such as gastric acid and pepsin, and protective factors, which include the alkaline duodenal secretions (bile, pancreatic juice, and duodenal secretion from Brunner's glands) and the duodenal epithelium (hydrogen for sodium exchange, bicarbonate secretion, blood flow, and release of antisecretory hormones such as secretin).

Several observations suggest that duodenal ulcer disease in many patients is a consequence of the secretion of acid in excess of the amount that can be efficiently disposed of by the duodenum. Such patients have an increased basal and stimulated acid secretory output. In addition, they have an augmented cumulative gastrin response to an ingested meal. They also have acidification of the duodenum for prolonged periods (pH < 2), an event rarely seen in normal patients. That hypersecretion of acid can cause duodenal ulceration has been well established in experimental animal models. Furthermore, as mentioned above, patients with hypersecretion of acid on the basis of hypergastrinemia from a pancreatic tumor have a severe ulcer diathesis that subsides when acid secretion is controlled by antisecretory agents. The usual forms of duodenal ulcer also heal when gastric acid is either neutralized by ingestion of antacids or inhibited by antisecretory agents.

There is abundant evidence that reduction of duodenal buffers contributes to ulceration. An example is the removal of bile from the duodenum by biliary diversion into a limb of jejunum. Another is the reduction in the flow of pancreatic juice in chronic pancreatitis or following extensive pancreatic resection. Transposition of the bile and pancreatic secretions into the small intestine at a point where they cannot reflux into the duodenum in experimental animals uniformly leads to chronic duodenal ulceration.

The surgical treatment of peptic ulcer has as its rationale the reduction of acid secretory output to a point that will provide permanent cure for peptic ulcer. There has been a gradual evolution of how this can best be accomplished. Initial efforts were directed toward diversion of acid from the duodenum (gastroenterostomy) and reduction of the acid secretory mass by extensive resection. Knowledge that acid secretion is under vagal control has led to vagotomy as a simpler operative approach with less immediate and late morbidity.

CLINICAL MANIFESTATIONS. Chronic duodenal ulcer disease can present in a number of ways. It usually has its onset in early or midadult life and occurs more frequently in males than in females (4 to 1). The clinical stereotype of an intense, compulsive, cigarette-smoking, alcohol-drinking executive has not been well established in careful epidemiologic studies, but such individuals do represent a high-risk group. There may also be genetic factors other than those that relate to families with gastrinoma or hyperparathyroidism as a component of a multiple endocrine neoplasia syndrome (MEN).

Abdominal Pain. The most common feature of duodenal ulcer is a gnawing, sometimes sharp, well-localized midepigastric pain. The pain is tolerable and usually relieved by alkali or milk. It is for this reason that many patients do not seek medical advice until they have had the disease for many years. In addition, the pain is episodic, coming and going over periods of months for unknown reasons. There appears to be a spring and fall seasonal occurrence and a relapse during periods of extreme stress. The development of constant pain is a sign of deep penetration. Referral of pain to the back is often associated with penetration into the pancreas. Generalized severe abdominal pain is a sign of free perforation.

Bleeding. Gastrointestinal bleeding is a common manifestation of duodenal ulcer. This is not surprising, since the duodenal wall has an abundant blood supply, and there are several large blood vessels posterior to the duodenal bulb. In fact, most cases of massive upper gastrointestinal hemorrhage are secondary to a posterior ulcer that has penetrated into the gastroduodenal artery or one of its branches. Most ulcers are more superficial or are located on the duodenal wall that is not adjacent to large blood vessels. This is the reason why most duodenal ul-

cers present with only minor bleeding episodes, usually detected by melenic (black) or guaiac positive feces.

Obstruction. Duodenal ulcer during a period of activity is often associated with delayed gastric emptying characterized by anorexia, or nausea, or vomiting. These symptoms may be a consequence of pylorospasm or obstruction to the gastric outlet by an inflammatory mass. In cases of protracted vomiting, patients may become dehydrated and develop a hypokalemic, hypochlorhydric alkalosis from the loss of large amounts of gastric juice that is rich in hydrogen, chloride, and potassium ions. Therapy, therefore, includes intravenous restitution of these losses and nasogastric suction for control and assessment of replacement needs. Until the chloride and potassium deficits have been replaced, the kidney is unable to correct the metabolic alkalosis.

Long-standing duodenal ulcer, with recurrent episodes of healing and repair, may lead to cicatricial stenosis of the lumen of the duodenum. Patients with pyloric obstruction on this basis usually have painless vomiting of large volumes of undigested food once or twice a day. The stomach in this condition is usually massively dilated and has lost its muscular tone. This form of obstruction may be associated with marked weight loss and malnutrition. Treatment is always surgical after appropriate metabolic and nutritional preparation that may include a period of parenteral hyperalimentation.

Perforation. Penetration of an ulcer through the duodenal wall is usually accompanied by an effort at containment by the greater omentum or adjacent viscera. Occasionally (about 5 percent of the time), a penetrating ulcer will perforate into the free peritoneal cavity. This is a dramatic clinical event, characterized by severe generalized abdominal pain, fever, tachycardia, dehydration, and ileus. This complication represents a surgical emergency. The diagnosis is easily made by palpation of the abdomen, which almost always reveals exquisite tenderness, rigidity, and rebound. Percussion demonstrates loss of liver dullness. An upright radiograph of the chest will usually demonstrate free air beneath the diaphragm. Operation to close the perforation and clean the peritoneal cavity should be carried out within a few hours after the patient enters the emergency department. Operation should be delayed only for appropriate fluid resuscitation. Early intervention will usually reveal sterile exudate within the abdomen; delay will most certainly be associated with a subsequent septic complication. A prompt operation may also provide an opportunity for performing an acid-reducing procedure if indicated.

Zollinger-Ellison Syndrome. The description of an association between a pancreatic tumor and severe ulcer disease by Zollinger and Ellison in 1955 initiated a new era in the study and treatment of acid-peptic disease of the duodenum. Their observation was made before the isolation and characterization of gastrin and the ability to measure its presence in the bloodstream by radioimmunoassay. Gastrointestinal endoscopy was in its early phase of development, and medical treatment for ulcer disease centered on antacids. A great deal of knowledge about peptic ulcer has derived from the study of the Zollinger-Ellison

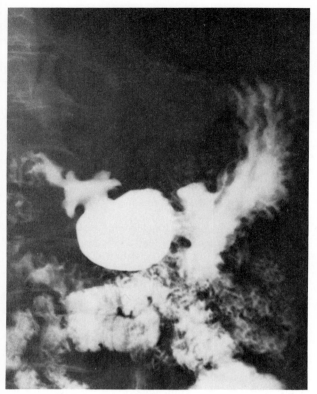

Fig. 26-12. Barium radiograph demonstrating the classic cloverleaf appearance of a deformed duodenal bulb due to the scarring of chronic ulcer disease. *(Courtesy of FA Mann, MD.)*

syndrome, a disease characterized clinically by flagrant duodenal ulcer disease, high basal acid secretory outputs, and a pancreatic tumor. Serum gastrin levels are usually in excess of 1000 pg/mL, but in some cases, the serum gastrin may be only mildly elevated for reasons not yet known. In the latter cases, serum gastrin levels can be increased by provocation with the intravenous administration of calcium or secretin. Increase in serum gastrin to above 350 pg/mL when calcium is infused at a rate of 4 μg/(kg · h) is indicative of a gastrinoma. An increase of serum gastrin in excess of 150 pg/mL in response to a bolus dose of 2 μg/kg of secretin is also considered to be a positive response. The true value of these tests is still being studied.

The pancreatic tumor of Zollinger-Ellison disease is a true neoplasm. In fact, approximately half of the patients have metastases to adjacent pancreatic nodes or the liver at the time of the discovery of the disease. Fortunately, the neoplasm has a slow growth pattern, and survival, even with proved metastases, is in the range of decades rather than months or years, as is true of most gastrointestinal malignancies.

DIAGNOSIS. Active ulcer disease of the duodenum can usually be detected by a directed history and careful physical examination. When epigastric pain and tenderness are the only findings, a clinical trial of antacid or antisecretory therapy may be sufficient to provide symp-

tomatic relief, healing, and in some instances a cure. This is especially true when symptoms are of an acute nature and related to environmental stress. In most cases, however, there is a history of chronic dyspepsia, and activity is manifested by bleeding or incapacitating pain. These symptoms require endoscopic examination of the duodenum to determine the precise nature of the lesion. Examination of the upper gastrointestinal tract by barium radiography is also a useful study to determine the location and depth of penetration of the ulcer, as well as the extent of deformation from chronic fibrosis (Fig. 26-12). Unfortunately, superficial ulceration will not be detected by this technique. False negatives in the range of 50 percent have been documented by follow-up endoscopy when ulcer symptoms are present and barium radiographs are negative. Pyloric obstruction is easily diagnosed by an upright radiograph of the abdomen; perforation is best detected by a chest x-ray also performed in the upright position (Fig. 26-13*A* and *B*).

TREATMENT. Medical. The medical therapy of duodenal ulcer is based upon the premise that it is a chronic, incurable disease. Treatment, therefore, is directed toward symptomatic relief during periods of acute exacerbation. This is best accomplished by a 6-week course of the H_2 blocker, cimetidine, in a dose of 300 mg four times a day. The frequent (every-hour) ingestion of antacids is as effective as antisecretory therapy for symptomatic relief, but the H_2 blockers shorten the period of complete healing. Furthermore, patient compliance appears to be higher on H_2 blockers in view of the ease of taking a pill and the avoidance of the undesirable intestinal symptoms (diarrhea or constipation) associated with antacid ingestion. Tranquilizers and diets have not proved to be efficacious, although both are employed on an empiric basis by most clinicians. A six-feeding bland diet may help to reduce the gastric phase of acid secretion. Tranquilizers themselves have a modest antisecretory effect. A new generation of H_2 blockers (ranitidine) are now available that are more potent and associated with even fewer side effects than cimetidine. A highly specific inhibitor of the hydrogen-potassium ATPase is also undergoing human trials (omeprazole). These advances will offer not only the possibility of providing symptomatic relief during activity but also the possibility of protection against recurrences. Knowledge derived from their mechanisms of action may also lead to an understanding of the pathogenesis of the disease and its ultimate prevention. There is no question that acid antisecretory agents have made a profound impact on the treatment of this common disease.

Surgical. Surgical therapy for chronic duodenal ulcer has two purposes: (1) to salvage patients from the life-threatening complications of perforation, massive hemorrhage, and gastric outlet obstruction and (2) to provide cure for the disease in the form of protection from recurrence. The indications for surgery, therefore, include perforation, obstruction, massive bleeding, and intractable abdominal pain.

The objective of therapy for perforation is early recognition of the complication and prompt closure of the opening in the duodenum. This procedure, termed "plica-

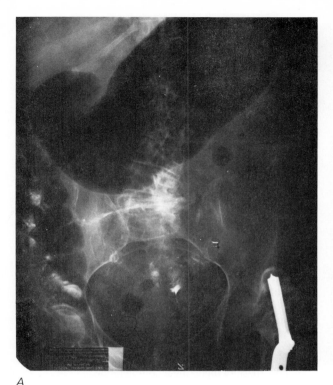

A

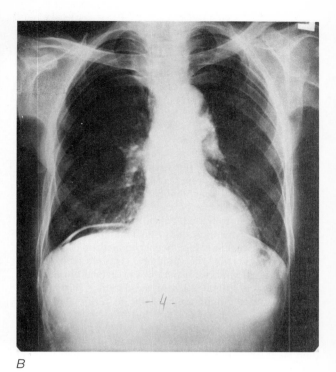

B

Fig. 26-13. *A*. Plain abdominal film demonstrating massive gastric distention. *B*. Erect chest film demonstrating free air under the right hemidiaphragm.

tion,'' is accomplished through an upper midline incision. Usually three or four silk (00) sutures placed in seromuscular fashion across the site of perforation is sufficient for secure closure. It is customary to tie in a tag of omentum with these sutures to provide a biologic buttress, a procedure termed a "Graham patch." Thorough cleansing of the peritoneal cavity by irrigation is an essential part of the operation. A major decision relates to whether an acid-reducing procedure should be performed as part of the therapy. The criteria for this approach include long-standing ulcer symptoms, a perforation of less than 6 h duration, and a patient whose condition is conducive to a longer operation than is associated with simple plication. The procedure of choice is a truncal vagotomy and Heineke-Mikulicz pyloroplasty (Fig. 26-14) with excision of the ulcer that is almost always on the anterior surface of the first part of the duodenum.

Pyloric obstruction can be treated by either a partial gastrectomy or vagotomy and drainage procedure. The former is preferred when the stomach is massively dilated. By this approach, the potentially deleterious effects of vagotomy on gastric emptying are avoided. Truncal vagotomy with pyloroplasty or gastroenterostomy, however, conserves the gastric reservoir and can be done with a lower risk in these patients who may have incompletely corrected fluid and electrolyte imbalance or malnutrition. A newer and more rational approach is the per-

Fig. 26-14. Diagram of the most frequently used drainage procedures: *A*. Heineke-Mikulicz pyloroplasty. *B*. Finney pyloroplasty. *C*. Jaboulay pyloroplasty. *D*. Gastroenterostomy.

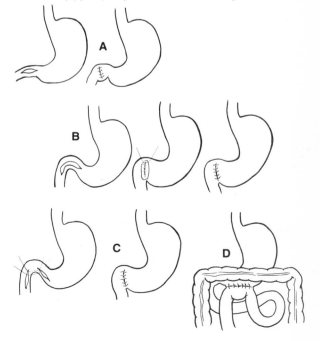

Table 26-2. RESULTS OF OPERATIONS FOR
DUODENAL ULCER

	Mortality	Morbidity	Recurrence
Partial gastrectomy	3%	10%	5%
Vagotomy and antrectomy	2%	12%	1%
Vagotomy and drainage	1%	15%	10%
Proximal gastric vagotomy	0.5%	5%	15%

formance of a proximal gastric vagotomy with either a pyloroplasty or gastroenterostomy (Fig. 26-14). This operation allows for preservation of the antral pump, thereby reducing the incidence of dumping, gastric stasis, and bile reflux gastritis.

Rapid, uncontrolled bleeding from a duodenal ulcer (usually posterior) requires surgical intervention once the intravascular volume has been reconstituted. Immediately upon entering the abdomen, the surgeon incises through the midanterior aspect of the distal 3 cm of stomach and the proximal 2 cm of duodenum. This incision provides direct visualization of the posterior wall of the duodenum, the ulcer crater, and the spurting vessel within its base. Bleeding can be controlled by compression with the left index finger, and the open vessel can then be easily secured by undersewing the finger with 00 silk on a stout needle. Sutures should be placed above and below this point in order to ensure complete encirclement of the gastroduodenal artery in this area. It may be necessary to place sutures deep at all four quadrants of the lesion. Some surgeons prefer a horizontal mattress stitch to encompass the bleeding vessel. Careful suture ligature of the vessel is essential if rebleeding is to be avoided. The operation is completed by a truncal vagotomy and pyloroplasty. A gastric resection should not be attempted because of the possibilities of pancreatic injury, anastomotic leak, or blown duodenal stump, complications that account for the majority of deaths in ulcer surgery.

The management of a medically controlled major bleed, or recurrent minor bleed, is controversial. Availability of effective antisecretory agents has introduced an element of uncertainty in these complications that were considered to be indications for operation in the recent past. Proximal gastric vagotomy is the preferred approach for reasons that will be discussed below.

Intractable pain is no longer a common indication for ulcer surgery. It has been reasonably well demonstrated that patients with intractable pain are usually poorly compliant in their antacid therapy. Antisecretory therapy has improved compliance of medical therapy and may account for the remarkable decrease in the number of cases of intractable pain referred for surgical therapy during the past 5 to 10 years. An operative approach is necessary in truly noncompliant patients or in those who cannot bear the expense or inconvenience of prolonged or repeated courses of H_2 blockage. These individuals should have a proximal gastric vagotomy as the next step in the treatment of their disease.

The relative advantages of the various operations for duodenal ulcer are shown in Table 26-2. Notice that proximal gastric vagotomy has a remarkably low morbidity and mortality but has a recurrence rate that is comparable with or even higher than truncal vagotomy and drainage. Antrectomy and vagotomy provide the best assurance of a low recurrence rate but at a mortality and morbidity that would be unacceptable for patients with easily controllable ulcer symptoms, which represents the majority. Candidates for vagotomy and antrectomy include patients who are to undergo an elective operation for a major complication of their ulcer and who are at high risk for recurrence. These would include individuals in high-stress situations, heavy smokers, chronic alcoholics, and patients who have known high acid secretory rates unrelated to hypergastrinemia. Such patients are usually middle-aged, heavy-set, aggressive, reasonably successful males.

There is some evidence that females do not tolerate truncal vagotomy as well as males. The availability of proximal gastric vagotomy offers an excellent alternative to partial gastrectomy for use in females needing surgery for peptic ulcer. The surgical therapy for duodenal ulcer, other than Zollinger-Ellison syndrome and the exceptions listed above, is based upon the reduction of the acid secretory response by vagotomy. This can be accomplished by division of the vagi above their major abdominal branches, thereby incurring a complete vagal denervation of the intraabdominal viscera. Selective vagotomy, whereby the major trunks are divided below the hepatic and celiac branches to include transection of the nerves of Laterjet, provides for total gastric denervation. Proximal gastric vagotomy, wherein the small branches of the nerves of Laterjet to the fundus are divided close to the gastric wall, leaves the vagal innervation undisturbed to the antrum and other intraabdominal viscera. Truncal vagotomy is currently the most popular method of gastric denervation because of its simplicity. Selective vagotomy is the best way to denervate the gastric remnant following antrectomy, but it does not reduce the incidence of postgastrectomy sequelae. Because of its low early and late morbidity, proximal gastric vagotomy has emerged as the preferred operation for duodenal ulcer when drainage is not required.

Truncal and selective vagotomy may lead to gastric stasis and therefore must be accompanied by a drainage procedure. Three types of pyloroplasty (Heineke-Mikulicz, Finney, and Jaboulay) are recommended for this purpose. They differ in the way in which the pylorus is reconstructed or bypassed, as shown in Fig. 26-14. A gastroenterostomy is also an acceptable way to prevent stasis following truncal gastric vagotomy, but it is more complex than pyloroplasty and therefore used when the latter cannot be easily performed.

Gastric resections are described by the amount of stomach removed: antrectomy (one-third), hemigastrectomy (one-half), partial gastrectomy (two-thirds), subtotal gastrectomy (three-fourths), and total gastrectomy. Except as described below for gastric cancer and the Zollinger-Ellison syndrome, attempts are made to preserve antral function and the gastric reservoir. When resection

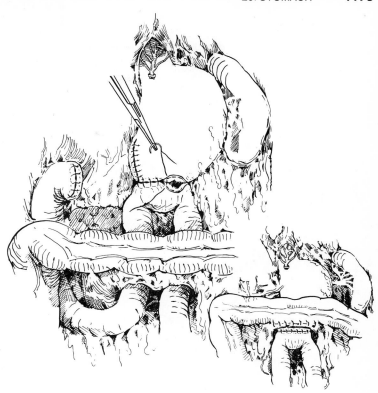

Fig. 26-15. Diagram of a Billroth II gastrojejunostomy placed behind the transverse colon. For cancer, the anastomosis is usually done in front of the colon away from areas of possible recurrence.

is required for benign ulcer of the duodenum or stomach, the gastric remnant is usually anastomosed to the duodenum (Billroth I), whereas resection for neoplasm is usually followed by a gastrojejunostomy (Billroth II) in order to avoid obstruction from tumor recurrence at the anastomosis (Fig. 26-15).

The surgical treatment of the Zollinger-Ellison syndrome has undergone dramatic change in recent years since the introduction of the H_2 blocker, cimetidine. Patients who are refractory to cimetidine or ranitidine usually respond to omeprazole. Dosages of cimetidine in the range of 600 mg four times a day have been effective in controlling the severe ulcer diathesis associated with the syndrome. Unfortunately, medical control precludes staging of the extent of the neoplastic process within the pancreas and adjacent lymph nodes and viscera. In addition, there are increasing numbers of reports documenting that many patients with a gastrinoma gradually become refractory to cimetidine and require total gastrectomy for control of ulcer disease. More recently it has been observed that proximal gastric vagotomy serves as a useful adjunct to cimetidine therapy by rendering the acid secretory cells more sensitive to lower doses of the drug. Another advantage to utilizing proximal gastric vagotomy as a component of initial pharmacologic therapy is the opportunity that it provides for assessing the extent of tumor. Occasionally (<5 percent of the time), the gastrinoma consists of a single tumor mass located within the distal pancreas that is readily accessible to excision and permanent cure. It is generally agreed that Zollinger-

Ellison patients should not have partial gastric resections, since recurrences in this situation can be catastrophic. Total gastrectomy with esophagojejunostomy in Roux en Y fashion (Fig. 26-16) is a safe operation that is well tolerated in the Zollinger-Ellison patient.

Peptic Ulcer—Stomach

ACUTE EROSIVE GASTRITIS

The gastric epithelium is constantly at risk of injury from ingestants in combination with its own secretions. Acute mucosal injury, called *erosive gastritis*, is the most common cause of upper gastrointestinal bleeding and by far the most frequent pathologic process within the stomach. The clinical problem is compounded by its relatively frequent occurrence in the setting of severe illness, or following physical or thermal injury, sepsis, or shock. Stress erosive gastritis has been of particular interest to the surgeon since it may require a surgical intervention in an already critically ill patient. Fortunately, advances in the understanding of the pathogenesis of the disease have led to a variety of ways to prevent its occurrence or progression.

MECHANISMS. The pathogenesis of erosive gastritis involves five variables: (1) acid secretion, (2) rate of back-diffusion of H^+ ions (the gastric barrier), (3) gastric mucosal blood flow, (4) mucus and alkaline secretion, and (5) submucosal buffers. Obviously, many other factors are involved in maintaining normal epithelial function,

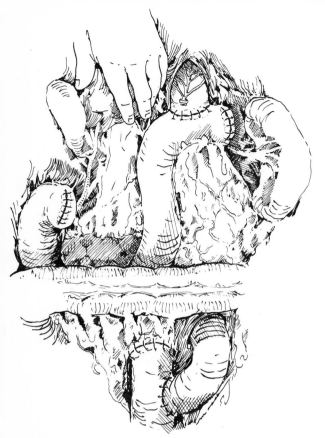

Fig. 26-16. Roux en Y reconstruction after total gastrectomy.

but their role in the pathogenesis of erosive gastritis has not yet been identified.

The dictum "no acid, no ulcer" clearly applies to erosive gastritis. This has been well established in experimental models and in the clinical situation. In fact, it represents the basis for modern therapy of the disease.

The precise role of H^+ ions in ulcerogenesis is not known. It has been well established, however, that the gastric epithelium is relatively impervious to H^+ ions, thereby accounting for their millionfold gradient from blood to gastric lumen. A disruption of this cation barrier leads to an influx of H^+ ions and an efflux of Na^+ ions, bicarbonate, and water. Breaking of the barrier by noxious agents such as aspirin, alcohol, or bile salts may lead to acute erosions within the superficial layers of the gastric epithelium. A variety of protective mechanisms attempt to counteract this possibility. Mucus and an alkaline secretion are produced by the surface epithelial cells in an attempt to wash away and neutralize the effects of the barrier breaker and H^+ ions by dilution and alkalinization. These functions of the surface cell represent the first line of defense against external injury.

Gastric mucosal blood flow maintains the epithelial integrity by delivery of buffers and nutrients to the gastric cells. Substrates for oxidative metabolism such as oxygen play a key role in this regard. Curiously, even prolonged intervals of hypoxia or hypoperfusion do not induce injury in the absence of H^+ ions and chemical disruption of the barrier. A critical relationship exists between the rate of hydrogen ion back diffusion, gastric mucosal blood flow, and extent of mucosal injury.

The role of mucus and buffer secretion by surface cells is only now being studied in a comprehensive way. Knowledge of these events is much too new to make a clear statement of their importance in the pathogenesis of acute lesions. It is possible that thickening of the mucus coat on the luminal side of the surface cell may provide an unstirred layer that allows entrapment and a titration sink for H^+ ions. This theory is currently under study in several laboratories.

Another area of intense inquiry relates to the fate of H^+ ions once they permeate the surface cell layer. It has been well established that acidification of the lamina propria can lead to surface cell injury, and that neutralization of this process by parenteral alkalinization can prevent cell loss. For example, the secreting stomach is less prone to experimental injury, possibly as a consequence of the delivery of alkali to the lamina propria following its discharge into the gastric venous effluent after the secretion of an H^+ ion into the stomach. The importance of this concept to the clinical problem has yet to be defined.

DIAGNOSIS. Painless upper gastrointestinal bleeding is the clinical hallmark of erosive gastritis. It may be characterized by hematemesis, bloody nasogastric aspirate, melena, or anemia associated with the detection of occult blood in the stool. Pain is uncommon and, when present, is a sign of a penetrating ulcer. Small amounts of blood in the nasogastric aspirate of patients in a critical care setting are so common that they provide enough evidence for making a presumptive working diagnosis without further work-up. Massive hematemesis requires gastric lavage for cleansing and endoscopic examination to determine the anatomic lesion. Superficial erosions rarely bleed rapidly; vomiting of large volumes of blood is an indication of penetration of an erosion into a large blood vessel within the submucosa or the presence of a chronic gastric or duodenal ulcer. Barium studies are not useful in this disease.

TREATMENT. The therapy of erosive gastritis is directed toward intravascular volume replacement and early control of hemorrhage by nonsurgical means. Gastric lavage with room temperature solutions such as water or saline is an important first step in therapy. The stomach must be completely evacuated of its blood contents in order to reduce fibrinolysis at bleeding sites. In addition, the stomach will be stimulated to secrete acid if the antrum is distended by clots. More than 80 percent of patients stop bleeding with this simple maneuver.

The third step in management is to provide for intragastric neutralization. This may be accomplished by inhibiting acid secretion with cimetidine (300 mg I.V. every 6 h) or the instillation of antacids (30 to 60 mL/h) into the stomach, checking its effectiveness by assessing gastric neutrality (pH > 5) by pH-sensitive paper at the end of each hour. The latter process must be pursued diligently if further penetration of erosions with rebleeding is to be avoided. Furthermore, antacid therapy must be included when cimetidine is used in the treatment of erosive gastritis.

If bleeding persists or recurs, the patient should be treated by transendoscopic bipolar electrocautery or by laser photocoagulation. Pharmacologic control by the selective infusion of pitressin into the left gastric artery is also effective, since it induces spasm and thrombosis of the bleeding artery. The associated decrease in mucosal perfusion does not lead to further ulceration if the gastric contents are carefully alkalinized during therapy. Transluminal occlusion of the left gastric artery by a gel forms a clot, or a coil is also an effective way to control bleeding from a branch of this vessel.

Bleeding that recurs or persists, requiring more than 6 units of blood (3000 mL), is an indication for operation. Since most erosions occur in the fundus of the stomach, a long anterior gastrotomy is made in this area. The gastric lumen is cleared of blood, and the mucosal surface is inspected for bleeding points in deeply penetrating lesions. These are secured with silk (00) by a figure-of-eight stitch taken deep within the gastric wall. Each actively bleeding site should be secured in this way. The majority of superficial erosions will not be actively bleeding and do not require ligature unless a blood vessel can be felt or seen at its base. The operation is completed by closure of the anterior gastrotomy and the performance of a truncal vagotomy and pyloroplasty. The incidence of rebleeding is less than 5 percent if bleeding points are carefully looked for and secured.

Some surgeons prefer a liberal partial gastrectomy and vagotomy. In fact, near-total gastrectomy even has its advocates because of concern over the possibilities of rebleeding. This radical surgical approach has no justification except in the rare instance in which suture ligature with vagotomy and pyloroplasty fails.

PREVENTION. An understanding of the importance of intragastric neutralization in erosive gastritis has provided a rationale for the prevention of the disease in critically ill patients. The efficacy of alkalinization has been established by randomized controlled trials. Inhibition of acid secretion by cimetidine has emerged as a useful adjunct to antacid therapy, since it reduces the need for instillation of large volumes of buffer that can lead to undesirable side effects. Cimetidine alone, however, does not provide adequate protection.

Prostaglandins of the E series have emerged as a potentially important group of compounds that may in themselves offer protection to the gastric epithelium. Their mechanism of action is not precisely known, but they may work through stimulation of mucus and alkaline secretion, enhancement of mucosal blood flow, or inhibition of acid secretion. The importance of the latter biologic property of prostaglandins has been challenged, since prostaglandins provide cytoprotection at dosages below those that inhibit acid secretion, and noninhibitory prostaglandins can also prevent experimentally induced gastritis. Prostaglandins have not yet been made available for clinical use because of undesirable side effects.

CHRONIC GASTRIC ULCER

DIFFERENTIAL DIAGNOSIS. Chronic gastric ulceration presents a unique challenge in diagnosis since malignant and benign lesions share many clinical and pathologic features. The advent of endoscopic biopsy and brush cytology has reduced uncertainty in this area, but a significant false-negative rate (5 to 10 percent), i.e., the lesion is neoplastic but the biopsies are benign, still exists. It is for this reason that patients with gastric ulcer require careful follow-up by radiographs and repeat endoscopy with biopsy if the ulcer persists. Gastric analysis can also be helpful since achlorhydria to maximal histamine stimulation excludes the possibility of a peptic ulcer.

The pathogenesis of a benign gastric ulcer remains unknown. Several prominent contributing factors are age (>forty), sex (female/male, 2/1), ingestion of barrier-breaking drugs such as aspirin, and malnutrition. Numerous attempts have been made to implicate chronic gastric ischemia, but with little success. The occurrence of the lesions on the lesser curvature at the junction of the antral and fundic mucosa suggests the possibility of a breakdown of mucosal protective factors at that site, but there is no evidence to support this speculation. It has been well demonstrated, however, that patients with gastric ulcer have an epithelium that is "leaky" to H^+ ions. This observation has suggested that regurgitation of bile acids and other barrier breakers within the duodenal succus may play an important role in the disease. Against this possibility is the fact that the experimental rerouting of bile through the stomach by a cholecystogastrostomy does not cause ulceration. Furthermore, chronic gastric ulceration is uncommon in patients with a gastroenterostomy, a situation in which bile is constantly bathing the mucosa of the gastric antrum. The most compelling evidence that the disease is acid-peptic in origin relates to the rapid healing that follows antacid therapy or vagotomy, even when the lesion-bearing portion of the stomach is left intact.

Ulceration within a gastric cancer is somewhat easier to explain. This lesion is most likely a consequence of local ischemia and malnourishment of the tissues within the center of the neoplastic process. It is easy to visualize how this might occur as the younger cells at the advancing edge of the penetrating neoplasm deprive the older cells within its center of nutrients and oxygen. The bulk lesion and infiltration of the gastric wall as revealed by barium radiographs provide the major diagnostic clues of the neoplastic nature of malignant ulcers. Furthermore, achlorhydria precludes peptic digestion of devitalized cells within the ulcer bed, resulting in an irregular, shaggy appearance in contrast to the clean, well-demarcated base of a benign peptic ulcer.

SYMPTOMS. Lack of appetite with vague upper abdominal distress following a meal is a common presenting complaint of patients with a benign gastric ulcer. This form of dyspepsia usually is accompanied by a gradual loss of weight as a consequence of a decrease in the intake of food. Severe pain is an unusual manifestation of the disease, except when the ulcer is located within the distal stomach or pyloric channel. Ulcers in this location assume the characteristics of a duodenal ulcer in that they are associated with increased rates of acid secretion, epigastric pain during the interdigestive period, and prompt relief with antacid ingestion. Gastric ulcers in the proximal stomach have less dramatic symptomatology and consequently may assume a large size and extensive depth of penetration before their detection.

Massive hemorrhage is an unusual event in chronic gastric ulceration; melena, or the detection of occult blood in the stool, is common. Gastric outlet obstruction as manifested by nausea and vomiting is also a rare finding, while delayed gastric emptying is frequent and the likely source of the vague ''indigestion'' experienced by this patient population.

DIAGNOSIS. Radiography. The upper gastrointestinal barium radiograph is the first step in diagnosis after a careful history and physical examination have focused attention on the stomach as the likely source of the patient's complaints. This is a simple, safe, convenient study that provides a great deal of diagnostic information in the hands of a well-trained radiologist. The radiographic characteristics of a benign gastric ulcer are shown in Fig. 26-17. A common mistake in the diagnostic approach is the utilization of endoscopic visualization of the lesion without obtaining a barium study. The two procedures complement each other. Their order of performance is obvious; barium examination performed first serves to identify the presence and location of a lesion

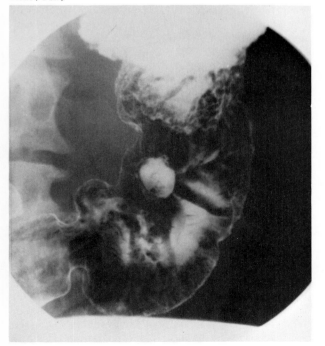

Fig. 26-17. This air contrast barium radiograph shows an ulcer with smooth margins. The rugal folds radiate toward the ulcer crater. This is the typical appearance of a benign ulcer. *(Courtesy of FA Mann, MD.)*

and the probability of its benign or malignant nature; subsequent endoscopy with biopsy provides a histologic diagnosis.

Endoscopy. The endoscopic appearance of a gastric ulcer offers information about its pathologic identity. Benign lesions usually have a well-demarcated, ''punched-out'' appearance, with a smooth base and a sharp, flat margin. Malignant ulcers usually have an irregular, ''heaped-up'' margin and a rough, necrotic-appearing base. Unfortunately, there is overlap, especially between benign ulcers and ulcerating cancers early in their genesis. This is why careful endoscopic biopsy at multiple sites at the margin of all gastric ulcers is a mandatory diagnostic procedure. It should not be omitted even when the radiograph and the eye suggest that the lesion is benign in appearance.

TREATMENT. Medical. The initial therapy for a benign gastric ulcer is a so-called medical trial. Unfortunately, there is no specific therapy for a gastric ulcer, since its etiology is unknown. The empiric use of antacid therapy appears to hasten the rate of ulcer healing. H_2 blockers such as cimetidine may also be a useful adjunct, but they were not found to be more effective than antacid therapy in ulcer healing. There has been a great deal of interest in diet manipulation that includes abstention from alcohol, spicy foods, and large meals that might aggravate symptoms associated with delayed gastric emptying. A six-feeding bland gastric diet is usually recommended for this reason. Aspirin and other barrier-breaking drugs (nonsteroidal, anti-inflammatory agents) must be stopped during the period of therapy. Sulfated glycoproteins (sucralfate), a new generation of antiulcer agents, appear to hasten the healing rate of gastric ulcer by binding to the devitalized tissues within the ulcer bed and thereby protecting it from further peptic digestion. Cytoprotective agents such as the prostaglandins of the E series may also play a role in the future of patients who must take barrier-threatening drugs on a chronic basis. This is currently an active area of investigation.

Unfortunately, some gastric ulcers, even when benign, fail to heal at a satisfactory rate (6 weeks) to provide symptomatic relief or assurance that they are not neoplastic. This situation requires a period of hospitalization for further evaluation and careful supervision of medical therapy. Since gastric ulcers are notorious for their tendency to recur even after a successful course of medical therapy, an operative approach should be considered early in patients with recalcitrant or recurrent benign gastric ulcers or when malignancy is even a remote possibility.

Surgical. The indications for surgical management of benign gastric ulcer are fairly clear-cut and include persistent bleeding, perforation, obstruction, failure to heal, recurrence, and suspicion of malignancy. Combined gastric and duodenal ulcer is also best treated by an acid-reducing procedure such as truncal vagotomy and antrectomy to include resection of the gastric ulcer. In fact, it is important to keep in mind that the surgical treatment of gastric ulcer must include a consideration of the presence of duodenal ulcer disease, since the rate of anastomotic ulcer is high (50 percent) if only a distal gastrectomy is used for this purpose.

The most popular operation for a benign lesser curvature gastric ulcer is a distal gastrectomy (antrectomy) to include the ulcer. Gastroduodenostomy is preferred since it reduces the risk of bile gastritis, iron deficiency, and afferent loop syndrome. The recurrence rate and incidence of undesirable side effects are low with this approach in the absence of duodenal ulcer disease or an overlooked cancer.

High-lying gastric ulcers near the esophagogastric junction present a special challenge in management. These can be locally excised or left in place in conjunction with a truncal vagotomy and pyloroplasty. Giant (>4 cm) benign ulcers are also a problem, since they may require an extensive gastric resection. Usually they occur in a malnourished, elderly patient who may have an underlying chronic disease. These patients are best managed by a period of hospitalization, parenteral hyperalimentation, and interval surgery (4 to 6 weeks) if inability to eat persists. Usually the ulcer reduces to a small size or heals during this period. Distal gastric and pyloric channel ulcers should be treated as a duodenal ulcer, since they usually are similar in their clinical presentation and relationship to acid hypersecretion.

Gastric Neoplasia

MALIGNANT TUMORS

The vast majority of gastric tumors are malignant, and of these, adenocarcinoma of the stomach is by far the most common (95 percent). Lymphomas (4 percent) and leiomyosarcomas (1 percent) constitute the rest, except for rare lesions such as squamous cell carcinoma, angiosarcoma, carcinosarcoma, and metastasis from adjacent or distant primary sites.

Cancer

Epidemiology. Gastric cancer is a biologically aggressive disease that is virtually incurable when discovered in its symptomatic phase. While it is worldwide in occurrence, its frequency varies greatly. Chile, Japan, and Iceland have the highest incidence. The disease is rarely encountered in Malaysia. The United States has experienced a rapid decline in stomach cancer deaths from a rate of 30 per 100,000 in 1930 to 8 per 100,000 today. The reason for this favorable trend is not known. Nor is the high incidence in some geographic areas understood, although a high consumption of smoked fish appears to be a characteristic common to these high-risk populations. Patients with pernicious anemia and blood group A also have an increased incidence of the disease, suggesting that genetic as well as environmental factors play a role. An important clue to pathogenesis is the high incidence of gastric cancer observed in the gastric remnant following operation for duodenal ulcer. This lesion is presumed to have its origins within the bile-induced gastritis so commonly found in this patient population.

Symptoms and Signs. Anorexia with weight loss is the most common sign of gastric cancer (>95 percent). Unfortunately, patients are relatively asymptomatic until there is extensive involvement of the gastric wall and adjacent viscera, or widespread metastases. Massive hematemesis occurs in less than 5 percent of patients, although the finding of occult blood in the stool is common. Nausea and vomiting may occur when distal lesions encroach upon the pylorus. Dysphagia is a dominant symptom when cancer arises within the cardia of the stomach. Pain is a late and uncommon complaint. While abdominal tenderness is a rare finding, a palpable abdominal mass is common (50 percent). Hepatomegaly is also a frequent finding and must arouse suspicion of liver metastases. Peritoneal seeding may cause massive ascites or involvement of the ovaries (Krukenberg tumor) or pelvic cul-de-sac (Bloomer's shelf) by gravitational metastases. These manifestations of advanced gastric cancer may lead to pelvic pain and constipation. A palpable lymph node in the left supraclavicular space (Virchow's node) is also a sign of advanced malignancy.

Pathologic Features. Gastric cancer may involve the stomach in a variety of ways (Table 26-3), even though each type usually originates from the progenitor cells at the base of the gastric pits. The most favorable form of the disease is superficial spreading carcinoma. In that condition, the neoplastic process does not penetrate through the muscularis mucosa, nor is it associated with a breakdown of the epithelium and chronic ulceration. Early detection by endoscopic biopsy and gastrectomy is associated with a good prognosis (75 percent with 10-year survival). Lesions of this type are usually detected by mass screening of high-risk populations by endoscopic visualization or photography.

Most symptomatic gastric cancers are infiltrating lesions that penetrate deep into the gastric wall. The luminal portion of the neoplastic process may be represented by a bulky tumor mass, a polypoid excrescence, or a flat, ulcerating lesion. Large cancers of this type are easily detected by radiography or endoscopy. Linitis plastica is an extensive infiltration of the gastric wall without tumor or ulceration. This form of gastric cancer produces a peculiar "leather-bottle" appearance to the gastric radiograph because of the rigid, nondistensible stomach.

Gastric cancer may spread in four ways: (1) lymphatics, (2) bloodstream, (3) peritoneal seeding, and (4) direct extension. More than half of the patients already have tumor spread at the time they seek medical therapy. It, therefore, is important to recognize high-risk groups. A family history of gastric cancer, detection of pernicious anemia, unexplained weight loss, and gastric symptoms that have their onset many years after gastrectomy re-

Table 26-3. TYPES OF GASTRIC CANCER

Superficial spreading
Polypoid
Ulcerative
Scirrhous-linitus plastica

quire careful medical evaluation. There is concern that chronic hypochlorhydria, even when obtained by H_2 blockers, may present a high-risk situation since bacterial overgrowth within the stomach may allow a buildup of oncogenic substances such as nitrosoureas.

Natural History. The tendency for gastric cancer to be advanced at the time of its detection has led to considerable therapeutic nihilism. This is not entirely justified, since gastric resection can provide excellent palliation in most patients and an occasional cure when the cancer is confined to the gastric epithelium. The latter form of the disease mimics chronic gastric ulcer. Even when such neoplastic ulcers are neglected, patients with them may survive for prolonged periods of time.

Chronic wasting and progressive weakness and cachexia constitute the usual mode of death. Liver and pulmonary metastases are common. Metastases to bone are uncommon; therefore, pain is usually not a major problem in management. Nutrition becomes the rate-limiting step in maintaining function due to mechanical or functional gastric obstruction caused by the cancer.

Therapeutic Alternatives. The therapy of gastric cancer is primarily surgical. Radiation and chemotherapy have little to offer even in the way of palliation. Except in advanced cases of carcinomatosis, a palliative subtotal gastrectomy should be done to provide a route for oral alimentation. When there is no evidence of distal spread, a radical subtotal gastrectomy should be performed for cure. This operation includes resection of the gastrocolic omentum and ligation of the right gastric, right gastroepiploic, and left gastric arteries at their origin. Approximately 4 cm of the proximal duodenum is included in the resection. More than 85 percent of the stomach is removed, and gastrointestinal continuity is reestablished by a gastrojejunostomy. Splenectomy and even total gastrectomy may be required when the lesion is large or within the proximal portion of the stomach.

Gastric resection usually provides a symptom-free interval of 1 or 2 years. Recurrences may respond to chemotherapy, although such responses are usually of short duration. The reported 5-year survival rate when gastric resection is performed for cure is less than 10 percent. Clearly, efforts must be directed toward early detection and prevention if survival statistics are to be improved. Mass screening in Japan by gastroscopy has established the validity of an aggressive public health approach. Cure rates are reported in the range of 85 percent at 5 years when gastric cancer is discovered in an early stage, when it is still confined to the epithelial surface of the stomach.

Lymphoma (Lymphosarcoma)

Gastric lymphoma may occur as an isolated neoplasm confined to the stomach, or it may be a manifestation of widespread infiltrative disease. The lesion may present as a tumor mass or, more commonly, as a thickening of the rugal epithelial folds secondary to lymphocytic infiltration within the submucosa. Anorexia and weight loss are the most common presenting complaints. Early satiety may also be a prominent symptom as the gastric wall becomes thickened, and the lumen is progressively compromised by the neoplastic infiltrate. Bleeding is uncommon.

Definitive diagnosis is made by endoscopic biopsy. Bulky lesions, with associated gastric outlet obstruction, are best treated by subtotal gastric resection and postoperative irradiation. Radiation therapy alone, however, provides a long-standing remission that is equal to that obtained by gastric resection in most cases. Radiation, in fact, has emerged as the treatment of choice because of its low morbidity. A combined approach is associated with an 85 percent, 5-year survival when the process is limited to the stomach. Involvement of the stomach by generalized lymphosarcoma is usually treated by radiation or chemotherapy. Gastrectomy in such cases is undertaken only when complications ensue or when the stomach is the major source of disabling symptoms, e.g., obstruction.

Leiomyosarcoma

This tumor of smooth muscle origin is the least common of gastric malignancies. Unfortunately, it usually grows to a very large size before detection because of its outward growth away from the gastric lumen. Distal spread, however, is late, and even massive tumors that become adherent to the liver or pancreas can be resected with prolonged survival. Leiomyosarcomas are not responsive to radiation or chemotherapy. They usually are detected following a gastrointestinal hemorrhage from a breakdown of overlying epithelium or as a consequence of malnutrition secondary to compromise of gastric storage capacity. They often are palpable on abdominal examination when they present in this way. Preoperative assessment can be enhanced by visceral angiography in order to determine mesenteric or hepatic vascular interrelationships to the tumor. Cleansing and chemical preparation of the large intestine are also useful, since resection of its transverse portion or splenic flexure may be required in order to encompass the tumor. Resection is the preferred treatment, even when all the tumor cannot be safely removed, since long-term survival is usual even in this incurable situation.

BENIGN TUMORS

Polyps

Papillary excrescences of the gastric epithelium (polyps) are the most common benign tumors of the stomach of clinical significance. They are of two types—inflammatory and adenomatous. While the latter are less common, they represent the more important lesion, since they are true neoplasms and may have a malignant potential. They can be distinguished from inflammatory polyps because of their long stalk and tendency to occur in the atrophic mucosa of patients with pernicious anemia. Occasionally, adenomatous polyps will arise in the stomach in conjunction with the multiple small bowel polyposis of the Peutz-Jeghers syndrome or the familial polyposis of Gardner's syndrome.

Inflammatory polyps are usually sessile excrescences within the antrum or fundus of the stomach. They are asymptomatic, except when they are adjacent to and prolapse through the pylorus. Hypertrophic gastritis

(Menetrier's disease) may also be associated with multiple inflammatory polypoid lesions within the fundic area of the stomach. These lesions can be distinguished from multiple gastric adenomatous polyposis by biopsy and histologic examination. They do not require surgical extirpation.

Gastric polyps should be biopsied and excised by ensnarement through the endoscope when their adenomatous nature has been determined. Malignant polyps should be treated as a gastric cancer by a partial gastrectomy. Patients with pernicious anemia require careful monitoring by gastric barium radiograph or endoscopy in order to detect neoplastic polyps early in their genesis.

Leiomyoma

Small, benign leiomyomas are commonly found within the smooth muscle of the gastric wall at autopsy or during palpation of the stomach at laparotomy. They are of little clinical significance until they enlarge to greater than 4 cm in diameter. At this point, they begin to compromise the blood supply to the overlying gastric epithelium. This leads to ulceration and proteolytic digestion of the core of the neoplasm that itself may have undergone central necrosis. This process culminates in a massive upper gastrointestinal hemorrhage that may require emergency gastric resection for control. Such lesions when large cannot be distinguished from their malignant counterparts and therefore should be treated by distal gastrectomy with a liberal margin (4 cm) proximally. Smaller lesions (<4 cm) can be shelled out of the gastric wall or removed by a wedge resection.

Fig. 26-18. Gross appearance of hypertrophic gastritis (Menetrier's disease).

Lipoma

Lipomas of the stomach are asymptomatic submucosal lesions that are a radiographic curiosity, distinguished by their smooth contour. Endoscopy will reveal their submucosal position. They need not be biopsied or excised.

Ectopic Pancreas

Rarely, a pancreatic rest will reside within the antrum of the stomach. While this lesion is usually submucosal, it often will present within the gastric lumen as an umbilicated dimple. It may require excision if there is a question about its nature or when patients present with unremitting dyspeptic symptoms that are refractory to antiulcer therapy.

Other Gastric Lesions

HYPERTROPHIC GASTRITIS (MENETRIER'S DISEASE)

Menetrier's disease is a rare inflammatory disease of the gastric epithelium that is characterized by massive gastric folds within the proximal stomach. In advanced stages, the epithelium assumes the appearance of large multiple polypoid excrescences as shown in Fig. 26-18. Histologic examination reveals that the thickened folds consist of a hypertrophy of the gastric glandular epithelium as well as a remarkable increase in the size of the submucosa that is edematous and contains a large number of small round cells. The latter finding has suggested that the disease may have an autoimmune component.

Menetrier's disease is characterized clinically by the massive amount of plasma proteins that can be lost through an epithelium that ordinarily is extremely tight to large molecules. The reason for this extraordinary event

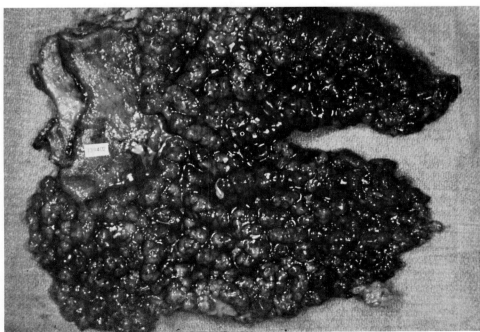

is not known. The immunologic aspects of the disease have not yet been studied.

Most cases of hypertrophic gastritis can be managed nonoperatively with treatment directed toward maintaining good nutrition and symptomatic relief of the vague gastric complaints offered by these patients. Rarely, loss of plasma proteins is so persistent and rapid that hypoproteinemia ensues. If left unrecognized, a state of severe protein deprivation may develop (kwashiorkor), with its attendant hepatic dysfunction, ascites, and peripheral edema. Cases with massive protein loss should have a total gastrectomy following a period of parenteral hyperalimentation. Individuals with less severe forms of the disease should be followed carefully by barium or endoscopic examination in view of the high incidence of gastric cancer reported in some series.

MALLORY-WEISS TEAR

Violent retching can lead to a disruption of the gastric mucosa high on its lesser curve at the esophagogastric junction. The usual story is that of retching after ingestion of solid food, which is followed shortly thereafter by bright red hematemesis. The mucosal tear often extends deep into the submucosa where a large arteriole is encountered as the source of bleeding. However, this lesion is associated with massive upper gastrointestinal bleeding in only 10 percent of cases. Alcoholics with portal hypertension may have as their source of bleeding a submucosal gastric or esophageal varix.

The diagnosis is suspected by history and confirmed by esophagogastroscopy. Rapidly bleeding lesions require immediate operation following reconstitution of intravascular volume. Nonactively bleeding tears can be safely observed and usually proceed to complete healing without symptoms or further evidence of bleeding.

The operation for persistent bleeding from a Mallory-Weiss tear is carried out through an upper midline incision. The lesion at the esophagogastric junction is approached through a long anterior gastrotomy. This provides a full view of the bleeding site which is secured by several deep 2-0 silk ligatures placed in such a way that the mucosal edges are reapproximated in an anatomic fashion. A supplemental antisecretory operation is not necessary. Extension of the tear into the lower end of the esophagus may require mobilization of the esophagogastric junction in order to approximate the margins of the esophageal component of tear. The operation is completed by a fundoplication whereby the upper part of the stomach is wrapped around the lower end of the esophagus. This provides protection to the closure. Furthermore, lesions of this type often occur in association with reflux esophagitis and direct hiatal hernia.

GASTRIC MUCOSAL PROLAPSE

There is uncertainty about whether the prolapse of antral gastric mucosa through the pylorus can lead to gastrointestinal symptoms. Unfortunately, it is observed as a radiologic finding in some patients with symptoms of acid-peptic disease who otherwise have no other findings to explain them. It is unlikely that the nonspecific complaints offered by such patients are a consequence of this radiographic curiosity.

ACUTE GASTRIC DILATATION

Sudden rapid distention of the stomach is associated with a vagovagal response characterized by pallor, sweating, bradycardia, hypotension, and abdominal pain in the nonsedated patient. Unfortunately, many patients develop this problem early after an operative procedure when they are under the influence of anesthetics and analgesics. If left unrecognized, gastric dilatation may lead to vomiting with aspiration, tissue decompensation from hypoxia, or bleeding from stress erosive gastritis. Treatment consists of nasogastric aspiration which can be dramatic in providing relief of associated symptoms. The stomach often requires a period of 24 to 48 h to regain normal emptying. Nasogastric aspiration should be maintained throughout this period of recovery.

GASTRIC VOLVULUS

Torsion of the stomach is an uncommon, serious complication that occurs in association with a paraesophageal hiatal hernia. In this condition, the stomach, which is located within the mediastinum in an orad-caudad reversal (upside-down stomach), can rotate in a clockwise manner, thereby entrapping ingestants, air, and gastric juice. The associated distention and venous obstruction lead to ischemic gangrene of the gastric wall and subsequent perforation. It is for this reason that patients with the otherwise relatively asymptomatic condition of paraesophageal hiatal hernia are advised to have an operative repair. The procedure usually involves returning the stomach to the abdominal cavity and closure of the large opening within the diaphragm adjacent to the right crus.

FOREIGN BODIES AND BEZOARS

The stomach becomes a repository for objects other than food that are taken into the mouth. Infants and those who are mentally deranged represent those most vulnerable to this complication. Children most commonly swallow coins, small parts of toys, or their diaper pins when they are very young. As a rule of thumb, blunt objects that enter the stomach will usually pass on through the intestinal tract. Sharp objects should be retrieved by endoscopy. If this cannot be easily accomplished, the progress of the object should be followed radiographically while carefully observing the patient for signs of perforation. Adults may ingest numerous large objects that make endoscopic retrieval both time-consuming and difficult. These cases usually require operative evacuation. Bulky, solid, nondigestible objects, retained for prolonged periods of time, may, even when single, require operative extraction.

Bezoars are conglomerates of nondigestible materials usually of vegetable origin. Persimmon peels or pits, orange or grapefruit pulp, or fruit pits are the usual offenders, especially in the postgastrectomy stomach. Patients of this type must be advised to avoid foodstuffs that have a great deal of cellulose or other vegetable fiber. Bezoars are associated with vague upper abdominal discomfort, nausea, and vomiting. A barium radiograph will reveal a mass lesion within the lumen of the stomach. Treatment consists of dissolution of the undigested bolus by ingestion of proteolytic enzymes such as papain or by mechanical fragmentation via the endoscope. Recurrence can be prevented by dietary management.

ATROPHIC GASTRITIS

Pernicious anemia is associated with a gradual thinning of the gastric epithelium of the proximal stomach and a complete loss of parietal cells. This results in achlorhydria and a loss of the secretion of intrinsic factor which is responsible for the absorption of vitamin B_{12}. A deficiency of this vitamin will develop within 3 or 4 years if it is not provided by monthly replacement (1000 μg I.M.). Atrophic gastritis itself does not produce symptoms. Its major significance is a high risk for gastric malignancy.

EOSINOPHILIC ANTRITIS

Rarely, eosinophils may infiltrate beneath the submucosa of the antrum, producing a nodular deformity. Patients with this lesion usually present with ill-defined complaints. The diagnosis can be confirmed by endoscopic biopsy. The pathogenesis and natural history of these lesions are unknown. Careful follow-up and observation are therefore essential if for no other reason than to learn what the clinical significance of this lesion might be.

CORROSIVE GASTRITIS

The ingestion of strong alkali or acid may lead to gastric as well as esophageal injury. Lye remains a principal cause of this problem even though alterations in packaging of caustic materials have decreased the frequency of accidental ingestion. Suicide attempts by ingestion of large volumes of liquid lye lead to severe erosive esophagitis and gastritis. The subsequent healing process may be associated with gastric outlet obstruction as well as esophageal stricture. Gastric perforation, however, is unusual.

The ingestion of strong acid (sulfuric or hydrochloric) may lead to a full-thickness perforation of the stomach. History of this form of caustic injury requires endoscopic visualization of the gastric epithelium. The identification of large areas of epithelial necrosis should lead to immediate exploration and resection of the involved stomach.

GASTRIC PROCEDURES FOR MORBID OBESITY

RATIONALE. Morbid obesity is a condition wherein people exceed twice their ideal weight. This physical state is not associated with symptoms or disease in early life. By midlife, however, the morbidly obese may develop hypertension, carbohydrate intolerance (adult-onset diabetes), degenerative arthritis, cardiopulmonary dysfunction, or gallstones. Possibly of equal importance is the fact that afflicted individuals are forced to live a suboptimum life since our culture is designed for slim people.

The pathogenesis of morbid obesity is poorly understood. Of the many factors involved, probably the most dominant is a combination of a genetic predisposition and an affluent society where there is an abundance of food. Childhood or teenage onset obesity appears to have this background. However, obesity that starts in midlife does not usually reach massive proportions. Obesity has been presumed to be an inequality of energy intake versus expenditure. Recent results from both animal and human studies suggest that body weight is not always directly related to the amount of food one eats. Some obesity may result from an inability to burn off excess calories as heat, leading to storage of these calories as fat. It is speculated that this disturbance in thermogenesis is due to a decreased amount of brown adipose tissue.

It is generally agreed that morbid obesity is refractory to medical therapy. Jejuno-ileal bypass, wherein the length of the small bowel is shortened, has been an effective way to induce weight loss in the morbidly obese. Its efficacy has been based upon the malabsorption of excess food. Diarrhea associated with overeating also contributes to a reduction in food intake. Unfortunately, the operation which involves anastomosis of the jejunum 14 in. beyond the ligament of Treitz to the ileum, 4 in. from the ileocecal valve, requires bypass of the majority of the small bowel. The bypassed segment in some way contributes to the development of liver disease in 5 to 10 percent of patients. Malabsorption is associated with fluid and electrolyte abnormalities in an additional 5 percent. Over 50 percent of jejuno-ileal bypass patients develop oxalate kidney stones. Bloating with crampy abdominal pain is also a common complaint. These side effects have led to an abandonment of the procedure.

OPERATIONS. Gastric operations for morbid obesity are designed to reduce the daily intake of food to less than 800 cal until weight reduction has been achieved. A variety of such operations have been developed and evaluated by Edward Mason and his colleagues at the University of Iowa. These procedures are depicted in Fig. 26-19. Gastric bypass, which consists of constructing a small proximal pouch that is drained into a loop or Roux en Y limb of jejunum, is the oldest and still the most popular procedure. Its disadvantages include a high operative morbidity, a 5 percent incidence of stomal ulcer, and uncertainties as to the future problems associated with bypass of the lower stomach and duodenum.

Attempts to gain and maintain weight loss by gastroplasty (gastric partition) have been less successful even though perioperative mortality and complications have been less. This procedure is accomplished by placing staples across the upper portion of the stomach. The size of the proximal pouch and stoma is usually similar to that employed in gastric bypass. Stomas have been placed on

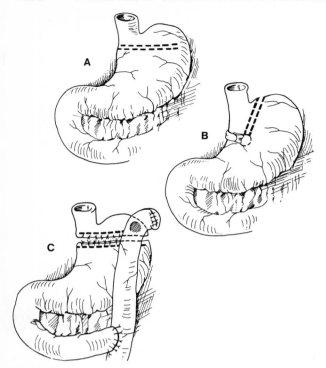

Fig. 26-19. Most common procedures designed to reduce gastric capacity and induce weight loss. *A.* Horizontal gastric partition. *B.* Vertical banded gastroplasty. *C.* Gastric emptying.

Table 26-4. MAJOR COMPLICATIONS OF GASTRIC BYPASS*

Wound infection	14%
Wound hernia	6%
Splenectomy	2%
Subphrenic abscess	2%
Gastric leak	5%
Pouch ulcer	3%
Pouch obstruction	5%
Bile gastritis	1%
Pneumonia	2%
Atelectasis	3%
Embolism	1%
Early reoperation	7%
Readmission for vomiting	5%
Postoperative death	
Pulmonary embolus	0.6%
Peritonitis	2%

* Adapted from Mason EE: Surgical treatment of obesity, in Ebert PA (ed): *Major Problems in Clinical Surgery*. Philadelphia, Saunders, 1981, vol XXVI, p 154.

either curvature of the stomach or its middle with comparable results. This procedure, called *gastric partition* or *stapling,* has a low morbidity and allows for subsequent visualization of the lower stomach and duodenum by radiography or endoscopy. In addition, the potential harmful side effects of antral and duodenal bypass can be avoided. Unfortunately, many patients ultimately lose the feeling of early satiety that they experienced in the early postoperative period (12 to 18 months). As they increase their intake, they stretch the pouch and the stoma. Ultimately, they are able to eat larger meals and slowly regain weight. Attempts to overcome this problem include use of a circumferential suture to prevent stomal dilatation, vertical rather than horizontal stapling to utilize the lesser curve as a nonelastic or less stretchable portion of the stomach, and gastric wrapping whereby the lumen is compromised by infolding of the gastric wall. These variations are currently under investigation.

RESULTS. There is no ideal operation for chronic morbid obesity. In fact, it may be an incurable disease at this stage because of our lack of understanding of its origins. For this reason safety and avoidance of long-term side effects must take precedence over efficacy as it might relate to a long-term cure. While gastric partition provides the best chance for safe palliation and retention of the integrity of the upper gastrointestinal tract, it does not provide for the rapid, extensive weight reduction that accompanies gastric bypass. However, gastric partition is still in the early phase of perfection and evaluation.

Mason and his colleagues have reported the largest and best studied series of patients undergoing gastric bypass. Their mortality and morbidity are shown in Table 26-4. More recently, they have abandoned gastric bypass in favor of gastric partitioning, currently performed by fashioning a 30-mL pouch along the proximal lesser curvature that communicates with the main stomach by a 1-cm conduit that is encircled by a Teflon ring. This is called a *vertical banded gastroplasty* since staples are placed in a vertical manner from the angle of His caudad in order to fashion the proximal pouch. Mason feels that this is the ultimate in gastric procedures for morbid obesity. However, the follow-up is too short for his results to support this contention. The need for performing an operation so deforming to the gastric outlet to gain dietary compliance is further testimony to the complex nature of the disease for which it is designed. The development of a multidisciplinary team approach has strengthened the follow-up and improved the results in most series. Dietary counseling, motivational support, exercise instruction, and social rehabilitation through a self-help group have greatly enhanced the effectiveness of the surgical approach.

Mason has pointed out that all forms of gastric capacity reduction will provide a 50 percent loss of excess weight in 75 percent of patients so treated. The remaining problem is that of long-term weight containment, which can be achieved only by a lifetime of dieting. For most patients with morbid obesity, this means 1000 cal or less each day for the rest of their lives.

Bibliography

History

Beaumont W: *Experiments and Observations on the Gastric Juice and the Physiology of Digestion.* New York, Dover, 1959.

Blalock JB Jr: History and evolution of peptic ulcer surgery. *Am J Surg* 141:317, 1981.

Jordan PH Jr: Duodenal ulcers and their surgical treatment: Where did they come from? *Am J Surg* 149:2, 1985.

Wagensteen OH, Wagensteen SD: Gastric surgery, in *The Rise of Surgery*. Minneapolis, University of Minnesota Press, 1978.

Zollinger RM: Reflections on gastric surgery. *Am J Surg,* 139:10, 1980.

Anatomy

Griffith CA: Anatomy, in Harkins HN, Nyhus LM (eds): *Surgery of the Stomach and Duodenum*. Boston, Little, Brown, 1969, p 25.

Lillibridge CB: The fine structure of normal human gastric mucosa. *Gastroenterology* 47:269, 1964.

McGuigan JE: Gastric mucosal intracellular localization of gastrin by immunofluorescence. *Gastroenterology,* 55:315, 1968.

Michels NA: Blood supply of the stomach and the esophagus, in *Blood Supply and Anatomy of the Upper Abdominal Organs*. Philadelphia, Lippincott, 1955, p 248.

Schofield GC: Anatomy of muscular and neural tissues in the alimentary canal, in Code CF (ed): *Handbook of Physiology*. Washington, DC, American Physiological Society, 1968, sec 6, p 1579.

Physiology

Card WI, Marks IN: The relationship between the acid output of the stomach following "maximal" histamine stimulation and the parietal cell mass. *Clin Sci* 19:147, 1960.

Cooke AR: Control of gastric emptying and motility. *Gastroenterology* 68:804, 1975.

Davenport HW: Gastric secretion, in *Physiology of the Digestive Tract*. Chicago, Year Book Medical Publishers, 1971, p 95.

Davenport HW: Why the stomach does not digest itself. *Sci Am* 226:86, 1972.

Davenport HW, et al: Functional significance of gastric mucosal barrier to sodium. *Gastroenterology* 57:142, 1964.

Debas HT, Hollinshead J, et al: Vagal control of gastrin release in the dog: Pathways for stimulation and inhibition. *Surgery* 95:34, 1984.

Dragstedt LR: The physiology of the gastric antrum. *Arch Surg* 75:552, 1957.

Edkins JS: The chemical mechanism of gastric secretion. *J Physiol* 34:183, 1906.

Flemstrom G: Gastroduodenal mucosal secretion of bicarbonate and mucus. Physiologic control and stimulation by prostaglandins. *Am J Med* 81:18, 1986.

Fordtran JS, Walsh JH: Gastric acid secretion rate and buffer control of the stomach after eating: Results in normal subjects and in patients with duodenal ulcer. *J Clin Invest* 52:645, 1973.

Gregory RA: Memorial lecture: The isolation and chemistry of gastrin. *Gastroenterology* 51:953, 1966.

Gregory RA, Tracy HJ: The constitution and properties of two gastrins extracted from hog antral mucosa. *Gut* 5:103, 1964.

Grossman MI: Neural and hormonal stimulation of gastric secretion of acid, in Code CF (ed): *Handbook of Physiology*. Washington, DC, American Physiological Society, 1967, sec 6, vol II, p 835.

Grossman MI, et al: Candidate hormones of the gut. *Gastroenterology* 67:730, 1974.

Heading RC, et al: Gastric emptying rate measurement in man. A double isotope scanning technique for simultaneous study of liquid and solid components of a meal. *Gastroenterology* 71:45, 1976.

Hunt JN, Knox MT: Regulation of gastric emptying, in Code CF (ed): *Handbook of Physiology*. Washington, DC, American Physiological Society, 1968, sec 6, vol IV, p 1917.

Hunt JN, Stubbs DF: The volume and energy content of meals as determinants of gastric emptying. *J Physiol (London)* 245:209, 1975.

Ippoliti AF, et al: Demonstration of the intestinal phase of gastric acid secretion in man. *Gastroenterology* 70:896, 1976.

Jeffries GH: Gastric secretion in intrinsic factor, in Code CF (ed): *Handbook of Physiology*. Washington, DC, American Physiological Society, 1967, sec 6, vol II, p 919.

Johnson LR: Progress in gastroenterology: The trophic action of gastrointestinal hormones. *Gastroenterology* 70:278, 1976.

Kelly KA, Code CF: Canine gastric pacemaker. *Am J Physiol* 220:112, 1971.

Kleibeuker JH, Eysselein VE, et al: Role of endogenous secretin in acid-induced inhibition of human gastric function. *J Clin Invest* 73:526, 1984.

Makhlouf GM, et al: A quantitative statement of the two component hypothesis of gastric secretion. *Gastroenterology* 51:149, 1966.

Malagelada JR, et al: Measurement of gastric function during digestion of ordinary solid meals in man. *Gastroenterology* 70:203, 1976.

Meyer JH, Mayer EA, et al: Gastric processing and emptying of fat. *Gastroenterology* 90:1176, 1986.

Nyhus LM, et al: The control of gastric release: An experimental study illustrating a new concept. *Gastroenterology* 39:582, 1960.

Richardson CT, et al: Studies on the role of cephalic-vagal stimulation in the acid secretory response to eating in normal human subjects. *J Clin Invest* 60:435, 1977.

Samloff IM: Pepsinogens, pepsins and pepsin inhibitors. *Gastroenterology* 69:586, 1971.

Sircus W: The intestinal phase of gastric secretion. *Q J Exp Physiol* 38:91, 1953.

Thompson JC: Gastrointestinal hormones—introduction to symposium on gastrointestinal hormones. *World J Surg* 3:389, 1979.

Uvnas B: Role of duodenum in inhibition of gastric acid secretion. *Scand J Gastroent* 6:113, 1971.

Walsh JH, Grossman MI: Gastrin. *N Engl J Med* 292:1324, 1975.

White CM, Poxon V, et al: The importance of the distal stomach in gastric emptying of liquids in man. *Surg Gastroenterol* 3:13, 1984.

Wolf S, Wolff HG: *Human Gastric Function*. London, Oxford University Press, 1943.

Woodward ER: The role of the gastric antrum in the regulation of gastric secretion. *Gastroenterology* 38:7, 1960.

Gastric Dysfunction

Alexander-Williams J: Alkaline reflux gastritis: A myth or a disease? *Am J Surg* 143:17, 1982.

Barnes AD, Cox AG: Diarrhea, in Williams JA, Cox AG (eds): *After Vagotomy*. London, Butterworth, 1969, p 211.

Baron JH: The clinical use of gastric function tests. *Scand J Gastroent Suppl* 6:9, 1970.

Becker JM, Sava P, et al: Intestinal pacing for canine postgastrectomy dumping. *Gastroenterology* 84:383, 1983.

Condon JR, et al: The cause and treatment of postvagotomy diarrhea. *Br J Surg* 62:309, 1975.

Fiore AC, et al: Surgical management of alkaline reflux gastritis. *Arch Surg* 117:689, 1982.

Goldberg J, et al: A clinical evaluation of the maximal histalog test. *Am J Dig Dis* 12:468, 1967.

Gustavsson S, et al: Scintigraphic assessment of biliary reflux into the residual stomach after subtotal gastrectomy and gastrojejunostomy. *Acta Radiol [Diagn] (Stockh)* 21:639, 1980.

Halpern NB, et al: Failure to achieve success with remedial gastric surgery. *Am J Surg* 125:108, 1973.

Herrington JL Jr, Sawyers JL: Surgical management of alkaline reflux gastritis and esophagitis. *Surg Annu* 13:341, 1981.

Herrington JL Jr, et al: Surgical management of reflux gastritis. *Ann Surg* 180:526, 1974.

Hirschowitz BI, et al: Demonstration of a new gastroscope, the "Fiberscope." *Gastroenterology* 35:50, 1958.

Isenberg JI, et al: Pentagastrin vs betazole as stimulant of gastric secretion. *JAMA* 206:2897, 1968.

Johnstone FR, et al: Postgastrectomy problems in patients with personality defects: The "albatross" syndrome. *Can Med Assoc J* 96:1559, 1967.

Jordon GL: Surgical management of postgastrectomy problems. *Arch Surg* 102:251, 1971.

Kelly KA: Gastric motility in health and after gastric surgery. *Viewpoints, Dig Dis* 8:1, 1976.

Kennedy T: The failures of gastric surgery. *Br J Surg* 68:677, 1981.

Laufer I: A simple method for routine double constrast study of the upper gastrointestinal tract. *Radiology* 117:513, 1975.

Laufer I, et al: The diagnostic accuracy of barium studies of the stomach and duodenum—correlation with endoscopy. *Radiology* 115:569, 1975.

LeQuesne LP, et al: The dumping syndrome—1. Factors responsible for the symptoms. *Br Med J* 1:141, 1960.

Lundh G: Intestinal digestion and absorption after gastrectomy. *Acta Chir Scand Suppl* 231:1, 1958.

Martin LF, Larson GM, et al: Bleeding from stress gastritis. Has prophylactic pH control made a difference? *Am Surg* 5:189, 1985.

Mathias JR, Fernandez A, et al: Nausea, vomiting, and abdominal pain after Roux en Y anastomosis: Motility of the jejunal limb. *Gastroenterology* 88:101–107.

Metzger WH, et al: Effect of metoclopramide in chronic gastric retention after gastric surgery. *Gastroenterology* 71:30, 1976.

Phillips JC, et al: Gastric leiomyosarcoma; Roentgenologic and clinical findings. *Am J Dig Dis* 15:239, 1970.

Reasbeck PG, Van Rij AM: The effect of somatostatin on dumping after gastric surgery: A preliminary report. *Surgery* 99:462, 1986.

Reber HA, Way LW: Surgical treatment of late postgastrectomy syndromes. *Am J Surg* 129:71, 1975.

Sakita T, Oguro Y: Endoscopic diagnosis of early gastric cancer, in Berry LH (ed): *Gastrointestinal Pan-Endoscopy.* Springfield, IL, Charles C Thomas, 1974, p 278.

Sawyers JL, et al: Remedial operation for alkaline reflux gastritis and associated postgastrectomy syndromes. *Arch Surg* 115:519, 1980.

Seaman WB: Non-neoplastic diseases of the stomach, in Margulis AR, Burhenne HJ (eds): *Alimentary Tract Roentgenology.* St Louis, CV Mosby, 1973, vol 1, p 607.

Shaffer EA: The effect of vagotomy on gallbladder function and bile composition in man. *Ann Surg* 195:413, 1982.

Sheiner HJ, et al: Gastric motility and emptying in normal and post-vagotomy subjects. *Gut* 21:753, 1980.

Shirakabe H, et al: *Atlas of X-ray Diagnosis of Early Gastric Cancer.* Philadelphia, Lippincott, 1966.

Tovey FI, Clark CG: Anaemia after partial gastrectomy: A neglected curable condition. *Lancet* 1:956, 1980.

van Heerden JA, et al: Postoperative reflux gastritis. *Am J Surg* 129:82, 1975.

Vogel SB, Vair DB, et al: Alterations in gastrointestinal emptying of 99m-technetium-labeled solids following sequential antrectomy, truncal vagotomy and Roux Y gastroenterostomy. *Ann Surg* 198:506, 1983.

Wormsley KG, Grossman MI: Maximal histalog test in control subjects and patients with peptic ulcer. *Gut* 6:427, 1965.

Yalow RS, Berson SA: Radioimmunoassay of gastrin. *Gastroenterology* 58:1, 1970.

Zboralske FF: Gastric ulcer, in Margulis AR, Burhenne HJ (eds): *Alimentary Tract Roentgenology.* St Louis, CV Mosby, 1967, vol 1, p 475.

Gastric and Duodenal Disease

Adami H, Enander L, et al: Recurrences one to ten years after highly selective vagotomy in prepyloric and duodenal ulcer. *Ann Surg* 199:393, 1984.

Adkins RB Jr, DeLozier JB III, et al: The management of gastric ulcers: A current review. *Ann Surg* 201:741, 1985.

Amdrup E: Recurrent ulcer. *Br J Surg* 68:679, 1981.

Amdrup E, Jensen HE: Selective vagotomy of the parietal cell mass preserving innervation of the undrained antrum. *Gastroenterology* 59:522, 1970.

Amdrup E, et al: Clinical results of parietal cell vagotomy (highly selective vagotomy) two to four years after operation. *Ann Surg* 180:279, 1974.

Amdrup E, et al: Parietal cell (highly selective or proximal gastric) vagotomy for peptic ulcer disease. *World J Surg* 1:19, 1977.

Anderson JR, et al: Cholelithiasis following peptic ulcer surgery: A prospective controlled study. *Br J Surg* 67:618, 1980.

Asbaugh D, et al: Gastroscopy in corrosive burn of the stomach. *JAMA* 216:1638, 1971.

Bader JP: The surgical treatment of peptic ulcer disease. A physician's view. *Dig Dis Sci* 30(11 suppl):52S, 1985.

Bardhan DD: Refractory duodenal ulcer. *Gut* 25:711–717, 1984.

Barragry TP, Blatchford JW, et al: Giant gastric ulcers, a review of 49 cases. *Ann Surg* 203:255, 1986.

Bergegardh S, et al: Gastric acid responses to graded I.V. infusion of pentagastrin and histalog in peptic ulcer patients before and after antrum-bulb resection. *Scand J Gastroent* 11:337, 1976.

Berne CJ, Rosoff L: Peptic ulcer perforation of the gastroduodenal artery complex. *Ann Surg* 169:141, 1969.

Binder HJ, et al: Cimetidine in the treatment of duodenal ulcer: A multicenter double-blind study. *Gastroenterology* 74:380, 1978.

Bittner R, Schirrow H, et al: Total gastrectomy: A 15-year experience with particular reference to the patient over 70 years of age. *Arch Surg* 120:1120, 1985.

Blumenthal IS: Digestive disease as a national problem. III. Social cost of peptic ulcer. *Gastroenterology* 54:86, 1968.

Bonfils S, et al: Cimetidine treatment of acute and chronic Zollinger-Ellison syndrome. *World J Surg* 3:597, 1979.

Bringaze WL III, Chappuis CW, et al: Early gastric cancer. *Ann Surg* 204:103, 1986.

Burgess JN, et al: Sarcomatous lesions of the stomach. *Ann Surg* 173:758, 1971.

Burhenne HJ: The postoperative stomach, in Margulis AR, Burhenne HJ (eds): *Alimentary Tract Roentgenology*. St Louis, CV Mosby, 1973, vol 1, p 740.

Castrini G, Pappalardo G: Carcinoma of the cardia: Tactical problem. *J Thorac Cardiovasc Surg* 82:190, 1981.

Cathcart PM, et al: Tumors of gastric smooth muscle. *South Med J* 73:18, 1980.

Cello JP, Grendell JH: Endoscopic laser treatment for gastrointestinal vascular ectasias. *Ann Intern Med* 104:352, 1986.

Christiansen J, et al: Prospective controlled vagotomy trial for duodenal ulcer: Primary results, sequelae, acid secretion, and recurrence rates two to five years after operation. *Ann Surg* 193:49, 1981.

Chung R, DenBesten L: Fiberoptic endoscopy in treatment of corrosive injury of the stomach. *Arch Surg* 110:725, 1975.

Collen MJ, Howard JM, et al: Comparison of ranitidine and cimetidine in the treatment of gastric hypersecretion. *Ann Intern Med* 100:52, 1984.

Conn HO, et al: Intra-arterial vasopressin in the treatment of upper gastrointestinal hemorrhage. A prospective, controlled clinical trial. *Gastroenterology* 68:211, 1975.

Cooke AR: The role of the mucosal barrier in drug-induced gastric ulceration and erosions. *Am J Dig Dis* 21:155, 1976.

Cooperative Study Group: Omeprazole in duodenal ulceration: Acid inhibition, symptom relief, endoscopic healing, and recurrence. *Br Med J* 289:525, September 1984.

Cowley DJ, et al: Acid secretion in relation to recurrence of duodenal ulcer after vagotomy and drainage. *Br J Surg* 60:517, 1973.

Cox AJ Jr: Pathology, in Harkins HN, Nyhus LM (eds): *Surgery of the Stomach and Duodenum*, 2d ed. Boston, Little, Brown, 1969.

Cross S, et al: Carbenoxolone: Its protective action on gastric mucosa, in *Biologie et Gastroenterologie*. 9th International Congress of Gastroenterology, Paris, 5:568C, 1972.

Csendes A, Braghetto L, et al: Surgical treatment of high gastric ulcer. *Am J Surg* 149:765, 1985.

Czaja AJ, et al: Gastric acid secretion and acute gastroduodenal disease after burns. *Arch Surg* 111:243, 1976.

DeBakey M, Ochsner A: Bezoars and concretions. *Surgery* 4:934, 1938.

Diggory RT, Cuschieri A: R2/3 gastrectomy for gastric carcinoma: An audited experience of a consecutive series. *Br J Surg* 72:146, 1985.

Donovan AJ, et al: Selective treatment of duodenal ulcer with perforation. *Ann Surg* 189:627, 1979.

Dougherty SH, et al: Stomach cancer following gastric surgery for benign disease. *Arch Surg* 117:294, 1982.

Dragstedt LR, Owens FM Jr: Supradiaphragmatic secretion of vagus nerves in treatment of duodenal ulcer. *Proc Soc Exp Biol Med* 53:152, 1943.

DuPlessis DJ: Pathogenesis of gastric ulceration. *Lancet* 1:974, 1965.

Duthie HL, et al: Surgical treatment of gastric ulcers. Controlled

comparison of billroth-I gastrectomy and vagotomy and pyloroplasty. *Br J Surg* 57:784, 1970.

Elashoff JD, Van Deventer G, et al: Long-term follow-up of duodenal ulcer patients. *J Clin Gastroenterol* 5:509, 1983.

Ellis FH Jr: Esophagogastrectomy for carcinoma: Technical considerations based on anatomic location of lesion. *Surg Clin North Am* 60:265, 1980.

Emas S, Aly A: Acid and pepsin responses to graded doses of pentagastrin in duodenal and corporeal gastric ulcer patients before and after selective proximal vagotomy. *Am J Surg* 150:543, 1985.

Emas S, Fernstrom M: Prospective, randomized trial of selective vagotomy with pyloroplasty and selective proximal vagotomy with and without pyloroplasty in the treatment of duodenal, pyloric, and prepyloric ulcers. *Am J Surg* 149:236, 1985.

Engstrom PF, Lavin PT, et al: Postoperative adjuvant 5-fluorouracil plus methyl-CCNU therapy for gastric cancer patients: Eastern Cooperative Oncology Group Study (EST 3275). *Cancer* 55:1863, 1985.

Fakhry SM, Herbst CA Jr, et al: Complications requiring intervention after gastric bariatric surgery. *South Med J* 78:536, 1985.

Farris JM, Smith GK: Vagotomy and pyloroplasty: A solution to the management of bleeding duodenal ulcer. *Ann Surg* 152:416, 1960.

Feczko PJ, Halpert RD: Gastric polyps: Radiological evaluation and clinical significance. *Radiology* 155:581, 1985.

Finsberg HV, Pearlman LA: Surgical treatment of peptic ulcer in the United States. Trends before and after the introduction of cimetidine. *Lancet* 1:1305, 1981.

Fleischer D: Endoscopic laser therapy for gastrointestinal neoplasms. *Surg Clin North Am* 64:947, 1984.

Fleming ID, et al: The role of surgery in the management of gastric lymphoma. *Cancer* 49:1135, 1982.

Fordtran JS, et al: In vivo and in vitro evaluation of liquid antacids. *N Engl J Med* 288:293, 1973.

Foster JH, et al: Factors influencing mortality following emergency operation for massive upper gastrointestinal hemorrhage. *Surg Gynecol Obstet* 117:257, 1963.

Fraser AG, Brunt PW, et al: Comparison of highly selective vagotomy with truncal vagotomy and pyloroplasty: One surgeon's results after 5 years. *Br J Surg* 70:485, 1983.

Fraser GM, Earnshaw PM: Double-contrast barium meal: Correlation with endoscopy. *Clin Radiol* 34:121, 1983.

Friedman GD, et al: Cigarettes, alcohol, coffee and peptic ulcer. *N Engl J Med* 290:469, 1974.

Gall FP, Hermanek P: New aspects in the surgical treatment of gastric carcinoma—a comparative study of 1636 patients operated on between 1969 and 1982. *Eur J Surg Oncol* 11:19, 1985.

Gentsch HH, et al: Results of surgical treatment of early gastric cancer in 113 patients. *World J Surg* 5:103, 1981.

Gilbert DA, Surawicz CM, et al: Prevention of acute aspirin-induced gastric mucosal injury by 15-R-15 methyl prostaglandin E_2: Endoscopic study. *Gastroenterology* 86:339, 1984.

Gledhill T, Buck M, et al: Cimetidine or vagotomy? Comparison of the effects of proximal gastric vagotomy, cimetidine, and placebo on nocturnal intragastric acidity and acid secretion in patients with cimetidine-resistant duodenal ulcer. *Br J Surg* 70:7043, 1983.

Goldstein F, Kline TS, et al: Early gastric cancer in a United States hospital. *Am J Gastroenterol* 78:715, 1983.

Goligher JC: A technique for highly selective (parietal cell or proximal gastric) vagotomy for duodenal ulcer. *Br J Surg* 61:337, 1974.

Goligher JC, et al: Controlled trial of vagotomy and gastroenterostomy, vagotomy and antrectomy and subtotal gastrectomy in elective treatment of duodenal ulcer: Interim report. *Br Med J* 1:455, 1964.

Goligher JC, et al: Five to eight year results of truncal vagotomy and pyloroplasty for duodenal ulcer. *Br Med J* 1:7, 1972.

Gough KR, Korman MG, et al: Rantidine and cimetidine in prevention of duodenal ulcer relapse: Double-blind, randomized, multicenter, comparative trial. *Lancet* 2:659, 1984.

Graffner HO, Liedberg GF, et al: Parietal cell vagotomy in the surgical treatment of chronic duodenal, pyloric and prepyloric ulcer disease. *Int Surg* 70:139, 1985.

Graffner HO, Liedberg GF, et al: Recurrence after parietal cell vagotomy for peptic ulcer disease. *Am J Surg* 150:336, 1985.

Greenall MJ, Lehnert T: Vagotomy or gastrectomy for elective treatment of benign gastric ulceration? *Dig Dis Sci* 30:353, 1985.

Greenall MJ, et al: Long term effect of highly selective vagotomy on basal and maximal acid output in man. *Gastroenterology* 68:1421, 1975.

Gregory RA, et al: Extraction of gastrin-like substance from pancreatic tumor in case of Zollinger-Ellison syndrome. *Lancet* 1:1045, 1960.

Griffith CA, Harkins HN: Partial gastric vagotomy. An experimental study. *Gastroenterology* 32:96, 1957.

Grossman MI: Some minor heresies about vagotomy. *Gastroenterology* 67:1016, 1974.

Grossman MI, et al: A new look at peptic ulcer. *Ann Intern Med* 84:57, 1976.

Grossman MI, et al: Peptic ulcer: New therapies, new diseases. *Ann Intern Med* 95:609, 1981.

Hallenbeck GA, et al: Proximal gastric vagotomy: Effects of two operative techniques on clinical and gastric secretory results. *Ann Surg* 184:435, 1976.

Hastings PR, et al: Mallory-Weiss syndrome, review of 69 cases. *Am J Surg* 142:560, 1981.

Herrington JL, et al: A twenty-five year experience with vagotomy-antrectomy. *Arch Surg* 106:469, 1973.

Hirschowitz BI, Luketic GC: Endoscopy in the post-gastrectomy patient: An analysis of 580 patients. *Gastrointest Endosc* 18:27, 1971.

Hunt PS: Surgical management of bleeding chronic peptic ulcer: A 10-year prospective study. *Ann Surg* 199:44, 1984.

Hunt PS, et al: The management of bleeding gastric ulcer: A prospective study. *Aust NZ J Surg* 50:41, 1980.

Iishi H, Tatsuta M, et al: Enoscopic diagnosis of minute gastric cancer of less than 5 mm in diameter. *Cancer* 56:655, 1985.

Inberg MV, et al: Total and proximal gastrectomy in the treatment of gastric carcinoma: A series of 305 cases. *World J Surg* 5:249, 1981.

Ippoliti AF, et al: Cimetidine versus intensive antacid therapy for duodenal ulcer: A multicenter trial. *Gastroenterology* 74:393, 1978.

Isenberg JI, Peterson WL, et al: Healing of benign gastric ulcer with low-dose antacid or cimetidine: A double-blind randomized, placebo-controlled trial. *N Engl J Med* 308:1319, 1983.

Ivy AC, et al: *Peptic Ulcer*. Philadelphia, Blakiston, 1950.

Jaffin BW, Kaye MD: The prognosis of gastric outlet obstruction. *Ann Surg* 201:176, 1985.

Johnston D, Wilkinson AR: Highly selective vagotomy without a drainage procedure in the treatment of duodenal ulcer. *Br J Surg* 57:289, 1970.

Jordan GL Jr, et al: Surgical management of perforated peptic ulcer. *Ann Surg* 179:628, 1974.

Jordan PH Jr, Condon RE: A prospective evaluation of vagotomy-pyloroplasty and vagotomy-antrectomy for treatment of duodenal ulcer. *Ann Surg* 172:547, 1970.

Klein TS, Goldstein F: Malignant lymphoma involving the stomach. *Cancer* 32:961, 1973.

Knauer CM: Mallory-Weiss syndrome. Characterization of 75 Mallory-Weiss lacerations in 528 patients with upper gastrointestinal hemorrhage. *Gastroenterology* 71:5, 1976.

Koga S, et al: Results of total gastrectomy for gastric cancer. *Am J Surg* 140:636, 1980.

Koo J, Lam SK, et al: Proximal gastric vagotomy, truncal vagotomy with drainage, and truncal vagotomy with antrectomy for chronic duodenal ulcer: A propsective, randomized controlled trial. *Ann Surg* 197:265, 1983.

Kuster GGR, et al: Gastric cancer in pernicious anemia and in patients with and without achlorhydria. *Ann Surg* 175:783, 1972.

Lamers, CBHW, Lind T, et al: Omeprazole in Zollinger–Ellison syndrome: Effects of a single dose and of long-term treatment in patients resistant to histamine H_2-receptor antagonists. *N Engl J Med* 310:758, 1984.

Laurence BH, et al: Endoscopic laser photocoagulation for bleeding peptic ulcers. *Lancet* 1:124, 1980.

Lieberman DA, Keller FS, et al: Arterial embolization for massive upper gastrointestinal tract bleeding in poor surgical candidates. *Gastroenterology* 86:376, 1984.

Littman A (ed): The Veterans Administration cooperative study on gastric ulcer. *Gastroenterology* 61:567, 1971.

Longmire WP Jr: Gastric carcinoma: Is radical gastrectomy worthwhile? *Ann R Coll Surg Engl* 62:25, 1980.

Lucas CE, et al: Natural history and surgical dilemma of "stress" gastric bleeding. *Arch Surg* 102:266, 1971.

Lunde OC, Liavag I, et al: Proximal gastric vagotomy and pyloroplasty for duodenal ulcer with pyloric stenosis: A thirteen-year experience. *World J Surg* 9:165, 1985.

Lygidakis NJ: Gastric stump carcinoma after surgery for gastroduodenal ulcer. *Ann R Coll Surg Engl* 63:203, 1981.

Lygidakis NJ: Total gastrectomy for gastric carcinoma: A retrospective study of different procedures and assessment of a new technique of gastric reconstruction. *Br J Surg* 68:649, 1981.

McCarthy DM: Report of the United States experience with cimetidine in the Zollinger-Ellison syndrome and other hypersecretory states. *Gastroenterology* 74:453, 1978.

McCarthy E, et al: H_2-histamine receptor blocking agents in the Zollinger-Ellison syndrome. *Ann Intern Med* 87:668, 1977.

MacLeod LA, Mills PR, et al: Neodymium-yttrium-aluminum-garnet laser photocoagulation for a major hemorrhage from peptic ulcers and single vessels: A single-blind controlled study. *Br Med J* 286:345, 1983.

Madsen P, Kronborg O: Recurrent ulcer $5\frac{1}{2}$–8 years after highly selective vagotomy without drainage and selective vagotomy with pyloroplasty. *Scand J Gastroenterol* 15:193, 1980.

Malagelada JR: Medical versus surgical therapy for duodenal ulcer: Making the right choices. *Mayo Clin Proc* 55:25, 1980.

Malagelada JR, Ahlquist DA, et al: Defects in prostaglandin synthesis and metabolism in ulcer disease. *Dig Dis Sci* 31(suppl 2):20S, 1986.

Malagelada J, Edis AJ, et al: Medical and surgical options in the management of patients with gastrinoma. *Gastroenterology* 84:1524, 1983.

Malagelada J, Phillips SF, et al: Postoperative reflux gastritis: Pathophysiology and long-term outcome after Roux en Y diversion. *Ann Intern Med* 103:178, 1985.

Mallory GK, Weiss S: Hemorrhages from lacerations of cardiac orifice of the stomach due to vomiting. *Am J Med Sci* 178:506, 1929.

Marshak RH, Lindner AE: The Zollinger-Ellison syndrome, in *Radiology of the Small Intestine*. Philadelphia, Saunders, 1970, p 88.

Mekelvey STD: Gastric incontinence and postvagotomy diarrhea. *Br J Surg* 57:741, 1970.

Mendeloff AI: What has been happening to duodenal ulcer? *Gastroenterology* 67:1020, 1974.

Menetrier P: Des polyadenomes gastriques et de leurs rapports avec le cancer de l'estomac. *Arch Physiol Norm Path* 1:32, 226, 1888.

Menguy R: Pathophysiology of peptic ulcer. *Am J Surg* 120:282, 1970.

Menguy R, et al: Mechanism of stress ulcer: Influence of hypovolemic shock on energy metabolism in the gastric mucosa. *Gastroenterology* 66:46, 1974.

Menguy R, et al: The surgical management of acute gastric mucosal bleeding. Stress ulcer, acute erosive gastritis, and acute hemorrhagic gastritis. *Arch Surg* 99:198, 1969.

Messer J, Reitman D, et al: Association of adrenocorticosteroid therapy and peptic ulcer disease. *N Engl J Med* 309:21, 1983.

Mizuno H, et al: Endoscopic followup of gastric polyps. *Gastrointest Endosc* 21:112, 1975.

Moertel CG, et al: Sequential and combination chemotherapy of advanced gastric cancer. *Cancer* 38:678, 1976.

Monaco AP, et al: Adenomatous polyps of the stomach. A clinical and pathological study of 153 cases. *Cancer* 15:456, 1962.

Moody FG: Role of mucosal blood flow in the pathogenesis of gastric ulcers, in Holton P (ed): *International Encyclopedia of Pharmacology and Therapeutics*. Oxford, Pergamon, 1973, sec 39A, vol 1.

Moody FG, et al: Stress and the acute gastric mucosal lesion. *Am J Dig Dis* 21:148, 1976.

Nicosia J, et al: Surgical management of corrosive gastric injuries. *Ann Surg* 180:139, 1974.

Norton JA, Doppman JL, et al: Aggressive resection of metastatic disease in selected patients with malignant gastrinoma. *Ann Surg* 203:352, 1986.

Nyhus LM: Gastric ulcer, in Harkins HN, Nyhus LM (eds): *Surgery of the Stomach and Duodenum*, 2d ed. Boston, Little, Brown, 1969, p 203.

O'Brien JJ, Burakoff R, et al: Early gastric cancer: Clinicopathologic study. *Am J Med* 78:195, 1985.

Ochsner A, et al: Cancer of the stomach. *Am J Surg* 141:10, 1981.

Oi M, et al: The location of gastric ulcer. *Gastroenterology* 36:45, 1959.

O'Neill JA, et al: Studies related to the pathogenesis of Curling's ulcer. *J Trauma* 7:275, 1967.

Orlando R III, Welch JP: Carcinoma of the stomach after gastric operation. *Am J Surg* 141:487, 1981.

O'Rourke IC: Elective surgery for peptic ulcer: A five-year review. *Med J Aust* 143:13, 1985.

Overholt BF, Jeffries GH: Hypertrophic, hypersecretory protein-losing gastropathy. *Gastroenterology* 58:80, 1970.

Palmer ED: The vigorous diagnostic approach to upper gastrointestinal tract hemorrhage. *JAMA* 207:1477, 1969.

Pellegrini CA, Patti MG, et al: Alkaline reflux gastritis and the effect of biliary diversion on gastric emptying of solid food. *Am J Surg* 150:166, 1985.

Primrose JN, Ratcliffe JG, et al: Differences between peptic ulcer and control patients on the basis of the response to secretion. *Digestion* 32:249, 1985.

Richardson CT, Peters MN, et al: Treatment of Zollinger–Ellison syndrome with exploratory laparotomy, proximal gastric vagotomy, and H_2-receptor antagonists: A prospective study. *Gastroenterology* 89:357, 1985.

Richardson CT, Walsh JH: The value of a histamine H_2-receptor antagonist in the management of patients with the Zollinger-Ellison syndrome. *N Engl J Med* 294:133, 1976.

Ritchie WP Jr: Alkaline reflux gastritis, late results on a controlled trial of diagnosis and treatment. *Ann Surg* 203:537, 1986.

Romanus ME, Neal JA, et al: Comparison of four provocative tests for the diagnosis of gastrinoma. *Ann Surg* 198:608, 1983.

Rossi RL, et al: Parietal cell vagotomy for intractable and obstructing duodenal ulcer. *Am J Surg* 141:482, 1981.

Rotter JL, et al: Genetics of peptic ulcer disease: Segregation of serum group I pepsinogen concentrations in families with peptic ulcer disease. *Clin Res* 25:114A, 1977.

Sakita T, et al: Observations on the healing of ulcerations in early gastric cancer. The life cycle of the malignant ulcer. *Gastroenterology* 60:835, 1971.

Sawyers JL, Scott HW Jr: Selective gastric vagotomy with antrectomy or pyloroplasty. *Ann Surg* 174:541, 1971.

Schafer LW, Larson DE, et al: Risk of development of gastric carcinoma in patients with pernicious anemia: A population-based study in Rochester, Minnesota. *Mayo Clinic Proc* 60:444, 1985.

Scott, HW Jr, Adkins RB Jr, et al: Results of an aggressive surgical approach to gastric carcinoma during a twenty-three-year period. *Surgery* 97:55, 1985.

Shepherd AF, Allan RN, et al: The surgical treatment of gastroduodenal Crohn's disease. *Ann R Coll Surg Engl* 67:382, 1985.

Shimm DS, Dosoretz DE, et al: Primary gastric lymphoma: An analysis with emphasis on prognostic factors and radiation therapy. *Cancer* 52:2044, 1983.

Sirinek KR, et al: Simple closure of perforated peptic ulcer. Still an effective procedure for patients with delay in treatment. *Arch Surg* 116:591, 1981.

Stabile BE, Passaro E Jr: Recurrent peptic ulcer. *Gastroenterology* 70:124, 1976.

Stanten A, Peters H Jr: Enzymatic dissolution of phytobezoars. *Am J Surg* 130:259, 1975.

Stempien SJ, et al: Hypertrophic hypersecretory gastropathy. *Am J Dig Dis* 9:471, 1964.

Swain CP, Storey DW, et al: Nature of the bleeding vessel in recurrently bleeding gastric ulcers. *Gastroenterology* 90:595, 1986.

Tanphiphat C, Tanprayoon T, et al: Surgical treatment of perforated duodenal ulcer: A prospective trial between simple closure and definitive surgery. *Br J Surg* 72:370, 1985.

Thomas WE, et al: The long-term outcome of billroth I partial gastrectomy for benign gastric ulcer. *Ann Surg* 195:189, 1982.

Thomsen F, et al: Cimetidine treatment of recurrent ulcer after vagotomy. *Acta Chir Scand* 146:35, 1980.

Vallon AG, et al: Randomized trial of endoscopic argon laser photocoagulation in bleeding peptic ulcers. *Gut* 22:228, 1981.

Wara P: Endoscopic management of the bleeding ulcer. *Danish Med Bull* 33:1, 1986.

Wastell C, Ellis H: Volvulus of the stomach. *Br J Surg* 58:557, 1971.

Weaver RM, Temple JG: Proximal gastric vagotomy in patients resistant to cimetidine. *Br J Surg* 72:177, 1985.

Weiland D, et al: Gastric outlet obstruction in peptic ulcer disease: An indication for surgery. *Am J Surg* 143:90, 1982.

Weinberg JA: Treatment of the massively bleeding duodenal ulcer by ligation. Pyloroplasty and vagotomy *Am J Surg* 102:158, 1961.

Wermer P: Multiple endocrine adenomatosis: Multiple hormone producing tumors, a familial syndrome. in Bonfils S (ed): *Endocrine-Secreting Tumours of the Gastrointestinal Tract*. Philadelphia, Saunders, 1974, p 671.

Wilson SD, Ellison EH: Survival in patients with Zollinger-Ellison syndrome treated by total gastrectomy. *Am J Surg* 111:787, 1966.

Wilson WS, et al: Superficial gastric erosions. Response to surgical treatment. *Am J Surg* 126:133, 1973.

Wyllie JH, et al: Effect of cimetidine on surgery for duodenal ulcer. *Lancet* 1:1307, 1981.

Yalow RS, Berson SA: Size and charge distinctions beween endogenous human plasma gastrin in peripheral blood and heptadecapeptide gastrins. *Gastroenterology* 58:609, 1970.

Yan CJ, Brooks JR: Surgical management of gastric adenocarcinoma. *Am J Surg* 149:771, 1985.

Zollinger RM: Gastrinoma: Factors influencing prognosis. *Surgery* 97:49, 1985.

Zollinger RM, Ellison EH: Primary peptic ulcerations of the jejunum associated with islet cell tumors of the pancreas. *Ann Surg* 142:709, 1955.

Gastric Procedures for Morbid Obesity

Agha FP, Eckhauser FE, et al: Mason's vertical banded gastroplasty for morbid obesity: Surgical procedure and radiographic evaluation. *Radiology* 150:825, 1984.

Buckwalter JA: Clinical trial of jejunoileal and gastric bypass for the treatment of morbid obesity: Four-year progress report. *Am Surg* 46:377, 1980.

Flickinger EG, Pories WJ, et al: The Greenville gastric bypass: Progress report at 3 years. *Ann Surg* 199:555, 1984.

Flickinger EG, Sinar DR, et al: The bypassed stomach. *Am J Surg* 149:151, 1985.

Freeman JB, Burchett HJ: A comparison of gastric bypass and gastroplasty for morbid obesity. *Surgery* 88:433, 1980.

Gannon MX, Pears DJ, et al: The effect of gastric partitioning on gastric emptying in morbidly obese patients. *Br J Surg* 72:952, 1985.

Gentry K, Halverson JD, et al: Psychologic assessment of morbidly obese patients undergoing gastrc bypass: A comparison of preoperative and postoperative adjustment. *Surgery* 95:215, 1984.

Gomez CA: Gastroplasty in the surgical treatment of morbid obesity. *Am J Clin Nutr* 33(2 suppl):406, 1980.

Griffen WO Jr, et al: Experiences with conversion of jejunoileal bypass to gastric bypass: Its use for maintenance of weight loss. *Arch Surg* 116:320, 1981.

Halverson JD, et al: Gastric bypass for morbid obesity: A medical-surgical assessment. *Ann Surg* 194:152, 1981.

Halverson JD, Koehler RE: Assessment of patients with failed gastric operations for morbid obesity. *Am J Surg* 145:357, 1983.

Jones KB Jr: Horizontal gastroplasty: A safe, effective alternative to gastric bypsss in the surgical management of morbid obesity. *Ann Surg* 50:128, 1984.

Laws HL, Piantadosi S: Superior gastric reduction procedure for morbid obesity: A prospective, randomized trial. *Ann Surg* 193:334, 1981.

MacLean LD, et al: Gastroplasty for obesity. *Surg Gynecol Obstet* 153:200, 1981.

Makarewicz PA, Freeman JB, et al: Vertical banded gastroplasty: Assessment of efficacy. *Surgery* 98:700, 1985.

Mason EE: Vertical banded gastroplasty for obesity. *Arch Surg* 117:701, 1982.

Mason EE, et al: Gastric bypass in morbid obesity. *Am J Clin Nutr* 33(2 suppl):395, 1980.

O'Leary JP: Partition of the lesser curvature of the stomach in morbid obesity. *Surg Gynecol Obstet* 154:85, 1982.

Sugarman HJ, Fairman RP, et al: Gastric surgery for respiratory insufficiency of obesity. *Chest* 90:81, 1986.

Villar HV, et al: Mechanisms of satiety and gastric emptying after gastric partitioning and bypass. *Surgery* 90:229, 1981.

Chapter 27

Small Intestine

Courtney M. Townsend, Jr., and James C. Thompson

INTRODUCTION

Considered teleologically, the small bowel is the *raison d'être* for the entire gut. The esophagus brings food to the stomach, which prepares it for digestion. The exocrine secretions of the liver and pancreas make digestion possible. Digestion is achieved in the lumen of the small bowel, and food is absorbed through the small bowel mucosa; the colon disposes of whatever is left.

In addition to its vital function in nutrition, the small bowel has other important roles. It is the largest endocrine organ in the body. It has tremendous defenses against infection and is one of the most, if not the most, important organ in immune defense. It is a marvel of efficiency and works so well that, excepting the proximal 3 cm of the duodenum, it is not a common site for disease. We are supplied with a great excess of small bowel and can exist on far less than one-half of the absorptive surface provided.

Until recently, the small intestine had been relatively inaccessible for nonoperative diagnostic procedures compared to the stomach or colon. Several diagnostic techniques are now available for specific diseases of the small bowel. Mucosal biopsies obtained with the peroral biopsy capsule are often diagnostic in diffuse mucosal diseases. Enteroclysis is a more sensitive radiographic technique than the conventional barium follow-through examination of the small bowel. Selective mesenteric angiography is often helpful in cases of discrete lesions with abnormal vascular patterns, such as neoplasms, vascular malformations, or actively bleeding lesions. Scintigraphy may be helpful in localizing sites of bleeding. Fiberoptic endoscopy of the duodenum, proximal jejunum, and distal ileum are routinely employed.

Some diseases affecting the small intestine are discussed in other chapters: intestinal obstruction (Chap.

24), mesenteric vascular disease (Chap. 35), diseases of the intestine in infancy and childhood (Chap. 39), the intestine in trauma (Chap. 6), and duodenal and gastrojejunal peptic ulcer (Chap. 26).

ANATOMY

The most impressive thing about the small bowel is its immense mucosal surface area, which is responsible for the organ's tremendously efficient digestion of food. Several layers of muscle, combined with actin and myosin components in the microstructures, provide great motility, so that not only is there great surface area, but the interface between the surface and the luminal contents, presented for absorption, is in constant motion as well.

Gross Anatomy

The small bowel extends from the pylorus to the cecum. The length of the small intestine depends entirely upon the state of bowel activity at the time of measurement. Careful estimates provide a duodenal length of 20 cm, a jejunal length of 100 to 110 cm, and an ileal length of 150 to 160 cm. The jejunoileum extends from the peritoneal fold that supports the duodenal-jejunal junction (the ligament of Treitz) downward to the ileocecal valve. The jejunoileum is estimated to comprise 60 percent of the entire length of the gut and to be approximately 160 percent of the body height, so that the small bowel, of couse, is considerably longer in a 7-ft basketball player than it is in a 5-ft jockey.

Generally, the jejunum occupies the upper abdomen, especially on the left, and is in contact with the pancreas, spleen, colon, and left kidney and adrenals. Affliction of these organs may affect the jejunum; pancreatitis, for example, may cause local ileus (the "sentinel loop") of the jejunum.

The jejunum has a larger circumference and is thicker than the ileum, and it may be identified at operation because of this and also because the mesenteric vessels usually form only one or two arcades and send out long straight vasa recta to the mesenteric border of the bowel. By contrast, the blood supply to the ileum may have four or five separate arcades, the vasa recta are shorter, and, most importantly, there is usually much more fat in the mesentery of the ileum than in the jejunum (Fig. 27-1). The jejunal mesentery may be transparent, but mesenteric fat will usually reach all the way to the bowel in the ileum. The ileum occupies the lower abdomen, especially on the right, and the pelvis. It is smaller in diameter and somewhat more mobile.

Except for the duodenum, the small bowel is entirely covered with visceral peritoneum (the serosa) and is tethered only by its attachment to the mesentery, through which course arteries, veins, and lymphatics. The mesentery is obliquely attached to the posterior body wall, beginning superiorly well to the left of the second lumbar vertebra and ending obliquely downward and to the right to overlie the right sacroiliac joint. The mesentery is normally covered with glistening peritoneum, which is nonadherent, but after trauma (external, chemical, septic, or operative), it may become adherent to other surfaces (mesenteric, visceral, or parietal) and greatly limit bowel mobility.

Except for the proximal duodenum, which is supplied by branches of the celiac axis, the blood supply of the small bowel is entirely from the superior mesenteric artery, which is the second major branch of the infradiaphragmatic aorta. The superior mesenteric artery also supplies the appendix, cecum, and ascending and proximal transverse colons. There is an abundant collateral supply to the small bowel, provided by the vascular arcades in the mesentery. In spite of this collateral supply, occlusion of a major branch of the superior mesenteric artery, or of the superior mesenteric artery itself, will lead to bowel death if not quickly corrected. Venous drainage of the segments of the small bowel is in parallel with the arterial supply. The superior mesenteric vein joins the splenic behind the neck of the pancreas to form the portal vein. The relatively high oxygen content of the blood leaving the gut provides a significant portion of the oxygen supply to the liver.

Fig. 27-1. Jejunum contrasted with ileum. Note the larger jejunal diameter, the thicker wall, prominent plicae circulares, one or two arterial arcades, long vasa recta, and translucent (fat-free) areas at the mesenteric border. The ileum is smaller, thinner walled, has few plicae, multiple vascular arcades with short vasa recta, and abundant mesenteric fat.

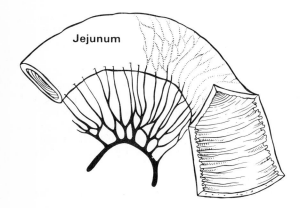

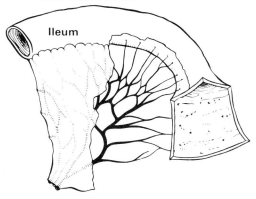

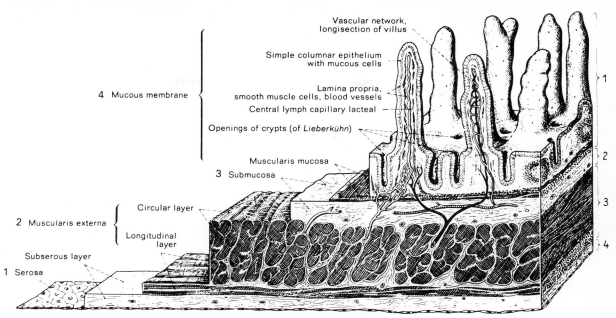

Fig. 27-2. Layers of the small intestine: A large surface is provided by villi for the absorption of required nutriments. The solitary lymph follicles in the lamina propria of the mucous membrane (not labeled). In the stroma of both sectioned villi are shown the central chyle vessels (lacteal) or the villous capillaries. (From: *Sabotta/ Figge: Atlas of Human Anatomy. New York, Hafner, 1974, with permission.*)

If the mesentery is not greatly infiltrated by fat, and if there are no peritoneal adhesions, the bowel is extraordinarily mobile on its vascular tether, and in some individuals, jejunal segments may be sufficiently mobilized to allow anastomosis in the neck to replace the cervical esophagus.

The small bowel contains major deposits of lymphatic tissue, particularly in the Peyer's patches of the ileum. There is a rich lymphatic drainage of the entire small bowel, and this plays a major role in fat absorption. Lymphatic drainage proceeds from the mucosa through the wall of the bowel to a set of nodes adjacent to the bowel in the mesentery. Drainage continues to a group of regional nodes adjacent to the mesenteric arterial arcades and then to a group at the base of the superior mesenteric vessels. From there, lymph goes to the cisterna chyli and from thence up the thoracic ducts to empty into the venous system in the neck. The lymphatics of the gut play a major role in immune defense and also in the spread of cells arising from neoplasms in the gut.

The small bowel mucosa is characterized by transverse folds (plicae circulares or valves of Kerckring), but actually these are absent in the duodenal bulb and in the distal ileum. They are more prominent in the distal duodenum and jejunum, where they may reach 1 cm in height and form interlocking transverse ridges (Fig. 27-1). The small bowel mucosa has a pink velvet-like appearance with a glistening surface. It is usually thicker in the jejunum than in the ileum, where there may be no folds and the surface may be entirely smooth, except for small scattered lymphatic nodules.

The innervation of the small bowel comes from both sympathetic and parasympathetic systems. Parasympathetic fibers come from the vagus and traverse the celiac ganglia. They affect secretion and motility and probably all phases of bowel activity. Vagal afferent fibers are present but apparently do not carry pain impulses. The sympathetic fibers come from the three sets of splanchnic nerves and have their ganglion cells usually in a plexus around the base of the superior mesenteric artery. Their motor impulses affect blood vessel motility and probably gut secretion and motility. Pain from the intestine is mediated through general visceral afferent fibers in the sympathetic system.

Histology

The wall of the small bowel has four layers, the serosa, the muscularis, the submucosa, and the mucosa (Fig. 27-2).

SEROSA. The serosa is the outermost layer and consists of visceral peritoneum that encircles the jejunoileum, but that covers the duodenum only anteriorly. It consists of a single layer of flattened mesophelial cells overlying loose connective tissue.

MUSCULARIS. The muscularis consists of a thin outer longitudinal layer and a thicker inner circular layer of smooth muscle. Specialized gaps in the muscle-cell membranes permit cell-to-cell communication, which facilitates the ability of the muscle layer to function as an electrical syncytium. Ganglion cells from the myenteric (Auerbach's) plexus are interposed between the two muscle layers and send fibers into both layers.

SUBMUCOSA. The submucosa is a layer of fibroelastic connective tissue containing blood vessels and nerves. It

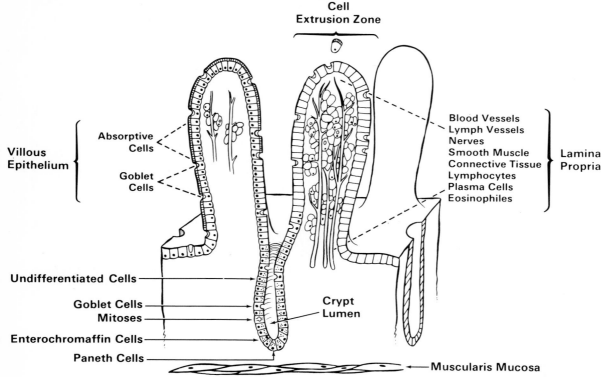

Fig. 27-3. Schematic diagram of two sectioned villi and a crypt of Lieberkühn illustrating the histologic organization of the small intestine mucosa. [Adapted and redrawn from: *Trier JS et al*, in *Sleisenger MH, Fordtran JS (eds): Gastrointestinal Disease. Pathophysiology, Diagnosis, Management. Philadelphia, Saunders, 1983, chap 48, with permission.*]

is the strongest component of the bowel wall and must, therefore, be included in placing sutures through the bowel. It contains elaborate networks of lymphatics and arterioles and venules and an extensive plexus of nerve fibers and ganglion cells (Meissner's plexus). Although frequently subdivided, the nerves from the mucosa, submucosa, and muscle layers are interconnected by small nerve fibers, and cross-connections between adrenergic and cholinergic elements have been described.

MUCOSA. Looked upon as a device to increase absorptive surface, the small bowel mucosa is an architectural marvel. The gross transverse folds, the finger-like villi protruding into the lumen of the bowel, the microvilli (brush border) covering the cells, and the glycocalyx fuzz covering the microvilli each tremendously increase the surface area exposed to luminal contents. Villi protrude $\frac{1}{2}$ to 1 mm into the lumen, are tallest in the distal duodenum and proximal jejunum, and become progressively shorter towards the terminal ileum.

The mucosa can be divided into three layers, the muscularis mucosae, lamina propria, and the epithelium. The deepest of these, the muscularis mucosae, is a thin sheet of muscle separating mucosa from submucosa. The lamina propria is a continuous layer of connective tissue between the epithelium and the muscularis mucosae. It extends into the villi and around the pitlike crypts of Lieberkühn (Fig. 27-3). The lamina propria contains, additionally, a variety of cells—plasma cells, lymphocytes, mast cells, eosinophils, macrophages, fibroblasts, smooth muscle cells—and noncellular connective tissue. The

lamina propria is the architectural base upon which the epithelium lies, but it also has important functions of its own and apparently serves protectively to combat microorganisms that penetrate the overlying epithelium. The plasma cells are an active site of synthesis of immunoglobulins.

Epithelium. The innermost mucosal layer is a continual sheet, one layer thick, of epithelial cells covering the villi and lining the crypts of Lieberkühn (see Fig. 27-3). The crypts contain four types of cells, goblet cells that secrete mucus, enterochromaffin cells whose endocrine function is unknown, Paneth cells that secrete zymogen granules and whose function is also unknown, and undifferentiated epithelial cells whose function is to provide for cell renewal. The epithelium of the small intestine is rapidly proliferating tissue in which old cells are discarded into the lumen and are replaced by newly-formed cells that appear to march up from the crypt into the villus in orderly sequence. This trip takes 5 to 7 days in the proximal small bowel, but in the ileum, labeled cells may travel from crypt to villous tip in 3 days.

The epithelium covering the villi consists of scattered endocrine cells, goblet cells, and absorptive cells. The major known functions of the villi are digestion and absorption. These functions are carried out by the absorp-

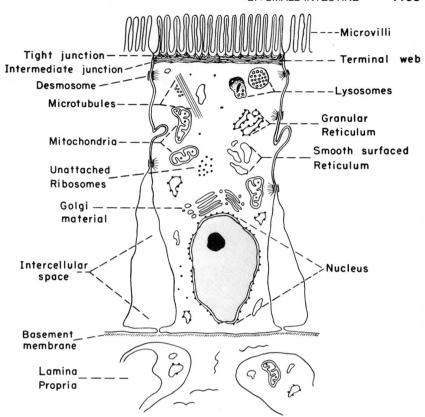

Fig. 27-4. Schematic diagram of an intestinal absorptive cell. [From: *Trier JS et al, in Sleisenger MH, Fordtran JS (eds): Gastrointestinal Disease. Pathophysiology, Diagnosis, Management. Philadelphia, Saunders, 1983, chap 48, with permission.*]

tive cells, tall columnar cells resting on a thin basement membrane that separates them from the lamina propria. Their luminal surface is covered by microvilli that rest on a terminal web (Fig. 27-4). The microvillar projections multiply the cell surface exposed to the lumen 30 times. The microvilli are covered in turn by a fuzzy coat of glycoprotein, the glycocalyx (Fig. 27-5). The microvilli participate actively in absorption and digestion: they contain enzymes for digestion of disaccharides and peptides, and certain cells may contain specific receptors that facilitate absorption (for example, certain ileal cells have receptors for vitamin B_{12} on their microvilli).

The plasma (or cell) membranes of the epithelial cells consist of three layers and are thicker over the microvilli than over the lateral and basal portions of the cell (Fig. 27-5). The lateral portion of the plasma membrane is also specialized. There are tight junctions between epithelial cells that prevent communication between intercellular spaces and the lumen. Immediately underneath the tight junction is a narrow space called an intermediate junction and beneath that is a desmosome, which provides tight attachments of adjacent membrane, by binding adjacent cells together. The depths of the tight junctions are greater between adjacent absorptive cells than between adjacent undifferentiated crypt cells. The permeability of the barrier between the intestinal lumen and the space between cells may vary from one location to another.

Fig. 27-5. Schematic illustration of the specializations of the apical cytoplasm of the plasma membrane of intestinal absorptive cells. [From: *Tier JS et al, in Sleisenger MH, Fordtran JS (eds): Gastrointestinal Disease. Pathophysiology, Diagnosis, Management. Philadelphia, Saunders, 1983, chap 48, with permission.*]

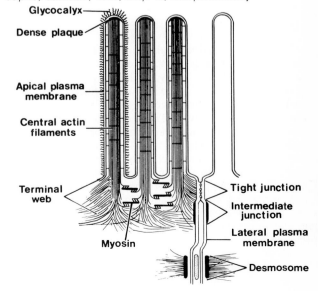

The cytoplasm immediately beneath the microvilli consists of fine filaments, known as the terminal web. This interconnects with filaments forming the core of the microvilli, which contain actin (Fig. 27-5). Myosin may also be present at the base of the microvilli, and these contractile proteins may allow for movement and contraction of the microvilli.

The processes of digestion and absorption within the epithelial cells are carried out by specific organelles (Fig. 27-4). The mitochondria participate in intracellular oxidation and provide energy for metabolism. The lysosomal sacs contain cytotoxic substances and intracellular waste products. The endoplasmic reticulum is the main synthesizing element within the cell and appears to be responsible for at least two major processes in fat absorption, the resynthesis of triglycerides from absorbed fatty acid fragments and the synthesis of the lipoprotein coat for chylomicrons. It is also the major synthetic site for intracellular digestive enzymes. The Golgi apparatus segregates, stores, and chemically modifies material that is absorbed and synthesized by the cell.

It may be useful to follow the path of a food element absorbed from the intestinal lumen. Initial contact is with the glycocalyx coating the microvilli, where some digestion may occur. Products of this digestion may go through the microvillous membrane, traversing the terminal web into the cytoplasm. The absorbed material may then either go laterally into the intracellular spaces or enter the channels of the endoplasmic reticulum, where it may be biochemically modified and transmitted to the Golgi material, where it may be stored. Eventually the material leaves the cell by crossing either the lateral or basal plasma (cell) membrane. It penetrates the basal lamina to enter the lamina propria, where it traverses the lymphatic or capillary endothelial cells to gain access to lymph or blood.

PHYSIOLOGY

Motility

Food is propelled through the small bowel by a complex series of muscular contractions. Motility patterns in the small bowel vary greatly in the fed and fasting state. Pace-setter potentials, probably originating in the duodenum, initiate a series of contractions that propel food through the small bowel. These contractions are of two types, segmentation and peristalsis. Contractions of the circular muscle divide the bowel into segments that are moved to and fro over the column of bowel contents for a short distance. The contents of adjacent segments then combine, and the process is repeated. About 40 percent of contractions are segmental. The circular muscle also initiates peristalsis, circular contractions migrating in an aboral direction propelling intestinal contents onward. The peristaltic reflex may function independently of extrinsic nerves. Abnormal waves of powerful contractions (*peristaltic rushes*) may rapidly traverse the entire segment of small intestine during episodes of enteritis.

During the interdigestive (fasting) period between meals, the bowel is regularly swept by a series of contractions initiated by the migrating myoelectric complex (MMC). The MMC is under neural and humoral control and initiates a triphasic series of contractions, phase I of which is resting, phase II intermittent contractions of moderate amplitude, and phase III the activity front that consists of a brief series of high-pressure waves. The MMC in man is stimulated by some (but not all) fluctuating increases in serum concentrations of motilin.

Small bowel motility is modulated by neural and humoral influences. Extrinsic nerves to the small bowel are vagal and sympathetic. Vagal fibers have two functionally different effects, one is cholinergic and excitatory and the other is peptidergic and probably inhibitory. Sympathetic fibers from the splanchnics appear chiefly to modulate the activity of intrinsic nerves.

Although gut peptides clearly influence bowel motility, their physiologic function is uncertain, except for the role of motilin in initiating MMC activity. Gastrin, cholecystokinin, and motilin are known to stimulate muscle contraction, whereas muscle activity is inhibited by secretin and often by glucagon (Table 27-1). Cholecystokinin may be physiologically important, since ingestion of a fatty meal may stimulate peristaltic contraction.

Digestion and Absorption

Liters of water and hundreds of grams of food move across the intestinal mucosa from the lumen to the blood stream each day. The process is remarkably efficient, nearly all food is absorbed unless protected by indigestible cellulose. There is no apparent governor; food absorption is just as efficient in the corpulent as it is in the starving.

FAT. Most individuals in Western Europe and North America consume 60 to 100 g of fat per day in the form of triglycerides. Fat digestion and absorption occurs in the small intestine, where triglycerides are partially hydrolyzed by pancreatic lipase, which splits off the two exposed fatty acids to leave a single central fatty acid still combined with glycerol (beta monoglyceride) plus two fatty acids (Fig. 27-6). Both are poorly soluble in water but combine with bile salts to form micelles. A mixed micelle is composed of bile salts, fatty acids, and the beta monoglyceride, and may also include phospholipids, cholesterol, and fat-soluble vitamins. The micelle must traverse three diffusion barriers in the passive process of entry into the intestinal epithelial cell. These are the unstirred water layer, the mucous coat overlying the brush border, and finally the lipid bilayer membrane making up the brush border. The micelle may release its fatty acid and monoglyceride component in traversing these barriers. After disaggregation of the micelle, bile salts remain within the intestinal lumen to enter into the formation of other micelles, and the released fatty acids and monoglycerides traverse the plasma membrane into the epithelial cell. The major metabolic pathway within the cell is initiated by reformation of the triglyceride through the interactions of intracellular enzymes (see Fig. 27-6) that are associated with the endoplasmic reticulum.

The triglycerides then combine with cholesterol and

Table 27-1. EFFECTS OF GASTROINTESTINAL HORMONES ON SMALL BOWEL MOTILITY

Gastrin — ↑[a]	Neurotensin — ↑
CCK — ↑[a]	Somatostatin — ↕[c]
Secretin — ↓[a]	Bombesin — ↕
Vasoactive intestinal peptide (VIP) — ↕	Enkephalins — ↕[c]
Glucagon — ↕[a]	Pancreatic polypeptide — ↑
Motilin — ↑[b,c]	Peptide YY (PYY) — ↓
Substance P — ↑	

↑ Increased
↓ Decreased
[a] Induction of fed pattern of motility from fasting
[b] Possible physiologic role
[c] Induction of migrating motor complexes
SOURCE: Adapted from: Sakamoto T, Guo Y-S, Thompson JC: Motility: gut and biliary, in Thompson JC, Greeley GH Jr, Rayford PL, Townsend CM Jr (eds): *Gastrointestinal Endocrinology.* New York, McGraw-Hill, 1987, pp 123–136.

phospholipids and apoproteins to form chylomicrons. These consist of an inner core containing almost all triglycerides with a membranous outer coat of phospholipids and apoproteins. The chylomicron exits the cell from the basolateral region and preferentially enters the central lacteal of the villus from whence it moves to the thoracic duct. Small fatty acids with chain lengths of C_{10} and less

may move directly through the cell into capillaries to flow into the portal vein. The bulk of chylomicron assimilation from the intestinal cell is via lymphatics, but some direct transfer to the portal vein may take place, particularly during periods between meals.

Bile salts are resorbed into the enterohepatic circulation from the distal ileum, in one of the examples of selective sites of resorption (Table 27-2). The total bile salt pool in man is about 5 g, and it recirculates about 6 times every 24 h (the enterohepatic circulation of bile salts). Only about 0.5 g is lost in the stool every day, and this is replaced by resynthesis from cholesterol. All ingested fat

Fig. 27-6. Diagrammatic representation of fat digestion and absorption. Abbreviated structures and names are given. DG = diglyceride; C_{10} and C_{15} = carbon chain length of amino acids. [From: *Gray GM, in Sleisenger MH, Fordtran JS (eds): Gastrointestinal Disease. Pathophysiology, Diagnosis, Management. Philadelphia, Saunders, 1983, chap 51, with permission.*]

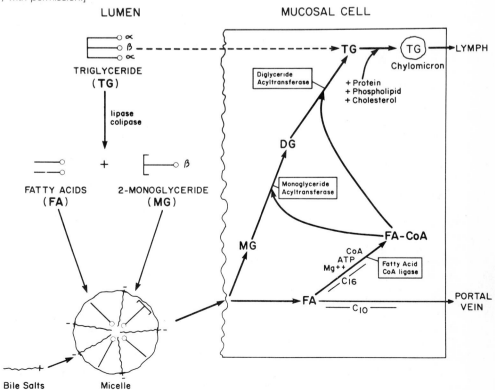

Table 27-2. DIFFERENTIAL SITES OF ABSORPTION FROM THE JEJUNOILEUM

Proximal	Distal
Calcium	Bile salts
Fat (absorbed mainly in jejunum)	Vitamin B$_{12}$
Folate	
Iron	

is usually absorbed, and the small amount appearing in the stool comes from sloughed cells and bacteria.

PROTEIN. Protein digestion is initiated in the stomach, where gastric acid denatures proteins, and proteolysis is initiated by activated pepsin. Little actual digestion takes place, however, until protein enters the duodenum and upper jejunum, when proteins come under the influence of pancreatic proteases. Pancreatic trypsinogen is activated by the duodenal mucosal enzyme, enterokinase, and then activated trypsin further activates all proteases. Endopeptidases (trypsin, elastase, chymotrypsin) act on peptide bonds at the interior of the protein molecule, producing peptides that are substrates for exopeptidases (carboxypeptidases), which serially remove a single amino acid at a time from the carboxy-terminal end of the peptide. The final products are amino acids and peptides of 2–6 amino acid residues. The intraluminal action of pancreatic proteases is efficient and yields 70 percent short-chain peptides and 30 percent amino acids. Short peptides are optimal substrates for the peptide transport mechanism that brings di- and tripeptides into the cell. Of peptides that are assimilated intact, at least 90 percent are hydrolyzed to free amino acids by cytosol peptidases, before delivery to the portal venous system.

CARBOHYDRATE. Western men and women take in about 400 g of carbohydrates a day, 60 percent as starch, 30 percent as sucrose, and 10 percent as lactose. Carbohydrates comprise about half the calories ingested in our society, but in underdeveloped countries they may provide a much higher proportion.

Starch is a polysaccharide consisting of long chains of glucose molecules. Amylose makes up 20 percent of starch in the diet and has an alpha glucose-to-glucose bridge. Amylopectin (80 percent of dietary starch) has branching points every 25 molecules along the straight glucose chains. Both have an alpha$_{1-4}$ glucose-linked chain. Alpha amylase attacks the alpha$_{1-4}$ linkage and converts amylose to maltotriose and maltose. Amylase converts amylopectin to shorter dextrins. Intraluminal digestion of starch in the duodenum is rapid because of the huge amounts of pancreatic amylase, and digestion is often complete by the time the starch enters the jejunum.

The enzyme responsible for final surface digestion is concentrated in the brush border of the luminal surface (Fig. 27-7). After dietary carbohydrate is reduced to monosaccharides by surface digestion, transport of the released hexoses (glucose, galactose, or fructose) is carried out by a specific process. Glucose and galactose are actively transported across the intestinal membrane,

whereas fructose is absorbed by facilitated diffusion. The rate-limiting phenomenon for most carbohydrate absorption occurs during transport through the intestinal cell, but luminal hydrolysis of lactose is slower than its transport capacity, so that surface hydrolysis of lactose is rate-limiting.

WATER AND ELECTROLYTES. In addition to ingested water, salivary, gastric, biliary, pancreatic, and intestinal fluids add up to 8 to 10 L of water per day, of which all but about 0.5 L per day is resorbed proximal to the ileocecal valve. The small bowel secretes and absorbs huge amounts of water. Net absorption is the algebraic sum of two fluxes going in opposite directions. Water may simply diffuse in or out of the cell or may be drawn through by osmotic or hydrostatic pressures. The osmotic pressures result from active transport of sodium glucose or amino acids into cells. Diffusion occurs through pores in plasma cell membranes. Jejunal pores are larger (7 to 9 Å) than those in the ileum (3 to 4 Å). Hypertonic solutions in the duodenum and upper jejunum are rapidly equilibrated to isotonicity by the influx of large amounts of water.

Sodium and chloride are absorbed from the small bowel by active transport, by coupling to organic solutes and cotransport by carriers of neutral sodium chloride. A small portion of sodium absorption in the jejunum is by active transport, but the bulk is by coupling to organic solutes. In the ileum, sodium is absorbed against deep gradients and is not stimulated by glucose, galactose, or bicarbonate. Bicarbonate is absorbed by a sodium-hydrogen exchange, so that one bicarbonate ion is released into interstitial fluid for every hydrogen ion secreted. Calcium is absorbed by active transport, particularly in the duodenum and jejunum. Absorption appears to be facilitated by an acid environment and is enhanced by vitamin D and parathormone. Potassium appears to be absorbed by passive diffusion.

Endocrine Function

The mucosa of the small bowel is the primary source of regulatory peptides of the gut, and the muscle wall of the small bowel is rich in peptidergic nerves containing neuroendocrine peptides. Although we often call these agents hormones, they do not always function in a truly endocrine fashion, that is, the active peptides are not always discharged into blood vessels to act upon some distant site. Sometimes they are discharged and act locally in a paracrine fashion [for example, bombesin (gastrin-releasing peptide) and somatostatin], or they may serve as neurotransmitters, or they may be discharged into blood vessels after nerve stimulation in a true neuroendocrine manner. We will briefly describe some of these agents.

SECRETIN. The discovery of secretin in 1902 gave birth to the entire field of endocrinology. Secretin is a 27-amino acid, helical peptide that is present in specialized cells in the small bowel mucosa and is released by acidification or by contact with bile and perhaps fat. It acts to stimulate release of water and bicarbonate from pancreatic ductal cells, and when this combination flows into the duodenal lumen, the bicarbonate neutralizes gastric acid. The

LUMEN

INTESTINAL CELL

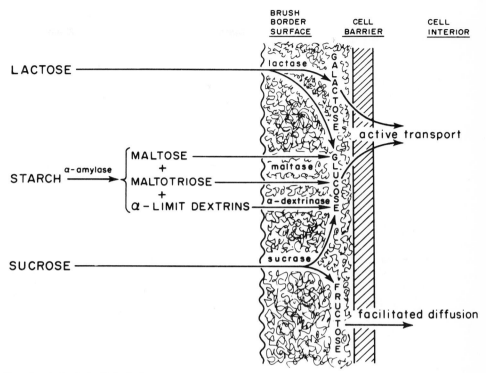

Fig. 27-7. The digestion and absorption of carbohydrate. Note that only starch is digested in the lumen; other dietary saccharides are hydrolyzed by constitutive enzymes of the intestinal surface. The final monosaccharide products are then transported by their specific mechanisms. [From: *Gray GM, in Sleisenger MH, Fordtran JS (eds): Gastrointestinal Disease. Pathophysiology, Diagnosis, Management. Philadelphia, Saunders, 1983, chap 51, with permission.*]

amount of pancreatic bicarbonate released after a meal closely approximates the amount of acid secreted by the stomach. Secretin also acts to stimulate the flow of bile and to inhibit gastrin release, gastric acid secretion, and gastrointestinal motility. Secretin has the unique ability to release gastrin from gastrinomas, and intravenous secretin is used as a diagnostic test in patients with the Zollinger-Ellison syndrome.

CHOLECYSTOKININ. Cholecystokinin (CCK) is released from small bowel mucosa by contact with certain amino acids (especially tryptophan and phenylalanine) and medium- to long-chain fatty acids. It has two major actions, one to stimulate contractions of the gallbladder and relaxation of the sphincter of Oddi and the other to stimulate the secretion of enzymes by pancreatic acinar cells. CCK also stimulates growth of bowel mucosa and pancreas, it stimulates bowel motility, and it releases insulin. CCK exists in multiple molecular forms (CCK-8, CCK-33, CCK-39, among others), and the larger forms contain the smaller ones. CCK and gastrin share the identical C-terminal tetrapeptide (Trp-Met-Asp-Phe-NH$_2$), which explains many of the similarities in their action.

OTHER PEPTIDES. Largely through the efforts of Viktor Mutt and colleagues at the Karolinska Institute, several active agents have been isolated from the mucosa of the small bowel that greatly influence physiologic activities of the gut. Of these, only *gastric inhibitory polypeptide* (GIP) has satisfied rigid criteria for hormonal status, but others will be discussed as well. GIP is a 43-amino acid peptide member of the secretin-glucagon family that is released by glucose and by fat. Although it was initially studied for its properties of inhibition of gastric secretion, later studies showed that it was a prime incretin candidate because it greatly stimulated insulin release when levels of glucose were elevated. Glucose-stimulated release of intestinal GIP apparently solves the conundrum posed by the fact that oral ingestion of a fixed amount of glucose releases more insulin than the intravenous administration of the same amount. A family of peptides reacting with glucagon antibodies is present in small bowel mucosa, and it has been given a variety of names. *Enteroglucagon* is a term used to designate all such gut peptides. It inhibits bowel motility, and it apparently stimulates mucosal growth. *Vasoactive intestinal peptide* (VIP) is a 28-amino acid basic peptide of the secretin-glucagon family that appears to function chiefly as a neuropeptide. VIP is a potent vasodilator and stimulates pancreatic and intestinal secretion and inhibits gastric acid secretion. It is the chief agent in the watery diarrhea syndrome caused by pancreatic endocrine tumors. *Motilin* is a 22-amino acid

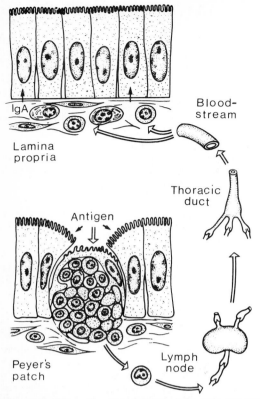

Fig. 27-8. Schematic representation of the pathways involved in the secretory immune system. Lymphocytes in Peyer's patches exposed to antigens from the gut lumen migrate to regional lymph nodes and thence to the bloodstream. Circulating in the blood, they home into the lamina propria of the gut and there develop into plasma cells secreting IgA, which acquires a secretory piece in the epithelium and is released into the gut lumen. (From: *Fawcett DW: A Textbook of Histology. Philadelphia, Saunders, 1986, with permission.*)

peptide widely distributed through the gut. It causes contraction of intestinal smooth muscle, including the gallbladder, and appears to be involved in the interdigestive pattern of gut motility. *Bombesin* is a 14-amino acid peptide first isolated from frog skin. It has the capacity to release probably all gut peptides except secretin. Its mammalian equivalent, gastrin-releasing peptide, is present in small bowel mucosa, where it probably serves as an "on" switch regulating release of gastrointestinal hormones. *Somatostatin* is a 14-amino acid peptide first isolated from the brain that is also widely distributed in the gut, where it probably functions in a paracrine fashion as an "off" switch. *Peptide YY* (PYY) is a 36-amino acid peptide in the distal ileum and colon. It inhibits gastric and pancreatic secretion but has no effect on gallbladder motility. PYY is released by perfusion of the colon with fat and may be involved in the physiologic inhibition of pancreatic secretion.

Immune Function

We ingest thousands of bacteria and parasites and viruses every day. Only a few of these are pathogenic, but the huge surface of the small bowel mucosa represents a massive potential portal of entry. An important component of bowel defense is the secretory immune system that produces a special group of antibodies that resist bacterial proliferation, neutralize virus, and minimize the penetration of enterotoxins.

The small bowel is a major source of immunoglobulin A (IgA). Cells of the lamina propria of the small intestine contain plasma cells that produce IgA. The population of cells producing IgA (the secretory immunoglobulin) is ten times greater than that producing IgG (the antibody mediating general humoral immunity).

Antigens from the intestinal lumen crossing the mucosal barrier contact M cells overlying lymphoid nodules. These cells are specialized for uptake and transport of antigen, which they convey to the underlying lymphoblasts that produce IgA. After interacting with the antigen, the lymphoblasts migrate to the regional lymph nodes from which they enter the systemic circulation. They then are returned to the intestine, where they are widely distributed in the lamina propria (Fig. 27-8). In the lamina propria, they differentiate into plasma cells that produce a specific IgA antibody directed to the absorbed antigen. This IgA antibody traverses the epithelial cell to the lumen by means of a protein carrier (the secretory component) that not only transports the IgA, but also protects it against the intracellular lysosomes. The antibodies at the free surface of the cell collect in the glycocalyx where they are in a strategic position to combat new antigens, preventing their attachment to the cell membrane, achieving immune exclusion.

INFLAMMATORY DISEASES

Crohn's Disease

Crohn's disease is a chronic granulomatous disease of the alimentary tract first described as regional ileitis by Crohn, Ginzburg, and Openheimer in 1932. In the introduction to their landmark paper, they stated

We propose to describe, with pathologic and clinical details, a disease of the terminal ileum affecting mainly young adults, characterized by a subacute or chronic necrotizing and cicatrizing inflammation. The ulceration of the mucosa is accompanied by a disproportionate connective tissue reaction of the remaining walls of the involved intestine, a process which frequently leads to stenosis of the lumen of the intestine, associated with the formation of multiple fistulas.

This disease has never been more elegantly, accurately, or completely described. Many different terms have been used to describe this disease, but because of its multiple clinical appearances and because the disease is not confined to the terminal ileum, Crohn's disease has been universally accepted as its name.

Since 1932, we have learned a great deal about the disease; unfortunately, we still do not know the etiology, and curative treatment has not been devised. We have learned, however, that extensive surgical resection, in an attempt at cure, plays no role in the management of patients with Crohn's disease. Our discussion will be limited to Crohn's disease of the small intestine.

Crohn's disease is a chronic inflammatory disease characterized by spontaneous remissions and acute exacerbations. There is a peak age of onset between the second and fourth decades. The typical patient is a young adult with a long history of chronic abdominal pain, diarrhea, and weight loss. The diagnosis is often delayed; an average of 3 years has elapsed between the onset of symptoms and the time the diagnosis is established. The abdominal pain is usually cramping, and often becomes constant. Diarrhea is intermittent, explosive, associated with meals, and frequently nocturnal. Weight loss usually appears later and is the result of decreased food intake, as well as nutritional abnormalities that develop as a result of defects of digestion and absorption in the diseased bowel.

Crohn's disease is the most common surgical disease of the small intestine. The incidence of Crohn's disease is greatest in North America and Northern Europe and is still increasing. For example, the incidence increased from 1.8 to 3.7 per 100,000 from 1963 to 1973 in the United States. There is a familial association with Crohn's disease, but no specific pattern of inheritance has been described. The risk for Crohn's disease is increased 30 times in siblings of patients with the disease and 13 times for all first-degree relatives. Although surgical resection is not curative, 75 percent of patients studied in the National Cooperative Crohn's Disease Study (NCCDS) required one or more surgical procedures within 20 years of onset of the disease. Operations are used only to treat complications. Recurrence rates after operation are high; surgical cure is not possible.

PATHOLOGY. The usual sequence in discussion of a disease is etiology, pathogenesis, and pathology. This sequence is here reversed in order to relate pathologic findings, which are well known, to hypotheses concerning pathogenic and etiologic factors, which are not known.

Microscopic features of Crohn's disease vary, but some histologic features occur with sufficient consistency to create a pattern that, while not specific, is at least characteristic of the disease. Some understanding of pathogenesis may be gained by observing the progression of changes from early to late phases of regional enteritis.

Intense mucosal and submucosal edema may be seen microscopically before any gross changes are apparent. The earliest gross pathologic lesion is a superficial aphthous ulcer. As the disease progresses, the ulceration becomes more pronounced and complete transmural inflammation results. The inflammatory reaction is characterized by extensive edema, hyperemia, lymphangiectasia, an intense infiltration of mononuclear cells, and hyperplasia of lymphoid follicles. The ulcers are characteristically linear. As the disease progresses, linear ulcers may coalesce to produce transverse clefts and sinuses that result in the characteristic cobblestone appearance of the mucosa. There is thickening and hypertrophy of the submucosa and the muscularis, which results in narrowing of the gut lumen; obliterative lymphangitis occurs; the bowel wall becomes thickened and edematous and quite rigid. Granulomas appear later and are found in the bowel wall and in regional lymph nodes. These are noncaseating granulomas with Langhans' giant cells. As the transmural inflammation progresses, the mesentery becomes involved in the inflammatory reaction and becomes thickened and shortened. At operation, one observes thickened, grayish pink or dull purple-red loops of bowel with areas of thick, gray-white exudate or fibrosis of the serosa. Areas of diseased bowel separated by areas of grossly normal bowel, called skip areas, are commonly encountered. A striking finding of Crohn's disease at operation is extensive fat-wrapping, caused by circumferential growth of the mesenteric fat around the wall of the bowel. The thickened bowel wall is very firm, rubbery, and virtually incompressible. The uninvolved proximal bowel is often dilated because of the considerable degree of obstruction present in the diseased segment. Involved segments are often adherent to adjacent loops or other viscera, or several loops may be matted together into a bulky conglomerate mass. Internal fistulas are common in such adherent areas. The mesentery of the segment is characteristically greatly thickened, dull, and rubbery, and contains masses of lymph nodes up to 3 or 4 cm in size.

Crohn's disease is a chronic granulomatous disease of unknown etiology. Despite years of trials, no animal model has been developed for Crohn's disease. Theories that have been put forth to suggest causative factors in the development of the disease have included immunologic abnormalities or the presence of transmissible agents.

Immunologic abnormalities that have been found in patients have included both humoral and cell-mediated immune reactions directed against gut cells, suggesting autoimmunity. However, there has been no direct correlation between these abnormalities, immunologic reactivity, and the development of Crohn's disease; they are probably epiphenomena.

A transmissible agent was first suggested in 1970 by Mitchell and Rees who inoculated the foot pads of mice with extracts of diseased bowel from patients; granulomatous lesions were produced in the footpads. These lesions were proposed as evidence of transmissable agents causing Crohn's disease. Other workers have failed to confirm these findings. Cytotrophic agents, or viruses, have been found by some investigators in diseased human tissue; however, there is controversy as to whether their findings represent true viruses. Electron microscopic analysis of large numbers of specimens has failed to reveal any viruses. Mycobacteria (*Mycobacterium kansasii*) have also been implicated, but presently, no etiologic agent has been found.

CLINICAL MANIFESTATIONS. A typical patient is a young adult with a long history of recurring and persistent abdominal pain, diarrhea, and weight loss. About one-third of patients have fever. There are three patterns of involvement: the small bowel is involved alone in 30 percent of patients; ileocolitis is present in 55 percent of patients; and 15 percent of patients have involvement of only the colon. These findings from the NCCDS differ from some British and Australian series in which as many as 50 percent of patients have only colonic involvement. The site of involvement is an indicator of prognosis; ileocolitis has the highest incidence of recurrence after resection.

Perianal disease (fissure, fistula, stricture, or abscess) is common, occurring in 25 percent of patients with small intestinal disease, 41 percent of patients with ileocolitis, and 48 percent of patients with exclusively colonic involvement. Perianal disease may be the sole presenting feature in 5 percent of patients and may precede the onset of intestinal disease by months to years. Any patient with multiple, chronic, recurrent perianal fistulas should be suspected of Crohn's disease. Extraintestinal manifestations of Crohn's disease include arthritis and arthralgia, uveitis and iritis, hepatitis and pericholangitis, and erythema nodosum and pyoderma gangrenosum.

In the majority of patients, the onset of disease is insidious, with a slow, protracted course. There are symptomatic periods of abdominal pain and diarrhea interspersed with varying intervals of remission; but over time, symptomatic periods gradually become more frequent and more severe and long-lasting. Pain (the most common symptom) is usually intermittent and cramping early in the course of the disease, but may develop into persistent, dull aching abdominal pain, most prominent in the lower abdomen.

Diarrhea is the next most frequent symptom and is present, at least intermittently, in 85 percent of patients. The frequency of stools is not great compared with ulcerative colitis, numbering two to five daily, and, unlike ulcerative colitis, the stools rarely contain mucus, pus, or blood.

Fever is present in about one-third of these patients; moderate weight loss, loss of strength, and easy fatigability, in over one-half. Frank nutritional disorders and steatorrhea are uncommon before surgical treatment.

DIAGNOSIS. Patients with chronic, recurring episodes (often of long duration) of abdominal pain, diarrhea, and weight loss should be suspected of having Crohn's disease. Diagnosis is confirmed by barium radiographic studies of the small bowel. The most accurate technique of examination is radiographic enteroclysis. Although numerous findings have been described for Crohn's disease, the most common findings noted in the NCCDS survey were a nodular contour, diffuse narrowing of the lumen, sinuses, clefts, and linear ulcers, separation of bowel loops, and asymmetrical involvement of the bowel wall. One-half of patients had a cobblestone mucosal pattern composed of linear ulcers and transverse sinuses and clefts. This study showed that the radiographic features of Crohn's disease of the small bowel did not correlate with clinical symptoms or response to drug therapy. Therefore, there is no need for ritual, periodic radiographic examination of the small bowel in patients with established Crohn's disease, except in one of the following situations: (1) evaluating the appearance of Crohn's disease in a patient with severe clinical exacerbation, looking particularly for evidence of stricture with obstruction or fistula; (2) preoperative evaluation of patients undergoing planned resection; or (3) evaluation of post-operative patients who develop clinical symptoms of recurrence.

TREATMENT. Patients presenting with signs and symptoms of acute intestinal obstruction are common; however, complete obstruction is unusual. Most patients with these findings will improve on a conservative program of intravenous fluids, nasogastric suction, and medications. Complete obstruction is uncommon compared to partial obstruction. The acute obstruction is produced by intense edema and inflammation of the bowel wall. Emergency operation for obstruction per se is usually not necessary, since most patients respond rather quickly to nonoperative measures. Elective operative treatment for high-grade partial obstruction (characterized by Kantor's string sign on barium radiographic studies, (Fig. 27-9) is usually indicated, however, as soon as the patient can be prepared.

Medical treatment of Crohn's disease is largely symptomatic and empiric and is usually followed by remissions and exacerbations until a complication that requires surgical intervention supervenes. Goals of medical therapy are relieving abdominal pain, controlling diarrhea, treating infection, and correcting any nutritional deficiencies.

Intraluminal antibiotics, particularly sulfasalazine (Azulfidine), do have significant beneficial effects in certain patients. Corticosteroids are also useful in effecting re-

Fig. 27-9. This radiograph demonstrates Kantor's string sign (arrows). The string sign is the result of narrowing of the lumen due to mucosal ulceration, extensive thickening, and rigidity of the bowel wall.

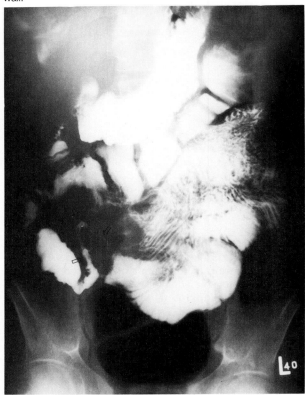

mission of symptoms during acute exacerbations of ileitis, and a combination of sulfasalazine and steroids may be used to maintain patients for a short period of time after resolution of an acute inflammatory episode. Long-term maintenance therapy, with either agent alone or in combination, however, has not been shown to be of benefit in preventing recurrence of the disease. Although there have been implications of immunologic abnormality in Crohn's disease, immunosuppressive treatment with azathioprine and 6-mercaptopurine have not been conclusively shown to be of advantage when compared to placebo. Systemic antibiotics are valuable in the management of infectious complications, but have no effect on the primary disease process and should not be considered to be therapeutic.

Elemental diets and total parenteral nutrition have been touted as being beneficial, even curative, in patients with acute Crohn's disease or in patients with complications such as enterocutaneous fistulas. There is no specific therapeutic benefit in any dietary measure. The provision of adequate nutrition is much more important in preparing patients for operation than it is for cure.

There is a subgroup of patients with acute abdominal signs and symptoms in whom the usual preoperative diagnosis is acute appendicitis. At operation, the appendix is found to be normal, but the terminal ileum is edematous and beefy red, having a thickened mesentery with enlarged lymph nodes. The condition is acute ileitis, a self-limiting disease, which does not lead to subsequent development of Crohn's disease. The precise etiology of acute ileitis is unknown; however, some patients have been found to have *Yersinia* or *Campylobacter* infections.

Although in the past, performance of appendectomy has been controversial in this setting, the place of appendectomy now seems clear. In the absence of acute inflammatory involvement of the appendix or the cecum, appendectomy should be performed. This removes the possibility of acute appendicitis in the differential diagnosis of any subsequent abdominal complaints in these patients. In the few patients who have developed enterocutaneous fistulas after appendectomy, the fistulas have all originated from the ileum.

Although medical management is certainly indicated during acute exacerbations of disease, the majority of patients with chronic Crohn's disease will require operation sometime during the course of their illness. In patients with more than 20 years of disease, the NCCDS reported that the cumulative probability of operation was 78 percent.

Cure of patients with Crohn's disease is not possible by either medical or surgical therapy. Indications for operation are limited to complications, including: obstruction, abscess, fistula, free perforation, urologic complications, hemorrhage, cancer, perianal disease, and growth retardation.

Patients with Crohn's disease who have had a previous abdominal operation and who develop signs of mechanical bowel obstruction pose a difficult problem. The most likely cause is progressive disease, but the obstruction may be caused by postoperative adhesions. In this setting, the historical sequence of symptoms becomes most important. A history of increasing pain, diarrhea, and fever over days to weeks points toward a recrudescence of Crohn's disease. A short history (hours) of the acute onset and rapid progression of cramping abdominal pain, nausea, and vomiting, without an antecedent history of increasing disease activity, usually means adhesions.

At operation, only the segment of the bowel involved in the obstructive process should be resected. Even if adjacent areas of bowel are clearly diseased, they should be ignored unless also obstructed. Early in the history of surgical treatment of Crohn's disease, many surgeons tended towards wide resection in an attempt to effect cure. Repeated wide resections lead to the short bowel syndrome, a devastating surgical complication. In the past, the most common cause of the short bowel syndrome was repeated resections for Crohn's disease. We and most other surgeons have, for at least the past two decades, concluded that it is extremely difficult surgically to eradicate this disease, and we have, for example, given up frozen-section study of the resected margin because we generally limit our resection to areas that are grossly involved adjacent to sites of obstruction or fistulization. We ignore microscopic evidence of involvement.

Fistulas in patients with Crohn's disease are usually enteroenteral or enterocutaneous. The presence of a radiographically demonstrable enteroenteral fistula without any signs of sepsis or other complication is not in itself an indication for operation. However, the vast majority of patients who have radiographic demonstration of enteroenteral fistulas will develop later complications, most commonly sepsis, and will require resection of the fistula. Enterocutaneous fistulas are rarely spontaneous, but follow resections or external drainage of intraabdominal abscesses. All enterocutaneous fistulas associated with active Crohn's disease must be treated by resection of the involved segment of the bowel, in addition to closure of the fistula. The formation of enteroenteric or enterovesicle fistulas usually involves either a previous intestinal perforation with formation of a walled-off abscess that finally perforates or the adherence of one diseased loop of bowel to another diseased loop of bowel or an adjacent normal organ. If the fistula forms between two or more adjacent loops of diseased bowel, the entire involved segment should be excised. On the other hand, if the fistula involves an adjacent normal organ, such as the bladder or the colon, only the segment of the diseased small bowel and fistulous track should be resected, and the defect that is left in the normal organ is simply closed. Block and Schraut have shown that the majority of patients with ileosigmoid fistulas do not require resection of the sigmoid because the disease is confined to the small bowel. If the segment of sigmoid involved in an ileosigmoid fistula is found to have Crohn's disease, it should be resected, along with the segment of diseased small bowel.

Perforation into the free peritoneal cavity is not common, but occurs occasionally. Free perforation usually occurs in a diseased segment of bowel but can also occur in bowel proximal to an obstruction. The segment should be resected back to relatively good bowel on each side of the perforation, and no attempt should be made to eradicate all diseased bowel. If generalized peritonitis is present, an anastomosis should not be done because of the high rate of anastomotic dehiscence; an ileostomy should be performed until intraabdominal sepsis is controlled. Later restoration of intestinal continuity can be carried out safely.

The most common urologic complication is ureteral obstruction, which is usually due to ileocolic disease with retroperitoneal abscess. Periureteric fibrosis may be present and may require extensive ureteral lysis.

Although anemia from chronic blood loss is common, life-threatening hemorrhage is rare. When it occurs, the segment involved should be resected and intestinal continuity restored. Up to one-fourth of children with Crohn's disease may have significant growth retardation that may precede the appearance of active bowel disease. In these children, bowel resection, in the absence of other common indications, is indicated and will often result in restoration of normal growth.

Treatment of perianal disease should be conservative, and wide excisions of abscesses or fistulas are not indicated. Definitive fistulotomy is indicated in the majority of patients, although one must recognize that some degree of anal stenosis may occur as a result of the chronic inflammation. Fissures are usually lateral, relatively painless, large and indolent, and will usually respond to conservative management. Abscesses should be drained, but large excisions of tissue should not be carried out.

The optimum treatment of complications of Crohn's disease is surgical resection of the involved segment with restoration of intestinal continuity. Current evidence indicates that results are not improved by increasing the margins of normal tissue proximal and distal to the diseased intestine. Thus, the proximal margin should be through soft, pliable bowel—dilatation does not necessarily indicate disease—and microscopic control of margins with frozen sections is not helpful and is often confusing. With disease in the terminal ileum, the distal line of resection should be in the ascending colon, although the standard right colectomy is technically easier. No attempt should be made to remove all enlarged mesenteric lymph nodes, since this does not change the rate of recurrence and may endanger the blood supply to otherwise normal intestine. In selected patients with obstruction caused by strictures (either single or multiple), many surgeons utilize strictureplasty as an alternative to resection. The technique involves longitudinal incision of the stricture, including one centimeter of bowel on either side of the stricture. The incision is then closed transversely. This technique is said to be associated with no increased incidence of leaks or recurrence of disease compared to resection. We do not use this method. No one should be confused; the standard surgical treatment is limited resection and anastomosis of diseased bowel.

In the past, bypass procedures were commonly used, but today, bypass with exclusion is now only used in elderly, poor-risk patients; in patients who have had several prior resections and can ill afford to lose any more bowel; and in patients in whom resection would necessitate entering an abscess or endangering normal structures. The reasons for this are twofold: the disease often persists in the bypassed segment with development of intraabdominal sepsis, and cancer may occur in the bypassed segment.

PROGNOSIS. The occurrence of cancer in Crohn's disease has been well documented. Cancer is reported to be 60 to 300 times more frequent in patients with Crohn's ileitis than in patients the same age without Crohn's disease. Cancer arising in the small bowel afflicted with Crohn's disease is different than small bowel cancer in patients without Crohn's disease. The cancers occur more commonly in the ileum, they occur more often in men, they have a worse prognosis, and Crohn's disease patients are younger.

There is no surgical cure for Crohn's disease. It is now clear that a substantial proportion of patients who have had one operation will require another operation for complications of Crohn's disease. In one study, the cumulative recurrence rates were reported to be 29 percent at 5 years, 52 percent at 10 years, 64 percent at 15 years, and 84 percent at 25 years. No important differences were noted between disease location and the type of operation. One cannot predict which patients will develop recurrent disease. Sex, age, duration of disease, granulomas, enteral or perirectal fistulas, the length of resection, the length of diseased gut, and the proximal resection margin had no significant influence on the rate of recurrent disease or functional outcome. The most common site of recurrence is the small bowel proximal to the site of previous resection. Recurrence is five times more likely to involve the adjacent or remote colon in patients with ileocolitis compared to ileitis. Few patients with ileitis eventually require ileostomy, whereas one-third of patients with ileocolitis or colitis often may require permanent ileostomy.

Crohn's disease gradually burns out with advancing age. Active disease is unusual between the ages of 50 and 55, but gradual cicatrization with healing may cause bowel obstruction in old patients.

Tuberculous Enteritis

Tuberculosis of the gut is now rare in Western countries, but is still a significant problem in India and developing countries. Tuberculosis of the gastrointestinal tract occurs in two forms. Primary infection is usually due to the bovine strain of *Mycobacterium tuberculosis* and results from ingesting infected milk. This now accounts for less than 10 percent of reported cases. Secondary infection, due to the human strain, results from the swallowing of bacilli by patients with active pulmonary tuberculosis. Chemotherapy has greatly decreased the incidence of secondary tuberculous enteritis, so that it now occurs in only about 1 percent of patients with pulmonary tuberculosis.

The ileocecal region is the site of involvement in about 85 percent of patients with tuberculous enteritis, presumably because of the abundance of lymphoid tissue in this area. Three patterns of involvement are seen: hypertrophic, ulcerative, or ulcerohypertrophic.

Occasionally, a hypertrophic reaction produces contracture and stenosis of the lumen of distal ileum, which requires resection. The diagnosis is not often made pre-operatively; only 50 percent of patients have evidence of active pulmonary tuberculosis; 45 percent of patients have negative skin tests. If the diagnosis is suspected pre-operatively, chemotherapy, best given as a combination of isoniazid, 100 mg three times a day, with either rifam-pin (600 mg daily) or ethanibutol (15 mg/kg daily), should be administered for about 2 weeks before operation. If unsuspected tuberculosis is found at operation, chemo-therapy should be started, and in both instances, drugs should be continued for 1 year after the patient has be-come asymptomatic. Surgical therapy of hypertrophic tuberculous enteritis is usually inadvisable unless bowel obstruction due to high-grade stenosis requires relief. Resection and anastomosis should be performed unless extensive disease is present, otherwise ileocolic bypass is the safer procedure.

Symptoms of the more common ulcerative form of tu-berculous enteritis include alternating constipation and diarrhea associated with crampy lower abdominal pain. At times, the diagnosis may only be made by radiographic intestinal examination of patients with pulmonary tuber-culosis. In severe cases, diarrhea is persistent, and anemia and inanition are progressive. Clinical confirma-tion of a presumptive diagnosis may be obtained by a prompt response to antituberculous chemotherapy. Sur-gical therapy is contraindicated except for the rare com-plications of perforation, obstruction, or hemorrhage.

Typhoid Enteritis

Typhoid enteritis is an acute, systemic infection of sev-eral weeks' duration, caused by *Salmonella typhosa*. There is hyperplasia and ulceration of Peyer's patches of the intestine, mesenteric lymphadenopathy, splenomeg-aly, and parenchymatous changes in the liver. Confirma-tion of diagnosis is obtained by culturing *S. typhosa* from blood or feces or by finding a high titer of agglutinins against the O and H antigens.

Typhoid fever is still a major disease in areas of the world that have not yet attained high public health stand-ards, but it is now rare in the West. The death rate, for-merly about 10 percent, is now about 2 percent, in large part because of the specific antimicrobial chlorampheni-col, introduced in 1948.

There is some disagreement as to whether chloram-phenicol remains the drug of choice, however, because of the emergence of resistant strains, high relapse rate, and risk of marrow toxicity. Trimethoprim-sulfamethoxazole has emerged as the best successor to chloramphenicol. Trimethoprim-160 mg and sulfamethoxazole-800 mg are given, either orally or parenterally, twice daily for 2 weeks. Amoxycillin is also effective and should be given intravenously or intramuscularly in doses of 1 g every 6 h for 2 weeks.

Gross hemorrhage occurs in 10 to 20 percent of hospi-talized patients, even while on adequate therapy. Trans-fusion is indicated and usually suffices. Every effort should be made to avoid operation, since the bleeding is often from multiple ulcers and the bowel is exceedingly friable. Rarely, laparotomy must be done for uncontrolla-ble, life-threatening hemorrhage.

Perforation, through ulcerated Peyer's patches, is usu-ally single and found in the terminal ileum, and occurs in about 2 percent of cases. Operative treatment is indicated unless the patient is moribund, since localization or walling-off of the perforation is uncommon. Simple clo-sure of the perforation is successful in the majority of patients. With multiple perforations, which occur in about one-fourth of patients, resection with primary anas-tomosis or a temporary ileostomy is preferred. The mor-tality rate of those with free perforation is about 10 per-cent.

NEOPLASMS

General Considerations

Primary neoplasms of the small bowel are extremely rare, despite the much greater mucosal surface area and rapidity of cell turnover of the small bowel compared to the stomach and colon; neoplasms are 40 times more common in the colon; the reasons for this difference are not clear. Several theories have been proposed as possi-ble explanations: rapid transit time decreases the time for contact of carcinogens with the mucosa; the local immune system of the small bowel mucosa; the alkaline pH of the *succus entericus*; the absence of bacteria that might con-vert certain ingested products to carcinogens; and the presence of mucosal enzymes that destroy certain car-cinogens.

Primary small bowel neoplasms are either benign or malignant and may arise from any of the cells of the small bowel. The frequency of benign and malignant neoplasms is reported to be equal in surgical series, whereas benign neoplasms far exceed malignant neoplasms in autopsy series. Malignant neoplasms (75 to 80 percent) more often produce symptoms than benign neoplasms.

Symptoms associated with small bowel neoplasms are often vague; they include epigastric discomfort, nausea, vomiting, abdominal pain (often intermittent and col-icky), diarrhea, and bleeding (often manifest as symptoms of anemia). Symptoms may be present for months to years prior to operation. Bleeding is usually occult; hematochezia or hematemesis may occur, although life-threatening hemorrhage is not common. The most com-mon indications for operation in patients with neoplasms of the small bowel are obstruction, bleeding, and pain. The mechanism of obstruction differs, depending upon whether it is caused by a benign or malignant neoplasm. Benign neoplasms are the most common cause of intus-susception in the adult; whereas malignant neoplasms commonly cause obstruction by circumferential growth or kinking of the bowel due to longitudinal, intramural growth.

Because of their relative infrequency and the vague symptoms they produce, the diagnosis of small bowel neoplasms requires informed suspicion. Endoscopy is useful in evaluating the duodenum and possibly the most proximal jejunum, just beyond the ligament of Treitz. The

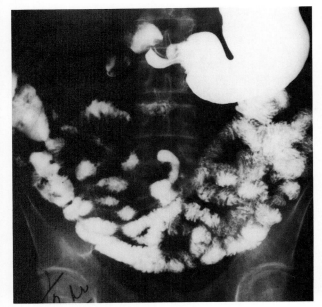

A

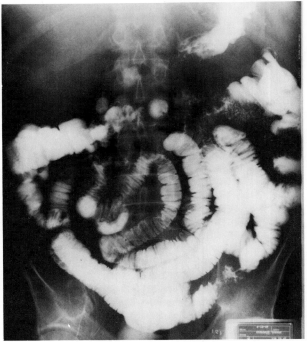

B

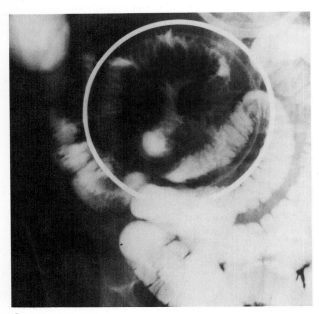

C

Fig. 27-10. Enteroclysis compared to small bowel follow-through. *A.* An overhead view obtained one-half hour after administration of barium in a small bowel follow-through examination. Note the incomplete filling and poor distention of bowel loops. The lesion in the ileum was not found. *B.* An overhead view from an enteroclysis examination in the same patient. The entire small bowel is nicely distended, except for ileal loops in the right abdomen. Each loop is individually examined by compression. *C.* This is a compression film of the involved ileal loops. These loops exhibit thickened, irregular mucosal folds; the thickening and kinking of the bowel wall are characteristic of an infiltrating carcinoid tumor.

great majority of the small bowel is not accessible to endoscopic scrutiny. Barium contrast radiography is therefore required.

Hypotonic duodenography employing glucagon to produce temporary paralysis of the duodenum allows excellent visualization of the duodenal mucosa; exquisite detail can be obtained and accurate diagnoses rendered.

For the small bowel distal to the ligament of Treitz, however, traditionally, the motor meal, or small bowel follow-through, examination was employed. This was accomplished by taking overhead radiographs every 15 to 30 min after ingestion of barium until barium reached the cecum. Compression films of the terminal ileum were also obtained. This method is limited by low diagnostic sensitivity. Intubation infusion for small bowel examination, termed *enteroclysis*, has recently been widely employed. The availability of better intubation techniques, improved mixtures of barium, and improved results have increased its use.

In performing enteroclysis, the tip of a naso-small bowel tube is placed just beyond the ligament of Treitz, and dilute barium sulfate is instilled at a constant flow rate by an electric pump. The examination is complete when the barium reaches the cecum; this usually occurs within 10 to 15 min. Enteroclysis (Fig. 27-10) is superior to small bowel follow-through for detection of small filling defects and for determination of changes in mucosal pattern; the diagnostic accuracy of enteroclysis approaches 90 percent. The sensitivity and accuracy of enteroclysis has led to its acceptance by more gastrointestinal radiologists as the examination of choice for radiographic study of the small bowel.

Benign Neoplasms

PATHOLOGY. Benign tumors of the small bowel may either be of epithelial or of connective tissue origin. The most common lesions are adenomas, leiomyomas, and lipomas. Other benign lesions include hamartomas, fibromas, angiomas, lymphangiomas, neurofibromas, and hemangiomas. Adenomas are the most common benign tumors reported in autopsy series; however, leiomyomas are the most common benign small bowel lesions that produce symptoms.

Histologic types of benign small bowel tumors and their relative incidence are shown in Table 27-3. The incidence of these tumors varies, depending upon whether they are reported from autopsy or clinical series.

CLINICAL MANIFESTATIONS. An appreciable number of small bowel benign tumors apparently cause no serious symptoms during life and are incidental findings at autopsy. The diagnosis is delayed or missed in many patients because symptoms may be absent or vague or nonspecific until significant complications have developed. Physical examination rarely provides any clue unless intestinal obstruction is present, and radiographic studies of the small bowel and selective angiography, the only specific diagnostic aids, may fail to demonstrate an existing tumor, even though it is suspected clinically. In only about one-half of small bowel tumors found at operation has the correct diagnosis been made preoperatively.

The two most common clinical manifestations of small bowel tumors are bleeding and obstruction. Rarely, perforation of the bowel wall occurs, resulting in abscess or internal fistula formation, peritonitis, or pneumatosis cystoides intestinalis. Bleeding occurs in about one-third of patients but is rarely gross hemorrhage. More commonly, bleeding is occult and intermittent, producing guaiac-positive stools and iron-deficiency anemia. Leiomyomas and hemangiomas are the lesions that most often cause bleeding.

TREATMENT. Surgical treatment of benign tumors is nearly always indicated because of the risk of subsequent complications and because the diagnosis of benign disease cannot be made without microscopic evaluation.

Table 27-3. TYPES AND RELATIVE FREQUENCY OF SMALL BOWEL BENIGN NEOPLASMS

Neoplasms	Percent
Leiomyomas	17
Lipomas	16
Adenomas	14
Polyps	14
Polyposis, Peutz-Jeghers	3
Hemangiomas	10
Fibromas	10
Neurogenic tumors	5
Fibromyomas	5
Myxomas	2
Lymphangiomas	2
Fibroadenomas	1
Others	1

Complications of benign neoplasms most often requiring treatment are bleeding and obstruction. Segmental resection and primary reanastomosis is most commonly used except for very small lesions that may be excised by enterotomy. The entire small bowel should be searched for other lesions since they are often multiple.

ADENOMA

Adenomas are of three primary types: true adenomas, villous adenomas, or Brunner's gland adenomas. Twenty percent of adenomas are found in the duodenum, 30 percent in the jejunum, and 50 percent in the ileum. The majority of adenomas are asymptomatic, single, and are most commonly found incidentally at autopsy. If adenomas cause symptoms, they usually are associated with bleeding or obstruction. Villous adenomas of the small bowel are rare but do occur and are most commonly found in the duodenum. Their presence may be suspected by the characteristic "soap bubble" appearance on contrast radiography. They may attain large size (greater than 5 cm in diameter) and are usually found because of pain or bleeding. Obstruction may also occur. There have been no reports of secretory diarrhea associated with villous tumors of the small bowel; however, the malignant potential of these lesions is reportedly between 35 and 55 percent.

Brunner's gland adenomas are hyperplastic proliferations of normal exocrine glands located in the duodenum. Brunner's gland adenomas may produce symptoms that mimic those of peptic ulcer disease or may cause obstruction. Diagnosis can be made by endoscopy and biopsy, and symptomatic lesions in an accessible region should be resected. There is no malignant potential for Brunner's gland adenomas, and a radical resection should not be employed.

LEIOMYOMA

The most common symptomatic benign lesions of the small bowel are leiomyomas. Leiomyomas are benign tumors of smooth muscle that are most common in the jejunum. They are usually single, although multiple tumors may occur. The incidence is equal in men and women. Two growth patterns are noted: (1) the tumor may grow primarily intramurally and cause obstruction; (2) both intramural and extramural growth occurs and produces a dumbbell-shaped mass. These tumors may attain considerable size, outgrowing their blood supply, and tumor necrosis with bleeding may occur. The most common indication for operation on leiomyomas is bleeding. Angiography may provide the correct preoperative diagnosis.

LIPOMA

Lipomas are most common in the ileum and are single intramural lesions, submucosal in location, and usually small. Less than one-third of lipomas are found at operation and, when found, usually are the cause of obstruction, most commonly as the lead point of an intussuscep-

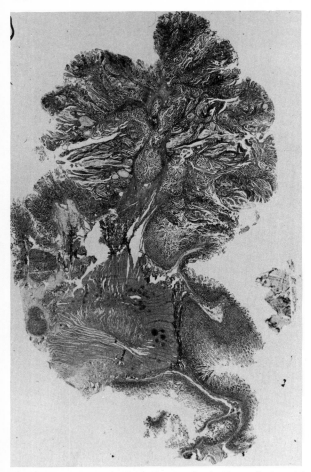

Fig. 27-11. Low-power photomicrograph of a Peutz-Jeghers jejunal polyp. Instead of one predominant cell, as seen in most intestinal polyps, these contain all cells of normal intestinal mucosa interspersed within bands of smooth muscle. They are hamartomas.

tion. Bleeding may occur from ulceration of the overlying mucosa. Lipomas do not possess malignant potential and, therefore, when found incidentally, should be removed only if the resection is simple. Pedunculated lipomas should be excised.

Peutz-Jeghers Syndrome

This is an inherited syndrome of mucocutaneous melanotic pigmentation and gastrointestinal polyps. The pattern of inheritance is simple mendelian dominant, with a high degree of penetrance. A single pleiotropic gene is responsible for both polyps and melanin spots. The classic pigmented lesions are small, 1 to 2 mm brown or black spots, located on the circumoral region of the face, buccal mucosa, forearms, palms of the hands, soles of the feet, the digits, and the perianal area. The syndrome was first reported in 1921 by Peutz. Jeghers et al. redescribed it in 1949. Multiple pigmented lesions may be noted or only a single buccal lesion may be present. Pigmentation appears in childhood. All cutaneous lesions may fade, leaving only buccal lesions. Pigmentation with polyposis and polyposis without pigmentation have been reported. The entire jejunum and ileum are the most frequent portions of the gastrointestinal tract to be involved with multiple polyps. Fifty percent of patients may, in addition, have rectal and colonic polyps, and one-fourth of the patients may have gastric polyps. The chief point to note is that if a patient with multiple rectal, colonic, or gastric polyps is found to have hamartomas rather than adenomas, a search for small bowel polyposis and pigmented lesions should be carried out.

The lesions are not true polyps but are hamartomas and, as such, are not premalignant (Fig. 27-11). However, there have been a few reported cases of malignant tumors of the gastrointestinal tract associated with Peutz-Jeghers syndrome. Some of these adenomatous and carcinomatous changes were noted in the hamartomatous polyps. It is not clear, however, whether this represents a coincidence or a true malignant transformation of this syndrome.

The most common symptom is recurrent colicky abdominal pain, due to intermittent intussusception. Lower abdominal pain associated with palpable mass has been reported to occur in one-third of patients. Hemorrhage occurs less frequently and is most commonly manifested by insidious involvement of anemia. Acute life-threatening hemorrhage is uncommon but may occur.

Surgical therapy is required only for obstruction or persistent bleeding. The resection should be limited to the segment of bowel that is producing complications, that is, polypectomy or limited resection. Because of the widespread nature of intestinal involvement, cure is not possible and extensive resections are not indicated.

Malignant Neoplasms

The most common malignant neoplasms of the small bowel are adenocarcinomas, carcinoids, sarcomas, and lymphomas, in about that order of frequency.

CLINICAL MANIFESTATIONS. Rochlin and Longmire called attention to three distinct clinical presentations of patients with malignant small bowel neoplasms: diarrhea, with large amounts of mucus and tenesmus; obstruction, with nausea, vomiting, and cramping abdominal pain; and chronic blood loss, with anemia, weakness, guaiac-positive stools, and occasionally melena or hematochezia. As with benign neoplasms, symptoms of malignant neoplasms are often present for many months before the diagnosis is made, emphasizing their insidious nature.

TREATMENT. The treatment for malignant neoplasms of the small bowel is wide resection, including regional lymph nodes. This may require a radical pancreatoduodenectomy (Whipple operation) for duodenal lesions. Because of the extent of the disease at the time of operation, curative resection may not be possible. Palliative resection should be performed when possible to prevent further complications of bleeding, obstruction, and perforation. However, if that is not possible, bypass of the involved segment is an alternative that may provide worthwhile relief of symptoms. If this is used, the proximal end of the bypassed segment should be brought out as a mucous fistula to prevent development of a closed loop.

PROGNOSIS. The overall survival of malignant neoplasms of the small bowel is not good. The highest survival rates are reported for duodenal periampullary carcinomas (about 30 to 40 percent), whereas adenocarcinomas occurring elsewhere in the small bowel have a 5-year survival of 20 percent or less. Leiomyosarcomas of the small bowel have a 5-year survival of between 30 to 40 percent. Radiation and chemotherapy play little role in treatment of patients with adenocarcinomas of the small bowel. There may be some improvement in survival when radiation therapy is employed in patients with sarcomas. Determinants of survival for patients with lymphomas is the cell type and extent of disease. Radiation therapy and chemotherapy, combined with surgical excision, provide the best survivals for patients with lymphomas. Five-year survivals have been reported to range between 10 and 50 percent, with an average of about 30 percent.

CARCINOMA

Carcinomas comprise about 50 percent of the malignant tumors of the small bowel in most reported series and are twice as common in men as in women. The average age at diagnosis is 50 years. Adenocarcinomas are more common in the duodenum and proximal jejunum than in the remainder of the small bowel. The reasons for this are unclear. About half of duodenal carcinomas involve the ampulla of Vater.

The location in the small bowel often determines the presenting symptoms. For example, periampullary adenocarcinomas are associated with intermittent jaundice, whereas carcinomas of the jejunum usually produce symptoms of mechanical small bowel obstruction (Fig. 27-12). The presence of jaundice, often intermittent, and a positive stool test for guaiac should immediately call to mind the possibility of a periampullary carcinoma.

As with carcinomas arising in other organs, survival of patients with small bowel carcinomas is related to the stage of disease at the time of diagnosis. Diagnosis is often delayed, and disease is often far advanced at the time of operation. The delay in diagnosis is due to a combination of factors, including lack of suspicion because of the relative rarity of the lesions, vagueness of symptoms, and absence of physical findings.

Fig. 27-12. Malignant tumors. *A.* Adenocarcinomas produce a typical apple core or napkin ring deformity of the small bowel. *B.* The operative specimen illustrates a fungating intraluminal mass that is typical of adenocarcinoma.

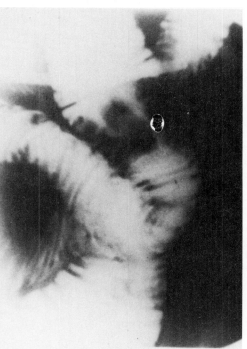

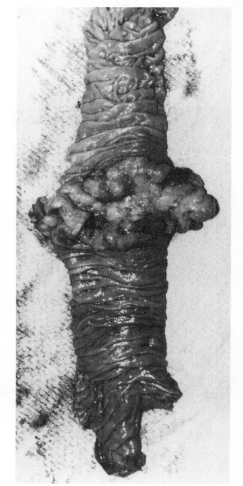

A

B

SARCOMA

Sarcomas comprise about 20 percent of malignant neoplasms of the small bowel, and the most common by far is the leiomyosarcoma. Leiomyosarcomas are evenly distributed throughout the small bowel, the incidence between men and women is equal, and the most common age at diagnosis is the sixth decade. The most common indications for operation are bleeding and obstruction, although free perforation due to hemorrhagic necrosis in large tumor masses may occur. Leiomyosarcomas are spread by direct invasion of adjacent structures, by hematogenous dissemination, or by transperitoneal seeding producing sarcomatosis.

LYMPHOMA

Lymphomas comprise about 10 to 15 percent of small bowel malignant tumors and are most commonly found in the ileum, where the greatest concentration of gut-associated lymphoid tissue is present. Lymphomas may be primary or part of a generalized disease. Dawson and colleagues have devised criteria to determine whether lymphoma of the small bowel is primary. These include: (1) absence of peripheral lymphadenopathy; (2) normal chest x-ray without evidence of mediastinal lymph node enlargement; (3) normal white blood cell count, total and differential; (4) at operation, the bowel lesion must predominate and the only involved nodes are associated with the bowel lesion; and (5) absence of disease in the liver and spleen. Even when these criteria are employed, one-third or more of patients with lymphomatous involvement of the small bowel will be found to have generalized lymphoma.

There are three syndromes of small bowel lymphoma. Western lymphoma is a disease predominantly of adults, typically found in the western hemisphere and associated with severe malabsorption in 5 to 10 percent of patients. Another form, known as "Mediterranean," is a malignant lymphoma first noted in non-Ashkenazi Jews and Arabs in Israel, which has subsequently been reported in other countries and in other ethnic groups, including Hispanic Americans. Since this disease is not confined to the Mediterranean basin, the term *immunoproliferative small intestinal disease* has been used. One-third of the patients may be found to have an abnormal fragment of IgA heavy-chain in their serum, which is produced by plasma cells infiltrating the small bowel. This variant is known as "heavy-chain disease."

The third intestinal manifestation of lymphoma is childhood abdominal lymphoma. This is a group of lymphomas including American (nonendemic) Burkitt's lymphoma, undifferentiated non-Burkitt's lymphoma, and diffuse histiocytic lymphoma.

CARCINOID

Carcinoids of the small bowel arise from the enterochromaffin, or Kulchitsky, cells found in the crypts of Lieberkühn. These cells are also known as argentaffin cells because of their staining by silver compounds. Carcinoids of the small bowel occur with almost the same frequency as adenocarcinoma and together they make up the preponderance of malignant neoplasms of the small bowel. Carcinoids have variable malignant potential and are composed of multipotential cells with the ability to secrete numerous humoral agents, the most prominent of which are serotonin and substance P. Although the carcinoid syndrome, characterized by episodic attacks of cutaneous flushing, bronchospasm, diarrhea, and vasomotor collapse occurs in fewer than 5 percent of the patients with malignant carcinoids, it is quite dramatic and has been extensively described and discussed with fascination by many authors.

The primary importance of carcinoid tumors is not, however, the carcinoid syndrome, but the malignant potential of the tumors themselves. Oberndorfer coined the term *karzinoide* to denote that this tumor was carcinomalike, and to emphasize the assumed lack of malignant potential. By 1930, this concept was no longer supported, since many patients with metastatic carcinoid tumors had been reported. In 1953 and 1954, the carcinoid syndrome was described.

PATHOLOGY. Carcinoids may arise in organs derived from the foregut, midgut, and hindgut. In the gastrointestinal tract, the appendix is most frequently involved (46 percent), followed by the ileum (28 percent), and rectum (17 percent). Other locations are shown in Table 27-4. The malignant potential, thus the ability to metastasize, appears to be related to the site of origin and the size of the primary tumor. Only about 3 percent of appendiceal carcinoids metastasize, but about 35 percent of ileal carcinoids are associated with metastasis. Seventy-five percent of gastrointestinal carcinoids are less than 1 cm in diameter; only 2 percent of this group metastasize. About 20 percent of primary tumors are 1 to 2 cm in diameter,

Table 27-4. DISTRIBUTION OF GASTROINTESTINAL CARCINOIDS: INCIDENCE OF METASTASES AND OF CARCINOID SYNDROME

Site	Cases	Average metastasis, %	Cases of carcinoid syndrome
Esophagus	1	—	0
Stomach	93	23	8
Duodenum	135	20	4
Jejunoileum	1032	34	91
Meckel's diverticulum	42	19	3
Appendix	1686	2	6
Colon	91	60	5
Rectum	592	18	1
Ovary	34	6	17
Biliary tract	10	30	0
Pancreas	2	—	1
	3718		136

SOURCE: From Wilson JM, Cheek RC, et al: 1970, with permission.

and 50 percent of this group metastasize. Only about 5 percent are over 2 cm in diameter; 80 to 90 percent of these metastasize. Multiple carcinoids of the small bowel occur in 30 percent of cases but are rare in the appendix. This tendency to multicentricity exceeds that of any other malignant neoplasm of the gastrointestinal tract. An unusual observation that is yet unexplained is the frequent coexistence of a second primary malignant neoplasm of a different histologic type; a second primary neoplasm was reported in 25 percent of patients in one large series.

Carcinoids present grossly as a slightly elevated, smooth, rounded, hard nodule, covered with normal mucosa. On cut section, they have a characteristic yellow-gray or tan appearance. Extensive fibrosis of the mesentery and of the bowel wall, due to an intense desmoplastic reaction, may be present. This fibrosis may produce mechanical bowel obstruction from kinking or matting of loops of small bowel together. Obstruction is rarely due to direct tumor encroachment on the lumen of the bowel. In addition to the desmoplastic reaction apparently produced by humoral agents elaborated by the tumor, metastases to mesenteric nodes also result in kinking and fixation by large, metastatic tumor deposits. An often remarked upon finding is that of a small primary tumor associated with massive mesenteric metastases.

CLINICAL MANIFESTATIONS. In the absence of the malignant carcinoid syndrome, symptoms of patients with carcinoid tumors of the small bowel are similar to those of patients with small bowel tumors of other histologic types. The most common symptoms are abdominal pain, bowel obstruction, diarrhea, and weight loss. In the majority of patients (in the absence of the malignant carcinoid syndrome), the diarrhea is due to partial bowel obstruction, rather than secretory diarrhea. On rare occasions, malignant carcinoid tumors of the ampulla of Vater may be found in patients with disseminated neurofibromatosis (von Recklinghausen's disease).

DIAGNOSTIC FINDINGS. Radiographic studies of the small bowel may exhibit multiple filling defects sometimes due to tumors but more often due to kinking and fibrosis of the bowel, mesenteric calcifications, and fixed rigid loops of intestine. Mesenteric vascular angiography may reveal abnormal arrangement of mesenteric arteries, and narrowing of peripheral branches together with poor accumulation of contrast and poor venous drainage of the tumor area. Tumor staining during angiography may be enhanced by administration of norepinephrine. Angiography is the most sensitive diagnostic test to detect hepatic metastasis, particularly diffuse metastatic disease with fine nodular distribution. Hepatic metastases are hypervascular and intensely stained during arteriography.

TREATMENT. The treatment of patients with small bowel carcinoid tumors is based upon size and site of the tumor and the presence or absence of metastatic disease. For primary tumors less than 1 cm in diameter without evidence of regional lymph node metastasis, a segmental intestinal resection is adequate. For lesions greater than 1 cm, for patients with multiple tumors, and in the presence of regional lymph node metastasis regardless of the size of the primary tumor, wide excision of bowel and mesentery is required. Since the majority of small bowel carcinoids are found in the ileum, wide excision usually entails a right hemicolectomy. Malignant carcinoid tumors of the duodenum may require radical pancreatoduodenectomy.

Treatment of Carcinoid Tumors of the Appendix.

Simple appendectomy is curative for patients with tumors less than 1 cm in diameter without gross evidence of metastasis. Because of the potential for metastasis, right hemicolectomy should be performed for tumors greater than 2 cm. Intramural lymphatic invasion, serosal involvement, or microscopic involvement of the mesoappendix associated with tumors less than 2 cm is not an indication for extensive resection.

PROGNOSIS. Survival for small bowel carcinoid tumors has been reported to be 75 percent for those tumors staged as local, 59 percent for regional tumors, and 19 percent for tumors with distant spread. The overall survival rate is 54 percent. Attempts to relate microscopic growth patterns to prognosis suggests that, as the site of origin of carcinoid tumor is an independent predictor of outcome, the growth pattern is likewise an independent predictor of outcome. Decreasing order of median survival time of the various growth patterns is illustrated: mixed insular plus glandular, 4.4 years; insular, 2.9 years; trabecular, 2.5 years; mixed insular plus trabecular, 2.3 years; glandular growth pattern, 0.9 years; and undifferentiated, 0.5 years.

When widespread metastatic disease precludes cure, extensive resection for palliation is indicated. Since these tumors are often indolent and slow growing, long-term palliation often results. Bypass procedures may be used in poor-risk patients with extensive disease. The overall 5-year survival rate after resection of intestinal carcinoids is about 50 percent. If "curative resection" is done, 70 percent of patients live 5 years. Chemotherapy has not been entirely successful; however, treatment with streptozocin and 5-fluorouracil (5-FU) may provide significant palliation. Up to 25 percent of patients with palliative resections survive 5 years.

MALIGNANT CARCINOID SYNDROME

This rare syndrome is widely described but rarely seen. The infrequent occurrence of this syndrome is emphasized when one considers that 30 to 70 percent of carcinoid tumors of the gut are metastatic at the time of diagnosis, but that only 6 to 9 percent of patients with metastatic disease will develop manifestations of the malignant carcinoid syndrome. By far the most commonly associated primary tumor is located in the small bowel, and massive hepatic replacement by metastatic tumor is usually found.

CLINICAL MANIFESTATIONS. The syndrome is characterized by hepatomegaly, diarrhea, and flushing in 80 percent of patients, right heart valvular disease in 50 percent, and asthma in 25 percent. Malabsorption and pellagra (dementia, dermatitis, and diarrhea) may infrequently be present and are thought to be due to excessive diversion of dietary tryptophan to meet the metabolic requirements of the tumor.

Diarrhea is episodic, often occurring after meals, and is due to elevated circulating levels of serotonin, which stimulates secretion of small bowel fluid and electrolytes, and increases intestinal motility. Some patients may present with acute abdominal symptoms, characterized by severe abdominal cramping without mechanical bowel obstruction. This has been called "carcinoid abdominal crisis." The mechanism of this crisis is thought to be intestinal ischemia, caused by the vasoactive substances elaborated by the tumor, combined with decreased mesenteric blood supply due to perivascular fibrosis.

Flushing is not temporally related to diarrhea, and although both may be present, either may be present without the other. The lack of relationship between flushing and diarrhea suggests that these two manifestations of the syndrome are due to different mediators. Although substance P produces all of the vasomotor phenomena associated with the flush, it has been questioned as the primary mediator. Besides serotonin and substance P, other substances that have been implicated include bradykinin and prostaglandins E and F.

Valvular heart disease is due to irreversible endocardial fibrosis, which is similar in genesis to the fibrosis noted in the gut wall, retroperitoneum, and around the mesenteric blood vessels. It occurs in patients with hepatic metastases and is limited to tricuspid and pulmonary valves. The reason that the right side valvular lesions predominate is that they are exposed to high levels of serotonin. The pulmonary filter deactivates serotonin, thereby preventing left sided valvular lesions.

Asthma is due to bronchoconstriction, which may be produced by serotonin, bradykinin, or substance P. Treatment of asthma associated with carcinoid syndrome must be carried out very carefully, since use of adrenergic drugs may cause release of humoral agents that may cause status asthmaticus.

Although the syndrome is seen in patients with high circulating levels of serotonin and often substance P, these are probably not the only mediators of all components of the syndrome. The malignant enterochromaffin cells produce 5-hydroxytryptamine, also called serotonin (5-HT). Circulating serotonin is metabolized in the liver and in the lung to 5-hydroxyindoleacetic acid (5-HIAA), which is pharmacologically inactive. Elevated levels of 5-HIAA are only seen in patients with metastasis. However, not all patients with metastasis have increased levels of 5-HIAA. The majority of patients who exhibit malignant carcinoid syndrome have massive hepatic replacement by their metastatic disease. Tumors that bypass the hepatic filter, specifically ovarian and retroperitoneal carcinoids, may produce the syndrome in the absence of liver metastasis.

DIAGNOSTIC FINDINGS. The diagnosis is most reliably established by repeated determination of urinary 5-HIAA. A single determination may be normal in the presence of metastatic disease. Provocative testing to reproduce symptoms has employed injection of pentagastrin, calcium, or epinephrine. The pentagastrin test is by far the most reliable and safest provocative test. During times of testing for increased levels of 5-HIAA, the patient must avoid foods rich in serotonin, such as bananas, tomatoes, walnuts, pineapples and certain drugs, including phenothiazines, glycerol guaiacolate, or reserpine.

TREATMENT. Treatment of the carcinoid syndrome would require removal of all tumor; this is rarely possible. Hepatic resection, however, even when known tumor is left behind, may result in significant relief of symptoms due to removal of the mass of tumor. When resection is not possible, hepatic dearterialization or embolization of the hepatic arterial branches may provide some relief. The duration of response after resection was 6 months compared to 4.8 months for hepatic artery ligation.

Drug therapy for prevention or relief of symptoms is directed at blockade of the effects of humoral agents elaborated by the tumor. Interferon has provided some symptomatic improvement in a small group of patients. Somatostatin or the long-acting analogue of somatostatin (SMS 201-995, Sandoz) prevents diarrhea and flushing in the majority of patients with the syndrome. Chemotherapeutic attacks on the tumor itself have been disappointing, although streptozocin, alone or combined with 5-FU, appears to be the most effective.

Treatment of carcinoid tumors remains wide surgical resection of the small bowel and regional lymph nodes. In addition, significant palliation may be achieved with aggressive hepatic resection in patients with malignant carcinoid syndrome.

DIVERTICULAR DISEASE

Diverticula of the small bowel may either be congenital or acquired. A congenital diverticulum is a true diverticulum; it is composed of all layers of the bowel wall. An acquired diverticulum is a false diverticulum; only mucosa and submucosa protrude through a defect in the muscle coat of the bowel wall. Diverticula may occur in any portion of small intestine. Duodenal diverticula are the most common acquired diverticula of the small bowel. Meckel's diverticulum is the most common true diverticulum of the small bowel.

Duodenal Diverticula

The true incidence of duodenal diverticula is unknown and varies depending upon whether they are found clinically (by x-ray, endoscopy, or operation) or at autopsy. It has been reported that between 1 to 5 percent of upper gastrointestinal x-ray examinations will reveal duodenal diverticula; between 9 to 20 percent of upper gastrointestinal endoscopic examinations show them. This is compared to a 10 to 20 percent incidence reported from autopsy series. More than 90 percent of these diverticula are clearly asymptomatic, and less than 5 percent will require operation due to a complication of the diverticulum itself. The ratio of appearance in men to women is about 1:2. Duodenal diverticula are rare in patients under 40 years of age, and the incidence increases with increasing age.

Two-thirds to three-fourths of duodenal diverticula are found in a periampullary region and project from the medial wall of the duodenum (Fig. 27-13). Duodenal diverticula are clinically important for two reasons: they may occasionally produce symptoms related to the diverticulum, including obstruction, perforation, or bleeding, and the presence of the diverticulum may cause recurrent pancreatitis, cholangitis, or recurrent common-duct stones after cholecystectomy.

Only those diverticula associated with the ampulla of Vater have significant relationship to complications of cholangitis, pancreatitis, and stone disease. In patients with these diverticula, the ampulla most often enters the duodenum at the superior margin of the diverticulum, rather than through the diverticulum itself. The mechanism proposed for the increased incidence of complications of the biliary tract is the location of the periviaterian diverticula, which may produce mechanical distortion of the common bile duct as it enters the duodenum, resulting in partial obstruction and stasis. Bile stasis allows proliferation of bacteria and subsequent formation of stones. The incidence of bactibilia is significantly increased in patients with periviaterian diverticula compared to diverticula located in other parts of the duodenum. The bacteria isolated from the bile duct and from the diverticula are identical. There is also evidence that dysfunction of the choledochal sphincter is produced by presence of diverticula. In one study of 101 patients who had undergone cholecystectomy more than 2 years previously, a significantly increased incidence of recurrent calculi was noted in patients with diverticula compared to patients without. A causal relationship of duodenal diverticula and biliary tract stones, however, has not been demonstrated. The great majority of duodenal diverticula cause no trouble and should be left alone unless they can be closely related to disease.

Fewer than 60 patients have been reported with intraluminal duodenal diverticula. These diverticula, which probably originate from incomplete duodenal webs, are lined both inside and out with duodenal mucosa, have a characteristic picture of a barium-filled wind sock on contrast radiography, and most often have required operation because of duodenal obstruction or recurrent pancreatitis. In these diverticula the common bile duct and pancreatic duct usually enter the diverticulum, and a second orifice is present that allows drainage of the biliary-pancreatic secretions into the lumen of the gut.

Symptoms related to duodenal diverticula, in the absence of any other demonstrable disease, are usually nonspecific epigastric complaints. Bleeding, perforation, and diverticulitis are all rare. The morbidity and mortality caused by complications of diverticula are nonetheless high because of delay in diagnosis due to the lack of suspicion of the underlying condition. Diagnosis is seldom made preoperatively.

TREATMENT. Treatment of complications of the diverticulum are directed toward the control of the complication. In those patients who have bleeding or symptoms that are related to the duodenal diverticulum, several operative procedures have been described. The most

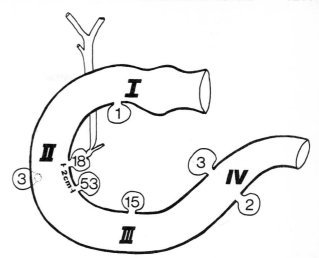

Fig. 27-13. Distribution of 95 duodenal diverticula within the four portions of the duodenum. (From: *Eggert A, Wittmann DH: Surg Gynecol Obstet 154:62, 1982, with permission.*)

common and most effective treatment in this situation is diverticulectomy. This is most easily accomplished by performing a wide Kocher maneuver that exposes the diverticulum. The diverticulum can then be excised, and the duodenum is closed in a transverse or longitudinal manner, whichever technique produces the least amount of luminal obstruction. For those diverticula embedded deep within the head of the pancreas, lateral duodenotomy is performed, and the diverticulum is invaginated into the lumen and excised, and the wall closed. An alternative method that has been described for the duodenal diverticula associated with the ampulla of Vater is an extended sphincteroplasty through the common wall of the ampulla and the diverticulum.

A perforated diverticulum may cause great trouble. When found, the perforated diverticulum should be excised and the duodenum closed with a serosal patch from the jejunal loop. If the inflammation is severe, it may be necessary to divert enteric flow away from the site of the perforation, with either a gastrojejunostomy or, preferably, a duodenojejunostomy if possible. It may be possible to interrupt duodenal countinuity proximal to the perforated diverticulum with a row of staples. Great care should be taken if the perforation is adjacent to the papilla. In one early perforation, we were able simply to invert the diverticulum, close the duodenal wall, and reinforce this with a serosal patch.

Because of the relationship of the common bile duct and pancreatic duct in patients with intraluminal diverticula associated with the ampulla of Vater, subtotal resection of the diverticulum should be carried out to protect the entry of the biliary-pancreatic ducts. If an intraluminal diverticulum arises at a site distant from the ampulla, complete excision may be possible.

Although fascinating, the vast majority of duodenal diverticula are asymptomatic, boringly benign, and, when found incidentally, should not be resected.

Jejunal and Ileal Diverticula

Diverticula of the jejunum and ileum are much less common than duodenal diverticula, with an incidence between 0.5 and 1 percent on small bowel x-ray examination. Jejunal diverticula are more common and are larger than those in the ileum. Multiple diverticula are more common in the jejunum and ileum than in the duodenum. These are false diverticula, usually protrude from the mesenteric border of the bowel, and may be overlooked at operation because they are embedded within the small bowel mesentery. When jejunal and ileal diverticula give trouble, the symptoms are usually due to imcomplete bowel obstruction, acute diverticulitis, hemorrhage, or malabsorption due to bacterial overgrowth within the diverticulum. A specific syndrome of intestinal pseudoobstruction or jejunal dyskinesia is characterized by symptoms of intermittent partial bowel obstruction. On enteroclysis examination, barium may be seen to pass back and forth from the intestinal lumen into the diverticulum, rather than move normally through the bowel. This condition may be associated with hypertrophy and dilatation of the bowel proximal to the diverticulum. A recent study found that the condition may be associated with one of three syndromes: systemic sclerosis, visceral myopathy, or visceral neuropathy. If this condition is the only finding, resection of a large segment of jejunum containing diverticula should be avoided. Treatment of complications of obstruction, bleeding, and perforation is by intestinal resection and end-to-end anastomosis. Patients with malabsorption due to production of the blind loop syndrome by bacterial overgrowth within the diverticulum can usually be treated with antibiotics. Asymptomatic diverticula require no treatment.

Meckel's Diverticulum

The most common true diverticulum of the gastrointestinal tract is Meckel's diverticulum. This is a congenital diverticulum that results from incomplete closure of the omphalomesenteric or vitelline duct. Meckel's diverticula are located usually within 2 to 3 ft of the ileocecal valve and vary in length from 1 to 12 cm. Heterotopic gastric or pancreatic tissue is often found in Meckel's diverticula. The great majority of symptomatic Meckel's diverticula will be found in childhood, and the most common symptom in childhood is bleeding. A 2 percent incidence of Meckel's diverticula in the general population is based upon reports of several autopsy series. In adults, most Meckel's diverticula are found incidentally by radiographic examination of the small bowel. Enteroclysis has a very high incidence of accurate diagnosis. Another technique for detection of Meckel's diverticulum in symptomatic patients is radionuclide scanning, using ^{99m}Tc-pertechnetate. The basis for this is the uptake of radioisotope by the heterotopic gastric mucosa within the diverticulum. The diagnostic accuracy of this scanning technique may be increased by administration of pentagastrin (6 mg/kg subcutaneously) 15 min before the scan, which enhances the uptake of the radioisotope by the gas-

tric mucosa. It has been shown, however, that the parietal cells do not specifically accumulate pertechnetate and are not essential for detection purposes. The scan is not nearly so useful in adults as it is in children.

Complications of Meckel's diverticulum in adults include intestinal obstruction, bleeding, acute diverticulitis, or the presence of a diverticulum in a hernia sac (Littre's hernia). Obstruction may be produced by one of two mechanisms. The most common is volvulus or kinking around a band running from the tip of the diverticulum to the umbilicus, abdominal wall, or mesentery. The diverticulum may also cause obstruction by intussusception. Bleeding is the second most common complication and is usually found only in those patients who have heterotopic gastric mucosa within the diverticulum. The bleeding ulcer is found not in the diverticulum, but in the ileum adjacent to the diverticulum.

Meckel's diverticulitis, which is clinically indistinguishable from appendicitis, is the third most common complication in adults. The incidence of perforation or peritonitis with Meckel's diverticulitis is about 50 percent.

A Meckel's diverticulum should be considered in the differential diagnosis of patients who present with a mechanical bowel obstruction, with low small bowel hemorrhage, or with signs and symptoms of inflammation or peritonitis. Treatment is prompt surgical intervention with resection of the diverticulum or resection of the segment of ileum bearing the diverticulum. Segmental intestinal resection is required for treatment of patients with bleeding, because the bleeding site is usually in the ileum adjacent to the diverticulum.

Removal of an asymptomatic Meckel's diverticulum found incidentally at laparotomy in adults should not be performed. Soltero and Bill have estimated that the likelihood of Meckel's diverticulum becoming symptomatic in an adult is 2 percent or less and that morbidity from incidental removal (reported to be as high as 12 percent) far exceeds the potential for prevention of disease.

MISCELLANEOUS PROBLEMS

Small Bowel Ulcerations

The majority of ulcerations of the small bowel have definable causes, which include the following: drug-induced (enteric-coated potassium chloride tablets or corticosteroids), vascular (occlusion or vasculitis), Crohn's disease, syphillis, typhoid fever, tuberculosis, lymphoma, heterotopic gastric mucosa (Meckel's diverticulum), and ulcers associated with gastrinoma. This discussion is limited to those ulcerations of the small intestine in which no etiologic agent can be identified.

Patients with discrete isolated ulcers of the small bowel, without any identifiable underlying disease, have nonspecific ulcers. Ulcers are more common in the terminal ileum. These appear to be self-limited and do not recur after bowel resection.

These patients usually present with a single ulceration,

although multiple ulcers may be present. Indications for operation are for complications of the ulcers, including perforation, bleeding, or stricture. Recurrence of ulceration in the small bowel distal to the duodenum is rare. A review of 59 patients studied from 1956 to 1979 reports the overall incidence of 4 patients per 100,000 new patients seen at the Mayo Clinic. These investigators noted that the yearly rate fell from 3.6 new cases per year from 1960 to 1969 to 1.2 cases per year from 1970 to 1979. They believe, despite the absence of a documented underlying etiology, that the decrease in incidence was directly related to the removal of enteric-coated potassium chloride tablets.

The ulcers are discrete, vary in size from 0.3 to 5 cm in diameter, are sharply demarcated, and the surrounding mucosa is perfectly normal. They occur more frequently on the antimesenteric border and may be associated with fibrous scar formation, which produces the obstruction. The characteristic microscopic findings include acute granulation tissue and inflammatory cells at the base of the ulcer, local hyperplasia of the muscularis mucosae, and pyloric metaplasia of the adjacent mucosa. Varying degrees of edema and fibrosis, depending upon the chronicity of the ulcer, are noted. There is no evidence of vascular disease associated with the ulcer. With time, the ulcers may increase in size, become annular, and, with healing, may produce fibrous strictures of the intestine, which may produce obstruction.

Diagnosis is rarely if ever made before operation; the majority of patients present with complications. In a Mayo Clinic series, 63 percent of patients had intermittent small bowel obstruction, while 25 percent had bleeding, and 12 percent had symptoms of acute abdominal inflammation caused by perforation. With the increasing use of enteroclysis, the diagnosis of small bowel ulcer may be made more frequently, and an asymptomatic solitary ulcer does not require treatment.

TREATMENT. The treatment of small bowel ulcers depends upon the complications encountered at the time of diagnosis. Mechanical bowel obstruction and bleeding should be treated by segmental resection. Although excision and primary closure of perforated ulcers has been advocated by some, high recurrence rates have been associated with this technique. Resection of the ulcerated segment of bowel should be done.

Ingested Foreign Bodies

A great variety of objects that are capable of penetrating the wall of the gut are swallowed, usually accidentally, but sometimes intentionally by the mentally deranged. These include glass and metal fragments, pins, needles, cocktail toothpicks, fish bones, coins, whistles, toys, and broken razor blades.

Treatment is expectant, since the vast majority pass without difficulty. If the object is radiopaque, progress can be followed by serial plain films. Catharsis is contraindicated.

Sharp, pointed objects such as sewing needles may penetrate the bowel wall. If abdominal pain, tenderness,

fever or leukocytosis occur, immediate surgical removal of the offending object is indicated. Abscess or granuloma formation are the usual outcomes without surgical therapy.

Small Bowel Fistulas

The vast majority of small bowel fistulas are due to operation; less than 2 percent are associated with granulomatous disease of the bowel (Crohn's disease) or trauma. In some patients, there are contributing factors, such as preoperative radiotherapy, intestinal obstruction, inflammatory bowel disease, mesenteric vascular disease, and intraabdominal sepsis. But in the majority, surgical misadventures are the primary cause. These include anastomotic leak, injury of bowel or blood supply at operation, laceration of bowel by wire mesh or retention sutures, and retained sponges. We have seen fistulas result from injury by suction catheters and from erosion by abscesses.

The major complications associated with small bowel fistulas include sepsis, fluid and electrolyte depletion, necrosis of the skin at the site of external drainage, and malnutrition. Successful management of patients with small bowel fistulas requires meticulous attention to detail and a logical, stepwise plan of management. One must establish controlled drainage, manage sepsis, prevent fluid and electrolyte depletion, protect the skin, and provide for adequate nutrition.

Mortality for patients with intestinal fistulas remains high, 20 percent or greater, even with the use of total parenteral nutrition (TPN). Although TPN has not been shown to reduce mortality significantly, it is the single most important advance in the management of patients with enterocutaneous fistulas. Fluid, electrolyte, and nutritional status may be maintained from the time the fistula becomes apparent and throughout the time required for control of sepsis. The key to successful management of intestinal fistulas is control of sepsis and prevention of malnutrition.

Diagnosis of small bowel fistula is usually not difficult. When the damaged area of the small bowel breaks down and discharges its contents, dissemination may occur widely in the peritoneal cavity, producing generalized peritonitis. More commonly, however, the process is more or less walled-off to the immediate area of the leak, with formation of an abscess. This usually underlies the operative incision, so that when a few skin sutures are removed to ascertain why the incision is becoming red and tender, contents of the abscess are discharged and the fistula established. The discharge may initially be purulent or bloody, but this is followed, sometimes immediately, sometimes within a day or two, by drainage of obvious small bowel contents. If the diagnosis is in doubt, confirmation can be obtained by oral administration of a nonabsorbable marker such as charcoal or Congo red.

Small bowel fistulas are classified according to their location and volume of daily output, since these factors dictate treatment as well as morbidity and mortality rates. In general, the more proximal the fistula in the intestine, the more serious the problem. Proximal fistulas have a greater fluid and electrolyte loss, the drainage has a greater digestive capacity, and an important (distal) segment is not available for food absorption. High-output fistulas are those which discharge 500 mL or more each 24 h. It is important, therefore, as soon as the patient's condition is stabilized, to identify the site of the fistula, to determine the extent of the associated abscess cavity by fistulogram, and to ascertain whether there is distal obstruction, since fistulas will not close in the presence of distal obstruction. Upper gastrointestinal series with small bowel follow-through and barium enema studies usually provide this information.

TREATMENT. Control of sepsis is aided by sump suction, which provides drainage of the associated intraabdominal abscess cavity and prevents accumulation of intestinal contents. Control of fistula output is most easily accomplished by percutaneous intubation of the fistula track. Protection of the skin around the fistulous opening is important. In the past, frequent applications of zinc oxide, aluminum paste ointment, or karya powder were required; excoriation and destruction of skin still occurred. The advent of stomahesive appliances used for colostomy and ileostomy bags greatly improved and facilitated protection of the skin at the site of fistula. The stomahesive appliance should be cut so that the opening just fits over the fistulous opening and no unprotected skin remains. The suction catheter can be brought out through the end of the bag which is fixed firmly about the tube. This allows for collection of all the drainage and accurate quantitation of the lost volume.

The volume depletion that occurs from a proximal small bowel fistula may present a formidable problem. Patients with volume losses exceeding 5 L/day are not uncommon. Agents that inhibit gut motility (codeine, Lomotil, or loperamide) are not generally helpful. Somatostatin inhibits both intestinal secretion and motility. We have successfully used a long-acting analog of somatostatin (SMS-201995 Sandoz) to stop fistula output in three patients. Somatostatin, however, is a general ''off'' switch, and ileus can be a problem. In none of our patients was spontaneous healing effected, but the analog ameliorated the problems associated with massive volume loss. Systemic antibiotics should be administered until sepsis is controlled. At the same time, TPN should be instituted because a prolonged course of inability to use the gut for nutrition is likely.

Several factors may prevent spontaneous closure of fistulas. Fistulas will not close spontaneously if there is high output (>500 mL/24 h) or severe disruption of intestinal continuity (>50 percent of the circumference of the bowel involved in the fistula). A fistula will not close spontaneously if it arises from a segment of bowel involved with active granulomatous disease, cancer, or radiation enteritis, if there is distal obstruction, or if there is an undrained abscess cavity. If a foreign body is in the track, if the fistulous track is less than 2.5 cm in length, or if there is epithelialization of the track, spontaneous closure will not occur. Radiographic investigation of the fistula by means

of injection of water soluble contrast material through the fistulous track should be carried out early to delineate the presence and extent of any abscess cavities and obtain information about the length of the track and the extent of bowel wall disruption. A diligent search by means of contrast studies for distal obstruction should be performed. CT will often reveal undrained collections of fluid.

When any of the conditions noted above are present, spontaneous closure is unlikely; therefore, management should be directed toward obtaining prompt control of sepsis, maintaining positive nitrogen balance, and early operation.

Conservative treatment for up to 3 months with TPN has been advocated by some to allow spontaneous closure of the fistula. We do not believe that the results support this plan. Fewer than 30 percent of all small bowel fistulas will close spontaneously. In patients with low output fistulas, particularly those located in the distal small bowel without any of the conditions that will prevent spontaneous closure, a wait of up to 6 weeks may be indicated. The patient can usually wait at home. When we reviewed reported series that advocate conservative therapy for longer than 6 weeks, we found that the majority of fistulas that close spontaneously do so within 3 weeks after their appearance. After 3 weeks, if sepsis has been controlled and adequate nutritional status has been achieved, operative control of the fistula should be carried out promptly. Delay only produces delay. TPN simplifies management of patients, but it does not cure fistulas. The single most important determinant in successful treatment of fistulas is sepsis. If sepsis is not controlled, the patient will die. After sepsis has been controlled, one should not wait endlessly for a fistula to spontaneously close simply because malnutrition can be avoided by use of TPN. The proper role of TPN is prevention or treatment of malnutrition prior to operative closure of fistulas.

Operation is most easily accomplished by entering the previous abdominal wound. The wound should be reopened with great care to avoid needless reinjury to the bowel. The fistulous track is excised, the bowel should be completely mobilized, and the portion of bowel involved in the fistula resected. The technique of excision and fistula closure must be precise and accurate, and all rigid or diseased bowel must be resected. Simple closure of the fistula after removing the fistulous track and minimal mobilization of the bowel almost always results in recurrence of the fistula.

If an unexpected abscess is encountered or if the bowel wall is rigid and distended over a large distance, a proximal enterostomy should be performed. Later, resection of the bowel involved in the fistula will be required for successful closure. Side-to-side bypass should not be done.

The overall mortality rate in enterocutaneous fistulas of the small bowel is still greater than 20 percent. It is higher in jejunal fistulas and significantly lower in ileal fistulas. Successful treatment of the majority of patients with small bowel fistulas requires control of sepsis, provision of adequate nutrition, and operative closure.

Pneumatosis Cystoides Intestinalis

This is an uncommon condition manifested by multiple gas-filled cysts of the gastrointestinal tract. The cysts are either submucosal or subserosal and vary in size from microscopic to several centimeters in diameter. The jejunum is most frequently involved, followed by the ileocecal region and colon. Gas cysts are associated with other lesions of the gastrointestinal tract in about 85 percent of cases. Pneumatosis not associated with other lesions (15 percent of cases) is called "primary."

Grossly, the cysts resemble cystic lymphangiomas or hydatid cysts. On section, the involved portion has a honeycomb appearance. The cysts are thin-walled and break easily. Spontaneous rupture gives rise to pneumoperitoneum.

Symptoms are nonspecific and in "secondary" pneumatosis may be those of the associated disease. In primary pneumatosis, symptoms, when present, resemble those of irritable bowel syndrome. The diagnosis is usually made radiographically (Fig. 27-14). No treatment is necessary unless one of the very rare complications supervenes, such as rectal bleeding, cyst-induced volvulus, or tension pneumoperitoneum. Prognosis in most patients is that of the underlying disease. When pneumatosis occurs in infants with necrotizing enterocolitis, it does not make the outlook any worse. The cysts may disappear spontaneously or may persist for prolonged periods without serious symptoms.

Blind Loop Syndrome

This is a rare clinical syndrome manifested by diarrhea, steatorrhea, anemia, weight loss, abdominal pain, multiple vitamin deficiencies, and neurologic disorders. The underlying cause is not a blind loop per se, but bacterial overgrowth in stagnant areas of small bowel produced by stricture, stenosis, fistulas, blind pouch, or diverticula (Table 27-5). The bacterial flora are altered in the stagnant area, both in number and in kind. Bacteria compete successfully for vitamin B_{12}, producing a systemic deficiency of B_{12} and megaloblastic anemia. Steatorrhea also occurs; bacteria in the stagnant area deconjugate bile salts, causing disruption of micellar solubilization of fats. There may also be absorptive defects of other macro- and micronutrients, probably caused by direct injury of the mucosal cells.

The syndrome can be confirmed by a series of laboratory investigations. First, a Schilling test (^{60}Co-labeled B_{12} absorption) is performed; this should reveal a pattern of urinary excretion of vitamin B_{12} resembling pernicious anemia (that is, a urinary loss of 0 to 6 percent of vitamin B_{12}, compared with the normal of 7 to 25 percent). The test is then repeated with the addition of intrinsic factor. In true pernicious anemia, the excretion should rise to normal; in the blind loop syndrome, the addition of intrinsic factor will not increase the excretion of B_{12}. Next, the patient is given a course of tetracycline for 3 to 5 days, and the Schilling test is repeated. With blind loop syn-

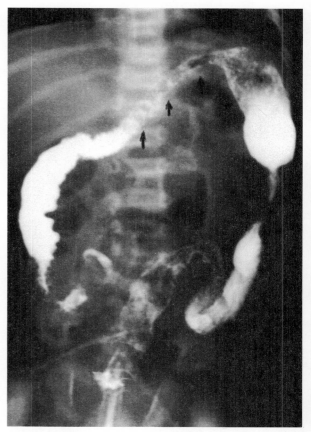

Fig. 27-14. Barium enema radiograph of an infant with pneumatosis cystoides coli. Arrows point to several submucosal gas cysts.

Table 27-5. CLINICAL CONDITIONS PREDISPOSING TO BACTERIAL OVERGROWTH WITHIN THE SMALL BOWEL

Gastric proliferation
    Achlorhydria, especially when combined with motor or anatomic disturbance
Small intestinal stagnation
    Anatomic
    Afferent loop of Billroth II partial gastrectomy
    Duodenal/jejunal diverticulosis
    Surgical blind loop (end-to-side anastomosis)
    Surgical recirculating loop (side-to-side anastomosis)
    Obstruction (stricture, adhesion, inflammation, cancer)
Motor
    Diabetic autonomic neuropathy
    Scleroderma
    Idiopathic intestinal pseudoobstruction
    Absence of "intestinal housekeeper"
Abnormal communication between proximal and distal gastrointestinal tract
    Gastrocolic or jejunocolic fistula
    Resection of ileocecal valve

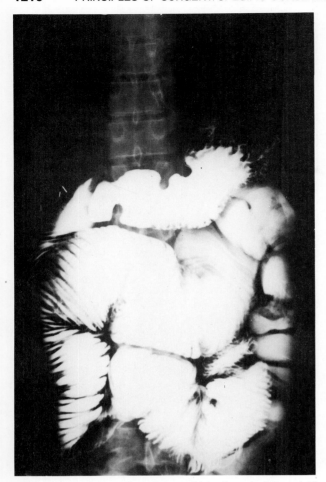

Fig. 27-15. This picture illustrates small intestine adaptation at 18 months after massive bowel resection.

drome, absorption of ^{60}Co-labeled B$_{12}$ returns to normal; this does not occur in the macrocytic anemia due to steatorrhea. Patients with the blind loop syndrome respond to tetracycline and parenteral B$_{12}$ therapy. Medical treatment is not definitive, but should be employed to prepare patients for operation. Surgical correction of the condition producing stagnation and blind loop syndrome effects a permanent cure and is indicated.

Short Bowel Syndrome

Emergency massive resection of the small bowel must sometimes be done when extensive gangrene precludes revascularization. Mesenteric occlusion, midgut volvulus, and traumatic disruption of the superior mesenteric vessels are the most frequent causes. Short bowel syndrome may result from such massive resections; it may also be produced by several bowel resections in patients with severe recurrent Crohn's disease.

The short bowel syndrome is a group of signs and symptoms that result from a length of small bowel that is inadequate to support nutrition. The clinical hallmarks of the short bowel syndrome include diarrhea, fluid and electrolyte deficiency, and malnutrition. The small bowel has two primary functions, digestion and absorption of nutrients. Problems that result from extensive resection of the small bowel can be divided into two types: (1) those related to the extent of small bowel loss and (2) those related to the specific area of bowel removed.

Although there is considerable individual variation, resection of up to 70 percent of the small bowel can usually be tolerated if the terminal ileum and ileocecal valve are preserved. Length alone, however, is not the only determining factor of complications of small bowel resection. For example, if the distal two-thirds of the ileum, including the ileocecal valve, are resected, significant abnormalities of absorption of bile salts and B$_{12}$ may occur, although only 25 percent of the total length of the small bowel has been removed. Proximal bowel resection is tolerated much better than distal resection.

Digestion and absorption in the small bowel depend upon the presence of brush border enzymes, an adequate number of enterocytes for absorption, and normal intestinal motility. With massive resection of the small bowel, there is reduced absorption of all nutrients, including electrolytes, water, carbohydrates, protein, fat, trace elements, and vitamins. The proximal small bowel is the primary site of absorption of iron, folate, and calcium, whereas the distal small bowel is the site of absorption of bile salts and vitamin B$_{12}$ (Table 27-2).

The bowel has an intrinsic capacity to adapt after small bowel resection, and in many instances, this process of intestinal adaptation effectively prevents severe complications due to the reduced surface area of the small bowel available for absorption and digestion. Any adaptive mechanism can be overwhelmed; maximum adaptation will be inadequate if sufficient small bowel is lost. Intestinal adaptation is characterized by increased absorptive surface due to hyperplasia of the remaining enterocytes. The villi lengthen (but do not increase in number), more cells are produced, and there is increased cell renewal and migration to the villous tip. This allows for a total increase in absorptive surface. Although there are more cells, individual cells do not increase their life span (they must migrate farther) or their capacity to synthesize digestive enzymes or to increase absorptive processes, so the overall net increase in digestive efficacy is not great (Fig. 27-15).

Mechanisms responsible for intestinal adaptation have been studied widely in animals. Multiple factors are responsible and are required for development of successful intestinal adaptation. For reasons that are not known, the ileum exhibits a much greater adaptive response than the jejunum. Luminal nutrients, trophic gut hormones, and pancreatic and biliary secretions are all required for complete adaptation to occur. In animals maintained on TPN after extensive small bowel resection, nutrition may be maintained, but intestinal adaptation does not occur. The trophic gut peptides studied most intensively in small bowel adaptation are gastrin, CCK, secretin, and enteroglucagon. We now know that, although hypergastrinemia is associated with the short bowel syndrome, gastrin does not play a major role in the adaptive response after resection. CCK and secretin may have direct effects on enterocyte replication; however, their primary importance in intestinal adaptation may be in stimulation of pancreaticobiliary secretions rather than in directly stimulating enterocyte proliferation. Enteroglucagon has been recently emphasized as the primary trophic stimulus for intestinal adaptation. This idea is based upon the findings of increased numbers of cells containing enteroglucagon in the intestinal mucosa and measured increases of plasma enteroglucagon after bowel resection. Direct analysis of the effects of enteroglucagon on intestinal growth have not been possible because of the lack of pure peptide for such studies.

In man, the adaptive responses to massive resection have been found to be increased caliber of the remaining small bowel, hypertrophy of the gut wall, increased villous height, and increased numbers of enterocytes. This process often takes weeks to months to complete after small bowel resection. With time, absorptive function increases. This increase is characterized by decreasing stool losses of water and electrolyte and increased absorption of glucose and vitamin B_{12}.

Hypergastrinemia and gastric hypersecretion occur after massive small bowel resection and have been widely studied in experimental animals; some information has come from man. Diarrhea associated with gastric hypersecretion is caused by (1) delivery of a massive volume of fluid and electrolytes to the shortened small bowel, (2) steatorrhea due to failure of lipolysis by pancreatic lipase, which requires an intraluminal pH greater than 5.0 for activity (pancreatic secretion of lipase is not affected), and (3) acid enteritis. Although acid hypersecretion was at one time thought to be of prime importance in producing diarrhea after extensive small bowel resection, both hypergastrinemia and hypersecretion of acid are transient. Acid hypersecretion is now easily managed by H_2-receptor antagonists. Control of acid secretion controls diarrhea to a great extent during the early phase. Several operations, including vagotomy and pyloroplasty, or vagotomy and antrectomy, have been employed with treatment of the short bowel syndrome to control acid hypersecretion. Since the problem is self-limited, however, these procedures are not indicated and should not be done.

Resection of specific segments of the small bowel leads to specific problems. Resection of the distal small bowel results in diarrhea, steatorrhea, and malabsorption. Conjugated bile salts, essential for normal fat absorption, are almost totally absorbed in the distal ileum by active transport mechanisms. Resection of the ileum results in disruption of the enterohepatic circulation of bile salts and may lead to two types of diarrhea. If less than 100 cm of small bowel is resected, excessive amounts of bile salts enter the colon and produce a chemical enteritis; this type of diarrhea has been termed *cholerrheic*. The toxic effects of bile acids on colonic epithelial cells are twofold: bile salts inhibit absorption of water and electrolytes in the colon, and the injured colonic cells secrete excessive amounts of water and electrolytes. The response to de-

creased absorption of bile salts is increased hepatic production of bile salts, and this leads to perpetuation of diarrhea.

When more than 100 cm of ileum has been resected, the loss of bile salts is so great that hepatic synthesis cannot compensate. In addition to the direct toxic effects of bile salts on the colonic epithelium, fat malabsorption (steatorrhea) occurs. Differentiation of the two types of diarrhea associated with distal resection is important because treatment is different. Measurement of stool fat content, vitamin B_{12} absorptive capacity, and fecal bile salt concentrations are important for accurate determination of deficits produced. For those patients who have cholerrheic diarrhea, agents that bind bile acids (cholestyramine) may alleviate diarrhea. If steatorrhea is present, then medium-chain triglycerides that do not require micelle formation for absorption should also be used.

Another factor contributing to diarrhea after ileal resection is loss of the ileocecal valve. The ileocecal valve has two important actions. It prolongs intestinal transit time, and it prevents retrograde passage of colonic bacteria into the small bowel, which, if not prevented, causes bacterial enteritis.

Other complications associated with alteration of enterohepatic circulation of bile acids include gallstones and anemia. The changes in the bile salt pool produce lithogenic bile; the incidence of gallstones in patients with ileal resection is three to four times greater than that of the normal population. The ileum is the specific site for transport mechanisms for intrinsic-factor–mediated vitamin B_{12} absorption, and with total ileal resection, stores of vitamin B_{12} are depleted, and anemia will result.

TREATMENT. The most important principle in treatment of short bowel syndrome is prevention. This means that at operation, when intestinal viability is questionable, the smallest possible resections should be performed, and "second look" operations 24 to 48 h later should be carried out to allow the ischemic bowel to demarcate. Delay may prevent unnecessary, extensive resection of bowel. In patients with Crohn's disease, the devastating complications of the short bowel syndrome have led all students of the disease to recognize that only limited resections should be performed.

After massive small bowel resection, the program for treatment may be properly divided into early and late. Early on, treatment is primarily directed at the control of diarrhea, replacement of fluid and electrolytes, and the prompt institution of total parenteral nutrition. Volume losses may exceed 5 L/day, and vigorous monitoring of intake and output with adequate replacement must be carried out. Depletion of fluid volume caused by diarrhea, especially in the early phase, is often a formidable problem. Judicious use of agents that inhibit gut motility (codeine, Lomotil, loperamide) may be helpful. These drugs may cause profound ileus if used excessively, and you simply trade volume lost through the gut for volume lost through nasogastric suction. In addition, prolonged ileus with dilatation and edema of the bowel wall may result.

As intestinal adaptation progresses, and gut absorption increases, the stool volume gradually decreases. Once patients have completely adapted to an oral diet, semi-formed stools may appear, but these patients will likely never have the normal number or consistency of stools.

As soon as the patient has recovered from the acute phase, he or she should begin enteral nutrition, so that intestinal adaptation may begin early and proceed successfully. The most common types of enteral diets are either elemental diets (Vivonex, Flexical) or polymeric diets (Isocal, Ensure). Each presents problems with increased osmolality and may contain foodstuffs that may not be absorbed due to enzyme deficiency (for example, deficiency of lactase). Milk products should be avoided, and diets should be begun at isoosmolar concentrations and with small volumes (50 mL/h), even though the full nutrient value may not be obtained. As the gut adapts, the osmolality volume and caloric content may be increased.

Reduction of dietary fat has long been considered to be important in the treatment of patients with the short bowel syndrome. High-carbohydrate, high-protein, low-fat diets have been prescribed. Fat has more than twice as many calories per gram as protein and carbohydrate and is important for maintenance of proper nutrition. Supplementation of the diet with 100 g or more of fat should be carried out. Often this requires the use of medium-chain triglycerides, which may be absorbed in the proximal bowel without micelle formation. Vitamins, especially fat-soluble vitamins, as well as calcium, magnesium and zinc supplementation, must also be provided. H_2-receptor antagonists may greatly diminish the diarrhea that is largely caused by the early, transient acid hypersecretion. Measurement of intragastric pH can be used to guide the dose of drugs required. Antacids are not useful because they may aggravate diarrhea or bind essential ions. In no case should gastric resection or vagotomy be used for the treatment of the short bowel syndrome.

Since the dysfunction of massive small bowel resection is caused by decreased absorptive surface and rapid transit time, most attempts at surgical treatment have been directed toward increasing the absorptive surface or slowing the intestinal transit time. These operations have included serosal patches of the colon in order to stimulate neomucosal growth, longitudinal small bowel division and lengthening, construction of valves (artificial sphincters), reversed segments of small bowel or colon, or insertion of isoperistaltic colonic segments. None of these surgical operations has been found effective, and they should not be performed.

The present treatment of the short bowel syndrome is palliative and is directed toward control of diarrhea and prevention of dehydration and malnutrition. Only with the development of successful allotransplantation of the gut will the short bowel syndrome be cured.

Intestinal Bypass

MORBID OBESITY

Surgical procedures to treat morbid obesity (defined as more than 100 lb over ideal weight) have become popular because the long-term success rate of nonsurgical treatment of this condition is only 1 percent. The original procedure designed to create a short-gut malabsorption syndrome, jejunocolostomy, had to be abandoned because of an unacceptable rate of complications. It was succeeded by jejunoileostomy, either end-to-side (Payne procedure) or end-to-end (Scott procedure). Many thousands of these procedures have been done in the United States. These too have been abandoned. An alternative method of operative therapy of obesity is the gastric bypass or partition. This method limits food intake by reducing the reservoir capacity of the stomach to 5 to 10 percent of normal.

Jejunoileal bypass produces very significant weight loss in the majority of patients, with the heaviest patients losing the most weight. Weight loss goes on for 12 to 18 months and then plateaus at a level that is still considerably above the ideal, but well below the preoperative weight. Despite the effectiveness of jejunoileal bypass in producing weight loss, there is widespread disenchantment with the procedure, principally due to very serious long-term complications, and it has been abandoned by most surgeons.

The operative mortality rate of jejunoileostomy is 2 to 5 percent. The morbidity, as always in operations on very obese patients, is appreciable and includes atelectasis, pneumonia, wound infection and dehiscence, and thromboembolism.

The late mortality rate has been about 10 percent, one-half the deaths being from liver failure. Late complications are many and formidable; they include hepatic steatosis, cirrhosis, and failure; hyperoxaluria and calcium oxalate urinary tract calculi; hyperbilirubinemia and gallstones; electrolyte imbalances, including hypocalcemia, hypomagnesemia, and hypokalemia; avitaminoses; psychologic problems and emotional upsets; loss of hair; polyarthropathy; pancreatitis; blind loop syndrome; pneumatosis cystoides intestinalis; colonic pseudo-obstruction; intussusception of bypassed jejunum; and bypass enteritis. Although many morbidly obese (and some not so morbidly obese) patients are eager to submit to these procedures and many surgeons appear eager to comply, these procedures are metabolically unsound.

Fifteen to 25 percent of patients in whom jejunoileal bypass has been performed have had the shunt reversed. The morbidity and mortality of the reanastomosis is not inconsequential in patients who are often nutritionally and metabolically crippled. The principal indications have been hepatic failure, unmanageable electrolyte and metabolic imbalances, persistent uncontrollable diarrhea or associated severe anorectal problems, excessive or excessively rapid weight loss, and inadequate weight loss.

Alpers has pointed out three major problems with operations for morbid obesity: lack of criteria for proper patient selection, lack of clear superiority for any operative procedure, and the lack of any long-term benefit of decreased mortality.

HYPERLIPIDEMIA

Surgical bypass of a portion of the small intestine is a useful method of treating hypercholesterolemia and hypertriglyceridemia. The operation, designed by Buchwald and Varco, short-circuits either the distal 200 cm or one-third of the small intestine length, whichever is greater. This operation, though occasionally associated with diarrhea, does not cause significant weight loss and is not associated with the undesirable side effects of the jejuno-ileal bypass.

This procedure lowers serum cholesterol level through two mechanisms: by interfering with the absorption of cholesterol by short-circuiting the usual site of absorption, and by increasing cholesterol and bile acid excretion, which accelerates cholesterol turnover.

Clinical metabolic studies have demonstrated a 60 percent decrease in cholesterol absorption, a 40 percent reduction in serum cholesterol, and a more than 50 percent reduction in plasma triglycerides. About 70 percent of patients with angina have had improvement or total remission of symptoms after this operation. Thus, partial ileal bypass, when employed for the correction of hyperlipidemia, appears to be an effective method of lipid reduction. It is obligatory in its actions, safe, and is associated with minimal side effects.

Bibliography

Anatomy

Fawcett DW (ed): Intestines, in *A Textbook of Histology*. Philadelphia, Saunders, 1986, pp 641–660.

Grand RJ, Watkins JB, et al: Development of the human gastrointestinal tract. *Gastroenterology* 70:790, 1976.

Hirsch J, Ahrens EH Jr, et al: Measurement of the human intestinal length in vivo and some causes of variation. *Gastroenterology* 31:274, 1956.

Trier JS: Morphology of the epithelium of the small intestine, in Code CF (ed): *Handbook of Physiology*, sect 6. Washington, DC, American Physiological Society, 1968, pp 1125–1175.

Trier JS: Diagnostic value of peroral biopsy of the proximal small intestine. *N Engl J Med* 285:1470, 1971.

Trier JS, Krone CL, et al: Anatomy, embryology, and developmental abnormalities of the small intestine and colon, in Sleisenger MH, Fordtran JS (eds): *Gastrointestinal Disease. Pathophysiology, Diagnosis, Management*. Philadelphia, Saunders, 1983, pp 780–811.

Physiology

Alpers DH: Absorption of water-soluble vitamins, folate, minerals, and vitamin D, in Sleisenger MH, Fordtran JS (eds): *Gastrointestinal Disease. Pathophysiology, Diagnosis, Management*. Philadelphia, Saunders, 1983, pp 830–844.

Becker JM, Duff WM, et al: Myoelectric control of gastrointestinal and biliary motility: A review. *Surgery* 89:466, 1981.

Binder HJ: Absorption and secretion of water and electrolytes by small and large intestine, in Sleisenger MH, Fordtran JS (eds): *Gastrointestinal Disease. Pathophysiology, Diagnosis, Management*. Philadelphia, Saunders, 1983, pp 811–829.

Code CF (ed): *Handbook of Physiology*, sect 6. Washington, DC, American Physiological Society, 1968.

Cohen S, Snape WJ Jr: Movement of the small and large intestines, in Sleisenger MH, Fordtran JS (eds): *Gastrointestinal Disease. Pathophysiology, Diagnosis, Management*. Philadelphia, Saunders, 1983, pp 859–873.

Davenport HW (ed.): Intestinal secretion, in *Physiology of the Digestive Tract*. Chicago, Yearbook Medical Publishers, 1982, pp 174–178.

Hofmann AF: A physicochemical approach to the intraluminal phase of fat absorption. *Gastroenterology* 50:56, 1966.

Gangl A, Ockner RK: Intestinal metabolism of lipids and lipoproteins. *Gastroenterology* 68:167, 1975.

Gray GM: Mechanisms of digestion and absorption of food, in Sleisenger MH, Fordtran JS (eds): *Gastrointestinal Disease. Pathophysiology, Diagnosis, Management*. Philadelphia, Saunders, 1983, pp 844–858.

Scratcherd T, Grundy D: The physiology of intestinal motility and secretion. *Br J Anaesth* 56:3, 1984.

Thompsom JC, Greeley George H Jr, et al (eds): *Gastrointestinal Endocrinology*, New York, McGraw-Hill, 1987.

Thompson JC, Marx M: Gastrointestinal hormones. *Curr Probl Surg* 21:1, 1984.

Inflammatory Diseases

Alexander-Williams J, Haynes IG: Up-to-date management of small-bowel Crohn's disease. *Adv Surg* 20:245, 1987.

Aston NO, de Costa AM: Tuberculous perforation of the small bowel. *Postgrad Med J* 61:251, 1985.

Bartlett JG: *Clostridium difficile* and inflammatory bowel disease. *Gastroenterology* 80:863, 1981.

Beart RW Jr, McIlrath DC, et al: Surgical management of inflammatory bowel disease. *Curr Probl Surg* 17(10):533, 1980.

Block GE, Enker WE, et al: Significance and treatment of occult obstructive uropathy complicating Crohn's disease. *Ann Surg* 178:322, 1973.

Block GE, Schraut WH: The operative treatment of Crohn's enteritis complicated by ileosigmoid fistula. *Ann Surg* 196:356, 1982.

Bluth EI, McVay LV III, et al: Ultrasonic characteristics of ileal tuberculosis. *Dis Colon Rectum* 28:613, 1985.

Broe PJ, Bayless TM, et al: Crohn's disease: Are enteroenteral fistulas an indication for surgery? *Surgery* 91:249, 1982.

Chouhan MK, Pande SK: Typhoid enteric perforation. *Br J Surg* 69:173, 1982.

Collier PE, Turowski P, et al: Small intestinal adenocarcinoma complicating regional enteritis. *Cancer* 55:516, 1985.

Crohn BB, Ginzburg L, et al: Regional enteritis. A pathologic and clinical entity. *JAMA* 99:1323, 1932.

Eggleston FC, Santoshi B, et al: Typhoid perforation of the bowel. *Ann Surg* 190:31, 1979.

Eustache J-M, Kreis DJ Jr: Typhoid perforation of the intestine. *Arch Surg* 118:1269, 1983.

Farmer RG, Hawk WA, et al: Indications for surgery in Crohn's disease: Analysis of 500 cases. *Gastroenterology* 71:245, 1976.

Fresko D, Lazarus SS, et al: Early presentation of carcinoma of the small bowel in Crohn's disease ("Crohn's carcinoma"). *Gastroenterology* 82:783, 1982.

Gilinsky NH, Marks IN, et al: Abdominal tuberculosis. A 10-year review. *SA Med J* 64:849, 1983.

Gitnick G: Is Crohn's disease a mycobacterial disease after all? *Dig Dis Sci* 29:1086, 1984.

Goldberg HI, Caruthers SB Jr, et al: Radiographic findings of the National Cooperative Crohn's Disease Study. *Gastroenterology* 77:925, 1979.

Greenstein AJ, Janowitz HD, et al: The extraintestinal manifestations of Crohn's disease and ulcerative colitis: A study of 700 patients. *Medicine* (Balt) 55:401, 1976.

Greenstein AJ, Meyers S, et al: Surgery and its sequelae in Crohn's colitis and ileocolitis. *Arch Surg* 116:285, 1981.

Greenstein AJ, Sachar D, et al: Cancer in Crohn's disease after diversionary surgery. A report of seven carcinomas occurring in excluded bowel. *Am J Surg* 135:86, 1978.

Greenstein AJ, Sachar DB, et al: Patterns of neoplasia in Crohn's disease and ulcerative colitis. *Cancer* 46:403, 1980.

Gryboski JD, Spiro HM.: Prognosis in children with Crohn's disease. *Gastroenterology* 74:807, 1978.

Hamilton SR, Reese J, et al: The role of resection margin frozen section in the surgical management of Crohn's disease. *Surg Gynecol Obstet* 160:57, 1985.

Hawker PC, Givel JC, et al: Management of enterocutaneous fistulae in Crohn's disease. *Gut* 24:284, 1983.

Heuman R, Boeryd B, et al: The influence of disease at the margin of resection on the outcome of Crohn's disease. *Br J Surg* 70:519, 1983.

Homan WP, Dineen P: Comparison of the results of resection, bypass, and bypass with exclusion for ileocecal Crohn's disease. *Ann Surg* 187:530, 1978.

Homan WP, Tank C-K, et al: Acute massive hemorrhage from intestinal Crohn's disease: Report of seven cases and review of the literature. *Arch Surg* 111:901, 1976.

Janowitz HD: Crohn's disease—50 years later. *N Engl J Med* 304:1600, 1981.

Kakar A, Aranya RC, et al: Acute perforation of small intestine due to tuberculosis. *Aust NZ J Surg* 53:381, 1983.

Kendall GPN, Hawley PR, et al: Strictureplasty. A good operation for small bowel Crohn's disease? *Dis Colon Rectum* 29:312, 1986.

Kewenter J, Hulten L, et al: The relationship and epidemiology of acute terminal ileitis and Crohn's disease. *Gut* 15:801, 1974.

Khanna AK, Misra MK: Typhoid perforation of the gut. *Postgrad Med J* 60:523, 1984.

Kim J-P, Oh S-K, et al: Management of ileal perforation due to typhoid fever. *Ann Surg* 181:88, 1975.

Kirschner BS, Voinchet O, et al: Growth retardation in inflammatory bowel disease. *N Engl J Med* 306:775, 837, 1982.

Knutson L, Arosenius K-E: Tuberculosis of the large bowel. Report of two cases. *Acta Chir Scand* 150:345, 1984.

Korelitz BI, Present DH: Favorable effect of 6-mercaptopurine on fistulae of Crohn's disease. *Dig Dis Sci* 30:58, 1985.

Lennard-Jones JE: Azathioprine and 6-mercaptopurine have a role in the treatment of Crohn's disease. *Dig Dis Sci* 26:364, 1981.

Lennard-Jones JE, Singleton JW: The Azathioprine controversy. *Dig Dis Sci* 26:364, 1981.

Lizarralde AE: Typhoid perforation of the ileum in children. *J Pediatr Surg* 16:1012, 1981.

Lock MR, Farmer RG, et al: Recurrence and reoperation for Crohn's disease: The role of disease location in prognosis. *N Engl J Med* 304:1586, 1981.

Mayberry JF, Rhodes J: Epidemiological aspects of Crohn's disease: A review of the literature. *Gut* 25:886, 1984.

Mekhjian HS, Switz DM, et al: Clinical features and natural history of Crohn's disease. *Gastroenterology* 77:898, 1979.

Mekhjian HS, Switz DM, et al: National Cooperative Crohn's Disease Study: Factors determining recurrence of Crohn's disease after surgery. *Gastroenterology* 77:907, 1979.

Menguy R: Surgical management of free perforation of the small intestine complicating regional enteritis. *Ann Surg* 175:178, 1972.

Meyers S, Walfish JS, et al: Quality of life after surgery for Crohn's disease: A psychosocial survey. *Gastroenterology* 78:1, 1980.

Nugent FW, Richmond M, et al: Crohn's disease of the duodenum. *Gut* 18:115, 1977.

Pennington L, Hamilton SR, et al: Surgical management of Crohn's disease: Influence of disease at margin of resection. *Ann Surg* 192:311, 1980.

Present DH, Korelitz BI, et al: Treatment of Crohn's disease with 6-mercaptopurine: A long-term, randomized, double-blind study. *N Engl J Med* 302:981, 1980.

Prior P, Gyde S, et al: Mortality in Crohn's disease. *Gastroenterology* 80:307, 1981.

Rankin GB, Watts HD, et al: National Cooperative Crohn's Disease Study: Extraintestinal manifestations and perianal complications. *Gastroenterology* 77:914, 1979.

Rombeau JL, Barot LR, et al: Preoperative total parenteral nutrition and surgical outcome in patients with inflammatory bowel disease. *Am J Surg* 143:139, 1982.

Sachar DB, Auslander MO: Missing pieces in the puzzle of Crohn's disease. *Gastroenterology* 75:745, 1978.

Sachar DB, Auslander MO, et al: Aetiological theories of inflammatory bowel disease. *Clin Gastroenterol* 9:231, 1980.

Sachar DB, Wolfson DM, et al: Risk factors for postoperative recurrence of Crohn's disease. *Gastroenterology* 85:917, 1983.

Seashore JH, Hillemeier AC, et al: Total parenteral nutrition in the management of inflammatory bowel disease in children: A limited role. *Am J Surg* 143:504, 1982.

Shorter RG, Huizenga KA, et al: A working hypothesis for the etiology and pathogenesis of nonspecific inflammatory bowel disease. *Am J Dig Dis* 17:1024, 1972.

Simpson S, Traube J, et al: The histologic appearance of dysplasia (precarcinomatous change) in Crohn's disease of the small and large intestines. *Gastroenterology* 81:492, 1981.

Singleton JW: The National Cooperative Crohn's Disease Study. *Gastroenterology* 77:825, 1979.

Singleton JW: Azathioprine has a very limited role in the treatment of Crohn's disease. *Dig Dis Sci* 26:368, 1981.

Sleisenger MH: How should we treat Crohn's disease? *N Engl J Med* 302:1024, 1980.

Stead WW, Dutt AK: Chemotherapy for tuberculosis today. *Am Rev Respir Dis* 125:94, 1982.

Strobel CT, Byrne WJ, et al: Home parenteral nutrition in children with Crohn's disease: An effective management alternative. *Gastroenterology* 77:272, 1979.

Summers RW, Switz DM, et al: National Cooperative Crohn's Disease Study: Results of drug treatment. *Gastroenterology* 77:847, 1979.

Tandon HD, Prakash A: Pathology of intestinal tuberculosis and its distinction from Crohn's disease. *Gut* 13:260, 1972.

Trnka YM, Glotzer DJ, et al: The long-term outcome of restorative operation in Crohn's disease. *Ann Surg* 196:345, 1982.

Vaidya MG, Sodhi JS: Gastrointestinal tract tuberculosis: A study of 102 cases including 55 hemicolectomies. *Clin Radiol* 29:189, 1978.

Vantrappen G, Ponette E, et al: Yersinia enteritis and enterocolitis: Gastroenterological aspects. *Gastroenterology* 72:220, 1977.

Weakley FL, Turnbull FL: Recognition of regional ileitis in the operating room. *Dis Colon Rectum* 14:17, 1971.

Wolff BG, Beart RW Jr, et al: The importance of disease-free margins in resections for Crohn's disease. *Dis Colon Rectum* 26:239, 1983.

Wolfson DM, Sachar DB, et al: Granulomas do not affect postoperative recurrence rates in Crohn's disease. *Gastroenterology* 83:405, 1982.

Neoplasms

Ahlman H, Dahlstrom A, et al: The pentagastrin test in the diagnosis of the carcinoid syndrome. Blockade of gastrointestinal symptoms by Ketanserin. *Ann Surg* 201:81, 1985.

Akwari OE, Dozois RR, et al: Leiomyosarcoma of the small and large bowel. *Cancer* 42:1375, 1978.

Awrich AE, Irish CE, et al: A twenty-five year experience with primary malignant tumors of the small intestine. *Surg Gynecol Obstet* 151:9, 1980.

Bancks NH, Goldstein HM, et al: The roentgenologic spectrum of small intestinal carcinoid tumors. *Am J Roentgenol* 123:274, 1975.

Barclay THC, Schapira DV: Malignant tumors of the small intestine. *Cancer* 51:878, 1983.

Beaton H, Homan W, et al: Gastrointestinal carcinoids and the malignant carcinoid syndrome. *Surg Gynecol Obstet* 152:268, 1981.

Boddie AW Jr, Mullins JD, et al: Extranodal lymphoma: Surgical and other therapeutic alternatives. *Curr Probl Cancer* 6:1, 1982.

Bremer EH, Battaile WG, et al: Villous tumors of the upper gastrointestinal tract. Clinical review and report of a case. *Am J Gastroenterol* 50:135, 1968.

Darling RC, Welch CE: Tumors of the small intestine. *N Engl J Med* 260:397, 1959.

Davis GR, Camp RC, et al: Effect of somatostatin infusion on jejunal water and electrolyte transport in a patient with secretory diarrhea due to malignant carcinoid syndrome. *Gastroenterology* 78:346, 1980.

Davis Z, Moertel CG, et al: The malignant carcinoid syndrome. *Surg Gynecol Obstet* 137:637, 1973.

Dawson IMP, Cornes JS, et al: Primary malignant lymphoid tumours of the intestinal tract. Report of 37 cases with a study of factors influencing prognosis. *Br J Surg* 49:80, 1961.

Emson PC, Gilbert RFT, et al: Elevated concentrations of substance P and 5-HT in plasma in patients with carcinoid tumors. *Cancer* 54:715, 1984.

Godwin JD II: Carcinoid tumors. An analysis of 2837 cases. *Cancer* 36:560, 1975.

Goedert M, Otten U, et al: Dopamine, norepinephrine, and serotonin production by an intestinal carcinoid tumor. *Cancer* 45:104, 1980.

Halpert RD, Feczko PJ, et al: Enteroclysis for the examination of the small bowel. *Henry Ford Hosp Med J* 33:116, 1985.

Herbsman H, Wetstein L, et al: Tumors of the small intestine. *Curr Probl Surg* 17(3):121, 1980.

Jeghers H, McKusick VA, et al: Generalized intestinal polyposis and melanin spots on the oral mucosa, lips and digits. *N Engl J Med* 241:993, 1949.

Johnson LA, Lavin P, et al: Carcinoids: The association of histologic growth pattern and survival. *Cancer* 51:882, 1983.

Kvols LK, Moertel CG, et al: Treatment of the malignant carcinoid syndrome. Evaluation of a long-acting somatostatin analogue. *N Engl J Med* 315:663, 1986.

Long RG, Peters JR, et al: Somatostatin, gastrointestinal peptides, and the carcinoid syndrome. *Gut* 22:549, 1981.

Maglinte DDT, Hall R, et al: Detection of surgical lesions of the small bowel by enteroclysis. *Am J Surg* 147:225, 1984.

Martin JK Jr, Moertel CG, et al: Surgical treatment of functioning metastatic carcinoid tumors. *Arch Surg* 118:537, 1983.

McAllister AJ, Richards KF: Peutz-Jeghers syndrome: Experience with twenty patients in five generations. *Am J Surg* 134:717, 1977.

McDermott WV, Hensle TW: Metastatic carcinoid to the liver treated by hepatic dearterialization. *Ann Surg* 180:305, 1974.

Moertel CG, Dockerty MB, et al: Carcinoid tumors of the vermiform appendix. *Cancer* 21:270, 1968.

Moertel CG, Sauer WG, et al: Life history of the carcinoid tumor of the small intestine. *Cancer* 14:901, 1961.

Nagorney DM, Sarr MG, et al: Surgical management of intussusception in the adult. *Ann Surg* 193:230, 1981.

Oates JA: The carcinoid syndrome. *N Engl J Med* 315:702, 1986.

Pagtalunan RJG, Mayo CW, et al: Primary malignant tumors of the small intestine. *Am J Surg* 108:13, 1964.

Perzin KH, Bridge MF: Adenomatous and carcinomatous changes in hamartomatous polyps of the small intestine (Peutz-Jeghers syndrome): Report of a case and review of the literature. *Cancer* 49:971, 1982.

Rao AR, Kagan AR, et al: Management of gastrointestinal lymphoma. *Am J Clin Oncol* 7:213, 1984.

River L, Silverstein J, et al: Benign neoplasms of the small intestine. A critical comprehensive review with reports of 20 new cases. *Intl Abst Surg* 102:1, 1956.

Rochlin DB, Longmire WP Jr: Primary tumors of the small intestine. *Surgery* 50:586, 1961.

Salem PA, Nassar VH, et al: Mediterranean abdominal lymphoma, or immunoproliferative small intestinal disease. Part I: Clinical aspects. *Cancer* 40:2941, 1977.

Schulten MF Jr, Oyasu R, et al: Villous adenoma of the duodenum. A case report and review of the literature. *Am J Surg* 132:90, 1976.

Starr GF, Dockerty MB: Leiomyomas and leiomyosarcomas of the small intestine. *Cancer* 8:101, 1955.

Stothert JC Jr, Riaz MA, et al: Preoperative angiographic diagnosis of small bowel leiomyomas. *Arch Surg* 113:643, 1978.

Strodel WE, Talpos G, et al: Surgical therapy for small-bowel carcinoid tumors. *Arch Surg* 118:291, 1983.

Stubenbord WT, Thorbjarnarson B: Intussusception in adults. *Ann Surg* 172:306, 1970.

Weingrad DN, DeCosse JJ, et al: Primary gastrointestinal lymphoma: A 30-year review. *Cancer* 49:1258, 1982.

Wilson H, Cheek RC, et al: Carcinoid syndrome. *Curr Probl Surg* 36:41, 1970.

Wilson JM, Melvin DB, et al: Primary malignancies of the small bowel: A report of 96 cases and review of the literature. *Ann Surg* 180:175, 1974.

Wilson JM, Melvin DB, et al: Benign small bowel tumor. *Ann Surg* 181:247, 1975.

Zollinger RM Jr, Sternfeld WC, et al: Primary neoplasms of the small intestine. *Am J Surg* 151:654, 1986.

Diverticular Disease

Adams DB: Management of the intraluminal duodenal diverticulum: Endoscopy or duodenostomy? *Am J Surg* 151:524, 1986.

Brian JE Jr, Stair JM: Noncolonic diverticular disease. *Surg Gynecol Obstet* 161:189, 1985.

Critchlow JF, Shapiro MD, et al: Duodenojejunostomy for the pancreaticobiliary complications of duodenal diverticulum. *Ann Surg* 202:56, 1985.

DeBartolo HM Jr, van Heerden JA: Meckel's diverticulum. *Ann Surg* 183:30, 1976.

Eckhauser FE, Zelenock GB, et al: Acute complications of jejuno-ileal pseudodiverticulosis: Surgical implications and management. *Am J Surg* 138:320, 1979.

Economides NG, McBurney RP, et al: Intraluminal duodenal diverticulum in the adult. *Ann Surg* 185:147, 1977.

Eggert A, Teichmann W, et al: The pathologic implication of duodenal diverticula. *Surg Gynecol Obstet* 154:62, 1982.

Griffin M, Carey WD, et al: Recurrent acute pancreatitis and intussusception complicating an intraluminal duodenal diverticulum. *Gastroenterology* 81:345, 1981.

Haugh DC, McBee MH: Perforation of duodenal diverticula. *Contemp Surg* 25:72, 1984.

Howard JM, Wynn OB, et al: Intraluminal duodenal diverticulum: An unusual cause of acute pancreatitis. *Am J Surg* 151:505, 1986.

Kaminsky HH, Thompson WR, et al: Extended sphincteroplasty for juxtapapillary duodenal diverticulum. *Surg Gynecol Obstet* 162:280, 1986.

Karoll MP, Ghahremani GG, et al: Diagnosis and management of intraluminal duodenal diverticulum. *Dig Dis Sci* 28:411, 1983.

Kellum JM, Boucher JK, et al: Serosal patch repair for benign duodenocolic fistula secondary to duodenal diverticulum. *Am J Surg* 131:607, 1976.

Kilpatrick ZM, Aseron CA: Radioisotope detection of Meckel's diverticulum causing acute rectal hemorrhage. *N Engl J Med* 287:653, 1972.

Krishnamurthy S, Kelly MM, et al: Jejunal diverticulosis. A heterogenous disorder caused by a variety of abnormalities of smooth muscle or myenteric plexus. *Gastroenterology* 85:538, 1983.

Leinkram C, Roberts-Thomson IC, et al: Juxtapapillary duodenal diverticula. Association with gallstones and pancreatitis. *Med J Aust* 1:209, 1980.

Løtveit T, Osnes M: Duodenal diverticula. *Scand J Gastroenterol* 19:579, 1984.

Løtveit T, Osnes M, et al: Studies of the choledocho-duodenal sphincter in patients with and without juxtapapillary duodenal diverticula. *Scand J Gastroenterol* 15:875, 1980.

Løtveit T, Osnes M, et al: Recurrent biliary calculi. Duodenal diverticula as a predisposing factor. *Ann Surg* 196:30, 1982.

Manny J, Muga M, et al: The continuing clinical enigma of duodenal diverticulum. *Am J Surg* 142:596, 1981.

Mendelson RM, Shepherd HA, et al: "Inverted" diverticulum mimicking an ulcerated duodenal tumour. *Br J Radiol* 57:426, 1984.

Scudamore CH, Harrison RC, et al: Management of duodenal diverticula. *Can J Surg* 24:311, 1982.

Soltero MJ, Bill AH: The natural history of Meckel's diverticulum and its relation to incidental removal. A study of 202 cases of diseased Meckel's diverticulum found in King County, Washington, over a fifteen-year period. *Am J Surg* 132:168, 1976.

Williams RA, Davidson DD, et al: Surgical problems of diverticula of the small intestine. *Surg Gynecol Obstet* 152:621, 1981.

Ulcers

Boydstun JS Jr, Gaffey TA, et al: Clinicopathologic study of nonspecific ulcers of the small intestine. *Dig Dis Sci* 26:911, 1981.

Guest JL: Nonspecific ulceration of the intestine: Collective review. *Surg Gynecol Obstet* 117:409, 1963.

McMahon FG, Akdamar K: Gastric ulceration after "slow-K." *N Engl J Med* 295:733, 1976,

Thomas WEG, Williamson RCN: Enteric ulceration and its complications. *World J Surg* 9:876, 1985.

Foreign Bodies

Goldman AL: Foreign bodies of the gastrointestinal tract. *Contemp Surg* 18:45, 1981.

McCanse DE, Kurchin A, et al: Gastrointestinal foreign bodies. *Am J Surg* 142:335, 1981.

Schwartz JT, Graham DY: Toothpick perforation of the intestines. *Ann Surg* 185:64, 1977.

Fistulas

Blackett RL, Hill GL: Postoperative external small bowel fistulas: A study of a consecutive series of patients treated with intravenous hyperalimentation. *Br J Surg* 65:775, 1978.

Chapman R, Foran R, et al: Management of intestinal fistulas. *Am J Surg* 108:157, 1964.

Coutsoftides T, Fazio VW: Small intestine cutaneous fistulas. *Surg Gynecol Obstet* 149:333, 1979.

Edmunds LH, Williams GM, et al: External fistulas arising from the gastrointestinal tract. *Ann Surg* 152:445, 1960.

Hill GL: Operative strategy in the treatment of enterocutaneous fistulas. *World J Surg* 7:495, 1983.

Jones SA, Gazzaniga AB, et al: The serosal patch: A surgical parachute. *Am J Surg* 126:186, 1973.

Kingsnorth AN, Moss JG, et al: Failure of somatostatin to accelerate closure of enterocutaneous fistulas in patients receiving total parenteral nutrition. *Lancet* 1:1271, 1986.

Knighton DR, Burns K, et al: The use of stomahesive in the care of the skin of enterocutaneous fistulas. *Surg Gynecol Obstet* 143:449, 1976.

Malangoni MA, Madura JA, et al: Management of lateral duodenal fistulas: A study of fourteen cases. *Surgery* 90:645, 1981.

McIntyre PB, Ritchie JK, et al: Management of enterocutaneous fistulas: A review of 132 cases. *Br J Surg* 71:293, 1984.

McLean GK, Mackie JA, et al: Enterocutaneous fistulae: Interventional radiologic management. *AJR* 138:615, 1982.

Reber HA, Roberts C, et al: Management of external gastrointestinal fistulas. *Ann Surg* 188:460, 1978.

Soeters PB, Ebeid AM, et al: Review of 404 patients with gastrointestinal fistulas. Impact of parenteral nutrition. *Ann Surg* 190:189, 1979.

Webster MW Jr, Carey LC: Fistulae of the intestinal tract. *Curr Probl Surg* 13(6):1, 1976.

Zera RT, Bubrick MP, et al: Enterocutaneous fistulas. Effects of total parenteral nutrition and surgery. *Dis Colon Rectum* 26:109, 1983.

Enterocutaneous fistulas—Encouraging trends. *Lancet* 2:204, 1984 (Editorial.)

Blind Loop Syndrome

Fromm D: Ileal resection, or disease, and the blind loop syndrome: Current concepts of pathophysiology. *Surgery* 73:639, 1973.

Kern L: Bacterial contamination syndrome of the small bowel. *Clin Gastroenterol* 8:397, 1979.

King CE, Toskes PP: Small intestine bacterial overgrowth. *Gastroenterology* 76:1035, 1979.

Short Bowel Syndrome

Boeckman CR, Traylor R: Bowel lengthening for short gut syndrome. *J Pediatr Surg* 16:996, 1981.

Bristol JB, Williamson RCN: Postoperative adaptation of the small intestine. *World J Surg* 9:825, 1985.

Cortot A, Fleming CR, et al: Improved nutrient absorption after cimetidine in short-bowel syndrome with gastric hypersecretion. *N Engl J Med* 300:79, 1979.

Fleming CR, Beart RW Jr, et al: Home parenteral nutrition for management of the severely malnourished adult patient. *Gastroenterology* 79:11, 1980.

Gladen HE, Kelly KA: Electrical pacing for short bowel syndrome. *Surg Gynecol Obstet* 153:697, 1981.

Grosfeld JL, Rescorla FJ, et al: Short bowel syndrome in infancy and childhood. Analysis of survival in 60 patients. *Am J Surg* 151:41, 1986.

Hyman PE, Everett SL, et al: Gastric acid hypersecretion in short bowel syndrome in infants: Association with extent of resection and enteral feeding. *J Pediatr Gastroenterol Nutr* 5:191, 1986.

Koretz RL, Meyer JH: Elemental diets—facts and fantasies. *Gastroenterology* 78:393, 1980.

Krejs GJ: Intestinal resection. *Clin Gastroenterol* 8:373, 1979.

McIntyre PB: The short bowel. *Br J Surg* 72:592, 1985.

Mitchell A, Watkins RM, et al: Surgical treatment of the short bowel syndrome. *Br J Surg* 71:329, 1984.

Murphy JP Jr, King DR, et al: Treatment of gastric hypersecretion with cimetidine in the short-bowel syndrome. *N Engl J Med* 300:80, 1979.

Postuma R, Moroz S, et al: Extreme short-bowel syndrome in an infant. *J Pediatr Surg* 18:264, 1983.

Ricotta J, Zuidema GD, et al: Construction of an ileocecal valve and its role in massive resection of the small intestine. *Surg Gynecol Obstet* 152:310, 1981.

Ricour C, Duhamel JF, et al: Enteral and parenteral nutrition in the short bowel syndrome in children. *World J Surg* 9:310, 1985.

Russell RI: Intestinal adaptation to an elemental diet. *Proc Nutr Soc* 44:87, 1985.

Sheldon GF: Role of parenteral nutrition in patients with short bowel syndrome. *Am J Med* 67:1021, 1979.

Tepas JJ III, MacLean WC Jr, et al: Total management of short gut secondary to midgut volvulus without prolonged total parenteral alimentation. *J Pediatr Surg* 13:622, 1978.

Thompson JS: Surgical therapy for the short bowel syndrome. *J Surg Res* 39:81, 1985.

Weser E: Short bowel syndrome. *Gastroenterology* 77:572, 1979.

Williams RCN: Medical progress: Intestinal adaptation. Part 1, Structural, functional and cytokinetic changes. Part 2, Mechanisms of control. *N Engl J Med* 298:1393, 1444, 1978.

Williams NS, Evans P, et al: Gastric acid secretion and gastrin production in the short bowel syndrome. *Gut* 26:914, 1985.

Winchester DP, Dorsey JM: Intestinal segments and pouches in gastrointestinal surgery. *Surg Gynecol Obstet* 132:131, 1971.

Ziegler MM: Short bowel syndrome in infancy: Etiology and management. *Clin Perinatol* 13:163, 1986.

Intestinal Bypass

Alpers DH: Surgical therapy for obesity. *N Engl J Med* 308:1026, 1983.

Buchwald H, Moore RB, et al: Ten years clinical experience with partial ileal bypass in management of the hyperlipidemias. *Ann Surg* 180:384, 1974.

Griffen WO Jr, Young VL, et al: A prospective comparison of gastric and jejunoileal bypass for morbid obesity. *Ann Surg* 186:500, 1977.

Halverson JD: Obesity surgery in perspective. *Surgery* 87:119, 1980.

Ravitch MM, Brolin RE: The price of weight loss by jejunoileal shunt. *Ann Surg* 190:382, 1979.

Terry BE: Surgical management of morbid obesity. *Bull Am Col Surg* 67:3, 1982.

Index